The New York School of Regional Anesthesia

Textbook of Regional Anesthesia and Acute Pain Management

Notice

Medicine is an ever-changing science. As new research and clinical experience broaden our knowledge, changes in treatment and drug therapy are required. The authors and the publisher of this work have checked with sources believed to be reliable in their efforts to provide information that is complete and generally in accord with the standards accepted at the time of publication. However, in view of the possibility of human error or changes in medical sciences, neither the authors nor the publisher nor any other party who has been involved in the preparation or publication of this work warrants that the information contained herein is in every respect accurate or complete, and they disclaim all responsibility for any errors or omissions or for the results obtained from use of the information contained in this work. Readers are encouraged to confirm the information contained herein with other sources. For example and in particular, readers are advised to check the product information sheet included in the package of each drug they plan to administer to be certain that the information contained in this work is accurate and that changes have not been made in the recommended dose or in the contraindications for administration. This recommendation is of particular importance in connection with new or infrequently used drugs.

The New York School of Regional Anesthesia

Textbook of Regional Anesthesia and Acute Pain Management

Editor

Admir Hadzic, MD, PhD
Director of Regional Anesthesia
St. Luke's–Roosevelt Hospital Center
Professor of Anesthesiology
College of Physicians and Surgeons
Columbia University
New York, New York

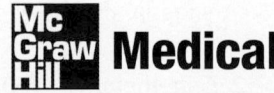

New York   Chicago   San Francisco   Lisbon   London   Madrid   Mexico City   Milan
New Delhi   San Juan   Seoul   Singapore   Sydney   Toronto

Textbook of Regional Anesthesia and Acute Pain Management

6 7 8 9 0   CTP/CTP   17 16 15 14 13

ISBN-13: 978-0-07-144906-9
ISBN-10: 0-07-144906-X

This book was set in Minion by TechBooks.
The editors were Joe Rusko, Robert Pancotti, and Peter J. Boyle.
The production supervisor was Catherine H. Saggese.
The indexer was Coughlin Indexing Services, Inc.
China Translation & Printing Services, Ltd., was printer and binder.

Library of Congress Cataloging-in-Publication Data

Textbook of regional anesthesia and acute pain management / editor, Admir Hadzic.
      p. ; cm.
   Includes bibliographical references and index.
   ISBN 0-07-144906-X (alk. paper)
   1. Conduction anesthesia.   2. Nerve block.   3. Analgesia.   I. Hadzic, Admir.   II. New
York School of Regional Anesthesia.
   [DNLM: 1. Anesthesia, Conduction–methods.   2. Pain–therapy.   WO 300 R33385 2007]
   RD84.R4224 2007
   617.9'64–dc22   2006048185

This work is dedicated to the loving memory of Dennis Hadzic
(December 6, 1995 – March 8, 1998)

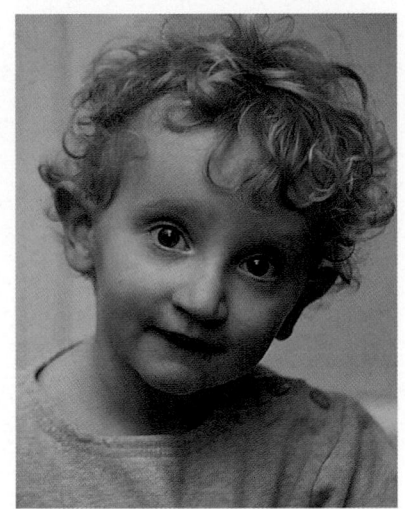

Contents

Contents

Contents

Contributors

Marina Allen, MD
Regional Anesthesiologist
St. Luke's-Roosevelt Hospital Center
Assistant Professor of Anesthesiology
College of Physicians and Surgeons
Columbia University
New York, New York

Anna Barczewska-Hillel, MD
Pain Management Specialist
Staff Anesthesiologist
St. Luke's-Roosevelt Hospital Center
Assistant Professor of Anesthesiology
College of Physicians and Surgeons
Columbia University
New York, New York

Alton Barron, MD
Associate Professor of Orthopedic Surgery
Staff Orthopedic Surgeon
St. Luke's-Roosevelt Hospital Center
College of Physicians and Surgeons
Columbia University
New York, New York

James Beckman, MD
Attending Anesthesiologist
Clinical Assistant Professor of Anesthesiology
Department of Anesthesiology
Hospital for Special Surgery
Weill Medical College of Cornell University
New York, New York

Honorio T. Benzon, MD
Professor of Anesthesiology
Chief, Division of Pain Medicine
Feinberg School of Medicine
Northwestern University
Chicago, Illinois

David J. Birnbach, MD
Professor of Anesthesiology
Miller School of Medicine
University of Miami
Miami, Florida

Stephan Blumenthal, MD
Consultant
Department of Anesthesiology
Orthopedic University Hospital Balgrist
Zurich
Switzerland

André P. Boezaart, MB ChB, MPraxMed, DA(SA), FFA(SA), MMed(Anaesth), PhD
Professor
Department of Anesthesia
University of Iowa Hospitals and Clinics
Director of Regional Anesthesia Study Center of Iowa (RASCI)
Director of Orthopaedic Anesthesia
Director of Regional Anesthesia Fellowship Program
Iowa City, Iowa

Steven C. Borene, MD
Anesthesiologist
North Iowa Anesthesia Associates
Mason City, Iowa

Alain Borgeat, MD
Professor and Chief of Staff
Department of Anesthesiology
Orthopedic University Hospital Balgrist
Zurich
Switzerland

Hervé Bouaziz, MD
Professor of Anesthesiology
Hôpitaux de Ville

Centre Hospitalier Universitaire de Nancy
Nancy
France

Chester C. Buckenmaier III, MD
Chief, Army Regional Anesthesia and Pain Management
Assistant Professor, Uniformed Services
Walter Reed Army Medical Center
Washington, DC

John Butterworth, MD
Robert K. Stoelting Professor
Chairman, Department of Anesthesia
Indiana University School of Medicine
Indianapolis, Indiana

Kenneth D. Candido, MD
Associate Professor of Anesthesiology
Chief, Division of Pain Management
Loyola University Medical Center
Maywood, Illinois

Andrea Casati
Associate Professor of Anesthesiology
Department of Anesthesia and Pain Therapy
University of Parma
Policlinico di Parma
Parma
Italy

Gregory M. Casey, DDS
Department of Oral and Maxillofacial Surgery
St. Luke's-Roosevelt Hospital Center
New York, New York

Louis Catalano, MD
Hand Surgeon
Assistant Professor of Surgery
St. Luke's-Roosevelt Hospital Center
College of Physicians and Surgeons
Columbia University
New York, New York

Vincent Chan, MD, FRCPC
Professor
Department of Anesthesia
Toronto Western Hospital
University Health Network
University of Toronto
Toronto, Ontario
Canada

Olivier Choquet, MD
Regional Anesthesiologist
La Conception Hospital
Marseille
France

Laura Lowrey Clark, MD
Associate Professor
Department of Anesthesia and Perioperative Medicine
University of Louisville
Louisville, Kentucky

Stacy A. Coffin, MD
Anesthesiologist
St. Luke's Hospital Duluth
Duluth, Minnesota

Adam Cohen, MD
Assistant Professor, Orthopedic Surgery
College of Physicians and Surgeons
Columbia University
New York, New York

Cliff P. Connery, MD
Chief, Division of Thoracic Surgery
St. Luke's-Roosevelt Hospital Center
Assistant Professor of Clinical Surgery
College of Physicians and Surgeons
Columbia University
New York, New York

Elyad Davidson, MD
Department of Anesthesiology
Miller School of Medicine
University of Miami
Miami, Florida

José De Andrés, MD, PhD
Associate Professor of Anesthesia
Valencia University Medical School
Chairman of Anesthesia Department
Director, Multidisciplinary Pain Management Center
Department of Anesthesia
Valencia University General Hospital
Valencia
Spain

Oscar de Leon, MD
Chief, Pain Medicine
Department of Anesthesiology and Pain Medicine
Roswell Park Cancer Institute
Professor of Anesthesiology
School of Medicine and Biomedical Sciences
State University of New York at Buffalo
Buffalo, New York

Robert Della Rocca, MD
Professor of Ophthalmology
St. Luke's-Roosevelt Hospital Center
College of Physicians and Surgeons
Columbia University
New York, New York

Rick J. Delmonte, DPM
Attending Podiatrist
Department of Orthopedic Surgery
St. Luke's-Roosevelt Hospital Center
New York, New York

Bonnie Deschner, MD
Regional Anesthesiologist
Assistant Professor of Clinical Anesthesiology
St. Luke's-Roosevelt Hospital Center
New York, New York

Steven Deschner, MD, PhD
Neurologist and Research Fellow
Department of Anesthesia
Division of Regional Anesthesia
St. Luke's-Roosevelt Hospital Center
New York, New York

Faruk Dilberovic, MD, PhD
Professor of Anatomy
Faculty of Medicine
University of Sarajevo
Sarajevo
Bosnia and Herzegovina

Benaifer D. Dubash, DMD
Department of Oral and Maxillofacial Surgery
St. Luke's-Roosevelt Hospital
New York, New York

Clint E. Elliott, MD
Department of Anesthesiology
Ochsner Clinic Foundation
New Orleans, Louisiana

F. Kayser Enneking, MD
Professor
Departments of Anesthesiology, and Orthopedics
    and Rehabilitation
University of Florida
Gainesville, Florida

Vicente Roqués Escolar, MD
Department of Anesthesiology
Hospital Universitario Virgen de la Arrixaca
Murcia, Spain

Holly Evans, MD, FRCP(C)
Associate
Department of Anesthesiology
Division of Ambulatory Anesthesiology
Duke University Medical Center
Durham, North Carolina

Elisabeth Fouché, MD
Designer
Advanced Data Network
Sainte Foy les Lyon
France

Carlo D. Franco, MD
Chairman Orthopedic Anesthesiology
John H. Stroger, Jr. Hospital of Cook County
Associate Professor
Departments of Anesthesiology and Anatomy
    and Cell Biology
Rush University Medical Center
Chicago, Illinois

Michael Fredrickson, MD
Specialist in Pediatric Anesthesia
Starship Children's Hospital
Park Road, Grafton
Honorary Clinical Senior Lecturer in Anesthesiology
The University of Auckland
Auckland
New Zealand

Jeffrey Gadsden, MD, FRCPC
Assistant Professor
Bond University Faculty of Health Sciences and Medicine
Consultant Anesthetist
Gold Coast Hospital
Queensland
Australia

Elizabeth Gaertner, MD
Department of Anesthesiology
Hautpierre Hospital
Strasbourg
France

Philippe Gautier, MD
Wezembeek-Oppem
Belgium

J. C. Gerancher, MD
Associate Professor and Section Head
Regional Anesthesia and Acute Pain Management
Wake Forest University School of Medicine
Winston-Salem, North Carolina

Steven Z. Glickel, MD
Associate Professor of Surgery
Hand Surgeon
Department of Orthopedic Surgery
St. Luke's-Roosevelt Hospital Center
New York, New York

Andrew T. Gray, MD, PhD
Department of Anesthesia and Perioperative Care
University of California, San Francisco
San Francisco General Hospital
San Francisco, California

Paul M. Greenburg, DPM
Podiatric Surgeon
Department of Orthopedic Surgery
St Luke's-Roosevelt Hospital
New York, New York

Roy A. Greengrass, MD, FRCP(C)
Professor
Department of Anesthesiology
Mayo Clinic Jacksonville
Jacksonville, Florida

Admir Hadzic, MD, PhD
Director of Regional Anesthesia
St. Luke's-Roosevelt Hospital Center
Professor of Anesthesiology
College of Physicians and Surgeons
Columbia University
New York, New York

Brian E. Harrington, MD
Anesthesiologist
Billings, Montana

William Harrop-Griffiths, MB BS, FRCA
Department of Anesthesia and Perioperative Medicine
Royal Brisbane and Women's Hospital
Herston, Queensland
Australia

Adam T. Hershkin, DMD
Department of Oral and Maxillofacial Surgery
St. Luke's-Roosevelt Hospital
New York, New York

Loreen A. Herwaldt, MD
Department of Internal Medicine
Carver College of Medicine
University of Iowa
Program of Hospital Epidemiology
University of Iowa Hospitals and Clinics
Iowa City, Iowa

Anthony M.-H. Ho, MSc, MD, FRCPC, FCCP, FHKCA, FHKAM
Professor
Department of Anaesthesia and Intensive Care
The Chinese University of Hong Kong
Prince of Wales Hospital
Shatin, New Territories
Hong Kong
People's Republic of China

Paul Hobeika, MD
Assistant Professor of Orthopedic Surgery
Staff Orthopedic Surgeon
St. Luke's-Roosevelt Hospital
College of Physicians and Surgeons
Columbia University
New York, New York

Brian M. Ilfeld, MD
Associate Professor of Anesthesiology
University of California San Diego
San Diego, California

Giorgio Ivani, MD
Pediatric Anesthesiologist
Chairman, Division of Pediatric Anesthesia and
    Intensive Care
Regina Margharita Children's Hospital
Torino
Italy

Tagashige Iwata, MD
Research Fellow in Regional Anesthesia
St. Luke's-Roosevelt Hospital Center
New York, New York

Rasha S. Jabri, MD
Instructor of Anesthesiology
Feinberg School of Medicine
Northwestern University
Chicago, Illinois

Rehana Jan, MD
Anesthesiologist
Thomas Jefferson University
Philadelphia, Pennsylvania

Edward Jew, MD
Surgeon
Department of Obstetric and Gynecologic Surgery
St. Luke's-Roosevelt Hospital Center
Assistant Professor of Clinical Obstetric and Gynecologic
    Surgery
College of Physicians and Surgeons
Columbia University
New York, New York

Stephan Kapral, MD
Professor of Anesthesia
Department of Anesthesia and Intensive Care Medicine
Medical University Vienna
Austrian Regional Anaesthesia Group (ARAG)
Vienna
Austria

Eldan Kapur, MD
Assistant Professor of Anatomy
Department of Anatomy
Medicine School
University of Sarajevo
Sarajevo
Bosnia and Herzegovina

Manoj K. Karmakar, MD, FRCA, DA (UK), FHKCA, FHKAM
Associate Professor
Department of Anaesthesia and Intensive Care
The Chinese University of Hong Kong
Prince of Wales Hospital
Shatin, New Territories
Hong Kong
People's Republic of China

Joseph Kay, MD, FRCPC
Assistant Professor of Anesthesiology
Department of Anesthesia
Sunnybrook and Women's College HSC
University of Toronto
Toronto, Ontario
Canada

Stephen M. Klein, MD
Associate Professor
Department of Anesthesiology
Division of Ambulatory Anesthesiology
Duke University Medical Center
Durham, North Carolina

Zbigniew J. Koscielniak-Nielsen, MD, PhD, FRCA
Assistant Professor
Head of Orthopaedic Anaesthesia
Rigshospital
Copenhagen
Denmark

Sabine Kost-Byerly, MD
Clinical Director, Pediatric Pain Management
Assistant Professor
Department of Anesthesiology/Critical Care Medicine and
    Pediatrics
The Johns Hopkins Hospital
Baltimore, Maryland

Maxine M. Kuroda, PhD, MPH
Statistician
Children's Memorial Research Center
Chicago, Illinois

Suzanne Lenart, RN
Thomas Jefferson University
Philadelphia, Pennsylvania

Gregory A. Liguori, MD
Attending Anesthesiologist
Clinical Associate Professor of Anesthesiology
Chair, Department of Anesthesiology
Hospital for Special Surgery

Weill Medical College of Cornell University
New York, New York

Spencer S. Liu, MD
Staff Anesthesiologist
Virginia Mason Medical Center
Clinical Professor of Anesthesiology
University of Washington School of Medicine
Department of Anesthesiology
Virginia Mason Medical Center
Seattle, Washington

Navin A. Mallavaram, MD
Department of Anesthesiology
St. Luke's-Roosevelt Hospital Center
New York, New York

Peter Marhofer, MD
Professor of Anesthesia
Medical University Vienna
Department of Anesthesia and Intensive Care Medicine
Austrian Regional Anaesthesia Group (ARAG)
Vienna
Austria

Joseph Marino, MD
Anesthesiologist
Greenlawn, New York

Colin J. L. McCartney, MB ChB, FRCA, FCARCSI, FRCPC
Assistant Professor and Director of Regional Anesthesia
Toronto Western Hospital
University of Toronto
Toronto, Ontario
Canada

Susan B. McDonald, MD
Staff Anesthesiologist
Virginia Mason Medical Center
Seattle, Washington

Patrick M. McQuillan, MD
Professor, Anesthesiology and Pediatrics
Associate Chair for Clinical Affairs
Director, Acute Pain Management and Regional Anesthesia
Department of Anesthesiology
Milton S. Hershey Medical Center
Pennsylvania State University
Hershey, Pennsylvania

Kenneth Merhige, MD
Associate Professor of Ophthalmology
St. Luke's-Roosevelt Hospital Center
College of Physicians and Surgeons
Columbia University
New York, New York

David Misita, MD
Assistant Professor of Anesthesiology
St. Luke's-Roosevelt Hospital Center
College of Physicians and Surgeons
Columbia University
New York, New York

Zakira Mornjaković, MD, PhD
Professor and Chair, Institute of Histology
Medical School of the University of Sarajevo
Sarajevo
Bosnia and Herzegovina

Michael F. Mulroy, MD
Staff Anesthesiologist
Virginia Mason Medical Center
University of Washington
Seattle, Washington

Joseph M. Neal, MD
Staff Anesthesiologist
Virginia Mason Medical Center
Clinical Professor of Anesthesiology
University of Washington
Seattle, Washington

Karen C. Nielsen, MD
Associate Professor
Department of Anesthesiology
Division of Ambulatory Anesthesiology
Duke University Medical Center
Durham, North Carolina

Anahi Perlas, MD, FRCPC
Assistant Professor
Department of Anesthesia
Toronto Western Hospital
University Health Network
University of Toronto
Toronto, Ontario
Canada

Geofrey J. Pollack, MD
Head and Neck Surgeon
Facial Plastic Surgery
Department of Otolaryngology
St. Luke's-Roosevelt Hospital Center
Clinical Instructor in Otolaryngology
College of Physicians and Surgeons
Columbia University
New York, New York

Jean M. Pottinger, RN, MA
Program of Hospital Epidemiology
University of Iowa Hospitals and Clinics
Iowa City, Iowa

Marta Putzu, MD
Anesthesia Fellow
Department of Anesthesia and Pain Therapy
University of Parma
Parma, Italy

Jayanthi Sudharma Ranasinghe, MD, FFARCSI
Department of Anesthesiology
Miller School of Medicine
University of Miami
Miami, Florida

James P. Rathmell, MD
Director, MGH Pain Center
Department of Anesthesia and Critical Care
Massachusetts General Hospital
Boston, Massachusetts

Narinder Rawal, MD, PhD
Department of Anesthesiology and Intensive Care
Orebro University Hospital
Orebro
Sweden

Elizabeth M. Renehan, MD, MSc, FRCPC
Fellow in Regional Anesthesia
Department of Anesthesiology
University of Florida
Gainesville, Florida

Scott S. Reuben, MD
Anesthesiologist
Department of Anesthesiology
Baystate Medical Center
Springfield, Massachusetts

Jacques Ripart, MD, PhD
Staff Anesthesiologist
Department of Anesthesiology, Pain Management, and
    Intensive Care
Centre Hospitalier Universitaire Nimes
Nimes
France

Christopher Robards, MD
Regional Anesthesiologist
Assistant Professor of Anesthesia
Mayo Clinic
Jacksonville, Florida

Xavier Sala-Blanch, MD
Assistant Professor of Anesthesiology
University of Barcelona
Barcelona
Spain

Francis V. Salinas, MD
Staff Anesthesiologist
Virginia Mason Medical Center
Seattle, Washington

Alan C. Santos, MD
Professor and Chair
Department of Anesthesiology
Ochsner Clinic Foundation
New Orleans, Louisiana

Leslie Schechter, PharmD
Thomas Jefferson University
Philadelphia, Pennsylvania

Robert J. Schlosser, MD
Department of Anesthesiology
Froedtert East Clinics
Milwaukee, Wisconsin

Sebastian Schulz-Stübner, MD, PhD
Department of Anesthesia
University of Iowa Hospitals and Clinics
Iowa City, Iowa

Paul J. Seider, DMD
Department of Oral and Maxillofacial Surgery
St. Luke's-Roosevelt Hospital
New York, New York

François J. Singelyn, MD, PhD
Associate Professor
Department of Anesthesiology
Université Catholique de Louvain School of Medicine
St Luc Hospital
Brussels
Belgium

Ilija Škrinjarić
Professor of Pediatric Dentistry
Department of Pediatric Dentistry
School of Dental Medicine
University of Zagreb
Zagreb
Croatia

Lakshmanasamy Somasundaram, MD
Research Fellow in Regional Anesthesia
St. Luke's-Roosevelt Hospital Center
New York, New York

Susan M. Steele, MD
Professor
Department of Anesthesiology
Division of Ambulatory Anesthesiology
Duke University Medical Center
Durham, North Carolina

Santhanam Suresh, MD, FAAP
Director of Research
Children's Memorial Hospital
Associate Professor of Anesthesiology and Pediatrics
Feinberg School of Medicine
Northwestern University
Chicago, Illinois

Leroy Sutherland, MD
Assistant Professor of Clinical Anesthesiology
Instructor of Difficult Airway Management
Pain Management Specialist
St. Luke's-Roosevelt Hospital Center
College of Physicians and Surgeons
Columbia University
New York, New York

Leslie C. Thomas, MD
Department of Anesthesiology
Ochsner Clinic Foundation
New Orleans, Louisiana

Daniel M. Thys, MD
Department of Anesthesiology
St. Luke's-Roosevelt Hospital Center
New York, New York

Knox H. Todd, MD, MPH
Professor of Emergency Medicine
Director, Pain and Emergency Medicine Institute
Department of Emergency Medicine
Beth Israel Hospital
Albert Einstein College of Medicine
New York, New York

Tony Tsai, MD
Assistant Professor of Anesthesiology
Regional Anesthesiologist
St. Luke's-Roosevelt Hospital
College of Physicians and Surgeons
Columbia University
New York, New York

Ban C. H. Tsui, Dip. Engineering, BSc (Mathematics), BSc (Pharmacy), MSc, MD, FRCP(C)
Pediatric and Adult Anesthesiologist
Director of Clinical Research
Alberta Heritage Clinical Investigator
Assistant Professor
Department of Anesthesiology and Pain Medicine
University of Alberta
Edmonton, Alberta
Canada

Contributors

Marcy S. Tucker, MD, PhD
Department of Anesthesiology
Division of Ambulatory Anesthesiology
Duke University Medical Center
Durham, North Carolina

Tetsu Uejima, MD, FAAP
Assistant Professor of Anesthesiology
Children's Memorial Hospital
Feinberg School of Medicine
Northwestern University
Chicago, Illinois

Douglas Unis, MD
Assistant Professor of Orthopedic Surgery
St. Luke's-Roosevelt Hospital Center
College of Physicians and Surgeons
Columbia University
New York, New York

William F. Urmey, MD
Associate Professor of Clinical Anesthesiology
Hospital for Special Surgery
Weill Medical College of Cornell University
Department of Anesthesiology
Hospital for Special Surgery
New York, New York

Bernadette Veering, MD, PhD
Associate Professor
Department of Anesthesiology
Leiden University Medical Center
Leiden
The Netherlands

Eugene R. Viscusi, MD
Associate Professor of Anesthesiology
Thomas Jefferson University
Philadelphia, Pennsylvania

Jerry D. Vloka, MD, PhD
Associate Professor of Anesthesiology
St. Luke's-Roosevelt Hospital Center
College of Physicians and Surgeons
Columbia University
New York, New York

Daniel T. Warren, MD
Anesthesia Pain Management Fellow
Department of Anesthesiology
Virginia Mason Medical Center
Seattle, Washington

Paul F. White, PhD, MD, FANZCA
Professor and Holder of the Margaret Milam McDermott
Distinguished Chair in Anesthesiology
Department of Anesthesiology and Pain Management
University of Texas Southwestern Medical Center at Dallas
Dallas, Texas

Brian A. Williams, MD, MBA
Associate Professor of Anesthesiology
University of Pittsburgh
Director, Outpatient Regional Anesthesia Service
University of Pittsburgh Medical Center South Side
Pittsburgh, Pennsylvania

Paul H. Willoughby, MD
Associate Professor
Director, Acute Pain Service
Department of Anesthesiology
Health Sciences Center
State University of New York at Stony Brook
Stony Brook, New York

Alon P. Winnie, MD
Professor Emeritus
Department of Anesthesiology
Northwestern University
Feinberg School of Medicine
Chicago, Illinois

Chi Wong, MS
Anatomy Fellow
New York College of Osteopathic Medicine
Old Westbury, New York

Christopher L. Wu, MD
Associate Professor
Department of Anesthesiology and Critical Care Medicine
The Johns Hopkins University
Baltimore, Maryland

Myron Yaster, MD
Richard J. Traystman Professor
Departments of Anesthesiology/Critical Care Medicine and
    Pediatrics
The Johns Hopkins Hospital
Baltimore, Maryland

Foreword

The use of regional anesthesia for surgery and as part of a multimodal analgesic strategy for the management of acute perioperative pain has evolved over the last 20 years, from its start as an eclectic practice of selective nerve blocks championed by a relatively small group of devoted practitioners to its current position as a standard part of nearly every procedure involving anesthesia. In the past, regional anesthesia was largely synonymous with spinal or epidural anesthesia. Subsequently, with advances in functional regional anesthesia anatomy and with development of better equipment for nerve localization, major nerve blocks were made available to practitioners. Presently, regional anesthetic techniques involving peripheral nerve blocks have become an essential part of monitored anesthetic care (MAC) and many general anesthetic techniques. Regional anesthesia is also a key component of many multimodal analgesic regimens used for postoperative pain management. Not surprisingly, regional anesthesia and acute pain management are among the most rapidly growing areas in our specialty.

In this comprehensive textbook of 83 chapters on the current state of knowledge in regional anesthesia and acute pain management, the reader is provided with detailed evidence-based information covering diverse topics such as the embryologic origins of the nervous system and the relevant anatomic, histologic, and pathologic considerations involved in the functional aspects of the nervous system. The relevant chapters on neurophysiology and pharmacology of analgesic drugs are essential to understanding the optimal approaches to using regional anesthetic techniques during surgery and preventing postoperative pain as well as managing complex patients with acute and chronic pain syndromes. Understanding the impact of co-existing diseases and aging on the practice of regional anesthesia is essential to administering safe and effective regional anesthesia and optimizing pain management for these higher-risk patient populations. The use of opioid and non-opioid analgesic drugs as a part of a multimodal approach to pain management is also discussed because it is essential to achieving improved patient outcomes.

Recent advances in the equipment used to administer regional anesthesia (eg, stimulating needles, constant-current nerve stimulators, ultrasound devices, and disposable catheter-based local anesthetic delivery systems), which have made it possible for practitioners to improve the accuracy of nerve blocks, to extend the duration of analgesia by using continuous infusion techniques, and to minimize complications (eg, nerve injury and infections), are extensively discussed. Similarly, chapters are devoted to the use of regional anesthesia in specific practice settings (eg, for ambulatory [outpatient] surgery, the elderly, obstetrical patients, and in chronic pain clinics and emergency departments). Finally, essential information for incorporating regional anesthetic techniques into acute pain management services and information on academic teaching (and research) programs is also provided.

Although a number of "how to" textbooks in anesthesiology have been published in the past, this comprehensive multi-authored textbook on the principles and practice of regional anesthesia and acute pain management is unique because it incorporates both the theoretical and the practical aspects of regional anesthesia in the context of everyday clinical practice. As a direct result of the tremendous efforts and dedication of the editor, Admir Hadzic, MD, PhD, and a highly selective group of contributors who are opinion leaders in their own subspecialty areas, this book is destined to become a classic in its field and the standard against which all future texts in regional anesthesia will be compared. The scope of this book reaches far beyond the typical regional anesthesia text: it provides both the novice and the experienced practitioner with exhaustive and well-organized practical information on how to improve patient outcome by incorporating regional anesthetic techniques into clinical practice. It is noteworthy that several chapters are written on the use of regional anesthesia in various subspecialty fields by paired teams of contributors (eg, surgeons with anesthesiologists). As a result, the information in this book will be of value not only to anesthesiologists, but also to surgeons, perioperative physicians, emergency department physicians, oromaxillar surgeons, and many others.

It was indeed an honor for me to participate in this project with one of the most progressive young academic anesthesiologists in the world. In my opinion, this book will become a standard text for experienced practitioners of anesthesiology and pain management as well as for postdoctoral anesthesia trainees. This textbook should find a prominent place in the libraries of anesthesiologists and other specialists who use local or regional anesthesia in their clinical practice.

Paul F. White, PhD, MD, FANZCA
Professor and Holder of the Margaret Milam McDermott
Distinguished Chair in Anesthesiology
Department of Anesthesiology and Pain Management
University of Texas Southwestern Medical Center at Dallas
Dallas, Texas

Preface

Medicine is a dynamic and constantly changing art. However, regional anesthesia, as a discipline, has often lagged behind the progress and developments of other subspecialties of anesthesiology. This is due, in part, to the fact that regional anesthesia is both the oldest and, in some respects, the youngest discipline of anesthesiology. It is the oldest because the introduction of cocaine for ocular surgery by Karl Koller in 1884 marked the beginning of what could be called *modern anesthesiology*. It is the youngest because, despite its 150-year-long history, it has only recently begun to acquire the means and technology necessary to make it as reproducible and objective as other medical subspecialties.

This lack of objectivity in regional anesthesia stems from the fact that most procedures have relied on subjective "feel" rather than an objective, quantifiable methodology. "Feel" techniques traditionally have been taught by a relatively small number of enthusiastic, charismatic, and uniquely capable "masters." While regional anesthesia, throughout the 20th century, depended almost entirely on *subjective* methods, general anesthesia advanced substantially through *technologic* and *pharmacologic* developments as well as via *objective* physiologic monitoring. Taken together, these factors conspired to use and teach objective and reproducible *general anesthetic techniques* rather than *regional anesthesia techniques*. Although neuraxial regional anesthesia has been in widespread use (especially in obstetric anesthesia), peripheral nerve block techniques were almost forgotten until a resurgence in the 1990s, which continues today.

Research efforts, data on improved patient outcomes with regional anesthesia and better pain management, and the rapid growth of ambulatory surgery have come together to provide an exciting environment for a renaissance of regional anesthesia and its role in perioperative management of acute pain. That being so, there is probably no better time for the publication of this book because it coincides with what must be one of the most exciting periods in the development of modern regional anesthesia.

Today, regional anesthesia and acute pain management are undoubtedly among the most discussed, researched, and lectured areas of clinical anesthesiology. Ongoing research in functional regional anesthesia anatomy, wider availability of training in regional anesthesia, and rapid development of better techniques and equipment for regional anesthesia have fueled the interest and the development of this field and have made techniques much more reproducible. For example, continuous perineural catheters; sophisticated nerve stimulators; depth-coded, insulated, stimulating needles; injection pressure monitoring; and real-time, ultrasound-guided peripheral nerve blocks are now commonly available. Contrary to conventional practice, in which the practitioner chooses either regional anesthesia or pharmacologic management of pain, it has become clear today that management of acute pain is a multimodal approach. This book aims to provide the anatomic, physiologic, and pharmacologic bases for the practice of regional anesthesia and its integration into pharmacologic management of acute pain. To accomplish this aim, I have recruited key opinion leaders from within the United States and abroad and have asked them not only to share the in-depth science that is their area of expertise but also to present their practical approaches to managing a spectrum of scenarios in clinical practice of regional anesthesia and acute pain management.

The book consists of 83 chapters. The first part of the book discusses the history of regional anesthesia, its roots, and its early developments. Readers should realize, however, that the history of regional anesthesia does not end with these events of the past. Au contraire, the history of *modern* regional anesthesia is being created by the pioneers of the 1990s onward.

The chapter on embryology provides substantial background regarding dermatomes, osteotomes, and myotomes as well as relevant information necessary for understanding the development of nerves and plexi. The chapters on anatomy, pharmacology, and electrophysiology are written to give the reader insight into the basic principles, techniques, pharmacologic issues, and instruments used in regional anesthesia.

Part III, "Clinical Practice of Regional Anesthesia," begins with a chapter on local anesthesia. Because local anesthesia is administered more often by surgeons than by anesthesiologists, I have invited surgical colleagues to contribute the expertise that they rely upon in their everyday practice. To provide authentic, solid, and practical information, the same principle has been followed in all chapters: that is, practical information from practicing physicians was favored over purely academic, theoretical discussions.

Neuraxial anesthesia comprises spinal, epidural, and caudal anesthesia; separate, in-depth chapters are provided covering a wide range of neuraxial techniques. Following the introductory remarks and the chapter on equipment for peripheral nerve blocks, chapters on a variety of peripheral nerve block techniques are organized according to body regions. Each chapter begins with a brief historical review, followed by the indications and contraindications, discussion of the relevant anatomy, and various aspects of the techniques and perioperative management. As is the case for other chapters in the book, the information here focuses primarily on practical aspects. Substantial information and literature review also are devoted to the recent developments in the field, outcome data, variations in the techniques, and complications and their prevention.

Subsequent parts of the book focus on new developments in the instrumentation and monitoring used in regional anesthesia, ultrasound-assisted techniques for nerve blocks in both adult and pediatric populations, and the use of regional anesthesia in the obstetric patient.

When applied skillfully and for correct indications, regional anesthesia can improve patient outcomes. However, this may not be the case in patients with concomitant medical or surgical disease. For this reason, substantial information is provided on the implications and use of regional anesthesia in patients with cardiac and other medical diseases. The use of regional anesthesia in special patient populations or in special settings must be tailored to the specific needs of such patients in these special scenarios. Several chapters are devoted to the use of regional anesthesia in pediatrics, community practice, austere environments, critically ill patients, and emergency settings.

Because the risk of complications is one of the major factors impeding the wider use of regional anesthesia, separate chapters provide information on etiology, prevention, and management of complications related to the use of regional anesthesia. These comprise chapters on systemic, infectious, and neurologic complications of neuraxial anesthesia and peripheral nerve blocks. Similarly, the widespread perioperative use of potent anticoagulants mandates careful consideration of their effects on the safety of regional anesthesia techniques. Separate chapters are devoted to managing patients on anticoagulants.

Part XIII, "Regional Anesthesia & Acute Patient Management," includes chapters on pre-emptive analgesia, acute pain management, and integration of regional anesthesia into modern pain management pathways. Part XIV, "Documentation & Training of Regional Anesthesia," includes chapters on documenting regional anesthesia procedures and residency and fellowship training in regional anesthesia. The book ends with a chapter focusing on research design in regional anesthesia. This last chapter has been prepared to acquaint the young investigator with specific research methodologic issues and methods of importance to designing and conducting quality research in regional anesthesia. A separate section of this chapter presents the reader with practical examples of common mistakes encountered in manuscripts submitted for publication in major anesthesia journals.

As can be seen from the table of contents, this textbook is intended as both an in-depth reference text for academicians, teachers, and scholars of regional anesthesia and a down-to-earth practical guide for the practicing clinician. It is my hope that its content will promote the more widespread use of regional anesthesia techniques and foster research for its improvement for future generations.

Admir Hadzic, MD, PhD

Acknowledgments

The completion of this book would have been impossible without a number of special people who contributed enormously to this book with their encouragement, wisdom, or intellectual input.

Foremost, I would like to thank Alen and Gorica Hadzic for their unselfish support and understanding while I was grinding through the massive information that makes up this volume. Your patience, love, and support meant so much to me through the years. Many thanks to my parents Safeta and Junuz Hadzic as well as to Admira, Nermin, Emma, and Harris for their unconditional love and for forgiving me all the time I deprived them of my company while accomplishing the writing and editing tasks.

I would like to thank my chairman, Dr. Daniel Thys. Without his unmatched wisdom, encouragement, and academic advice, I may never have had the chance to successfully pursue my academic goals and this book may never have seen the light of day. Daniel is an exemplary academic chairperson and an incredible human being. Daniel, I am proud to have worked for you during much of my career and I consider it a privilege to call you my friend.

Many thanks to my research staff and colleagues at St. Luke's–Roosevelt Hospital Center, all of whom contributed hugely, in one way or another, to this book: Richard Claudio, Lakshman Sundharadam, Steven and Bonnie Deschner, Marina Allen, Alen Santos, Thomas Kurian, Paul Hobeika, George and Doug Unis, Jeff Dermeksian, Vincent Fietti, John Lantis, David Fox, Paul Greenberg, Rick Delmonte, Tarek Mardambey, Alton Baron, Andrea Valicenti, Beklan Kerimoglu, Pelin Emine Karaca, Daquan Xu, Henri Shih, Toni Tsai, Jeff Gadsden, Natasha Ortiz, and many others who also deserve to be mentioned here. A special thank you to all the contributors, most of whom are not only exemplary academicians and practitioners of the subspecialty, but also my close friends and colleagues.

I would also like to thank some great people at McGraw-Hill for their work on this gigantic undertaking. Many thanks to my chief editor, Joe Rusko, and to Robert Pancotti, Peter Boyle, Marc Strauss, Linda Davoli, Alison Kelley, and Andrea Ralya. I have been hugely helped by this incredible team of high-level professionals spread across two floors of the building above Madison Square Garden in New York.

A big thank you to Jerry Vloka, my long-time academic partner and friend, whose unfortunate accident unjustly forced him to leave medicine. Jerry has been a source of inspiration for me through the years and has left an academic influence that has been an essential ingredient in many of my aspirations. Jerry, I have sorely missed you all these years. You should know that this book has your stamp on every page.

Finally, special thanks to Lejla Hadzic for dedicating her enormous artistic talent to this project. Besides being my favorite cousin, Lejla is a graduate of the School of Fine Arts and Architectural Faculty at the University of Sarajevo. She also holds several postgraduate degrees from some of the most prestigious European universities. She is currently associated with Foundation Cultural Heritage Without Borders, based in Stockholm, Sweden. Lejla, I am eternally grateful to you for your dedication to this book and the many nights you spent burning the midnight oil working on the illustrations, always with a smile on your face.

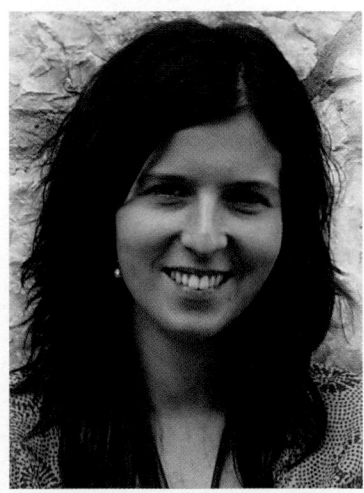

The New York School of Regional Anesthesia

Textbook of Regional Anesthesia and Acute Pain Management

History

The History of Local Anesthesia

Bonnie Deschner, MD • Christopher Robards, MD • Lakshmanasamy Somasundaram, MD •
William Harrop-Griffiths, MD

INTRODUCTION

The history of local anesthesia suffers, if it suffers from any-thing, from the lack of a distinct *Eureka moment*. It is arguable that we do not have in our history a pivotal day that signi-fied the wholesale change from an era before local anesthesia to the dawn of a new and wonderful age that included parts of the body being rendered insensate for therapeutic reasons. We do not have the equivalent of 16 October 1846 and the trembling hands of William Thomas Green Morton. What we have is a remarkably slow concatenation of the three ele-ments necessary for the administration of the vast majority of local anesthetics: a syringe, a needle, and a local anesthetic

drug. Many, however, would argue that to these three need be added several other factors: a detailed knowledge of anatomy and an appreciation of the body's pain mechanisms and more objective methods to localize peripheral nerves and monitor administration of local anesthetics. The authors make no ex-cuse for concentrating in this chapter on the early history of local anesthesia in order to dissect the development of these three vital components.

BEFORE COCAINE

The origins of the first attempts at some form of local anal-gesia or anesthesia are lost in the mists of time. Direct nerve

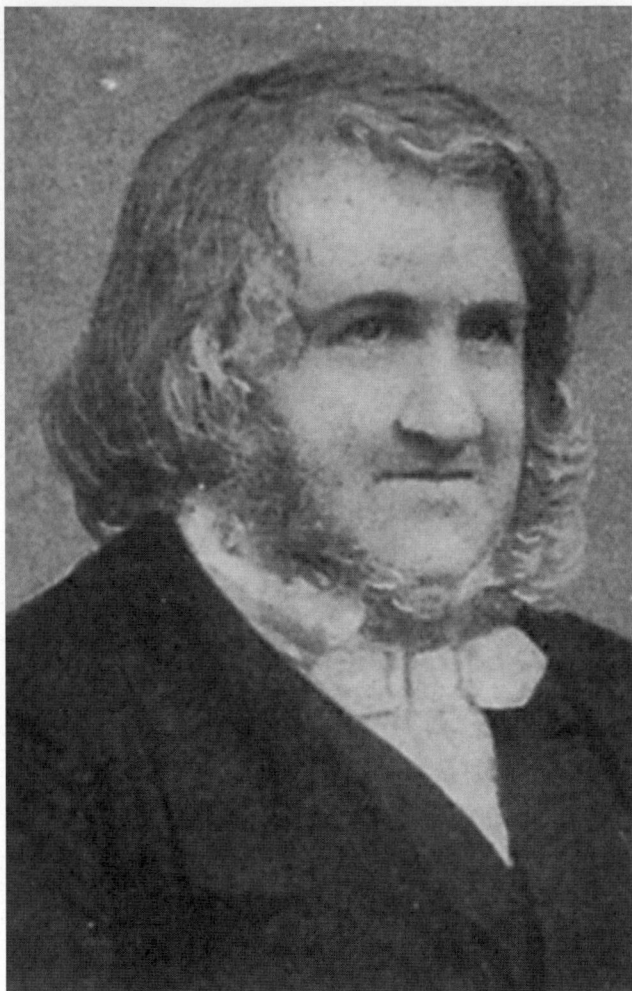

Figure 1–1. James Young Simpson.

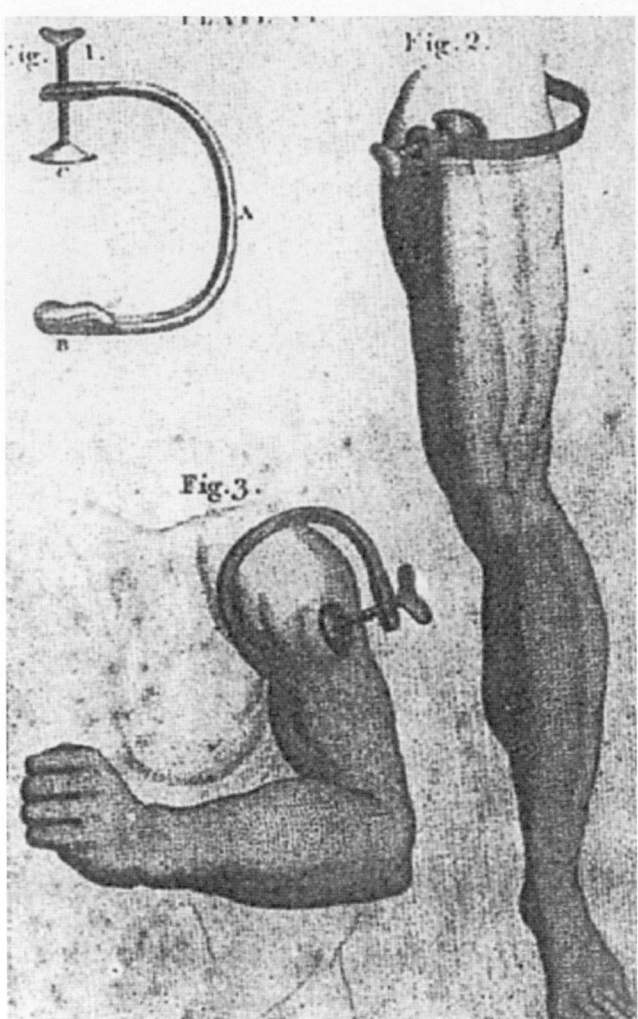

Figure 1–2. Nerve compression technique.

compression and the direct application of ice to peripheries before surgery have distant origins but were certainly in regular use from the latter half of the eighteenth century. The first detailed appreciation of the benefits of local anesthesia was written by James Young Simpson and published in 1848, decades before local anesthesia became a practical possibility (Figure 1–1). In this paper, he also described his own unsuccessful experiments with the topical application of a variety of liquids and vapors in an attempt to produce local anesthesia. The paper was published less than 2 years after Oliver Wendell Holmes had coined the term *anesthesia,* and it therefore almost certainly represents the first use of the term *local anesthesia,* although Simpson would have used the (arguably more correct) English spelling *anaesthesia.* However, Simpson was well aware that his were far from being the first attempts to produce peripheral insensibility, for he refers to some ancient methods, which he considered 'apocryphal,' and also to Moore's method of nerve compression (Figure 1–2).[1]

Another distinguished British physician and president of the Medical Society of London in 1868 was Sir Benjamin Ward Richardson. He spent many years in the attempt to alleviate pain by modifying substances capable of producing general or local anesthesia. He brought into use no fewer than

14 anesthetics and invented the first double-valved mouthpiece for the administration of chloroform. He initially experimented with electricity before turning to the effects of cold as an anesthetic. Cold was known to produce a numbing effect and was used as far back as Napoleon's time when his surgeon, Baron Larrey, used its effects to alleviate pain. He introduced a method of producing local insensibility by freezing the part with an *ether spray,* which became the most practical method of using local anesthesia until cocaine's actions became apparent. The ether spray was utilized as a local agent until it was replaced by ethyl chloride in 1880[2] (Figure 1–3).

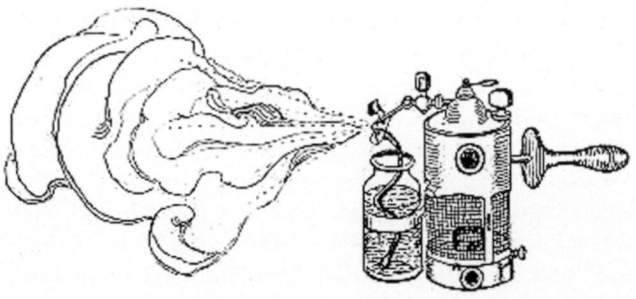

Figure 1–3. Ether spray.

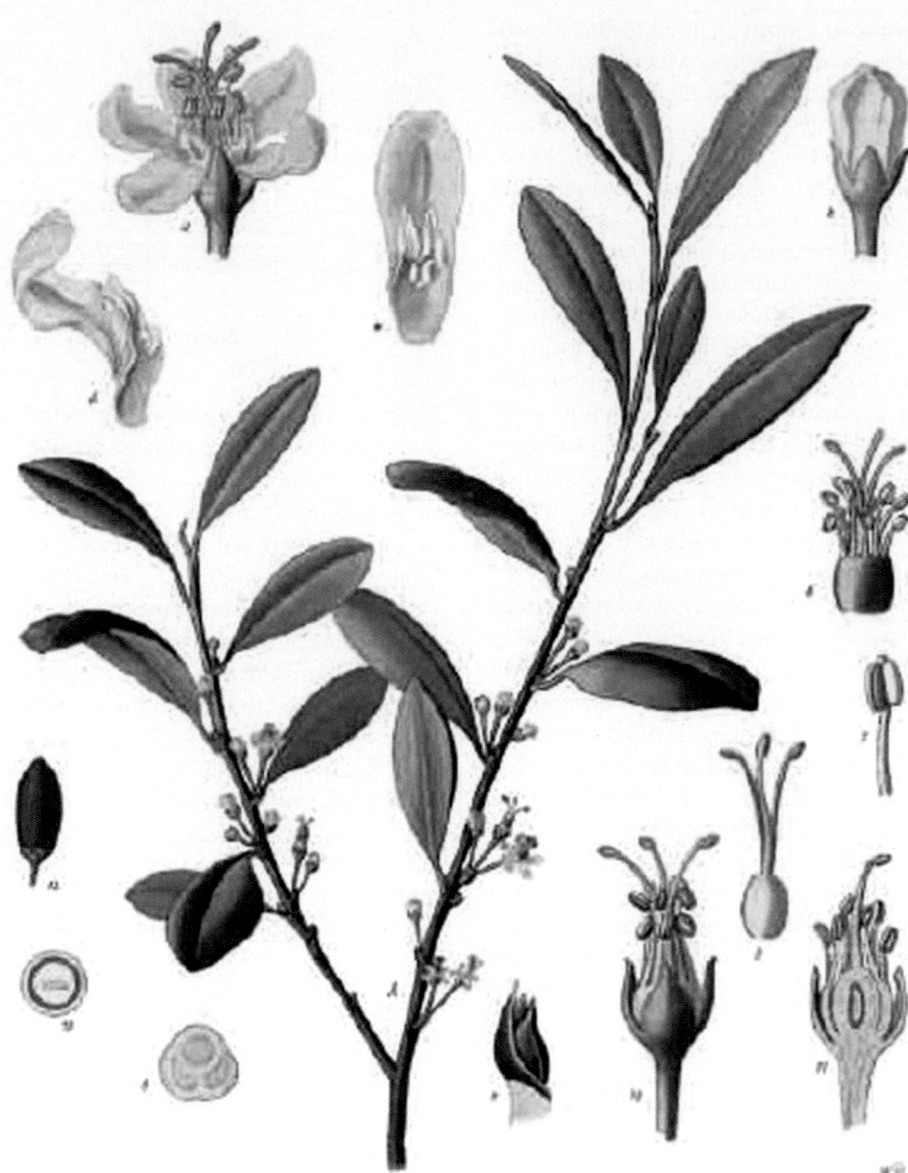

Figure 1–4. Coca leaf.

COCAINE ANESTHESIA

The Origins

If local anesthesia has a Eureka moment, then it may have happened in the forests of South America. Centuries ago, an unnamed inhabitant of these climates may have been experimenting by putting leaves of various plants into his mouth and giving them a good chew. We can imagine that this would be a largely unrewarding hobby, but let us focus on the moment when he first placed a coca leaf into his mouth and masticated vigorously. Did he fall to his knees and shout in wonderment: "My lips have gone numb—surely this is the dawn of a new age of painless surgery!". Almost certainly not—although he might have later told his friends that he felt somewhat excited, energetic, and euphoric while he chewed the leaves.

For thousands of years, South American peoples have chewed the coca leaf. It is a remarkable plant in that it contains

vital nutrients as well as numerous alkaloids, most notably cocaine. The coca leaves are taken from a shrub of the genus *Erythroxylon coca,* named by Patrico Browne because of the reddish hue of the wood of the main species.[3] Many species of this genus have been grown in Nicaragua, Venezuela, Bolivia, and Peru since pre-Columbian times. *Erythroxylon coca* contains the highest concentration of the alkaloid known as cocaine in its leaves[3,4] (Figure 1–4).

Traditionally, the leaves were chewed for social, mystical, medicinal, and religious purposes. The Florentine cartographer Amerigo Vespucci (1451–1512) was arguably the first European to document the human use of the coca leaf.[5,6] In his account of his voyage to America on the second expedition of Alonso de Ojeda and Juan de la Cosa from 1499 to 1500, he reported that the inhabitants of the Island of Margarita chewed certain herbs containing a white powder.[7] Among sixteenth-century Spanish chroniclers, the appearance of coca is associated with Francisco Pizarro's (1475–1541) conquest of the Inca or Tawantinsuyo Empire in 1532. Pedro Pizarro (1515–1571), Francisco Pizarro's cousin who played a leading role in the capture of the last king of the Incas, described coca consumption by the nobles and high officials of the Inca Empire.[8] After the fall of the Inca Empire in the early 1500s, coca consumption spread to the population at large, creating a drastic change in the entire social system.

When the Spaniards conquered South America, they initially ignored the aboriginal claims that the leaf gave them vigor and liveliness. They self-righteously declared the practice of chewing the leaf the "work of the Devil."[5] But once they found that the claims of the natives were true, they not only legalized the leaf, but they taxed it—taking 10% of the value of each crop! The taxes were then used to support the Roman Catholic Church—the main source of revenue for the church to thrive. In 1609, Padre Blas Valera wrote: "Coca protects the body from many ailments, and our doctors use it in powdered form to reduce the swelling of wounds, to strengthen broken bones, to expel cold from the body or prevent it from entering, and to cure rotten wounds or sores that are full of maggots. And if it does so much for outward ailments, will not its singular virtue have even great effect in the entrails of those who eat it?"[9] If the padre was blessed with the ability to foresee the future, perhaps his enthusiasm would have been redirected toward limiting the use of the leaf, and the field of anesthesia might have taken a different turn.

Another member of the clergy, Bernabé Cobo, who spent his life bringing Christianity to the Incas, is the first to describe the anesthetic effects of coca. In a 1653 manuscript, he mentioned that toothaches could be alleviated by chewing the coca leaves. In 1859, an Italian physician by the name of Paolo Mantegazza had witnessed the use of coca by the natives in Peru. He wrote a paper describing the medicinal use in the treatment of "a furred tongue in the morning, flatulence and whitening of the teeth."[10]

Needles & Syringes

If local anesthetic drugs are the bullets used when fighting pain, the gun needed to fire it is made up of a syringe and a needle. Without the bullets, the gun is useless and, just as certainly, without the gun, the bullets will have little effect. The development of the hypodermic syringe and needle was therefore an important prerequisite for the use of cocaine for anything but topical application. A thorough sifting of the available historical evidence and independent reexamination of the sources support the following outline of the facts. In 1845, Francis Rynd described the idea of introducing a solution of morphine hypodermically in the neighborhood of a peripheral nerve to alleviate neuralgic pain.[11] He introduced the solution by means of gravity, passively through a cannula once the trocar had been removed.

Several centuries past before the development of a syringe to deliver medicine was described by Alexander Wood (Figure 1–5). Wood, a contemporary of James Young Simpson, was, in 1855, the first to combine needle and syringe for hypodermic medication. He used the equipment manu-

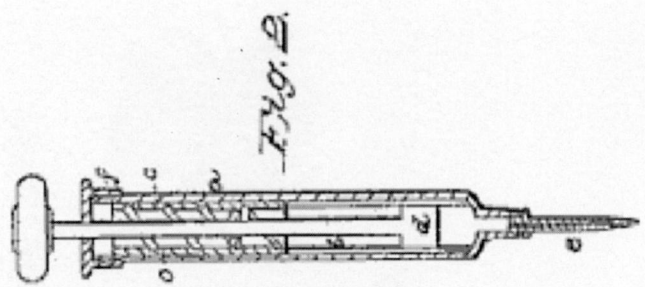

Figure 1–5. Early syringe.

factured by a gentleman by the name of Ferguson who had developed the graduated glass syringe and hollow needle for the purpose of treating aneurysms by injecting ferric perchloride into the aneurysm to form a coagulated mass. Wood, a physician interested in the treatment of neuralgia, reasoned that morphine might be more effective if it were injected close to the nerve supplying the affected area. Although morphine may have some peripheral actions, and the effect of Wood's morphine was almost certainly central, he was nevertheless the first to think of the possibility of producing nerve blockade by direct drug injection. Thus he has been called the "father-in-law" of local anesthesia—all he lacked was an agent that worked locally. Wood's contribution was therefore his procedure of subcutaneous injection. This technique was subsequently adopted by C. Hunter and renamed hypodermic injection presumably because Hunter's purpose was to provide systemic absorption of medications injected.[12,13]

The Introduction of Cocaine

The growth in Western science and technology exploded during the nineteenth century. Six years after Charles Darwin's controversial book, *On the Origin of Species by Means of Natural Selection,* Joseph Lister was an important figure in changing the face of surgery. He applied Pasteur's principles of bacterial growth in eliminating sepsis in the operating theatre. Other prominent figures contributed to the understanding of human physiology, eg, Sydney Ringer's discovery of the need for calcium and potassium to maintain cardiac excitability, significantly advancing medical care. And then there was cocaine.

Although the stimulant and hunger-suppressant effects of coca had been known for years, the isolation of the cocaine alkaloid was not achieved until 1855. Scientists attempted to isolate cocaine, but none were successful for two reasons: coca did not grow in the colder environment of Europe, and the chemistry involved was unknown at that time. Finally in 1855, the German chemist Friedrich Gaedcke was able to isolate the cocaine alkaloid and publish the description in the journal *Archieves de Pharmacie.* In 1856, Friedrich Wöhler asked a colleague to bring him a large amount of coca leaves from South America. Wöhler then gave the leaves to Albert Niemann, a PhD student at the University of Göttingen in Germany, who then developed an improved purification process. His dissertation, *On a New Organic Base in the Coca*

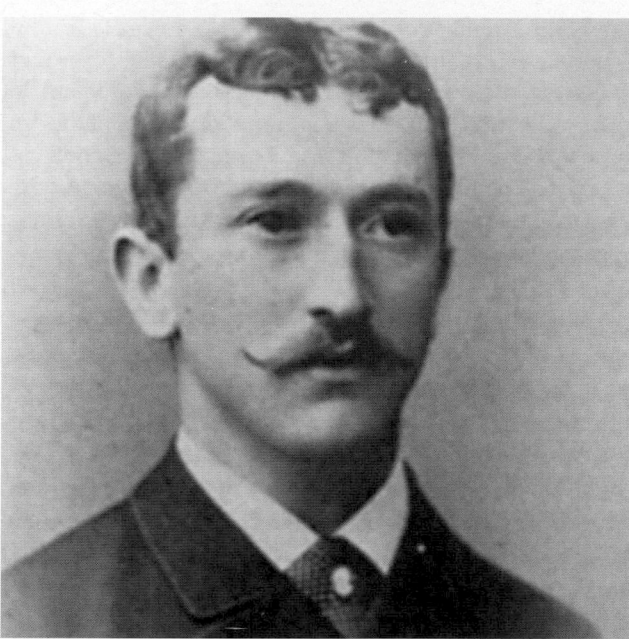

Figure 1–6. Carl Koller.

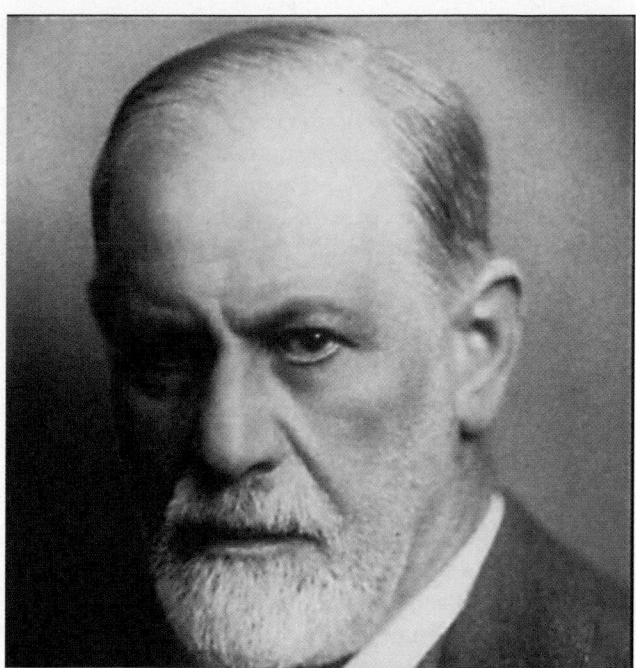

Figure 1–7. Sigmund Freud.

Leaves, published in 1860, earned him his doctoral degree. Of interest, he described cocaine as having "a bitter taste, promotes the flow of saliva, and leaves a peculiar numbness, followed by a sense of cold when applied to the tongue."[14,15] Following Niemann, the first experimental study on cocaine was conducted by a former naval surgeon from Peru, Thomas Moreno y Maiz. He discovered that the injection of cocaine solutions caused insensitivity in rats, guinea pigs, and frogs. But it wasn't until 1880 when Basil Von Anrep experimented on himself, that the application of cocaine for surgery was appreciated. Von Anrep injected a small amount of cocaine under the skin on his arm and noted that the area became insensitive to pinpricks. He did the same to his tongue with the same effect. He published his findings with the caveat "the animal experiments have no practical application; nevertheless I would recommend trying cocaine as a local anesthetic in persons of melancholy disposition."[16]

The groundwork was in place, but the final step toward the clinical use of cocaine had yet to be taken. Viennese ophthalmologist Karl Koller (1857–1944) rose to the challenge (Figure 1–6). Koller was an intern working in the Viennese General Hospital, where he was befriended by Sigmund Freud[17] (Figure 1–7). Freud wanted to know more about the stimulating action of cocaine, which he hoped might prove useful in curing one of his close friends of morphine addiction. This friend was a pathologist and had developed an agonizingly painful thenar neuroma secondarily to cutting himself during the performance of an autopsy. Freud was able to obtain a supply of cocaine from the pharmaceutical firm, Merck. He shared it with Koller, who helped him investigate its effects on the nervous system during the spring of 1884.[18]

Koller had dreams of achieving an appointment to assistant, and knew his chances would be greatly enhanced by

the creation of a respectable piece of research. The research he produced proved worthy enough, but interpersonal animosity intervened, and he was not awarded the position. Deeply disappointed, he moved first to the Netherlands, then to the United States.[19] In July 1884, Freud published a review of cocaine and his experiments with the drug, again noting, but without lending any particular attention to, the alkaloid's anesthetic effect on mucous membranes.[20] It was Koller who grasped the importance of this observation. His discovery was no accident, for he was keenly aware of the limitations of general anesthesia in ophthalmic surgery. Koller understood what others had failed to recognize because of his past experience in the field of ophthalmology. Many eye surgeries at that time were still being performed without anesthesia. Almost four decades after the discovery of ether, general anesthesia by mask had a number of limitations for ophthalmic surgery, eg, the anesthetized patient could not cooperate with his surgeon, the anesthesiologist's apparatus interfered with surgical access. At that time, many surgical incisions in the eye were not closed, as fine sutures were not yet available. Vomiting from chloroform or ether threatened to cause extrusion of the internal contents of the globe, markedly increasing the risk of permanent blindness. As a medical student, Koller had worked in a laboratory searching for a topical ophthalmic anesthetic to overcome the restrictions posed by general anesthesia. The medications available at that time had proved to be ineffective.

One day, Freud gave Koller a small sample of cocaine in an envelope, which he slipped into his pocket (an everyday occurrence in many American and European cities to this day). When the envelope leaked, a few grains of cocaine stuck to Koller's finger, which he casually licked with his tongue. His tongue became numb—if he had been able to mouth the word *Eureka* with a numb tongue, he may well have done so at this precise instant. At that moment, Koller realized that he had found what he had been searching for. He immediately created a suspension of cocaine crystals in his laboratory.[2] Koller realized that this had been noted by all who had worked with cocaine and that "in the moment it flashed upon me that I was carrying in my pocket the local anesthetic for which I had searched some years earlier".[1] In Freud's absence, he and another colleague, Joseph Gartner, dissolved a trace of the white powder in distilled water and instilled the solution into the conjunctival sac of a frog. After a minute or so, "the frog allowed his cornea to be touched and he also bore injury to the cornea without a trace of reflex action or defense." Koller wrote: "One more step had yet to be taken. We trickled the solution under each other's lifted eyelids. Then we placed a mirror before us, took pins, and with the head tried to touch the cornea. Almost simultaneously we were able to state 'I can't feel anything'".[21,22] Then, he experimented with dog and guinea pig corneas with 2 to 5% cocaine solutions.[23]

Koller soon achieved the extraordinary notoriety he had longed for when in September of 1884 he performed the first ophthalmologic surgical procedure on a patient with glaucoma using local anesthesia. The German Ophthalmologist Society Congress was to meet in Heidelberg in September of 1884 where Koller was going to present his findings. Unfortunately, he was unable to attend. He asked Dr. Joseph Brettauer, an ophthalmologist from Trieste, to present his paper at the Congress. The effect of his work was immediate. Koller was able to present his findings in October of that year to the Viennese Medical Society. He published his findings in late 1884.[21]

Physicians in the United States soon heard about Koller's amazing work. Dr. Henry Noyes of New York, an attendee of the Heidelberg Congress, published a summary of Koller's work in the New York Medical Record.[24] Another American physician, Dr. Bloom, translated Koller's article into English and published it in *The Lancet* in December of that same year. Koller's work was the trigger for the development of regional/local anesthesia. In the subsequent year, more than 60 publications on local anesthesia with cocaine appeared in the United States and Canada.

One of the most significant publications was that of N. J. Hepburn, an ophthalmologist from New York.[15] Self-experimentation was the standard for drug trials in those days. To determine whether a drug was safe or effective, the researcher or physician commonly tried the drug on himself. It takes courage to try a new drug on a patient, but it takes a particular and much greater form of courage to try that drug on yourself. Hepburn was no different from his colleagues. He gave himself a succession of subcutaneous injections of 0.4 mL (8 mg) of cocaine at 5-min intervals. By the eighth injection, the stimulating effects of the drug were strong enough that he decided it was best to stop. Unfortunately, Hepburn didn't stop with those initial injections. He repeated the "experiment" 2 days later and 4 days after that, each time increasing the total amount of cocaine injected. Most likely by this time he was hopelessly addicted.

By November of 1884, the ophthalmologist C. S. Bull reported that he had been able to use cocaine to produce anesthesia of the cornea and conjunctiva in more than 150 cases.[25] He was enthusiastic about the advantages of the drug in that he saved time required for complete anesthesia with ether; patients were less nauseated, the engorgement of the ocular blood vessels (caused by ether) was eliminated, and he was less hampered by the anesthesia equipment required for inhalation anesthesia. Cocaine revolutionized eye, nose, and mouth surgery. Operations that had been exceedingly difficult or painful became routine when topical or injectable cocaine was used. Koller didn't forget the contribution of his friend, Freud. He gave him the credit as his muse. Despite his disillusionment at not being foremost with the discovery, Freud is considered by many to be the founder of psychopharmacology because of his initial use of cocaine. He is considered the predecessor in the discovery and experimentation with mescaline, LSD, and amphetamines to modify behavior and to attempt to cure mental illness.[20]

Dangers of Cocaine

The "wonder drug" cocaine was soon sold everywhere and in almost everything. Following its isolation from the coca leaf, cocaine emerged as an ingredient in wine both in the United States and in Europe in amounts up to 7 mg/oz. In the original recipe for Coca-Cola (1866), coca leaves were included in the ingredients. It wasn't until 1906 when the Pure Food and Drug Act was passed that the Coca-Cola company began using decocainized leaves.[14] Until 1916, cocaine could be purchased over the counter at Harrods in London. It was found in tonics, toothache cures, and medicines (Figure 1–8). Coca cigarettes were sold with the promise of lifting depression. Those who purchased cocaine were promised in ads by the pharmaceutical firm Parke-Davis, that it could "make the coward brave, the silent eloquent, and render the sufferer insensitive to pain." In the operatic world, it became commonplace to use cocaine to ease the pain of sore throats and to shrink nasal mucous membranes to enable the singers to improve the resonation of their voices.

Had cocaine's use been restricted to enhancing opera singing and local anesthesia, it would have become the achievement of nineteenth-century medicine. As had happened earlier with brandy, tobacco, morphine, and other drugs, cocaine was administered in too high concentrations and with too few precautions. In 1886 William Hammond, a former US Army Surgeon General, assured an audience of physicians that cocaine addiction did not exist. Based on self-experimentation, he concluded that regular use of cocaine was as easy to stop as quitting coffee. It did not have the addictive qualities of drugs like opium. But when Hammond finished his lecture, an addiction specialist named Jansen Mattison offered a rebuttal. He related incidences of fierce addictions in patients under his care. He described cocaine's damaging effect on nerves and its ability to produce hallucinations, delusions, and emaciation. Many other practitioners began to encounter serious side effects.[26,27]

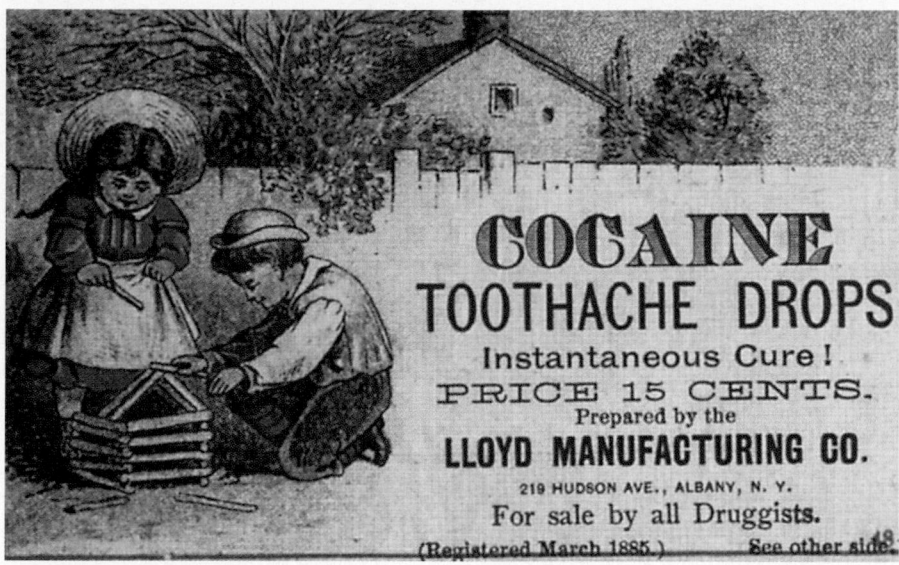

Figure 1–8. Cocaine toothache drops.

Mattison knew what he was talking about. Over the next several years, medical journals published hundreds of case reports of "cocainism." Unfortunately, many of the addicts were medical practitioners who had experimented on themselves, most notably Freud and William Stewart Halsted.[28,29] The opiate addicts, promised a cure for their addiction, switched to cocaine, but continued to use both drugs, further compromising their health.

Several researchers deserve the credit for making the infiltration of cocaine safer. Maximillian Oberst, Ludwig Pernice, and Carl Ludwig Schleich, all from Germany, described the use of low concentrations of cocaine as effective means of local anesthetic.[30] The Parisian surgeon Paul Reclus described the use of very low concentrations of cocaine as effective anesthesia without harmful side effects for tooth extractions and pulpotomies.[31]

About the same time, Halsted was experimenting with low concentrations of cocaine applied by compression devices. Unfortunately, he too became addicted to both cocaine and morphine and could not publish his results.[12,17,29] Over time, the maximum "safe" cocaine dosage for infiltration anesthesia was established at 50 mg.

◼ AFTER COCAINE

As the undesirable effects of cocaine, most notably addiction and toxicity, gradually became known, new anesthetic drugs were sought to replace it. Local methods to provide anesthesia had to await the development of less toxic drugs. As part of the purification process of cocaine, Niemann had hydrolyzed benzoic acid from cocaine. Once the clinical usefulness of cocaine became evident, efforts were made by various researchers to identify the active portion of the cocaine molecule and to create new substances that possessed local anesthetic activity without the adverse side effects. Most of

the chemical work involving the creation of local anesthetics took place in Germany from 1900 to 1930.[32]

Niemann, in his pioneer work, had hydrolyzed benzoic acid from cocaine. In the search for other benzoic acid esters with local anesthetic properties, amylocaine (stovaine) was introduced in 1903. It became popular for spinal anesthesia until it was shown to be an irritant. But it was the development of procaine in 1904 by the German chemist Alfred Einhorn that revolutionized local anesthetics.[33] On November 27 1904, Einhorn (1856–1917) patented 18 *para*-aminobenzoic acid derivatives that had been developed in the Meister Lucius and Brüning plants at Höchst, in Hesse, Germany. His compound Number Two was to bring about a radical change in local anesthetic practice. He named the new anesthetic, Novocain.[11] Procaine (Novocain) was introduced into clinical practice by Professor Heinrich Braun in 1905. Braun published a study comparing this new anesthetic to stovaine and alypine, two other promising local anesthetics.[34] Procaine was found to be safe and quickly became the standard local anesthetic drug. Within a short time, procaine completely replaced cocaine as the most commonly used local anesthetic. But because of the short duration of action and prominent allergic potential limiting its clinical effectiveness, the search for longer lasting compounds continued.[11,18,26,35]

In the years that followed, several local anesthetics were synthesized and used in clinical practice until side effects or other unfavorable characteristics were noted. In 1925 Karl Meischer synthesized dibucaine and in 1928 Otto Eisleb synthesized tetracaine. Both were effective local anesthetics and had the desirable qualities of longer duration and potency, but systemic toxic effects limited their usefulness for regional techniques other than for spinal anesthesia. Most of the compounds developed during this time were amino ester derivatives, similar to cocaine, with similar allergic potential.

A major breakthrough came in the mid 1940s when the Swedish chemists, Nils Löfgren and Bengt Lundquist, developed a new local anesthetic they called lidocaine. Lidocaine was an amino amide derivative, a stable compound not influenced by exposure to high temperatures, and, most importantly, one that did not have the allergic potential of the ester-type local anesthetics. With the development of this amide-type anesthetic drug, a whole new class of new local anesthetics were synthesized. In 1957 Af Ekenstam developed mepivacaine and bupivacaine, and in 1969 Löfgren and Claes Tegnér developed prilocaine. Prilocaine's synthesis began because of a desire to produce a local anesthetic with a potency similar to that of lidocaine but without lidocaine's systemic toxic effects. Unfortunately, it was soon discovered that large doses of prilocaine produced a metabolite that caused methemoglobinemia. Although probably not clinically significant, this discovery severely limited its use in clinical practice.[36] In 1972 etidocaine was introduced to the clinical scene, but was soon discovered to lack a differential sensory–motor blockade. Its clinical usefulness was therefore limited.

The only new ester local anesthetic developed in more recent times was chloroprocaine. Its rapid hydrolysis reduced the possibility of systemic toxicity, but its usefulness was restricted to procedures of short duration that did not produce a high degree of postoperative pain. In modern regional practices it has been used both in spinal anesthesia and in nerve blocks for short, relatively painless procedures.

After the development of etidocaine, a pause in the development of newer local anesthetics occurred. One of the goals of modern pharmaceutical research is modification in the delivery of the most commonly used local anesthetics rather than the development of completely new drugs. For example, liposomal delivery systems that allow slow release of commonly used local anesthetics deposited at specific sites may make the practice of indwelling peripheral nerve block catheters obsolete in the foreseeable future.

LOCAL ANESTHESIA TECHNIQUES

Infiltration Anesthesia

In 1895, a then novel approach, termed *infiltration anesthesia*, had been promoted by Karl Ludwig Schleich (1859–1922).[35] Schleich applied the principle that pure water has a weak anesthetic effect but is painful on injection, whereas physiologic saline is not. In 1869, Pierre Carl Edouard Potain first observed that the subcutaneous injection of water produced local anesthesia. Halsted, a surgeon at Roosevelt hospital in New York City, in a frank letter to the editor of the *New York Medical Journal* in 1885, declared that the "skin can be completely anesthetized to any extent by cutaneous injections of water."[37] In his own practice, Halsted had begun using water instead of cocaine in skin incisions, noting that the anesthesia did not subside completely when hyperemia reappeared.

In the belief that there was a solution capable of performing as a useful anesthetic that would not cause pain on injection, Schleich mixed 0.2% sodium chloride with 0.02%

cocaine. He used the mixture to produce cutaneous anesthesia for sebaceous cystectomy, hemorrhoidectomies, and small abscesses. Although Braun dismissed Schleich's solutions as "nonphysiologic," Schleich's work was important in advancing the application of small quantities of local anesthetics for surgical procedures. Because of the reported serious toxic reactions and fatalities reported with cocaine, enthusiasm for the utilization of local anesthesia had waned considerably. Paul Reclus undoubtedly understood that the cause of death from local anesthetics was related to overdose from excessively high doses. He was able to demonstrate that absorption could be limited with lower concentrations of cocaine, a fact that Schleich obviously supported and implemented.[31] Schleich's approach still seems to be relevant, particularly with the recent European enthusiasm for *tumescent anesthesia*, in which sometimes huge volumes of very dilute local anesthetic are used for surface surgery.

Conduction Anesthesia

With the excitement generated by Koller's report of cocaine anesthesia in 1884, several US surgeons concurrently entertained the idea of injecting cocaine directly into tissues to render them insensitive. William Burke injected five drops of 2% cocaine solution close to a metacarpal branch of the ulnar nerve and then painlessly removed a bullet from the base of his patient's little finger.[38] However, it was William Stewart Halsted (1852–1922; Figure 1–9) and his associate

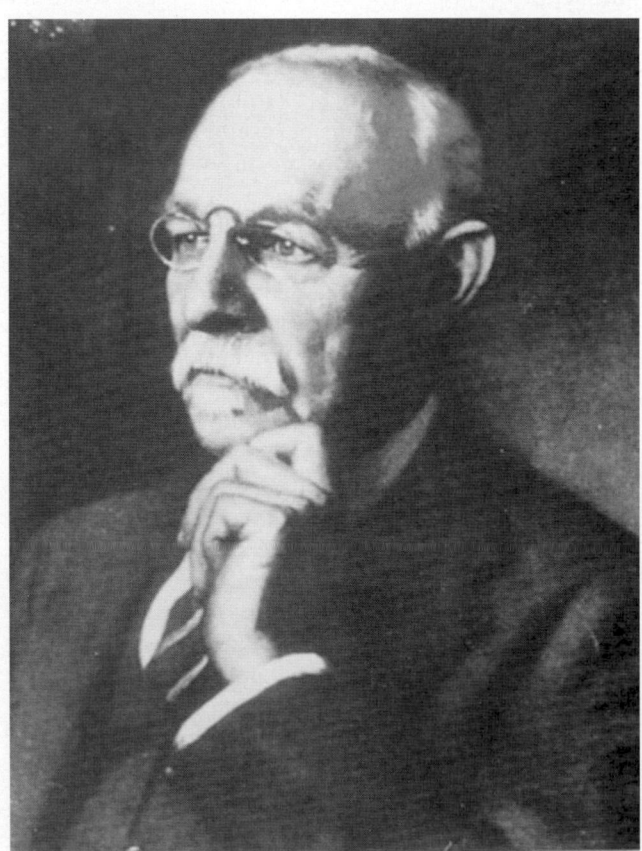

Figure 1–9. William Stewart Halsted.

John Hall at Roosevelt Hospital in New York City, who most clearly saw the great possibilities of conduction block.[39] Hall experimented on himself by blocking a cutaneous branch of the ulnar nerve in his own forearm.[40] He and Halsted did not stop with upper extremity injections; they also successfully injected the musculocutaneous (superficial peroneal) nerve of the leg. Hall described the manifestation of systemic symptoms such as giddiness, severe nausea, cold perspiration, and dilated pupils, but these symptoms did not stop these daring scientists from further self-experimentation. Halsted blocked Hall's supratroclear nerve to remove a congenital cystic tumor. One can assume that both Halsted and Hall had run out of minor surgical ailments in themselves and therefore had to look to others on whom they could experiment. In the days long before ethics committees and informed consent, one is tempted to speculate about the true "volunteer" status of the poor, and most likely, unsuspecting, medical students. Hall's report was unequivocal in predicting that this mode of administration of cocaine would find wide application in outpatient surgery once the limits of safety had been determined—remarkably prescient of him![40]

Although the conduction blocks were successful, unfortunately, several members of their group became addicted to cocaine. No further publications about the usefulness of cocaine anesthesia for surgical procedures were presented. It is one of the great sadnesses of the development of analgesic drugs in the history of humankind that two of the most effective agents, morphine and cocaine, are wickedly addictive. They deprived medicine of many of the potential discoveries of its most gifted sons and daughters. However, that Hall and Halsted were the true progenitors of conduction anesthesia can scarcely be doubted.[17,26]

In 1891, François-Franck was the first to apply the term *blocking* to the infiltration of a nerve trunk in any part.[41] He correctly discovered that the effect of the blocking drug was not limited to sensory fibers, but provided blockade of all nerves, both motor and sensory. He noted that sensory anesthesia became apparent more rapidly than the motor paralysis, a fact confirmed by von Anrep's observations in 1880.[16] François-Frank described the action of cocaine as transitory and noninjurious, "physiologic and segmental" anesthesia. He may well have borrowed part of it from J. Leonard Corning, who in 1886 wrote that "the thought of producing anaesthesia by abolishing conduction in sensory nerves, by suitable means, should have been rife in the minds of progressive physicians".[42] Corning most likely got the idea from Halsted, because he had frequently observed Halsted and Hall's work at Roosevelt Hospital in New York.

The advantage of utilizing cocaine as a local anesthetic was that it anesthetized only the section of the body where surgery was to be performed, the goal of because regional techniques in modern practice. But the price to be paid was in the duration of action and toxicity, not to mention the more commonly recognized problem of addiction. The dose of cocaine was limited to 30 mg because of rapid absorption. Unfortunately, the duration of anesthesia was therefore to no more than 15 min. Corning, in 1885, began researching means of prolonging the local anesthetic action of cocaine for surgery. He believed that once cocaine was injected beneath the skin, capillary circulation was responsible for distributing, diluting, and removing the anesthetic substance. In one experiment, he injected 0.3 mL of a 4% solution of cocaine into a cutaneous nerve of the arm and produced immediate anesthesia of the skin of the forearm. By compressing the extremity proximal to the site of injection with an Esmarch bandage, he was able to intensify and prolong the anesthesia to the forearm.[43]

Corning's successes with prolonging the action of local anesthetic with a physical tourniquet inspired Heinrich F. W. Braun to substitute epinephrine, a "chemical tourniquet," for the Esmarch tourniquet.[44] John Jacob Abel had isolated the pure form from the suprarenal medulla in 1897, and it had been subsequently used in ophthalmology to limit hemorrhage and in the treatment of glaucoma.[45] During its use in ophthalmology and subsequently in ear, nose, and throat surgeries, it was discovered that epinephrine prolonged the effect of cocaine, thereby allowing a reduction in dose and limiting side effects. Braun determined the optimal solution of epinephrine with cocaine by once again experimenting on himself. He discovered that the maximal dose that he could tolerate without side effects was 0.5 mg (0.5 mL of a 1:1000 solution of epinephrine). He coined the term *conduction anesthesia* when publishing the results of his experimentation.[46]

Intravenous Regional Anesthesia

The first reported use of intravenous regional anesthesia can be traced back to August Karl Gustav Bier (Figure 1–10), the originator of the infamous **Bier block**. Bier, a German surgeon (1861–1949), influenced surgery, anesthesia, and general medicine with his contributions through the decades. Intravenous regional anesthesia (IVRA) was first described by Bier in 1908. His method consisted of occluding the circulation in a segment of the arm with two tourniquets. He then injected a solution of dilute procaine through a venous cut-down in the isolated segment. The injected solution diffused through the entire section of the limb quickly producing **direct vein anesthesia** in just a few minutes.[47] The anesthesia lasted as long as the upper tourniquet was in place. Recovery of sensation was rapid after the tourniquet was removed.[48] Despite his successes, IVRA was not widely used until the technique was reintroduced by C. M. Holmes in the 1960s.[49]

Spinal Anesthesia

Soon after its introduction in 1884, local anesthesia became very popular with surgeons, particularly those in France, Germany, and the United States.[18] This was in large part due to concerns about the safety of inhalational anesthesia which, increased by the introduction of chloroform, had given rise to significant worries about toxicity. General anesthetic mortality was high at this time, and there was a distinct shortage of personnel trained to administer general anesthesia.[50] In a bizarre twist, the first spinal anesthetic was given some whether masturbation played any role in local anesthesia—this question can now be answered in the affirmative. Corning administered one dose without effect and then, after a second dose had been given, the patient's legs "felt sleepy." The man had impaired sensibility in his lower extremity after about 20 minutes. He left Corning's office "none the worse for the experience"—although this experience itself may well have put him off his penchant for onanism. Corning had injected a total of 120 mg of cocaine, about four times the potentially lethal dose, in a period of 8 min. What he achieved in this patient was probably what is now called *epidural,* or *extradural,* anesthesia. The dog probably received a spinal anesthetic with approximately 13 mg of cocaine as a spinal anesthetic, as judged by the rate of onset described.

Although Corning most assuredly had an innovative idea, his results were not more than a lucky accident because he injected a fatal dose of cocaine into the man. A direct communication between the extradural capillaries and the spinal cord does not exist. Based on the education that Corning received at the time, he was probably unaware of the existence of the subarachnoid space and cerebrospinal fluid.

Lumbar Puncture/Spinal Anesthesia

Heinrich Irenaeus Quincke (Figure 1–11) is credited with the introduction and popularization for the lumbar puncture. It was developed as a treatment for hydrocephalus in children

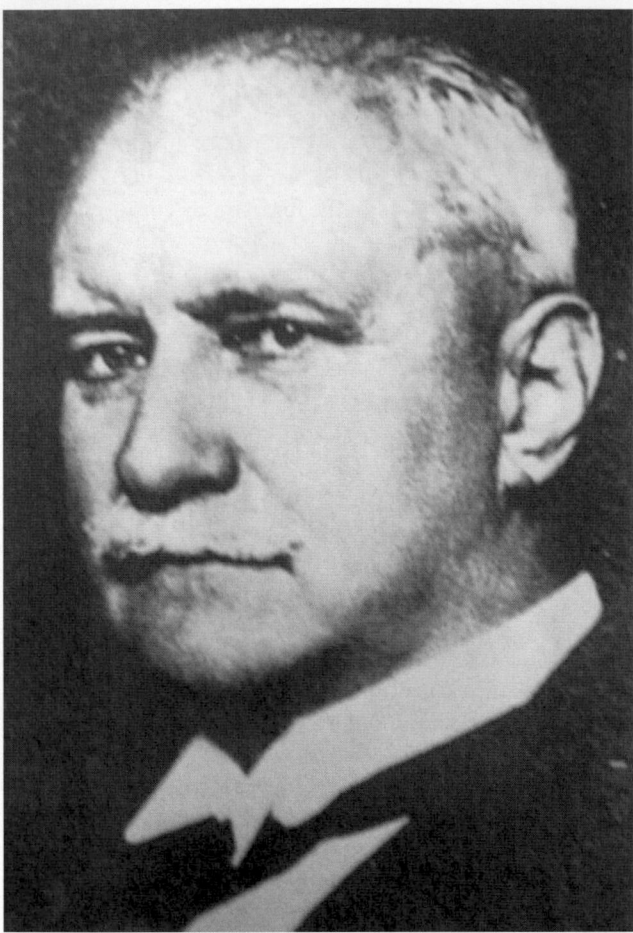

Figure 1–10. August Bier.

5 years before the first lumbar puncture. The term *spinal anesthesia* was introduced by Corning, a neurologist, in his famous paper of 1885 entitled "Spinal Anaesthesia and Local Medication of the Cord with Cocaine."[42] He theorized that interspinal blood vessels would carry the local anesthetic (cocaine) to communicating vessels into the spinal cord. He did not mention anything about cerebrospinal fluid or the depth of the needle insertion into the spinal space. It is speculated that he was aiming directly at the spinal cord as he introduced a needle between the eleventh and twelfth vertebrae. In his paper he wrote: "I reasoned that it was highly probably that, if the anesthetic was placed between the spinous processes of the vertebrae, it would be rapidly transported by the blood to the substance of the cord and would give rise to anaesthesia of the sensory and perhaps also of the motor tracts of the same. To be more explicit, I hoped to produce artificially a temporary condition of things analogous in its physiological consequences to the effects observed in transverse myelitis or after total section of the cord."[42]

Corning's report was based on a series of two injections: one human and one animal (a dog). After first assessing its action in a dog, producing a blockade of rapid onset that was confined to the animal's rear legs, he administered cocaine to a man who was "addicted to masturbation." It may be that many anesthesiologists have spent much time wondering

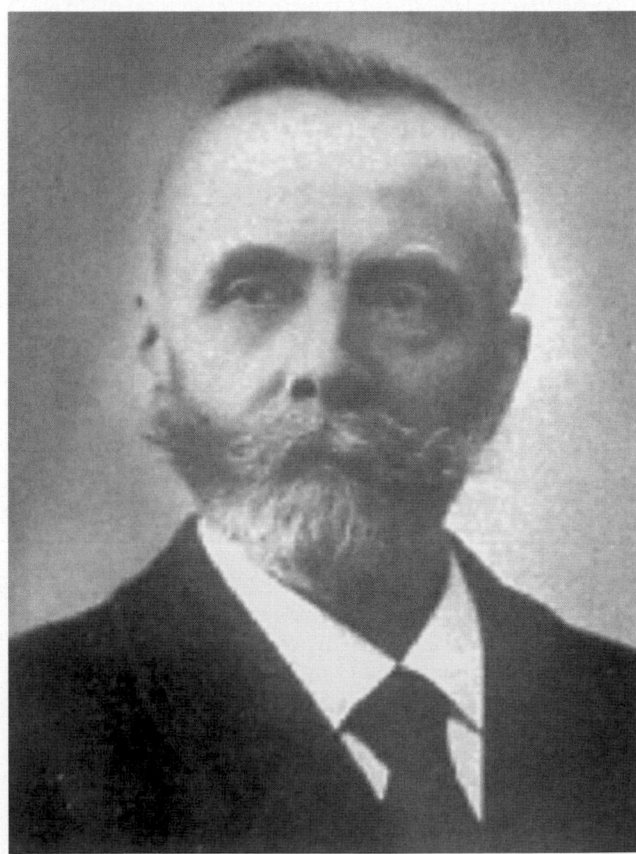

Figure 1–11. Heinrich Irenaeus Quincke.

with tubercular meningitis, then later as a diagnostic method for certain central nervous system diseases.[51] He based his approach on sound anatomic knowledge of the subarachnoid space and spinal cord. He used needles with an internal diameter of 0.5 to 1.2 mm and entered the subarachnoid space via a paravertebral approach. Interestingly, he prescribed bedrest for 24 h following the puncture.

Despite the strides made by Quincke, utilizing his technique for spinal anesthesia did not occur for 8 years after Quincke's first publication. Bier published his renowned paper on spinal anesthesia in 1899. Bier had the good fortune to work at the same institution as Quincke and was most likely familiar with his work. His intention was to use spinal anesthesia with cocaine for major operations. He realized that he could produce a profound block with a minimum amount of the drug, thereby eliminating the majority of the adverse side effects noted by his colleagues. In his experiments, he noted that the extent of anesthesia produced was not always predictable. As was popular with his colleagues, he experimented on himself. He had his assistant, August Hildebrandt, perform lumbar punctures on him. In the first attempt, Hildebrandt was unable to administer an appreciable amount of cocaine before a large volume of cerebrospinal fluid leaked out of Bier. Because of the poor response, they were close to abandoning the experiment. Hildebrandt then offered to be the next "guinea pig" instead. Bier successfully placed the spinal anesthetic and proceeded to "punish" Hildebrandt with blows to the tibia, pulling on his testicle, and even putting out a cigar on Hildebrandt's thigh.[52,53] Unfortunately, both men developed violent headaches that lasted for days, leading Bier to recommend the following practices that are still being followed today: preventing the excessive loss of cerebrospinal fluid, using very fine (small) needles, and strict bedrest if significant loss of CSF cannot be avoided.[54] Intelligent prescience was at work again.

Bier was able to demonstrate that small amounts of local anesthetic (cocaine) injected into the subarachnoid space could provide surgical anesthesia for over 67% of the body. The anesthetic condition lasted approximately 45 min, an adequate time for many surgical procedures. His work provided the basis of spinal anesthesia as we practice it in modern medicine. Coincidentally, the practice of wearing rubber gloves emerged as a part of aseptic technique prior to Bier's work on spinal anesthesia, thus preventing many of the serious complications that could have occurred without this prophylactic measure.[55]

So who deserves the laurels for the first spinal anesthetic? The history of anesthesiology is similar to that of other medical branches in that it has had its share of quarrels concerning priority. International disputes between the surgeon August Bier and his former colleague, August Hildebrandt regarding the question of who was the actual inventor of spinal anesthesia are well-documented. Although Hildebrandt and other colleagues frequently give credit to Corning, Bier insisted that he administered and described the technique of spinal anesthesia. In an extensive review (in the original language) of Corning's publication and those of Bier of Germany,

the author compared key factors, ie, the mention of cerebrospinal fluid, dose of injected cocaine, onset of action, and height of sensory analgesia. He noted that Corning's dose of local anesthetic was eight times higher than the dose given by Bier, yet the onset of analgesia was slower with a lower sensory block. Cerebrospinal fluid was not mentioned in Corning's paper. Bier concluded that Corning's injection was extradural, and that he (Bier) deserved to be acknowledgement for introducing spinal anesthesia.[53,56–58]

After Bier's work in spinal anesthesia (published in 1899), interest in spinal anesthesia spread rapidly. Within 2 years of Bier's work, it has been estimated that more than 1000 papers were published relating to spinal anesthesia. Frederick Dudley Tait and Guido Caglieri in San Francisco were the first Americans to use true spinal anesthesia clinically.[59] Rudoph Matas, head of the Department of Surgery at the University of Louisiana (later known as Tulane University), was the first American to report on spinal anesthesia. In his description of spinal anesthesia, Matas initially dissolved cocaine in water, creating a hypobaric solution. Later he changed his "standard" mixture to cocaine with morphine, making him a pioneer in the use of spinal opioids to enhance central neuraxial anesthesia.[59]

With the vast interest in spinal anesthesia, serious complications from its application were soon observed. F. Gumprecht published a report of 15 cases of sudden death after spinal anesthesia.[60] Multiple cases of respiratory arrest and hypotension, following Harvey Cushing's introduction of blood pressure measurement, were also reported leading to spinal anesthesia falling into disfavor.[61,62] Several pioneers sought to determine the causes of the variations in blood pressure from spinal anesthesia. Several theories emerged that have shaped our understanding of physiology today. L. G. Gray and H. T. Parsons of England did an extensive study to evaluate the causes for the changes in blood pressure after spinal anesthesia. They concluded that the decrease in arterial blood pressure was attributed to the diminished negative intrathoracic pressure during inspiration. High spinal anesthesia paralyzed the abdominal and thoracic muscles necessary to maintain that negative pressure.[63] With the understanding that hypotension was a primary danger with spinal anesthesia, G. Smith and W. Porter determined in 1915 that the fall in blood pressure was related to paralysis of the vasomotor fibers in the splanchnic area that regulated the tone of the blood vessels. They concluded that for spinal anesthesia to be effective without serious drops in blood pressure, cephalad diffusion of the local anesthetic should be avoided.[64] Gastan Labat contended that the serious adverse effects of spinal anesthesia were related to cerebral ischemia, not hypotension. He recommended that the patient should be placed in the Trendelenburg position after the spinal injection to keep the brain supplied with blood, therefore avoiding respiratory embarrassment.[65] Rather than looking at the position of the patient during injection, Arthur E. Barker promoted the idea that the baricity of the solution was instrumental in determining the cephalad spread. He made the injected solution stovaine, less toxic than cocaine but more irritating, hyperbaric with 5% glucose.[66] Barker was also a strong advocate for using sterile equipment and medication for spinal techniques. In 1934, Pitkin and Etherington-Wilson experimented with hypobaric solutions and changes in patient position to maintain control of the spread of the anesthetic.[32] Although there were other proponents of hypobaric spinal anesthesia, most had to deal with serious adverse effects, such as respiratory impairment and profound blood pressure changes requiring resuscitative maneuvers. It was not until 1920 that W. G. Hepburn and Lincoln Sise revived Barker's methods. Sise, an anesthesiologist at the Lahey Clinic in Boston, used hyperbaric tetracaine, rather than stovaine.

Because of the irritating qualities of stovaine, Sise was interested in finding other local anesthetics that would provide sufficient length of anesthesia with limited side effects—something modern anesthesiologists can relate to in our daily practice. He was frustrated by the short duration of action of Novocaine, "the ending of a spinal anesthesia in the midst of an operation is always disturbing and annoying, but when this takes place in the midst of an abdominal operation, with the belly open, it may be dangerous as well."[67] He began using tetracaine because of its longer duration of action, but was concerned about controlling the height of the block. Following Barker's recommendations regarding hyperbaric solutions, he added 10% glucose with success. He applied the same technique to tetracaine in 1935.[67,68]

The most negative consequence of spinal anesthesia came from a trial in 1953. Two healthy young men had received spinal anesthesia on the same day in a hospital in England. Both developed *permanent* painful spastic paresis. Although the exact cause of the neurologic injury was never proven, it was suspected to be caused by contamination of the local anesthetic solution.[69,70] Several other cases of paralysis after spinal anesthesia followed, casting a dark shadow on the future application of this anesthetic technique. Fortunately, a follow-up analysis of over 10,000 spinal anesthetics was published by L. D. Vandam and R. D. Dripps. "The most gratifying result was the failure to discover persistent, progressive major neurological disease," providing the way for spinal anesthesia to again emerge as a safe, effective means of providing anesthesia.[71]

The recurring problem of the inadequate duration of single-injection spinal anesthesia led a Philadelphia surgeon, William Lemmon, to report the development of an apparatus for continuous spinal anesthesia in 1940.[72] Lemmon began with the patient in the lateral position. The spinal tap was performed with a malleable silver needle that was left in position. As the patient was turned supine, the needle was positioned through a hole in the mattress and table. Additional injections of local anesthetic could be administered as required. Malleable silver needles also found a less cumbersome and more common application in 1942 when Waldo Edwards and Robert Hingson encouraged the use of Lemmon's needles for continuous caudal anesthesia in obstetrics. In 1944, Edward Tuohy of the Mayo Clinic introduced important modifications of the continuous spinal techniques. He developed the now-familiar Tuohy needle as a means of improving the ease

of passage of lacquered silk ureteral catheters through which he injected incremental doses of local anesthetic.[73]

Obstetric & Epidural Anesthesia

The origin of epidural analgesia began with Jean Enthuse Sicard, a neurologist, who introduced cocaine through the sacral hiatus for the treatment of sciatica and tabes. Independently, Fernand Cathelin used the same technique for surgical anesthesia.[74,75] In 1921, the Spanish surgeon Fidel Pagés-Miravé used a lumbar approach to the epidural space for surgical patients. His greatest contribution to the field of anesthesia was the introduction of *segmental anesthesia*, thereby eliminating some of the serious side effects of complete neuraxial blocks. Unfortunately, he died in an automobile accident before his methods could be shared by the students he worked with at the time. In 1931, Achille Dogliotti published a report on epidural injection of local anesthetics without knowledge of Pagés-Miravé's work. One of the most important features of Dogliotti's work was his identification of the epidural space. He produced a textbook of his technique that was both reproducible and easy to learn.[76] The limitation of epidural anesthesia was similar to that of spinal anesthesia—the duration of anesthesia provided. In 1947, Manuel Martinez Curbelo of Cuba is credited with using the Tuohy needle and a small ureteral catheter to provide continuous lumbar epidural analgesia.[77]

In the practice of obstetrics, religious beliefs obstructed the progress of pain relief for women in labor. It was commonly believed that providing anesthesia for the woman in labor went against God's will. James Young Simpson is credited with providing the first ether anesthetic for a complex obstetric delivery in 1847. He was severely criticized by both his peers and the clergy, but many women, most conspicuously Queen Victoria, began requesting anesthesia for the delivery of their children. There wasn't much progress in the field of obstetric analgesia/anesthesia from 1860 to 1940 until John Bonica, chief of anesthesia at the University of Washington, took over the management of his wife's anesthesia (and probably saved her life) during labor in 1943. She had a near fatal complication during open drop ether anesthesia. From the time that he intervened in his wife's care, he devoted his career to the advancement of anesthetic care of the mother and fetus.[78]

When Bonica was chief of anesthesia, caudal anesthesia was the primary means used for providing labor analgesia. This followed a report by W. B. Edwards and R. A. Hingson that analgesia for labor and delivery could be satisfactorily achieved with caudal injections of tetracaine through a needle left in place within the sacral canal.[79] When commercially available catheters became available in the 1970s, continuous epidural analgesia gained popularity. In the years following Bonica's contributions, epidural anesthesia for obstetrics has become the norm. Modifications of the techniques and the introduction of either spinal or epidural opioids have made labor and delivery a most pleasant experience for expecting mothers.

A FEW THOUGHTS ON PAIN

Fundamental to modern neural blockade is the concept that pain is a sensory warning conveyed by specific nerve fibers, amenable, at least in principle, to modulation or interruption anywhere in the nerve's pathway. This outlook may be traced back to developments in the study of physiology that finally supplanted the view, first expressed by Plato and Aristotle, that pain, like pleasure, is a passion of the soul, ie, an emotion and not one of the senses. Philosophical changes growing out of the great revolutions of the eighteenth century and the birth of biology as a science gradually, although not entirely, effaced the religious connotations of pain in Western civilization. The doctrine of specific energies of the senses was first promulgated by Johannes P. Müller (1801–1858) in 1826.[80] This doctrine, although not specific for the conduction of pain, initiated the movement of scientific thought toward analysis and classification of the specific characters of different nerves. The theory that pain was a separate and distinct sense was first definitively developed by Moritz S. Schiff (1823–1896) in 1858. By examining the effect of incisions in the spinal cord, Schiff was able to demonstrate that touch and pain were independent sensations. On animals, he demonstrated that injury to specific sections of the spinal cord resulted in loss of one modality without affecting the other.[81] Müller's theories led Erasmus Darwin (grandfather of Charles Darwin) to suggest the *intensive theory of pain*. Darwin felt that the sensation of pain was not a separate modality, but resulted from "whenever the sensorial motions are stronger than usual." Basically it is a theory of sensory overload leading to pain.[82] The theories of pain remained controversial throughout the early twentieth century, but by the midtwentieth century, the specificity theory (each sensory modality is transmitted along an independent pathway), became universally accepted as the most credible.

Applying drugs to transmitting nerves to alleviate neuralgic pain was first introduced by Francis Rynd in the early 1800s. Rynd's ideas possibly influenced the later development of both nerve blocks and opioid regional anesthesia.[81] When Carl Koller discovered the utility of cocaine as a surgical local anesthetic, a vast new world of local and regional analgesic therapy began. Corning is credited with the concept of direct application of an analgesic to the spinal cord for alleviation of pain, but it was not until the mechanism of pain was more fully understood that pain therapy could be focused on interrupting pain pathways. Unfortunately, by believing that pain pathway interruption was the complete answer to blocking pain, researchers focused only on that aspect, closing their minds to other related aspects of pain development. When Jean Joseph Emile Letievant described specific neurectomy techniques in the late nineteenth century, a myriad of surgical interventions, such as, rhizotomy, cordotomy and, tractotomy emerged to treat pain.[83] Unfortunately, most of these techniques were atrocious failures that often created more intense pain than was present prior to the procedure. Ronald Melzack and Patrick Wall's hypothesis that a spinal gate controls the cephalad transmission of nociception led to the modern introduction of electrical stimulation as a method of treating chronic pain. The concept proposed in the theory, that pain perception could be lessened by increasing activity in neural structures not associated with pain, led to chronic stimulation of the deep brain and spinal cord as a modality for the management of chronic pain. Consequently, both the brain and spinal structures emerged as targets for neuroaugmentation.[84,85] Although great strides have been made in our understanding of pain development and treatment, it is only through continued research that our understanding of preemptive pain control, such as those methods used in regional anesthesia, can be complete.

TWENTIETH-CENTURY REGIONAL ANESTHESIA

Orthopedic surgery has always lent itself to regional anesthesia techniques because of the ability to isolate anesthesia to the extremity being operated on. Initially, general anesthesia and nerve blocks were combined (still a somewhat common practice today). Harvey Cushing is credited with coining the name *regional anesthesia* for his method of blocking a nerve plexus under direct vision during general anesthesia. His goal was to decrease the anesthetic requirements and to provide postoperative pain relief. It's amazing to consider that he developed this technique in 1902, more than 100 years ago. A similar approach had been proposed by George Crile, 15 years earlier, to decrease the stress of surgery. Upper extremity anesthesia by blocking the brachial plexus percutaneously was achieved by many of our early colleagues. G. Hirschel is credited with developing the "blind" axillary brachial plexus block and D. Kulenkampff the supraclavicular technique, both in 1911. Because the risk of pneumothorax was high with the technique described by Kulenkampff, it was subsequently modified by A. Mulley using a lateral paravertebral approach. Mulley's approach is most likely the precursor of what is now commonly referred to as the "Winnie block" for the brachial plexus.

The spread of regional anesthesia in the United States was greatly facilitated by the work of Gaston Labat (Figure 1–12). Recruited to work at the Mayo Clinic in Rochester, Minnesota, Labat published his influential textbook, *Regional Anesthesia,* in which he described his techniques to the next generation of physicians, most notably Hippolite Wertheim, John Lundy, Ralph Waters, and Emery Rovenstine. Labat worked at the Mayo Clinic, then moved to Bellevue Hospital in New York City where he worked with Wertheim. Together, they formed the first American Society of Regional Anesthesia. Labat's successor, Emery A Rovenstine, was recruited to Bellevue to continue Labat's work. It was Rovenstine who was responsible for creating the specialty of anesthesiology in the 1920s and 1930s. He also is responsible for the creation of the first American clinic for the treatment of chronic pain, where he and his associates refined techniques of both lytic and therapeutic injections. Rovenstine and his successors used the American Society of Regional Anesthesia to educate

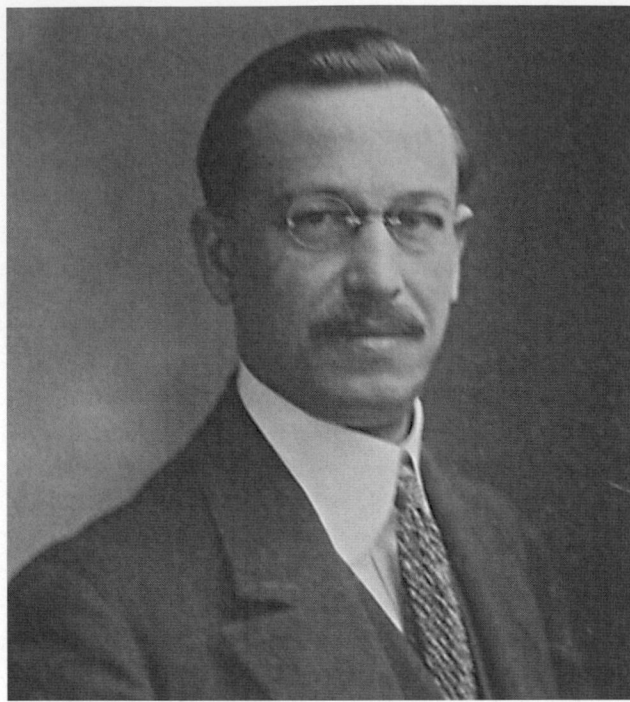

Figure 1–12. Gaston Labat.

physicians about pain management throughout the United States.[86]

The development of the multidisciplinary pain clinic was one of many contributions to anesthesiology made by John J. Bonica, a renowned teacher of regional techniques. During his periods of military, civilian, and university service at the University of Washington, John Bonica formulated a series of improvements in the management of chronic pain. His text, *The Management of Pain*, is regarded as a classic of the literature.[87,88]

THE POPULARITY & USE OF LOCAL ANESTHESIA

Ever since Koller's original work, the popularity of local anaesthesia has waxed and waned, like that of many other medical developments. The announcement of his work produced a massive wave of enthusiasm, which was tempered as the problems of cocaine became increasingly appreciated. The first resurgence of interest came with the introduction of safer drugs at the beginning of the twentieth century, and the second as a result of the efforts of Labat, Lundy, Maxson, Odom, and Pitkin in the United States in the years between the two World Wars.

In Britain, general anesthesia has traditionally been administered by qualified doctors (though not always by specialists who practiced anesthesia exclusively). Standards have usually been high because the conduct of general anesthesia has been their entire responsibility. By contrast, local and regional techniques, if they were used at all, were performed by the surgeon, whose interest and attention were divided between anesthetic and operation. Regional anesthesia was not seen always to be to the patient's best advantage under such circumstances. Nevertheless, when the examination for the Diploma in Anaesthesia was instituted in 1935, the curriculum included local anesthesia. This, together with the establishment of anesthesia as an independent specialty within the UK National Health Service in 1948, did much to encourage local anesthetic techniques. Unfortunately, the years between 1950 and 1955 saw a sharp decrease in the use of local, and particularly spinal, anesthesia in the UK and in the United States. The many advances in general anesthesia then taking place were partly responsible, since they encouraged the belief that a local technique was unnecessary. More important though was the fear of severe neurologic damage. The report entitled "The Grave Spinal Cord Paralyses Caused by Spinal Anesthesia" written in 1950 in New York by a British-trained neurologist, Foster Kennedy, was followed by the Woolley and Roe case and lead to a virtual extinction of the use of regional techniques (see discussion in the section on Spinal Anesthesia).[70] After a number of reports of the safe use of local anesthetics for surgical procedures emerged, regional anesthesia techniques once again began to slowly emerge.

Local anesthetic techniques are of value in blocking afferent stimuli even in major surgery because of the reduction in the pain and stress suffered by the patient. This approach is now extending even to cardiac surgery, but the concept is far from new. As early as 1902, Harvey Cushing was advocating the combination of local with general anesthesia to decrease "surgical shock," a concept that was further developed by Crile. The term *balanced anaesthesia* is very common today and implies a triad of sleep produced by either inhalational or intravenous route, profound analgesia with opioid drugs, and muscle relaxation by neuromuscular block. But interestingly, when Lundy first used the term in 1926, he intended that the second and third parts of the triad would be produced by a local anesthetic block, something proponents of regional anesthesia are implementing in modern anesthesia practice.

Other advances, although more difficult to quantify, have directly or indirectly helped the cause of local anesthesia. For example, developments in the field of medical plastics have resulted in safe and reliable syringes, catheters, and filters, and the anesthesiologist can select from a wide variety of sedative and anxiolytic drugs that, when carefully used, can greatly improve the patient's acceptance of a nerve block. Of great importance has been the understanding of the effects and treatment of sympathetic block. Ephedrine became available in 1924 and was first used to treat hypotension during spinal anesthesia in 1927, but readily available intravenous fluids and equipment for their administration are more recent developments.

Most currently used techniques of regional anesthesia were devised during that first decade of the twentieth century: brachial plexus block, axillary and supraclavicular approaches; intravenous regional anesthesia; celiac plexus block; caudal anesthesia; hyperbaric and hypobaric techniques of spinal anesthesia, and all the presently employed nerve blocks for the head and neck as applied in dentistry and plastic surgery. Thereafter, aside from technical innovation and understanding of some of the physiologic and toxicologic responses to local anesthetics, the great impetus to regional anesthesia came from the synthesis of the amide local anesthetics and an understanding of their pharmacodynamic and especially pharmacokinetic properties.[32]

In present-day practice, more advanced techniques of regional anesthesia (eg, continuous catheters, combination blocks, deep plexus blocks) have evolved because of the groundwork put in place by those earlier pioneers. With the advent of the Internet providing easier access to current medical practice, patients are better educated and are becoming advocates for regional anesthetic techniques.

It is appropriate to conclude by mentioning the organizations that seek to promote education and training in the use of regional anesthetic techniques. The American Society of Regional Anesthesia was reborn in 1975 and became firmly established. Its European counterpart (the European Society of Regional Anaesthesia and Pain Medicine) is younger, but is now equally well established, and similar societies are flourishing in many other parts of the world. Other important educational entities, such as the New York Society of Regional Anesthesia (founded in 1994, by Drs. Hadzic and Vloka), have been developed to continue to promote the safe and effective practice of regional anesthesia.

THE TWENTY-FIRST CENTURY & BEYOND

The history of local and regional anesthesia did not end in the first half of the twentieth century. In fact, it is often said, "we are making history every day." For instance, important techniques developed in the last few decades have refined our ability to identify peripheral nerves accurately. With the increasingly enthusiastic introduction of the use of ultrasound for nerve location, the rate of development in this area of regional anesthetic practice will increase at a greater pace. Perhaps the most important role for the regional anesthesiologists who will make history in the next few decades will be to document the clinical advantages and benefits of local and regional anesthesia. This endeavor will not just manifest itself as enthusiasm and skill, but will be based on the generation of convincing data through careful clinical research and academic cooperation within the regional anesthesia community. Books such as this are a vital part of building the future of regional anesthesia and in themselves will form a part of the history of local and regional anesthesia.

References

1. Vandam L: Early American anesthetists: The origins of professionalism in anesthesia. Anesthesiology 1973;38:264–274.
2. Greene N: A consideration of factors in the discovery of anesthesia and their effects on its development. Anesthesiology 1971;38:264–274.
3. Cadwell J, Sever P: The biochemical pharmacology of abused drugs: I. Amphetamines, cocaine, and LSD. Clin Pharmacol Ther 1974;16:625–638.
4. Loza-Balsa G: *Monografia sobre la Coca.* Edita Sociedad Geografica de la Paz 1991, pp. 9–15.
5. Van Dyke C, Byck R: Cocaine. Sci Am 1982;246:128–141.
6. Guerra F: *The Pre-Columbian Mind.* Seminar Press 1971;1:47, 52, 126, 191
7. Vespucci A: Cartas de viaje. Introduccion y notas de Luciano Formisano. Alianza Editorial SA 1986;48:102–137.
8. Romero C: Descubrimiento y conquista del Peru por Pedro Pizarro conquistador y poblador de este reino. Biografia de Pedro Pizarro 1917;VI:1–187.
9. Ruetsch Y, Boni T, Borgeat A: From cocaine to ropivacaine: The history of local anesthetic drugs. Curr Topics Med Chem 2001;1:175–182.
10. Lossen W: Über das cocain. Ann Chem Pharmacol 1865;133:351–371.
11. Link W, Einhorn A: Inventor of novocaine. Dent Radiogr Photogr 1959;32:20.
12. Fink B: Leaves and needles: The introduction of surgical local anesthesia. Anesthesiology 1985;63:77.
13. Howard-Jones N: A critical study of the origins and early development of hypodermic medications. J Hist Med 1947;2:201.
14. Blejer-Prieto H: Coca leaf and cocaine addiction—some historical notes. Can Med Assoc J 1965;93:700–704.
15. Niemann A: Über eine neue organische Base in den Cocablattern. Arch Pharmacol 1860;153:129–155, 291–308.
16. von Anrep B: Über die physiologische Wirkung des Cocain. Pflugers Arch 1880;21:38.
17. Matas R: Local and regional anesthesia: A retrospect and prospect. American Journal of Surgery 1934; 25: 189–96.
18. Koller K: Historical notes on the beginning of local anesthesia. JAMA 1928;90:1742–1743.
19. Buess H: Über die Anwendung der Koka und des Kokains in der Medizin. Ciba Z 1944;8:3362–3365.
20. Freud S: Über Coca. Centralbl Gesamte Ther 1884:289–314.
21. Koller C: On the use of cocaine for producing anaesthesia on the eye. Lancet 1884;2:990.
22. Becker H: Carl Koller and cocaine. Psychoanal Q 1963;32:309.
23. Koller K: Über die Verwendung des Cocain zur Aanasthesirung am Auge. Wien Med Wochenschr 1884;34:1276–1278.
24. Willstatter R, Wolfes D, Mader H: Synthese des naturlichen Cocains. Justus Liebigs Ann Chem 1923;434:111–139.
25. Hurtado P: *Indianos cacerenos. Notas biograficas de los hijos de la Alta Extremadura que sirvieron en America durante el primer siglo de su conquista.* Tipografia Luis Tasso 1892, pp. 38–39.
26. McAuley J: The early development of local anaesthesia. Br Dent J 1966;121:139–142.
27. Pernice L: Über Cocain anasthesie. Dtsch Med Wochenschr 1890;16:287–289.
28. Liljestrand G: Carl Koller and the development of local anesthesia. Acta Physiol Scand Suppl 1967;299:3–30.
29. Olch P, William S: Halsted and local anesthesia: Contributions and complications. Anesthesiology 1975;42:479–486.
30. Schleich C: Infiltration anasthesie (locale anasthesie) und ihr Verhaltniss zur allgemeinen Narcose (inhalation anasthesie). Verh Dtsch Ges Chiropractic 1892;21:121–127.
31. Reclus P: Analgesie locale par la cocaine. Rev Chiropr 1889;9:913.
32. Covino B: One hundred years plus two of regional anesthesia. Reg Anesth 1986;11:105.
33. Link W: Alfred Einhorn, Sc.D: Inventor of novocaine. Dent Radiogr Photogr 1959;32:1, 20.
34. Braun H: Über einige neue ortliche anaesthetica. Dtsch Med Wochenschr 1905;31:1667–1671.
35. Benedict H, Clark S, Freeman C: Studies in local anesthesia. J Am Dent Assoc 1932;19:2087–2105.
36. Ritchie J, Ritchie B, Greengard P: The active structure of local anesthetics. J Pharmacol Exp Ther 1965;150:152–159.
37. Halsted W: Water as a local anesthetic. N Y Med J 1885;42:327.

38. Burke W: Hydrochlorate of cocaine in minor surgery. N Y Med J 1884;40:616.

39. Halsted W: Practical comments on the use and abuse of cocaine; suggested by its invariably successful employment in more than a thousand minor surgical operations. N Y Med J 1885;42:327.

40. Hall R: Hydrochlorate of cocaine. N Y Med J 1884;40:643.

41. Francois-Frank C: Action patalysant locale de la cocaine sur les nerfs et les centres nerveux: Applications a la technique experimentale. Arch Physiol 1900;24:562.

42. Corning J: Spinal anaesthesia and local medication of the cord with cocaine. N Y Med J 1885;42:483.

43. Esmarch F: Über kunsstliche Blutleere. Arch Klin Chiropractic 1874;17:292.

44. Braun H: Über den Einfluss der Vitalitat der Gewebe auf die ortlichen und allgemeinen Giftwirkungen localanasthesirender Mittel und über die Bedeutung des Adrenalins für die Localanasthesie. Arch Klin Chiropr 1903;69:541.

45. Abel J: On the blood pressure raising constituent of the suprarenal capsule. Johns Hopkins Hosp Bull 1897;8:151.

46. Braun H: *Local Anesthesia: Its Scientific Basis and Practical Use,* 3rd ed. Lea & Febiger, 1914, pp. 541.

47. Rodola F, Vagnoni S, Ingletti S: An update on intravenous regional anaesthesia of the arm. Eur Rev Med Pharmacol Sci 2003;7:131–138.

48. Brill S, Middleton W, Brill G, et al: Bier's block; 100 years old and still going strong! Acta Anaesthesiol Scand 2004;48:117–122.

49. Holmes G: Intravenous regional anesthesia: A useful method of producing analgesia of the limbs. Lancet 1963;1:245–247.

50. Greene N: Anesthesia and the development of surgery (1846–1896). Anesth Analg 1979;58:5–12.

51. Quincke H: Die Lumbalpunction des Hydrocephalus. Ber Klin Wochenschr 1891;28:929.

52. Bier A: Versuche über Cocainisirung des Ruckenmarkes. Dtsch Z Chir 1899;5151:361.

53. Marx G: The first spinal anesthesia. Who deserves the laurels? Reg Anesth 1994;19:429–430.

54. Bier A: Über einen neuen Weg Localanasgthesie an den Gliedmassen zu erzeugen. Arch Klin Chiropr 1908;86:1007.

55. Halsted W: *Surgical Papers by William Steward Halsted.* Johns Hopkins Press, 1924, pp 37–39.

56. Goerig M, Beck H: Priority conflict concerning the discovery of lumbar anesthesia between August Bier and August Hildebrandt. Anasthesiol Intensivemed Notfallmed Schmerzther 1996;31:111–119.

57. Goerig G, Esch J: In memory of August Bier (1861–1949). Anasthesiol Intensivemed Notfallmed Schmerzther 1999;34:463–474.

58. Goerig M, Agarwal K, Schulte-Steinberg O, et al: The versatile August Bier (1861–1949), father of spinal anesthesia. J Clin Anesth 2000;12:561–569.

59. Matas R: Local and regional anesthesia with cocaine and other analgesic drugs, including the subarachnoid method, as applied in general surgical practice. Phila Med J 1900;6:820–843.

60. Gumprecht F: Gefahren der Lumbalpunktion: Plotzliche Todesfalle danach. Dtsch Med Wochenschr 1900;27:386–389.

61. Cushing H: On routine determinations of arterial tension in operating room and clinic. Boston Med Surg J 1903;148:250–256.

62. Thorsen G: Neurologic complications after spinal anesthesia and results from 2493 follow-up cases. Acta Chir Scand 1950;(Suppl)121:385–398.

63. Gray H, Parsons L: Blood pressure variations associated with lumbar puncture and the induction of spinal anesthesia. Q J Med 1912;5:339.

64. Smith G, Porter W: Spinal anesthesia in the cat. Am J Physiol 1915;38:108.

65. Labat G: Circulatory disturbances associated with subarachnoid nerve block. Long Island Med J 1927;21:573.

66. Barker A: Clinical experiences with spinal analgesia in 100 cases and some reflections on the procedure. BMJ 1907;I:665.

67. Sise L: Pontocain-Glucose solution for spinal anesthesia. In Faulconer A, Keys T (eds): *Foundations of Anesthesiology.* Charles C. Thomas, 1965, pp 874–882.

68. Sise L: Spinal anesthesia for upper and lower abdominal operations. New Engl J Med 1928;199:61.

69. Cope R: The Wooley and Roe case. Anaesthesia 1954;9:249–270.

70. Kennedy F, Effron A, Perry G: The grave spinal cord paralysis caused by spinal anesthesia. Surg Gynecol Obstet 1950;91:385–398.

71. Vandam L, Dripps R: Long-term Follow-up of patients who received 10,098 spinal anesthetics. In Faulconer A, Keys T (eds): *Foundations of Anesthesiology.* Charles C. Thomas, 1965, pp 901–913.

72. Lemmon W: A method for continuous spinal anesthesia, A Preliminary Report. In Faulconer A, Keys T (eds): *Foundations of Anesthesiology.* Charles C. Thomas, 1965, pp 883–900.

73. Tuohy E: Continuous spinal anesthesia: Its usefulness and technic involved. Anesthesiology 1944;5:142.

74. Sicard M: Les injections medicamenteuses extradurales par voie sacro-coccygienne. C R Soc Dev Biol 1901;53:396–398.

75. Cathelin M: Une nouvelle voie d'injection rachidienne. Methodes des injections epidurales par le precede du canal sacre. C R Soc Dev Biol 1901;53:452–453.

76. Dogliotti A: Eine neue Methode der regionaren Anasthesie: Die peridurale segmentaire Anasthesie. Zentralbl Chir 1931;58:3141–3145.

77. Curbelo M: Continuous peridural segemental anesthesia by means of a ureteral catheter. Anesth Analg 1949;28:13–23.

78. Chadwick H: Obstetric anesthesia—Then and Now. Minerva Anestesiol 2005;71:517–520.

79. Edwards W, Hingson R: Continuous caudal anesthesia in obstetrics. Am J Surg 1942;57:459–464.

80. Wade N: *Muller's Elements of Physiology,* Thoemmes Continuum: The History of Ideas, 2003, pp 1–11.

81. Bonica J: Evolution of pain concepts and pain clinics. Clin Anesthesiol 1985;3:1.

82. Darwin E: *Zoonomia, or the Laws of Organic Life.* J. Johnson, 1794.

83. Spicher C, Kohut G: Jean Joseph Emile Letievant: A review of his contributions to surgery and rehabilitation. J Reconstr Microsurg 2001;17:169–177.

84. Gildenberg P: History of neuroaugmentative procedures. Neurosurg Clin North Am 2003;14:327–337.

85. Stanton-Hicks M, Salamon J: Stimulation of the central and peripheral nervous system for the control of pain. J Clin Neurophysiol 1997;14:46–62.

86. Bacon D: Gaston Labat, John Lundy, Emery Rovenstine, and the Mayo Clinic: The spread of regional anesthesia in American between the World Wars. J Clin Anesth 2002;14:315–320.

87. Bonica J: *The Management of Pain,* 2nd ed. Lea and Febiger, 1953.

88. Benedetti C, Chapman C: John J. Bonica. A biography. Minerva Anestesiol 2005;71:391–396.

Foundations of Regional Anesthesia

Embryology

Patrick M. McQuillan, MD

INTRODUCTION

A thorough understanding of the underlying anatomy is fundamental to a logical approach to the techniques used in regional anesthesia. An appreciation for the embryologic development of tissues and structures can significantly add to the understanding of functional anatomy as it relates to regional anesthesia. In this chapter I emphasize the embryologic development of the brain, spinal cord, peripheral and autonomic nervous systems, as well as the musculoskeletal system as it pertains to regional anesthesia. Many excellent comprehensive texts on embryology are available. For this chapter, I have relied heavily on information from primary texts and refer the reader to them for a complete discussion of all embryologic development. The first two, *Langman's Medical Embryology*[1] and *Basic Concepts in Embryology*,[2] are valuable for their ease of readability, clarity of figures, and clinical correlations. *Human Embryology and Developmental Biology*[3] is a good contemporary, comprehensive explanation of the molecular genetics of embryologic development. *The Developing Human: Clinically Oriented Embryology*[4] is the time-tested standard text of embryology.

GENERAL EMBRYOLOGY

The prenatal period is divided into two major periods: the embryonic period, from fertilization through 2 months,

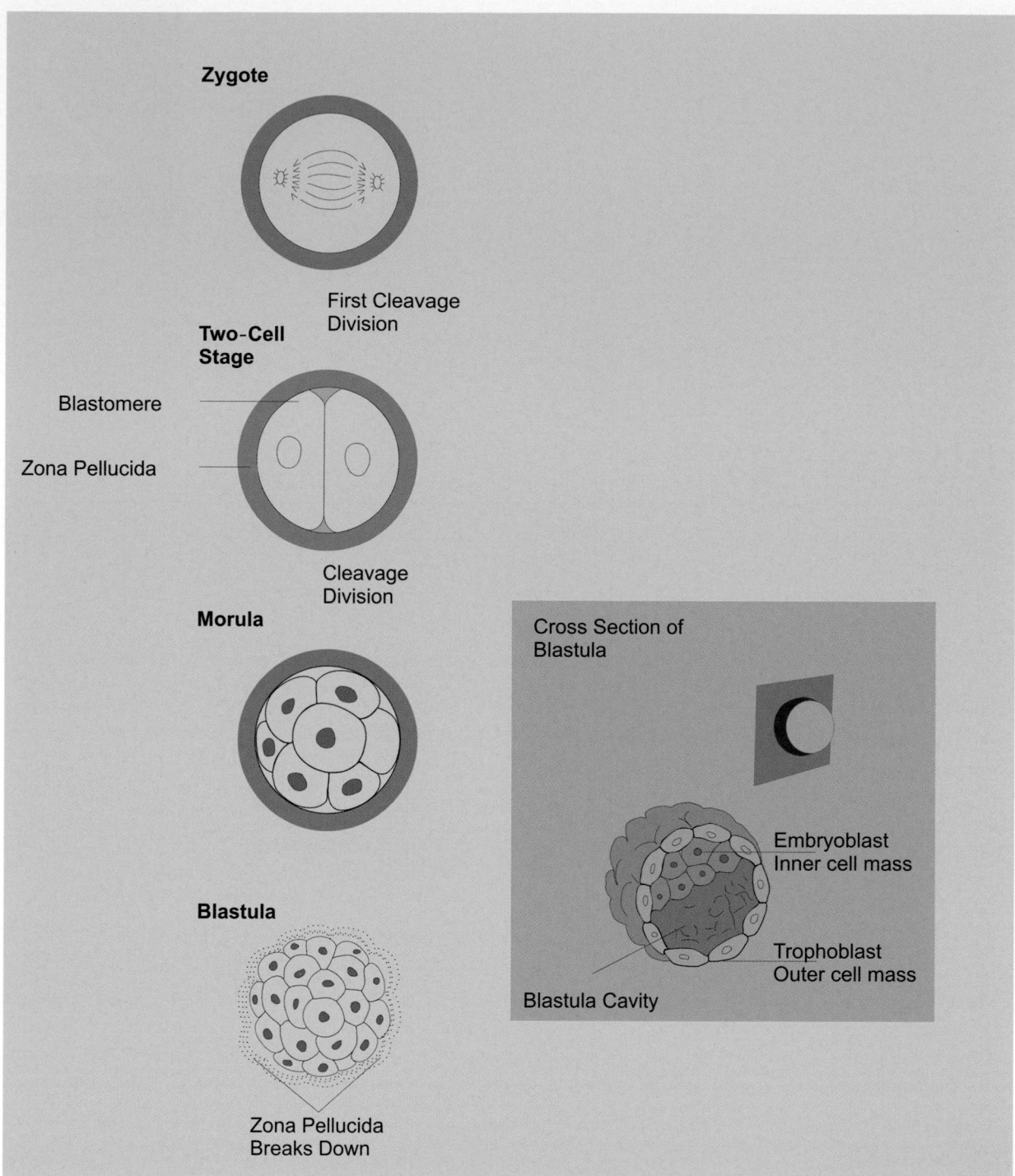

Figure 2–1. Formation of the blastocyst

and the fetal period, from the third month through birth.

Embryonic Period

The embryonic period is the time when all tissue is formed and, particularly during the second month, when all organs are formed. The fetal period is a time of organ growth.[2]

Embryologic development begins with fertilization, the process by which the male and female gametes unite to give rise to a zygote. Approximately 3 days after fertilization cells of the compacted embryo divide to form a **morula,** which is composed of an inner and outer cell mass. The inner cell mass gives rise to the tissues of the **embryoblast,** and the outer cell mass forms the **trophoblast,** which later contributes to the placenta. After a period of cell division, during which time the morula enters the uterine cavity, the **blastocoele** forms, and the embryo is known as a **blastocyst** (Figure 2–1).

By the eighth day of development the blastocyst is partially embedded in the endometrium. At this time the trophoblast differentiates into an inner and an outer layer. Lacunae develop in the outer layer, maternal sinusoids are eroded, and by the end of the second week a primitive uteroplacental circulation begins to develop.

The inner cell mass, or embryoblast, differentiates into two layers, the **epiblast** and the **hypoblast,** which together form the bilaminar germ disk.

The most characteristic event occurring during the third week of gestation is **gastrulation.** This is the process that establishes all three germ layers: **endoderm, ectoderm,** and **mesoderm** in the embryo (Figure 2–2). Gastrulation begins with the formation of the **primitive streak** on the surface of the epiblast portion of the bilaminar germ disk. Cells migrate toward the primitive streak, detach from the epiblast, and slip beneath it. This inward movement is known as **invagination.** Once the cells have invaginated, some displace the hypoblast, creating the new embryonic endoderm. Other cells come to lie between the epiblast and the newly created endoderm to form the mesoderm. Cells remaining in the epiblast then form the ectoderm. Through the process of gastrulation, the epiblast therefore, becomes the source of all the germ layers in the embryo.[1] Developments during the first 3 weeks of the embryonic period therefore produce an embryo with: one germ layer (week 1), two germ layers (week 2) and three germ layers with a recognizable three-dimensional body form (week 3[2] (Figure 2–3).

In general terms the **ectoderm** germ layer gives rise to organs and structures that allow us to maintain contact with the outside world.[4] It gives rise to the central and peripheral nervous systems; the sensory epithelium of the eye, ear and nose; the epidermis and its appendages; hair and nails, mammary glands; the hypophysis, subcutaneous glands; and the enamel of the teeth.

The **mesoderm** gives rise to supporting structures of the body, such as cartilage, bone, and connective tissue; striated and smooth muscle; the heart, blood, lymph vessels, and cells; the kidneys, gonads, and serous membranes lining the body cavities, spleen, and the cortex of the adrenal gland.

The **endoderm** produces the epithelial lining of the gastrointestinal and respiratory tracts, as well as the epithelial lining of the bladder and urethra, tympanic cavity, antrum, and auditory tube. It also engenders the parenchyma of the tonsils, thyroid, parathyroid thymus, liver, and pancreas.

As the embryo forms, it rapidly develops along several axes,[2] the first of which is the craniocaudal axis. It is established while the embryo is still a flat disk or sheet of cells. This axis runs from the future head to future tail of the body form. The dorsoventral axis is the next to be established. This occurs as the body folds and defines the future front and back sides of the body form.

Establishment of the body axes takes place prior to and during the period of gastrulation. Cells at the posterior margin of the embryonic disk signal the craniocaudal axis. The dorsoventral orientation of tissue is controlled by a complex interaction of proteins and growth factors.

This early orientation of cells in the body is a result of the expression of Hox genes. There are four Hox gene complexes in vertebrates: *Hoxa, b, c,* and *d.* Each consists of a group of between 9 and 11 genes arranged sequentially along a particular chromosome. A cascade of genes producing signaling factors also orchestrates left–right asymmetry, which is established early in development. As a result of complex interactions, for example, the heart and spleen lie on the left side of the body and the main lobe of the liver lies on the right.

Regions of the epiblast that migrate and ingress through the primitive streak have been mapped and their ultimate fates determined. Mesoderm cells that ingress through the cranial region of the primitive node become the notochord, those migrating at the lateral edges of the primitive node and from the cranial end of the primitive streak become the paraxial mesoderm. Cells migrating through the midstreak region become the intermediate mesoderm, and those migrating through the caudal part of the streak form the lateral plate mesoderm. This orientation of the mesoderm is important in understanding limb development.

The embryonic disc, initially flat and almost round, gradually becomes elongated, with a broad cephalic and a narrow caudal end. Expansion of the embryonic disk occurs mainly in the cephalic region. This growth in elongation is caused by continuous migration of cells from the primitive streak region in a cephalad direction. Invagination and migration forward and laterally of surface cells in the primitive streak continue until the end of the fourth week. Germ cell layers in the cephalic region begin their specific differentiation by the middle of the third week, whereas those in the caudal part differentiate beginning by the end of the fourth week. This causes the embryo to develop in a cephalocaudal direction (Figure 2–4).

At the beginning of the third week of development the ectodermal germ layer has the shape of the disk. The ectoderm gives rise to two subdivisions: neuroectoderm, which forms all neural tissue, and the epidermal covering of the body.[2] Appearance of the notochord and prechordal mesoderm induces the overlying ectoderm to thicken and form the neural plate (Figure 2–5). Cells of the neural plate make up the neuroectoderm, and their induction represents the initial event in the process of **neurulation.** By the end of the third week the lateral edges of the neural plate become elevated to form neural folds, and the depressed midregion forms the neural groove. Gradually, the neural folds approach each other in the midline where they fuse, resulting in formation of the neural tube. Neurulation is then complete, and the central nervous system is represented by a closed tubular structure with a narrow caudal portion, the spinal cord, and a much broader cephalic portion characterized by a number of dilations, the brain vesicles. As the neural folds elevate and fuse, cells at the lateral border begin to dissociate from their neighbors. This cell population, called the **neural crest,** will undergo a transition as they leave the neuroectoderm to enter the underlying mesoderm.

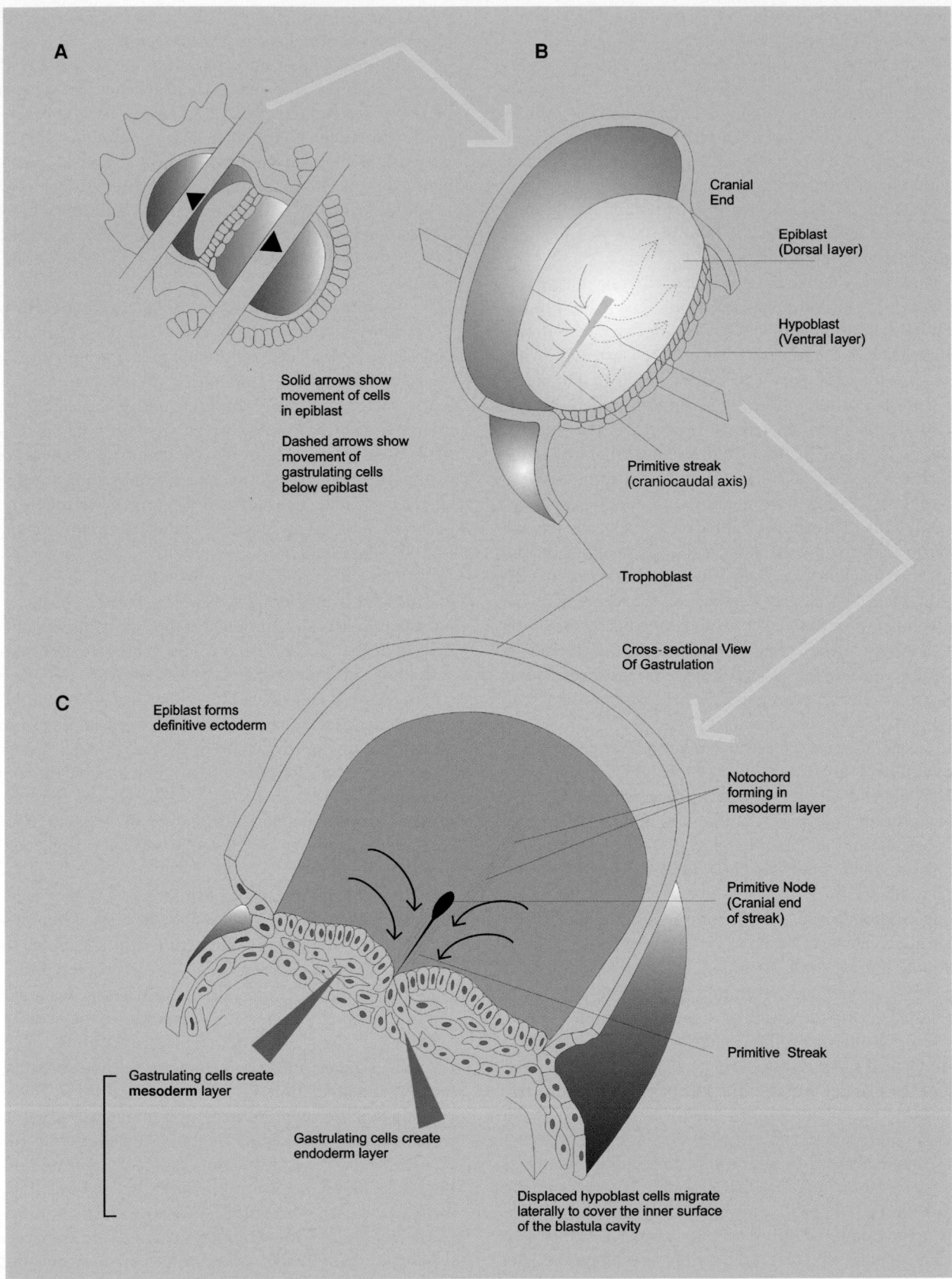

Figure 2–2. Establishment of the three basic germ layers: endoderm, ectoderm, and mesoderm in the embryo. **A:** Trophoblast with the shell removed. **B:** Gastrulation viewed from the dorsal surface. Solid arrows show movement of cells in epiblast; dashed arrows show movement of gastrulating cells below the epiblast. **C:** Differentiation of the basic germ layers

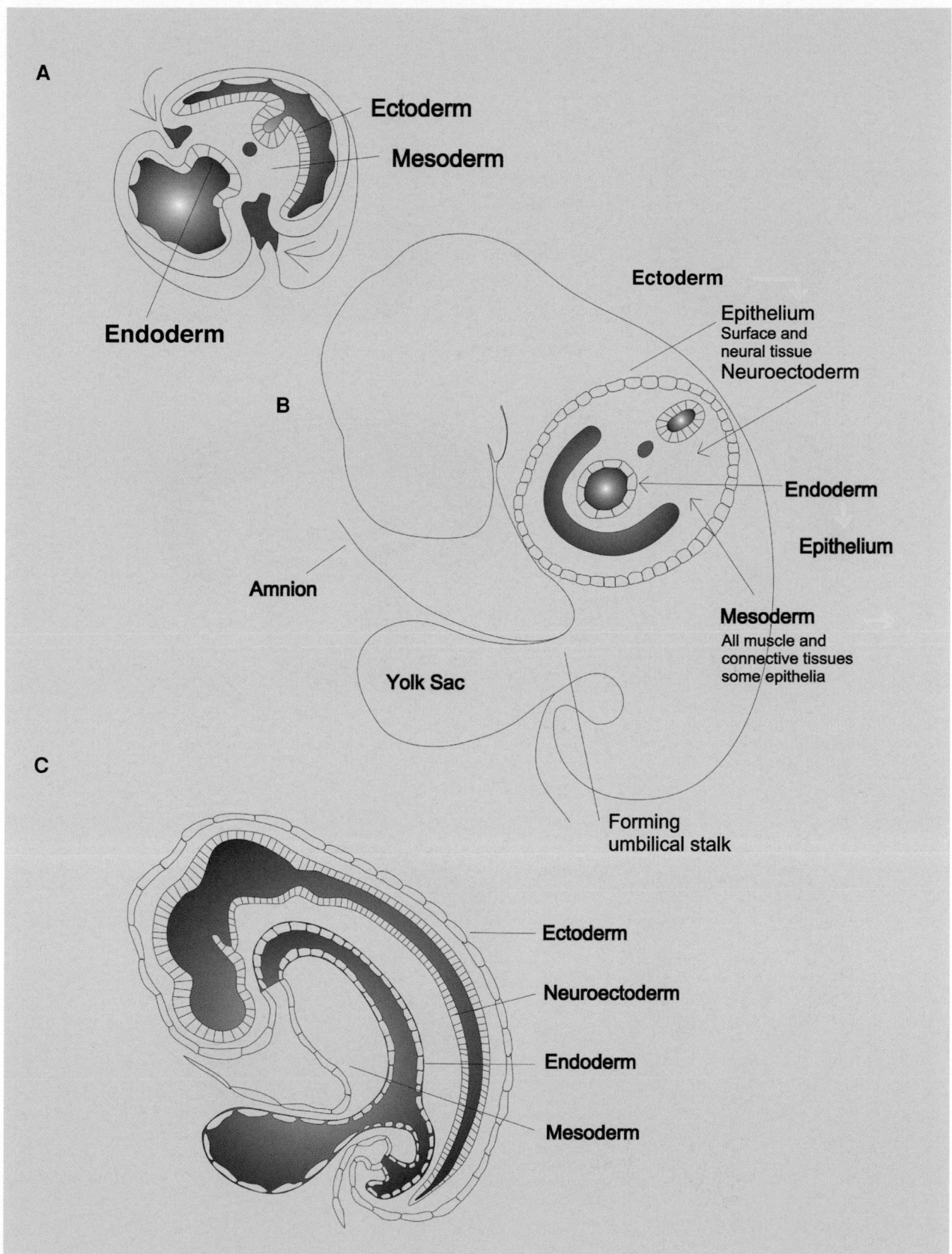

Figure 2–3. Cross section of germ layers as they appear during embryonic folding. **A:** Cross section. **B:** Cross section of germ layers after folding is completed. **C:** Longitudinal section

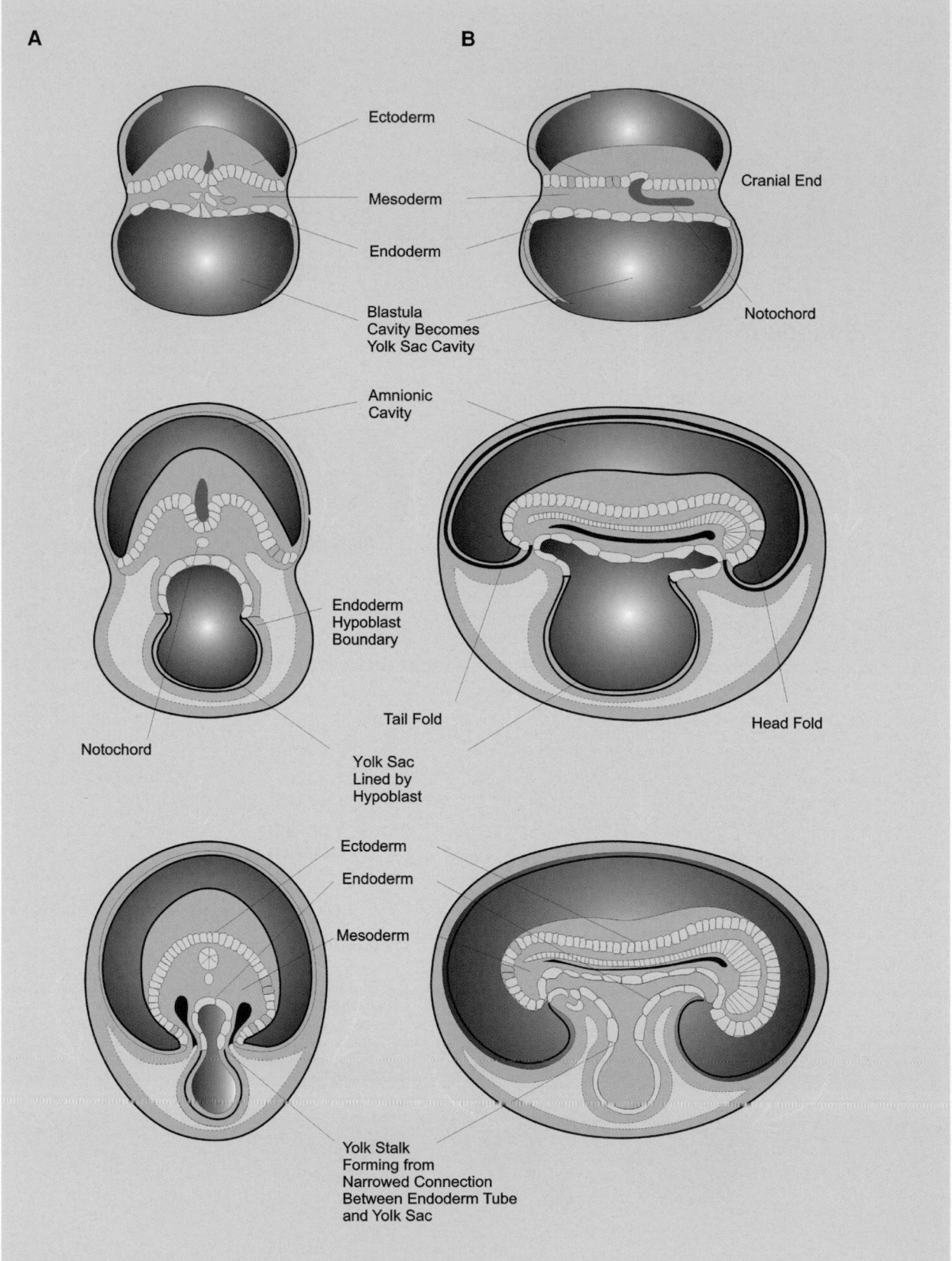

Figure 2–4. Development of the embryo in a cephalocaudal direction. **A:** Lateral body folds, cross-sectional views. **B:** Craniocaudal body folds, longitudinal views

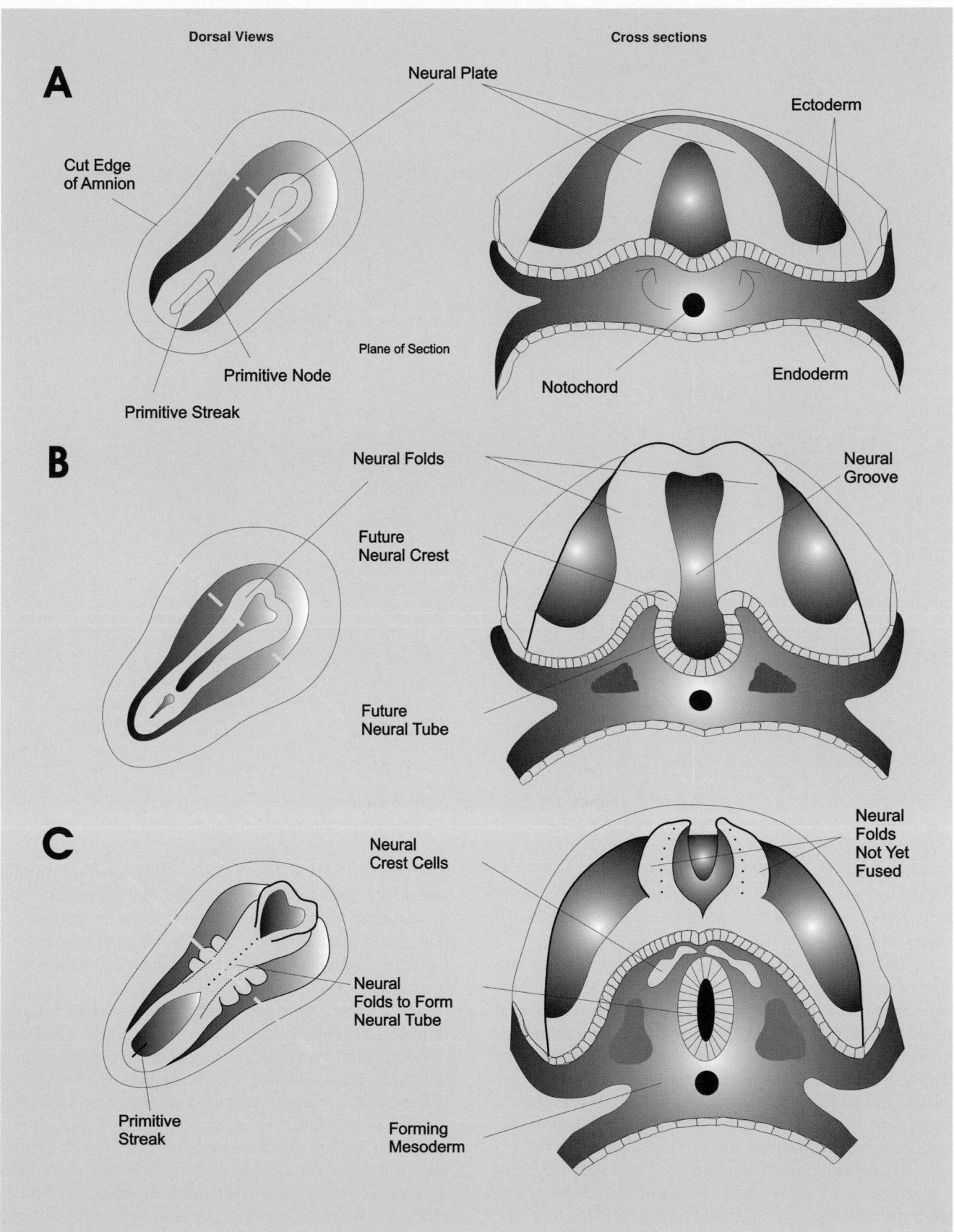

Figure 2–5. Formation of the neural plate. **A:** Formation of the neural plate. **B:** Formation of the neural folds and neural groove. **C:** Completion of neurulation, the creation of the neural tube

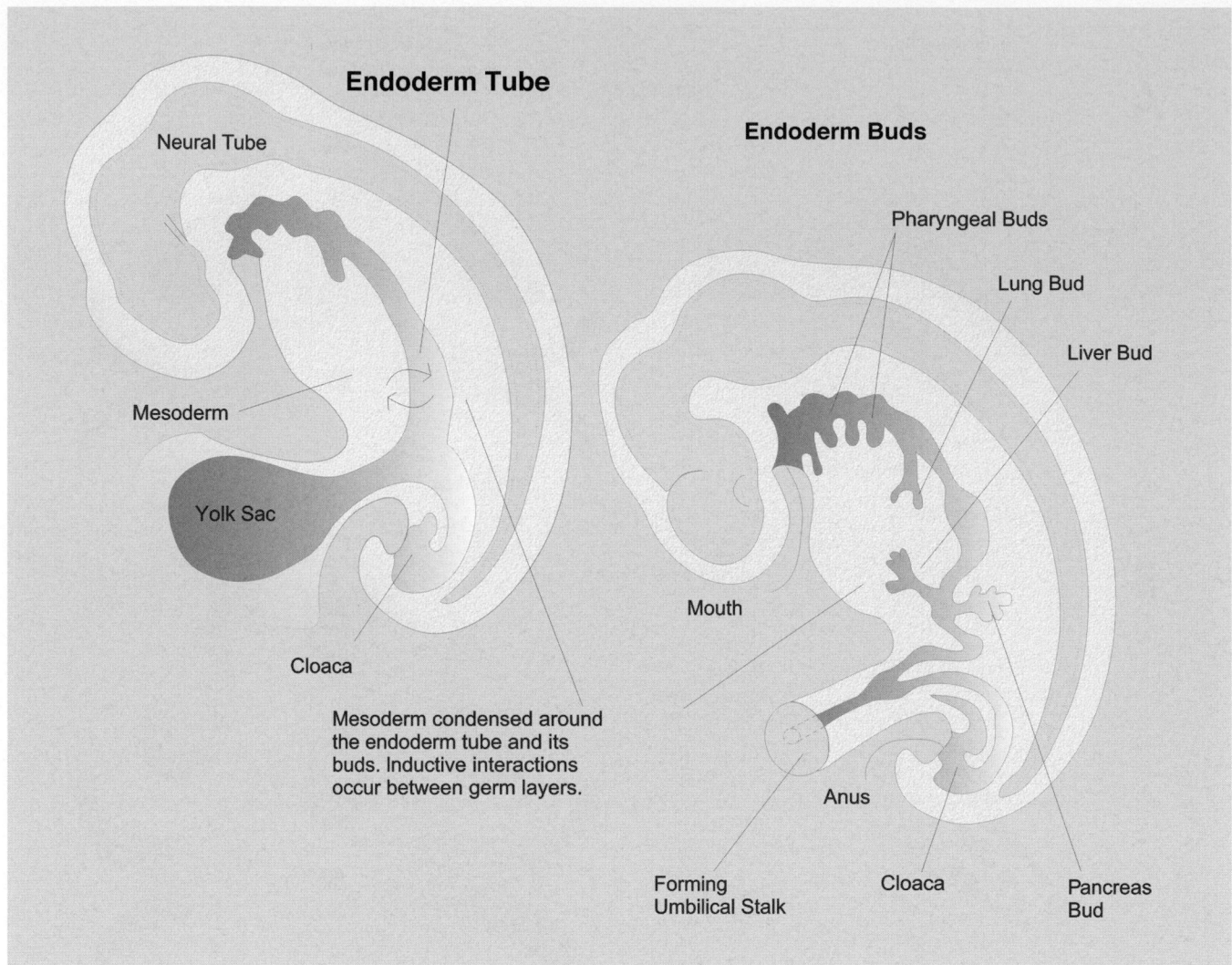

Figure 2–6. Formation of the endoderm

During the body-folding process, the endoderm is formed into an epithelial tube, which runs the length of the body. The derivatives of the endoderm tube are all epithelial tissues (Figure 2–6).

Initially cells of the mesoderm germ layer form a thin sheet of tissue on each side of the midline.[1] These cells proliferate and form a thick end plate of tissue known as paraxial mesoderm (Figure 2–7). More laterally the mesoderm remains thin and is known as the lateral plate. This lateral plate divides into two layers: a somatic, or parietal, mesoderm layer and a splanchnic, or visceral, mesoderm layer. Together these layers form the intraembryonic cavity. Intermediate mesoderm connects the paraxial and lateral plate mesoderm.

By the beginning of the third week, paraxial mesoderm is organized into segments. These segments are known as **somitomeres.** They first appear in the cephalic region of the embryo, and their formation proceeds in a craniocaudal direction. In the head region, somitomeres transition, in association with segmentation of the neural plate, into neuromeres.

From the occipital region caudally, somitomeres further organize into **somites.** Somites give rise to the **myotome** (ultimately muscle tissue), **sclerotome** (ultimately cartilage and bone), and **dermatome** (ultimately subcutaneous tissue of the skin). Collectively, these are all supporting tissues of the body (Figure 2–8).

Signaling for this somite differentiation arises from surrounding structures, including the notochord, neural tube, epidermis, and lateral plate mesoderm. By the beginning of the fourth week cells forming the ventral and media walls of the somite lose their compact organization and shift their position to surround the notochord (the dense cord of mesoderm that induces neuroectoderm). These cells, collectively known as the sclerotome, form a loosely woven tissue called the mesenchyme. They will surround the spinal cord and notochord to form the vertebral column. Cells at the dorsolateral portion of the somite also migrate as precursors of limb and body wall structures. Following migration of these muscle cells and cells of the sclerotome, cells at the dorsomedial

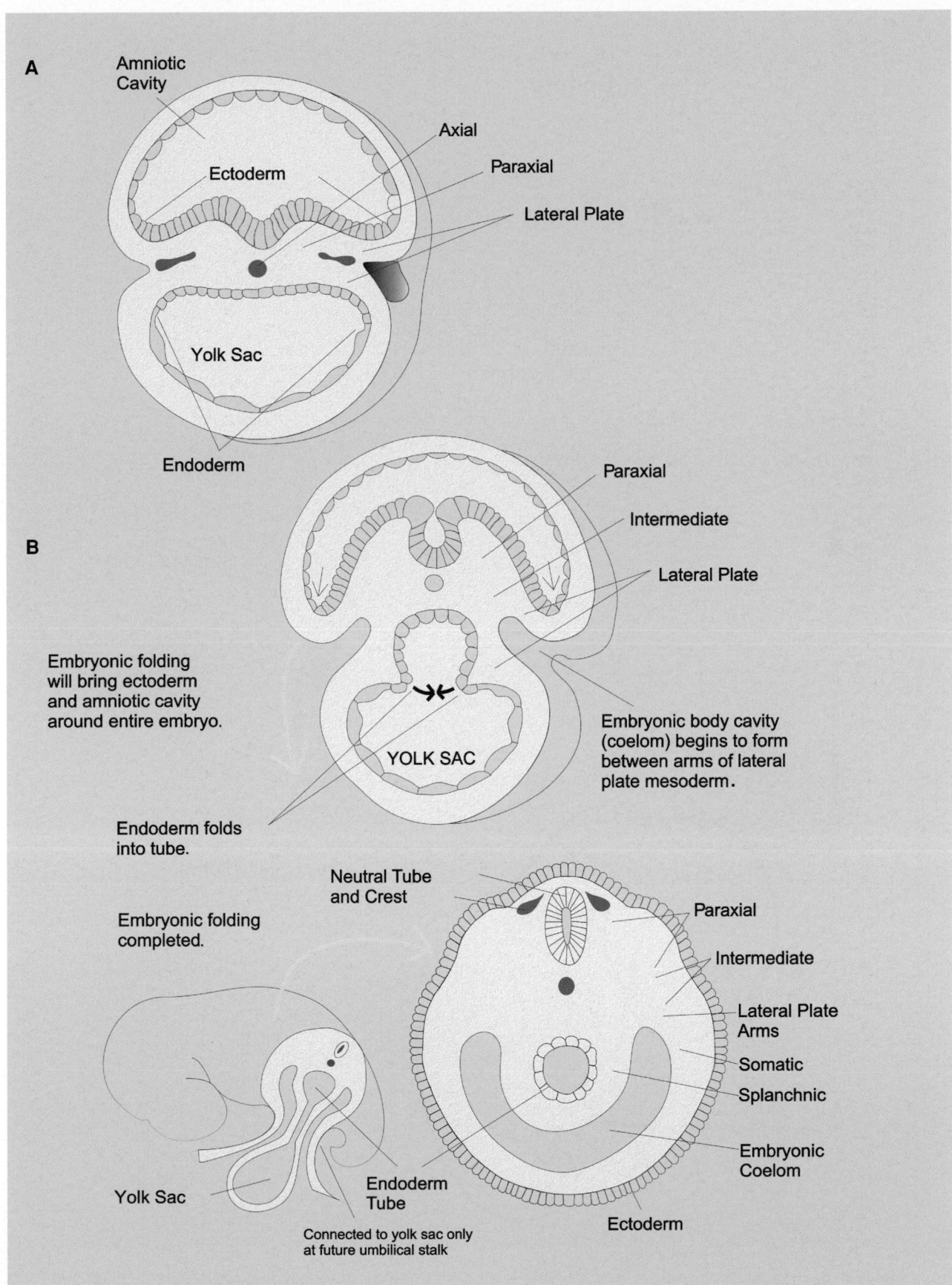

Figure 2–7. Formation of paraxial mesoderm (**A**), embryonic cavity (**B**), and embryonic folding (**C**)

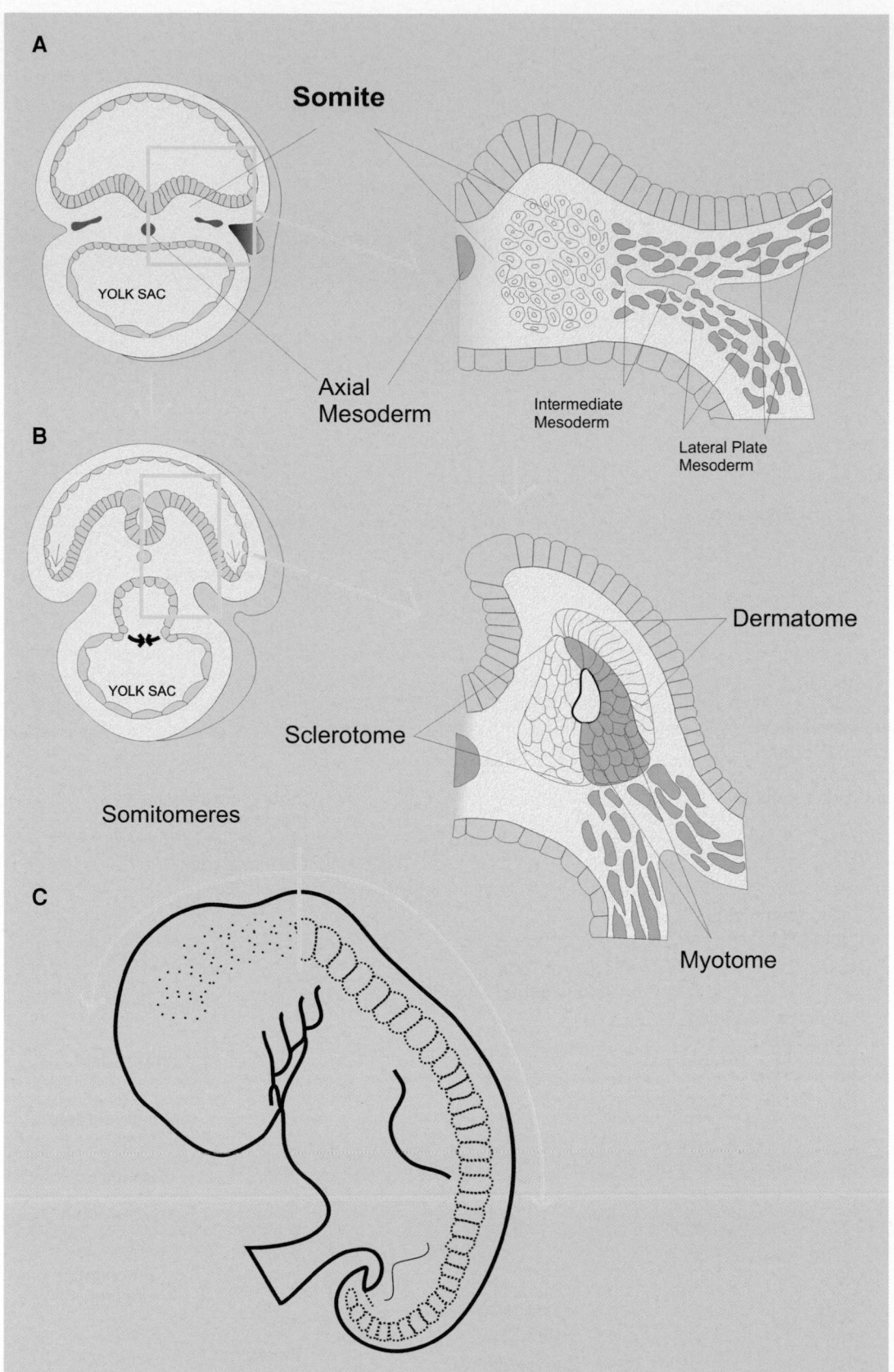

Figure 2–8. Development of the supporting tissues of the body myotome (muscle tissue), sclerotome (cartilage and bone), and dermatome (subcutaneous tissue). **A:** Paraxial mesoderm condenses to form the somite. **B:** Somite forms three regions. **C:** Somitomeres develop into somites

portion of the somite proliferate and migrate down the ventral side of the remaining dorsal epithelium of the somite to form a new layer, the myotome. The remaining dorsal epithelium forms the dermatome, and together these layers constitute the dermomyotome. Each segmentally arranged myotome contributes to muscles of the back, whereas the dermatomes disperse to form the dermis and subcutaneous tissue of the skin. Each myotome and dermatome retains its innervation from the segment of origin, no matter where the cells migrate to. Therefore, each somite forms its own sclerotome, the cartilage and bone component; its own myotome, providing the segmental muscle component; and its own dermatome, the segmental skin component. Each myotome and dermatome also has its owns segmental nerve component (Figure 2–9).

During the second month, the external appearance of the embryo is changed greatly by the enormous size of the head and formation of the limbs, face, ears, nose, and eyes.[1] By the beginning of the fifth week, fore- and hindlimbs appear as paddle-shaped buds (Figure 2–10). The forelimbs are located dorsal to the pericardial swelling at the level of the fourth cervical to first thoracic somites, which explains their innervation by the brachial plexus. Hindlimb buds appear slightly later just caudal to the attachment of the umbilical stock at the level of the lumbar and uppers sacral somites. With further growth the terminal portions of the buds flatten, and a circular constriction separates them from the proximal, more cylindrical segment. Soon four radial grooves separating five slightly thicker areas appear on the distal portion of the buds. This development foreshadows formation of the digits. These grooves, known as rays, appear in the hand region first, and shortly afterward, in the foot because the upper limb is slightly more advanced in development than the lower limb. While fingers and toes are being formed, a second constriction divides the proximal portion of the buds into two segments, and the three parts characteristic of the adult extremities can be recognized.

Fetal Period

The period from the beginning of the ninth week to the end of the intrauterine life is known as the fetal period.[1] It is characterized by maturation of tissues and organs and rapid growth of the body growth in length. This is particularly striking during the third, fourth, and fifth months, and increasing weight are most striking during the last 2 months of gestation. During the third month the face becomes more human-looking, and the limbs reach their relative length in comparison with the rest of the body, although the lower limbs are still a little shorter and less well developed than the upper extremities. Primary ossification centers are present in the long bones and the skull by the twelfth week.

Skeletal System: Limb Growth & Development

The skeletal system develops from paraxial and lateral plate mesoderm as well as neural crest tissue.[1] The somites (as previously described) differentiate into a ventromedial component called the sclerotome and a dorsolateral component called the dermomyotome. This organization of cells forms a loosely woven tissue called the mesenchyme. The mesenchyme migrates and differentiates into fibroblasts, chondroblasts, and osteoblasts.

At the end of the fourth week of development limb buds become visible as out-pocketings of the ventrolateral body wall.[1] Initially they consist of a mesenchymal core derived from the somatic layer of lateral plate mesoderm that will form the bones and connective tissue of the limb, covered by a layer of ectoderm. Ectoderm at the distal border of the limb thickens and forms a specialized inducing tissue known as the **apical ectodermal ridge (AER).** The AER exerts an inductive influence on the adjacent mesenchyme, causing it to remain as a population of undifferentiated, rapidly proliferating cells called the **progress zone.** As the limb grows, cells farther from the influence of the AER begin to differentiate into cartilage and muscle. In this manner of development of the limb proceeds proximodistally. In 6-week-old embryos, the terminal portion of the limb buds become flattened to form hand and footplates and are separated from the proximal segment by a circular constriction. Later a second constriction divides the proximal portions into two segments, and the main parts of the extremities can be recognized.[1] Fingers and toes are formed when programmed cell death in the AER separates this ridge into five parts. Further formation of the digits depends on their continued outgrowth under the influence of the five remaining segments of ridge ectoderm. This results in condensation of the mesenchyme to form cartilaginous digital rays. Development of the upper and lower limbs is similar except that morphogenesis of the lower limb is approximately 1–2 days behind that of the upper limb.

During the seventh week of gestation a key event occurs that is critical in understanding the final orientation and innervation of the limbs. The limbs rotate in opposite directions. The upper limb rotates 90 degrees **laterally** so that the extensor muscles lie on the lateral and posterior surface and the thumbs lie laterally. The lower limb rotates approximately 90 degrees **medially,** placing the extensor muscles on the anterior surface and the great toe medially.[1] This explains why *homologous joints* of the upper and lower extremities (knees and elbows) *point in opposite directions.* This limb rotation results in:[2]

1. The final orientation of the limbs
2. The final location and orientation of muscle groups (because the muscles are connected to the limb bones prior to rotation)
3. The patterns of sensory innervation of the skin (also because nerve fibers are connected with the dermis layer of the skin prior to rotation and are pulled along)

While the external shape is being established, mesenchyme in the buds begins to condense, and by the sixth week of development the first hyaline cartilage models can be recognized. Ossification of the bones of the extremities begins by the end of the embryonic period. Primary ossification centers

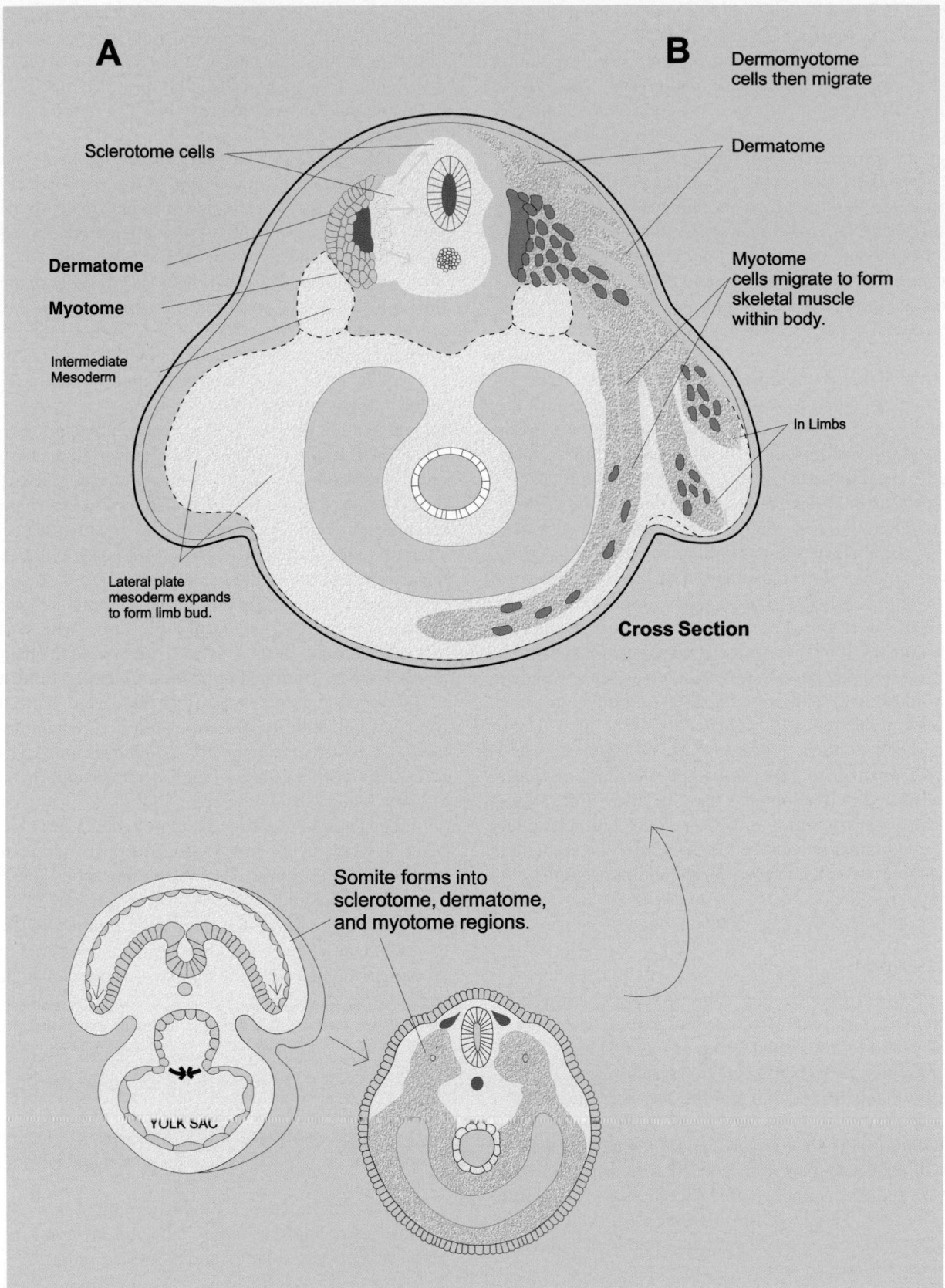

Figure 2–9. Cells of each somite region migrate separately to target destinations before forming specific tissues. Each somite forms its own sclerotome, myotome, and dermatome. **A:** Sclerotome cells migrate medially to form bones (vertebrae and ribs). **B:** Dermatome cells then migrate under ectoderm to form connective tissue of skin (dermis)

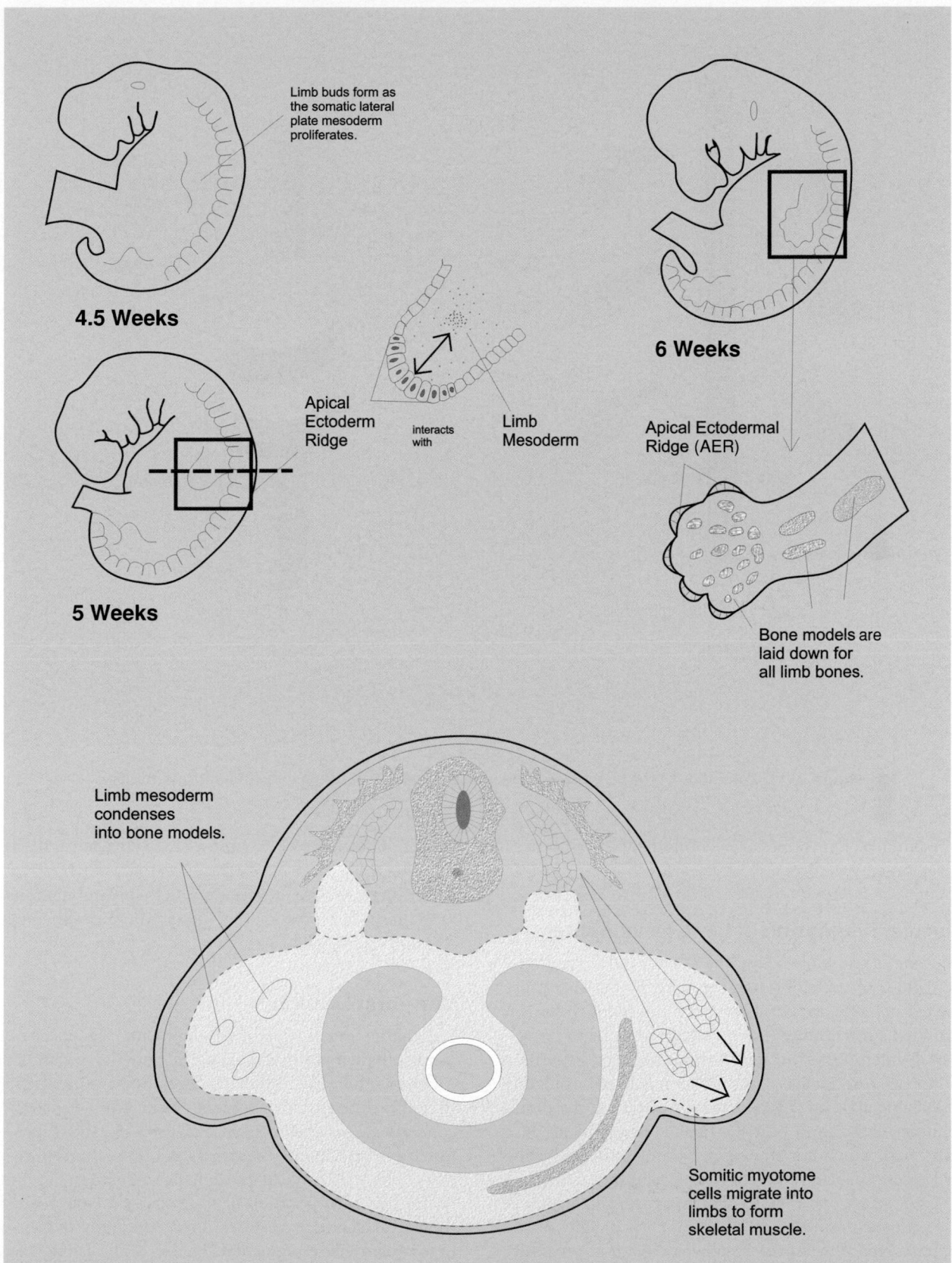

Figure 2–10. During the second month of development, the external appearance of the embryo greatly changes by rapid appearance of the large size of the head and formation of the limbs, face, ears, nose, and eyes. By the beginning of the fifth week, forelimbs and hindlimbs appear as paddle-shaped buds

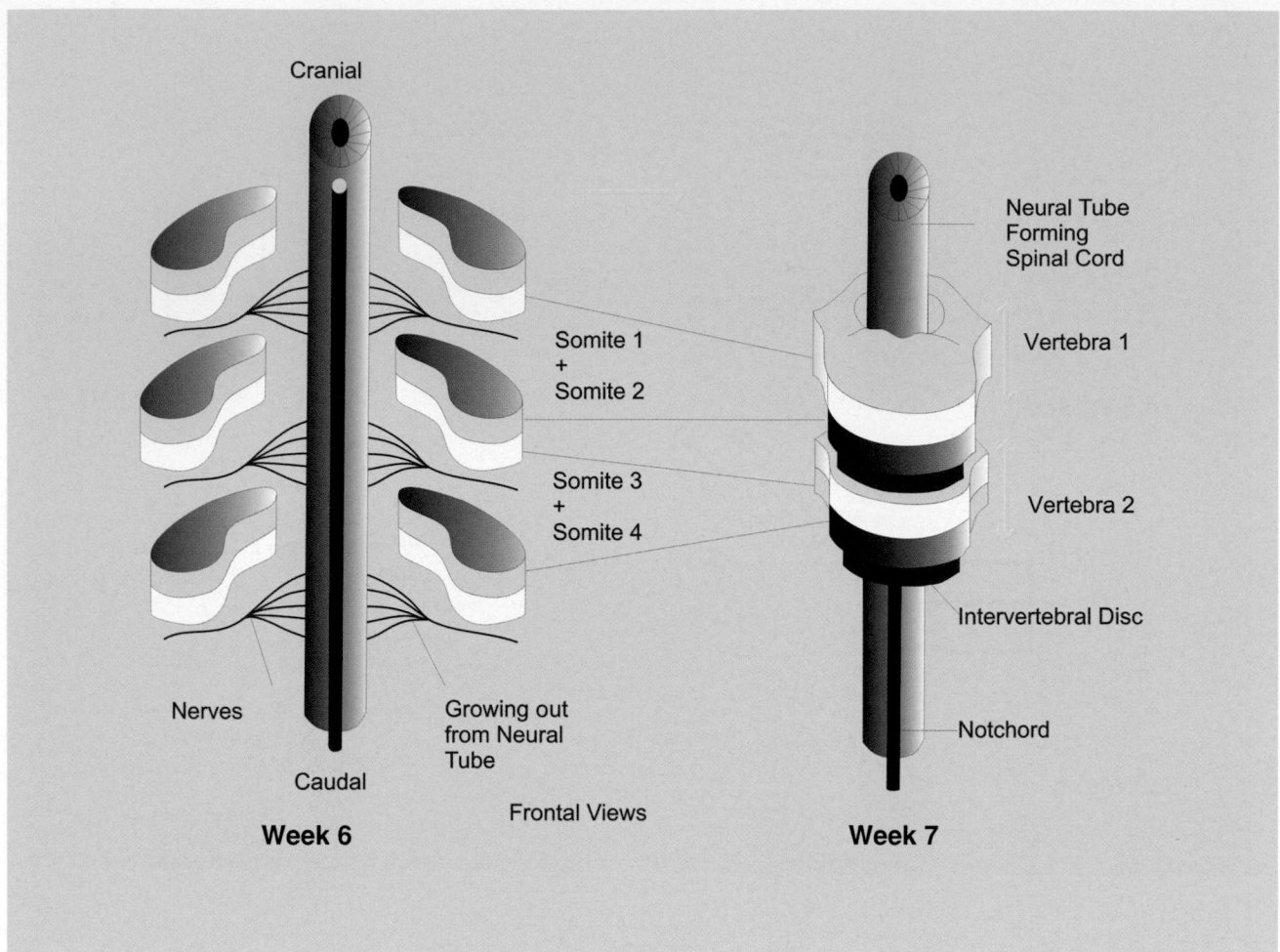

Figure 2–11. Formation of the vertebrae by fusion of sclerotome cells from two different somite levels

are present in all long bones of the limbs by the twelfth week of development.

Molecular Regulation of Limb Development

Positioning of the limbs along the craniocaudal axis in the flank regions of the embryo is regulated by the Hox genes expressed along this axis.[1] Once positioning along this axis is determined, growth must also be regulated along the proximodistal, anteroposterior, and dorsoventral axes. Patterning of the anteroposterior axis of the limb is regulated by the **zone of polarizing activity (ZPA),** a cluster of cells at the posterior border of the limb near the flank. These cells produce retinoic acid, which initiates expression of **sonic hedgehog (Shh),** a secreted factor that regulates development along this axis.[1] This regulation results in digits appearing in the proper order, with the thumb on the radial (anterior) side. As the limb grows, the ZPA moves distally to remain in proximity to the posterior border of the AER. The dorsoventral axis is patterned in a similar fashion by the dorsal ectoderm of the limb.

Although patterning genes for the limb axes have been predetermined, it is the Hox genes that regulate the types and

shapes of the bones of the limbs. These Hox genes are nested in overlapping patterns of expression that somehow regulate patterning.[1] As a result, variations in their combinations create patterns of expression that may account for differences in fore and hind limb structures.

Vertebral Column

During the fourth week of development, cells of the sclerotome shift their position to surround both the spinal cord and the notochord.[1] During further development, the caudal portion of each sclerotome segment proliferates extensively and condenses. This proliferation is so extensive that it proceeds into the subjacent intersegmental tissue and binds the caudal half of one sclerotome to the cephalic half of the adjacent sclerotome. By incorporation of this intersegmental tissue into the precartilaginous vertebral body, the body of the vertebrae becomes intersegmental (Figure 2–11). Hox genes also control this patterning. Mesenchymal cells between cephalic and caudal parts of the original sclerotome form the intervertebral disk. Although the notochord regresses entirely in the region of the vertebral bodies, it persists and enlarges in the region of the intervertebral disk. Here it contributes to the nucleus pulposus, which is later surrounded by circular fibers of the anulus fibrosus. Together these structures form the intervertebral disk.[1]

Muscular & Peripheral Nervous Systems

With the exception of some smooth muscle tissue, the muscular system develops from the mesoderm germ layer.[1] Skeletal muscle is derived from paraxial mesoderm, which forms somites from the occipital to sacral regions and somitomeres in the head. The somites and somitomeres form the musculature of the axial skeleton body wall, limbs, and head. From the occipital region caudally, somites form and differentiate into this sclerotome, dermatome, and two muscle forming regions. One of these is in the dorsolateral region of the somite and provides progenitor cells (myoblasts) for the limb and body wall musculature. The other region lies dorsomedially, migrates ventrally to cells that form the dermatome, and forms the myotome. Patterns of muscle formation are under the influence of the surrounding connective tissue in to which myoblasts migrate. In the head region, this connective tissue is derived from neural crest cells. In cervical and occipital regions muscles differentiate from somitic mesoderm, whereas in the body wall and limbs they originate from the somatic mesoderm. By the end of the fifth week prospective muscle cells are collected into two parts: a small dorsal portion, the **epimere,** and a larger ventral part called the **hypomere.**[1] Nerves innervating segmental muscles are also divided into a dorsal primary ramus for the epimere and a ventral primary ramus for the hypomere. These nerves remain with their original muscle segment throughout its migration. Myoblasts of the epimere form extensor muscles of the vertebral column, and those of the hypomere is give rise to the muscles of the limbs and body wall. The first indication of limb musculature is observed in the seventh week of development as a condensation of mesenchyme near the base of the limb buds. This mesenchyme is derived from dorsolateral cells of the somites that migrate into the limb bud to form the muscles. This connective tissue dictates the pattern of muscle formation and is derived from somatic mesoderm, which also gives rise to the bones of the limb.[1]

With elongation of the limb buds the muscles tissue splits into flexor and extensor components. The upper limb bud lies opposite the lower five cervical and upper two thoracic segments. The lower limb buds lie opposite the lower four lumbar and upper two sacral segments. As soon as the buds form, ventral primary rami from the appropriate spinal nerves penetrate into the mesenchyme (Figure 2–12). At first, each ventral ramus enters with isolated dorsal and ventral branches, but soon these branches unite to form large dorsal and ventral nerves. Thus, in the upper extremity, the radial nerve supplies all the extensor musculature and is formed by a combination of dorsal segmental branches. The ulnar and median nerves, which supply all the flexor muscles, are formed by a combination of the ventral branches[1] (Figure 2–13). Immediately after the nerves have entered the limb buds they establish contact with the differentiating mesoderm

condensations. This early contact is a prerequisite for their complete functional differentiation. Spinal nerves therefore play an important role in differentiation and motor innervation of the limb musculature, as well as providing sensory innervation for the dermatomes. Although the original dermatomal pattern changes with growth of the extremities, an orderly sequence can still be recognized in the adult.

Central Nervous System

The central nervous system (CNS) originates in the ectoderm and appears as the **neural plate** at the middle of the third week[1] (Figure 2–14). After the edges of the plate fold, the **neural folds** approach each other in the midline to fuse, forming the **neural tube.** The CNS then forms as a tubular structure with a broad cephalic portion (the brain) and a long caudal portion (the spinal cord). A basal plate, containing the motor neurons, and an alar plate, containing the sensory neurons, characterize the spinal cord, which forms the caudal end of the CNS.

The walls of the recently closed neural tube consist of neuroepithelial cells. These cells give rise to another type of cell, the **neuroblasts,** which are primitive nerve cells. They form a **mantle layer** around the neuroepithelial layer. This mantle layer later forms the gray matter of the spinal cord. The outermost layer of the spinal cord, called the **marginal layer,** contains nerve fibers emerging from neuroblasts in the mantle layer. As a result of myelination, this layer takes on a white appearance and is called the white matter of the spinal cord.[1] As a result of continuous addition of neuroblasts to the mantle layer, each side of the neural tube shows ventral and dorsal thickening. The ventral thickening—the basal plates—contains ventral motor horn cells. The dorsal thickening—the alar plates—forms the sensory areas. A group of neurons accumulate between these two areas, forming a small intermediate horn, which contains neurons of the sympathetic portion of the autonomic nervous system and is present only at thoracic and upper lumbar levels of the spinal cord[1] (Figure 2–15).

Spinal Nerves

Motor nerve fibers begin to appear in the fourth week, arising from nerve cells in the basal plates of the spinal cord.[4] They collect into bundles known as a ventral nerve roots. Likewise dorsal nerve roots form as collections of fibers originating from cells in dorsal root ganglia. Central processes from these ganglia form processes that grow into the spinal cord opposite the dorsal horns, and distal processes join the ventral nerve roots to form a spinal nerve. Spinal nerves divide into dorsal and ventral primary rami. Dorsal rami innervate dorsal axial musculature, vertebral joints, and the skin of the back. Ventral primary rami innervate the limbs and ventral body wall and form the major nerve plexuses.[1]

In the third month of development, the spinal cord extends the entire length of the embryo, and spinal nerves pass through the intervertebral foramina at their level of origin.

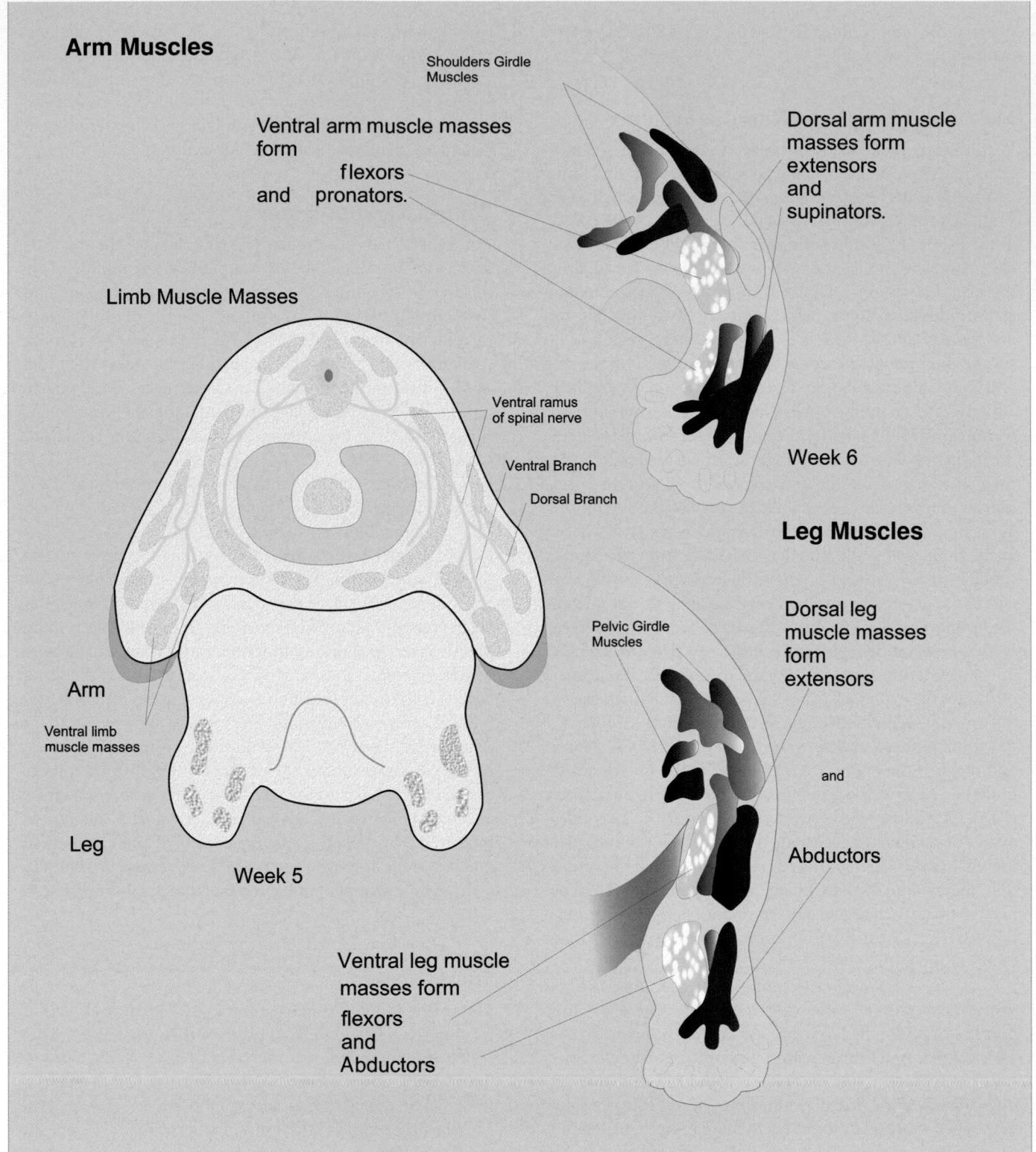

Arm Muscles

Shoulders Girdle Muscles

Ventral arm muscle masses form

flexors

and   pronators.

Dorsal arm muscle masses form extensors and supinators.

Limb Muscle Masses

Ventral ramus of spinal nerve

Ventral Branch

Dorsal Branch

Week 6

Arm

Ventral limb muscle masses

Leg

Week 5

Leg Muscles

Pelvic Girdle Muscles

Dorsal leg muscle masses form extensors

and

Abductors

Ventral leg muscle masses form

flexors and Abductors

Figure 2–12. Formation of the spinal nerves

With increasing age, the vertebral column and dura lengthen more rapidly than the neural tube, resulting in the terminal end of the spinal cord gradually shifting to a higher level. At birth, this level is at the third lumbar vertebra. In the adult the spinal cord terminates at the level of L2 to L3, whereas the du-ral sac and subarachnoid space extends to S2. As a result of this disproportionate growth, spinal nerves run obliquely from their segment of origin in the spinal cord to the corresponding level of the vertebral column. Below L2 to L3 a thread-like ex-tension of the pia mater forms the filum terminale, which

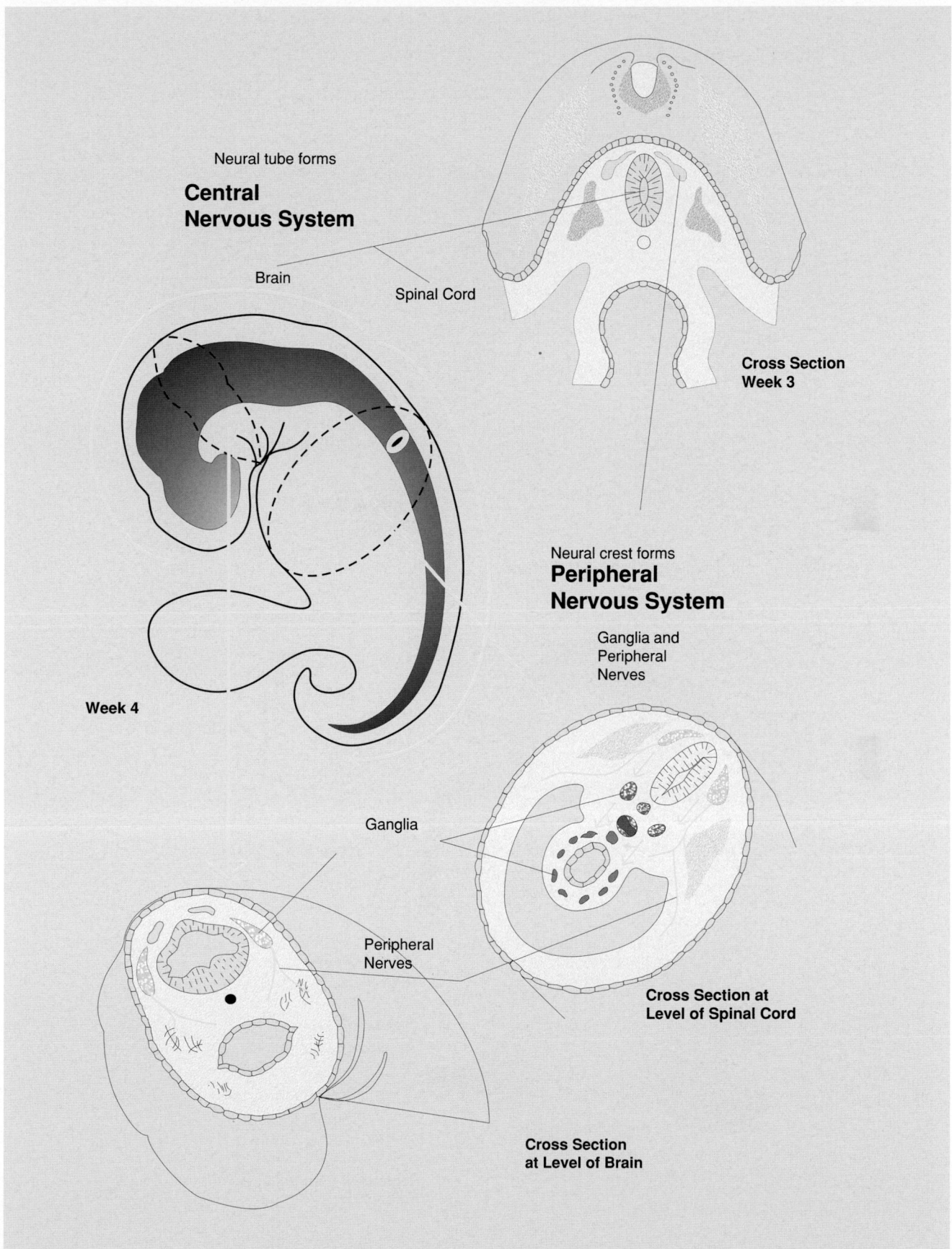

Figure 2–13. Development of the peripheral nervous system

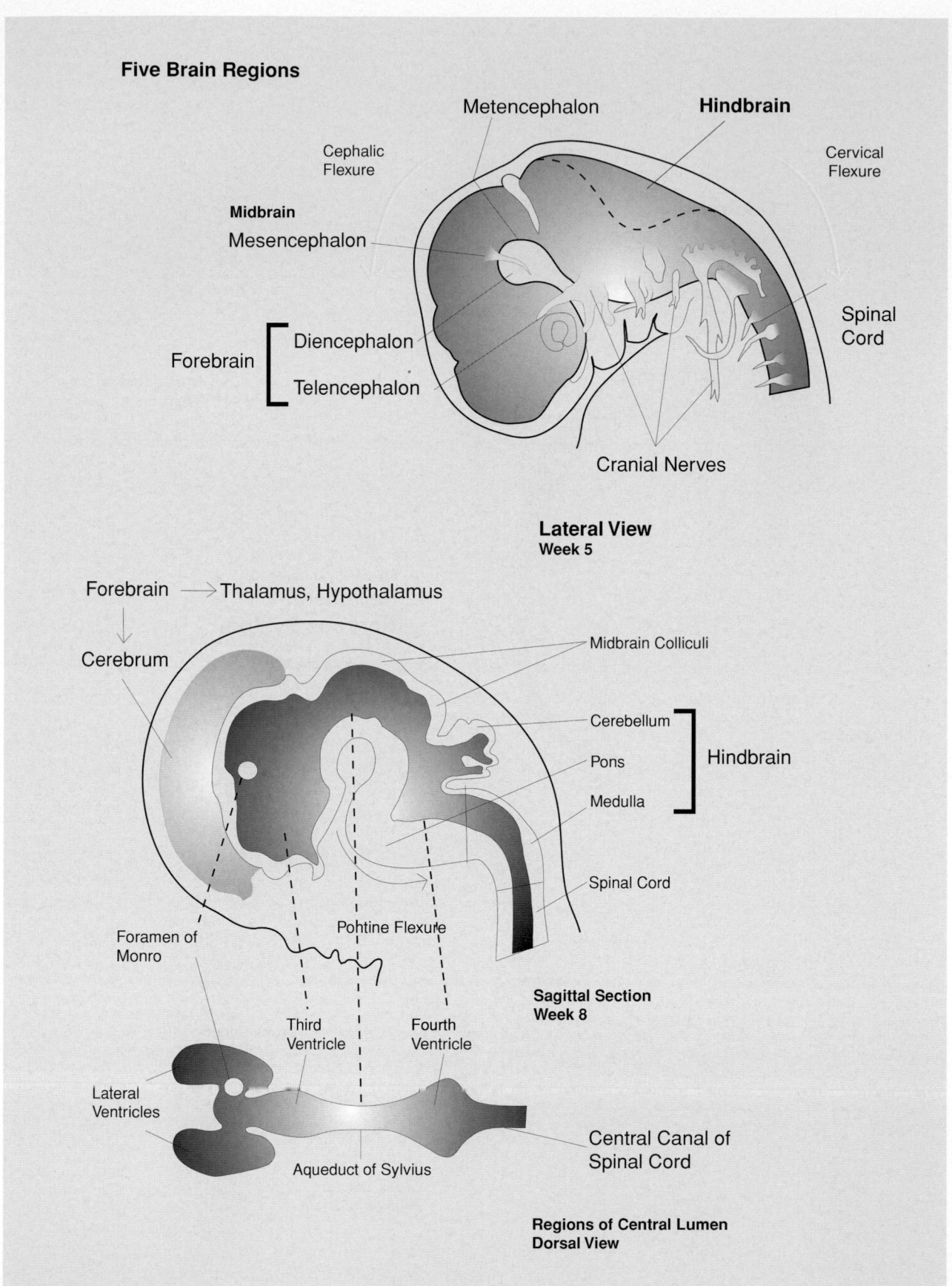

Figure 2–14. Development of the central nervous system

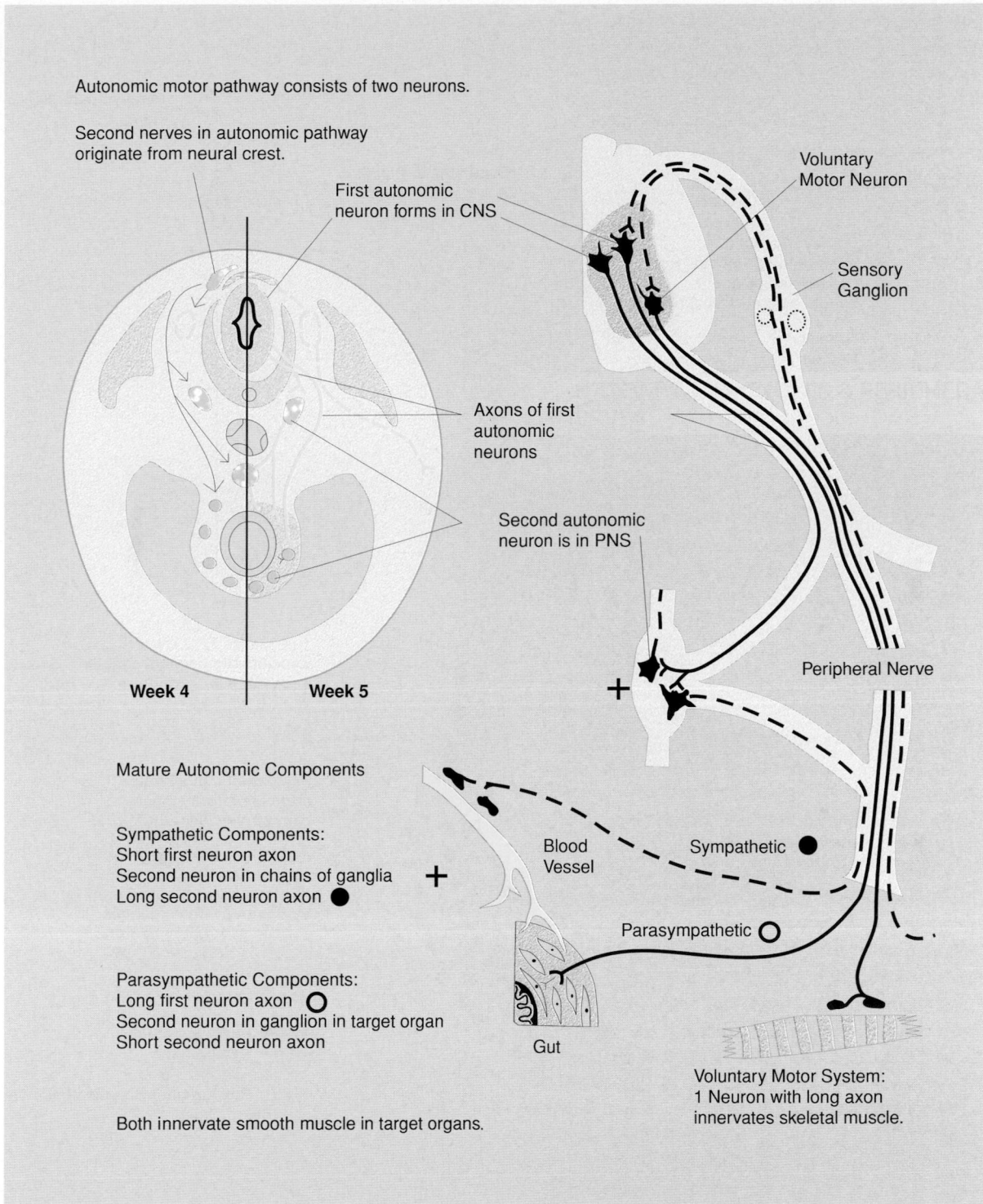

Autonomic motor pathway consists of two neurons.

Second nerves in autonomic pathway originate from neural crest.

First autonomic neuron forms in CNS

Voluntary Motor Neuron

Sensory Ganglion

Axons of first autonomic neurons

Second autonomic neuron is in PNS

Peripheral Nerve

Week 4   Week 5

Mature Autonomic Components

Sympathetic Components:
Short first neuron axon
Second neuron in chains of ganglia
Long second neuron axon ●

+

Blood Vessel

Sympathetic ●

Parasympathetic ○

Parasympathetic Components:
Long first neuron axon ○
Second neuron in ganglion in target organ
Short second neuron axon

Gut

Voluntary Motor System:
1 Neuron with long axon innervates skeletal muscle.

Both innervate smooth muscle in target organs.

Figure 2–15. Development of autonomic nervous system

is attached to the periosteum of the first coccygeal vertebra and marks the tract of regression of the spinal cord.[1]

The Brain

The brain consists originally of three vesicles: the **rhombencephalon** (hindbrain), **mesencephalon** (midbrain), and **prosencephalon** (forebrain). The rhombencephalon will ultimately form the medulla oblongata, pons, and cerebellum. The mesencephalon resembles the spinal cord with its basal and alar plates. It will contain the anterior and posterior colliculi, forming the relay stations for visual and auditory reflex centers. The prosencephalon will ultimately give rise to the thalamus and hypothalamus as well as the cerebral hemispheres.[1]

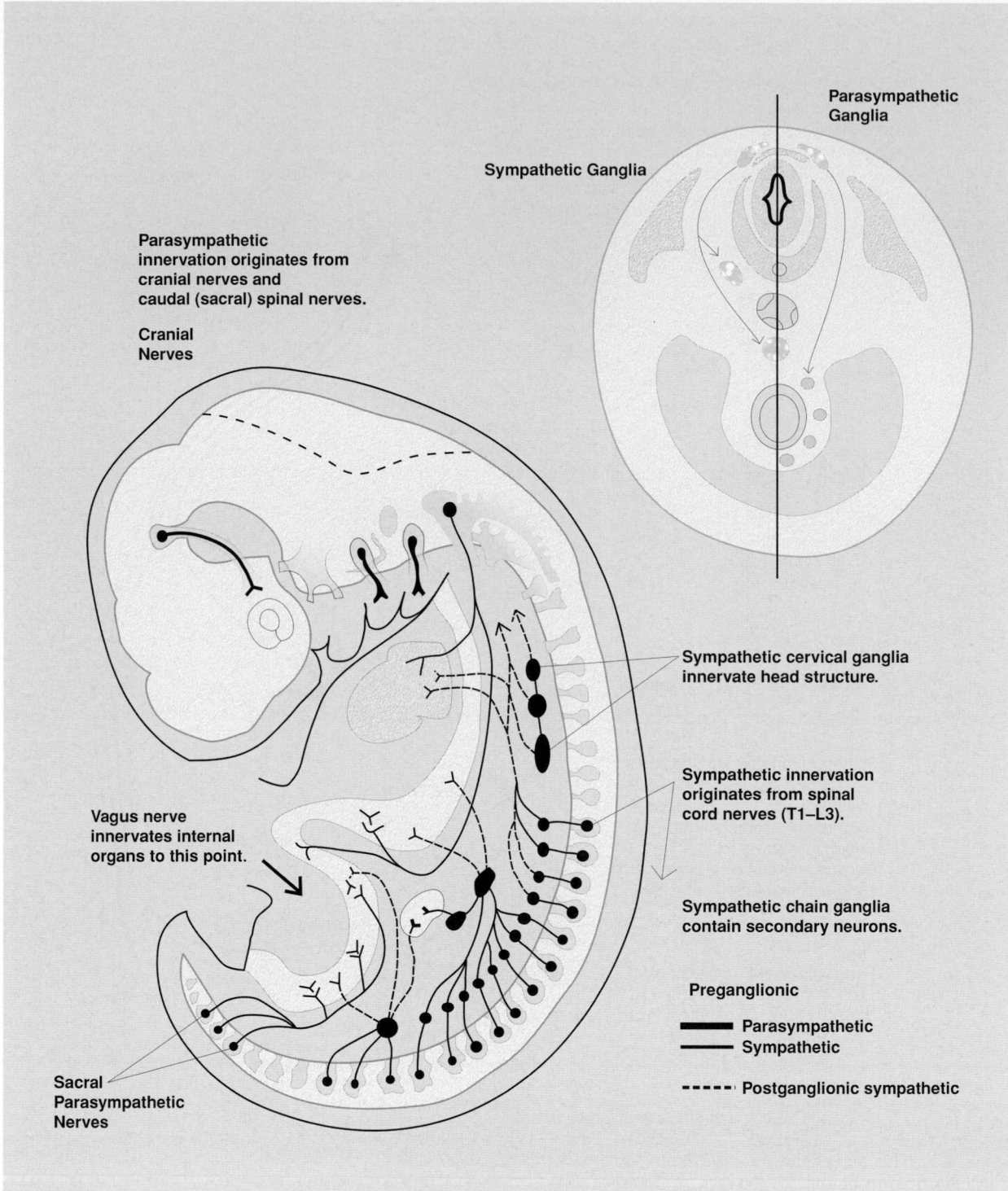

Figure 2–16. Development of autonomic nervous system: pre- and postganglionic neurons

Autonomic Nervous System

Functionally the autonomic nervous system can be divided into two parts: a sympathetic portion in the thoracolumbar region, and a parasympathetic portion in the cephalic and sacral regions. Both components of the autonomic nervous system consist of two tiers of neurons: pre- and postganglionic (Figures 2–16).

Sympathetic Nervous System

Preganglionic neurons of the sympathetic nervous system arise from the intermediate horn of the gray matter in the spinal cord.[3] At levels from T1 to L2 their myelinated axons grow from the cord *through* the ventral roots, paralleling the motor axons that supply the skeletal musculature. Shortly after the dorsal and ventral roots of the spinal nerve join, the preganglionic sympathetic axons, derived from the neuroepithelium of the neural tube, leave the spinal nerve via a **white communicating ramus.** They soon enter one of a series of sympathetic ganglia to synapse with neural crest-derived postganglionic neurons. The sympathetic ganglia, the bulk of which are organized as two chains running ventrolateral to the vertebral bodies, are laid down by neural crest cells that migrate from the closing neural tube along a special pathway. Once the migrating sympathetic neuroblasts have reached the site at which the sympathetic chain ganglia form, they spread both cranially and caudally until the extent of the chains approximates that seen in the adult. Some of the sympathetic neuroblasts migrate farther ventrally than the level of the chain ganglion to form a variety of other collateral ganglia. The adrenal medulla can be broadly viewed as a highly modified sympathetic ganglion. The outgrowing preganglionic sympathetic neurons either terminate within the chain ganglia or pass through on their way to more distant sympathetic ganglia to form synapses with the cell bodies of the second-order, or postganglionic, sympathetic neuroblasts. Axons of some postganglionic neuroblasts, which are unmyelinated, leave the chain ganglion as a parallel group and reenter the nearest spinal nerve through the **gray communicating ramus.** Once in the spinal nerve, these axons continue to grow until they reach their peripheral targets.

During the fifth week of development cells originating in the neural crest of the thoracic region migrate on each side of the spinal cord toward the region immediately behind the dorsal aorta.[1] Here they form a bilateral chain of segmentally arranged sympathetic ganglia interconnected by longitudinal nerve fibers. Together they form the sympathetic chains on each side of the vertebral column. From their position in the thorax neuroblasts migrate toward the cervical and lumbosacral regions, extending the sympathetic chains to their full length. Some sympathetic neuroblasts migrate in front of the aorta to form preaortic ganglia such as the celiac and mesenteric ganglia. Other sympathetic cells migrate to the heart, lungs, and gastrointestinal tract, where they give rise to sympathetic organ plexuses. Once the sympathetic chains have been established, nerve fibers originating in the intermediate horn of the thoracolumbar segments of the spinal cord penetrate the ganglia of the chain. They are known as preganglionic fibers, have a myelin sheath, and stimulate sympathetic ganglion cells. Passing from spinal nerves to the sympathetic ganglia, they form the **white communicating rami.** Axons of the sympathetic ganglion cells, the postganglionic fibers, have no myelin sheath. They either pass to other levels of the sympathetic chain or extend to the heart, lungs, and intestinal tract. Other fibers, the gray communicating rami, which are found at all levels of the spinal cord, pass from the sympathetic chain to spinal nerves and from there to peripheral blood vessels, hair, and sweat glands.

Parasympathetic Nervous System

Neurons in the brainstem and the sacral region of the spinal cord give rise to preganglionic parasympathetic fibers.[1]

Although also organized on a preganglionic and postganglionic basis, the parasympathetic nervous system has a distribution quite different from that of the sympathetic system. Like those of the sympathetic nervous system preganglionic parasympathetic neurons originate in the intermediate column of the CNS. However, the levels of origin of these neuroblasts are the mid- and hindbrain and in the second to fourth sacral segments of the developing spinal cord. Axons from these preganglionic neuroblasts grow long distances before they meet the neural crest-derived postganglionic neurons. These are typically embedded in small, scattered ganglia or plexuses in the walls of the organs they innervate.

CLINICAL RELEVANCE

Functional Analysis of the Brachial Plexus

The separation of the trunks of the brachial plexus into anterior and posterior divisions places the nerves into relation with muscles formed from primitive anterior and posterior mesoderm masses during the development of the limbs. Once these relationships are established they are never reversed, and the same fundamental correlation exists in the adult.[5,6] The anterior divisions of the trunks unite to form the lateral and medial chords of the brachial plexus and the posterior divisions joined to form the single posterior cord. Thus, all branches of the lateral and medial chords carry nerve bundles derived from the anterior divisions of the trunks, and the branches of the posterior cord conduct exclusively fibers from the posterior divisions. The discrete compartments of the upper extremity contain muscle groups of similar and related functions as well as the blood vessels and nerves that supply them. This concept is emphasized in the word *preaxial* to designate the component and structures anterior to the bone and fascial plane or axis of the limb and the word *postaxial* to designate structures behind the bony and facial axis. With the limb in the anatomical position, those parts anterior to the bony axis are all in a continuous plane down the front of the limb, with the ventral axial line extending along the anterior surface of the arm and forearm. The postaxial parts are positioned continuously down the back of the limb.

The branches of the lateral and medial chords are all preaxial and innervate the preaxial muscles of the limb, whereas the posterior cord branches are postaxial and innervate the postaxial musculature. The radial nerve, being the only postaxial nerve below the shoulder, supplies all the postaxial muscles in the remainder of the limb. The median, musculocutaneous, and ulnar nerves share preaxial innervation.

The musculocutaneous nerve is muscular in the arm and cutaneous in the forearm, and it is the sole preaxial muscular nerve in the arm. The preaxial median and ulnar nerves are nerves of passage in the arm, but in the forearm and hand each contributes to innervation, the median nerve more heavily in the forearm, the ulnar nerve more heavily in the hand.

In the shoulder region, many of the supra- and infraclavicular branches of the brachial plexus arise from recognizable pre- and postaxial cords or divisions. Their origins have the same significance as the major anterior and posterior divisions of the trunks. An example of this is the clavicle and the scapula. The clavicle is an anterior and the scapula a posterior bone. An exception to this designation involves the scapula because its coracoid process has a phylogenetic history as a separate bone and fuses with the scapula. Therefore, all muscles arising from the scapula, exclusive of the coracoid process (pectoralis minor, coracobrachialis, and short head of biceps), belong to a postaxial group at the shoulder, and those from the clavicle and coracoid belong to a preaxial group. The nerve–muscle correlation is maintained in that all muscles of scapular origin are supplied by postaxial branches of the brachial plexus, and all muscles derived from the clavicle and coracoid are supplied by preaxial branches.

Functional Analysis of the Lumbosacral Plexus

The innervation of the lower extremity follows the same pattern of pre- and postaxial orientation as described for the upper extremity. The primordial dermatomal pattern has disappeared, but an orderly sequence of dermatomes can still be recognized. Most of the original ventral surface of the lower limb lies on the back of the adult limb. The ventral axial line extends along the medial side of the thigh and knee to the posteromedial aspect of the leg to the heel.

As previously described this results from the medial rotation of the lower limb at the end of the embryonic period. The lumbar plexuses are formed by the ventral rami of the first three lumbar nerves and part of the fourth lumbar nerve. The primary preaxial components are the genitofemoral nerve, which derives from L1 and L2, and obturator and accessory obturator nerves, which are derived from L2 and L3, respectively. The primary postaxial components are the lateral femoral cutaneous nerve, derived from L2 and L3, and the femoral nerve, derived from L2 through L4. The sacral plexus combines the ventral rami of part of L4 and L5 and S1 through S3, as well as part of S4. All these nerves, except S4, divide into anterior and posterior branches. Like the brachial plexus the anterior branches form preaxial nerves related to preaxial muscle masses in skin areas, and the posterior branches form similarly related postaxial nerves. The principal nerve of the sacral plexus is the sciatic, which is composed of a preaxial nerve (the tibial nerve) and a postaxial nerve (the common peroneal), which is enclosed within a single sheath.

SUMMARY

In summary, regional anesthesia may be considered as a practice of applied anatomy. Successful neuraxial and peripheral nerve blockade alike require a logical approach to the anatomic principles. A knowledge of the embryologic development of tissues and neural structures can significantly add to the understanding of functional anatomy as it relates to regional anesthesia.

References

1. Sadler TW: *Langman's Medical Embryology,* 9th ed. Lippincott Williams & Wilkins, 2003.
2. Sweeney LJ: *Basic Concepts in Embryology: A Student's Survival Guide.* McGraw-Hill, 1998.
3. Carlson B: *Human Embryology and Developmental Biology,* 3rd ed. Mosby, 2004.
4. Moore KL: *The Developing Human: Clinically Oriented Embryology,* 7th ed. W. B. Saunders, 2003.
5. Woodburne RT: *Essentials of Human Anatomy,* 6th ed. Oxford University Press, 1978.
6. Larsen WJ: *Human Embryology,* 2nd ed. Churchill Livingstone, 1997.

3

Functional Regional Anesthesia Anatomy

Faruk Dilberovic, MD • Eldan Kapur, MD • Chi Wong, MS • Admir Hadzic, MD

INTRODUCTION

It is often said that the practice of regional anesthesia is the practice of applied anatomy. Indeed, the practice of regional anesthesia is inconceivable without a sound knowledge of the basic anatomic facts that pertain to the individual anesthesia techniques. However, just as surgeons rely on surgical anatomy or pathologists rely on pathologic anatomy, the anatomic information necessary for the practice of regional anesthesia must be specific to this application. In the past, many new nerve block techniques and "me-too" approaches were devised by academicians merely relying on idealized anatomic diagrams and schematics, rather then on functional anatomy. Ultimately, many of these techniques have only introduced unnecessary confusion in the field and been of negligible relevance to clinical practice. Indeed, once the anatomic layers and tissues sheets are dissected, the fully exposed nerve structures are almost irrelevant to the practice of regional anesthesia. This is because accurate placement of the needle and the spread of the local anesthetic after an injection depends on the interplay between neurologic structures and the neighboring tissues where local anesthetic pools and accumulates, rather than on the mere anatomic organization of the nerves and plexuses. However, much research by regional

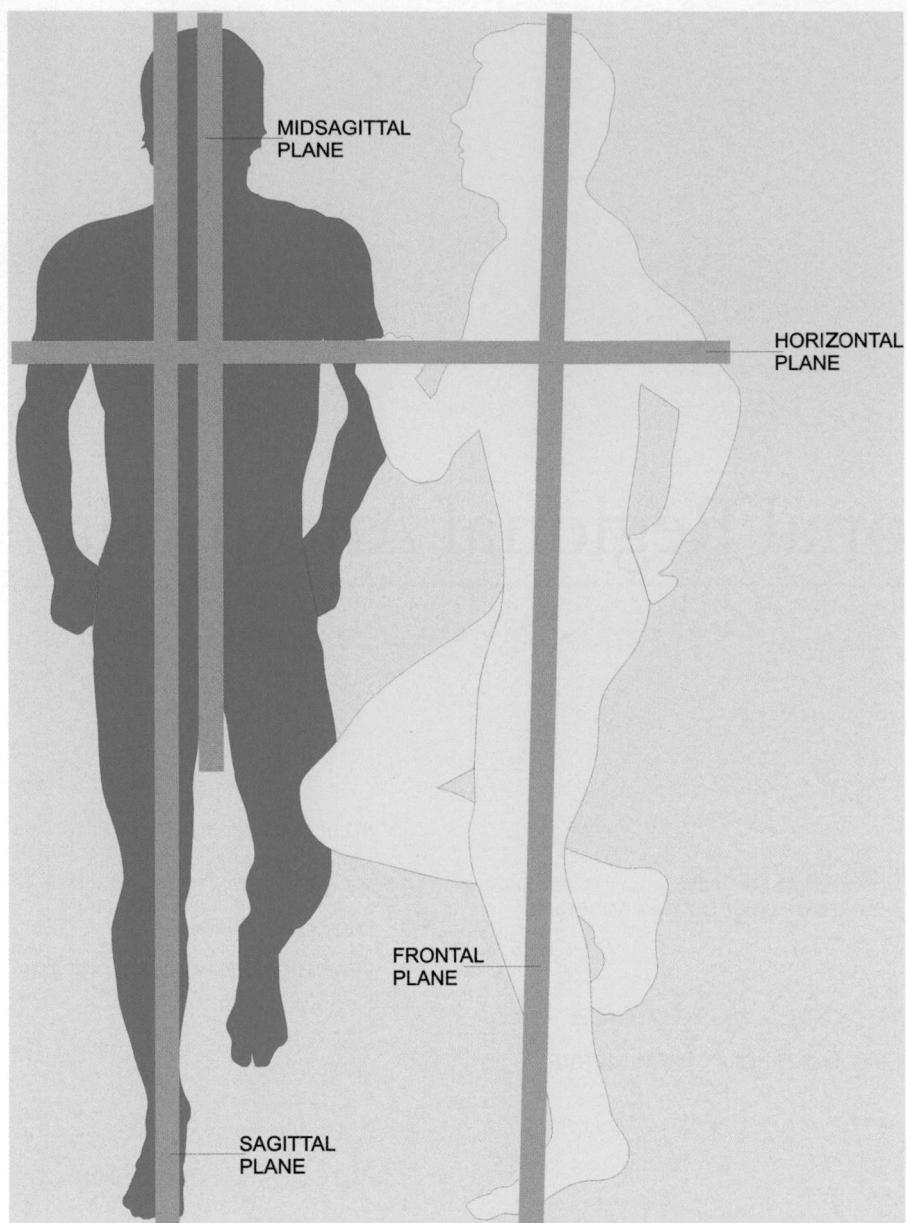

Figure 3–1. Conventional body planes.

anesthesiologists has been done in the past 10–15 years on this subject, and many myths of the past have been dispelled. The reader should note that specific anatomic discussions pertaining to individual regional anesthesia techniques are detailed in their respective chapters. The purpose of this chapter is to provide a generalized and rather concise overview of anatomy relevant to the practice of regional anesthesia. The reader is referred to Figure 3–1 for an easier orientation of the body planes discussed throughout the book.

ANATOMY OF PERIPHERAL NERVES

All peripheral nerves are similar in structure. The **neuron** is the basic functional neuronal unit responsible for the

conduction of nerve impulses. Neurons are the longest cells in the body, many reaching a meter in length. Most neurons are incapable of dividing under normal circumstances and have a very limited ability to repair themselves after injury. A typical neuron consists of a cell body (soma) that contains a large nucleus. The cell body is attached to several branching processes, called dendrites, and a single axon. Dendrites receive incoming messages; axons conduct outgoing messages. Axons vary in length, and there is one only per neuron. In peripheral nerves, axons are very long and slender. They are also called nerve fibers. The peripheral nerve (PN) is composed of three parts: (1) somatosensory or afferent neurons, (2) motor or efferent neurons, and (3) autonomic neurons.

Individual nerve fibers bind together, somewhat like individual wires in an electric cable (Figure 3–2). In a peripheral

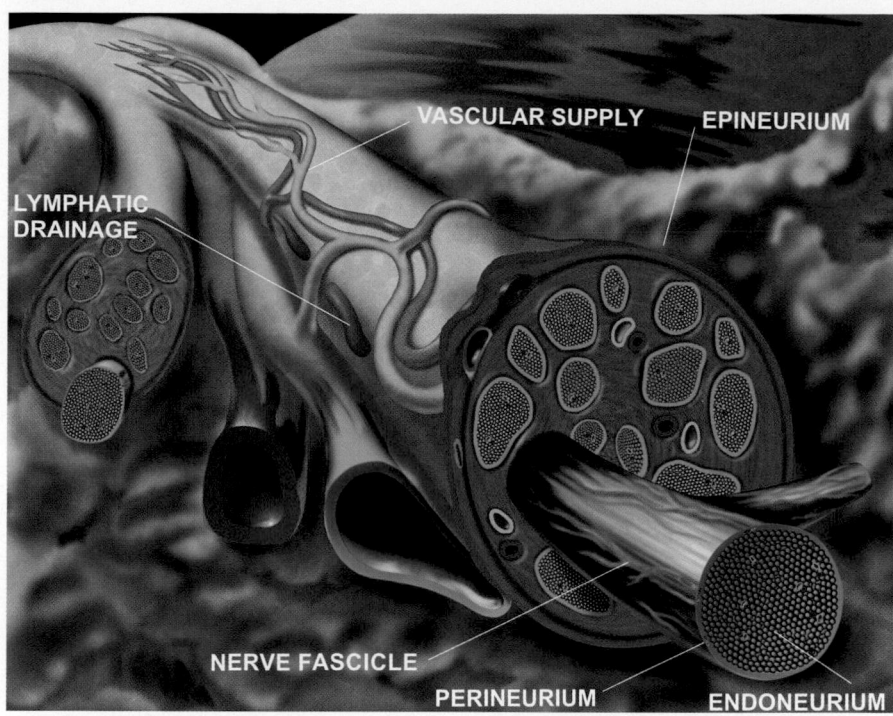

Figure 3–2. Organization of the peripheral nerve.

nerve, individual axons are enveloped in a loose connective tissue, the endoneurium. The **endoneurium** is a delicate layer of connective tissue around each nerve that is embedded within the **perineurium.** Small groups of axons are closely associated within a bundle called a nerve fascicle, which imparts mechanical strength to the peripheral nerve. In surgical procedures, the perineurium holds sutures without tearing. In addition to its mechanical strength, the perineurium functions as a diffusion barrier to the fascicle, isolating the endoneural space around the axon from the surrounding tissue.[1] This barrier helps to preserve the ionic milieu of the axon and functions as a blood–nerve barrier. Several fascicles together form fascicular bundles within an extensive multilaminated perineurium. The **perineurium** surrounds each fasciculus and splits with it at each branching point. The fascicular bundles in turn, collectively form the peripheral nerve that is embedded in loose connective tissue called the epineurium. The **epineurium** surrounds the entire nerve and holds it loosely to the connective tissue through which it runs. This layer also sends septa into the nerve that divide the nerve fibers into bundles (fasciculi or funiculi) of varying sizes.

Of note, the fascicular bundles are not continuous throughout the peripheral nerve. They divide and anastomose with one another as frequently as every few millimeters.[1] However, the axons within a small set of adjacent bundles redistribute themselves so that the axons remain in approximately the same quadrant of the nerve for several centimeters. This arrangement is a practical concern to the surgeons trying to repair a severed nerve. If the cut is clean, it may be possible to suture individual fascicular bundles together. In such a scenario, the probability is good that the distal segment

of nerves synapsing with the muscles will be sutured to the central stump of motor axons; the same is true for sensory axons. In such cases, good functional recovery is possible. If a short segment of the nerve is missing, however, the fascicles in the various quadrants of the stump may no longer correspond with one another, good axial alignment may not be possible, and functional recovery is greatly compromised or improbable.[1] This arrangement of the peripheral nerve helps explain why intraneural injections result in disastrous consequences as opposed to clean needle nerve cuts which tend to heal much more readily and regularly.

The connective tissue of a nerve is tough, compared with the nerve fibers themselves. The connective tissue of a nerve permits a certain amount of stretch without damage to the nerve fibers. The nerve fibers are somewhat "wavy," and when they are stretched, the connective tissue around them is also stretched—giving it some protection. This feature, perhaps, plays a "safety" role in nerve blockade by allowing the nerves to be "pushed" rather than pierced by the advancing needle during nerve localization. For this reason, it is prudent to avoid stretching the nerves and nerve plexuses during nerve blockade (eg, in axillary brachial plexus blocks and some approaches to the sciatic block).

Nerves receive blood from the adjacent blood vessels running along their course. These feeding branches to larger nerves are macroscopic in size and irregularly arranged, forming anastomoses to become longitudinally running vessel(s) that supply the nerve and give off subsidiary branches. Although the connective tissue sheath enveloping nerves serves to protect the nerves from stretching, it is also believed that neuronal injury after nerve blockade may be due, at least

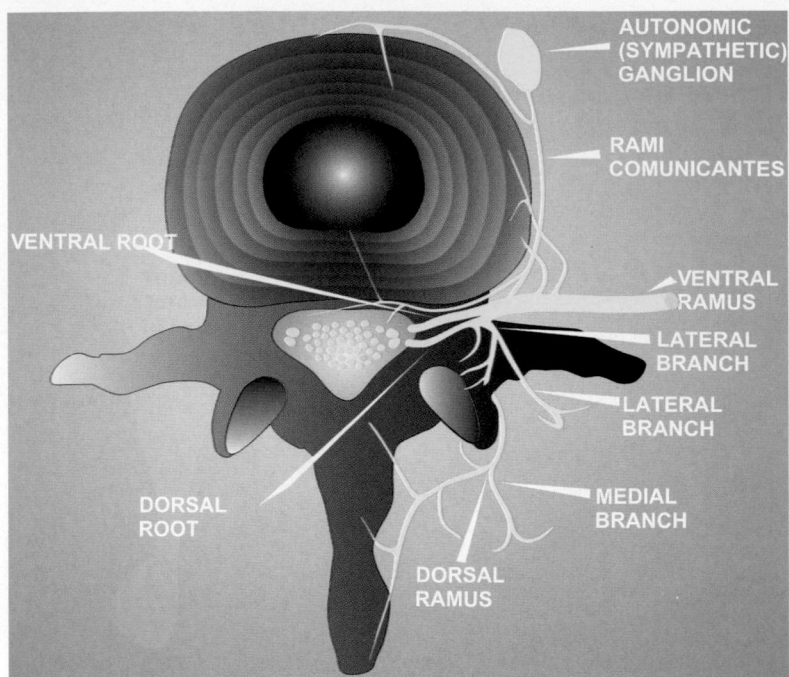

Figure 3–3. Anatomy of the spinal nerve.

partly, to the pressure or stretch within connective sheaths that do not stretch well and the consequent interference with the vascular supply to the nerve.

Communication Between the Central & Peripheral Nervous Systems

The functional boundary between the central (CNS) and the peripheral nervous system (PNS) lies at the junction where oligodenodrocytes meet Schwann cells along the axons that form the cranial and spinal nerve. The PNS, as opposed to the CNS, is not surrounded by bone and is therefore accessible for neural blockade, but it is also quite susceptible to physical injury. The CNS communicates with the body through spinal nerves. Spinal nerves have both sensory and motor components (Figure 3–3). The **sensory fibers** arise from neurons in the dorsal root ganglia. Fibers enter the dorsolateral aspect of the spinal cord to form the dorsal root. The **motor fibers** arise from neurons in the ventral horn of the spinal cord. The fibers pass through the ventrolateral aspect of the spinal cord and form the ventral root. The dorsal and ventral roots converge in the intervertebral foramen to form a spinal nerve. After passing through the intervertebral foramen, the spinal nerve divides into dorsal and ventral rami. The dorsal ramus innervates muscle, bones, joints, and the skin of the back. The ventral ramus innervates muscle, bones, joints, and the skin of the anterior neck, thorax, abdomen, pelvis, and the extremities.

Spinal Nerves

There are 31 pairs of spinal nerves. The spinal nerves are enumerated by region: 8 cervical, 12 thoracic, 5 lumbar, 5 sacral, and 1 coccygeal. Spinal nerves pass through the vertebral column at the intervertebral foramina. The first cervical nerve (C1) passes superior to the C1 vertebra (atlas). The second cervical nerve (C2) passes between the C1 (atlas) and C2 (axis) vertebrae. This pattern continues down the cervical spine. A shift in pattern occurs at the C8 nerve because there is no C8 vertebra. The C8 nerve passes between the C7 and T1 vertebrae. The T1 nerve passes between the T1 and T2 vertebrae. This pattern continues down the through the remainder of the spine. The vertebral arch of the fifth sacral and first coccygeal vertebrae is rudimentary. Because of this, the vertebral canal opens inferiorly at the sacral hiatus. The fifth sacral and first coccygeal nerves pass through the sacral hiatus. Because the inferior end of the spinal cord (conus medullaris) in adults is located at the L1 to L2 vertebral level, roots of spinal nerves must descend through the vertebral canal before exiting the vertebral column through the appropriate intervertebral foramen. Collectively, these roots are called the cauda equina (Figure 3–4).

Outside the vertebral column, ventral rami from different spinal levels coalesce to form intricate networks called plexuses. From the plexuses, nerves extend into the neck, the arms, and the legs.[1,2]

DERMATOMES, MYOTOMES, & OSTEOTOMES

Dermatomal, myotomal, and osteotomal innervation are often emphasized in regional anesthesiology texts as important for the application of nerve blocks. However, it is more practical to think in terms of which block techniques provide adequate analgesia and anesthesia for specific surgical procedures, rather than trying to match nerves and spinal segments to the dermatomal, myotomal, and osteotomal territory.

vertebrae extend as a series of bands from the midline of the trunk posteriorly into the limbs. It should be noted that considerable overlapping occurs between adjacent dermatomes, that is, each segmental nerve overlaps the territories of its neighbors.[3]

A **myotome** is the segmental innervation of skeletal muscle by the ventral (motor) root(s) of the spinal nerve(s). Major myotomes, their function, and corresponding spinal levels are represented in Figure 3–7. The innervation of the bones (**osteotome**) often does not follow the same segmental pattern as the innervation of the muscles and other soft tissues (Figure 3–8).

ANATOMY OF PLEXUSES & PERIPHERAL NERVES

Cervical Plexus

The cervical plexus innervates muscles, joints, and skin in the anterior neck (Table 3–1). It is formed by the ventral rami of C1 through C4 (Figures 3–9 and 3–10). The rami form a loop called the ansa cervicalis that sends branches to the infrahyoid muscles. In addition, the rami form nerves that pass directly to several structures in the neck and thorax, including the scalene muscles, diaphragm, clavicular joints, and skin covering the anterior neck.

Ansa Cervicalis

The ventral ramus of C1 attaches to the ventral rami of C2 to C3. The attachment forms a loop called the ansa cervicalis, which sends branches to the infrahyoid muscles. The infrahyoid muscles consist of the omohyoid, sternohyoid, and sternothyroid muscles. They attach to the anterior surface of the hyoid bone or to the thyroid cartilage. Contraction of these muscles moves the hyoid bone or thyroid cartilage downward, effectively opening the laryngeal aditus. This promotes inspiration. The C1 component also sends fibers to the thyrohyoid and geniohyoid muscles. Contraction of these muscles moves the anterior hyoid bone superiorly, closing the laryngeal aditus. Closure of the laryngeal aditus is necessary for swallowing to occur safely. This is one of the reasons why high levels of spinal anesthesia result in airway compromise and the risk of aspiration.

Nerves to Scalene Muscles

The ventral rami of C2 to C4 send branches directly to the scalene muscles, which attach between the cervical spine and ribs. When the cervical spine is stabilized, contraction elevates the ribs. This promotes inspiration. Interscalene block may result in block of the scalene muscles in addition to the phrenic block. This is typically asymptomatic in healthy patients but may result in acute respiratory insufficiency in patients with borderline pulmonary function or in those with an exacerbation of asthma or chronic obstructive bronchitis. It is recommended that more distal approaches to a brachial

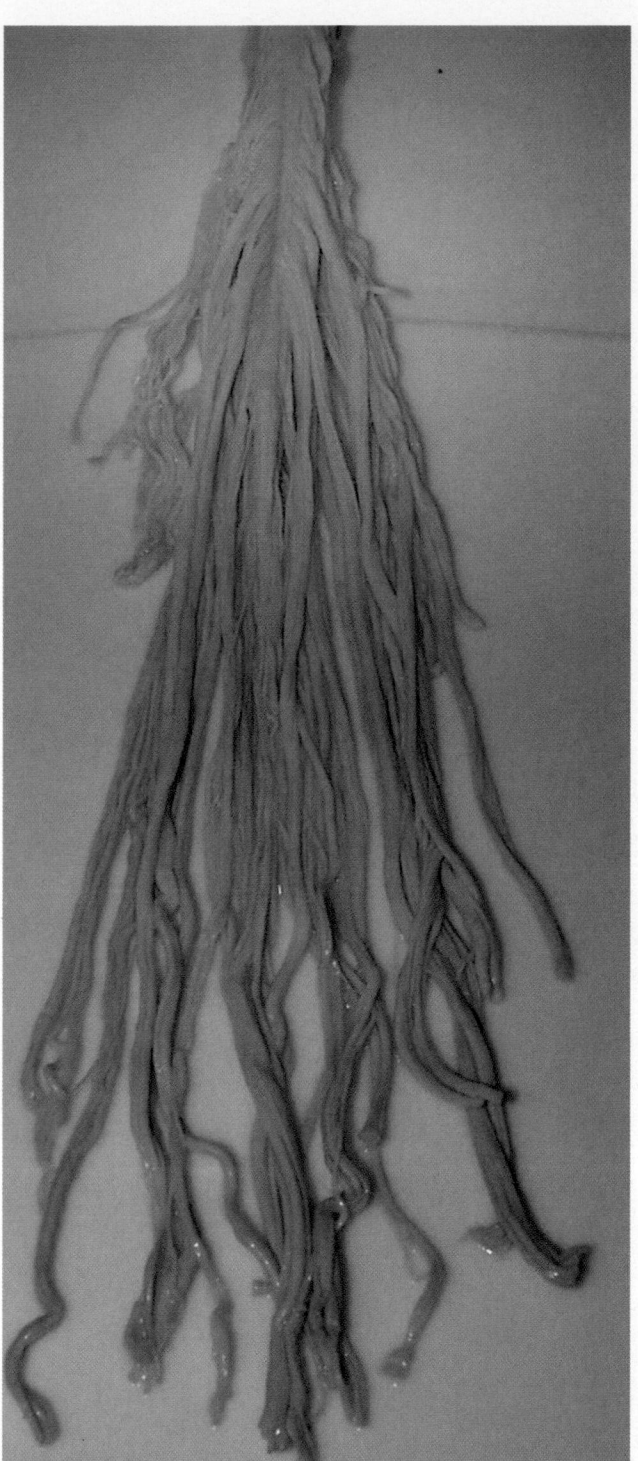

Figure 3–4. Cauda equina.

Nevertheless, their description is of didactic importance in regional anesthesia and is briefly presented here.

A **dermatome** is an area of the skin supplied by the dorsal (sensory) root of the spinal nerve (Figures 3–5 and 3–6). In the head and trunk, each segment is horizontally disposed, except C1, which does not have a sensory component. The dermatomes of the limbs from the fifth cervical to the first thoracic nerve and from the third lumbar to the second sacral

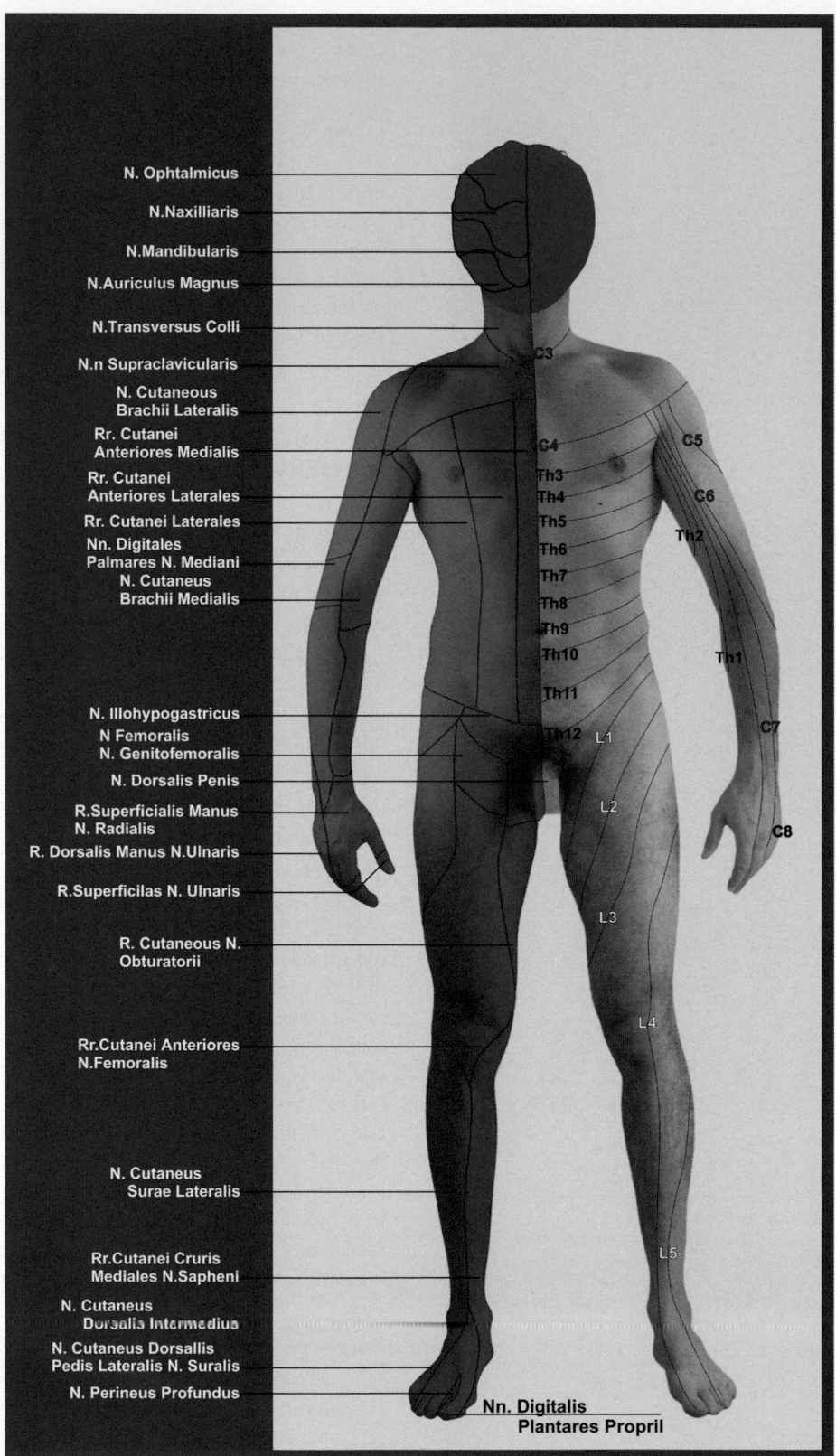

N. Ophtalmicus

N.Naxilliaris

N.Mandibularis

N.Auriculus Magnus

N.Transversus Colli

N.n Supraclavicularis

N. Cutaneous
Brachii Lateralis

Rr. Cutanei
Anteriores Medialis

Rr. Cutanei
Anteriores Laterales

Rr. Cutanei Laterales

Nn. Digitales
Palmares N. Mediani

N. Cutaneus
Brachii Medialis

N. Illohypogastricus

N Femoralis
N. Genitofemoralis

N. Dorsalis Penis

R.Superficialis Manus
N. Radialis

R. Dorsalis Manus N.Ulnaris

R.Superficilas N. Ulnaris

R. Cutaneous N.
Obturatorii

Rr.Cutanei Anteriores
N.Femoralis

N. Cutaneus
Surae Lateralis

Rr.Cutanei Cruris
Mediales N.Sapheni

N. Cutaneus
Dorsalis Intermedius

N. Cutaneus Dorsallis
Pedis Lateralis N. Suralis

N. Perineus Profundus

C3

C4

Th3

Th4

Th5

Th6

Th7

Th8

Th9

Th10

Th11

Th12 L1

C5

C6

Th2

Th1

C7

C8

L2

L3

L4

L5

**Nn. Digitalis
Plantares Propril**

Figure 3–5. Dermatomes, anterior.

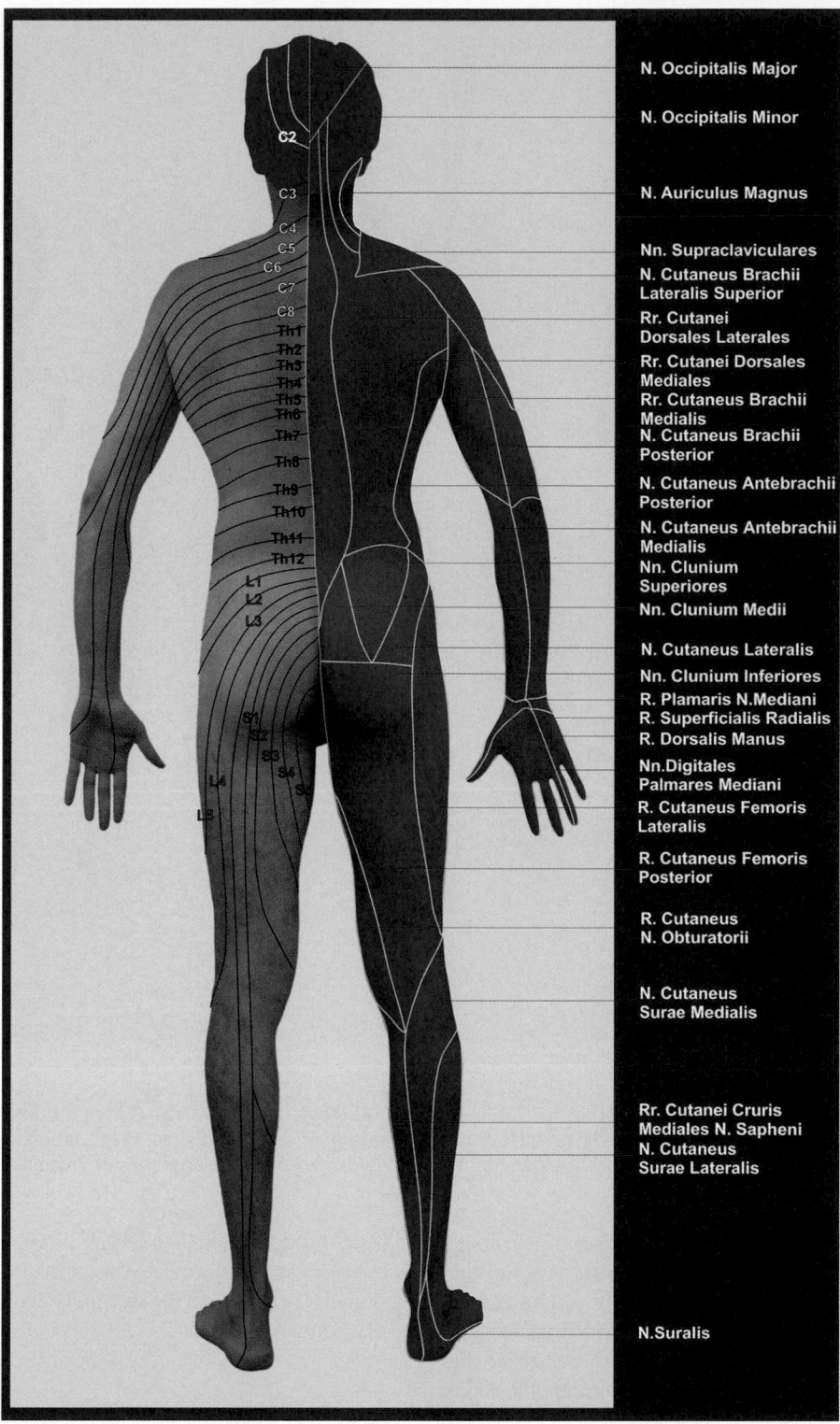

Figure 3–6. Dermatomes, posterior.

plexus block and smaller injection volumes be used to limit the cephalad extension of the block, as well as shorter acting local anesthetics to avoid prolonged blockade in case of respiratory insufficiency.

Phrenic Nerve

The phrenic nerve is formed by junction of fibers from C3 to C5, and it innervates the diaphragm. The phrenic nerve descends through the neck on the anterior surface of the anterior

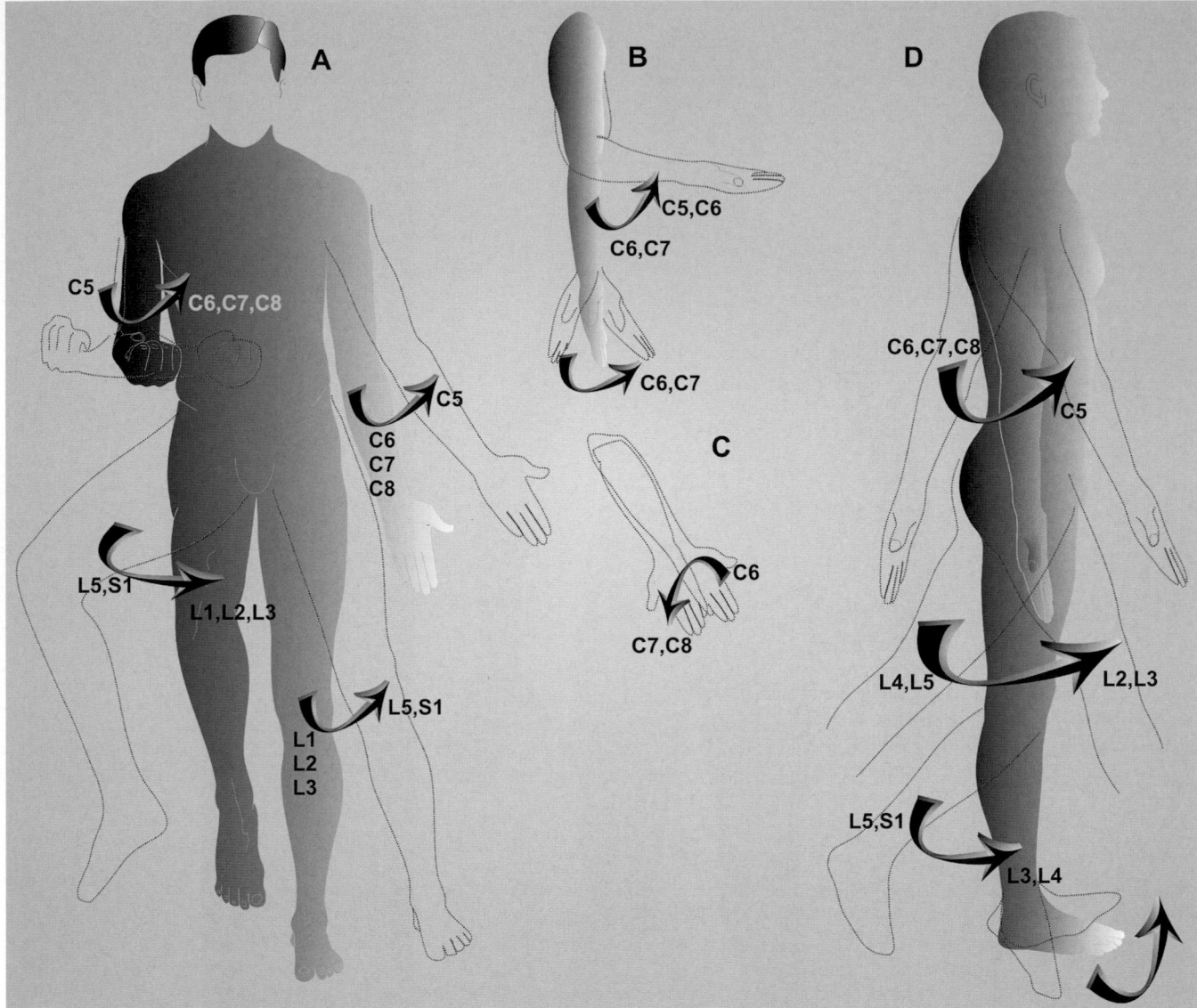

Figure 3–7. Functional innervation of the muscles (myotomes): **A:** Medial and lateral rotation of shoulder and hip. Abduction and adduction of shoulder and hip. **B:** Flexion and extension of elbow and wrist. **C:** Pronation and supination of forearm. **D:** Flexion and extension of shoulder, hip, and knee. Dorsiflexion and plantar flexion of ankle, lateral views.

scalene muscle, passing through the superior thoracic aperture and descending on the walls of the mediastinum to the diaphragm. In addition to muscular fibers, the phrenic nerve transmits sensory fibers to the superior and inferior surfaces of the diaphragm. All approaches to the block of the brachial plexus above the clavicle result in phrenic blockade (Figure 3–11).

Cutaneous Nerves of the Anterior Neck

Cutaneous sensory nerves arise from the cervical plexus, pass around the posterior margin of sternocleidomastoid, and terminate in the scalp and anterior neck. The minor occipital nerve passes to the posterior auricular region of the scalp (Figure 3–12). The major auricular nerve passes to the auricle of the ear and to the region of the face anterior to the tragus. The transverse cervical nerve supplies the anterior neck. A

series of supraclavicular nerves innervate the region covering the clavicle. Furthermore, the supraclavicular nerves provide articular branches to the sternoclavicular and acromioclavicular joints.[4]

Brachial Plexus

The brachial plexus innervates muscles, joints, and the skin of the upper extremity (Table 3–2). It is formed by ventral rami of C5 to T1 (Figure 3–13). In the posterior cervical triangle between the anterior and middle scalene muscles, the ventral rami join to form trunks. C5 and C6 join to form the superior trunk. C7 forms the middle trunk. C8 and T1 join to form the inferior trunk. All trunks branch into anterior and posterior divisions. All the posterior divisions join to form the posterior cord. The anterior divisions of the superior and

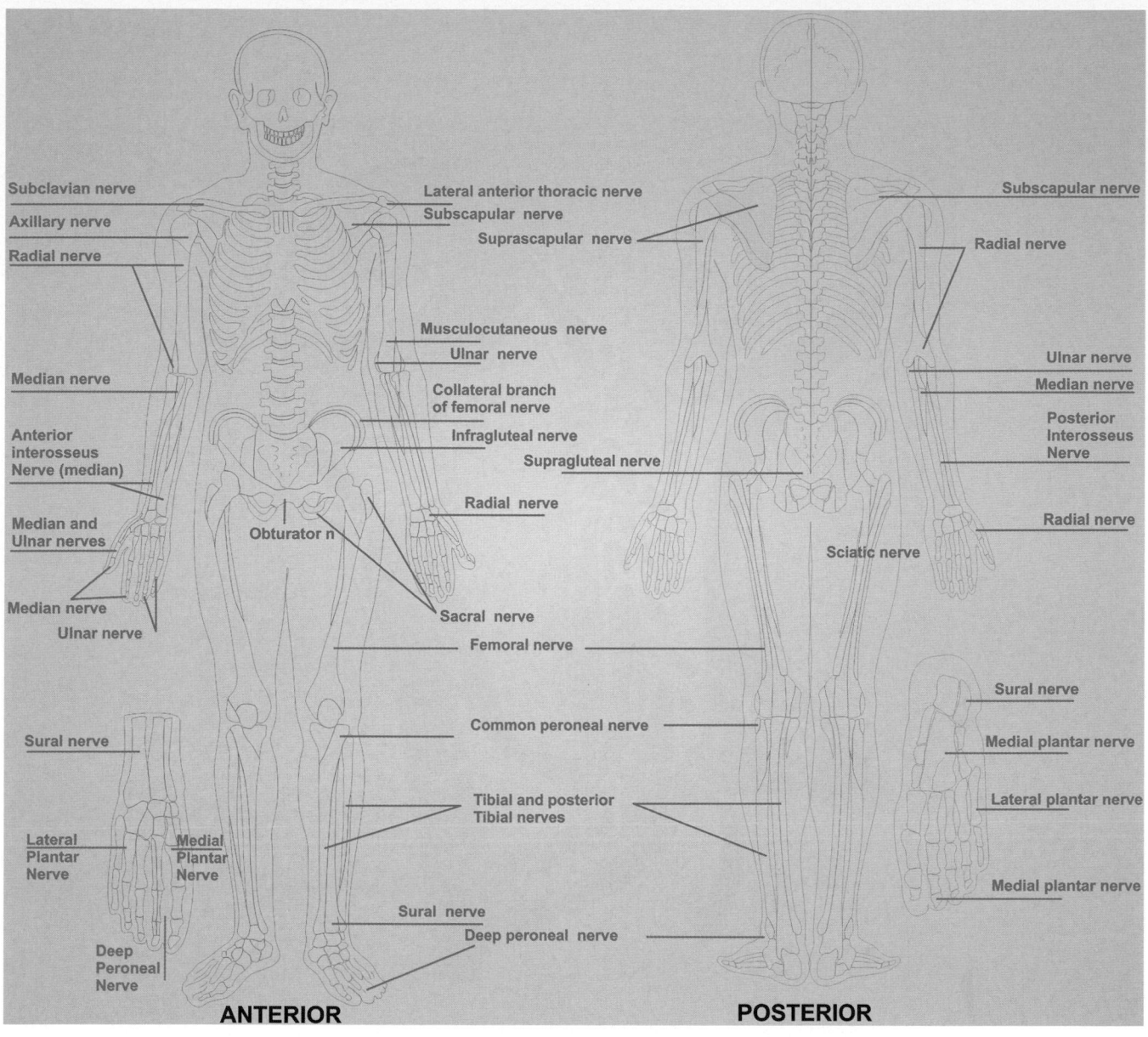

Figure 3–8. Innervation of the major bones (osteotomes).

Table 3–1.

Organization and Distribution of the Cervical Plexus

Nerves	Spinal Segments	Distribution
Ansa cervicalis (superior and inferior branches)	C1 to C4	Five of the extrinsic laryngeal muscles (sternothyroid, sternohyoid, omohyoid, geniohyoid and thyrohyoid) by way of CN XII
Lesser occipital, transverse cervical, supraclavicular, and greater auricular nerves	C2 to C3	Skin of upper chest, shoulder, neck and ear
Phrenic nerve	C3 to C5	Diaphragm
Cervical nerves	C1 to C5	Levator scapulae, scalenes, sternocleidomastoid, and trapezius muscles (with CN XI)

CN = cranial nerve.

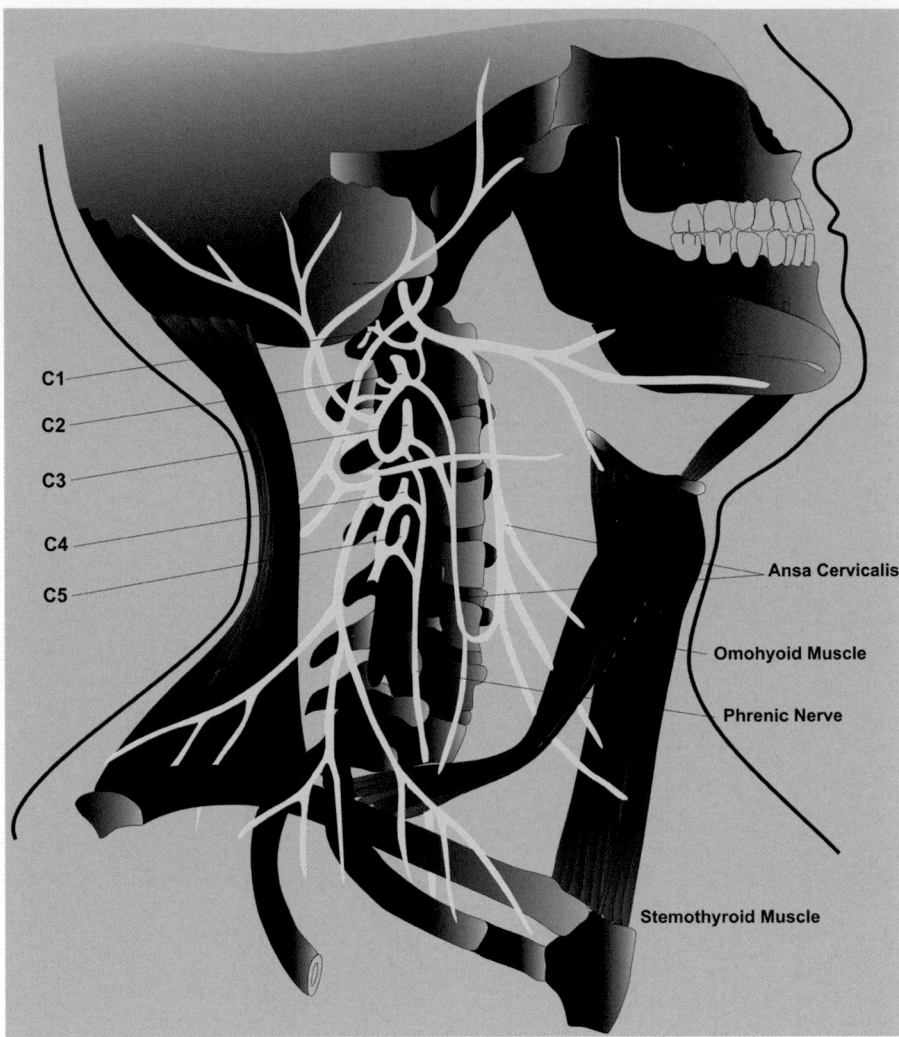

C1

C2

C3

C4

C5

Ansa Cervicalis

Omohyoid Muscle

Phrenic Nerve

Sternothyroid Muscle

Figure 3–9. Cervical plexus.

middle trunks join to form the lateral cord. The anterior division of the inferior trunk forms the medial cord. Several terminal nerves arise within the posterior cervical triangle. Because they arise superior to the clavicle, they are called supraclavicular branches. The supraclavicular branches include the dorsal scapular nerve, the long thoracic nerve, the suprascapular nerve, and the nerve to subclavius.[5–7]

Supraclavicular Branches

Dorsal Scapular Nerve

The dorsal scapular nerve arises from the ventral ramus of C5. It follows the levator scapula muscle to the scapula and descends the medial border of the scapula on the deep surface of the rhomboid muscles. In its route, the dorsal scapular nerve innervates the levator scapula and rhomboid muscles.

Long Thoracic Nerve

The long thoracic nerve arises from the ventral rami of C5 to C7. It descends along the anterior surface of the middle scalene to the first rib and then transfers onto the serratus anterior muscle, which it innervates.

Suprascapular Nerve

The suprascapular nerve arises form the superior trunk. It follows the inferior belly of the omohyoid muscle to the scapula, passes through the superior notch into the supraspinatus fossa, where it innervates the supraspinatus muscle, and continues around the scapular notch (lateral margin of the scapular spine) to the infraspinatus fossa, where it innervates the infraspinatus muscle. In addition to muscle, the suprascapular nerve innervates the glenohumeral joint.

Nerve to Subclavius

The nerve to subclavius arises from the superior trunk. It passes anteriorly a short distance to innervate the subclavius muscle and the sternoclavicular joint.

The cords of the brachial plexus leave the posterior cervical triangle and enter the axilla through the axillary inlet. The remainder of the terminal branches arise within the axilla from the cords.

Posterior Cord Branches

The posterior cord forms the upper and lower subscapular nerves, thoracodorsal nerve, axillary nerve, and radial nerve.

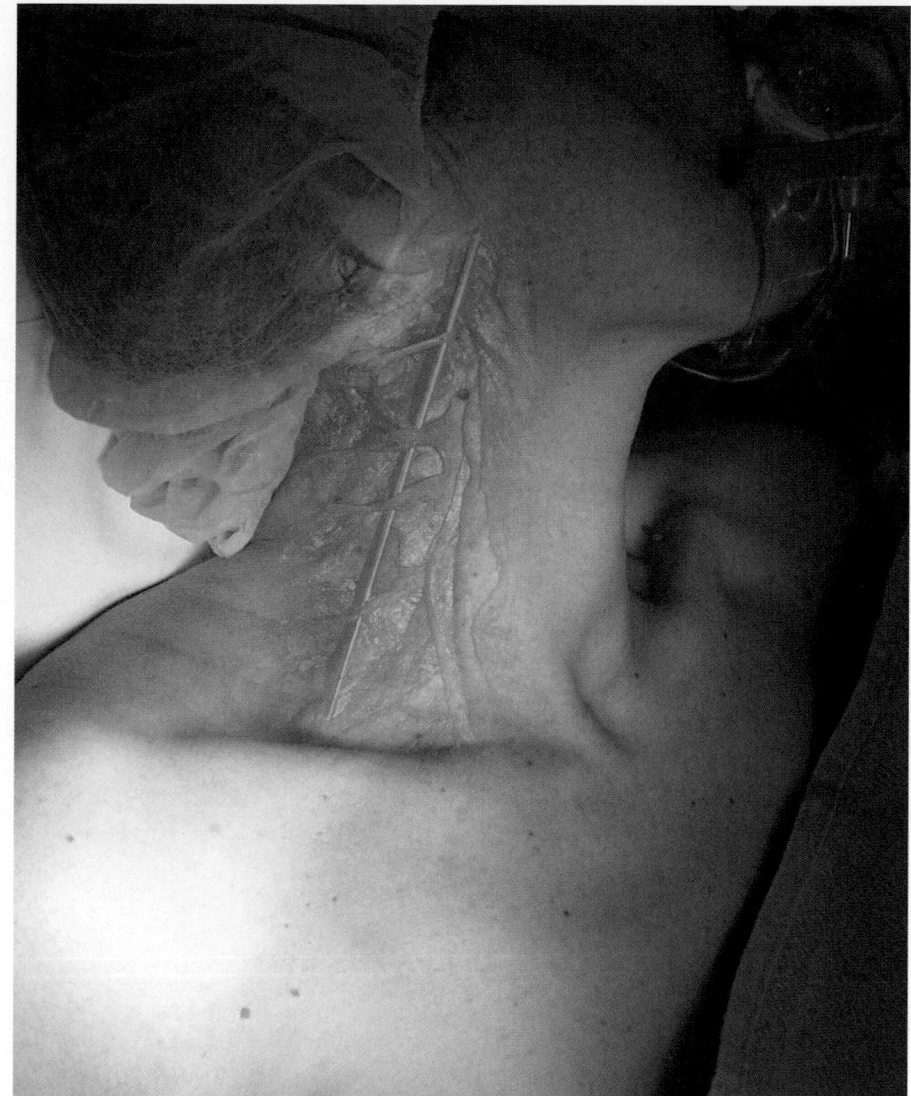

Figure 3–10. Roots of the cervical plexus.

Anterior

Cephalad

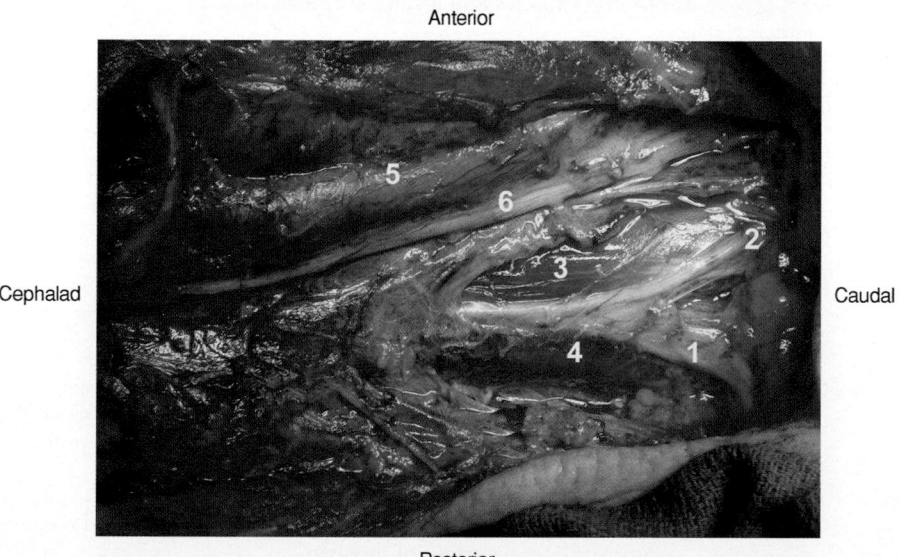

Caudal

Posterior

Figure 3–11. Anatomy of the neck after removal of the sternocleidomastoid muscle (Body is horizontal). Shown are: (1) brachial plexus between the (3) anterior and (4) middle scalene muscles, and the (2) phrenic nerve, (5) carotid artery, and (6) vagus nerve.

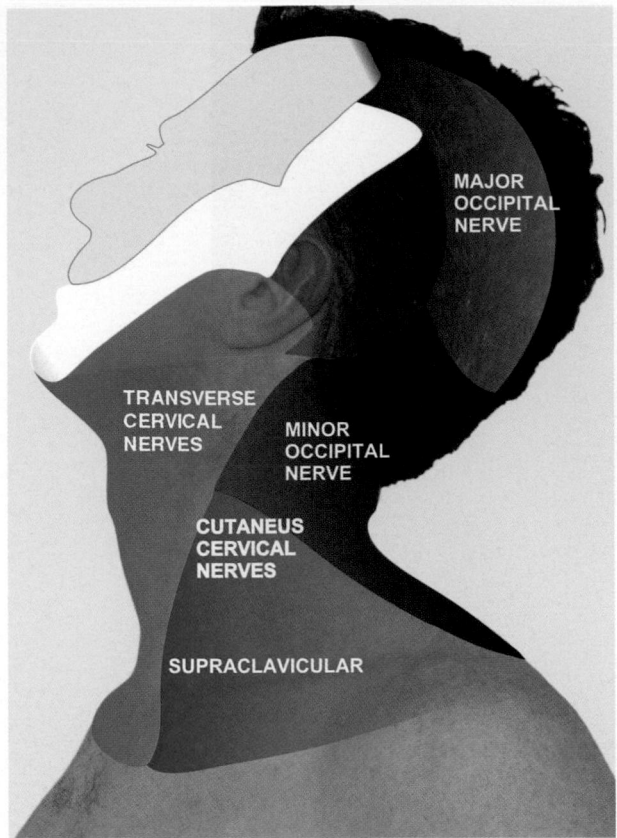

Figure 3–12. Sensory innervation of the cervical plexus.

Table 3–2.

Organization and Distribution of the Brachial Piexus

Nerves(s)	Spinal Segments	Distribution
Nerves to subclavius	C4 to C6	Subclavius muscle
Dorsal scapular nerve	C5	Rhomboid muscles and levator scapulae muscle
Long thoracic nerve	C5 to C7	Serratus anterior muscle
Suprascapular nerve	C5, C6	Supraspinatus and infraspinatus muscles
Pectoralis nerve (median and lateral)	C5 to T1	Pectoralis muscles
Subscapular nerves	C5, C6	Subscapularis and teres major muscles
Thoracodorsal nerve	C6 to C8	Latissimus dorsi muscle
Axillary nerve	C5, C6	Deltoid and teres minor muscles; skin of shoulder
Radial nerve	C5 to T1	Extensor muscle of the arm and forearm (triceps brachii, extensor carpi radialis, supinator and aneoneus muscles, and extensor carpi ulnaris muscles) and brachioradialis muscle; digital extensors, and abductor pollicis muscle; skin over the posterolateral surface of the arm
Musculocutaneous nerve	C5 to C7	Flexor muscles on the arm (biceps brachii, brachiallis, and coracobrachialis muscles); skin over lateral surface of forearm
Median nerve	C6 to T1	Flexor muscles on the forearm (flexor carpi radialis and palmaris longus muscles); pronator quadratus and pronator teres muscles; digital flexors (through the palmar interosseous nerve); skin over anterolateral surface of hand
Ulnar nerve	C8, T1	Flexor carpi ulnaris muscle, adductor pollicis muscle and small digital muscles; medial part of flexor digitorum profundus muscle; skin over medial surface of the hand

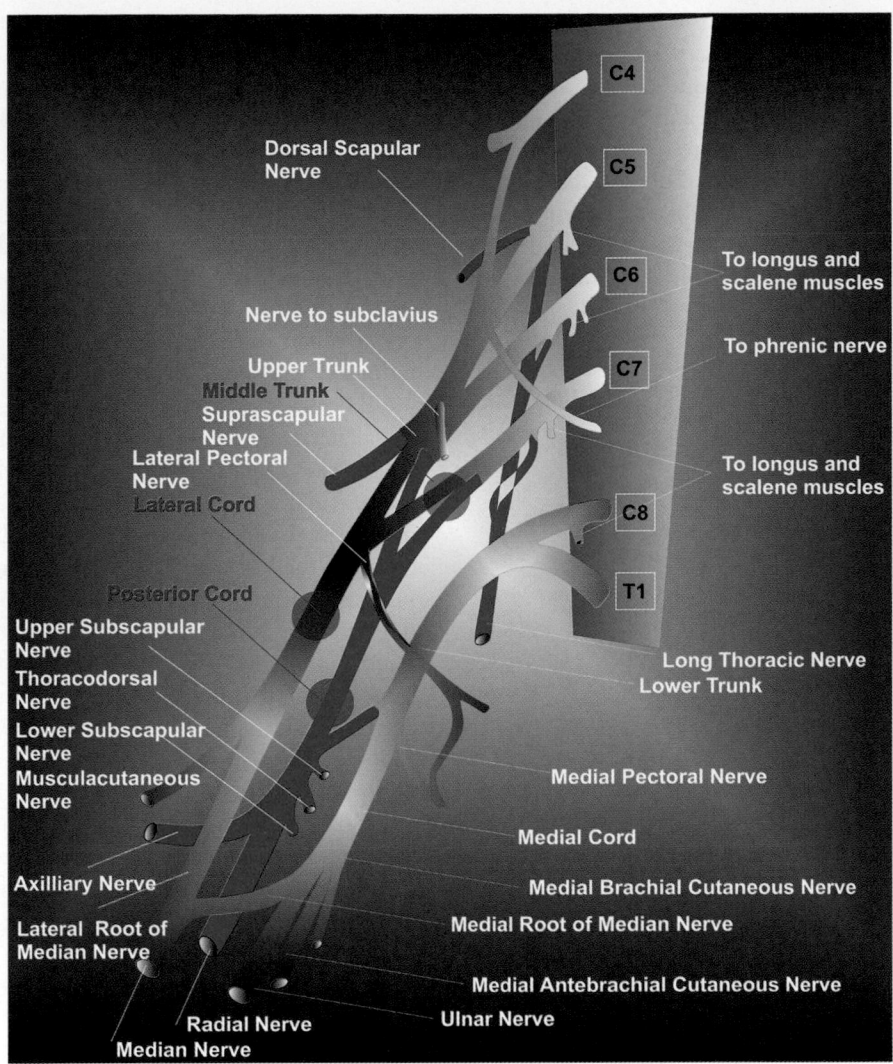

Figure 3–13. Organization of the brachial plexus.

Subscapular Nerves

The subscapular nerves are formed by fibers from C5 to C6. The upper subscapular nerve is the first nerve to arise from the posterior cord. It passes onto the anterior surface of the sub- scapularis muscle, which it innervates. The lower subscapular nerve arises more distally. It descends across the anterior sur- face of the subscapularis muscle to the teres major muscle and innervates both the subscapularis and teres major muscles.

Thoracodorsal Nerve

The thoracodorsal nerve is formed by fibers from C5 to C7. It arises from the posterior cord, usually between the subscapu- lar nerves, and descends across the subscapularis and teres major muscle to the latissimus dorsi muscle. It innervates latissimus dorsi.

Axillary Nerve

The axillary nerve is formed by fibers from C5 to C6 (Box 3–1). It passes from the axilla into the shoulder between

Box 3–1.

Axillary Nerve (C5 to C6)

Muscular branches

- Adduction, flexion, or extension of shoulder
- Deltoid
- Lateral rotation the shoulder. Stabilization of gleno- humeral joint.
- Teres minor

Articular branches

- Acromioclavicular joint
- Glenohumeral joint

Cutaneous branch

- Superior lateral brachial cutaneous nerve

the teres major and minor muscles. It innervates the teres minor. The nerve continues posterior to the surgical neck of the humerus to innervate the deltoid muscle. The superior lateral brachial cutaneous branch of the axillary nerve passes around the posterior margin of the deltoid to innervate the skin covering the deltoid. In addition to muscle and skin, the axillary nerve innervates the glenohumeral and acromioclavicular joints. Throughout it coarse, the nerve is associated with the posterior circumflex humeral artery and its branches.

Radial Nerve

The radial nerve is formed by fibers from C5 to T1 (Box 3–2). It passes from the axilla into the arm through the triangular

---

Box 3–2.

Radial Nerve

Muscular branches

- Extension of shoulder
  - Triceps brachii—long head
- Extension of elbow
  - Triceps brachii—long, lateral, medial heads
  - Anconeus
- Supination of forearm
  - Supinator
- Extension of wrist
  - Extensor carpi radialis—longus and brevis
  - Extensor carpi ulnaris
  - Extensor muscles of fingers and thumb listed below
- Extension of fingers (metacarpophalangeal and interphalangeal joints)
  - Extensor digitorum communis (index, middle, ring, little fingers)
  - Extensor indicis (index finger)
  - Extensor digiti minimi (little finger)
- Extension of thumb
  - Extensor pollicis longus (metacarpophalangeal and interphalangeal)
  - Extensor pollicis brevis (metacarpophalangeal joint)
- Abduction of thumb
  - Abductor pollicis longus

Articular branches

- Elbow (humeroradial and humeroulnar joints)
- Radioulnar joints—proximal and distal
- Radiocarpal joint

Cutaneous branches

- Posterior brachial cutaneous nerve
- Inferior lateral brachial cutaneous nerve
- Posterior antebrachial cutaneous nerve
- Superficial branch of the radial nerve

---

space. The triangular space is located inferior to the teres major between the long head of triceps brachii and the humerus. The radial nerve innervates the long head of the triceps muscle and sends a posterior brachial cutaneous branch to the skin covering this muscle. It descends along the shaft of the humerus (Figure 3–14) in the spiral groove in association with the deep radial artery. In the spiral groove, the radial nerve innervates the medial and lateral heads of the triceps brachii as well as the anconeus muscles. In addition to innervating these muscles, it sends an inferior lateral brachial cutaneous nerve to the skin covering the posterior arm and a posterior antebrachial cutaneous branch to the skin covering the posterior surface of the forearm. The radial nerve pierces the lateral intermuscular septum and crosses the elbow anterior to the lateral epicondyle between the brachialis and brachioradialis muscles. Here it divides into a superficial and deep branch. The superficial branch descends the forearm on the deep surface of brachioradialis. Proximal to the wrist, it enters the skin providing innervation over the dorsum of the hand onto the thumb, index, middle, and ring fingers to the level of the distal interphalangeal joint. The deep branch pierces the supinator muscle and descends the forearm along the interosseous membrane as the posterior interosseous nerve. En route, it innervates the brachioradialis, extensor carpi radialis longus and brevis, supinator, extensor digitorum communis, extensor digiti minimi, extensor carpi ulnaris, extensor indicis, extensor pollicis longus and brevis, and abductor pollicis muscles. In addition, it innervates the elbow, radioulnar, and wrist joints.[8]

Branches from the Lateral Cord

The lateral cord forms the lateral pectoral nerve, musculocutaneous nerve, and part of the median nerve.

Lateral Pectoral Nerve

The lateral pectoral nerve is formed by fibers from C5 to C7. It crosses the axilla deep to the pectoralis minor muscle and penetrates the deep surface of pectoralis major muscle, which it innervates. In addition, it innervates the glenohumeral joint.

Musculocutaneous Nerve

The musculocutaneous nerve is formed by fibers from C5 to C7 (Box 3–3). It pierces the coracobrachialis muscle and descends between the brachialis and biceps brachii muscles (see Figure 3–14). En route, it innervates all of these muscles. At the elbow, the musculocutaneous nerve becomes the lateral antebrachial cutaneous nerve and descends along the superficial surface of the brachioradialis muscle, innervating the skin covering that muscle. In addition to muscle and skin, the musculocutaneous nerve innervates the elbow and proximal radioulnar joints.

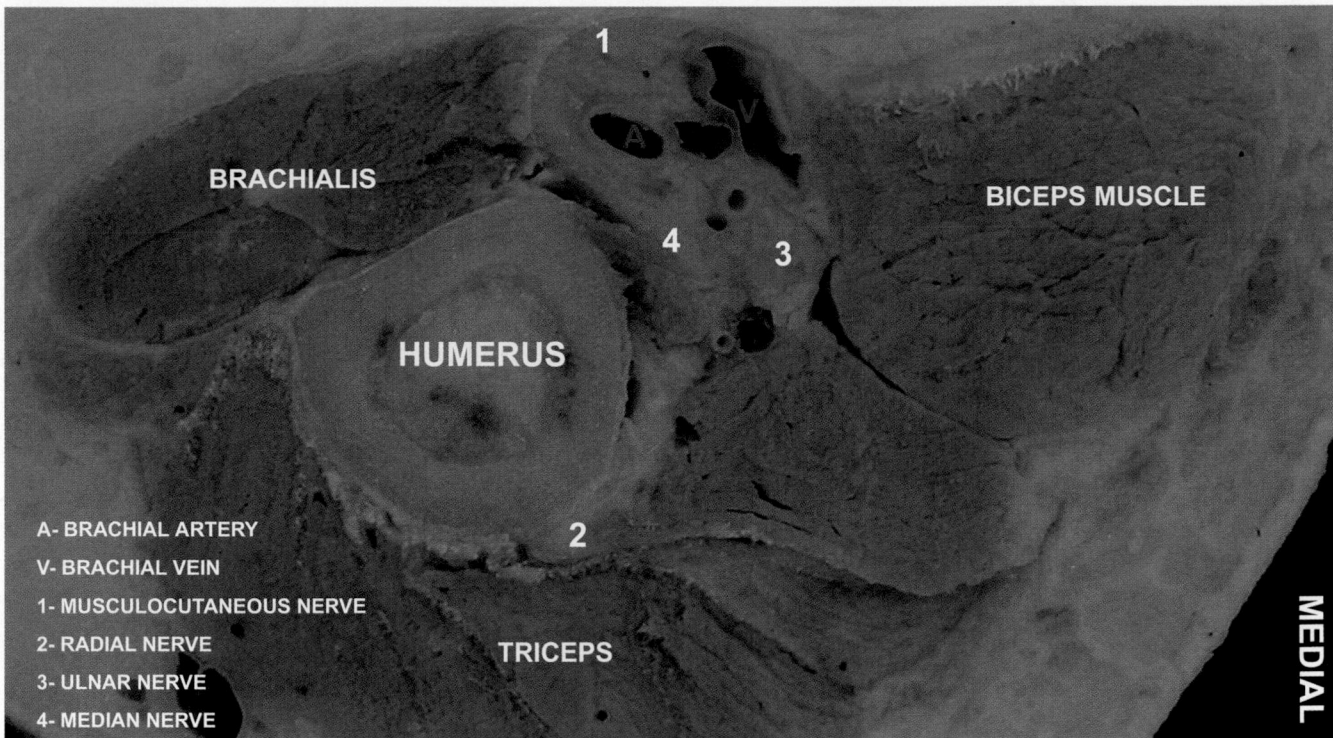

Figure 3–14. Cross-sectional anatomy and position of the nerves of the brachial plexus at the upper arm level.

Median Nerve

The median nerve is formed by junction of branches from the lateral and medial cords (Box 3–4). It descends the arm in association with the brachial artery and crosses the cubital fossa medial to the artery (see Figure 3–14). At the elbow, it innervates the pronator teres, flexor carpi radialis, and palmaris longus muscles. It passes into the forearm between the humeral and radial heads of the pronator teres muscle and descends in the space between the flexor digitorum superficialis and profundus muscles. En route, it innervates the flexor digitorum superficialis, the lateral part of flexor digitorum profundus (fibers to the index and middle fingers), the flexor pollicis longus, and the pronator quadratus muscles. In addition, the median nerve sends a palmar cutaneous branch to the skin covering the thenar eminence. At the wrist, the median nerve passes through the carpal tunnel deep to the flexor retinaculum. In the hand, the median nerve sends branches to the thenar muscles, which are the abductor pollicis brevis, flexor pollicis brevis, and opponens pollicis. The median nerve divides into three common palmar digital branches, which innerve the lateral two lumbrical muscles. The common palmar branches divide into proper palmar branches that innervate the skin of the thumb, index, middle, and ring (lateral half) fingers. The innervation covers the palmar surface and the nailbeds. In addition to muscle and skin, the median nerve innervates the elbow and all joints distal to it.[9,10]

Box 3–3.

Musculocutaneous Nerve (C5 to C7)

Muscular branches

- Flexion of the shoulder
  - Biceps brachii—long head
  - Coracobrachialis
- Flexion of elbow
  - Brachialis (humeroulnar joint)
  - Biceps brachii—long and short heads (humeroulnar joint)
- Supination of forearm
  - Biceps brachii—long and short heads

Articular branches

- Elbow (humeroulnar and humeroradial joints)
- Proximal radioulnar joint

Cutaneous branch

- Lateral antebrachial cutaneous nerve

Medial Cord Branches

The medial cord forms the medial pectoral nerve, medial brachial cutaneous nerve, medial antebrachial cutaneous nerve, and ulnar nerve and sends fibers to the median nerve.

Box 3–4.

Median Nerve

Muscular branches

- Flexion of the elbow
  - Flexor carpi radialis
  - Pronator teres
- Pronation of forearm
  - Pronator teres
  - Pronator quadratus
- Flexion of wrist
  - Flexor carpi radialis
  - Palmaris longus
  - Flexor digitorum superficialis and profundus
  - Flexor pollicis longus
- Flexion of fingers
  - Flexor digitorum superficialis (index, middle, ring, little fingers)
  - Flexor digitorum profundus (index, middle fingers)
- Flexion of metacarpophalangeal and extension of interphalangeal joints
  - Lumbricals (index, middle finger)
- Flexion of thumb
  - Flexor pollicis longus
  - Flexor pollicis brevis
- Abduction of thumb
  - Abductor pollicis brevis
- Opposition of thumb
  - Opponens pollicis

Articular branches

- Elbow (humeroulnar and humeroradial joints)
- Radioulnar joints—proximal and distal
- All joints of the wrist and hand

Cutaneous branches

- Palmar branch of median nerve
- Proper palmar digital nerves

Medial Pectoral Nerve

The medial pectoral is formed by fibers from C8 to T1. It pierces the pectoralis minor and ends by branching on the deep surface of the pectoralis major, both of which muscles it innervates. Contraction of the pectoralis minor in conjunction with the serratus anterior and rhomboid muscles pulls the pectoral girdle (clavicle and scapula) against the chest wall when load is applied to the upper extremity. Without this stabilization of the proximal joints, movement of the distal joint in the upper extremity would collapse.

Medial Brachial and Antebrachial Cutaneous Nerves

Both nerves descend in the arm associated with the brachial artery. The medial brachial cutaneous nerve distributes fibers to the skin covering the medial surface of the arm. Occasionally, the medial brachial nerve joins the lateral cutaneous branch of the second intercostal nerve to form the intercostobrachial nerve. The medial antebrachial cutaneous nerve crosses the cubital fossa and enters the skin to innerve the medial aspect of the forearm.[4]

Ulnar Nerve

The ulnar nerve is formed by fibers from C8 to T1 (Box 3–5). It descends the arm in association with the brachial artery (see Figure 3–14), pierces the medial intermuscular septum, and crosses the elbow posterior to the medial epicondyle. After crossing the elbow, the ulnar nerve descends the forearm between the flexor carpi ulnaris and flexor digitorum

Box 3–5.

Ulnar Nerve (C8 to T1)

Muscular branches

- Flexion of wrist
  - Flexor carpi ulnaris
  - Flexor digitorum profundus
- Flexion of fingers
  - Flexor digitorum profundus (ring, little finger)
  - Flexor digiti minimi (little finger)
- Flexion of knuckles and extension of fingers
  - Lumbricals (ring, little finger)
  - Interosseous muscles (index, middle, ring, little fingers)
- Adduction of fingers (metacarpophalangeal joint)
  - Palmar interosseous muscles (index, middle, ring, little finger)
- Abduction of fingers
  - Dorsal interosseous muscles (index, middle, ring finger)
  - Abductor digiti minimi (little finger)
- Opposition of little finger
  - Opponens digiti minimi
  - Palmaris brevis
- Adduction of thumb
  - Adductor pollicis
- Flexion of thumb
  - Flexor pollicis brevis

Articular branches

- Ulnocarpal joint
- All joints of the hand except interphalangeal joint of the thumb

Cutaneous branches

- Dorsal branch of the ulnar nerve
- Palmar branch of the ulnar nerve
- Proper palmar digital branches

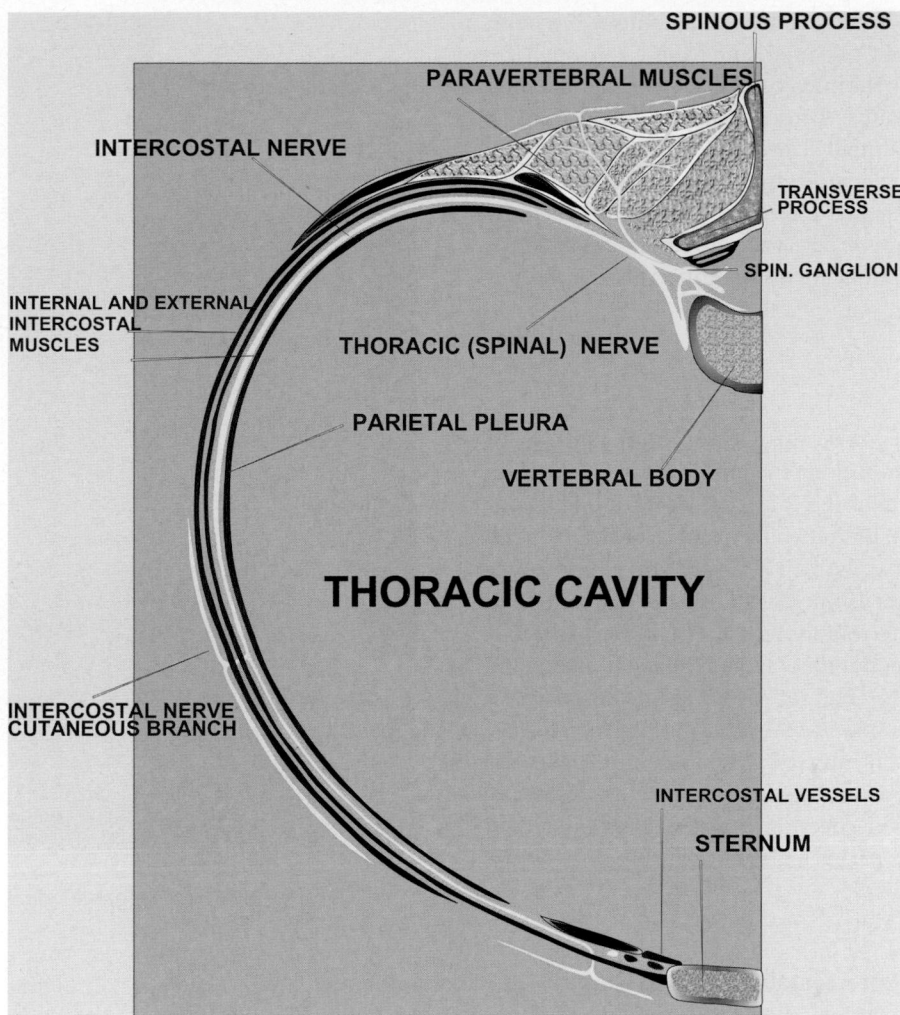

Figure 3–15. Organization and distribution of the spinal nerves at the thoracic level.

profundus, both of which muscles it innerves. The ulnar innervation of the flexor digitorum is limited to fibers affecting
the ring and little fingers. Proximal to the wrist, the ulnar
nerve sends a palmar branch to the skin covering the hypothenar eminence and a dorsal branch to the skin covering
the dorsal and medial surface of the hand and the skin covering the dorsal surface of the ring and little fingers. The ulnar
nerve passes through Guyon's canal (deep to the transverse
carpal ligament) to enter the hand. It divides into a superficial
and deep branch. The superficial branch sends branches to all
muscles of the hypothenar eminence, including the abductor
digiti minimi, flexor digiti minimi, and opponens digiti minimi. Then, it divides into common palmar digital branches,
which in turn divide into proper palmar digital branches.
These branches innervate the skin covering the palmar surface of ring and little fingers. The innervation continues onto
the nailbeds of these fingers. The deep branch of the ulnar
nerve passes beneath the adductor pollicis muscle, which it
innervates. The ulnar nerve sends fibers to the all interosseous
muscles in the hand and to the lumbrical muscles affecting
the ring and little fingers. The ulnar nerve ends by innervating
the deep head of the flexor pollicis brevis muscle.[9,10]

Thoracic Spinal Nerves

Thoracic spinal nerves innervate the muscles, joints, skin,
and pleuroperitoneal lining of the thoracic and abdominal
walls. Because the nerves travel within the intercostal spaces,
they are called intercostal nerves. The intercostal nerves comprise the anterior rami of the upper 11 thoracic spinal nerves.
Each intercostal nerve enters the neurovascular plane posteriorly and gives a collateral branch that supplies the intercostal muscles of the space. Except for the first, each intercostal nerve gives off a lateral cutaneous branch that pierces
the overlying muscle near the midaxillary line. This cutaneous nerve divides into anterior and posterior branches,
which supply the adjacent skin (Figure 3–15). The intercostal
nerves of the second to the sixth spaces enter the superficial
fascia near the lateral border of the sternum and divide into
medial and lateral cutaneous branches. Most of the fibers of
the anterior ramus of the first thoracic spinal nerve join the
brachial plexus for distribution to the upper limb. The small
first intercostal nerve is the collateral branch and supplies
only the muscles of the intercostal space, not the overlying
skin.

The intercostal nerves can be divided into two groups. One group is formed by nerves arising from T1 through T5. These nerves remain in the intercostal spaces throughout their coarse. The second group is formed by nerves arising from T6 to T12. These nerves initially travel in the intercostal spaces, but then cross the costal margin and terminate in the abdominal wall. This subgroup of intercostals nerves is called the thoracoabdominal nerves. The ventral ramus of T12 forms the subcostal nerve. This nerve travels entirely in the abdominal wall.

Intercostal Nerves

The intercostal nerves arise form the ventral rami of T1 through T11. They travel along the inferior margin of the rib of corresponding number (eg, T1 nerve travels along the inferior margin of rib 1). En route, the nerve is located between the deepest (transverse thoracis muscle) and intermediate layer (internal intercostals muscle) of muscle. It is associated with the intercostal arteries and veins. From the top to the bottom, the neurovascular bundle is arranged as vein, artery, and nerve (mnemonic VAN) (Figure 3–16). The intercostal nerves send branches to the transverse thoracis, internal intercostals, and external intercostal muscles. They innervate the costal joints. Through lateral and anterior cutaneous branches, they innervate the skin covering the respective intercostal spaces as well as the parietal pleura lining the intercostal spaces.

Thoracoabdominal (Intercostals T6 to T11) Nerves

The T6 through T11 intercostal (thoracoabdominal) nerves begin as typical intercostal nerves, but then send branches across the costal margin into the muscles of the anterior

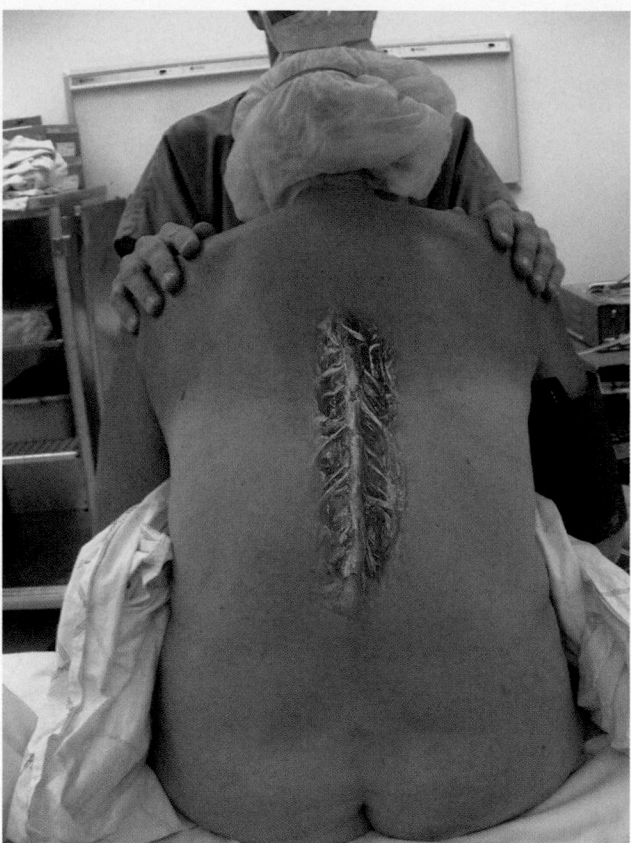

Figure 3–17. Thoracoabdominal spinal nerves.

abdominal wall (Figure 3–17). These branches innervate the transverse abdominis, internal abdominal oblique, external abdominal oblique, and rectus abdominis muscles. In addition, they innervate the skin of the anterior wall in a metameric manner from the xiphoid process to the umbilicus.

Subcostal Nerve

The T12, or subcostal, nerve never enters an intercostal space. It travels through the abdominal wall, terminating between the umbilicus and the pubic symphysis. It innervates muscle and skin along its coarse.

Lumbosacral Plexus

The lumbosacral plexus innervates the muscles, joints, skin, and peritoneal lining of the abdominopelvic wall[11,12] (Tables 3–3 and 3–4).

It also innervates the inferior extremities. It is formed by the ventral rami of L1 to S5 (Figure 3–18). The ventral rami join to form the terminal nerves. Between the L2 and S3 levels, the plexus is more complex. The ventral rami divide into anterior and posterior divisions that join to form the terminal nerves. The plexus is located in the posterior abdominal wall between the psoas major and quadratus lumborum muscles (Figure 3–19).

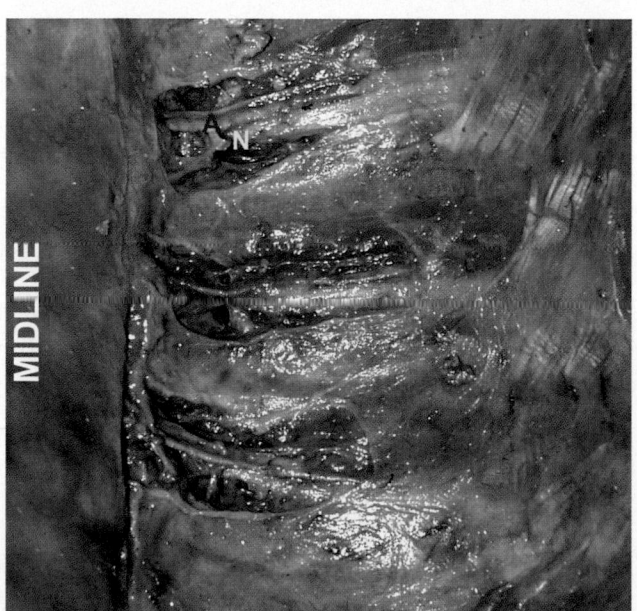

Figure 3–16. Intercostal nerves. V = vein; A = artery; N = nerve.

Table 3–3.

Organization and Distribution of the Lumbar Plexus

Nerves(s)	Spinal Segments	Distribution
Iliohypogastric nerve	T12 to L1	Abdominal muscles (external and internal oblique muscles, transverse abdominis muscles); skin over inferior abdomen and buttocks
Ilioinguinal nerve	L1	Abdominal muscles (with iliohypogastric nerve); skin over superior, medial thigh and portions of external genitalia
Genitofemoral nerve	L1, L2	Skin over anteromedial surface of thigh and portions over genitalia
Lateral femoral cutaneous nerve	L2, L3	Skin over anterior, lateral, and posterior surfaces of thigh
Femoral nerve	L2 to L4	Anterior muscles of thigh (sartorius muscle and quadriceps group); adductor of thigh (pectineus and iliopsoas muscles); skin over anteromedial surface of thigh, medial surface of leg, and foot
Obturator nerve	L2 to L4	Adductors of thigh (adductors magnus, brevis, and longus); gracilis muscle; skin over medial surface of thigh
Saphenous nerve	L2 to L4	Skin over medial surface of leg

Iliohypogastric Nerve

The iliohypogastric nerve arises from the ventral ramus of L1 and travels in the abdominal wall to the level of the pubic symphysis (Figures 3–18 and 3–20). It innervates the muscle, skin, and parietal peritoneum along its coarse.

Ilioinguinal Nerve

The ilioinguinal nerve (see Figures 3–18 and 3–20) arises from the ventral rami of L1, travels in the abdominal wall, pierces in the posterior wall of the inguinal canal, passes through the superficial inguinal ring, and terminates on the anterior

Table 3–4.

Organization and Distribution of the Sacral Plexus

Nerves(s)	Spinal Segments	Distribution
Gluteal nerves: Superior Inferior	L4 to S2	Abductors of thigh (gluteus minimus, gluteus medius, and tensor fasciae latae) Extensor of thigh (gluteus maximus)
Posterior femoral cutaneous nerve	S1 to S3	Skin of perineum and posterior surface of thigh and leg
Sciatic nerve: Tibial nerve Common peroneal nerve	L4 to S3	Three of the hamstrings (semitendinosus and semimembrenosus long head of biceps femoris); adductor magnus (with obturator nerve) Flexor of knee and plantar flexors of ankle (popliteus, gastrocnemius, soleus plantaris, and tibialis posterior muscles and long head of biceps femoris muscle); flexors of toes; skin over posterior surface of leg, plantar surface of foot Biceps femoris muscle (short head); fibularis (brevis and longus) and tibialis anterior muscles; extensors of toes, skin over anterior surface of leg and dorsal surface of foot; skin over lateral portion of foot (through the sural nerve)
Pudendal nerve	S2 to S4	Muscles of perineum, including urogenital diaphragm and external anal and urethral sphincter muscles; skin of external genitalia and related skeletal muscles (bulbospongiosus, ischiocavernosus muscles)

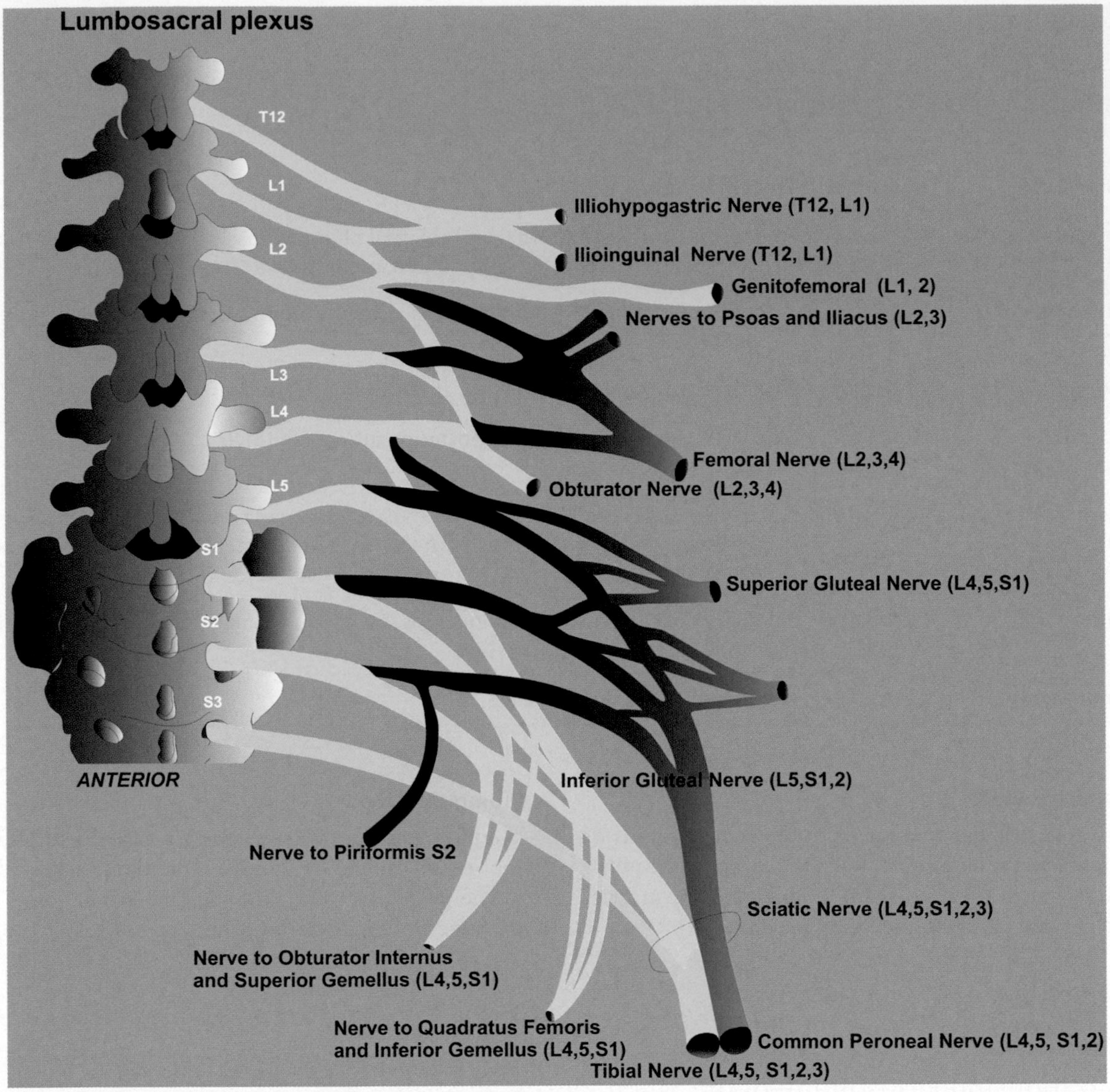

Lumbosacral plexus

T12

L1

L2

L3

L4

L5

S1

S2

S3

ANTERIOR

Illiohypogastric Nerve (T12, L1)

Ilioinguinal Nerve (T12, L1)

Genitofemoral (L1, 2)

Nerves to Psoas and Iliacus (L2,3)

Femoral Nerve (L2,3,4)

Obturator Nerve (L2,3,4)

Superior Gluteal Nerve (L4,5,S1)

Inferior Gluteal Nerve (L5,S1,2)

Nerve to Piriformis S2

Sciatic Nerve (L4,5,S1,2,3)

Nerve to Obturator Internus
and Superior Gemellus (L4,5,S1)

Nerve to Quadratus Femoris
and Inferior Gemellus (L4,5,S1)

Common Peroneal Nerve (L4,5, S1,2)

Tibial Nerve (L4,5, S1,2,3)

Figure 3-18. Organization of the lumbosacral plexus.

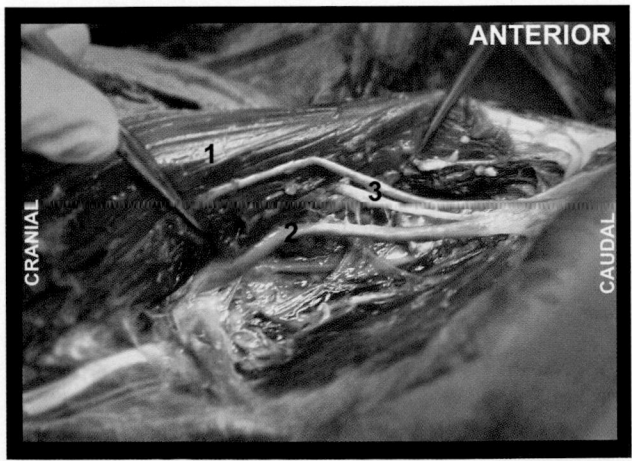

Figure 3-19. Lumbar plexus. Shown are nerves of the lumbar plexus (2, and 3) as they emerge from or underneath the iliopsoas muscle (1).

scrotum or labia majora. It innervates the muscle, skin, and parietal peritoneum along its coarse.

Genitofemoral Nerve

The genitofemoral nerve arises from the ventral rami from L1 and L2. It travels in the abdominal wall and passes through the deep inguinal ring into the inguinal canal. A femoral branch pierces the anterior wall of the canal and innervates the skin covering the femoral hiatus in the crural fascia. The genital branch passes through the superficial inguinal ring to innervate the skin on the scrotum or labia majora. En route, it innervates the cremaster muscle. Contraction of the cremaster elevates the scrotum.

Nerve to the Coccygeus and Levator Ani

The nerve to the coccygeus and levator ani muscles arises from the posterior division of the ventral rami at S3 to S4. It

Inferior Gluteal Nerve

The inferior gluteal nerve arises from the posterior division of the ventral rami at L5 to S2. It passes from the pelvis through the greater sciatic foramen into the gluteal region. It enters the gluteal region inferior to the piriformis muscle and terminates on the deep surface of the gluteal maximus muscle, which it innervates.

Nerve to Piriformis

The nerve to piriformis arises from the posterior division of the ventral rami at S1 to S2 and passes onto the deep surface of the piriformis muscle, which it innervates.

Nerve to Obturator Internus and Superior Gemellus

The nerve to the obturator internus and superior gemellus muscles arises form the anterior division of the ventral rami at L5 and S1. It passes from the pelvis through the greater sciatic foramen into the gluteal region. In enters the gluteal region inferior to the piriformis muscle and passes along the deep surface of the superior gemellus to the obturator internus, innervating these last two muscles.

Nerve to the Quadratus Femoris and Inferior Gemellus

The nerve to the quadratus femoris and inferior gemellus muscles arises from the anterior division of the ventral rami at L4 to L5. It passes from the pelvis through the greater sciatic foramen to the gluteal region and enters the gluteal region inferior to piriformis, passing deep to obturator internus to terminate in the inferior gemellus and quadratus femoris muscles. As indicated by its name, the nerve innervates the inferior gemellus and quadratus femoris muscles.

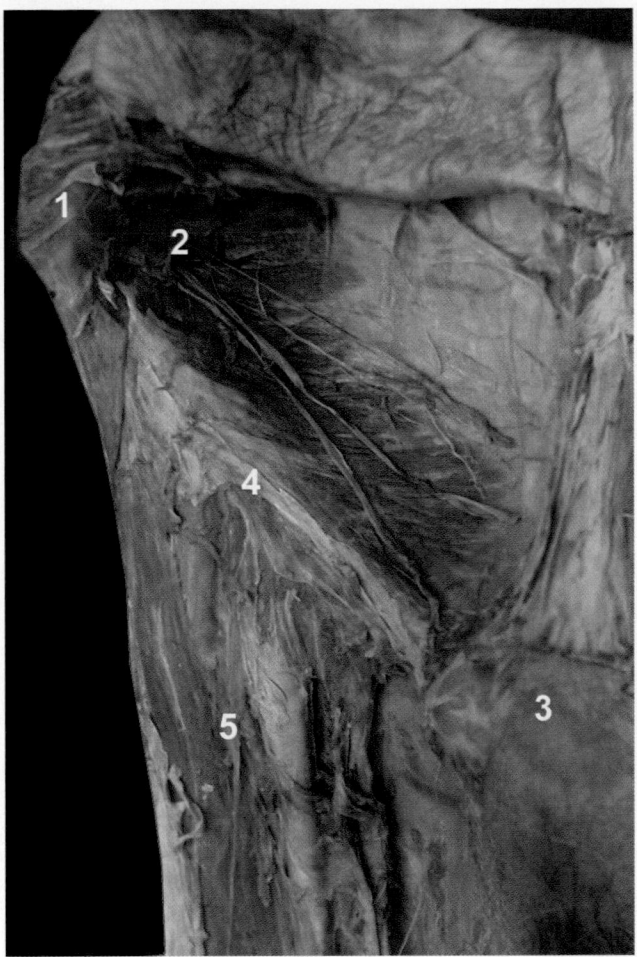

Figure 3–20. Ilioinguinal and iliohypogastric nerves. Shown are: (1) anterosuperior iliac spine, (2) ilioinguinal and iliohypogastric nerves, (3) pubic tubercle, (4) inguinal ligament, and (5) laterofemoral cutaneous nerve.

travels anteriorly onto the superior surface of the coccygeus and levator ani.

Pudendal Nerve

The pudendal nerve arises from the anterior division of the ventral rami from S2 to S4. It passes from the pelvis through the greater sciatic foramen into the gluteal region. It enters the gluteal region inferior to the piriformis muscle, passes posterior to the ischial spine, then enters the perineum by passing through the lesser sciatic foramen. It innervates the muscle and skin of the perineum.

Superior Gluteal Nerve

The superior gluteal nerve arises from the posterior division of the ventral rami at L4 to S1. It passes from the pelvis through the greater sciatic foramen to the gluteal region. It enters the gluteal region superior to the piriformis muscle, passes in the plane between gluteal medius and minimus muscles, and terminates in the tensor fascia lata muscle. En route, it innervates the gluteus medius and minimus muscles as well as the tensor fascia lata.

Box 3–6.

Obturator Nerve

Muscular branches

- Adduction of hip
  - Adductor magnus, longus, and brevis
  - Gracilis
- Flexion of hip
  - Adductor magnus (anterior fibers)
  - Adductor longus and brevis
- Extension of hip
  - Adductor magnus (posterior fibers)

Articular branches

- Hip
- Knee

Cutaneous branches

- Medial femoral cutaneous branches

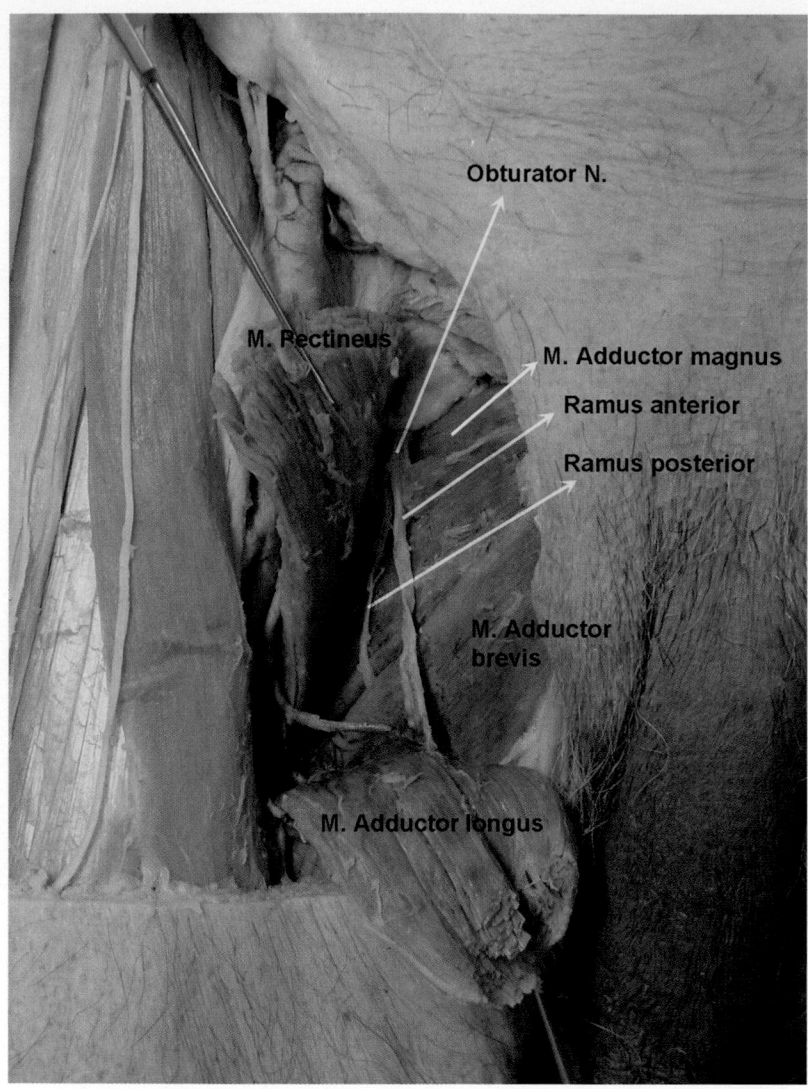

Figure 3–21. Anatomy of the obturator nerve.

Lateral Femoral Cutaneous Nerve

The lateral femoral cutaneous nerve arises form the posterior divisions of the ventral rami at L2 to L3. It descends the posterior abdominal wall, crosses the iliac crest into the pelvis where it descends on the iliacus muscle, passes deep to the inguinal ligament at the anterior iliac spine, and distributes cutaneous innervation on the lateral aspect of the thigh to the level of the knee (see Figure 3–20).

Posterior Femoral Cutaneous Nerve

The posterior femoral cutaneous nerve arises from the anterior and posterior divisions of the ventral rami at S1 to S3. It passes from the pelvis through the greater sciatic foramen into the gluteal region. It enters the gluteal region inferior to the piriformis muscle, descends in the muscle plane between gluteus maximus posteriorly and obturator internus anteriorly, and passes into the posterior thigh where it supplies cutaneous innervation from the hip to the midcalf.[4]

Obturator Nerve

The obturator nerve (see Box 3–6) arises from the anterior division of the ventral rami at L2 to L4 (see Figure 3–18). It descends through the pelvis medial to the psoas major muscle, crosses the superior pubic ramus inferiorly, passes through the obturator foramen into the medial compartment of the thigh where it divides into posterior and anterior branches (Figure 3–21). The posterior branch descends superficial to the adductor magnus muscle, which it innervates. The anterior branch passes superficial to the obturator externus muscle, descends the thigh in the muscle plane between the adductor brevis and adductor longus, and terminates in the gracilis muscle. En route, it innervates all of these muscles. Furthermore, it provides articular branches to the hip and cutaneous branches to the skin covering the medial thigh.

Femoral Nerve

The femoral nerve arises from the posterior division of the ventral rami at L2 to L4 (Box 3–7). It descends through the

Box 3–7.

Femoral Nerve

Muscular branches

- Flexion of hip
  - Iliacus
  - Psoas major
  - Pectineus
  - Rectus femoris
  - Sartorius
- Lateral rotation of hip
  - Sartorius
- Extension of knee
  - Rectus femoris
  - Vastus lateralis
  - Vastus intermedius
  - Vastus medialis
- Flexion of knee
  - Sartorius

Articular branches

- Hip
- Knee

Cutaneous branches

- Anterior femoral cutaneous nerves
- Saphenous branch of the femoral nerve

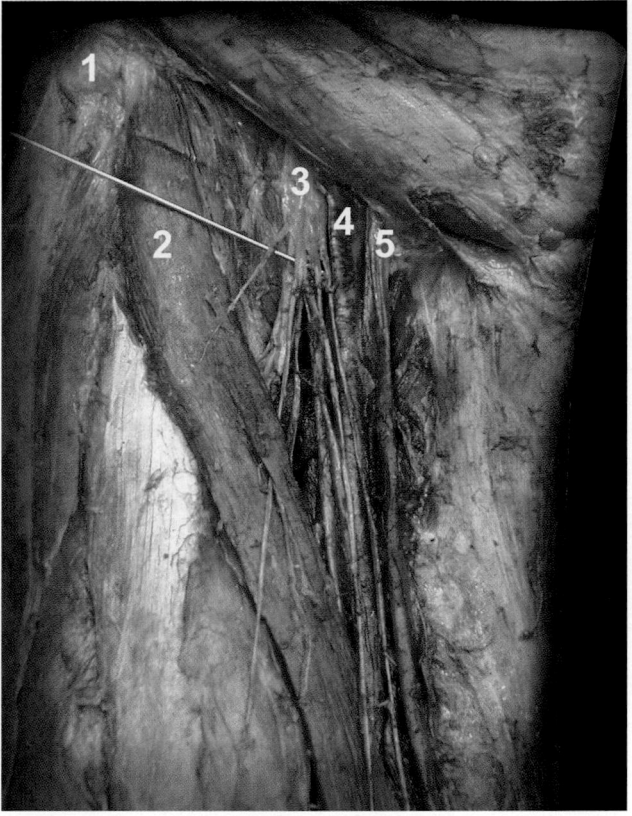

Figure 3–22. Anatomy of the femoral triangle. Shown are: (1) Anteriosuperior iliac spine, (2) sartorius muscle, (3) femoral nerve, (4) femoral artery, and (5) femoral vein.

pelvis lateral to the psoas major muscle, passes deep to the inguinal ligament, and enters the anterior compartment of the thigh where it divides into multiple branches supplying the muscle, joints, and skin in that region. In the femoral crease-inguinal area, the nerve is positioned lateral to the femoral artery and vein (mnemonic: NAVEL) (Figure 3–22). Muscular branches innervate the iliacus, psoas major, pectineus, rectus femoris, vastus lateralis, vastus intermedius, vastus medialis, and sartorius muscles. Articular branches innervate the hip and knee.[13] Of note, the femoral nerve bellow the inguinal ligament consists of an anterior and a posterior part. The anterior part contains branches to the sartorius muscle and the posterior contains the saphenous nerve (most medial part) and branches to the individual heads of the quadriceps muscle.[14]

Saphenous Nerve and Other Cutaneous Branches of the Femoral Nerve

The superficial branches of the femoral nerve supply the skin covering the anterior thigh. One cutaneous branch follows the deep surface of the sartorius muscle to its attachment on the tibia. Here, it passes onto the skin, providing innervation of the medial leg from knee to the arch of the foot (Figure 3–23). En route, the nerve is accompanied by the saphenous vein, so it is called the saphenous branch of the femoral nerve.

As previously mentioned, the saphenous nerve is the most medial part of the femoral nerve at the inguinal (femoral) crease.[14]

Sciatic Nerve

The sciatic nerve is formed by the junction of the tibial and common peroneal nerves (Box 3–8). The tibial nerve arises from the anterior division of the ventral rami at L4 to S3 (see Figure 3–18). The common peroneal nerve arises from the posterior division of the ventral rami at L4 to S2. The sciatic nerve passes from the pelvis through the greater sciatic foramen into the gluteal region. It enters the gluteal region inferior to the piriformis muscle, descends in the muscle plane between the gluteus maximus posteriorly and the obturator internus anteriorly, and passes lateral to the ischial tuberosity to enter the posterior thigh (Figure 3–24). In the posterior thigh, it passes between the adductor magnus and the long head of the biceps femoris. It descends in the groove between the biceps femoris medially and the semitendinosus and semimembranosus laterally. En route, it innervates the adductor magnus, biceps femoris, semitendinosus, and semimembranosus muscles (Figure 3–25).[15] Posterior to the knee the sciatic nerve descends into the popliteal fossa, where it diverges into the tibial and common peroneal nerves (Figure 3–26).[16] Of note, these two branches are distinct from the onset and travel together enveloped in the same tissue sheath.[17]

Box 3–8.

Sciatic Nerve

Muscular branches

- Extension of hip—sciatic nerve
  - Biceps femoris—long head
- Flexion of knee—sciatic nerve
  - Biceps femoris—long and short heads
  - Semimembranosus
  - Semitendinosus
  - Popliteus—tibial division only
  - Gastrocnemius—tibial division only
- Plantarflexion of ankle—tibial nerve
  - Soleus
  - Gastrocnemius
  - Tibialis posterior
  - Flexor digitorum longus
  - Flexor hallucis longus
  - Peroneus longus and brevis—superficial peroneal nerve
- Dorsiflexion of ankle—deep peroneal nerve
  - Tibialis anterior
  - Extensor digitorum longus
  - Extensor hallucis longus
- Inversion of ankle—deep peroneal nerve
  - Tibialis anterior
- Eversion of ankle—superficial peroneal nerve
  - Peroneus longus and brevis

- Adduction of toes—tibial nerve
  - Plantar interosseus muscles
- Abduction of toes—tibial nerve
  - Dorsal interosseous muscles
  - Abductor hallucis
  - Abductor digiti minimi
- Flexion of toes—tibial nerve
  - Flexor digitorum longus and brevis
  - Flexor hallucis longus and brevis
- Extension of toes—deep peroneal nerve
  - Extensor digitorum longus and brevis
  - Extensor hallucis longus and brevis

Articular branches

- Knee
- Ankle
- Foot—all joints

Cutaneous branches

- Superficial peroneal
- Sural
- Calcaneal branches—medial and lateral
- Plantar nerves—medial and lateral

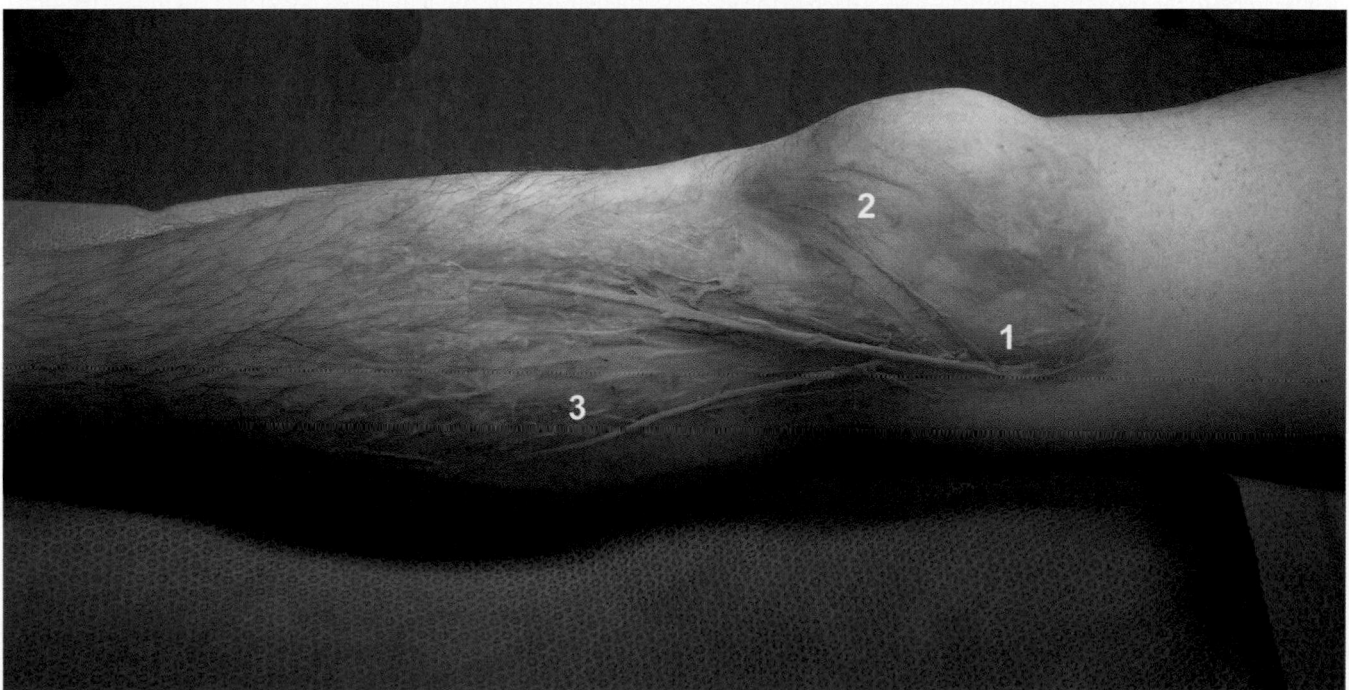

Figure 3–23. Saphenous nerve and its branches as the nerve emerges through the lower sartorius muscle. Shown are (1) main trunk of the saphenous nerve, (2) subpatellar branch of the saphenous nerve, and (3) branches of the saphenous nerve on the medial skin bellow the knee.

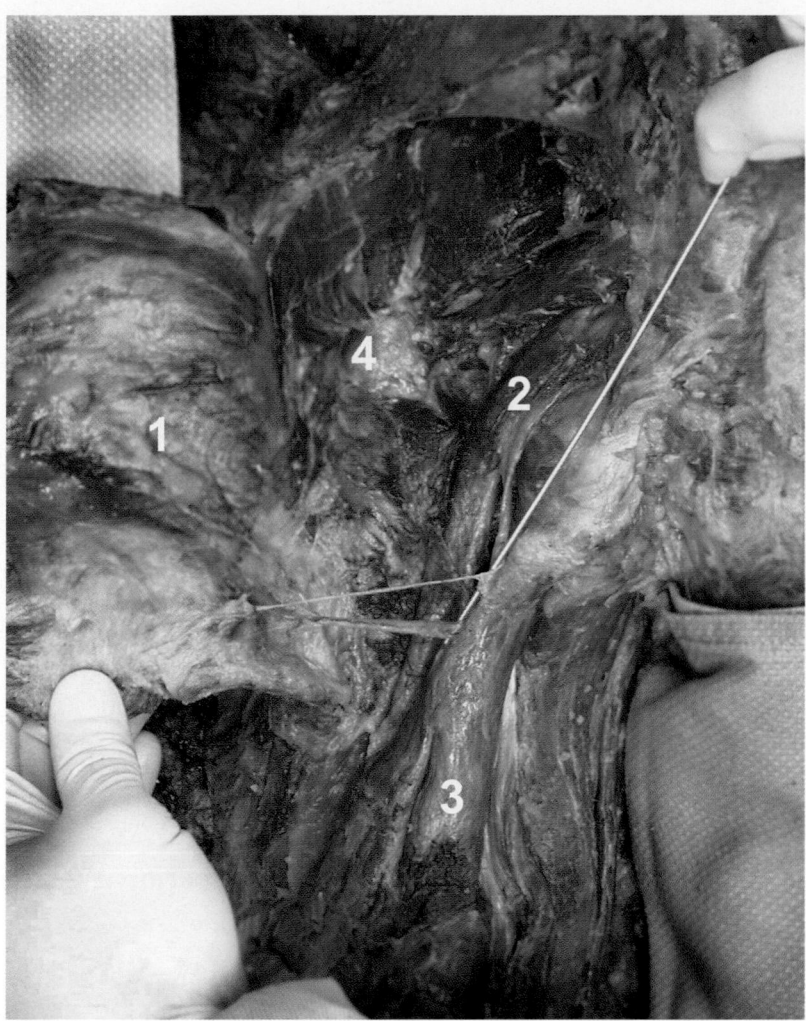

Figure 3–24. Anatomy of the sciatic nerve. Shown are (1) gluteus muscle, (2) sciatic nerve, (3) biceps femoris muscle, and (4) ischial spine.

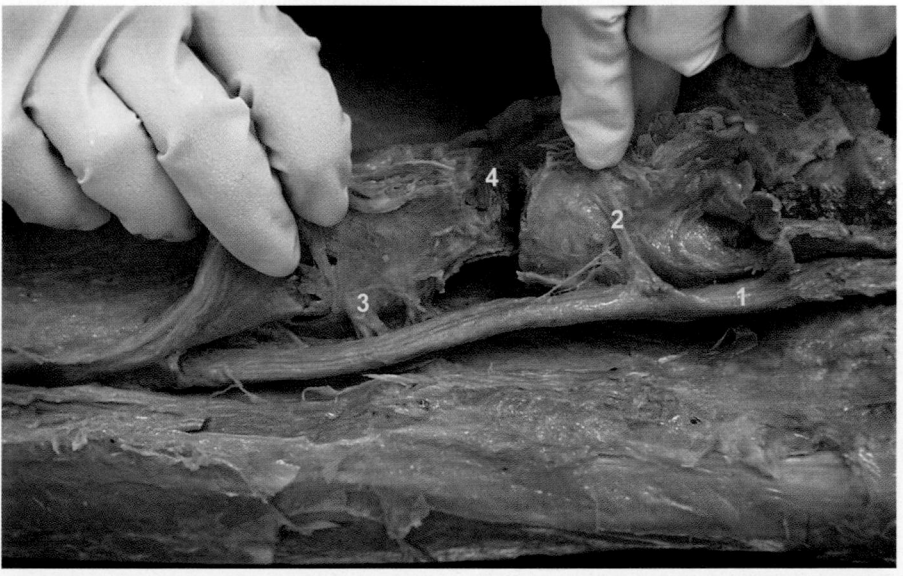

Figure 3–25. Sciatic nerve shown in the posterior compartment of the leg. Shown are (1) the sciatic nerve and (2–3) its branches to the (4) hamstrings muscles.

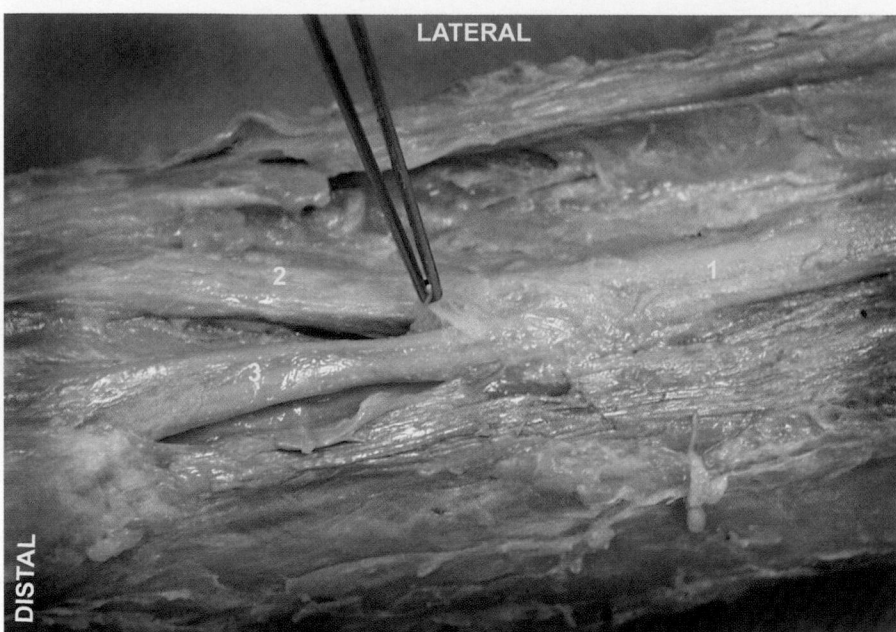

Figure 3–26. Anatomy of the sciatic nerve at the popliteal fossa. Shown are the (1) sciatic nerve in the popliteal fossa, (2) common peroneal, and (3) tibial nerve.

The tibial nerves exits the popliteal fossa passing between the heads of the gastrocnemius muscle into the superficial posterior compartment of the leg. Here, it descends deep to the plantaris and superficial to popliteus muscles. It passes between the tibial and fibular heads of the soleus muscle to enter the deep posterior compartment. The nerve passes posterior to the medial malleolus, where it enters the foot and divides into medial and lateral plantar nerves that innervate the muscle and skin on the plantar surface of the foot. The common peroneal nerve follows the tendon of the biceps femoris to its attachment on the fibula. The nerve passes inferior to the neck of the fibula and divides into superficial and deep branches. The superficial branch enters the lateral compartment of the leg, where it innervates the peroneus longus and brevis muscles. The nerve terminates as cutaneous fibers on the dorsal and lateral surface of the foot. The deep peroneal nerve enters the anterior compartment of the leg, where is innervates the tibialis anterior, extensor digitorum longus, and extensor hallucis longus muscles. It crosses the anterior surface of the ankle into the foot, where it innervates the extensor digitorum brevis and extensor hallucis brevis muscles. It terminates as cutaneous fibers supplying skin between the hallux and second toe.[18]

SENSORY INNERVATION OF THE MAJOR JOINTS

Much of the practice of peripheral nerve blocks involves orthopedic and other joint surgery. Consequently, knowledge of the sensory innervation of the major joints is important to the better understanding of the neuronal components that need to be anesthetized to achieve anesthesia for or analgesia after joint surgery. Tables 3–5 and 3–6

Table 3–5.

Innervation of Joints in the Superior Extremity

Joint	Innervation
Sternoclavicular	Medial supraclavicular, nerve to subclavius
Acromioclavicular	Axillary, lateral pectoral, lateral supraclavicular
Shoulder (glenohumeral)	Axillary, suprascapular, lateral pectoral
Elbow (humeroulnar, humeroradial)	Radial, musculocutaneous, ulnar
Radioulnar—proximal and distal	Median, radial, musculocutaneous
Wrist (radiocarpal, ulnocarpal)	Median, ulnar, radial
Intercarpal	Median, ulnar
Carpometacarpal	Median, ulnar, radial
Knuckle (metacarpophalangeal)	Median, ulnar
Interphalangeal—proximal and distal	Median, ulnar
Interphalangeal joint of the thumb	Median

Table 3–6.

Innervation of Joints of the Inferior Extremity

Joint	Innervation
Hip (acetabulofemoral)	Femoral, obturator, superior gluteal, nerve to quadratus femoris and inferior gemellus
Knee (tibiofemoral)	Sciatic, femoral, obturator
Ankle (tibiotalar, talocalcaneal)	Tibial, deep peroneal
Metatarsophalangeal	Tibial
Interphalangeal	Tibial

summarize the sensory innervation of the major joints of the upper and lower extremity. Tables 3–7 and 3–8 summarize the innervation and kinetic function of the major muscle groups of the upper (see Table 3–7) and lower (see Table 3–8) extremity.

Shoulder Joint

Innervation to the shoulder joints stems mostly from the axillary and suprascapular nerves. The skin over most medial parts of shoulder receives nerves from the cervical plexus. Such an arrangement explains why a brachial plexus block at the interscalene level is the most appropriate technique to achieve anesthesia to the shoulder (Figure 3–27).

Elbow Joint

Nerve supply to the elbow joint includes branches of all major nerves of the brachial plexus: musculocutaneous, radial, median, and ulnar nerves (Figure 3–28).

Table 3–7.

Summary of Movement by Joint—Upper Extremity

Shoulder (Glenohumeral) Joint

Flexion	Biceps brachii—long head	Musculocutaneous nerve
	Coracobrachialis	
	Deltoid	Axillary nerve
	Pectoralis major	Medial and lateral pectoral nerve
Extension	Triceps brachii—long head	Radial nerve
	Latissimus dorsi	Thoracodorsal nerve
	Deltoid	Axillary nerve
Adduction	Latissimus dorsi	Thoracodorsal nerve
	Pectoralis major	Medial and lateral pectoral nerves
	Teres major	Lower subscapular nerve
	Subscapularis	Upper and lower subscapular nerve
Abduction	Supraspinatus	Suprascapular nerve
	Deltoid	Axillary nerve
Medial rotation	Pectoralis major	Medial and lateral pectoral nerve
	Latissimus dorsi	Thoracodorsal nerve
	Teres major	Lower subscapular nerve
	Subscapularis	Upper and lower subscapular nerves
Lateral rotation	Teres minor	Axillary nerve
	Infraspinatus	Suprascapular nerve

Elbow (Humeroulnar, Humeroradial) Joint

Flexion	Brachialis	Musculocutaneous
	Biceps brachii—long and short heads	
	Flexor carpi radialis	Median nerve

(continued)

Table 3–7.

(Continued)

Extension	Triceps brachii—long lateral, medial head Anconeous	Radial nerve
Radioulnar Joints		
Supination	Biceps brachii—long and short head Supinator	Musculocutaneous Radial nerve
Pronation	Pronator teres Pronator quadratus	Median nerve
Wrist (Radiocarpal, Ulnocarpal) Joint		
Flexion	Flexor carpi radialis Palmaris longus Flexors of fingers listed below Flexor carpi ulnaris	Median nerve Ulnar nerve
Extension	Extensor carpi radialis longus and brevis Extensors of fingers listed below Extensor carpi ulnaris	Radial nerve
Carpometacarpal Joints		
Opposition	Opponen pollicis Opponens digiti minimi	Median nerve Ulnar nerve
Matacarpophalangeal Joints		
Flexion	Flexor digitorum superficialis Flexor digitorum profundus Flexor pollicis longus and brevis Interosseus Lumbricals	Median nerve Median and ulnar nerves Median nerve Ulnar nerve Median and ulnar nerves
Extension	Extensor digitorum communis Extensor indicis Extensor digiti minimi	Radial nerve
Adduction	Palmar interosseous Abductor pollicis	Ulnar nerve
Abduction	Dorsal interosseous Abductor digiti minimi Abductor pollicis longus Abductor pollicis brevis	Ulnar nerve Radial nerve Median nerve
Interphalangeal Joints		
Flexion	Flexor digitorum superficialis Flexor digitorum profundus Flexor pollicis longus and brevis	Median nerve Median and ulnar nerves Median nerve
Extension	Extensor digitorum communis Extensor indicis Extensor digiti minimi Lumbricals (index, middle fingers) Lumbricals (ring, little fingers) Interosseous muscles	Radial nerve Median nerve Ulnar nerve

Table 3–8.

Summary of Movement by Joints—Lower Extremity

Hip (Acetabulofemoral) Joint

Flexion	Iliacus/Psoas major	Femoral nerve
	Pectineus	
	Rectus femoris	
	Sartorius	
	Adductor magnus	Obturator nerve
	Adductor longus and brevis	
	Tensor fascia lata	Superior gluteal nerve
Extension	Biceps femoris—long head	Sciatic nerve
	Semimembranosis	
	Semitendinosis	
	Gluteus maximus	Inferior gluteal nerve
	Adductor magnus	Obturator nerve
Adduction	Adduct magnus, longus, brevis	Obturator nerve
	Gracilis	
	Pectineus	Femoral nerve
Abduction	Gluteus minimus	Superior gluteal nerve
	Gluteus medius	
	Tensor fascia lata	
Medial rotation	Gluteus minimus	Superior gluteal nerve
	Gluteus medius	
	Tensor fascia lata	
Lateral rotation	Piriformis	Nerve to piriformis
	Obturator internus	Nerve to obturator internus
	Superior gemilli	Nerve to obturator internus
	Inferior gemelli	Nerve to quadratus femoris
	Quadratus femoris	Nerve to quadratus femoris
	Sartorius	Femoral nerve

Knee (Tibiofemoral) Joint

Flexion	Bicep femoris—long and short heads	Sciatic nerve
	Semitendinosis	
	Semimembranosis	
	Popliteus	Tibial nerve
	Gastrocnemius	
	Sartorius	Femoral nerve
Extension:	Rectus femoris	Femoral nerve
	Vastus lateralis	
	Vastus intermedius	
	Vastus medialis	
Medial rotation	Popliteus	Tibial nerve
	Semimembranosis	Sciatic nerve
	Semitendinosis	
Lateral rotation	Biceps femoris	Sciatic nerve

Ankle (Talocrural) Joint

Plantarflexion	Soleus	Tibial nerve
	Gastronemius	
	Tibialis posterior	
	Flexor digitorum longus	
	Flexor hallucis longus	
	Peroneus longus and brevis	Superficial peroneal nerve

(continued)

Table 3–8.		
(Continued)		
Dorsiflexion	Tibialis anterior Extensor digitorum Extensor hallucis longus	Deep peroneal nerve
Subtalar Joint		
Inversion	Tibialis anterior	Deep peroneal nerve
Eversion	Peroneus longus and brevis	Superficial peroneal nerve
Metatarsophalangeal Joints		
Flexion	Flexor digitorum longus and brevis Flexor hallucis longus and brevis Flexor digiti minimi Lumbricals Interosseous muscles	Tibial nerve
Extension	Extensor digitorum longus and brevis Extensor hallucis longus and brevis	Deep peroneal nerve
Adduction	Plantar interosseous muscles Adductor hallucis	Tibial nerve
Abduction	Dorsal interosseous Abductor hallucis Abductor digiti minimi	Tibial nerve
Intephalangeal Joints		
Flexion	Flexor digitorum longus and brevis Flexor hallucis longus and brevis	Tibial nerve
Extension	Extensor digitorum longus and brevis Extensor hallucis longus and brevis	Deep peroneal nerve
	Lumbricals Interosseous muscles	Tibial nerve

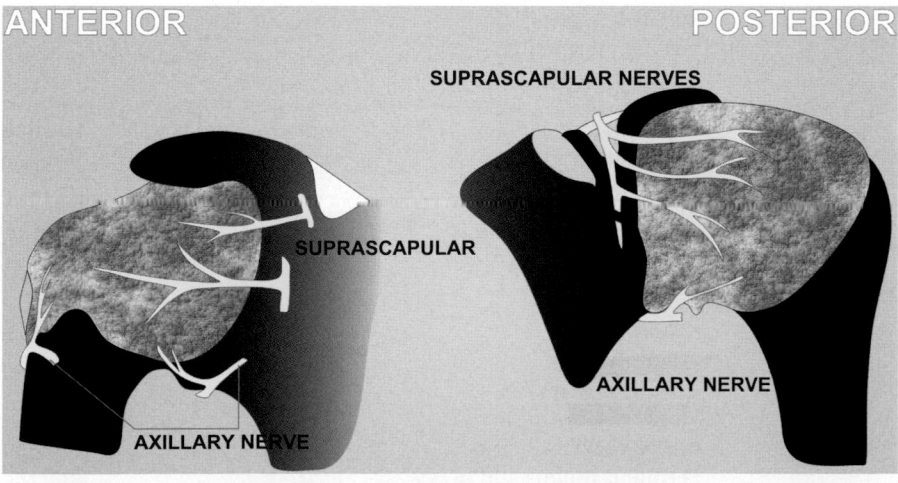

Figure 3–27. Shoulder joint—sensory innervation.

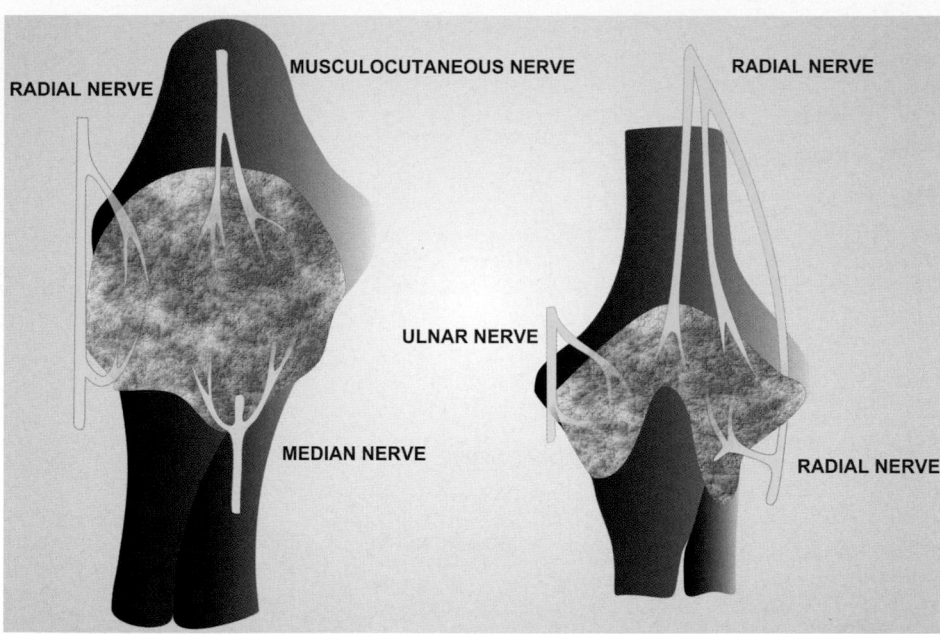

Figure 3–28. Elbow joint—sensory innervation.

Wrist Joint

The wrist is innervated by the radial, ulnar and median nerves (Figures 3–29 and 3–30).

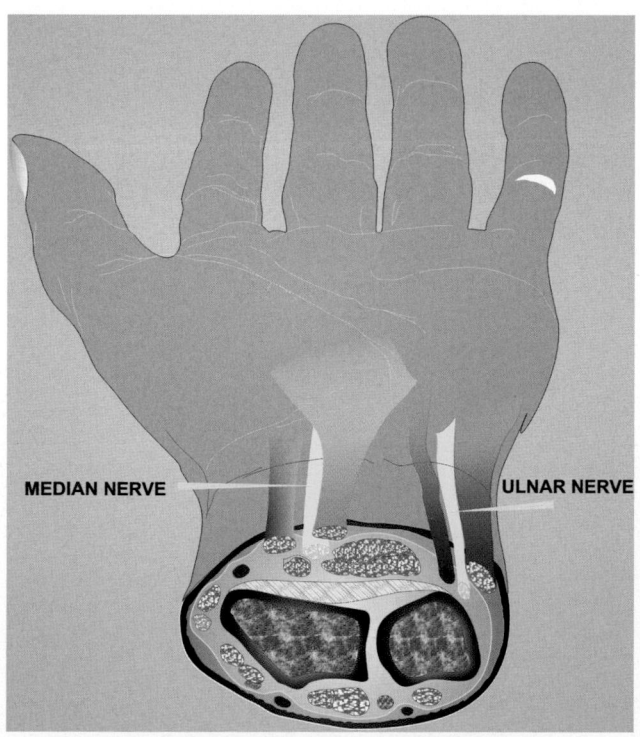

Figure 3–29. Innervation of the wrist joint.

Hip Joint

Nerves to the hip joint include the nerve to the rectus femoris from the femoral nerve, branches from the anterior division of the obturator nerve, and the nerve to the quadratus femoris from the sacral plexus (Figure 3–31).

Knee Joint

Knee innervation is obtained from branches from the femoral, obturator, and sciatic nerves (Figure 3–32). Articular branches from the tibial and common peroneal divisions of the sciatic nerve, together with fibers from the posterior division of the obturator nerve, may also contribute to the innervation of the joint.

Ankle Joint

The innervation of the ankle joint is quite complex and involves the terminal branches of the peroneal (deep and superficial peroneal nerves), tibial (posterior tibial nerve), and femoral nerves (saphenous nerve). A more simplistic view is that the entire innervation of the ankle joint stems from the sciatic nerve, with the exception of the skin on the medial aspect around the medial malleolus (saphenous nerve, a branch of the femoral nerve (Figure 3–33).

AUTONOMIC COMPONENT OF SPINAL NERVES

All spinal nerves transmit autonomic fibers to glands and smooth muscle in the region they innervate. The autonomic

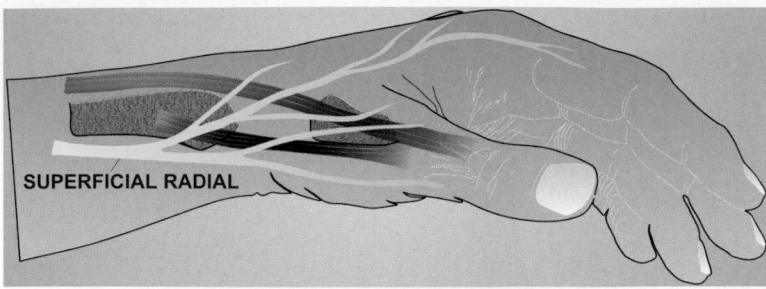

Figure 3–30. Innervation of the wrist joint.

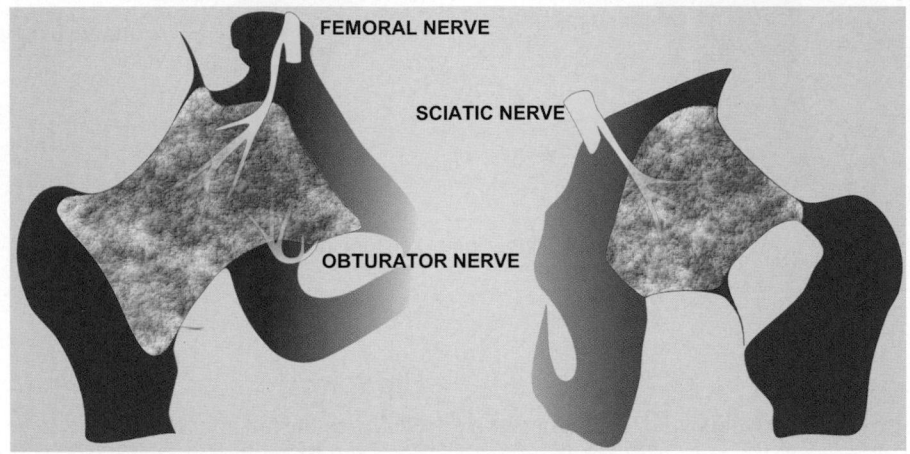

Figure 3–31. Hip joint—sensory innervation.

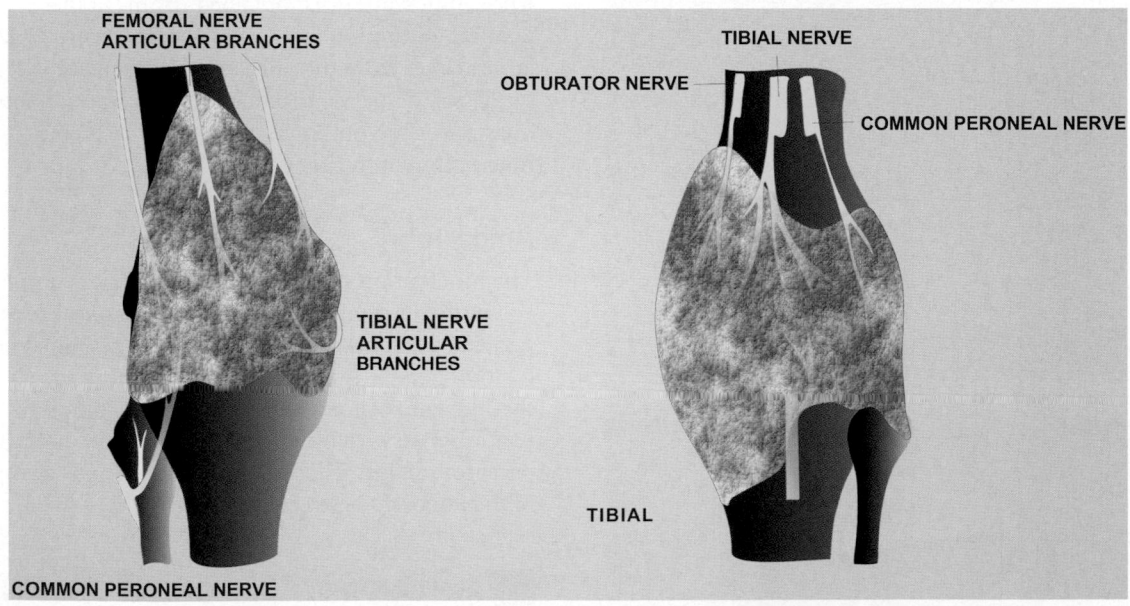

Figure 3–32. Knee joint—sensory innervation.

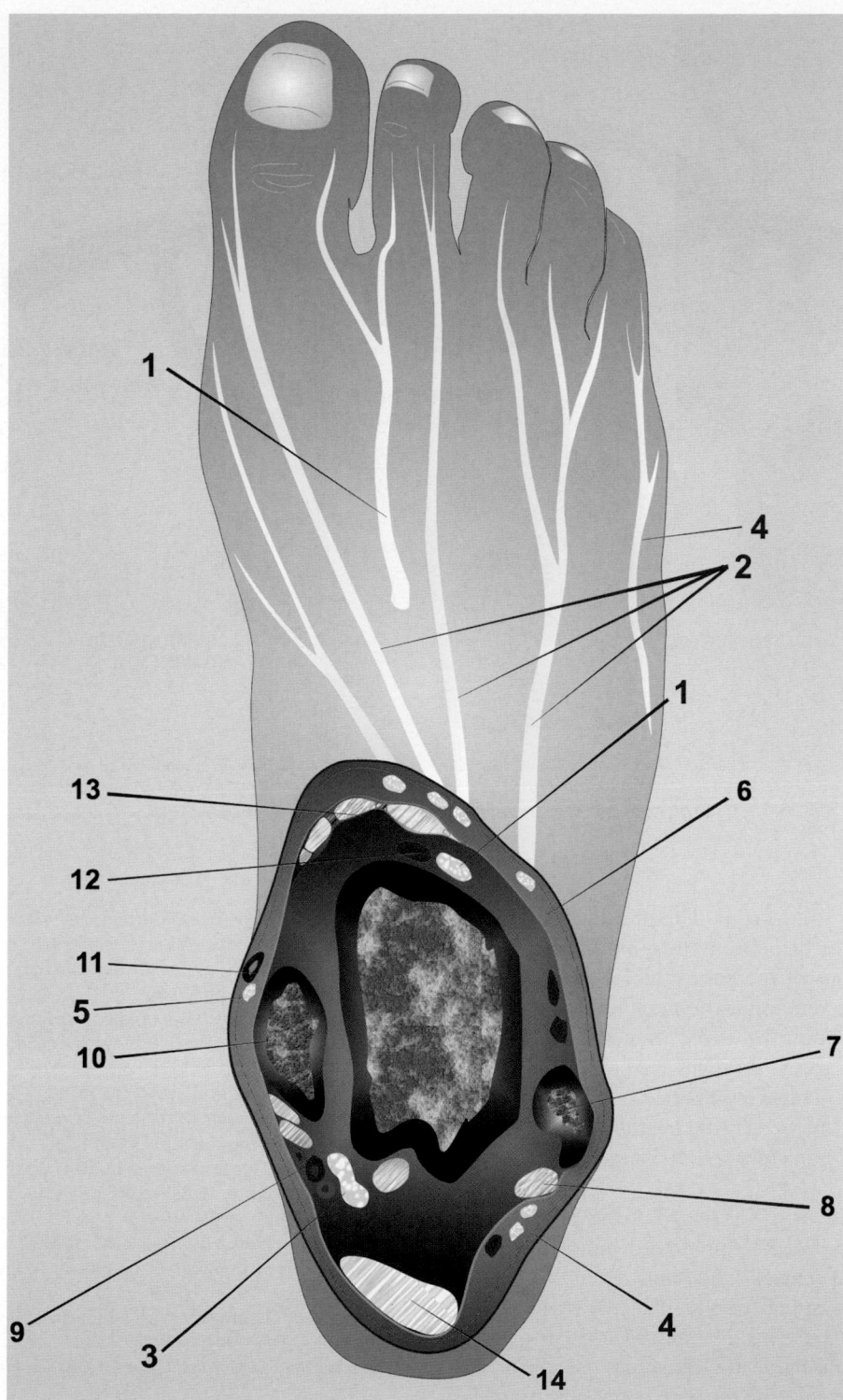

Figure 3–33. Innervation of the foot. (1) Deep peroneal nerve, (2) superficial peroneal nerve, (3) posterior tibial nerve, (4) sural nerve, (5) saphenous nerve, (6) dorsalis pedis fascia, (7) lateral malleolus, (8) tendon of the peroneus brevis muscle, (9) posterior tibial vessels, (10) medial malleolus, (11) great saphenous vein, (12) anterior tibial artery, (13) extensor hallucis longus tendon, (14) Achilles' tendon.

fibers are sympathetic. There are no parasympathetic fibers in spinal nerves. Sympathetic fibers originate in the spinal cord between T1 and L2. They pass from the spinal cord through the ventral roots of the T1 to L2 spinal nerves. They depart from the spinal nerve through white rami communicans to enter the sympathetic trunk. The sympathetic trunk is formed by a series of interconnected paravertebral ganglia, which are adjacent to the vertebral bodies and extend from the

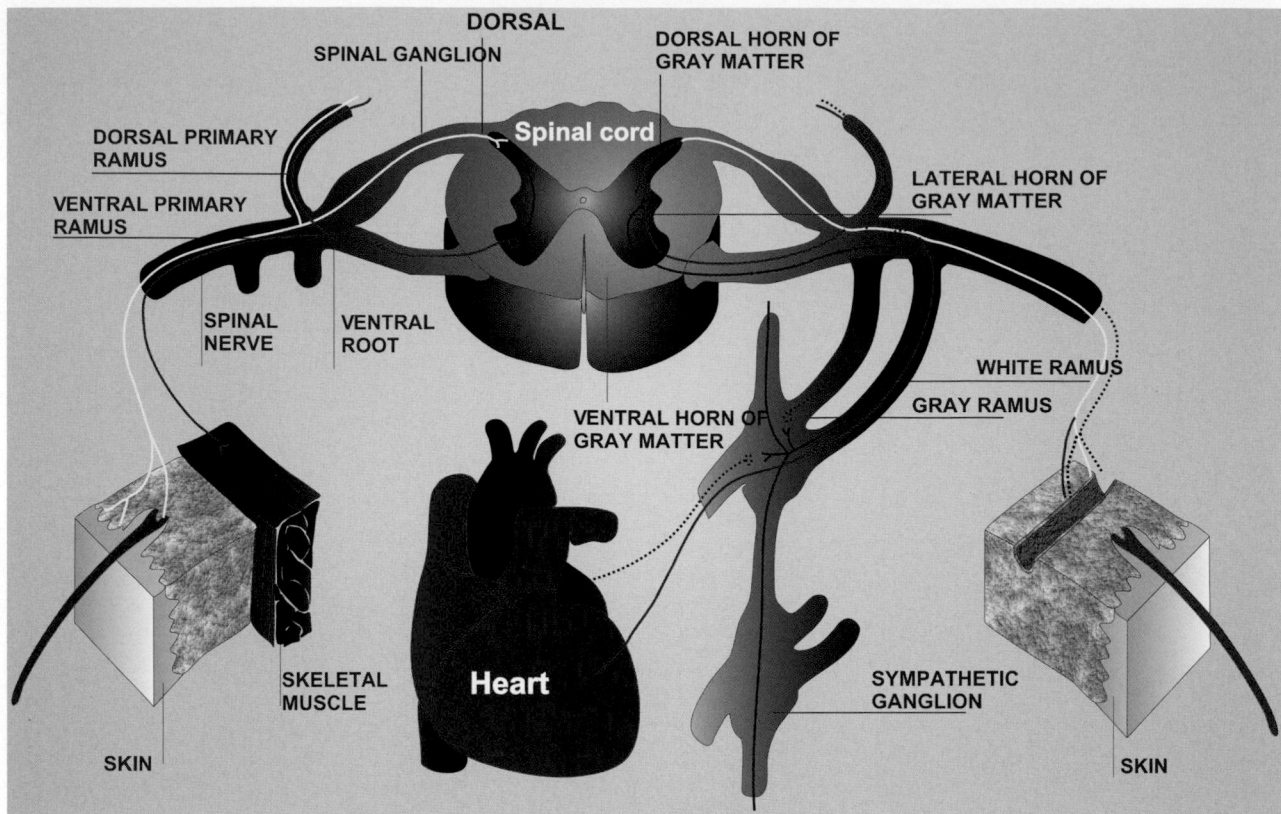

Figure 3–34. Organization of the autonomic nervous system.

axis (C2 vertebra) to the sacrum. The preganglionic fibers synapse on cell bodies of neurons forming the paravertebral ganglia. The axons of the paravertebral ganglia (postganglionic fibers) can remain at the same level or they can change level by ascending or descending the trunk. The fibers pass from the trunk through gray rami communicans to spinal nerves. The sympathetic trunk sends a gray ramus to every spinal nerve. The sympathetic nerves travel along branches of the spinal nerve to the target destination[19] (Figure 3–34).

Parasympathetic fibers arise from the lumbosacral plexus. They originate in the spinal cord between S2 and S4, pass through the ventral roots, and enter the ventral rami of the S2 to S4 spinal nerves. The parasympathetic fibers separate from the ventral rami and form the pelvic splanchnic nerve. This nerve travels across the pelvic diaphragm (formed by levator ani and coccygeus muscles) to synapse on intramural ganglia in the wall of the pelvic viscerae.[20,21]

References

1. Kingsley R (ed): *The Gross Structure of the Nervous System, Concise Text of Neuroscience.* Lippincott Williams & Wilkins, 2000, pp 1–90.
2. Moore K, Dalley A: *Introduction to Clinically Oriented Anatomy.* Lippincott Williams & Wilkins, 1999, p 42.
3. Fix J: Neurohistology. In Baltimore KS (ed): *Neuroanatomy.* Williams & Wilkins, 1992, pp 59–69.
4. Gardner E, Bunge R: Gross anatomy of the peripheral nervous system. In Dyck P, Thomas P (eds): *Peripheral Neuropathy.* Elsevier Saunders, 2005, pp 11–34.
5. Spinal nerves. In Williams P, Bannister L, Berry M, et al (eds): *Gray's anatomy: The anatomical basis of medicine and surgery,* 38th ed. Churchill-Livingstone, 1995, pp. 1258–1292.
6. Foerster O: The dermatomes in man. Brain 1933:1–8.
7. Fix J: Spinal cord. In Baltimore KS (ed): *Neuroanatomy.* Williams & Wilkins, 1992, pp 59–69.
8. Moore K: Neck. In Moore K, Dalley A: *Introduction to Clinically Oriented Anatomy.* Lippincott Williams & Wilkins, 1999, p 42.
9. Harris W: The true form of the brachial plexus and its motor distribution. J Anat 1904;38:399.
10. Harris W: *The Morphology of the Brachial Plexus.* Humprey Milford, 1939.
11. Kerr A: The brachial plexus of nerves in man, the variations in its formation and branches. Am J Anat 1918;23:285.
12. Sunderland S: The metrical and non-metrical features of the muscular branches of the radial nerve. J Comp Neurol 1946; 85:93.
13. Sunderland S, Ray L: Metrical and nonmetrical features of the muscular branches of the median nerve. J Comp Neurol 1946;85:191.
14. Sunderland S, Hughes E: Metrical and nonmetrical features of the muscular branches of the ulnar nerve. J Comp Neurol 1946;85:113.

15. Moore K: Thorax and abdomen. In Moore K, Dalley A: *Introduction to Clinically Oriented Anatomy.* Lippincott Williams & Wilkins, 1999, p 85.

16. MHorwitz M: The anatomy of the lumbosacral nerve plexus—Its relationship to vertebral segmentation and the posterior sacral nerve plexus. Anat Rec 1939;74:91.

17. Webber R: Some variations in the lumbar plexus of nerves in man. Acta Anat 1961:44:336–345.

18. Chung K: Abdomen. In Chung K (ed): *Gross Anatomy,* 3rd ed. Williams & Wilkins, 1995, pp 177–178.

19. Alast R: Innervation of the limbs. J Bone Joint Surg [Br] 1949;31:452.

20. Keegan J, Garrett F: The segmental distribution of the cutaneous nerves in the limbs of man. Anat Rec 1948;102:409.

21. Langley J: *The Autonomic Nervous System.* Heffer, 1926.

4

Histology of Peripheral Nerves

Zakira Mornjaković, MD • Steven Deschner, MD

INTRODUCTION

Knowledge of histology is vital to understanding cell function and the composition of the tissue layers and planes, as well as being relevant to clinical practice of regional anesthesia. The primary objective of this chapter is to provide a basic understanding of the structure, classification, and organization of peripheral nerves.

MORPHOLOGIC ORGANIZATION OF PERIPHERAL NERVOUS SYSTEM

The peripheral nervous system consists of sensory afferent (centripetal) nerve fibers connecting receptors to the central nervous system (CNS) and motor efferent (centrifugal) nerve fibers connecting the CNS to muscle or glands. The system includes somatic and autonomic nerves, as well as their associated Schwann cells and connective tissue sheaths. All lie peripheral to the pial covering of the CNS, through which the central and peripheral nerve fibers are continuous.[1]

The connection between the CNS and the peripheral structures derived from the somites and neural crest is formed by axon growth from the dorsal root ganglia into the alar plate of the neural tube and by axon outgrowth from neurons in the basal plate. These distally growing motor axons join the peripherally growing sensory axons of the dorsal root ganglia to form nerves innervating the somite at the same level, Figure 4–1. Nerves formed in this fashion at spinal level are the spinal nerves; those formed at the posterior fossa

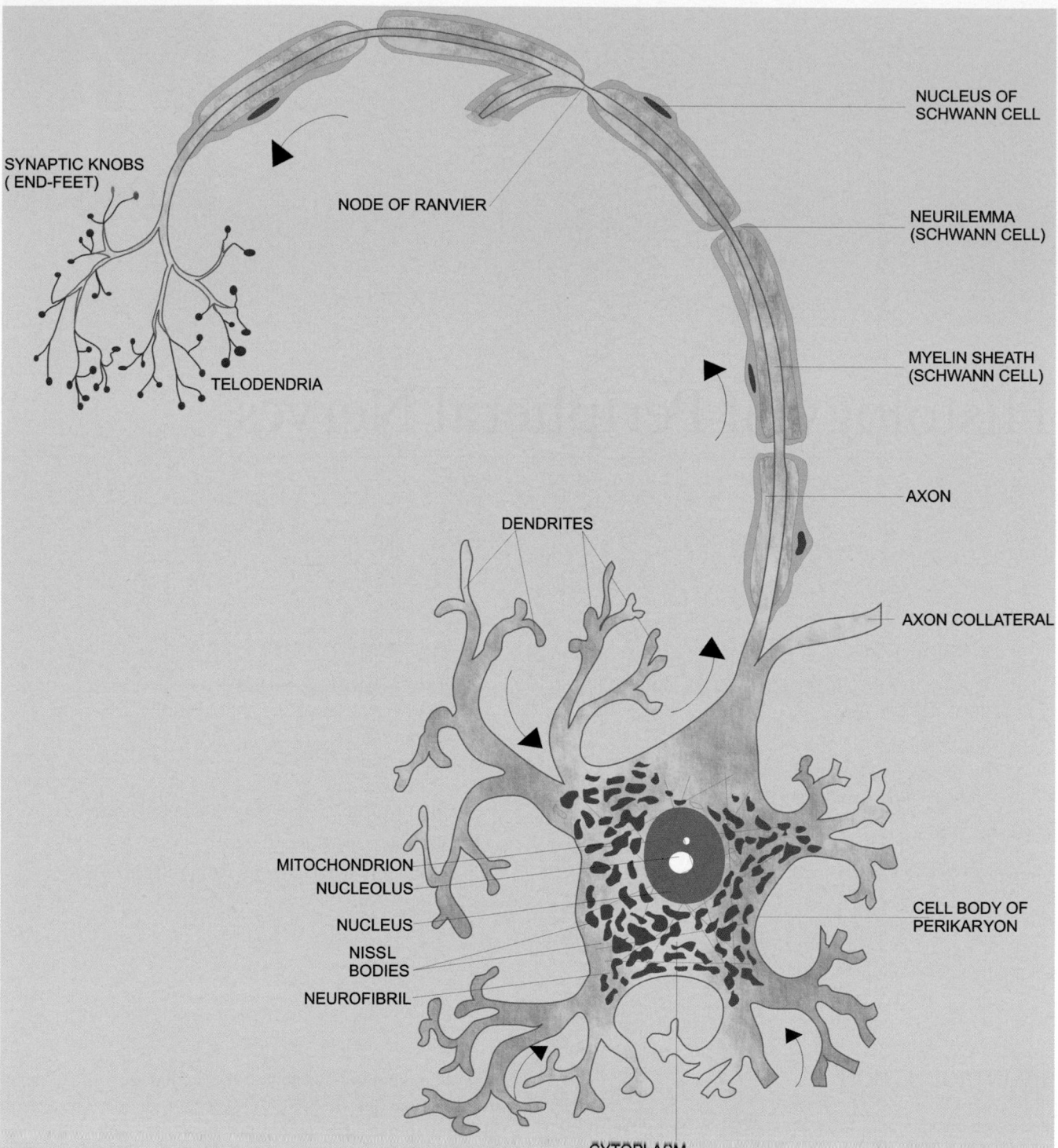

Figure 4–1. Anatomy of the peripheral nerve. Shown are the cell body, axon with its myelin sheath, nodes of Ranvier, synaptic terminals, and the direction of the transmission.

and supratentorial levels are the cranial nerves. Both types are composed of sensory and motor axons. Motor axons from the CNS innervate the muscles and autonomic ganglia, whereas sensory axons innervate receptors in the skin, muscle, bone, and viscerae. As the embryo develops and cells forming bone, muscles, skin, and internal organs migrate to their adult locations, these neural processes will follow suit in order to establish the peripheral nerves' innervation pattern. Fibers innervating tissue derived from somites (muscles and skin) are described as somatic; fibers innervating endodermal or other mesodermal derivatives (internal organs) are called visceral.

Axons are guided to their targets by apical growth cones. The growth cone, which is thought to move by means of filopodia, is believed to guide the axon to its destination by sensing molecular markers that designate the correct route. This activity of the growth cone is called path finding. Once the growth cone reaches its target, it halts and forms a synapse. Numerous mechanisms have been proposed to explain the ability of neurons to establish correct connections with each other and with end organs.[2]

Clinical Pearls

MOTOR AXONS

- The motor axons can arise from either the somatic or autonomic system. Somatic motor neurons innervate skeletal muscle.

- Alpha motor neurons innervate the extrafusal fibers. Smaller γ motor neurons innervate the intrafusal fibers. The perikarya of these neurons are located in specific brainstem nuclei or the ventral horn of the spinal cord.

- Autonomic motor neurons innervate cardiac muscle, smooth muscle, or glands. The autonomic motor neurons can be either sympathetic and parasympathetic.

- Peripheral nerves transmit both preganglionic and postganglionic sympathetic fibers. Preganglionic fibers arise from neurons in the intermediolateral column of the spinal cord between the T1 and L2 level. The fibers travel along peripheral nerves to synapse on paravertebral or preaortic ganglia. From the ganglia, postganglionic fibers travel to cardiac muscle, smooth muscle, or glands.

- In the parasympathetic system, only preganglionic fibers are transmitted on peripheral nerves. The fibers arise from nuclei within the brainstem or sacral spinal cord. They travel along peripheral nerves to synapse on intramural ganglia in the wall of target organs.

SENSORY AXONS

- Sensory axons are either somatic or visceral. The perikarya of all sensory neurons are located in the dorsal root ganglia or sensory ganglia of the cranial nerves.

- Somatic sensory neurons transmit proprioceptive information from skeletal muscle and joints or they transmit information about touch, temperature, or pain from receptors in the body wall.

- Visceral sensory neurons transmit information about pressure or chemicals adjacent to the wall of viscerae. The axons of these neurons travel along the autonomic motor fibers, pass through the gray rami communicans, and enter the dorsal root of the spinal nerves.

Similarly to the organization of the CNS tracts, both myelinated and unmyelinated fibers occur peripherally too.[3,4]

A myelinated nerve fiber is surrounded by the plasma membrane of Schwann cell (lemmocyte). The plasma membrane spirals around the axon arranging the membranes in concentric layers. The structure is called a myelin sheath. In the myelinated nerve fiber a single axon is enclosed by a series of Schwann cells arranged along its length. The region where two adjacent Schwann cells abut and the myelin is interrupted is referred to as a node of Ranvier (Figure 4–2). Individual axons, generally less than 1.0 μm in diameter, that indent the surface of the Schwann cell and become embedded in separate troughs are known as unmyelinated nerve fibers. Each Schwann cell can sheathe many axons in this way. However, a single Schwann cell does not sheathe the entire length of a group of axons. Instead the sheath is formed by a chain of Schwann cells, the axons being passed on from cell to cell. Thus all axons in the peripheral nervous system are invaginated into Schwann cell surfaces, but myelin sheaths only form around larger axons, which represent only a small portion of peripheral nerve fibers.[1,3]

Nerve trunks and their principal branches (Figures 4–3 and 4–4) consist of parallel bundles of nerve fibers (nerve fascicles, fasciculi). The size, number, and pattern of fasciculi vary in different nerves and at different levels along their paths. The axon-associated surface glycoprotein neurofascin is implicated in axonal growth and fasciculation as revealed by antibody perturbation experiments. We will examine the basic organization of the peripheral nerves using the sural nerve as an example. The sural nerve includes 9–21 fascicles and comprises 4600–9600 myelinated nerve fibers and 19,000–45,000 unmyelinated axons[5,6] depending, on age of the nerve.

Peripheral nerves have three separate connective tissue sheaths.[3] On the outside of each peripheral nerve there is a dense irregular connective tissue sheath, the **epineurium. Perineurium** surrounds each fascicle of nerve fibers. Individual nerve fibers are embedded in a loose, delicate connective tissue (**endoneurium**), filling the space bounded by the perineurium. The connective tissue sheaths support nerve fibers and their associated blood and lymphatic vessels (see Figure 4–3).

Both central and peripheral fibers present challenges for light microscopists because of the small size of unmyelinated fibers (Figure 4–5) and a disruption of sheaths of myelinated fibers that commonly occurs due to treatment with lipid solvents prior to sectioning. Various methods have been devised to overcome these problems. It is electron microscopy, however, that has added to our knowledge perhaps more than any method.

NERVE FIBERS

As axons course through body tissues, they are associated with Schwann cells. The axon with its associated Schwann cells forms a nerve fiber. A nerve fiber is the basic structural and functional unit of peripheral nerves (Figure 4–6).

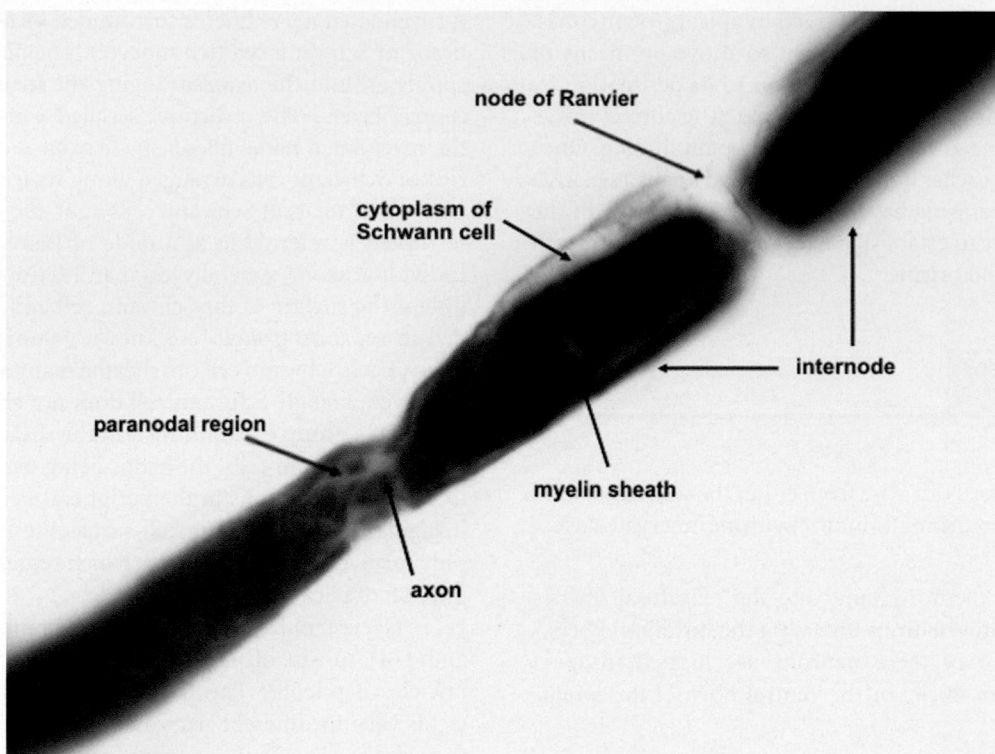

Figure 4–2. Nodes of Ranvier.

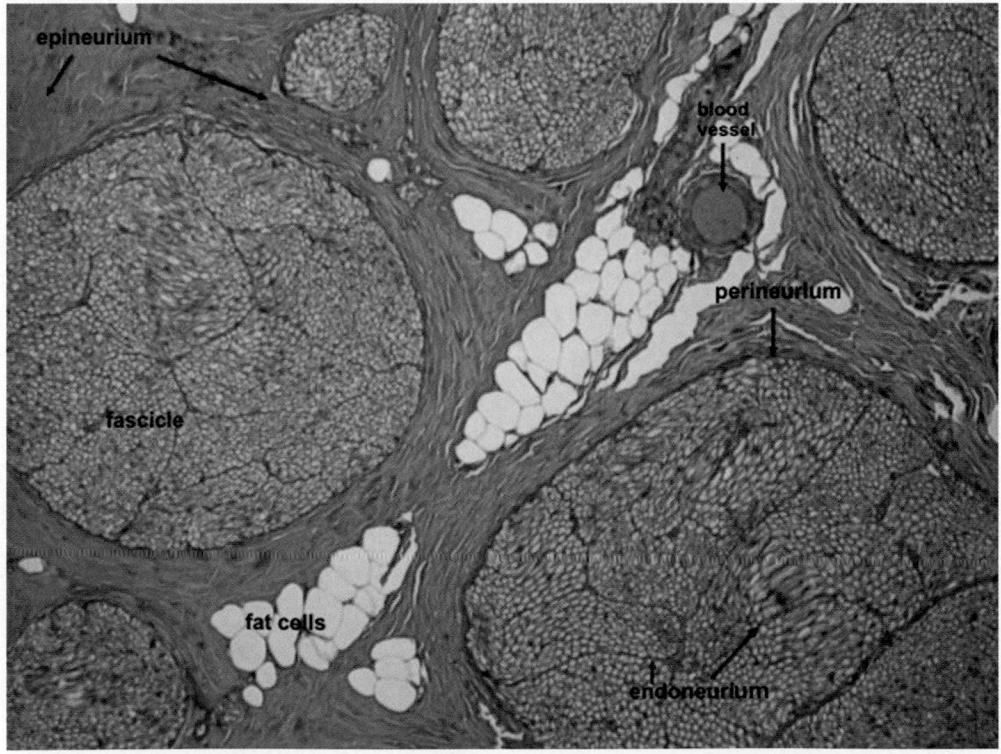

Figure 4–3. Connective tissue sheaths and fascicles of the human ulnar nerve as seen on light microscopy (Hematoxylin–eosin × 400).

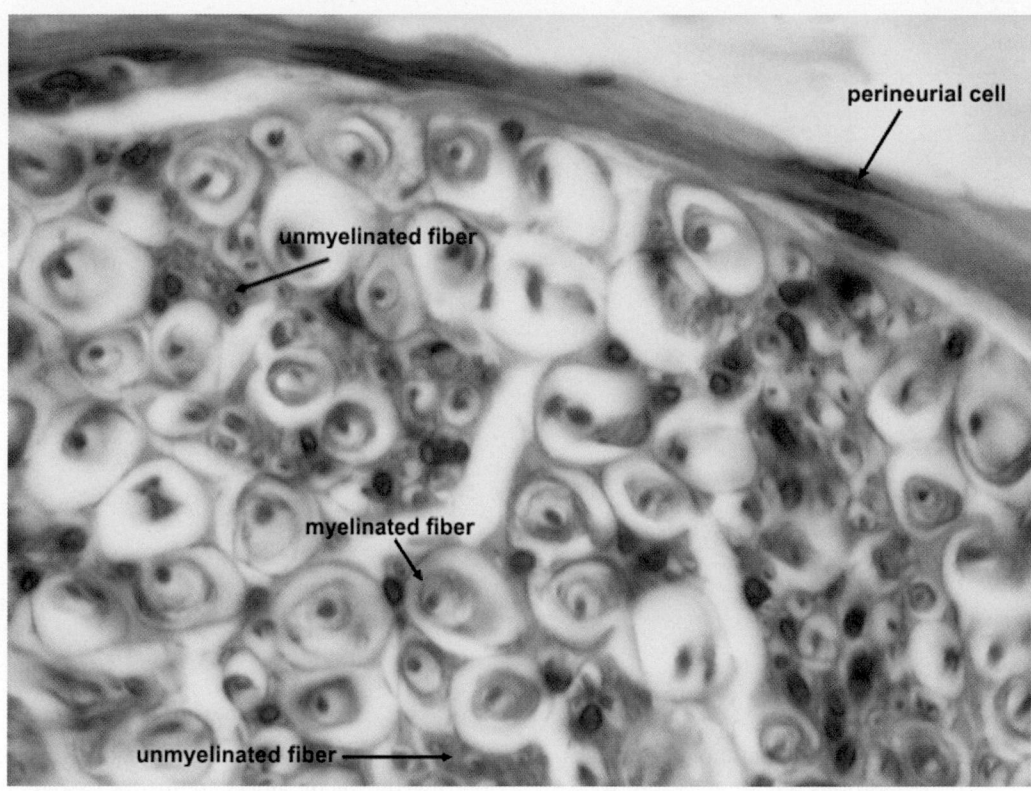

Figure 4–4. Myelinated and unmyelinated nerve fibers bundled in a fascicle by perineurial membrane. Light microscopic image of rat sciatic nerve in cross section (Hematoxylin–eosin × 400).

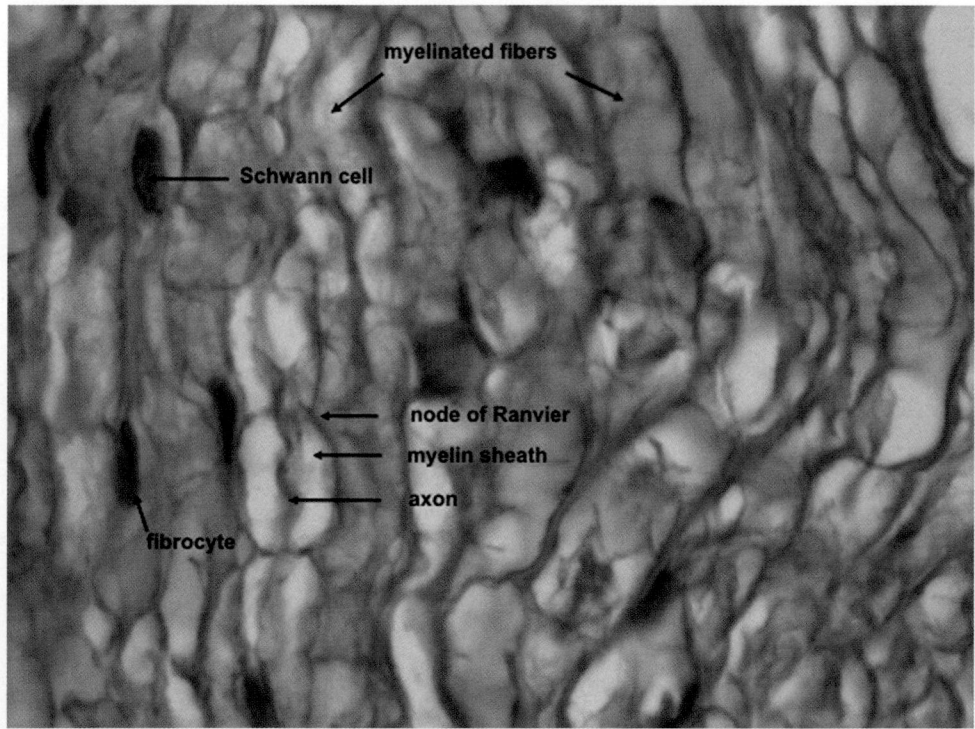

Figure 4–5. Organization of the nerve shown in longitudinal section (Bodian × 400).

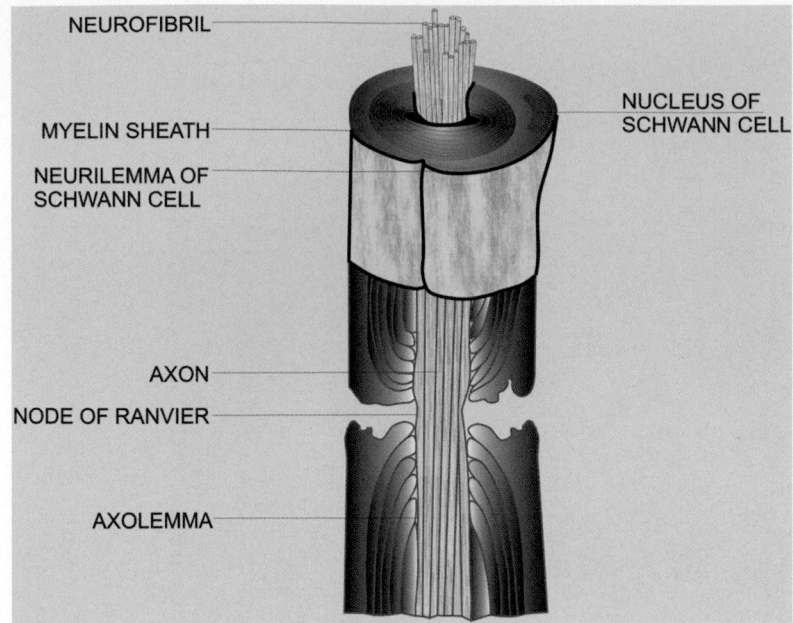

NEUROFIBRIL

NUCLEUS OF
SCHWANN CELL

MYELIN SHEATH

NEURILEMMA OF
SCHWANN CELL

AXON

NODE OF RANVIER

AXOLEMMA

Figure 4–6. Schematic diagram of an axon with its accompanying connective tissue sheaths.

Fresh myelinated fibers appear as homogeneous, glistening tubes. In stained preparations (Figure 4–7) appearance of various constituents of the nerve fiber differs according to the technique applied (Table 4–1). Motor nerve fibers of the skeletal muscles are thick and heavily myelinated; those of visceral smooth muscle are thin, lightly myelinated, or without myelin. Tactile fibers are medium-sized and moderately myelinated, whereas pain and taste fibers are thinner, with less myelin or none at all. In comparison, olfactory nerve filaments are always unmyelinated.[1,3]

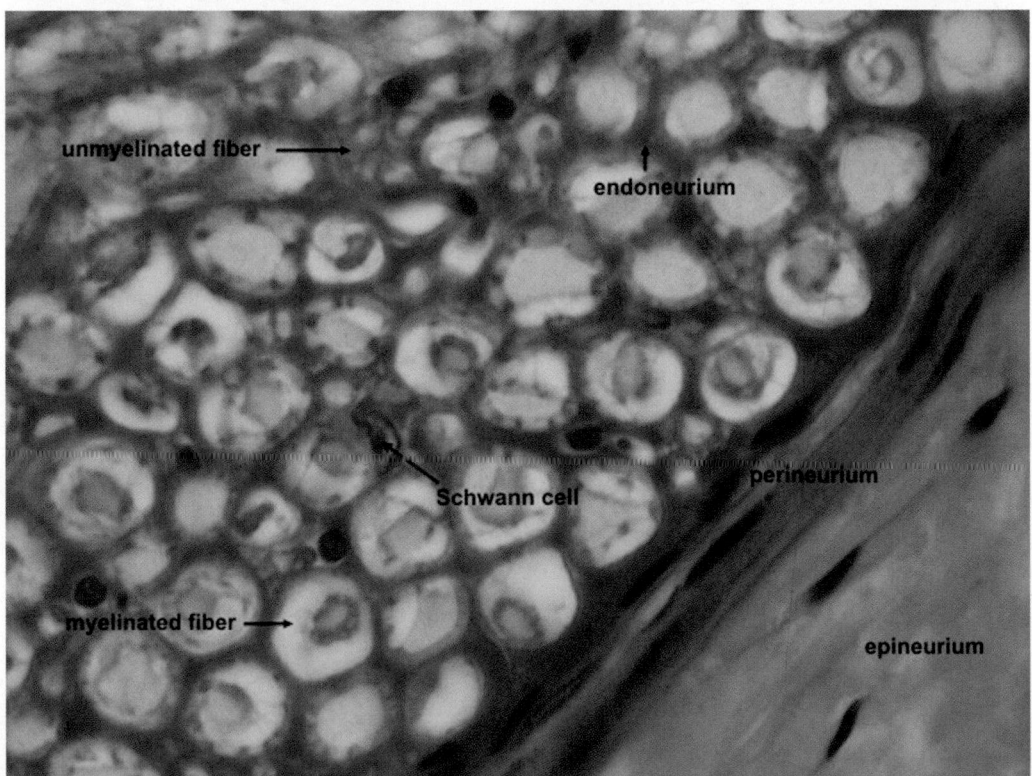

Figure 4–7. Exaggerated Schwann cells shown in cross section (×400).

Table 4–1.

Histological Techniques for Peripheral Nerves

Technique	Application
General	
Hematoxylin and eosin	Myelin and axons
Hematoxylin van Giesen	Myelin, black; collagen, red
Reticulin stains	Basement membrane of Schwann cells
Toluidine blue	Mast cells; general stain for semithin resin sections
Stains for Myelin	
Luxol-fast blue	Myelin, blue
Osmium	Myelin, black
Loyez	Myelin, black
Periodic acid Virgule Schiff (PAS)	Myelin, bright pink
Marchi	Normal myelin, unstained
Oil red O (frozen sections)	Normal myelin, pink
Stains for Axons	
Palmgren or Bodian (silver stains)	Axons, black
Semithin resin sections	
Toluidine blue and carbol fuchsin	Myelin, black; axons, unstained; Schwann cells and other cells, pink/blue;
Toluidine blue	Myelin, black; axons, unstained; Schwann cells, blue;
Immunocytochemistry	
S–100 protein	Schwann cells
Leu-7	Schwann cells
Epithelial membrane antigen	Perineurium
Neurofilament proteins	Axons
Teased Fibers	
Osmium	Myelin; nodes of Ranvier; de- and remyelination
Enzyme histochemistry	
Mitochondrial enzymes	Schwann cell; axoplasm
Acid phosphatase	Lysosomes
Lipid histochemistry	
Sudan black B	Myelin, black
Oil red O	Myelin, red
Electron Microscopy	Ultrastructural characteristics

Classification of Nerve Fibers: Axon Diameter, Myelination, & Conduction Velocity

The diameter of axons ranges between 0.5 and 20 μm. The larger axons are myelinated. Myelination allows for saltatory conduction, which accelerates the rate of signal transmission along an axon. Therefore, larger axons transmit signal at a faster rate. Myelinated axons are designated as A fibers. The diameter of myelinated axons can range between 2 and 20 μm. Within this group, axons of larger diameter conduct signal more rapidly. The A fibers come from somatic motor and sensory neurons. The axons of α motor neurons are larger and conduct more rapidly than the axons of γ motor neurons. With sensory neurons, axon diameter is related to modality. Axons transmitting proprioception are the largest. They are followed by axons relaying perception of fine touch and finally axons transmitting thermal or pain sensation. In addition to somatic neurons, preganglionic sympathetic fibers supplying the sympathetic chain are myelinated. They form the white rami communicans. Unmyelinated axons are designated as C fibers, which come from visceral motor and sensory neurons. The autonomic fibers are unmyelinated distal to the sympathetic trunk. In addition to axons from visceral neurons, some somatic neurons sensitive to crude touch, temperature, and pain send information through C fibers.

Myelination has been used to classify axons into types A and C. The type A fibers are then further subdivided into α, β, γ, δ. Type A fibers are the typical myelinated fibers of spinal nerves. In contrast, type C are the small, unmyelinated nerve fibers that conduct impulses at low velocities. The C fibers constitute more than one half the sensory fibers in most peripheral nerves as well as all the postglanglionic autonomic fibers. Figure 4–8 illustrates the sizes, velocities of conduction, and functions of the different nerve fibers found in human body. It should be noted that there is a substantial difference in the speed of conduction among different fibers. For instance, some large fibers can conduct as fast as 120 m/sec, whereas smaller fibers may conduct at only 0.5 m/sec. In other words, information from the periphery to the spinal cord or brain can be transmitted in a split second with larger fibers, whereas with slow conducting fibers it may take up to 2 sec of delay.

The reader should know that other systems of classification besides the one presented here are occasionally used in physiologic studies (eg, sensory physiologists). Further discussion on this topic, however, is beyond the intended scope of this chapter.

AXONS

The processes of a nerve cell, often called neurites, may be divided into dendrites and axons, (see Figure 4–1) The axon (or axis cylinder) is the longest process of a nerve cell body, and it carries the response of the neuron in the form of a propagated action potential. The axons of many nerve cells have a prominent sheath of material called myelin.

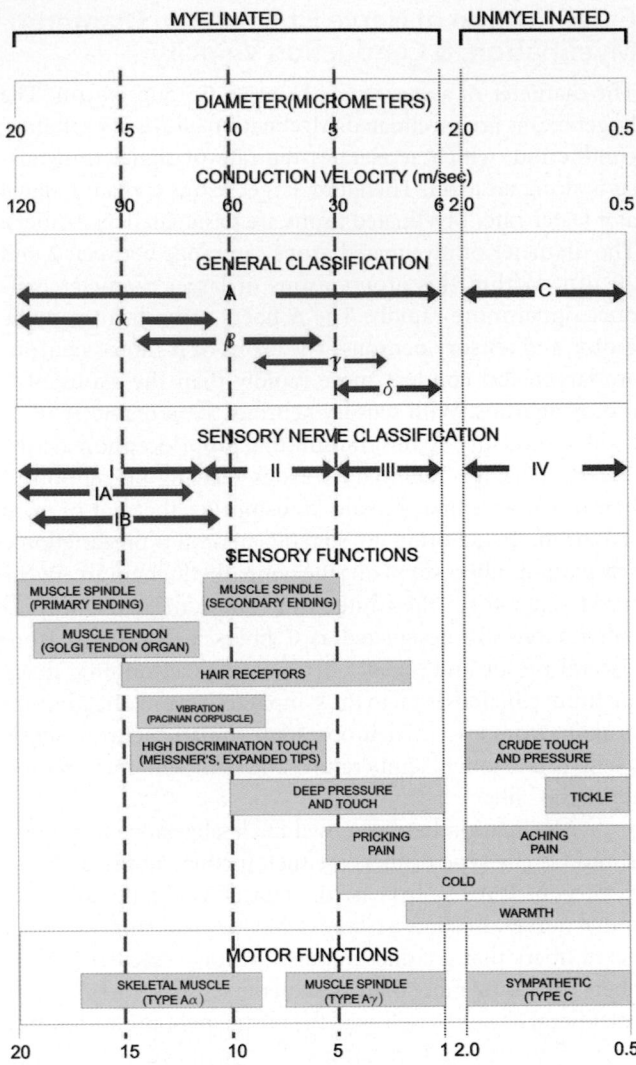

Figure 4–8. Classification and function of peripheral nerves.

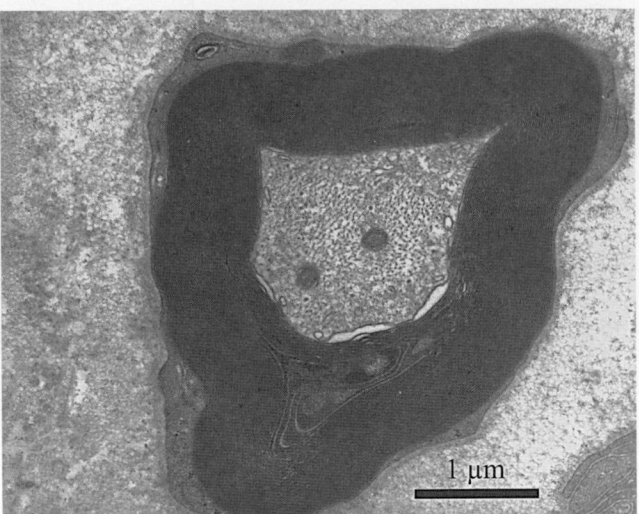

Figure 4–9. Electromicrograph of the Schwann cell.

The myelin and the Schwann sheath appear distinct with the light microscopy and were formerly considered separate structures. It should be noted that Schwann cells are considered to be electrically silent satellite cells, although they exhibit ionic channels, some of which are similar to those employed by axons for the generation and transmission of nerve impulses. Schwann cells generate, in response to a short and gentle electrical stimulus, a long-lasting depolarizing potential, slowly propagating along the Schwann cell. This electrical signal, which might be generated by the Schwann cells in response to the axonal electrical activity, constitutes in the peripheral glia a form of long-range intercellular signaling, which may be involved in the regulation and modulation of the axonal excitability.[7]

Electron microscopy shows that myelin is actually part of the Schwann cell (Figure 4–9), consisting of spirally wrapped layers of its surface membrane.[4,8,9] The presence or absence of myelin exerts an important influence on the physiologic properties of the neuron. Because it is associated only with axons, it provides a criterion for recognizing them—

except, of course, for those axons that are devoid of a myelin sheath (unmyelinated axons).

The axon[4,8–10] is smooth in outline, usually of constant diameter, and surrounded by a plasma membrane (7–8 nm thick) called the axolemma. Modifications of the basic axolemmal structure occur in the following sites: at nodes of Ranvier, in the paranodal region, in chemical synapses (synaptic complex), and in electronic synapses (gap junction). The axon cytoplasm is called the axoplasm.

The axoplasm contains cisternae of smooth endoplasmic reticulum (composed of two subsystems: (1) the central portion extending through most of the axoplasm as a complex of rather narrow and long tubules and irregularly shaped sacs, oriented parallel to the long axis; and (2) the peripheral portion, just beneath the axolemma in the form of tubules and flattened sacs), mitochondria (thin and often several micrometers long, oriented parallel to the length of the axon, may have longitudinally arranged cristae), peroxisomes, glycogen granules, and vesicles containing neurotransmitters. In some axons, there is a small numbers of free ribosomes.[11–15]

The axon diameter varies considerably with different neurons; those of larger diameter conduct impulses rapidly.[3] Morphometric alterations of myelinated axons exist with aging.[16] Normal axons narrow at the nodes of Ranvier. When fibers branch, they do so at nodes. The distal ends of the terminal branches (called terminals) are often enlarged and have specific structural characteristics.

SCHWANN CELLS

Schwann cells participate[17–19] in supplying metabolites and trophic factors to axons, in maintaining the ionic state of the periaxonal space, in siting of sodium channels along the axolemma, and in distributing neurotransmitters, etc. Conversely, Schwann cells depend on axons for many aspects of their biology (size of the cell territories, cell differentiation

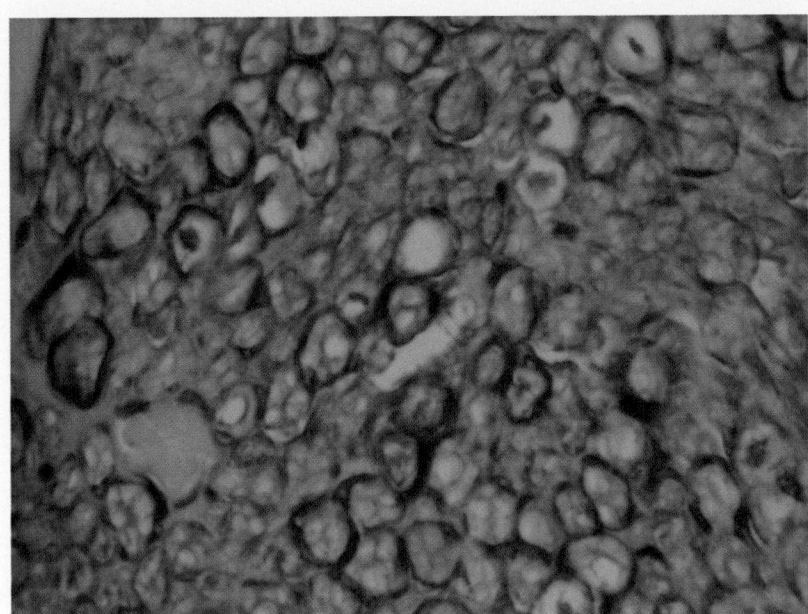

Figure 4–10. Immunohistologic image of peripheral nerve depicting Schwann cells on light microscopy.

and mitotic activity). Experimental evidence also suggests that continued axon regeneration depends on the presence of Schwann cells.[20] In a study of early forelimb development, Noakes and Bennett[21] used the antibody HNK-1 to identify Schwann cells. They have found HNK-1-positive Schwann cells in forelimb myotomes before motor axons arrived and suggest that Schwann cells might have "path finder" and guidance functions for growing axons. Schwann cells are derived from the neural crest[2] and as they associate with axons, they move along with them, become spindle-shaped, and acquire a basal lamina. The migratory Schwann cells grow in number by mitotic division and form a complete layer on the outside of the fiber bundle. Also, they start to invade between the axons. Their processes subdivide the axons into groups. While moving, Schwann cells are ovoid, have several long processes ending in blunt expansions, but they lack a basal lamina. Different Schwann cell phenotypes are caused by no axonal contact, contact with multiple small axons, contact with a single large axon, or contact with degenerating axons. Schwann cell phenotypes are characterized by distinct morphologies[4,22] and the differential expression of myelin proteins, cell adhesion molecules, receptors, enzymes, intermediate filament proteins, ion channels, and extracellular matrix proteins.[23] Schwann cells can be identified in paraffin sections by immunocytochemistry Figure 4–10.

MYELINATED AXONS

As maturation continues, some Schwann cells[4,8,9,22–25] become related to only a single axon, these usually being the axons of larger diameter. Axons below 1.0 μm in diameter do not appear to stimulate myelin formation. The Schwann cell rotates around the axon and may form 50 or more spirals, resulting in formation of the myelin sheath. By electron microscopy it is seen as regularly repeating lamellated structure

with a 12- to 18-nm periodicity. As the Schwann cell enwraps the axon, it leaves a 20-nm-wide periaxonal space of Klebs. This space is in continuity with the extracellular space at the node of Ranvier.

One Schwann cell is responsible for the formation of one internodal length of myelin. In the adult nerve, normal Schwann cells may extend up to 1.5 mm in length along myelinated fibers (the internodal distance varies directly with the diameter of fiber from 150 to 1500 μm). The internodal segments are shorter in the terminal portion of the fiber. Each myelin lamella ends in contact with the paranodal axolemma as an expanded loop containing spiraling microtubules and dense cytoplasm. The external paranodal cytoplasm of Schwann cells sends a number of digital processes curving to contact the naked nodal axolemma; these fingers are numerous in large fibers, but few in smaller ones.

During their growth, the compact myelin sheath and the persisting cytoplasm are contained in a series of small helical pockets—the Schmidt–Lanterman clefts, or myelin incisures. The incisures of Schmidt–Lanterman are seen on longitudinal sections of myelinated nerve fibers as oblique interruptions in compacted myelin lamellae. The number of Schmidt–Lanterman clefts correlates with the axon diameter; the larger the fiber, the more clefts in the Schwann cell. The cytoplasmic layer on the inside of the myelin is usually quite thin, but on the outside it is much thicker. Cytoplasm in the clefts contains membrane-bound dense bodies, lysosomes, and a single microtubule running circumferentially around the fiber.

The elongated Schwann cells nuclei forming myelin segments are located at the midpoint between adjacent nodes of Ranvier and are closely related to the myelin sheath. Therein the Schwann cell nucleus and its surrounding organelles form a bulge. The Schwann cytoplasm is rich in mitochondria, polyribosomes, Golgi cisterns, and rough endoplasmic reticulum. The cells include vimentin intermediate filaments.

With increasing age, Schwann cells accumulate lipofuscin and in the paranuclear cytoplasm pi granules of Reich (lamellated, osmiophilic, rich in acid phosphatase).

Schwann cells produce basement membrane composed of laminin, fibronectin, and entactin, heparin sulfate, collagens type III, IV, and V, and protein BM-40. There is a rich reticulin network investing each cell.

The close interrelation of axons and Schwann cells is confirmed by their mutual reactions to injury. Any disturbance of either structure results in cellular alterations. Any metabolic or chemical damage that may primarily affect Schwann cells results in demyelination or hypomyelination, but not always in axonal degeneration.[17]

UNMYELINATED AXONS

Each axon, usually less than 1.0 μm in diameter, indents the surface of the Schwann cell. As many as 15 or more axons may share a single Schwann cell. Axons are embedded in Schwann cells, and they run from one cell to another, with a series of such cells occurring along their lengths. There are no nodes of Ranvier. Axons are usually separated from one another by tongues of Schwann cell cytoplasm, but are sometimes further isolated by separate processes of cytoplasm converging in the perinuclear region. The periaxonal space is 10–15 nm wide. The endoneurial tissue fluid reaches the periaxonal space between the mesaxonal membranes. (The line of axonal invagination during development is marked by a mesaxon.)

Schwann cells associated with unmyelinated fibers grow in length to reach approximately 250 μm (in sural nerve between 200 and 500 μm). On Schwann cell extremities, their cytoplasmic processes interdigitate. The cytoplasm contains rough endoplasmic reticulum, Golgi apparatuses, mitochondria, lysosomes, microtubules, microfilaments, and an oval nucleus with one or more prominent nucleoli.

Pi granules are not present. Schwann cells associated with unmyelinated axons lack myelin-associated glycoprotein (MAG), which is necessary for segregation and myelination of axons.

The collagen fibers may be invaginated into the surface of Schwann cells associated with unmyelinated fibers and be separated from cells by a layer of basement membrane. The basement membrane appears deeply black in silver preparations due to the presence of reticular fibers, and it stains red after periodic acid/Schiff for its polysaccharides.

Connective Tissue Sheaths of Peripheral Nerves

On the outside of each peripheral nerve there is a collagenous epineurium and beneath it a perineurium, which surrounds each fascicle of nerve fibers (see Figure 4–3). Individual nerve fibers are embedded in endoneurium, which completely fills the space bounded by the perineurium. These three connective tissue sheaths surround the larger peripheral nerves composed of numerous fascicles of nerve fibers. As the peripheral nerve divides and the number of fascicles is reduced, the connective tissue sheaths become progressively thinner. Around monofascicular nerves the epineurium is lacking, intermittent, or merged with the perineurium. Before the individual nerve fibers terminate, their connective tissue sheaths become attenuated and dispersed and are no longer distinguishable from the general connective tissue.[1,3,4,22,24,25]

Epineurium

This outermost sheath consists of moderately dense connective tissue binding nerve fascicles (see Figures 4–3, 4–4, and Figure 4–7). It merges with adipose tissue surrounding peripheral nerves, particularly in subcutaneous tissue. The amount of epineurial tissue varies and is more abundant in nerves adjacent to joints. The epineurium is lacking around monofascicular nerves.

The epineurium contains fibroblasts, connective tissue fibers, mast cells, small lymphatics, as well as blood vessels and some small nerve fibers innervating the vessels. Fibroblasts are ultrastructurally identical to fibroblasts elsewhere in the body. Scattered throughout the epineurium these cells form the epineurial collagen, the most prominent component of the epineurium. Collagen fibrils are mainly oriented longitudinally. Collagen is a protein that stains with most acid dyes. In sections stained with hematoxylin and eosin, collagen fibers stain weakly pink with eosin; they stain red with hematoxylin van Giesen's stain, and blue with Mallory's trichrome stain. Collagen fibers are green or blue in Masson's trichrome, depending on the modification used, ie, whether the stain contains light green or aniline blue. The electron microscope fibrils of mature collagen have periodic cross bandings. Elastin fibers are also present, and these are much stouter than collagen fibrils. They stain weak pink in sections stained with hematoxylin and eosin, brown with orcein, and blue-purple with resorcin-fuchsin. In electron micrographs elastin fibers are usually most darkly stained at their peripheries and embedded in a ground substance containing finer elastin filaments.

Mast cells are rounded or spindle-shaped, and their cytoplasm is packed with granules staining metachromatically with basic aniline dyes. Mast cells are distributed throughout connective tissue and tend to be situated close to small blood vessels.

Vasa nervorum supplying peripheral nerves are derived from a series of branches from associated regional arteries. Branches from these arteries enter the epineurium to form an intercommunicating or anastomosing plexus. From the plexus, vessels obliquely penetrate the perineurium and enter the endoneurium as arterioles and capillaries. In nerves consisting of several fascicles, one or more arteries, veins, and lymphatics run longitudinally parallel to nerve fascicles.

Perineurium

Each nerve fiber fascicle is surrounded by a connective tissue sheath, the perineurium. The perineurium consists of concentric layers of flattened cells separated by layers of collagen (see Figures 4–3 through 4–5). The number of perineurial cell layers seems to depend on the size of the sheathed nerve fascicle and its proximity to the CNS. As many as 10 concentric layers (sleeves of cells) may be present around large nerve fascicles, but a single layer of perineurial cells surrounds fine distal nerve branches. In larger peripheral nerves, the concentric cell layers alternate with layers of collagen fibrils arranged longitudinally like those of the epineurium. The collagen fibrils are rather thinner than those of the epineurium, and only a few elastic fibers are scattered among them. Perineurial cells have a basal lamina on each side. Sometimes this basal lamina may be quite thick, and, at sites known as hemidesmosomes, the perineurial cell plasma membrane strongly adheres to the basal lamina.

Under the electron microscope, perineurial cells are seen as thin sheets of cytoplasm containing small amounts of endoplasmic reticulum, filaments, and numerous endocytotic vesicles. Tight junctions (zonulae occludentes) and gap junctions between adjacent cells within the same layer of perineurium are also observed. Similar zonulae may also occur between successive layers of the perineurium when their cells are in close approximation (in the delicate nerves of the eye muscles the amount of collagen is quite small; the concentric layers of perineurial cells, which can be as thin as 0.1 μm, become closely approximated). Tight junctions in the inner layers of the perineurium and tight junctions in endoneurial capillaries form a blood–nerve barrier. The blood–nerve barrier is not equivalent to the blood–brain barrier.[26] The blood–brain barrier includes astrocytes. Astrocytes are involved in regulating the flow of multiple compounds between blood and the brain.

Endoneurium

The endoneurium immediately surrounds Schwann cells (sheath of Schwann) and completely fills the space bounded by the perineurium (see Figure 4–3). This peripheral nerve connective tissue sheath contains collagen fibers, fibroblasts, capillaries, and a few mast cells and macrophages. The collagen fibrils are concentrated in a zone beneath the perineurium and around nerve fibers and blood vessels. The collagen fibrils surrounding myelinated and unmyelinated nerve fibers may form two distinct layers. The outer endoneurial layer (the outer endoneurial sheath of Key and Retzius) consists of predominantly longitudinally oriented collagen fibrils that are closely packed together. The inner endoneurial layer (the inner endoneurial sheath of Plenk and Laidlaw) consists of fine collagen fibers randomly oriented. The endoneurial sheaths around smaller myelinated fibers and around some unmyelinated axons are not as well organized.

Fibroblasts are one of the most numerous cell types of the endoneurium. They are responsible for fiber formation, and there is evidence that they form the ground substance. When sectioned transversely, endoneurial fibroblasts have triangular or rectangular perikarya. Extending from the perikarya are processes interweaving with collagen fibrils and interdigitating with processes of other fibroblasts. The appearance of the fibroblast varies depending on its functional activity. When the cell is actively producing intercellular materials, as it is the case in normal development and in tissue regeneration after injury, the nucleus is larger, nucleoli are more prominent, and the cytoplasm stains more deeply and is basophilic in contrast with the lightly staining, slightly acidophilic cytoplasm of a relatively inactive cell. Like those in the epineurium, fibroblasts in the endoneurium lack a basal lamina.

Mast cells occur in varying numbers, being especially numerous along blood vessel courses. Mast cell granules are soluble in water and are therefore not very visible in most routinely prepared hematoxylin and eosin-stained sections. After appropriate fixation the granules stain with most basic dyes and are metachromatic after certain dyes such as toluidine blue. Electron micrographs show that the secretory granules are membrane-bounded and that, in humans, the granule matrices have varying densities and characteristic scroll-resembling patterns. Macrophages are also found in the endoneurium, frequently in the perivascular location.

Blood Supply to the Nerves (Vasa Nervorum)

In recent decades many methods (injection of various dyes, plastics, and vital microscopic methods) have become available, allowing a more complete description of the vascular architecture of peripheral nerves. These studies[1,3,4,25–27] showed that a peripheral nerve is a well-vascularized structure, with two integrated but functionally independent microvascular systems, extrinsic and intrinsic. The **extrinsic system** is composed of segmentally arranged vessels, varying in number and size, which originate from nearby large arteries and veins as well as from smaller adjacent muscular and periostal vessels. When the local nutrient vessels reach the epineurium they divide into ascending and descending branches and anastomose with intraneural intrinsic system (see Figure 4–3).

The intrinsic system is composed of the epineurial, perineurial, and endoneurial plexuses and their communicating vessels. In the epineurial plexus a large number of arterioles and venules form numerous anastomoses in all directions, as well as arteriovenular shunts. Epineurial blood vessels also have communications with plexuses in the perineurim and endoneurium. Blood vessels penetrate the perineurium obliquely and enter the endoneurium, forming the intrafascicular endoneurial vascular bed, which extends along the whole length of the nerve and consisting mainly of capillaries. Like capillaries elsewhere, those of the endoneurium have their associated pericytes, and, as usual, these cells are completely enclosed in a basal lamina. Tight junctions between the endothelial cells of the endoneurial capillaries constitute the blood–nerve barrier.

TRANSITION ZONE

All spinal nerves have zones of transition where the cells that myelinate axons change from oligodendrocytes to Schwann cells. Where the transition occurs, astrocytes invaginate into the node of Ranvier to form a glia limitans. This barrier may be reinforced along a single axon at several nodes. In the transition zone, the numbers of nodes is increased and the internodal distance is decreased. To prevent nodal cross-talk, individual axons are isolated from one another by astrocytes. Furthermore, nodes are offset. The transition occurs on the roots of spinal nerves near the surface of the spinal cord. As the roots pass through the vertebral canal, the axons are surrounded by Schwann cells and enclosed in pia mater. Pia mater consists of one or two layers of squamous to cuboidal cells attached by desmosomes and gap junctions. This cell layer has a basal lamina composed of loose connective tissue that expands in the nerve roots to form endoneurium. As the root approaches the intervertebral foramen, the pia mater joins the arachnoid. The cells forming the arachnoid are similar to those found in the pia mater; however, there are many more layers of cells and the cells are attached differently. In the outer layers of the arachnoid, cells are attached by tight junctions. This type of junction forms a fluid barrier to cerebrospinal fluid. The arachnoid divides into two parts at the intervertebral foramen. One part continues into the peripheral nerve as the perineurium. As described earlier, the perineurium contains cells attached by tight junctions that form a blood–nerve barrier. The second part of the arachnoid reflects onto the inner surface of the dura mater. The dura mater is a thick layer of dense irregular connective tissue that passes over the surface of the spinal cord. At the intervertebral foramina, it reflects onto the spinal nerve and becomes confluent with the epineurium (Figure 4–11).

Histologic Techniques for Peripheral Nerves

Information about selection of nerves for biopsy and techniques of excision and preparation is given by several authors.[28–30] Application of most frequent histologic techniques for normal peripheral nerves is illustrated in Table 4–1.[24]

Nerve fibers are prone to numerous artifacts if not properly excised, oriented, fixed or frozen, or embedded, cut, and stained. Semithin sections of plastic (epoxy resin)-embedded nerves are most informative. Glutaraldehyde fixation is essential for semithin sections but not for paraffin

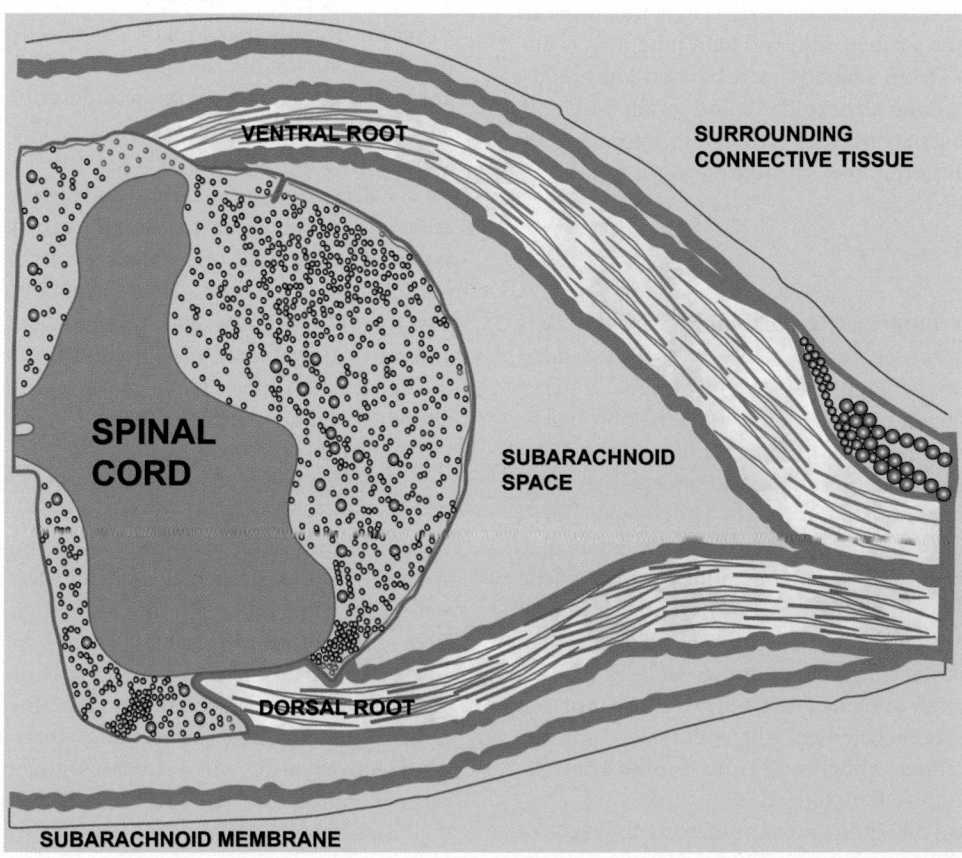

Figure 4–11. Transition of connective tissue from the spinal cord to the peripheral (spinal) nerves.

sections (paraffin blocs become too hard and difficult to cut, and it usually abolishes antigenicity for immune reactions). Paraffin sections of formalin-fixed nerve segments are still needed for measurement of fascicular diameters or areas, immunohistochemical determination of cellular infiltrates and macrophages, and for immunocytochemistry. Paraffin-embedded, fresh or frozen nerve biopsies can be used for DNA extraction. Deep-frozen nerve specimens are essential for immunohistochemical identification of components with low tissue concentration. Teased fiber preparations are good for enzyme and lipid histochemistry, as well as for examination of demyelination and remyelination (see Figure 4–1). Electron microscopic examination is extremely useful for identifying normal or abnormal ultrastructural characteristics of peripheral nerves (see Figures 4–10 and 4–11). Assay for nerve growth factor receptor (NGFR)-mRNA may be utilized as a rapid and simple method to screen for peripheral neurotoxicity. NGFR expression is also a sensitive indicator of less profound perturbation in normal axon/Schwann cell interactions.[31]

References

1. *Gray's Anatomy,* 37th ed. Churchill Livingstone, 1989, pp 896–917.
2. Larsen WJ: *Human Embryology,* 3rd ed. Churchill Livingstone, 2001, pp 113–131.
3. Boyd IA, Davey MR: Composition of Peripheral Nerves. Churchill Livingstone, 1968.
4. Peters A, Palay SL, Webster HF: *The Fine Structure of the Nervous System: Neurons and Their Supporting Cells,* 3rd ed. Oxford University Press, 1991.
5. Schröder JM, Gibbels E: Marklose nervenfasern im senium und im spatstadium der thalidomid—Polyneuropathie: Quantitativ—elektronenmikroskopische untersuchungen. Acta Neuropathol (Berl) 1977; 39:271–280.
6. Jacobs JM, Love S: Qualitative and quantitative morphology of human sural nerve at different ages. Brain 1985;108:897–924.
7. Brunet PC, Jirounek P: Long-range intercellular signalling in glial cells of the peripheral nerve. Neuroreport 1994;5(5):635–638.
8. Angevine JB: The nervous tissue. In Bloom W, Fawcett DW (eds): *A Textbook of Histology,* 10th ed. WB Saunders, 1975, pp 333–382.
9. Bischoff A: The peripheral nerves. In Vincents Johannessen (ed): *Electron Microscopy in Human Medicine.* McGraw-Hill, 1979, pp 137–236.
10. Jones EG: *The Nervous Tissue, Cell and Tissue Biology,* 6th ed. Weiss L (ed). Urban & Schwarzenberg, 1988.
11. Holenbeck PJ: The transport and assembly of the axonal cytoskeleton. J Cell Biol 1989;108:223–227.
12. Matus A: Stiff microtubules and neuronal morphology. Trends Neurosci 1994;17(1):19–22.
13. Xu Z, Marszalek JR, Lee MK, et al: Subunit composition of neurofilaments specifies axonal diameter. J Cell Biol 1996;133(5):1061–1069.
14. Starr R, Attema B, DeVries GH, et al: Neurofilament phosphorylation is modulated by myelination. J Neurosci Res 1996;44(4):328.
15. Forsman DS: Axonal transport: Visualization by light microscopy. In Adelman G (ed): *Encyclopedia of Neuroscience.* Birkhauser, 1987, p 104.
16. Knox CA: Morphometric alterations of rat myelinated fibers with aging. J Neuropathol Exp Neurol 1989;42:119–139.
17. Bunge RP: Expanding roles for the Schwann cell: Ensheathment, myelination, trophism and regeneration. Curr Opin Neurobiol 1993;3(5):805–809.
18. Orkand RK, Opava SC: Glial function in homeostasis of the neuronal microenvironment. NIPS 1994;9:265–267.
19. De Waegh SM, Lee VMY, Brady ST: Local modulation of neurofilament phosphorylation, axonal caliber and slow axonal transport by myelinating Schwann cells. Cell 1992;68:451–463.
20. Nadim W, Anderson PN, Turmaine M: The role of Schwann cells and basal lamina tubes in the regeneration of axons through long lengths of freeze-killed nerve graft. Neuropathol Appl Neurobiol 1990;16:419–429.
21. Noakes PG, Bennett MR: Growth of axons into developing muscle of the chick forelimb in preceded by cells that stain with Schwann cell antibodies. J Comp Neurol 1987;259:330–347.
22. Thomas PK, Ochoa J: Microscopic anatomy of peripheral nerve fibers. In Dyck PJ, Thomas PK, Lambert EH, et al (eds): *Peripheral Neuropathy,* 2nd ed. WB Saunders, 1984, pp 34–96.
23. Mezei C: Myelination in the peripheral nerve during development. In Dyck PJ, Thomas PK, Lambert EH, et al (eds): *Peripheral Neuropathy.* WB Saunders, 1993, pp 267–281.
24. Ortiz-Hidalgo C, Weller RO: Peripheral nervous system. In Sternberg SS: *Histology for Pathologists.* Raven Press, 1992, pp 169–193.
25. Bischoff A: The peripheral nerves. In Vincents Johannessen J: *Electron Microscopy in Human Medicine.* McGraw-Hill, 1979, 137–236.
26. Kiernan JA: Vascular permeability in the peripheral autonomic and somatic nervous systems: Controversial aspects and comparisons with the blood-brain barrier. Microsc Res Tech 1996;35(2):122–136.
27. Lundborg G: Structure and function of the intraneural microvessels as related to trauma, edema formation, and nerve function. J Bone Joint Surg 1975;57-A (7):938–947.
28. Downing AE: Neuropathological histotechnology. In Prophet EB, Mills B, Arrington JB, et al (eds): *Laboratory Methods in Histotechnology.* American Registry of Pathology, 1992, pp 81–108.
29. Schröder JM: *Pathology of Peripheral Nerves: An Atlas of Structural and Molecular Pathological Changes.* Springer, 2001, pp 1–307.
30. Evans SM, Nyengaard JR: General introduction. In Evans SM, Janson AM, Nyengaard JR (eds): *Quantitative Methods in Neuroscience a Neuroanatomical Approach.* Oxford University Press, 2004, pp 1–15.
31. Roberson MD, Toews AD, Bouldin TW, et al: NGFR-mRNA expression in sciatic nerve: A sensitive indicator of early stages of axonopathy. Brain Res Mol Brain Res 1995;28(2):231–238.

5

Peripheral Nerve Stimulators & Electrophysiology of Nerve Stimulation

Ban C. H. Tsui, MD • Admir Hadzic, MD

INTRODUCTION

Eliciting paresthesia or nerve stimulation are commonly used methods for localizing nerves prior to the injection of local anesthetic. Paresthesia is thought to result from mechanical stimulation of the nerve, resulting in a sensory feeling described as "an electric current" or "shock" in the sensory distribution of the nerve that is being touched. As such, paresthesia can indicate that the needle is in close proximity to the nerve and may be a warning sign of impending mechanical injury, should the needle be further advanced. In contrast, nerve stimulation techniques rely on the use of electric current to elicit motor stimulation of nerves and confirm the proximity of the needle to the nerve.

Electrical nerve stimulation is currently the most common technique for localizing nerves prior to the injection of local anesthetic. Depolarizing the nerve membrane results in contraction of the effector muscles (motor fibers) or in paresthesias (sensory fibers) in the distribution of the nerve. These responses can be used to confirm the proximity of a needle or catheter to the nerve. This localization technique for nerve blocks was first described by von Perthes in 1912; however, it has only gained wider acceptance in regional anesthesia over the last two decades.[1] Subsequently, a number of researchers

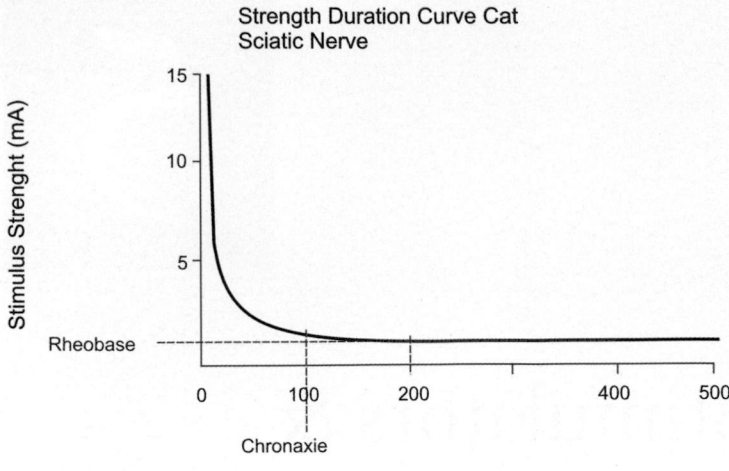

Figure 5–1. Strength–duration curve. The curve illustrates the relationship between the threshold current intensity and pulse duration. (Adapted, with permission, from Pither CE, Raj PP, Ford DJ: The use of peripheral nerve stimulators for regional anaesthesia: A review of experimental characteristics, technique, and clinical applications. Reg Anesth 1985;10:49–58).

have further improved and developed this technique. Pearson introduced the concept of using an insulated needle for the localization of nerves;[2] however, Montgomery and colleagues later demonstrated that ordinary uninsulated needles could also be used to localize nerves, albeit with a higher current.[3] The use of a portable transistorized nerve stimulator with a variable current output was first introduced by Greenblatt and Denson.[4] Ford and associates further emphasized the important characteristics of electrical nerve stimulators and the differences between insulated and uninsulated needles.[5,6] In recent years, the same electrical stimulation principles have been applied for new uses such as percutaneous electrode guidance (PEG),[7–10] confirmation of epidural catheter placement,[11–13] and peripheral catheter placement for continuous regional anesthesia.[14] The clinical relevance of the duration of the stimulating current and optimal placement of the return (skin) electrode have also been determined.[15]

In order to use nerve stimulation effectively a basic knowledge of the electrophysiologic principles is necessary. The following discussion is based on the commonly accepted theoretical and practical concepts of nerve stimulation. However, our understanding of the mechanisms of nerve stimulation is still incomplete. Thus, the reader should remain cognizant of the fact that current literature still has conflicting concepts and recommendations regarding several aspects of nerve stimulation.[16]

CHARACTERISTICS OF ELECTRICAL IMPULSE: INTENSITY, DURATION, & RATE OF CHANGE

Clinical Pearls

- Uncomfortable motor response to nerve stimulation can be avoided by using a low-intensity stimulating current with a short pulse width.
- However, when a higher current is used, preferential stimulation of the motor nerve may be lost

- Therefore, the best method to avoid discomfort on nerve stimulation is to limit the energy (E) or current intensity (I) during nerve localization.

Electrical impulses excite nerves by inducing a flow of ions through the nerve membrane, which then initiates an action potential. The characteristics of the electrical impulse affect its ability to stimulate motor and sensory nerve fibers. The quality of stimulation is also influenced by the polarity and the type of electrode, the distance between the stimulating needle and the nerve, and the interactions at the tissue–needle interface.

Intensity

A total charged (Q) applied to a nerve is equal to the product of the intensity (I) of the applied current and the duration (t) of the square pulse of the current:

$$Q = I \times t$$

The minimum current intensity (I) required to produce an action potential can be expressed by the relationship $I = Ir\,(1 + C/t)$, with three important parameters (Figure 5–1). In this equation: (t) is the duration of the applied pulse (Ir), or **rheobase,** is the minimum current intensity required to depolarize the nerve and (C), or **chronaxy** is the minimum duration of the pulse required to depolarize the nerve when the current intensity is twice the rheobase.

Chronaxy measures the stimulation threshold of the different types of nerve fibers.[17] The larger the fiber, the shorter its chronaxy and the easier it is to stimulate.[18,19] Varying the electrical pulse width can stimulate different types of nerve fibers. Large A-α motor fibers with chronaxies of 50–100 μsec can be stimulated without stimulating the smaller A-δ and C sensory fibers with chronaxies of about 150 μsec and 400 μsec, respectively.[20,21] A painless motor response to nerve stimulation can be elicited using a low-intensity stimulating current and a short pulse width because sensory fibers require a longer pulse for stimulation. The

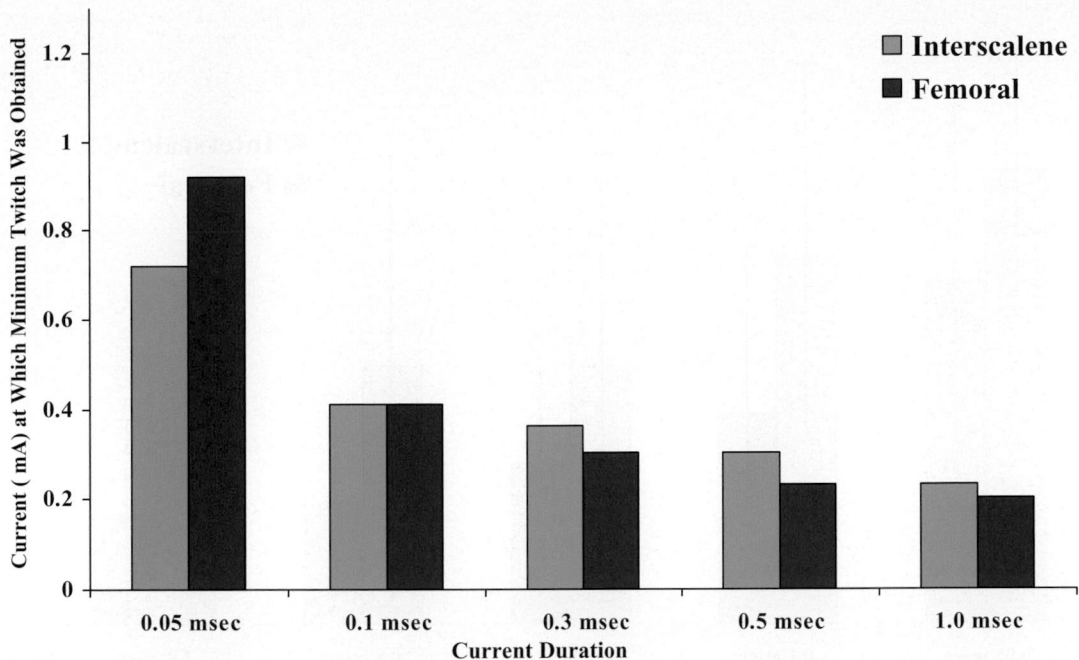

Figure 5–2. Intensity of the stimulating current required to obtain specific visible motor response during interscalene (biceps contractions) and femoral block (quadriceps contractions). Current of longer duration elicits motor response at significantly lower current intensity.

current intensity required to obtain a clinically discernable motor response is shown in Figure 5–2. However, recent data have demonstrated that choosing the pulse width to achieve sensory–motor differentiation and avoid discomfort to the patient during peripheral nerve stimulation may not be applicable in clinical practice as previously thought.[22,23] Rather, the main causes of discomfort are related to the withdrawal and repositioning of the stimulating needle,[24] maintain the strength of elicited muscle contractions, and the high-intensity of the stimulating current.[22] The discomfort on nerve stimulation occurs mainly when an exaggerated (violent) motor response to motor response is elicited, regardless of the current intensity, Figure 5–3.[15] Therefore, when the current intensity is properly selected (and appropriately low current intensity is used), one can avoid discomfort on nerve stimulation with current of any duration (0.05–1.0 msec). By and large, using a longer pulse width of at least 300 µsec to 1 msec and low-intensity current, one may still preferentially stimulate sensory nerves and elicit a radiating paresthesia in the distribution of the nerve with every pulse.[20,24]

A narrow pulse width may be superior to a long pulse width in estimating the relative distance between needle and nerve.[5] This is illustrated in Figure 5–4 where the current intensity necessary to produce a twitch is plotted against the pulse width. The narrower the pulse width, the greater the intensity required. When the needle tip is in contact with the nerve, the pulse width of the stimulus has only a moderate effect on the minimal intensity required. However, when the needle tip is far away from the nerve, the influence of the pulse duration becomes a more important variable. For instance, when the needle tip is 1 cm away from the nerve, compared with the needle directly contacting the nerve, there is a 10-fold increase in the threshold current with a 40-µsec

pulse. If the pulse width is lengthened to 1 msec, the required current increase is only two fold.

Rate of Change

A prolonged subthreshold stimulus or a slowly rising current may reduce nerve excitability by inactivating sodium conductance before the depolarization reaches its threshold.[25] Under these circumstances, it may be impossible to stimulate a nerve fiber even with a strong stimulus, if it is applied too slowly. This phenomenon is described as the "accommodation" of nerve fibers. To avoid accommodation in clinical practice, a square wave of current with a sharp rising time is typically used.

POLARITY OF STIMULATING & RETURNING ELECTRODES

Clinical Pearls

- During nerve stimulator-assisted nerve localization, the cathode ("−") should be connected to the stimulating electrode (needle) and anode ("+") to the patient's skin (return electrode).
- Most newer nerve stimulators have a foolproof connectors to the skin and needle electrodes.
- The following mnemonic is helpful when connecting a nerve stimulator:
  1. Negative pole (N for **N**eedle), also often labeled as "black"
  2. Positive electrode (P for **P**atient), also often labeled as "red"

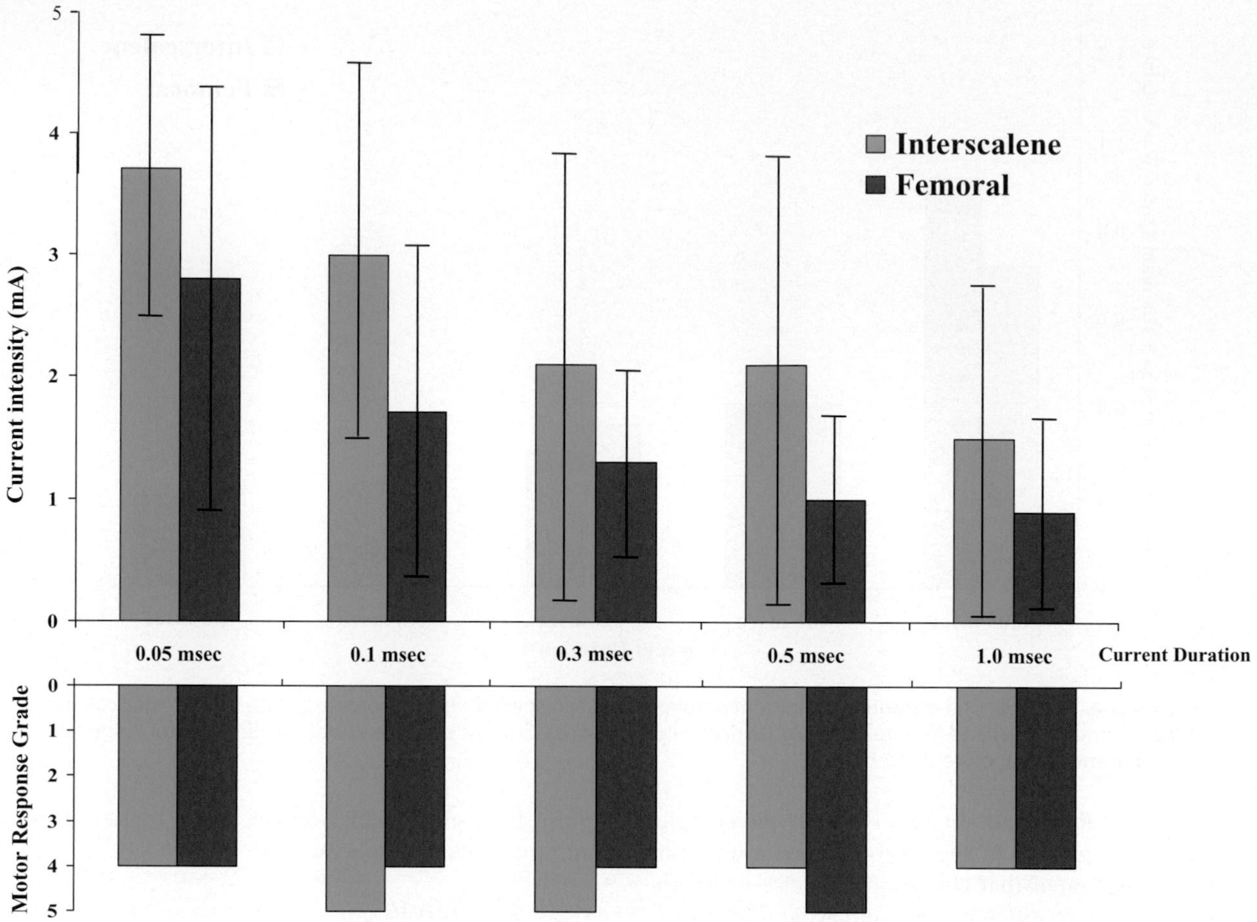

Figure 5–3. Intensity of the stimulating current at which a painful motor response (VAS ≫ 3) is elicited during interscalene brachial plexus (biceps muscle) and femoral nerve (quadriceps muscle) stimulation is obtained. The discomfort on stimulation occurs at a significantly lower current intensity with currents of longer rather than shorter duration. However, the discomfort occurs only with the exaggerated (violent) motor response, regardless of the current intensity. Therefore, the main factor in determining the discomfort during nerve stimulation is the energy ($E = I(mA) \times t(sec)$) delivered to the tissue.

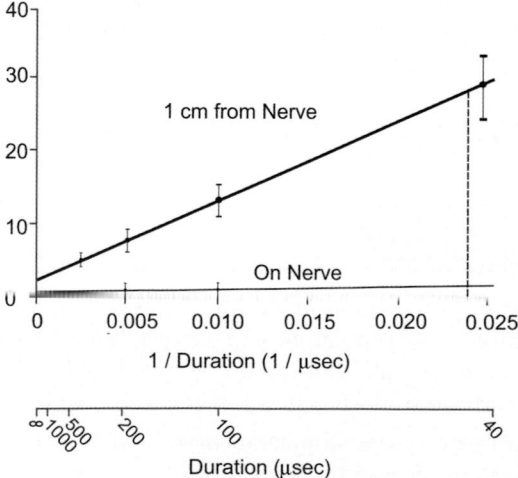

Figure 5–4. Distance–pulse duration curve. A short pulse duration is a better discriminator of the distance between needle and nerve. (Adapted, with permission, from Pither CE, Raj PP, Ford DJ: The use of peripheral nerve stimulators for regional anaesthesia: A review of experimental characteristics, technique, and clinical applications. Reg Anesth 1985;10:49–58.)

The polarity of the stimulating current is an important aspect of nerve stimulation. Preferential cathodal stimulation refers to the fact that when the cathode (negative electrode) is used as the stimulating electrode, rather than the anode (positive electrode), significantly less current (three to four times) is required to elicit a motor response.[5,21,26,27] Thus, the negative electrode is typically connected to the stimulating needle/catheter and the positive electrode to the patient's skin as the returning electrode. The negative current from the cathode reduces the voltage immediately outside the membrane. As a result, the voltage gradient across the membrane is decreased, causing an area of depolarization and resulting in an action potential (Figure 5–5). Hyperpolarization and a decrease in excitability occurs if the polarity of the stimulating and returning electrodes are reversed. It was previously suggested that the returning electrode (anode) had to be positioned at least 20 cm away from the site of stimulation in order to prevent the direct stimulation of muscles via a local flow of the current.[28] However, recent reports have demonstrated that the anode site is not critical when using a constant-current output nerve stimulator.[21]

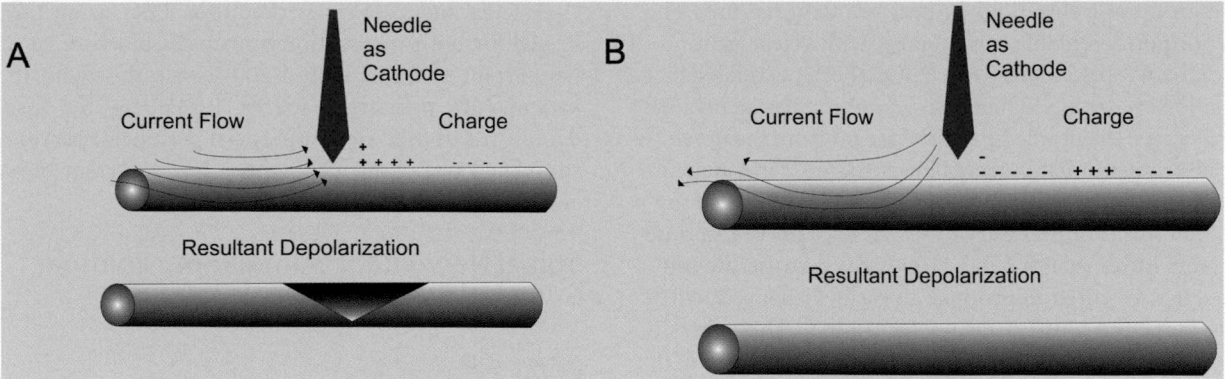

Figure 5–5. Preferential cathodal stimulation. **A.** Cathode stimulation favors depolarization **B.** Anode stimulation results in hyperpolarization and requires higher current for depolarization. (Adapted, with permission, from Pither CE, Raj PP, Ford DJ: The use of peripheral nerve stimulators for regional anaesthesia: A review of experimental characteristics, technique, and clinical applications. Reg Anesth 1985;10:49–58.)

DISTANCE–CURRENT INTENSITY RELATIONSHIP

Clinical Pearls

- The threshold current relationship is the inverse of the square of the distance. As the stimulating electrode moves away from the nerve, an exponentially higher current is required to maintain the motor response.

- This principle is applied clinically to peripheral nerve blocks, percutaneous electrode guidance (PEG), and spinal nerve root stimulation (the epidural stimulation test).

Peripheral Nerve Blocks

The relationship between the current intensity required for excitation and the distance from the nerve is governed by Coulomb's law:

$$I = k(i/r^2)$$

where (I) is the current required, (k) is a constant, (i) is the minimal current, and (r) is the distance from the nerve. Since the current relationship is the inverse of the square of the distance, a very high stimulus current is required as the stimulating electrode moves away from the nerve (Figure 5–6).[20] In clinical practice, an initial stimulating current of 1–2 mA with a pulse of 100 to 200 μsec is used to elicit a response. The stimulating needle is then advanced until it reaches a distance close enough to the nerve to elicit contractions of the appropriate

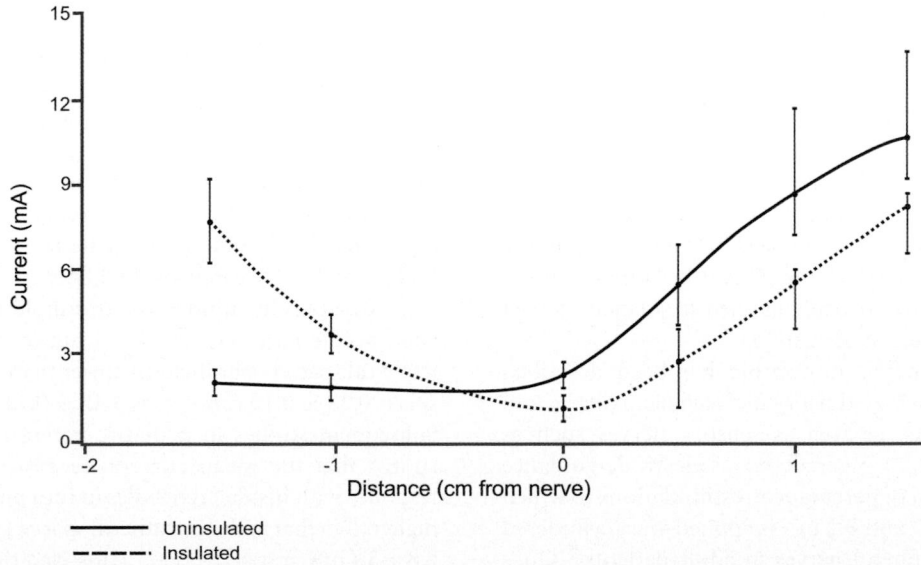

Uninsulated
------- Insulated

Figure 5–6. Distance–current relationship for insulated and uninsulated needles. (Adapted, with permission, from Pither CE, Raj PP, Ford DJ: The use of peripheral nerve stimulators for regional anaesthesia: A review of experimental characteristics, technique, and clinical applications. Reg Anesth 1985;10:49–58.)

muscle group at a threshold current less than 0.5 mA. The most common acceptable current range with a clear motor response is between 0.2 and 0.5 mA.[29] It has been postulated that stimulation at currents higher than 0.5 mA may result in block failure because the needle tip may be too far from the nerve,[30] whereas stimulation at currents lower than 0.2 mA may increase the risk of intraneural injection.[21] It has been also suggested that it was unnecessary to search for a nerve response at currents lower than 0.2 mA (100 μsec) because the minimal current required to produce an easily visualized twitch was about 0.3 mA with a 100-μsec duration.[20] These threshold currents may not apply to all patients, particularly elderly patients or those patients with underlying neuropathies or diabetes, as these patients may have slower nerve conduction velocities and lower motor response amplitudes.[31,32]

Percutaneous Electrode Guidance

Clinical Pearls

- Peripheral nerves and plexuses that are anatomically positioned relatively close to the skin can be stimulated percutaneously with a current between 2 and 5 mA (1.0 msec).
- Percutaneous stimulation to localize nerves can be used clinically to estimate the location of the nerves before introducing the needle.

Percutaneous location of nerves using electrical stimulation has recently been introduced to identify the optimal point on the skin for insertion of the block needle.[7–10] This method is a modification of needle nerve stimulation and as such, it is based on the same distance–current relationship to trace the path of a nerve. Different types of cutaneous stimulating electrodes have been described, including a modified (0.5-cm diameter) electrocardiograph electrode,[33] the negative electrode of the nerve stimulator,[24] and a stub needle.[7] Cutaneous electrodes may also serve as a direct guide for the block needle.[8,9] The smaller the stimulating electrode, the greater the current density applied to the skin and the greater the effect on the tissue. However, this may also increase the risk of causing discomfort to the patient because of an excessive amount of current being applied to a small contact surface area (high "current density").

Percutaneous nerve stimulation has been described for locating motor nerves during interscalene, axillary, and femoral nerve blocks, as well as sensory nerves such as the saphenous nerve.[7–9,34] Percutaneous electrode guidance (PEG) is an extension of percutaneous stimulations in which a current between 1.3 and 8.2 mA is applied via a cylindered probe to locate peripheral nerves in adult patients.[9] Once the electrolocation is accomplished, a needle is introduced to electrolocate at a lower current intensity and inject local anesthetic (see Chapter 45, Percutaneous Nerve Localization).

Capdevila and colleagues described PEG using the same needle for both prelocation and nerve blockade at an initial current of 5 mA with a 200-μsec pulse width in adult patients.[8] In pediatric patients, Bosenberg and associates demonstrated that most superficial peripheral nerves can be stimulated percutaneously with a lower current between 2 and 3.5 mA.[7]

Spinal Nerve Root Stimulation: Epidural Stimulation Test

Clinical Pearls

- Proper epidural catheter placement is indicated by a motor response elicited with a current between 1 and 10 mA.
- A misplaced subarachnoid or subdural catheter is indicated by any response observed with a lower threshold current (<1 mA).
- If no motor response is obtained with a current ≥= 10 mA, the catheter is probably in the subcutaneous tissue.

The previously discussed principle of the distance–current relationship can also be applied to safely, reliably, and conveniently monitor and confirm placement of epidural catheters[11,12] and to guide the placement of epidural catheters from lower spinal levels to specific higher thoracic or cervical levels.[13,35,36]

During epidural stimulation test (Tsui test), the spinal nerve roots (not the spinal cord) are stimulated by an electric current that is conducted through normal saline in the epidural space via an electrically conducting catheter.[37] Since the typical epidural catheter is anatomically situated 1–2 cm from the nerve root, correct placement of the epidural catheter is indicated by a motor response elicited with a current between 1 and 10 mA.[11–13] A response observed with a significantly lower threshold current (≤1 mA) may indicate that a catheter is in the subarachnoid or subdural space, or placed very close to a nerve root.[11,38,39] In these rare, but clinically important instances, a significantly lower threshold current is required because the stimulating needle is very close to the nerve roots or because the stimulating needle is in direct contact with highly conductive cerebrospinal fluid.

In a porcine model, the threshold current of an insulated needle required to elicit a motor response in the intrathecal space is significantly lower than that in the epidural space, 0.38 ± 0.19 mA versus 3.45 ± 0.73 mA, respectively.[40] Subsequent studies in pediatric patients have also demonstrated that the mean current necessary to elicit a motor response with insulated needles in the epidural space is much higher than that in the intrathecal space (11.1 ± 3.1 mA versus 0.8 ± 3.1 mA, respectively).[41] Thus, electrical stimulation may be a useful means of distinguishing entry of a needle into the epidural space from entry into the intrathecal space. It should be noted, however, that the mean threshold current required to elicit a motor response is significantly higher with insulated needles than with epidural catheters in pediatric patients.[13,41] It has been suggested that this may be because the needle tip is placed farther from the nerve roots compared with the tip of the threaded epidural catheter.[41]

CURRENT DENSITY

Clinical Pearls

- The smaller the conductive area for current flow at the needle tip, the higher the current density and the lower the threshold current for a motor response.
- Electric current density depends on the conductive surface area and current intensity applied.
- The smaller the conductive area for current flow at the needle tip, the higher the current density and the lower the threshold current for a motor response. Therefore, current density is sensitive to changes that occur at the needle/catheter–tissue interface (ie, changing the type of needle or injecting fluid).

PERIPHERAL NERVE STIMULATORS

Peripheral nerve stimulators have become indispensable in the practice of modern regional anesthesia. A more in-depth understanding of how they function is required so that their full potential will be realized in a clinical setting. In this section, we review some basic engineering principles behind nerve stimulators and provide tips on how to choose one for your practice and make the most of it. Although the use of peripheral nerve stimulators (PNS) for regional anesthesia

was first suggested by von Perthes in 1912, it has only gained wider acceptance concurrent with the resurgence of interest in regional anesthesia over the last two decades. The manufacturers met the demand for devices that are more accurate in determining the nerve location prior to the injection of local anesthetic. A number of makes and models are commercially available. Though the newer models are inherently more accurate, they often include a plethora of functions with controls that may not be intuitive. Figure 5–7 demonstrates the essential components of a nerve stimulator.

Clock Reference

The clock reference functions as a synchronizing mechanism for the PNS. Generally, it is a crystal oscillator that produces a very accurate, high-frequency clock signal. This clock signal is then fed as an input to the microcontroller and used to control all functions. The specific frequency of the oscillator depends on the type of microcontroller used in the design.

Microcontroller

The microcontroller functions as the brain of the nerve stimulator. Most nerve stimulators run on battery power, so choosing a low-power microcontroller is of the utmost importance. The microcontroller receives an input from the controls and, according to the instructions received, changes the value of the current, frequency, or pulse width. In addition to changing the value, it also relays that value to the display so that the user knows what the new setting is.

Constant-Current Generator

The constant-current generator can be modeled as a reference current (Box 5–1). An ideal constant-current source could deliver the same current regardless of the value of the impedance (resistance) load connected to it. Since ideal constant-current source intensity does not exist, a clinically acceptable

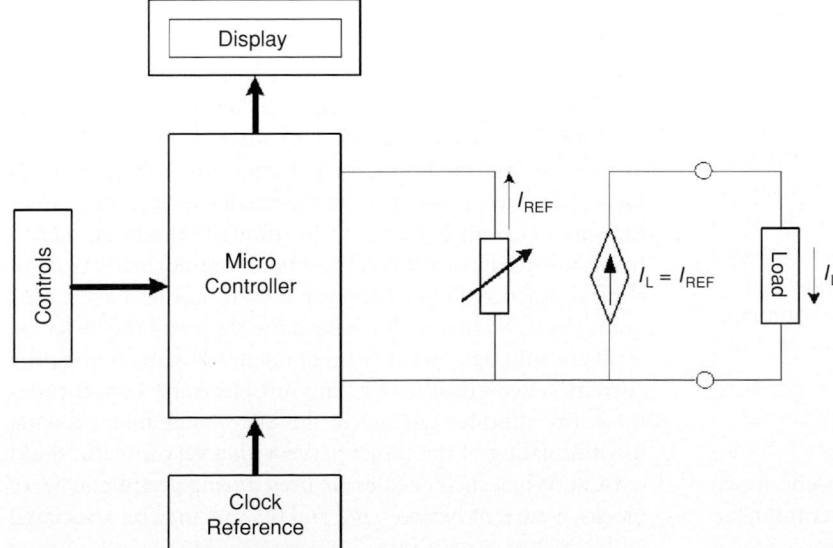

Figure 5–7. Anatomy of a Nerve Stimulator. This is a standard block circuit of a constant-current nerve stimulator. The circuit has six main parts as seen in the block diagram: (1) Clock reference, (2) Microcontroller, (3) Controls, (4) Display, (5) Current reference generator, and (6) Constant-current generator.

Box 5–1.

Important Features of Nerve Stimulators

- **Constant-current output**—The impedance of tissues, needles, connecting wires, and grounding electrodes may vary. A constant-current design incorporates automatic compensation in voltage output for changes in tissue or connection impedance during nerve stimulation, ensuring accurate delivery of the specified current within a clinically relevant range of impedance loads.
- **Accurate current display**—The ability to read the current being delivered is of utmost importance for both the success and safety of nerve blocks.
- **Conveninet means of current intensity control**—Current may be controlled using either a digital means or an analog dial. Alternatively, current intensity can be controlled using a remote controller, such as a foot pedal, allowing a single operator to perform the procedure and contraol the current output. The stimulator design should allow for change in the current intensity in increments of 0.01 mA in the range of 0.00 to 0.50 mA.
- **Pulse width**—A short pulse width (100–200 μsec), corresponding to the chronaxies of A-α fibers, appears to be the most suitable for nerve localization. Although some units give the user the ability to change the current duration, the clinical utility for such a feature is not well defined.
- **Stimulating frequency**—A stimulating frequency of 2 Hz to 2.5 Hz appears optimal for nerve localization. When using older units with 1-Hz stimulation (one stimulus per second), the needle must be advanced very slowly to avoid missing the nerve between the stimuli.
- **Disconnect and malfunction indicator**—This is an essential feature, since the anesthesiologist should know when the stimulus is not being delivered due to malfunctions (eg, disconnect, poor electrical connection, battery failure, etc).

compromise can be achieved using a current generator to provide a stable current over the clinically expected range of impedance loads. This is achieved by generating progressively higher voltage output as the impedance between the electrodes is increased. For instance, when set to deliver a current of 1 mA and the tissue impedance between the two electrodes is 1 kΩ, the nerve stimulator will deliver 1 V. If the impedance between the electrodes is 5 kΩ, the stimulator will deliver 5 V to maintain the same set current of 1 mA ($I = U/R$).

Current Reference Generator

The current reference generator is based on a precisely known voltage source and a low-tolerance digital potentiometer. A voltage regulator usually supplies the voltage source. A low-tolerance digital potentiometer is very similar to a standard potentiometer in that it changes resistance over its entire range. It is controlled by the microcontroller using a series of command pulses that tell it to increase or decrease the value. Unlike the analog types, digital potentiometers adjust values in discrete increments, so it is important to choose one with enough steps. Generally, a 10-bit potentiometer, giving 1024 steps, is sufficient for the application.

Display

A typical PNS has a standard liquid crystal display (LCD) that uses less current and is more versatile than seven-segment light-emitting diode (LED) displays. Most displays show the set value of current, frequency, and pulse width. Other indicators, like low battery level and probe disconnect, can also be included.

Controls

Three sets of controls are usually found on a typical PNS: frequency, pulse width, and current. The controls can be analog or digital. Each control increases or decreases the value of the controlled parameter. Once the user sets a value, the microcontroller changes the value of the desired parameter. A remote foot pedal or a hand controller can be used to facilitate quick current adjustment, thereby allowing a single operator to perform the nerve block procedure (Figure 5–8).

TYPES OF ELECTRODES (NEEDLES)

Two types of stimulating needles can be used for this purpose: (1) electrically insulated or (2) electrically uninsulated. The properties of insulated and uninsulated needles and the geometries of the electric fields they produce are quite different (Figure 5–9).[6,42] A recently introduced stimulating catheter is another form of the stimulating electrode.

Insulated Needles

Insulated needles are coated with a layer of nonconducting material (eg, polytetrafluoroethylene [Teflon] or silicon) over the entire length of the needle, with the exception of the needle tip. Upon stimulation, the pattern of the current density focuses on the uncoated tip of the needle. As a result, a low threshold current is sufficient to stimulate the target nerve. Insulated needles with a cutting bevel are normally used in clinical practice. Other commonly used needles have a pinpoint electrode tip, in which both the shaft and the bevel are insulated and only the very tip of the needle can conduct the current. Theoretically, the pinpoint electrode concentrates the entire stimulus current in this very small area, allowing for stimulating of the target nerve with a very low threshold current. When such needles are used during peripheral nerve blocks, a current between 0.2 and 0.5 mA may be associated with a higher success rate.[29]

catheter.[14,43] However, the mean current required to stimulate motor nerves with stimulating catheters was significantly higher following the injection of saline compared with the mean current required when using insulated needles alone (see section on Types of Injectates).[44]

Uninsulated Needles

Uninsulated needles are bare metallic needles that transmit the current throughout the entire length of their shaft (see Figure 5–9). Compared with insulated needles, uninsulated needles have a much larger conducting area. Therefore, when the total current remains constant but the conductive area increases, the current density at the tip of the needle decreases. This explains why higher threshold currents, generally in excess of 1 mA, are required to excite a nerve with uninsulated needles.[6] With these needles, it may be more difficult to accurately localize a target nerve, especially when a current of low intensity is used.

TYPES OF INJECTATES

Clinical Pearl

The injection of a nonconducting solution (D_5W) maintains or augments a motor response elicited by 0.5 mA or less by decreasing the conductive surface area and therefore increasing the current density at the needle tip.

A small volume of local anesthetic or normal saline typically abolishes the muscle twitch induced by a low current (0.5 mA) during nerve stimulation. This phenomenon, commonly known as the **Raj test** is used by some to confirm the needle being close to the target nerve.[28] However, the electrophysiologic effect of injectates on nerve stimulation was never fully explained. Previously, the cause of this muscle twitch dissipation was thought to be a result of the physical displacement of the nerve from the stimulating needle tip by the injected fluid.[5] However, this mechanism appears to be best explained in electrical terms and is not due to the sole physical displacement of the nerve.[45] For instance, in a porcine model, the injection of a 0.9% NaCl solution abolished the motor response, whereas a subsequent injection of 5% dextrose re-established a motor response during PNS.[45] An accompanying in vitro experiment showed that injections of solutions, such as 0.9% NaCl, cause a change in the electric field at the needle–tissue interface (Figure 5–10). It was concluded that the injection of electrically conducting solutions (saline or local anesthetic) increases the conductive area surrounding the stimulating needle tip, leading to a decrease in the current density surrounding a target nerve. As a result, the needle tip no longer has enough current density to stimulate the desired nerve.[45] This suggests that effective nerve stimulation is sensitive to changes that occur at the needle–tissue

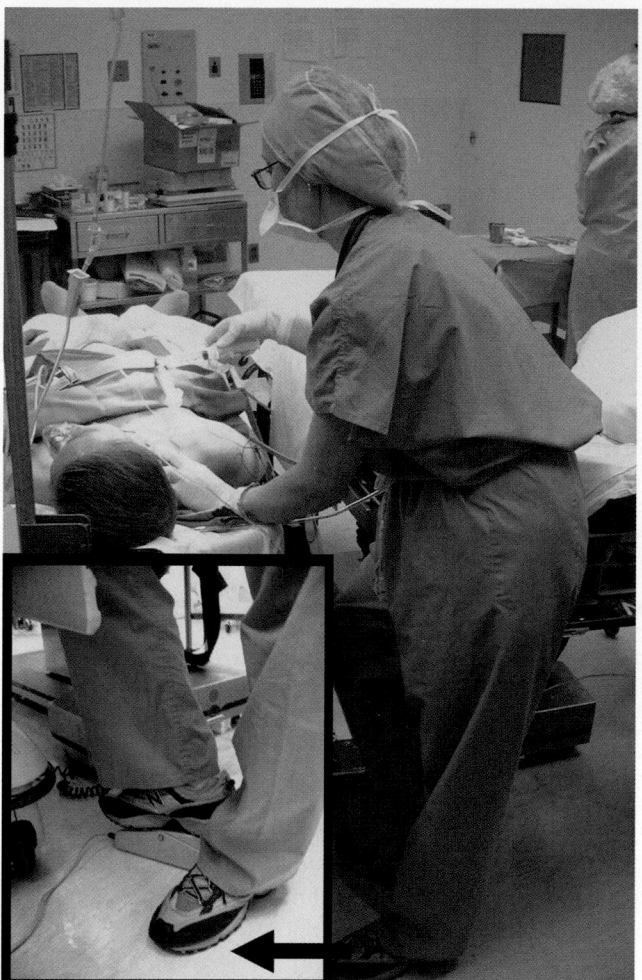

Figure 5–8. Nerve stimulators with foot or hand control of the current intensity (*inset*) allow quick and convenient change of the current intensity by a single operator.

Stimulating Catheter

Clinical Pearl

Stimulating catheters function like insulated needles. However, the threshold current will be much higher using stimulating catheters following the injection of saline.

Similar to insulated needles, stimulating catheters are covered with a layer of nonconducting materials over the entire length of the catheter, with the exception of the catheter tip. Thus, the stimulating catheter behaves likes a soft flexible insulated needle. The ability to elicit a motor response with a stimulating catheter is a great advantage because it allows "real-time" observation of motor responses as the catheter is advanced along the axis of the target nerve. Reports in which stimulating catheters were threaded without the use of saline to dilate the perineural space demonstrated similar threshold currents for both the needle and the stimulating

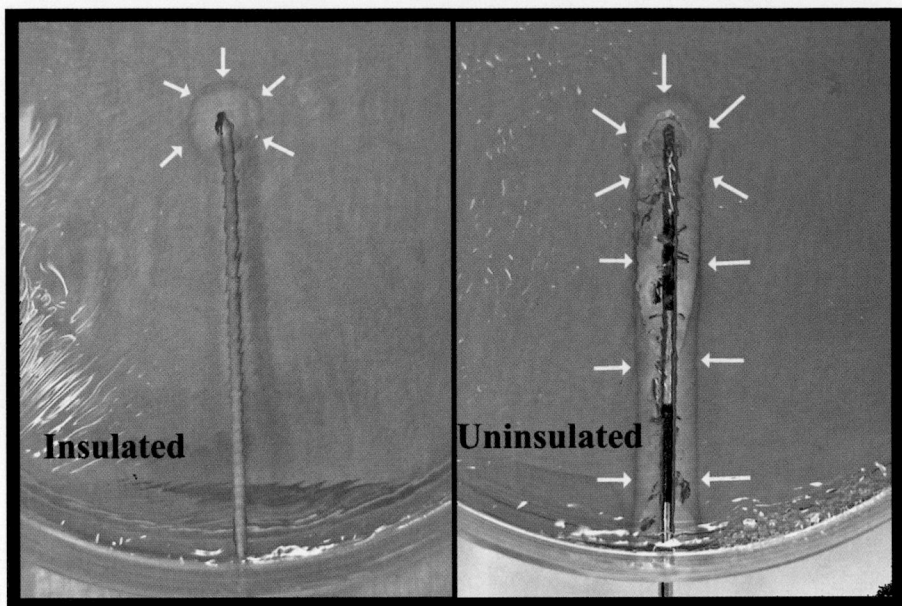

Figure 5–9. Gel electrophoresis: Changes in the electric field with insulated and uninsulated needles. Arrows show the margin of the clear zone/electric field. *Left:* An insulated needle. *Right:* An uninsulated needle. (Reprinted, with permission, from Tsui BC, Wagner A, Finucane B: Electrophysiologic effect of injectates on peripheral nerve stimulation. Reg Anesth Pain Med 2004;29:189–193.)

interface, such as a change in the angle of the needle or injection of local anesthetic. The net effect appears to affect the current density at the tip of the needle or a path of the electric current, ultimately resulting in a change in the quality of the motor response.[16] This phenomenon has also recently been reported in a clinical setting.[46,47]

In a clinical study, the mean currents required to stimulate the intersternocleidomastoid, axillary, femoral, and sciatic nerves, using an insulated needle were 0.6, 0.5, 0.7, and 0.5 mA, respectively.[15,44] In contrast, the mean currents required to stimulate these same nerves using a stimulating catheter following the injection of normal saline were much

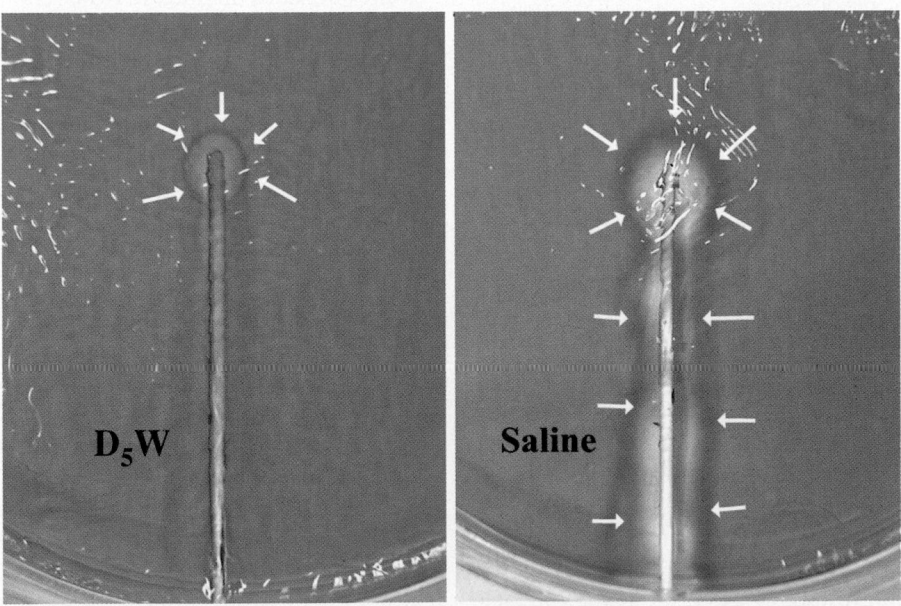

Figure 5–10. Gel electrophoresis: Changes in the electric field with injection of nonionic (D_5W) and ionic (saline) solutions. Arrows show the margin of the clear zone/electric field. *Left:* An uninsulated needle after D_5W injection). *Right:* An insulated needle after normal saline injection. (Reprinted, with permission, from Tsui BC, Wagner A, Finucane B: Electrophysiologic effect of injectates on peripheral nerve stimulation. Reg Anesth Pain Med 2004;29:189–193.)

higher (1.5, 1.5, 2, and 3 mA, respectively).[43] On the other hand, reports in which stimulating catheters were threaded without the use of saline did not demonstrate such discrepancies between the threshold currents of the needle and the catheter.[14,43] These clinical observations suggest that when saline is used to dilate the perineural space during continuous peripheral nerve blocks, the loss of motor response may require additional efforts to confirm the catheter placement. This can be avoided by using a nonconducting solution, such as D_5W, instead of saline to dilate the perineural space.[45] More studies are indicated to determine the clinical merit of this technique.[46,47]

SUMMARY

The main advantages of nerve stimulation is that the motor response can be elicited without the need to establish a direct nerve contact.[4,9,48] Nerve stimulation can provide objective responses without relying on a patient's report when localizing motor or mixed nerves. Intuitively, one would then expect that nerve stimulation should increase the success rate of regional nerve blocks and decrease the risk of direct nerve trauma and intraneural injections. However, no compelling evidence supports this widespread belief. Nonetheless, nerve stimulation has been reported to be superior over other regional techniques in small isolated studies. For instance, compared with a paresthesia technique, nerve stimulator-assisted sciatic nerve blocks resulted in a higher success rate.[49,50] Similarly, the multistimulation technique of axillary blockade of the brachial plexus results in a higher success rate than transarterial or paresthesia techniques.[23,51–54]

More recent studies have examined the relationship between nerve stimulation and paresthesia.[5,55–57] Paresthesia presumably occurs when the needle mechanically excites the nerve by making direct contact with the nerve but it can also occur from pressure exerted on the nerve from surrounding tissues. Current controversy surrounds the question of why a motor response may not be elicited with a current intensity of 1 mA in up to 70% of patients at the position in which paresthesia is elicited or when intimate needle–nerve location is verified by using ultrasound.[55–57] As discussed in the previous section, the motor response elicited by electrical stimulation is sensitive to changes in the electric field at the needle–tissue interface (ie, electrical conduction interference from surrounding tissue, blood, or interstitial fluid).[45,58] This may partly account for the observed dissociation between paresthesia and motor nerve stimulation.[45] Obviously, many aspects of nerve stimulation are not well understood, and more studies are clearly needed to clarify some of the principles of nerve stimulation and the factors that influence its clinical application in peripheral nerve blocks.

References

1. von Perthes G: Über leitungsanasthesis unter zuhilfenahme elektrischer reizung. Munch Med Wochenschr 1912;47:2545–2548.

2. Pearson RB: Nerve block in rehabilitation: A technique of needle localization. Arch Phys Med Rehabil 1955;36:631–633.

3. Montgomery SJ, Raj PP, Nettles D, et al: The use of the nerve stimulator with standard unsheathed needles in nerve blockade. Anesth Analg 1973;52:827–831.

4. Greenblatt GM, Denson JS: Needle nerve stimulatorlocator: Nerve blocks with a new instrument for locating nerves. Anesth Analg 1962;41:599–602.

5. Ford DJ, Pither CE, Raj PP: Electrical characteristics of peripheral nerve stimulators: Implication for nerve localization. Regional Anesth 1984;9:73–77.

6. Ford DJ, Pither C, Raj PP: Comparison of insulated and uninsulated needles for locating peripheral nerves with a peripheral nerve stimulator. Anesth Analg 1984;63:925–8.

7. Bosenberg AT, Raw R, Boezaart AP: Surface mapping of peripheral nerves in children with a nerve stimulator. Paediatr Anaesth 2002;12:398–403.

8. Capdevila X, Lopez S, Bernard N, et al: Percutaneous electrode guidance using the insulated needle for prelocation of peripheral nerves during axillary plexus blocks. Reg Anesth Pain Med 2004;29:206–211.

9. Urmey WF, Grossi P: Percutaneous electrode guidance: A noninvasive technique for prelocation of peripheral nerves to facilitate peripheral plexus or nerve block. Reg Anesth Pain Med 2002;27:261–267.

10. Urmey WF, Grossi P: Percutaneous electrode guidance and subcutaneous stimulating electrode guidance: Modifications of the original technique. Reg Anesth Pain Med 2003;28:253–255.

11. Tsui BC, Gupta S, Finucane B: Confirmation of epidural catheter placement using nerve stimulation. Can J Anaesth 1998;45:640–644.

12. Tsui BC, Guenther C, Emery D, et al: Determining epidural catheter location using nerve stimulation with radiological confirmation. Reg Anesth Pain Med 2000;25:306–309.

13. Tsui BC, Seal R, Koller J, et al: Thoracic epidural analgesia via the caudal approach in pediatric patients undergoing fundoplication using nerve stimulation guidance. Anesth Analg 2001;93:1152–1155.

14. Boezaart AP, De Beer JF, du Toit C, et al: A new technique of continuous interscalene nerve block. Can J Anaesth 1999;46:275–281.

15. Hadzic A, Vloka JD, Claudio RE, et al: Effects of surface electrode placement and duration of the stimulus on motor response. Anesthesiology 2004;100:1526–1530.

16. Hadzic A: Peripheral nerve stimulators: Cracking the code-one at a time. Reg Anesth Pain Med 2004;29:185–188.

17. Lapicque L: *L'excitabilite en Fonction du Temps: La Chronaxie, sa Signification et sa Mesure.* Paris, Presses Universitaires de France, 1926, p 365.

18. Ganong WF: Excitable tissues: Nerve. In: *Review of Medical Physiology,* 19 ed. Lange, 1999, pp 47–59.

19. Guyton AC, Hall JE: Membrane potentials and action potentials, *Textbook of Medical Physiology,* 9th ed. WB Saunders, 1996, pp 57–71.

20. Pither CE, Raj PP, Ford DJ: The use of peripheral nerve stimulators for regional anaesthesia: A review of experimental characteristics, technique, and clinical applications. Reg Anesth 1985;10:49–58.

21. Hadzic A, Vloka JD, Claudio RE, et al: Electrical nerve localization: Effects of cutaneous electrode placement and duration of the stimulus on motor response. Anesthesiology 2004;100:1526–1530.

22. Koscielniak-Nielsen ZJ, Rassmussen H, Jepsen K: Effect of impulse duration on patients' perception of electrical stimulation and block effectiveness during axillary block in unsedated ambulatory patients. Reg Anesth Pain Med 2001;26:428–433.

23. Sia S, Bartoli M, Lepri A, et al: Multiple-injection axillary brachial plexus block: A comparison of two methods of nerve localization-nerve stimulation versus paresthesia. Anesth Analg 2000;91:647–651.

24. Shannon J, Lang SA, Yip RW, et al: Lateral femoral cutaneous nerve block revisited. A nerve stimulator technique. Reg Anesth 1995;20:100–104.

25. Kimura J: Facts, Fallacies, and Fancies of Nerve Stimulation Techniques. In Kimura J (eds): *Electrodiagnosis in Diseases of Nerve and Muscle: Principles and Practice,* 2nd ed. FA Davis, 1989, pp 139–166.

26. Hodgkin AL: The subthreshold potentials in a crustacean nerve fiber. Proc R Soc Lond 1938;126:87.

27. Tulchinsky A, Weller RS, Rosenblum M, et al: Nerve stimulator polarity and brachial plexus block. Anesth Analg 1993;77:100–103.

28. Raj PP: Peripheral nerve stimulators for nerve blocks. In Raj PP, De Andres J, Grossi P, et al (eds): *Textbook of Regional Anesthesia,* 1st ed. Churchill Livingstone, 2002, pp 251–268.

29. Hadzic A, Vloka J: Peripheral nerve stimulators and nerve stimulation. In Hadzic A, Vloka J (eds): *Peripheral Nerve Blocks: Principles and Practice,* 1st ed. McGraw-Hill, 2004, pp 43–50.

30. Magora F, Rozin R, Ben-Menachem Y, et al: Obturator nerve block: An evaluation of technique. Br J Anaesth 1969;41:695–698.

31. Kimura J: Principles of nerve conduction studies. In Kimura J et al (eds): *Electrodiagnosis in Diseases of Nerve and Muscle: Principles and Practice,* 2nd ed. FA Davis, 1989, pp 78–102.

32. Kimura J: Polyneuropathies. In Kimura J et al (eds): *Electrodiagnosis in Diseases of Nerve and Muscle: Principles and Practice,* 2nd ed. FA Davis, 1989, pp 462–494.

33. Ganta R, Cajee RA, Henthorn RW: Use of transcutaneous nerve stimulation to assist interscalene block. Anesth Analg 1993;76:914–915.

34. Stone BA: Transcutaneous stimulation of the saphenous nerve to locate injection site. Reg Anesth Pain Med 2003;28:153–154.

35. Tsui BC, Seal R, Entwistle L: Thoracic epidural analgesia via the caudal approach using nerve stimulation in an infant with CATCH22. Can J Anaesth 1999;46:1138–1142.

36. Tsui BC, Bateman K, Bouliane M, et al: Cervical epidural analgesia via a thoracic approach using nerve stimulation guidance in an adult patient undergoing elbow surgery. Reg Anesth Pain Med 2004;29:355–360.

37. Tsui BCH, Finucane B: Epidural stimulator catheter. Reg Anesth Pain Med 2002;6:150–154.

38. Tsui BC, Gupta S, Finucane B: Detection of subarachnoid and intravascular epidural catheter placement. Can J Anaesth 1999;46:675–678.

39. Tsui BC, Gupta S, Emery D, et al: Detection of subdural placement of epidural catheter using nerve stimulation. Can J Anaesth 2000;47:471–473.

40. Tsui BC, Wagner A, Finucane B: The threshold current in the intrathecal space to elicit motor response is lower and does not overlap that in the epidural space: A porcine model. Can J Anaesth 2004;51:690–695.

41. Tsui BC, Wagner A, Cave D, et al.: Threshold current for an insulated epidural needle in pediatric patients. Anesth Analg 2004;99:694–696.

42. Bashein G, Haschke RH, Ready LB: Electrical nerve location: Numerical and electrophoretic comparison of insulated vs uninsulated needles. Anesth Analg 1984;63:919–924.

43. Sutherland ID: Continuous sciatic nerve infusion: Expanded case report describing a new approach. Reg Anesth Pain Med 1998;23:496–501.

44. Pham-Dang C, Kick O, Collet T, et al: Continuous peripheral nerve blocks with stimulating catheters. Reg Anesth Pain Med 2003;28:83–88.

45. Tsui BC, Wagner A, Finucane B: Electrophysiologic effect of injectates on peripheral nerve stimulation. Reg Anesth Pain Med 2004;29:189–193.

46. Tsui BC, Kropelin B, Ganapathy S, et al: Dextrose 5% in water: Fluid medium for maintaining electrical stimulation of peripheral nerves during stimulating catheter placement. Acta Anaesthesiol Scand 2005; 49:1562–1565.

47. Tsui BC, Kropelin B: Electrophysiological effect of dextrose 5% in water on single-shot peripheral nerve stimulation. Anesth Analg 2005; 100:1837–1839.

48. Raj PP, Rosenblatt R, Montgomery SJ: Use of the nerve stimulator for peripheral blocks. Reg Anesth 1980;5:14–21.

49. Smith BL: Efficacy of a nerve stimulator in regional analgesia; experience in a resident training programme. Anaesthesia 1976;31:778–782.

50. Smith BE, Allison A: Use of a low-power nerve stimulator during sciatic nerve block. Anaesthesia 1987;42:296–298.

51. Baranoswski AP, Pither CE: A comparison of three methods of axillary brachial plexus anaesthesia. Anaesthesia 1990;45:362–365.

52. Bouaziz H, Narchi P, Mercier FJ, et al: Comparison between conventional axillary block and a new approach at the midhumeral level. Anesth Analg 1997;84:1058–1062.

53. Goldberg ME, Gregg C, Larijani GE, et al: A comparison of three methods of axillary approach to brachial plexus blockade for upper extremity surgery. Anesthesiology 1987;66:814–816.

54. Lavoie J, Martin R, Tetrault JP: Axillary plexus block using a peripheral nerve stimulator: Single or multiple injections. Can J Anaesth 1990;37:S39.

55. Bollini CA, Urmey WF, Vascello L, et al: Relationship between evoked motor response and sensory paresthesia in interscalene brachial plexus block. Reg Anesth Pain Med 2003;28:384–388.

56. Choyce A, Chan VW, Middleton WJ, et al: What is the relationship between paresthesia and nerve stimulation for axillary brachial plexus block? Reg Anesth Pain Med 2001;26:100–104.

57. Urmey WF, Stanton J: Inability to consistently elicit a motor response following sensory paresthesia during interscalene block administration. Anesthesiology 2002;96:552–554.

58. Hogan Q: Finding nerves is not simple. Reg Anesth Pain Med 2003;28:367–371.

6

Clinical Pharmacology of Local Anesthetics

John Butterworth, MD

INTRODUCTION

Local and regional anesthesia, defined as the selective numbing of a specific nerve distribution or region of the body to facilitate surgery, appear to be undergoing a renaissance, as judged by attendance at specialty meetings and numbers of published manuscripts. In contrast to general anesthesia, in which the molecular mechanism remains the subject of speculation, the site at which local anesthetic drugs bind to produce nerve blocks has been cloned and mutated. This chapter will focus on mechanisms of anesthesia and toxicity, especially as knowledge of these mechanisms will assist the clinician in conducting safer and more effective regional anesthetics.

PREHISTORY & HISTORY

The Incas regarded coca as a gift from the son of the sun god and limited its use to the "upper crust" of society.[1] The Incas recognized and used the medicinal properties of cocaine long before the compound was brought back to Europe for its properties to be "discovered." The Incas sometimes treated persistent headaches with trepanation (Figure 6–1), and coca was sometimes a part of this procedure. Local anesthesia was accomplished by having the operator chew coca leaves and apply the mascerated pulp to the skin and wound edges while using a tumi knife (Figure 6–2) to bore through the bone.

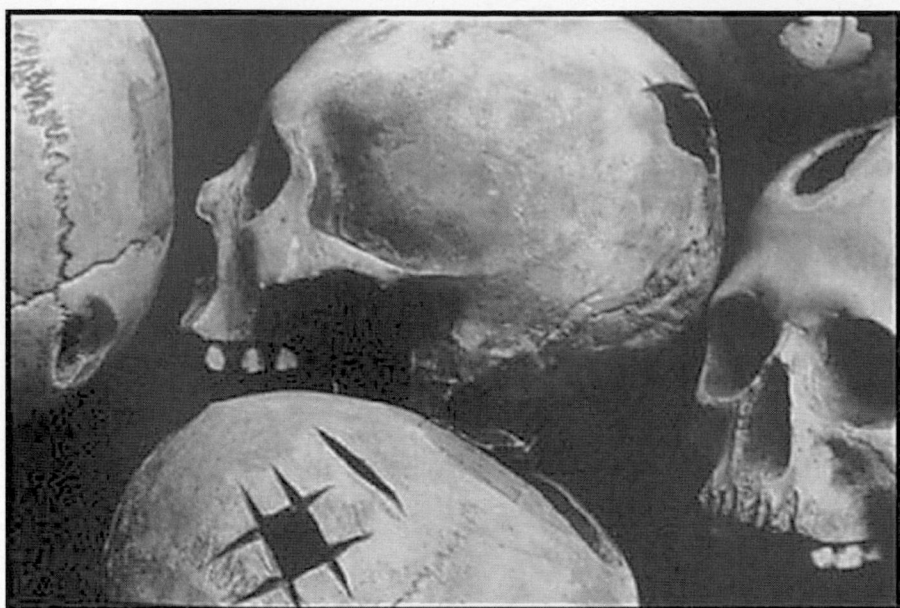

Figure 6–1. Skulls showing knife marks from ritual trepanning. This procedure was intended to release spirits causing headaches and other cranial ailments. (Photograph © Rosamond Purcell. Originally published in Mütter Museum calendar, College of Physicians, Philadelphia, PA, 1993.)

By the sixteenth century, the conquistadors had disrupted Incan society and began paying laborers with cocaine paste. The laborers generally rolled the cocaine leaves into balls (called *cocadas*), bound together by guano or cornstarch.[1,2] These cocadas released the free-base cocaine as a consequence of the alkalinity of the guano and of the practice of chewing the cocadas with ash or lime (such alkaline compounds increase pH, favoring the free-base cocaine form over the positively charged hydrochloride salt). This practice probably marks the birth of "free-basing" cocaine and is the historic antecedent of the "rock" or "crack" cocaine so often abused in Western societies.

Cocaine was brought back to Vienna by an explorer/physician named Scherzer.[1] In Vienna, the chemist Albert Niemann isolated and crystallized the pure cocaine hydrochloride in 1860. The Merck Company distributed batches of this agent to physicians for investigational purposes. Sigmund Freud was the most prominent of these cocaine experimenters. Freud reviewed his experimental work in a monograph devoted to cocaine titled *Über Coca*. Freud and Carl Koller (an ophthalmology trainee) took cocaine orally and noticed that the drug rendered their tongues insensible. Koller and Joseph Gartner began a series of experiments using cocaine to produce topical anesthesia of the conjunctiva. The birth of local and regional anesthesia dates from 1884 when Koller and Gartner reported their success at producing topical cocaine anesthesia of the eye in the frog, rabbit, dog, and human.[2–4]

The use of local anesthesia quickly spread around the world. The American surgeon William Halsted at Roosevelt Hospital in New York reported using cocaine to produce mandibular nerve block in 1884 and to produce brachial plexus block less than a year later.[5] These blocks were accomplished by surgically exposing the nerves, then injecting them under direct vision. Leonard Corning injected cocaine near the spine of dogs, producing what was likely the first epidural in 1885. Spinal anesthesia was first accomplished in 1898 by August Bier. Caudal epidural anesthesia was introduced in 1902 by Sicard and Cathelin.[5] Cocaine spinal anesthesia was used to treat cancer pain in 1898. Bier described intravenous regional anesthesia in 1909. In 1911, Hirschel reported the first three percutaneous brachial plexus anesthesias. Fidel Pages reported using epidural anesthesia for abdominal surgery in 1921.

Cocaine was incorporated into many other products, including the original formulation of Coca-Cola devised by Pemberton in 1886. Wine tonics and other "patent" medicines of the day commonly contained cocaine (Figure 6–3), until the early 1990s when governments began regulating the use of cocaine.

MEDICINAL CHEMISTRY

All local anesthetics (LAs) contain an aromatic ring and an amine at either end of the molecule, separated by a hydrocarbon chain, and either an ester or an amide bond (Figure 6–4).[3,4,6,7] Cocaine is the archetypical ester LA and is the only naturally occurring one. Procaine, the first synthetic ester LA, was introduced by Einhorn in 1904 (Table 6–1).[2] The introduction of the amide LA lidocaine in 1948 was transformative. Lidocaine quickly became used for all forms of regional anesthesia. Other amide LAs based on the lidocaine structure (prilocaine, etidocaine) subsequently appeared. A related series of amide LAs based on 2′, 6′-pipecoloxylidide was introduced (mepivacaine, bupivacaine, ropivacaine, and

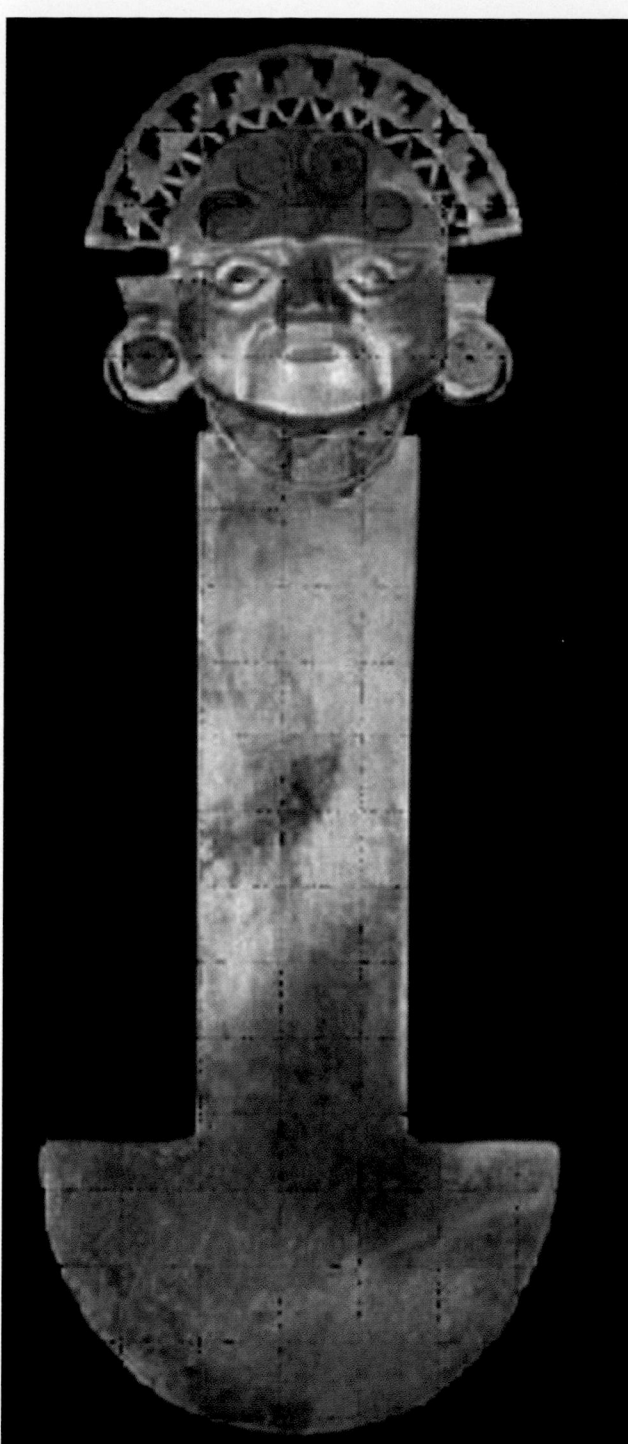

Figure 6–2. A ceremonial tumi knife of the same shape and size as the less ornate ones that were used by the Incas to bore holes through the skull (trepanning). (Reprinted, with permission, from Sabbatini RME: Brain & Mind Magazine, 1997, June.)

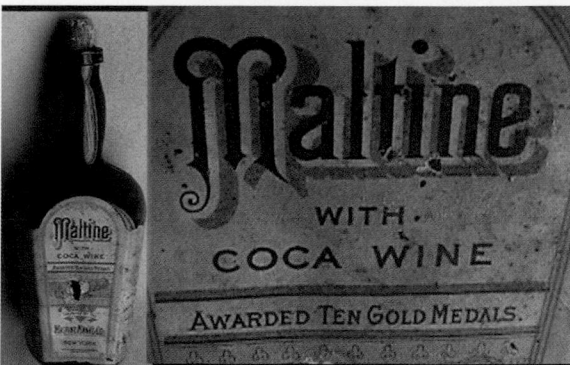

A

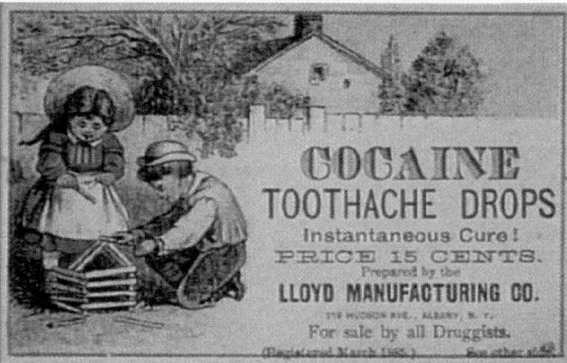

B

Figure 6–3. Examples of products that incorporated cocaine during the time before it became a controlled substance. Wines fortified with cocaine were particularly popular as "tonics." (Reprinted, with permission, from Addiction Research Unit, University of Buffalo.)

Clinical Pearls

- All LAs contain an aromatic ring and an amine at either end of the molecule, separated by a hydrocarbon chain, and either an ester or an amide bond.

BIOPHYSICS OF VOLTAGE-GATED Na CHANNELS & LAs

Studies of the mechanisms of LA action on nerves are studies of interactions between LAs and voltage-gated Na channels, since Na channels contain the LA binding site. Na channels are integral membrane proteins that initiate and propagate action potentials in axons, dendrites, and muscle tissue; initiate and maintain membrane potential oscillations in specialized heart and brain cells; and shape and filter synaptic inputs. Na channels share structural features with other voltage-gated ion channels in their genetic "superfamily," wich includes voltage-gated Ca and K channels. Na channels contain one larger α-subunit and one or two smaller β-subunits, depending on the species and the tissue of origin. The

levobupivacaine). Ropivacaine and levobupivacaine are the only single-enantiomer (single optical isomer) LAs. Both are S(−)-enantiomers, which avoid the increased cardiac toxicity associated with racemic mixtures and the R(+)-isomers (this will be discussed in a subsequent section). All other LAs either exist as racemates or have no asymmetric carbons.

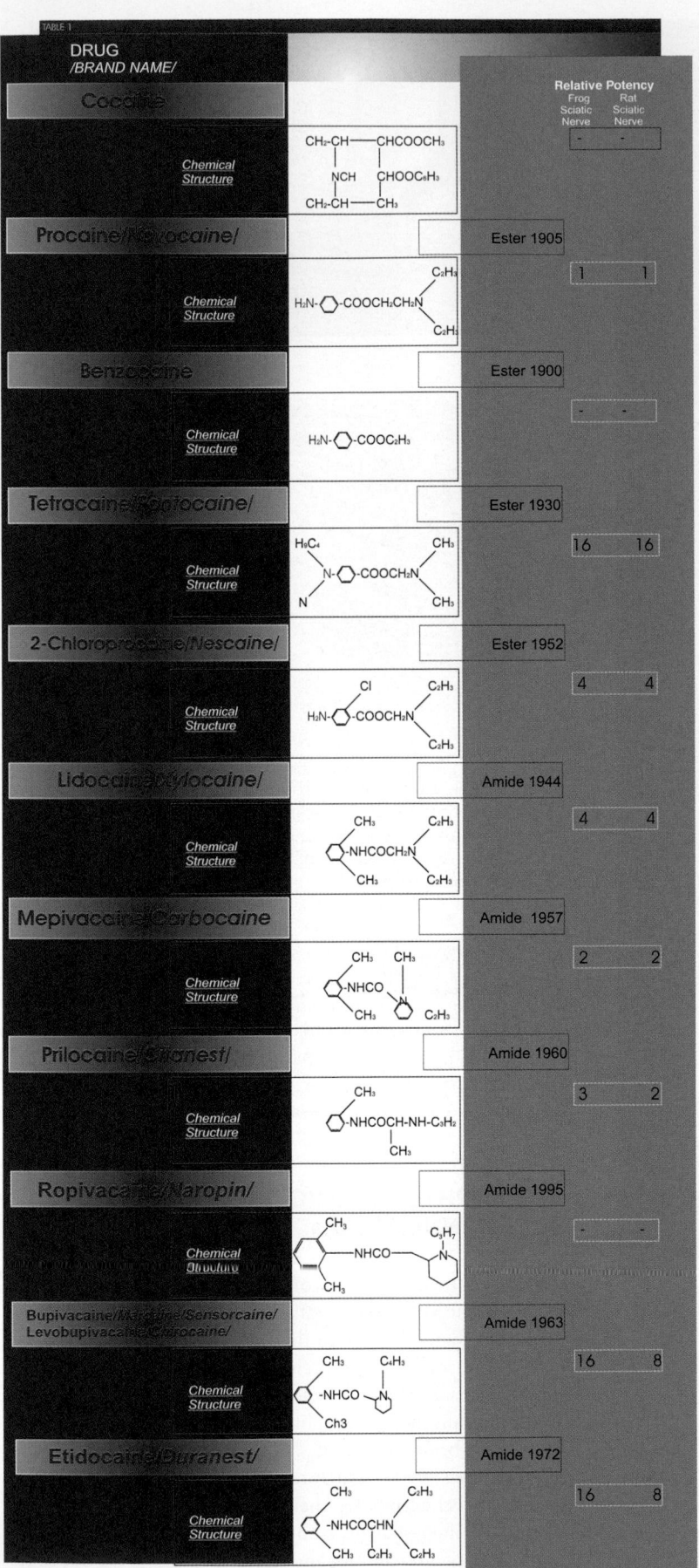

Figure 6–4. Structures of commonly used local anesthetics.

Table 6–1.

Chronology of Amide Local Anesthetic Development

Agent	Initial Investigator	Date Introduced
Cocaine	Niemann	1860
Benzocaine	Salkowski	1895
Procaine	Einhorn	1904
Dibucaine	Meischer	1925
Tetracaine	Eisler	1928
Lidocaine	Lofgren, Lundquist	1943
Chloroprocaine	Marks, Rubin	1949
Mepivacaine	Ekenstam	1956
Bupivacaine	Ekenstam	1957
Etidocaine	Adams, Kronberg, Takman	1972
Ropivacaine	Ekenstam, Sandberg	1996
Levobupivacaine	Ekenstam and others	1999

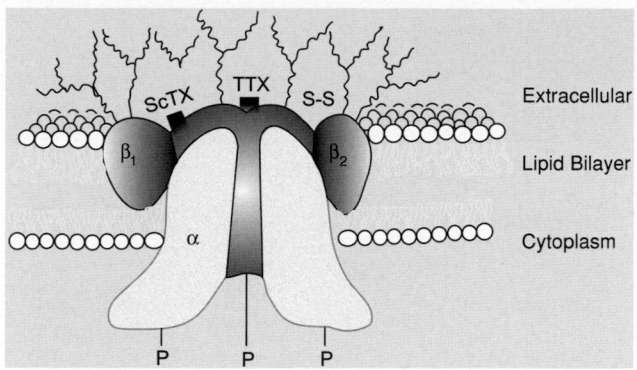

Figure 6–6. Cartoon of a Na channel in the plasma membrane. Note that all three subunits are heavily glycosylated. In contrast to local anesthetics, note that both scorpion toxins (ScTX) and tetrodotoxin (TTX) have binding sites on the external surface of the channel. Note also that the cytoplasmic side of the channel is phosphorylated. (Reprinted, with permission, from Catterall WA: Cellular and molecular biology of voltage-gated sodium channels. Physiol Rev 1992;72(Suppl):S15–S48.)

α-subunit, the site of ion conduction and LA binding, has four homologous domains each with six α-helical membrane-spanning segments (Figure 6–5).[8,9] The external surface of the α-subunit is heavily glycosylated, which serves to orient the channel properly within the plasma membrane (Figure 6–6).

Invertebrates have only one or two Na channel α-subunit genes. Humans, in contrast, have nine active Na channel α-subunit genes on four chromosomes, with cell-specific expression and localization of gene products. The Na_v 1.4 gene (by convention, geneticists refer to voltage-gated Na-channel isoforms as Na_v 1.x) supplies channels to skeletal muscle, and the Na_v 1.5 gene supplies channels to cardiac muscle, leaving seven Na_v isoforms in neural tissue (Table 6–2). Defined genes contribute specific Na channel forms to each of unmyelinated axons, nodes of Ranvier in motor axons, and small dorsal root ganglion nociceptors.[10] Whereas all Na channel α-subunits will bind local anesthetics similarly, not all of them will bind neurotoxins with the same affinity.

Na channel α- and β-subunit mutations lead to muscle, cardiac, and neural diseases.[11] For example, inherited mutations in Na_v 1.5 have been associated with congenital long QT syndrome, Bruguda syndrome, and other conduction system diseases.[11] It has been shown that certain Na_v isoforms proliferate in animal models of chronic pain. The existence of specific Na_v gene α-subunit products offers the enticing possibility that inhibitors may some day be developed for each specific Na_v α-subunit form. Such

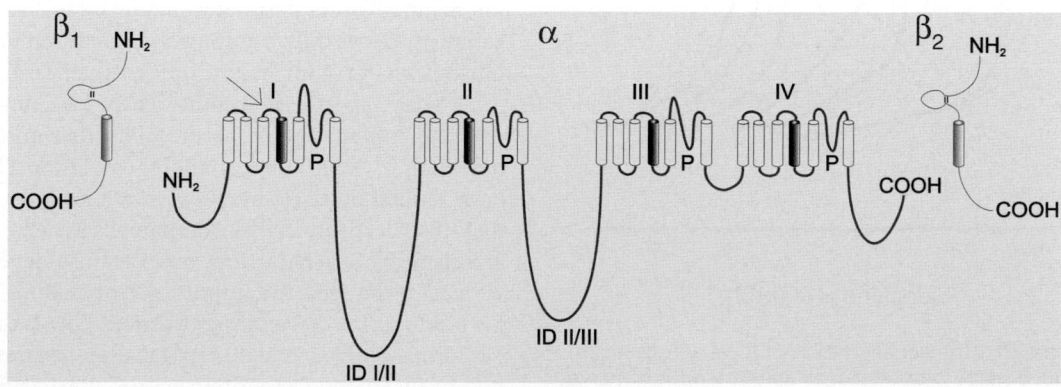

Figure 6–5. Structure of Na channel subunits. Note that the α-subunit has four domains that each contain six membrane-spanning segments. (Reprinted, with permission, from Plummer NW, Meisler MH: Evolution and diversity of mammalian sodium channel genes. Genomics 1999;57:323–331.)

Table 6–2.							
Voltage-Gated Na Channel–Neural Isoforms							
	Na$_v$1.1	**Na$_v$1.2**	**Na$_v$1.3**	**Na$_v$1.6**	**Na$_v$1.7**	**Na$_v$1.8**	**Na$_v$1.9**
Chromosome	2	2	2	12	2	3	3
Where identified	CNS, DRG	CNS	CNS upregulated after injury	DRG (large and small), CNS, Ranvier node	DRG (large and small)	DRG (small)	DRG (small)
Inactivation	Fast	Fast	Fast	Fast	Fast	Slow	Slow
TTX	Sensitive	Sensitive	Sensitive	Sensitive	Sensitive	Insensitive	Insensitive

CNS = central nervous system; DRG = dorsal root gamglion; TTX = tetrodotoxin.
Adapted, with permission, from Novakovic SD, et al. Regulation of Na$^+$ channel distribution in the nervous system. Trends Neurosci 2001;24:473–478) (Table 1, page 474).

developments could revolutionize the treatment of chronic painful conditions.

Blocking of impulses in a nerve fiber requires that a defined length of nerve become nonexcitable (to prevent the impulse from "jumping over" the blocked segment). Thus, as the LA concentration increases, it must need inhibit a shorter length of nerve to prevent impulse conduction, as is shown in Figure 6–7. Both normal conduction and LA inhibition of conduction differs between myelinated and unmyelinated nerve fibers. Conduction in myelinated fibers proceeds in jumps from one Ranvier node to the next, a process termed saltatory conduction. To block impulses in myelinated nerve fibers, it is generally necessary for LAs to inhibit channels in three successive Ranvier nodes (Figure 6–8). Unmyelinated fibers, lacking the saltatory mechanism, conduct much more slowly than myelinated fibers. Unmyelinated fibers are

relatively resistant to local anesthesia, despite their smaller diameter, due to dispersal of Na channels throughout their plasma membranes. These differences among nerve fibers arise during development when Na channels begin to cluster at Ranvier nodes in myelinated axons. Nodal clustering of channels, essential for high-speed signal transmission, is initiated by Schwann cells in the peripheral nervous system and by oligodendrocytes in the central nervous system.[12] It is the loss of clustering of Na channels in axons that underlies the electrophysiologic consequences of multiple sclerosis.

Na channels exists in at least three native conformations: "resting," "open," and "inactivated," first described by Hodgkin and Huxley.[13] During an action potential, neuronal Na channels open briefly, allowing extracellular Na ions to flow into the cell, depolarizing the plasma membrane. After only a few milliseconds, Na channels inactivate (whereupon the Na current ceases). Na channels return to the resting conformation with membrane repolarization. The process by which channels change from conducting to nonconducting forms is termed *gating*. Gating is assumed to result from movements of dipoles in response to changes in potential. The process by which voltage-gated channels operate likely involves movements of paddle-shaped voltage sensors within the channel's outer perimeter (Figure 6–9).[14,15] The speed of gating processes differs among Na$_v$ α-subunit forms: skeletal muscle and nerve forms gate quicker than cardiac forms.

Local anesthesia results when LAs bind Na channels and inhibit the Na permeability that underlies action potentials.[6,13] Our understanding of LA mechanisms has been refined by several key observations. Taylor confirmed that LAs selectively inhibit Na channels in nerves under voltage clamp.[16] Strichartz first observed use-dependent block with LAs, showing the importance of channel opening for LA binding. *Use-dependence* describes how LA inhibition of Na currents increases with repetitive depolarizations. Repetitive trains of depolarizations increase the likelihood that an LA will encounter an Na channel that is open or inactivated, both of which forms have greater LA affinity than do resting channels (Figure 6–10).[6,13,17] Thus, membrane potential

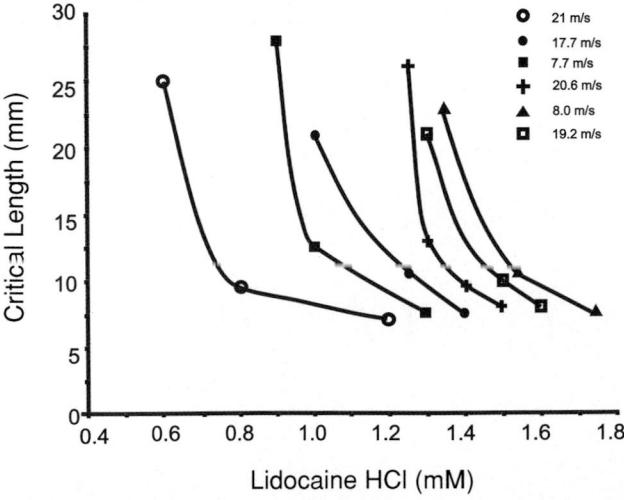

Figure 6–7. Note that the concentration of local anesthetic required to produce nerve block declines as the length of nerve exposed to the local anesthetic increases. (Reprinted, with permission, from Raymond SA, Steffensen SC, Gugino LD, et al: The role of length of nerve exposed to local anesthetics in impulse blocking action. Anesth Analg 1989;68:563–570.)

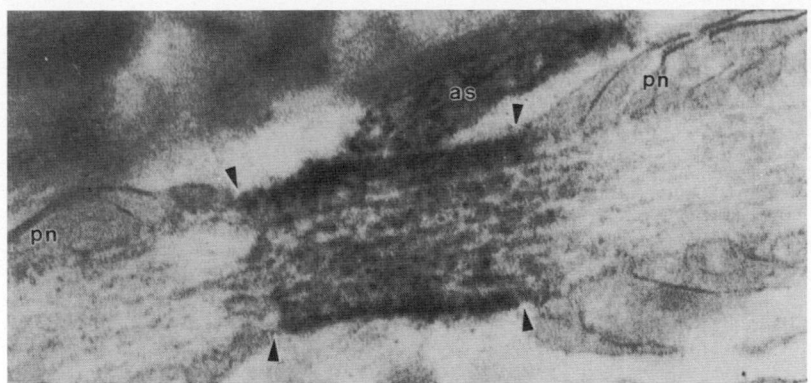

Figure 6–8. Electron micrograph of a node of Ranvier. Na channels have been immunolabeled and appear as dense granules between the four arrows. The paranodal region is indicated by pn," and an astrocyte is indicated by as." (Reprinted, with permission, from Black JA, Friedman B, Waxman SG, et al: Immunoultrastructural localization of sodium channels at nodes of Ranvier and perinodal astrocytes in rat optic nerve. Proc R Soc Lond B Biol Sci 1989;238:39–51.)

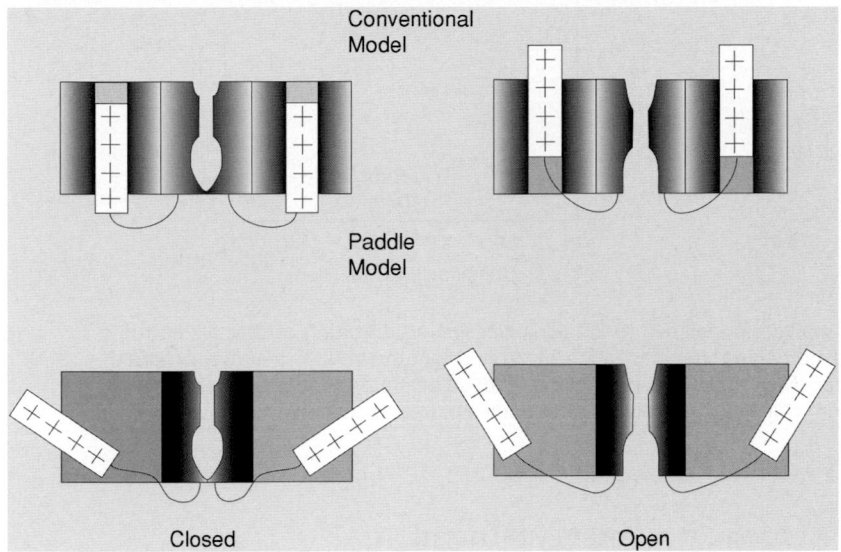

Conventional Model

Paddle Model

Closed

Open

Figure 6–9. In the conventional model for voltage-gating the voltage-sensing part of the channel slides in and out" of the membrane. More recent x-ray diffraction studies of the channel suggest that a more appropriate mechanism is that of paddle-like structures sliding diagonally through the plasma membrane. (Reprinted, with permission, from Århem P: Voltage sensing in ion channels: A 50-year-old mystery resolved? Lancet 2004;363:1221.)

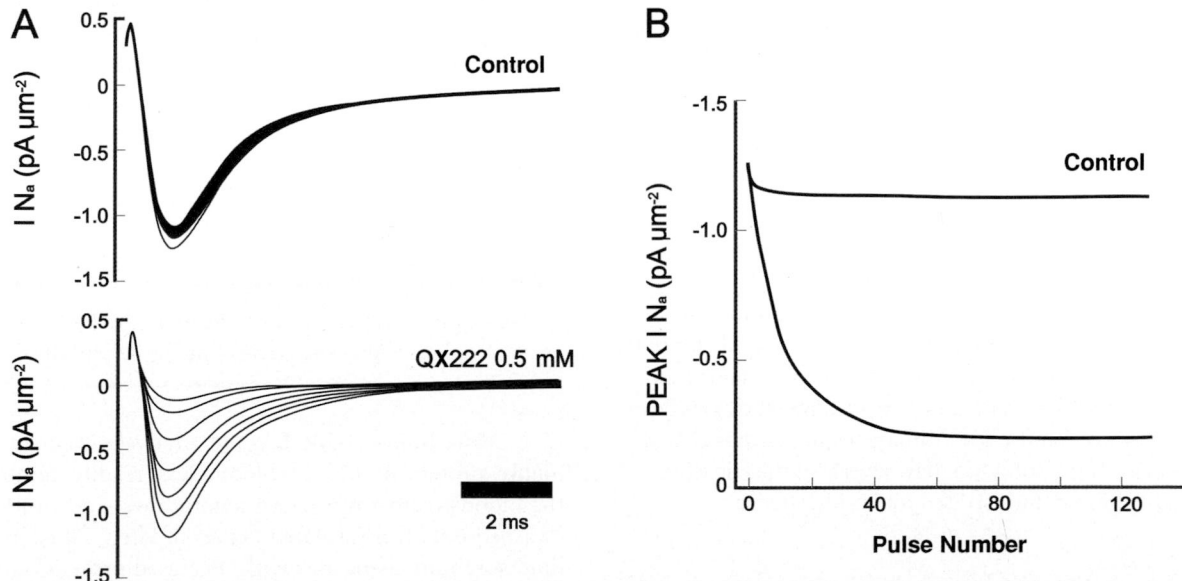

Figure 6–10. Use-dependent block of Na currents in Purkinje fibers. Under control conditions each of a train of impulses results in identical currents. In the presence of the local anesthetic QX222, the first impulse is nearly the same size as under control conditions. Each succeeding impulse is smaller (reduced peak I_{Na}), reflecting accumulating block of Na channels, until a nadir is reached. (Reprinted, with permission, from Hanck DA, Makielski JC, Sheets MF: Kinetic effects of quaternary lidocaine block of cardiac sodium channels: A gating current study. J Gen Physiol 1994;103: 19–43.)

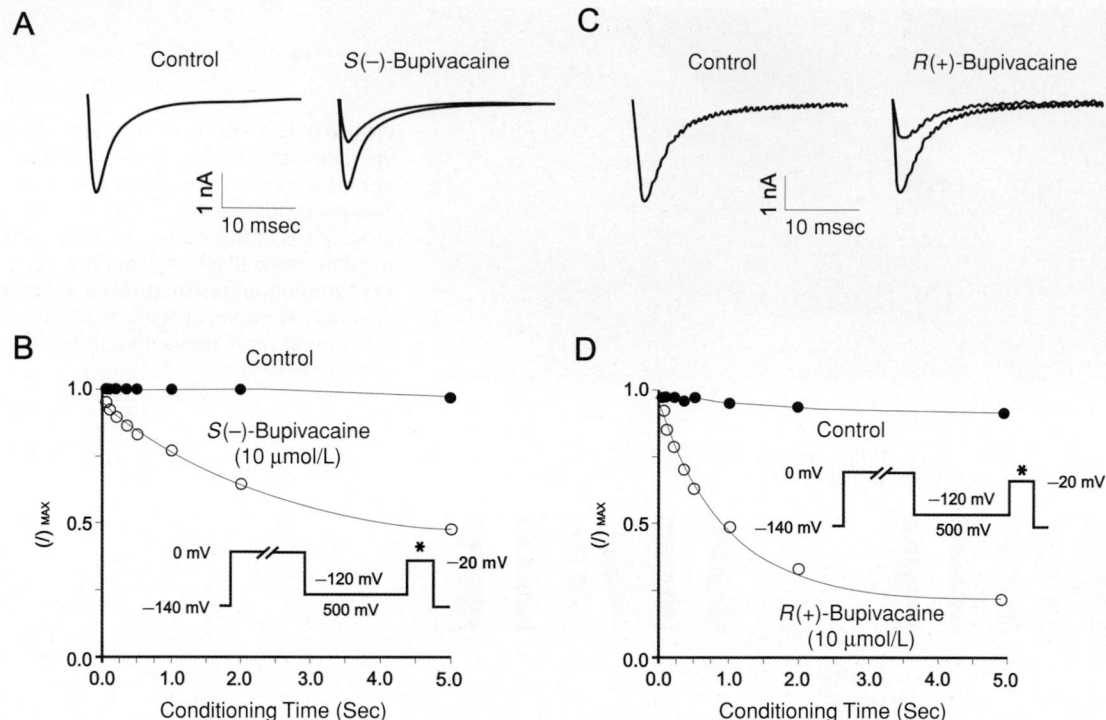

Figure 6–11. Reduced potency of $S(-)$-bupivacaine relative to $R(+)$-bupivacaine at inhibiting cardiac Na currents under voltage clamp. After a standard conditioning" depolarization of varying lengths, the $S(-)$-isomer produces less reduction of I/I_{max} than the $R(+)$-isomer. (Reprinted, with permission, from Valenzuela C, Snyders DJ, Bennett PB, et al: Stereoselective block of cardiac sodium channels by bupivacaine in guinea pig ventricular myocytes. Circulation 1995;92:3014–3024.)

influences both Na channel conformation and Na channel affinity for LAs. Use-dependent block appears important for LAs functioning as antiarrhythmics and may also underlie the effectiveness of reduced LA concentrations in managing pain. Finally, using site-directed mutagenesis, Ragsdale and Wang have localized LA binding to specific amino acids in D4S6 of Na$_v$ 1.2 and Na$_v$ 1.4.[18,19]

Some LA optical isomers confer greater apparent safety than their opposite enantiomer. For example, under voltage clamp, the $R(+)$-bupivacaine isomer more potently inhibits cardiac Na currents than the $S(-)$-bupivacaine (levobupivacaine) isomer (Figure 6–11).

Many other types of chemicals will also bind and inhibit Na channels, including general anesthetics, substance P inhibitors, α_2-adrenergic agonists, tricyclic antidepressants, and nerve toxins.[6,20–22] The latter two chemical classes have undergone animal and early human testing as possible replacements for LAs. Unfortunately, several of the tricyclic antidepressants have demonstrated toxic side effects.

LA PHARMACODYNAMICS

In clinical practice LAs are typically described by their potency, duration of action, speed of onset and tendency for differential sensory nerve block. These properties do not sort independently.

Potency & Duration

Nerve-blocking potency of LAs increases with increasing molecular weight and increasing lipid solubility.[23,24] Larger, more lipophilic LAs permeate nerve membranes more readily and bind Na channels with greater affinity. For example, etidocaine and bupivacaine have greater lipid solubility and potency than lidocaine and mepivacaine, to which they are closely related chemically.

Clinical Pearl

■ Nerve-blocking potency of LAs increases with increasing molecular weight and increasing lipid solubility.

More lipid-soluble LAs are relatively water-insoluble, highly protein-bound in blood, less readily removed by the bloodstream from nerve membranes, and more slowly "washed out" from isolated nerves in vitro. Thus, increased lipid solubility associates with increased protein binding in blood, increased potency, and longer duration of action. Extent and duration of anesthesia can be correlated with LA content of nerves in animal experiments.[25,26] In animals, blocks of greater depth and longer duration arise from smaller volumes of more concentrated LA, compared wth larger volumes of less concentrated LA.[27]

Table 6–3.

Characteristics of Local Anesthetics

Physical and Chemical
  Increasing lipid solubility
  Increased protein binding

Pharmacologic and Toxicologic
  Increasing potency
  Prolonged onset time
  Prolonged duration of action
  Increasing tendency to produce severe cardiovascular
    toxicity

In general, all tend to sort together

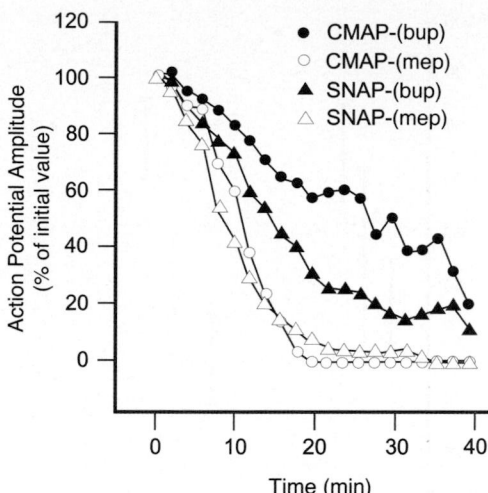

Figure 6–12. Differential onset of median nerve block with bupivacaine 0.3% (bup), but not with mepivacaine 1% (mep). Note that the compound motor action potential (CMAP) is inhibited less than the sensory nerve action potential (SNAP) during onset of bupivacaine block in these normal volunteer subjects. At steady state (20 min) CMAP and SNAP are comparably inhibited. On the other hand, mepivacaine produced faster inhibition of both CMAP and SNAP, and there was no differential onset of block. (Reprinted, with permission, from Butterworth J, Ririe DG, Thompson RB, et al: Differential onset of median nerve block: Randomized, double-blind comparison of mepivacaine and bupivacaine in healthy volunteers. Br J Anaesth 81:515–521, 1998.)

Speed of Onset

Many textbooks and review articles assert that the onset of anesthesia in isolated nerves decreases with increasing LA lipid solubility and increasing pK_a (Table 6–3). At any pH, the percentage of LA molecules present in the uncharged form, largely responsible for membrane permeability, decreases with increasing pK_a.[23,24] However, of the two LAs of fastest onset, etidocaine is highly lipid-soluble and chloroprocaine has a pK_a greater than that of other LAs. Finally, LA rate of onset associates with aqueous diffusion rate, which declines with increasing molecular weight.[28]

Differential Sensory Nerve Block

Regional anesthesia and pain management would be transformed by an LA that would selectively inhibit pain transmission while leaving other functions intact. However, sensory anesthesia sufficient for skin incision usually cannot be obtained without motor impairment.[3,4,6] As was first demonstrated by Gasser and Erlanger in 1929, all LAs will block smaller (diameter) fibers at lower concentrations than are required to block larger fibers of the same type.[29,30] As a group, unmyelinated fibers are resistant to LAs compared with larger myelinated A-δ fibers.[29,30] Bupivacaine and ropivacaine are relatively selective for sensory fibers. Bupivacaine produces more rapid onset of sensory than motor block, whereas the closely related chemical mepivacaine demonstrates no differential onset during median nerve blocks (Figure 6–12).[31] True differential anesthesia may be possible when Na_v isoform-selective antagonists become available. Certain Na_v isoforms have been found to be prevalent in dorsal root ganglia, and (as previously noted) the relative populations of various Na_v isoforms can change in response to various pain states.[32]

Other Factors Influencing LA Activity

Many factors influence the ability of a given LA to produce adequate regional anesthesia, including the dose, site of administration, additives, temperature, and pregnancy. As the

LA dose increases, the likelihood of success and the duration of anesthesia increase, while the delay of onset and tendency for differential block decrease. In general, the fastest onset and shortest duration of anesthesia occur with spinal or subcutaneous injections; a slow onset and long duration are obtained with plexus blocks.[33]

Clinical Pearl

- The effectiveness of a given LA is influenced by the dose, site of administration, additives, temperature, and pregnancy.

Epinephrine is frequently added to LA solutions to cause vasoconstriction and to serve as a marker for intravascular injection.[4,7] Epinephrine and other α_1-agonists increase LA duration largely by prolonging and increasing intraneural concentrations of LAs.[26] Blood flow is decreased only briefly, and the block will persist long after the α_1-adrenergic effect on blood flow has disipated.[34] Other popular LA additives include clonidine, $NaHCO_3$, opioids, neostigmine, and hyaluronidase.

LAs have greater apparent potency at basic pH, where an increased fraction of LA molecules are uncharged, than at more acidic pH (Figure 6–13).[35] Uncharged LA bases diffuse across nerve sheaths and membranes more readily than charged LAs, hastening onset of anesthesia. Not surprisingly,

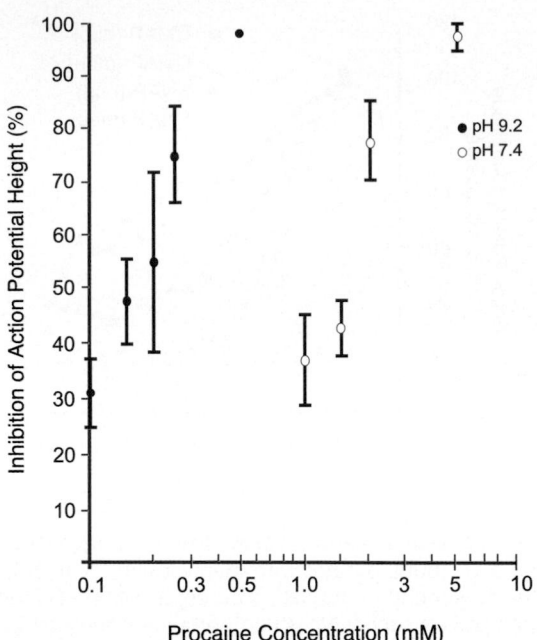

Figure 6–13. The potency of procaine at inhibiting compound action potentials in isolated frog sciatic nerves is dramatically increased at pH 9.2 as compared with pH 7.4. (Reprinted, with permission, from Butterworth JF 4th, Lief PA, Strichartz, GR: The pH-dependent local anesthetic activity of diethylaminoethanol, a procaine metabolite. Anesthesiology 1988;68:501–506.)

some clinical studies show that the addition of sodium bicarbonate to LAs speeds the onset of nerve blocks.[4,7] Bicarbonate has an inconsistent action during clinical nerve block, however, in that not all studies demonstrate a faster onset of anesthesia. One might anticipate that bicarbonate would have its greatest effect when added to LA solutions to which epinephrine was added by the manufacturer. Such solutions are more acidic than "plain" (epinephrine-free) LA solutions so as to increase shelf life. Bicarbonate shortens duration of lidocaine in animals.[27] Curiously, once LAs gain access to the cytoplasmic side of the Na channel, H^+ ions potentiate use-dependent block.[6,13]

Clinical Pearl

■ Pregnancy increases neural susceptibility to LAs.

Pregnant women and pregnant animals demonstrate increased neural susceptibility to LAs.[36–38] In addition, spread of neuraxial anesthesia likely increases during pregnancy due to decreases in thoracolumbar cereborspinal fluid volume.

BLOOD CONCENTRATIONS & PHARMACOKINETICS

Peak LA concentrations vary by the site of injection (Figure 6–14). With the same LA dose, intercostal blocks consistently produce greater peak LA concentrations than

epidural or plexus blocks.[4,7,33,39] As has been recently discussed by others, it makes little sense to speak of "maximal" doses of local anesthetics except in reference to a specific nerve block procedure.[40]

In blood, all LAs are partially protein-bound, primarily to α_1-acid glycoprotein and secondarily to albumin.[3,4,7] Affinity for α_1-acid glycoprotein correlates with LA hydrophobicity and decreases with protonation.[41] Extent of protein binding is influenced by the concentration of α_1-acid glycoprotein. Both protein binding and protein concentration decline during pregnancy.[42] During longer term infusion of LA and LA–opioid combinations, concentrations of serum binding proteins progressively increase.[43] There is considerable first-pass uptake of LAs by the lungs,[44] and animal studies suggest that patients with right-to-left cardiac shunting may be expected to demonstrate LA toxicity after smaller intravenous bolus doses.[45]

Clinical Pearls

■ Recommendations on maximal doses of LAs commonly found in pharmacology texts are not directly applicable to the practice of regional anesthesia.

■ The serum concentrations of LAs depend on the injection technique, place of injection, and addition of additives to LA.

■ Any recommendation on the maximal doses can be valid only in reference to a specific nerve block procedure

Esters undergo rapid hydrolysis in blood, catalyzed by pseudocholinesterase.[3,4,7] Procaine and benzocaine are metabolized to *para*-aminobenzoic acid (PABA), the species underlying anaphylaxis to these agents.[4] The amides undergo metabolism in the liver. Lidocaine undergoes oxidative N-dealkylation (by the cytochromes CYP 1A2 and CYP 3A4 to monoethyl glycine xylidide and glycine xylidide).[3,4,7] Bupivacaine, ropivacaine, mepivacaine, and etidocaine also undergo N-dealkylation and hydroxylation.[3,4,7] Prilocaine is hydroxylized to *o*-toluidine, which causes methemoglobinemia.[4,24] Prilocaine doses >8 mg/kg may be expected to produce sufficient methemoglobin concentrations to cause clinical cyanosis. Amide LA clearance is highly dependent on hepatic blood flow, hepatic extraction, and enzyme function, and is reduced by factors that decrease hepatic blood flow, such as β-adrenergic receptor or H_2-receptor blockers, and by heart or liver failure.[3,4,7]

Disposition of amide LAs is altered in pregnancy due to increased cardiac output, hepatic blood flow, and clearance, as well as the previously mentioned decline in protein binding. Renal failure tends to increase volume of distribution of amide LAs and to increase the accumulation of metabolic byproducts of ester and amide local anesthetics.

Theoretically, cholinesterase deficiency and cholinesterase inhibitors should increase the risk of systemic toxicity from ester local anesthetics; however, there are no confirmatory data from patients.

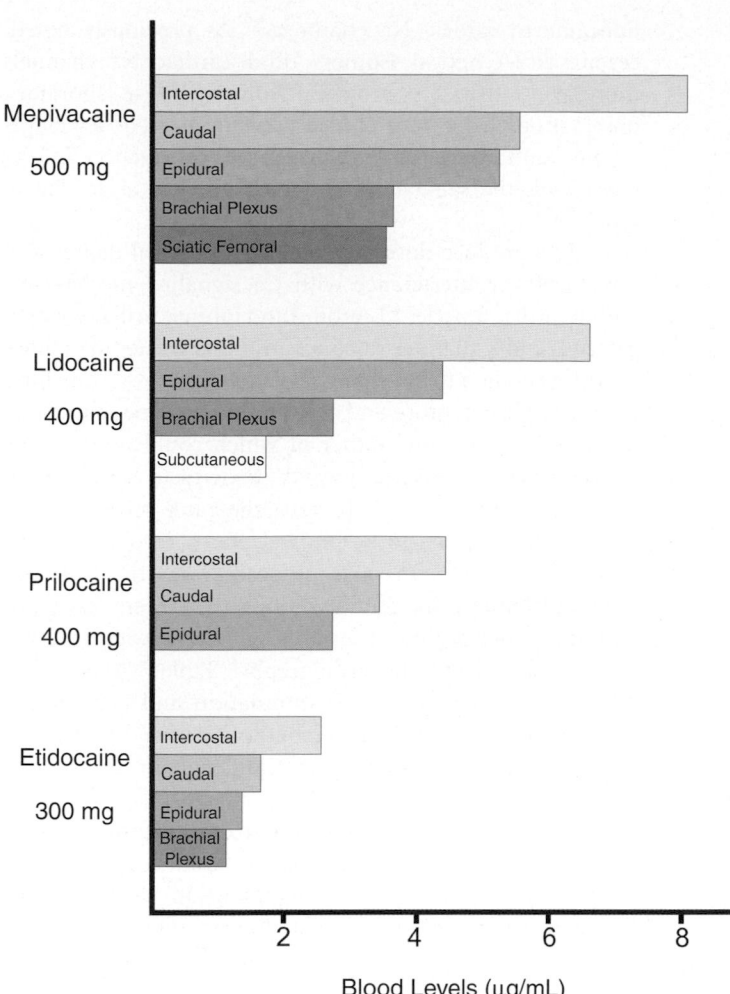

Figure 6-14. Peak blood concentrations of local anesthetics after various forms of regional anesthesia. Note that intercostal blocks consistently results in the greatest local anesthetic concentrations in blood, plexus blocks result in the least local anesthetic concentrations in blood, and that epidural/caudal techniques are in between. (Reprinted, with permission, from Covino BG, Vassallo HG: *Local Anesthetics: Mechanisms of Action and Clinical Use.* Grune & Stratton, 1976.)

Some drugs inhibit various cytochromes responsible for LA metabolism; however, the importance of cytochrome inhibitors varies depending on the specific LA species. β-Blockers and H_2-receptor blockers inhibit CYP 2D6, which may contribute to reduced amide LA metabolism. Itraconazole has no effect on hepatic blood flow, but inhibits CYP 3A4 and bupivacaine elimination by 20–25%.[46] Ropivacaine is hydroxylated by CYP 1A2 and metabolized to 2′, 6′-pipecoloxylidide by CYP 3A4.[47,48] Fluvoxamine inhibits CYP 1A2 and reduces ropivacaine clearance by 70%. On the other hand, coadministration with strong inhibitors of CYP 3A4 (ketoconazole, itraconazole) has only a small effect on ropivacaine clearance.

DIRECT TOXIC SIDE EFFECTS

It is a common, but misguided, assumption that all LA actions including toxic side effects arise from interaction with voltage-gated Na channels. There is abundant evidence that LAs will bind many other targets aside from Na channels, including voltage-gated K and Ca channels, HERG channels, K_{ATP} channels, enzymes, *N*-methyl-D-aspartate receptors, β-adrenergic receptors, G-protein-mediated modulation of K and Ca channels, and nicotinic acetylcholine receptors.[6,49,50]

LA binding to any one or all of these other sites could underlie LA production of spinal or epidural analgesia and could contribute to toxic side effects.[6,13,51]

Central Nervous System Side Effects

LA central nervous system (CNS) toxicity arises from inhibition of excitatory pathways in the CNS, producing a stereotypical sequence of signs and symptoms as the LA concentration in blood gradually increases (Table 6–4).[3,4,7,33] With increased LA doses, seizures may arise in the amygdala.[3,4] With further LA dosing, CNS excitation progresses to CNS depression, and eventual respiratory arrest. More potent (at nerve block) LAs produce seizures at lower blood concentrations and at lower doses than less potent LAs. In a study of cats, both metabolic and respiratory acidosis decreased the convulsive dose of lidocaine.[52]

Cardiovascular Toxicity

In laboratory experiments most LAs will not produce cardiovascular (CV) toxicity until the blood concentration exceeds three times that ncessary to produce seizures; however, there are clinical reports of simultaneous CNS and CV toxicity with bupivacaine (Table 6–5).[3,4,7] In dogs, supraconvulsant doses of bupivacaine more commonly produce arrhythmias than

Table 6–4.

Progression of Signs and Symptoms of Toxicity as the Local Anesthetic Dose (or Concentration) Gradually Increases

Vertigo

Tinnitus

Ominous feelings

Circumoral numbness

Garrulousness

Tremors

Myoclonic jerks

Convulsions

Coma

Cardiovascular collapse

supraconvulsant doses of ropivacaine and lidocaine.[53] LAs produce CV signs of CNS excitation (increased heart rate, arterial blood pressure, and cardiac output) at lower concentrations than those associated with cardiac depression. Hypocapnia reduces ropivacaine-induced changes in ST segments and left-ventricular contractility.[54]

Clinical Pearl

- In laboratory experiments most LAs will not produce CV toxicity until the blood concentration exceeds three times that ncessary to produce seizures.

LAs bind and inhibit cardiac Na channels (Na$_v$ 1.5 isoform).[3,13] Bupivacaine binds more avidly and longer than lidocaine to cardiac Na channels.[55] As previously noted, certain $R(+)$ optical isomers bind cardiac Na channels more avidly than $S(-)$ optical isomers. These laboratory observations led to the clinical development of levobupivacaine and ropivacaine. LAs inhibit conduction in the heart with the same rank order of potency as for nerve block.[56,57]

LAs produce dose-dependent myocardial depression, possibly from interference with Ca signaling mechanisms within cardiac muscle.[56] LAs bind and inhibit cardiac voltage-gated Ca and K channels at concentrations greater than those at which binding to Na channels is maximal.[6,13,58] LAs bind β-adrenergic receptors and inhibit epinephrine-stimulated cyclic-AMP formation, either of which could underlie the refractoriness of bupivacaine CV toxicity to standard resuscitation measures.[59,60] In rats, the rank order for cardiac toxicity appears to be bupivacaine > levobupivacaine > ropivacaine.[61–63] In dogs, lidocaine was the least potent, and bupivacaine and levobupivacaine were more potent than ropivacaine at inhibiting left-ventricular function as assessed by echocardiography (Table 6–6). In dogs, both programmed electrical stimulation and epinephrine resuscitation elicited more arrhythmias after bupivacaine and levobupivacaine than after lidocaine or ropivacaine administration.[64–66]

The mechanism by which CV toxicity is produced may depend on which LA has been administered. When LAs were given to the point of extreme hypotension, dogs receiving lidocaine could be resuscitated, but required continuing infusion of epinephrine to counteract LA-induced myocardial depression. Conversely, many dogs receiving bupivacaine or levobupivacaine to the point of extreme hypotension could not be resuscitated. After bupivacaine, levobupivacaine, or ropivacaine, dogs that could be defibrillated often required no additional therapy.[64–66] Similarly in pigs, comparing lidocaine with bupivacaine, the ratio of potency for myocardial depression was 1:4; whereas that for arrhythmogenesis was 1:16.[67] LAs produce dilation of vascular smooth muscle at clinical concentrations.[68] Cocaine is the only LA that consistently produces local vasoconstriction.

Table 6–5.

Margin of Safety Between Convulsive and Lethal Dose of Local Anesthetics Observed in Anesthetized Dogs

	Lidocaine	Etidocaine	Bupivacaine	Tetracaine
Dose producing convulsions in all animals (mg/kg)	22	8	5	4
Dose producing lethality in all animals (mg/kg)	76	40	20	27

Data sources: Reg Anesth 1982;7:14–19; Anesth Analg 1982;61:317–322; and Anesth Analg 1983;62:375–379.

Table 6–6.

Effects of Local Anesthetics on Indices of Myocardial Function Measured in Dogs

Local Anesthetic	LVEDP (EC$_{50}$ for 125% base) (mcg/mL)	dP/dt$_{max}$ (EC$_{50}$ for 65% base) (mcg/mL)	%FS (EC$_{50}$ for 65% base) (mcg/mL)
Bupivacaine	2.20 (1.15–4.4)	2.30 (1.73–3.05)	2.12 (1.47–3.08)
Levobupivacaine	1.65 (0.87–3.13)	2.42 (1.88–3.12)	1.26 (0.89–1.79)
Ropivacaine	3.98 (2.1–7.54)[a]	4.03 (3.13–5.19)[b]	2.95 (2.07–4.19)[a]
Lidocaine	6.75 (2.96–15.4)[c]	7.95 (5.74–11.02)[d]	5.54 (3.52–8.72)[d]

Note: Data represented are EC estimates and 95% confidence intervals.
[a] *Ropivacaine > levobupivacaine, p < .05.*
[b] *Ropivacaine > bupivacaine, levobupivacaine, p < .05.*
[c] *Lidocaine > bupivacaine, levobupivacaine, p < .01.*
[d] *Lidocaine > bupivacaine, levobupivacaine, ropivacaine, p < 0.01.*

EC$_{50}$, effective concentration for 50% of population; base, baseline; LVEDP = left-ventricular end-diastolic pressure; dP/dt$_{max}$ = maximal rate-of-change of developed pressure (inotropy); %FS = percent fractional shortening.
Reproduced, with permission, from Tech Reg Anesth Pain Manage 2001;5:48–55.

Allergic Reactions

Clinical Pearls

- True immunologic reactions to LAs are generally rare.
- True allergic reactions to preservative-free amide-type local anesthetics are so rare that they are not reportable.
- True anaphylaxis appears more common with ester LAs that are metabolized directly to PABA than to other LAs.
- Accidental intravenous injections of LAs or preservative/epinephrine-containing LA are often misdiagnosed as allergic reactions.
- Some patients may react to preservatives, such as methylparaben, included with LAs.

True immunologic reactions to LAs are rare.[69] Accidental intravenous injections of LAs are sometimes misdiagnosed as allergic reactions. True anaphylaxis appears more common with ester LAs that are metabolized directly to PABA than to other LAs. Some patients may react to preservatives, such as methylparaben, included with LAs. In the allergy and immunology literature, several recent studies have shown that patients referred for evaluation of apparent LA allergy, even after exhibiting signs or symptoms of anaphylaxis, almost never demonstrate true allergy to the LA that was administered.[69,70]

Neurotoxic Effects

During the 1980s, 2-chloroprocaine (at that time formulated with sodium metabisulfite at a relatively acidic pH) occasionally produced cauda equina syndrome when large doses were accidentally injected into spinal fluid during attempted epidural administration.[4,6,71–73] Reports of neurotoxicity virtually disappeared when the compound was reformulated, but have now returned following the introduction of generic products containing the original metabisulfite and pH.[73] Whether the toxin is 2-chloroprocaine or metabisulfite remains unsettled: 2-chloroprocaine is now being tested as a substitute for lidocaine in human spinal anesthesia,[74] and a series of publications suggest that it may be safe and effective. At the same time, other investigators have linked neurotoxic reactions in animals to large doses of 2-chloroprocaine rather than to metabisulfite.[75] Presently, there is controversy about transient neurologic symptoms and persistent sacral deficits after lidocaine spinal anesthesia. These reports have persuaded many physicians to abandon lidocaine spinal anesthesia. Unlike other spinal LA solutions, lidocaine 5% permanently interrupts conduction when applied to isolated nerves or to isolated neurons.[76] This may be the result of lidocaine-induced increases in intracellular calcium and does not appear to involve Na channel blockade.[77] We await those studies that will determine whether chloroprocaine, or perhaps mepivacaine, will prove to be appropriate lidocaine substitutes for brief spinal anesthesias.

Treatment of Local Anesthetic Toxicity

Treatment of adverse LA reactions depends on their severity. Minor reactions can be allowed to terminate spontaneously. LA-induced seizures should be managed by maintaining a patent airway and by providing oxygen. Seizures may be terminated with intravenous thiopental (1–2 mg/kg), midazolam (0.05–0.10 mg/kg), propofol (0.5–1.5 mg/kg), or

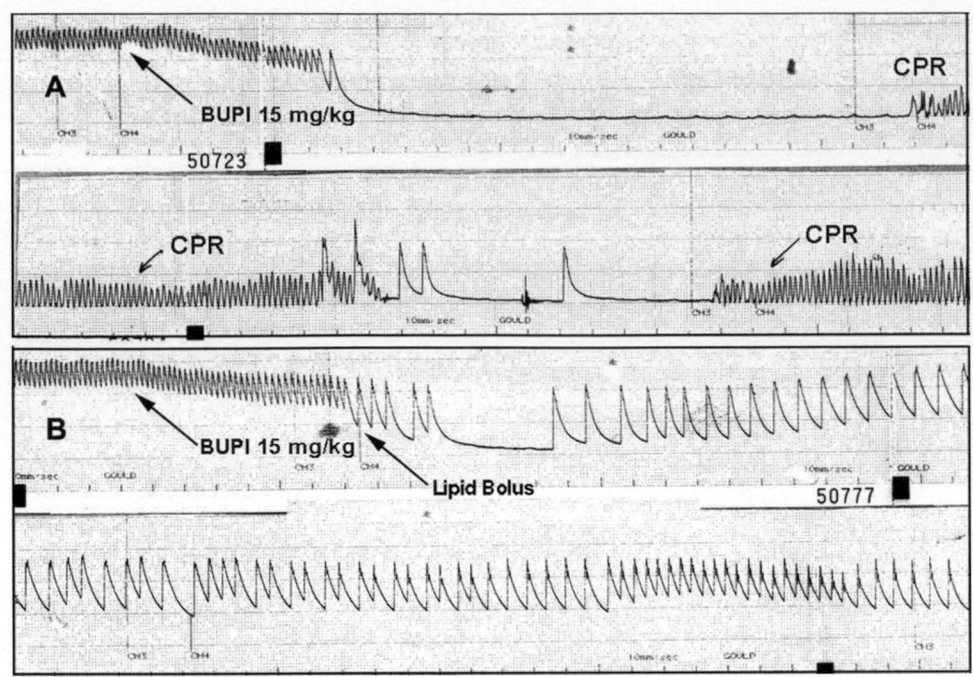

Figure 6–15. **A:** An anesthetized rat is given bupivacaine 15 mg/kg as indicated. The arterial blood pressure rapidly declines to cardiac arrest. CPR is given but no arterial pressure is observed when CPR is discontinued. **B:** The same experiment is conducted, but a bolus of lipid is given, note that the arterial pressure is never lost (despite the same dose of bupivacaine being used) and that cardiac arrest does not ensue. (Reprinted, with permission, from Weinberg GL: Current concepts in resuscitation of patients with local anesthetic cardiac toxicity. Reg Anesth Pain Med 2002;27: 568–575.)

a paralytic dose of succinylcholine (0.5–1 mg/kg) followed by mask ventilation or tracheal intubation.[4] If LA CV depression is manifested by moderate hypotension, it may be treated by infusion of intravenous fluids and vasopressors (phenylephrine 0.5–5 mcg/kg/min, norepinephrine 0.02–0.2 mcg/kg/min, or vasopressin 40 mcg IV). If myocardial failure is present, epinephrine (1–15 mcg/kg IV bolus) may be required. When toxicity progresses to cardiac arrest, the guidelines for advanced cardiac life support are reasonable;[78] however, I suggest that amiodarone and vasopressin be substituted for lidocaine and epinephrine, respectively.[79–81] With unresponsive bupivacaine cardiac toxicity, intravenous lipid or cardiopulmonary bypass should be considered.[82] Recent animal experiments demonstrate the remarkable ability of lipid infusion to resuscitate animals from bupivacaine overdosage, even after 10 min of unsuccessful "conventional" resuscitative efforts (Figure 6–15).[83–85] We now have a report showing that lipid infusion can resuscitate an LA-intoxicated human.[86] Given the nearly nontoxic status of lipid infusion, one could not make a convincing argument to withhold this therapy from a patient experiencing difficult resuscitation from LA intoxication.

SUMMARY

After nearly 120 years of use in Western medicine, LAs remain important tools for the twenty-first-century physician.

Peripheral nerve blocks are almost certainly the result of LA inhibition of voltage-gated Na channels in neuronal membranes. The mechanisms of spinal and epidural anesthesia remain poorly defined. The appropriate and safe dose of LAs is defined by the specific nerve block procedure that is to be undertaken. The mechanisms by which differing LAs produce CV toxicity likely vary: the more potent agents (eg, bupivacaine) may produce arrhythmias through a Na channel action, whereas the less potent agents (eg, lidocaine) may produce myocardial depression through other pathways.

References

1. Vandam LD: Some aspects of the history of local anesthesia. In Strichartz GR, ed: *Local Anesthetics: Handbook of Experimental Pharmacology.* Springer-Verlag, 1987, pp 1–19.
2. Calatayud J, Gonzalez A: History of the development and evolution of local anesthesia since the coca leaf. Anesthesiology 2003;98:1503–1508.
3. Strichartz GR: *Local Anesthetics: Handbook of Experimental Pharmacology.* Springer-Verlag, 1987.
4. de Jong RH: *Local Anesthetics.* Mosby-Year Book, 1994.
5. Keys TE: *The History of Surgical Anesthesia.* Wood Library, Museum of Anesthesiology, 1996.
6. Butterworth JF IV, Strichartz GR: Molecular mechanisms of local anesthesia: A review. Anesthesiology 1990;72:711–734.
7. Tetzlaff J: *Clinical Pharmacology of Local Anesthetics.* Butterworth-Heinemann, 2000.
8. Wang SY, Nau C, Wang GK: Residues in Na(+) channel D3-S6 segment modulate both batrachotoxin and local anesthetic affinities. Biophys J 2000;79:1379–1387.

9. Wang SY, Barile M, Wang GK: Disparate role of Na(+) channel D2-S6 residues in batrachotoxin and local anesthetic action. Mol Pharmacol 2001;59:1100–1107.

10. Lopreato GF, Lu Y, Southwell A, et al: Evolution and divergence of sodium channel genes in vertebrates. Proc Natl Acad Sci USA 2001;98:7588–7592.

11. Viswanathan PC, Balser JR: Inherited sodium channelopathies: A continuum of channel dysfunction. Trends Cardiovasc Med 2004;14:28–35.

12. Rasband MN, Shrager P: Ion channel sequestration in central nervous system axons. J Physiol 2000;525:63–73.

13. Hille B: *Ionic Channels of Excitable Membranes,* 3rd ed. Sinauer Associates, 2001.

14. Jiang Y, Lee A, Chen J, et al: X-ray structure of a voltage-dependent K+ channel. Nature 2003;423:33–41.

15. Jiang Y, Ruta V, Chen J, et al: The principle of gating charge movement in a voltage-dependent K+ channel. Nature 2003;423:42–48.

16. Taylor CP. Na$^+$ currents that fail to activate. Trends Neurosci 1993;16:455–460.

17. Hanck DA, Makielski JC, Sheets MF: Kinetic effects of quaternary lidocaine block of cardiac sodium channels: A gating current study. J Gen Physiol 1994;103:19–43.

18. Ragsdale DS, McPhee JC, Scheuer T, et al: Molecular determinants of state-dependent block of Na$^+$ channels by local anesthetics. Science 1994;265:1724–1728.

19. Wang GK, Quan C, Wang S: A common local anesthetic receptor for benzocaine and etidocaine in voltage-gated mu1 Na$^+$ channels. Pflugers Arch 1998;435:293–302.

20. Sudoh Y, Cahoon EE, Gerner P, et al: Tricyclic antidepressants as long-acting local anesthetics. Pain 2003;103:49–55.

21. Kohane DS, Lu NT, Gokgol-Kline AC, et al: The local anesthetic properties and toxicity of saxitonin homologues for rat sciatic nerve block in vivo. Reg Anesth Pain Med 2000;25:52–59.

22. Butterworth JF IV, Strichartz GR: The alpha 2-adrenergic agonists clonidine and guanfacine produce tonic and phasic block of conduction in rat sciatic nerve fibers. Anesth Analg 1993;76:295–301.

23. Sanchez V, Arthur GR, Strichartz GR: Fundamental properties of local anesthetics. I. The dependence of lidocaine's ionization and octanol:buffer partitioning on solvent and temperature. Anesth Analg 1987;66:159–165.

24. Strichartz GR, Sanchez V, Arthur GR, et al: Fundamental properties of local anesthetics. II. Measured octanol:buffer partition coefficients and pK$_a$ values of clinically used drugs. Anesth Analg 1990;71:158–170.

25. Popitz-Bergez FA, Leeson S, Strichartz GR, et al: Relation between functional deficit and intraneural local anesthetic during peripheral nerve block. A study in the rat sciatic nerve. Anesthesiology 1995;83:583–592.

26. Sinnott CJ, Cogswell III LP, Johnson A, et al: On the mechanism by which epinephrine potentiates lidocaine's peripheral nerve block. Anesthesiology 2003;98:181–188.

27. Nakamura T, Popitz-Bergez F, Birknes J, et al: The critical role of concentration for lidocaine block of peripheral nerve in vivo: Studies of function and drug uptake in the rat. Anesthesiology 2003;99:1189–1197.

28. Brouneus F, Karami K, Beronius P, et al: Diffusive transport properties of some local anesthetics applicable for iontophoretic formulation of the drugs. Int J Pharm 2001;218:57–62.

29. Gissen AJ, Covino BG, Gregus J: Differential sensitivities of mammalian nerve fibers to local anesthetic agents. Anesthesiology 1980;53:467–474.

30. Raymond SA, Gissen AJ: Mechanisms of differential nerve block. In Strichartz GR, ed: *Handbook of Experimental Pharmacology: Local Anesthetics.* Springer-Verlag, 1987, pp 95–164.

31. Butterworth J, Ririe DG, Thompson RB, et al: Differential onset of median nerve block: Randomized, double-blind comparison of mepivacaine and bupivacaine in healthy volunteers. Br J Anaesth 1998;81:515–521.

32. Novakovic SD, Eglen RM, Hunter JC: Regulation of Na$^+$ channel distribution in the nervous system. Trends Neurosci 2001;24:473–478.

33. Covino BG, Vasallo HG: *Local Anesthetics.* Grune & Stratton, 1976.

34. Kohane DS, Lu NT, Cairns BE, et al: Effects of adrenergic agonists and antagonists on tetrodotoxin-induced nerve block. Reg Anesth Pain Med 2001;26:239–245.

35. Butterworth JF IV, Lief PA, Strichartz GR: The pH-dependent local anesthetic activity of diethylaminoethanol, a procaine metabolite. Anesthesiology 1988;68:501–506.

36. Fagraeus L, Urban BJ, Bromage PR: Spread of epidural analgesia in early pregnancy. Anesthesiology 1983;58:184–187.

37. Butterworth JF IV, Walker FO, Lysak SZ: Pregnancy increases median nerve susceptibility to lidocaine. Anesthesiology 1990;72:962–965.

38. Popitz-Bergez FA, Leeson S, Thalhammer JG, et al: Intraneural lidocaine uptake compared with analgesic differences between pregnant and nonpregnant rats. Reg Anesth 1997;22:363–371.

39. Scott DB, Jebson PJ, Braid DP, et al: Factors affecting plasma levels of lignocaine and prilocaine. Br J Anaesth 1972;44:1040–1049.

40. Rosenberg PH, Veering BTh, Urmey WF: Maximum recommended doses of local anesthetics: A multifactorial concept. Reg Anesth Pain Med 2004;29:564–575.

41. Taheri S, Cogswell LP III, Gent A, et al: Hydrophobic and ionic factors in the binding of local anesthetics to the major variant of human alpha$_1$-acid glycoprotein. J Pharmacol Exp Ther 2003;304:71–80.

42. Fragneto RY, Bader AM, Rosinia F, et al: Measurements of protein binding of lidocaine throughout pregnancy. Anesth Analg 1994;79:295–297.

43. Thomas JM, Schug SA: Recent advances in the pharmacokinetics of local anaesthetics. Long-acting amide enantiomers and continuous infusions. Clin Pharmacokinet 1999;36:67–83.

44. Rothstein P, Arthur GR, Feldman HS, et al: Bupivacaine for intercostal nerve blocks in children: Blood concentrations and pharmacokinetics. Anesth Analg 1986;65:625–632.

45. Bokesch PM, Castaneda AR, Ziemer G, et al: The influence of a right-to-left cardiac shunt on lidocaine pharmacokinetics. Anesthesiology 1987;67:739–744.

46. Palkama VJ, Neuvonen PJ, Olkkola KT: Effect of itraconazole on the pharmacokinetics of bupivacaine enantiomers in healthy volunteers. Br J Anaesth 1999;83:659–661.

47. Oda Y, Furuichi K, Tanaka K, Hiroi T, Imaoka S, Asada A, Fujimori M, Funae Y: Metabolism of a new local anesthetic, ropivacaine, by human hepatic cytochrome P450. Anesthesiology 1995;82:214–220.

48. Ekstrom G, Gunnarsson UB: Ropivacaine, a new amide-type local anesthetic agent, is metabolized by cytochromes P450 1A and 3A in human liver microsomes. Drug Metab Dispos 1996;24:955–961.

49. Hirota K, Browne T, Appadu BL, et al: Do local anaesthetics interact with dihydropyridine binding sites on neuronal L-type Ca^{2+} channels? Br J Anaesth 1997;78:185–188.

50. Olschewski A, Olschewski H, Brau ME, et al: Effect of bupivacaine on ATP-dependent potassium channels in rat cardiomyocytes. Br J Anaesth 1999;82:435–438.

51. Sugimoto M, Uchida I, Fukami S, et al: The alpha and gamma subunit-dependent effects of local anesthetics on recombinant GABA(A) receptors. Eur J Pharmacol 2000;401:329–337.

52. Englesson S, Grevsten S: The influence of acid–base changes on central nervous system toxicity of local anaesthetic agents. II. Acta Anaesthesiol Scand 1974;18:88–103.

53. Feldman HS, Arthur GR, Covino BG: Comparative systemic toxicity of convulsant and supraconvulsant doses of intravenous ropivacaine, bupivacaine, and lidocaine in the conscious dog. Anesth Analg 1989;69:794–801.

54. Porter JM, Markos F, Snow HM, et al: Effects of respiratory and metabolic pH changes and hypoxia on ropivacaine-induced cardiotoxicity in dogs. Br J Anaesth 2000;84:92–94.

55. Chernoff DM: Kinetic analysis of phasic inhibition of neuronal sodium currents by lidocaine and bupivacaine. Biophys J 1990;58:53–68.

56. Feldman HS, Covino BM, Sage DJ: Direct chronotropic and inotropic effects of local anesthetic agents in isolated guinea pig atria. Reg Anesth 1982;7:149–156.

57. Reiz S, Nath S: Cardiotoxicity of local anaesthetic agents. Br J Anaesth 1986;58:736–746.

58. McCaslin PP, Butterworth J: Bupivacaine suppresses [Ca(2+)](i) oscillations in neonatal rat cardiomyocytes with increased extracellular K+ and is reversed with increased extracellular Mg(2+). Anesth Analg 2000;91:82–88.

59. Butterworth JF IV, Brownlow RC, Leith JP, et al: Bupivacaine inhibits cyclic-3',5'-adenosine monophosphate production. A possible contributing factor to cardiovascular toxicity. Anesthesiology 1993;79:88–95.

60. Butterworth J, James RL, Grimes J: Structure-affinity relationships and stereospecificity of several homologous series of local anesthetics for the beta$_2$-adrenergic receptor. Anesth Analg 1997;85: 336–342.

61. Ohmura S, Kawada M, Ohta T, et al: Systemic toxicity and resuscitation in bupivacaine-, levobupivacaine-, or ropivacaine-infused rats. Anesth Analg 2001;93:743–748.

62. Dony P, Dewinde V, Vanderick B, et al: The comparative toxicity of ropivacaine and bupivacaine at equipotent doses in rats. Anesth Analg 2000;91:1489–1492.

63. Chang DH, Ladd LA, Copeland S, et al: Direct cardiac effects of intracoronary bupivacaine, levobupivacaine and ropivacaine in the sheep. Br J Pharmacol 2001;132:649–658.

64. Groban L, Deal DD, Vernon JC, et al: Ventricular arrhythmias with or without programmed electrical stimulation after incremental overdosage with lidocaine, bupivacaine, levobupivacaine, and ropivacaine. Anesth Analg 2000;91:1103–1111.

65. Groban L, Deal DD, Vernon JC, et al: Cardiac resuscitation after incremental overdosage with lidocaine, bupivacaine, levobupivacaine, and ropivacaine in anesthetized dogs. Anesth Analg 2001;92: 37–43.

66. Groban L, Deal DD, Vernon JC, et al: Does local anesthetic stereoselectivity or structure predict myocardial depression in anesthetized canines? Reg Anesth Pain Med 2002;27:460–468.

67. Nath S, Haggmark S, Johansson G, et al: Differential depressant and electrophysiologic cardiotoxicity of local anesthetics: An experimental study with special reference to lidocaine and bupivacaine. Anesth Analg 1986;65:1263–1270.

68. Carpenter RL, Kopacz DJ, Mackey DC: Accuracy of laser Doppler capillary flow measurements for predicting blood loss from skin incisions in pigs. Anesth Analg 1989;68:308–311.

69. deShazo RD, Nelson HS: An approach to the patient with a history of local anesthetic hypersensitivity: Experience with 90 patients. J Allergy Clin Immunol 1979;63:387–394.

70. Berkun Y, Ben-Zvi A, Levy Y, et al: Evaluation of adverse reactions to local anesthetics: experience with 236 patients. Ann Allergy Asthma Immunol 2003;91:342–345.

71. Gissen AJ, Datta S, Lambert D: The chloroprocaine controversy. I. A hypothesis to explain the neural complications of chloroprocaine epidural. Reg Anesth 1984;9:124–134.

72. Gissen AJ, Datta S, Lambert D: The chloroprocaine controversy. II. Is chloroprocaine neurotoxic? Reg Anesth 1984;9:135–145.

73. Winnie AP, Nader AM: Santayana's prophecy fulfilled. Reg Anesth Pain Med 2001;26:558–564.

74. Kouri ME, Kopacz DJ: Spinal 2-chloroprocaine: A comparison with lidocaine in volunteers. Anesth Analg 2004;98:75–80.

75. Taniguchi M, Bollen AW, Drasner K: Sodium bisulfite: Acapegoat for chloroprocaine neurotoxicity? Anesthesiology 2004;100:85–91.

76. Lambert LA, Lambert DH, Strichartz GR: Irreversible conduction block in isolated nerve by high concentrations of local anesthetics. Anesthesiology 1994;80:1082–1093.

77. Gold MS, Reichling DB, Hampl KF, et al: Lidocaine toxicity in primary afferent neurons from the rat. J Pharmacol Exp Ther 1998;285:413–421.

78. Guidelines 2000 for Cardiopulmonary Resuscitation and Emergency Cardiovascular Care. Circulation 2000;102(Suppl 1):I-1–I-384.

79. Simon L, Kariya N, Pelle-Lancien E, et al: Bupivacaine-induced QRS prolongation is enhanced by lidocaine and by phenytoin in rabbit hearts. Anesth Analg 2002;94:203–207.

80. Krismer AC, Hogan QH, Wenzel V, et al: The efficacy of epinephrine or vasopressin for resuscitation during epidural anesthesia. Anesth Analg 2001;93:734–742.

81. Mayr VD, Raedler C, Wenzel V, et al: A comparison of epinephrine and vasopressin in a porcine model of cardiac arrest after rapid intravenous injection of bupivacaine. Anesth Analg 2004;98:1426–1431.

82. Soltesz EG, van Pelt F, Byrne JG: Emergent cardiopulmonary bypass for bupivacaine cardiotoxicity. J Cardiothorac Vasc Anesth 2003;17:357–358.

83. Weinberg GL, VadeBoncouer T, Ramaraju GA, et al: Pretreatment or resuscitation with a lipid infusion shifts the dose-response to bupivacaine-induced asystole in rats. Anesthesiology 1998;88:1071–1075.

84. Weinberg G, Ripper R, Feinstein DL, et al: Lipid emulsion infusion rescues dogs from bupivacaine-induced cardiac toxicity. Reg Anesth Pain Med 2003;28:198–202.

85. Groban L, Butterworth J: Lipid reversal of bupivacaine toxicity: Has the silver bullet been identified? Reg Anesth Pain Med 2003;28:167–169.

86. Rosenblatt, MA, Abel M, Fischer GW, et al: Successful use of a 20% lipid emulsion to resuscitate a patient after a presumed bupivacaine-related cardiac arrest. Anesthesiology 2006;105:217–218.

7

Newer Amide Local Anesthetics & Sustained-Release Local Anesthetics

Clint E. Elliott, MD • Leslie C. Thomas, MD • Alan C. Santos, MD

NEWER AMIDE LOCAL ANESTHETICS

Introduction

The use of regional anesthesia has been increasing not only in obstetrics, where it is the predominant anesthetic technique used, but also during surgery and for acute postoperative pain management. This has been partly due to the safety of regional anesthesia because of better injection techniques and equipment, increased attention to detecting (preventing) misplaced injection, greater vigilance/monitoring, and the introduction of newer long-acting amide local anesthetics. The increasing demand for regional anesthesia is nowhere more true than in obstetric anesthesia, where local anesthetics have become the most frequently administered drugs for obstetric pain relief or cesarean delivery. When injected epidurally or intrathecally, local anesthetics provide effective labor analgesia that is superior to that of systemic opioids and without the attendant risks of maternal sedation and neonatal depression. Regional anesthesia is now the most frequently used technique for cesarean section delivery in the U.S.[1]

Historical Perspective

Why the need for new amide local anesthetics? The answer is partly related to the history of bupivacaine use, particularly in North America and Europe. After its introduction into clinical practice, bupivacaine quickly became very popular for several reasons, particularly for use in obstetrics. It has a longer duration of action than 2-chloroprocaine and lidocaine and thus requires less frequent supplemental doses, a feature that is less important now with the widespread use of continuous epidural infusion techniques. More important and in contrast to other local anesthetics, bupivacaine has a motor-sparing effect; it produces less motor block for a comparable degree of sensory analgesia. This is particularly true at the low concentrations used for labor epidural analgesia and acute postoperative pain management. Furthermore, bupivacaine has excellent compatibility with neuraxial opioids, and this allows for concentrations as low as 0.03% and 0.04% bupivacaine to be used successfully so that many patients are pain-free and even able to ambulate during labor or with regional analgesia after surgery. Less motor block also improves expulsive efforts during the second stage of labor and may reduce the need for an instrumental vaginal or abdominal delivery.[2] The ability of bupivacaine to provide good sensory analgesia with little motor block is essential for management of postoperative, during which early mobilization may decrease the risk of deep venous thrombosis and result in better respiratory mechanics. Nonetheless, despite its many advantages, there have been some concerns regarding bupivacaine, particularly in obstetric anesthesia.

Clinical Pearls

- In contrast to other shorter-acting amide local anesthetics, bupivacaine, levobupivacaine, and ropivacaine have a motor-sparing effect; they produce less motor block for a comparable degree of sensory analgesia.
- This feature is particularly true at the low concentrations used for labor epidural analgesia and acute postoperative pain management.

Clinical experience has been that cardiac arrest after unexpected intravascular injection of clinical doses of local anesthetics could be prevented by prompt oxygenation, ventilation, and, if necessary, cardiovascular support. However, in 1979, George Albright[3] alerted anesthesia practitioners to a cluster of six anecdotal cases of sudden cardiac arrest after unexpected intravascular injection of what then were the newer amide local anesthetics, bupivacaine and etidocaine. In his editorial, Albright[3] suggested that intoxication with bupivacaine (and etidocaine), in contrast to lidocaine and mepivacaine, could result in almost simultaneous onset of convulsions and circulatory collapse without antecedent hypoxia and acidosis.

Since then, bupivacaine has been shown to have a narrower margin of safety than lidocaine and mepivacaine.[4–6] The ratio of the doses or plasma concentrations required to produce cardiovascular collapse compared with those associated with convulsions is lower for bupivacaine than for the other two drugs.[5,6] Also, in contrast to the intermediate-acting local anesthetics, bupivacaine intoxication is associated with malignant ventricular arrhythmias, which may be difficult to treat.[5,6] This is because unlike other amide local anesthetics, bupivacaine dissociates from blocked sodium channels at a much slower rate, resulting in a prolongation of the maximal rate of depolarization (V_{max}) and creating the potential for reentrant-type ventricular arrhythmias.[7]

The epidemic of bupivacaine-related cardiac arrests, particularly among parturients in the U.S., directed interest toward discovering whether pregnancy itself enhances the arrhythmogenicity of bupivacaine.[8] Indeed, in vitro studies conducted on rabbit heart preparations have demonstrated that myocardial muscle treated with progesterone and exposed to bupivacaine showed greater depression of V_{max} than those exposed to lidocaine, thus increasing susceptibility to malignant reentrant-type ventricular arrhythmias.[9]

In vivo experiments have been less conclusive. In an early study using a small number of animals given a continuous intravenous infusion of bupivacaine, circulatory collapse occurred at lower doses and lower plasma drug concentrations in pregnant than in nonpregnant ewes.[5] However, a subsequent study involving a larger group of animals and the use of blinding and randomization failed to confirm these findings.[10] Cardiac arrest also occurred in surgical patients after intoxication with bupivacaine, but less frequently.

Some suggested that the disproportionate number of cardiac arrests among parturients compared with surgical patients was not related to increased sensitivity to the drug during pregnancy but to the widespread use of bupivacaine in obstetrics and, in some instances, to inadequate cardiopulmonary resuscitation.[11] In many of these cases that were fatal, the fetus had not been delivered immediately, thus hampering efforts to restore maternal circulation as a result of aortocaval compression.[11]

Nonetheless, the U.S. and Drug Administration (FDA) proscribed the use of the higher concentration of bupivacaine, that is,. 0.75%, in pregnant women; by clinical practice, this was extended to surgical patients as well. Since then, anesthesiologists have perceived a need for alternative amide local anesthetics with the beneficial blocking properties of bupivacaine but with a greater margin of safety.

Chirality

Amide local anesthetics of the mepivacaine homologue type are known as chiral drugs because they can exist in isomeric (enantiomeric) forms, which are mirror images of each other (Figure 7–1). The isomers are defined according to the direction that a molecule rotates polarized light: dextrorotary (+ or rectus) and levorotary (− or sinister). Isomers of the same compound may have different biologic activities. For instance, it was suggested in early studies, that the levo-isomers of amide local anesthetics tend to produce greater vasoconstriction but have lower systemic toxicity than the dextro form of the drug.[12–14]

However, until the 1990s, the formulations of amide local anesthetics used in clinical practice contained a racemic

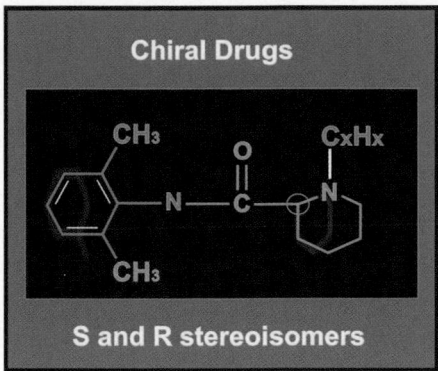

Figure 7–1. Levo- and dextro-stereoisomer configuration of amide local anesthetics.

Table 7–1.

Physical Characteristics of Local Anesthetics

	Mepivacaine	Ropivacaine	Bupivacaine
Weight	246	274	288
Pkb	7.6	8.0	8.1
Solubility	1.0	2.8	3.0
%Bound	75	90–95	95

mixture (approximately 50:50) of both the levo- and the dextro-isomers because single-isomer preparations were costly to produce. Fortunately, with technologic advances and an interest in a less toxic alternative to bupivacaine, single-isomer preparations of local anesthetics are now available. The first to be approved for clinical use was ropivacaine, followed shortly by levobupivacaine.

Physicochemical Properties

Ropivacaine (1-propyl-2′, 6′-pipecoloxylidide) is a homologue of mepivacaine and bupivacaine (Figure 7–2). It differs from bupivacaine in having a propyl rather than a butyl group attached to the pipechol ring). Ropivacaine is formulated as the single levo-isomer (99.5% purity) rather than as a racemic mixture. As would be expected, ropivacaine's physicochemical properties are intermediate between those of mepivacaine and bupivacaine[15] (Table 7–1). Ropivacaine, like other amide local anesthetics, is used in its water-soluble form as the hydrochloride monohydrate salt (molecular weight [MW] 329) of the base (MW 275).[15] The pK_B value of ropivacaine is 8.07 and similar to that of bupivacaine (8.1). Ropivacaine, like bupivacaine, is highly protein-bound at 94% and thus has a long duration of action. However, it is considerably less lipid-soluble than bupivacaine.[15] This may be important for two reasons. It may explain why bupivacaine has greater

motor-blocking effects than ropivacaine because the greater lipid solubility of the former may result in enhanced penetration into the heavily myelinated, large motor neurons. Second, it raises the question as to whether ropivacaine is truly equipotent to bupivacaine.

Levobupivacaine (Chirocaine, Chiroscience, Ltd) is the other single levorotary isomer formulation of local anesthetic available for clinical use. Its physicochemical characteristics are virtually indistinguishable from those of bupivacaine[15] (see Table 7–1). Unfortunately, although a promising drug, financial and economic considerations have resulted in levobupivacaine no longer being available for use in North America, although it is available in other parts of the world. The advantage of levobupivacaine is that it may be closer in its in vitro potency and efficacy to the currently used clinical formulation of racemic bupivacaine,[12,16] whereas ropivacaine is 20–30% less potent.[17,18] Thus, in contrast to ropivacaine, any expected benefits to be gained from the lower cardiotoxicity of levobupivacaine do not appear to be at the expense of potency.

Pharmacokinetics

Ropivacaine

Generally speaking, ropivacaine has lower lipid solubility and slightly lower protein binding than racemic bupivacaine[15] (see Table 7–1). Note that the elimination half-life ($T_{\{1/2\}B}$) of ropivacaine is shorter than that of bupivacaine after intravenous administration to animals and humans.[19–21] The shorter elimination half-life of ropivacaine has been

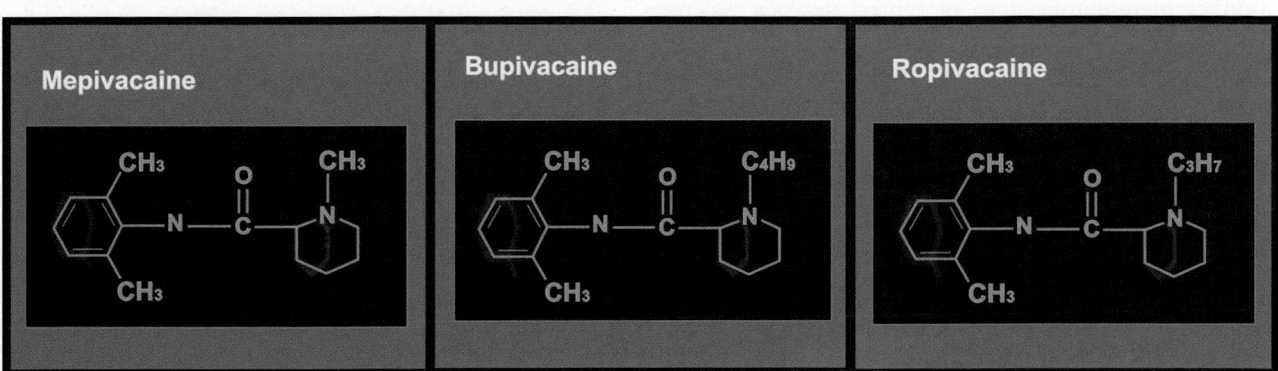

Figure 7–2. Chemical structure of mepivacaine, ropivacaine, and bupivacaine.

attributed to a faster clearance and shorter mean residence time than bupivacaine.[21]

In sheep, pregnancy is associated with smaller volumes of distribution during the terminal phase of drug elimination and steady state and a slower clearance for both drugs.[21] In pregnant animals, ropivacaine also had shorter elimination half-life and mean residence times and a faster clearance than bupivacaine.[21] Similarly, ropivacaine has been shown to have a lower $T_{\{1/2\}B}$ value than bupivacaine in women having epidural anesthesia for cesarean section delivery.[22]

Levobupivacaine

Levobupivacaine has similar protein binding and lipid solubility to those of racemic bupivacaine[15] (see Table 7–1). However, there are differences between the two optically active isomers of bupivacaine. Levobupivacaine exhibits a slightly greater degree of protein binding, lower volume of distribution, higher plasma clearance, and shorter elimination half-life than the dextrorotary form of the drug.[23] However, in pregnant women given levobupivacaine or bupivacaine for epidural anesthesia during cesarean section delivery, there was no significant difference between the two drugs in the maximum concentration of drug in the plasma and the area under concentration versus time curve.[24]

Systemic Toxicity

Ropivacaine

In vitro studies using isolated rabbit Purkinje fibers have shown that ropivacaine depresses electrophysiologic parameters such as V_{max}, much less than does bupivacaine.[25] A number of studies performed in laboratory animals have also demonstrated that ropivacaine has a greater margin of safety than bupivacaine. In dogs, the margin of safety, defined as the ratio between the dose required to produce cardiovascular collapse and the dose associated with convulsions, was greater for ropivacaine than for bupivacaine.[26] In another study, almost twice the dose of ropivacaine compared with bupivacaine was necessary to prolong the QRS interval after intravenous administration to pigs.[27] In sheep, the mean fatal dose of ropivacaine was greater than that of bupivacaine at 60 and 45 mg, respectively.[28]

In human volunteers, the doses of ropivacaine required to produce premonitory signs of central nervous system (CNS) toxicity during slow intravenous infusion were approximately 25% greater than for bupivacaine.[29,30] Furthermore, bupivacaine depressed cardiac conduction and contractility at lower dosages and plasma concentrations than did ropivacaine.[29]

Pregnancy does not enhance the systemic toxicity of ropivacaine. In vitro studies have shown that progesterone has little effect on myocardial sensitivity to ropivacaine.[31] In sheep, the doses and plasma concentrations required to produce convulsions and circulatory collapse were similar in pregnant and nonpregnant animals.[10,32] However, in pregnant animals, the doses required to produce circulatory collapse were approximately 40–50% greater for ropivacaine

than for bupivacaine, but the corresponding serum concentrations of the two drugs were similar.[10] This has been attributed to a shorter elimination half-life and faster clearance of ropivacaine.[21]

Clinical Pearls

- Pregnancy does not enhance the systemic toxicity of ropivacaine.
- In vitro studies have shown that progesterone has little effect on myocardial sensitivity to ropivacaine.

Levobupivacaine

Levobupivacaine has less of an inhibitory effect on inactivated cardiac sodium channels than dextro or racemic drug.[33] Using isolated perfused rabbit hearts, Mazoit et al.[34] demonstrated that levobupivacaine caused less QRS widening and less severe ventricular arrhythmias than dextro or racemic bupivacaine. Similarly, levobupivacaine produced less atrial–ventricular conduction delay and second-degree heart block in isolated perfused guinea pig hearts than the other two forms of the drug.[35]

In vivo toxicity also appears to be less with levobupivacaine than with bupivacaine. For instance, the convulsant dose range for levobupivacaine was greater (75–100 mg) than for the racemate (50–75 mg) in sheep given graded intravenous doses of the drug.[36] Levobupivacaine was also associated with a lower incidence of cardiac arrhythmias, whereas 43% of sheep given racemic bupivacaine died as a result of irreversible malignant ventricular arrhythmias.[36]

In healthy male volunteers, intravenous infusion of levobupivacaine until premonitory symptoms of toxicity resulted in a smaller reduction in mean stroke index, acceleration index, and ejection fraction than racemic bupivacaine.[37]

Comparative Systemic Toxicity

The most useful studies compare the systemic toxicity of bupivacaine, levobupivacaine, and ropivacaine under a single methodology. For the most part, the results of these studies indicate that bupivacaine has a narrower margin of safety compared with that of ropivacaine, with levobupivacaine being intermediate. In vitro studies performed on isolated and perfused rabbit heart preparations suggest that bupivacaine, levobupivacaine, and ropivacaine prolong the duration of the QRS interval in a potency ratio of 1.0:0.4:0.3.34).

Clinical Pearls

- In sheep, CNS-directed (carotid artery) infusion of all three amide local anesthetics resulted in increased arrhythmias, but the overall rank order of potency was ropivacaine < levobupivacaine < bupivacaine

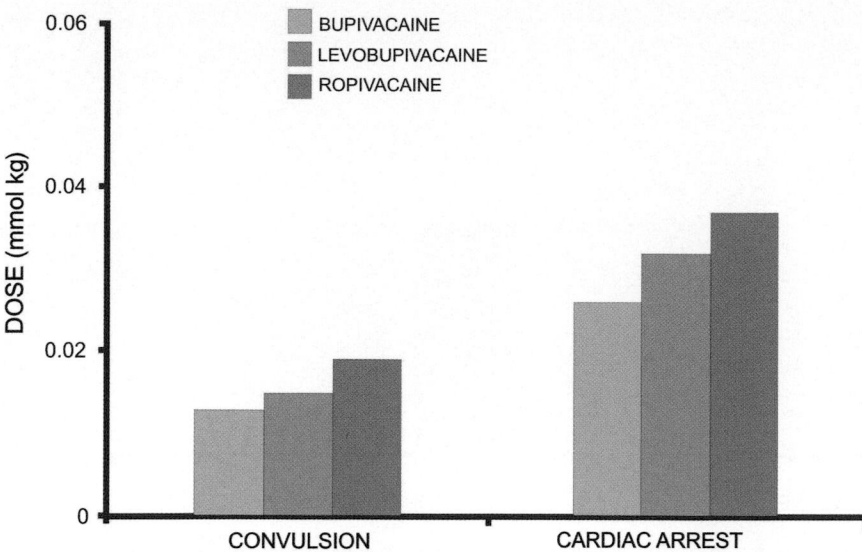

Figure 7–3. Dose (mean) required to produce convulsions and circulatory collapse with bupivacaine, levobupivacaine, and ropivacine. (Adapted from Santos AC, DeArmas P: Systemic toxicity of levobupivacaine, bupivacaine and ropivacaine during continuous intravenous infusion to nonpregnant and pregnant ewes. Anesthesiology 2001;95:1256–1264.)

Studies comparing the three drugs have also been performed using various laboratory animals. In one study, chronically prepared sheep were randomized to receive a constant intravenous infusion of bupivacaine, levobupivacaine, or ropivacaine at an equal rate until circulatory collapse occurred.[38] The cumulative dose of local anesthetic required to produce convulsions and circulatory collapse was lowest for bupivacaine and highest for ropivacaine, with levobupivacaine being intermediate[38] (Figure 7–3). The incidence of ventricular arrhythmias as the terminal event, was similar among the three drugs. In another study, anesthetized swine were given an intracoronary injection of one of the three local anesthetics.[39] The lowest lethal dose occurred with bupivacaine, with ropivacaine and levobupivacaine being somewhat greater.[39] Application of high concentrations of local anesthetics to specific areas of the brainstem can result in ventricular arrhythmias. In sheep, CNS-directed (carotid artery) infusion of all three local anesthetics resulted in increased arrhythmias, but the overall rank order of potency was ropivacaine < levobupivacaine < bupivacaine.[40]

The Controversy Regarding Systemic Toxicity

It is well accepted that lipid solubility usually goes hand in hand with local anesthetic potency. All things being equal, greater lipid solubility is related to increasing length of the aliphatic chain on the amino ring. Structurally, ropivacaine has one less carbon on the aliphatic chain (C3) than bupivacaine, which has four carbons (see Figure 7–2). This difference in the length of the aliphatic chain between the two drugs renders bupivacaine approximately 10 times more lipid-soluble than ropivacaine[15] (see Table 7–1). In vitro studies performed on rat sciatic nerve indicate that bupivacaine is approximately 25% more potent in blocking conduction than ropivacaine.[12,13] However, the argument has been made that although bupivacaine is slightly more potent than ropivacaine, the two drugs would be equieffective in producing clinical regional anesthesia. Because of this, most of the

studies of systemic toxicity have compared equal doses of the two drugs. Thus, these studies did not resolve the controversy as to whether ropivacaine is truly less cardiotoxic than bupivacaine because it is also 20–30% less potent. However, this would be of clinical significance only if greater doses of ropivacaine than bupivacaine would be needed to produce a comparable level of regional blockade. In fact, we now know that in some situations bupivacaine and ropivacaine are not equieffective. For instance, the median local analgesic concentration of local anesthetic for epidural analgesia in laboring woman is approximately 40% greater for ropivacaine compared with bupivacaine[18] (Figure 7–4).

In a recent study, the median analgesic (effective) dose for intrathecal labor analgesia was lowest for bupivacaine (2.37 mg) and highest for ropivacaine (3.64 mg), with levobupivacaine being intermediate (2.94 mg).[41] In other studies, greater doses of ropivacaine compared with bupivacaine were required to produce comparable surgical spinal anesthesia.[42] This is important because if larger doses of ropivacaine compared with bupivacaine are required to produce comparable regional anesthesia, then the anticipated benefit of lower cardiotoxicity with ropivacaine compared with bupivacaine may be reduced. However, the results of a recently published study performed in rats suggests that ropivacaine is still less cardiotoxic than bupivacaine, even when given at equipotent doses.[43]

Clinical Pearls

- It is well accepted that lipid solubility usually goes hand in hand with local anesthetic potency. All things being equal, greater lipid solubility is related to increasing length of the aliphatic chain on the amino ring

Regardless of the controversy, our belief is that these new single-isomer preparations of long-acting local

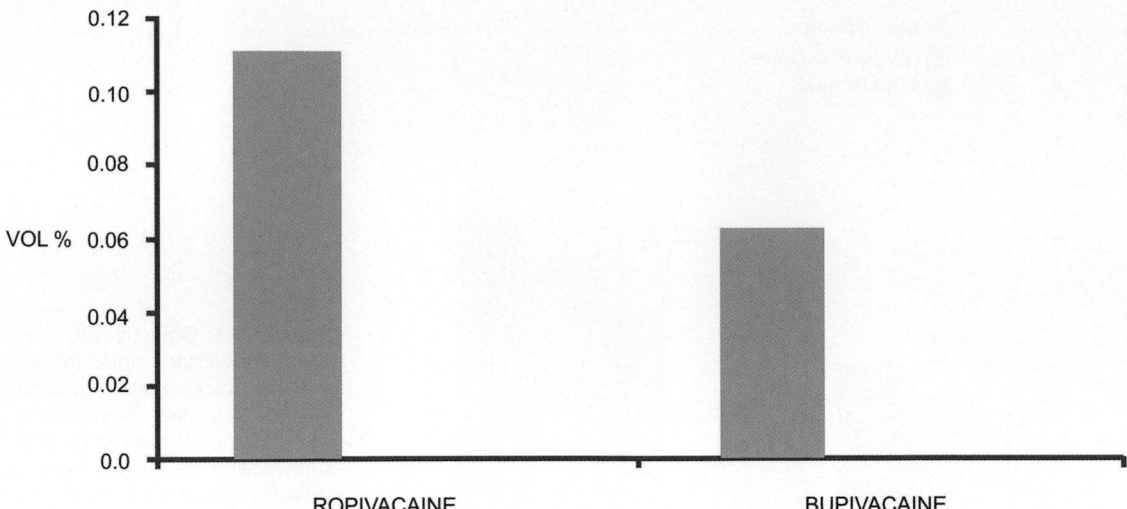

Figure 7–4. Median local analgesic concentrations of ropivacaine and bupivacaine for epidural analgesia during labor. (Adapted from Polley LS, Columb MO, Wagner S, Naughton NN: Relative analgesia potencies of ropivacaine and bupivacaine for epidural analgesia in labor: Implications for therapeutic indexes. Anesthesiology 1999;90:944–950.)

anesthetics, namely, ropivacaine and levobupivacaine, are very potent, and, if injected intravenously or with a relative overdose, can cause severe manifestations of cardiotoxicity, though easier to treat than with racemic bupivacaine. Indeed, there already have been three published reports of cardiac arrest following intoxication with ropivacaine.[44–46] In contrast to the reported cases of bupivacaine cardiotoxicity in humans,[3] two patients[44,45] had progressive bradycardia and asystole rather than a lethal ventricular arrhythmia, and all patients were able to be resuscitated easily.[44–46] Nonetheless, there is no substitute for adhering to maximum recommended dosage guidelines, using appropriate test doses to identify misplaced needles/catheters, always fractionating the total dose of local anesthetic, and carrying out heightened monitoring and vigilance in preventing toxic reactions with local anesthetics.[47]

Ease of Resuscitation

Two studies, performed in animals, suggest that cardiac resuscitation after intoxication with the newer amide local anesthetics is easier than with bupivacaine.[48,49] In the first study, Groban et al.[48] administered incremental doses of bupivacaine, ropivacaine, or levobupivacaine to anesthetized dogs until cardiac arrest. At the point of cardiovascular collapse, the dogs were treated with epinephrine, open chest cardiac massage, and an advanced life support protocol. Mortality was greatest at 50% with bupivacaine, followed by levobupivacaine at 30%, ropivacaine at 10%, and lidocaine at 0%. Unfortunately, these differences did not achieve statistical significance because of the small number of dogs studied. In another study, anesthetized rats given an infusion of bupivacaine, ropivacaine, or levobupivacaine until cardiovascular collapse were resuscitated with epinephrine and closed-chest cardiac massage.[49]

Although the total number of successful resuscitations did not differ among the groups, less epinephrine was required with ropivacaine compared with the other two drugs. It is interesting that in the two aforementioned case reports of cardiac arrest after ropivacaine intoxication, one patient was resuscitated easily with atropine 1 mg and ephedrine 12 mg, and the other with epinephrine 1 mg.[44,45]

Effects on Uterine Blood Flow & Placental Transfer

All local anesthetics can reduce uterine blood flow at plasma levels that greatly exceed those occurring during routine obstetric anesthesia.[50] However, because the levo-isomers of amide local anesthetics tend to produce vasoconstriction at clinically relevant plasma concentrations, there has been an added concern that their use could result in a decrease in uteroplacental perfusion. It is reassuring that neither bupivacaine, ropivacaine, nor levobupivacaine affected uterine tone or blood flow during intravenous infusion to pregnant sheep.[51,52] Furthermore, even at relatively high drug concentrations, fetal heart rate, blood pressure, and acid–base state were not affected by the three drugs.[52] In humans, Doppler velocimetry studies have shown that ropivacaine has negligible effects on the uteroplacental circulation during epidural anesthesia for cesarean section delivery.[53]

The placental transfer of levobupivacaine and ropivacaine is similar to that of bupivacaine.[52] Intravenous infusions of ropivacaine, levobupivacaine, or bupivacaine for 1 hour to pregnant sheep resulted in steady-state maternal plasma concentration of 1.5–1.6 mcg/mL and fetal concentrations of approximately 0.25 mcg/mL (Figure 7–5).[52] More important, there was no significant difference in brain and myocardium drug concentrations among the three drugs[52] (Figure 7–6).

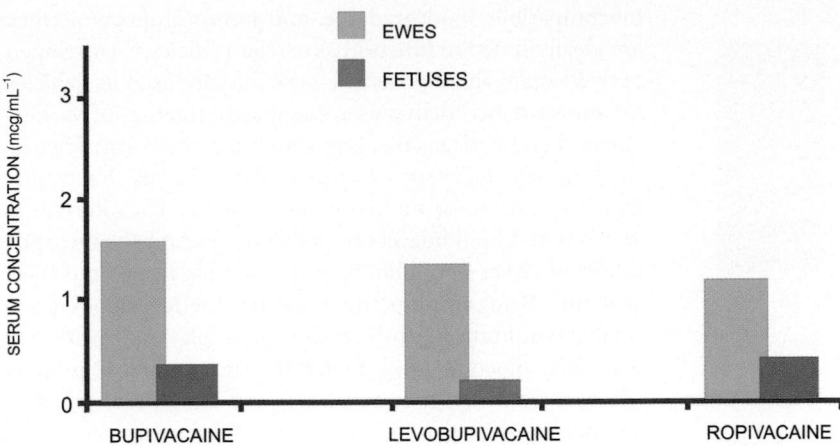

Figure 7–5. Maternal and fetal serum concentrations of bupivacaine, levobupivacaine and ropivacaine (mcg/mL) after maternal infusion to chronically instrumented pregnant sheep. Differences are not statistically significant. (Adapted from Santos AC, Karpel B, Noble G: The placental transfer and fetal effects of levobupivacaine, racemic bupivacaine and ropivacaine. Anesthesiology 1999;90:1698–1703.)

Clinical Use

The clinical use of each drug is covered in chapters pertaining to specific regional techniques. Generally speaking, there are two important advantages of the newer amide local anesthetics. First, they tend to produce less motor than sensory block compared with racemic bupivacaine, particularly at the low concentrations used for pain management and obstetrics.[54,55] This is important in allowing patients with continuous epidural/peripheral nerve block to ambulate, thus decreasing the potential for deep venous thrombosis. It is also important in obstetric patients, by allowing ambulation during labor and more effective expulsive efforts during the second stage of labor. Indeed, the ratio of the median local anesthetic concentration to achieve a Bromage score less than 4 was 0.66 for ropivacaine:bupivacaine and 0.87 for levobupivacaine:bupivacaine. This indicates that bupivacaine produced greater motor block than either ropivacaine or levobupivacaine.[54,55] Second, as mentioned earlier, the levorotary isomers of local anesthetics tend to produce

vasoconstriction rather than vasodilation[56] (Figure 7–7). This could be useful in some clinical scenarios in prolonging the duration of block.[23]

Summary

The introduction of stereospecific levorotary isomers of the amide local anesthetics, ropivacaine and levobupivacaine, is important because these drugs, although more costly, appear to have a wider margin of safety but blocking properties similar to the currently available formulation of racemic bupivacaine. Because studies have compared the systemic toxicity of these local anesthetics at equal doses with that of bupivacaine, this would apply only if equal concentrations of drug are used clinically across the board. Although this may hold true with levobupivacaine and bupivacaine, it appears that in clinical use, anesthesiologists are using higher concentrations of ropivacaine (0.75%). Regardless, it is noteworthy that, even before the introduction of ropivacaine and levobupivacaine, modifications in clinical practice, such as the use of appropriate test

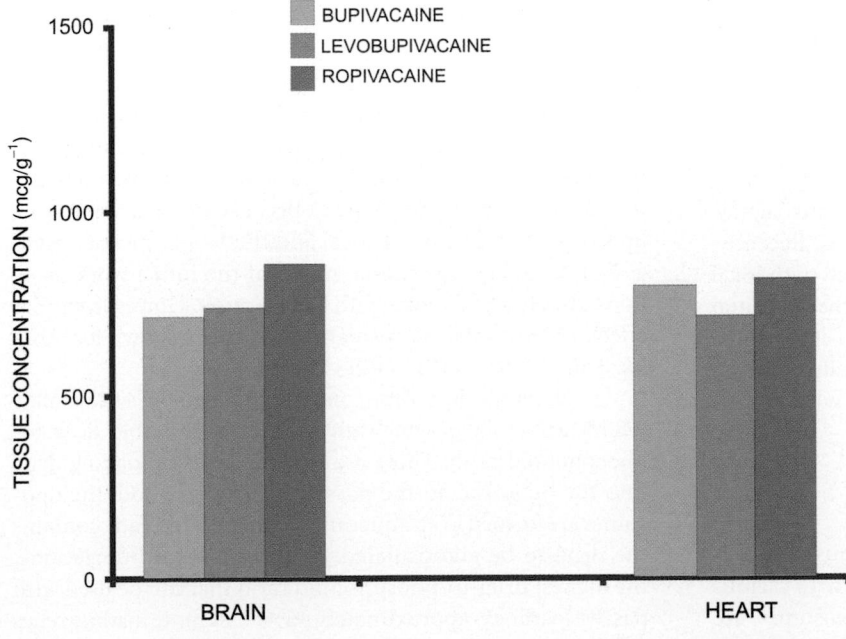

Figure 7–6. Fetal brain and heart concentrations (mcg/mg) of bupivacaine, levobupivacaine and ropivacaine after maternal infusion of drug to chronically instrumented pregnant ewes. Differences are not statistically significant. (Adapted from Santos AC, Karpel B, Noble G: The placental transfer and fetal effects of levobupivacaine, racemic bupivacaine and ropivacaine. Anesthesiology 1999;90:1698–1703.)

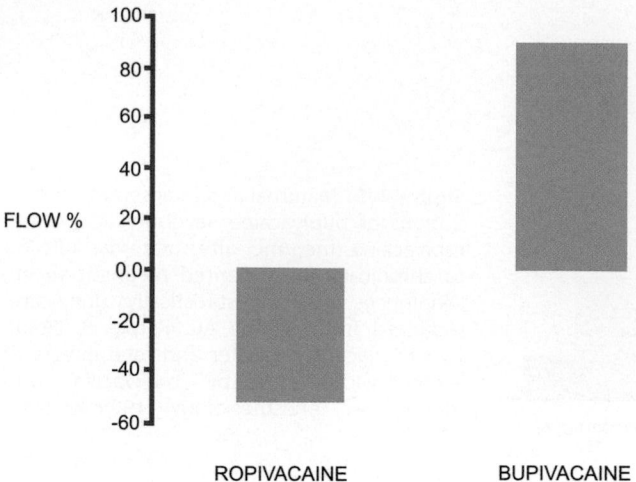

Figure 7–7. Mean change in capillary blood flow after administration of 0.25% ropivacaine or 0.25% bupivacaine to pigs. (Data from Kopacz DJ, Carpenter RL, Mackey DC: Effect of ropivacaine on cutaneous capillary blood flow in pigs. Anesthesiology 1989;71:69–74.)

doses and fractionation of the therapeutic dose, have made regional anesthesia a very safe procedure.[57] In no situation should a greater margin of safety be a substitute for proper technique.

LIPOSOMAL PREPARATIONS OF LOCAL ANESTHETICS

General Considerations

Local anesthetics temporarily block neural transmission and are used extensively for surgery and obstetrics. In addition, local anesthetics are an important component of the management of acute postoperative and chronic pain conditions.[58] Unfortunately, even the longest-acting local anesthetics have a short duration of action relative to the prolonged analgesia that is required for acute and chronic pain management. Adjuvants such as vasoconstrictors and opioids have been added to local anesthetics in an attempt to prolong their effects, but with limited success. Continuous delivery systems using infusion catheters have been successfully used, but these have limitations, for instance, in the patient having anticoagulation prophylaxis against deep venous thrombosis. Recently, there has been interest in using liposomes loaded with local anesthetics to provide sustained analgesia/anesthesia. Initial testing suggests that liposome encapsulation of local anesthetic offers a simple, economical, and theoretically nontoxic delivery system to prolong local anesthetic effect with a single injection of drug.

Chemistry

Liposomes are lipid vesicles that contain an aqueous compartment. The aqueous compartments can be loaded with various drugs, including local anesthetics. Because liposomes are

biocompatible, biodegradable, and nonimmunogenic, they are ideally suited to function as carrier vehicles.[59] Developed over 30 years ago, liposomes were initially used as vehicles for the sustained delivery or enhanced targeting of various chemotherapeutic agents. Liposomes may be constructed as small unilamellar vesicles, large unilamellar vesicles, multi-lamellar vesicles, or multivesicular vesicles. The alternating aqueous and lipid bilayers of liposomes permit the incorporation of either lipophilic or water-soluble drugs into their structure. Being amphipathic, local anesthetics can be encapsulated within the aqueous and/or lipid bilayers.[60] Naturally occurring biocompatible materials, such as phospholipids (derived from soy or egg sources) and cholesterol typically are used to construct the lipid bilayer. Because liposomes are composed of these naturally occurring materials, liposomes resemble biologic membranes, which render them neither antigenic nor toxic.[58]

Preparation

Liposomes are microscopic spheres containing an aqueous core surrounded by a phospholipid bilayer.[61] Typically, a phospholipid moiety is first dissolved in a solvent that is subsequently evaporated. This leaves a residual lipid film into which lipophilic active agents can be dissolved. For incorporation of aqueous drug, the lipid film is reconstituted, and the aqueous drug becomes trapped between the concentric phospholipid layers. Liposomes take on a spherical shape through several thawing/freezing cycles.[62,63] For a liposomal formulation to be suitable for use in humans, the drug-to-phospholipid ratio is crucial. A higher drug-to-phospholipid ratio allows more of the drug to be delivered with less liposome, whereas a low drug-to-phospholipid ratio requires administration of a very large lipid load to achieve the desired drug effect. The large lipid mass of the latter would make this formulation unsuitable for use in a defined area, such as injection into subcutaneous tissue.[59] Because the major goal of a liposomal formulation of local anesthetic is to prolong analgesia rather than anesthesia, much of the initial work using liposomes has been done with bupivacaine. However, similar effects of liposomal encapsulation have been shown for other local anesthetics, such as lidocaine.[62]

Currently, liposomes are formulated to encapsulate ~80% active drug, which gives them a desirable drug-to-phospholipid ratio. There are two methods of loading drug into the liposome. In the passive loading method, the liposomes are formed in an aqueous solution that already contains the drug to be encapsulated. With liposomal bupivacaine, the highest drug-to-phospholipid ratio that can be used with passive loading is approximately 36%.[59] Remote loading relies on a transmembrane pH gradient to encapsulate bupivacaine within a preexisting liposomal carrier. By using a pH gradient, 64–82% of bupivacaine can be loaded in a large unilamellar vesicle.[61] The use of large multivesicular vesicles and remote loading enable the encapsulation of large amounts of bupivacaine within a relatively small total volume.[59]

Liposomes have also been loaded with tetracaine for topical anesthesia of the skin. This formulation enhances drug delivery to the dermis by increasing the rate of dermal penetration of tetracaine and is highly effective. For instance, in one study, liposome-encapsulated tetracaine was compared with EMLA (eutectic mixture of local anesthetic) for the prevention of discomfort related to intravenous catheterization in healthy adult volunteers.[64] In this study, patients reported lower visual analog pain scores during intravenous cannulation on the arm treated with liposome-encapsulated tetracaine than on the arm treated with EMLA.[64]

Pharmacokinetics

Liposomes prolong neural blockade or spinally mediated opioid effects by extending and controlling the release of local anesthetic or opioid.[58] Liposomes provide a depot from which the local anesthetic can be released into the surrounding tissues, since they are cleared slowly after intradermal or subcutaneous injection.[61] Furthermore, liposomal preparations encapsulate high drug concentrations and maximize the active release of drug in a controlled–sustained manner.[61] Plain liposomes are devoid of inherent pharmacologic activity[65–68] and are unable to cross the blood–brain barrier or blood–nerve barrier.[69]

Early trials used relatively simple liposomal delivery systems, such as multilamellar vesicles , or small unilamellar vesicles. Multilamellar vesicles tend to remain in the epidural space longer than small unilamellar vesicles.[61] Within these early liposomes, the local anesthetic was either partially encapsulated in the aqueous core or associated hydrophobically as the free base within the liposomal bilayer. Because of this simple construction, no mechanism existed to control drug release rates, and therefore duration of action. The advantage of large unilamellar vesicles over multilamellar vesicles is that they contain a relatively large trapping volume, thus allowing greater quantities of drug to be encapsulated.[61] Large unilamellar vesicles with a pH gradient can be efficiently loaded with a high mass of bupivacaine, because the drug is both amphipathic and a weak base. In addition, the larger size of large unilamellar vesicles compared with the multilamellar vesicles causes them to remain at the site of injection for longer periods.[61] Large unilamellar vesicles are typically greater than 300 nm, whereas small liposomes are usually 80–90 nm. Moreover, the latter may drain into the blood via the lymphatic system after subcutaneous injection, whereas vesicles of larger diameter (greater than 120 nm) have not been detected in the blood to any appreciable extent.[70]

More recently, technologic advances that result in an increase in the drug-to-phospholipid ratio have yielded a large multivesicular vesicle. These vesicles are much larger than the large unilamellar vesicles (mean size 2,439 ± 544 nm) and have a fivefold greater drug-to-phospholipid ratio.[59] The pharmacodynamic effects of liposomal-encapsulated local anesthetic is related to the release of active drug from the liposomal matrix rather than from neural uptake of the combined liposomal–drug moiety.[69]

Plasma levels after epidural injection of liposome-encapsulated local anesthetic may exhibit a brief initial peak, regardless of the size of the vesicle used to encapsulate the drug. This initial peak in drug concentration has been attributed to free drug contained within the diluent/liposome solution[62] and to drug residing on the surface of the liposome.[58] Onset of action after subcutaneous injection of liposomal bupivacaine is similar to that of aqueous bupivacaine. However, after injection of subcutaneous liposomal bupivacaine, there is a delay in achieving peak plasma levels. These levels are approximately 20% lower than those observed with plain bupivacaine.[66] The initial bupivacaine plasma level achieved remains constant for a short period of time before gradually rising as residual drug is released from the liposome and absorbed into the plasma. In contrast, injection with plain bupivacaine results in a significantly higher peak plasma level that occurs rapidly, and systemic absorption of drug is complete within 60 minutes of injection.[66]

Liposomes are cleared by the lymphatic system and macrophages. Intravascular liposomes are cleared by several processes, including circulating monocytes, the reticular endothelial system, and high-density lipoproteins. Cholesterol is added to phospholipids during liposome construction to enhance stability by counteracting the effects of high-density lipoproteins.[62,63]

Clinical Effects

Liposome-encapsulated local anesthetics have been shown to produce prolonged nerve blockade in animals owing to the controlled, sustained release of local anesthetic.[58] Sensory block lasted five times longer after subcutaneous injection of multivesicular vesicle bupivacaine in rats—447 ± 29 minutes compared with 87 ± 7 minutes with plain bupivacaine.[66] Similarly, local anesthetic duration of bupivacaine was three times longer in guinea pigs given intradermal liposomal bupivacaine compared with plain bupivacaine[61] and nearly two times longer when injected into the root of mice tails compared with bupivacaine plus epinephrine.[71] In rabbits, motor block was nearly two times longer after intracisternal injection of liposomal bupivacaine than plain bupivacaine (126 versus 70 minutes, respectively).[72]

Other than topical administration, there are only four published reports of liposome administration in humans for regional analgesia/anesthesia.[58] An open-label, nonrandomized trial compared postoperative epidural administration of 0.5% liposomal bupivacaine (14 patients) with aqueous 0.5% bupivacaine with epinephrine (12 patients) for pain relief after various major surgeries.[73] The onset of block and visual analog pain scores were similar between the two preparations of bupivacaine, but the duration of analgesia was almost two times longer in patients receiving liposomal bupivacaine compared with plain bupivacaine and nearly four times greater in a small subset of patients undergoing abdominal surgery.[73] Multilamellar vesicle bupivacaine has been successfully used for brachial plexus block using a supraclavicular approach for chronic arm pain in a single patient.[74]

In another patient with lung cancer-related pain, liposomal bupivacaine was administered through a thoracic epidural and provided 11 hours of complete pain relief compared with only 4 hours after the administration bupivacaine with epinephrine.[75] In this patient, no motor block was detected with the liposomal bupivacaine injection, whereas a grade 1 (Bromage scale) motor block was observed with the plain bupivacaine/epinephrine injection.[75] Using bupivacaine and large multivesicular vesicles, analgesia is prolonged in a dose-dependent manner.[59] For instance, six healthy male volunteers were given injections of 0.5% plain bupivacaine or liposomal 0.5%, 1%, and 2% bupivacaine. The median duration of analgesia after each was 1 hour, 19 hours, 38 hours, and 48 hours, respectively.[59]

Systemic Toxicity

Local anesthetics can produce both CNS and cardiovascular toxicity. Bupivacaine is known to cause both CNS and cardiovascular toxic effects. However, in contrast to other local anesthetics, cardiovascular toxicity with bupivacaine can be particularly serious.[3] Liposomal encapsulation of bupivacaine appears to offer some protection against the CNS and cardiovascular toxic effects when the drug is injected intravascularly. For instance, in a study using rabbits,[76] the lethal dose of a continuous infusion of 0.25% plain bupivacaine was 15.7 ± 2.5 mg/kg, compared with 22.43 ± 2.63 mg/kg of bupivacaine in multilamellar vesicles. Some of this "protection" may be related to the fact that multilamellar vesicles are unable to cross the blood–brain barrier; however, more work needs to be done in this area.[77]

Tissue Toxicity

Liposomes are created using naturally occurring phospholipids and cholesterol. In theory, these should not cause neurotoxic effects. Bupivacaine 0.75%, encapsulated in Multilamellar vesicles, has not been shown to cause neurotoxicity when injected into the brachial plexus of rabbits.[78] After injection, the brachial plexus was dissected on either day 2 or day 7 and examined histologically. Light microscopy demonstrated weak perineural inflammation, but electron microscopy did not show any changes of the myelin sheath.[78] A single rat study has associated demyelination with the intrathecal administration of lysophosphatidyl choline.[79] Neurotoxicity, if any, with liposomes may be related to the choice of lipid used to formulate the liposomes, and further study is required.[58]

SUMMARY

Liposome encapsulation may become useful in prolonging the duration of action of local anesthetics and perhaps diminishing some toxic effects. However, there is no FDA-approved formulation of liposomal local anesthetic at this time. Clinical experience with recent FDA approval and clinical use of a sustained-release liposomal preparation of morphine have been encouraging. Although initial studies suggest that sustained, controlled-release local anesthetic formulations are possible using liposomes, their ultimate contribution to clinical anesthesia remains to be determined.[58]

References

1. Hawkins JL, Gibbs CP, Orleans M, et al: Obstetric anesthesia workforce survey. 1981 versus 1992. Anesthesiology 1997;87:135–143.
2. Chestnut DH, Owens CL, Bates BN, et al: Continuous infusion of epidural analgesia during labor: A randomized, double-blind comparison of 0.0625% bupivacaine/0.0002% fentanyl versus 0.125% bupivacaine. Anesthesiology 1988;68:754–759.
3. Albright GA: Cardiac arrest following regional anesthesia with etidocaine or bupivacaine. Anesthesiology 1979;51:285–287.
4. de Jong RH, Ronfeld RA, DeRosa RA: Cardiovascular effects of convulsant and supraconvulsant doses of amide local anesthetics. Anesth Analg 1982;61:3–9.
5. Morishima HO, Pedersen H, Finster M, et al: Bupivacaine toxicity in pregnant and nonpregnant ewes. Anesthesiology 1982;63:134–139.
6. Santos AC, Pedersen H, Harmon TW, et al: Does pregnancy alter the systemic toxicity of local anesthetics. Anesthesiology 1989;70:991–995.
7. Clarkson CW, Hondeghem LM: Mechanism for bupivacaine depression of cardiac conduction: Fast block of sodium channels during the action potential with slow recovery from block during diastole. Anesthesiology 1985;62:396–405.
8. Marx GF: Cardiotoxicity of local anesthetics: The plot thickens. Anesthesiology 1984;60:3–5.
9. Moller RA, Datta S, Fox J, et al: Effects of progesterone on the cardiac electrophysiologic action of bupivacaine and lidocaine. Anesthesiology 1990;76:604–608.
10. Santos AC, Arthur GR, Wlody D, et al: Comparative systemic toxicity of ropivacaine and bupivacaine in nonpregnant and pregnant ewes. Anesthesiology 1995;82:734–740.
11. Marx GF: Cardiopulmonary resuscitation of late-pregnant women. Anesthesiology 1982;56:156.
12. Aberg G: Toxicological and local anaesthetic effects of optically active isomers of two local anaesthetic compounds. Acta Pharmacol et Toxicol 1972;31:273–286.
13. Akerman B, Hellenberg I, Trossvik C: Primary evaluation of the local anaesthetic properties of the amino amide agent ropivacaine (LEA 103). Acta Anaesthesiol Scand 1988;32:571–578.
14. Aps C, Reynolds F: An intradermal study of the local anesthetic and vascular effects of the isomers of bupivacaine. Br J Clin Pharmacol 1978;6:63–68.
15. de Jong RH: 1995 Gaston Labat lecture—ropivacaine—white knight or dark horse? Anesthesiology 1995;20:474–481.
16. Bardsley H, Gristwood R, Watson N, Nimmo W: The local anesthetic activity of levobupivacaine does not differ from racemic bupivacaine (Marcain): First clear evidence. Expert Opin Investig Drugs 1997;6:1883–1885.
17. Van Kleef JW, Veering BY, Burm AGL: Spinal anesthesia with ropivacaine: A double-blind study on the efficacy and safety of 0.5% and 0.75% solutions on patients undergoing minor lower limb surgery. Anesth Analg 1994;78:1125–1130.

18. Polley LS, Columb MO, Wagner S, Naughton NN: Relative analgesia potencies of ropivacaine and bupivacaine for epidural analgesia in labor: Implications for therapeutic indexes. Anesthesiology 1999;90:944–950.

19. Arthur GR, Feldman HS, Covino BG: Comparative pharmacokinetics of bupivacaine and ropivacaine, a new amide local anesthetic. Anesth Analg 1988;67:1053–1058.

20. Lee A, Fagan D, Lamont M, et al: Disposition kinetics of ropivacaine in humans. Anesth Analg 1989;69:736–738.

21. Santos AC, Arthur GR, Lehning EJ, Finster M: Comparative pharmacokinetics of ropivacaine and bupivacaine in nonpregnant and pregnant ewes. Anesth Analg 1997;85:87–93.

22. Datta S, Camann W, Bader A, VanderBurgh L: Clinical effects on maternal and fetal plasma concentrations of epidural ropivacaine versus bupivacaine for cesarean section. Anesthesiology 1995;82:1346–1352.

23. Thomas JM, Schug SA: Recent advances in the pharmacokinetics of local anaesthetics. Long-acting amide enantiomers and continuous infusions. Clin Pharmacokinet 1999;36:67–83.

24. Bader AM, Tsen LC, Camann WR, et al: Clinical effects and maternal and fetal plasma concentrations of 0.5% epidural levobupivacaine versus bupivacaine for cesarean delivery. Anesthesiology 1999;90:1596–601.

25. Moller RA, Covino BG: Cardiac electrophysiologic properties of bupivacaine and lidocaine compared with those of ropivacaine, a new amide local anesthetic. Anesthesiology 1990;72:322–329.

26. Feldman HS, Arthur GR, Covino BG: Comparative systemic toxicity of convulsant and supraconvulsant doses of intravenous ropivacaine, bupivacaine and lidocaine in the conscious dog. Anesth Analg 1989;69:794–801.

27. Reiz S, Haggmark S, Johansson G, Nath SW: Cardiotoxicity or ropivacaine: A new amide local anesthetic agent. Acta Aaesthesiol Scand 1989;33:93–98.

28. Rutten AT, Nancarrow C, Mather LE: Hemodynamic and central nervous system effects of intravenous bolus doses of lidocaine, bupivacaine and ropivacaine in sheep. Anesth Analg 198;69:291–299.

29. Scott DB, Lee A, Fagan D, et al: Acute toxicity of ropivacaine compared with that of bupivacaine. Anesth Analg 69:563–569.

30. Knudsen K, Suurkula MB, Blomberg S, et al: Central nervous and cardiovascular effects of i.v. infusions of ropivacaine, bupivacaine, and placebo in volunteers. Br J Anaesth 1997;78:507–514.

31. Moller RA, Covino BG: Effects of progesterone on the cardiac electrophysiologic alterations produced by ropivacaine and bupivacaine. Anesthesiology 1992;77:735–741.

32. Santos AC, Arthur GR, Pedersen H, et al: Systemic toxicity of ropivacaine during ovine pregnancy. Anesthesiology 1991;75:137–141.

33. Valenzuela C, Snyders DJ, Bennett PB, et al: Stereoselective block of cardiac sodium channels by bupivacaine in guinea-pig ventricular myocytes. Circulation 1995;92:3014–3024.

34. Mazoit JX, Boico O, Samii K: Myocardial uptake of bupivacaine: II. Pharmacokinetics and pharmacodynamics of bupivacaine enantiomers in the isolated perfused rabbit heart. Anesth Analg 1993;77:477–482.

35. Graf BM, Martin E, Bosnjak ZJ, Stowe DF: Stereospecific effect of bupivacaine isomers on atrioventricular conduction in the isolated perfused guinea-pig heart. Anesthesiology 1997;86:110–119.

36. Huang YF, Mather LM, Pryor ME Veering BT: Cardiovascular and central nervous system effects of intravenous bupivacaine and levobupivacaine in sheep. Anesth Analg 1998;86:797–804.

37. Bardsley H, Gristwood R, Baker H, et al: A comparison of the cardiovascular effects of levobupivacaine and racemic bupivacaine following intravenous administration to healthy volunteers. Br J Clin Pharmacol 1998;46:245–249.

38. Santos AC, DeArmas P: Systemic toxicity of levobupivacaine, bupivacaine and ropivacaine during continuous intravenous infusion to nonpregnant and pregnant ewes. Anesthesiology 2001;95:1256–1264.

39. Morrison SG, Dominguez JJ, Frascarolo P, Reiz S: A comparison of the electrocardiographic and cardiotoxic effects of racemic bupivacaine, levobupivacaine, and ropivacaine in anesthetized swine. Anesth Analg 2000;90:1308–1314.

40. Ladd LA, Chang DH, Wilton KA, et al: Effects of CNS site-directed carotid arterial infusion of bupivacaine, levobupivacaine and ropivacaine in sheep. Anesthesiology 2002;97:418–428.

41. Camorcia M, Capogna G, Columb MO: Minimum local analgesic doses of ropivacaine, levobupivacaine, and bupivacaine for intrathecal labor analgesia. Anesthesiology 2005, 102:646–650.

42. McDonald SB, Liu SS, Kopacz DJ, Stephenson CA: Hyperbaric spinal ropivacaine: A comparison to bupivacaine in volunteers. Anesthesiology 1999;90:971–977.

43. Dony P, Dewinde V, Vanderich B, et al: The comparative toxicity of ropivacaine and bupivacaine at equipotent doses in rats. Anesth Analg 2000;91:1489–1492.

44. Huet O, Eyrolle LJ, Mazoit JX, Ozier YM: Cardiac arrest after injection of ropivacaine for posterior lumbar plexus blockade. Anesthesiology 2003;99:1451–1452.

45. Chazalon P, Tourtier JP, Villevielle T, et al: Ropivacaine-induced cardiac arrest after peripheral nerve block: Successful resuscitation. Anesthesiology 2003;99:1449–1450.

46. Klein SM, Pierce T, Rubin Y, et al: Successful resuscitation after ropivacaine-induced ventricular fibrillation. Anesth Analg 2003;97:901–903.

47. Polley LS, Santos AC: Cardiac arrest following regional anesthesia with ropivacaine: Here we go again! Anesthesiology 2003;99:1253–1254.

48. Groban L, Deal DD, Vernon JC, et al: Cardiac resuscitation after incremental overdosage with lidocaine, bupivacaine, levobupivacaine, and ropivacaine in anesthetized dogs. Anesth Analg 2001;92:37–43.

49. Ohmura S, Kawada M, Ohta T, et al: Systemic toxicity and resuscitation in bupivacaine-, levobupivacaine-, or ropivacaine-infused rats. Anesth Analg 2001;93:743–748.

50. Fishburne JI, Greiss FC, Hopkinson R, Rhyne AL: Responses of the gravid uterine musculature to arterial levels of local anesthetic agents. Am J Obstet Gynecol 1979;133:753–761.

51. Santos AC, Arthur GR, Roberts DJ, et al: Effects of ropivacaine and bupivacaine on uterine blood flow in pregnant ewes. Anesth Analg 1992:74:62–67.

52. Santos AC, Karpel B, Noble G: The placental transfer and fetal effects of levobupivacaine, racemic bupivacaine and ropivacaine. Anesthesiology 1999;90:1698–1703.

53. Alahuhta S, Rasanen J, Jouppila P, et al: The effects of epidural ropivacaine and bupivacaine for cesarean section on uteroplacental and fetal circulation. Anesthesiology 1995;83:23–32.

54. Lacassie HJ, Columb MO, Lacassie HP, Lantadilla RO: The relative motor blocking potencies of epidural bupivacaine and ropivacaine in labor. Anesth Analg 2002;95:204–208.

55. Lacassie HJ, Columb MO: The relative motor blocking potencies of bupivacaine and levobupivacaine in labor. Anesth Analg 2003;97:1509–1513.

56. Kopacz DJ, Carpenter RL, Mackey DC: Effect of ropivacaine on cutaneous capillary blood flow in pigs. Anesthesiology 1989;71:69–74.

57. Hawkins JL, Koonin LM, Palmer SK, Gibbs CP: Anesthesia-related deaths during obstetric delivery in the United States, 1979–1990. Anesthesiology 1997;86:277–284.

58. Rose, JS, Neal, JM, Kopacz, DJ: Extended-duration analgesia: Update on microspheres and liposomes. Reg Anesth Pain Medicine 2005;30:275–285.

59. Grant, GJ, Barenholz, Y, Bolotin EM, et al: A novel liposomal bupivacaine formulation to produce ultralong-acting analgesia. Anesthesiology 2004;101:133–137.

60. Gupta RK: Drug targeting in cancer chemotherapy: A clinical prospective. J Pharm Sci 1990;79:949–963.

61. Mowatt JJ, Mok MJ, MacLeod BA, Madden TD: Liposomal bupivacaine. Extended duration nerve blockade using large unilamellar

vesicles that exhibit a proton gradient. Anesthesiology 1996;85:635–643.

62. Mashimo T, Uchida I, Pak M, et al: Prolongation of canine epidural anesthesia by liposome encapsulation of lidocaine. Anesth Analg 1992;74:827–834.

63. Gregoriadis G, Florence AT: Liposomes in drug delivery. Clinical, diagnostic, and ophthalmic potential. Drugs 1993;45:15–28.

64. Hung O, Comeau L, Riley MR, et al: Comparative topical anesthesia of EMLA and liposome encapsulated tetracaine. Can J Anesth 1997;44:707–711.

65. Grant GJ, Vermeulen K, Zakowski MI, et al: Prolonged analgesia and decreased toxicity with liposomal morphine in a mouse model. Anesth Analg 1994;79:706–709.

66. Yu H, Shyh-Dar L, Sun P: Kinetic and dynamic studies of liposomal bupivacaine and bupivacaine solution after subcutaneous injection in rats. J Pharm Pharmacol 2002;54:1221–1227.

67. Bernards CM, Luger TJ, Malmberg AB, et al: Liposome encapsulation prolongs alfentanil spinal analgesia and alters systemic redistribution in the rat. Anesthesiology 1992;77:529–535.

68. Grant GJ, Cascio M, Zakowski MI, et al: Intrathecal administration of liposomal morphine in a mouse model. Anesth Analg 1995;81:514–518.

69. Boogaerts JG, Lafont ND, Carlinos, et al: Biodistribution of liposome associated bupivacaine after extradural administration in rabbits. Br J Anaesth 1995;75:319–325.

70. Allen TM, Hansen CB, Guo LS: Subcutaneous administration of liposomes: A comparison with intravenous and intraperitoneal routes of injection. Biochem Biophys Acta 1993;1150:9–16.

71. Grant GJ, Piskoun B, Bansinath M: Analgesic duration and kinetics of liposomal bupivacaine after subcutaneous injection in mice. Clin Exp Pharmacol Physiol 2003;30:966–968.

72. Malinovsky J-M, Benhamou D, Alafandy M, et al: Neurotoxicological assessment after intracisternal injection of liposomal bupivacaine in rabbits. Anesth Analg 1997;85:1331–1336.

73. Boogaerts JG, Lafont ND, Declercq AG, et al: Epidural administration of liposome-associated bupivacaine for the management of postsurgical pain: A first study. J Clin Anesth 1994;6:315–320.

74. Lafont ND, Legros FJ: Use of liposome-associated bupivacaine in a cancer pain syndrome. Anaesthesia 1996;51:578–579.

75. Lafont ND, Boogaerts JG, Legros FJ: Use of liposome-associated bupivacaine for the management of a chronic pain syndrome (correspondence). Anesth Analg 1994;79:818.

76. Boogaerts JG, Declerq A, Lafont N, et al: Toxicity of bupivacaine encapsulated into liposomes and injected intravenously: Comparison with plain solutions. Anesth Analg 1993;76:553–555.

77. Tokes ZA, Kulscar St. Peteri A, Todd JA: Availability of liposome content to the nervous system. Liposomes and the blood-brain barrier. Brain Res 1980;188:282–286.

78. Boogaerts JG, Lafont N, Donnay M, et al: Motor blockade and absence of local nerve toxicity induced by liposomal bupivacaine injected into the brachial plexus of rabbits. Acta Anaesthesiol Belg 1995;46:19–24.

79. Hall SM: The effect of injections of lysophosphatidyl choline into white matter of the adult mouse spinal cord. J Cell Sci 1972;10:535–546.

8

Analgesic Adjuvants in Neuraxial Anesthesia

Daniel T. Warren, MD • Spencer S. Liu, MD

INTRODUCTION

The ease of practice and relative predictability of neuraxial anesthesia, coupled with its potential to provide multiple benefits to patients in the perioperative period has led to its widespread popularity. Nevertheless, concern of potential failed blocks and untoward effects still limits the acceptance of these techniques. Much effort has been put forth to minimize these undesirable events and optimize the patient experience. The addition of adjuvant medications to local anesthetic preparations has been one avenue pursued to attain these goals.

As early as 1900, Matas[1] was combining morphine and cocaine for subarachnoid injection. Morphine was added in an attempt to prolong the effects of cocaine and to provide sedation. It was not until the 1970s, after the demonstration of opiate receptors in the spinal cord, that neuraxial opioids again began to enter routine use as part of modern regional anesthesia. As the percentage of surgeries performed in the ambulatory setting increases, interest has shifted to finding adjuncts that will provide faster recovery without compromising anesthetic reliability. Many substances have been investigated for use in the subarachnoid and epidural space as an attempt to improve the way that we care for patients (Tables 8–1 and 8–2).

OPIOIDS

Since the identification of opioid receptors in the spinal cord, the potent analgesic effects of neuraxial opioids have been exploited to improve perioperative analgesia and reduce the supraspinal side effects of sedation and respiratory depression seen with systemic opioids. This technique is still limited by dose-dependent pruritis, nausea, and urinary retention.

Pharmacology

Whether administered in the epidural or subarachnoid space, opioids that diffuse into the spinal cord exert spinal analgesia by modulating A-δ and C fibers to decrease afferent nociceptive input.[2] Both μ- and δ-receptor agonists act presynaptically by inhibiting Ca^{2+} influx. Postsynaptically, μ-receptor agonists increase K^+ conductance and hyperpolarize ascending neurons.[3] Opioids have minimal effect on dorsal root axons and somatosensory-evoked potentials.

Cardiovascular Effects

Intrathecal opioids have been shown to have a synergistic interaction with local anesthetics, which allows for enhanced analgesia without increased motor or sympathetic blockade.[4] Thus neuraxial opioids are considered to maintain cardiovascular stability better than equally analgesic doses of local anesthetics. However, neuraxial opioids can reduce sympathetic outflow, via opioid receptors in the sympathetic ganglia, thereby eliciting hypotension. Furthermore, Curatolo and coworkers[5] identified the addition of fentanyl to local anesthetics as a factor associated with hypotension with epidural blockade. They proposed that this reaction may be secondary to a faster onset of blockade exceeding the rate of compensatory mechanisms.

Epidural Space

Given its delayed onset, the addition of morphine to epidural anesthetics may not reduce the intraoperative requirement for volatile anesthetics.[6] This is typically done in an effort to provide postoperative analgesia with prolonged effect. The use of the lipophilic opioid fentanyl intraoperatively for epidural administration can reduce requirements for volatiles more than intravenous fentanyl (more than twofold at 2 mcg/kg).[7] The method of delivery of epidural fentanyl may be important for optimal effect. Ginosaur and colleagues[8] have presented evidence that when epidural fentanyl is given as a bolus, it imparts segmental analgesia consistent with spinal level of action. On the other hand, if given as an infusion, the analgesia is mediated through systemic uptake and supraspinal effect. Similar findings have been reported for sufentanil and alfentanil.[9]

Clinical Pearl

- Intraepidurally administered opioids (eg, fentanyl) reduce intraoperative requirements for volatile anesthetics significantly more than their intravenous administration. This indicates site-specific action in the epidural space.

Subarachnoidal Space

Owing to its hydrophilic nature, intrathecal morphine provides highly selective, prolonged spinal analgesia, but is not typically used to augment intraoperative anesthesia.

The lipophilic opioids are more suited for intraoperative use in the intrathecal space due to their rapid onset and modest duration. Additionally, with more timely clearance from the CSF, the risk of delayed respiratory depression from these drugs is much lower than morphine. Exploiting the synergy between local anesthetics and opioids, the addition of 10 to 25 mcg fentanyl to low-dose lidocaine and bupivacaine spinal anesthetics dramatically improves anesthetic success, without delaying achievement of discharge criteria for ambulatory patients.[4,10] Pruritis remains a concern with intrathecal fentanyl, especially when administered with procaine or 2-chloroprocaine.[11] Furthermore, when used with the ultrashort-acting spinal anesthetic 2-chloroprocaine, fentanyl can slightly delay discharge (95 vs 104 min) as shown by Vath and Kopacz.[11] Nevertheless, fentanyl remains one of the most useful analgesic adjuncts for ambulatory spinal anesthesia.

VASOCONSTRICTORS

Vasoconstricting agents are commonly added to local anesthetic solutions and have a long history of clinical use. Epinephrine is by far the most commonly employed vasoconstrictor in neuraxial anesthesia for prolonging the anesthetic effect, but it can also reduce peak blood levels, provide more reliable block, and intensify anesthesia and analgesia.[12–15] All of these benefits can result in a reduction in the amount of local anesthetic necessary and consequently decrease the potential for toxicity in a given clinical situation. It had long been thought that the effects of epinephrine are solely due to its vasoconstricting effects, but we now know that it exerts presynaptic adrenergic receptor activity that directly contributes to analgesia.[16]

Phenylephrine is a synthetic α-adrenergic agonist typically used to prolong spinal anesthesia. Currently it is far less commonly used clinically than epinephrine.

Pharmacology

Epinephrine is an endogenous catacholamine that produces a dose-related pharmacologic profile that is linked to its affinity for various adrenergic receptors. At low doses, epinephrine stimulates β_2-receptors, producing arterial vasodilation. Higher doses cause arterial vasoconstriction by stimulating α_1-and α_2-receptors. Vasoconstriction, and thus decreased blood flow, can reduce uptake of local anesthetics into the circulation, thus maintaining concentrations at the site of injection and reducing peak plasma concentrations. The intrinsic analgesic effects of epinephrine are exerted via stimulation of presynaptic α_2-adrenoreceptors found at the terminals of primary afferents. These receptors are also found centrally on neurons in the superficial laminae of the spinal cord and several brainstem nuclei that participate in analgesic mechanisms.

Epinephrine is metabolized rapidly by monoamine oxidase (MAO) and cataechol-*O*-methyl transferase, resulting in the end product vanillylmandelic acid (VMA). These enzymes are present in the plasma, kidneys, and liver. They are also present in the central nervous system and show particularly high activity in the arachnoid mater.[17,18] Due to the rapid inactivation of epinephrine by these enzymes, the duration of the clinical effect of epinephrine is dependent on the rate of exposure to these enzymes.

Cardiovascular Effects

With the typical dose range used for epidural anesthesia, systemic levels of epinephrine remain low. This usually produces mild vasodilation and increased heart rate and myocardial contractility. Ward and coworkers[19] evaluated the cardiovascular effects of epidural blockade to T5 using lidocaine with and without epinephrine. Mean arterial pressure decreased 20% in the epinephrine group, compared with 10% in the group receiving plain lidocaine. However, the group with epinephrine also showed a 20–30% increase in cardiac output. Bonica suggested that the systemic β-adrenergic effects of epinephrine administered epidurally might prevent the potential cardiovascular collapse from epidural blockade.[20] Higher than normal doses or situations that result in increased vascular uptake can result in peripheral alpha stimulation, thus increasing peripheral vascular resistance. Exceeding a

total dose of 0.25 mg of epinephrine may be associated with cardiac arrhythmias.[21]

When phenylephrine is added to epidural solutions, the systemic absorption results in increased vascular resistance without the benefit of increased contractility or chronotropy seen with epinephrine. Bearing this is mind, anesthesiologists typically only use phenylephrine in the subarachnoid space.

Epidural Space

The typical concentration of epinephrine for epidural anesthesia is 1:200,000, or 5 mcg/mL. The commercially available premixed solutions of local anesthetics with epinephrine are more acidic in an effort to preserve the potency of the epinephrine. This lower pH will slow the onset of blockade and inhibit the vasoconstricting actions of epinephrine; therefore, adding "fresh" epinephrine to local anesthetic solutions at the time of use is preferred.

The clinical effect of epinephrine on duration of anesthesia depends on the local anesthetic used. Epinephrine is more effective at prolonging the anesthetic duration of shorter acting agents, such as lidocaine and 2-chloroprocaine. Adding 1:200,000 epinephrine to 2% lidocaine will nearly double the time to resolution of blockade.[22] Agents with longer duration of action show much less prolongation of anesthesia with the addition of epinephrine. Adding epinephrine to ropivacaine will intensify the block, but will not prolong the duration of epidural anesthesia or affect plasma levels.[13] This is likely due to the inherent vasoconstricting effects of ropivacaine. Other agents do show reduction of plasma levels when epinephrine is added.[12,14] Epinephrine 1:200,000 will decrease plasma lidocaine and chloroprocaine levels by 20% to 30%, but will decrease plasma bupivacaine levels only by 10% to 20%. The effect of epinephrine on plasma levels of local anesthetics has long been thought to be due to constriction of the epidural venous plexus and therefore leads to reduced blood flow and slower uptake of local anesthetics. More recent evidence implies that reduced dural blood flow and increased hepatic clearance may be more important in this phenomenon.[23] Its potential to prolong discharge times and delay bladder function limits the utility of adding epinephrine to epidural agents for ambulatory surgery.

Subarachnoidal Space

Both epinephrine and phenylephrine will prolong spinal anesthesia and provide a more intense and reliable block in a dose-related fashion. Epinephrine is much more commonly employed with a typical dose of 0.2 mg, although doses of 0.1 to 0.6 mg have been described. Adding 0.2 mg of epinephrine to a bupivacaine spinal anesthetic will typically increase time of regression to L2 by 25%.[24,25]

The use of vasoconstrictors in ambulatory spinal anesthesia is quite problematic. Adding epinephrine to spinal anesthetics will prolong motor blockade and delay the return of bladder function, thus preventing patients from achieving discharge criteria. Chiu and coworkers[26] showed in volunteers that adding 0.2 mg epinephrine to 50 mg hyperbaric lidocaine prolonged surgical anesthesia (as demonstrated by tolerance of transcutaneous electrical stimulation) by 30 min, and time to void and discharge time increased by 80 min.

In clinically relevant doses intrathecal epinephrine by itself does not carry a risk of neurotoxicity. Spinal cord blood flow is well maintained in the dog and cat model in doses up to 0.5 mg.[27] However, it is suggested that epinephrine may contribute to the neurotoxicity of local anesthetics and has been associated with a case report of cauda equina syndrome after single-shot lidocaine spinal anesthesia.[28]

Clinical Pearls

- The value of vasoconstrictors in ambulatory spinal anesthesia is controversial.
- Adding epinephrine to spinal anesthetics will prolong motor blockade and delay the return of bladder function, thus preventing patients from achieving discharge criteria.
- In clinically relevant doses intrathecal epinephrine by itself does not carry a risk of neurotoxicity.
- However, epinephrine may contribute to the neurotoxicity of local anesthetics and has been associated with a case report of cauda equina syndrome after single-shot lidocaine spinal anesthesia

Phenylephrine may increase the risk of transient neurologic symptoms as suggested by Sakura and coworkers in a study of tetracaine spinal anesthesia.[29] A recent volunteer study with spinal 2-chloroprocaine reported consistent flu-like symptoms when epinephrine was added.[30]

ALPHA$_2$-ADRENERGIC AGONISTS

Alpha$_2$-agonists have been gaining popularity in the field of regional anesthesia. Clonidine was first injected intrathecally in humans in 1984, but other α_2-agonists had been used in veterinary anesthesia for many years. Clonidine can be useful in enhancing neuraxial analgesia with a different side effect profile than opioids. A preservative-free preparation of clonidine is commercially available in the United States.

Pharmacology

Clonidine binds to α_2-adrenoreceptors on primary afferent, substantia gelatinosa, and several brainstem nuclei attributed to analgesic mechanisms. Clonidine is thought to exert its effects by attenuating A-δ and C-fiber nociception and producing conduction blockade via increased potassium conductance.[30,31] Clonidine has been shown to increase acetylcholine and norepinephrine in the CSF and to inhibit the release of substance P and modulate wide dynamic range neurons in the dorsal horn of the spinal cord.[32] Clonidine is rather lipophilic and thus is rapidly redistributed systemically to the periphery after epidural or spinal administration.

However, neuraxially administered clonidine imparts analgesia through spinal mechanisms rather than systemic absorption as evidenced by the lack of correlation between time of analgesia and peripheral blood levels. The analgesic effects of clonidine have been shown to be reversed by yohimbine, an α_2-adrenergic antagonist.[33] Clonidine is an extremely stable compound and has undergone extensive testing for neurotoxicity and safety in several animal models without histopathologic or behavioral evidence of detriment.

Cardiovascular Effects

Neuraxially administered clonidine exerts hemodynamic effects through not only central means, but also peripheral action due to its rapid systemic absorption. The effect of clonidine on blood pressure is the result of potentially opposing actions at multiple sites. Neuraxially administered clonidine directly inhibits preganglionic sympathetic neurons in the spinal cord.[34] When injected in the low thoracic or lumbar region, or even the cervical epidural space, the effect on blood pressure is not significantly different from intravenous injection.[35] However, when given in the mid or upper thoracic epidural space, a much more profound drop in blood pressure is observed.[36] This is thought to be due to the upper thoracic dermatomes supplying the heart and the relative concentration of noradrenergic innervation of sympathetic preganglionic neurons.

In the brainstem, activation of α_2-adrenoreceptors of the locus ceruleus and nucleus tractus solitarius decreases sympathetic drive. Clonidine will also bind to nonadrenergic imidazoline-prefering receptors in the nucleus reticularis lateralis and impart both hypotensive and antiarrhythmogenic actions.[37,38] In the periphery, clonidine activates presynaptic α_2-receptors and inhibits the release of norepinephrine from the terminals of sympathetic nerves, thus promoting vasoconstriction and reducing chronotropic drive. However, at higher concentrations of circulating clonidine, the direct α_2-/α_1-agonist action begins to promote vasoconstriction and thus opposes the presynaptic and brainstem effects. Thus the dose–response curve for neuraxially or systemically administered clonidine is U-shaped, reflecting the central sympatholysis being offset by peripheral vasoconstriction at higher doses.[39]

Clonidine reduces heart rate by not only inhibiting norepinephrine release, but also through a vagomimetic effect. This, as with afterload-reducing effects, decreases myocardial oxygen demand. The resulting effect of clonidine on cardiac output varies from patient to patient depending on the predominance of either its vasoactive or chronotropic influences. The hemodynamic effect of clonidine peaks after 1 to 2 h and lasts 6–8 h after a single bolus. The addition of clinical doses clonidine to local anesthetics for neuraxial anesthesia is unlikely to increase the degree of resulting hypotension or significantly alter responsiveness to resuscitation drugs.[40–43]

Epidural Space

Clonidine produces segmental hypoalgesia when administered in the epidural space.[35,44] Doses ranging from 100 to 900 mcg have been studied and shown to produce analgesic effects that begin about 20 min after administration and peak at around 1 h.[45] The quality of analgesia produced by epidural clonidine has been said to be comparable with that from epidural morphine.[46] Side effects of sedation and dry mouth are usually dose-related.

Although clonidine has been studied as a sole agent for epidural administration,[47] it is typically used in combination with local anesthetics or opiates in clinical practice. When clonidine is used in combination with opiates, the analgesic effects have been shown to be additive, but not synergistic.[48–51] Thus, patients require a smaller total dose of the narcotic and have a decreased incidence of oxygen desaturation with equivalent analgesia.

Clinical Pearls

- Clonidine produces segmental hypoalgesia when administered in the epidural space.
- Doses ranging from 100 to 900 mcg have been studied and shown to produce analgesic effects that begin about 20 min after administration and peak at around 1 h.
- The quality of analgesia produced by epidural clonidine has been said to be comparable with that from epidural morphine.
- When clonidine is used in combination with opiates, the analgesic effects have been shown to be additive, but not synergistic. Thus, patients require a smaller total dose of narcotic and have a decreased incidence of oxygen desaturation with equivalent analgesia.
- Adding clonidine to local anesthetics intensifies and prolongs epidural blockade and can reduce local anesthetic dose requirement.
- The side effects of neuraxially administered clonidine include sedation and dry mouth are usually dose-related.

Adding clonidine to local anesthetics intensifies and prolongs epidural blockade and can reduce local anesthetic dose requirement.[52,53] When adding clonidine to local anesthetics, the typical dose for epidural bolus administration is 150 mcg, or 2 mcg/kg.[54–56] Klimscha and colleagues showed that the addition of 150 mcg of clonidine to 10 mL of 0.5% bupivacaine for epidural anesthesia in patients undergoing hip surgery increased the mean duration of anesthesia from 1.8 to 5.3 h.[55] This dose is associated with decreased intraoperative anesthetic and analgesic requirements,[56] reduced pain scores,[54–58] increased time to first analgesic request[51,54,56–58] and increased patient satisfaction.[57] These benefits usually persist for around 3 h and can be achieved without increasing hemodynamic instability more than would occur from local anesthetic alone.

Subarachnoid Space

Intrathecal clonidine produces dose-dependent analgesia without the concerns of pruritis and respiratory depression seen with opioids. Malinovsky and coworkers[59] investigated intrathecal clonidine, in doses of 75 to 450 mcg, as the sole anesthetic for transurethral resection of the prostate. All but two patients required general anesthesia, but prolonged analgesia was evident in all patients. The majority of the clinical use of intrathecal clonidine occurs in combination with a variety of local anesthetics, in which it produces dose-dependent prolongation of both sensory and motor blockade.[60–63] Side effects of sedation, hypotension, and bradycardia are seen with intrathecal clonidine and are also dose-dependent. Less urinary retention is seen with intrathecal clonidine than with intrathecal morphine.[64]

Low-dose intrathecal clonidine has a promising role in ambulatory anesthesia. De Kock and coworkers[65] demonstrated that the addition of 15 mcg of clonidine to 8 mg of ropivacaine for spinal anesthesia in patients undergoing knee arthroscopy increased anesthetic success from 70 to 90% without significant effect on recovery time. However, when the dose of clonidine was increased to 45 mcg, resolution of motor and sensory blockade and time to voiding increased from 170 to 215 min.

ALKALINIZATION & CARBONATION

Local anesthetics are weak bases consisting of a lipophilic benzene ring linked to a hydrophilic group, usually a tertiary amine, that can exist in ionized and nonionized forms. To promote aqueous solubility, these compounds are typically prepared in the form of their hydrochloride salts resulting in an acidic solution (pH ranging from 3.4 to 6.4). Commercially available solutions containing epinephrine are prepared at an even lower pH (usually with bisulfite), ranging from 3.2 to 4.2, in efforts to preserve the epinephrine. Alkalinizing solutions to raise the pH closer to the pK_a of the local anesthetic and thus increase the proportion of the nonionized form available to cross cell membranes, is thought to speed the onset

Table 8–1.

Commonly Recommended Volumes of 8.4% Sodium Bicarbonate for Alkalinization of Local Anesthetic Solutions

Local Anesthetic	8.4% NaHCO₃/10 mL of solution	Final pH
2-Chloroprocaine	0.3 mL	6.8
Lidocaine	1 mL	7.2
Mepivacaine	1 mL	7.2
Bupivacaine	0.1 mL	6.4
Ropivacaine	Not recommended due to risk of precipitation	

Reprinted, with permission, from Mulroy MF: Regional Anesthesia: An Illustrated Procedural Guide, 3rd ed. Lippincott Williams & Wilkins, 2002.

of anesthesia. Although this is well demonstrated, in vitro[66] studies attempting to demonstrate this in epidural anesthetics are sometimes conflicting.

Most studies show that alkalinization speeds onset of epidural blockade with lidocaine,[67–72] bupivacaine,[67,73,74] mepivacaine,[67,75,76] and chloroprocaine[77,78] by up to 10 min. Ropivacaine seems to not show faster onset with alkalinization,[79] but like the other drugs, there is evidence that alkalinization can intensify epidural anesthesia and improves spread to sacral dermatomes.[68,71,72,80] One noted trend is that the effects of alkalinization are greatest on solutions containing epinephrine, whether freshly added or prepackaged. This is perhaps due to pH-dependent vasoconstrictive actions of epinephrine.

It should be noted that the degree of alkalinization is limited by precipitation. Table 8–1 shows the commonly recommended amounts of sodium bicarbonate to be added to each local anesthetic solution, but all preparations should be inspected for precipitation before administration. Alternatively, the carbonate salts of local anesthetics have been shown to have more rapid onset of epidural blockade than standard hydrochloride preparations.[81] However, carbonated drugs are of limited availability and may be more prone to induce hypotension with epidural administration.[5]

UNCOMMON ADJUNCTS

Neostigmine

The acetylcholinesterase inhibitor neostigmine has been investigated as a neuraxial analgesic adjunct due to its ability to provide analgesia without hemodynamic depression. However, enthusiasm for clinical use of neostigmine is limited by its tendency to induce nausea and delay recovery from neuraxial blockade.

Pharmacology

Intrathecal neostigmine inhibits the breakdown of acetylcholine in the spinal cord via reversible inhibition of acetylcholinesterase. Animal models have suggested that acetylcholine plays a role in spinal analgesia through stimulation of cholinergic receptors in the substantia gelatinosa and superficial laminae of the dorsal horn of the spinal cord[82–84] and perhaps through stimulating nitric oxide production in the spinal cord.[85] Although intrathecal injection of cholinergic agonists will stimulate all receptors of a particular class, neostigmine increases endogenous acetylcholine in a manner dependent on the tonic production of this neurotransmitter within each particular region of the spinal cord.

Cardiovascular Effects

Intrathecal neostigmine has been shown to counteract hypotension resulting from bupivacaine spinal anesthesia in rats,[86] but these effects are not reproducible in human subjects.[87] Volunteers receiving high doses of intrathecal neostigmine developed increased heart rate and respiratory rate—responses that have been attributed to the concomitant severe nausea and vomiting.[88] Low and moderate doses are considered to have little or no cardiovascular effects.

Epidural Space

Lauretti and coworkers[89] studied the analgesic effect of epidural neostigmine in doses from 1 to 4 mcg/kg added to epidural lidocaine and showed a dose-independent analgesic effect, increasing time to first analgesic request from 3.5 to 8 h. Other studies have reported similar results with doses in the range of 1 to 10 mcg/kg, without report of increased nausea,[90–95] but some suggestion of sedation.[94]

Subarachnoid Space

Subsequent to reassuring toxologic studies in animals, Hood and colleagues[88] evaluated safety, analgesic efficacy, and side effects of intrathecal neostigmine in volunteers. All doses produced analgesia without sedation, pruritis, respiratory depression, hypotension, or bradycardia; however, dose-related motor weakness, decreases in deep tendon reflexes, urinary incontinence, genitourinary stimulation, and nausea and vomiting did occur. Further studies in patients revealed similar responses of nausea and vomiting that proved to be prolonged and difficult to treat.[96–100] Liu and coworkers[100] showed that when added to low-dose (7.5 mg) bupivacaine spinal anesthetics, 50 mcg of neostigmine enhanced motor and sensory blockade, but delayed achievement of discharge criteria. Doses of 6.25 and 12.5 mcg did not prolong anesthesia but still elicited nausea and delayed discharge.

Ketamine

Many studies have demonstrated the involvement of *N*-methyl-D-aspartate (NMDA) receptors in analgesia,[101–107] central sensitization,[102,103,106–108] and opioid tolerance.[104,105,107] Ketamine is a noncompetitive antagonist of

Table 8–2.

Adjuvants for Neuraxial Anesthesia

Opioids

Epidural
   Morphine 40 mcg/kg for postoperative analgesia—risk of respiratory depression
   Fentanyl 1–2 mcg/kg bolus (infusions act via systemic uptake)
   Sufentanil probably acts via systemic uptake—no advantage over IV administration

Spinal
   Morphine 100–200 mcg for postoperative analgesia up to 24 h—risk of delayed respiratory depression
   Fentanyl 10–25 mcg
      Improves quality and duration of spinal anesthetics without delaying recovery
      Useful for ambulatory spinal anesthesia
      Increased pruritus with procaine and 2-chloroprocaine
   Sufentanil probably acts via systemic uptake

Vasoconstrictors

Epidural
   Epinephrine 5 mcg/ml (1:200,000). Total dose not to exceed 0.25 mg
      Effective prolongation of block and recovery with lidocaine and 2-chloroprocaine, and reduced plasma levels of lidocaine
      Will intensify block and reduce plasma levels of bupivacaine, but less effect on duration
      Minimal effect with ropivacaine
      Phenylephrine may result in systemic uptake and reduced cardiac output

Spinal
   Epinephrine 0.2 mg will intensify block, prolong duration of blockade
   Less effect on duration of high dose bupivacaine
   Not advantageous in ambulatory settings due to prolongation of recovery and delay of discharge times
   Do not use with 2-chloroprocaine
   Phenylephrine can have profound effect on duration of blockade, but may increase risk of TNS

Clonidine

Epidural
   Typical dose of 150 mcg or 2 mcg/kg for 6–8 h of analgesia
   Additive analgesia when combined with opiates
   More profound hypotension when used in upper thoracic epidural space
   Cardiovascular effects are not significantly greater than local anesthetic alone
   Less oxygen desaturation and urinary retention compared to opioids, but can produce sedation

Spinal
   15 mcg for low-dose/ambulatory spinal anesthetics
   Higher doses will prolong motor block and recovery time
   Doses up to 150 mcg have been used, but with increasing sedation and cardiovascular depression

Sodium Bicarbonate

See Table 8–1 for recommended doses
More effective on speed of onset with lidocaine and mepivacaine than with bupivacaine or ropivacaine epidural anesthesia
Effect on speed of onset may not be clinically relevant
Can intensify epidural blockade, especially in sacral dermatomes
May be associated with hypotension
Monitor solution for precipitation

Neostigmine

Epidural doses of 1–2 mcg/kg seems to be beneficial
Main concern is protracted nausea
Clinical utility in spinal anesthesia is yet to be determined due to high incidence of nausea

Depot Formulations, Ketamine, Ketorolac, Adenosine, Midazolam

Some evidence of potential benefit
Clinical safety and utility is yet to be determined

TNS = transient neurologic symptoms

NMDA receptors, but also has actions at monoaminergic receptors, opioid receptors, voltage-sensitive Ca channels, muscarinic receptors, and local anesthetic actions through Na channel blockade.[109] Commercially available as a racemic mixture, the *S*-enantiomer is far more potent at NMDA receptors.[110] Animal models suggest that preservative-free ketamine lacks neurotoxicity.[111]

Epidural administration of ketamine at 0.5 to 1 mg/kg has been shown to reduce intraoperative[112] and postoperative[112–115] analgesic requirements without increased side effects. Ozyalcin and coworkers demonstrated decreased pinprick hyperalgesia and touch allodynia in thoracotomy patients receiving epidural versus intramuscular ketamine.[115]

Ketamine was first used intrathecally as a sole anesthetic by Bion in 1984.[116] Hawksworth and coworkers reported intolerable rate of anesthetic failure and psychometric side effects at doses of 0.7 to 0.95 mg/kg.[117] Other investigators found similar problems when combining with bupivacaine for spinal anesthesia.[118] Further work continues to delineate potential applications for ketamine in the treatment of chronic neuropathic pain, as a preemptive analgesia, and in the modulation of opioid tolerance.[119,120]

Ketorolac

Eisenach and coworkers have demonstrated involvement of spinal cyclooxygenase (COX) enzymes in postoperative hypersensitivity and pain.[121,122] Ketorolac tromethamine is a nonselective, but COX-1-preferring, nonsteroidal antiinflammatory drug that has been investigated in multiple animal models for intrathecal administration and has demonstrated antinociception and lack of neurotoxicity.[121–128] There is evidence that ketorolac may enhance analgesic effects of intrathecal clonidine[127] and have analgesic synergy with intrathecal morphine[128] in rat models. A phase I safety study of preservative-free ketorolac in healthy volunteers using single bolus doses of 0.5 to 2 mg showed no immediate or delayed neurologic detriment.[129] This study revealed no significant effect on blood pressure or motor function, but also showed no decrease in pain with heat stimuli. Further human investigations are underway and will it is hoped identify the clinical role of intrathecal ketorolac.

Other Agents and Future Considerations

Researchers continue to investigate various compounds in the hope of improving neuraxial anesthesia. One avenue of research is in liposomal and polymer-encapsulated compounds. Thus far, liposomal morphine is the only agent on the market and intended for single-shot epidural analgesia lasting up to 48 h. It should be noted that it must not be administered with epidural local anesthetics. Doing so can cause early and uncontrolled release of the drug.

Eisenach and coworkers are investigating the role of adenosine in spinal analgesia.[130] The potential benefits appear to be in treating chronic neuropathic pain rather than for acute analgesia.

Although previous animal studies had shown inconsistent evidence of neurotoxicity,[131,132] further evidence is gathering to suggest that intrathecal midazolam may be a safe and promising adjunct to spinal anesthesia.[133,134] The analgesic benefits appear to be greatest when combined with intrathecal opioids,[135] but the appropriate clinical role is still to be determined.

SUMMARY

The use of analgesic adjuvants in neuraxial anesthesia has improved the care we can provide by improving the reliability and quality of neuraxial blockade, reducing local anesthetic dose and systemic plasma levels, and providing postoperative analgesia. This area continues to be a rich source of future research into the ways of optimizing ambulatory anesthesia, and potentially affecting preemptive analgesia and central sensitization.

References

1. Matas R: Local and regional anesthesia with cocaine and other analgesic drugs, including the subarachnoid method, as applied in general surgery practice. Philadelphia Med J 1900;6:820–843.
2. Hamber EA, Viscomi CM: Intrathecal lipophilic opioids as adjuncts to surgical spinal anesthesia. Reg Anesth Pain Med 1999;24: 255–263.
3. Schneider SP, Eckert WA, Light AR: Opioid-activated postsynaptic, inward rectifying potassium currents in whole cell recordings in substantia gelatinosa neurons. J Neurophysiol 1998;80:2954–2962.
4. Liu S, Chiu AA, Carpenter RL, et al: Fentanyl prolongs lidocaine spinal anesthesia without prolonging recovery. Anesth Analg 1995;80:730–734.
5. Curatolo M, Scaramozzino P, Venuti FS, et al: Factors associated with hypotension and bradycardia after epidural blockade. Anesth Analg 1996;83(5):1033–1040.
6. Koo M, Sabate A, Dalmau A, et al: Sevoflurane requirements during coloproctologic surgery: Difference between two different epidural regimens. J Clin Anesth 2003;15(2):97–102.
7. Harukuni I, Yamaguchi H, Sato S, et al: The comparison of epidural fentanyl, epidural lidocaine, and intravenous fentanyl in patients undergoing gastrectomy. Anesth Analg 1995;81(6):1169–1174.
8. Ginosar Y, Riley ET, Angst MS. The site of action of epidural fentanyl in humans: the difference between infusion and bolus administration. Anesth Analg 2003;97(5):1428–1438.
9. Coda BA, Brown MC, Schaffer R, et al: Pharmacology of epidural fentanyl, alfentanil, and sufentanil in volunteers. Anesthesiology 1994;81(5):1149–1161.
10. Ben-David B, Solomon E, Levin H, et al: Intrathecal fentanyl with small-dose dilute bupivacaine: Better anesthesia without prolonging recovery. Anesth Analg 1997;85:560–565.
11. Vath JS, Kopacz DJ: Spinal 2-chloroprocaine: The effect of added fentanyl. Anesth Analg 2004;98(1):89–94.
12. Burm, AG, van Kleef JW, Gladines MP, et al: Epidural anesthesia with Lidocaine and bupivacaine: Effects of epinephrine on plasma concentration profiles. Anesth Analg 1986;65:1281–1284.
13. Lee BB, Ngan Kee WD, Plummer JL, et al: The effect of the addition of epinephrine on early systemic absorption of epidural ropivacaine in humans. Anesth Analg 2002;95(5):1402–1407.
14. Niemi G, Breivik H: Epinephrine markedly improves thoracic epidural analgesia produced by a small-dose infusion of ropivacaine, fentanyl, and epinephrine after major thoracic or abdominal surgery: A randomized, double-blinded crossover study with and without epinephrine. Anesth Analg 2002;94:1598–1605.

15. Sakura S, Sumi M, Morimoto N, et al: The addition of epinephrine increases intensity of sensory block during epidural anesthesia with lidocaine. Reg Anesth Pain Med 1999;24(6):541–546.

16. Curatolo M, Petersen-Felix S, Arendt-Nielsen L, et al: Epidural epinephrine and clonidine. Segmental analgesia and effects on differential pain modalities. Anesthesiology 1997;87:785–794.

17. Bernards CM, Shen DD, Sterling ES, et al: Epidural, cerebrospinal fluid, and plasma pharmacokinetics of epidural opioids (part 2): effect of epinephrine. Anesthesiology 2003;99(2):466–475.

18. Kern C, Mautz DS, Bernards CM: Epinephrine is metabolized by the spinal meninges of monkeys and pigs. Anesthesiology 1995;83:1078–1081.

19. Ward RJ, Bonica JJ, Freund FG, et al: Epidural and subarachnoid anesthesia. Cardiovascular and respiratory effects. JAMA 1965;191:275–278.

20. Bonica JJ, Akamatsu TJ, Berges PU et al: Circulatory effects of epidural block: II. Effects of epinephrine. Anesthesiology 1971;34:514.

21. Katz RL, Bigger JT: Cardiac arrhythmias during anesthesia and operation. Anesthesiology 1970;33:193.

22. Liu SS, Hodgson PS: Local anesthetics, in Barash PG, Cullen BF, Stoelting RF (eds): *Clinical Anesthesia*. Lippincott-Raven, Philadelphia, 2001, pp 449–472.

23. Sharrock N, Go G, Mineo R: Effect of IV low-dose adrenaline and phenylephrine infusions on plasma concentrations of bupivacaine after lumbar extradural anaesthesia in elderly patients. Br J Anaesth 1991;67:694–698.

24. Moore JM, Liu SS, Pollock JE, et al: The effect of epinephrine on small-dose hyperbaric bupivacaine spinal anesthesia: Clinical implications for ambulatory surgery. Anesth Analg 1998;86:973–977.

25. Kito K, Kato H, Shibata M, et al: The effect of varied doses of epinephrine on duration of lidocaine spinal anesthesia in the thoracic and lumbosacral dermatomes. Anesth Analg 1998;86:1018–1022.

26. Chiu AA, Liu S, Carpenter RL, et al: The effects of epinephrine on lidocaine spinal anesthesia: A cross-over study. Anesth Analg 1995;80:735–739.

27. Kozody R, Palahniuk RJ, Wade JG, et al: The effect of subarachnoid epinephrine and phenylephrine on spinal cord blood flow. Can Anaesth Soc J 1984;31:503–508.

28. Gerancher JC: Cauda equine syndrome following single spinal administration of 5% hyperbaric lidocaine through a 25-gauge Whitacre needle. Anesthesiology 1997;87:687–689.

29. Sakura S, Sumi, M, Sakaguchi Y, et al: The Addition of Phenylephrine Contributes to the Development of Transient Neurologic Symptoms after Spinal Anesthesia with 0.5% Tetracaine. Anesthesiology 1997;87:771–778.

30. Smith KN, Kopacz DJ, McDonald SB: Spinal 2-chloroprocaine: a dose-ranging study and the effect of added epinephrine. Anesth Analg 2004;98(1):81–88.

31. Gaumann DM, Brunet PC, Jirounek P: Hyperpolarizing afterpotentials in C fibers and local anesthetic effects of clonidine and lidocaine. Pharmacology 1994;48:21–29.

32. De Kock M, Eisenach J, Tong C, et al: Analgesic doses of intrathecal but not intravenous clonidine increase acetylcholine in cerebrospinal fluid in humans. Anesth Analg 1997;84(4):800–803.

33. Liu N, Bonnet F, Delaunay L, et al: Partial reversal of the effects of extradural clonidine by oral yohimbine in postoperative patients. Br J Anaesth 1993;70:515–518.

34. Guyenet PG, Cabot JB: Inhibition of sympathetic preganglionic neurons by catecholamines and clonidine: Mediation by an a-adrenergic receptor. J Neurosci 1981;1:908–917.

35. De Kock M, Crochet B, Morimont C, et al: Intravenous or epidural clonidine for intra- and postoperative analgesia. Anesthesiology 1993;79:525–531.

36. De Kock M: Site of hemodynamic effects of alpha sub 2 -adrenergic agonists. Anesthesiology 1991;75:715–716.

37. Bruban V, Estato V, Schann S, et al: Evidence for synergy between alpha (2)-adrenergic and nonadrenergic mechanisms in central blood pressure regulation. Circulation 2002;105(9):1116–1121.

38. De Vos H, Bricca G, De Keyser J, et al: Imidazoline receptors, non-adrenergic idazoxan binding sites and alpha sub 2-adrenoceptors in the human central nervous system. Neuroscience 1994;59:589–598.

39. Langer SZ, Duval N, Massingham R: Pharmacologic and therapeutic significance of alpha-adrenoceptor subtypes. J Cardiovasc Pharmacol 1985;7(Suppl 8):S1–S8.

40. De Kock M, Versailles H, Colinet B, et al: Epidemiology of the adverse hemodynamic events occurring during "clonidine anesthesia": A prospective open trial of intraoperative. J Clin Anesth 1995;7:403–410.

41. Nishikawa T, Kimura T, Taguchi N, et al: Oral clonidine pre-anesthetic medication augments the pressor responses to intravenous ephedrine in awake or anesthetized patients. Anesthesiology 1991;74:705–710.

42. Nishikawa T, Dohi S: Oral clonidine blunts the heart rate response to intravenous atropine in humans. Anesthesiology 1991;75:217–222.

43. Inomata S, Nishikawa T, Kihara S, et al: Enhancement of pressor response to intravenous phenylephrine following oral clonidine medication in awake and anaesthetized patients. Can J Anaesth 1995;42:119–125.

44. Curlato M, Petersen-Felix S, Arendt-Nielsen L, et al: Epidural epinephrine and clonidine: Segmental analgesia and effects on different pain modalities. Anesthesiology 1997;87:785–794.

45. Eisenach JC, Lysak SZ, Viscomi CM: Epidural clonidine analgesia following surgery. Anesthesiology 1989;71:640–646.

46. Tamsen A, Gordh T: Epidural clonidine produces analgesia. Lancet 1984;28;2(8396):231–232.

47. De Kock M, Wiederkher P, Laghmiche A, et al: Epidural clonidine used as the sole analgesic agent during and after abdominal surgery. A dose-response study. Anesthesiology 1997;86(2):285–292.

48. Capogna G, Celleno D, Zangrillo A, et al: Addition of clonidine to epidural morphine enhances postoperative analgesia after cesarean delivery. Reg Anesth 1995;20(1):57–61.

49. Murga G, Samso E, Valles J, et al: The effect of clonidine on intra-operative requirements of fentanyl during combined epidural/general anaesthesia. Anaesthesia 1994;49(11):999–1002.

50. Eisenach JC, D'Angelo R, Taylor C, et al: An isobolographic study of epidural clonidine and fentanyl after cesarean section. Anesth Analg 1994;79(2):285–290.

51. Delaunay L, Leppert C, Dechaubry V, et al: Epidural clonidine decreases postoperative requirements for epidural fentanyl. Reg Anesth 1993;18(3):176–180.

52. Aveline C, El Metaoua S, Masmoudi A, et al: The effect of clonidine on the minimum local analgesic concentration of epidural ropivacaine during labor. Anesth Analg 2002;95(3):735–740.

53. Landau R, Schiffer E, Morales M, et al: The dose-sparing effect of clonidine added to ropivacaine for labor epidural analgesia. Anesth Analg 2002;95(3):728–734.

54. Bouguet D: Caudal clonidine added to local anesthetics enhances post-operative analgesia after anal surgery in adults (Abst). Anesthesiology 1994;81:A942.

55. Klimscha W, Chiari A, Krafft P, et al: Hemodynamic and analgesic effects of clonidine added repetitively to continuous epidural and spinal blocks. Anesth Analg 1995;80:322–327.

56. Wu CT, Jao SW, Borel CO, et al: The effect of epidural clonidine on perioperative cytokine response, postoperative pain, and bowel function in patients undergoing colorectal surgery. Anesth Analg 2004;99(2):502–509.

57. O'Meara ME, Gin T: Comparison of 0.125% bupivacaine with 0.125% bupivacaine and clonidine as extradural analgesia in the first stage of labour. Br J Anaesth 1993;71:651–656.

58. Jellish WS, Abodeely A, Fluder EM, et al: The effect of spinal bupivacaine in combination with either epidural clonidine and/or 0.5%

bupivacaine administered at the incision site on postoperative outcome in patients undergoing lumbar laminectomy. Anesth Analg 2003;96(3):874–880.

59. Malinovsky JM, Bernard JM: Spinal clonidine fails to provide surgical anesthesia for transurethral resection of prostate. A dose-finding pilot study. Reg Anesth 1996;21(5):419–423.

60. Bonnet F, Buisson VB, Francois Y, et al: Effects of oral and subarachnoid clonidine on spinal anesthesia with bupivacaine. Reg Anesth 1990;15(4):211–214.

61. Ota K, Namiki A, Iwasaki H, et al: Dose-related prolongation of tetracaine spinal anesthesia by oral clonidine in humans. Anesth Analg 1994;79(6):1121–1125.

62. Strebel S, Gurzeler JA, Schneider MC, et al: Small-dose intrathecal clonidine and isobaric bupivacaine for orthopedic surgery: a dose-response study. Anesth Analg 2004;99(4):1231–1238.

63. Davis BR, Kopacz DJ: Spinal 2-chloroprocaine: The effect of added clonidine. Anesth Analg 2005;100(2):559–565.

64. Gentili M, Bonnet F: Spinal clonidine produces less urinary retention than spinal morphine. Br J Anaesth 1996;76(6):872–873.

65. De Kock M, Gautier P, Fanard L, et al: Intrathecal ropivacaine and clonidine for ambulatory knee arthroscopy: A dose-response study. Anesthesiology 2001;94(4):574–578.

66. Wong K, Strichartz GR, Raymond SA: On the mechanisms of potentiation of local anesthetics by bicarbonate buffer: Drug structure-activity studies on isolated peripheral nerve. Anesth Analg 1993;76(1):131–143.

67. Capogna G, Celleno D, Laudano D, et al: Alkalinization of local anesthetics. Which block, which local anesthetic? Reg Anesth 1995;20(5):369–377.

68. Curatolo M, Petersen-Felix S, Arendt-Nielsen L, et al: Adding sodium bicarbonate to lidocaine enhances the depth of epidural blockade. Anesth Analg 1998;86(2):341–347.

69. Difazio CA, Carron H, Grosslight KR, et al: Comparison of pH-adjusted lidocaine solutions for epidural anesthesia. Anesth Analg 1986;65:760–764.

70. Fernando R, Jones HM: Comparison of plain and alkalinized local anaesthetic mixtures of lignocaine and bupivacaine for elective extradural caesarean section. Br J Anaesth 1991;67(6):699–703.

71. Benzon HT, Toleikis JR, Dixit P, et al: Onset, intensity of blockade and somatosensory evoked potential changes of the lumbosacral dermatomes after epidural anesthesia with alkalinized lidocaine. Anesth Analg 1993;76(2):328–332.

72. Arakawa M, Aoyama Y, Ohe Y: Block of the sacral segments in lumbar epidural anaesthesia. Br J Anaesth 2003;90(2):173–178.

73. McMorland GH, Douglas MJ, Jeffery WK, et al: Effect of pH-adjustment of bupivacaine on onset and duration of epidural analgesia in parturients. Can Anaesth Soc J 1986;33(5):537–541.

74. McMorland GH, Douglas MJ, Axelson JE, et al: The effect of pH adjustment of bupivacaine on onset and duration of epidural anaesthesia for caesarean section. Can J Anaesth 1998;35(5):457–461.

75. Capogna G, Celleno D, Tagariello V: The effect of pH adjustment of 2% mepivacaine on epidural anesthesia. Reg Anesth 1989;14(3):121–123.

76. Capogna G, Celleno D, Varrassi G, et al: Epidural mepivacaine for cesarean section: effects of a pH-adjusted solution. J Clin Anesth 1991;3(3):211–214.

77. Stevens RA, Chester WL, Schubert A, et al: pH-adjustment of 2-chloroprocaine quickens the onset of epidural anaesthesia. Can J Anaesth 1989;36(5):515–518.

78. Ackerman WE, Denson DD, Juneja MM, et al: Alkalinization of chloroprocaine for epidural anesthesia: Effects of pCO_2 at constant pH. Reg Anesth 1990;15(2):89–93.

79. Ramos G, Pereira E, Simonetti MP: Does alkalinization of 0.75% ropivacaine promote a lumbar peridural block of higher quality? Reg Anesth Pain Med 2001;26(4):357–362.

80. Gosteli P, Van Gessel E, Gamulin Z: Effects of pH adjustment and carbonation of lidocaine during epidural anesthesia for foot or ankle surgery. Anesth Analg 1995;81(1):104–109.

81. Siler JN, Rosenberg H: Lidocaine hydrochloride versus lidocaine bicarbonate for epidural anesthesia in outpatients undergoing arthroscopic surgery. J Clin Anesth 1990;2(5):296–300.

82. Seybold VS: Distribution of histaminergic, muscarinic and serotonergic binding sites in cat spinal cord with emphasis on the region surrounding the central canal. Brain Res 1985;342:219–296.

83. Yaksh TL, Dirksen R, Harty GJ: Antinociceptive effects of intrathecally injected cholinomimetic drugs in the rat and cat. Eur J Pharmacol 1985;117:81–88.

84. Bartolini A, Ghelardini C, Fantetti L, et al: Role of muscarinic receptor subtypes in central antinociception. Br J Pharmacol 1992;105:77–82.

85. Chiari A, Eisenach JC: Spinal anesthesia: Mechanisms, agents, methods, and safety. Reg Anesth Pain Med 1998;23(4):357–362.

86. Pan HL, Song HK, Eisenach JC: Intrathecal cholinergic agonists lessen bupivacaine spinal-block-induced hypotension in rats. Anesth Analg 1994;79(1):112–116.

87. Lauretti GR, Reis MP: Subarachnoid neostigmine does not affect blood pressure or heart rate during bupivacaine spinal anesthesia. Reg Anesth 1996;21(6):586–591.

88. Hood DD, Eisenach JC, Tuttle R: Phase I safety assessment of intrathecal neostigmine methylsulfate in humans. Anesthesiology 1995;82:331–343.

89. Lauretti GR, de Oliveira R, Reis MP, et al: Study of three different doses of epidural neostigmine coadministered with lidocaine for postoperative analgesia. Anesthesiology 1999;90(6):1534–1538.

90. Lauretti GR, de Oliveira R, Perez MV, et al: Postoperative analgesia by intraarticular and epidural neostigmine following knee surgery. J Clin Anesth 2000;12(6):444–448.

91. Kirdemir P, Ozkocak I, Demir T, et al: Comparison of postoperative analgesic effects of preemptively used epidural ketamine and neostigmine. J Clin Anesth 2000;12(7):543–548.

92. Nakayama M, Ichinose H, Nakabayashi K, et al: Analgesic effect of epidural neostigmine after abdominal hysterectomy. J Clin Anesth 2001;13(2):86–89.

93. Omais M, Lauretti GR, Paccola CA: Epidural morphine and neostigmine for postoperative analgesia after orthopedic surgery. Anesth Analg 2002;95(6):1698–1701.

94. Kaya FN, Sahin S, Owen MD, et al: Epidural neostigmine produces analgesia but also sedation in women after cesarean delivery. Anesthesiology 2004;100(2):381–385.

95. Roelants F, Lavand'homme PM: Epidural neostigmine combined with sufentanil provides balanced and selective analgesia in early labor. Anesthesiology 2004;101(2):439–444.

96. Krukowski JA, Hood DD, Eisenach JC, et al: Intrathecal neostigmine for post-cesarean section analgesia: Dose response. Anesth Analg 1997;84:1269–1275.

97. Lauretti GR, Reis MP, Prado WA, et al: Dose-response study of intrathecal morphine versus intrathecal neostigmine, their combination, or placebo for postoperative analgesia in patients undergoing anterior and posterior vaginoplasty. Anesth Analg 1996;82:1182–1187.

98. Lauretti GR, Mattos AL, Reis MP, et al: Intrathecal neostigmine for postoperative analgesia after orthopedic surgery. J Clin Anesth 1997;9:473–477.

99. Yegin A, Yilmaz M, Karsli B, et al: Analgesic effects of intrathecal neostigmine in perianal surgery. Eur J Anaesthesiol 2003;20(5):404–408.

100. Liu SS, Hodgson PS, Moore JM et al: Dose-response effects of spinal neostigmine added to bupivacaine spinal anesthesia in volunteers. Anesthesiology 1999;90(3):710–717.

101. Fürst S: Transmitters involved in antinociception in the spinal cord. Brain Res Bull 1999;48:129–141.

102. Dickenson AH: Spinal cord pharmacology of pain. Br J Anaesth 1995;75:193–200.

103. Woolf CJ, Thompson SW: The induction and maintenance of central sensitization is dependent on N-methyl-ᴅ-aspartate acid receptor activation: implication for the treatment of post-injury pain hypersensitivity states. Pain 1991;44:293–299.

104. Trujillo KA, Akill H: Inhibition of morphine tolerance and dependence by the NMDA receptor antagonist MK-801. Science 1991;251:85–87.

105. Trujillo KA, Akill H: Inhibition of opiate tolerance by non-competitive N-methyl-ᴅ-aspartate receptor antagonists. Brain Res 1994;633:178–188.

106. Silva E, Cleland CL, Gebhart GF: Contributions of glutamate receptors to the maintenance of mustard oil-induced hyperalgesia in spinalized rats. Exp Brain Res 1997;117:379–388.

107. Dickenson AH, Chapman V, Green GM: The pharmacology of excitatory and inhibitory amino acid-mediated events in the transmission and modulation of pain in the spinal cord. Gen Pharmacol 1997;28:633–638.

108. Yaksh TL, Hua XY, Kalcheva I, et al: The spinal biology in humans and animals of pain states generated by persistent small afferent input. Proc Natl Acad Sci USA 1999;96:7680–7686.

109. Hirota K, Lambert DG: Ketamine: its mechanism(s) of action and unusual clinical uses. Br J Anaesth 1996;77(4):441–444.

110. Joó G, Horvath G, Klimscha W, et al: The effects of ketamine and its enantiomers on the morphine- or dexmedetomidine-induced antinociception after intrathecal administration in rats. Anesthesiology 2000;93:231–241.

111. Malinovsky JM, Lepage JY, Cozian A, et al: Is ketamine or its preservative responsible for neurotoxicity in the rabbit? Anesthesiology 1993;78(1):109–115.

112. Xie H, Wang X, Liu G, et al: Analgesic effects and pharmacokinetics of a low dose of ketamine preoperatively administered epidurally or intravenously. Clin J Pain 2003;19(5):317–322.

113. Subramaniam K, Subramaniam B, Pawar DK, et al: Evaluation of the safety and efficacy of epidural ketamine combined with morphine for postoperative analgesia after major upper abdominal surgery. J Clin Anesth 2001;13(5):339–344.

114. Chia YY, Liu K, Liu YC, et al: Adding ketamine in a multimodal patient-controlled epidural regimen reduces postoperative pain and analgesic consumption. Anesth Analg 1998;86:1245–1249.

115. Ozyalcin NS, Yucel A, Camlica H, et al: Effect of pre-emptive ketamine on sensory changes and postoperative pain after thoracotomy: comparison of epidural and intramuscular routes. Br J Anaesth 2004;93(3):356–361.

116. Bion J: Intrathecal ketamine for war surgery. A preliminary study under field conditions. Anaesthesia 1984;39:1023–1028.

117. Hawksworth C, Serpell M: Intrathecal anaesthesia with ketamine. Reg Anesth Pain Med 1998;23:283–288.

118. Togal T, Demirbilek S, Koroglu A, et al: Effects of S(+) ketamine added to bupivacaine for spinal anaesthesia for prostate surgery in elderly patients. Eur J Anaesthesiol 2004;21(3):193–197.

119. Mao J, Price DD, Hayes RL, et al: Intrathecal treatment with dextrorphan or ketamine potently reduces pain-related behaviors in a rat model of peripheral mononeuropathy. Brain Res 1993;605:164–168.

120. Miyamoto H, Saito Y, Kirihara Y, et al: Spinal coadministration of ketamine reduces the development of tolerance to visceral as well as somatic antinociception during spinal morphine infusion. Anesth Analg 2000;90(1):136–141.

121. Ma W, Du W, Eisenach JC: Role for both spinal cord COX-1 and COX-2 in maintenance of mechanical hypersensitivity following peripheral nerve injury. Brain Res 2002;937(1–2): 94–99.

122. Zhu X, Conklin D, Eisenach JC: Cyclooxygenase-1 in the spinal cord plays an important role in postoperative pain. Pain 2003;104(1–2):15–23.

123. Yaksh TL, Horais KA, Tozier N, et al: Intrathecal ketorolac in dogs and rats. Toxicol Sci 2004;80(2):322–334.

124. Korkmaz HA, Maltepe F, Erbayraktar S, et al: Antinociceptive and neurotoxicologic screening of chronic intrathecal administration of ketorolac tromethamine in the rat. Anesth Analg 2004;98(1):148–152.

125. Gallivan ST, Johnston SA, Broadstone RV, et al: The clinical, cerebrospinal fluid, and histopathologic effects of epidural ketorolac in dogs. Vet Surg 2000;29(5):436–441.

126. Kang YJ, Vincler M, Li X, et al: Intrathecal ketorolac reverses hypersensitivity following acute fentanyl exposure. Anesthesiology 2002;97(6):1641–1644.

127. Conklin DR, Eisenach JC: Intrathecal ketorolac enhances antinociception from clonidine. Anesth Analg 2003;96(1):191–194.

128. Martin TJ, Zhang Y, Buechler N, et al: Intrathecal morphine and ketorolac analgesia after surgery: Comparison of spontaneous and elicited responses in rats. Pain 2005;113(3):376–385.

129. Eisenach JC, Curry R, Hood DD, et al: Phase I safety assessment of intrathecal ketorolac. Pain 2002;99(3):599–604.

130. Eisenach JC, Curry R, Hood DD: Dose response of intrathecal adenosine in experimental pain and allodynia. Anesthesiology 2002;97(4):938–942.

131. Erdine S, Yucel A, Ozyuvaci E, et al: Neurotoxicity of midazolam in the rabbit. Pain 1999;80:419–423.

132. Svensson BA, Welin M, Gordh T, et al: Chronic subarachnoid midazolam (Dormicum) in the rat: Morphologic evidence of spinal cord neurotoxicity. Reg Anesth 1995;20:426–434.

133. Johansen MJ, Gradert TL, Satterfield WC, et al: Safety of continuous intrathecal midazolam infusion in the sheep model. Anesth Analg 2004;98(6):1528–1535.

134. Tucker AP, Lai C, Nadeson R: Intrathecal midazolam I: A cohort study investigating safety. Anesth Analg 2004;98(6):1512–1520.

135. Tucker AP, Mezzatesta J, Nadeson R, et al: Intrathecal midazolam II: Combination with intrathecal fentanyl for labor pain. Anesth Analg 2004;98(6):1521–1527.

9

Analgesic Adjuvants in the Peripheral Nervous System

Colin J. L. McCartney, MD

INTRODUCTION

Peripheral nerve blocks provide many benefits for patients, including superior pain control and reduction in general anesthesia-related side effects. In order to optimize pain relief while reducing the total dose of local anesthetic it would be of use to add a drug that both speeds onset and prolongs sensory blockade or analgesic effect. Improvements in our knowledge of peripheral nervous system pain mechanisms allow us to develop methods of prolonging analgesia while reducing central and peripherally mediated adverse effects.

In the last 20 years a number of drugs have been tested, and several have proven clinically useful when added to local anesthetic for peripheral nerve block or when used for local infiltration or intraarticular analgesia. These drugs are known as analgesic adjuvants.

This chapter examines the rationale and current evidence base for use of analgesic adjuvants and summarizes the best strategies for optimizing pain control and reducing adverse effects after surgery under peripheral nerve block, local infiltration, or injection of drugs in the intraarticular space.

RATIONALE FOR USE

Pain transmission in the central and peripheral nervous systems involves a complex array of neurotransmitters and pathways that are not easily blocked by one drug type or technique

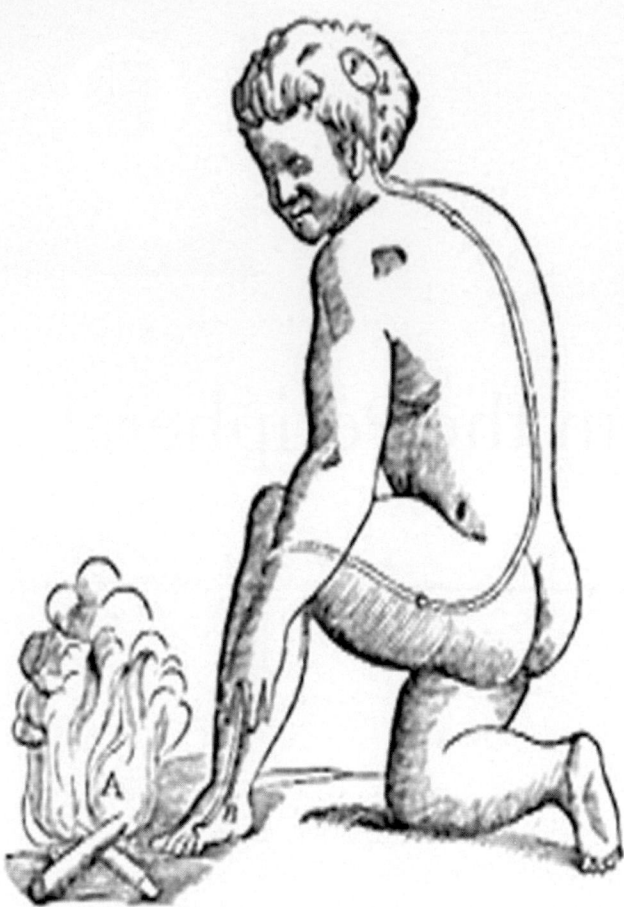

Figure 9–1. Descartes model of pain transmission in the peripheral nervous system.

alone. Involvement of several classes of neurotransmitter at the injury site, peripheral nerve, dorsal horn of the spinal cord, and supraspinal sites are responsible for the transmission of nociception. Use of agonists at inhibitory receptors and antagonists at excitatory receptors allows a "multimodal" approach with optimization of pain control and reduction of adverse effects.[1]

In 1645 Descartes proposed a mechanism for pain transmission, suggesting that a peripheral pain impulse was transmitted directly from the periphery to the brain by a "hard-wired" system without any intermediate modulation (Figure 9–1). This theory of pain transmission was widely held as true until as recently as 40 years ago.

In 1965 Melzack and Wall proposed their groundbreaking gate-control theory of pain that suggested that pain could be modulated or "gated" at a number of points in the pain pathway. Subsequent research identified the dorsal horn (lamina II) of the spinal cord as an important site of potential modulation, and subsequent treatments for acute and chronic pain have utilized this knowledge to good effect. Treatments such as the use of spinal opioids and transcutaneous electrical nerve stimulation (TENS) have both been developed in the light of this knowledge. The gate theory also changed many (often unsuccessful) pain management strategies from techniques where we tried to ablate pain pathways either chemically or surgically to more recent modulation techniques where we attempt to inhibit excitatory influences and enhance inhibitory influences within the pain pathway.

In the last few decades important advances have also occurred in our knowledge of how pain is generated and transmitted from the peripheral nervous system (PNS) to the central nervous system (CNS). Modulation of pain in the PNS also involves numerous transmitters and mechanisms that both excite and inhibit nociceptive pathways.

In the PNS under normal physiologic conditions nociceptive signals are produced when A-α and C fibers are stimulated by heat, pressure, or several chemicals produced by tissue damage and inflammation (potassium, histamine, bradykinin, prostaglandins, adenosine triphosphate [ATP]).[2] Nociceptive signals are transmitted to the superficial layers of lamina II of the dorsal horn in the spinal cord where they are modulated at both the presynaptic and postsynaptic level and also by excitatory and inhibitory descending control pathways form the brainstem (Figure 9–2)[3]. Signals that are successful in crossing this gate travel on to the brainstem and thalamus before reaching the cerebral cortex to produce a pain stimulus.

A wide array of chemical mediators are produced in the the PNS and have both excitatory and inhibitory influences on peripheral sensory nerve transmission[4] both in the acute and chronic phase of injury (Figure 9–3)[5]. These can directly activate the nerve (ATP, glutamate, 5-hydroxytryptamine [5-HT], histamine, bradykinin), enhance depolarization by sensitizing the nerve to other stimuli (prostaglandins, prostacyclin, and cytokines such as interleukins) or provide a regulatory role on the sensory neuron, inflammatory cells, and sympathetic fibers (bradykinin, tachykinin, and nerve growth factor).

RATIONALE FOR USE OF ANALGESIC ADJUVANTS

As previously noted pain transmission in the central and peripheral nervous systems involves a complex array of neurotransmitters and pathways that are not easily blocked by one drug type or technique alone. A number of drugs in the anesthesiologist's armamentarium, including opioids, nonsteroidalantiinflammatory drugs (NSAIDs), α_2-agonists, and N-methyl-D-aspartate (NMDA) antagonists, have activity at these sites of action and may have benefit if applied in the PNS.

This knowledge can aid the regional anesthesiologist in a number of ways:

1. In the selection of adjuvants to local anesthetics in order to speed onset, prolong effect, and reduce total required dose.
2. Suggest agents that can enhance postoperative analgesia without prolonging adverse effects of local anesthetics.

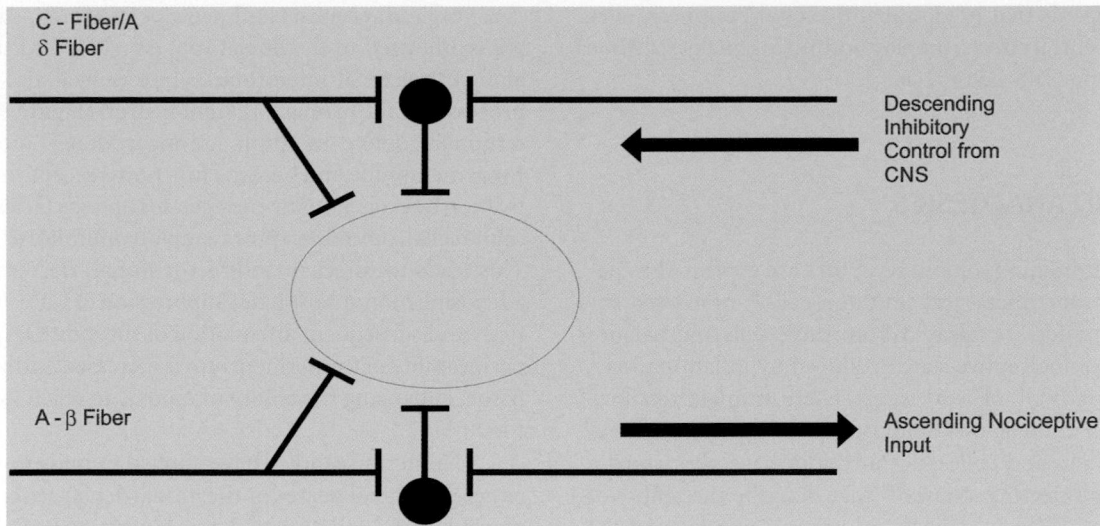

Figure 9–2. The gate theory proposed that small (C) fibers activated excitatory systems (black neuron) that subsequently excited output cells—these latter cells had their activity controlled by the balance of large fibers (A-β)-mediated inhibitions (mediated by endogenous opioids) and also by descending control systems from the central nervous system (mediated by norepinephrine and serotonin). (Reprinted, with permission, from: Dickenson AH: Gate control theory of pain stands the test of time. Br J Anaesth 2002;88:755–757.)

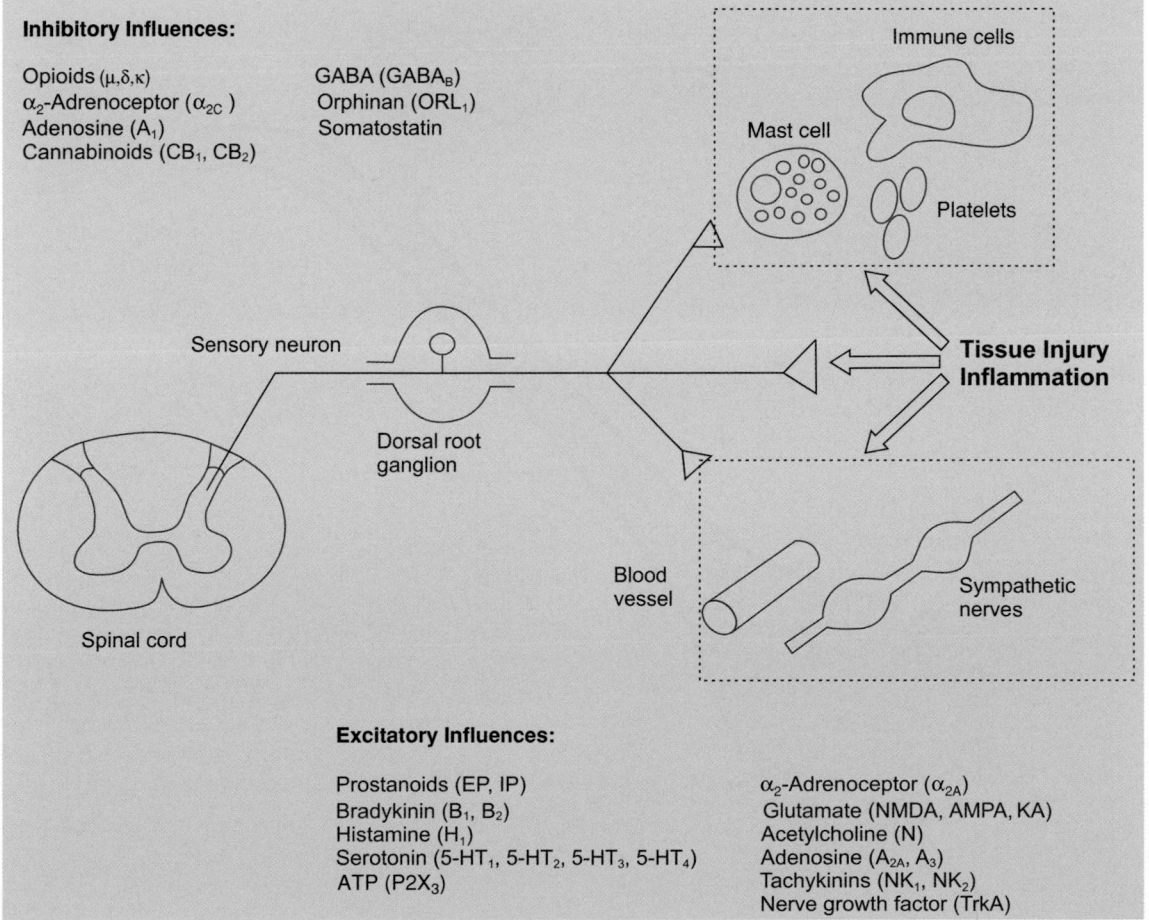

Figure 9–3. Excitatory and inhibitory influences on peripheral nerve activity by mediators released by tissue injury and inflammation and by a variety of agents acting on neuroreceptors. (Reprinted, with permission, from Sawynok J: Topical and peripherally acting analgesics. Pharmacol Rev 2003;55:1–20.)

3. Suggest agents that predominantly act at peripheral sites without central effects, thereby optimizing analgesia while minimizing CNS side effects.

OPIOID ANALGESICS

During inflammation, opioid receptors are expressed in peripheral sensory fibers and immune cells,[6] moreover endogenous opioids are released from these cells and balance the increased nociceptive state produced by inflammation.[7] An increasing body of work suggests an intimate relationship between endogenous opioids and the immune system. Christoph Stein and colleagues in Berlin have performed a number of pioneering studies[8,9] that describe the ability of the immune system to deliver endogenous opioids and the ability of inflammation to stimulate movement of opioid receptors to the site of injury, thereby allowing antinociception to occur. However these changes do not occur immediately after injury and can take up to 96 h to occur.[10]

Opioid receptors and neuropeptides (eg, substance P) are synthesized in the dorsal root ganglion and transported along intraaxonal microtubules into central and peripheral processes of the primary afferent neuron (Figure 9–4). At the terminals, opioid receptors are incorporated into the neuronal membrane and become functional receptors. Upon activation by exogenous or endogenous opioids (released by immune cells), opioid receptors couple to inhibitory G-proteins. This leads to direct or indirect (through decrease of cyclic adenosine monophosphate) suppression of Ca^{2+} or Na^+ currents and subsequent attenuation of substance P release. The permeability of the perineurium is increased within inflamed tissue, enhancing the ability of opioids to reach target receptors.

Numerous studies have applied opioids in the PNS to either peripheral nerves or the intraarticular space. Although many studies claim an analgesic benefit of peripherally applied opioids, few studies incorporated a control group with a systemically applied opioid for comparison. Without inclusion of a control it is impossible to interpret whether the peripheral opioid is having a true peripheral effect or is instead

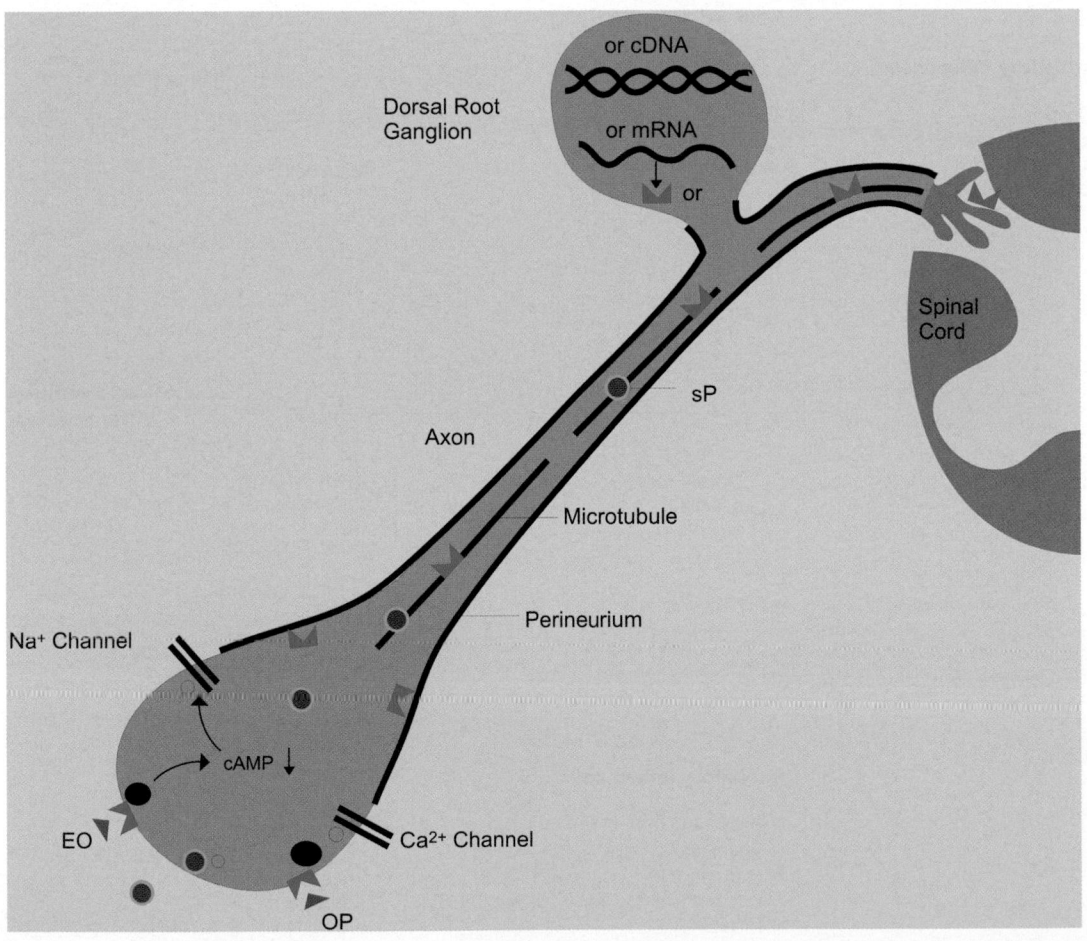

Figure 9–4. Opioid receptor transport and signaling in primary afferent neurons. (Adapted, with permission, from Stein C: Nature Med 2003;9(8):1003). OR = opioid receptor; sP = substance P, EO = exogenous opioids; OP = endogenous opioid peptides; $G_{i/o}$ = inhibitory G proteins; cAMP = cyclic adenosine monophosphate.

being carried to the CNS to induce analgesia. True peripherally mediated opioid analgesia may be beneficial if this is associated with improved analgesia or reduced adverse effects compared with systemic administration. If the effect is mediated centrally then there is no clear benefit over systemic administration.

Perineural Opioids

Opioid receptors identified on primary afferent fibers are transported from the dorsal root ganglion to the site of inflammation; however, while they are undergoing axonal transport they may not be easily reached by opioid agonists. This may explain the reason that two recent systematic reviews published in 1997 and 2000[11,12] found little evidence for the benefit of adding opioids to local anesthetics in peripheral nerve blockade. An updated table of studies examining perineuronal administration of opioids[13–16] (excluding buprenorphine and tramadol) shows that analgesic benefit remains equivocal (Table 9–1). In addition Peng and Choyce[17] reviewed the use of opioids in intravenous regional anesthesia (IVRA) with similar disappointing conclusions.

Despite these disappointing results, the two opioid agonists that have demonstrated analgesic efficacy when administered perineuronally are buprenorphine and tramadol. Buprenorphine is a partial μ-receptor agonist with a very high receptor affinity compared with fentanyl (24-fold) or morphine (50-fold). In addition it has intermediate lipid solubility, which allows it to cross the neural membrane.[18–19]

Table 9–1.

Outcomes of Studies[12–16] Examining the Effect of Perineuronal Opioids (excluding tramadol and buprenorphine)

Total Studies	Overall Outcomes	Systemic Control Outcomes
15 studies	8 supportive	6 systemic control: 4 supportive 2 negative
	7 negative	9 no systemic control: 4 supportive 5 negative

Candido and colleagues[20] added 0.3 mg buprenorphine (a partial opioid agonist) to a combination of mepivacaine and tetracaine in axillary block and found an almost 100% increase in the duration of analgesia compared with the administration of axillary block plus the same dose of intramuscular buprenorphine with no significant increase in adverse effects. This supports the peripheral analgesic effect of buprenorphine and also the earlier findings of two studies that examined buprenorphine without a systemic control group.[21,22] Studies examining buprenorphine are examined in greater detail in Table 9–2.

Table 9–2.

Studies Examining Buprenorphine as an Analgesic Adjuvant with Local Anesthetics

Author/Date	Patients/ Groups	Block Type	Dose	Local Anesthetic	Systemic Control	Results
Viel[22] 1989	20/2	Supraclavicular	3 mcg/kg	Bupivacaine 0.5% 40 mL	No	Prolonged analgesia compared to morphine group (35 vs 18.25 h). No difference in sensory block.
Bazin[23] 1997	89/4	Supraclavicular	3 mcg/kg	Bupivacaine 0.5% Lidocaine 1%	No	Prolonged analgesia compared to control group (20 vs 11.5 h)
Candido[21] 2001	40/2	Supraclavicular	0.3 mg	Mepivacaine 1% Tetracaine 0.2%	No	Prolonged analgesia compared to control group (17.4 vs 5.3 h)
Candido[20] 2002	60/3	Axillary	0.3 mg	Mepivacaine 1% Tetracaine 0.2%	Yes IM	The mean duration of postoperative analgesia was 22.3 h in axillary group vs 12.5 h in IM group, and 6.6 h in placebo group.

IM = intramuscular

Clinical Pearls

- Buprenorphine (0.3 mg) enhances anesthesia and prolongs analgesia when added to local anesthetic for peripheral nerve block.

Tramadol is a weak opioid agonist with some selectivity for the μ-receptor that also inhibits norepinephrine reuptake and stimulates serotonin release in the intrathecal space. Norepinephrine and serotonin are transmitters for the descending control pathway in the spinal cord and enhance analgesia.[23,24] Kapral and coworkers[25] used a 100-mg dose of tramadol as an adjuvant to mepivacaine in axillary brachial plexus block. They divided 60 patients into three groups, one group received mepivacaine 1% with 2 mL saline, the second group received mepivacaine 1% with 100 mg tramadol, and the third group received mepivacaine 1% with 2 mL saline and 100 mg tramadol intravenously. This study demonstrated an increased duration of motor and sensory blockade in the axillary tramadol group that significantly ($p < 0.01$) outlasted both an intravenous and placebo group. Robaux and colleagues[26] subsequently performed a dose-response study with placebo, and 40-, 100-, and 200-mg doses of tramadol added to a fixed dose of mepivacaine 1.5% in axillary block and found that the 200-mg dose provided best analgesia with no increased adverse effects.

Clinical Pearls

- Tramadol (200 mg) enhances anesthesia and prolongs analgesia when added to local anesthetic for peripheral nerve block.

Intraarticular Opioids & Other Peripheral Routes of Administration

Opioid agonists administered into inflamed tissue will bind to opioid receptors on sensory terminals and induce analgesia. Animal studies indicate that these peripheral opioid receptors are expressed 96 h after the initial inflammatory injury.[10] Intraarticular (IA) administration of opioids will therefore only produce analgesia in patients with preexisting inflammation. Kalso and coworkers[27] systematically examined the role of IA opioids in 1997 and established that there existed evidence for a prolonged benefit from IA morphine without significant adverse effects, at doses of 1 to 5 mg. No dose response was detected. Recent articles support this finding and show the benefit of IA morphine[28,29] tramadol,[30] buprenorphine[31] and sufentanil.[32]

Clinical Pearl

- Morphine in doses up to 5 mg provides significant analgesia when injected intraarticularly but does require a preexisting inflammatory site of action.

A recent interesting study by Reuben and colleagues[33] investigated the use of morphine (5 mg) injected into the iliac crest bone graft donor site during cervical spine fusion surgery. Morphine significantly reduced both acute pain and the incidence of development of chronic pain (assessed 1 year after surgery) compared with patients who had intramuscular morphine or placebo (5% vs 37 and 33%).

Clinical Pearls

PERIPHERAL OPIOIDS SUMMARY

- Tramadol 200 mg or buprenorphine 0.3 mg both enhance local anesthetic effect and prolong analgesia when used for peripheral nerve block.
- Morphine in doses up to 5 mg provides significant analgesia when injected intraarticularly but does require a pre-existing inflammatory site of action.
- Morphine 5 mg injected into the donor site during bone graft harvest may reduce acute and chronic bone graft site pain.

ALPHA$_2$-AGONISTS & CLONIDINE

Clonidine is an α_2-agonist with some α_1-stimulatory effects. It has traditionally been used as an antihypertensive agent and has been noted to have sedative and analgesic effects for many years. More recently it was determined that α_2-receptors exist in the dorsal horn of the spinal cord, and stimulation of these receptors produces analgesic effects by inhibiting the presynaptic release of excitatory transmitters, including substance P and glutamate.[34-36] Intrathecal clonidine mediates analgesia by increasing acetylcholine levels, which in turn stimulates muscarinic receptors. Muscarinic excitation increases γ-amino butyric acid levels onto the primary afferent fiber inhibiting the release of the excitatory neurotransmitter, glutamate.[37]

Clonidine injected close to peripheral nerves with or without local anesthetic drugs appears to mediate analgesia in a number of ways. Clonidine has local anesthetic properties[38] and tonically inhibited compound action potentials of C fibers greater then A-α fibers in rat sciatic nerve and was comparable to lidocaine in its ability to inhibit C fibers in rabbit vagus nerve.[38,39] Clonidine also has a pharmacokinetic effect on local anesthetic redistribution mediated by a vasoconstrictor effect at the α_1-receptor.[40] Recent animal models have demonstrated and supported earlier work that clonidine predominantly facilitates peripheral nerve block through hyperpolarization-activated cationic current and that this effect is independent of any vasoconstrictor effect.[41]

A more recent addition to the selection of α_2-agonists is dexmedetomidine, which is selective for the α_2-receptor and which at present is mainly studied as a sedative agent in intensive care units. Dexmedetomidine may be expected to produce more profound analgesia but also greater adverse effects because of the selectivity of action.

Stimulation of the α_2-receptor produces hypotension, bradycardia, and sedation at higher doses, and these effects may outweigh any analgesic benefits produced by the use of these agents.

Perineuronal Application

Over 30 studies in humans are now examining the effect of clonidine on local anesthetics in peripheral nerve block. There is good evidence from these studies that clonidine in doses up to 1.5 mcg/kg prolongs sensory block and analgesia when administered with local anesthetics for peripheral nerve block. This supports the early opinion of Murphy and colleagues[12] that clonidine is a beneficial adjuvant when added to peripheral nerve block and that the effect is most likely mediated in the PNS.

Although a number of studies are examining the effect of clonidine added to peripheral nerve block, only a few have controlled for a systemic effect of clonidine. Singelyn and coworkers[42] evaluated 30 patients receiving an axillary brachial plexus block with 40 mL of 1% mepivacaine plus epinephrine 5 mcg/mL. Patients were randomized to three groups and received: (1) local anesthetic alone, (2) local anesthetic plus 150 mcg of clonidine administered subcutaneously, or (3) 150 mcg of clonidine in the brachial plexus block with local anesthetic. Clonidine added to the axillary brachial plexus block delayed the onset of pain twofold, without adverse effects when compared with systemic control. Hutschala and coworkers[43] have recently demonstrated the peripheral analgesic effect of clonidine in volunteers when added to brachial plexus block with 0.25% bupivacaine. However, other recent studies demonstrate no overall benefit of adding clonidine to long-acting local anesthetics such as bupivacaine and ropivacaine.[44]

The addition of clonidine to continuous peripheral nerve blocks is not beneficial. Ilfeld and colleagues[45,46] have demonstrated in two studies that both 0.1 and 0.2 mcg/mL of clonidine added to continuous infusion of ropivacaine 0.2% failed to reduce pain scores or oral analgesic use after upper extremity surgery.

Intravenous Regional Anesthesia

Intravenous regional anesthesia (IVRA) is a useful, simple regional anesthetic technique especially for minor peripheral upper limb procedures that are limited by tourniquet tolerance and poor postoperative analgesia. Clonidine has been demonstrated in a number of studies to improve onset time[47] and intraoperative tourniquet tolerance.[48–50]

Only one study has demonstrated improved postoperative analgesia in the early postoperative period compared with placebo. Reuben and coworkers[49] randomized 45 patients to 40 mL 0.5% lidocaine with clonidine 1 mcg/kg, lidocaine alone with intravenous clonidine, and lidocaine alone with intravenous saline. Patients who were given clonidine with lidocaine experienced significantly less pain and requested fewer analgesics then patients in the other two groups. Higher doses of clonidine (150 mcg) produce significantly more sedation and incidence of hypotension.[48]

To date only one study has used dexmedetomidine in IVRA. Memis and colleagues[51] added 0.5 mcg/kg of dexmedetomidine to 0.5% lidocaine and demonstrated reduction in onset time and improvement in postoperative analgesia compared with placebo with no significant adverse effects.

Intraarticular Techniques

The intraarticular effect of clonidine has been examined when administered with[52,53] and without local anesthetic[54–56] and been found to have beneficial effects on postoperative analgesia. The addition of morphine and clonidine may be expected to have additive effects. Two studies have examined this question with one demonstrating improved analgesia[54] and the other no difference.[56]

Preclinical trials have demonstrated that, similar to opioids, clonidine-mediated analgesia is enhanced by inflammation although at the present time the mechanism is not evident.[57]

Clinical Pearls

ALPHA$_2$-AGONISTS SUMMARY

- Clonidine (1–2 mcg/kg) prolongs sensory block and analgesic effect when added to local anesthetic after peripheral nerve block.
- Clonidine (1 mcg/kg) or dexmedetomidine (0.5 mcg/kg) added to IVRA speeds onset, reduces tourniquet pain, and improves postoperative analgesia.
- Intraarticular clonidine improves postoperative analgesia and is equivalent to that produced by intraarticular morphine.

N-METHYL-D-ASPARTATE ANTAGONISTS

Within the dorsal horn of the spinal cord both ionotropic (N-methyl-D-aspartate (NMDA), α-amino-3-hydroxy-5-methylisoxazole-4-propionic acid (AMPA), kainic acid (KA), and metabotropic glutamate receptors are involved in nociceptive signaling and central sensitization in conditions of chronic pain.[58–60] Recently, multiple glutamate receptors have been found in peripheral nerve terminals and may contribute to peripheral pain signaling.[61] Injection of the NMDA receptor agonist, glutamate, into masseter muscle produces pain in both rats and humans.[62,63] Subsequent injection of NMDA receptor antagonists such as ketamine and dextromethorphan attenuates the pain.[64]

A number of studies have examined the effect of NMDA antagonists in producing peripherally mediated analgesia in patients. Tverskoy and colleagues[65] infiltrated bupivacaine with 0.3% ketamine or placebo for patients having inguinal herniorraphy and found that ketamine significantly enhanced the anesthetic and analgesic actions of a local anesthetic administered for infiltration anesthesia. Ketamine has been used as the sole anesthetic in IVRA, but patients suffered excessive adverse effects on tourniquet deflation.[66] Other workers have added ketamine (0.1 mg/mL) or clonidine (1 mcg/kg) to lidocaine for IVRA.[67] Patients in the ketamine group had best pain control although both clonidine and ketamine significantly reduced analgesic consumption compared with lidocaine alone with mild psychomimetic side effects in the ketamine group.

Two studies have examined the use of intraarticular ketamine. Dal and coworkers[68] randomized patients to intraarticular ketamine (0.5 mg/kg), neostigmine, bupivacaine, or placebo. Patients receiving all three drugs had similar improvements in analgesia with knee flexion compared with placebo; however, the ketamine group had longest duration of analgesia. However, Brill and colleagues[69] performed a dose-response study using up to 1 mg/kg intraarticular ketamine after knee arthroscopy and found that the analgesic benefit only occurred in the first hour after surgery compared with placebo.

Magnesium has NMDA-blocking effects and blocks the ion channel on the NMDA receptor during normal physiologic states. Persistent nociceptive input in the dorsal horn of the spinal cord removes magnesium allowing calcium influx and intracellular changes leading to persistent pain states.[60]

Turan et al[70] exploited this analgesic potential in the PNS by adding 1.5 g magnesium to lidocaine 0.5% for IVRA. Magnesium reduced onset time and significantly prolonged analgesic effect up to 6h after surgery with no difference in adverse effects.

Overall NMDA antagonists may have significant potential for producing peripherally mediated analgesia in the future although currently available agents (except magnesium in IVRA) have limited effects and at higher doses produce excessive adverse effects.

Clinical Pearls

NMDA RECEPTOR ANTAGONISTS SUMMARY

- NMDA receptors exist in the peripheral nervous system and are involved in hypersensitivity and prolonged pain states.
- Several studies have demonstrated an analgesic benefit of injecting NMDA antagonists in the PNS.
- Preliminary work suggests magnesium has significant benefit when added to lidocaine for IVRA.
- Further studies are required, however, to determine best route and most effective dose with other agents.

CYCLOOXYGENASE INHIBITION

Prostaglandins sensitize peripheral nerve endings to the effects of endogenous chemical mediators released during tissue injury. NSAIDs inhibit the production of prostaglandins through their well known effect of inhibiting cyclooxygenase (COX). Application of NSAIDs directly in the PNS would therefore appear to make sense as a means of reducing pain by peripheral mechanism.

Intravenous Regional Anesthesia

A number of authors have added ketorolac to IVRA in doses from 5 to 60 mg, producing an improvement in intraoperative tourniquet tolerance and postoperative analgesia.[70] Steinberg and colleagues[71] performed a dose-response study with ketorolac in IVRA using placebo, 5-, 10-, 15-, 20-, 30-, and 60-mg doses of ketorolac. It was found that 20 mg was the ideal dose, with lower doses producing less analgesia and higher doses being no more effective.

Lysine acetylsalicylic acid 90 mg (equivalent to 50 mg acetylsalicylic acid) has been added to prilocaine for IVRA with prolongation of postoperative analgesia.[72]

■ Ketorolac (20 mg) added to lidocaine for IVRA prolongs postoperative analgesia.

Intraarticular

The use of ketorolac alone, with local anesthetic or local anesthetic and morphine, is no more effective then local anesthetic alone when administered in the intraarticular space.

Infiltration

Ketorolac has been successfully infiltrated in a dose of 30 to 60 mg following hernia repair, giving an effect similar to infiltration with bupivacaine. However, local infiltration was found to be no more effective then systemic administration.[73–77]

CHOLINERGIC ANALGESIA

Muscarinic receptors mediate analgesia in the dorsal horn of the spinal cord, and neostigmine has produced analgesia when administered to both the intrathecal and epidural space.

Neostigmine has also been applied in the PNS in a number of studies, with generally disappointing results. Van Elstraete and coworkers[78] and Bone and colleagues[79] have both added neostigmine 500 mcg to local anesthetic in axillary brachial plexus block. One study demonstrated no difference,[77] and the other found only significant reduction in pain at 24 h with no difference at other time points.[78]

Neostigmine added to local anesthetic for IVRA has also been disappointing. Turan and coworkers[80] added 500 mcg neostigmine to prilocaine 0.5% and found improvement in sensory and motor block onset and offset with prolonged time to first analgesic request. However, McCartney and colleagues[81] performed a similar study using Neostigmine 1mg added to lidocaine 0.5% with no differences found between groups. Overall neostigmine appears disappointing as an analgesic adjuvant for peripheral nervous block or IVRA.

Neostigmine has however been used successfully as an analgesic adjuvant for intraarticular use after knee arthroscopy.[68,81–83] Yang and coworkers[82] performed a dose-response study and found 500 mcg to be most effective, which was more effective than 2 mg of intraarticular morphine.

■ Neostigmine (500 mcg) injected in the intraarticular space following knee arthroscopy provides prolongation of analgesia without significant adverse effects.

The effectiveness of the intraarticular cholinergic analgesic pathway compared with the poor results with perineuronal application may be related to the presence of the inflammatory response in the intraarticular space, increasing the analgesic efficacy of acetylcholine by an as yet undefined mechanism.

PERIPHERAL CHOLINERGIC ANALGESICS SUMMARY

■ Neostigmine 500 mcg injected in the intraarticular space following knee arthroscopy provides prolongation of analgesia. Neostigmine added to peripheral nerve block or IVRA is ineffective.

SUMMARY

Peripheral nerve blocks provide significant anesthetic and analgesic benefits for our patients. Analgesic adjuvants such as opioids, α_2-agonists, NMDA receptor antagonists, and other agents can be added to local anesthetics both to facilitate onset and to prolong anesthetic and analgesic effects by mechanisms existing in the PNS. Several agents are effective when administered in the perineuronal or intraarticular space and when given in IVRA or local infiltration (Table 9–3).

Our evolving knowledge of nociceptive mechanisms in the PNS will allow novel techniques to be developed in the future to further improve pain management.

Table 9–2.

Best Analgesic Adjuvants in the Peripheral Nervous System by Route of Administration

Route	Agent and Dose
Perineuronal	Buprenorphine 0.3 mg[20] Clonidine 1–2 mcg/kg[42] Tramadol 200 mg[26]
IVRA	Clonidine 1 mcg/kg[49] Dexmedetomidine 0.5 mcg/kg[51] Ketorolac 20 mg[72] Magnesium 1.5 g[70]
Intraarticular	Clonidine 150 mcg[56] Morphine 5 mg[27] Neostigmine 0.5 mg[81]
Local Infiltration	Ketamine 3 mg/mL[65] Morphine 5 mg (to bone graft site)[33]

IVRA = intravenous regional anesthesia

References

1. Kehlet H, Dahl JB: The value of "multimodal" or "balanced analgesia" in postoperative pain treatment. Anesth Analg 1993;77:1048–1056.

2. Raja SN, Meyer RA, Ringkamp M, et al: Peripheral neural mechanisms of nociception. In Wall PD, Melzack R, eds: *Textbook of Pain*, 4th ed. Churchill-Livingstone, 1999, pp 11–57.

3. Dickenson AH: Gate control theory of pain stands the test of time. Br J Anaesth 2002;88:755–757.

4. Millan MJ: The induction of pain: An integrative review. Prog Neurobiol 1999;57:1–164.

5. Sawynok J: Topical and peripherally acting analgesics. Pharmacol Rev 2003;55:1–20.

6. Likar R, Mousa SA, Philippitsch G, et al: Increased numbers of opioid expressing inflammatory cells do not affect intra-articular morphine analgesia. Br J Anaesth 2004;93:375–380.

7. Brack A, Rittner HL, Machelska H, et al: Control of inflammatory pain by chemokine-mediated recruitment of opioid-containing polymorphonuclear cells. Pain 2004;112:229–238.

8. Machelska H, Cabot PJ, Mousa SA, et al: Pain control in inflammation governed by selectins. Nat Med 1998;4:1425–1428.

9. Stein C, Schafer M, Machelska H: Attacking pain at its source: New perspectives on opioids. Nat Med 2003;9:1003–1008.

10. Mousa SA, Zhang Q, Sitte N, et al: beta-Endorphin-containing memory-cells and mu-opioid receptors undergo transport to peripheral inflamed tissue. J Neuroimmunol 200;115:71–78.

11. Picard PR, Tramer MR, McQuay HJ, et al: Analgesic efficacy of peripheral opioids (all except intra-articular): A qualitative systematic review of randomised controlled trials. Pain 1997;72:309–318.

12. Murphy DB, McCartney CJ, Chan VW: Novel analgesic adjuncts for brachial plexus block: A systematic review. Anesth Analg 2000;90:1122–1128.

13. Fanelli G, Casati A, Magistris L, et al: Fentanyl does not improve the nerve block characteristics of axillary brachial plexus anaesthesia performed with ropivacaine. Acta Anaesthesiol Scand 2001;45:590–594.

14. Karakaya D, Buyukgoz F, Baris S, et al: Addition of fentanyl to bupivacaine prolongs anesthesia and analgesia in axillary brachial plexus block. Reg Anesth Pain Med 2001;26:434–438.

15. Likar R, Koppert W, Blatnig H, et al: Efficacy of peripheral morphine analgesia in inflamed, non-inflamed and perineural tissue of dental surgery patients. J Pain Symptom Manage 2001;21:330–337.

16. Nishikawa K, Kanaya N, Nakayama M, et al: Fentanyl improves analgesia but prolongs the onset of axillary brachial plexus block by peripheral mechanism. Anesth Analg 2000;91:384–387.

17. Choyce A, Peng P: A systematic review of adjuncts for intravenous regional anesthesia for surgical procedures. Can J Anaesth 2002;49:32–45.

18. Gutstein H, Akil H: Opioid analgesics. In Hardman J, Limbird L (eds): *Goodman & Gilman's The Pharmacologic Basis of Therapeutics*, 10th ed. McGraw-Hill, 2001, p 601.

19. Lanz E, Simko G, Theiss D, et al: Epidural buprenorphine—A double-blind study of postoperative analgesia and side effects. Anesth Analg 1984;63:593–598.

20. Candido KD, Winnie AP, Ghaleb AH, et al: Buprenorphine added to the local anesthetic for axillary brachial plexus block prolongs postoperative analgesia. Reg Anesth Pain Med 2002;27:162–167.

21. Candido KD, Franco CD, Khan MA, et al: Buprenorphine added to the local anesthetic for brachial plexus block to provide postoperative analgesia in outpatients. Reg Anesth Pain Med 2001;26:352–356.

22. Viel EJ, Eledjam JJ, De La Coussaye JE, et al: Brachial plexus block with opioids for postoperative pain relief: Comparison between buprenorphine and morphine. Reg Anesth 1989;14:274–278.

23. Bazin JE, Massoni C, Bruelle P, et al: The addition of opioids to local anaesthetics in brachial plexus block: The comparative effects of morphine, buprenorphine and sufentanil. Anaesthesia. 1997;52:858–862.

24. Alhashemi JA, Kaki AM: Effect of intrathecal tramadol administration on postoperative pain after transurethral resection of prostate. Br J Anaesth 2003;91:536–540.

25. Kapral S, Gollmann G, Waltl B, et al: Tramadol added to mepivacaine prolongs the duration of an axillary brachial plexus blockade. Anesth Analg 1999;88:853–856.

26. Robaux S, Blunt C, Viel E, et al: Tramadol added to 1.5% mepivacaine for axillary brachial plexus block improves postoperative analgesia dose-dependently. Anesth Analg 2004;98:1172–1177.

27. Kalso E, Tramer MR, Carroll D, et al: Pain relief from intra-articular morphine after knee surgery: A qualitative systematic review. Pain 1997;71:127–134.

28. Brandsson S, Karlsson J, Morberg P, et al: Intraarticular morphine after arthroscopic ACL reconstruction: A double-blind placebo-controlled study of 40 patients. Acta Orthop Scand 2000;71:280–285.

29. Rasmussen S, Larsen AS, Thomsen ST, et al: Intra-articular glucocorticoid, bupivacaine and morphine reduces pain, inflammatory response and convalescence after arthroscopic meniscectomy. Pain 1998;78:131–134.

30. Alagol A, Calpur OU, Kaya G, et al: The use of intraarticular tramadol for postoperative analgesia after arthroscopic knee surgery: A comparison of different intraarticular and intravenous doses. Knee Surg Sports Traumatol Arthrosc 2004;12:184–188.

31. Varrassi G, Marinangeli F, Ciccozzi A, et al: Intra-articular buprenorphine after knee arthroscopy. A randomised, prospective, double-blind study. Acta Anaesthesiol Scand 1999;43:51–55.

32. Vranken JH, Vissers KC, de Jongh R, et al: Intraarticular sufentanil administration facilitates recovery after day-case knee arthroscopy. Anesth Analg 2001;92:625–628.

33. Reuben SS, Vieira P, Faruqi S, et al: Local administration of morphine for analgesia after iliac bone graft harvest. Anesthesiology 2001;95:390–394.

34. Unnerstall JR, Kopajtic TA, Kuhar MJ: Distribution of alpha 2 agonist binding sites in the rat and human central nervous system: Analysis of some functional, anatomic correlates of the pharmacologic effects of clonidine and related adrenergic agents. Brain Res 1984;319:69–101.

35. Kuraishi Y, Hirota N, Sato Y, et al: Noradrenergic inhibition of the release of substance P from the primary afferents in the rabbit spinal dorsal horn. Brain Res 1985;359:177–182.

36. Fleetwood-Walker SM, Mitchell R, Hope PJ, et al: An alpha 2 receptor mediates the selective inhibition by noradrenaline of nociceptive responses of identified dorsal horn neurones. Brain Res 1985;334:243–254.

37. Baba H, Kohno T, Okamoto M, et al: Muscarinic facilitation of GABA release in substantia gelatinosa of the rat spinal dorsal horn. J Physiol 1998;508:83–93.

38. Butterworth JF 5th, Strichartz GR: The alpha 2-adrenergic agonists clonidine and guanfacine produce tonic and phasic block of conduction in rat sciatic nerve fibers. Anesth Analg 1993;76:295–301.

39. Gaumann DM, Brunet PC, Jirounek P: Clonidine enhances the effects of lidocaine on C-fiber action potential. Anesth Analg 1992;74:719–725.

40. Eisenach JC, Gebhart GF: Intrathecal amitriptyline. Antinociceptive interactions with intravenous morphine and intrathecal clonidine, neostigmine, and carbamylcholine in rats. Anesthesiology 1995;83:1036–1045.

41. Kroin JS, Buvanendran A, Beck DR, et al: Clonidine prolongation of lidocaine analgesia after sciatic nerve block in rats is mediated via the hyperpolarization-activated cation current, not by alpha-adrenoreceptors. Anesthesiology 2004;101:488–494.

42. Singelyn FJ, Dangoisse M, Bartholomee S, et al: Adding clonidine to mepivacaine prolongs the duration of anesthesia and analgesia after axillary brachial plexus block. Reg Anesth 1992;17:148–150.

43. Hutschala D, Mascher H, Schmetterer L, et al: Clonidine added to bupivacaine enhances and prolongs analgesia after brachial plexus block via a local mechanism in healthy volunteers. Eur J Anaesthesiol 2004;21:198–204.

44. Culebras X, Van Gessel E, Hoffmeyer P, et al: Clonidine combined with a long acting local anesthetic does not prolong postoperative analgesia after brachial plexus block but does induce hemodynamic changes. Anesth Analg 2001;92:199–204.

45. Ilfeld BM, Morey TE, Enneking FK: Continuous infraclavicular perineural infusion with clonidine and ropivacaine compared with ropivacaine alone: A randomized, double-blinded, controlled study. Anesth Analg 2003;97:706–712.

46. Ilfeld BM, Morey TE, Thannikary LJ, et al: Clonidine added to a continuous interscalene ropivacaine perineural infusion to improve postoperative analgesia: A randomized, double-blind, controlled study. Anesth Analg 2005;100:1172–1178.

47. Alayurt S, Memis D, Pamukcu Z: The addition of sufentanil, tramadol or clonidine to lignocaine for intravenous regional anaesthesia. Anaesth Intensive Care 2004;32:22–27.

48. Gentili M, Bernard JM, Bonnet F: Adding clonidine to lidocaine for intravenous regional anesthesia prevents tourniquet pain. Anesth Analg 1999;88:1327–1330.

49. Reuben SS, Steinberg RB, Klatt JL, et al: Intravenous regional anesthesia using lidocaine and clonidine. Anesthesiology 1999;91:654–8.

50. Lurie SD, Reuben SS, Gibson CS, et al: Effect of clonidine on upper extremity tourniquet pain in healthy volunteers. Reg Anesth Pain Med 2000;25:502–505.

51. Memis D, Turan A, Karamanlioglu B, et al: Adding dexmedetomidine to lidocaine for intravenous regional anesthesia. Anesth Analg 2004;98:835–840.

52. Reuben SS, Connelly NR: Postoperative analgesia for outpatient arthroscopic knee surgery with intraarticular clonidine. Anesth Analg 1999;88:729–733.

53. Joshi W, Reuben SS, Kilaru PR, et al: Postoperative analgesia for outpatient arthroscopic knee surgery with intraarticular clonidine and/or morphine. Anesth Analg 2000;90:1102–1106.

54. Tan PH, Buerkle H, Cheng JT, et al: Double-blind parallel comparison of multiple doses of apraclonidine, clonidine, and placebo administered intra-articularly to patients undergoing arthroscopic knee surgery. Clin J Pain 2004;20:256–260.

55. Gentili M, Juhel A, Bonnet F: Peripheral analgesic effect of intra-articular clonidine. Pain 1996;64:593–596.

56. Gentili M, Houssel P, Osman M, et al: Intra-articular morphine and clonidine produce comparable analgesia but the combination is not more effective. Br J Anaesth 1997;79:660–661.

57. Buerkle H, Schapsmeier M, Bantel C, et al: Thermal and mechanical antinociceptive action of spinal vs peripherally administered clonidine in the rat inflamed knee joint model. Br J Anaesth 1999;83:436–441.

58. Coderre TJ, Katz J, Vaccarino AL, et al: Contribution of central neuroplasticity to pathological pain: Review of clinical and experimental evidence. Pain 1993;52:259–285.

59. Price DD, Mao J, Mayer DJ: Central neural mechanisms of normal and abnormal pain states. In Fields HL, Liebskind JC (eds): *Progress in Pain Research and Management*. IASP Press, 2001.

60. Dickenson AH, Chapman V, Green GM: The pharmacology of excitatory and inhibitory amino acid-mediated events in the transmission and modulation of pain in the spinal cord. Gen Pharmacol 1997;28:633–638.

61. Alfredson H, Forsgren S, Thorsen K, et al: Glutamate NMDAR1 receptors localised to nerves in human Achilles tendons. Implications for treatment? Knee Surg Sports Traumatol Arthrosc 2001;9:123–126.

62. Cairns BE, Hu JW, Arendt-Nielsen L, et al: Sex-related differences in human pain and rat afferent discharge evoked by injection of glutamate into the masseter muscle. J Neurophysiol 2001;86:782–791.

63. Svensson P, Cairns BE, Wang K, et al: Injection of nerve growth factor into human masseter muscle evokes long-lasting mechanical allodynia and hyperalgesia. Pain 2003;104:241–247.

64. Cairns BE, Svensson P, Wang K, et al: Activation of peripheral NMDA receptors contributes to human pain and rat afferent discharges evoked by injection of glutamate into the masseter muscle. J Neurophysiol 2003;90:2098–2105.

65. Tverskoy M, Oren M, Vaskovich M, et al: Ketamine enhances local anesthetic and analgesic effects of bupivacaine by peripheral mechanism: A study in postoperative patients. Neurosci Lett 1996;215:5–8.

66. Amiot JF, Bouju P, Palacci JH, et al: Intravenous regional anaesthesia with ketamine. Anaesthesia 1985;40:899–901.

67. Gorgias NK, Maidatsi PG, Kyriakidis AM, et al: Clonidine versus ketamine to prevent tourniquet pain during intravenous regional anesthesia with lidocaine. Reg Anesth Pain Med 2001;26:512–517.

68. Dal D, Tetik O, Altunkaya H, et al: The efficacy of intra-articular ketamine for postoperative analgesia in outpatient arthroscopic surgery. Arthroscopy 2004;20:300–305.

69. Brill S, McCartney CJ, Sawyer R, et al: Intra-articular ketamine analgesia following knee arthroscopy: A dose finding study. Pain Clin 2005;17:25–29.

70. Turan A, Memis D, Karamanlioglu B, et al: Intravenous regional anesthesia using lidocaine and magnesium. Anesth Analg 2005;100:1189–1192.

71. Reuben SS, Steinberg RB, Kreitzer JM, et al: Intravenous regional anesthesia using lidocaine and ketorolac. Anesth Analg 1995;81:110–113.

72. Steinberg RB, Reuben SS, Gardner G: The dose-response relationship of ketorolac as a component of intravenous regional anesthesia with lidocaine. Anesth Analg 1998;86:791–793.

73. Corpataux JB, Van Gessel EF, Donald FA, et al: Effect on postoperative analgesia of small-dose lysine acetylsalicylate added to prilocaine during intravenous regional anesthesia. Anesth Analg 1997;84:1081–1085.

74. Reuben SS, Duprat KM: Comparison of wound infiltration with ketorolac versus intravenous regional anesthesia with ketorolac for postoperative analgesia following ambulatory hand surgery. Reg Anesth 1996;21:565–568.

75. Ben-David B, Katz E, Gaitini L, et al: Comparison of IM and local infiltration of ketorolac with and without local anaesthetic. Br J Anaesth 1995;75:409–412.

76. Connelly NR, Reuben SS, Albert M, et al: Use of preincisional ketorolac in hernia patients: Intravenous versus surgical site. Reg Anesth 1997;22:229–232.

77. Bosek V, Cox CE: Comparison of analgesic effect of locally and systemically administered ketorolac in mastectomy patients. Ann Surg Oncol 1996;3:62–66.

78. Van Elstraete AC, Pastureau F, Lebrun T, et al: Neostigmine added to lidocaine axillary plexus block for postoperative analgesia. Eur J Anaesthesiol 2001;18:257–260.

79. Bone HG, Van Aken H, Booke M, et al: Enhancement of axillary brachial plexus block anesthesia by coadministration of neostigmine. Reg Anesth Pain Med 1999;24:405–410.

80. Turan A, Karamanlyoglu B, Memis D, et al: Intravenous regional anesthesia using prilocaine and neostigmine. Anesth Analg 2002;95(5):1419–1422.

81. McCartney CJ, Brill S, Rawson R, et al: No anesthetic or analgesic benefit of neostigmine 1 mg added to intravenous regional anesthesia with lidocaine 0.5% for hand surgery. Reg Anesth Pain Med 2003;28:414–417.

82. Yang LC, Chen LM, Wang CJ, et al: Postoperative analgesia by intra-articular neostigmine in patients undergoing knee arthroscopy. Anesthesiology 1998;88:334–339.

83. Gentili M, Enel D, Szymskiewicz O, et al: Postoperative analgesia by intraarticular clonidine and neostigmine in patients undergoing knee arthroscopy. Reg Anesth Pain Med 2001;26:342–347.

10

Local Anesthetic Solutions for Continuous Nerve Blocks

Marta Putzu, MD • Andrea Casati, MD

INTRODUCTION

In the past few years progress has been made in understanding the mechanisms and pathways involved in the modulation of pain, as well as in developing new therapeutic tools to provide satisfactory pain relief after surgery. The relationship between the intensity of acute postoperative pain and the duration of the patient's recovery and functional outcome has been well established. For these reasons, the prevention and treatment of acute pain had become the focus of great interest for perioperative specialists. Postoperative pain differs from chronic pain by its shorter duration and its requirement for immediate relief, which dictate the devel-opment of suitable management protocols. Preemptive and preventive analgesia also represent concepts that only apply to acute postoperative pain. Finally, it is important to recognize the role of acute pain in the development of chronic pain syndrome.

Irrespective of its nature, pain is not an objective but rather a subjective symptom. In the surgical as well as medical environment, intrinsic and extrinsic factors affect individual pain thresholds. Accordingly, the clinician must be always aware that pain treatment must be approached using a multimodal and multipharmacologic approach; no one single technique by itself, including the use of continuous peripheral nerve block, provides adequate pain relief in all patients and in all circumstances. The first description of continuous peripheral nerve block was reported in 1946 by Paul Ansbro,[1] who described the placement at the supraclavicular level of a blunt needle secured to the patient's skin using a cork, through which the needle was inserted before block placement. This cumbersome apparatus allowed the incremental injection of local anesthetic in order to prolong the duration of anesthesia in patients undergoing upper extremity surgery. In their report the authors used a short-onset/intermediate-duration local anesthetic, like 1% procaine. After an initial 40-mL bolus the authors injected incremental doses based on the duration of surgery, up to a final volume ranging between 120 mL for 1.5-h surgery and 220 mL for 4-h surgery. During the following 3 decades continuous perineural infusion techniques continued to be developed, and their indications extended; initially they were mainly used for upper extremity blocks, afterward they were also employed for lower limb blocks.

In 1977 Selander[2] reported on the injection of 30 to 50 mL of mepivacaine to conduct a continuous axillary block in 137 patients undergoing hand surgery, and in 1979 Manriquez and Pallares[3] reported on the repeated injection of 20 mL of 0.25% bupivacaine every 6 h to prolong the sympathetic block and pain control for 4 days.

In 1982 Matsuda and colleagues[4] reported on the use of either 30 mL of 1% lidocaine with epinephrine followed by 15 mL intermittently (1.5–2.75 h) or 40 mL of a 0.5% bupivacaine and 1% lidocaine mixture followed by intermittent injection of 20 mL (1.25–4.3 h) in 50 patients undergoing upper extremity reimplantation. Subsequently most of the groups have focused their clinical protocols on the use of low concentrations (0.125–0.25%) of bupivacaine.[5–7]

More recently, with the introduction of new long-acting aminoamide local anesthetics, such as ropivacaine or levobupivacaine, the attention of clinicians has shifted to the evaluation of these new agents, often with interesting findings. Borgeat and coworkers[8] compared 0.2% ropivacaine and 0.15% bupivacaine (to account for the difference in potency between the two agents) in terms of their effects on motor function and demonstrated that they provided similar postoperative pain control, but 0.2% ropivacaine allowed for better preservation of motor function than bupivacaine. On the other hand, levobupivacaine at 0.125% concentration seems to provide the same level of motor preservation as 0.2% ropivacaine.[9]

The advantages of continuous block techniques have been largely demonstrated for major orthopedic surgery, implementing the rehabilitation of these patients after total arthroplasty allowing early, pain-free mobilization of the operated limb. Finally, the indication of this technique of pain control has also been expanded to outpatient procedures. In fact it is known that over 40% of ambulatory patients experience moderate to severe pain within the first 48 h after ambulatory orthopedic surgery. Although different therapeutic approaches have been advocated, none provide reliable

pain control, and pain remains a major concern. Most frequently patients are discharged with oral medication that has limited effects on pain relief. Intraarticular injections of narcotic analgesics or local anesthetics have also been used, but these techniques have been shown to provide only limited and short-lasting pain relief. In recent years several groups have evaluated the use of continuous nerve blocks in outpatients. Most of these investigators used solutions of 0.125% bupivacaine or 0.2% ropivacaine infused through either elastomeric or electronic patient-controlled (PCA) pumps, with relevant benefits not only in terms of quality of postoperative analgesia, but also in improved quality of life during the first postoperative days.[10–12]

NERVE ROOTS ANATOMY & CLASSIFICATION OF NERVE FIBERS

The nerve roots are divided into three types according to their anatomic and functional properties: A, B, and C fibers. The A fibers are responsible for motor efferent conduction and are divided in Aα, Aβ, and Aγ fibers. They are all myelinated, like the Aδ fibers, which are sensory fibers carrying pressure and distension information. The B fibers are constituted of the autonomic pregangl014 fibers, and the C fibers include all the amyelinic fibers of the posterior spinal roots as well as the postgangliar autonomic fibers.

Clinical Pearls

- Generally, the bigger the size of the nerve fibers the greater the amount of local anesthetic solution required to block conduction. Thus, fibers of small size are blocked sooner than those of larger diameter.
- The B fibers of the autonomic system constitute an exception of this rule: even though they are myelinated fibers a minimum concentration of local anesthetic solution is required to produce an effective blockade.
- This explains why the sympathetic blockade is observed before the onset of sensory or motor blockade.

In the myelinated nerve roots, the action potential conduction proceeds from one Ranvier node to the next (jumping, or saltatory, conduction). Because the size of the fibers is proportional to the length between one Ranvier node and the next, the speed of conduction of the action potential increases with the size of the fibers. Generally, the bigger the size of the nerve fibers, the greater the amount of local anesthetic solution required to block the conduction. Thus, the fibers of small size are blocked sooner than those of larger diameter. The B fibers of the autonomic system constitute an exception to this rule: even though they are myelinated fibers, a minimum concentration of local anesthetic solution

Table 10–1.

Onset and Recovery of Nerve Blockade in the Different Types of Nerve Fibers

Nerve Block Onset	Nerve Block Recovery
B	A-α
C; A-δ	A-β
A-γ	A-γ
A-β	C; A-δ
A-α	B

Clinical Pearls

- The onset time of local anesthetics is influenced by the molecule's pK_a (the higher the pK_a, the slower the onset time of the nerve block in a physiologic environment) and diffusibility.
- The ability to cross the cell membrane depends on the molecular weight and the liposolubility of the molecule.
- All local anesthetics have nearly the same molecular weight, but the diffusibility of the local anesthetic molecules from the injection site depends on its hydrophilicity.
- The nonionized form of the molecule is more lipid-soluble than the ionized one, therefore, it can more readily cross the cell membrane but diffuses less easily.

is required to produce an effective blockade. This property of B fibers explains why the sympathetic blockade is observed before the block of the other fibers (Table 10–1). The difference in sensitivity to neural blockade allows determination of the minimum concentration of local anesthetic that blocks only the small fibers, mainly responsible for nociception, with minimum or no block of the lager fibers. This in turn, allows neural blockade to accomplish analgesia with no or minimum motor block; the basis of the differential sensory–motor blockade.

CLINICAL PROPERTIES OF LOCAL ANESTHETIC SOLUTIONS

The choice for a local anesthetic solution for peripheral nerve blocks is based on

1. Onset time
2. Duration of blockade
3. Ability to produce a differential sensory–motor block
4. Potential for toxicity

The *onset time* of local anesthetics is influenced by the molecule's pK_a (the higher the pK_a the slower the onset time of the nerve block in a physiologic environment) and diffusibility.[13] On the other hand, the ability to cross the cell membrane depends on the molecular weight and the liposolubility of the molecule. All local anesthetics have nearly the same molecular weight, but the diffusibility of the local anesthetic molecules from the injection site depends on its hydrophilicity. The nonionized form of the molecule is more lipid-soluble than the ionized one, so it and can cross the cell membrane easier but diffuses less easily. The commercial solutions of local anesthetics have an acid pH, and the pK_a of the different local anesthetics range from 7.9 to 8.1. Accordingly, the ionized form, which is less lipophilic, is more represented than the nonionized one.

As onset time decreases, the dose, volume, or concentration of a given local anesthetic can be increased. Other strategies include the modification of the pK_a of the anesthetic solution by warming it or adding sodium bicarbonate to increase the number of nonionized local anesthetic molecules, especially with lidocaine and mepivacaine. The alkalinization of ropivacaine, bupivacaine, or levobupivacaine is much more difficult, because of their very high pK_a. Another important aspect deserving consideration is the pH of tissues; for example, the local tissue acidosis related to inflammation can increase the ionized form of local anesthetic, thereby reducing its efficacy. The potency of a local anesthetic is usually expressed as the minimum effective concentration (C_m): the minimum anesthetic concentration that reduces the action potential of a nerve fiber bathed in a solution with a 7.2–7.4 pH and stimulated with a 30-Hz current by 50% within 5 min. The potency of local anesthetics is strictly related to their lipid-solubility; the more lipid-soluble a local anesthetic is, the greater its potency and consequently the lower its C_m.

The C_m of a local anesthetic also changes according to the size of the nerve fiber. Although the total amount of local anesthetic affects the onset, degree, and duration of the nerve block, its concentration primarily influences the intensity of the blockade. The smallest fibers (A-δ, β, and C), with a slower conduction speed, are more sensitive to the blocking activity of the local anesthetic solution than are those with a larger diameter (A-β and A-α) and fast conduction. In other words, the smallest fibers need a lower C_m than those of larger size. This aspect is related to the number of anesthetic molecules available to block the conduction; when using low concentrations the small number of local anesthetic molecules available will block only the small fibers. A possible explanation is the need for blocking three consecutive Ranvier nodes in order to produce a complete nerve block. Since the distance between consecutive Ranvier nodes increases as the size of the nerve fiber increases, low concentrations of local anesthetics block three consecutive nodes only in the small nerve fibers and not

Table 10–2.

Chemical and Physical Properties of the Main Local Anesthetic Drugs, Including the Reported Equipotent Concentrations

	Lidocaine	Mepivacaine	Bupivacaine	Ropivacaine	Levobupivacaine
Molecular weight	234	246	288	274	288
pK_a	7.7	7.6	8.1	8.1	8.1
Liposolubility	4	1	30	2.8	30
Partition coefficient	2.9	0.8	28	9	28
Protein binding	65%	75%	95%	94%	95%
Equipotent concentration	2%	1.5%	0.5%	0.75%	0.5%

in the large ones. This is the basis for the differential sensory–motor blockade, which is more evident with the lipophilic agents with high pK_a, such as bupivacaine, ropivacaine, and levobupivacaine.

Clinical Pearl

- The duration of the action of local anesthetic solutions depends on the protein binding as well as the clearance from the injection site

The **duration of the action** of local anesthetic solutions depends on the protein binding as well as the clearance from the injection site.[13] Table 10–2 shows the main chemical/physical properties of the considered local anesthetics, as well as their reported equipotent concentrations.

Clinical Pearls

- The closer the pK_a of a local anesthetic is to physiologic pH, the shorter the onset time of the nerve block.
- Increasing the lipophilicity of a local anesthetic increases its potency and toxicity, whereas protein binding is proportional to the duration of action of the local anesthetic.
- Sensory–motor differentiation is based on the different size and myelinization of the nerve fibers involved in pain conduction (Aα and C) as compared with those involved in motor function (Aα)

GENERAL PRINCIPLES

Different local anesthetic solutions, including lidocaine, bupivacaine, ropivacaine, and more recently levobupivacaine,

have been used for continuous peripheral nerve blocks. When choosing a local anesthetic solution for continuous peripheral nerve blocks, two main aspects are considered:

1. The need for the surgical anesthesia and
2. Maintenance of the block through a perineural catheter

Ideally, the local anesthetic would provide a fast and reliable onset time for surgery; long duration, good differentiation in sensory–motor block during postoperative continuous infusion; and a safe toxicity profile without a risk of accumulation in the postoperative period.

SELECTING A LOCAL ANESTHETIC FOR SURGICAL ANESTHESIA

The choice of the best anesthetic solution to induce the nerve block should be tailored to patient characteristics as well as to the safe dose according to the type of block and effect desired (anesthesia versus analgesia). Local anesthetics with a short onset have the disadvantage of short duration that usually reduces their usefulness for painful procedures where prolonged postoperative analgesia is desirable. However, placing a catheter close to the nerve(s) allows for prolongation of the block with the same or another agent. Therefore, a short-onset/intermediate-duration anesthetic solution (eg, mepivacaine or lidocaine at concentrations ranging between 1.5% and 2%) can be used to initiate the block and accomplish surgical anesthesia. The block can then be extended with another agent as desired. Some authors use combinations of anesthetic solutions with different kinetic properties; the most frequent mixture is a combination of a short-onset anesthetic, like mepivacaine, with a long-duration one, such as bupivacaine, ropivacaine, or levobupivacaine. Theoretically, the advantage of mixing different anesthetics is that the risk of toxicity decreases with long-acting mixtures. However, injection of two anesthetic drugs results in competitive binding to the protein

Table 10–3.

Block Characteristics, Concentrations and Doses Suggested to Induce a Peripheral Nerve Block With the Considered Local Anesthetic Agents

Agent	Concentration (%)	Onset	Duration (h)	Maximum Dose (mg)	pH
Lidocaine	1.5–2	Fast	1–2	300 500 + epinephrine 500	6.5
Mepivacaine	1.5–2	Fast	2–3	600 + epinephrine 150	4.5
Bupivacaine	0.5	Slow	4–8	225 + epinephrine 300	4.5–6
Ropivacaine	0.75–1	Slow	2–6		4–6
Levobupivacaine	0.5–0.75	Slow	4–8	150	4–6

carriers and the free concentration of the more toxic local anesthetic is similar to that produced by using it alone in a volume similar to the total injected volume of the mixture. Consequently, it is questionable whether these mixtures reduce the overall toxicity.

The volumes and doses of local anesthetics depend on the type of surgery (eg, single block or combination of different blocks, such as for lower limb procedures), as well as on the use of additional anesthetic agents (eg, light general anesthesia) for intraoperative maintenance. Accordingly, the maximum doses suggested for each anesthetic drug should be always kept in mind (Table 10–3). It should be noted, however, that significantly larger doses of local anesthetics than those recommended for epidural administration may be safely used for peripheral nerve blocks.

POSTOPERATIVE MAINTENANCE OF NERVE BLOCK

In several fields of anesthesia the pharmaceutical research is focused on the development of very short acting agents to be used through continuous infusion in order to allow rapid titration of the effects and easy handling of the anesthesia plan, but peripheral nerve blocks are mainly conducted using longer acting agents.

Capdevila and colleagues[14,15] reported on the use of 1% lidocaine solution for continuous peripheral nerve blocks after major orthopedic surgery and demonstrated similar benefits to those obtained with bupivacaine and ropivacaine perineural infusions. Moreover, lidocaine also has the advantage of a reduced toxicity compared with bupivacaine, levobupivacaine, and even ropivacaine.[13] In addition, using short-acting agents to maintain continuous peripheral nerve block also has the theoretical advantage of allowing a faster recovery of normal neurologic function (when indicated) after

the infusion is stopped. Unfortunately, shorter acting anesthetic agents have been demonstrated to be less effective in providing a good differentiation between sensory and motor blocks. For instance, patient-controlled interscalene analgesia with 0.2% ropivacaine or 1% lidocaine after open shoulder surgery both result in a similar quality of pain relief.[16] However, a more efficient recovery of motor function occurs in patients receiving 0.2% ropivacaine than in those receiving 1% lidocaine. This finding is similar to a previous report with epidural analgesia and can be explained by the different physical-chemical properties of the two agents: lidocaine penetrates nerve roots easier than ropivacaine, because of the different pK_a and lipophilicity of the two agents.[15] This property can explain the less effective differentiation between sensory and motor blocks with lidocaine than occur with ropivacaine. Even though the mild sparing effect on motor block can be considered as a minor problem, it is of clinical interest because a differentiation in sensory and motor blocks is an important endpoint in improving postoperative patient rehabilitation.

It is for this reason that most authors prefer to use long-acting agents for continuous peripheral block techniques (eg, bupivacaine, ropivacaine, or levobupivacaine).

For the last 20 years, bupivacaine (0.125–0.25%) has been generally used for upper limb continuous peripheral nerve block; however, 0.2% ropivacaine provides a similarly effective analgesia with better preservation of motor function than an equipotent concentration of 0.15% bupivacaine.[8] Levobupivacaine at 0.125% concentration has been reported to be similarly effective in pain relief to 0.2% ropivacaine, with a comparable preservation of motor function, whereas the use of 0.2% levobupivacaine resulted in deeper motor block than both 0.2% ropivacaine and 0.125% levobupivacaine.[9,17] It is for these reasons that clinicians prefer to use low concentrations of long-acting agents to provide a postoperative analgesia with minimal impairment of motor function.

Concentrations as low as 0.125–0.25% bupivacaine, 0.125–0.2% levobupivacaine, or 0.2% ropivacaine are usually used.

The infusion rate is usually adjusted according to the block technique selected. Several infusion regimens have been suggested, ranging from an intermittent bolus technique to a patient-controlled continuous perineural infusion. In general, continuous infusion combined with patient-controlled bolus doses optimizes analgesia and decreases the need for oral analgesic use compared with basal- or bolus-only dosing regimens.[18–20]

USING ADDITIVES FOR CONTINUOUS PERIPHERAL NERVE BLOCKS

Addition of various additives to local anesthetics has been suggested to hasten the onset, decrease systemic absorption, and prolong neural blockade or analgesia. The most commonly used additives for peripheral nerve blocks are vasoactive agents, alkalinizing agents, clonidine, and opioids. Unfortunately, few properly conducted studies have focused on the specifically proposed advantages for continuous peripheral nerve blocks.

Vasoconstrictors

The duration of a local anesthetic agent depends on the duration of the contact between the anesthetic agent and the nerve fibers as well as on the number of local anesthetic molecules bound to the sodium channels. A more intense and longer lasting block can be achieved by increasing the concentration and dose of the local anesthetic solution or pharmacologically reducing the removal of local anesthetic from the nerve target. Epinephrine, in a dose range of 5 mcg/mL (1:200.000), reduces the absorption of local anesthetics, increasing their concentration at the intended target nerves or plexuses. In general, addition of epinephrine to solutions of lidocaine, mepivacaine, or bupivacaine used for peripheral nerve blocks increases the duration and intensity of the block. However, a vasoconstrictor reduces the perfusion of the vasa nervorum, which potentially increases the risk of an ischemic nerve injury. For these reasons the extensive use of epinephrine as an adjuvant to local anesthetic solutions for continuous peripheral nerve blocks is not recommended, especially if continuous infusion rather than an intermittent bolus technique is used to manage postoperative pain. In addition, it is probably prudent to limit the concentration of epinephrine to 1:300,000 in peripheral nerve blockade.

Alkalinization

The pH of commercially available solutions of local anesthetic ranges from 3 to 6.5, whereas their pK_a ranges from 7.6 to 8.9. The alkalinization of local anesthetic solutions, usually obtained by adding 1 mEq of sodium bicarbonate to 10 mL of lidocaine, mepivacaine, and chloroprocaine reduces the onset time of a nerve block induced with these agents. This, however, does not occur when sodium bicarbonate is added to bupivacaine or ropivacaine.[21,22] However, even though changing the pH of the anesthetic solution may shorten the onset time of the block, there are not clinically relevant advantages when a continuous peripheral nerve block is used. Importantly, the stability of anesthetic solutions with added bicarbonate is not well studied. Therefore, because the local anesthetic mixtures in the infusion are used for 24 h or longer, the use of sodium bicarbonate for continuous peripheral nerve blocks is not recommended.

Clonidine

The analgesic effects of μ_2-agonists have been well documented. For instance, the addition of clonidine to local anesthetic solutions is known to improve the duration and quality of analgesia with peripheral nerve blocks. Clonidine reduces the onset time, prolongs postoperative analgesia, and improves the efficacy of nerve block during surgery. Several authors have reported on the use of low doses of clonidine for continuous peripheral nerve blocks using a concentration as low as 1 mcg/mL. The rationale for adding clonidine is to minimize the doses of local anesthetic solution required to produce an effective postoperative analgesia and thus reduce the risks of local anesthetic-related side effects; nonetheless, only few controlled studies have investigated the efficacy of this practice to improve analgesia for continuous perineural local anesthetic.

Ilfeld and coworkers[23] evaluated the usefulness of adding 1 mcg/mL clonidine to 0.2% ropivacaine for a continuous infraclavicular brachial plexus block in 34 outpatients undergoing moderately painful upper extremity orthopedic surgery. The authors reported that adding clonidine resulted in a statistically significant decrease in the number of self-administered bolus doses on the first two postoperative days, but this decreased actual local anesthetic consumption by only 2–7 mL/day. In addition, no differences in any other investigated variable were reported, including sleep quality or oral analgesic requirements. Therefore, the clinical significance of this finding is questionable.

When clonidine is added to the initial bolus of local anesthetic (1 mcg/kg), or to both the initial bolus (1 mcg/kg) and the continuous infusion solution (1 mcg/mL) for continuous femoral nerve block after total knee arthroplasty, no differences were found among the groups in the degree of pain, total consumption of local anesthetic solution, sedation, and hemodynamic parameters during the first 48 h of infusion.[24] However, persistent motor function impairment after 48 h of infusion was observed in 27% of patients receiving clonidine in the infusion solution, but only 6% of cases in patients not receiving clonidine at all, or receiving it only with the initial bolus ($p = 0.05$). This finding may be of clinical significance because it could potentially delay the recovery of normal motor function, which is important in orthopedic patients undergoing early rehabilitation.

Similar results have been also reported during continuous epidural infusion of clonidine containing solutions of local anesthetics.[25]

Peripheral Opioids

Opioid agents are known to exert their analgesic activity directly in the neuraxis; the addition of opioids to local anesthetic solution improves the quality of anesthesia and postoperative analgesia during epidural and spinal block. Various biochemical and electrophysiologic studies have suggested and supported the existence and functional significance of opioid receptors on primary afferent neurons.[26] The existence of such peripheral receptors has been demonstrated both immunocytochemically[27] and functionally.[28] Occupation of these receptors has been suggested to result in the inhibition of either the propagation of action potentials or release of excitatory transmitters in primary afferent fibers. Adding small doses of opioids to local anesthetic solutions for peripheral nerve blocks has been suggested to result in an improvement in the onset time, quality, and duration of nerve block.[29] Small concentrations of either fentanyl (1–2 mcg/mL), sufentanil (0.1 mcg/mL), or morphine (0.03 mg/mL) have been suggested for continuous peripheral nerve blocks. However, there is no evidence that addition of opioids to local anesthetics in peripheral nerve blocks results in any clinically significant benefit.

Tramadol is a weak opioid receptor agonist and an interesting opioid agent for use as an additive to local anesthetic due to its inhibitory effects on the reuptake of serotonin and norepinephrine. Tramadol has a local anesthetic-like effect on peripheral nerves,[30,31] and this could potentially provide a synergistic effect during continuous peripheral infusion of local anesthetic solutions. However, its clinical use has not be reported.

Table 10–4 shows the concentration and regimens suggested for maintenance of continuous peripheral nerve blocks with the main anesthetic solutions used in the literature and in our clinical experience, as well as the concentrations of additives.

Clinical Pearls

- When a catheter is placed for postoperative analgesia, the induction of nerve block can be performed with a short-acting agent (mepivacaine 1.5%) or a combination of a short-acting (mepivacaine 1.5%) and a long-acting one (ropivacaine 0.75% or levobupivacaine 0.5%).
- Postoperative maintenance is best performed with low concentrations of a long-acting agent, like 0.2% ropivacaine, 0.125–0.2% levobupivacaine.
- The addition of vasoconstrictors or sodium bicarbonate is not recommended for postoperative continuous infusion.
- Always remember that postoperative analgesia must be a multimodal and multipharmacologic treatment. Thus *always* implement analgesia with NSAIDs at fixed times and oral or parenteral opioids at request for breakthrough pain.

COMPLICATIONS RELATED TO THE INJECTION & INFUSION OF LOCAL ANESTHETIC SOLUTIONS

Although rare, administration of local anesthetic drugs can results in allergic reaction. These are however, primarily related to the use of aminoester drugs, such as procaine and chloroprocaine. The allergic reaction is related to the *para*-aminobenzoic acid, a preservative commonly found in cosmetic preparations. However, even when using amide-type local anesthetic solutions, allergies can occur when solutions contain preservatives (multidose preparations) or antibacterial additives.

Local tissue toxicity reactions are rare when clinically relevant concentrations of the anesthetic solution are used. However, local anesthetics can result in neurotoxicity in cases of intraneural injection. To minimize the risk of incorrect

Table 10–4.

Concentrations and Infusion Rates Suggested for the Maintenance of Continuous Peripheral Nerve Blocks With the Considered Anesthetic Solutions

	Concentration (%)	Infusion Rate (mL/h)	Additives
Lidocaine	1	5–10	Clonidine, 1 μg/mL
Bupivacaine	0.125–0.25	5–10	Fentanyl, 1–2 μg/mL
Ropivacaine	0.20–0.30	5–10	Sufentanil, 0.1 μg/mL
Levobupivacaine	0.125–0.25	5–10	Morphine sulfate, 0.03 mg/mL

needle placement, much work on imaging-assisted nerve block placement and injection monitoring is underway. For instance, ultrasound scanning has been suggested to locate the nerve structures and more precisely place the perineural catheter.[32,33] Such technology may allow both a real-time monitoring of the catheter placement and reduction in the dose required to accomplish a successful nerve block.[34] Another important issue in decreasing the risk of intraneural injection is avoidance of high injection pressures during local anesthetic administration. Unintentional intraneural injection of local anesthetics is associated with resistance to injection and high injection pressures (>20 psi) and may result in mechanical injury and pressure ischemia of the nerve fascicles.[35] Perineural injections result in a "seamless" injection; consequently, the injection pressures are low (<5 psi). In contrast, most intraneural injections are associated with a resistance to injection and high injection pressures exceeding 20 psi at the beginning of the injection. Such injections are followed by persistent motor deficits with destruction of neural architecture and degeneration of axons at the histologic examination.[35] Accordingly, to minimize the risk of this type of **local anesthetic-related** toxicity we should avoid injection if high injection pressures are encountered.

Systemic toxicity of local anesthetics can occur in cases of overdose or in cases of inadvertent intravascular injection. The severity of these systemic reactions is related to the maximum concentration achieved in the blood and may vary from simple reports of agitation, drowsiness, and metallic taste, to seizures, coma, and cardiac arrest with increasing plasma levels. More discussion on systemic toxicity of local anesthetic can be found in Chapter 6 (Clinical Pharmacology of Local Anesthetics).

Theoretically, continuing infusion of a local anesthetic solution after surgery may be associated with a risk for drug accumulation. This can be especially troublesome in patients discharged home after surgery with an infusion of local anesthetic solution still running. Fortunately, however, pharmacokinetic studies during continuous peripheral nerve blocks reported on the safety of this technique, with unbound plasma concentrations of local anesthetic remaining well below threshold levels for systemic central nervous toxicity,[36–38] provided the catheter is located in the right position.[39]

Clinical Pearls

- Allergic reactions are rare and are associated with aminoester type local anesthetics.
- Local toxicity with neurotoxicity primarily occurs in cases of intraneural injection, rather than normal application of clinically relevant concentrations of local anesthetics.
- To decrease the risk of nerve injury, utmost care should be taken during nerve localization; excessively high concentrations of local anesthetic and high injection pressures should be avoided.

- Systemic toxicity can be associated with unwanted intravascular injection (early-onset) or systemic reabsorption with overdosing (late-onset). To minimize these complications the planned volume of local anesthetic should be injected only with frequent aspiration to reduce the risk of intravascular injection.

References

1. Ansbro FP: A method of continuous brachial plexus block. Am J Surg 1946;71:716–722.
2. Selander D: Catheter technique in axillary block. Acta Anaesth Scand 1977;21:324–329.
3. Manriquez RG, Pallares V: Continuous brachial plexus block for prolonged sympathectomy and control of pain. Anesth Analg 1978;57:128–130.
4. Matsuda M, Kato N, Hosoi M: Continuous brachial plexus block for reimplantation in the upper extremity. Hand 1982;14:129–134.
5. Tuominen M, Pitkanen M, Rosenberg PH: Postoperative pain relief and bupivacaine plasma levels during continuous interscalene brachial plexus block. Acta Anaesthesiol Scand 1987;31:276–8.
6. Haasio J, Tuominen M, Rosenberg PH: Continuous interscalene brachial plexus block during and after shoulder surgery. Ann Chir Gynaecol 1990;79:103–107.
7. Pere P, Pitkanen M, Rosenberg PH, et al: Effect of continuous interscalene brachial plexus block on diaphragm motion and on ventilatory function. Acta Anaesthesiol Scand 1992; 36:53–57.
8. Borgeat A, Kalberer F, Jacob H, et al: Patient-controlled interscalene analgesia with ropivacaine 0.2% versus bupivacaine 0.15% after major open shoulder surgery: The effects on hand motor function. Anesth Analg 2001;92:218–223.
9. Casati A, Borghi B, Fanelli G, et al: Interscalene brachial plexus anesthesia and analgesia for open shoulder surgery: A randomized, double-blinded comparison between levobupivacaine and ropivacaine. Anesth Analg 2003;96:253–259.
10. Ilfeld BM, Morey TE, Wright TW, et al: Continuous interscalene brachial plexus block for postoperative pain control at home: A randomized, double-blinded, placebo-controlled study. Anesth Analg 2003;96:1089–1095.
11. White PF, Issioui T, Skrivanek GD, et al: The use of a continuous popliteal sciatic nerve block after surgery involving the foot and ankle: Does it improve the quality of recovery? Anesth Analg 2003;97:1303–1309.
12. Zaric D, Boysen K, Christiansen J, et al: Continuous popliteal sciatic nerve block for outpatient foot surgery—A randomized, controlled trial. Acta Anaesthesiol Scand 2004;48:337–341.
13. Covino BG. Pharmacology of local anaesthetic agents. Br J Anaesth 1986;58:701–716.
14. Capdevila X, Barthelet Y, Biboulet P, et al. Effects of perioperative analgesic technique on the surgical outcome and duration of rehabilitation after major knee surgery. Anesthesiology 1999;91: 8–15.
15. Capdevila X, Biboulet P, Bouregba M, et al: Bilateral continuous 3-in-1 nerve blockade for postoperative pain relief after bilateral femoral shaft surgery. J Clin Anesth 1998;10:606–609.
16. Casati A, Vinciguerra F, Scarioni M, et al: Lidocaine versus ropivacaine for continuous interscalene brachial plexus block after open shoulder surgery. Acta Anaesthesiol Scand 2003;47:355–360.
17. Casati A, Vinciguerra F, Cappelleri G, et al: 0.2% or 0.125% levobupivacaine for continuous sciatic nerve block: A prospective, randomized, double-blind comparison with 0.2% ropivacaine. Anesth Analg 2004;99:919–923.

18. Ilfeld BM, Morey TE, Enneking FK: Infraclavicular perineural local anesthetic infusion: A comparison of three dosing regimens for postoperative analgesia. Anesthesiology 2004;100:395–402.

19. Ilfeld BM, Thannikary LJ, Morey TE, et al: Popliteal sciatic perineural local anesthetic infusion: A comparison of three dosing regimens for postoperative analgesia. Anesthesiology 2004;101:970–977.

20. Ilfeld BM, Morey TE, Wright TW, et al: Interscalene perineural ropivacaine infusion: A comparison of two dosing regimens for postoperative analgesia. Reg Anesth Pain Med 2004;29:9–16.

21. Capogna G, Celleno D, Laudano D, et al: Alkalinization of local anesthetics. Which block, which local anesthetic? Reg Anesth 1995;20:369–377.

22. Milner QJ, Guard BC, Allen JG: Alkalinization of amide local anaesthetics by addition of 1% sodium bicarbonate solution. Eur J Anaesthesiol 2000;17:38–42.

23. Ilfeld BM, Morey TE, Enneking FK: Continuous infraclavicular perineural infusion with clonidine and ropivacaine compared with ropivacaine alone: A randomized, double-blinded, controlled study. Anesth Analg 2003;97:706–712.

24. Casati A, Vinciguerra F, Cappelleri C, et al: Adding clonidine to the induction bolus and postoperative infusion during continuous femoral nerve block delays recovery of motor function after total knee arthroplasty. Anesth Analg 2004;100:866–872.

25. Milligan KR, Convery PN, Weir P, et al: The efficacy and safety of epidural infusions of levobupivacaine with and without clonidine for postoperative pain relief in patients undergoing total hip replacement. Anesth Analg 2000;91:393–397.

26. Fields HL, Emcen PC, Leigh BK, et al: Multiple opiate receptor sites on primary afferent fibers. Nature 1980;284:351–353.

27. Stein C, Hassan AHS, Przewlocki R, et al: Opioids from immunocytes interacts with receptors on sensory nerves to inhibit nociception in inflammation. Proc Nat Acad Sci USA 1990;87:5935–5939.

28. Barthò L, Stein C, Herz A: Involvement of capsaicin-sensitive neurones in hyperalgesia and enhanced opioid antinociception in inflammation. Naunyn-Schmiedebergs Arch Pharmacol 1980;342:666–670.

29. Murphy DB, McCartney CJ, Chan VW: Novel analgesic adjuncts for brachial plexus block: a systematic review. Anesth Analg 2000;90:1122–1128.

30. Mert T, Gunes Y, Guven M, et al: Differential effects of lidocaine and tramadol on modified nerve impulse by 4-aminopyridine in rats. Pharmacology 2003;69:68–73.

31. Kapral S, Gollmann G, Waltl B, et al: Tramadol added to mepivacaine prolongs the duration of an axillary brachial plexus blockade. Anesth Analg 1999;88:853–856.

32. Williams SR, Chouinard P, Arcand G, et al: Ultrasound guidance speeds execution and improves the quality of supraclavicular block. Anesth Analg 2003;97:1518–1523.

33. Chan VW: Applying ultrasound imaging to interscalene brachial plexus block. Reg Anesth Pain Med 2003;28:340–343.

34. Marhofer P, Schrogendorfer K, Wallner T, et al: Ultrasonographic guidance reduces the amount of local anesthetic for 3-in-1 blocks. Reg Anesth Pain Med 1998;23:584–588.

35. Hadzic A, Dilberovic F, Shah S, et al: Combination of intraneural injection and high injection pressure leads to fascicular injury and neurologic deficits in dogs. Reg Anesth Pain Med 2004;29:417–423.

36. Pere P, Tuominen M, Rosenberg PH: Cumulation of bupivacaine, desbutylbupivacaine and 4-hydroxybupivacaine during and after continuous interscalene brachial plexus block. Acta Anaesthesiol Scand 1991;35:647–650.

37. Rosenberg PH, Pere P, Hekali R, et al: Plasma concentrations of bupivacaine and two of its metabolites during continuous interscalene brachial plexus block. Br J Anaesth 1991;66:25–30.

38. Ekatodramis G, Borgeat A, Huledal G, et al: Continuous interscalene analgesia with ropivacaine 2 mg/mL after major shoulder surgery. Anesthesiology 2003;98:143–150.

39. Tuominen MK, Pere P, Rosenberg PH: Unintentional arterial catheterization and bupivacaine toxicity associated with continuous interscalene brachial plexus block. Anesthesiology 1991;75:356–358.

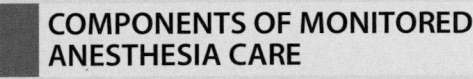

Sedation–Analgesia during Local & Regional Anesthesia

Paul F. White, PhD, MD

I. INTRODUCTION

II. COMPONENTS OF MONITORED ANESTHESIA CARE

III. USE OF ADJUNCTIVE SEDATIVE–HYPNOTIC DRUGS

IV. ROLE OF OPIOID & NONOPIOID ANALGESICS

V. MISCELLANEOUS TECHNIQUES USED TO SUPPLEMENT LOCAL ANESTHESIA

VI. COSTS AND BENEFITS OF MONITORED ANESTHESIA CARE

INTRODUCTION

During local and regional anesthesia, it is a common practice to administer both sedative and analgesic medications to enhance patient comfort during the operation. Use of local anesthetic infiltration and peripheral nerve blocks (PNBs) techniques in combination with intravenous (IV) sedative–hypnotic and analgesic drugs is commonly referred to as monitored anesthesia care (MAC). In many centers around the world, over 50% of all ambulatory (day-surgery) procedures are performed utilizing these techniques (Table 11–1).[1] When patients undergo surgical procedures under local anesthesia with IV sedation—analgesia in the operating room (OR), the old terminology used to describe the care of these patients as "conscious sedation." As the term implies, conscious sedation was a minimally depressed level of consciousness that retained the patient's ability to main-

tain an airway independently and continuously and to respond appropriately to physical stimulation and verbal commands. The American Society of Anesthesiologists (ASA) avoids this term in their *Practice Guidelines for Sedation and Analgesia by Non-anesthesiologists*[2] because it is imprecise and instead refers to this practice of anesthesia as MAC.

COMPONENTS OF MONITORED ANESTHESIA CARE

According to the ASA,[2] MAC is the term used to describe the administration of local anesthesia alone or the use of anesthetic drugs for a patient undergoing diagnostic or therapeutic procedures with or without local anesthesia. The ASA defines MAC "as instances in which an anesthesiologist has

Table 11–1.

Surgical Procedures Commonly Performed Under Local Anesthesia with Intravenous Sedation–Analgesia Techniques

Peripheral nerve blocks

Ilioinguinal/hypogastric (eg, herniorrhaphy)
Paracervical (eg, dilation/curettage, cone biopsy)
Dorsal penile (eg, circumcision)
Peroneal/femoral/saphenous/tibial/sural
  (eg, podiatric)
 Femoral/obturator/lateral
  femoral cutaneous/sciatic (eg, leg)
Brachial plexus/axillary/ulnar/median/radial
  (eg, arm/hand)
Peribulbar/retrobulbar (eg, ophthalmologic
  procedures)
Mandibular/maxillary (eg, oral surgery)
Intravenous regional (Bier block) (eg, arms, legs)
Intercostal/paravertebral (eg, breast surgery)

Tissue infiltration and wound instillation

Cosmetic procedures (eg, blepharoplasty, nasal,
  septum, endosinus)
Excision of masses and biopsies (eg, breast, axilla,
  lipomas)
Field blocks or instillation technique (eg, hernia
  repair, vasovasotomy)
Laparoscopic procedures (eg, cholecystectomy,
  tubal ligation)
Arthroscopic procedures (eg, knee, shoulder, wrist,
  ankle)

Topical analgesia

Eutectic mixture of local anesthetics (EMLA)
  (eg, skin lesions)
Lidocaine spray (eg, bronchoscopy, endoscopy,
  hernia repair)
Lidocaine gel or cream (eg, circumcision, urologic,
  oral surgery)
Lidocaine–bupivacaine (Duocaine) (eg, cataract
  surgery)
Tetracaine (eg, cataract and plastic surgery)
Cocaine paste (eg, nasal, endosinus surgery)

should be the same as for patients undergoing general anesthesia or central neuroaxial blockade and should include a complete preoperative assessment, intraoperative monitoring, and postoperative care in the recovery room prior to discharge.

Vigilant monitoring is required because patients may rapidly progress from a "light" level of sedation to "deep" sedation and ultimately, unconsciousness (Figure 11–1).[1] As a result, patients may be at risk for airway obstruction, oxygen desaturation, and even aspiration.[3] Therefore, supplemental oxygen is commonly administered with end-expiratory CO_2 monitoring for assessing ventilatory rate, presence of airway obstruction, and apnea.[4] Although cerebral monitoring (eg, electroencephalographic [EEG] bispectral index [BIS]) has been used successfully to assess the sedative effects of both midazolam[5] and propofol[6] during procedures performed using local anesthesia and PNBs, the confounding effects of the surgical stimulus and patient discomfort on the cerebral index can make it difficult to interpret the findings.[7] In addition, background noise in the OR can affect the cerebral index at "light" levels of sedation.[8] Nevertheless, some investigators have suggested that the BIS is useful for monitoring the central nervous system during surgery under local or regional anesthesia with IV sedation.[9]

A wide variety of pharmacologic agents are commonly administered during administration of local anesthesia or PNBs, as well as during surgical procedures under local anesthesia (or PNBs) to produce sedation, analgesia, and anxiolysis, while optimizing the surgical conditions and ensuring cardiorespiratory stability and a rapid recovery of cognitive functioning without untoward side effects (Table 11–2).[10] Systemic opioid and nonopioid analgesics are used to reduce discomfort associated with injection of local anesthetics and prolonged immobilization, as well as procedure-related pain that is not amendable to local anesthesia (eg, endoscopy).

Clinical Pearl

- Sedative–hypnotic drugs as well as narcotics are commonly used perioperatively to make regional anesthesia more tolerable for patients by reducing anxiety and providing an appropriate degree of sedation, amnesia, and analgesia.

been called upon to provide specific anesthesia services to a particular patient undergoing a planned procedure in connection with which a patient receives local anesthesia or, in some cases, no anesthesia at all. In such a case, the anesthesiologist is providing specific services to the patient, is in control of his or her vital signs, and is available to administer anesthetics or provide other medical care as appropriate." The standard of care for patients receiving MAC

Sedative–hypnotic drugs are also commonly used to make procedures more tolerable for patients by reducing anxiety and providing an appropriate degree of intraoperative sedation and amnesia. During longer surgical procedures, patients may become restless, bored, or uncomfortable when forced to remain immobile. Therefore, sedative–hypnotic drugs, as well as nonpharmacologic approaches (eg, music), may prove beneficial because they allow patients to rest during the operation. Patients' anxiety can be reduced by using

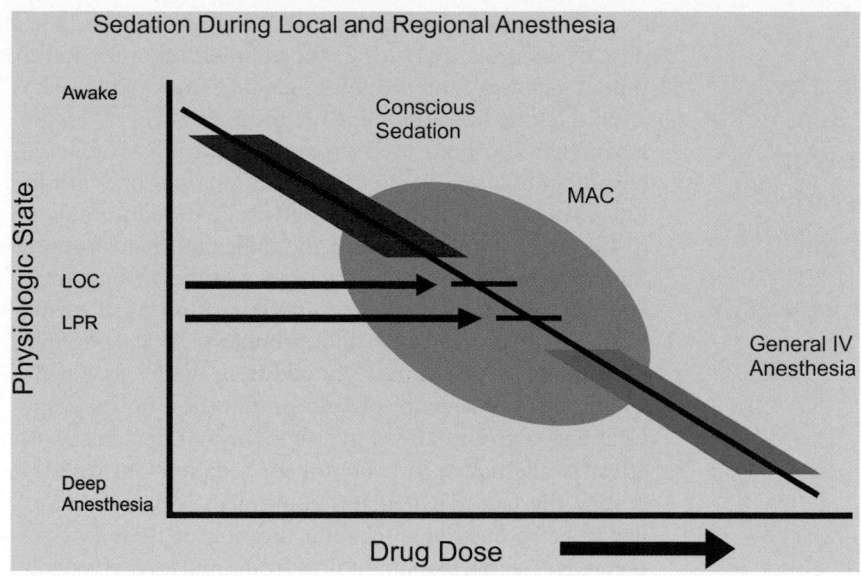

Figure 11–1. The dose-dependent spectrum of central nervous system depression produced by sedative–hypnotic drugs. MAC = monitored anesthesia care; LOC = loss of consciousness; LPR = loss of protective reflexes.

benzodiazepines, as well as by good preoperative communication, keeping the patient warm and covered, and allowing the patient to listen to relaxing music during the procedure. This chapter will discuss the commonly used adjunctive techniques to enhance patient comfort during local and regional anesthesia.

USE OF ADJUNCTIVE SEDATIVE–HYPNOTIC DRUGS

Many different sedative–analgesic drugs have been used for premedication (including barbiturates, benzodiazepines, opioid analgesics, and α_2-agonists) (Table 11–3).[10] Midazolam remains the most popular premedication because of its predictable sedative, anxiolytic, and amnestic properties irrespective of the route of administration (ie, oral, topical, or parenteral).[11–14] In addition, midazolam decreases the seizure threshold (as do other benzodiazepines). A wide variety of drug delivery systems such as intermittent boluses, variable-rate infusions, and target-controlled infusions, as well as patient-controlled sedation–analgesia techniques have been utilized during procedures under local and regional anesthesia.[15,16]

Although benzodiazepines (eg, diazepam, midazolam) were formerly the most popular sedatives for "conscious sedation,"[17,18] their use has declined with the introduction of more titratable IV sedative–hypnotics (eg, methohexital, etomidate, propofol) and analgesics (eg, alfentanil, remifentanil).[15,19] Methohexital, a shorter acting barbiturate than thiopental, was the IV sedative–hypnotic of choice prior to the introduction of propofol. Etomidate, a popular IV induction agent for cardiovascular surgery, can be administered by continuous infusion (5–20 mcg/kg/min) and may be particularly useful for sedation of elderly patients and those with significant underlying cardiac disease because to its minimal

cardiovascular depressant properties. However, when combined with opioid analgesics, etomidate is associated with an increased risk of postoperative nausea and vomiting (PONV).

Clinical Pearl

- Propofol is probably the IV sedative–hypnotic of choice for intraoperative sedation for many patients having surgery under regional anesthesia.

Propofol, the current IV sedative–hypnotic of choice, has been found to be equivalent to both midazolam and methohexital in providing adequate sedation and amnesia during superficial procedures under local anesthesia and PNBs.[20–23] Importantly, compared with other available sedative–hypnotic drugs, use of propofol is associated with less residual postoperative sedation, amnesia, and nausea and vomiting. Propofol facilitates fast-tracking (ie, bypassing the postanesthesia care unit), which requires reduced recovery time and an earlier "home readiness" state. Use of the benzodiazepine antagonist, flumazenil, also reduces the residual sedative–amnestic effects of midazolam and allows for the early recovery profile after midazolam sedation, which compares favorably with propofol.[24] However, the short duration of action of the reversal drug can lead to varying degrees of resedation in the postdischarge period.

Clinical Pearl

- The most popular sedative technique consists of a small dose of midazolam (1–2 mg) for premedication (or induction of sedation), and propofol (0.5–0.75 mg/kg followed by a variable-rate infusion at 25–100 mcg/kg/min).

Table 11–2.

Sedative–Analgesic Drugs and Nonpharmacologic Techniques Used for Premedication to Minimize Perioperative Discomfort During Local and Regional Anesthesia

Sedative–hypnotics

Midazolam, 1–5 mg PO/IM/IV
Thiopental, 75–150 mg IV
Methohexital, 20–50 mg IV
Etomidate, 10–15 mg IV
Propofol, 50–100 mg IV

Local anesthetics

Lidocaine, 0.5–2% SQ/IV
Bupivacaine, 0.12–0.5% SQ
Levobupivacaine, 0.125–0.5% SQ
Ropivacaine, 0.25–0.75% SQ
EMLA cream, lidocaine 25 mg/g, prilocaine 25 mg/g, topical

Opioid analgesics

Fentanyl, 0.75–1.5 mcg /kg, IV
Alfentanil, 10–20 mcg /kg, IV
Remifentanil, 0.5–1 mcg /kg, IV
Sufentanil, 0.1–0.2 mcg /kg IV
Dextromethorphan, 40–120 mg PO/IM/IV

Nonsteroidal antiinflammatory drugs

Ketorolac, 15–30 mg PO/IM/IV
Diclofenac, 50–100 mg PO/IM/IV
Ibuprofen, 300–800 mg PO
Naproxen, 25–500 mg PO
Celecoxib, 200–400 mg PO

Miscellaneous compounds

Acetaminophen, 0.5–2 g PO/PR/IV
Propacetamol, 1–2 g IV
Ketamine, 10–20 mg PO/IM/IV
Clonidine, 0.1–0.2 mg PO/TC/IM/IV
Dexmedetomidine, 0.5–1 mcg /kg, IM/IV
Gabapentin, 600–1200 mg bid PO
Pregabalin, 75–150 mg bid PO

Nonpharmacologic techniques

Music and "white" noise
Electroanalgesia, TENS

Routes of administration: PO = oral, IM = intramuscular, IV = intravenous, SQ = subcutaneous/tissue, TENS = transcutaneous electrical nerve stimulation, and PR = per rectum.
Reprinted, with permission, from White PF: Perioperative Drug Manual, Elsevier/Saunders Publishers, 2005.

The most popular sedative technique consists of a small dose of midazolam (1–2 mg) for premedication (or induction of sedation), and propofol (0.5–0.75 mg/kg followed by a variable-rate infusion at 25–100 mcg/kg/min).[20,25] Methohexital has also been used successfully during MAC by intermittent boluses (10–20 mg) or as a variable-rate infusion (20–60 mcg/kg/min).[19,26] Although residual sedation appears to be somewhat greater with methohexital than propofol, there were no differences in the recovery times to ambulating and discharge home when comparing infusions of methohexital (40 mcg/kg/min) and propofol (50 mcg/kg/min) during a MAC technique.[26] In addition, there was a significantly higher incidence of pain on injection in the propofol infusion group. Therefore, methohexital remains a cost-effective alternative to propofol for sedation during MAC despite the fact that it is less convenient to use because it has to be reconstituted. Careful titration of these IV anesthetics is essential to maintaining the desired level of sedation while avoiding ventilatory depression during surgery and to ensuring a prompt recovery of cognitive functioning after surgery.

In an effort to enhance patient comfort, both opioid and nonopioid analgesics have been used to supplement the sedative–hypnotics.[27–31] Although fentanyl remains the most commonly used opioid analgesic, remifentanil has become increasingly popular because its faster onset and recovery characteristics may minimize the potential for adverse drug interactions in the postoperative period. However, to avoid ventilatory depression and apnea, careful titration is necessary when remifentanil is combined with midazolam and propofol.[30–35] Of interest, some investigators have suggested that remifentanil fails to improve the quality of propofol sedation[36] A variety of nonsteroidal antiinflammatory drugs (NSAIDs) (eg, ibuprofen, ketorolac, piritramide, celecoxib) may also prove useful in preventing pain and discomfort that is refractory to local anesthetics.[37–40] However, with effective local anesthesia, the addition of an NSAID provides only minimal intraoperative improvement in the local analgesic effect.[27,38,41]

ROLE OF OPIOID & NONOPIOID ANALGESICS

Opioid analgesics are routinely administered to alleviate the discomfort associated with injection of the local anesthetic solution and to treat pain not amenable to local anesthesia.[28] In addition, the concomitant use of opioid analgesics reduces the sedative–hypnotic dosage requirement and thereby minimizes residual sedation. Avramov and White[29] first described the combined use of alfentanil (0.3–0.4 mcg/kg/min) and propofol (25, 50, or 75 mcg/kg/min) infusions for MAC. Compared with the opioid alone, concomitant use of propofol significantly reduced the alfentanil dosage requirement (30–50%) and the incidence of PONV. Comparing alfentanil (0.25 mcg/kg/min) and remifentanil (0.05 mcg/kg/min) infusions when administered as an adjuvant to propofol, Dilger

Table 11–3.

Sedative–Anxiolytic Drugs Used for Premedication in Patients Undergoing Local and Regional Anesthesia

	Dosage Range (and route)	Onset (min)	Key Points
Barbiturates			
Amobarital	100–200 mg PO	10–20	Delays early recovery
Butalbital	50–100 mg PO	20–40	Variable response
Chloral hydrate	0.5–1 g PO	20–40	Variable response
Secobarbital	200–300 mg PO	15–30	Delays early recovery
Zaleplon	5–20 mg PO	20–40	Variable response
Zolpidem	5–10 mg PO	15–30	Variable response
Benzodiazepines			
Midazolam	7.5–15 mg PO	15–30	Large first-pass effect
	5–7 mg IM	5–10	Water-soluble, nonirritating
	1–2 mg IV	1–3	Rapid-onset, excellent amnesia
Diazepam	5–10 mg PO	30–60	Long-acting metabolites
Temazepam	15–3 mg PO	15–30	Similar to midazolam
Triazolam	0.12–0.25 mg PO	15–30	Prominent sedation
Lorazepam	1–2 mg PO	45–90	Prolonged amnestic effect
Opioid analgesics			
Alfentanil	250–500 mcg	2–3	Minimal residual analgesia
Fentanyl	50–100 mcg	3–5	Mild sedation
Remifentanil	40–80 mcg	<2	No residual analgesia
α_2-Adrenergic agonists			
Clonidine	0.1–0.3 mg PO	30–60	Prolonged sedative effect
Dexmedetomidine	50–70 mcg IM	10–20	Bradycardia and hypotension
	50 mcg IV	5–10	Reduced anesthetic and analgesic requirements

Reprinted, with permission, from White PF: Perioperative Drug Manual, Elsevier/Saunders Publishers, 2005.

and colleagues[30] reported that the remifentanil group required fewer "rescue" doses of local anesthetic during MAC for breast surgery.

Clinical Pearl

- Opioid analgesics are routinely administered to alleviate the discomfort associated with injection of the local anesthetic solution.

When administered in combination with small doses of midazolam an infusion of remifentanil (0.05–0.15 mcg/kg/min) can provide adequate sedation and analgesia during minor surgical procedures performed with the patient under local anesthesia.[31,32] Sá Rêgo and coworkers[35] compared the use of intermittent remifentanil boluses (25 mcg) vs a continuous variable-rate infusion (0.025–0.15 mcg/kg/min) when administered to patients receiving a MAC technique involving midazolam (2 mg) and propofol (25–50 mcg/kg/min). Patient comfort was higher during the procedure when remifentanil was administered by a variable-rate infusion. However, the patients receiving the propofol–remifentanil infusion also experienced a higher incidence of desaturation (30% vs 0%) compared with those receiving small intermittent boluses of remifentanil during a propofol infusion.

In direct comparisons of remifentanil and propofol administered by continuous infusion after premedication with midazolam, there was a decreased level of intraoperative sedation and a greater degree of respiratory depression with remifentanil (vs propofol) administration.[33,34] Therefore, remifentanil infusions must be carefully titrated to avoid excessive respiratory depression in the presence of midazolam or propofol (or both). Using remifentanil in combination with local anesthetics obviates the disadvantage associated with the minimal residual analgesia when remifentanil is used during painful procedures. Unfortunately, even the short-acting opioid analgesic remifentanil can increase PONV and the need for antiemetic prophylaxis.[42]

Given the increased risk of ventilatory depression when opioid analgesics are combined with sedative–hypnotics, a variety of nonopioid analgesics have been evaluated during MAC. Ketorolac, a potent, parenterally active NSAID, has been used as an analgesic supplement to propofol sedation during local anesthesia.[27,37–39] Use of ketorolac was associated with a lower incidence of pruritus, nausea, and vomiting than fentanyl. However, when used with propofol sedation, ketorolac-treated patients required higher intraoperative doses of propofol and more supplemental opioid analgesia compared with those given fentanyl.[27,37] Piritramide, 0.05 mg/kg IV, prior to PNBs can reduce pain perception and the endocrine stress response during cataract surgery.[40]

Low-dose ketamine (0.25–0.75 mg/kg) combined with either midazolam or propofol has also been administered before injection of local anesthetics in outpatients undergoing a variety of surgical procedures.[18,43–47] Ketamine has the advantage over opioid analgesics of producing less ventilatory depression and PONV while providing better intraoperative analgesia than the NSAIDs, when it is combined with propofol as part of a MAC technique. Importantly, both midazolam and propofol are highly effectively in attenuating the dysphoric and psychomimetic side effects associated with ketamine administration.[18,45,46] When used for sedation during local anesthesia, newer formulations of propofol may reduce pain on injection (eg, propofol-MCT/LCT,[48] a propofol prodrug [fospropofol disodium] called Aquavan)[49] and the risk of hyperlipidemia (eg, Ampofol) during prolonged sedation.[50]

The α_2-agonists reduce central sympathetic outflow and have been shown to produce both anxiolysis and sedation.[10] Kumar and colleagues[51] demonstrated that oral clonidine (300 mcg) provided effective anxiolysis for elderly patients undergoing ophthalmic surgery under local anesthesia and also decreased the incidence of intraoperative hypertension and tachycardia. Dexmedetomidine, a more selective and potent α_2-agonist, significantly decreased anxiety levels and reduced the requirements for supplemental opioid analgesic medications when given before IV regional anesthesia for hand surgery.[52] When comparing dexmedetomidine with midazolam for sedation, Aho and coworkers[53] described a faster recovery from sedation when dexmedetomidine was followed by reversal with the specific α_2-antagonist atipamezole. Unfortunately, the midazolam-treated patients did not receive the reversal drug flumazenil. In the early studies, administration of dexmedetomidine during local anesthesia was associated with severe bradycardia. However, more recent studies[54,55] involving lower dosages have been associated with good intraoperative hemodynamic stability and reduced patient discomfort during local anesthesia compared with midazolam and propofol.

Other nonopioid analgesics that may be useful adjuvants to local anesthesia in the future include novel compounds like gabapentin and pregabalin,[56–58] as well as adenosine[59] and compounds that can elevate levels of this endogenous compound. For example, pregabalin (300 mg) produced a significantly longer duration of analgesia than ibuprofen (400 mg) after oral surgery under local anesthesia.[57] Although lacking any intrinsic analgesic properties, dexamethasone has been found to facilitate an earlier discharge after MAC independent of its well-known antiemetic properties.[60] Perhaps one of the most intriguing new analgesic compounds in development is capsaicin (ALGRX 4975) for injection, as well as a gel formulation for intraoperative topical applications. Although capsaicin causes transient discomfort on administration, it can produce prolonged analgesia by producing localized degradation of the C-neuron endings. Topical treatment with capsaicin may offer other clinical advantages over existing analgesic drugs used to prevent postoperative pain in combination with local anesthetics (eg, by reducing tissue swelling).[61]

MISCELLANEOUS TECHNIQUES USED TO SUPPLEMENT LOCAL ANESTHESIA

Several investigators have evaluated the use of patient-controlled sedation–analgesia.[62–67] Although self-administration of midazolam and propofol can be an effective alternative to MAC in selected patients, careful monitoring is required to optimize surgical conditions and patient safety.[62] Osborne and colleagues[65] reported that patient-controlled sedation with propofol was preferred by the patients over a standard propofol infusion during MAC. Nevertheless, many patients prefer to have an expert in charge of sedative–analgesic drug administration during surgery.[62] Interestingly, patient-controlled sedation requirements were similar for cataract surgery under topical and retrobulbar anesthesia.[66] Use of intraoperative patient-controlled analgesia with potent opioids can produce significant ventilatory depression when patients are also receiving sedative–hypnotic drugs.[62] However, a recent study suggested patient-controlled remifentanil administration in combination with midazolam sedation is "a safe and reliable" method in conjunction with local anesthesia for oral surgery.[67]

Subanesthetic concentrations of inhaled anesthetics (eg, N_2O, 30–50% in oxygen or sevoflurane 0.3–0.6% inspired) can also be used to supplement local and regional anesthesia.[68,69] However, this technique did not offer any significant advantages over IV midazolam[70] or propofol.[71] The primary concerns in using inhaled anesthetics are the ease with which the patient can drift into an unconscious state or develop upper airway obstruction, as well as the issue of OR air pollution. Therefore, volatile anesthetics are rarely used, and N_2O is only used to supplement inadequate local anesthesia or PNBs not well-controlled by potent parenteral opioid analgesics.

Table 11–4.

Potential Side Effects of Sedative–Hypnotic, Opioid and Nonopioid Analgesic Drugs Used During Local and Regional Anesthesia

Sedative–hypnotics

Respiratory and cardiovascular depression
Cognitive dysfunction
Agitation
Amnesia
Sedation and dizziness

Opioid analgesics

Respiratory and cardiovascular depression
Nausea, vomiting, and retching
Constipation and ileus
Urinary hesitancy and retention
Pruritus and skin rash
Sedation and dizziness
Acute tolerance

Local anesthetics

Residual motor weakness
Peripheral nerve irritation
Cardiac arrhythmias
Allergic reactions
Sympathomimetic effects (due to vasoconstrictors)

Nonsteroidal antiinflammatory drugs and COX-2 inhibitors

Operative-site bleeding
Gastrointestinal bleeding
Renal tubular dysfunction
Allergic reactions (eg, Steven–Johnson syndrome)
Bronchospasm
Hypertension
Pedal edema

Acetaminophen

Gastrointestinal upset
Sweating
Hepatotoxicity
Agranulocytosis

Ketamine and NMDA antagonists

Hypertension
Diplopia and nystagmus
Dizziness and confusion
Cardiac arrhythmias
Nausea and vomiting
Psychomimetic reactions

Miscellaneous drugs

Somnolence, dizziness and peripheral edema (gabapentin)
Dizziness, somnolence, weight gain (pregabalin)
Nausea and vomiting (neostigmine)
Muscle weakness and sedation (magnesium)
Transient injection pain (capsaicin)

COX-2 = Cyclooxygenase-2; NMDA = N-Methyl-D-aspartate. Data taken, with permission, from White PF: The changing role of nonopioid techniques in the management of postoperative pain. Anesth Analg 2005; 101:S5–S22.

Finally, nonpharmacologic therapies like music,[72,73] electroanalgesia,[74,75] and hypnosis[76] may also prove useful in enhancing patient comfort and in reducing the sedative and analgesic requirements during surgical procedures under local anesthesia in the future. If effective, these nonpharmacologic approaches have the potential of reducing drug-related side effects and adverse drug interactions during the perioperative period (Table 11–4).[77]

COSTS AND BENEFITS OF MONITORED ANESTHESIA CARE

Due to the presence of an anesthesia provider, the cost for MAC is obviously higher than for OR nurse-administered "conscious sedation." Although some studies have suggested that patient outcomes are comparable for the two methods,[78] these findings have been seriously questioned because of flaws in the study design.[70] Although so-called "unmonitored" local anesthesia can be used as an alternative to MAC for minor surgical procedures,[71] most patients (and surgeons) prefer the presence of an anesthesia provider to ensure optimal sedation and analgesia during surgery under local anesthesia.[79] From a cost–benefit perspective, local anesthesia and PNBs with or without sedation offer significant advantages in addition to reduced costs compared with general and central neuroaxial anesthesia.[79] One study found that when MAC was used for assisted reproductive procedures the patients' experienced improved pregnancy rates compared with the same procedures performed under general anesthesia.[80]

In women undergoing laparoscopic tubal sterilization with a MAC technique, the anesthetic drug costs were found to be significantly reduced relative to general anesthesia (US $21 vs $46, respectively).[81] The MAC technique was also associated with less time in the OR, a higher degree of alertness on the evening of the day of surgery, as well as decreased postoperative pain (33% vs 80%) and sore throats (3% vs 70%), contributing to a significant reduction in the overall perioperative costs. Patel and coworkdes[82] reported that the use of MAC sedation resulted in a 6- to 7-min decrease in OR exit time compared with general anesthesia with desflurane, contributing to enhanced turnover of cases. Similarly, comparative studies involving general endotracheal anesthesia, central neuroaxial blockade, and MAC techniques for inguinal herniorrhaphy (Table 11–5)[83] and anorectal (Table 11–6)[84] procedures have consistently found improved recovery profiles, decreased side effects, greater patient satisfaction, and reduced anesthetic costs with MAC.[83–85] More recent studies[86–88] involving outpatients undergoing orthopedic procedures have also found superior recovery profiles with PNB compared with those for general anesthesia, contributing to a more favorable cost–benefit profile. The use of topical local anesthetics has also offered significant advantages for outpatients undergoing ophthalmologic

Table 11–5.

Patient Demographic Characteristics, Anesthesia, Surgery, and Recovery Times for Local Anesthesia with Sedation, General Anesthesia, or Spinal Anesthesia for Inguinal Herniorrhaphy Procedures.

Demographic Characteristic	Local Anesthesia with Sedation	General Anesthesia	Spinal Anesthesia
Age (y)	42 ± 18	36 ± 16	39 ± 14
Weight	73 ± 9	75 ± 10	73 ± 14
Surgery time (min)	86 ± 21	93 ± 31	91 ± 22
Anesthesia time (min)	109 ± 23	119 ± 29	116 ± 22
Recovery times (min)			
Awakening	3 ± 2	5 ± 2*	0†
Orientation	5 ± 4	11 ± 5*	1 ± 2*†
Phase 1 PACU (min)	5 ± 14	40 ± 13*	35 ± 22*
Phase 2 DSU (min)	153 ± 67	168 ± 58	276 ± 86*†
Home-readiness (min)	133 ± 68	171 ± 40*	280 ± 80*†
Actual discharge (min)	158 ± 71	208 ± 56*	309 ± 83*†
Postoperative side effects [n(%)]			
Backache	0	0	6(24)*†
Drowsiness	4(14)	15(54)*	3(12)†
Nausea and/or vomiting	2(7)	17(61)*	3(12)†
Pruritus	0	0	6(24)*†
Sore throat	0	6(22)*	2(8)†
Urine retention	0	0	5(20)*†
Maximum nausea score (mm)	1 ± 5	27 ± 27*	4 ± 1†
Maximum pain score (mm)	15 ± 14	39 ± 28*	34 ± 32*
Oral analgesics [n(%)]	16(57)	18(64)	17(68)
Highly satisfied [n(%)]	21(75)	10(36)*	16(64)

* $p < 0.05$ *vs local anesthesia and spinal anesthesia.*

† $p < 0.05$ *vs local anesthesia.*

Reprinted, with permission, from Song D, Greilich NB, White PF, Watcha MF, et al: Recovery profiles and costs of anesthesia for outpatient unilateral inguinal herniorrhaphy. Anesth Analg 2000;91: 876–81.

(eg, cataract)[66] and plastic (eg, facial laser resurfacing) surgery procedures.[89] The effect of the anesthetic technique on cost and recovery time is an increasingly important consideration in today's clinical practice environment because of the heavy emphasis on "fast-tracking" recovery processes.

In summary, the use of local (infiltration) or regional anesthesia with IV sedation–analgesia is the anesthetic technique of choice for providing cost-effective anesthetic care for patients undergoing superficial (noncavitary) surgical procedures (Table 11–7).[1,90] The most important factors in

Table 11–6.

Patient Demographic Characteristics, Surgical, Anesthetic, and Recovery Times for the Three Anesthetic Techniques Used for Anorectal Procedures

	Local Anesthesia with Sedation	Spinal Anesthesia	General Anesthesia
Age(y)	40 ± 9	43 ± 10	41 ± 9
Weight (kg)	83 ± 18	82 ± 16	82 ± 22
Duration of surgery (min)	26 ± 14	26 ± 13	26 ± 15
Duration of anesthesia (min)	40 ± 15	$72 \pm 17^*$	$75 \pm 19^*$
Phase 1 PACU stay (min)	0	$52 \pm 18^*$	$44 \pm 27^*$
Phase 2 DSU stay (min)	71 ± 17	$135 \pm 113^*$	$120 \pm 52^*$
Time to oral intake (min)	12 ± 5	$59 \pm 18^*$	$60 \pm 29^*$
Time to Aldrete score of 10 (min)	0	$19 \pm 7^*$	$30 \pm 19^{*\dagger}$
Time to home-readiness (min)	76 ± 17	$193 \pm 112^*$	$171 \pm 58^*$
Duration of hospital stay (min)	116 ± 21	$266 \pm 112^*$	$247 \pm 65^*$
Side effects [n(%)]			
Hypotension	0	2(6)	2(6)
Pain medication requested	6(19)	6(19)	14(45)*
Nausea	0	1(3)	8(26)*
Vomiting	0	1(3)	1(3)
Urinary retention	0	2(6)	1(3)
Supplemental oxygen in recovery	0	4(13)	27(87)*
Overnight hospitalization	0	0	1(3)
Acceptable surgical conditions (%)	100	100	100
Highly satisfied	21(68)	18(58)	12(39)†

Values are numbers (n) and percentages (%).
* p < 0.05 vs local anesthesia and spinal anesthesia.
† p < 0.05 vs local anesthesia.
PACU = postanesthesia care unit; DSU = day surgery unit.
Reprinted, with permission, from Li S, Coloma M, White PF, Watcha MF, et al: Comparison of the costs and recovery profiles of three anesthetic techniques for ambulatory anorectal surgery. Anesthesiology 2000;93:1225–30.

achieving the desired clinical outcome and highest patient satisfaction are achieving effective local analgesia and carefully titrating intravenous sedative and analgesic medications to avoid ventilatory depression and to ensure a prompt recovery of cognitive functioning following surgery. The recommended loading and maintenance doses of the most commonly used IV-selective analgesic drugs are summarized in Table 11–8.[90]

In conclusion, use of sedation–analgesia techniques in combination with local anesthesia and regional anesthesia achieve the *best outcome* for the patient at the lowest cost to the health care system. When properly applied, the use of MAC techniques can provide excellent operating conditions while optimizing patient comfort and safety during the operation, while ensuring a prompt resumption of normal activities of daily living after surgery.

Table 11–7.

Summary of Commonly Used Monitored Anesthesia Care (MAC) Techniques and Overall Advantages Compared with General Endotracheal Anesthesia and Central Neuroaxial Blockade

Techniques

Use of local anesthetic infiltration or peripheral nerve blocks
Use of intravenous adjuvants (e.g. sedative- hypnotics. amnesiacs. analgesics and sympatholytic drugs)
Level of sedation varies from minimal (e.g. patient- controiled) to profound (e.g. intravenous anesthesia)

Advantages

Minimizes postoperative pain
Low incidence of postoperative nausea and vomiting
Reduces incidence of airway complications, backaches, and headaches
Provides for an earlier discharge
Cost-effective technique

Table 11–8.

Recommended Dosages of Commonly Used Parenteral Sedative and Analgesic Drugs During Local Anesthesia and Peripheral Nerve Blocks

Drug	Loading Dosage*	Maintenance Infusion
Sedative–anxiolytics		
Diazepam	5–10 mg	N/A
Midazolam	2.5–7.5 mg (alone)	1–2 mcg/kg/min
	1–2 mg (with propofol)	
Etomidate	5–15 mg	5–10 mcg/kg/min
Propofol	25–100 mg	25–75 mcg/kg/min
Thiopental	50–150 mg	
Methohexital	10–20 mg	20–60 mcg/kg/min
Sedative-analgesics		
Ketamine	10–20 mg	5–15 mcg/kg/min
Dexmedetomidine	25–75 mcg	0.01–0.02 mcg/kg/min
Analgesics		
Alfentanil	0.25–0.50 mg	0.5 1 mcg/kg/min
Fentanyl	25–50 mcg	N/A
Remifentanil	12.5–25 mcg	0.02–0.1 mcg/kg/min
Ketorolac	30–60 mg	N/A
Parecoxib	20–40 mg	N/A

In the elderly population, lower initial dosages of the sedative–analgesic drugs should be administered. N/A = not applicable.
Reprinted, with permission, from White PF: Perioperative Drug Manual. Elsevier/Saunders, 2005.

References

1. Sa Rego MM, Watcha MF, White PF: The changing role of monitored anesthesia care in the ambulatory setting. Anesth Analg 1997;85:1020.
2. American Society of Anesthesiologists: *Position on Monitored Anesthesia Care.* Directory of Members. American Society of Anesthesiologists, 1997, p 413.
3. Smith I, White PF: Use of intravenous adjuvants during local and regional anesthesia. Curr Rev Clin Anesth 1992;12:145–152.
4. Soto RG, Fu ES, Vila H Jr, et al: Capnography accurately detects apnea during monitored anesthesia care. Anesth Analg 2004;99:379–382.
5. Liu J, Singh H, White PF: EEG bispectral analysis predicts the depth of midazolam-induced sedation. Anesthesiology 1996;84:64–9.
6. Liu J, Singh H, White PF: Electroencephalographic bispectral index correlates with intraoperative recall and depth of propofol-induced sedation. Anesth Analg 1997;84:185–189.
7. Sakai T, Matsuki A, White PF, et al: Use of an EEG-bispectral closed-loop system for administering propofol. Acta Anaesthesiol Scand 2000;44:1007–1010.
8. Kim DW, Kil HY, White PF: The effect of noise on the bispectral index during propofol sedation. Anesth Analg 2001;93:1170–1173.
9. Buyukkocak U, Ozcan S, Daphan C, et al: A comparison of four intravenous sedation techniques and bispectral index monitoring in sinonasal surgery. Anaesth Intensive Care 2003;31:164–171.
10. White PF: *Perioperative Drug Manual.* Elsevier/Saunders Publishers, 2005.
11. van Vlymen JJ, Sa Rego MM, White PF: Benzodiazepine premedication: Can it improve outcome in patients undergoing breast biopsy procedures? Anesthesiology 1999;90:740–747.
12. al-Rakaf H, Bello LL, Turkustani A, et al: Intra-nasal midazolam in conscious sedation of young paediatric dental patients. Int J Paediatr Dent 2001;11:33–40.
13. Cote CJ, Cohen IT, Suresh S, et al: A comparison of three doses of a commercially prepared oral midazolam syrup in children. Anesth Analg 2002;94:37–43.
14. Habib NE, Mandour NM, Balmer HG: Effect of midazolam on anxiety level and pain perception in cataract surgery with topical anesthesia. J Cataract Refract Surg 2004;30:437–443.
15. White PF: Clinical uses of intravenous anesthetic and analgesic infusions. Anesth Analg 1989;68:161–171.
16. Newson C, Joshi GP, Victory R, et al: Comparison of propofol administration techniques for sedation during monitored anesthesia care. Anesth Analg 1995;81:486–491.
17. Hegarty JE, Dundee JW: Sequelae after the intravenous injection of three benzodiazepines—diazepam, lorazepam, and flunitrazepam. Br Med J 1977;2:1384–1385.
18. White PF, Vasconez LO, Mathes SA, et al: Comparison of midazolam and diazepam for sedation during plastic surgery. J Plast Reconstr Surg 1988;81:703–712.
19. Urquhart ML, White PF: Comparison of sedative infusions during regional anesthesia—methohexital, etomidate, and midazolam. Anesth Analg 1989;68:249–254.
20. White PF, Negus JB: Sedative infusions during local and regional anesthesia: A comparison of midazolam and propofol. J Clin Anesth 1991;3:32.
21. Pratila MG, Fischer ME, Alagesan R, et al: Propofol vs midazolam for monitored sedation: A comparison of intraoperative and recovery parameters. J Clin Anesth 1993;5:268.
22. Smith I, Monk TG, White PF, et al: Propofol infusion during regional anesthesia: Sedative, amnestic, and anxiolytic properties. Anesth Analg 1994;79:313–319.
23. Ferrari LR, Donlon JV: A comparison of propofol, midazolam, and methohexital for sedation during retrobulbar and peribulbar block. J Clin Anesth 1992;4:93–96.
24. Ghouri AF, Ramirez Ruiz MA, White PF: Effect of flumazenil on recovery after midazolam and propofol sedation. Anesthesiology 1994;81:333–339.
25. Taylor E, Ghouri AF, White PF: Midazolam in combination with propofol for sedation during local anesthesia. J Clin Anesth 1992;4:213.
26. Sá Rêgo MM, Inagaki Y, White PF: The cost-effectiveness of methohexital versus propofol for sedation during monitored anesthesia care. Anesth Analg 1999;88:723–728.
27. Ramirez-Ruiz M, Smith I, White PF: Use of analgesics during propofol sedation: A comparison of ketorolac, dezocine, and fentanyl. J Clin Anesth 1995;7:481–485.
28. Gesztesi Z, Sa Rego MM, White PF: The comparative effectiveness of fentanyl and its newer analogs during extracorporeal shock wave lithotripsy under monitored anesthesia care. Anesth Analg 2000;90:567–570.
29. Avramov MN, White PF: Use of alfentanil and propofol for outpatient monitored anesthesia care. Determining the optimal dosing regimen. Anesth Anlag 1997;85:566–572.
30. Dilger JA, Sprung J, Maurer W, et al: Remifentanil provides better analgesia than alfentanil during breast biopsy surgery under monitored anesthesia care. Can J Anaesth 2004;51:20–24.
31. Avramov MN, Smith I, White PF: Interactions between midazolam and remifentanil during monitored anesthesia care. Anesthesiology 1996;85:1283–1289.
32. Gold MI, Watkins WD, Sung YF, et al: Remifentanil versus remifentanil/midazolam for ambulatory surgery during monitored anesthesia care. Anesthesiology 1997;87:51–57.
33. Smith I, Avramov MN, White PF: A comparison of propofol and remifentanil during monitored anesthesia care. J Clin Anesth 1997;9:148–154.
34. Krenn H, Deusch E, Jellinek H, et al: Remifentanil or propofol for sedation during carotid endarterectomy under cervical plexus block. Br J Anaesth 2002;89:637–640.
35. Sa Rego MM, Inagaki Y, White PF: Remifentanil administration during monitored anesthesia care: Are intermittent boluses an effective alternative to a continuous infusion? Anesth Analg 1999;88:518–522.
36. Moerman AT, Struys MM, Vereecke HE, et al: Remifentanil used to supplement propofol does not improve quality of sedation during spontaneous respiration. J Clin Anesth 2004;16:237–243.
37. Bosek V, Smith DB, Cox C: Ketorolac or fentanyl to supplement local anesthesia? J Clin Anesth 1992;4:480–483.
38. Coloma M, White PF, Huber PJ, et al: The effect of ketorolac on recovery after anorectal surgery: Intravenous versus local administration. Anesth Analg 2000;90:1107–1110.
39. Place RJ, Coloma M, White PF, et al: Ketorolac improves recovery after outpatient anorectal surgery. Dis Colon Rectum 2000;43:804–808.
40. Reinhardt S, Burkhardt U, Nestler A, et al: Use of piritramide for analgesia and sedation during peribulbar nerve block for cataract surgery. Ophthalmologica 2002;216:256–260.
41. Clerc S, Vuilleumier H, Frascarolo P, et al: Is the effect of inguinal field block with 0.5% bupivacaine on postoperative pain after hernia repair enhanced by addition of ketorolac or S(+) ketamine? Clin J Pain 2005;21:101–105.
42. Burmeister MA, Standl TG, Wintruff M, et al: Dolasetron prophylaxis reduces nausea and postanesthesia recovery time after remifentanil infusion during monitored anaesthesia care for extracorporeal shock wave lithotripsy. Br J Anaesth 2003;90:194–198.
43. White PF: Use of ketamine for sedation and analgesia during injection of local anesthetics. Ann Plast Surg 1985;15:53–56.
44. Blakeley KR, Klein KW, White PF, et al: A total intravenous anesthetic technique for outpatient facial laser resurfacing. Anesth Analg 1998;87:827–829.
45. Monk TG, Rater JM, White PF: Comparison of alfentanil and ketamine infusions in combination with midazolam for outpatient lithotripsy. Anesthesiology 1991;74:1023–1028.
46. Badrinath S, Avramov MN, Shadrick M, et al: The use of a ketamine-propofol combination during monitored anesthesia care. Anesth Analg 2000;90:858–862.

47. Mortero RF, Clark LD, Tolan MM, et al: The effects of small-dose ketamine on propofol sedation: Respiration, postoperative mood, perception, cognition, and pain. Anesth Analg 2001;92:1465–1469.

48. Adam S, van Bommel J, Pelka M, et al: Propofol-induced injection pain: Comparison of a modified propofol emulsion to standard propofol with premixed lidocaine. Anesth Analg 2004;99:1076–1079.

49. Fechner J, Ihmsen H, Hatterscheid D, et al: Comparative pharmacokinetics and pharmacodynamics of the new propofol prodrug GPI 15715 and propofol emulsion. Anesthesiology 2004;101:626–639.

50. Song D, Hamza MA, White PF, et al: Comparison of a lower-lipid propofol emulsion with standard emulsion for sedation during monitored anesthesia care. Anesthesiology 2004;100:1072–1075.

51. Kumar A, Bose S, Bhattacharya A, et al: Oral clonidine premedication for elderly patients undergoing intraocular surgery. Acta Anaesthesiol Scand 1992;36:159–164.

52. Jaakola ML: Dexmedetomidine premedication before intravenous regional anesthesia in minor outpatient hand surgery. J Clin Anesth 1994;6:204–211.

53. Aho MS, Erkola O, Kallio A, et al: Comparison of dexmedetomidine and midazolam sedation and antagonism of dexmedetomidine with atipamezole. J Clin Anesth 1993;5:194–203.

54. Arain SR, Ebert TJ: The efficacy, side effects, and recovery characteristics of dexmedetomidine versus propofol when used for intraoperative sedation. Anesth Analg 2002;95:461–466.

55. Hall JE, Uhrich TD, Barney JA, et al: Sedative, amnestic, and analgesic properties of small-dose dexmedetomidine infusions. Anesth Analg 2000;90:699–705.

56. Turan A, Memis D, Karamanlioglu B, et al: The analgesic effects of gabapentin in monitored anesthesia care for ear-nose-throat surgery. Anesth Analg 2004;99:375–378.

57. Hill CM, Balkenohl M, Thomas DW, et al: Pregabalin in patients with postoperative dental pain. Eur J Pain 2001;5:119–124.

58. Dahl JB, Mathiesen O, Moiniche S: "Protective premedication": An option with gabapentin and related drugs? A review of gabapentin and pregabalin in the treatment of post-operative pain. Acta Anaesthesiol Scand 2004;48:1130–1136.

59. Zarate E, Sa Rego MM, White PF, et al: Comparison of adenosine and remifentanil infusions as adjuvants to desflurane anesthesia. Anesthesiology 1999;90:956–963.

60. Coloma M, Duffy LL, White PF, et al: Dexamethasone facilitates discharge after outpatient anorectal surgery. Anesth Analg 2001;92:85–88.

61. Zheng C, Wang Z, Lacroix JS: Effect of intranasal treatment with capsaicin on the recurrence of polyps after polypectomy and ethmoidectomy. Acta Otolaryngol 2000;120:62–66.

62. Ghouri AF, Taylor E, White PF: Patient-controlled drug administration during local anesthesia: A comparison of midazolam, propofol and alfentanil. J Clin Anesth 1992;4:476–479.

63. Osborne GA, Rudkin GE, Curtis NJ, et al: Intra-operative patient-controlled sedation. Comparison of patient-controlled propofol with anaesthetist-administered midazolam and fentanyl. Anaesthesia 1991;46:553–556.

64. Rudkin GE, Osborne GA, Finn BP, et al: Intra-operative patient-controlled sedation. Comparison of patient-controlled propofol with patient-controlled midazolam. Anaesthesia 1992;47:376–381.

65. Osborne GA, Rudkin GE, Jarvis DA, et al: Intra-operative patient-controlled sedation and patient attitude to control. A crossover comparison of patient preference for patient-controlled propofol and propofol by continuous infusion. Anaesthesia 1994;49:287–292.

66. Balkan BK, Iyilikci L, Gunene F, et al: Comparison of sedation requirements for cataract surgery under topical anesthesia or retrobulbar block. Eur J Ophthalmol 2004;14:473–477.

67. Esen E, Ustun Y, Balcioglu YO, et al: Evaluation of patient-controlled remifentanil application in third molar surgery. J Oral Maxillofac Surg 2005;63:457–463.

68. Ibrahim AE, Ghoneim MM, Kharasch ED, et al: Speed of recovery and side-effect profile of sevoflurane sedation compared with midazolam. Anesthesiology 2001;94:87–94.

69. Ibrahim AE, Taraday JK, Kharasch ED: Bispectral index monitoring during sedation with sevoflurane, midazolam, and propofol. Anesthesiology 2001;95:1151–1159.

70. White PF, Coleman JE: Commentary on comparing intravenous "conscious" sedation with monitored anesthesia care (MAC) for aesthetic surgery. Plast Reconstr Surg 2003;112:1690–1691.

71. Callesen T, Bech K, Kehlet H: One-thousand consecutive inguinal hernia repairs under unmonitored local anesthesia. Anesth Analg 2001;93:1373–1376.

72. Cruise CJ, Chung F, Yogendran S, et al: Music increases satisfaction in elderly outpatients undergoing cataract surgery. Can J Anaesth 1997;44:43.

73. Koch ME, Kain ZN, Ayoub C, Rosenbaum SH: The sedative and analgesic sparing effect of music. Anesthesiology 1998;89:300–306.

74. Baghdadi ZD: A comparison of parenteral and electronic dental anesthesia during operative procedures in children. Gen Dent 2000;48:150–156.

75. White PF, Li S, Chiu JW: Electroanalgesia: Its role in acute and chronic pain management. Anesth Analg 2001;92:505–513.

76. Hermes D, Turebger D, Hakim SG, et al: Tape recorded hypnosis in oral and maxillofacial surgery—Basics and first clinical experience. J Craniomaxillofac Surg 2005;33:123–129.

77. White PF: The changing role of non-opioid analgesic techniques in the management of postoperative pain. Anesth Analg 2005;101: S5–S22.

78. Hasen KV, Samartzis D, Casas LA, et al: An outcome study comparing intravenous sedation with midazolam/fentanyl (conscious sedation) versus propofol infusion (deep sedation) for aesthetic surgery. Plast Reconstr Surg 2003;112:1683–1689.

79. Kehlet H, White PF: Optimizing anesthesia for inguinal herniorrhaphy: General, regional, or local anesthesia? Anesth Analg 2001;93:1367–1369.

80. Wilhelm W, Hammadeh ME, White PF, et al: General anesthesia versus monitored anesthesia care with remifentanil for assisted reproductive technologies: Effect on pregnancy rate. J Clin Anesth 2002;14:1–5.

81. Bordahl PE, Raeder JC, Nordentoft J, et al: Laparoscopic sterilization under local or general anesthesia? A randomized study. Obstet Gynecol 1993;81:137.

82. Patel N, Smith CE, Pinchak AC, et al: Desflurane is not associated with faster operating room exit times in outpatients. J Clin Anesth 1996;8:130–135.

83. Song D, Greilich NB, White PF, et al: Recovery profiles and costs of anesthesia for outpatient unilateral inguinal herniorrhaphy. Anesth Analg 2000;91:876–881.

84. Li S, Coloma M, White PF, et al: Comparison of the costs and recovery profiles of three anesthetic techniques for ambulatory anorectal surgery. Anesthesiology 2000;93:1225–1230.

85. Sungurtekin H, Sungurtekin U, Erdem E: Local anesthesia and midazolam versus spinal anesthesia in ambulatory pilonidal surgery. J Clin Anesth 2003;15:201–205.

86. Hadzic A, Arliss J, Kerimoglu B, et al: A comparison of infraclavicular nerve block versus general anesthesia for hand and wrist day-case surgeries. Anesthesiology 2004;101:127–132.

87. Hadzic A, Karaca PE, Hobeika P, et al: Peripheral nerve blocks result in superior recovery profile compared with general anesthesia in outpatient knee arthroscopy. Anesth Analg 2005;100:976–981.

88. Williams BA, Kentor ML, William JP, et al: Process analysis in outpatient knee surgery: Effects of regional and general anesthesia on anesthesia-controlled time. Anesthesiology 2000;93:529–538.

89. Kilmer SL, Chotzen V, Zelickson BD, et al: Full-face laser resurfacing using a supplemented topical anesthesia protocol. Arch Dermatol 2003;139:1279–1283.

90. White PF: Choice of peripheral nerve block for inguinal herniorrhaphy: Is better the enemy of good? Anesth Analg 2006;102, 1073.

Clinical Practice of Regional Anesthesia

12

Local Infiltration Anesthesia

Tony Tsai, MD • Jeffrey Gadsden, MD • Cliff Connery, MD

▮ INTRODUCTION

Many procedures can be performed with the use of local anesthetic alone, instilled at or near the site of surgery. Often this can be done by the surgeon without the use or assistance of an anesthesiologist. Local infiltration is also technically easy to perform and requires minimal postoperative care. Together, these factors contribute to its popularity and nearly ubiquitous application as a means of anesthesia for small minimally invasive procedures and operations. This technique is relatively safe as well, but does require an understanding of basic local anesthetic pharmacology, especially with respect to dosing and toxicity, as well as skill for successful application.

History of Local Anesthesia

There are several references throughout history of efforts to produce local anesthesia by various means.[1] Ancient Egyptians believed that the fat of the crocodile could induce anesthesia if placed on the skin of a patient. The same people also believed that the stone of Memphis could produce local anesthesia if rubbed on the skin with vinegar. Chinese physicians were known to use a mixture of jimson weed, marijuana, deadly nightshade, and mandrake placed into calamus leaves and burned over the operative or painful site to produce anesthesia. In the sixteenth century, Marco Aurelio Severino, an Italian anatomist and surgeon, advocated the use of cold to decrease pain, and this principle was frequently put to use by Napoleon's military surgeons. Other methods of inducing anesthesia locally included electrical current and superficial application of volatile liquids. The first clinical use of a local anesthetic was in 1884, when Austrian ophthalmologist Carl Koller used raw cocaine topically to anesthetize a patient's eye. After this, the use of local anesthetics spread quickly, especially with the synthesis of less toxic compounds such as procaine and lidocaine.[2]

General Principles of Local Infiltration Anesthesia

The aim of local infiltration is to anesthetize nerve endings in a finite area of tissue by the injection of local anesthetics nearby. This stands in contrast to peripheral nerve blocks, in which nerve axons are the target and the injection may take place in an area removed from the surgical site (eg, brachial plexus block for hand surgery). The depth of the area to be operated on typically determines the required extent of infiltration. For superficial skin procedures such as suturing of lacerations and skin biopsies, subcutaneous or intradermal infiltration is sufficient. More extensive operations may demand infiltration into muscle, fascia, and other deep tissues.

Two general approaches exist for anesthetizing skin and subcutaneous tissue. The first involves injecting local anesthetic directly into the line of incision and nearby tissues, effectively flooding the individual local nerve endings to produce anesthesia. This can be very effective, but may require large volumes of local anesthetic to achieve complete coverage.

In contrast, field or ring blocks encircle the site of incision with walls of local anesthetic solution through which nerve fibers must pass before branching into terminal nerve endings (Figure 12–1). Field blocks carry several advantages over direct injection into the incision line. First, although discrete nerves are not specifically blocked, less solution is usually required. Furthermore, because the solution is not injected directly in the wound, no anatomic distortion is produced at the surgical site. Wound healing is not affected by field block because it may be from local edema of infiltration. Finally, field blocks are useful when direct injection into the surgical site may be troublesome or harmful (eg, to avoid rupturing a cyst or spreading malignant cells).

Field blocks can also be performed using a single line of local anesthesia "upstream" from the incision site, thereby anesthetizing any skin distal to the injection. For example, a 5- to 6-cm line of subcutaneous local anesthetic extending across the lateral styloid process at the wrist effectively anesthetizes any superficial terminal branches of the radial nerve beyond the wrist. Clearly, this requires a working knowledge of peripheral nerve anatomy.

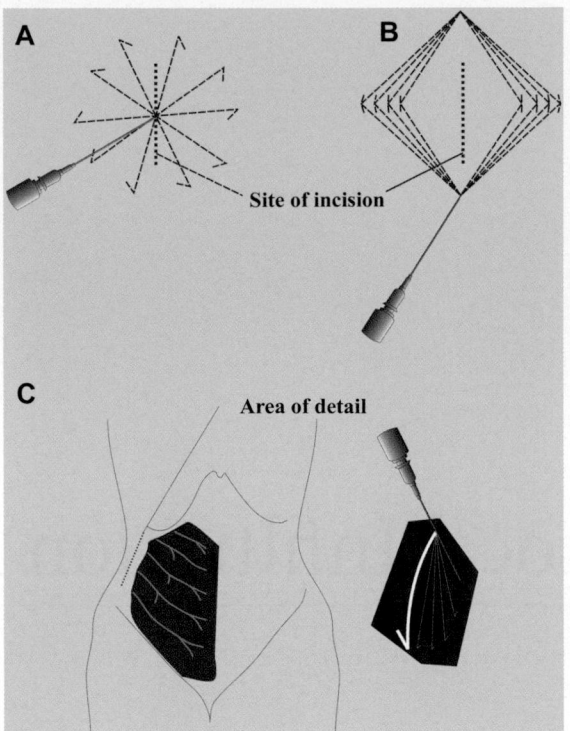

Figure 12–1. Skin and subcutaneous tissues can be anesthetized by (**A**) injecting local anesthetic directly into the line of incision and nearby tissues or (**A** and **B**) field or ring blocks that encircle the site of incision with walls of local anesthetic solution through which nerve fibers must pass before branching into terminal nerve endings. **C:** Area of detail.

Clinical Pearls

Two general approaches exist for anesthetizing skin and subcutaneous tissue:
- Injection of local anesthetic directly into the line of incision and nearby tissues effectively floods the local nerve endings to produce anesthesia. This can be very effective, but may require large volumes of local anesthetic to achieve complete coverage.
- Field or ring blocks encircle the site of incision with walls of local anesthetic solution through which nerve fibers must pass before branching into terminal nerve endings

Choice of Local Anesthetic Solutions

The choice of local anesthetic agent depends on the size of the area to be anesthetized and on the desired duration of action. If a large surface is involved, large volumes of diluted agents should be used to avoid exceeding the maximum dosage limits of the various agents (Table 12–1).

Maximum safe dosages of local anesthetics for local and infiltrational anesthesia are controversial. Traditionally, manufacturers have cited these in the form of a single dose (eg, 300 mg for lidocaine) or a weight-related dose (eg, 3 mg/kg

Table 12–1.

Dosages and Duration of Commonly Used Local Anesthetics for Infiltration

Anesthetic	Duration Without Epinephrine (min)	Duration With Epinephrine (min)	Maximum Dose Without Epinephrine (mg/kg)	Maximum Dose With Epinephrine (mg/kg)
Ester-Type Local Anesthetic				
Procaine	15–30	30–90	7	8.5
Chloroprocaine	30–60	40–70	11	14
Amide-Type Local Anesthetic				
Lidocaine	60–120	90–180	4.5	7
Mepivacaine	60–120	60–120	4.5	7
Bupivacaine	180–360	300–480	3	3
Ropivacaine	180–360	180–360	3	3

for bupivacaine). However, the rate of systemic uptake differs markedly for different injection sites and is related to both the vascularity at the site of administration and the tissue binding of the local anesthetic.[3] For instance, local anesthetic administered via an intercostal block results in significantly higher peak plasma concentrations when compared with the epidural or brachial plexus routes. Subcutaneous infiltration appears to produce relatively low plasma levels of local anesthetic compared with equivalent doses used via the epidural, caudal, brachial plexus, and intercostal routes. For example, to produce the same peak plasma level of lidocaine, twice as much local anesthetic is required via the subcutaneous route than for the epidural route. This should not be seen as an invitation to administer subcutaneous local anesthetic without regard for toxicity issues, as systemic toxicity has been described.[4,5] Rather, it highlights the need for further study into site and agent-specific dosing guidelines. More discussion on pharmacology of local anesthetics can be found in Chapter 6.

Epinephrine is often added to aid in hemostasis, prolong duration of anesthesia, and reduce the absorption rate of local anesthetic, thereby reducing the risk of systemic toxicity when higher doses of local anesthesia are used.[6] The usefulness of this adjuvant depends on the intrinsic vasoactive properties of a particular local anesthetic. For example, lidocaine in clinical doses is a potent vasodilator and is therefore amenable to the vasoconstrictive properties of epinephrine. In fact, epinephrine 5 mcg/mL (1:200 000) has been shown to reduce peak plasma levels after subcutaneous infiltration by 50%.[7] On the other hand, ropivacaine is itself a mild vasoconstrictor, and the addition of epinephrine provides a smaller advantage in this context. Bupivacaine, a vasodilator, increases capillary blood flow significantly when injected in the skin.[8] Typical concentrations of epinephrine added to

local anesthetic solution range from 1:200,000 to 1:500,000. Epinephrine is often avoided when local anesthetic solutions are used for extremities such as fingers, toes, nose, or penis to avoid ischemic tissue damage, although such risk remains controversial.

Although the duration of action varies for various agents, the onset of action is almost immediate for most local anesthetics when administered subcutaneously. In contrast to peripheral nerve blocks, even dilute solutions can provide excellent analgesia and operating conditions. For example, lidocaine 0.5% is a common concentration used to maximize the available volume without exceeding toxic limits.

Clinical Pearls

Strategies to lessen the degree of pain on injection include:
- The use of a small-gauge needle (eg, 25- to 30-gauge)
- Slow administration of the local anesthetic
- Buffering of local anesthetic solutions (except bupivacaine and ropivacaine) with sodium bicarbonate (1 mEq/mL of $NaHCO_3$ to 10 mL of lidocaine)

Communication with the patient is an important aspect of local infiltration. Frequent reassessment of the quality of anesthesia is reassuring to the patient and helps to prevent unexpected movement as a result of painful stimuli. In addition to the discomfort of a needle puncture, injection of local anesthetic itself can be painful.[9] Patients often describe an initial burning sensation, which is felt to be due in part to the acidic nature of these solutions or a mechanical pressure to the nerve endings.[10,11] Certain agents such as etidocaine are associated with more severe pain, whereas lidocaine is perceived as less painful.[12] Strategies to lessen the degree of pain on injection include the use of a small needle (eg, 25- to 30-gauge) and slow administration of the local anesthetic.[13] Buffering of lidocaine solutions with sodium bicarbonate is also effective at reducing the sting of injection and is accomplished by adding 1 mL of an 8.4% solution (1 mEq/mL) to 10 mL of lidocaine.[14]

Complications & Side Effects

Complications due to local infiltration fall into two broad categories: allergic reactions and systemic toxicity. True allergy to local anesthetics is rare. Not infrequently a patient may report an "allergy" to local anesthesia when in fact what was experienced was a vagal reaction or a response to intravascular injection of the anesthetic or epinephrine. Genuine allergic reactions typically produce rash, urticaria, and/or upper airway edema.[9] False-positives also occur and are much more common. For instance, a nonallergic reaction to a local anesthetic injection that produced life-threatening airway swelling was later found on testing to be angioedema secondary to C1-esterase inhibitor deficiency.[15] Allergies to local anesthetics are almost always due to the metabolite para-aminobenzoic acid (PABA) in ester anesthetics or the preservative methylparaben in amide anesthetics.[16] These patients may have a history of allergy to various cosmetic preparations (PABA is a common ingredient). If in doubt regarding a patient allergy, it is safest to administer a preservative-free amide anesthetic.

The toxic profile of local anesthetics primarily affects the central nervous system (CNS) and cardiovascular systems. The risk of toxicity is for the most part related to the potency of the anesthetic (eg, bupivacaine is more potent and therefore more toxic than lidocaine), the total dose administered, and the rate of systemic absorption. Clearance of local anesthetic rarely plays a role in toxicity unless continuous infusions are used. Symptoms of CNS toxicity range from mild complaints such as dizziness, perioral numbness, and a metallic taste to more severe neurologic signs such as restlessness, excitability, and disinhibition, aphasia, and finally seizures and/or coma. Cardiovascular toxicity is due to blockade of sodium channels in cardiac muscle and is manifested by ventricular dysrhythmias, bradycardia, depressed myocardial contractility, and cardiovascular collapse.

Despite the often-memorized range of symptoms, systemic toxicity can present without warning, and resuscitation equipment must be immediately available wherever local anesthetics are used. This includes oxygen, a bag-valve-mask and other airway management devices, and a cardiac defibrillator—either automated or manual. Benzodiazepines should also be on hand for treatment of seizures, as well as the equipment and medications for advanced cardiac life support medications. More in-depth discussions of the toxicity of local anesthetics can be found in Chapter 6.

TECHNIQUES FOR COMMON INDICATIONS

Wound & Laceration Closure

Infiltration of local anesthetic solution into wound edges is usually sufficient to permit cleansing, debridement, and suture repair. Lacerations are typically irrigated with sterile saline or washed with surgical soap before infiltration of local anesthetic solution, but this can be uncomfortable. A more thorough cleansing can be performed after anesthesia. The infiltration of local anesthetic from inside the wound is less painful than injection through intact skin.[17] The somatosensory innervation of skin is multifaceted and comprises both nociceptive free nerve endings and specialized receptors that transduce mechanical, thermal, and chemical stimuli.[18] It was once thought that the epidermis was not innervated, but this outermost layer is in fact rich in small, unmyelinated nociceptive fibers[19] (Figure 12–2). When anesthetizing skin, it is important to deposit local anesthetic in or just under the dermal layers because administration too deep in the subcutaneous fat may miss some of the more shallow fibers. Adipose tissue is generally poorly innervated, and placing local anesthetic deep in subcutaneous fat simply wastes drug while increasing the total dose administered—hence the risk of systemic toxicity.

Clinical Pearls

- Adipose tissue is generally poorly innervated.
- Injecting local anesthetic into the adipose tissue increases the total dose administered without significant analgesic/anesthetic benefit.

Infiltration of the wound at the end of the operation is an effective method of postoperative pain relief, especially when used as a component of multimodal analgesia.[20] This has been demonstrated for a wide variety of procedures, including laparoscopy,[21] laparotomy,[22] thyroid surgery,[23] and craniotomy.[24] For this to be successful, all layers of the wound, including muscles in fascial sheaths, must be injected with local anesthesia. Bupivacaine 0.25% can provide good quality pain control for 6 hours or more, depending on the site of the wound and the volume used to infiltrate the site. The anesthetic effect of wound infiltration may be prolonged by continuous infusion of local anesthesia through an implanted subcutaneous catheter system or by irrigation of the wound drain. Occasional reports of the use of this approach have appeared, but this technique has not achieved widespread popularity.[25,26]

In an animal model of wound infection, local anesthetic infiltration reduced wound bacterial counts by more than 70% over controls.[27] The addition of epinephrine to the anesthetic solution decreases bleeding from the wound edges, but may be associated with an increased rate of wound infection. When epinephrine is used for wound closure, a

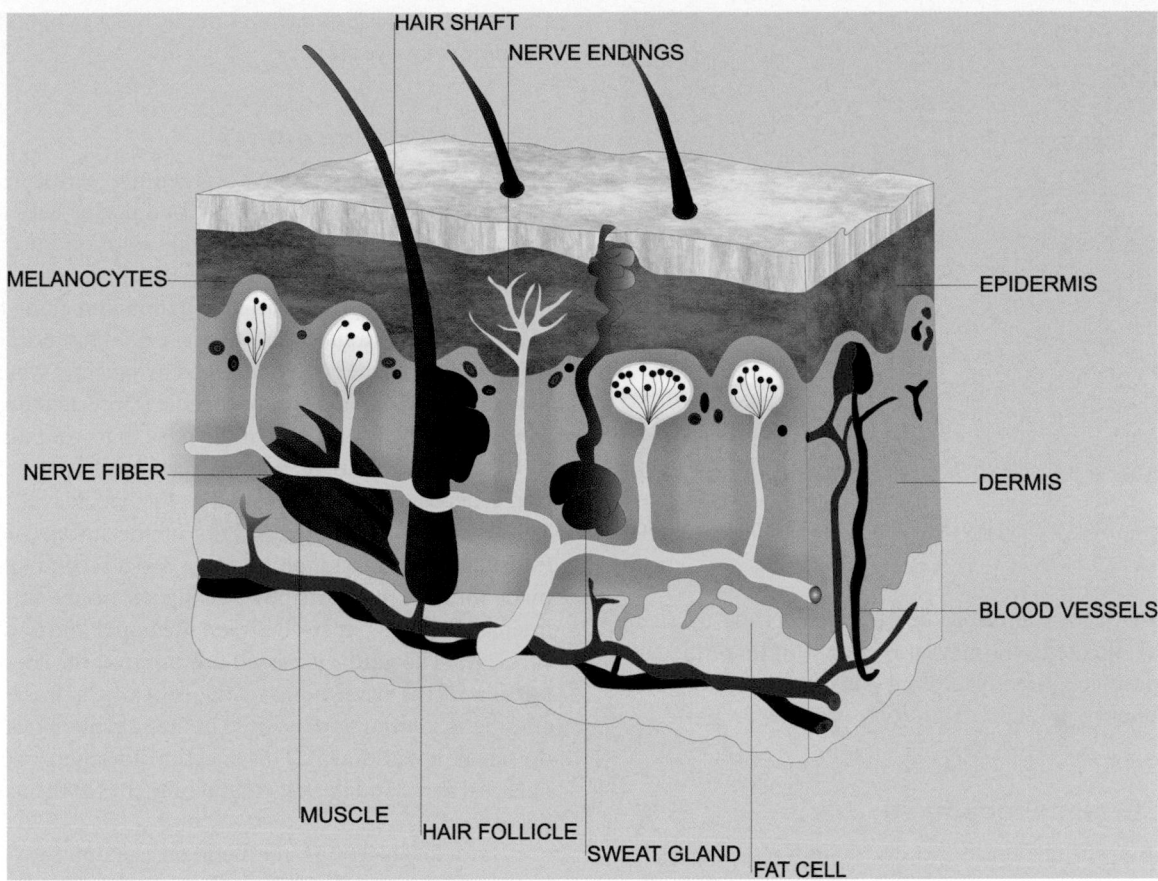

Figure 12–2. Anatomy of the skin and subcutaneous tissues. When anesthetizing skin, it is important to deposit local anesthetic in or just under the dermal layers because too deep of an administration in the subcutaneous fat may miss some of the more shallow fibers.

clinician may mistakenly believe that adequate hemostasis has been achieved owing to vasoconstriction. For this reason, it is often prudent practice to examine wounds for hematomas up to 24 hours after closure in these instances to ensure that bleeding has not recommenced after the drug effect has worn off.

Routine closure of linear scalp lacerations can be accomplished in the emergency room if the area is anesthetized with local anesthesia. Because of the rich vascularity of the scalp, careful attention to dosages of local anesthetics must be taken. Sedation should be used with caution in instances of an associated head injury. Local anesthetic solutions containing epinephrine are particularly helpful both in controlling troublesome scalp bleeding and in prolonging anesthesia. Regional and field blocks are useful for larger injuries, but direct infiltration of the margins of small lacerations provides, adequate analgesia for closure of the wound.

Hemostasis is particularly important when closing a facial wound, and attention must be paid to potentially serious bleeders when epinephrine has been used in the local anesthetic solution. Certain regions of the face, because of their unique anatomic or functional characteristics, require special consideration when injured. Lacerations of both the upper and lower lip are common. Small lacerations do not require

suturing and heal spontaneously. Through-and-through injuries are repaired in layers and if the laceration crosses the skin vermilion border, correct anatomic alignment of this border is important to promote proper healing and a good cosmetic result. The vermilion margin is marked with a dye (methylene blue, brilliant green, or India ink) before the injection of local anesthetic, because the local anesthetic solution blanches and distorts both skin and mucosa and makes recognition of the border difficult.

Excision of Superficial Lesions

Biopsies of tumors of skin, soft tissue, oral cavity, and lymph tissue can be performed under local anesthesia. Gentle aspiration should be performed before any injection to guard against intravascular injection. Topical sprays can be used occasionally, but the best anesthesia is achieved with injection at the surgical site. A 25-gauge needle is used to raise the skin wheal next to the biopsy site, followed by infiltration of the deeper tissues. It is preferable in this case to use the field block technique and avoid direct injection into the tumor (Figure 12–3).

Incision and drainage of hematomas or abscesses can be exquisitely painful without anesthesia, but can be effectively

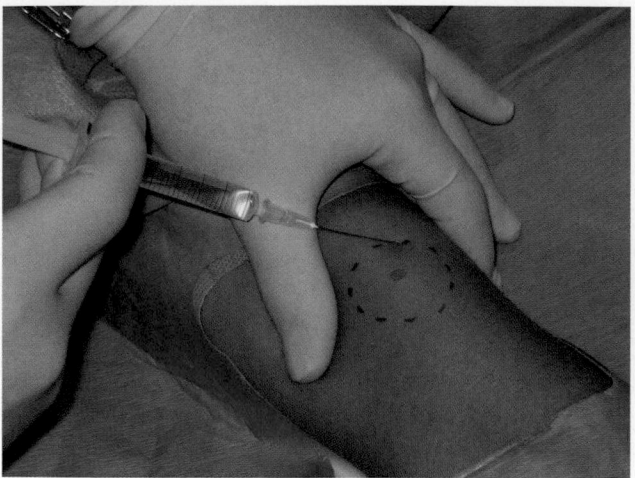

Figure 12–3. Ring or field block for excision of a small skin lesion.

managed with local infiltration.[28] Field blockade in a ring around the affected area may cause less pain than injection of local anesthetic directly into the skin overlying the abscess or hematoma.

Plastic Surgery Procedures

Many skin-grafting procedures are done under general or neuraxial anesthesia, especially if the donor and graft sites are remote from each other. However, it is possible to perform skin harvesting under local anesthesia. A large field block is effective for this purpose. For instance, a graft that is 2 cm^2 requires a donor area of approximately 4 cm^2 to be anesthetized via subcutaneous infiltration using a 2-inch needle and injecting approximately 10 mL of 0.5% lidocaine with epinephrine.

Although local anesthesia, even with epinephrine, is commonly used on "safe" flaps with good blood supply as in rhytidectomy, there is a reluctance to use this type of anesthesia on flaps with a somewhat compromised circulation. This is based on the empirical belief that vasoconstriction, needle puncture, and fluid infiltration may negatively influence flap survival. Local infiltrative anesthesia, even with epinephrine in a concentration of 1:200,000, probably has no harmful effect on the survival of primarily raised skin flaps.[29] For hemostasis, even lower doses of epinephrine can be used. Epinephrine in 1:800,000 dilution provides hemostasis comparable to higher, more commonly used concentrations. Epinephrine in concentrations of 1:100,000 or greater may be detrimental to flap survival.

Many cosmetic procedures are performed under local infiltration. Blepharoplasty, the removal of excess skin around the eye and orbit, is an example. After appropriate preoperative examination of the eye, including the lacrimal drainage system, muscle tone of the orbicularis oculi, and fundoscopic examination, the patient is lightly sedated. Infiltration is often carried out with 1% lidocaine with epinephrine, and the previously determined skin and periorbital fat are removed.

Chapter 21 describes various nerve block and infiltration techniques for eye surgery.

Head & Neck Procedures

Reduction of *nasal fracture* is sometimes performed under local anesthesia. One effective method begins with inserting cotton packs soaked with 4% cocaine solution into the nose. These packs should be placed along the course of the anterior nerves over the sphenopalatine ganglion and along the floor of the nose. Infiltration anesthesia with 1% lidocaine containing epinephrine is then initiated by raising a wheal lateral to each ala. A 2-inch, 27-gauge needle is inserted through the wheal along the lateral wall of the nose to its root just medial to the inner canthus of the eye. The local anesthetic solution is deposited along this tract as the needle is withdrawn. This injection anesthetizes fibers of the infratrochlear, infraorbital, and anterior alveolar nerves. A second injection is made through the nostril by passing the needle through the intercartilaginous sulcus between the upper and lower lateral cartilages. The needle is passed upward over the lateral dorsal portion of the nasal bone to the root of the nose, and the anesthetic solution is deposited in the subcutaneous tissue as the needle is withdrawn. This injection anesthetizes the external nasal nerve and the trigeminal branches of the nasociliary nerve.

Similar injections are made on the opposite side. The membranous septum and nasal spine are injected on each side, and the previously inserted nasal packs are removed. This technique, when performed properly, gives excellent anesthesia to the nose and allows the surgeon to manipulate the nose with little discomfort for the patient.

Many surgical *operations on structures in the neck* can be carried out under local anesthesia. Spanknebel and colleagues[30] reported a series of over 1000 patients in whom thyroidectomy was carried out with local anesthetic infiltration. Parathyroidectomy has been similarly performed in the same manner.[31] Occasionally, local anesthesia is the safest method of managing neck lesions such as tumors and hematomas that are compromising a patient's airway, especially if an awake endotracheal intubation cannot be performed. Prophylactic tracheostomy under local anesthesia is sometimes indicated when less invasive methods of airway management are expected to be unsuccessful or have already failed.[32] Manoppo[33] described the use of local anesthesia for the successful resection of an enormous goiter (75 × 60 × 45 cm), which was accomplished in the prone position because of the patient's dyspnea. The skin of the anterolateral neck is supplied by branches of the cervical plexus, which can be blocked as it emerges from under the lateral aspect of the sternocleidomastoid muscle, or alternatively a field block can be performed more medially. Note that some nerve fibers from the cervical plexus cross the midline to provide innervation to the contralateral side. For this reason, it is often useful to perform a subcutaneous midline injection from the thyroid cartilage to the sternal notch when unilateral anesthesia of the neck is desired. Figure 12–4 demonstrates infiltration

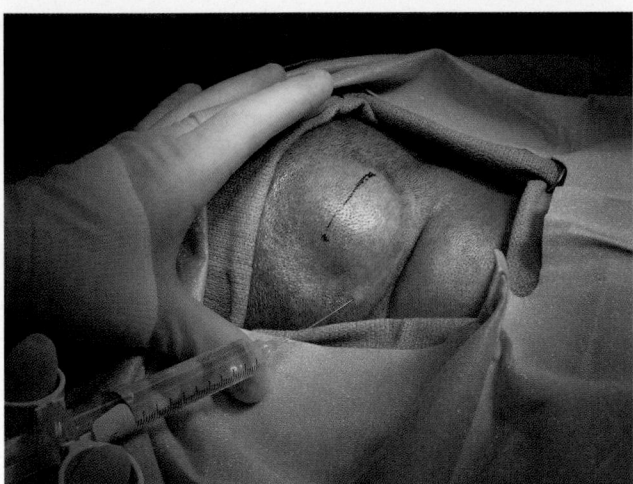

Figure 12–4. Infiltration anesthesia for removal of the lipoma on the back of the neck. Another superficial infiltration should be made along the incision line.

anesthesia for removal of the lipoma on the back of the neck; this helped prevent the need for general endotracheal anesthesia in the prone position for a relatively minor ambulatory procedure.

Preauricular cysts and accessory auricles are frequently excised under local anesthesia. The posterior aspect of the ear may be anesthetized by infiltration close to the posterior aspect of the auricle over the mastoid process with 5–10 mL of local anesthetic. The auriculotemporal nerve is blocked by infiltration of 5–10 mL of local anesthetic anterior to the ear, beginning at the zygoma. Clinically, this infiltration provides adequate anesthesia for procedures such as otoplasty, reconstruction of pinna, and excision of cysts. Occasionally, anesthesia of the concha may be inadequate, but this area can be blocked with subcutaneous infiltration of 2–3 mL of local anesthetic posteriorly through the conchal cartilage.

Procedures on the Trunk

Superficial or minor surgical procedures of the truncal area, such as excision of superficial lesions, central venous catheter placement, minor incision and drainage procedures, and excisional breast biopsies, may be performed under local, intercostal, or field block.

Adequate anesthesia of the chest wall for thoracic procedures (eg, thoracocentesis, thoracostomy, pleural biopsy) may be accomplished by infiltration of the skin, rib periosteum intercostal muscle, and parietal pleura with local anesthetic. In addition, for chest tube placement an intercostal nerve block can enhance the pain control (see Chapter 44). The visceral pleura is not innervated by somatic nerves.

An abdominal field block can be performed by subcutaneous infiltration of the anterolateral chest and abdominal wall. Below the costal margin, the field block can be extended along the anterior axillary line until the anterior superior iliac spine of the iliac bone is encountered; this is also known as the costoiliac block.

The tough fibrous anterior rectus sheath requires a more specialized *rectus field block* for midline incisions. Because there are tendinous intersections within the rectus muscle itself, two to six sites may need to be injected, depending on the location and size of the surgical incision. With the patient lying supine, at points 3 cm from the midline bilaterally, a short-bevel 5-cm, 22-gauge needle is passed posteriorly through the skin and subcutaneous tissue until firm resistance of the anterior rectus sheath is encountered. If this sheath is not demonstrated convincingly, the block should be discontinued. With controlled steady pressure, a definitive pop is felt as the needle penetrates this sheath.

As the needle is further advanced through the softer belly of the muscle, it approaches the posterior rectus sheath, which is apparent as the second firm resistance. At this point, 10 mL of local anesthetic are injected. Blocks above the umbilicus should be performed first, and needle depth should be noted before attempting blocks below the umbilicus, where injection is made just after the loss of first resistance, signifying the anterior sheath.

Rectus block is used in the management of surgical pain after incisional and umbilical hernias, postpartum and laparoscopic tubal ligation, cesarean section delivery when a midline incision is used, and outpatient laparoscopy.[34,35] Infiltration and field blocks are also helpful in diagnosing abdominal nerve entrapment syndromes and localized myofascial problems.

Orthopedic Procedures

Superficial procedures of the hand or foot may be amenable to local infiltration, although a digital, wrist, or ankle block is often a more efficacious method with less use of local anesthetic. Epinephrine-containing local anesthetics should be avoided when infiltrating into distal extremities.

Certain operations for decompression of subcutaneously located peripheral nerves can be carried out safely in the outpatient clinic. Transverse carpal ligament section for median nerve entrapment (carpal tunnel syndrome) and ulnar nerve transposition for ulnar nerve entrapment (tardy ulnar palsy) can both be performed under local infiltration.

Local anesthesia for *knee arthroscopy* is often used for simple arthroscopies (Figure 12–5). Both sites of port insertion are infiltrated with local anesthetic. The bulk of the anesthesia is provided by an intraarticular injection of local anesthetic, which anesthetizes the synovium, the most sensitive aspect of the joint capsule. Often 0.5% bupivacaine is used for its postoperative duration of action. The needle is inserted into the skin beneath the patella and above the joint fat pad. A loss of resistance or "give" is often appreciated when the needle enters the joint space, allowing the local to be injected freely. Injection into the fat pad should be avoided because this causes it to swell, obscuring the field of view during arthroscopy. The two portal sites can be infiltrated with 5–6 mL each of lidocaine 1% with epinephrine. The meniscus cartilage has only a sparse sensitive nerve supply, and surgery on the meniscus is typically not painful. The intraarticular

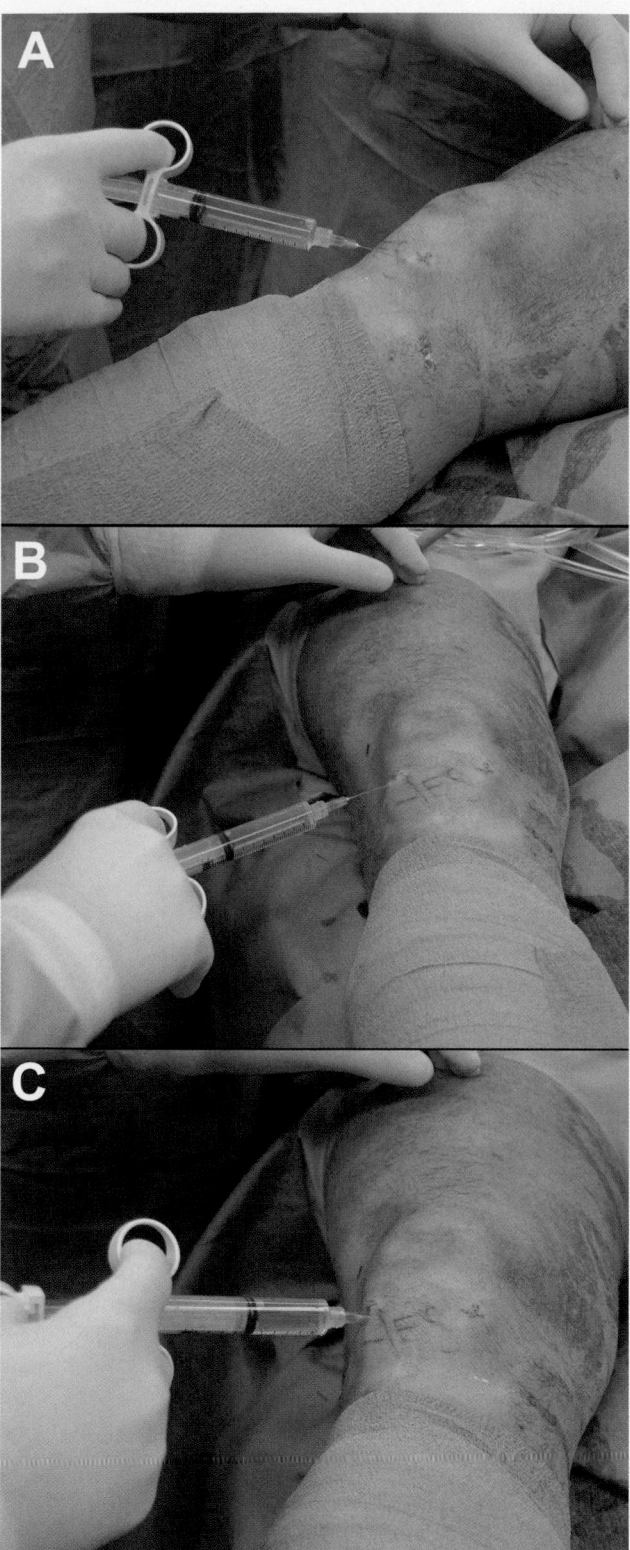

Figure 12–5. Local anesthesia for knee arthroscopy is often used for simple arthroscopies. **A** and **B:** Both sites of port insertion are infiltrated with local anesthetic. **C:** Local anesthetic (typically 20 mL of 0.25%–0.5% bupivacaine) is then injected intraarticularly.

injection of local anesthetic is often supplemented with intraarticular NSAIDs or opioids.[36]

Shoulder arthroscopy and subacromial decompression have also been described using a similar technique.[37] Local anesthetic infiltrated into the skin and underlying tissues as well as into the glenohumeral and subacromial joint provides adequate anesthesia for this operation.

Manipulation or examination of a painful or frozen joint can sometimes be achieved with an intraarticular injection of local anesthetic. Approximately 10 mL of 1% lidocaine usually provide good analgesia for large joints such as the knee or shoulder. Pain due to a rotator cuff tear can often be neutralized by a subacromial bursa injection of 1% lidocaine.

Breast Surgery

Infiltration anesthesia can be used for a wide variety of breast surgeries. Breast mass biopsy, reduction mammoplasty, simple mastectomy, and gynecomastia surgery all can be performed with local anesthetic infiltration and sedation. The large number of cutaneous nerve branches around the breast requires it to be completely encircled with local anesthetic solution to produce complete skin anesthesia. Nerves penetrating the lateral and inferior margins of the breast are anesthetized by blocking the second to sixth intercostal nerves. Thoracic epidural or paravertebral block can be performed to cover these same dermatomes. Medial nerve branches, overlapping from the opposite side, require skin infiltration along the entire sternum from the sternal notch to the xiphoid process. Superior branches from the supraclavicular nerves of the superficial cervical plexus require infiltration along the inferior edge of the clavicle from the acromion to the sternal notch. Branches arising from the deep tissues can be anesthetized by infiltration into the retromammary space between the pectoralis major muscle and the breast and by infiltration posterior to the pectoral muscles, where they are innervated by the medial and lateral pectoral nerves.

For biopsy of a breast mass, the mass is stabilized with one hand, and skin and subcutaneous tissue are infiltrated with 1% lidocaine. For an incisional breast biopsy, an incision site is chosen, and the area of proposed incision is infiltrated with lidocaine.

When performing reduction mammoplasty, local infiltration of 0.5% lidocaine with epinephrine (1:200,000) is administered along with intravenous sedation and analgesia. The "superwet infiltration method" with 240 mL per breast of 1:1,000,000 epinephrine has been shown to reduce blood loss, operative time, and sponge use without increasing complications in breast reduction surgery compared with standard infiltration along incision lines (25 mL per breast of 1:100,000 epinephrine).[38] Although not common, reduction mammoplasty can be performed under local anesthesia and sedation as an outpatient procedure.[39]

One technique for infiltrating the breast for simple mastectomy is to inject local anesthetic along the proposed skin incision intradermally with further infiltration into the pectoral fascia. More local anesthetic is injected as needed into

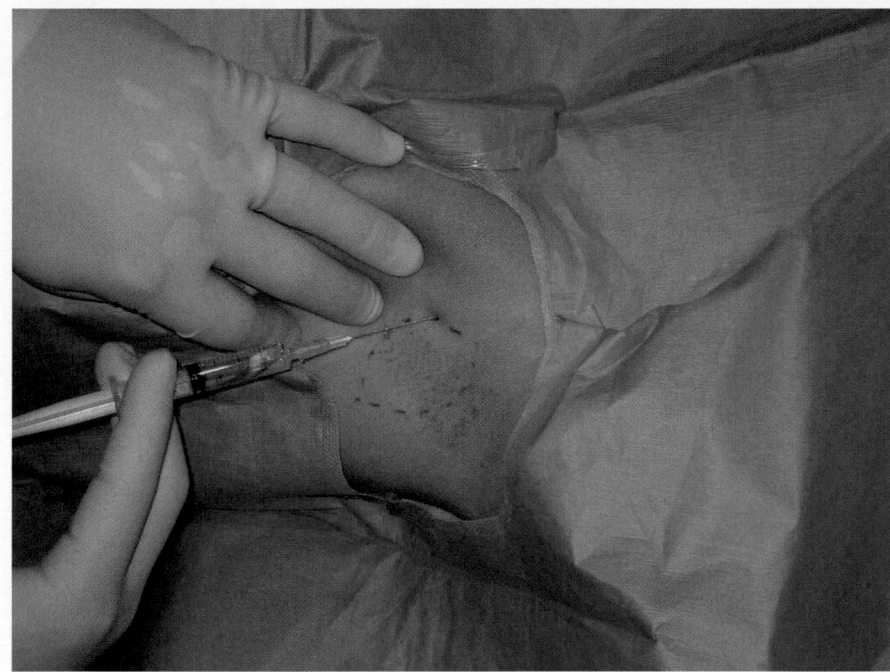

Figure 12–6. Field block in the axilla for lymph node biopsy.

the surrounding tissues. Alternatively, a field block lateral to the breast can anesthetize much of the skin, allowing for less tissue deformation if this is desired. When injecting the area of prepectoral breast, the pleural cavity is well protected by the pectoralis muscle. However, when injecting the area of the inframammary crease, the surgeon has to be careful to insert the needle superficially to avoid inadvertent entry into the pleural cavity.

Although the likelihood of a clinically significant pneumothorax occurring with a 25-gauge needle is small, it is best to exercise caution when injecting in this area. Local anesthesia of the breast, especially for deep lesions, requires a generous amount of anesthetic. For this reason, it is probably more appropriate to perform thoracic paravertebral or thoracic epidural anesthesia for bilateral operations, so as to avoid local anesthetic systemic toxicity.

Because the histology of the axillary lymph node is the most important prognostic indicator of breast cancer, performing a *sentinel lymph node biopsy* is a common operation.[40] Sentinel lymph node biopsy can be performed as an outpatient procedure under local anesthesia with or without sedation. After locating the sentinel lymph node with a gamma probe, the area is marked on the skin, and local anesthesia is infiltrated along the incision line[41] (Figure 12–6). Additional local anesthetic is injected as necessary into the surrounding tissues. Using local anesthesia allows early diagnosis of the lymph node pathology, acquired on an outpatient basis with minimal discomfort to the patient.[42]

Inguinal Hernia Repair

Local infiltration is a very common method of anesthesia for inguinal hernia repair.[43] Block of afferent nociceptive signals from the surgical site decreases postoperative analgesic re-

quirements and may have a preemptive analgesic effect manifested by decreased long-term pain.[44] The resulting analgesia involves a limited area and does not interfere with the function of other organs. Muscle relaxation is limited to the area of operation and does not interfere with ventilation, and there is considerably less postoperative nausea, retching, and vomiting when regional anesthesia is used. Local or regional field block has been associated with a lower incidence of urinary retention compared with general or spinal anesthesia[45] and is also associated with decreased costs associated with general anesthesia and recovery room time.[46] Unlike spinal anesthesia, local or regional field anesthesia is not associated with hypotension. In addition, the immediate postanesthetic period is pain-free, especially if a longer-acting local anesthetic is used. All of these factors permit early ambulation and resumption of oral intake and require minimal postoperative care.

The technique of local infiltration first developed by Harvey Cushing consists of successive infiltration and incision of the various layers of the abdominal wall and direct application of local anesthetic to the ilioinguinal nerve when it is exposed. After the surgical field is prepared, a series of intracutaneous injections with a 22- to 25-gauge needle is made along the course of the proposed incision site (Figure 12–7). Subcutaneous infiltration is next carried out with a long needle (Figure 12–8). A total of 10–15 mL of solution is injected while the needle is being advanced and withdrawn along the line of incision. Except in very obese people, it is relatively easy to feel the needle as it is directed beneath the skin. Analgesia may be expected within 1–2 minutes because very small, virtually unprotected nerves are involved. After anesthesia has been ascertained by pinching the skin with an Allis forceps, the incision is made from the skin down to the aponeurosis of the external oblique muscle. The edges of the

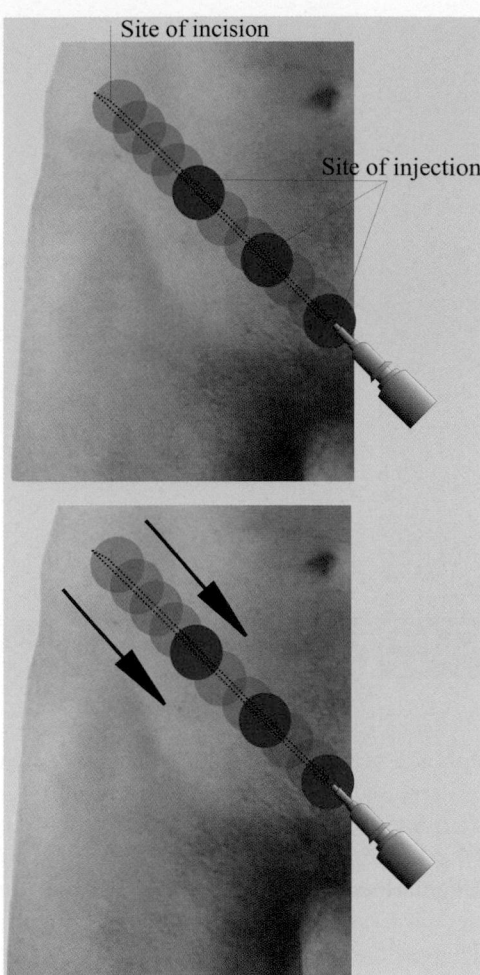

Figure 12–7. Local infiltration for inquinal hernia repair. After the surgical field is prepared, a series of intracutaneous injections with a 25-gauge needle is made along the course of the proposed incision site.

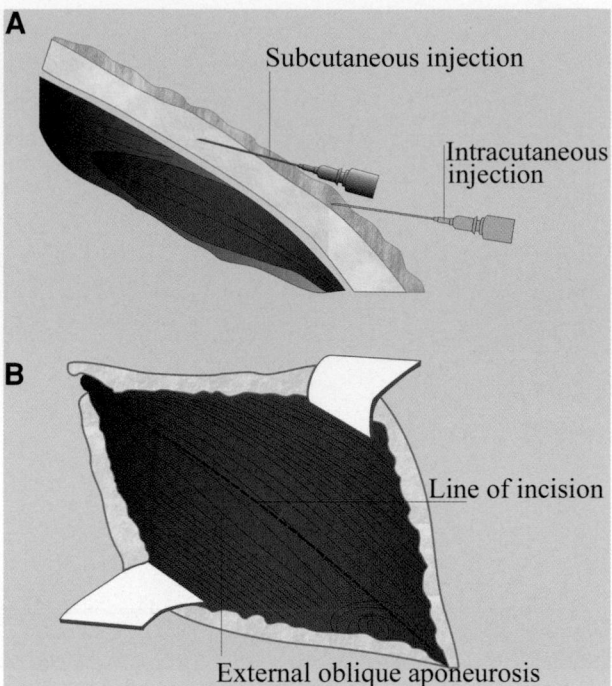

Figure 12–8. Local infiltration for inguinal hernia repair. A series of intracutaneous injections are made along the line of the incision, followed by a subcutaneous injection (*A*). **B:** Additional infiltration is performed along the site of incision through the muscle layer.

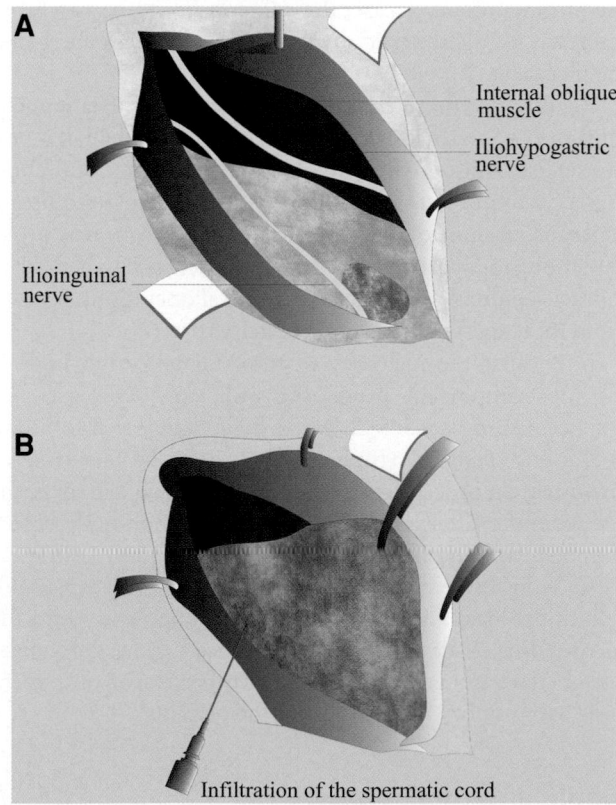

Figure 12–9. A: Location of the ilioinguinal and inguinal branch of iliohypogastric nerves with the herniorrhaphy exposure. **B:** Injection of the spermatic cord can be carried out under direct vision.

incision are gently separated to visualize this layer, and the infiltration is carried out along the line of next incision with 10 mL of anesthetic solution (see Figure 12–8). After 2–3 minutes, the aponeurosis is incised, exposing the spermatic cord and the internal oblique muscles. The ilioinguinal and the inguinal branch of iliohypogastric nerve are found at the lateral edge of the incision. Two to three mL of the local anesthetic solution are infiltrated around each of these nerves, with care being taken to avoid intraneural injection or traction. If the internal oblique muscle is to be incised for better visualization of the internal ring, it is infiltrated with an additional 8–10 mL of local anesthetic solution (Figure 12–9).

The final step is to inject 5–10 mL of solution into the region of the internal inguinal ring to block the genitofemoral nerve and the sensory fibers of spermatic plexus (see Figure 12–9). As the local anesthetic penetrates the area, it readily diffuses into the spermatic cord. Therefore, no attempt should be made to infiltrate the spermatic cord in order to prevent injury to the vessels of the cord and serious hematomas. If the hernia is not reducible, the edges of the hernia sac are carefully infiltrated. Tension or torsion of strangulated intestine or omentum that becomes adherent to the hernia sac causes pain, and this area must be blocked.

This infiltration method provides analgesia but little or no muscle relaxation. If the surgery involves suture of the lacunar and Cooper ligaments, these structures should be infiltrated before suturing. Local anesthetic should be infiltrated over the pillars of the external ring because branches from the 12th thoracic nerve (T-12) occasionally reach this point. This technique usually requires less than the published maximum doses of anesthetic agents.

In infants and children, local infiltration and general anesthesia are often used in combination to reduce general anesthesia–related side effects and to provide superior postoperative pain relief. In the pediatric population, caudal anesthesia, local wound infiltration, and ilioinguinal and iliohypogastric nerve block all have been demonstrated to decrease postoperative pain compared with placebo or general anesthesia alone.[47] Regional anesthesia is often used as an alternative to general anesthesia in formerly premature infants who are at risk for apneic spells.[48]

Urologic & Gynecologic Procedures

Local infiltration of the skin, subcutaneous tissues, and muscle layers of the anterior abdominal wall produces sufficient anesthesia for short operative procedures on the bladder, such as cystostomy and suprapubic catheter insertion. It is also common to perform penile circumcision under local infiltration by using a circumferential subcutaneous wheal around the base of the penis.

Infection of Bartholin's duct may lead to obstruction and abscess formation. To prevent recurrence, Bartholin's gland is marsupialized. After cleansing, 1% lidocaine is infiltrated at the intended line of incision at the musculocutaneous junction of the affected labium minus.

Cesarean section delivery can be performed under local infiltration.[49] This is usually done in countries or regions with limited health resources or where anesthesia personnel and/or equipment are unavailable. It is also occasionally used for patients for whom general or regional anesthesia is contraindicated or deemed unsafe. For a transverse suprapubic (Pfannenstiel) incision, simple subcutaneous infiltration is all that is required to anesthetize the skin. The underlying fascia can be injected directly or anesthetized by performing bilateral rectus sheath blocks. The parietal peritoneum can be difficult to adequately anesthetize and may require 15–20 mL of local anesthetic injected in a fan-like manner before and after the peritoneal incision. The visceral peritoneum and uterus do not need local infiltration. Because this is a high-volume infiltrational technique, most practitioners advocate dilute solutions (eg, 0.5% lidocaine). Epinephrine is usually added to reduce peak plasma levels of local anesthetic. An additional consideration is the potential for fetal systemic toxicity, which is increased with fetal acidosis. Ester local anesthetics such as chloroprocaine 1% have been used for their safety profile, because they are metabolized quickly in both maternal and fetal plasma.

Infiltration with local anesthetic can be used to anesthetize the perineum before episiotomy or repair of a perineal tear. Lidocaine 1% is the agent of choice, and care must be taken with the total dose administered in this extremely vascular area, especially if the patient is already receiving continuous local anesthetic infusion via an epidural catheter.

Anorectal Procedures

Patients presenting with a *thrombosed external hemorrhoid* stand a good chance of instant relief if the lesion is evacuated within 24–48 hours after onset of pain. Local infiltration is an acceptable alternative to general anesthesia for this procedure. To do so, the skin and subcutaneous tissues around and beneath the hematoma are infiltrated with a 1% lidocaine solution containing epinephrine. Anesthesia for management of an anal fissure, pilonidal sinus, or fulguration of anal condylomata can be achieved in a similar manner.

Rectal prolapse is a condition that primarily affects the elderly. The Thiersch procedure, which involves inserting a band of elastic material around the outside of the anal muscle, is performed on patients who are generally unfit for a more definitive operation to treat rectal prolapse. This procedure is carried out under local anesthetic by infiltration of the perianal tissues with 1% lidocaine containing epinephrine.

SUMMARY

Many surgical procedures are suitable for anesthesia by local infiltration. One common reason to choose this method is the desire to avoid side effects associated with general anesthesia such as nausea and vomiting, increased postoperative pain, and delayed home discharge. Other and perhaps more important reasons include ease of administration, lack of a requirement for special anesthetic equipment or personnel, and outstanding postoperative analgesia that is a norm with this anesthesia. The ability to produce a blockade of sensation to areas of surgical manipulation with local anesthetic solution is a powerful tool that all physicians should be able to use.

Although many techniques are presented in this chapter, the knowledge of basic anatomy and principles of use of local anesthesia are the basis of their successful application.

References

1. Braun H: *Local Anesthesia: Its Scientific Basis and Practical Use.* Lea & Febiger, 1914.
2. Ball C, Westhorpe R: Local anaesthesia after cocaine. Anaesth Intensive Care 2004;32:157.
3. Rosenberg PH, Veering BT, Urmey WF: Maximum recommended doses of local anesthetics: A multifactorial concept. Reg Anesth Pain Med 2004;29:564–575.
4. Rao RB, Ely SF, Hoffman RS: Deaths related to liposuction. N Engl J Med 1999;340:1471–1475.
5. Palmisano JM, Meliones JN, Crowley DC, et al: Lidocaine toxicity after subcutaneous infiltration in children undergoing cardiac catheterization. Am J Cardiol 1991;67:647–648.

6. Tucker GT, Mather LE: Clinical pharmacokinetics of local anaesthetics. Clin Pharmacokinet 1979;4:241–278.

7. Braid DP, Scott DB: Effect of adrenaline on the systemic absorption of local anaesthetic drugs. Acta Anaesthesiol Scand 1966;23(Suppl):334–346.

8. Kopacz DJ, Carpenter RL, Mackey DC: Effect of ropivacaine on cutaneous capillary blood flow in pigs. Anesthesiology 1989;71:69–74.

9. Morris R, McKay W, Mushlin P: Comparison of pain associated with intradermal and subcutaneous infiltration with various local anesthetic solutions. Anesth Analg 1987;66:1180–1182.

10. Quaba O, Huntley JS, Bahia H, McKeown DW: A user's guide for reducing the pain of local anaesthetic administration. Emerg Med J 2005;22:188–189.

11. McKay W, Morris R, Mushlin P: Sodium bicarbonate attenuates pain on skin infiltration with lidocaine, with or without epinephrine. Anaesth Analg 1987;66: 572–574.

12. Howe NR, Williams JM: Pain of injection and duration of anesthesia for intradermal infiltration of lidocaine, bupivacaine, and etidocaine. J Dermatol Surg Oncol 1994;20:459–464.

13. Scarfone RJ, Jasani M, Gracely EJ: Pain of local anesthetics: Rate of administration and buffering. Ann Emerg Med 1998;31:36–40.

14. Crystal CS, Blankenship RB: Local anesthetics and peripheral nerve blocks in the emergency department. Emerg Med Clin North Am 2005;23:477–502.

15. Wong DT, Gadsden JC: Acute upper airway angioedema secondary to acquired C1 esterase inhibitor deficiency: A case report. Can J Anaesth 2003;50:900–903.

16. Aldrete JA, Johnson DA: Allergy to local anesthetics. JAMA 1969;207:356–357.

17. Bartfield JM, Sokaris SJ, Raccio-Robak N: Local anesthesia for lacerations: Pain of infiltration inside vs outside the wound. Acad Emerg Med 1998;5:100–104.

18. Oaklander AL, Siegel SM: Cutaneous innervation: Form and function. J Am Acad Dermatol 2005;53:1027–1037.

19. Hilliges M, Wang L, Johansson O: Ultrastructural evidence for nerve fibers within all vital layers of the human epidermis. J Invest Dermatol 1995;104:134–137.

20. Dahl JB, Moiniche S, Kehlet H: Wound infiltration with local anaesthetics for postoperative pain relief. Acta Anaesthesiol Scand 1994;38:7–14.

21. Gupta A: Local anaesthesia for pain relief after laparoscopic cholecystectomy: A systematic review. Best Pract Res Clin Anaesthesiol 2005;19:275–292.

22. Updike GM, Manolitsas TP, Cohn DE, et al: Pre-emptive analgesia in gynecologic surgical procedures: Preoperative wound infiltration with ropivacaine in patients who undergo laparotomy through a midline vertical incision. Am J Obstet Gynecol 2003;188:901–905.

23. Bagul A, Taha R, Metcalfe MS, et al: Pre-incision infiltration of local anesthetic reduces postoperative pain with no effects on bruising and wound cosmesis after thyroid surgery. Thyroid 2005;15:1245–1248.

24. Law-Koune JD, Szekely B, Fermanian C, et al: Scalp infiltration with bupivacaine plus epinephrine or plain ropivacaine reduces postoperative pain after supratentorial craniotomy. J Neurosurg Anesthesiol 2005;17:139–143.

25. LeBlanc KA, Bellanger D, Rhynes VK, Hausmann M: Evaluation of continuous infusion of 0.5% bupivacaine by elastomeric pump for postoperative pain management after open inguinal hernia repair. J Am Coll Surg. 2005;200:198–202.

26. Levack I, Holmes J, Robertson GS: Abdominal wound perfusion for the relief of postoperative pain. Br J Anaesth 1986;58:615–619.

27. Stratford AF, Zoutman DE, Davidson JS: Effect of lidocaine and epinephrine on *Staphylococcus aureus* in a guinea pig model of surgical wound infection. Plast Reconstr Surg 2002;110:1275–1279.

28. Tandon S, Roe J, Lancaster J: A randomized trial of local anaesthetic in treatment of quinsy. Clin Otolaryngol Allied Sci 2004;29:535–537.

29. Atabey A, Galdino G, El-Shahat A, Ramirez OM: The effects of tumescent solutions containing lidocaine and epinephrine on skin flap survival in rats. Ann Plast Surg 2004;53:70–72.

30. Spanknebel K, Chabot JA, DiGiorgi M, et al: Thyroidectomy using local anesthesia: A report of 1,025 cases over 16 years. J Am Coll Surg 2005;201:375–385.

31. Biertho L, Chau C, Inabnet WB: Image-directed parathyroidectomy under local anaesthesia in the elderly. Br J Surg 2003;90:738–742.

32. Gerig HJ, Schnider T, Heidegger T: Prophylactic percutaneous transtracheal catheterisation in the management of patients with anticipated difficult airways: A case series. Anaesthesia 2005;60:801–805.

33. Manoppo AE: Resection of an unusually large goitre. Br J Surg 1977;64:158–159.

34. Templeton T: Rectus block for postoperative pain relief. Reg Anesth 1993;18:258–260.

35. Smith BE, Suchak M, Siggins D, Challands J: Rectus sheath block for diagnostic laparoscopy. Anaesthesia 1988;43:947–948.

36. Hultin J, Hamberg P, Stenstrom A: Knee arthroscopy using local anesthesia. Arthroscopy 1992;8:239–241.

37. Karkabi S, Besser M, Zinman C: Arthroscopic subacromial decompression performed under local anesthesia. Arthroscopy 2005;21:1404.

38. Armour AD, Rotenberg BW, Brown MH: A comparison of two methods of infiltration in breast reduction surgery. Plast Reconstr Surg 2001;108:343–347.

39. Mottura AA: Local anesthesia in reduction mastoplasty for outpatient surgery. Aesthetic Plast Surg 1992;16:309–315.

40. Fisher B, Bauer M, Wickerham DL, et al: Relation of number of positive axillary nodes to the prognosis of patients with primary breast cancer. An NSABP update. Cancer 1983;52:1551–1557.

41. Smidt ML, Janssen CM, Barendregt WB, et al: Sentinel lymph node biopsy performed under local anesthesia is feasible. Am J Surg 2004;187:684–687.

42. Luini A, Gatti G, Zurrida S, et al: The sentinel lymph node biopsy under local anesthesia in breast carcinoma: Experience of the European Institute of Oncology and impact on quality of life. Breast Cancer Res Treat 2005;89:69–74.

43. Amid PK, Shulman AG, Lichtenstein IL: Local anesthesia for inguinal hernia repair step-by-step procedure. Ann Surg 1994;220:735–737.

44. Narchi P, Carry PY, Catoire P, et al: Postoperative pain relief and recovery with ropivacaine infiltration after inguinal hernia repair. Ambulatory Surg 1998;6:221–226.

45. Finley RK Jr, Miller SF, Jones LM: Elimination of urinary retention following inguinal herniorrhaphy. Ann Surg 1991;57:486–488.

46. Behnia R, Hashemi F, Stryker SJ, et al: A comparison of general versus local anesthesia during inguinal herniorrhaphy. Surg Gynecol Obstet 1992;174:277–280.

47. Cross GD, Barrett RF. Comparison of two regional techniques for postoperative analgesia in children following herniotomy and orchidopexy. Anaesthesia 1987;42:845–849.

48. Warner LO, Teitelbaum DH, Caniano DA, et al: Inguinal herniorrhaphy in young infants: Perianesthetic complications and associated preanesthetic risk factors. J Clin Anesth 1992;4:455–461.

49. Cooper MG, Feeney EM, Joseph M, McGuinness JJ: Local anaesthetic infiltration for caesarean section. Anaesth Intensive Care 1989;17:198–201.

13

Spinal Anesthesia

Tony Tsai, MD • Roy Greengrass, MD

INTRODUCTION WITH GENERAL CONSIDERATIONS & BRIEF HISTORY

Carl Koller, an ophthalmologist from Vienna, first described the use of topical cocaine for analgesia of the eye in 1884.[1] William Halsted and Richard Hall, surgeons at Roosevelt Hospital in New York City, took the idea of local anesthesia a step further by injecting cocaine into human tissues and nerves in order to produce anesthesia for surgery.[2] James Leonard Corning, a neurologist in New York City, described the use of cocaine for spinal anesthesia in 1885.[3] Since Corning was a frequent observer at Roosevelt Hospital, the idea of using cocaine in the subarachnoid space may have come from observing Halsted and Hall performing cocaine injections. Corning first injected cocaine intrathecally into a dog and within a few minutes the dog had marked weakness in the hindquarters.[4] Next, Corning injected cocaine into a man at the T11-T12 interspace into what he thought was the subarachnoid space. Since Corning did not notice any effect after 8 min, he repeated the injection. Ten minutes after the second injection, the patient complained of sleepiness in his legs, but was able to stand and walk. Because Corning made no mention of cerebrospinal fluid (CSF) efflux, most likely he inadvertently gave an epidural rather than a spinal injection to the patient.

Dural puncture was described by Essex Wynter in 1891[5] followed shortly by Heinrich Quincke 6 months later.[6] Augustus Karl Gustav Bier, a German surgeon, used cocaine intrathecally on six patients for lower extremity surgery in 1898.[7,8] In true scientific fashion, Bier decided to experiment on himself and developed a postdural puncture headache (PDPH) for his efforts. His assistant, Dr. Otto Hildebrandt, volunteered to have the procedure performed after Bier was unable to continue due to the PDPH. After injection of spinal cocaine into Hildebrandt, Bier conducted experiments on the lower half of Hildebrandt's body. Bier described needle pricks and cigar burns to the legs, incisions on the thighs, avulsion of pubic hairs, strong blows with an iron hammer to the shins, and torsion of the testicles. Hildebrandt reported minimal to no pain during the experiments; however, afterward he suffered nausea, vomiting, PDPH, and bruising and pain in his legs. Bier attributed the PDPH to loss of CSF and felt the use of small-gauge needles would help prevent the headache.[9]

Dudley Tait and Guido Caglieri performed the first spinal anesthetic in the United States in San Francisco in 1899. Their studies included cadavers, animals, and live patients in order to determine the benefits of lumbar puncture, especially in the treatment of syphilis. Tait and Caglieri injected mercuric salts and iodides into the CSF, but worsened the condition of one patient with tertiary syphilis.[10] Rudolph Matas, a vascular surgeon in New Orleans, described the use of spinal cocaine on patients and possibly was the first to use morphine in the subarachnoid space.[11,12] Matas also described the complication of death after lumbar puncture. Theodore Tuffier, a French surgeon in Paris, studied spinal anesthesia and reported on it in 1900. Tuffier felt that cocaine should not be injected until cerebrospinal fluid was recognized.[13] Tuffier taught at the University of Paris at the same time that Tait was a medical student there and most likely was one of Tait's mentors. Tuffier's demonstrations in Paris helped popularize spinal anesthesia in Europe.

Arthur Barker, a professor of surgery at the University of London, reported on the advancement of spinal techniques in 1907, including the use of a hyperbaric spinal local anesthetic, emphasis of sterility, and ease of midline over paramedian dural puncture.[14] Advancement of sterility and the investigation of decreases in blood pressure after injection helped make spinal anesthesia safer and more popular. Gaston Labat was a strong proponent of spinal anesthesia in the United States and performed early studies on the effects of Trendelenburg position on blood pressure after spinal anesthesia.[15] George Pitkin attempted to use a hypobaric local anesthetic to control the level of spinal block by mixing procaine with alcohol.[16] Lincoln Sise, an anesthesiologist at the Lahey Clinic in Boston, used Barker's technique of hyperbaric spinal anesthesia with both procaine and tetracaine.[17–19]

Spinal anesthesia became more popular as new developments occurred, including the introduction of saddle block anesthesia by Adriani and Roman-Vega in 1946.[20] The height of spinal anesthesia's popularity in the United States occurred in the 1940s, but fears of neurologic deficits and complications caused anesthesiologists to discontinue the use of spinal anesthesia. The development of novel intravenous anesthetic agents and neuromuscular blockers coincided with the decreased use of spinal anesthesia. In 1954 Dripps and Vandam described the safety of spinal anesthetics in more than 10,000 patients,[21] and spinal anesthesia was revived.

The early development of spinal needles paralleled the early development of spinal anesthesia. Corning chose a gold needle that had a short bevel point, flexible cannula, and set screw that fixed the needle to the depth of dural penetration. Corning also used an introducer for the needle, which was right-angled. Quincke used a beveled needle that was sharp and hollow. Bier developed his own sharp needle that did not require an introducer. The needle was larger bore (15-gauge or 17-gauge) with a long, cutting bevel. The main problems with Bier's needle were pain on insertion and the loss of local anesthetic due to the large hole in the dura after dural puncture. Barker's needle did not have an inner cannula, was made of nickel, and had a sharp, medium-length bevel with a matching stylet. Labat developed an unbreakable nickel needle that had a sharp, short-length bevel with a matching stylet. Labat believed that the short bevel minimized damage to the tissues when inserted into the back.

Herbert Greene realized that loss of CSF was a major problem in spinal anesthesia and developed a smooth tip, smaller gauge needle that resulted in a lower incidence of PDPH.[22] Barnett Greene described the use of a 26-gauge spinal needle in obstetrics with a decreased incidence of PDPH.[23] The Greene needle was very popular until the introduction of the Whitacre needle. Hart and Whitacre used a pencil-point needle to decrease PDPH from 5–10% to 2%.[24] Sprotte modified the Whitacre needle and published his trial of over 34,000 spinal anesthetics in 1987.[25] Modifications of the Sprotte needle occurred the 1990s to produce the needle that is in use today.[26]

Spinal anesthesia has progressed greatly since 1885 and has become standard technique in a number of different clinical situations. However, anatomy, choice of local anesthetic, physiologic effects of spinal anesthesia, patient positioning, and the approach to spinal anesthesia must all be considered. The patient should be educated about the possible side effects and complications that can occur from performing a spinal anesthetic in order to obtain informed consent before the procedure. Spinal anesthesia is an invaluable technique that all anesthesiologists should have in their armamentarium.

CONTRAINDICATIONS TO SPINAL ANESTHESIA

There are absolute and relative contraindications to spinal anesthesia. The only absolute contraindications include patient refusal, infection at the site of injection, hypovolemia, indeterminate neurologic disease, severe coagulopathy, and increased intracranial pressure, except in cases of pseudotumor cerebri. Relative contraindications include sepsis distinct from the anatomic site of puncture (eg, chorioamnionitis or lower extremity infection) and unknown duration of surgery. In the former case, if the patient is treated with antibiotics and the vital signs are stable, spinal anesthesia may be considered.

Prior to placing a spinal anesthetic, the anesthesiologist should examine the patient's back to look for any signs of local skin infection, which may carry the risk of CNS infection. Preoperative hemodynamic instability or hypovolemia increase the risk of hypotension after placement of a spinal anesthetic. High intracranial pressure increases the risk of uncal herniation when CSF is lost through the needle. Coagulation abnormalities increase the risk of hematoma formation. It is also important to communicate with the surgeon to determine the amount of time needed to complete the operation before inducing spinal anesthesia. If the duration of surgery is unknown, the spinal anesthetic given may not last long enough to cover the surgery. Knowing the duration of surgery helps the anesthesiologist determine the local anesthetic that will be used, addition of additives such as epinephrine, and whether a spinal catheter will be necessary.

Clinical Pearls

Absolute contraindications to spinal anesthesia:

- Patient refusal
- Sepsis at the site of injection
- Hypovolemia
- Coagulopathy
- Indeterminate neurologic disease
- Increased intracranial pressure

Relative contraindications:

- Infection distinct from the site of injection
- Unknown duration of surgery

Performing spinal anesthesia in patients with neurologic diseases, such as multiple sclerosis, is controversial. In vitro experiments that suggest that demyelinated nerves are more susceptible to local anesthetic toxicity. However, no clinical study has convincingly demonstrated that spinal anesthesia worsens a preexisting neurologic disease. Indeed, perioperative pain, stress, fever, and fatigue can all exacerbate these diseases; therefore, a stress-free central neuraxial block may be preferred for surgery.[27–31] Significant cardiac disease when sensory levels above T6 are required may present a relative contraindication to spinal anesthesia.[32,33] Aortic stenosis, once considered to be an absolute contraindication for spinal anesthesia, does not always preclude a carefully conducted spinal anesthetic.[34–36] Severe deformities of the spinal column can increase the difficulty in placing a spinal anesthetic. Arthritis, kyphoscoliosis, and previous lumbar fusion surgery do not contraindicate a spinal anesthetic. It is essential to examine the patient's back to determine any anatomic abnormality before attempting a spinal anesthetic.

FUNCTIONAL ANATOMY OF SPINAL BLOCKADE

In reviewing the functional anatomy of spinal blockade, an intimate knowledge of the spinal column, spinal cord, and spinal nerves must be present. This chapter reviews briefly the curvature of the vertebral column, the ligaments of the spinal column, membranes and length of the spinal cord, and passage of the spinal nerves from the spinal cord.

The vertebral column consists of 33 vertebrae: 7 cervical, 12 thoracic, 5 lumbar, 5 sacral, and 4 coccygeal segments. The vertebral column usually contains three curves. The cervical and lumbar curves are convex anteriorly, and the thoracic curve is convex posteriorly. The vertebral column curves, along with gravity, baricity of local anesthetic, and patient position, influence the spread of local anesthetics in the subarachnoid space. Figure 13–1 depicts the spinal column, vertebrae, and intervertebral discs and foramina.

Five ligaments hold the spinal column together (Figure 13–2). The supraspinous ligaments connect the apices of the spinous processes from the seventh cervical vertebra (C7) to the sacrum. The supraspinous ligament is known as the ligamentum nuchae in the area above C7. The interspinous ligaments connect the spinous processes together. The ligamentum flavum, or yellow ligament, connects the laminae above and below together. Finally, the posterior and anterior longitudinal ligaments bind the vertebral bodies together.

Clinical Pearls

When performing a spinal anesthetic using the midline approach, the layers of anatomy that are traversed (from posterior to anterior) are:

- Skin
- Subcutaneous fat
- Supraspinous ligament
- Interspinous ligament
- Ligamentum flavum
- Dura mater
- Subdural space
- Arachnoid mater
- Subarachnoid space

When performing a spinal anesthetic using the paramedian approach, the spinal needle should traverse:

- Skin
- Subcutaneous fat
- Ligamentum flavum
- Dura mater
- Subdural space
- Arachnoid mater
- Subarachnoid space

The three membranes that protect the spinal cord are the dura mater, arachnoid mater, and pia mater (Figure 13–3). The dura mater, or "tough mother", is the outermost layer. The dural sac extends to the second sacral vertebra (S2). The arachnoid mater is the middle layer, and the subdural space lies between the dural mater and arachnoid mater. The arachnoid mater, or cobweb mother, also ends at S2, like the dural sac. The pia mater, or soft mother, clings to the surface of the spinal cord and ends in the filum terminale, which helps to hold the spinal cord to the sacrum. The space between the arachnoid and pia mater is known as the subarachnoid space, and spinal nerves run in this space, as does CSF.

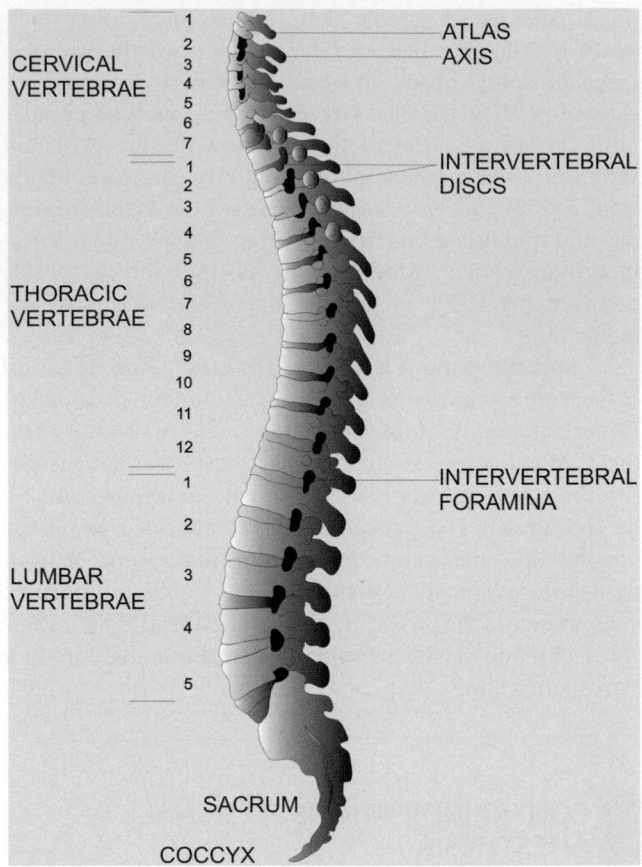

Figure 13–1. The spinal column is seen from a lateral view. All of the vertebrae, intervertebral discs, and intervertebral foraminae are shown.

Figure 13–3 depicts the spinal cord, dorsal root ganglia and ventral rootlets, spinal nerves, sympathetic trunk, rami communicantes, and pia, arachnoid, and dura mater.

When performing a spinal anesthetic using the midline approach, the layers of anatomy that are traversed (from posterior to anterior) are skin, subcutaneous fat, supraspinous ligament, interspinous ligament, ligamentum flavum, dura mater, subdural space, arachnoid mater, and finally the subarachnoid space. When the paramedian technique is used, the spinal needle should traverse the skin, subcutaneous fat, ligamentum flavum, dura mater, subdural space, arachnoid mater, and then pass into the subarachnoid space.

The length of the spinal cord varies according to age. In the first trimester, the spinal cord extends to the end of the spinal column, but as the fetus ages, the vertebral column lengthens more than the spinal cord. At birth, the spinal cord ends at approximately L3 and in the adult, the cord ends at approximately L1 with 30% of people having a cord that ends at T12 and 10% at L3. Figure 13–4 shows a cross section of the lumbar vertebrae and spinal cord. The position of the conus medullaris, cauda equina, termination of the dural sac, and filum terminale are shown. A sacral spinal cord in an adult has been reported, though this is extremely rare.[37] The length of the spinal cord must always be kept in mind

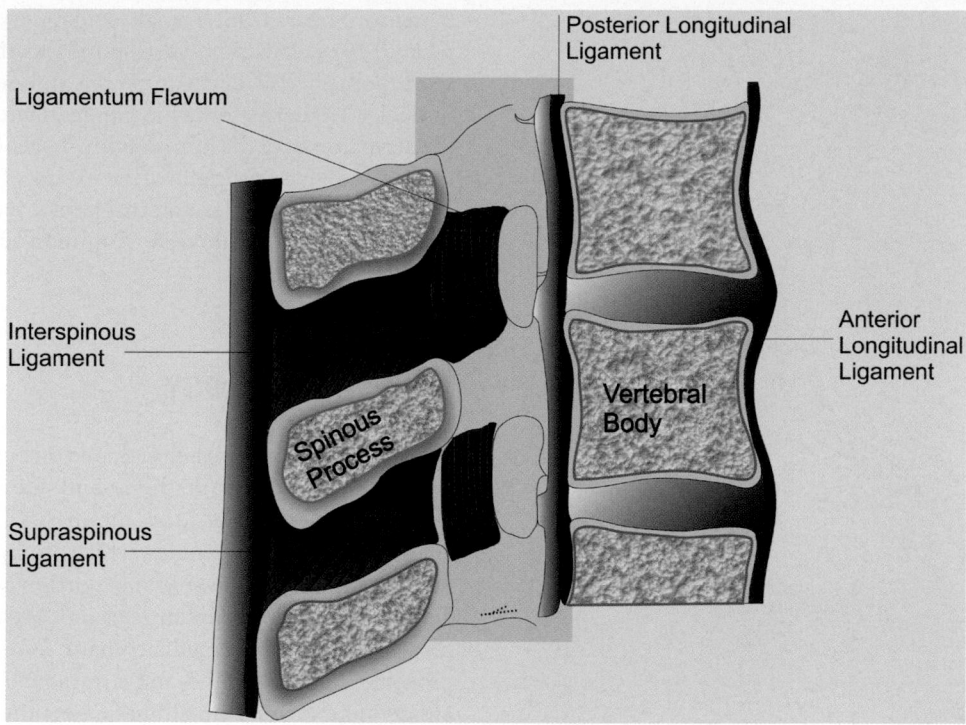

Figure 13–2. A cross section of the spinal canal is shown with the ligaments, vertebral body, and spinous processes.

when a neuraxial anesthetic is performed, as injection into the spinal cord can result in severe neurologic complications or in paralysis.[38]

Spinal nerves in the cervical region are named according to the upper cervical vertebral body from which they exit, with the exception of the eighth cervical nerve, which exits from below the seventh cervical vertebral body. This method of naming then continues in the thoracic and lumbar regions. The spinal nerve roots and spinal cord serve as the target sites for spinal anesthesia.

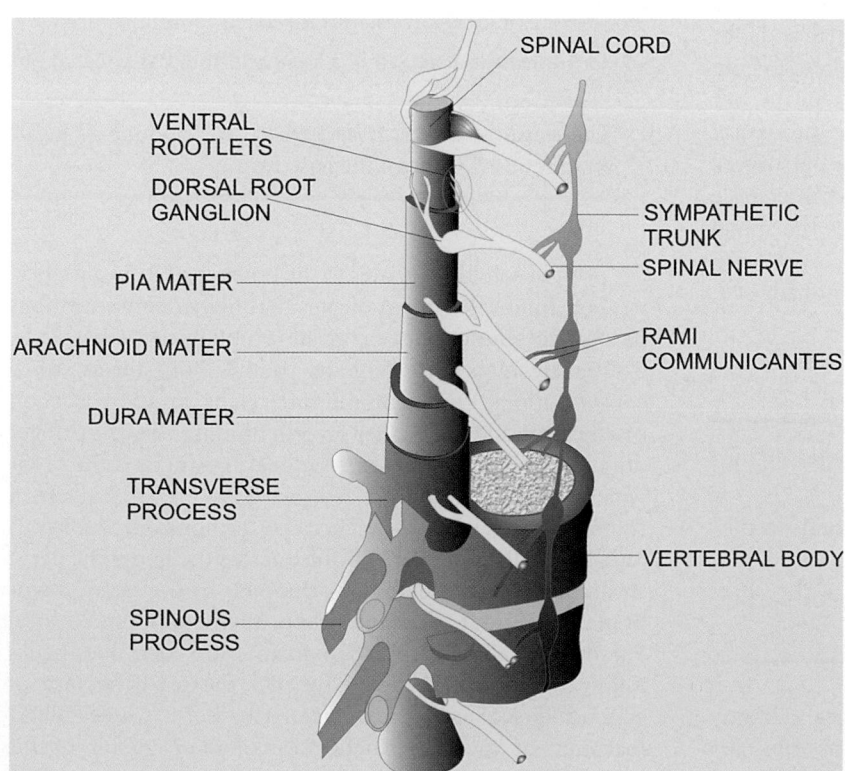

Figure 13–3. The spinal cord is shown along with the dorsal root ganglia and ventral rootlets, spinal nerves, sympathetic trunk, rami communicantes, and pia, arachnoid, and dura mater.

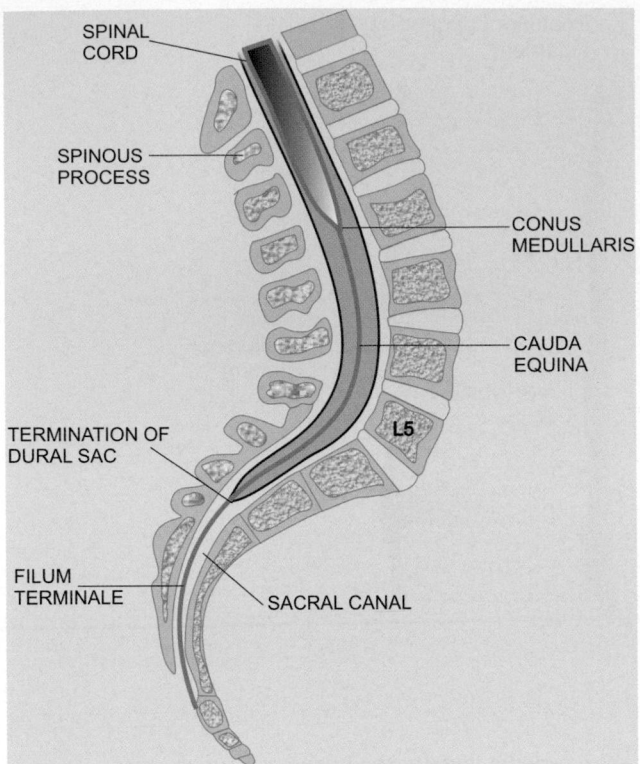

Figure 13–4. A cross section of the lumbar vertebrae and spinal cord. The position of the conus medullaris, cauda equina, termination of the dural sac, and filum terminale are shown.

Surface Anatomy

When preparing for spinal anesthetic blockade, it is important to accurately identify landmarks on the patient. The iliac crests usually mark the interspace between the fourth and fifth lumbar vertebrae; a line can be drawn between them to help locate this interspace. Care must be taken to feel for the soft area between the spinous processes to locate the interspace. Depending on the level of anesthesia necessary for the surgery and the ability to feel for the interspace, the L3-4 interspace or the L4-5 interspace can be used to introduce the spinal needle. Because the spinal cord ends at the L1 to L2 level, spinal anesthesia at or above this level is usually not advised.

Clinical Pearls

- The tenth thoracic (T10) dermatome corresponds to the umbilicus.
- The sixth thoracic (T6) dermatome corresponds to the xiphoid.
- The fourth thoracic (T4) dermatome corresponds to the nipples.

It would be incomplete to discuss surface anatomy without mentioning the dermatomes that are important for spinal anesthesia. A dermatome is an area of skin innervated

by sensory fibers from a single spinal nerve. The tenth thoracic (T10) dermatome corresponds to the umbilicus, the sixth thoracic (T6) dermatome the xiphoid, and the fourth thoracic (T4) dermatome the nipples. Figure 13–5 illustrates the dermatomes of the human body. To achieve surgical anesthesia for a given procedure, the extent of spinal anesthesia must reach a certain dermatomal level. Dermatomal levels of spinal anesthesia, required for common surgical procedures are listed in Table 13–1.

PHARMACOLOGY

The choice of local anesthetic is based on potency of the agent, onset and duration of anesthesia, and side effects of the drug. Two distinct groups of local anesthetics are used in spinal anesthesia, esters and amides, which are characterized by the bond that connects the aromatic portion and the intermediate chain. Esters contain an ester link between the aromatic portion and the intermediate chain, and examples include procaine, chloroprocaine, and tetracaine. Amides contain an amide link between the aromatic portion and the intermediate chain, and examples include bupivacaine, ropivacaine, etidocaine, lidocaine, mepivacaine, and prilocaine. Although metabolism is important for determining activity of local anesthetics, lipid solubility, protein binding, and pK_a also influence activity.[39]

Clinical Pearls

- Potency of local anesthetics is related to lipid solubility.
- The duration of action of a local anesthetic is affected by the protein binding.
- The onset of action is related to the amount of local anesthetic available in the base form.

Lipid solubility relates to the potency of local anesthetics. Low lipid solubility indicates that higher concentrations of local anesthesia must be given to obtain nerve blockade. Conversely, high lipid solubility produces anesthesia at low concentrations. Protein binding affects the duration of action of a local anesthetic. Higher protein binding results in longer duration of action. The pK_a of a local anesthetic is the pH at which ionized and nonionized forms are present equally in solution, which is important because the nonionized form allows the local anesthetic to diffuse across the lipophilic nerve sheath and reach the sodium channels in the nerve membrane. The onset of action relates to the amount of local anesthetic available in the base form. Most local anesthetics follow the rule that the lower the pK_a, the faster the onset of action and vice versa. Please refer to Chapter 6 (Clinical Pharmacology of Local Anesthetics) for more discussion of this topic.

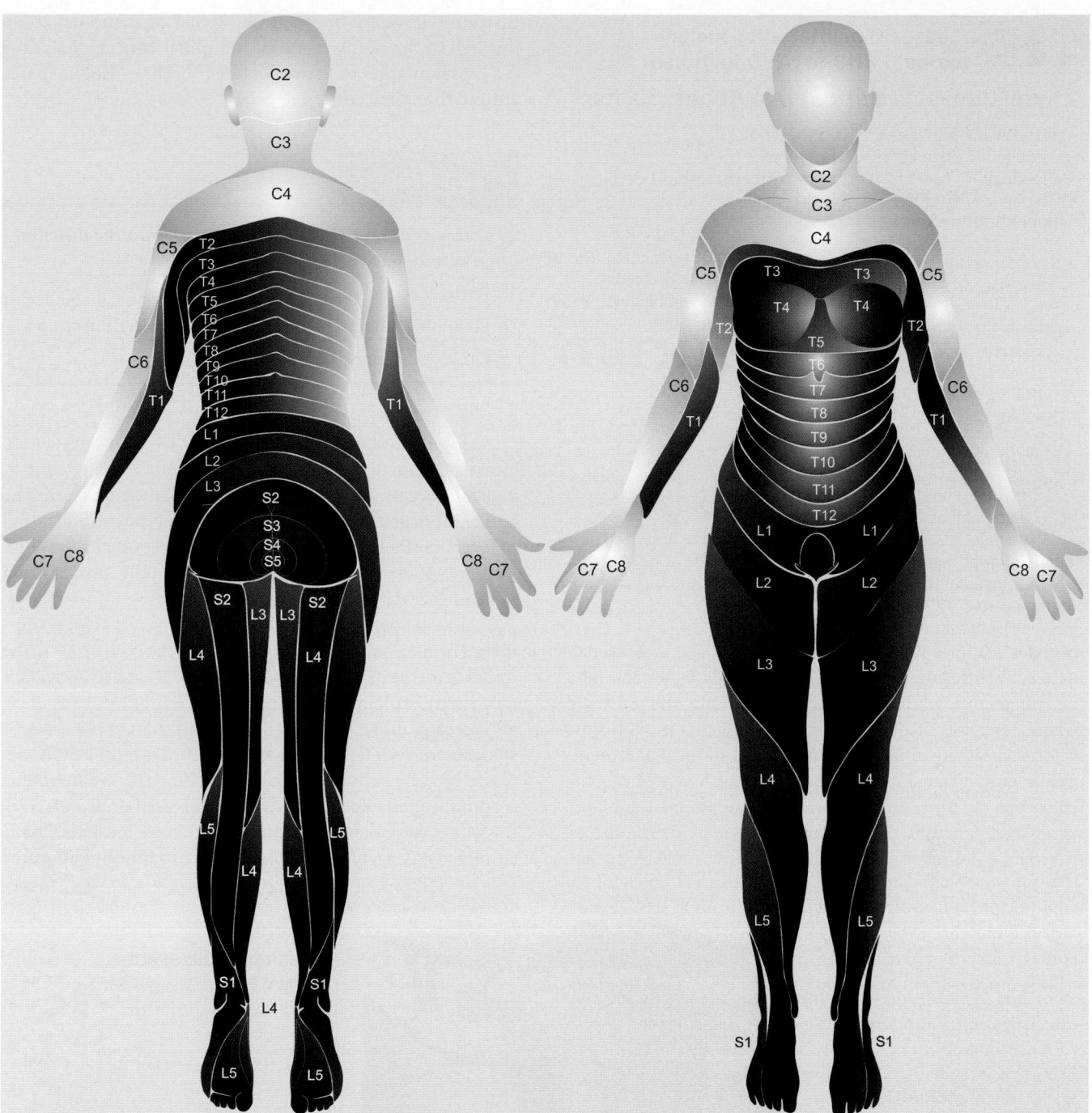

Figure 13–5. The dermatomes of the human body.

Pharmacokinetics of Local Anesthetics in the Subarachnoid Space

Pharmacokinetics of local anesthetics includes uptake and elimination of the drug. Four factors play a role in the uptake of local anesthetics from the subarachnoid space into neuronal tissue, (1) concentration of local anesthetic in CSF, (2) surface area of nerve tissue exposed to CSF, (3) lipid content of nerve tissue, and (4) blood flow to nerve tissue.[40,41]

The uptake of local anesthetic is greatest at the site of highest concentration in the CSF and is decreased above and below this site. As discussed previously, uptake and spread of local anesthetics after spinal injection are determined by multiple factors including dose, volume, and baricity of local anesthetic and patient positioning.

Both the nerve roots and the spinal cord take up local anesthetics after injection into the subarachnoid space. The more surface area of the nerve root exposed, the greater the uptake of local anesthetic.[42–45] The spinal cord has two

Table 13–1.

Dermatomal Levels of Spinal Anesthesia for Common Surgical Procedures

Procedure	Dermatomal Level
Upper abdominal surgery	T4
Intestinal, gynecologic, and urologic surgery	T6
Transurethral resection of the prostate	T10
Vaginal delivery of a fetus, and hip surgery	T10
Thigh surgery and lower leg amputations	L1
Foot and ankle surgery	L2
Perineal and anal surgery	S2 to S5 (saddle block)

surround nerve cell bodies in the spinal cord and penetrate through to the deeper areas of the spinal cord. Figure 13–6 is a representation of the periarterial Virchow–Robin spaces around the spinal cord.

Clinical Pearls

The three most important factors in determining distribution of local anesthetics:

- Baricity of the local anesthetic solution
- Position of the patient during and just after injection
- Dose of the anesthetic injected

mechanisms for uptake of local anesthetics. The first mechanism is by diffusion from the CSF to the pia mater and into the spinal cord, which is a slow process. Only the most superficial portion of the spinal cord is affected by diffusion of local anesthetics. The second method of local anesthetic uptake is by extension into the spaces of Virchow–Robin, which are the areas of pia mater that surround the blood vessels that penetrate the central nervous system. The spaces of Virchow–Robin connect with the perineuronal clefts that

Lipid content determines uptake of local anesthetics. Heavily myelinated tissues in the subarachnoid space contain higher concentrations of local anesthetics after injection. The higher the degree of myelination, the higher the concentration of local anesthetic, as there is a high lipid content in myelin. If an area of nerve root does not contain myelin, an increased risk of nerve damage occurs in that area.[46]

Blood flow determines the rate of removal of local anesthetics from spinal cord tissue. The faster the blood flow in the spinal cord, the more rapid the anesthetic is washed away. This may partly explain why the concentration of local anesthetics is greater in the posterior spinal cord than in the anterior spinal cord, even though the anterior cord is more readily accessed by the Virchow–Robin spaces. After a spinal anesthetic is administered, blood flow may be increased or decreased to the spinal cord, depending on the particular local anesthetic administered, eg, tetracaine increases cord flow but lidocaine

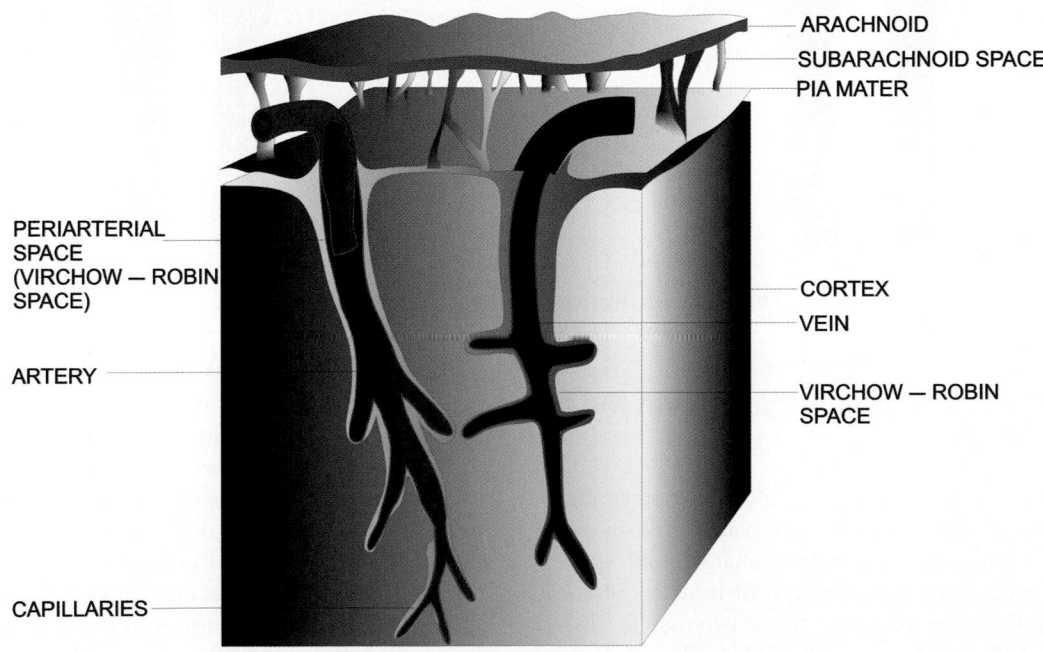

Figure 13–6. A representation of the periarterial Virchow–Robin spaces around the spinal cord.

and bupivacaine decrease it, which affects elimination of the local anesthetic.[47–49]

Elimination of local anesthetic from the subarachnoid space is by vascular absorption in the epidural space and the subarachnoid space. Local anesthetics travel across the dura in both directions. In the epidural space, vascular absorption can occur, just as in the subarachnoid space. Vascular supply to the spinal cord consists of vessels located on the spinal cord and in the pia mater. Because vascular perfusion to the spinal cord varies , the rate of elimination of local anesthetics varies.[40]

Distribution

The distribution and decrease in concentration of local anesthetics is based on the area of highest concentration, which can be independent of the injection site. Many factors affect the distribution of local anesthetics in the subarachnoid space. Table 13–2 lists some of these factors.[50]

The three most important factors for determining spread of local anesthesia in the subarachnoid space are baricity of the local anesthetic solution, position of the patient during and just after injection, and dose of the anesthetic injected.

Baricity plays an important role in determining the spread of local anesthetic in the spinal space and is equal to the density of the local anesthetic divided by the density of the CSF at 37°C.[51–58] Local anesthetics can be hyperbaric, hypobaric, or isobaric when compared to CSF, and baricity is the main determinant of how the local anesthetic is distributed when injected into the CSF. Table 13–3 compares the density, specific gravity, and baricity of different substances and local anesthetics.[50,51,53,59,60]

Table 13–2.

Determinants of Local Anesthetic Spread in the Subarachnoid Space

Properties of local anesthetic solution
    Baricity
    Dose
    Volume
    Specific gravity

Patient characteristics
    Position during and after injection
    Height (extremely short or tall)
    Spinal column anatomy
    Decreased CSF volume (increased intraabdominal
        pressure due to increased weight, pregnancy, etc.)

Technique
    Site of injection
    Needle bevel direction

CSF = cerebrospinal fluid.

Hypobaric solutions are less dense than CSF and tend to rise against gravity. Isobaric solutions are as dense as CSF and tend to remain at the level at which they are injected. Hyperbaric solutions are more dense than CSF and tend to follow gravity after injection.

Hypobaric solutions have a baricity of less than 1.0 relative to CSF and are usually made by adding distilled sterile water to the local anesthetic. Tetracaine, dibucaine, and bupivacaine have all been used as hypobaric solutions in spinal

Table 13–3.

Density, Specific Gravity, and Baricity of Different Substances and Local Anesthetics

		Density	Specific Gravity	Baricity
Water		0.9933	1.0000	0.9930
CSF		1.0003	1.0069	1.0000
Hypobaric				
Tetracaine	0.33% in water	0.9980	1.0046	0.9977
Lidocaine	0.5% in water	N/A	1.0038	0.9985
Isobaric				
Tetracaine	0.5% in 50% CSF	0.9998	1.0064	0.9995
Lidocaine	2% in water	1.0003	1.0066	1.0003
Bupivacaine	0.5% in water	0.9993	1.0059	0.9990
Hyperbaric				
Tetracaine	0.5% in 5% dextrose	1.0136	1.0203	1.0133
Lidocaine	5% in 7.5% dextrose	1.0265	1.0333	1.0265
Bupivacaine	0.5% in 8% dextrose	1.0210	1.0278	1.0207
Bupivacaine	0.75% in 8% dextrose	1.0247	1.0300	1.0227

anesthesia. Patient positioning is important after injection of a hypobaric spinal anesthetic because it is the first few minutes that determine the spread of anesthesia. If the patient is in Trendelenburg position after injection, the anesthetic will spread in the caudal direction and if the patient is in reverse Trendelenburg position, the anesthetic will spread cephalad after injection. If a procedure were to be performed in the perineal or anal area in the prone, jackknife position, a hypobaric spinal anesthetic would be an excellent choice to avoid the need for waiting for the anesthetic to "set in" and repositioning the patient after injection.

Clinical Pearls

The three most important factors in determining distribution of local anesthetics:

- Baricity of the local anesthetic solution
- Position of the patient during and just after injection
- Dose of the anesthetic injected

The baricity of isobaric solutions is equal to 1.0. Tetracaine and bupivacaine have both been used with success for isobaric spinal anesthesia, and patient positioning does not affect spread of the local anesthetic, unlike the case with hyperbaric or hypobaric solutions. Injection can be made in any position, and then the patient can be placed into the position necessary for surgery. Gravity dose not play a role in the spread of isobaric solutions, unlike with hypo- or hyperbaric local anesthetics.

Hyperbaric solutions in spinal anesthesia have baricity greater than 1.0. A local anesthetic solution can be made hyperbaric by adding dextrose or glucose. Bupivacaine, lidocaine and tetracaine have all been used as hyperbaric solutions in spinal anesthesia. Patient positioning affects the spread of the anesthetic. A patient in Trendelenburg position would have the anesthetic travel in a cephalad direction and vice versa.

Dose and volume both play a role in the spread of local anesthetics after spinal injection, although dose has been shown to be more important than volume.[61] Concentration of local anesthetic before injection has no bearing on distribution because after injection, due to the mixing of the CSF and local anesthetic, there is a new concentration.

Effects of the Volume of the Lumbar Cistern on Block Height

CSF is produced in the brain at 0.35 mL/min and fills the subarachnoid space. This clear, colorless fluid has an approximate volume of 150 mL in adults, half of which is in the cranium and half in the spinal canal. However, CSF volume varies considerably, and decreased CSF volume

can result from obesity, pregnancy, or any other cause of increased abdominal pressure.[62] This is partly due to compression of the intervertebral foramen, which displaces the CSF.

Clinical Pearl

- Due to the wide variability in CSF volume, the ability to precisely predict the level of the spinal blockade after local anesthetic injection is poor, even if body mass index is calculated and used.

Multiple factors affect the distribution of local anesthesia after spinal blockade,[50] one being CSF volume. Carpenter showed that lumbosacral CSF volume correlated with peak sensory block height and duration of surgical anesthesia.[63] The density of CSF is related to peak sensory block level, and lumbosacral CSF volume correlates to peak sensory block level, and onset and duration of motor block.[64] However, due to the wide variability in CSF volume the ability to predict the level of the spinal blockade after local anesthetic injection is very poor, even if body mass index (BMI) is calculated and used.

Local Anesthetics

Cocaine was the first spinal anesthetic used, and procaine and tetracaine soon followed. Spinal anesthesia with lidocaine, bupivacaine, tetracaine, mepivacaine, and ropivacaine have also been introduced in clinical use over the last several decades. Some of the more common local anesthetics used for spinal anesthesia will be discussed in this portion of the chapter. In addition, there is a growing interest in medications that produce anesthesia and analgesia while limiting side effects. A variety of medications, including vasoconstrictors, opioids, α_2-adrenergic agonists, and acetylcholinesterase inhibitors, have been added to spinal medications to enhance analgesia while reducing the motor blocade with local anesthetics.

Lidocaine was first used as a spinal anesthetic in 1945, and it had been one of the most widely used spinal anesthetics since. Onset of anesthesia occurs in 3 to 5 min with a duration of anesthesia that lasts for 1 to 1.5 h. Lidocaine spinal anesthesia can be used for short to intermediate length operating room cases. One drawback of lidocaine has been the association with transient neurologic symptoms (TNS), which present as low back pain and lower extremity dysesthesias with radiation to the buttocks, thighs, and lower limbs after recovery from spinal anesthesia. TNS occurs in about 14% of patients receiving lidocaine spinal anesthesia.[65-67] Because of the risk of TNS associated with lidocaine, other intermediate-acting local anesthetics with lower risk of TNS are being used instead of lidocaine in many practices.

Table 13–4.

Dose, Duration, and Onset of Local Anesthetics Used in Spinal Anesthesia

	Dose (mg)		Duration (min) Plain	With 0.2 mg Epinephrine	Onset (min)
	to T10	to T4			
Commonly Used					
Lidocaine 5%*	50–75	75–100	60–70	75–100	3–5
Bupivacaine 0.75%	8–12	14–20	90–110	100–150	5–8
Less Commonly Used					
Tetracaine 0.5%	6–10	12–16	70–90	120–180	3–5
Mepivacaine 2%	N/A	60–80	140–160	N/A	2–4
Ropivacaine 0.75%	15–17	18–20	140–200	N/A	3–5
Levobupivacaine 0.5%	10–15	N/A	135–170	N/A	4–8
Chloroprocaine 3%	30	45	80–120	130–170	2–4

* *Lidocaine has been less commonly used in the last decade due to the association with TNS.*

Clinical Pearls

- Bupivacaine is a popular alternative to lidocaine for spinal anesthesia and has been used frequently with lower incidence of TNS.

- Onset of anesthesia occurs in 5 to 8 min with bupivacaine and a duration of anesthesia that lasts from 90 to 150 min, thus it is appropriate for a wide range of surgical procedures.

Bupivacaine is a viable alternative to lidocaine for spinal anesthesia and has been used frequently with very little incidence of TNS.[68–70] Onset of anesthesia occurs in 5 to 8 min with a duration of anesthesia that lasts from 90 to 150 min; thus it is appropriate for intermediate to long operating room cases. For outpatient spinal anesthesia, small doses of bupivacaine are recommended to avoid prolonged discharge time due to offset of block. Bupivacaine has almost replaced lidocaine as the most commonly used spinal local anesthetic in the United States. Bupivacaine is often packaged as 0.75% in 8.25% dextrose. Other forms of spinal bupivacaine include 0.5% with or without dextrose and 0.75% without dextrose.

Tetracaine has an onset of anesthesia within 3 to 5 min and a duration of 70 to 180 min, and like bupivacaine, is used for cases that are intermediate to longer duration. The 1% solution is often mixed with 10% glucose in equal parts to form a hyperbaric spinal anesthetic that is used for perineal and abdominal surgery. With tetracaine, TNS occurs at a lower rate than with lidocaine spinal anesthesia. The addition of phenylephrine however, may play a role in the development of TNS.[71–73]

Mepivacaine is similar to lidocaine and has been used since the 1960s for spinal anesthesia. The incidence of TNS reported after mepivacaine spinal anesthesia varies widely, with rates from 0% to 30%.[74–76] Ropivacaine was introduced in 1996. For applications in spinal anesthesia, ropivacaine has been found to be less potent than spinal bupivacaine. Ropivacaine has significantly less risk of TNS than spinal lidocaine. Studies comparing ropivacaine to bupivacaine in spinal anesthesia are in progress.[77–79]

Table 13–4 shows some of the local anesthetics used for spinal anesthesia and dosage duration, and concentration for different levels of spinal blockade.[79–88]

Additives to Local Anesthesia

Vasoconstrictors are often added to local anesthetics, and both epinephrine and phenylephrine have been studied. Anesthesia is intensified and prolonged with smaller doses of local anesthetics when epinephrine or phenylephrine is added. Tissue vasoconstriction is produced, thus limiting the systemic reabsorption of the local anesthetic and prolonging the duration of action by keeping the local anesthetic in contact with the nerve fibers. However, ischemic complications can occur after the use of vasoconstrictors in spinal anesthesia. In some studies, epinephrine was implicated as the cause of cauda equina syndrome because of anterior spinal artery ischemia. Regardless, most studies did not demonstrate an association between the use of vasoconstrictors for spinal anesthesia and the incidence of cauda equina.[89,90] Phenylephrine has been shown to increase the risk of TNS.[73,91]

Epinephrine is thought to work by decreasing local anesthetic uptake and thus prolonging the spinal blockade of local anesthetics. However, vasoconstrictors can cause ischemia, and there is a theoretical concern of spinal cord ischemia when epinephrine is added to spinal anesthetics. Animal models have not shown any decrease in spinal cord blood flow or increase in spinal cord ischemia when epinephrine is given for spinal blockade, even though some neurologic complications associated with the addition of epinephrine exist.[47,49,92,93]

Clinical Pearls

- Adding 0.1 mL of epinephrine to 10 mL of local anesthetic yields a 1:100,000 concentration of epinephrine.
- Adding 0.1 mL of epinephrine to 20 mL of local anesthetic yields a 1:200,000 concentration, and so on (0.1 mL in 30 mL = 1:300,000).

Epinephrine comes packaged as 1 mg in 1 mL, which is a 1:1000 solution. The dosage of epinephrine added to local anesthetics is 0.1 to 0.5 mg, meaning 0.1 mL to 0.5 mL is added to the local anesthetic solution. Adding 0.1 mL of epinephrine to 10 mL of local anesthetic yields a 1:100,000 concentration of epinephrine. Adding 0.1 mL of epinephrine to 20 mL of local anesthetic yields a 1:200,000 concentration, and so on (0.1 mL in 30 mL = 1:300,000). Calculation of epinephrine concentration does not need to be complex if this simple formula is remembered.

Epinephrine prolongs the duration of spinal anesthesia.[94–96] In the past, it was thought that epinephrine had no effect on hyperbaric spinal bupivacaine using two-segment regression to test neural blockade.[97] However, a recent study showed that epinephrine prolongs the duration of hyperbaric spinal bupivacaine when pinprick, transcutaneous electrical nerve stimulation (TENS) equivalent to surgical stimulation (at umbilicus, pubis, knee, and ankle), and tolerance of a pneumatic thigh tourniquet were used to determine neural blockade.[98] Currently there is controversy regarding prolongation of spinal bupivacaine neural blockade when epinephrine is added.[99–102] The same controversy exists about the prolongation of spinal lidocaine with epinephrine.[103–107]

All three types of opioid receptors are found in the dorsal horn of the spinal cord and serve as the target for intrathecal opioid injection. Receptors are located on spinal cord neurons and terminals of afferents originating in the dorsal root ganglion. Fentanyl, sufentanil, meperidine, and morphine have all been used intrathecally. Side effects that may be seen include pruritus, nausea and vomiting, and respiratory depression.[108–112]

Alpha$_2$-adrenergic agonists can be added to spinal injections of local anesthetics in order to enhance pain relief and prolong sensory block and motor block. Enhanced postoperative analgesia has been demonstrated in cesarean deliveries, fixation of femoral fractures, and knee arthroscopies when clonidine was added to the local anesthetic solution. Clonidine prolongs the sensory and motor blockade of a local anesthetic after spinal injection.[113–115] Sensory blockade is thought to be mediated by both presynaptic and postsynaptic mechanisms. Clonidine induces hyperpolarization at the ventral horn of the spinal cord and facilitates the

action of the local anesthetic, thus prolonging motor blockade when used as an additive. However, when used alone in intrathecal injections, clonidine does not cause motor block or weakness.[116] Side effects can occur with the use of spinal clonidine, and include hypotension, bradycardia, and sedation. Currently, neuraxial clonidine is approved by the Food and Drug Administration (FDA) for intractable neuropathic pain.[117,118]

Acetylcholinesterase inhibitors prevent the breakdown of acetylcholine and produce analgesia when injected intrathecally. The antinociceptive effects are due to increased acetylcholine and generation of nitric oxide. It has been shown in a rat model that diabetic neuropathy can be alleviated after intrathecal neostigmine injection.[119] Side effects of intrathecal neostigmine include nausea and vomiting, bradycardia requiring atropine, anxiety, agitation, restlessness, and lower extremity weakness.[120–122] Although spinal neostigmine provides extended pain control, the side effects that occur do not allow its widespread use.

PHARMACODYNAMICS OF SPINAL ANESTHESIA

The pharmacodynamics of spinal injection of local anesthesia are wide-ranging.

Hepatic blood flow correlates to arterial blood flow. There is no autoregulation of hepatic blood flow, thus, as arterial blood flow decreases after spinal anesthesia, so does hepatic blood flow.[123] If the mean arterial pressure (MAP) after placing a spinal anesthetic, is maintained hepatic blood flow will also be maintained. Patients with hepatic disease must be carefully monitored and their blood pressure must be controlled during anesthesia to maintain hepatic perfusion. No studies have conclusively shown the superiority of regional or general anesthesia in patients with liver disease.[124–128] In patients with liver disease either regional or general anesthesia can be given, as long as the MAP is kept close to baseline.

Clinical Pearls

- If mean blood pressure is maintained after placing a spinal anesthetic, neither hepatic nor renal blood flow will decrease.
- Spinal anesthesia does not alter autoregulation of renal blood flow.

Renal blood flow is autoregulated. The kidneys remain perfused when the MAP remains above 50 mm Hg. Transient decreases in renal blood flow may occur when MAP is less than 50 mm Hg, but even after long decreases in MAP, renal function returns to normal when blood pressure returns to normal. Again, attention to blood pressure is important after placing a spinal anesthetic, and the MAP should be as close to baseline as possible. Spinal anesthesia does not affect autoregulation of renal blood flow. It has been shown in sheep that renal perfusion changed very little after spinal anesthesia.[129–132]

Cardiovascular Effects of Spinal Anesthesia

The sympathectomy produced by spinal anesthesia induces hemodynamic changes. The block height determines the extent of sympathetic blockade, which determines the amount of change in cardiovascular parameters. However, this relationship cannot be predicted. Hypotension and bradycardia are the most common side effects seen with sympathetic denervation.[133] Risk factors associated with hypotension include hypovolemia, preoperative hypertension, high sensory block height, age older than 40 years, obesity, combined general and spinal anesthesia, and addition of phenylephrine to the local anesthetic.[134–136] Chronic alcohol consumption, history of hypertension, elevated BMI, high level of sensory block height, and urgency of surgery all increase the likelihood of hypotension after spinal anesthesia.[137] Hypotension occurs in about 33% of the nonobstetric population.[134] Figure 13–7 depicts changes in blood pressure and heart rate after injection of hyperbaric bupivacaine and tetracaine.[138]

Arterial and venodilation both occur in spinal anesthesia and combine to produce hypotension. Arterial vasodilation is not maximal after spinal blockade, and vascular smooth muscle continues to retain some autonomic tone after sympathetic denervation. Due to retention of autonomic tone, total peripheral vascular resistance (TPVR) decreases only by 15% to 18%, thus MAP decreases by 15% to 18% if cardiac output is not decreased. In patients with coronary artery disease, systemic vascular resistance can be decreased by up to 33% after spinal anesthesia.[139] However after spinal anesthesia, venodilation, is significant depending on the location of the veins. If the veins lie below the right atrium, gravity will cause pooling of the blood peripherally, and if the veins are above, there is back-flow of the blood into the heart. Venous return to the heart, or preload, therefore depends on patient positioning during spinal anesthesia.[140]

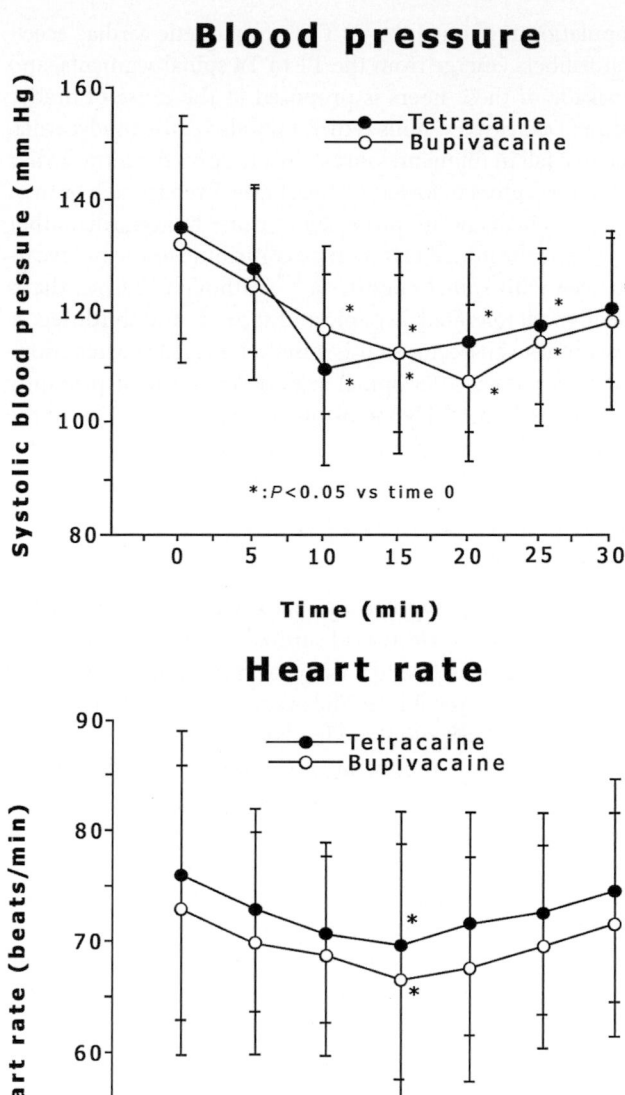

Figure 13–7. A graph depicting changes in blood pressure and heart rate after injection of hyperbaric bupivacaine and tetracaine. Blood pressure is shown in the upper graph and heart rate is shown in the lower graph with the mean ± SD. Time 0 is the time before spinal anesthetic placement and time 5 is 5 minutes after spinal anesthetic placement. Reproduced with permission from Nishiyama T, Komatsu K, Hanaoka K.: Comparison of hemodynamic and anesthetic effects of hyperbaric bupivacaine and tetracaine in spinal anesthesia. J Anesth., 17:219, 2003.

Clinical Pearls

- Spinal anesthesia denervates the sympathetic chain, which is the main mechanism of cardiovascular changes.
- The block height determines the level of sympathetic blockade, which determines the degree of change in cardiovascular parameters.

Because preload determines cardiac output and patient positioning is a major factor in determining preload, as long as a euvolemic patient is positioned with the legs elevated above the heart, there should be no significant changes in cardiac output after spinal anesthesia. The reverse Trendelenburg position, however, leads to large decreases in preload and thus large decreases in cardiac output.[141,142]

Most patients do not experience a significant change in heart rate after spinal anesthesia, but in young (age 1 < 50), healthy (ASA class 1) patients there is a higher risk of bradycardia. Beta-blocker use also increases the risk of bradycardia. The incidence of bradycardia in the nonpregnant population is about 13%.[134] The sympathetic cardiac accelerator fibers emerge from the T1 to T4 spinal segments, and blockade of these fibers is proposed as the cause of bradycardia. Decreased venous return may also cause bradycardia, due to a fall in filling pressures. This triggers the intracardiac stretch receptors to lower the heart rate. Even though both of these mechanisms are proposed to cause bradycardia, other as yet undetermined factors may contribute to the bradycardia seen with spinal anesthesia.[143] Although bradycardia is usually well tolerated, asystole and second- and third-degree heart block can occur, so it is wise to be vigilant when monitoring a patient after spinal anesthesia and treat promptly and aggressively.[144] Hypotension occurs in about 33% of the nonobstetric population.[134]

Treatment of Hypotension After Spinal Anesthesia

To effectively treat hypotension, the cause of the hypotension must be corrected. Decreased cardiac output and venous return must be treated, and a bolus of crystalloid is often used to enhance venous volume. The practice of prehydration with 500 to 1500 mL of crystalloid has been shown to decrease hypotension in some studies, but not in others.[145–147] No reliable method to prevent hypotension after spinal blockade exists. Treatment of hypotension, however, remains essential so that the myocardium and brain remain perfused. If a patient without major target organ disease is asymptomatic, decreases in blood pressure up to 33% need not be treated. Careful monitoring of blood pressure as well as supplemental oxygen should be implemented when performing spinal anesthesia. Fluid bolus should be carefully monitored as excess fluid may cause patients to go into congestive heart failure, pulmonary edema, or both, and also may necessitate bladder catheterization after surgery. Bladder catheterization can lead to its own set of problems, including urinary tract infections.

If pharmacologic treatment of hypotension is indicated, vasopressors remain the mainstay of treatment. Combined α- and β-adrenergic agonists may be better than pure α-agonists for treating blood pressure depression, and ephedrine is currently the drug of choice.[148,149] Cardiac output and peripheral vascular resistance are increased by ephedrine, which restores blood pressure. However, physiologic treatment of hypotension centers on restoration of preload. The most effective and simple way to achieve this is by positioning the patient in the Trendelenburg, or head down, position.[150] This position should not exceed 20 degrees because extreme Trendelenburg can lead to a decrease in cerebral perfusion and blood flow due to increases in jugular venous pressure. If the level of spinal anesthesia is not fixed, the Trendelenburg position can alter the level of spinal anesthesia and cause a high level of spinal anesthesia in patients receiving hyperbaric local anesthetic solutions.[151] This can be minimized by raising the upper part of the body with a pillow under the shoulders while keeping the lower part of the body elevated above heart level. Figure 13–8 shows an algorithm for the treatment of hypotension after spinal anesthesia.

The Bezold–Jarisch Reflex

The Bezold–Jarisch reflex (BJR) has been implicated as a cause of bradycardia, hypotension, and cardiovascular collapse after central neuraxial anesthesia, and in particular spinal anesthesia.[152,153] The BJR is a cardioinhibitory reflex and consists of the triad of symptoms, bradycardia, hypotension, and cardiovascular collapse, seen after intravenous injection of *Veratrum* alkaloids in animals.[154] The BJR is usually not a dominant reflex and the association with spinal anesthesia is probably weak.[154,155] Blood pressure regulation is multimodal and complex, and while the BJR likely plays a role in this regulation, the dominant reflex in regulation of blood pressure is the baroreceptor reflex. The BJR is also not a vasovagal reflex, although BJR has been blamed for bradycardia after spinal anesthesia, especially after hemorrhage.[156] No studies have yet defined this relationship. The definitive role of BJR as the cause of bradycardia, hypotension, and circulatory collapse after spinal anesthesia has not been fully established.

Respiratory Effects of Spinal Anesthesia

In patients with normal lung physiology, spinal anesthesia has very little effect on pulmonary function.[157] Lung volumes, resting minute ventilation, dead space, arterial blood gas tensions, and shunt fraction show minimal change after spinal anesthesia. The main respiratory effect of spinal anesthesia occurs during high spinal blockade when active exhalation is affected due to paralysis of abdominal and intercostal muscles. During high spinal blockade, expiratory reserve volume, peak expiratory flow, and maximum minute ventilation are reduced. Patients with obstructive pulmonary disease that rely on accessory muscle use for adequate ventilation should be monitored carefully after spinal blockade. Patients with normal pulmonary function and a high spinal block may complain of dyspnea, but if they are able to speak clearly in a normal voice, ventilation is usually normal. The dyspnea is usually due to the inability to feel the chest wall move during respiration, and simple assurance is usually effective in allaying the patient's distress.

Clinical Pearls

- Arterial blood gas measurements do not change during high spinal anesthesia in patients who are spontaneously breathing room air.
- Since a high spinal usually does not affect the cervical area, sparing of the phrenic nerve and normal diaphragmatic function occurs, and inspiration is minimally affected.

Arterial blood gas measurements do not change during high spinal anesthesia in patients who are spontaneously breathing room air. The main effect of high spinal anesthesia is on expiration, as the muscles of exhalation are impaired. Since a high spinal usually does not affect the cervical area,

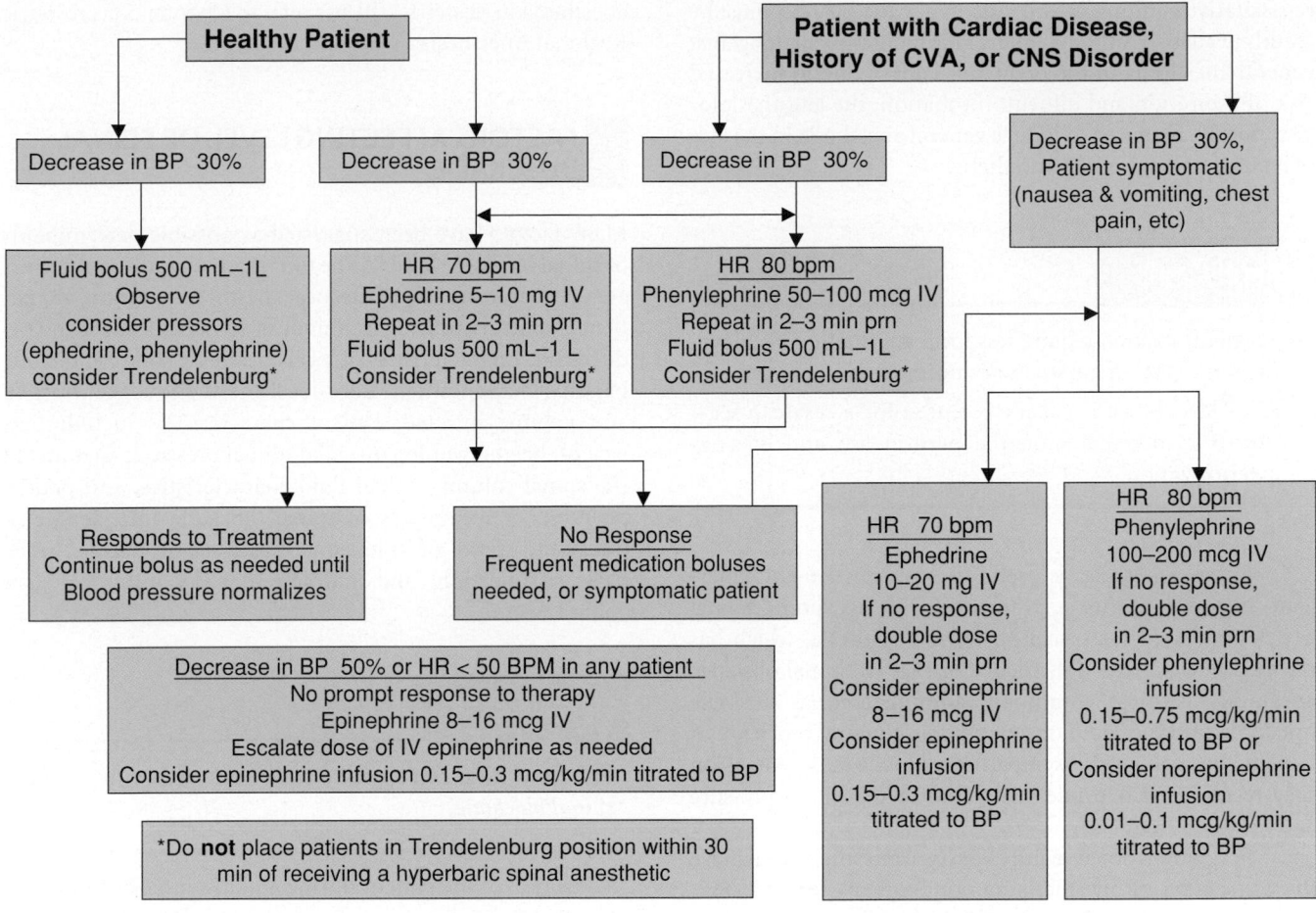

Figure 13–8. Treatment of hypotension after spinal anesthesia. CVA = cardiovascular accident, CNS = central nervous system, BP = blood pressure, HR = heart rate, bpm = beats per minute.

sparing of the phrenic nerve and normal diaphragmatic function occurs, and inspiration is minimally affected. Although Steinbrook and colleagues found that spinal anesthesia was not associated with significant changes in vital capacity, maximal inspiratory pressure, or resting end-tidal P_{CO_2}, an increased ventilatory responsiveness to CO_2 with bupivacaine spinal anesthesia was seen.[158]

Gastrointestinal Effects of Spinal Anesthesia

The sympathetic innervation to the abdominal organs arises from T6 to L2. Due to sympathetic blockade and unopposed parasympathetic activity after spinal blockade, secretions increase, sphincters relax, and the bowel becomes constricted.

Clinical Pearls

- Increased vagal activity after sympathetic block causes increased peristalsis of the gastrointestinal tract, which leads to nausea.
- Atropine is useful for treating nausea after high spinal blockade.

Nausea and vomiting occur after spinal anesthesia approximately 20% of the time, and risk factors include blocks higher than T5, hypotension, opioid administration, and a history of motion sickness.[134] Increased vagal activity after sympathetic block causes increased peristalsis of the gastrointestinal tract, which leads to nausea. Accordingly, atropine is useful for treating nausea after high spinal blockade.[149]

THE USE OF SPINAL ANESTHESIA IN OBSTETRICS

In 1901, Kreis described the first spinal anesthetic for vaginal delivery.[159] Spinal anesthesia for labor and delivery has progressed greatly since that time. When contemplating induction of anesthesia in the pregnant patient, many factors play a role. The anesthesiologist must perform a complete preanesthetic evaluation, including past medical and surgical history, past reactions to anesthesia, any difficulties during the pregnancy, maternal airway and back anatomy, and fetal assessment. In addition, the anesthesiologist must obtain informed consent for both regional and general anesthesia. Before performing a spinal anesthetic on the labor floor, resuscitative equipment and emergency medication must be readily available. Although many arguments are made against general anesthesia in the pregnant woman due to increased risk of aspiration and difficult intubation, the anesthesiologist must be prepared to induce general anesthesia in the face of a failed or total spinal anesthetic.

Clinical Pearls

- Pregnant women require less local anesthetic to achieve the same level of anesthesia as nonpregnant women.
- A T4 level block is usually required for a cesarean section due to traction on the peritoneum and uterine exteriorization.

Spinal anesthesia is useful in both elective and emergent cesarean sections. Noncutting, pencil-point spinal needles are used for spinal obstetric anesthesia, which has resulted in a decreased incidence of PDPH. Spinal obstetric anesthesia is most commonly administered as a single injection, and the rapid onset and dense neural block are of benefit. Because of the sympathetic blockade, hypotension may result, so it is prudent to monitor the blood pressure carefully and frequently.

Pregnant women require less local anesthetic to achieve the same level of anesthesia as nonpregnant women. This observation is likely due to both hormonal and mechanical factors. Procaine, tetracaine, lidocaine, bupivacaine, ropivacaine, and levobupivacaine have all been used for obstetric anesthesia, but the preferred local anesthetic is bupivacaine. Dosing is generally done either with a fixed amount of local anesthetic or changing the amount according to the height and weight of the patient. If hyperbaric bupivacaine is used, 12 mg is generally given, with a decreased dose for short patients and an increased dose if the spinal is given in the sitting position. Fentanyl 10–20 mcg can be added to enhance the quality of the block. Prior to placement of a spinal anesthetic, the pregnant patient should receive 30 mL of 0.3 M sodium citrate orally to decrease the stomach acidity, and a bolus of Ringer's lactate 15–20 mL/kg.

After the spinal anesthetic is given, the patient should be in the supine position with left uterine displacement. Fetal heart rate should be monitored by Doppler or fetal scalp electrocardiogram (ECG). Blood pressure and heart rate should be monitored repeatedly for at least 10 min, and prompt treatment should be given for decreases in blood pressure. A T4 level block is usually required for a cesarean section due to traction on the peritoneum and uterine exteriorization. Some patients complain of dyspnea due to abdominal and intercostal motor blockade, but if the patient is able to speak clearly, assurance is usually enough to calm the patient until delivery. Once the fetus is delivered, the uterus no longer causes upward pressure on the diaphragm, and the patient is able to breathe more easily. For more information on spinal anesthesia in obstetrics, please refer to Chapter 53 (Obstetric Regional Anesthesia).

FACTORS AFFECTING LEVEL OF SPINAL BLOCKADE

Many factors have been suggested as possible determinants of spinal blockade level.[50] The four main categories of factors are (1) characteristics of the local anesthetic solution, (2) patient characteristics, (3) technique of spinal blockade, and (4) diffusion. Characteristics of local anesthetic solution include baricity, local anesthetic dose, local anesthetic concentration, and volume injected. Patient characteristics include age, weight, height, gender, intraabdominal pressure, anatomy of the spinal column, spinal fluid characteristics, and patient position.[160] Techniques of spinal blockade include site of injection, speed of injection, direction of needle bevel, force of injection, and addition of vasoconstrictors (see Table 13–1).

Clinical Pearls

The three most important factors in determining level of spinal blockade:
- Baricity of the local anesthetic solution
- Position of the patient during and just after injection
- Dose of the anesthetic injected

Although all these factors have been postulated as affecting spinal spread of anesthetic, not many have been shown to change the distribution of blockade when all other factors that affect blockade are kept constant. Site of injection, age, position of the patient during and after injection, dosage and volume of anesthetic solution injected, baricity of local anesthetic, anatomy of the spine, direction of the needle during injection, volume of CSF, and increased intraabdominal pressure can all influence the spread of spinal blockade.

Site of Injection

The site of injection of local anesthetics for spinal anesthesia can determine the level of blockade. In some studies, isobaric spinal 0.5% bupivacaine produces sensory blockade that is reduced by two dermatomes per interspace when injection at L2-3, L3-4, and L4-5 interspaces are compared.[161,162]

Clinical Pearl

- Site of injection and baricity appear to be correlated in determining the level of spinal blockade.

However, no difference in block height exists when hyperbaric bupivacaine or dibucaine is injected as a spinal anesthetic in different interspaces.[163–165]

Age

Some studies have reported changes in block height after spinal anesthesia in the elderly patient as compared with the young patient, but other studies have reported no difference in block height.[166–169] These studies were performed with both isobaric and hyperbaric 0.5% bupivacaine.

Clinical Pearl

- Baricity plays a major role in determining block height after spinal anesthesia in older populations.

Isobaric bupivacaine appears to increase block height, and hyperbaric bupivacaine does not appear to change block height with increasing age. If there is a correlation between increasing age and spinal anesthesia height, it is not strong enough by itself to be a reliable predictor in the clinical setting.[170,171] Just as with site of injection, it appears that baricity plays a major role in determining block height after spinal anesthesia in older populations and age is not an independent factor.

Position

Positioning of the patient is very important for determining level of blockade after hyperbaric and hypobaric spinal anesthesia, but not for isobaric solutions. Sitting, Trendelenburg, and prone jackknife positions can greatly change the spread of the local anesthetic due to effect of gravity.[172–174] Gravity and baricity are interrelated when position is involved in determining spinal block height.

Clinical Pearl

- Positioning of the patient is very important for determining level of blockade after hyperbaric and hypobaric spinal anesthesia, but not for isobaric solutions.

The combination of baricity of the local anesthetic solution and patient positioning determines spinal block height level.[175] The sitting position in combination with a hyperbaric solution can produce analgesia in the perineum. Trendelenburg positioning will also affect spread of hyperbaric and hypobaric local anesthetics due to the effect of gravity.[151,176] Prone jackknife positioning is used for rectal, perineal, and lumbar procedures with a hypobaric local anesthetic.[59,177] This prevents rostral spread of the spinal blockade after injection and positioning in the jackknife position.

Speed of Injection

Speed of injection has been reported to affect spinal block height, but the data available in the literature are conflicting.[178]

Clinical Pearl

- Even though spinal block height does not change with speed of injection, use a smooth, slow injection when giving a spinal anesthetic.

In studies using isobaric bupivacaine, there is no difference in spinal block height with different speeds of injection.[179–181] Even though spinal block height does not change with speed of injection, a smooth, slow injection should be used when giving a spinal anesthetic. If a forceful injection is given and the syringe is not connected tightly to the spinal needle, the needle might disconnect from the syringe with loss of local anesthetic.

Volume, Concentration, & Dose of Local Anesthetic

It is difficult to maintain volume, concentration, or dose of local anesthetic constant without changing any of the other variables, thus it is difficult to produce high-quality studies that investigate these variables singly. Axelsson and associates showed that volume of local anesthetic can affect spinal block height and duration when equivalent doses are used.[182]

Clinical Pearl

- When performing a spinal anesthetic, be cognizant of not only the dose of local anesthetic, but also the volume and concentration so as not to overdose or underdose the patient.

Peng and coworkers showed that concentration of local anesthetic is directly related to dose when determining effective anesthesia.[183] However, dose of local anesthetic plays the greatest role in determining spinal block duration, as neither volume nor concentration of isobaric bupivacaine or tetracaine alter spinal block duration when the dose is held constant.[184,185] Studies have repeatedly shown that spinal block duration is longer when higher doses of local anesthetic are given.[54,61,182,186,187] When performing a spinal anesthetic, be cognizant of not only the dose of local anesthetic, but also the volume and concentration so as not to overdose or underdose the patient.

The use of hyperbaric solutions minimizes the importance of dose and volume except when doses of hyperbaric bupivacaine equal to or less than 10 mg are used. In those cases, there is less cephalad spread and a shorter duration of action.[173] A dose of hyperbaric bupivacaine between 10 and

20 mg results in similar block height.[163] When using hyperbaric solutions, it is important to note that patient positioning and baricity are the most influential factors on block height, except when low doses of hyperbaric bupivacaine are used.

CHOICE OF LOCAL ANESTHETIC

The choice of local anesthetic determines the duration of the spinal blockade. The shortest acting local anesthetic for spinal use is preservative-free 2-chloroprocaine.[188] Procaine is the next shortest acting local anesthetic, followed by lidocaine. The long-acting local anesthetics include bupivacaine, ropivacaine, and tetracaine. Even though chloroprocaine is not currently approved by the FDA for the specific indication of intrathecal use, results from recent clinical trials have shown preservative-free 2-chloroprocaine to be safe, short-acting, and acceptable for outpatient surgery, with some episodes of flu-like symptoms and low back pain associated with the addition of epinephrine.[88] Chronic neurologic deficits have been reported in rabbits when sodium bisulfite is injected into the lumbar subarachnoid space, but when preservative-free 2-chloroprocaine was injected, no permanent neurologic sequelae were noted.[189] Onset time is very fast, and the duration is around 60 min for surgical anesthesia. The dose ranges from 20 to 60 mg, with 40 mg as a usual dose.

Procaine, commonly known as Novocain, is a short-acting ester local anesthetic. Procaine has an onset time of 3 to 5 min and a duration time of 50 to 60 min. However, there is a 14% incidence of block failure associated with procaine 10%.[190] A dose of 50 to 100 mg is suggested for perineal and lower extremity surgery. Concerns about the neurotoxicity of procaine have limited its use, but there appears to be less risk of TNS and transient radicular irritation (TRI).[191–193] For all these reasons, particularly its short duration, procaine is nowadays rarely used for spinal anesthesia.

Clinical Pearls

- The shortest acting local anesthetic for spinal use is preservative-free 2-chloroprocaine.
- Procaine is the next shortest acting local anesthetic, followed by lidocaine.
- The long-acting local anesthetics include bupivacaine, ropivacaine, and tetracaine.

Lidocaine, an amide local anesthetic, also provides an onset time of 3 to 5 min with a duration time of 60 to 90 min. As described previously, there is a strong association between lidocaine and TNS, which limits the usefulness of lidocaine.[65–67] For perineal surgery and saddle-block anesthesia, a dose of 25 to 50 mg is given.

Tetracaine, a long-acting ester local anesthetic, provides anesthesia within 3 to 6 min and lasts 70 to 180 min. The duration of anesthesia is much longer than with the other ester anesthetics and also much longer than with lidocaine. The suggested dose is 5 mg for perineal and lower extremity surgery. Tetracaine is used for intermediate to long lasting cases.

Bupivacaine, another amide local anesthetic, has an onset time of 5 to 8 min with a duration time of 90 to 150 min, which is similar to tetracaine. The suggested dose is 8–10 mg for perineal and lower extremity surgery and 15–20 mg for abdominal surgery. Bupivacaine is one of the most widely used local anesthetics for spinal anesthesia and provides adequate anesthesia and analgesia for intermediate to long duration operating room cases.

Number & Frequency of Local Anesthetic Injections

In the majority of cases, a single-shot injection of local anesthetic is given when a spinal anesthetic is performed. However, a continuous spinal anesthetic can be utilized with an infusion pump continuously providing medication though a spinal catheter or by giving boluses through a spinal catheter.

Clinical Pearl

- When dosing a spinal catheter, if the spinal blockade level is lower than T10, half the initial dose of local anesthetic can be given through the catheter.

When a bolus of local anesthetic is given through a spinal catheter for surgical anesthesia, the onset time and efficacy of anesthesia are similar to injection through a needle.[194] The level of neural blockade should be checked prior to giving a bolus through the catheter. When the spinal blockade level recedes below T10, half the initial dose of local anesthetic can be given through the catheter.

EQUIPMENT FOR SPINAL ANESTHESIA

In the past, most institutions had reusable trays for spinal anesthesia. These trays required preparation by anesthesiologists or anesthesia personnel to ensure that bacterial and chemical contamination would not occur. The contents of the trays did not differ from those currently available commercially, but strict attention to sterility must be maintained to ensure patient safety while using the trays.

Clinical Pearl

- Resuscitation equipment must be available when performing a spinal anesthetic.

Currently, commercially prepared, disposable spinal trays are available and are in use by most institutions. Most

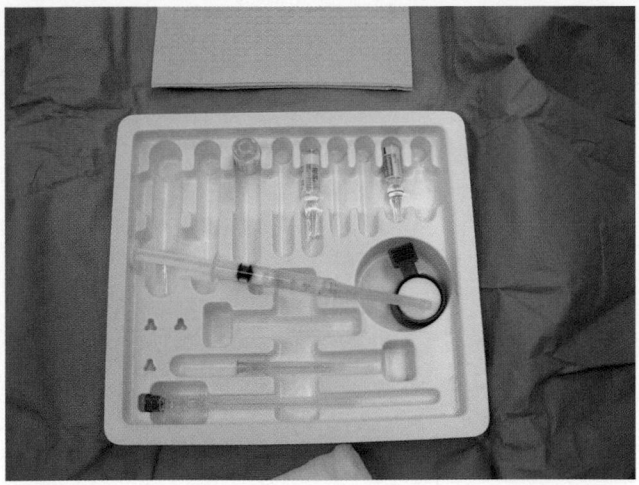

Figure 13–9. The contents of a standard, commercially prepared spinal anesthesia tray.

of these trays contain the same items: a paper towel, fenestrated drape, gauze sponges, prep solution well and sponges, medicine well, ampules of lidocaine 1% and epinephrine, standard or pencil-point needles, introducers, syringes and needles, a filter straw, povidone-iodine solution packet, needle block foam with holder, and an ampule of local anesthetic for spinal injection. These trays are portable, sterile, and easy to use. Familiarity with the contents of the spinal tray is essential to placing a spinal anesthetic quickly. Figure 13–9

shows the contents of a standard, commercially prepared spinal anesthetic tray.

Resuscitation equipment must be available whenever a spinal anesthetic is performed. This includes medication for sedation and induction of general anesthesia (propofol, fentanyl, midazolam, succinylcholine), medication for support of cardiac function (ephedrine, epinephrine, atropine), an oropharyngeal airway, a laryngoscope with blade, an endotracheal tube with stylet and cuff syringe, tape for securing the endotracheal tube, a tongue depressor, a suction apparatus, an oxygen source, and an Ambu bag and facemask. The patient should be monitored during the placement of the spinal anesthetic with a pulse oximeter, blood pressure cuff, and ECG. All of these precautions are necessary to assure administration of spinal anesthesia.

Needles

Needles of different diameters and shapes have been developed for spinal anesthesia. The ones currently used have a close-fitting, removable stylet, which prevents skin and adipose tissue from plugging the needle and possibly entering the subarachnoid space. Figure 13–10 shows the different types of needles used along with the type of point at the end of the needle.

The pencil-point needles (Sprotte and Whitacre) have a rounded, noncutting bevel with a solid tip. The opening is located on the side of the needle 2–4 mm proximal to the

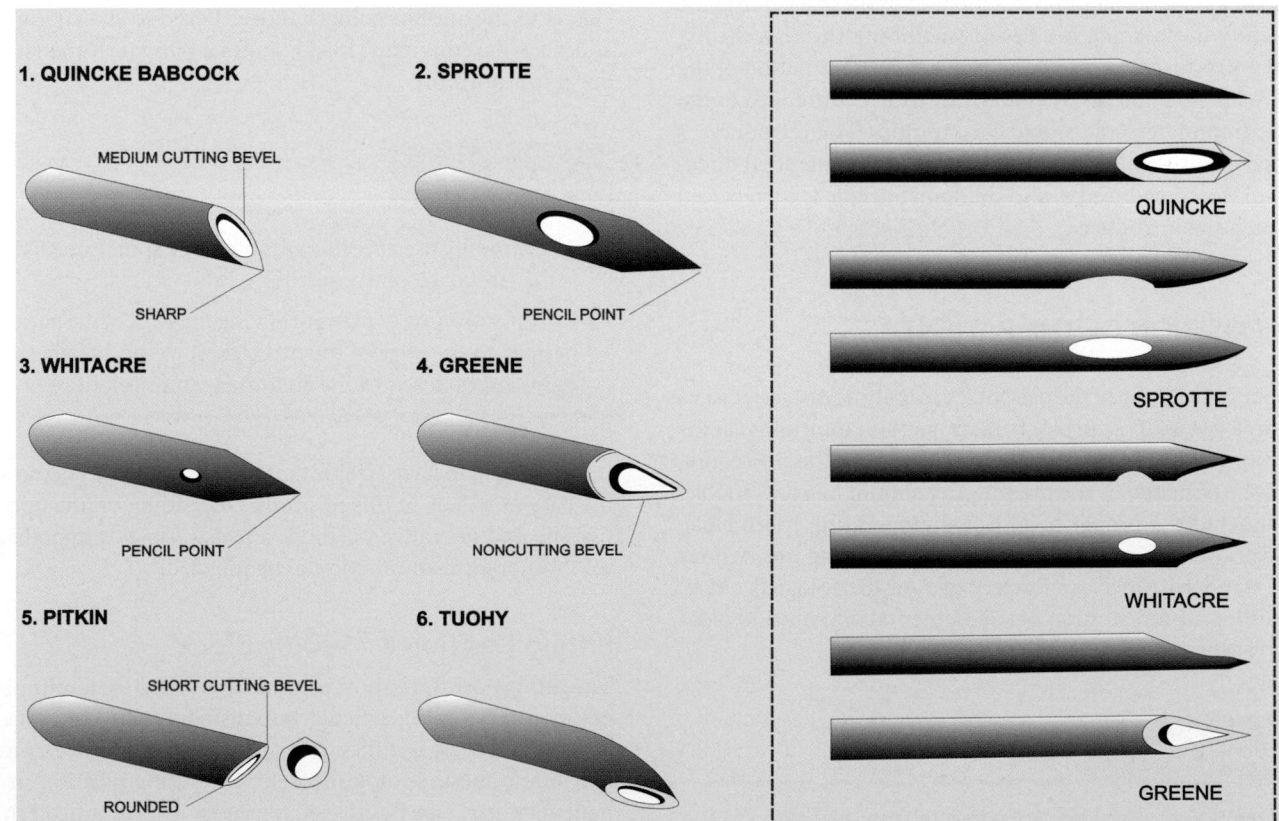

Figure 13–10. The different types of needles used for spinal anesthesia along with the type of point at the end of each type of needle.

tip of the needle. The needles with cutting bevels include the Quincke and Pitkin needles. The Quincke needle has a sharp point with a medium-length cutting needle, and the Pitkin has a sharp point and short bevel with cutting edges. Finally, the Greene spinal needle has a rounded point and rounded noncutting bevel. If a continuous spinal catheter is to be placed, a Tuohy needle can be used to find the subarachnoid space before placement of the catheter.

Pencil-point needles provide a better tactile sensation of the layers of ligament encountered but require more force to insert than bevel-tip needles. The bevel of the needle should be directed longitudinally to decrease the incidence of PDPH.[195]

Clinical Pearls

- Pencil-point needles provide a better tactile sensation of the layers of ligament encountered but require more force to insert than bevel-tip needles.
- The bevel of the needle should be directed longitudinally to decrease the incidence of PDPH.

Larger gauge needles and needles with rounded, noncutting bevels also decrease the incidence of PDPH, but are more easily deflected than smaller gauge needles.

Introducers have been designed to assist with the placement of spinal needles into the subarachnoid space due to the difficulty in directing needles of small bore through the tissues. Introducers also serve to prevent contamination of the CSF with small pieces of epidermis, which could lead to the formation of dermoid spinal cord tumors. The introducer is placed into the interspinous ligament in the intended direction of the spinal needle, and the spinal needle is then placed through the introducer.

POSITION OF THE PATIENT

Proper positioning of the patient for spinal anesthesia is essential for a fast, successful block. Many factors come into play for positioning of the patient. Before beginning the procedure, both the patient and the practitioner should be comfortable. This includes a proper height of the operating room table, blankets or covers for the patient, a functioning intravenous line, standard American Society of Anesthesiologists (ASA) monitors, administration of supplemental oxygen, and sedation for the patient.

Clinical Pearls

- The patient should be appropriately premedicated to assure comfort during the procedure.

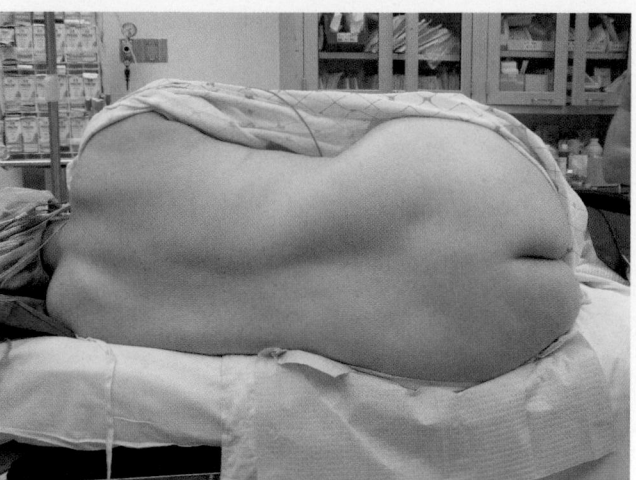

Figure 13–11. A patient in the lateral decubitus position.

A trained assistant should be available to help optimize patient position. Alternatively, special positioning devices can be used. There are three main positions for administering a spinal anesthetic: the lateral decubitus, sitting, and prone position.

Lateral Decubitus Position

A commonly used position for placing a spinal anesthetic is the lateral decubitus position. Ideal positioning consists of having the back of the patient parallel to the edge of the bed closest to the anesthesiologist, knees flexed to the abdomen, and neck flexed. Figure 13–11 shows a patient in the lateral decubitus position.

Clinical Pearls

- A commonly used position for placing a spinal anesthetic is the lateral decubitus position.
- Ideal positioning consists of having the back of the patient parallel to the edge of the bed closest to the anesthesiologist, knees flexed to the abdomen, and neck flexed.

It is beneficial to have an assistant to help hold and encourage the patient to stay in this position. Depending on the operative site and operative position, a hypo-, iso-, or hyperbaric solution of local anesthetic can be injected.

Sitting Position & "Saddle Block"

The sitting position is most commonly utilized for low lumbar or sacral anesthesia, particularly in instances when the patient is obese and there is difficulty in finding the midline. In practice, many anesthesiologists prefer the sitting position in all patients who can be positioned for the ease of identification of the landmarks. Using a stool for a footrest and a pillow for the patient to hold can be valuable in this position. The patient

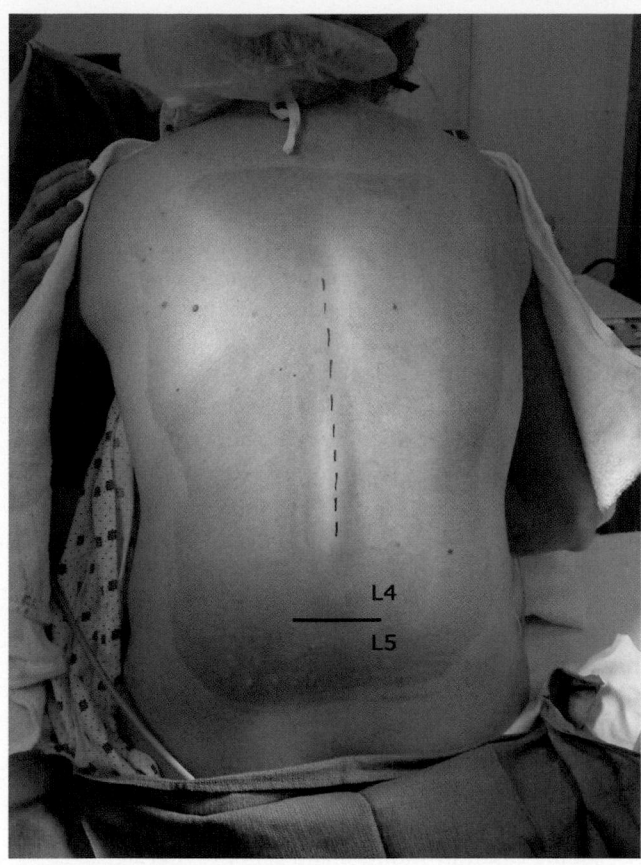

Figure 13–12. A patient in the sitting position with the L4/L5 interspace marked.

should have the neck flexed and the lower back pushed out to open up the lumbar vertebral space. Figure 13–12 depicts a patient in the sitting position and the L4-5 interspace is marked.

Clinical Pearls

- The sitting position is commonly used for low lumbar or sacral anesthesia and in instances when the patient is obese and there is difficulty in finding the midline in the lateral position.
- When performing a saddle block, the patient should remain in the sitting position for at least 5 min after a hyperbaric spinal anesthetic is placed to allow the spinal to settle into that region.

When performing a saddle block (hyperbaric solutions), the patient should remain in the sitting position for at least 5 min after a hyperbaric spinal anesthetic is placed to allow the spinal to settle into that region. If a higher level of blockade is necessary, the patient should be placed supine immediately after spinal placement and the table adjusted accordingly to allow the hyperbaric solution layer alongside the thoracic kyphosis.

Prone Position

The prone position can be utilized for induction of spinal anesthesia if the patient needs to be in this position for the surgery, such as for rectal, perineal, or lumbar procedures. A hypobaric or isobaric solution of local anesthetic is preferred in the prone jackknife position for these procedures.

Clinical Pearl

- The prone position can be utilized for spinal anesthesia if the patient needs to be in this position for the surgery, such as for rectal, perineal, or lumbar procedures.

This avoids rostral spread of the local anesthetic and decreases the risk of high spinal anesthesia.

Another, less elegant solution is to inject a hyperbaric solution of local anesthetic with the patient in the *sitting* position and wait until the spinal anesthesia "sets-in," which is typically 15–20 min after injection. The patient is then positioned in the prone position with vigilant monitoring, including frequent verbal communication with the patient.

TECHNIQUE OF LUMBAR PUNCTURE

When performing a spinal anesthetic, appropriate monitors should be placed, and airway and resuscitation equipment should be readily available. All equipment for the spinal blockade should be ready for use, and all necessary medications should be drawn up prior to positioning the patient for spinal anesthesia. Adequate preparation for the spinal reduces the amount of time needed to perform the block and assists with making the patient comfortable.

Proper positioning is the key to making the spinal anesthetic quick and successful. Once the patient is correctly positioned, the midline should be palpated. The iliac crests are palpated, and a line is drawn between them in order to find the body of L4 or the L4-5 interspace. Other interspaces can be identified, depending on where the needle is to be inserted.

Clinical Pearls

- When performing a spinal anesthetic, appropriate monitors should be placed, and airway and resuscitation equipment should be readily available.
- All equipment for the spinal blockade should be ready for use, and all necessary medications should be drawn up prior to positioning the patient for spinal anesthesia.

The skin should be cleaned with sterile cleaning solution, and the area should be draped in a sterile fashion. A small wheal of local anesthetic is injected into the skin at the site of insertion. More local anesthetic is then administered along the intended path of the spinal needle insertion to a depth of

1 to 2 in. This serves a dual purpose: additional anesthesia for the spinal needle insertion and identification of the correct path for spinal needle placement.

Midline Approach

If the midline approach is used, palpate the desired interspace and inject local anesthetic into the skin and subcutaneous tissue. The introducer needle is placed with a slight cephalad angle of 10 to 15 degrees. Next the spinal needle is passed through the introducer. The needle passes through the subcutaneous tissue, supraspinous ligament, interspinous ligament, ligamentum flavum, epidural space, dura mater, and subarachnoid mater in order to reach the subarachnoid space.

Resistance changes as the spinal needle passes through each level on the way to the subarachnoid space. Subcutaneous tissue offers less resistance to the spinal needle than ligaments. When the spinal needle goes though the dura mater, a "pop" is often appreciated. Once this pop is felt, the stylet should be removed from the introducer to check for flow of CSF. For spinal needles of small gauge (26–29 gauge), this may take 5–10 sec, but in some patients, it can take a minute or longer. If there is no flow, the needle might be obstructed and rotating it 90 degrees may be helpful. Debris can obstruct the orifice of the spinal needle and, if necessary, withdraw the needle and clear the orifice before attempting the spinal anesthetic again. Finally, the spinal needle may not be in the correct position if CSF does not flow freely and the needle should be repositioned.

If the spinal needle contacts bone, note the depth of the needle and reinsert the needle more cephalad. If the bone is contacted again, compare the needle depth with that of the last bone contact to determine what structure is being contacted. For instance, if bone contact is deeper to the first insertion, redirect the needle more cephalad to avoid the inferior spinous process. If bone contact is at the same depth as the original insertion, reassess the insertion point to avoid the vertebral lamina. If bone contact is more shallow than the original insertion, redirect the needle more caudad to avoid the superior spinous process.

Clinical Pearls

- As the spinal needle passes through the dura mater, a "pop" is often appreciated.
- Once this pop is felt, the stylet should be removed from the introducer to check for flow of CSF.
- For spinal needles of small gauge (26–29 gauge), this usually takes 5–10 sec, but in some patients, it can take longer (particularly in old or dehydrated patients).
- If there is no flow of CSF, the needle might be obstructed by a nerve root and rotating it 90 degrees may be helpful.

When the spinal needle needs to be reinserted, it is important to withdraw the needle back to the skin level before redirection. Only make small changes in the angle of direction when reinserting the spinal needle as small changes at the surface lead to large changes in direction when the needle reaches the meninges. Bowing and curving of the spinal needle when inserting through the skin also can steer the needle off course when attempting to contact the subarachnoid space.

Paresthesias may be elicited when passing a spinal needle. The stylet should be removed from the spinal needle, and if CSF is seen and the paresthesia no longer present, it is safe to inject the local anesthetic. Most likely a cauda equina nerve root was encountered. If there is no CSF flow, it is possible that the spinal needle has contacted a spinal nerve root traversing the epidural space. The needle should be removed and redirected toward the side opposite the paresthesia.

After free flow of CSF is established, inject the local anesthetic slowly at a speed of less than 0.5 mL/sec. Additional aspiration of CSF at the midpoint and end of injection can be attempted to confirm continued subarachnoid administration but may not always be possible when small needles are used. Once local anesthetic injection is complete, the introducer and spinal needle are removed as one unit from the back of the patient. The patient should then be positioned according to the surgical procedure and baricity of local anesthetic given. The table can be tilted either in the Trendelenburg or reverse Trendelenburg position as needed to adjust the height of the block after testing the sensory level. The anesthesiologist should carefully monitor and support vital signs.

Paramedian (Lateral) Approach

If the patient has a calcified interspinous ligament or difficulty in flexing the spine, a paramedian approach to achieve spinal anesthesia can be utilized. The patient can be in any position for this approach: sitting, lateral, or even prone jackknife. After identifying the correct level for spinal anesthesia placement, the spinous process is palpated. The needle should be inserted 1 cm lateral to this point and directed toward the middle of the interspace. The ligamentum flavum is usually the first resistance identified, but sometimes the lamina is contacted. If this is the case, redirection of the needle should be performed.

Clinical Pearls

For the paramedian approach:

- After identifying the correct level for spinal anesthesia placement, palpate the spinous process.
- The needle should be inserted 1 cm lateral and 1 cm inferior to this point and directed toward the middle of the interspace.
- The ligamentum flavum is usually the first resistance identified.

Another method is to insert the needle 1 cm lateral and 1 cm inferior to the interspace and contact the lamina. After

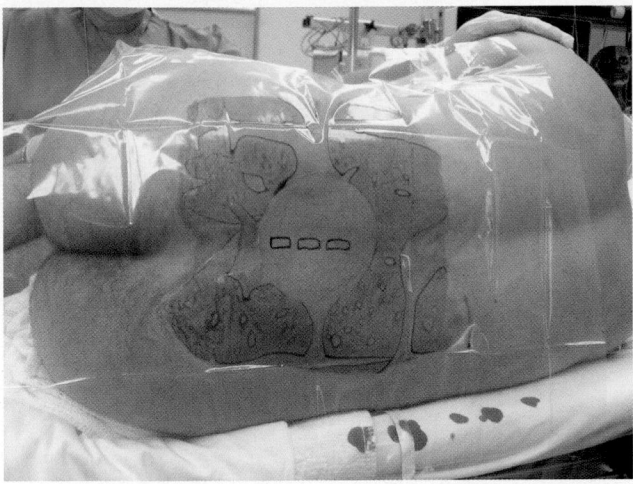

Figure 13–13. The landmarks used for a paramedian approach to spinal anesthesia. The patient is in the right lateral decubitus position and the spinous processes are marked.

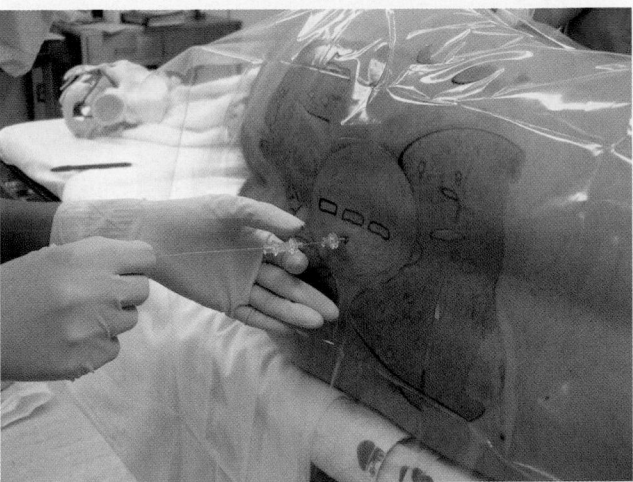

Figure 13–14. Successful performance of a paramedian spinal anesthetic. The needle is inserted 1 cm lateral to the spinous process and directed toward the middle of the interspace.

the bone is contacted, the needle should be walked off the lamina and into the subarachnoid space. Figure 13–13 shows the landmarks used for a paramedian approach to spinal anesthesia. Figure 13–14 depicts paramedian technique for spinal anesthesia.

Taylor Approach

The Taylor (or lumbosacral) approach to spinal anesthesia is a paramedian approach directed toward the L5-S1 interspace. Due to the fact that this is the largest interspace, the Taylor approach can be used when other approaches are not successful or cannot be performed. As with the paramedian approach, the patient can be in any position for this approach: sitting, lateral, or prone.

Clinical Pearls

For the Taylor approach:

■ The needle should be inserted 1 cm medial and inferior to the posterior superior iliac spine, then angled cephalad 45–55 degrees.

■ This should be medial enough to reach the midline at the L5 spinous process.

■ After needle insertion, the first significant resistance felt is the ligamentum flavum.

The needle should be inserted at a point 1 cm medial and inferior to the posterior superior iliac spine, then angled cephalad 45–55 degrees. This should be medial enough to reach the midline at the L5 spinous process. After needle insertion, the first significant resistance felt is the ligamentum flavum, and then the dura mater is punctured to allow free flow of CSF as the subarachnoid space is entered. Figure 13–15 shows the Taylor approach to spinal anesthesia.

CONTINUOUS CATHETER TECHNIQUES

An indwelling catheter can be placed for continuous spinal anesthesia. Local anesthetics can be dosed repeatedly through the catheter and the level and duration of anesthesia adjusted as necessary for the surgical procedure. Placement of a continuous spinal catheter occurs in a similar fashion as a regular spinal anesthetic except that a larger gauge needle, such as a Tuohy, is used to enable the passage of the catheter. After insertion of the Tuohy needle, the subarachnoid space is found and the spinal catheter is passed 2–3 cm into the subarachnoid space. If there is difficulty in passing the catheter, attempt to rotate the Tuohy needle 180 degrees. Never withdraw the catheter back into the needle shaft because there is a risk of shearing the catheter and leaving a piece of it in the subarachnoid space. If the catheter needs to be withdrawn, withdraw the catheter and needle together, and attempt the continuous spinal at another interspace.

Clinical Pearls

■ After insertion of the Tuohy needle, the subarachnoid space is entered, and the spinal catheter is passed 2–3 cm into the subarachnoid space.

■ If there is difficulty in passing the catheter, attempt to rotate the Tuohy needle 180 degrees.

Since the needle used to pass the spinal catheter is a large-bore needle, there is a much higher risk of PDPH, especially in young female patients. Cauda equina syndrome can occur with small spinal catheters, so the FDA has advised against using catheters smaller than 24 gauge for continuous spinal anesthetics.[196–199]

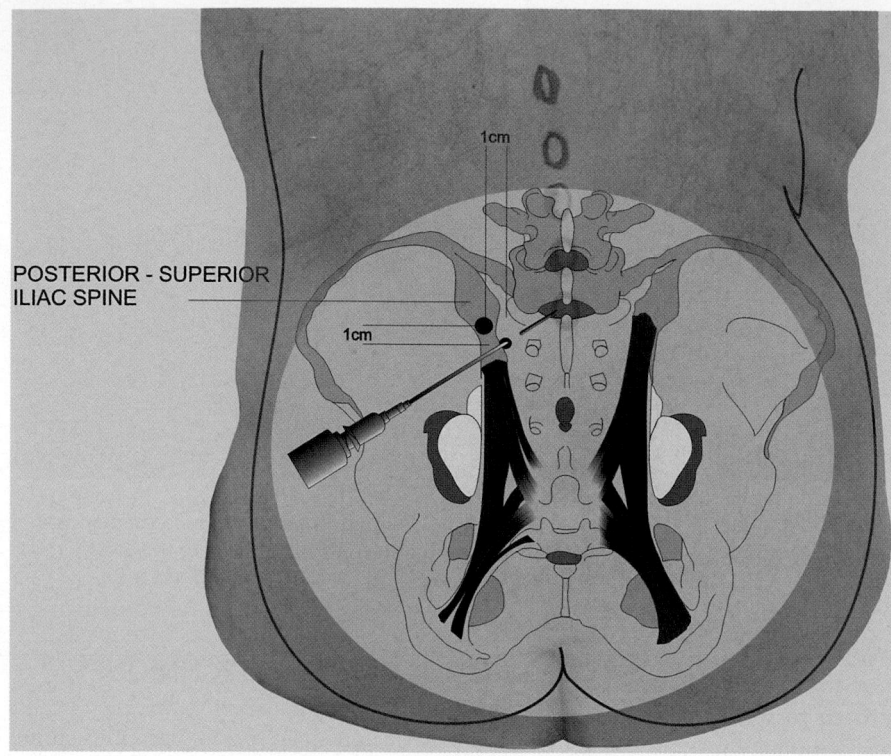

1cm

POSTERIOR - SUPERIOR
ILIAC SPINE

1cm

Figure 13–15. The Taylor approach to spinal anesthesia. The needle is inserted 1 cm medial and inferior to the posterior superior iliac spine, then angled cephalad 45–55 degrees.

INTRAOPERATIVE & POSTOPERATIVE MANAGEMENT

Depending on the baricity of the local anesthetic solution injected, the level of the spinal anesthetic may be adjusted by repositioning the patient during the first few minutes after injection is used. After injection of the spinal anesthetic, assess the cardiovascular status of the patient, as changes can occur up to 20 min after spinal anesthesia injection. Continued monitoring of the heart rate and frequent readings of the blood pressure are recommended to detect hypotension so that corrections can be made early and quickly.

Intraoperative management of spinal anesthesia is similar to intraoperative management of other forms of regional anesthesia. The patient may not feel operative pain but may still be uncomfortable. Supplemental benzodiazepines, hypnotics, or opioids can be given intravenously. Comforting words from a caring, empathetic anesthesiologist also go a long way toward a pleasant experience by the patient.

Clinical Pearl

- After injection of the spinal anesthetic, assess the cardiovascular status of the patient, as hemodynamic change can occur up to 20 min after spinal anesthesia injection.

Elderly patients can become confused with benzodiazepines. Propofol can be given as an infusion to assist with making the patient more comfortable, and opioids can assist with pain from an unanesthetized portion of the body. Oxygen should always be administered via facemask or nasal cannula.

Postoperatively the patient should be monitored until the spinal anesthetic recedes. In most circumstances the patient should void prior to being discharged from the postanesthesia care unit. Since the voiding mechanism is innervated by sacral autonomic fibers, which are the last to return to preoperative function, voiding may be delayed. The risk of discharging a patient from the recovery room prior to voiding includes complications involving a distended or ruptured bladder or a need for re-admission. Hypotension from continued blood volume redistribution as well as surgical bleeding should be monitored postoperatively.

COMPLICATIONS

Complications of spinal blockade include local anesthetic neurotoxicity, neurologic injury, PDPH, high spinal blockade, and cardiovascular collapse. Neurotoxicity studies performed in animal models producing neurologic deficits and changes in spinal cord histology were not seen with clinically useful concentrations of tetracaine, lidocaine, bupivacaine, or chloroprocaine in humans. High concentration tetracaine and lidocaine cause histopathologic changes and neurologic deficits in animal models.[200–202] Spinal cord blood flow is increased, and vasodilation occurs with intrathecal bupivacaine, lidocaine, mepivacaine, and tetracaine. Ropivacaine causes vasoconstriction and decreases spinal blood flow in a dose-dependent fashion. TNS may occur with spinal anesthesia, usually with lidocaine.

Neurologic Injury

Neurologic injury is a serious complication after spinal anesthesia. In a large, prospective survey in France, Auroy and colleagues reported 12 neurologic complications in a series of 35,439 spinal anesthetics.[203] Nine peripheral neuropathies and three cases of cauda equina were seen, which correlates to a 0.03% neurologic complication rate. Moen and coworkers reported similar complication rates after spinal anesthesia.[204] Neurologic injury can occur after needle introduction into the spinal cord or nerves, spinal cord ischemia, bacterial contamination of the subarachnoid space, or hematoma formation. Although the elicitation of paresthesias during spinal anesthesia has been implicated as a risk factor for persistent neurologic injury, it is not known whether an intervention after paresthesia can prevent development of neurologic complication.[205] It is also unknown as to whether the actual injection of local anesthesia after paresthesia is elicited causes permanent neurologic damage, similar to peripheral nerves when an injection is associated with high pressures during injection of local anesthetic solution.[206,207] It is possible that when paresthesia occurs, that a spinal nerve has been penetrated by the spinal needle; consequently, injection of local anesthetic into the spinal nerve may result in neurologic injury.

Cauda Equina Syndrome

Cauda equina syndrome has been reported with the use of continuous spinal microcatheters.[196–199] The use of hyperbaric 5% lidocaine for spinal anesthesia is also associated with an increased incidence of cauda equina syndrome,[208–210] although other local anesthetics have also been implicated.[204,211–213] Other risk factors for cauda equina syndrome include repeated dosing of local anesthetic solution through continuous spinal catheters and possibly multiple single-injection spinal anesthetics. Current suggestions for prevention of cauda equina syndrome from spinal anesthesia include aspiration of CSF before and after local anesthetic injection. When CSF cannot be aspirated after injection, some suggest that a full dose of local anesthetic not be injected. Limiting the amount of local anesthetic given in the subarachnoid space, and if a spinal anesthetic has to be repeated, use of a different local anesthetic also may help preventing cauda equina syndrome.

Clinical Pearls

To reduce neurologic complications after spinal anesthesia:

- Maintain strict sterility throughout the spinal block procedure.
- Ensure coagulation parameters are within normal limits.
- Follow the ASRA consensus conference guidelines on neuraxial anesthesia and anticoagulation.
- Use the lowest efficient dose of local anesthetic solution.

- Reevaluate after incomplete neural blockade prior to performing another spinal anesthetic.
- Avoid large volumes and repeated injections of hyperbaric lidocaine.
- Never use preservative-containing solutions in the subarachnoid space.

Arachnoiditis

Arachnoiditis can occur after spinal injection of local anesthetic solution, but is also known to occur after intrathecal steroid injection.[214–217] Causes of arachnoiditis include infection, myelograms from oil-based dyes, blood in the intrathecal space, neuroirritant, neurotoxic or neurolytic substances, surgical interventions in the spine, intrathecal corticosteroids, and trauma. Arachnoiditis has been reported after traumatic dural puncture, local anesthetics, detergents, antiseptics or other substances unintentionally injected into the spinal canal.[218]

Spinal Hematoma Formation

Spinal hematoma formation is rare complication after spinal anesthesia and infrequently occurs in the absence of trauma or anticoagulant therapy. Major spontaneous hemorrhagic complications have been reported after antithrombotic and thrombolytic therapy.[219] Risk factors for spinal hematoma formation include the intensity of the anticoagulant effect, increased age, female gender, history of gastrointestinal bleeding, concomitant aspirin use, and length of therapy.[220] Although most spinal hematomas occur in the epidural space due to the prominent epidural venous plexus, few reports have mentioned subarachnoid bleeding as the cause of neurologic deficits. The source of the bleeding can be from either an injured artery or vein. If new or progressive neurologic symptoms develop, an immediate neurosurgery consultation should be obtained and a magnetic resonance image (MRI) of the spine should be performed as soon as possible.

A recent study from Sweden showed that over a 10-year period from 1990 to 1999, out of 1,260,000 spinal anesthetics, eight spinal hematomas occurred, for an incidence of 0.00063%. Seven of the hematomas formed after single-shot spinal anesthesia and one formed after a continuous spinal blockade. A total of 33 spinal hematomas were noted in the study after (both) epidural and spinal blockade, and of these, 11 patients had evidence of coagulopathy or thromboprophylaxis administered soon before or after the central neuraxial blockade. In 10 patients who had spinal hematoma formation, difficulty in placing the epidural or spinal was noted, and in 5 patients symptoms of spinal hematoma appeared in the immediate postoperative period or shortly after removal of epidural catheter. Fourteen patients had delayed symptoms of spinal hematoma ranging from 6 h to 3 days after central neuraxial block was performed. In one patient, pain and paraparesis appeared 2 weeks after difficult spinal anesthetic placement. Of the 33 patients, 6 had full recovery, but 27 suffered permanent neurologic damage. Five of the six patients that had full recovery were treated conservatively, but one underwent laminectomy. Eleven of the patients who did not recover underwent laminectomy, and in a further six cases, laminectomy was considered, but, due to delay in diagnosis, was not performed. Thirteen patients suffered paraparesis, three had cauda equina syndrome, three were left with sensory deficit, three died, and five were reported only to have lack of recovery without more information.[204]

Meningitis

Meningitis, either bacterial or aseptic, can occur after spinal anesthesia is performed.[221] Sources of infection include contaminated spinal trays and medication, patient infection, and oral flora from the practitioner without a facemask. Povidone-iodine solution is most commonly chosen for skin antisepsis before initiation of epidural and spinal anesthesia, and single-use containers are suggested. Most cases of meningitis after spinal anesthesia in the first half of the twentieth century were aseptic and could be traced to chemical contamination and detergents.[222,223] Marinac showed that causes of drug- and chemical-induced meningitis include the nonsteroidal antiinflammatory drugs, certain antibiotics, radiographic agents, and muromonab-CD3. There also appears to be an association between the occurrence of the hypersensitivity-type reactions and underlying collagen vascular or rheumatologic disease.[224] Carp and Bailey performed lumbar puncture (LP) in bacteremic rats, and only those with a circulating *Escherichia coli* count of greater than 50 CFU/mL at the time of LP developed meningitis.[225] Although meningitis after LP has also been described in bacteremic children,[226] the incidence of meningitis after diagnostic LP is not significantly different in bacteremic patients compared with spontaneous incidence of meningitis.[227] Oral flora can contaminate the CSF when a spinal anesthetic is being performed. *Streptococcus salivarius, S. viridans, Staphylococcus aureus, Pseudomonas aeruginosa, Acinetobacter,* and *Mycobacterium tuberculosis* have all been isolated in cases of bacterial meningitis after spinal anesthesia or LP.[228–231] It is of utmost importance to use a strict aseptic technique when performing spinal anesthesia. Anyone standing behind the patient during spinal anesthetic administration should wear a cap and facemask to prevent seeding of the patient's CSF with oropharyngeal flora.

In general, to reduce neurologic complications after spinal anesthesia, strict sterility is maintained throughout the spinal block procedure. Check laboratory values of the patient and make sure coagulation parameters are within normal limits. Follow the second ASRA consensus conference guidelines on neuraxial anesthesia and anticoagulation.[232] When giving a spinal anesthetic, use the lowest efficient dose of local anesthetic solution. Incomplete neural blockade should not always necessitate repeat spinal injection of local anesthetic solution. Instead, reevaluate and attempt to change the level of the spinal block prior to repeat injection. Avoid large volumes and repeated injections of hyperbaric lidocaine. Never inject preservative-containing solutions into the subarachnoid space. The administration of new compounds in the subarachnoid space must be supported by data of spinal neuropharmacology and the lack of neurotoxicity must have been previously checked with animal studies.[233]

Postdural Puncture Headache

PDPH was first described by Dr. August Bier in 1898, after experimenting on himself. The incidence of PDPH is up to 25% after spinal anesthesia, and the main morbidity after PDPH is restriction of activities of daily living. The headache is characteristically worse when the head is elevated and becomes milder or completely relieved when the patient is supine. PDPH is due to loss of CSF. The subsequent low CSF pressure causes traction on nerve roots and intracranial structures when the patient stands upright. Pain after dural puncture is probably due to increase in cerebral blood flow (CBF). As CSF pressure decreases, CBF increases in order to maintain a constant intracranial volume. Cranial nerve symptoms such as diplopia and tinnitus may occur along with nausea and vomiting. Incidence of PDPH decreases with increasing age and use of small-diameter needles with noncutting, pencil-point needles.[234–236] Although most patients can be treated conservatively with fluids, caffeine, bed rest, analgesics, and sumatriptan, it can take anywhere from 1 to 6 weeks for symptoms to resolve spontaneously. Epidural blood patch remains the mainstay of invasive treatment for PDPH.[237] Effectiveness of blood patching ranges from 64% in obstetrical patients to 95% in the nonpregnant population. The proposed mechanism of action of blood patching is believed to be clot formation over the meningeal hole, preventing further leakage of CSF while the dural puncture heals. Symptoms usually resolve within 1 to 24 h. In patients who do not have symptomatic relief after the first epidural blood patch, a second epidural blood patch is effective 90% of the time. Complications may also arise after epidural blood patch. Reports of back pain, neck pain, lower extremity pain, transient temperature elevation, cranial nerve palsies, nerve root irritation, seizures, acute mental deterioration, subdural hematoma, permanent paresthesias, and cauda equina syndrome have been noted after an epidural blood patch was performed. The most common complication is back pain, which can occur in up to 35% of patients. However, an epidural blood patch is well tolerated if performed with attention to asepsis.[238] If any acute mental changes occur or a second blood patch fails to produce relief, a neurology consult should be immediately obtained.

Intravenous injection of 500 mg of caffeine results in better relief of PDPH than placebo.[234,239,240] One to two doses intravenously should be adequate. Three hundred milligrams of oral caffeine has also been shown to be better than placebo in relieving PDPH.[241] A cup of 150 mL of coffee contains 150 mg of caffeine. Because caffeine is a cerebral vasoconstrictor and a CNS stimulant, complications may occur after administration, including seizures and transient atrial fibrillation.

Sumatriptan is a serotonin agonist and causes cerebral vasoconstriction. Sumatriptan is used for the treatment of migraines; however, there are conflicting reports on the value of sumatriptan for PDPH.[242–244] Caution should be used for patients with coronary artery disease or Prinzmetal angina as sumatriptan can cause coronary artery vasospasm. Since sumatriptan is injected subcutaneously, pain at the injection site may occur. More studies need to be performed to determine the usefulness of sumatriptan in treating PDPH. The reader should refer to Chapter 73 (Postdural Puncture Headache) for more in-depth discussions on PDPH.

High Spinal Anesthesia

High spinal anesthesia can result in profound respiratory impairment, most likely due to brainstem ischemia from hypotension. If the blood pressure and cardiac output become too low due to vasodilation, cerebral blood flow can be impaired. This leads to ischemia of the medullary respiratory center. If blood pressure and cardiac output are restored, spontaneous respiration can quickly be restored. This illustrates the importance of monitoring the vital signs closely and acting quickly to correct them.

Cardiovascular Collapse

Cardiovascular collapse can occur after spinal anesthesia, although it is a rare event. Auroy and coworkers reported only 9 cardiac arrests in 35,439 spinal anesthetics performed.[203] Bradycardia usually precedes cardiac arrest,[143,153,245–247] and early, aggressive treatment of bradycardia is warranted. Treatment of bradycardia includes intravenous atropine, ephedrine, and epinephrine. In cases of cardiac arrest after spinal anesthesia, epinephrine should be used early, and the Advanced Cardiac Life Support (ACLS) protocol should be initiated.[248] There are a few theories as to why spinal anesthesia results in cardiac arrest. Respiratory depression, excessive sedation, and decrease in preload have all been implicated. Paradoxically hyperventilation, not hypoventilation occurs with spinal block levels up to T4.[249] Cardiac arrest after spinal anesthesia can occur with an oxygen saturation maintained above 95%, and hypoxemia cannot be blamed as the sole cause of cardiac arrest.[153,250] Excessive sedation has also been proposed as a reason for cardiac arrest, but with the use of pulse oximeters, it is unlikely that either excessive sedation or hypoxemia is a cause.[248] A decrease in preload likely leads to increased parasympathetic response that results in bradycardia.[248,251] Activation of three types of receptors have been proposed to cause bradycardia: the low-pressure baroreceptors in the right atrium, the receptors in the myocardial pacemaker, and the mechanoreceptors in the left atrium.[153] Other factors that can lead to more severe bradycardia after spinal anesthesia include high sympathetic blockade from the spinal anesthetic, hypercarbia, hypoxemia, excess sedation from medications given, and chronic medications that cause suppression of the sympathetic nervous system.

Several treatments have been advocated to decrease the incidence of and improve the survival after cardiac arrest due to spinal anesthesia. Prevention of a decrease in preload by volume loading prior to placement of the spinal and prompt replacement of fluid losses are key to lowering the risk of bradycardia and cardiac arrest. Treating even relatively mild decreases in heart rate with atropine and adding a vasopressor for aggressive vagolytic treatment can be beneficial.[245,246] Epinephrine should be administered early in cases of profound bradycardia or full cardiac arrest after spinal anesthesia. Cardiopulmonary resuscitation (CPR) can be ineffective after spinal anesthesia because of vasodilation, and successful CPR requires a coronary perfusion pressure gradient of 15 to 20 mm Hg. This amount of coronary perfusion pressure can be achieved with epinephrine 0.01–0.02 mg/kg IV initially with an increase to 0.1 mg/kg IV. IF these measures are unsuccessful, a larger dose of epinephrine may be needed and aggressive CPR may need to be instituted.[252]

OUTPATIENT SPINAL ANESTHESIA

Each year the number of surgeries increase and more are performed on an outpatient basis. As anesthesiologists, we are always looking for new ways to provide efficient anesthetic care that is safe, controls pain, allows the patient to be discharged home in a timely fashion as per postanesthesia care unit protocol, and is easily performed and reproducible. Spinal anesthesia fits well into the outpatient surgery model,[253] and techniques and medication cocktails are continuously improved.

Clinical Pearl

- Forty milligrams of spinal administration of 2-chloroprocaine produces a peak block height of T7, tourniquet tolerance of 46 min, and discharge within 104 min.

In the past, spinal administration of 2-chloroprocaine was associated with chronic neurologic deficits that were believed to be due to sodium bisulfite, an antioxidant used to prolong the shelf life of chloroprocaine.[189,200,254] Trials of spinal 2-chloroprocaine are being performed with new formulations that do not include sodium bisulfite.[186,188,255–260] Forty milligrams of spinal 2-chloroprocaine produces a peak block height of T7, tourniquet tolerance of 46 min, and discharge within 104 min. Forty milligrams of 2% isobaric lidocaine produces a peak block height of T8, tourniquet tolerance of 38 min, and discharge within 134 min. Slightly hyperbaric bupivacaine (1.00100; 7.5 mg) produces a peak block height of T9, tourniquet tolerance of 46 min, and ambulation within 191 min. Table 13–5 lists various choices of local anesthetics for spinal anesthesia, peak block height level and the duration of anesthesia. The reader is referred to Chapter 63 (Neuraxial Anesthesia in Outpatients) for more information on this topic.

Table 13–5.

Local Anesthetics Used for Outpatient Surgical Procedures

	Peak Height	Tourniquet Tolerance	Ambulation	Discharge
Spinal 2-Chloroprocaine				
40 mg	T7	46 min		104 min
Bupivacaine slightly hyperbaric (1.00100)				
7.5 mg	T9	52 min	191 min	
Lidocaine 2% isobaric				
40 mg	T8	38 min		134 min

COMMON CLINICAL PROBLEMS & DILEMMAS IN PRACTICE OF SPINAL ANESTHESIA

As with any other form of anesthesia, spinal anesthesia can present clinical problems. This includes inability to locate the subarachnoid space due to difficulties with patient positioning, a lower level of spinal blockade than required for surgery, and the use of spinal anesthesia for outpatient surgery.

Whenever there are problems with placing a spinal anesthetic, the anesthesiologist should check the position of the patient. In order to maximize the chances of success, optimal positioning of the patient should be sought. If the patient is in the sitting position, the shoulders should be placed in a down position, arms should be in front of the patient, neck should be flexed, and the lower back should be pushed out posteriorly so that the interspace can be maximally exposed to the anesthesiologist. A member of the operating room personnel who is trained to assist with patient positioning should be used. If the proposed interspace cannot be found by the midline technique, the paramedian technique can be attempted. The interspace above or below the original site of spinal injection can be attempted with adjustment to the local anesthetic that is injected.

Clinical Pearls

- To maximize the chances of success for spinal anesthesia, the patient should be in the optimal position.
- If the patient is sitting, place the shoulders down, arms in front, flex the neck, and push out the lower back posteriorly so that exposure of the interspace is maximal.
- When the sitting position cannot be used or is unsuccessful, attempt the lateral decubitus position.
- A repeat injection of local anesthetic could lead to a high level or total spinal anesthesia.

Positioning of the patient can also be enhanced with commercially available positioning devices. These devices can help maintain spinal flexion and create a stable support for the patient, which can be useful if no trained operating room personnel are available to assist with positioning. When the sitting position cannot be used or is unsuccessful, the lateral decubitus position can be used. Either the midline or lateral paramedian technique can be attempted. The largest interlaminar space is at L5, and this can be accessed via Taylor's approach, which is described previously in this chapter.

A repeat injection of local anesthetic could lead to high spinal blockade and possibly result in high or total spinal anesthesia. The alternatives include general anesthesia, peripheral nerve blockade, or infiltration of local anesthesia at the surgical site by the surgeon along with sedation. Different options are considered depending on the health status of the patient, the surgery being performed, use of a tourniquet, and other issues pertaining to the case. It is important to think through what will be best for the patient and the surgeon before choosing another plan of action.

In the past, spinal anesthesia was used sparingly in outpatient surgical procedures because of prolonged recovery room stays after a long-acting local anesthetic was given. Currently, spinal anesthesia is an accepted and sometimes preferred method of providing outpatient anesthesia. Short-acting local anesthetics, such as preservative-free 2-chloroprocaine, have been used with success for surgical procedures lasting an hour or less with no reports of TNS after surgery.[255]

RECENT DEVELOPMENTS IN SPINAL ANESTHESIA

Use of a unilateral spinal block for elderly patients and outpatient surgery has recently come into vogue. Unilateral spinal anesthesia was described in 1950 by Ruben and Kamsler. They reported 116 patients for surgical reduction of hip fracture performed under unilateral spinal blockade.[261] No deaths were reported and no increase in the hazard of operation was found. Recently, attention has returned to the use of unilateral spinal anesthesia in elderly patients[262] and for outpatient surgery.[263]

Use of unilateral spinal anesthesia results in lesser changes in systolic, mean and diastolic pressures, or oxygen saturation in elderly trauma patients (eg hip) fracture. Keeping the operative side up and using a hypobaric spinal solution in low dose for these cases results in excellent anesthesia and remarkable hemostability when the patient is kept in the lateral position for 5–10 min before repositioning supine.

Outpatient surgery using hyperbaric 0.5% bupivacaine takes about 16 minutes for development of surgical anesthesia from time of injection for unilateral spinal anesthesia compared to 13 minutes with traditional bilateral spinal anesthesia. Less hemodynamic changes are found in the unilateral spinal anesthesia group with quicker regression of the block and equal time to discharge home.[264]

In performing a unilateral spinal anesthesia, use of a Whitacre 25-gauge or 27-gauge needle with the bevel opening directed at the operative side is suggested. Low-dose bupivacaine should be used, with hyperbaric bupivacaine in outpatient surgery and hypobaric bupivacaine in the elderly trauma patient.[265] A slow injection rate should be used to produce laminar flow that will assist in producing a unilateral blockade. There is little evidence that keeping a patient in the lateral position for more than 15 min is helpful.

Clinical Pearls

- Use of unilateral spinal anesthesia results in fewer changes in systolic, mean and diastolic pressures, or oxygen saturation in elderly trauma patients.

- After low-molecular-weight heparin (LMWH) administration, delay spinal anesthesia for 10 to 12 h.

- In cases of continuous spinal anesthesia and accidental LMWH therapy, remove the catheter 10–12 h after the last dose of LMWH.

- Avoid spinal anesthesia for 14 days after the last dose of ticlopidine (Ticlid) and 7 days after clopidogrel (Plavix).

- Currently there are no specific concerns regarding spinal anesthesia in patients ingesting herbal medications.

As the population of older patients increases, novel methods of preventing deep venous thrombosis (DVT) and keeping these patients anticoagulated have been developed. Reports of spontaneous spinal and epidural hematoma formation were noted in the cardiology and neurosurgery literature in patients who were anticoagulated.[266–270] As spinal anesthesia was found to be useful in controlling pain postoperatively, such as in lower leg amputations, concern arose over complications occurring in such patients who may have been on concomitant anticoagulant therapy.[271–275]

The concerns of performing central neuraxial block on anticoagulated patients led to the second ASRA consensus conference on neuraxial anesthesia and anticoagulation.[232] There is a very limited risk of spinal hematoma when performing spinal anesthesia while a patient is on subcutaneous heparin. After LMWH administration, spinal anesthesia should be delayed 10–12 h. If blood is noted during needle placement, LMWH therapy should be delayed. In cases of continuous spinal anesthesia and accidental LMWH therapy, the catheter should be removed 10–12 h after the last dose of LMWH. Spinal anesthesia should not be performed for 14 days after the last dose of ticlopidine and 7 days after clopidogrel. Many patients ingest herbal medications; currently there are no specific concerns regarding spinal anesthesia in these patients. The reader is referred to Chapter 70 (Regional Anesthesia in Patients on Anticoagulants) for an in-depth discussion on the use of neuraxial anesthesia in the anticoagulated patient.

SUMMARY

Ever since the introduction of local anesthetics, physicians have investigated different methods of using them. Spinal anesthesia has enjoyed a long and successful history since the late nineteenth century and is currently enjoying significant popularity. Mastery of spinal anesthesia comes with practice; diligence; and knowledge of physiology, pharmacology, and anatomy. Patient safety must always be at the forefront when considering performing a spinal anesthetic. The ease of performance and versatility of spinal anesthesia will continue to result in its widespread popularity in both hospital and ambulatory surgical applications.

References

1. Koller C: Vorlaufige Mittheilung über locale Anasthesirung am Auge. Klin Mbl Augenheilk 1884;22:60–63.
2. Halsted WS: Practical comments on the use and abuse of cocaine; suggested by its invariably successful employment in more than a thousand minor surgical operations. NY Med J 1885;42:294.
3. Corning JL: Spinal anaesthesia and local medication of the cord. NY Med J 1885;42:483–485.
4. Gorelick PB, Zych D: James Leonard Corning and the early history of spinal puncture. Neurology 1987;37:672–674.
5. Wynter E: Four cases of tubercular meningitis in which paracentesis of the theca vertebralis was performed for relief of fluid pressure. Lancet 1891;981–982.
6. Ball C, Westhorpe R: Local anaesthesia—Early spinal anaesthesia. Anaesth Intensive Care 2003;31:493.
7. Bier A: Experiments regarding the cocainization of the spinal cord. Dtsch Z Chir 1899;51:361–369.
8. Marx GF: The first spinal anesthesia. Who deserves the laurels? Reg Anesth 1994;19:429–430.
9. Wulf HF: The centennial of spinal anesthesia. Anesthesiology 1998;89:500–506.
10. Larson MD: Tait and Caglieri: The First Spinal Anesthetic in America. Anesthesiology 1996;85:913–919.
11. Matas R: Local and regional anesthesia with cocaine and other analgesic drugs, including the subarachnoid method, as applied in the general surgical practice. Phil Med J 1900;6:820–843.
12. Vandam LD: On the origins of intrathecal anesthesia. Reg Anesth Pain Med 1998;23:335–339.
13. Tuffier T: Anesthesie medullaire chirurgicale par injection sous-arachnoidienne lombaire de cocaine; technique et resultats. Sem Med 1900;20:167.
14. Barker AE: A report on clinical experiences with spinal analgesia in 100 cases and some reflections on the procedure. BMJ 1907;1:665–674.
15. Labat G: Circulatory disturbances associated with subarachnoid nerve block. Long Island Med J 1927;21:573.
16. Pitkin G: Controllable spinal anesthesia. Am J Surg 1928;5:537.
17. Sise LF: Spinal anesthesia for upper and lower abdominal operations. N Engl J Med 1928;199:61.
18. Sise LF: Pontocainglucose for spinal anesthesia. Surg Clin North Am 1935;15:1501.
19. Brown DL, Fink BR: The history of neural blockade and pain management. In Cousins MJ, Bridenbaugh PO (eds): *Neural Blockade*, 3rd ed. Lippincott-Raven, 1998, pp 3–27.
20. Adriani J, Roman-Vega D: Saddle block anesthesia. Am J Surg 1946;71:12.
21. Dripps RD, Vandam LD: Long-term follow-up of patients who received 10,098 spinal anesthetics: failure to discover major neurologic sequelae. JAMA 1954;156:1486–1491.
22. Greene HM: Lumbar puncture and the prevention of postdural puncture headache. JAMA 1926;86:391–392.

23. Greene BA: A 26 gauge lumbar puncture needle: Its value in the prophylaxis of headache following spinal analgesia for vaginal delivery. Anesthesiology 1950;11:464–469.

24. Hart JR, Whitacre RJ: Pencil-point needle in prevention of postspinal headache. JAMA 1951;147:657–658.

25. Sprotte G, Schedel R, Pajunk H, et: An "atraumatic" universal needle for single-shot regional anesthesia: Clinical results and a 6 year trial in over 30,000 regional anesthesias. Reg Anaesth 1987;10:104–108.

26. Calthorpe N: The history of spinal needles: Getting to the point. Anaesthesia 2004;59:1231–1241.

27. Bamford C, Sibley W, Laguna J: Anesthesia in multiple sclerosis. Can J Neurol Sci 1978;5:41–44.

28. Kytta J, Rosenberg PH: Anaesthesia for patients with multiple sclerosis. Ann Chir Gynaecol 1984;73:299–303.

29. Bouchard P, Caillet JB, Monnet F, et al: Spinal anesthesia and multiple sclerosis. Ann Fr Anesth Reanim 1984;3:194–198.

30. Levesque P, Marsepoil T, Ho P, et al: Multiple sclerosis disclosed by spinal anesthesia. Ann Fr Anesth Reanim 1988;7: 68–70.

31. Vadalouca A, Moka E, Sykiotis C: Combined spinal-epidural technique for total hysterectomy in a patient with advanced, progressive multiple sclerosis. Reg Anesth Pain Med 2002;27:540–541.

32. Thompson RC, Liberthson RR, Lowenstein E: Perioperative anesthetic risk of noncardiac surgery in hypertrophic obstructive cardiomyopathy. JAMA 1985;254:2419–2421.

33. Loubser P, Suh K, Cohen S: Adverse effects of spinal anesthesia in a patient with idiopathic hypertrophic subaortic stenosis. Anesth Analg 1984;60:228–230.

34. McDonald SB: Is neuraxial blockade contraindicated in the patient with aortic stenosis? Reg Anesth Pain Med 2004;29:496–502.

35. O'Keefe JH Jr, Shub C, Rettke SR: Risk of noncardiac surgical procedures in patients with aortic stenosis. Mayo Clin Proc 1989;64:400–405.

36. Collard CD, Eappen S, Lynch EP, et al: Continuous spinal anesthesia with invasive hemodynamic monitoring for surgical repair of the hip in two patients with severe aortic stenosis. Anesth Analg 1995;81:195–198.

37. Reiman A, Anson B: Vertebral termination of the spinal cord with report of a case of sacral cord. Anat Rec 1944;88:127.

38. Bromage PR: Neurological complications of subarachnoid and epidural anaesthesia. Acta Anaesthesiol Scand 1997;41:439–444.

39. Covino B: Pharmacology of local anaesthetic agents. Br J Anaesth 1986;58:701–716.

40. Greene NM: Uptake and elimination of local anesthetics during spinal anesthesia. Anesth Analg 1983;62:1013–1024.

41. Stienstra R, Greene NM: Factors affecting the subarachnoid spread of local anesthetic solutions. Reg Anesth 1991;16:1–6.

42. Cohen EN: Distribution of local anesthetic agents in the neuraxis of the dog. Anesthesiology 1968;29:1002–1005.

43. Schell RM, Brauer FS, Cole DJ, et al: Persistent sacral nerve root deficits after continuous spinal anaesthesia. Can J Anaesth 1991;38:908–911.

44. Hogan Q: Size of human lower thoracic and lumbosacral nerve roots. Anesthesiology 1996;85:37–42.

45. Kaneko S, Matsumoto M, Tsuruta S, et al: The nerve root entry zone is highly vulnerable to intrathecal tetracaine in rabbits. Anesth Analg 2005;101:107–114.

46. Takenami T, Yagishita S, Asato F, et al: Neurotoxicity of intrathecally administered tetracaine commences at the posterior roots near entry into the spinal cord. Reg Anesth Pain Med 2000;25:372–379.

47. Kristensen JD, Karlsten R, Gordh T: Spinal cord blood flow after intrathecal injection of ropivacaine and bupivacaine with or without epinephrine in rats. Acta Anaesthesiol Scand 1998;42:685–690.

48. Dohi S, Matsumiya N, Takeshima R, et al: The effects of subarachnoid lidocaine and phenylephrine on spinal cord and cerebral blood flow in dogs. Anesthesiology 1984;61:238–244.

49. Kozody R, Palahniuk RJ, Cumming MO: Spinal cord blood flow following subarachnoid tetracaine. Can Anaesth Soc J 1985;32:23–29.

50. Greene NM: Distribution of local anesthetic solutions within the subarachnoid space. Anesth Analg 1985;64:715–730.

51. Horlocker TT, Wedel DJ: Density, specific gravity, and baricity of spinal anesthetic solutions at body temperature. Anesth Analg 1993;76:1015–1018.

52. Hallworth SP, Fernando R, Columb MO, et al: The effect of posture and baricity on the spread of intrathecal bupivacaine for elective cesarean delivery. Anesth Analg 2005;100:1159–1165.

53. McLeod GA: Density of spinal anaesthetic solutions of bupivacaine, levobupivacaine, and ropivacaine with and without dextrose. Br J Anaesth 2004;92:547–551.

54. Brown DT, Wildsmith JA, Covino BG, et al: Effect of baricity on spinal anaesthesia with amethocaine. Br J Anaesth 1980;52:589–596.

55. Siker ES, Wolfson B, Stewart WD, et al: Mepivacaine for spinal anesthesia: Effects of changes in concentration and baricity. Anesth Analg 1966;45:191–196.

56. Chambers WA, Edstrom HH, Scott DB: Effect of baricity on spinal anaesthesia with bupivacaine. Br J Anaesth 1981;53:279–282.

57. Denson DD, Bridenbaugh PO, Turner PA, et al: Comparison of neural blockade and pharmacokinetics after subarachnoid lidocaine in the rhesus monkey. II: Effects of volume, osmolality, and baricity. Anesth Analg 1983;62:995–1001.

58. Hare GM, Ngan JC: Density determination of local anaesthetic opioid mixtures for spinal anaesthesia. Can J Anaesth 1998;45:341–346.

59. Bodily MN, Carpenter RL, Owens BD: Lidocaine 0.5% spinal anaesthesia: A hypobaric solution for short-stay perirectal surgery. Can J Anaesth 1992;39:770–773.

60. Lui AC, Polis TZ, Cicutti NJ: Densities of cerebrospinal fluid and spinal anaesthetic solutions in surgical patients at body temperature. Can J Anaesth 1998;45:297–303.

61. Sheskey MC, Rocco AG, Bizzari-Schmid M, et al: A dose-response study of bupivacaine for spinal anesthesia. Anesth Analg 1983;62:931–935.

62. Hogan QH, Prost R, Kulier A, et al: Magnetic resonance imaging of cerebrospinal fluid volume and the influence of body habitus and abdominal pressure. Anesthesiology 1996;84: 1341–1349.

63. Carpenter RL, Hogan QH, Liu SS, et al: Lumbosacral cerebrospinal fluid volume is the primary determinant of sensory block extent and duration during spinal anesthesia. Anesthesiology 1998;89: 24–29.

64. Higuchi H, Hirata J, Adachi Y, et al: Influence of lumbosacral cerebrospinal fluid density, velocity, and volume on extent and duration of plain bupivacaine and spinal anesthesia. Anesthesiology 2004;100:106–114.

65. Schneider M, Ettlin T, Kaufmann M, et al: Transient neurologic toxicity after hyperbaric anesthesia with 5% lidocaine. Anesth Analg 1993;76:1154–1157.

66. Zaric D, Christiansen C, Pace NL, et al: Transient neurologic symptoms after spinal anesthesia with lidocaine versus other local anesthetics: A systematic review of randomized, controlled trials. Anesth Analg 2005;100:1811–1816.

67. Zaric D, Christiansen C, Pace NL, et al: Transient neurologic symptoms (TNS) following spinal anaesthesia with lidocaine versus other local anaesthetics. Cochrane Database Syst Rev 2005;100:1811 1816.

68. Hampl KF, Schneider MC, Ummenhofer W, et al: Transient neurologic symptoms after spinal anesthesia. Anesth Analg 1995;81:1148–1153.

69. Hampl KF, Heinzmann-Wiedmer S, Luginbuehl I, et al: Transient neurologic symptoms after spinal anesthesia: A lower incidence with prilocaine and bupivacaine than with lidocaine. Anesthesiology 1998;88:629–633.

70. Keld DB, Hein L, Dalgaard M, et al: The incidence of transient neurologic symptoms (TNS) after spinal anaesthesia in patients undergoing surgery in the supine position. Hyperbaric lidocaine 5% versus hyperbaric bupivacaine 0.5%. Acta Anaesthesiol Scand 2000;44:285–290.

71. Freedman JM, Li DK, Drasner K, et al: Transient neurologic symptoms after spinal anesthesia: an epidemiologic study of 1,863 patients. Anesthesiology 1998; 89: 633–41.

72. Sumi M, Sakura S, Kosaka Y: Intrathecal hyperbaric 0.5% tetracaine as a possible cause of transient neurologic toxicity. Anesth Analg 1996; 82: 1076–7.

73. Sakura S, Sumi M, Sakaguchi Y, et al: The addition of phenylephrine contributes to the development of transient neurologic symptoms after spinal anesthesia with 0.5% tetracaine. Anesthesiology 1997;87:771–778.

74. Liguori GA, Zayas VM, Chisholm MF: Transient neurologic symptoms after spinal anesthesia with mepivacaine and lidocaine. Anesthesiology 1998;88:619–623.

75. Salazar F, Bogdanovich A, Adalia R, et al: Transient neurologic symptoms after spinal anaesthesia using isobaric 2% mepivacaine and isobaric 2% lidocaine. Acta Anaesthesiol Scand 2001;45:240–245.

76. Eberhart LH, Morin AM, Kranke P, et al: Transient neurologic symptoms after spinal anesthesia. A quantitative systematic overview (meta-analysis) of randomized controlled studies. Anaesthesist 2002;51:539–546.

77. Ganapathy S, Sandhu HB, Stockall CA, et al: Transient neurologic symptom (TNS) following intrathecal ropivacaine. Anesthesiology 2000;93:1537–1539.

78. Buckenmaier CC 3rd, Nielsen KC, Pietrobon R, et al: Small-dose intrathecal lidocaine versus ropivacaine for anorectal surgery in an ambulatory setting. Anesth Analg 2002;95:1253–1257.

79. Breebaart MB, Vercauteren MP, Hoffmann VL, et al: Urinary bladder scanning after day-case arthroscopy under spinal anaesthesia: Comparison between lidocaine, ropivacaine, and levobupivacaine. Br J Anaesth 2003;90:309–313.

80. Bridenbaugh PO, Greene NM, Brull SJ: Spinal (subarachoid) neural blockade. In Cousins MJ, Bridenbaugh PO (eds): *Neural Blockade*, 3rd ed. Lippincott-Raven, 1998.

81. Brown DL: Spinal, Epidural, and Caudal Anesthesia. In Miller RD (ed): *Anesthesia*, 4th ed. Churchill Livingston, 1994, pp 1505–1533.

82. Pawlowski J, Sukhani R, Pappas AL, et al: The anesthetic and recovery profile of two doses (60 and 80 mg) of plain mepivacaine for ambulatory spinal anesthesia. Anesth Analg 2000;91:580–584.

83. Kallio H, Snall EV, Kero MP, et al: A comparison of intrathecal plain solutions containing ropivacaine 20 or 15 mg versus bupivacaine 10 mg. Anesth Analg 2004;99:713–717.

84. McNamee DA, Parks L, McClelland AM, et al: Intrathecal ropivacaine for total hip arthroplasty: Double-blind comparative study with isobaric 7.5 mg/mL and 10 mg/mL solutions. Br J Anaesth 2001;87:743–747.

85. Burke D, Kennedy S, Bannister J: Spinal anesthesia with 0.5% S(–)-bupivacaine for elective lower limb surgery. Reg Anesth Pain Med 1999;24:519–523.

86. Glaser C, Marhofer P, Zimpfer G, et al: Levobupivacaine versus racemic bupivacaine for spinal anesthesia. Anesth Analg 2002;94:194–198.

87. Alley EA, Kopacz DJ, McDonald SB, et al: Hyperbaric spinal levobupivacaine: A comparison to racemic bupivacaine in volunteers. Anesth Analg 2002;94:188–193.

88. Smith KN, Kopacz DJ, McDonald SB: Spinal 2-chloroprocaine: A dose-ranging study and the effect of added epinephrine. Anesth Analg 2004;9:81–88.

89. Tetzlaff JE, Dilger J, Yap E, et al: Cauda equina syndrome after spinal anaesthesia in a patient with severe vascular disease. Can J Anaesth 1998;45:667–669.

90. Lee DS, Bui T, Ferrarese J, et al: Cauda equina syndrome after incidental total spinal anesthesia with 2% lidocaine. J Clin Anesth 1998;10:66–69

91. Maehara Y, Kusunoki S, Kawamoto M, et al: A prospective multicenter trial to determine the incidence of transient neurologic symptoms after spinal anesthesia with phenylephrine added to 0.5% tetracaine. Hiroshima J Med Sci 2001;50:47–51.

92. Kozody R, Palahniuk RJ, Wade JG, et al: The effect of subarachnoid epinephrine and phenylephrine on spinal cord blood flow. Can Anaesth Soc J 1984;31:503–508.

93. Porter SS, Albin MS, Watson WA, et al: Spinal cord and cerebral blood flow responses to subarachnoid injection of local anesthetics with and without epinephrine. Acta Anaesthesiol Scand 1985;29:330–338.

94. Concepcion M, Maddi R, Francis D, et al: Vasoconstrictors in spinal anesthesia with tetracaine—A comparison of epinephrine and phenylephrine. Anesth Analg 1984;63:134–138.

95. Armstrong IR, Littlewood DG, Chambers WA: Spinal anesthesia with tetracaine—Effect of added vasoconstrictors. Anesth Analg 1983;62:793–795.

96. Rice LJ, DeMars PD, Whalen TV, et al: Duration of spinal anesthesia in infants less than one year of age. Comparison of three hyperbaric techniques. Reg Anesth 1994;19:325–329.

97. Chambers WA, Littlewood DG, Scott DB: Spinal anesthesia with hyperbaric bupivacaine: effect of added vasoconstrictors. Anesth Analg 1982;61:49–52.

98. Moore JM, Liu SS, Pollock JE, et al: The effect of epinephrine on small-dose hyperbaric bupivacaine spinal anesthesia: Clinical implications for ambulatory surgery. Anesth Analg 1998;86:973–977.

99. Racle JP, Poy JY, Benkhadra A, et al: Prolongation of spinal anesthesia with hyperbaric bupivacaine by adrenaline and clonidine in the elderly. Ann Fr Anesth Reanim 1988;7:139–144.

100. Vercauteren MP, Jacobs S, Jacquemyn Y, et al: Intrathecal labor analgesia with bupivacaine and sufentanil: The effect of adding 2.25 micrograms of epinephrine. Reg Anesth Pain Med 2001;26:473–477.

101. Goodman SR, Kim-Lo SH, Ciliberto CF, et al: Epinephrine is not a useful addition to intrathecal fentanyl or fentanyl-bupivacaine for labor analgesia. Reg Anesth Pain Med 2002;27:374–379.

102. Gautier PE, Debry F, Fanard L, et al: Ambulatory combined spinal-epidural analgesia for labor. Influence of epinephrine on bupivacaine-sufentanil combination. Reg Anesth 1997;22:143–149.

103. Chambers WA, Littlewood DG, Logan MR, et al: Effect of added epinephrine on spinal anesthesia with lidocaine. Anesth Analg 1981;60:417–420.

104. Chiu AA, Liu S, Carpenter RL, et al: The effects of epinephrine on lidocaine spinal anesthesia: A cross-over study. Anesth Analg 1995;80:735–739.

105. Racle JP, Benkhadra A, Poy JY: Subarachnoid anaesthesia produced by hyperbaric lignocaine in elderly patients. Prolongation of effect with adrenaline. Br J Anaesth 1988;60:831–835.

106. Spivey DL: Epinephrine does not prolong lidocaine spinal anesthesia in term parturients. Anesth Analg 1985;64:468–470.

107. Moore DC, Chadwick HS, Ready LB: Epinephrine prolongs lidocaine spinal: Pain in the operative site the most accurate method of determining local anesthetic duration. Anesthesiology 1987;67:416–418.

108. Glynn CJ, Mather LE, Cousins MJ, et al: Spinal narcotics and respiratory depression. Lancet 1979;2:356–357.

109. Cunningham AJ, McKenna JA, Skene DS: Single injection spinal anaesthesia with amethocaine and morphine for transurethral prostatectomy. Br J Anaesth 198355;:423–427.

110. Nordberg G, Hedner T, Mellstrand T, et al: Pharmacokinetic aspects of intrathecal morphine analgesia. Anesthesiology 1984;60:448–454.

111. Abouleish E, Rawal N, Rashad MN: The addition of 0.2 mg subarachnoid morphine to hyperbaric bupivacaine for cesarean delivery: A prospective study of 856 cases. Reg Anesth 1991;16:137–140.

112. Borgeat A, Singer T: Nausea and vomiting after spinal anaesthesia with morphine. Acta Anaesthesiol Scand 1998;42:1231.

113. Bonnet F, Buisson VB, Francois Y, et al: Effects of oral and subarachnoid clonidine on spinal anesthesia with bupivacaine. Reg Anesth 1990;15:211–214.

114. Dobrydnjov I, Axelsson K, Thorn SE, et al: Clonidine combined with small-dose bupivacaine during spinal anesthesia for inguinal herniorrhaphy: A randomized double-blinded study. Anesth Analg 2003;96:1496–503.

115. Strebel S, Gurzeler JA, Schneider MC, et al: Small-dose intrathecal clonidine and isobaric bupivacaine for orthopedic surgery: A dose-response study. Anesth Analg 2004;99:1231–1238.

116. Filos KS, Goudas LC, Patroni O, et al: Hemodynamic and analgesic profile after intrathecal clonidine in humans: A dose response study. Anesthesiology 1994;81:591–601.

117. Hassenbusch SJ, Gunes S, Wachsman S, et al: Intrathecal clonidine in the treatment of intractable pain: A phase I/II study. Pain Med 2002;3:85–91.

118. Ackerman LL, Follett KA, Rosenquist RW: Long-term outcomes during treatment of chronic pain with intrathecal clonidine or clonidine/opioid combinations. J Pain Symptom Manage 2003;26:668–77.

119. Chen SR, Khan GM, Pan HL: Antiallodynic effect of intrathecal neostigmine is mediated by spinal nitric oxide in a rat model of diabetic neuropathy. Anesthesiology 2001;95:1007–1012.

120. Ho KM, Ismail H, Lee KC, et al: Use of intrathecal neostigmine as an adjunct to other spinal medications in perioperative and peripartum analgesia: A meta-analysis. Anaesth Intensive Care 2005;33:41–53.

121. Yegin A, Yilmaz M, Karsli B, et al: Analgesic effects of intrathecal neostigmine in perianal surgery. Eur J Anaesthesiol 2003;20:404–408.

122. Tan P-H, Kuo J-H, Liu K, et al: Efficacy of intrathecal neostigmine for the relief of postinguinal hemiorrhaphy pain. Acta Anaesthesiol Scand 2000;44:1056–1060.

123. Nakayama M, Kanaya N, Fujita S, et al: Effects of ephedrine on indocyanine green clearance during spinal anesthesia: Evaluation by the finger piece method. Anesth Analg 1993;77:947–949.

124. Zinn SE, Fairley HB, Glenn JD: Liver function in patients with mild alcoholic hepatitis, after enflurane, nitrous oxide-narcotic, and spinal anesthesia. Anesth Analg 1985;64:487–490.

125. Igarashi M, Kawana S, Iwasaki H, et al: Anesthetic management for a patient with citrullinemia and liver cirrhosis. Masui 1995;44:96–99.

126. Fukuda T, Okutani R, Kono K, et al: Anesthetic management for cesarean section of a patient with transient diabetes insipidus and acute severe liver dysfunction. Masui 1993;42:1511–1516.

127. McNeill MJ, Bennet A: Use of regional anaesthesia in a patient with acute porphyria. Br J Anaesth 1990;64:371–373.

128. Consolo D, Ouardirhi Y, Wessels C, et al: Obstetrical anaesthesia and porphyrias. Ann Fr Anesth Reanim 2005;24:428–431.

129. Runciman WB, Mather LE, Ilsley AH, et al: A sheep preparation for studying interactions between blood flow and drug disposition. III: Effects of general and spinal anaesthesia on regional blood flow and oxygen tensions. Br J Anaesth 1984;56:1247–1258.

130. Runciman WB, Mather LE, Ilsley AH, et al: A sheep preparation for studying interactions between blood flow and drug disposition. IV: The effects of general and spinal anaesthesia on blood flow and cefoxitin disposition. Br J Anaesth 1985;57:1239–1247.

131. Runciman WB, Mather LE, Ilsley AH, et al: A sheep preparation for studying interactions between blood flow and drug disposition. VI: Effects of general or subarachnoid anaesthesia on blood flow and chlormethiazole disposition. Br J Anaesth 1986; 58: 1308–1316.

132. Mather LE, Runciman WB, Ilsley AH, et al: A sheep preparation for studying interactions between blood flow and drug disposition. V: The effects of general and subarachnoid anaesthesia on blood flow and pethidine disposition. Br J Anaesth 1986;58:888–896.

133. Bigler D, Hjortso NC, Edstrom H, et al: Comparative effects of intrathecal bupivacaine and tetracaine on analgesia, cardiovascular function and plasma catecholamines. Acta Anaesthesiol Scand 1986;30:199–203.

134. Carpenter RL, Caplan RA, Brown DL, et al: Incidence and risk factors for side effects of spinal anesthesia. Anesthesiology 1992;76:906–916.

135. Tarkkila P, Isola J: A regression model for identifying patients at high risk of hypotension, bradycardia and nausea during spinal anesthesia. Acta Anaesthesiol Scand 1992;36:554–558.

136. Klasen J, Junger A, Hartmann B, et al: Differing incidences of relevant hypotension with combined spinal-epidural anesthesia and spinal anesthesia. Anesth Analg 2003;96:1491–1495.

137. Hartmann B, Junger A, Klasen J, et al: The incidence and risk factors for hypotension after spinal anesthesia induction: An analysis with automated data collection. Anesth Analg 2002;94:1521–1529.

138. Nishiyama T, Komatsu K, Hanaoka K: Comparison of hemodynamic and anesthetic effects of hyperbaric bupivacaine and tetracaine in spinal anesthesia. J Anesth 2003;17:218–222.

139. Rooke GA, Freund PR, Jacobson AF: Hemodynamic response and change in organ blood volume during spinal anesthesia in elderly men with cardiac disease. Anesth Analg 1997;85:99–105.

140. Shimosato S, Etsten BE: The role of the venous system in cardiocirculatory dynamics during spinal and epidural anesthesia in man. Anesthesiology 1969;30:619–628.

141. Anzai Y, Nishikawa T: Heart rate responses to body tilt during spinal anesthesia. Anesth Analg 1991;73:385–390.

142. Bergenwald L, Freyschuss U, Kaijser L, et al: Cardiovascular response to spinal anaesthesia in elderly men: Effects of head-up tilt and dihydroergotamine administration. Clin Physiol 1981;1:453–460.

143. Caplan RA, Ward RJ, Posner K, et al: Unexpected cardiac arrest during spinal anesthesia: A closed claims analysis of predisposing factors. Anesthesiology 1988;68:5–11.

144. Bernards CM, Hymas NJ: Progression of first degree heart block to high-grade second degree block during spinal anaesthesia. Can J Anaesth 1992;39:173–175.

145. Graves CL, Underwood PS, Klein RL, et al: Intravenous fluid administration as therapy for hypotension secondary to spinal anesthesia. Anesth Analg 1968;47:548–556.

146. Venn PJ, Simpson DA, Rubin AP, et al: Effect of fluid preloading on cardiovascular variables after spinal anaesthesia with glucose-free 0.75% bupivacaine. Br J Anaesth 1989;63:682–687.

147. Coe AJ, Revanas B: Is crystalloid preloading useful in spinal anaesthesia in the elderly? Anaesthesia 1990;45:241–243.

148. Butterworth JF 4th, Piccione W Jr, Berrizbeitia LD, et al: Augmentation of venous return by adrenergic agonists during spinal anesthesia. Anesth Analg 1986;65:612–616.

149. Ward RJ, Kennedy WF, Bonica JJ, et al: Experimental evaluation of atropine and vasopressors for the treatment of hypotension of high subarachnoid anesthesia. Anesth Analg 1966;45:621–629.

150. Sidi A, Pollak D, Floman Y, et al: Hypobaric spinal anesthesia in the operative management of orthopedic emergencies in geriatric patients. Isr J Med Sci 1984;20:589–592.

151. Sinclair CJ, Scott DB, Edstrom HH: Effect of the Trendelenberg position on spinal anaesthesia with hyperbaric bupivacaine. Br J Anaesth 1982;54:497–500.

152. Ou CH, Tsou MY, Ting CK, et al: Occurrence of the Bezold-Jarisch reflex during Cesarean section under spinal anesthesia—a case report. Acta Anaesthesiol Taiwan 2004;42:175–178.

153. Mackey DC, Carpenter RL, Thompson GE, et al: Bradycardia and asystole during spinal anesthesia: A report of three cases without morbidity. Anesthesiology 1989;70:866–868.

154. Campagna JA, Carter C: Clinical relevance of the Bezold–Jarisch reflex. Anesthesiology 2003;98:1250–1260.

155. Lesser JB, Sanborn KV, Valskys R, et al: Severe bradycardia during spinal and epidural anesthesia recorded by an anesthesia information management system. Anesthesiology 2003;99:859–866.

156. Kinsella SM, Tuckey JP: Perioperative bradycardia and asystole: Relationship to vasovagal syncope and the Bezold–Jarisch reflex. Br J Anaesth 2001;86:859–868.

157. Greene NM, Brull SJ: *Physiology of Spinal Anesthesia*, 4th ed. Williams & Wilkins, 1981.

158. Steinbrook RA, Concepcion M, Topulos GP: Ventilatory responses to hypercapnia during bupivacaine spinal anesthesia. Anesth Analg 1988;67:247–252.

159. Schneider MC, Holzgreve W: 100 years ago: Oskar Kreis, a pioneer in spinal obstetric analgesia at the University Women's Clinic of Basel. Anaesthesist 2001;50:525–528.

160. Taivainen T, Tuominen M, Rosenberg PH: Influence of obesity on the spread of spinal analgesia after injection of plain 0.5% bupivacaine at the L3-4 or L4-5 interspace. Br J Anaesth 1990;64:542–546.

161. Tuominen M, Taivainen T, Rosenberg PH: Spread of spinal anaesthesia with plain 0.5% bupivacaine: Influence of the vertebral interspace used for injection. Br J Anaesth 1989;62:358–361.

162. Tuominen M, Kuulasmaa K, Taivainen T, et al: Individual predictability of repeated spinal anaesthesia with isobaric bupivacaine. Acta Anaesthesiol Scand 1989;33:13–14.

163. Sundnes KO, Vaagenes P, Skretting P, et al: Spinal analgesia with hyperbaric bupivacaine: Effects of volume of solution. Br J Anaesth 1982;54:69–74.

164. Konishi R, Mitsuhata H, Saitoh J, et al: The spread of subarachnoid hyperbaric dibucaine in the term parturient. Masui 1997;46:184–187.

165. Veering BT, Ter Riet PM, Burm AG, et al: Spinal anaesthesia with 0.5% hyperbaric bupivacaine in elderly patients: Effect of site of injection on spread of analgesia. Br J Anaesth 1996;77:343–346.

166. Cameron AE, Arnold RW, Ghorisa MW, et al: Spinal analgesia using bupivacaine 0.5% plain. Variation in the extent of the block with patient age. Anaesthesia 1981;36:318–322.

167. Pitkanen M, Haapaniemi L, Tuominen M, et al: Influence of age on spinal anaesthesia with isobaric 0.5% bupivacaine. Br J Anaesth 1984;56:279–284.

168. Veering BT, Burm AG, Vletter AA, et al: The effect of age on systemic absorption and systemic disposition of bupivacaine after subarachnoid administration. Anesthesiology 1991;74:250–257.

169. Racle JP, Benkhadra A, Poy JY, et al: Spinal analgesia with hyperbaric bupivacaine: Influence of age. Br J Anaesth 1988;60:508–514.

170. Schiffer E, Van Gessel E, Gamulin Z: Influence of sex on cerebrospinal fluid density in adults. Br J Anaesth 1999;83:943–944.

171. Pargger H, Hampl KF, Aeschbach A, et al: Combined effect of patient variables on sensory level after spinal 0.5% plain bupivacaine. Acta Anaesthesiol Scand 1998;42:430–434.

172. Povey HM, Jacobsen J, Westergaard-Nielsen J: Subarachnoid analgesia with hyperbaric 0.5% bupivacaine: Effect of a 60-min period of sitting. Acta Anaesthesiol Scand 1989;33:295–297.

173. Alston RP, Littlewood DG, Meek R, et al: Spinal anesthesia with hyperbaric bupivacaine: Effects of concentration and volume when administered in the sitting position. Br J Anaesth 1988;61:144–148.

174. Alston RP: Spinal anaesthesia with 0.5% bupivacaine 3 mL: Comparison of plain and hyperbaric solutions administered to seated patients. Br J Anaesth 1988;61:385–389.

175. Mitchell RW, Bowler GM, Scott DB, et al: Effects of posture and baricity on spinal anaesthesia with 0.5% bupivacaine 5 ml. A double-blind study. Br J Anaesth 1988;61:139–143.

176. Povey HM, Olsen PA, Pihl H: Spinal analgesia with hyperbaric 0.5% bupivacaine: effects of different patient positions. Acta Anaesthesiol Scand 1987;31:616–619.

177. Maroof M, Khan RM, Siddique M, et al: Hypobaric spinal anaesthesia with bupivacaine (0.1%) gives selective sensory block for ano-rectal surgery. Can J Anaesth 1995;42:691–694.

178. Tuominen M, Pitkanen M, Rosenberg PH: Effect of speed of injection of 0.5% plain bupivacaine on the spread of spinal anaesthesia. Br J Anaesth 1992;69:148–149.

179. Van Gessel EF, Praplan J, Fuchs T, et al: Influence of injection speed on the subarachnoid distribution of isobaric bupivacaine 0.5%. Anesth Analg 1993;77:483–487

180. Stienstra R, Van Poorten F: Speed of injection does not affect subarachnoid distribution of plain bupivacaine 0.5%. Reg Anesth 1990;15:208–210.

181. Bucx MJ, Kroon JW, Stienstra R: Effect of speed of injection on the maximum sensory level for spinal anesthesia using plain bupivacaine 0.5% at room temperature. Reg Anesth 1993;18:103–105.

182. Axelsson KH, Edstrom HH, Sundberg AE, et al: Spinal anaesthesia with hyperbaric 0.5% bupivacaine: Effects of volume. Acta Anaesthesiol Scand 1982;26:439–445.

183. Peng PW, Chan VW, Perlas A: Minimum effective anaesthetic concentration of hyperbaric lidocaine for spinal anaesthesia. Can J Anaesth 1998;45:122–129.

184. Alfonsi P, Brusset A, Levy R, et al: Spinal anesthesia with bupivacaine without glucose in the elderly: Effect of concentration and volume on the hemodynamic profile. Ann Fr Anesth Reanim 1991;10:543–547.

185. Pflug EA, Aasheim GM, Beck HA: Spinal anesthesia: bupivacaine versus tetracaine. Anesth Analg 1976;55:489–492.

186. Kopacz DJ: Spinal 2-chloroprocaine: Minimum effective dose. Reg Anesth Pain Med 2005;30:36–42.

187. Van Zundert AA, Grouls RJ, Korsten HH, et al: Spinal anesthesia. Volume or concentration—What matters? Reg Anesth 1996;21:112–118.

188. Gonter AF, Kopacz DJ: Spinal 2-chloroprocaine: a comparison with procaine in volunteers. Anesth Analg 2005;100:573–579.

189. Wang BC, Hillman DE, Spielholz NI, et al: Chronic neurological deficits and Nesacaine-CE—An effect of the anesthetic, 2-chloroprocaine, or the antioxidant, sodium bisulfite? Anesth Analg 1984;63:445–447.

190. Le Truong HH, Girard M, Drolet P, et al: Spinal anesthesia: a comparison of procaine and lidocaine. Can J Anaesth 2001;48:470–473.

191. Johnson ME: Neurotoxicity of spinal procaine—A caution. Reg Anesth Pain Med 2001;26:288.

192. Hodgson PS, Liu SS, Batra MS, et al: Procaine compared with lidocaine for incidence of transient neurologic symptoms. Reg Anesth Pain Med 2000;25:218–222.

193. Bergeron L, Girard M, Drolet P, et al: Spinal procaine with and without epinephrine and its relation to transient radicular irritation. Can J Anaesth 1999;46:846–849.

194. DeAndres JA, Febre E, Bellver J, et al: Continuous spinal anaesthesia versus single dosing. A comparative study. Eur J Anaesthesiol 1995;12:135–140.

195. Ross BK, Chadwick HS, Mancuso JJ, et al: Sprotte needle for obstetric anesthesia: Decreased incidence of post dural puncture headache. Reg Anesth 1992;17:29–33.

196. Ilias WK, Klimscha W, Skrbensky G, et al: Continuous microspinal anaesthesia: Another perspective on mechanisms inducing cauda equina syndrome. Anaesthesia 1998;53:618–623.

197. Rigler ML, Drasner K, Krejcie TC, et al: Cauda equina syndrome after continuous spinal anesthesia. Anesth Analg 1991;72:275–281.

198. Benson JS: U.S. Food and Drug Administration safety alert: Cauda equina syndrome associated with use of small-bore catheters in continuous spinal anesthesia. AANA J 1992;60:223.

199. Mollmann M, Holst D, Lubbesmeyer H, et al: Continuous spinal anesthesia: Mechanical and technical problems of catheter placement. Reg Anesth 1993;18(6 Suppl):469–472.

200. Ready LB, Plumer MH, Haschke RH, et al: Neurotoxicity of intrathecal local anesthetics in rabbits. Anesthesiology 1985;63:364–370.

201. Kirihara Y, Saito Y, Sakura S, et al: Comparative neurotoxicity of intrathecal and epidural lidocaine in rats. Anesthesiology 2003;99:961–968.

202. Takenami T, Yagishita S, Hoka S: Intrathecal 2% tetracaine causes mild histological lesions in the spinal cord without detectable sensory deficits on paw stimulation test in rats. Masui 2000;49:361–368.

203. Auroy Y, Benhamou D, Bargues L, et al: Major complications of regional anesthesia in France: The SOS Regional Anesthesia Hotline Service. Anesthesiology 2002;97:1274–1280.

204. Moen V, Dahlgren N, Irestedt L: Severe neurological complications after central neuraxial blockades in Sweden 1990–1999. Anesthesiology 2004;101:950–959.

205. Horlocker TT: Complications of spinal and epidural anesthesia. Anesthesiol Clin North America 2000;18:461–485.

206. Hadzic A, Dilberovic F, Shah S, et al: Combination of intraneural injection and high injection pressure leads to fascicular injury and

neurologic deficits in dogs. Reg Anesth Pain Med 2004;29:417–423.

207. Shah S, Hadzic A, Vloka JD, et al: Neurologic complication after anterior sciatic nerve block. Anesth Analg 2005;100:1515–1517.

208. Loo CC, Irestedt L: Cauda equina syndrome after spinal anaesthesia with hyperbaric 5% lignocaine: A review of six cases of cauda equina syndrome reported to the Swedish Pharmaceutical Insurance 1993–1997. Acta Anaesthesiol Scand 1999;43:371–379.

209. Panadero A, Monedero P, Fernandez-Liesa JI, et al: Repeated transient neurological symptoms after spinal anaesthesia with hyperbaric 5% lidocaine. Br J Anaesth 1998;81:471–472.

210. Pavon A, Anadon Senac P: Neurotoxicity of intrathecal lidocaine. Rev Esp Anestesiol Reanim 2001;48:326–336.

211. Akioka K, Torigoe K, Maruta H, et al: A case of cauda equina syndrome following spinal anesthesia with hyperbaric dibucaine. J Anesth 2001;15:106–107.

212. Lopez-Soriano F, Lajarin B, Verdu JM, et al: Cauda equina hemisyndrome after intradural anesthesia with bupivacaine for hip surgery. Rev Esp Anestesiol Reanim 2002;49:494–496.

213. Vianna PT, Resende LA, Ganem EM, et al: Cauda equina syndrome after spinal tetracaine: Electromyographic evaluation—20 years follow-up. Anesthesiology 2001;95:1290–1291.

214. Woods WW, Franklin RG: Progressive adhesive arachnoiditis following spinal anesthesia. Calif Med 1951;75:196–198.

215. Joseph SI, Denson JS: Spinal anesthesia, arachnoiditis, and paraplegia. JAMA 1958;168:1330–1333.

216. Parnass SM, Schmidt KJ: Adverse effects of spinal and epidural anaesthesia. Drug Saf 1990;5:179–194.

217. Roche J: Steroid-induced arachnoiditis. Med J Aust 1984;140:281–284.

218. Aldrete JA: Neurologic deficits and arachnoiditis following neuroaxial anesthesia. Acta Anaesthesiol Scand 2003;47:3–12.

219. Levine MN, Raskob G, Beyth RJ, et al: Hemorrhagic complications of anticoagulant treatment: The Seventh ACCP Conference on Antithrombotic and Thrombolytic Therapy. Chest 2004;126:287S–310S.

220. Horlocker TT: What's a nice patient like you doing with a complication like this? Diagnosis, prognosis and prevention of spinal hematoma. Can J Anaesth 2004;51:527–534.

221. Burke D, Wildsmith JA: Meningitis after spinal anaesthesia. Br J Anaesth 1997;78:635–636.

222. Goldman WW Jr, Sanford JP: An "epidemic" of chemical meningitis. Am J Med 1960;29:94–101.

223. Hurst EW: Adhesive arachnoiditis and vascular blockage caused by detergents and other chemical irritants: An experimental study. J Pathol Bacteriol 1955;70:167–178.

224. Marinac JS: Drug- and chemical-induced aseptic meningitis: A review of the literature. Ann Pharmacother 1992;26:813–22.

225. Carp H, Bailey S: The association between meningitis and dural puncture in bacteremic rats. Anesthesiology 1992;76:739–742.

226. Teele DW, Dashefsky B, Rakusan T, et al: Meningitis after lumbar puncture in children with bacteremia. N Engl J Med 1981;305:1079–1081.

227. Eng RH, Seligman SJ: Lumbar puncture-induced meningitis. JAMA 1981;245:1456–1459.

228. Conangla G, Rodriguez L, Alonso-Tarres C, et al: Streptococcus salivarius meningitis after spinal anesthesia. Neurologia 2004;19:331–333.

229. Pandian JD, Sarada C, Radhakrishnan VV, et al: Iatrogenic meningitis after lumbar puncture-a preventable health hazard. J Hosp Infect 2004;56:119–124.

230. Kocamanoglu IS, Sener EB, Tur A, et al: Streptococcal meningitis after spinal anesthesia: Report of a case. Can J Anaesth 2003;50:314–315.

231. Yaniv LG, Potasman I: Iatrogenic meningitis: An increasing role for resistant viridans streptococci? Case report and review of the last 20 years. Scand J Infect Dis 2000;32:693–696.

232. Horlocker TT, Wedel DJ, Benzon H, et al: Regional anesthesia in the anticoagulated patient: Defining the risks (the second ASRA Consensus Conference on Neuraxial Anesthesia and Anticoagulation). Reg Anesth Pain Med 2003;28:172–197.

233. Malinovsky JM, Pinaud M: Neurotoxicity of intrathecally administrated agents. Ann Fr Anesth Reanim 1996;15:647–658.

234. Morewood GH: A rational approach to the cause, prevention and treatment of postdural puncture headache. CMAJ 1993;149:1087–1093.

235. Halpern S, Preston R: Postdural puncture headache and spinal needle design. Metaanalyses. Anesthesiology 1994;81:1376–1383.

236. Lambert DH, Hurley RJ, Hertwig L, et al: Role of needle gauge and tip configuration in the production of lumbar puncture headache. Reg Anesth 1997;22:66–72.

237. Candido KD, Stevens RA: Post-dural puncture headache: pathophysiology, prevention and treatment. Best Pract Res Clin Anaesthesiol 2003;17:451–469.

238. Abouleish E, Vega S, Blendinger I, et al: Long-term follow-up of epidural blood patch. Anesth Analg 1975;54:459–463.

239. Choi A, Laurito CE, Cunningham FE: Pharmacologic management of postdural puncture headache. Ann Pharmacother 1996;30:831–839.

240. Yucel A, Ozyalcin S, Talu GK, et al: Intravenous administration of caffeine sodium benzoate for postdural puncture headache. Reg Anesth Pain Med 1999;24:51–54.

241. Camann WR, Murray RS, Mushlin PS, et al: Effects of oral caffeine on postdural puncture headache. A double-blind, placebo-controlled trial. Anesth Analg 1990;70:181–184.

242. Connelly NR, Parker RK, Rahimi A, et al: Sumatriptan in patients with postdural puncture headache. Headache 2000;40:316–319.

243. Carp H, Singh PJ, Vadhera R, et al: Effects of the serotonin-receptor agonist sumatriptan on postdural puncture headache: Report of six cases. Anesth Analg 1994;79:180–182.

244. Rohmer C, Le Bourlot G: Headache after spinal anesthesia treated with sumatriptan. Ann Fr Anesth Reanim 1995;14:237.

245. Lovstad RZ, Granhus G, Hetland S: Bradycardia and asystolic cardiac arrest during spinal anaesthesia: A report of five cases. Acta Anaesthesiol Scand 2000;44:48–52.

246. Geffin B, Shapiro L: Sinus bradycardia and asystole during spinal and epidural anesthesia: A report of 13 cases. J Clin Anesth 1998;10:278–285.

247. Pan PH, Moore CH, Ross VH: Severe maternal bradycardia and asystole after combined spinal-epidural labor analgesia in a morbidly obese parturient. J Clin Anesth 2004;16:461–464.

248. Pollard JB: Cardiac arrest during spinal anesthesia: Common mechanisms and strategies for prevention. Anesth Analg 2001;92:252–256.

249. Kennedy WF Jr, Bonica JJ, Akamatsu TJ, et al: Cardiovascular and respiratory effects of subarachnoid block in the presence of acute blood loss. Anesthesiology 1968;29:29–35.

250. Kreutz JM, Mazuzan JE: Sudden asystole in a marathon runner: The athletic heart syndrome and its anesthetic implications. Anesthesiology 1990;73:1266–1268.

251. Kopp SL, Horlocker TT, Warner ME, et al: Cardiac arrest during neuraxial anesthesia: Frequency and predisposing factors associated with survival. Anesth Analg 2005;100:855–865.

252. Rosenberg JM, Wahr JA, Sung CH, et al: Coronary perfusion pressure during cardiopulmonary resuscitation after spinal anesthesia in dogs. Anesth Analg 1996;82:84–87.

253. Capdevila X, Dadure C: Perioperative management for one day hospital admission: regional anesthesia is better than general anesthesia. Acta Anaesthesiol Belg 2004;55(Suppl:33–36.

254. Munnur U, Suresh MS: Backache, headache, and neurologic deficit after regional anesthesia. Anesthesiol Clin North Am 2003;21:71–86.

255. Yoos JR, Kopacz DJ: Spinal 2-chloroprocaine for surgery: An initial 10-month experience. Anesth Analg 2005;100:553–558.

256. Yoos JR, Kopacz DJ: Spinal 2-chloroprocaine: A comparison with small-dose bupivacaine in volunteers. Anesth Analg 2005;100:566–5672.
257. Drasner K: Chloroprocaine spinal anesthesia: Back to the future? Anesth Analg 2005;100:549–552.
258. Kouri ME, Kopacz DJ: Spinal 2-chloroprocaine: A comparison with lidocaine in volunteers. Anesth Analg 2004;98:75–80.
259. Vath JS, Kopacz DJ: Spinal 2-chloroprocaine: The effect of added fentanyl. Anesth Analg 2004;98:89–94.
260. Warren DT, Kopacz DJ: Spinal 2-chloroprocaine: The effect of added dextrose. Anesth Analg 2004;98:95–101.
261. Ruben JE, Kamsler PM: Unilateral spinal anesthesia for surgical reduction of hip fractures. Am J Surg 1950;79:312–317
262. Khatouf M, Loughnane F, Boini S, et al: Unilateral spinal anaesthesia in elderly patient for hip trauma: A pilot study. Ann Fr Anesth Reanim 2005;24:249–254
263. Cappelleri G, Aldegheri G, Danelli G, et al: Spinal anesthesia with hyperbaric levobupivacaine and ropivacaine for outpatient knee arthroscopy: A prospective, randomized, double-blind study. Anesth Analg 2005;101:77–82.
264. Fanelli G, Borghi B, Casati A, et al: Unilateral bupivacaine spinal anesthesia for outpatient knee arthroscopy. Italian Study Group on Unilateral Spinal Anesthesia. Can J Anaesth 2000;47:746–751.
265. Casati A, Fanelli G: Unilateral spinal anesthesia. State of the art. Minerva Anestesiol 2001;67:855–862.
266. Baron EM, Burke JA, Akhtar N, et al: Spinal epidural hematoma associated with tissue plasminogen activator treatment of acute myocardial infarction. Catheter Cardiovasc Interv 1999;48:390–396.
267. Sawin PD, Traynelis VC, Follett KA: Spinal epidural hematoma following coronary thrombolysis with tissue plasminogen activator. Report of two cases. J Neurosurg 1995;83:350–353.
268. Van Schaeybroeck P, Van Calenbergh F, Van De Werf F, et al: Spontaneous spinal epidural hematoma associated with thrombolysis and anticoagulation therapy: Report of three cases. Clin Neurol Neurosurg 1998;100:283–287.
269. Connolly ES Jr, Winfree CJ, McCormick PC: Management of spinal epidural hematoma after tissue plasminogen activator. A case report. Spine 1996;21:1694–1698.
270. Heppner PA, Monteith SJ, Law AJ: Spontaneous spinal hematomas and low-molecular-weight heparin. Report of four cases and review of the literature. J Neurosurg Spine 2004;1:232–236.
271. Sternlo JE, Hybbinette CH: Spinal subdural bleeding after attempted epidural and subsequent spinal anaesthesia in a patient on thromboprophylaxis with low molecular weight heparin. Acta Anaesthesiol Scand 1995;39:557–559.
272. Wysowski DK, Talarico L, Bacsanyi J, et al: Spinal and epidural hematoma and low-molecular-weight heparin. N Engl J Med 1998;338:1774–1775.
273. Chan L, Bailin MT: Spinal epidural hematoma following central neuraxial blockade and subcutaneous enoxaparin: A case report. J Clin Anesth 2004;16:382–385.
274. Litz RJ, Gottschlich B, Stehr SN: Spinal epidural hematoma after spinal anesthesia in a patient treated with clopidogrel and enoxaparin. Anesthesiology 2004;101:1467–1470.
275. Rainer JL, Gottschlich B, Stehr SN: Spinal epidural hematoma after spinal anesthesia in a patient treated with clopidogrel and enoxaparin. Anesthesiology 2004;101:1467–1470.

14

Epidural Blockade

Bonnie Deschner, MD • Marina Allen, MD • Oscar de Leon, MD

INTRODUCTION

Epidural blockade is one of the most useful and versatile procedures in modern anesthesiology. It is unique in that it can be placed at virtually any level of the spinal spine, allowing more flexibility in its application to clinical practice. It is more versatile than spinal anesthesia, giving the clinician the opportunity to provide anesthesia and analgesia, as well as enabling diagnosis and treatment of chronic disease syndromes. It can be used to supplement general anesthesia, decreasing the need for deep levels of general anesthesia, therefore providing a more hemodynamically stable operative course and faster emergence from general anesthesia. It provides better postoperative pain control and more rapid recovery from surgery. When combined with spinal anesthesia in a technique called a CSE (combined spinal-epidural), benefits of both techniques can be combined and shortcomings of each avoided.

Numerous studies have demonstrated the benefits of epidural blockade. Epidural anesthesia or analgesia can reduce the adverse physiologic responses to surgery such as autonomic hyperactivity, cardiovascular stress, tissue breakdown, increased metabolic rate, pulmonary dysfunction, and immune system dysfunction. Thoracic epidural analgesia has been shown to decrease the incidence of myocardial infarction[1] postoperative pulmonary complications[2,3] and to promote the return of gastrointestinal motility without compromising fresh suture lines in the GI tract.[4–6] Epidural anesthesia and analgesia reduces the incidence of hypercoagulability.[7,8] Well-conducted randomized trials have demonstrated the perioperative use of epidural anesthesia and analgesia may reduce overall mortality and morbidity by approximately 30% compared with general anesthesia using systemic opioids.[9]

This chapter aims to provide the information necessary to provide safe and effective epidural blockade. The reader is encouraged to review specific chapters in this text for a more detailed discussion on specialized topics such as local anesthetics, combined spinal-epidural anesthesia, obstetric anesthesia, and serious complications such as epidural hematomas.

Brief History

Two French physicians, Jean-Anthanase Sicard, a radiologist, and Ferdinand Cathelin have been credited with the intentional administration of caudal epidural anesthesia over a century ago in 1901. They found that injecting a dilute solution of cocaine through the sacral hiatus can provide an effective treatment for severe sciatic pain and suggested the technique for surgical procedures.[10] Nineteen years later, a Spanish military surgeon by the name of Fidel Pages Mirave, is credited with describing the lumbar approach to "peridural" anesthesia. Unfortunately he was killed in an accident at the early age of 37, and his work lay dormant for several years.[11] Then in 1931, an Italian surgeon, Archile Dogliotti, performed abdominal surgery using single-shot lumbar epidural anesthesia, popularizing the method for producing "segmental peridural anesthesia." He noted that a sufficient length of spinal nerves needed to be blocked with an anesthetic solution of sufficient quantity to provide adequate anesthesia. He correctly identified the epidural space by describing the sudden loss of resistance noted after the needle had crossed the ligamentum flavum.[12]

Aburel, Hingson, and Edwards all devised methods for continuous but cumbersome epidural blockade; however, Cuban anesthesiologist, Manual Martinez Curbelo, is credited with making the technique more practical. On a visit to the Mayo Clinic in 1947, he watched Edward Tuohy perform continuous spinal blocks. Tuohy had replaced sharp spinal needles with a curved tip design developed by Ralph Huber. Tuohy modified the needle by adding a stylet to decrease the risk of skin plugging during insertion. Curbelo then used the Tuohy needle with a silk ureteral catheter to provide continuous segmental lumbar "peridural" anesthesia.[13] Several modifications of the Tuohy–Huber epidural needle have been developed in the more recent past and are being utilized in modern anesthesia practice. The epidural catheters have undergone more major changes since the original 3.5 F silk catheter used by Curbelo. The silk catheters were difficult to sterilize and prone to causing serious infections. Polymers of nylon, Teflon, polyurethrane, and silicone are currently used by manufacturers to produce thin, kink-resistant catheters of appropriate tensile strength and stiffness.[10,14]

Combining spinal with epidural anesthesia (CSE) began shortly after epidural anesthesia was reintroduced by Dogliotti. In 1939, Dr. A. L. Soresi presented a paper in which he and his colleagues provided a combination of spinal and epidural anesthesia safely to over 200 patients. He used one needle to first enter the epidural space, injected local anesthesia, then used the same needle to enter the subarachnoid space, dosing the patient with a smaller amount of local anesthetic. He demonstrated that he was able to provide anesthesia to his patients for 24 to 48 h.[15] In 1979, a Swedish physician named. Curelaru was the first to describe a combined technique using separate intervertebral injections. Then in 1982, Coates from England and Mumtaz from Sweden published reports of the popular needle-through-needle approach[16,17] for combined spinal-epidural anesthesia. Since that time, modifications of the CSE needle delivery systems as well as the creation of special trays for the procedure have been developed and are being utilized in the practice of modern anesthesiology.

INDICATIONS, APPLICATIONS, CONTRAINDICATIONS

Indications

Epidural anesthesia has been typically limited to procedures involving the lower limbs, pelvis, perineum, and lower abdomen. As clinicians have become more experienced with its application, epidural anesthesia with or without sedation has been used as the sole anesthetic or in combination with general anesthesia for a larger variety of cases. Michalek reported the use of cervical epidural anesthesia at the C6–7 level for a total parathyroidectomy with parathyroid gland implantation into the forearm. He concluded that combined procedures involving the neck and upper limbs could be safely conducted under cervical epidural blockade.[18] Several studies have described the use of high thoracic epidural anesthesia for off-pump coronary revascularization[19,20] and even for minimally invasive aortic valve replacement,[21] although this has not become common practice in the United States. In patients in whom general anesthesia could lead to prolonged ventilatory care, such as those with diffuse interstitial lung disease, thoracic epidural anesthesia as the sole anesthetic has been described as a successful alternative.

Although it is intriguing to realize that epidural blockade can be performed for procedures that in the past were limited to general anesthesia, the decision about whether to use this form of neuraxial blockade should be determined by the needs of the patient. Physiologically, blocks above T5 have a far greater effect on patient hemodynamics than blocks at T10 or lower. However, if the benefits of epidural blockade outweigh the risks to the patient, and the sensory blockade needed for the particular procedure can be obtained, then it is indicated. This distinction is sometimes blurred in teaching institutions when the desire to "practice" overshadows the needs of the patient, or when impatient surgeons do not want to allow novice epiduralists the time to safely perform the procedure. By keeping the needs of the patient in the forefront, this should never be a problem in modern day clinical practice. Common applications for epidural blockade are listed in Table 14–1.

Contraindications

Contraindications to epidural blockade have been historically divided into absolute, relative, and controversial (Table 14–2).

Absolute

Absolute contraindications include patient refusal, severe, uncorrected hypovolemia (sympathectomy with hypovolemia may cause profound circulatory collapse), increased intracranial pressure (may predispose patient to brainstem herniation if accidental dural puncture occurs or if a large volume of anesthetic is rapidly injected into the epidural space), and infection at the site of injection.[22] True allergy to local anesthetics of both classes, although exceedingly rare, is also an absolute contraindication.

Relative

Coagulopathy, whether iatrogenic or idiopathic, previously an absolute contraindication, is now considered a relative contraindication.[23] Anticoagulants, however, should be withheld based on the mechanism of action and duration of the drug. The greatest concern with anticoagulant therapy and anticoagulation is the risk of an epidural hematoma (refer to epidural hematoma chapter). According to the consensus statements by the American Society of Regional Anesthesia and Pain Medicine,[23] epidural block can be placed 4 h after the last dose of subcutaneous heparin, and 12 h after the last dose of low-molecular-weight heparin. NSAIDs, including aspirin, are not contraindications to epidural placement provided that catheter placement is uncomplicated (one or two attempts). Other relative contraindications include uncooperative patient (therefore exposing neural structures to an unacceptable risk of injury), fixed cardiac output states (inability to increase cardiac output in response to sympathectomy), anatomic abnormalities of the vertebral column (making placement technically impossible), and *unstable* neurologic disease

Table 14–1.

Common Applications for Epidural Blockade

Orthopedic surgery	Major hip/knee surgery, pelvic fractures
Obstetrics	Cesarean section, labor analgesia
Gynecologic surgery	Procedures involving female pelvic organs
Urologic surgery	Prostate, bladder procedures
General surgery	Upper and lower abdominal procedures[a]
Pediatric procedures	Penile procedures, inguinal hernia repair, anal surgery, orthopedic procedures on the feet; supplement to GA, postoperative pain relief, orthopedic procedures on feet[b]
Vascular surgery	Vascular reconstruction of the lower limbs, amputations involving the lower extremities
Thoracic surgery	Postoperative analgesia, combination with GA to reduce GA requirements
Medical conditions	Known/suspected malignant hyperthermia
Diagnosis and management of chronic pain	Chronic pain

[a] *Height of block with side effects required for upper abdominal procedures, may make it difficult to avoid patient discomfort and increased risk.*[22]
[b] *Usually through a caudal epidural approach.*

(may mask exacerbation signs/symptoms).[24,25] Case reports have been published on patients undergoing epidural anesthesia safely with serious neurologic conditions such as neural tube defects, Guillain–Barré syndrome, and quadriplegia with autonomic hyperreflexia.[26–28] Careful evaluation and documentation of the patient's baseline neurologic status, a thorough discussion of risks as well as the benefits of epidural anesthesia and a multidisciplinary approach is required for these patients. The same approach should be taken with any patient with serious medical diseases prior to instituting epidural blockade.

Clinical Pearl

- Epidural blocks can be placed 4 h after the last dose of subcutaneous heparin, 12 h after the last dose of LMWH.

Table 14–2.

Contraindications: Epidural Blockade

Absolute	Relative	Controversial
Patient refusal	Coagulopathy	Inadequate training/experience
	Platelet count <100,000	
Uncorrected hypovolemia	Uncooperative patient	Elaborate tattoos at the needle insertion site
Increased ICP	Severe anatomic abnormalities of spine	Positioning that compromises respiratory status
Infection at site	Sepsis	Anesthetized patient (cervical/thoracic)
Allergic to amide/ester LA	Hypertension	Previous back surgery

ICP = intracranial pressure; LA = local anesthetic.

Controversial

The more controversial contraindications to epidural anesthesia include inability to communicate with the patient (placing an epidural in an anesthetized patient),[29] tattoos (potential risk of pigment-containing tissue coring into the epidural space),[30] complicated surgeries with major blood loss,[25] and in surgical maneuvers in which respiration may be compromised or the airway may be difficult to manage.

Clinical Pearls

- NSAIDs (including ASA) are *not* contraindications to epidural placement.
- LMWH should be held at least 12 h before placement of catheter and 2 h after removal.
- Epidural placement is relatively safe with internationalized ratio (INR) <1.5.
- If an epidural vein is punctured, subcutaneous heparin administration should be held at least 2 h, and LMWH held at least 24 h.
- GIIa/IIIb inhibitors should be withheld for at least 4 weeks after epidural placement.
- Epidural placement is best avoided for 7 days after clopidogrel and 14 days after ticlopidine.

ANATOMY

The key to safe and effective administration of an epidural blockade begins with a thorough understanding of the anatomy of the vertebral column, ligaments, and blood supply, the epidural space, spinal canal, and associated structures. A three-dimensional mental picture of surface structures as they relate to internal structures helps the clinician troubleshoot difficult epidural placement.

Vertebral Column

General Appearance

The vertebral column consists of 7 cervical, 12 thoracic, and 5 lumbar vertebrae. At the caudal end, the 5 sacral vertebrae are fused to form the sacrum, and the 4 coccygeal vertebrae are fused to form the coccyx (Figure 14–1). The primary functions of the vertebral column are to maintain erect posture, to encase and protect the spinal cord, and to provide attachment sites for the muscles responsible for movements of the head and trunk.[31] The normal spinal column is straight when viewed dorsally or ventrally. When viewed from the side, there are two ventrally convex curvatures in the cervical and lumbar regions, giving the spinal column the appearance of a double "C".

Structure of Vertebrae

Each vertebra is composed of a vertebral body and a bony arch. The arch consists of two anterior pedicles and two posterior laminae. The transverse processes are located at the junction of the pedicles and lamina, and the spinous process is located at the junction of the laminae. The spinous processes vary in their angulation in the cervical, thoracic, and lumbar regions. The spinous processes are almost horizontal in the cervical, lower thoracic, and lumbar regions, but become significantly more sharply angled in the midthoracic region (Figure 14–2). The greatest degree of angulation is found between the T3 and T7 vertebrae, making insertion of an epidural needle in the midline more difficult.

The shape and size of the vertebrae differ from the cervical to the lumbar region secondary to function. The vertebral bodies are smaller in the cervical region an become progressively larger in the lumbar area where they support the greatest amount of weight (Figure 14–2).

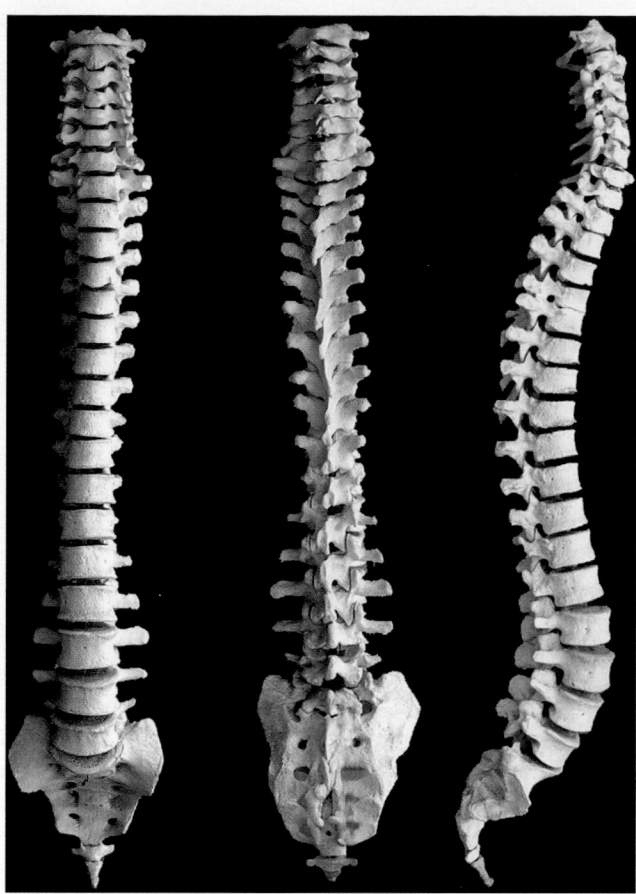

Figure 14–1. Anatomy of the vertebral column.

Joints of the Vertebral Column

The vertebrae articulate at the intervertebral and facet joints. The intervertebral joints are located between adjacent vertebral bodies. They maintain the strength of attachment between vertebrae. The facet joints form between articular processes. The facet joints are heavily innervated by the medial branch of the dorsal ramus of the spinal nerves. This innervation serves to direct contraction of muscle that moves the vertebral column.

Ligaments

The vertebrae are joined together by a series of ligaments and disks. Anteriorly, the vertebral bodies are separated by the intervertebral disks. The ligament connecting them runs from the base of the skull to the sacrum and is called the anterior longitudinal ligament. The posterior surface of the vertebral bodies is connected by the posterior longitudinal ligament, which also forms the anterior wall of the vertebral canal. The other ligaments of importance (Figure 14–3):

• Intertransverse ligament: connects transverse processes
• Supraspinous ligament: attaches to the apices of the spinous processes, extends from sacrum to skull where it becomes the ligamentum nuchae
• Interspinous ligament: connects spinous processes

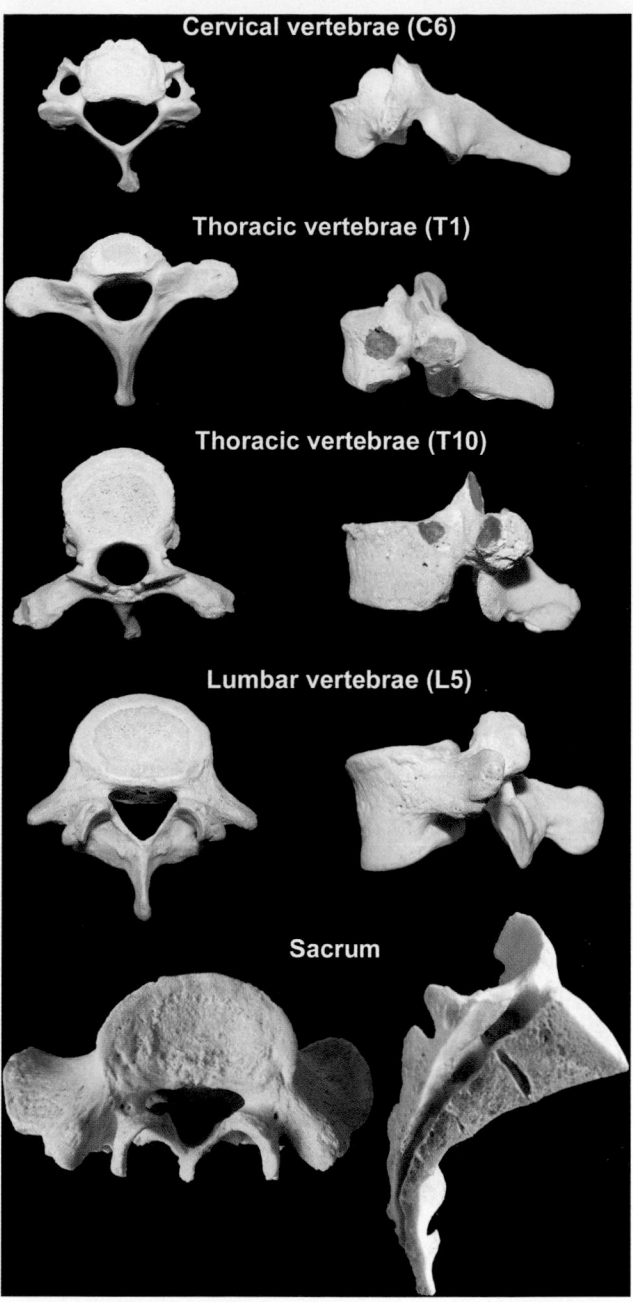

Figure 14–2. Comparison of cervical, thoracic, and lumbar vertebrae.

• Ligamentum flavum: thick, elastic ligament, connects the laminae, composed of a right and left ligament that joins in the middle forming an acute angle; narrows toward the articular processes

Spinal Cord/Spinal Canal

The spinal canal is formed by adjacent vertebral foramina. The canal provides support and protection to the spinal cord and its nerve roots. The spinal cord extends from the foramen magnum to the L1-2 vertebral level in adults, and L3 vertebral level in children before becoming the conus medullaris.

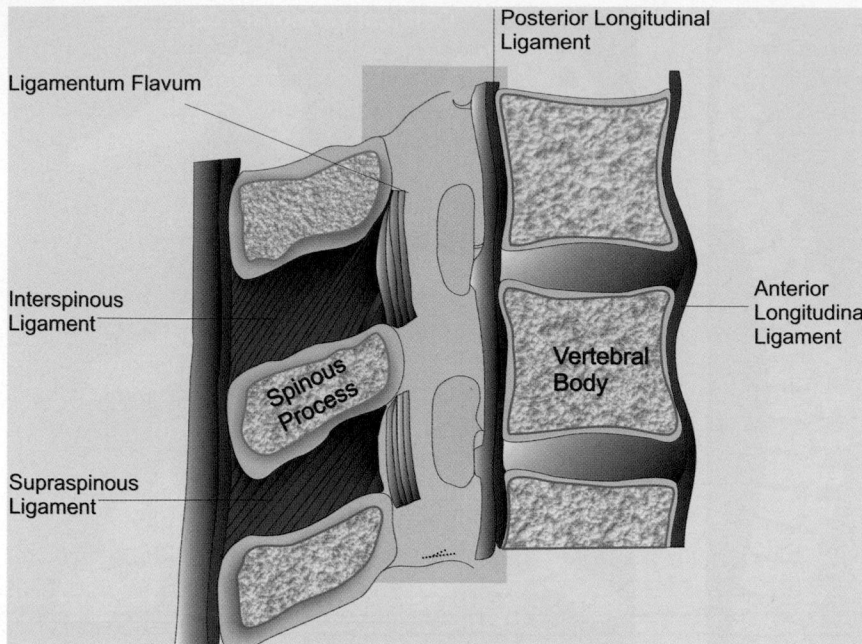

Figure 14–3. When performing an epidural, the needle passes through the following:
– skin
– subcutaneous fat
– supraspinous ligament
– interspinous ligament
– ligamentum flavum

From the spinal cord extends a series of dorsal and ventral roots that converge to form mixed spinal nerves. The mixed nerves contain motor, sensory, and in many cases, autonomic fibers. There are eight cervical, 12 thoracic, 5 lumbar, 5 sacral, and 1 coccygeal pairs of spinal nerves. The roots inferior to the conus medullaris become the cauda equina before exiting through the lumbar and sacral foramina. After the spinal nerves leave the spinal canal through the intervertebral foramina, they divide into the anterior and posterior primary rami. The posterior primary rami innervate the skin and muscles of the back. The anterior rami supply the rest of the trunk and the limbs. Each spinal nerve supplies a specific region of skin referred to as a dermatome (Figure 14–4). There is overlap between adjacent segmental nerves. Loss of a single spinal nerve will produce an area of altered sensation, but won't result in total sensory loss. For instance, destruction of at least three consecutive spinal nerves is required to produce a total sensory loss of the dermatome supplied by the middle nerve of the three.

Preganglionic fibers of the sympathetic nervous system originate from the spinal cord from T1 to L2. They travel with spinal nerves to form the sympathetic chain. This chain extends the entire length of the spinal column on the anterolateral aspects of the vertebral bodies. The chain gives rise to the stellate ganglion, splanchnic nerves, and the celiac plexus (Figure 14–5).

Simple surface landmarks can be used to indicate the level of dermatomal blockade, which correlates with the segmental spinal nerve (Figure 14–6). The degree and effect of sympathetic block depends on the height of the block (Table 14–3)

which attaches intimately to the surface of the spinal cord and roots of the spinal nerves. As the roots of the spinal nerves extend distally, the pia mater transforms into the second layer called the arachnoid. The aranchoid detaches from the roots and reflects back across the pia, enclosing the spinal cord within a cavity called the subarachnoid space. The space is filled with cerebrospinal fluid and transmits blood vessels to and from the spinal cord. Superficial to the arachnoid is the thick dura mater. The space between the arachnoid and dura is called the subdural space. Because the arachnoid is pushed against the dura mater by the pressure of the CSF, the subdural space is negligible. It contains a small amount of serous fluid which allows the dura and arachnoid to move over each other.[32] Because of its exceedingly small volume, it is referred to as a potential space.

Clinical Pearls

- Unintentional injection into the subdural space during epidural anesthesia explains the occasional patchy epidural, high epidural/spinal level or total spinal after epidural placement.

- Key features of a subdural injection: diffuse, spotty anesthesia with a delayed onset for 15 to 30 min, or clinical presentation of a high or total spinal.

- The subdural space extends into the skull, so LA injected into this space can affect higher levels in the brain than epidural medications—watch for neurologic changes.

Meninges/Meningeal Spaces

Surrounding the spinal cord and its roots are three layers of membranes. The innermost layer is called the pia mater,

Epidural Space

The epidural space is smaller than the subarachnoid space, extends from the base of the skull to the sacral hiatus, and

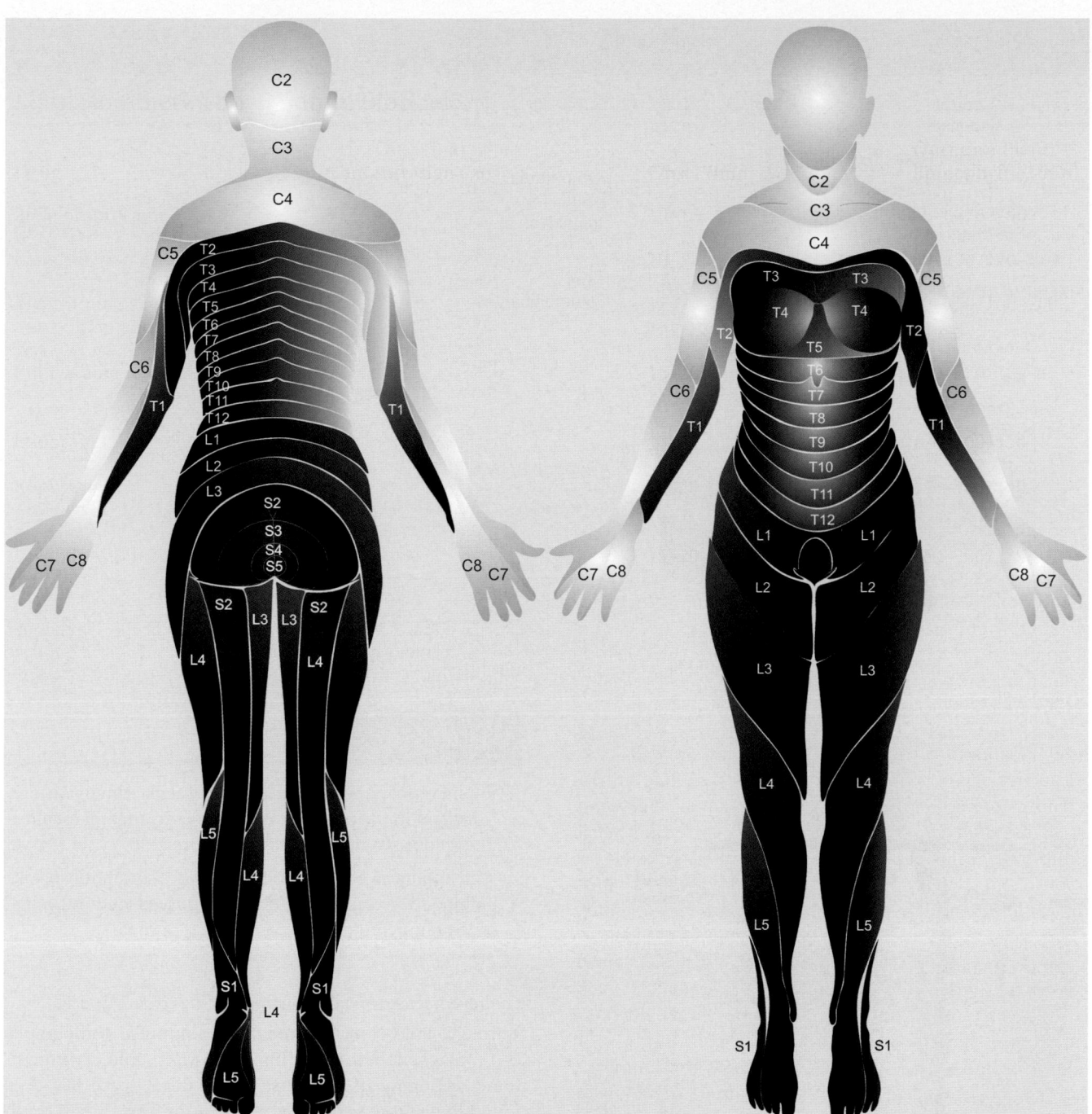

Figure 14–4. Body dermatomes.

surrounds the dura mater anteriorly, laterally, and posteriorly. The epidural space is bound posteriorly by the ligamentum flavum and laterally by the pedicles and the intervertebral foramina. It is filled with the fat, areolar tissue, lymphatics, veins, and nerve roots that traverse it, but there is no free fluid (Figure 14–7). The volume of fat is greater in obese individuals and less in the elderly. It is postulated that the decrease in epidural fat explains the age-related changes in epidural dose requirements.[32,33]

The epidural space is rich in blood vessels, including Batson's venous plexus. Batson's plexus is continuous with the iliac vessels in the pelvis and the azygos system in the abdominal and thoracic body walls (Figure 14–8). Because this plexus has no valves, blood from any of the connected systems can flow into the epidural vessels. This is especially important in obstetrics when compressed caval vessels can lead to engorgement of the epidural veins, increasing the risk of catheter entry into a vein. The engorgement is even greater at the intervertebral foramina where the vessels may bulge from the vertebral canal. Therefore, the incidence of penetrating a blood vessel with an "off-midline" needle insertion may be more likely.

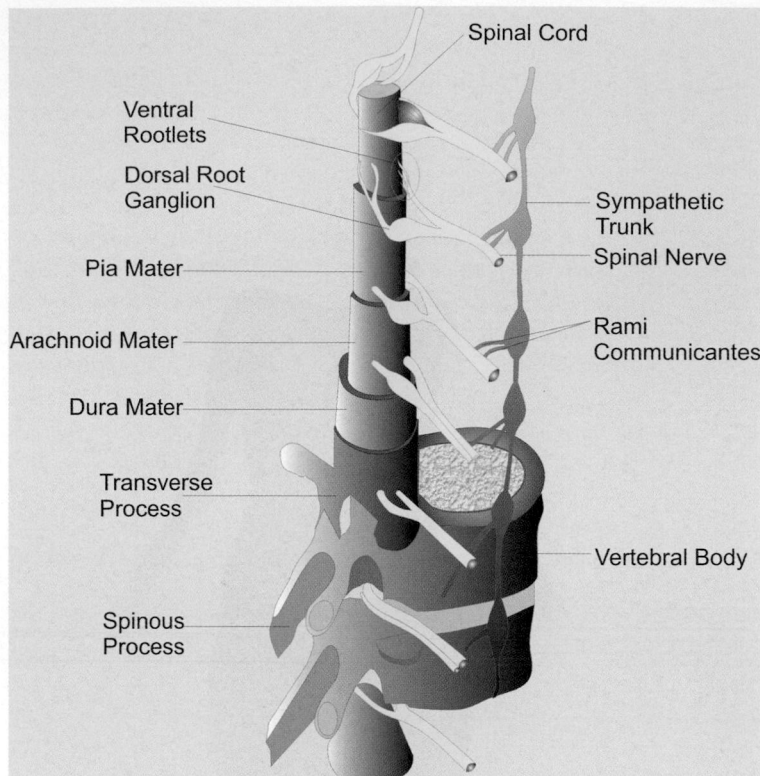

Spinal Cord

Ventral Rootlets

Dorsal Root Ganglion

Sympathetic Trunk

Spinal Nerve

Pia Mater

Arachnoid Mater

Rami Communicantes

Dura Mater

Transverse Process

Vertebral Body

Spinous Process

Figure 14–5. Preganglionic fibers of the sympathetic nervous system.

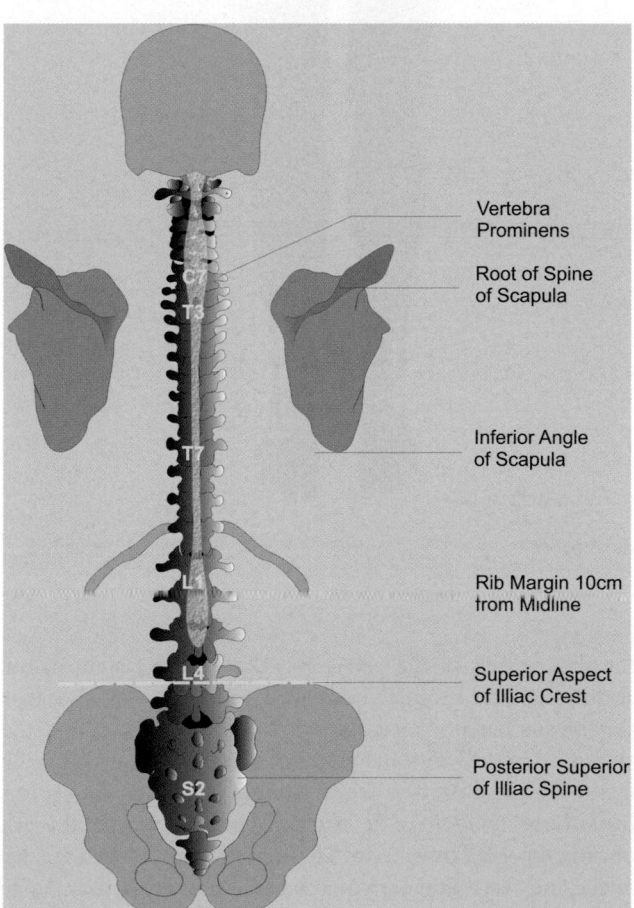

Vertebra Prominens

Root of Spine of Scapula

Inferior Angle of Scapula

Rib Margin 10cm from Midline

Superior Aspect of Illiac Crest

Posterior Superior of Illiac Spine

Figure 14–6. Surface landmarks for various dermatomal levels of epidural blockade.

Clinical Pearls

- Blood vessel puncture during epidural placement is more common in the pregnant patient due to engorgement of the epidural veins from caval compression.
- Off-midline needle insertion may more commonly result in blood vessel puncture due to engorged epidural veins converging into the intervertebral foramina.

Controversies Regarding the Anatomy of the Epidural Space

Through endoscopic examination, computed tomography (CT), magnetic resonance imaging (MRI), and cryomicrotome sectioning of cadavers, the epidural space has been found to be more segmented and less uniform[34] than traditionally taught (Figure 14–9). In a cadaver study, Blomberg[35] identified a midline band that he attributed to septations in the epidural space. This was later suggested by Hogan[36] to actually be an artifact of the midline posterior epidural fat pad. Between the epidural segments, the dura is adjacent but not adherent to the periosteum of the vertebra, making this space a potential space that can be dilated by the injection of fluid. It has been postulated that these anatomic variations in the epidural space account for the unilateral block or unpredictable epidural drug spread that is occasionally seen.[32,36]

Surface Anatomy, Structures Superficial to the Epidural Space

Surface structures assist the clinician in determining the level of entry into the epidural space. The spinous processes

Table 14–3.

Correlating Dermatomal Level to Surface Landmarks

Dermatomal Level	Surface Landmark	Comments
C8	Little finger	Cardioaccelerator fibers blocked (T1 to T4)
T1, T2	Inner aspect of the arm	Above fibers blocked but to lesser degree
T4	Nipple line, root of scapula	Cesarean section, Appendectomy, upper abdominal surgery
T7	Inferior border of scapula Tip of xiphoid	Splanchnic (T5 to L1) blockage; lower abdominal surgery; T5 to T7 for thoracotomy or fractured ribs (at relevant interspace)
T10	Umbilicus	Usual level for LE procedures, hip surgery, TURP, vaginal delivery
L2 to L3	Anterior thigh	Appropriate for knee, foot surgery
S1	Heel of foot	Part of sacral plexus, difficult to block

LE = lower extremity; TURP = transurethral prostatectomy.

help define the location of the midline as they are usually midline structures. The cervical and lumbar spinous processes are horizontally directed whereas the T4 through T9 thoracic spinous processes have a sharp caudal angulation (Figure 14–10).

Clinical Pearl

- Needle entry into the cervical and lumbar regions can be directed medially with a slight upward angulation, whereas in the upper thoracic region, a midline approach to the epidural space is more difficult because of the angulation of the spinous processes. A paramedian approach is usually more successful.

The safest point of entry into the epidural space is below the level of the spinal cord. In adults, this corresponds to the lower border of the L1 vertebrae, and in children, at the lower border of the L3 vertebrae. Epidural insertion in adults is commonly introduced at either the L3-4 interspinous space or one higher, L2-3. A line drawn between the superior aspect of the iliac crests crosses either the spinous process of L4 or the L4-5 interspace. The interspinous space above this point (L3-4 interspinous space) or one higher (L2-3) can safely be chosen for needle entry into the epidural space of adults (Figure 14–6). Some research has challenged the accuracy of the iliac crest in assessing the level, but this is still a generally accepted surface landmark.[37–39] By approximately the age of 8 years, the same interspaces can be chosen for children; however, under the age of 7, to avoid accidental cord injury the caudal approach to the epidural space is safer.

Anatomic landmarks used to identify vertebral levels prior to insertion of an epidural needle are summarized in Table 14–4.

Distance from Skin to Epidural Space

The last anatomic feature of clinical importance pertaining to the epidural space is the distance from the skin to the space. The depth varies depending on the body habitus. The distance is 4 cm in 50% of the population, and 4–6 cm in 80% of the population.[24,40,41] It is noteworthy that studies demonstrating skin-to-epidural space in extremes of weight have shown that in the thin patient, the distance can be less than 4 cm, and in the obese, greater than 8 cm.[24,42]

Clinical Pearl

- The distance from skin to epidural space in the midline is 4–6 cm in 80% of the population.
  This distance can be shorter in thin patients and longer in obese patients.

PHYSIOLOGIC EFFECTS OF EPIDURAL BLOCKADE

The primary site of action of local anesthetic solutions injected into the epidural space is the spinal nerve roots. The segmental nerve roots in the thoracic and lumbar regions are mixed nerves, containing somatic sensory, motor, and autonomic nerve fibers. Sensory blockade interrupts the transmission of both somatic and visceral painful stimuli, whereas motor blockade provides muscle relaxation with a varying degree of sympathetic blockade.[25] The injection site for epidural anesthesia should be close to the nerve roots of interest in order to obtain the best results with minimal amount of local anesthetic and decreased risk of side effects from systemic absorption of the local anesthetic (catheter/incision-congruent).[25,43]

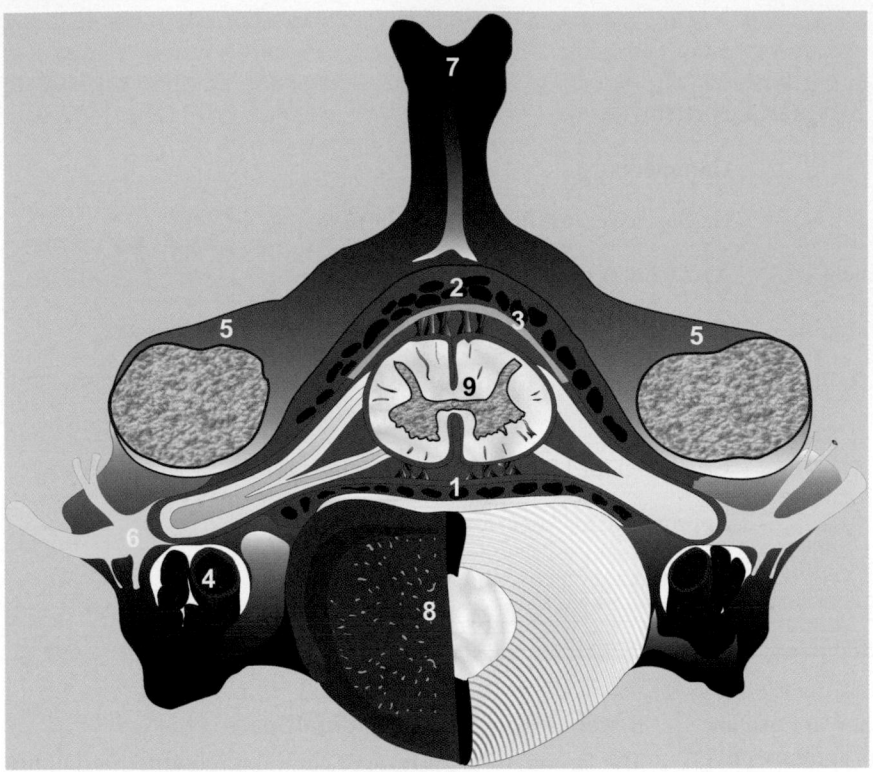

Figure 14–7. Epidural space: 1. Anterior epidural space, 2. Posterior epidural space, 3. Ligamentum flavum, 4. Blood vessels in the epidural space, 5. Pedicles, 6. Nerve roots, 7. Transverse process, 8. Vertebral body, 9. Spinal cord.

Differential nerve block, an important concept for epidural anesthesia, refers to the phenomenon in which nerve fibers with different functions demonstrate a varying sensitivity to the effects of local anesthetics. Sympathetic fibers are usually blocked first followed by pain/temperature, then proprioception, followed by motor blockade. After an epidural block, sympathetic blockade (temperature) may vary from zero to four segments higher than the sensory block level (pain/light touch), which is two segments higher than motor blockade. Regression of the block occurs in reverse order.

The physiologic effects of epidural blockade on organ systems depends on the spinal level and the number of spinal segments blocked. In general, high thoracic epidural blocks and extensive epidural blocks are associated with more

profound sympathetic block, resulting in a more profound physiologic effect in the cardiovascular system.

Cardiovascular

Block Below T4

The effect of epidural anesthesia on the cardiovascular system depends on the level and the degree of sympathetic blockade. Vasomotor tone is maintained by sympathetic fibers from T5 to L1 that innervate vascular smooth muscle. Blockade of these fibers cause venodilation with venous pooling as well as arterial vasodilation with decreased systemic vascular resistance. The venous pooling leads to a decrease in venous return, right atrial pressure, and subsequently, decrease in

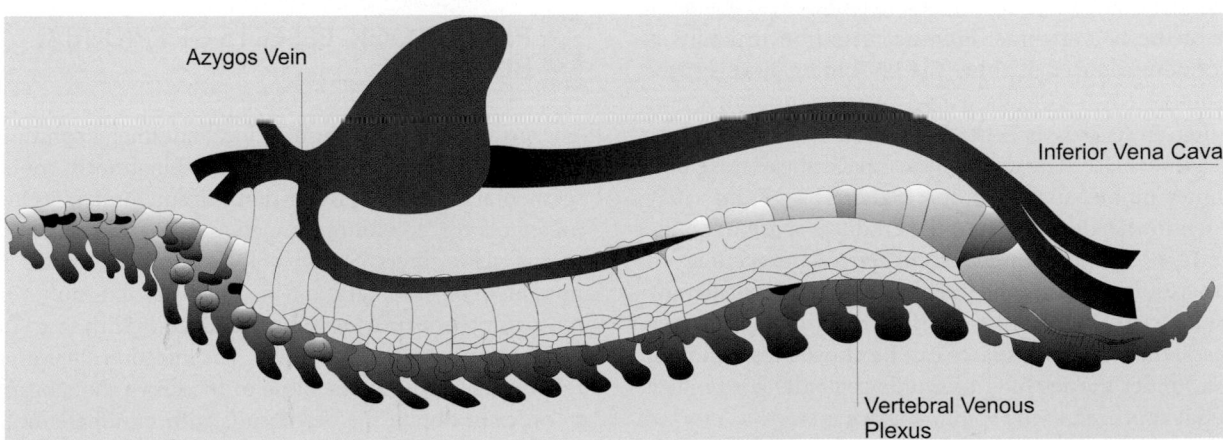

Figure 14–8. Blood vessels in the epidural space and their communication with systemic vessels.

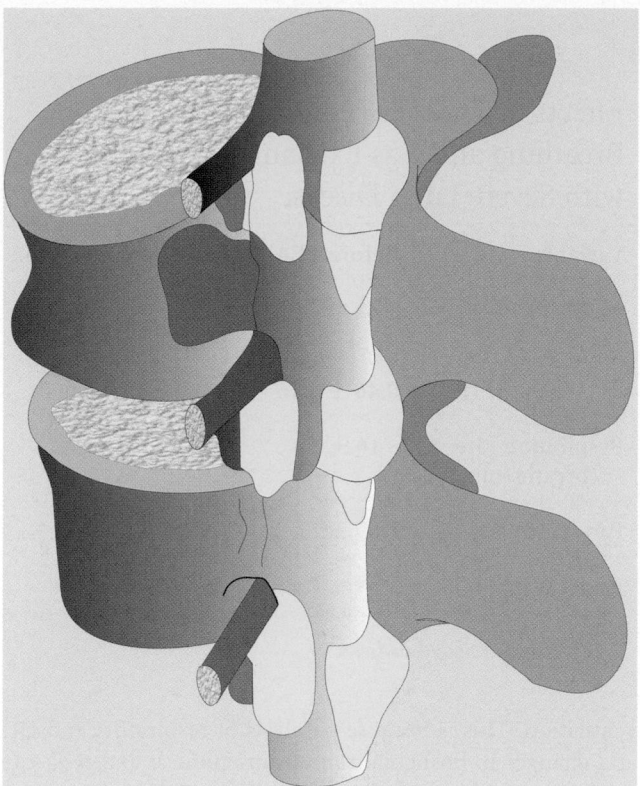

Figure 14–9. Segmentation of the epidural space. The yellow areas indicate various segments that may be inconsistently connected.

cardiac output. The decrease in venous return can also lead to an increase in cardiac vagal tone,[44] especially for blocks near the T5 level.

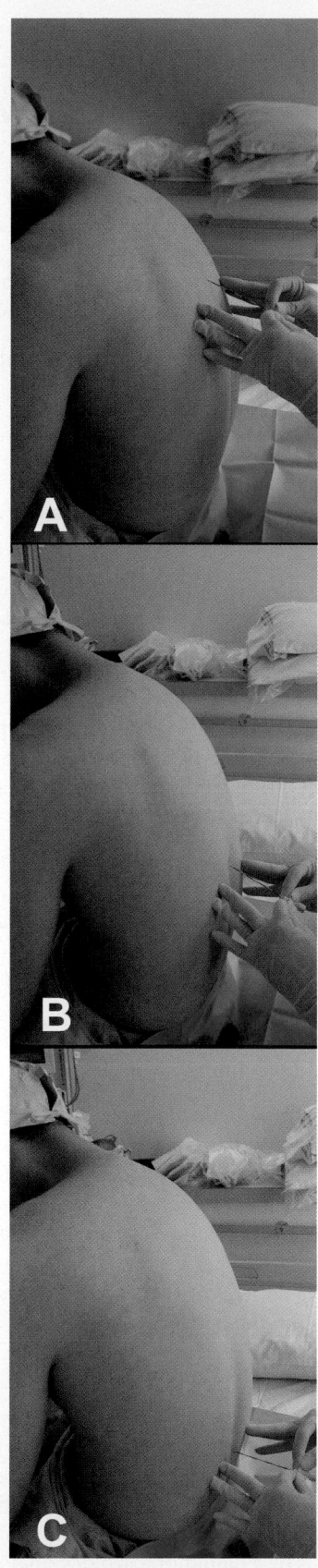

Clinical Pearl

- Upper body vasoconstriction with baroreceptor activation can lead to increased vagal tone, causing bradycardia *despite* the decrease in venous return.

The compensatory mechanism for the decrease in mean arterial pressure is a reflex increase in vasoconstriction above the level of the block as well as a release in catecholamines from the adrenal medulla. If normal cardiac output is maintained either by volume loading or by physiologic mechanisms, (ie, physiologic release of catecholamines, vasoconstriction in unblocked area), the total peripheral vascular resistance will only decrease by approximately 15%, a value well tolerated by a healthy patient. In an elderly patient with cardiovascular disease, a more significant decrease in blood pressure and the resultant need for vasopressor support.

Block Above T4

The cardiovascular effects of a block above T4 are the result of a high sympathetic block. The cardiac sympathetic fibers arise

Figure 14–10. Needle angulation required to accomplish thoracic blockade in the high thoracic/low thoracic/lumbar regions. **A:** High thoracic region. **B:** Low thoracic region. **C:** Lumbar region.

Table 14–4.

Anatomic Landmarks to Identify Vertebral Levels Before Epidural Injection

Anatomic Landmark	Features
C7	Vertebral prominence, the most prominent process in the neck
T3	Root of the spine of the scapula
T7	Inferior angle of the scapula
L4	Line connecting iliac crests
S2	Line connecting the posterior inferior iliac spines
Sacral hiatus	Groove or depression just above or between the gluteal clefts above the coccyx

Table 14–5.

Effects of Thoracic Epidural Analgesia on Breathing and Gas Exchange in Patients with Severe Lung Disease

Variable	Before TEA	After TEA	P Value
Minute ventilation (L)	7.5 ± 2.6	8.7 ± 2.1	0.04
Tidal volume (L)	0.46 ± 0.16	0.53 ± 0.14	0.003
Respiration rate (breaths/min)	16 ± 3	17 ± 3	0.63
Pao_2 (mm Hg)	69 ± 17	68 ± 9	0.79
$Paco_2$ (mm Hg)	39 ± 4	38 ± 5	0.04

TEA = thoracic epidural analgesia.

from T1 to T4, and when blocked, profound hypotension (the result of a decrease in cardiac contractility) and bradycardia can occur. In addition to the cardiac effects, a high level of sympathetic blockade causes:[24,45]

- Increased central venous pressure without an increase in stroke volume
- Compensatory vasoconstriction in the head, neck, and upper limbs
- Splanchnic nerve blockade with reduction in medullary secretion of catecholamines
- Blockade of vasoconstrictive effect on the capacitance vessels of the lower limbs

When a sympathetic block occurs at such a high level, the cardiovascular system may be left without its mechanisms for responding to low cardiac output states. This can be detrimental to a patient with limited cardiac reserve because profound hypotension with bradycardia and decreased contractility can result.[46] The anesthesiologist must be prepared to take over the control of the circulatory system until the block subsides and the patient stabilizes.

Respiratory

Epidural blockade to midthoracic levels have minimal effect on patients with adequate lung function. Lung volumes (tidal volume, vital capacity), resting minute ventilation, and dead space are basically unchanged even with a high thoracic epidural anesthesia. Even with abdominal or intercostal muscle paralysis by a high thoracic block, major alteration in pulmonary function is not seen.

There is concern regarding the use of epidural blockade in patients with severe chronic lung disease who may be dependent on accessory muscle function to maintain adequate

ventilation. This is because paralysis of respiratory muscles and changes in bronchial tone from epidural analgesia can occur. In a study by Gruber and colleagues, thoracic epidurals were placed in patients with end-stage chronic obstructive pulmonary disease undergoing lung volume reduction surgery. Thoracic epidural analgesia with 0.25% bupivacaine did not adversely affect ventilatory mechanics, breathing pattern, gas exchange, and inspiratory muscle force generation in these patients[47] (Tables 14–5 and 14–6).

Table 14–6.

Effects of Thoracic Epidural Analgesia on Ventilatory Mechanics in Patients with Severe Lung Disease

Variable	Before TEA	After TEA	P Value
Peak inspiratory flow rate (L/sec)	0.48 ± 0.17	0.55 ± 0.14	0.02
Peak expiratory flow rate (L/sec)	0.38 ± 0.17	0.40 ± 0.09	0.78
PEEP	4.8 ± 3.6	4.7 ± 3.9	0.67
Work of breathing (J/L)	1.5 ± 0.5	1.5 ± 0.6	0.79
Maximum inspiratory pressure (cm H_2O)	81.7 ± 25.5	76.8 ± 32	0.52

TEA = thoracic epidural analgesia; PEEP = positive end-expiratory pressure.

Rarely, respiratory arrest during high epidural blockade has been reported. Contrary to what may seem a logical explanation, the arrest is not due to the effects of sensory or motor blockade or any effect of the local anesthetic on the brain. The reported cause of rare instances of respiratory arrest is from the sympathetic block, leading to decreased cardiac output and subsequent reduction in blood flow to the brain and brainstem ischemia.

Gastrointestinal

The gastrointestinal effects of epidural anesthesia are largely the result of blockage of the sympathetic splanchnic fibers from the T5 through L1 level. Unopposed vagal dominance leads to an increase in secretions; peristalsis; and a smaller, contracted gut. Postoperatively, gastrointestinal motility returns more quickly when epidural analgesia with a local anesthetic is instituted. Several studies have demonstrated the beneficial effect of thoracic epidural anesthesia on visceral perfusion. Christopherson and colleagues used intramucosal pH measurements (pH_i) as an indicator of stable visceral perfusion during abdominal surgery. They suggested that thoracic epidural anesthesia prevented the decrease of intramucosal pH during major abdominal surgery as an effect of stable visceral perfusion.[48] When thoracic epidural anesthesia is used as an adjunct to general anesthesia for major thoracic, cardiac, or upper abdominal surgery, a segmental block of T1 through T5 is typically the goal. Segmental sympatholysis creating an increase of sympathetic activity in segments below the block leading to impaired splanchnic blood flow has been a concern. In a study in awake and anesthetized dogs, an upper thoracic epidural block had no compromising effect on gastrointestinal perfusion.[49]

Nausea is a relatively common problem following neuraxial anesthesia. It has been reported to occur in up to 20% of patients undergoing neuraxial blocks. It is thought to be related to increased gastric peristalsis secondary to unopposed vagal activity. It can be prevented by promptly treating hypotension with a fluid bolus, ephedrine, or phenylephrine. Atropine has been shown to be an effective treatment for nausea associated with a high thoracic block.[50,51]

Renal/Genitourinary

Since renal blood flow is maintained through autoregulation, epidural anesthesia has very little effect on renal function. Neuraxial blockade at the lumbar level has been postulated to impair control of bladder function secondarily to blockage of the S2 to S4 segments. Urinary retention may occur until the block wears off. The clinician should avoid administering an excessive volume of intravenous fluids if a urinary catheter is not in place. If a continuous epidural anesthesia/analgesia is used, then urinary catheterization may be necessary. However, more recent studies have questioned the validity of this belief.[32,52]

Neuroendocrine

Surgical stress produces a variety of changes in endocrine and metabolic function. Increased protein catabolism and oxygen consumption are common. Increased plasma concentrations of catecholamines, vasopressin, growth hormone, renin, angiotensin, cortisol, glucose, antidiuretic hormone, and thyroid-stimulating hormone have been documented and referred to as the surgical stress response. Perioperative manifestations of the stress response are demonstrated as hypertension, tachycardia, hyperglycemia, suppressed immune function, and altered renal function. Afferent sensory information from the surgical site is thought to play a pivotal role in the response.[53] This response can be abolished or reduced by an appropriate level of sensory blockade produced by epidural anesthesia. The inhibitory effect is greatest with lower abdominal and lower extremity surgery and less effective in upper abdominal and thoracic surgery, probably because the epidural anesthesia cannot completely block all nociceptive afferent pathways for these indications.[54]

The most critical effect of neuroendocrine activation in the perioperative period is the increase in plasma norepinephrine, which peaks about 18 h after the surgical stimulus is initiated. The increase in plasma norepinephrine is associated with activation of nitric oxide in the endothelium of patients with atherosclerotic disease, producing paradoxic vasospasm.[55] Thus, in patients with significant atherosclerotic disease, the combination of paradoxic vasospasm and the hypercoagulable state may be the factors modulated by the cardioprotective effects of thoracic epidural anesthesia and analgesia in patients with atherosclerotic cardiac disease.

PHARMACOLOGY OF EPIDURAL BLOCKADE

To be successful with epidural blockade, the clinician must understand the physiology of nerve conduction and the pharmacology of the local anesthetics. Potency and duration of the drugs, their ability to preferentially block sensory and motor fibers, as well as the anticipated duration of surgery or need for postoperative analgesia are factors that should be considered before instituting epidural blockade.

The principal site of action of local anesthetics after epidural injection is thought to be the spinal nerve roots, the spinal cord, and possibly the brain.[56] Nerve fibers with different features and function display varying sensitivity to local anesthetic blockade. For example, sympathetic fibers (thin, myelinated when entering the sympathetic trunk) tend to be blocked with the lowest concentration of drug, followed by pain, touch, and finally motor fibers.

Nerve Impulse Physiology

Nerve conduction involves the propagation of an electrical impulse created by the rapid movement of ions across the nerve cell membrane, creating an action potential. The principal ions involved in generating the action potential are sodium and potassium. The concentration of sodium is high extracellularly and low intracellularly. The opposite is true of potassium (high intracellularly, low extracellularly).

At rest, the cell is more permeable to the positively charged cation potassium. The leakage of a positively charged ion leaves the inside of the cell more negative than the outside of the cell, creating a negative resting membrane potential of −60 to −70 mV. The sodium–potassium pump actively transports sodium ions out of the cell and potassium into the cell to maintain the gradient at the resting level.

Once chemical, mechanical, or electrical excitation occurs, an impulse is conducted along the nerve axon, causing depolarization of the nerve cell membrane. If the depolarization exceeds the threshold level (membrane potential of −60 mV), ion channels in the cell membranes open, allowing a sudden influx of sodium. The rapid influx of positively charged sodium ions causes depolarization of the cell. The influx of positively charged ions alters the membrane potential to become positive (above +30 mV). When the membrane potential exceeds approximately −30 mV, the sodium channels close, abating the influx of sodium into the cell. Depolarization generates a current that causes further depolarization of adjacent segments of the nerve, allowing the action potential to spread along the entire length of the nerve. The cell attempts to return to its resting potential with the efflux of potassium, thereby making the membrane potential less positive (repolarization). Baseline concentration gradients are eventually reestablished by the sodium–potassium–ATP-ase pump.

The rapid influx of sodium that leads to depolarization of the nerve occurs through specific channels in the cell membrane. The sodium channel is a path that changes the nerve from nonconductive to conductive of an action potential (referred to as gated channels). If the change in conductance is created by electrical changes, the channel is called a voltage-gated channel. The voltage-gated sodium channel in the nerve is considered to be the site of action for local anesthetics.[57] (For more information on mechanisms of neural blockade, please refer to Chapter 20)

Action of Local Anesthetics

Local anesthetic binds to sodium channels, primarily in the inactivated state, preventing further channel activation. Sodium ion movement into the cell is prevented, effectively blocking the development of the action potential. The resulting resting membrane potential is unaffected by further nerve stimulation, referred to as **membrane stabilization** of local anesthetics.

Mechanism of Action of Local Anesthetics for Neuraxial Blockade

Within the dorsal horn, local anesthetics can block both sodium and potassium ion channels in the dorsal horn neurons, inhibiting the generation and propagation of pain signals (nociceptive electrical activity). Motor blockade oc-

curs from a similar action on the ventral horn neurons. Blockade of calcium ion channels in the spinal cord leads to resistance of electrical stimulation from nociceptive afferent nerves, creating an intense analgesic action seen in centrally administered local anesthetics.[58]

In addition to ion channel alterations in the central neuraxis, epidurally administered local anesthetics *indirectly* inhibit the release of substance P and other neurotransmitters involved in pain signal processing. Substance P is involved in pain transmission from the presynaptic terminals of dorsal root ganglionic cells. The putative effects of centrally administered local anesthetics on substance P and these other transmitters are linked to the presynaptic blockade of the voltage-gated calcium channel.[59,60] When calcium entry is blocked at the presynaptic level, release of these neurotransmitters (glutamate, substance P, calcitonin gene-related peptide [CGRP], neurokini-1 and -2 [NK1, NK2]) at the presynaptic level does not occur. Therefore, epidurally administered local anesthetics can indirectly inhibit pain signal transmission.

Choice of Local Anesthetics

Drugs used for epidural blockade can be categorized into short-, intermediate-, and long-acting local anesthetics. Onset of epidural blockade in the dermatomes immediately surrounding the site of injection can usually be detected within 5 or 10 min of injection of any of the local anesthetics. The time to peak effect varies with the type of local anesthetic chosen and the dose/volume administered. Table 14–7 summarizes the characteristics of the most commonly used local anesthetics for epidural anesthesia.

The shortest acting local anesthetic for neuraxial blockade is chloroprocaine (an ester). In the past, it was associated with adhesive arachnoiditis when large volumes were administered into the subarachnoid space.[61] When volumes greater than 25 mL were used in the epidural space, severe back pain most likely secondary to localized hypocalcemia introduced by the preservatives, ethylenediaminetetraacetic acid (EDTA) and bisulfites, in the solution. As of 1996, preservative-free chloroprocaine has been available and has not been associated with either neurotoxic effects or back pain. In ambulatory settings, utilizing the favorable characteristics of chloroprocaine with epidural catheter insertion provides excellent surgical anesthesia without delaying recovery room discharge.

The most commonly used intermediate-acting local anesthetic for surgical anesthesia via the epidural route is 2% lidocaine. When epinephrine is added to the solution (1:200,000), it prolongs the duration of action by 40 to 60%. However, the incidence of hypotension is increased in patients receiving lumbar epidural analgesia due to the beta effect of epinephrine-containing solutions that leads to peripheral vasodilation.

Long-acting local anesthetics used for epidural blockade are 0.5% bupivacaine, 0.5% levobupivacaine, and 0.5% ropivacaine. Of these, the most commonly used agent for epidural blockade is bupivacaine. Dilute concentrations can be used for analgesia, with more concentrated solutions

Table 14–7.

Local Anesthetics for Epidural Blockade

Drug	Concentration (%)	Onset (min)	Duration Plain/+ Epinephrine (min)
2-Chloroprocaine	3	10–15	45–60/60–90
Lidocaine	2	10–15	80–120/120–180
Mepivacaine	1	15	90–160/160–200
	2	15	Same
Bupivacaine	0.25	15–20	160–220/180+
	0.375–0.5		
Etidocaine	1	15–20	120–200/150+
Ropivacaine	0.5	15–20	140–180/150+
	0.6–0.75		
Levobupivacaine	0.5	15–20	160–220/180+

employed for surgical anesthesia. Epinephrine added to the solution can prolong its duration of action, but this is less consistent with the shorter acting agents. Accidental intravascular injection of bupivacaine has produced severe cardiotoxic reactions (hypotension, atrioventricular block, ventricular fibrillation) refractory to usual resuscitation methods. The rationale for the resistance to resuscitative measures lies in its high degree of protein binding and more pronounced effect on cardiac sodium channel blockade.[62,63] Levobupivacaine, the *S*-enantiomer of bupivacaine, has nearly an identical profile to bupivacaine but without the systemic cardiac toxic effects of bupivacaine. Ropivacaine, a mepivacaine analog, also has a similar profile of action to bupivacaine. In most studies, ropivacaine has demonstrated a slightly shorter duration of action than bupivacaine, with a less dense motor block when comparing equivalent doses. The only deterrent to a wider use of ropivacaine in clinical practice is its higher cost.[64,65]

Etidocaine, another long-acting amide local anesthetic, is infrequently used for epidural anesthesia. It produces a profound motor block that unfortunately can outlast the sensory block,[66] making it an undesirable choice for epidural anesthesia (see Table 14–7).

Onset/Duration of Local Anesthetics

Several investigators have attempted to find methods to speed up the onset or increase the duration of epidural blockade. Adding epinephrine to the local anesthetic can substantially increase the duration of action of some local anesthetics most likely by decreasing the vascular absorption. The effect is greatest with 2-chloroprocaine, lidocaine, and mepivacaine, and less effective with the longer acting agents. Other vaso-

constrictors, such as phenylephrine, have not been as effective in reducing the peak blood levels of local anesthetics as epinephrine.[67]

Alkalinization of the local anesthetic solution has been used to increase the speed of onset of local anesthetics. By increasing the concentration of the nonionic form of the drug, more drug is available to penetrate the lipid nerve cell membranes to produce more rapid intraneural diffusion. Adding sodium bicarbonate (1 mEq/10 mL of local anesthetic) immediately before injection of lidocaine, mepivacaine, or chloroprocaine produces a clinically significant faster onset of anesthesia and may provide a more complete block.[68,69] However, ropivacaine and bupivacaine will precipitate with the addition of bicarbonate unless a low concentration (0.1 mEq/10 mL of local anesthetics) is used. Combining long- and short-acting drugs to obtain a rapid onset as well as prolonged sensory block has not proven to be effective or predictably better. For example, mixing 2-chloroprocaine with bupivacaine for the rapid onset of the former and long duration of the latter resulted in shortening the duration and effectiveness of the bupivacaine.[70] Utilizing the additives currently available and using continuous techniques of drug administration rather than single-shot techniques obviates the need for mixing local anesthetics.

Novel Additives to Local Anesthetics in the Epidural Space

A variety of other classes of drugs have been studied more recently to try to improve the quality of neuraxial blockade, both in the epidural space and in the subarachnoid space. In addition to a variety of opioids (eg, fentanyl, sufentanil, and preparations of morphine), α-adrenergic agonists, cholinesterase inhibitors, semisynthetic opioid agonist–antagonists, ketamine, and midazolam have been studied with varied results.

Clonidine, the prototypical α_2-adrenoceptor agonist used in neuraxial blocks, has been studied extensively in combination with local anesthetics, as a primary agent, and in combination with a variety of other drugs. Clonidine is an α-adrenoreceptor agonist with selectivity for α_2-adrenoreceptors. The mechanism by which clonidine prolongs neuraxial anesthesia is unclear. Animal studies have shown that clonidine reduces regional spinal cord blood flow, therefore slowing the rate of drug elimination.[71] Kroin and colleagues demonstrated that the mechanism by which clonidine prolongs the duration of a block when mixed with local anesthetics is not mediated by an α-adrenergic mechanism but is more likely related to the hyperpolarization-activated cation current (I_h).[72]

Some of the benefits of the administration of clonidine in the epidural space include

1. Prolongs and intensifies the effects of epidural local anesthetics without increasing the degree of hypotension for epidural anesthesia and analgesia
2. Reduces the dose requirements of local anesthetics for labor epidural analgesia[73,74]
3. Produces analgesia without motor impairment and prolongs the duration of the local anesthetic analgesic effect[71]
4. Has a synergist effect when combined with opioids and opioid agonist–antagonists, allowing reduced doses and therefore side effects of both
5. Modulates the immune stress response to thoracic surgery[75]
6. Is superior in preserving preoperative lung function for thoracotomy patients[76]
7. May reduce cytokine response, therefore further reducing pain sensitivity[77]
8. Has possible antibacterial activity against *Staphylococcus aureus/epidermidis*

Side effects that are commonly associated with epidural clonidine include a dose-independent hypotension, bradycardia, sedation, and dry mouth. Combination of clonidine with other agents such as opioids, anticholinergics, opioid agonist–antagonists, and ketamine have been studied to enhance the beneficial effects of these drugs while limiting the adverse side effects.[78,79]

Neostigmine, a cholinesterase inhibitor, is a more recent addition to the list of epidural additives for selective analgesia. The mechanism of action for the analgesic effect of neostigmine appears to be the inhibition of the breakdown of acetylcholine and the indirect stimulation of muscarinic and nicotinic receptors into the spinal cord, inducing analgesia. By administering it via the epidural route, the gastrointestinal side effects (nausea/vomiting) noted with subaranchoid administration are reduced. It has been reported to provide postoperative pain relief without inducing respiratory depression, motor impairment, or hypotension.[78] When combined with other opioids, clonidine, and local anesthetics, it may provide benefits similar to clonidine without the side effect profile of any of the drugs given alone.[80-82]

Other agents such as ketamine, tramadol, droperidol, and midazolam have been studied with various effectiveness in epidural analgesia. Considerable controversy surrounds the use of midazolam intrathecally. Despite multiple publications recommending its use intrathecally,[83-85] recent studies have demonstrated that even a single dose of intrathecal midazolam may have neurotoxic effects on the neurons and myelinated axons.[86] Until its safety profile can be ensured in human subjects, it is not recommended for use intrathecally or epidurally at this time.[87]

One agent showing promise is a new, extended release formulation of one of the oldest opioids, morphine. Epidural morphine has proven analgesic efficacy with possibly less bothersome side effects of intravenous dosing. Pain relief with single epidural injection lasts less than 24 h, requiring the institution of alternate methods to provide pain relief. Depodur, the brand name for extended-release epidural morphine, uses a drug-release delivery system called Depofoam. Depofoam is composed of microscopic lipid-based particles with internal vesicles that contain the active drug and slowly release it. Recent studies of Depofoam have demonstrated effective pain relief with relatively minor side effects for up to 48 h when appropriately dosed.[88-90]

Other Factors Affecting Epidural Blockade

Injection Site

The epidural blockade is most effective when the block or the catheter is inserted in a location that corresponds to the dermatomes covered by the surgical incision. The most rapid onset and the densest block occurs at the site of injection. By inserting the catheter closer to the surgical site, a lower dose of drug can be given, thereby reducing side effects.[91,92] This concept is especially important when thoracic epidurals are used for postoperative analgesia.

After lumbar injection, analgesia–anesthesia spreads caudally and, to a greater degree, cranially. There is a delay at the L5 to S1 segments secondarily to the larger size of these nerve roots.[93] With thoracic injection, the local anesthetic spreads evenly from the site of injection, but because of the larger nerve roots, there is greater resistance to blockade. By controlling the dose in the thoracic region, a true segmental block can be placed, affecting only the thoracic region. Lumbar and sacral regions will be spared, therefore avoiding more extensive sympathetic blockade and subsequent associated hypotension and bladder dysfunction.

Dose, Volume, and Concentration

The dose of local anesthetics necessary for analgesia or anesthesia is a function of the concentration of the solution and the volume injected. Concentration of the drug affects the density of the block. The higher the concentration, the more profound the motor and sensory block. Lower concentrations can produce a more selective sensory block.[94]

Volume is the variable that affects the degree of distribution of the block. A larger volume will block a greater number of segments. A generally accepted guideline for dosing epidural anesthesia in adults is 1–2 mL per segment to be blocked. This guideline should be adjusted for shorter patients or for the very tall. For example, to achieve a T10 sensory level from an L3-4 injection, approximately 9–18 mL of local anesthetic should be administered. Below concentrations of the equivalent of 1% lidocaine, motor block is minimal, regardless of the volume of the local anesthetic injected, unless doses are given at repeating intervals.[57]

Clinical Pearls

- Volume is the key factor in determining the height of the block.
- The cookbook guideline for dosing an epidural in adults is 1–2 mL per segment to be blocked.
- Adjust the guideline for shorter patients (<5 ft 2 in.) or taller patients (>6 ft 2 in.).
- Example: T10 block from L3-4 injection: 9–18 mL of local anesthetic.

Time to repeat a dose of local anesthetics depends on the duration of the drug. Doses should be administered before the block regresses to the point where the patient experiences pain, commonly referred to as "time to two-segment regression." This is defined as the time it takes for the sensory block to regress by two dermatome levels. When two-segment regression has occurred, one-third to one-half of the initial loading dose can safely be administered to maintain the block. For example, the time to two-segment regression of lidocaine is 60–140 min[75] (Table 14–8).

Table 14–8.

Clinical Effects of Epidurally Injected Local Anesthetics

Drug (Concentration %)	Time to Two-Segment Regression (min)	Recommended Time for "Top-Up" Dose from Initial Activation Dose (min)
Chloroprocaine (3)	45–75	45
Lidocaine (2)	60–140	60
Mepivacaine (2)	90–160	90
Bupivacaine (0.5)	180–260	120
Ropivacaine (0.5–0.75)	180–260	120

Clinical Pearl

- When two-segment regression of the sensory block has occurred, administer 1/3 to 1/2 of the initial loading dose of local anesthetic to maintain the block.

Patient Position

The patient may be placed in either the lateral or sitting position depending on the patient's body habitus and medical conditions. The midline of the spine is easier to palpate when the patient is sitting, especially in the obese patient, therefore making the block technically easier. Whether the patient is sitting or in the lateral position, there is no significant difference in block height.[95] It has been suggested in a study by Seow and associates, that there is slightly faster onset time, duration, and density of motor block on the dependent side when the epidural in placed with the patient in the lateral position.[96]

Characteristics of the Patient: Age, Weight, Height, Pregnancy

With advancing age, the dose required to achieve the same level of block is reduced. The difference in block height with a fixed volume and concentration of local anesthetic in patients older than age 50 was between one to three segments higher (not considered clinically significant).[97,98] Greater spread in the elderly is theorized to be related to reduced size of the intervertebral foramina, therefore limiting the local anesthetic from leaving the epidural space. Decreased epidural fat, allowing more of the drug to bathe the nervous tissue; and changes in the compliance of the epidural space, leading to enhanced cephalad spread have also been suggested[99] (Table 14–9).

There is little correlation between the spread of analgesia and the weight of the patient. However, in morbidly obese patients, there may be compression of the epidural space secondarily to increased intraabdominal pressure, creating a higher block for a given dose of local anesthetic. Just as in the pregnant patient, venous engorgement in the epidural veins increases the risk of entry into a vessel.[94,100]

Table 14–9.

Effect of Aging on Sensory Segmental Spread of Local Anesthetic Administered via Lumbar Epidural Space

Age	Local Anesthetic Given at Lumbar Level	Sensory Level
20	0.5% Bupivacaine	L1 to T10
40	Same	T9 to T11
60	Same	T6 to T9
80	Same	T4 to T7

The correlation with height is usually not clinically significant. For short patients ($\leq$ 5 ft 2 in), the common practice has been to reduce the dose to 1 mL per segment to be blocked instead of 2 mL per segment. Bromage suggested a more precise dosing regime of increasing the dose of local anesthetic by 0.1 mL per segment for each 2 in. over 5 ft of height.[101] The safest practice is to use incremental dosing and monitor the effect to avoid excessively high anesthetic levels.

Clinical Pearls

- Reduce the dose of local anesthetic for the patient 5 ft 2 in. or less to 1 mL per segment to be blocked.
- Increase the dose of local anesthetic by 0.1 mL per segment for each 2 in. over 5 ft.

Pregnancy causes an increased sensitivity to both regional and general anesthetics, although the studies regarding the causes have been conflicting. The most recent studies attribute the sensitivity of pregnant women to regional and general anesthetics to levels of progesterone or increased concentrations of endorphins, causing an increase in the pain threshold.[102,103]

Intermittent vs Continuous Epidural Block

Whether the clinician chooses to use intermittent dosing after the initial activation dose or a continuous infusion, safe and effective epidural anesthesia can be provided. Advantages of continuous infusion include greater cardiovascular stability, less labor intensive, decreased incidence of tachyphylaxis, decreased frequency and severity of side effects related to bolus injections, less rostral spread, less potential risk of contamination, and the ability to achieve a steady-state of anesthesia. The advantages of intermittent bolus dosing is that it is simple and doesn't require additional equipment (infusion devices).

CLINICAL APPLICATION

Patient Evaluation

As with any neuraxial blockade, the risks and benefits of epidural placement need to be discussed with the patient. These should be explained in a thorough but appropriate manner in order to provide informed consent. The inability of the patient to speak English should not be a barrier to providing epidural placement as long as there is a mechanism in place for obtaining informed consent either through translation services in the hospital or through telephone systems.

Patients (particularly older patients) occasionally have misconceptions about epidural placement, such as:

- Permanent paralysis from the block
- Being awake during the operation
- Big needles puncturing the back while awake
- Epidural injection leads to back pain

These issues as well as any other concerns of the patient should be discussed prior to premedication. The level of awareness during the epidural placement and during the operation can be tailored to the patient's desires. The patient, as well as the surgical staff need to understand that the patient will have absent or reduced motor function after the block is placed until the block resolves.

The patient's medical history and medications should be evaluated to determine the presence of any condition that may increase the risks involved with epidural placement (ie, clotting abnormalities, platelet count, recent administration of anticoagulants).[23] Drug therapy that may influence the patient's physiologic response to epidural blockade should be noted to prepare the clinician for altered or exaggerated responses to dosing or test dosing (eg, beta-blockers, alpha-blockers). Medical conditions that may become more severe with reducing afterload or preload should be evaluated (eg, severe aortic stenosis, mitral stenosis, hypertrophic cardiomyopathy, congenital conditions requiring stable systemic vascular resistance such as ventricular septal defects). Other medical conditions that may become more severe with motor blockade (eg, myasthenia gravis, pulmonary fibrosis, severe chronic obstructive disease) require careful review of the patient's history, prior medical evaluations and testing, as well as a thorough physical examination. History of sensitivity to local anesthetics, adverse drug reactions, or prior history of complications related to epidural placement should be reviewed. Rather than eliminate these patients from receiving epidural anesthesia, a well-planned procedure with controlled initiation of the block can provide excellent anesthesia.

Physical examination should include an evaluation of the spine for evidence of scoliosis, focal infection or pain, scars, severely limited range of motion, or other findings that may make epidural placement more challenging or impossible. Obesity, especially central obesity, may obscure physical landmarks, making placement more difficult.

Baseline laboratory assessment of the patient's coagulation status and platelet count should be obtained when the patient has a history of coagulopathy or has recently received anticoagulants or any medications known to influence platelet quality or function. This includes an internationalized ration (INR) (or prothrombin time), activated partial thromboplastin time (aPTT), platelet count, and bleeding time (only if there is a specific concern). Many clinicians choose to obtain a hematocrit at the same time, especially when appreciable blood loss is expected.

The final consideration before placing the epidural is to determine the goal of the block. Epidural placement can be used for surgical anesthesia, as an adjunct to general anesthesia, or for postoperative analgesia. The advantage of epidural placement is the ability to provide **segmental blockade**, meaning that the block can cover as many or as few dermatomal levels as is clinically desired to meet the needs of the patient. Once the decision has been made as to the purpose and levels to be blocked, patient preparation can be initiated (Table 14–10).

Table 14–10.

Segmental Level for Epidural Block for Various Surgeries

Function	Type of Surgery (example)	Suggested Level of Entry
Surgical anesthesia	Hip surgery Lower extremity surgery Cesarean section	L2-3 or L3-4 interspace
Adjunct to general anesthesia	Lower abdominal surgery Upper abdominal surgery Thoracic surgery	Catheter should be placed at the intervertebral space corresponding to the middle of the planned surgical incision
Postoperative analgesia	Varied	Catheter should be placed at the midpoint of the surgical incision for thoracic or upper abdominal surgery, lumbar region for lower abdomen/LE surgery

LE = *lower extremity.*

Clinical Pearls

- Patient evaluation includes review of medications, medical conditions, and history.
- Pay attention to drug therapy that may obscure physiologic effects of block.
- Provide information appropriate to patient's ability to understand.
- Clear up common misconceptions about epidural anesthesia.
- Be prepared for airway management at a minimum.
- Do a quick spine examination to prepare you to make adjustments for potential problems with placement—scars, scoliosis, obesity-obscuring landmarks.

Patient Preparation

The key to providing safe epidural anesthesia is proper *preparation*. Intravenous access with a catheter large enough to administer fluids or emergency drugs should be in place

(ie, 18- to 20-gauge). Reversible conditions such as severe hypovolemia should be managed prior to block placement. However, routine fluid preloading of patients with crystalloids has been questioned and may prove to be harmful in patients with decreased serum colloid oncotic pressure (eg, those with burns, preeclamptic patients, patients on tocolytic therapy).[104,105] The type of monitoring and resuscitative equipment available depends on the purpose of the epidural block. Epidural blocks for analgesia, such as for labor or postoperative analgesia, require blood pressure and pulse oximetry ready access to vasopressors and positive pressure ventilation at a minimum. Drugs and equipment for life support, including airway management, must be readily available if the block is to be performed for surgical anesthesia or as an adjunct to general anesthesia (ASA Standard Monitors).

Controversies about placing the epidural block while the patient is awake or asleep continue to be addressed in the literature. The advantages to having the patient sedated or asleep are avoiding movement that could lead to injury to the spinal cord or neural tissue and alleviating the stress response associated with fear of pain or needles. The disadvantages are similar in that the patient is unable to verbalize when neural structures are encountered. For years, neuraxial blocks have been placed in children with heavy sedation or under general anesthesia without a preponderance of case reports on neural structure damage. Horlocker and colleagues at the Mayo Clinic recently published a report of over 4000 patients undergoing lumbar epidural placement under general anesthesia without any neurologic complications.[106] Sedating the patient with a benzodiazepam (eg, midazolam) and a narcotic (ie, alfentanil/fentanyl) allows the clinician to safely place the epidural catheter without undue stress to the patient. The choice of drugs for sedation depends on the patient's overall medical condition and age. An exception to the use of sedation is in the pregnant patient (potential of harming the fetus).

Clinical Pearls

- Adequate sedation is key to successful block placement.
- A combination of midazolam with fentanyl or alfentanil in a monitored patient is effective in allowing proper positioning and placement of the epidural catheter without undue stress to the patient.

Communication with the Surgical Staff

A discussion with the surgical staff to understand the operative approach, the desired positioning of the patient, and an estimated length of the surgical procedure is important for the anesthesiologist to determine the best choice of anesthetic. The anesthesiologist can decide if a simple epidural or a combined spinal-epidural with an initial more intense and faster onset motor block is indicated. Postoperative analgesia can be determined at the same time. Communicating with

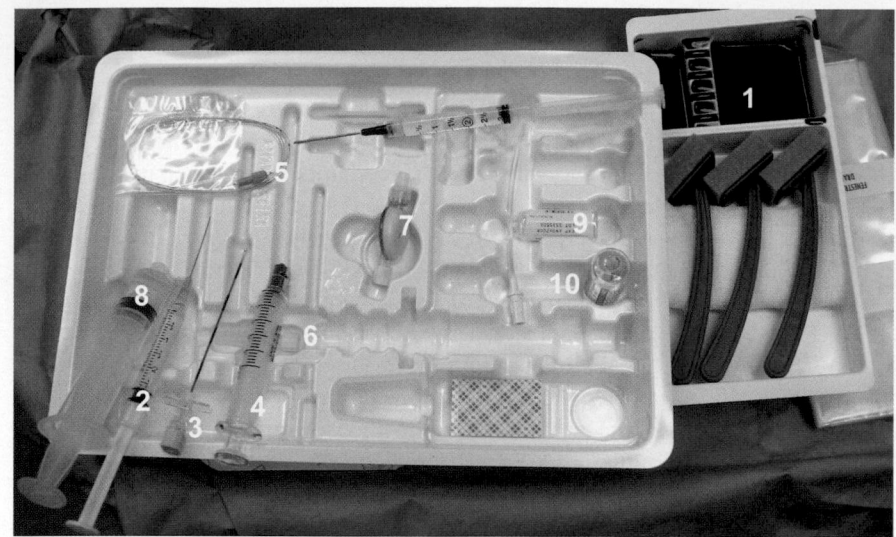

Figure 14–11. Prepared epidural tray. 1. Solution of antiseptic, 2. Syringe/needle for skin localization, 3. Epidural needle, 4. Glass syringe, 5. Epidural catheter, 6. Luer Lok attachment, 7. Glass filter, 8. Dosing syringe, 9. Local anesthetic, 10. Saline.

the nursing staff leads to better cooperation and assistance with the epidural block. If feasible, turnover time can be reduced by performing the block in the preoperative area or bringing the patient into the operating room and placing the epidural block while the nursing staff is still setting up the surgical equipment. Cooperation with the surgical staff improves when delays are not attributed to "anesthetic procedures."

Equipment

Commercially prepared, sterile disposable epidural trays are available and used by most institutions (Figure 14–11). All of the drugs included in the tray are preservative-free. A standard kit typically includes the following:

- Drapes: Paper towel, fenestrated plastic drape, one paper drape
- Small tray with prep sponges, 4 × 4 gauze sponges, packet of povidone-iodine solution
- Drugs: 10-mL ampule of 0.9% sodium chloride; 5-mL ampule of 1.5% lidocaine with epinephrine 1:200,000; 5-ml ampule of 1% lidocaine; 1-mL ampule of epinephrine 1:1000
- One filter straw
- Needles/Syringes: 25-gauge 1.5-in. needle, 18-gauge 1.5-in. needle, 18-gauge 3.5-in. Tuohy epidural needle with stylet, 3 mL/20 mL plastic syringes; 5-mL glass Luer Lok syringe 20-gauge calibrated epidural catheter

A styletted Tuohy epidural needle is typically 16 to 18 gauge, 8–10 cm in length, with surface markings at 1-cm intervals. It has a 15- to 30-degree curve at the tip with a blunt bevel. The curved tip is designed to prevent accidental dural puncture and to facilitate passage of the epidural catheter (Figure 14–12). At the junction of the needle shaft and hub are wings to allow better control as the needle is passed through tissue. Longer needles up to 10 cm in length are available for obese patients. A variety of needles are used for single-shot epidural blocks, but this practice is less common in modern

anesthesia because of the inability to redose if the initial block wears off.

Epidural catheters made of a durable, flexible plastic are designed to pass through the lumen of the Tuohy needle. They have either a single end hole or a number of side holes at the distal end. The 20-gauge catheters are calibrated for ease of determining the depth on insertion. The calibration markings, openings, and the flexibility of the catheter depend on the manufacturer. A more flexible catheter is designed to prevent forcing the catheter into a space other than the epidural space, but it can be more difficult to handle. The stiffer catheter is easier to pass, but can be forced into spaces or structures other than the epidural space. Some catheters include a reinforced, spring-loaded tip to prevent kinking. It is prudent for the clinician to become familiar with all of the trays and catheters used by the institution in the event that one particular tray is not available.

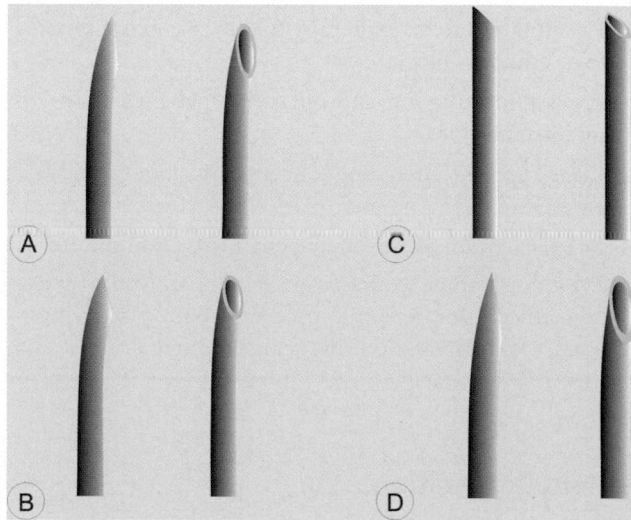

Figure 14–12. Common designs of epidural needles. **A:** Hustead 17-gauge, **B:** Hustead 18-gauge, **C:** Crawford, **D:** Tuohy.

The only additional equipment needed for placement is a dressing for the puncture site and tape to secure the catheter on the patient's back. Usually a large clear dressing with silk or cloth adhesive tape is sufficient to prevent catheter dislodgement and to keep the site clean. The tray should be prepared while an assistant is positioning the patient or prior to positioning out of sight of the patient to prevent increased anxiety especially for needle-phobic patients. The prep solution should not contaminate the epidural needles to prevent the rare possibility of chemical arachnoiditis.[107,108]

Clinical Pearl

■ Completely preparing the tray out of the patients sight and before positioning the patient reduces anxiety, saves time, and promotes efficient placement of the epidural catheter. The skin prep solution should be kept separate from the tray so as not to contaminate the needles with prep solution.

Patient Positioning

Careful attention to the patient's position is essential to successful placement of the epidural needle and catheter. Depending on the patient's medical status, weight, and ability to cooperate, the sitting or lateral decubitus position can be used. In general, it is technically easier to identify the midline in an obese patient in the sitting position, but this requires the assistance of a trained assistant to maintain the correct posture. Improper positioning can turn an otherwise easy epidural placement into a needlessly challenging one.

Monitoring equipment and oxygen can be attached to the patient before or after the patient is positioned. The operating table should be at a comfortable height for the clinician, blankets or covers should be available for the patient's comfort and privacy, a stool for the patient's feet to rest on (if sitting), and an assistant to support the patient in the correct posture should be ready prior to beginning the block. Intravenous sedation should be given to alleviate anxiety early in the preparation for the block. It is our practice to provide the patient with 2 mg of midazolam and 100 mcg of fentanyl IV for sedation purposes in most adult patients just prior to the procedure. Exceptions are pregnant mothers for labor and delivery or caesarian section. Administer oxygen via a face mask at 6 L/min in all patients. Likewise, pulse oximetry, and often, capnography are used during the procedure.

Sitting Position

If the sitting position is chosen, the patient should be assisted to sit on the table or bed with feet resting on a stool (or touching the floor if very tall). The patient should lean forward with elbows resting on a pillow or on the thighs. The back should be maximally flexed to open up the lumbar vertebral spaces.

Flexing the neck will help the patient to flex the lower spine (Figure 14–13). The assistant should help the patient to hold this position during the entire procedure. Special positioning devices also are available to maintain the position without assistants.

Lateral Decubitus Position

In the lateral decubitus position, the patient is placed on the side with the back at the edge of the operating table that is closest to the anesthesiologist. The spinous processes should be oriented parallel to the floor to prevent rotation of the spine. The thighs should be flexed on the abdomen with the knees drawn to the chest and the neck flexed so that the chin rests on the chest. Asking the patient to "assume the fetal position" or "touch your knees with your chin" may help with positioning during lumbar epidural placement. An assistant should be available to help with both positioning and maintenance of the proper position. Benefits of the lateral decubitus position are that sedation can be more liberally used, and that dependence on a well-trained assistant is not as important as for the sitting position.[32] Successful block placement depends on

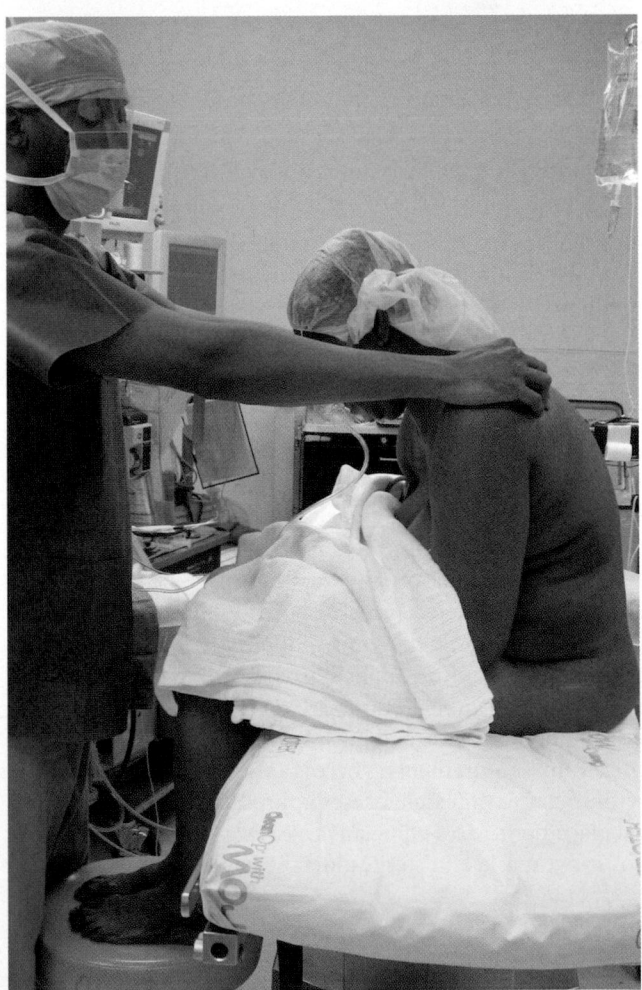

Figure 14–13. Patient in sitting position in preparation for epidural placement. Note the outward back-curving leg flexion and feet resting on the stool.

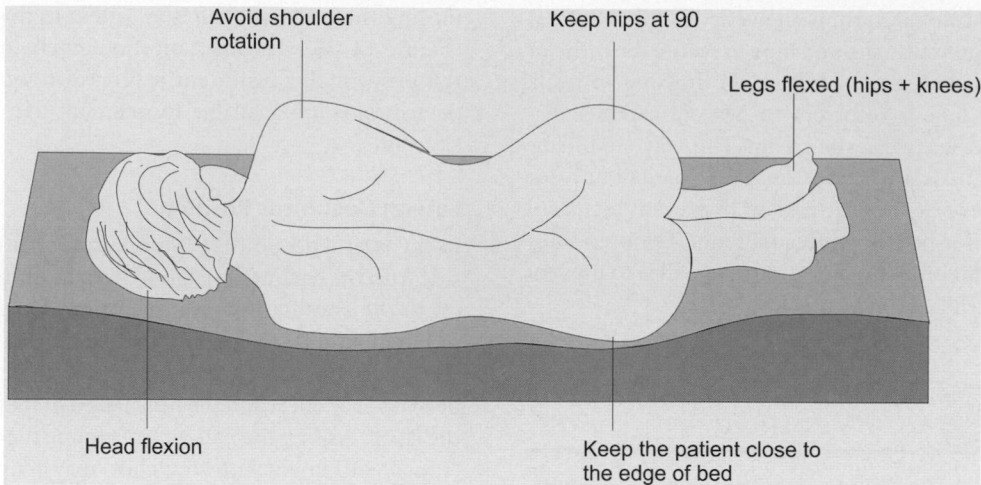

Figure 14–14. Patient positioning in lateral decubitus position.

keeping the spine parallel to the floor (Figure 14–14). Obese patients or those with larger hips may require additional pillows to maintain proper alignment of the spine.

Clinical Pearls

- Improper positioning can make simple epidural placement difficult.
- If a well-trained assistant is not available, the lateral position requires less dependability on the assistant.
- For the obese patient, the midline sitting approach is easier as midline structures are more easily estimated

Technique

The level of insertion and dosing of the epidural needle or catheter depends on the purpose of the epidural block. In pediatric cases, a single-shot caudal block is sometimes used, but in most adult cases, a catheter is placed so that either bolus dosing or a continuous infusion can be instituted. Preparation of the epidural tray and medications to be administered should be completed prior to positioning the patient. For epidural anesthesia, the same monitors required for general anesthesia should be applied. Oxygen by nasal cannula or mask should be in place prior to sedation. For epidural analgesia, blood pressure and pulse oximetry monitoring are the minimum requirements. There is a wide variation in practice with regard to the extent of aseptic precautions prior to epidural placement. Most clinicians agree that at a minimum, head covering, mask, and sterile gloves should be in place.[109–111]

Approach

Four common approaches to the epidural space are possible: midline, paramedian, Taylor (modified paramedian), and caudal. Each will be described in the following paragraphs. Clinical expertise in each of these techniques gives the anesthesiologist more flexibility when using an epidural block.

Midline Approach

This approach is most commonly used for epidural placement in the sitting position. After appropriate monitors are attached and the patient is positioned, the lumbar spine is prepped and draped in a sterile fashion (Figure 14–15A).

1. A *fully prepared* epidural tray should be placed to anesthesiologist's right for right-handed, left for left-handed clinician
2. Identify the vertebral level to be entered by surface landmarks (eg, crest of iliac spines L4 to L5, entry level usually L2-3 or L3-4.
3. Infiltrate skin with local anesthetic using 25-gauge $1\frac{1}{2}$-in. needle at midpoint between two adjacent vertebrae to raise a large skin wheel (Figure 14–15B).
4. Without removing needle, infiltrate deeper tissues to alleviate pain and to assist with locating midline.
5. Insert epidural needle with stylet through same skin puncture. The dorsum of the anesthesiologist's *noninjecting hand* rests on the patient's back with the thumb and index finger holding the hub of the epidural needle (Bromage grip).[112]
6. Advance the needle through the supraspinous ligament and into the interspinous ligament (approximately 2–3 cm depth) at which point the needle should sit firmly in the midline (see Figure 14–15C).
7. After the ligaments are penetrated, it is no longer possible to change the direction of the needle tip.[113] Without withdrawing the needle to the skin level.
8. Remove the stylet and attach the glass syringe to the hub of the needle. Lock it on firmly so that a false loss of resistance is not encountered (Figure 14–15D).

As a review, there are three alternative techniques to identify the epidural space: loss of resistance (LOR), hanging drop, and ultrasonography. Dogliotti described the first, using LOR to fluid.[12] This technique is based on the different densities of tissues as one passes a needle through the thickness of the ligamentum flavum into the epidural space.

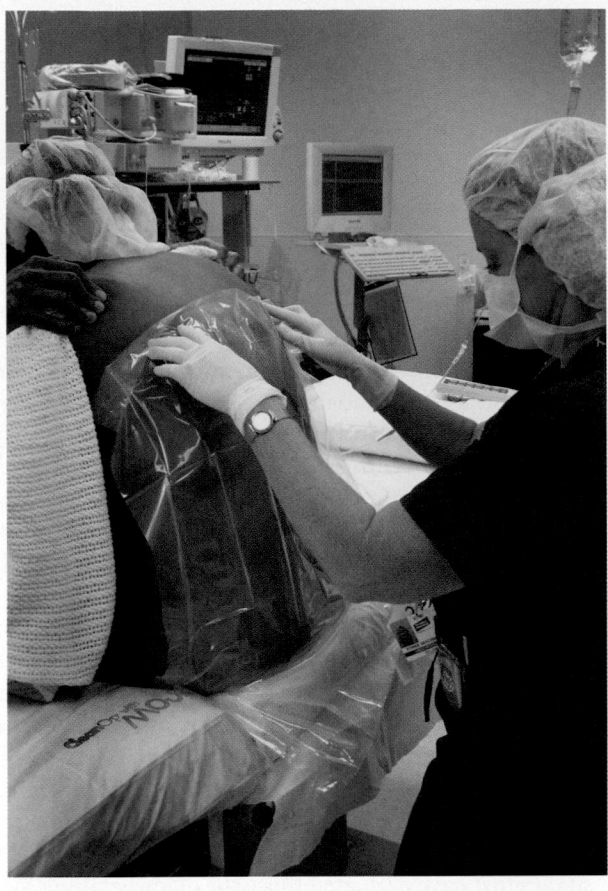

A

Figure 14–15A. Lumbar epidural block through the midline approach: Positioning and draping for midline approach.

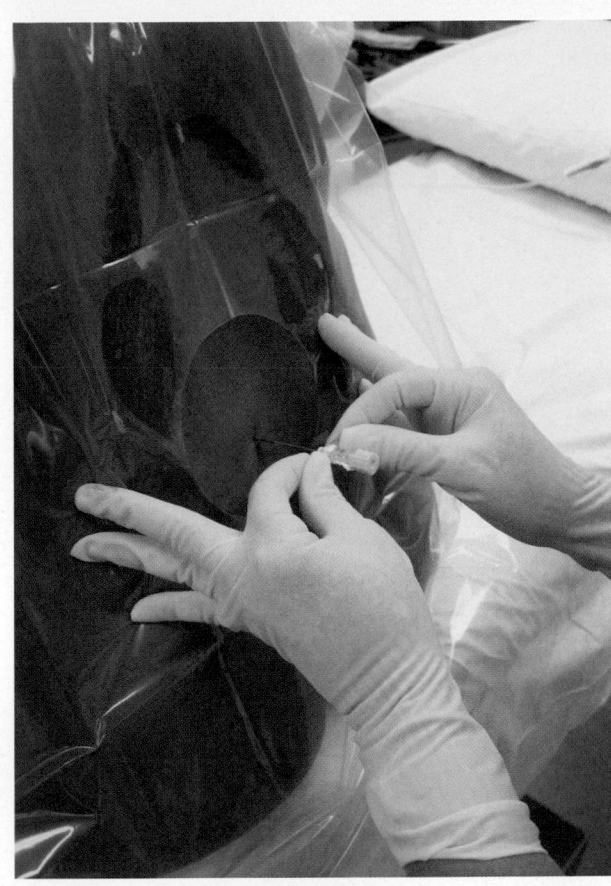

C

Figure 14–15C. Lumbar epidural block through the midline approach: Tuohy needle lodged in the interspinous ligament.

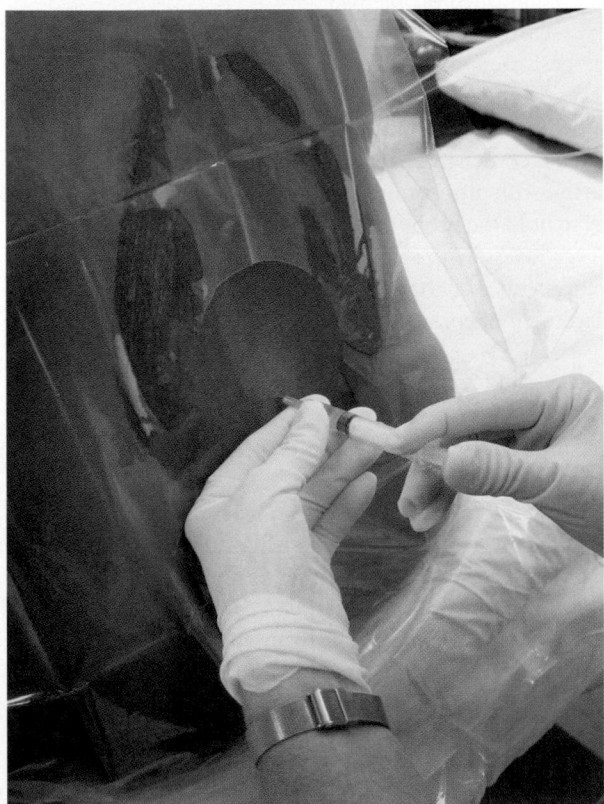

B

Figure 14–15B. Lumbar epidural block through the midline approach: Administration of local anesthesia to reduce pain during consequent epidural needle entry through the skin and subcutaneous tissues.

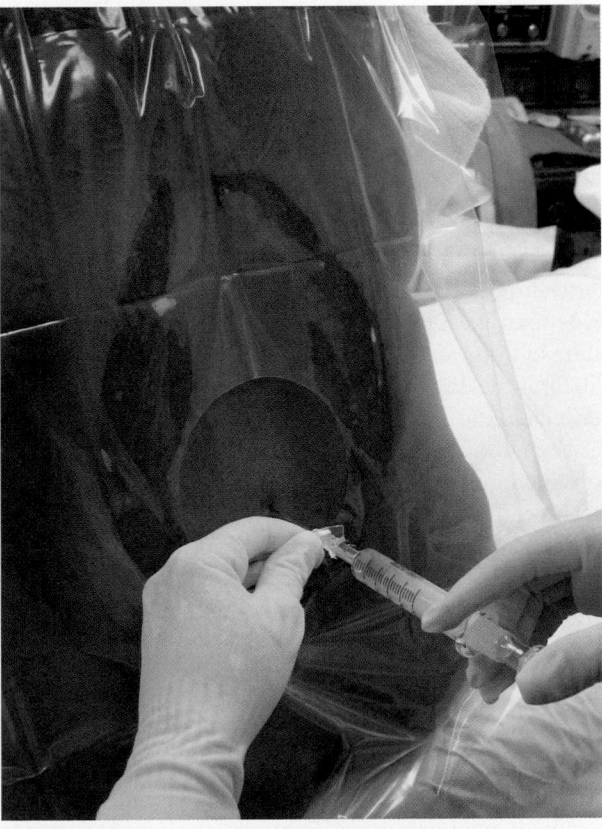

D

Figure 14–15D. Lumbar epidural block through the midline approach: Tuohy needle with glass syringe attached for testing the loss of resistance to air.

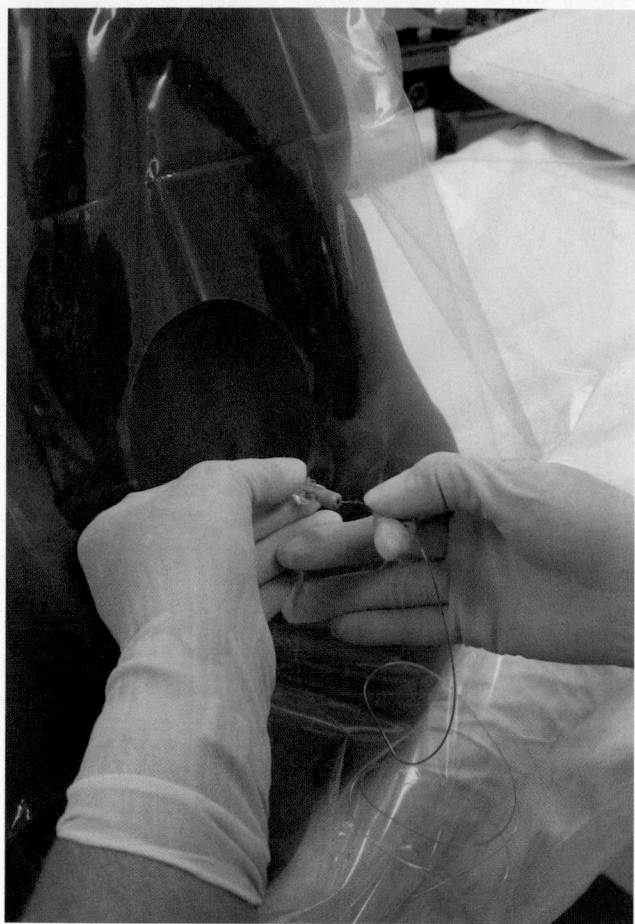

E

Figure 14–15E. Lumbar epidural block through the midline approach: After the loss of resistance to air is documented, indicating the proper position of the needle in the epidural space, the catheter is threaded while observing depth marks.

The technique has been modified so that both fluid and air are recognized as acceptable media for determining the LOR, with saline solution and air being the two most frequently used. We will limit the discussion to the advantages and disadvantages between saline and air for the loss of resistance. Controversy has been growing controversy regarding the use of air as the only medium to find the epidural space. First, air is compressible, thus the feeling in the plunger of the syringe might result in a false loss of resistance. Advocates of using air feel that it is easier to verify if the needle went too far and pierced the dura, in which case the practitioner could easily see cerebrospinal fluid (CSF) coming out. The use of air has come under scrutiny lately, by several authors who question its safety.

Air has been found to be less reliable than a combination of air and lidocaine to find the epidural space.[114] However, some argue that the use of air alone may cause pneumocephalus, which results in severe headaches, and it can cause venous air embolism.[115,116] The use of the loss of resistance to air technique to identify the epidural space has also been associated with an increased incidence of unblocked segments, and even persistent neurologic deficits when air bubbles were expanded by the use of nitrous oxide, causing either nerve root or, even worse, spinal cord compression.[117–119] It has also been suggested that the incidence of intravascular placement of epidural catheters is greater when air is used for LOR, but other researchers have not confirmed these claims.[114]

Few negative reports can be found in the literature related to the use of a fluid for LOR, one being the difficulty to verify if fluid obtained after placement of a catheter is either saline or CSF. To differentiate this, some practitioners check the contents of glucose and protein with a urine reagent strip, and if positive the diagnosis of CSF can be made.[120] Moreover, if a large volume of saline is used for LOR, this could produce an inadequate sensory block, probably due to dilution of the injected local anesthetic and a delay in the onset of the block supposedly due to the same reason.

Trainees learn different techniques from our preceptors during training. Under optimal conditions, trainees should be exposed to all the different techniques and then be able to choose the one they feel most comfortable with and which has less chance of negative side effects based on their experience and suggestions from the literature. Although the literature is supportive of the use of a fluid or a combination of a fluid and a small amount of air, there are limitations in the majority of studies that have evaluated this issue, namely sample size, and with it, the possibility of type I and type II errors. Thus, the best advice is to limit the volume of injected fluid and air in the epidural space to less than 2–3 mL to avoid the aforementioned problems.

Lastly, evidence in the literature is lacking concerning the best method to identify the epidural space in children. Recently, the use of ultrasound for the placement of epidural catheters in children has been advocated. However, the technique is somewhat cumbersome and requires significant expertise with ultrasound imaging as well as additional personnel to hold the probe and operate the ultrasound equipment. Nevertheless, with refinements in ultrasound technology, developments of better imaging probes may aid in the correct placement of epidural catheters in this population.

LOSS OF RESISTANCE TO AIR

1. Continue to hold the needle at the hub with the noninjecting hand.
2. Using the thumb of the *injecting* hand, lightly tap the end of the plunger of the needle while advancing the needle in a slightly cephalad direction.
3. Advance the needle *slowly with controlled motion* until the needle passes through the ligamentum flavum. As the needle enters the ligamentum flavum, there is usually a distinct sensation of increased resistance followed by a sudden loss of resistance to pressure exerted on the plunger. Avoid injecting greater than 1 mL of air.
4. Once the loss of resistance occurs, *do not advance the needle further without testing placement* as there is an increased risk of dural puncture. Experienced clinicians may elect to exert continuous pressure on the epidural needle plunger while advancing the needle until loss of resistance is noted.

Table 14–11.

Comparison of "Loss-of-Resistance" Techniques

Technique	Advantages	Disadvantages
LOR to air	*Theoretically*, more obvious identification of epidural space by "feeling" LOR. Not dependent on visual sign	During shock wave lithotripsy, may cause tissue damage at air–tissue interface.
	No timing with respiratory cycle required	Literature suggests several complications associated with its use
LOR to saline or hanging drip	Visual sign on entry into epidural space—not as dependent on "feel"	Plugged needle tip = low or no negative pressure
		Difficult to time advancement with inspiration (epidural space negative pressure maximal)

LOR = loss of resistance.

For the novice, the incidence of dural puncture is higher with this technique because of a lack of familiarity with structures encountered.

LOSS OF RESISTANCE TO SALINE WITH OR WITHOUT AIR BUBBLE

1. Instead of filling the glass syringe with 2 to 3 mL of air, the syringe is filled with saline, or with saline and a small air bubble (0.2–0.3 mL)
2. The needle is advanced in the same fashion as with air. Continuous pressure is exerted on the plunger of the needle. When using the combination of air and saline, if the air bubble cannot be compressed without injecting the saline, then the needle tip is probably not engaged in the ligamentum flavum (Table 14–11).
3. Once a loss of resistance to air or saline has occurred, the glass syringe is removed, and depth at which the epidural space was entered is noted. The noninjecting hand should continue to hold the needle in place.
4. For single-injection epidurals, local anesthetic can be injected through the needle.
5. For continuous epidurals, a small volume of sterile saline can be injected into the epidural space to dilate the space.

6. Note the depth of the needle at the skin. The marking on the needle at the skin is the depth from the skin to the epidural space.
7. Thread the catheter gently through the needle into the epidural space to approximately the 15–17 cm mark, then remove the needle without dislodging the catheter (Figure 14–15E).
8. Add the skin-to-epidural depth plus 3–5 cm. Withdraw the catheter to that point and secure. No more than 5 cm of catheter should be left in the epidural space to prevent displacement of the catheter laterally or into extradural structures.
   Example: Needle entered epidural space at 7 cm, the catheter should be withdrawn to 12-cm mark at the skin. This would allow 5 cm of the catheter in the epidural space.
9. Gently flush the catheter with a small amount of saline to ensure patency and aspirate to rule out intravascular (blood) or intrathecal (fluid) placement of the catheter.
10. A clear, occlusive dressing should be applied over the insertion site to allow inspection of the catheter. The catheter should be secured to the patient's back with the end at the shoulder for access in dosing. (See the section Activating the Thoracic Epidural for testing and dosing.)

Clinical Pearls

- Use the needle for skin infiltration to identify the midline structures (bone contact 1–2 cm from the skin-spinous process).
- In the lumbar area, insert the needle in a slightly cephalad direction.
- The needle will sit firmly in the midline once through the supraspinous ligament. If it does not, the insertion is most likely off-midline.
- Once the needle passes through the ligaments, the direction of the tip cannot be changed.
- The catheter should not be inserted >5 cm in the epidural space to prevent displacement of the catheter into other structures.

Paramedian Approach

It is essential for the anesthesiologist to become proficient with the paramedian approach to epidural placement as there are situations when it is the only technique feasible for epidural placement. This approach offers a much larger opening into the epidural space than the midline approach. Indications for this approach are:

- Patients who cannot be positioned easily or cannot flex the spine (trauma/arthritic) when inserting the needle into the lumbar epidural space
- Calcified interspinous ligament
- Spine deformities: kyphoscoliosis, prior lumbar surgery

• Entry level at T3 to T7: In the midthoracic spine, the angulation of the spinous processes is more oblique, the space between spinous processes is narrower, and the ligaments are less dense. False loss of resistance is much more common. Thus, the midline approach often proves difficult if not impossible.

1. The skin wheal is placed 1.5–2.0 cm lateral to the midline opposite the center of the selected interspace in the lumbar and lower thoracic levels (Figure 14–16A).
2. The epidural needle is advanced at that site perpendicular or slightly cephalad to the skin until the lamina is encountered (Figure 14–16B).
3. The needle is redirected and advanced at a 10–20-degree angle toward the midline and cephalad (Figure 14–16C).
4. If bone is encountered, the needle is "walked off" the bone into the ligamentum flavum.
5. The supraspinous and interspinous ligaments are midline structures. The paramedian approach is lateral to these ligaments. The epidural needle penetrates paraspinous muscles with little resistance before entering the ligamentum flavum.
6. The "feel" of the paramedian approach is completely different from that of the midline approach because of the difference in tissues penetrated.

Clinical Pearls

▪ Insert the needle 1.5–2.0 cm lateral to the midline of the center of the interspace.

▪ Advance the needle perpendicular or slightly cephalad to the skin until bone is encountered.

▪ "Walk off" the bone, advancing the needle at a 10 to 25-degree angle toward the midline and cephalad.

▪ The first resistance felt will be that of the ligamentum flavum.

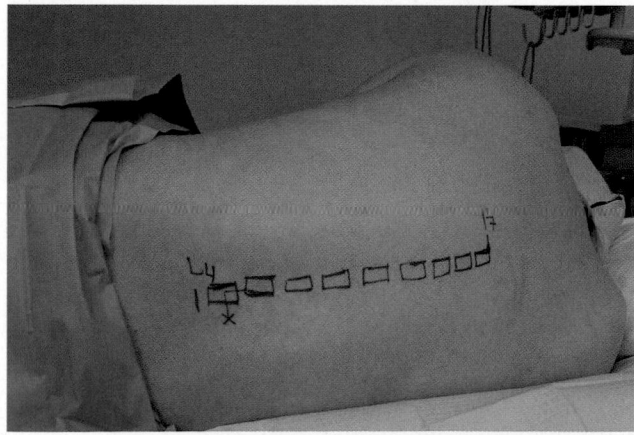

A

Figure 14–16A. Lumbar epidural block through the paramedian approach: The needle entry site is marked approximately 1.5–2 cm lateral and caudal to the desired level of blockade.

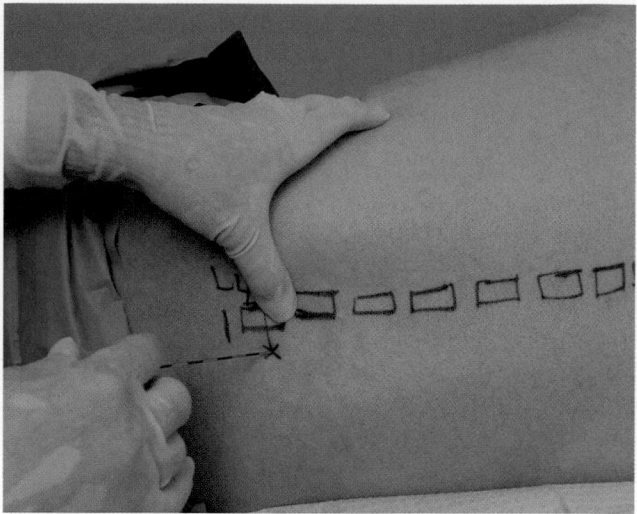

B

Figure 14–16B. Lumbar epidural block through the paramedian approach: Epidural needle angulation 45 degrees cephalad and very slightly medial.

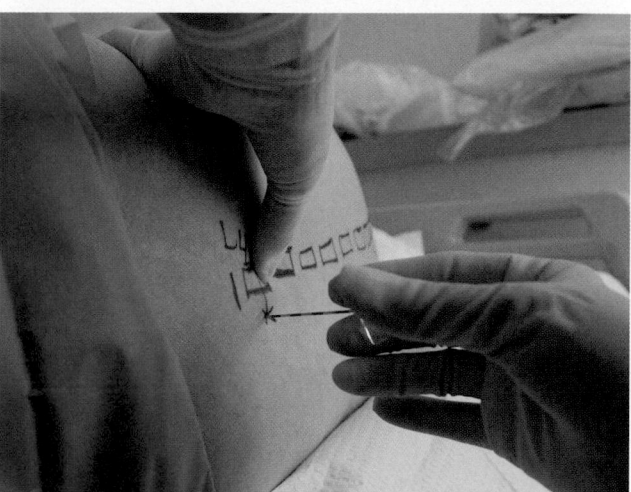

C

Figure 14–16C. Lumbar epidural block through the paramedian approach: When (if) the bone (lamina) is contacted during needle advancement, the cephalad needle angle is lowered to walk off the lamina.

MIDTHORACIC EPIDURAL PARAMEDIAN APPROACH: The T4-5 interspace is the injection site.

1. In the midthoracic level, the skin wheal is placed 1.5 to 2.0 cm lateral and inferior to the superior spinous process (Figure 14–17A). A 22-gauge "spinal needle" can be used to infiltrate the skin to lamina. Depth is noted to gauge the depth of epidural needle insertion.
2. Epidural needle is advanced perpendicularly and slightly cephalad through the skin at the same location until the lamina is contacted.
3. The needle is withdrawn approximately 2 cm, redirected at a 15- to 20-degree angle toward the midline cephalad.

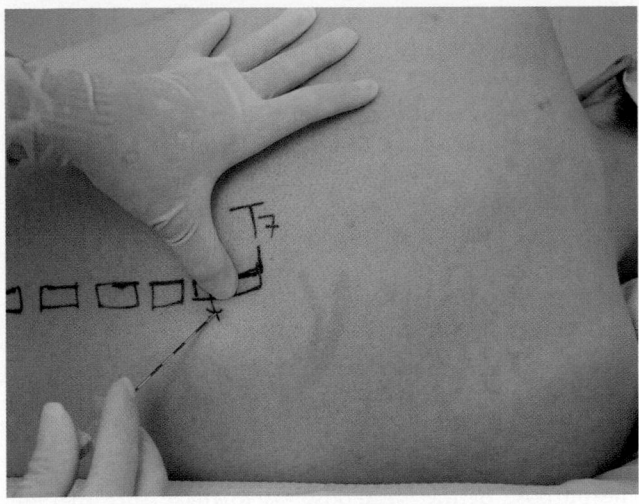

A

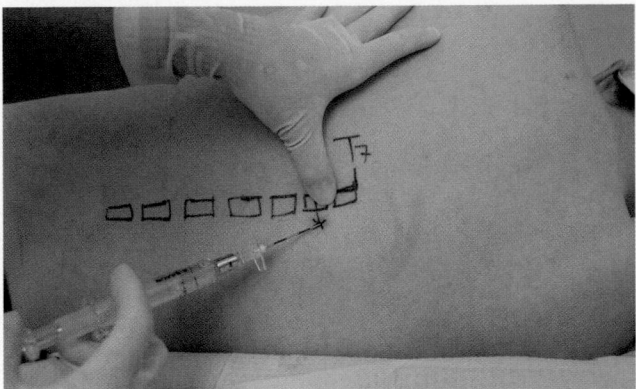

B

Figure 14–17B. Thoracic paramedian approach: Needle angle 55–60 degrees to the skin surface.

Figure 14–17A. Thoracic paramedian approach: Landmarks/initial needle insertion. Note the approximately 45-degree cephalad and medial needle angulation.

4. Each time bone is contacted, the needle is withdrawn 0.5 cm, then walked off the bone in a medial/cephalad direction[113] until the ligamentum flavum is entered (Figure 14–17B).

Taylor Approach

The Taylor approach[113,121] is a modified paramedian approach utilizing the large L5-S1 interspace. It is an excellent approach for patients needing hip surgery or for trauma patients needing lower extremity surgery who cannot tolerate the sitting position. Sometimes, it can provide the only available access to the epidural space in patients with ossified ligaments.

1. The skin wheal is placed 1 cm medial and 1 cm inferior to the posterior superior iliac spine (Figure 14–18).
2. The epidural needle is inserted into this site in a medial and cephalad direction at a 45- to 55-degree angle.
3. As in the classic paramedian approach, the first resistance felt is on entry to the ligamentum flavum.
4. If the needle contacts bone (usually the sacrum), the needle should be walked off the bone into the ligament, then into the epidural space using progressively more medial and cephalad redirections of the needle.

Caudal Approach

The caudal approach is commonly used in pediatrics for epidural catheter placement for postoperative analgesia. In adults, it is usually reserved for procedures requiring blockage of the sacral and lumbar nerves (eg, inguinal herniorrhaphy, cystoscopy), epidurography, and for lysis of adhesions in patients with low back pain with radiculopathy after spinal surgery.[122] Considering that the sacral hiatus is ossified in

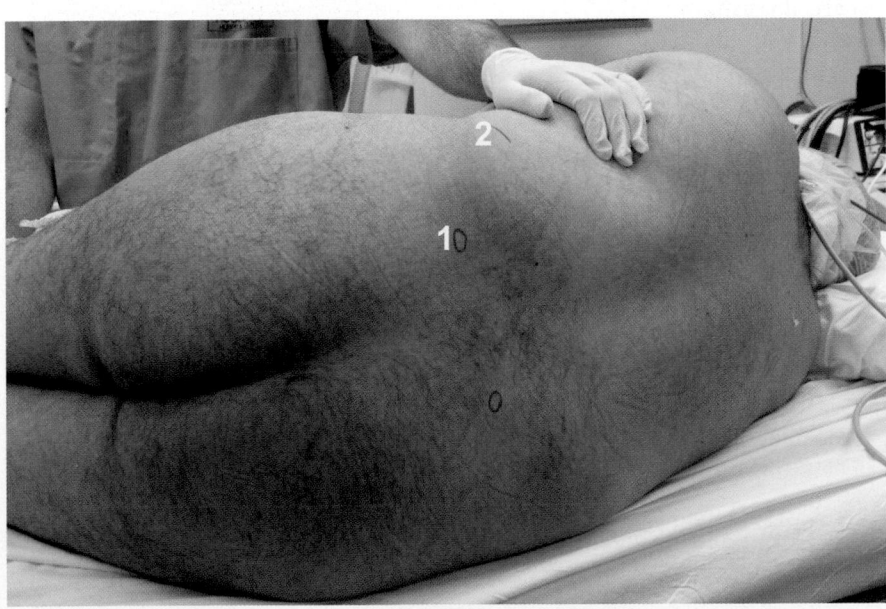

Figure 14–18. Taylor approach—landmarks: 1 = posterosuperior iliac spine, 2 = iliac crest (corresponds approximately to the L3-4 level).

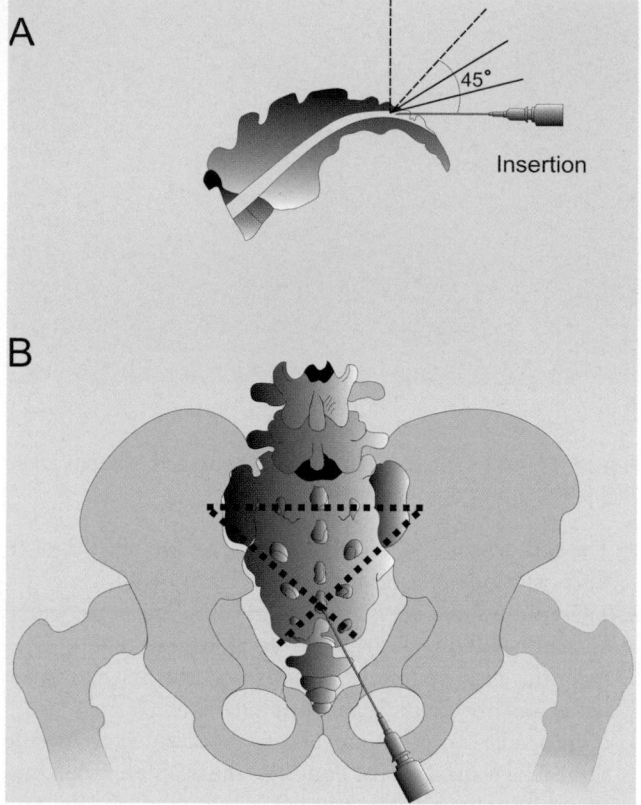

Figure 14–19. **A:** Caudal approach: Angle of needle insertion required to enter the caudal canal. **B:** Landmarks.

some patients, the use of fluoroscopy guidance is useful to decrease the incidence of needle and catheter malposition.

The sacrum is a triangular-shaped bone formed by the fusion of the five sacral vertebral. Nonfusion of the fifth sacral vertebral arch creates the structure known as the sacral hiatus. The hiatus is covered by the sacrococcygeal ligament (an extension of the ligamentum flavum). On its borders are the bony prominences known as the sacral cornu. The sacral hiatus is the point of access to the sacral epidural space. It is usually identified as a groove above the coccyx (Figure 14–19). If fluoroscopy is not used, there are two methods for identifying the hiatus: (1)Locate the posterior superior iliac spines. A line drawn between them becomes one side of a equilateral triangle. At the apex of the triangle is the sacral hiatus. (2)With firm pressure, identify the coccyx with the index finger. As the finger moves cephalad, the first pair of bony protuberances are the cornu, which surrounds the hiatus.

1. Prep and drape the skin in sterile fashion.
2. Patient is placed in a lateral or prone position (pillow under pelvis if prone).
3. Either a smaller gauge IV catheter (18- to 23-gauge) or a 20-gauge epidural needle is advanced at a 45-degree angle from the back with the bevel up (to avoid penetrating the anterior sacral wall).
4. A distinct "pop" or "snap" is felt when the needle pierces the sacrococcygeal membrane.

5. The needle angle is lowered to 160 degrees (almost flat) toward the back. It is advanced not more than 1.5 cm (usually between 5 and 7 mm) in adults and not more than 0.5 cm in children.
6. Aspirate for blood or CSF before injecting local anesthetic.
7. The epidural catheter can then be inserted through the needle to the desired level.

Implementing the Lumbar Epidural Block—Intraoperative Management

The volume and concentration of local anesthetic needed for epidural anesthesia is larger than that required for spinal anesthesia, therefore the catheter should be tested for evidence of proper placement in the epidural space. The purpose of the "test dose" is to make sure that the catheter is not in the subarachnoid, intravascular, or subdural space.

Test Dose

Although the validity of a test dose of local anesthetic with epinephrine in obstetrics and pediatrics has been questioned,[123,124] it is still suggested by many to decrease the risk of an intravascular injection.[125,126] The "classic" test dose combines 3 mL of 1.5% lidocaine with 15 mcg of epinephrine. The intrathecal injection of 45 mg of lidocaine will produce a significant motor block consistent with spinal anesthesia. A change in heart rate of 20% or greater is an indication of intravascular injection warranting the removal and replacement of the catheter. If the heart rate does not increase by 20% or greater, or if a significant motor block does not develop within 5 min of administering the test dose, it is considered negative. Exceptions to this rule have been observed in patients under general anesthesia with isoflurane, patients receiving β-adrenergic blocking agents with heart rates below 60 bpm, and obstetric patients in active labor.

In children and in obstetric patients, other methods of identifying intravascular placement of the epidural catheter have been advocated. Because children are anesthetized prior to epidural placement, interference with response to epinephrine under volatile general anesthetics creates a high percentage of false-negative test doses.[127] In the obstetric patient, if the test dose is injected during a contraction, the change in heart rate may be related to pain and not to the epinephrine. In this population, the test dose should be administered during uterine diastole, soon after a uterine contraction.[128] Changes in the P or T wave on the electrocardiogram in pediatrics or the use of nerve stimulators to confirm epidural placement in pregnant patients have been utilized.[129,130]

In patients on β-adrenergic blocking agents, heart rate changes may not be evident. Systolic blood pressure increases of greater than 20 mm Hg have been used as an indicator of intravascular injection.[131,132]

Clinical Pearls

- A change of 20% or greater in heart rate after the test dose indicates a probable intravascular injection—replace the catheter.

- A dense motor block within 5 min of a test dose should prompt a suspicion of a spinal block—monitor vital signs and block level repeatedly. Either convert to a continuous spinal anesthesia or replace the catheter.

- Peaked P waves or changes in the T wave in children indicate a vascular injection.

- Give the test dose to a pregnant patient after a contraction is over for a more accurate response to test dosing.

- A change in systolic blood pressure of >20 mm Hg in patients on beta-blocking agents is more indicative of an intravascular injection.

Dosing Regimen

After the epidural catheter has been aspirated to check for blood or CSF, and a negative test dose has been demonstrated, the catheter should be dosed to provide the level of surgical anesthesia desired. The maintenance of the desired level of anesthesia can be accomplished through intermittent or continuous dosing after the initial loading dose provides the level of anesthesia necessary for the surgical procedure.

As a general guideline, 1–2 mL per segment to be blocked in a lumbar epidural, 0.7 mL per segment for a thoracic epidural, and 3 mL per segment to be blocked for a sacral/caudal epidural is used as an initial loading dose. The loading dose is given in 5-mL aliquots through the catheter, repeated at 3- to 5-min intervals, giving the clinician time to assess the patient's response to dosing. If at any time the patient demonstrates an exaggerated response, further incremental doses should be withheld and the patient reassessed. The catheter should be removed and replaced if the following occurs: a large volume of local anesthetic is required to initiate the block or an incomplete, unilateral, or inadequate block results. Wasting time administering further doses of medication, repositioning the catheter, or other time-consuming measures leads to frustration for the patient, the surgical staff, and delays in the operative procedure. Moreover, these maneuvers rarely result in a successful block.

After the initial dose, one quarter to one third of the amount can be administered 10–15 min later to intensify the sensory block. The overall level of the block will not be significantly increased with this method.[120]

The level and duration of epidural anesthesia depends primarily on the injection site, and the volume and concentration of the drug. Other factors such as age, pregnancy, and sex are less important factors but need to be con-

sidered. The addition of fresh epinephrine and 8.4% sodium bicarbonate to lidocaine, mepivacaine, and chloroprocaine will decrease the latency, improve the quality, and prolong the duration of the block. Epinephrine is less effective with the long-acting local anesthetics. Adding bicarbonate to ropivicaine and in a dose greater than 0.05 mL/10 mL of bupivacaine will cause precipitation. The addition of opioids (eg, fentanyl) has been shown to improve the quality of the block without any effect on duration.[133]

Top-Up Dosing

Repeat doses, commonly referred to as "top-ups," need to be given *before* the level of the block has receded by more than two dermatomes. One half to two thirds of the original volume of local anesthetic should be given for each repeat dose. The anesthesiologist must have a working knowledge of the characteristics of the local anesthetic used to properly implement the redosing protocol so that the sedated patient does not have to be disturbed to check dermatomal levels for sensory block (Table 14–12).

A continuous infusion through the lumbar epidural catheter can be started after the initial bolus to maintain surgical anesthesia. Continuous infusions require the same diligent attention to the patient as any other anesthetic.[134] The usual infusion rate is between 4 and 15 mL/h. The wide range is usually dependent on the age, weight, and extension of the block desired in a particular patient. Thus, individualization is necessary, and a fixed rule cannot be applied for this purpose.

Clinical Pearls

DOSING REGIME: LUMBAR EPIDURAL

- The loading dose for epidural anesthesia is between 10 and 20 mL, given in increments of 5 mL. Wait 3–5 min between each increment to check patient response.

- If the block is incomplete, replace the catheter rather than waste time trying to reposition it or give a larger dose of local anesthetic.

- Inject one quarter to one third the initial dose 15 min after initial bolus to enhance the sensory block.

- Epinephrine and bicarbonate will speed up the onset and enhance the quality and duration of the block. Fentanyl will improve the quality of the block.

- Give the "top-up" dose before two-segment regression has occurred to maintain adequate anesthesia.

- A continuous infusion is an alternative to bolus dosing; it has the advantage of hemodynamic stability and can be continued postoperatively for analgesia.

Table 14–12.

Time to Two Dermatome Regression— Commonly Used Local Anesthetics

Local Anesthetic	Time to Two Dermatome Regression (min)	Time for Reinjection (min)
2–3% Chloroprocaine	50–70	30–45
2% Lidocaine	90–140	60
1.5–2.0% Mepivacaine	120–160	60
0.5 % Bupivacaine	200–280	120

Activating the Thoracic Epidural—Intraoperative Management

Epidural anesthesia is ideally suited for thoracic surgery. It is considered the gold standard for postthoracotomy analgesia because it produces better pain relief with fewer side effects than other commonly used methods.[135] When combined with general anesthesia, it prevents vagal reflexes and pain from traction on the diaphragm.[136]

Placement and activation are similar to lumbar epidural placement, with a few modifications. An epidural block provides the most intense block at the insertion site, so the tip of the catheter should be placed at midincision level, usually above T8. This will provide the best segmental analgesia. Because there is a greater incidence of false loss of resistance in the midline thoracic approach, the paramedian approach is the best technique to use for catheter placement.

The sharp angulation of the spinous processes especially in the midthoracic area can make the midline approach challenging even for the experienced clinicians.

1. Once the catheter is placed, it is aspirated for the presence of blood or CSF.
2. A test dose of 3 mL of 1.5% lidocaine with epinephrine 1:200,000 is given to (a) rule out intravascular catheter position and (b) provide a band of anesthesia before inducing general anesthesia.
3. If no anesthesia can be appreciated, the catheter should be replaced.
4. The patient should receive only light sedation for placement to alert the clinician to the development of paresthesias.

Dosing the Thoracic Epidural Catheter

Several dosing regimes have been suggested. All are effective means of providing surgical analgesia, allowing a "light general anesthesia" to be used and thereby reducing residual respiratory depressant effects.

After a negative aspiration and test dose:

1. An initial dose of 3 to 6 mL of dilute bupivacaine 0.125% to 0.25% or 0.1% to 0.2% ropivacaine with or without preservative-free morphine (1–2 mg) is administered, followed by 3 mL of 0.25% to 0.5% bupivacaine every 30 min.[137]
2. *Alternative regimen:* Administer a loading dose with 3 to 6 mL of bupivacaine (0.125%) or ropivacaine (0.1%–0.2%) with an opioid (fentanyl 2 mcg/mL or hydromorphone 20 mcg/mL) at least 30 min as tolerated before the end of the case. Start an infusion of bupivacaine 0.0625% or 0.1% ropivacaine with fentanyl or hydromorphone at 3 to 5 mL/h before the patient leaves the operating room.[138]

Clinical Pearls

THORACIC EPIDURALS

- The paramedian approach is easier especially in the midthoracic region.
- Expect more frequent false loss of resistance, especially if the midline approach is used.
- Lighter but adequate sedation should be given for placement because of the greater risk of injury to neural tissue.
- The test dose not only identifies intravascular injection, but also serves as a means of identifying placement as a band of anesthesia should develop in the segment where the local anesthetic was injected.
- Because of the proximity to cardiac accelerator fibers, smaller bolus doses of local anesthetic should be used and response checked carefully before redosing to prevent large drops in heart rate or blood pressure.
- Remember that hypotension can occur in nearly all patients with a high thoracic epidural blockade. In fact, it has been said that if there is no hypotension after an initial bolus in the high thoracic epidural space, it is likely that the epidural catheter is *not* in the epidural space.

Intraoperative Sedation

Intraoperative sedation can be provided to the level of the patient's comfort especially when the epidural is used as the primary anesthetic. If the patient prefers to be kept aware, then light sedation with an initial dose of a benzodiazepam and opioid on insertion can be effective. For those who prefer to be "asleep," a propofol infusion can be added to maintain sedation without respiratory impairment.

Clinical Pearls

- Appropriate sedation is the key to successful epidural placement and management.
- A great epidural anesthesia with poor sedation leads to an unpleasant operative experience.

Problem Solving

Problems with Epidural Placement

Epidural placement produces unique problems that are directly related to experience, body habitus of the patient, or disease states affecting the spine. Most of these problems can be overcome if the clinician recognizes the problem and knows how to make adjustments in technique (Table 14–13).

Problems with Epidural Function

An easily placed epidural catheter does not guarantee excellent function. Inadequate blocks, partial blocks, and unilateral blocks are some of the problems that can occur. Hypotension, often seen with epidural dosing, is a relatively common side effect that is easily managed if the clinician is prepared. Because of the discontinuous nature of the epidural space and variations in anatomy, sometimes these problems cannot be overcome. In the vast majority, careful evaluation of catheter placement, the dose and type of medication given, or administration of sedation can resolve these problems.

Hypotension

A decrease in blood pressure is common and expected with epidural anesthesia secondarily to the sympathectomy caused by local anesthetic action. The blood pressure should be maintained to within 20% of the patient's resting baseline.

ACTION. Bolus the patient with 500 to 1000 mL of a balanced salt solution.

- If necessary, small doses of ephedrine (10–20 mg) can be used in the pregnant or bradycardic patient after fluid bolus if the patient is still hypotensive.
- Phenylephrine (40–120 mcg) can be used to constrict peripheral blood vessels, thereby increasing venous return and blood pressure.

Unilateral Block

After an epidural has been adequately dosed, the patient may complain that one side is densely blocked, but pain and motor function is still intact on the opposite side. Because of the segmental and possibly septated nature of the epidural space, unilateral blocks can occur. The more common explanation for a unilateral block is incorrect catheter placement. If the catheter has been inserted >5 cm into the epidural space, the tip of the catheter may have entered the intervertebral foramen, exited the epidural space, or wrapped around a spinal nerve. The resultant block will be inadequate or unilateral

ACTION. Pull the catheter back 1–2 cm, leaving 3–4 cm in the epidural space.

- Turn the patient with the unblocked side down and redose the catheter with 3 to 5 mL of local anesthetic.
- If no effect, replace the catheter.

Inadequate Block: Breakthrough Pain Despite Adequate Block Height

This problem can be seen secondarily to inadequate sacral blockade. The sacral segment is larger, dense, and difficult to block.

ACTION. Raise the head of the bed and redose the catheter with a higher concentration of local anesthetic.

- Administration of 50 mcg of fentanyl to improve the quality of the block.

Questionable Quality of Epidural Catheter Placed for Analgesia, Fully Dosed. Patient Has to Go to Surgery.

This problem is often seen in obstetrics. An epidural is placed and dosed, but the patient is not fully comfortable. More local anesthetic is given with fair control of pain. Subsequently, the patient has to go urgently to the operating room for a cesarean section requiring dense block to a T4 level. The easiest way to prevent this problem is to replace a questionable epidural catheter.

ACTION. Take the patient to the operating room, remove the questionable catheter.

- Do a combined spinal-epidural (CSE) using a *lower* spinal dose.
- Use the new epidural catheter to raise the level of the block if necessary.
- Use general anesthesia if time does not permit placing the CSE.

Block is Dissipating Requiring Larger Doses of Local Anesthetic

This problem occurs for two potential reasons. If the epidural has been used for analgesia and has been dosed frequently, tachyphylaxis to the local anesthetic can occur. The other problem is catheter migration into a vessel.

ACTION. Check catheter to ensure it has not migrated into a blood vessel. If so, pull it back 1–2 cm, flush with saline. If no blood is aspirated, cautiously rebolus with incremental doses, being vigilant for systemic toxic signs.

- If blood is still in the catheter, replace.
- If the catheter has not migrated, rebolus the catheter with a higher concentration of local anesthetic and increase the infusion rate (if continuous). Add an opioid to enhance the quality of the block.

COMPLICATIONS OF EPIDURAL BLOCKADE

Any invasive procedure is associated with complications. The complications of epidural blockade can range from annoying to life-threatening. They can be classified as drug-related or procedure-related. Drug-related complications are the result of systemic toxicity of local anesthetics either injected directly into an epidural vein or from administration of excessively large doses. Procedure-related complications can

Table 14–13.

Problem Solving: Epidural Placement

Problem	Interpretation	Reason for Problem	Action
Needle floppy, angles laterally	Missed supraspinous ligament	Entry off midline	Reassess midline spinous processes, redirect needle
Contact hit bone at <2 cm	Contacted hit spinous process	Missed interspace; spine flexion inadequate	Identify interspace; needle entry should be more caudad
Contact hit bone 4 cm or >	Contacted hit lamina	Needle entry too lateral	Redirect needle to midline or use paramedian approach
Bony resistance in all midline approaches	Arthritic spine and ligaments	Ossification of ligaments	Use paramedian approach
Can't thread catheter	Narrow epidural space Missed epidural space, false loss of resistance	1. Space not dilated 2. Epidural needle too close to dura 3. Catheter not in epidural space	1. Dilate space with 20 mL sterile saline 2. Try rotating needle slightly to change direction of bevel 3. Reassess loss of resistance with glass syringe, advance needle into epidural space
Blood in catheter	Penetrated epidural vein	Possible too lateral entry (Hogan: epidural veins are scattered in the epidural space, not just laterally as commonly taught); engorged epidural veins	Withdraw 1–2 cm; flush with saline. Aspirate again—if still bloody—replace. If clear, use catheter cautiously with frequent aspirations; small incremental doses
Resistance to LA injection, difficulty passing catheter, clear fluid in catheter, cold	Drip back of LA	Fluid cold = LA; May be in subdural space	Will get widespread patchy block w/hemodynamic instability—replace catheter
Catheter passes easily, clear fluid in catheter, warm	Subarachnoid placement	Warm fluid/+ BS = CSF; catheter in subarachnoid space; missed epidural space/pierced dura	Two options; 1. Continuous spinal 2. Remove/replace at another interspace
Pain, paresthesia w/ catheter insertion	Catheter near nerve root	Too lateral an approach; too much catheter left in epidural space	If pain persists, replace catheter. Don't leave >5 cm in space, withdraw catheter if >5 cm
Can't palpate spinous processes	Adipose tissue or arthritic changes obscuring spinous processes	Obesity; severe arthritis	1. Try midline approach for obese 2. Use 5 cm, 22-gauge needle to find bony landmarks 3. If no luck with midline, try paramedian
Can't flex spine	Arthritis	Ossification of bony processes and ligaments	Try paramedian approach
Scapular "winging" Bone contact in multiple planes	Scoliosis	Lateral curvature of the spine, more commonly in thoracic region, females	Paramedian approach with visualization of curvature to direct needle entry

LA = local anesthetic, BS = buffered saline, CSF = cerebrospinal fluid.

further be classified as minor or major. Minor complications include back pain and headache (postdural puncture headache, PDPH). Major complications include subdural injection, subarachnoid injection, total or high spinal, meningitis, adhesive arachnoiditis, epidural abscess, and spinal cord or nerve root injury.

Drug-Related Complications

When an excessive dose of local anesthetics is injected into the epidural space or when a moderate dose is accidentally injected into an epidural vein, systemic toxicity can occur. The central nervous system is the first system affected. Symptoms include lightheadedness, tinnitus, circumoral numbness and tingling, numbness of the tongue, and blurred vision. Signs include muscle twitching, confusion, tremors of the facial muscles and extremities, and shivering. The patient may complain of feeling increasingly anxious.

Cardiovascular effects of local anesthetics range from mild changes in blood pressure and pulse to complete cardiovascular collapse. At low doses, a slight increase in blood pressure may be noted secondarily to an increase in cardiac output. At higher doses, a marked increase in blood pressure and heart rate will precede severe hypotension and cardiovascular collapse.

Treatment is supportive directed toward maintaining the airway, supporting ventilation, and cardiopulmonary resuscitation if necessary. It is of paramount importance to prevent hypoxia, hypercarbia, and acidosis to limit the cardiovascular toxic effects of systemically administered local anesthetics. If ventricular dysrhythmias occur, lidocaine should not be given as local anesthetic toxicity is additive. Amiodarone is the preferred antiarrhythmic. Epinephrine should be given early and in greater than usual doses especially if bupivacaine was the local anesthetic used. Because bupivacaine binds more tightly to the cardiac sodium channels, it is more difficult to displace it and therefore to treat dysrhythmias caused by it.[139] Calcium channel blockers must also be avoided as they will augment the cardiovascular effects of local anesthetics. (For in-depth discussion on local anesthetic toxicity and its treatment, refer to Chapter 6, Clinical Pharmacology of Local Anesthetics.)

Procedure-Related Complications

Minor Back Pain

The incidence of back pain after epidural anesthesia is between 20 and 30%. The incidence is higher and of longer duration than that arising from spinal or general anesthesia.[140] It is thought to be caused by injury to musculoskeletal structures of the spine from a larger needle. The pain is usually self-limiting. It should be treated with nonsteroidal antiinflammatory drugs, acetaminophen, or heat.[122]

Postdural Puncture Headache

Postdural puncture headache is a more common complication with spinal anesthesia than with epidural as the former

mechanism requires dural puncture. When a PDPH occurs after epidural placement, it usually occurs in the younger, female, pregnant patient.[141,142] In most instances, the clinician is aware that the dura has been pierced, but in many instances, no evidence of dural puncture exists.

The headache is thought to result from loss of CSF through the dural hole, causing lower CSF pressure. In the upright position, the brain tissue sags in the cranial vault, causing traction on cranial nerves and nerve roots. Traction on the cranial nerves causes the cranial nerve palsies that can be observed.[143]

The **key feature** of the headache is that it is mild or absent in the supine position, but intense when the head is elevated. Typically, the headache is bilateral, frontal or occipital, and extending into the neck. It is often described as throbbing or continuous. Cranial nerve signs (diplopia, tinnitus, nystagmus, hearing loss) may be present as well as nausea and vomiting. The onset of the headache is commonly 12–72 h following the procedure. Caution should be exercised if the headache occurs immediately after the procedure as this is more commonly due to excessive air used for loss-of-resistance techniques (air encephalogram).

The duration of the headache is typically 5 days with a range of 1 to 12 days.[144] Conservative treatment includes bedrest, analgesics, intravenous or oral fluids, and caffeine. Caffeine and hydration are used to stimulate the production of CSF and to constrict the intracranial vessels, thereby reducing the headache. The treatment of choice is an epidural blood patch. Uncontrolled studies report rapid recovery in between 90 to 95% of patients after blood patch.[145] Several studies have demonstrated that treatment with an epidural blood patch should occur early in the development of the headache although it is effective treatment as late as 5 days from presentation.[146] Treating the headache with the blood patch decreases the length of hospital stay and emergency room visits.[147]

The technique for the autologous blood patch is simple. Using sterile techniques, a needle is inserted into the epidural space at or one interspace below the prior level of dural puncture. Fifteen to 20 mL of the patient's blood (drawn aseptically) is slowly injected into the space. The injection should stop when the patient experiences focal back pain. The procedure can be repeated 24 h later and will provide equivalent success. Relatively few complications are reported from the procedure. Backache, neckache, and transient temperature elevation for 24 to 48 h may occur. Although rare, dural abscess has been reported after a blood patch. To prevent this complication, both the acquisition of autologous blood and the epidural needle placement should be done using aseptic technique.[148] (For in-depth discussion on this topic, refer to Chapter 73, Postdural Puncture Headache).

Subdural Injection

The subdural space is a potential space between the dura and arachnoid mater. Unlike the epidural space, the subdural space extends intracranially. A small dose of local anesthetic can have a profound effect. The space is wider in the cervical region and extends laterally over the nerve roots. Unintentional entry of an epidural needle or catheter is usually in this area. Although the incidence is low (0.82% of epidural injections), the effects are significant.[149] The clinical presentation varies, but is distinguished by a delayed onset by 10 to 15 min compared with a high spinal.

A key feature is a widespread sensory block with milder motor block. Sympatholysis out of proportion to the dose of local anesthetic occurs, causing moderate to severe hypotension. Treatment is similar to that of a high spinal—cardiovascular and respiratory support, including intubation and mechanical ventilation if necessary.

Subarachnoid Injection/High or Total Spinal Anesthesia

Accidentally puncturing the dura can occur with even the most careful placement of an epidural. If it is recognized during needle puncture, the needle should be removed and another interspace chosen. If it occurs after catheter insertion, either the procedure can be changed to a continuous spinal, or the catheter can be removed and the procedure repeated at another interspace.

A more serious complication occurs when the needle or catheter is advanced into the subarachnoid space and a large dose of local anesthetic is given directly into the CSF, causing total spinal anesthesia. Total spinal anesthesia occurs when local anesthetic spreads high enough to block the entire spinal cord and occasionally the brainstem. Because the anesthesia extends into the cervical levels, the cardioaccelerator fibers are affected. Profound hypotension, bradycardia, and apnea will occur. Unconsciousness follows as a result of the effect of local anesthetic action on the brainstem.

Treatment includes airway support and intubation, 100% oxygen, intravenous fluids and vasopressors to maintain hemodynamic stability. Epinephrine should be used early and in escalating doses to stabilize the heart rate and blood pressure. As the block recedes, the patient will regain consciousness and control of breathing followed by recovery of motor and sensory function.

Meningitis

Acute bacterial meningitis following epidural anesthesia is a rare event, but it has been reported.[150] Microorganisms can be transmitted via syringes, catheters, needles, and medications injected into the epidural space. They can come from the clinician or from the patient but are most commonly from localized infections in the skin and subcutaneous tissue. The most common infective microorganisms are *Staphylococcus* spp (coagulase-negative and *aureus*), followed by gram-negative bacilli and other species.[151]

Symptoms include fever, headache, lethargy, confusion, and the classic symptom, nuchal rigidity.[150] Because it is such a rare occurrence, diagnosis can be delayed due to assumption that a PDPH is present. Patients with meningitis have fever with mental status changes (lethargy at a minimum, confusion as disease progresses). The headache is not positional.

Treatment of bacterial meningitis includes emergent antibiotic therapy (usually ceftriaxone), head CT, and lumbar puncture with patient management by neurology. Fever, back pain, and nuchal rigidity is meningitis until proven otherwise.

Chronic Adhesive Arachnoiditis

Inflammatory changes in the subarachnoid space can cause the syndrome of chronic adhesive arachnoiditis. Strands of collagen begin to form between the nerve roots and the pia-arachnoid. Arachnoiditis ensues, characterized by collagen deposition and nerve root adherence. When the inflammatory process resolves, adhesive arachnoiditis develops. The collagen deposits encapsulate the nerve roots, creating nerve root atrophy as a result of the interruption of their blood supply.[152] It can follow trauma, surgery, infections, contaminants, tumors, or the subarachnoid administration of various medications.

The clinical picture is complex with varied symptomatology. The most common clinical features are:

- back pain that increases on exertion with or without leg pain
- bilateral leg pain
- hyporeflexia
- decreased range of motion of the trunk
- sensory abnormalities
- decreased straight leg raises
- urinary sphincter dysfunction

Unfortunately, the clinical symptoms can lead to a misdiagnosis of spinal stenosis, lumbar disk disease, spinal tumors, or other compressive lesions of the spine.[152]

Characteristic MRI findings show conglomerations of roots residing centrally in the dural sac, adhesions tethering the nerve roots peripherally, and soft tissue replacing the subarachnoid space.[153]

The link between epidural block or catheter placement and this disease is nebulous. Although a few case reports have suggested a connection, no prospective studies have yet linked epidurals to chronic adhesive arachnoiditis. Prospective studies have demonstrated that epidurals do not cause chronic backache.[154] Unfortunately, the neurologic deficits may progress to severe and permanent disability.

Spinal Cord/Nerve Root Injury

Serious neurologic injury is an extremely rare but feared complication of neuraxial anesthesia. The incidence of neurologic injury following neuraxial blocks is estimated to be 0.03–0.1%. It is prudent for the anesthesiologist to understand that a neurologic deficit in a patient who has had an epidural is *rarely caused by the epidural.* Horlocker and colleagues at the Mayo Clinic evaluated the records of over 4000 patients who had lumbar epidurals placed for thoracic surgery while asleep. No neurologic complications occurred, despite the epidurals being placed under general anesthesia.[29] In another extensive review of 45,000 patients undergoing epidural placement, only 40 cases arose of neurologic problems, 22 of

Table 14–14.

Neurologic Complications Associated with Epidural Anesthesia/Analgesia

Pathology	Cause	Onset	Clinical Features	Outcome
Spinal nerve neuropathy	Needle trauma	0–2 days	Pain with needle insertion and injection; paresthesia; numbness over spinal nerve distribution	Recovery 1–12 weeks
Anterior spinal artery syndrome	Hypotension Arteriosclerosis	Immediate	Painless paraplegia	Poor—painless paraplegia persists
Adhesive arachnoiditis	Trauma, surgery, infections Contaminants Irritant injectate	0–7 days	Pain on injection, back pain, bilateral leg pain, sensory abnormalities, hyporeflexia, progressive neurologic deficit with pain, paraplegia	Can progress to severe, permanent disability
Epidural hematoma	Coagulopathy	0–2 days	Severe backache with progressive sensory–motor deficits	Immediate surgery
Epidural abscess	IVDA, nonspinal infection; neurosurgical procedures	0–2 days	Fever, leukocytosis, >ESR Severe backache with sensory–motor deficits	Antibiotic therapy and immediate surgery

IVDA = intravenous drug abuse; ESR = erythrocyte sedimentation rate.

which had paresthesias.[155] There have been a few case reports of myelopathy and paraplegia occurring when thoracic epidurals were placed in anesthetized patients, but these complications are exceedingly rare.[156–158]

Neurologic deficits can be caused by direct trauma to the spinal cord or spinal nerves, from spinal cord ischemia, leading to anterior spinal artery syndrome, from accidental injection of neurotoxic drugs or chemicals, or from hematomas or abscesses.[107] Most peripheral neuropathies resolve spontaneously. Those that become permanent are usually limited to persistent paresthesias and limited motor weakness (Table 14–14).[122]

Cauda equina syndrome, a syndrome characterized by bowel and bladder dysfunction, patchy sensory deficits, pain, and paresis of the legs, was previously attributed to continuous subarachnoid infusions with microcatheters. The mechanism of injury was thought to be pooling of hyperbaric lidocaine, causing damage to the nerve roots of the cauda equina. The FDA withdrew the catheters from the market, but a few cases of cauda equina syndrome have been reported occurring with single-shot spinals. Much more rarely, the syndrome has been reported after caudal epidural anesthesia.

Trauma to epidural veins occurs in approximately 10% of epidural placement. It occurs more commonly in patients with engorged epidural veins (eg, pregnant patient). The bleeding that occurs is usually benign and self-limiting. But if the patient is thrombocytopenic, has received recent anticoagulant therapy, or is coagulopathic for other reasons, the incidence of bleeding leading to the development of epidural

hematoma is higher. The incidence of hematomas after epidural blocks is estimated at 1:150,000. No data support an increased risk of its development with aspirin therapy, but the incidence with the more potent antiplatelet drugs is yet to be determined.[159] These concerns led to the consensus statements developed at the Second ASRA Conference on Neuraxial Anesthesia and Anticoagulation.[23] These guidelines can be used to assist the anesthesiologist in determining the most appropriate and safest period for placing an epidural block.

Epidural hematomas can cause cord compression, cord ischemia, or myelopathy similar to that caused by a space-occupying tumor. It is prudent to remember that *most epidural hematomas are spontaneous and idiopathic.*[160] Symptoms range from mild sensory or motor deficits to devastating paraplegia and incontinence. The clinical features include severe back pain with progressive sensory and motor deficits and reappearance of resolving motor–sensory deficits. The onset of symptoms is usually between 0 and 2 days. Emergent surgical decompression is the treatment to avoid permanent neurologic injury.[161]

Epidural abscess is another rare, but potentially debilitating complication of epidural placement. Spinal epidural abscess can lead to irreversible complications and death if untreated.[162] The most common risk factors are *unrelated to anesthetic instrumentation.* Intravenous drug abuse, the presence of nonspinal infections, and neurosurgical procedures are the primary risk factors.[163] The most common presentation is back pain, radiculopathy, lower extremity weakness with sensory deficits, and decreased deep tendon reflexes. Fever, leukocytosis with a left shift, and an elevated erythrocyte sedimentation rate are usually present, but abscesses have been reported in normothermic patients with normal white blood counts. The average onset of symptoms is 2–5 days. It progresses from back pain that intensifies with palpation or percussion of the spine to paraplegia or paralysis.[164] The most common infective organism is *Staphylococcus aureus,* although multiple organisms have been implicated. MRIs of the spine will demonstrate the abscess as well as its progression into paraspinal structures.[165] Treatment is urgent surgical decompression or percutaneous drainage with fluoroscopic guidance. Antibiotics should be started immediately when abscess is suspected. Although successful therapy with antibiotics alone has been reported, urgent surgery is recommended, especially when neurologic deficits are present.[163]

Anterior spinal artery syndrome secondary to hypotension leading to spinal cord ischemia is a potentially life-threatening syndrome.[166] Theoretically, placement of high thoracic epidurals creating peripheral vasodilation and reduced blood flow to the spinal cord could cause the syndrome, but no reports have proved this occurrence. It is the most common neurologic complication after abdominal aortic surgery but has been reported after surgery on the thoracic spine.[167] Patients usually present with immediate, painless paraplegia. Prognosis is poor, with permanent and disabling neurologic deficits.[168]

SUMMARY

Epidural anesthesia is a time-proven, safe, effective means of providing surgical anesthesia or postoperative analgesia. It has the benefit of being used for segmental blocks or for more complete motor–sensory blocks necessary for surgery. It reduces the adverse physiologic responses to surgery, may decrease the incidence of myocardial infarctions and postoperative pulmonary sequelae, and can reduce the incidence of hypercoagulable events. Mastery of epidural placement comes with practice, attention to detail, and persistence. A thorough knowledge of anatomy, physiology, and the pharmacology of anesthetic agents is required for safe application. Patient satisfaction, efficient use of operating room time for anesthetic induction, and excellent postoperative pain management make epidural blockade an excellent choice of anesthetic management in many clinical scenarios.

References

1. Beattie WS, Badner NH, Choi P: Epidural analgesia reduces postoperative myocardial infarction: A meta-analysis. Anesth Analg 2001;93:853.
2. Ballantyne JC, Carr DB, DeFerranti S: The comparative effects of postoperative analgesic therapies on pulmonary outcome: Cumulative meta-analysis of randomized, controlled trials. Anesth Analg 1998;86:598
3. Rigg JR, Jamrozik K, Myles PS: Epidural anaesthesia and analgesia and outcome of major surgery: A randomized trial. Lancet 2002;359:1276.
4. Liu S, Carpenter R, Neal J: Epidural anesthesia and analgesia. Their role in postoperative outcome. Anesthesiology 1995;82:1474.
5. Holte K, Kehlet H: Epidural analgesia and risk of anastomotic leakage. Reg Anesth Pain Med 2001;26:111.
6. Scott A, Starling J, Ruscher AE et al: Thoracic versus lumbar epidural anesthesia's effect on pain control and ileus resolution after restorative proctocolectomy. Surgery 1996;120:688.
7. Tuman K, McCarthy R, March RJ: Effects of epidural anesthesia and analgesia on coagulation and outcome after major vascular surgery. Anesth Analg 1991;73:696.
8. Rosenfeld B: Benefits of regional anesthesia on thromboembolic complications following surgery. Reg Anesth 1996;21(Suppl):9.
9. Rodgers A, Walker N, Schug S: Reduction of postoperative mortality and morbidity with epidural or spinal anesthesia: Results from overview of randomised trials. BMJ 2000;321:1493.
10. Frolich MA, Caton D: Pioneers in epidural needle design. Anesth Analg 2001;93:215–220.
11. Cortes RC: Lumbar epidural anesthesia, 1931–1936: A second debut. Rev Esp Anestesiol Reanim 2005;52:159–168.
12. Dogliotti A: A new method of block: Segmental peridural spinal anesthesia. Am J Surg 1933;20:107–118.
13. Curbelo M: Continuous peridural segmental anesthesia by means of a ureteral catheter. Curr Res Anesth Analg 1949;28:12–23.
14. Yucesoy AY: The mechanical properties of intact and traumatized epidural catheters. Anesth Analg 2000;90:393–399.
15. Eldor JM: The evolution of combined spinal-epidural anesthesia needles. Reg Anesth 1997;22:294-296.
16. Coates M: Combined subarachnoid and epidural techniques: A single space technique for surgery of the hip and lower limb. Anaesthesia 1982;37:89–90.
17. Mumtaz M, Daz M, Kuz M: Combined subarachnoid and epidural techniques: Another single space technique for orthopaedic surgery. Anaesthesia 1982;37:90.
18. P Michalek, I David, M Adamec, et al: Cervical epidural anesthesia for combined neck and upper extremity procedures: A pilot study. Anesth Analg 2004;99:1833–1836.
19. Kirali K, Kocak T, Guzelmeric F, et al: Off-pump awake coronary revascularization using bilateral internal thoracic arteries. Ann Thorac Surg 2004;78:1602–1603.
20. Lucchetti V, Moscariello C, Catapano D, et al: Coronary artery bypass grafting in the awake patient: Combined thoracic epidural and lumbar subarachnoid block. Eur J Cardiothorac Surg 2004;26:658–659.
21. Klokocovnik T, Hollan J, Sostaric M, et al: Minimally invasive aortic valve replacement under thoracic epidural anesthesia in a conscious patient. Heart Surg Forum 2004;7:196–197.
22. LM Visser: *Epidural Anesthesia, Update in Anesthesia.* Ann Arbor, Michigan, CSEN: The global regional anesthesia website, 2001, pp 1–4.
23. Horlocker TT, Wedel DJ, Benzon H, et al: Regional anesthesia in the anticoagulated patient: Defining the risks (The Second ASRA Consensus Conference on Neuraxial Anesthesia and Anticoagulation). Reg Anesth Pain Med 2003;28:172–197.
24. Cousins M, Veering B: Epidural neural blockade. In Cousins M, Bridenbaugh P (eds): *Neural Blockade,* 3rd ed. Lippincott-Raven, 1998, pp 243–320.
25. Morgan GE Jr, Mikhail MSM, Murray MJM: *Clinical Anesthesiology,* 3rd ed. McGraw-Hill, 2002.
26. Burns R, Clark V: Epidural anesthesia for caesarean section in a patient with quadriplegia and autonomic hyperreflexia. Int J Obstet Anesth 2004;13:120–123.
27. Vassiliev DVM, Nystrom EUM, Leicht CHM: Combined spinal and epidural anesthesia for labor and cesarean delivery in a patient with Guillain-Barre Syndrome. Reg Anesth Pain Med 2001;28:174–176.
28. Tidmarsh MM: Epidural anesthesia and neural tube defects. Int J Obstet Anesth 1998;7:111–114.
29. Horlocker TM, Abel MD, Messick JM Jr, et al: Small risk of serious neurologic complications related to lumbar epidural catheter placement in anesthetized patients. Anesth Analg 2003;96:1547–1552.

30. Douglas MJM: Epidural anesthesia in three parturients with lumbar tattoos: A review of possible implications. Can J Anesth 2002;49:1057–1059.

31. Clemente CD: *Clemente Anatomy: A Regional Atlas of the Human Body*, 4th ed. Lippincott Williams & Wilkins, 1997.

32. Brown DL: Spinal, epidural, and caudal anesthesia. In Miller RD (ed): *Miller's Anesthesia*, 6th ed. Elsevier, 2005, pp 1653–1683.

33. Igarashi T, Hirabayashi Y, Shimizu R: The lumbar extradural structure changes with increasing age. Br J Anaesth 1997;78:149.

34. Hogan Q: Lumbar epidural anatomy: A new look by cryomicrotome section. Anesthesiology 1991;75:767.

35. Blomberg R: The dorsomedian connective tissue band in the lumbar epidural space of humans: An anatomic study using epiduroscopy in autopsy cases. Anesth Analg 1986;65:747.

36. Hogan Q: Distribution of solution in the epidural space; Examination by cryomicrotome section. Reg Anesth Pain Med 2002;27:150.

37. Kim J, Bahk J, Sung J: Influence of age and sex on the position of the conus medullaris and Tuffler's line in adults. Anesthesiology 2003;99:1359–1363.

38. Lee G, Lee J, Ko Y, et al: Comparison of the spinal level assumption by palpation of the iliac crest and posterior superior iliac spine. J Korean Acad Rehab Med 2004;28:596–600.

39. Tame S, Bursgtall R: Investigation of the radiological relationship between iliac crests, conus medullaris and vertebral level in children. Paediatr Anaesthesiol 2003;13:676–680.

40. Palmer S, Abram S, Maitra A, et al: Distance from the skin to the lumbar epidural space in an obstetric population. Anesth Analg 1983;62:944.

41. Rosenberg H, Keyhak M: Distance to epidural space in nonobese patients. Anesth Analg 1984;63:539–540.

42. Shiroyama K, Izumi H, Kubo T, et al: Distance from the skin to the epidural space at the first lumbar interspace in a Japanese obstetric population. Hiroshima J Med Sci 2003;52:27–29.

43. Wu C: Acute postoperative pain. In Miller RD (ed): *Miller's Anesthesia*, 6th ed. Elsevier, 2005, pp 2742–2743.

44. Baron J, Decaux-Jacolot A, Edouard A, et al: Influence of venous return on baro-reflex control of heart rate during lumbar epidural anesthesia in humans. Anesthesiology 1986;64:188.

45. Otton P, Wilson E: The cardiocirculatory effects of upper thoracic epidural analgesia. Can Anaesth Soc J 1966;13:541.

46. Bonica J, Kennedy W, Akamatsu T, et al: Circulatory effects of peridural block. Anesthesiology 1972;36:219.

47. Gruber E, Tschernko E, Kritzinger M, et al: The effects of thoracic epidural analgesia with bupivacaine 0.25% on ventilatory mechanics in patients with severe chronic obstructive pulmonary disease. Anesth Analg 2001;92:1015–1019.

48. Christopherson R, Beattie C, Frank SM, et al: Perioperative morbidity in patients randomized to epidural or general anesthesia for lower extremity vascular surgery. Anesthesiology 1993;79:422–434.

49. Meissner A, Weber T, Van Aken H, et al: Limited upper thoracic epidural block and splanchnic perfusion in dogs. Anesth Analg 1999;89:1378–1381.

50. Ramaioli F, DeAmici D: Central antiemetic effect of atropine: Our personal experience. Can J Anesth 1996;43:1079.

51. Ward R, Kennedy W, Bonnica J: Experimental evaluation of atropine and vasopressors for the treatment of hypotension during high subaranchnoid anesthesia. Anesth Analg 1966;45:621.

52. Walts L, Kaufman R, Moreland J, et al: Total hip arthroplasty: An investigation of factors related to postoperative urinary retention. Clin Orthop 1985;194:280.

53. Kehlet H: The stress response to surgery: Release mechanisms and the modifying effect of pain relief. Acta Chir Scan (Suppl) 1988;550:22.

54. Kehlet H: Surgical stress: The role of pain and analgesia. Br J Anaesth 1989;63:189.

55. Vanhoutte PM, Shimokawa H: Endothelium-derived relaxing factor and coronary vasospasm. Circulation 1989;80:1–9.

56. Bromage P: Mechanism of action of extradural analgesia. Br J Anaesth 1975;47:199.

57. DiFazio C, Woods A, Rowlingson J: Drugs commonly used for nerve blocking: Pharmacology of local anesthetics. In Raj PPM (ed): *Practical Management of Pain*, 3rd ed. Mosby, 2000, pp 558–563.

58. Xiong Z, Strichartz G: Inhibition of local anesthetics of Ca+ channels in rat anterior pituitary cells. Eur J Pharmacol 1998;363:8.

59. Smith F, Davis R, Carter R: Influence of voltage-sensitive Ca(++) channel drugs on bupivacaine in filtration anesthesia in mice. Anesthesiology 2001;95:1189–1197.

60. Liu B, Zhuang X, Li S, et al: Effects of bupivacaine and ropivacaine on high-voltage-activated calcium currents of the dorsal horn neurons in newborn rats. Anesthesiology 2001;95:139–143.

61. Moore D, Spierdijk J, VanKleef J, et al: Chloroprocaine neurotoxicity: Four additional cases. Anesth Analg 1982;61:155.

62. Lynch C: Depression of myocardial contractility in vitro by bupivacaine, etidocainem, and lidocaine. Anesth Analg 1986;65:551.

63. Graf B, Martin E, Bosnjak Z: Stereospecific effect of bupivacaine isomers on atrioventricular conduction in the isolated perfused guinea pig heart. Anesthesiology 1997;86:410.

64. McClure J: Ropivacaine. Br J Anaesth 1996;76:300.

65. Bader N, Datta A, Flanagan H, et al: Comparison of bupivacaine and ropivacaine induced conduction blockade in isolate rabbit vagus nerve. Anesth Analg 1989;68:724.

66. Axelsson K, Nydahl P, Philipson L, et al: Motor and sensory blockade after epidural injection of mepivacaine, bupivacaine, and etidocaine: A double-blind study. Anesth Analg 1989;69:739.

67. Stanton-Hicks M, Berges P, Bonica J: Circulatory effects of peridural block. Comparison of the effects of epinephrine and phenylephrine. Anesthesiology 1973;39:308.

68. Curatolo M, Petersen-Felix S, Arendt-Nielsen L: Adding sodium bicarbonate to lidocaine enhances the depth of epidural blockade. Anesth Analg 1998;86:341.

69. Mehta P, Theriot E, Mehrotra D, et al: A simple technique to make bupivacaine a rapid-acting epidural anesthetic. Reg Anesth 1987;12:135.

70. Corke B, Carlsonk C, Dettbarn W: The influence of 2-chloroprocaine on the subsequent analgesic potency of bupivacaine. Anesthesiology 1984;60:25.

71. Bouguet D: Caudal clonidine added to local anesthetics enhances post-operative analgesia after anal surgery in adults. Anesthesiology 1994;81:A942.

72. Kroin J, Buvanendran A, Beck D, et al: Clonidine prolongation of lidocaine analgesia after sciatic nerve block in rats is mediated via the hyperpolarization-activated cation current, not by alpha-adrenoreceptors. Anesthesiology 2004;101:488–494.

73. Landau R, Schiffer E, Morales M, et al: The dose-sparing effect of clonidine added to ropivacaine for labor epidural analgesia. Anesth Analg 2002;95:728–734.

74. Kyacan N, Arici G, Karsli B, et al: Patient-controlled epidural analgesia in labour: The addition of fentanyl or clonidine to bupivacaine. Agri 2004;16:59–66.

75. Novak-Jankovic V, Paver E, Iban A, et al: Effect of epidural and intravenous clonidine on the neuro-endocrine and immune stress response in patients undergoing lung surgery. Eur J Anaesthesiol 2000;17:50–56.

76. Matot I, Drenger B, Weissman C, et al: Epidural clonidine, bupivacaine and methadone as the sole analgesic agent after thoracotomy for lung resection. Anaesthesia 2004;59:861–866.

77. Wu C, Jao S, Borel CO: The effect of epidural clonidine on perioperative cytokine response, postoperative pain, and bowel function in patients undergoing colorectal surgery. Anesth Analg 2004;99:502–509.

78. Roelants F, Lavand'homme P, Mercier-Fuzier V: Epidural administration of neostigmine and clonidine to induce labor analgesia: Evaluation of efficacy and local anesthetic-sparing effect. Anesthesiology 2005;102:1205–1210.

79. Kayacan N, Arici G, Karsli B: Patient-controlled epidural analgesia in labour: The addition of fentanyl or clonidine to bupivacaine. Agri 2004;16:59–66.

80. Roelants F, Lavand'homme P: Epidural neostigmine combined with sufentanil provides balanced and selective analgesia in early labor. Anesthesiology 2004;101:439–444.

81. Omais M, Lauretti G, Paccola CA: Epidural morphine and neostigmine for postoperative analgesia after orthopedic surgery. Anesth Analg 2002;95:1698–1701.

82. Kirdemir P, Ozkocak I, Demir T: Comparison of postoperative analgesic effects of preemptively used epidural ketamine and neostigmine. J Clin Anesth 2000;12:543–548.

83. Johansen M, Gradert T, Sattefield W, et al: Safety of continuous intrathecal midazolam infusion in the sheep model. Anesth Analg 2004;98:1528–1535.

84. Bharti N, Madan R, Mohanty P, et al: Intrathecal midazolam added to bupivacaine improves the duration and quality of spinal anaesthesia. Acta Anaesthesiol Scand 2003;47:1101–1105.

85. Tucker A, Mezzatesta J, Nadeson R, et al: Intrathecal midazolam II: Combination with intrathecal fentanyl for labor pain. Anesth Analg 2004;98:1521–1527.

86. Ugur B, Basaloglu K, Yurtseven T, et al: Neurotoxicity with single dose intrathecal midazolam administration. Eur J Anaesthesiol 2005;22:907–912.

87. Yaksh T, Allen J: Preclinical insights into the implementation of intrathecal midazolam: A cautionary tale. Anesth Analg 2004;98:1509–1511.

88. Gambling D, Hughes T, Martin G, et al: A comparison of Depodur, a novel, single-dose extended-release epidural morphine, with standard epidural morphine for pain relief after lower abdominal surgery. Anesth Analg 2005;100:1065–1074.

89. Viscusi E, Martin G, Hartrick C, et al: 48 hours of postoperative pain relief after total hip arthroplasty with a novel, extended-release epidural morphine formulation. Anesthesiology 2005;102:1014–1022.

90. Carvalho B, Riley E, Cohen S, et al: Single-dose, sustained release epidural morphine in the management of postoperative pain after elective cesarean delivery: Results of a multicenter randomized controlled study. Anesth Analg 2005;100:1150–1158.

91. Magnusdottir H, Kimo K, Ricksten S: High thoracic epidural analgesia does not inhibit sympathetic nerve activity in the lower extremities. Anesthesiology 199;91:1299.

92. Basse L, Werner M, Kehlet H: Is urinary drainage necessary during continuous epidural anesthesia after colonic resection. Reg Anesthes Pain Med 2000;25:498.

93. Galindo A, Hernandez J, Benavides O, et al: Quality of spinal extradural anesthesia: The influence of spinal nerve root diameter. Br J Anaesthes 1975;47:41.

94. Duggan J, Bowler G, McClure J, et al: Extradural block with bupivacaine: Influence of dose, volume, concentration and patient characteristics. Br J Anaesthes 1988;61:324.

95. Hodgkinson R, Husain F: Obesity, gravity and the spread of epidural anesthesia. Anesth Analg 1981;60:421.

96. Seow L, Lips F, Cousins M: Effect of lateral position on epidural blockade for surgery. Anaesthes Intensive Care 1983;11:97.

97. Park W, Hagins F, Rivat E, et al: Age and epidural dose response in adult men. Anesthesiology 1982;56:318.

98. Park W, Massengale M, Kim S, et al: Age and spread of local anesthetic solutions in the epidural space. Anesth Analg 1980;9:768.

99. Hirabayashi Y, Shimizu R, Matsuda I: Effect of extradural compliance and resistance on spread of extradural analgesia. Br J Anaesthes 1990;65:508.

100. Cullen ML, Staren E, el-Ganzouri A, et al: Continuous epidural analgesia after major abdominal operations: A randomized prospective study. Surgery 1985;98:718–728.

101. Bromage P, Bufoot M, Crowell D, et al: Quality of epidural blockade. Influence of physical factors. Br J Anaesthes 1964;36:342.

102. Datta S, Migliozzi R, Flanagan H, et al: Chronically administered progesterone decreases halothane requirements in rabbits. Anesth Analg 1989;68:46–50.

103. Gintzler A: Endorphin-mediated increases in pain threshold during pregnancy. Science 1980;210:193–195.

104. Hofmeyr G, Cyna A, Middleton P: Prophylactic intravenous preloading for regional analgesia in labour. Cochrane Database System Review 2002;2:4.

105. Jackson R, Reid JA, Thorburn J: Volume preloading is not essential to prevent spinal-induced hypotension at Caesarean section. Br J Anaesthes 1995;75:262–265.

106. Horlocker TM, Abel M, Messick J, et al: Small risk of serious neurologic complications related to lumbar epidural catheter placement in anesthetized patients. Anesth Analg 2003;96:1547–1552.

107. Usubiaga J: Neurological complications following epidural anesthesia. Int Anaesthesiol 1975;13:2.

108. Gulve A, Eldabe S, Richardon J, et al: Obstetric epidural and chronic adhesive arachnoiditis. Br J Anaesthes 2004;92:765–767.

109. Sellors J, Cyna A, Simons S: Aseptic precautions for inserting an epidural catheter: A survey of obstetric anaesthetists. Anaesthesia 2002;57:593–596.

110. Sleth J: Evaluation of aseptic measures in the performance of epidural catheterization and perception of its risk of infection. Results of a survey in Languedoc-Roussilon. Ann French Anesthes Reanim 1998;17:408–414.

111. Schroter J, Wa Djamba D, Hoffman V, et al: Epidural abscess after combined spinal-epidural block. Can J Anaesthes 1997;44:235–238.

112. Bromage P: *Epidural Anesthesia.* WB Saunders, 1978.

113. McQuillan P: Central nerve blocks: Subarachnoid. In Raj PPM (ed): *Practical Management of Pain,* 3rd ed. Mosby, 2000, pp 631–636.

114. Evron S, Sessler D, Sadan O, et al: Identification of the epidural space: Loss of resistance with air, lidocaine, or the combination of air and lidocaine. Anesth Analg 2004;99:245–250.

115. Laviola S, Kirvela M, Spoto M: Pneumocephalus with intense headache and unilateral pupillary dilatation after accidental dural puncture during epidural anesthesia for cesarean section. Anesth Analg 1999;88:582–583.

116. Naulty J, Ostheimer G, Datta S: Incidence of venous air embolism during epidural catheter insertion. Anesthesiology 1982;57:410–412.

117. Dalens B, Bazin J, Haberer J: Epidural bubbles as a cause of incomplete analgesia during epidural anesthesia. Anesth Analg 1987;66:679–683.

118. Petty T, Stevens R, Erickson S: Inhalation of nitrous oxide expands epidural air bubbles. Reg Anesth 1996;21:144–148.

119. Hirsch M, Katz Y, Sasson A: Spinal cord compression by unusual epidural air accumulation after continuous epidural anesthesia. Am J Roentgenol 1989;153:887–888.

120. Gutsche B: *How to Make an Epidural Work.* American Society of Anesthesiologists. 2004, pp 1–7.

121. Gunter J: Thoracic epidural anesthesia via the modified Taylor approach in infants. Reg Anesth Pain Med 2000;25:555–557

122. McQuillan PM, Kafiluddi R, Halm MD. Central nerve blocks: Interventional techniques, In Raj PPM (ed): *Pain Medicine: A Comprehensive Review,* 2nd ed. Mosby, 2003, pp 212–222.

123. Moore D, Batra M, Bridenbaugh L, et al: Maternal heart rate changes with a plain epidural test dose—Validity of results open to question. Anesthesiology 1987;66:854.

124. Sethna N, McGowan F: Do results from studies of a simulated epidural test dose improve our ability to detect unintentional epidural vascular puncture in children. Pediatr Anaesthesiol 2005;15:711–715.

125. Steffek M, Owczuk R, Szlyk-Augustyn M, et al: Total spinal anesthesia as a complication of local anaesthetic test-dose administration through an epidural catheter. Acta Anaesthesiol Scand 2004;48:1211–1213.

126. Lee P, Kim J: Lumbar epidural blocks: A case report of a life-threatening complication. Arch Physician Med Rehab 2000;81:1587–15890.

127. Desparmet J, Mateo J, Esoffey C: Efficacy of an epidural test dose in children anesthetized with halothane. Anesthesiology 1990;72:249.

128. Rosen M, Hughes S, Levinson G: Regional anesthesia for labor and delivery. In Levinson SA (ed): *Anesthesia for Obstetrics.* Lippincott Williams & Wilkins, 2002, pp 123–148.

129. Tsui B, Gupta S, Finucane B: Confirmation of epidural catheter placement using nerve stimulation. Can J Anaesth 1998;45:640–644.

130. Sparks J, Seefelder C: Neonatal T-wave elevation from a positive epidural test dose. Pediatr Anaesthesiol 2005;15:706–707.

131. Moore D, Batra M: The components of an effective test dose prior to epidural block. Anesthesiology 1981;55:693.

132. Mackie K, Lam A: Epinephrine-containing test dose during beta blockade. J Clin Monitoring 1991;7:213.

133. Kasaba T, Yoshikawa G, Seguchi T: Epidural fentanyl improves the onset and spread of epidural mepivacaine analgesia. Can J Anesth 1996;43:1211.

134. Salim R, Nachum Z, Moscovici R, et al: Continuous compared with intermittent epidural infusion on progress of labor and patient satisfaction. Obstet Gynecol 2005;106:301–306.

135. Burgess F, Anderson D, Colonna D, et al: Thoracic epidural analgesia with bupivacaine and fentanyl for postoperative thoracotomy pain. J Cardiothorac Vasc Anesth 1994;8:420–424.

136. Bernards C: Epidural and spinal anesthesia. In Barash PG (ed): *Clinical Anesthesia.* Lippincott Williams & Wilkins, 201, pp 689–712.

137. Wilson W, Benumof J: Anesthesia for thoracic surgery, In Miller RD (ed): *Miller's Anesthesia,* 6th ed. Elsevier, 2005, pp 1907–1908.

138. Lui S, Carpenter R, Neal J: Epidural anesthesia and analgesia: Their role in postoperative outcome. Anesthesiology 1995;82:1474–1506.

139. Block A, Covino B: Effect of local anesthetic agents on cardiac conduction and contractility. Reg Anesth 1982;6:55.

140. Seeberger M, Lang M, Drewe J, et al: Comparison of spinal and epidural anesthesia in patients younger than 50 years of age. Anesth Analg 1994;78:667.

141. Rutter S, Shields F, Broadbent C, et al: Management of accidental dural puncture in labor with intrathecal catheters: An analysis of 10 years experience. Int J Obstet Anesth 2001;10:177–181.

142. Denny N, Masters R, Pearson D: Postdural puncture headache after continuous spinal anesthesia. Anesth Analg 1987;66:791.

143. Brownridge P: The management of headache following accidental dural puncture in obstetric patients. Anaesthesiol Intensive Care 1983;11:9.

144. Lybecker H, Djernes M, Schmidt J: Postdural puncture headache: Onset, duration, severity, and associated symptoms. Acta Anaesthesiol Scand 1995;39:605–612.

145. Oedit R, van Kooten F, Bakker S, et al: Efficacy of the epidural blood patch for the treatment of post lumbar puncture headaches: A randomized, observer-blind, controlled clinical trial. BMC Neurol 2005;5:12.

146. Vilming S, Kloster R, Sandvik L: When should an epidural blood patch be performed in postlumbar puncture headache? A theoretical approach based on a cohort of 79 patients. Cephalagia 2005;25:523–527.

147. Angle P, Tang S, Thompson D, et al: Expectant management of postdural puncture headache increases hospital length of stay and emergency room visits. Can J Anaesth 2005;52:397–402.

148. Collis R, Harries S: A subdural abscess and infected blood patch complicating regional anesthesia for labour. Int J Obstet Anesth 2005;14:246–251.

149. Lubenow T, Keh-Wong E, Kristof K, et al: Inadvertent subdural injection: A complication of epidural block. Anesth Analg 1988;67:175.

150. Berga S, Trierweiler M: Bacterial meningitis following epidural anesthesia for vaginal delivery: A case report. Obstet Gynecol 1989;74:437–439.

151. Ugeskr L: infections in connection with epidural catheterization. Ugeskr Laeger 1996;158:4403–4405.

152. Rice J, Wee M, Thomson K: Obstetric epidurals and chronic adhesive arachnoiditis. Br J Anaesth 2004;92:109–120.

153. Ross J, Masaryk T, Modic M, et. al: MR imaging of lumbar arachnoiditis. Am J Roentgenol 1987;149:1025.

154. Macarthur A, Macarthr C, Weeks S: Epidural anaesthesia and low back pain after delivery: A prospective cohort study. BMJ 1995;11:1336–1139.

155. Kane R: Neurologic deficits following epidural or spinal anesthesia. Anesth Analg 1981;60:150–161.

156. Kao M, Tsai S, Tsou M, et al: Paraplegia after delayed detection of inadvertent spinal cord injury during thoracic epidural catheterization in an elderly patient. Anesth Analg 2004;99:580–583.

157. Aldrete J, Ferrari H: Myelopathy with syringomyelia following thoracic epidural anesthesia. Anesth Intensive Care 2004;32:5967.

158. Lee B: Neuraxial complications after epidural and spinal anaesthesia. Acta Anaesthesiol Scand 2003;47:371–373.

159. Odom J, Sih I: Epidural analgesia and anticoagulant therapy: Experience with one thousand cases of continuous epidurals. Anesth Analg 1983;1980:72.

160. Hyderally H: Epidural hematoma unrelated to combined spinal-epidural anesthesia in a patient with ankylosing spondylitis receiving aspirin after a total hip replacement. Anesth Analg 2005;100:882–883.

161. Torres A, Acebes J, Cabiol J, et al: Spinal epidural hematomas. Prognostic factors in a series of 22 cases and a proposal for management. Neurocirugia (Astur) 2004;15:353–359.

162. Izci Y: Lumbosacral spinal epidural abscess caused by Brucella melitensis. Acta Neurochir J 2005;147:1207–1209.

163. Curry W, Hoh B, Amin-Hanjani S, et al: Spinal epidural abscess: Clinical presentation, management, and outcome. Surg Neurol 2005;63:364–371.

164. Brookman C, Rutledge M: Epidural abscess: Case report and literature review. Reg Anesth Pain Med 2000;25:428.

165. Volk T, Hebecker R, Ruecker G, et al: Subdural empyema combined with paraspinal abscess after epidural catheter insertion. Anesth Analg 2005;100:1222–1223.

166. Johnkura K, Joki H, Johmura Y, et al: Combination of infarctions in the posterior inferior cerebellar artery and anterior spinal artery territories. J Neurol Sci 2003;15:1–4.

167. Doita M, Marui T, Nishida K: Anterior spinal artery syndrome after total spondylectomy of T10, T11, and T12. Clin Orthop Rel Res 2002;405:175–181.

168. de la Barrera S, Barca-Buyo A, Montoto-Marques A, et al: Spinal cord infarction: Prognosis and recovery in a series of 36 patients. Spinal Cord 2001;39:520–525.

15

Caudal Anesthesia

Kenneth D. Candido, MD • Alon P. Winnie, MD

INTRODUCTION

Caudal anesthesia was first described at the turn of last century by two French physicians, Fernand Cathelin and Jean-Athanase Sicard. The technique predated the lumbar approach to epidural block by several years.[1] Caudal anesthesia, however, did not gain in popularity immediately following its inception. One of the major reasons caudal anesthesia was not embraced arose from the wide variety of arrangements of sacral bones encountered in the general population

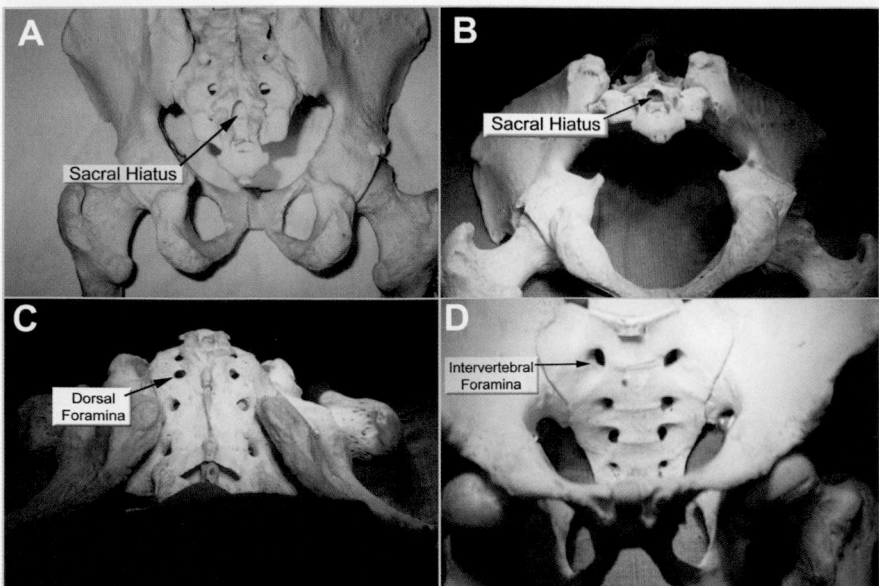

Figure 15–1. A: Skeletal model demonstrating the sacral hiatus and its relationship to the coccyx and sacrum. The fifth inferior articular processes project caudally and flank the sacral hiatus as sacral cornuae. **B:** Skeletal specimen viewed from inferior to the sacral hiatus. The hiatus is seen as the oval shaped opening at the 12 o'clock position in the photograph. **C:** Skeletal specimen of the sacrum viewed from craniad to caudad demonstrating the five dorsal foramina, situated bilaterally. **D:** Skeletal specimen of the sacrum demonstrating the ventral sacral surface. Note the five bilateral intervertebral foramina, paired on either side of the midline, defined by the retention screws used to hold the specimen together.

and the consequent high failure rate associated with attempts to locate the sacral hiatus. The failure rate of 5% to 10% made caudal epidural anesthesia unpopular until a resurgence of interest occurred in the 1940s led by Hingson and colleagues, who used it primarily in obstetrical anesthesia. Caudal epidural anesthesia has many applications, including surgical anesthesia in children and adults, as well as the management of acute and chronic pain conditions. Success rate of 98% to 100% can be achieved in infants and young children before the age of puberty, as well as in lean adults.[1] The technique of caudal epidural block in pain management has been greatly enhanced by the use of fluoroscopic guidance and epidurography, in which high success rates can be attained. Unfortunately, clinical indications, and especially therapeutic interventions for the relief of chronic pain in individuals with failed back surgery syndrome, are often most prevalent in patients with difficult caudal landmarks. It has been suggested that traditional lumbar peridural block should not be attempted employing an approach requiring needle placement through a spinal surgery scar, due to the likelihood of tearing the dura and the possibility of inducing hematoma formation over the cauda equina when blood from the procedure gets trapped between the layers of scar and connective tissues.[2] Under these circumstances, it is recommended that fluoroscopically guided caudal epidural block be performed in lieu of the traditional approach. The second resurgence in popularity of caudal anesthesia has paralleled the increasing need to find safe alternatives to conventional lumbar epidural block in selected patient populations, such as individuals with failed back surgery syndrome.

ANATOMIC CONSIDERATIONS

The sacrum is a large triangularly shaped bone formed by the fusion of the five sacral vertebrae. It has a blunted, caudal apex that articulates with the coccyx. Its superior, wide base articulates with the fifth lumbar vertebra at the lumbosacral angle (Figure 15–1A–D). Its dorsal surface is convex and has a raised interrupted median crest with four (sometimes three) spinous tubercles representing fused sacral spines. Flanking the median crest, the posterior surface is formed by fused laminae. Lateral to the median crest, four pairs of dorsal foramina lead into the sacral canal through intervertebral foraminae, each of which transmits the dorsal ramus of a sacral spinal nerve (see Figure 15–1B). Below the fourth (or third) spinous tubercle an arched sacral hiatus is identified in the posterior wall of the sacral canal, due to the failure of the fifth pair of laminae to meet, exposing the dorsal surface of the fifth sacral vertebral body. The caudal opening of the canal is the sacral hiatus (see Figure 15–1A and B), roofed by the firm elastic membrane, the sacrococcygeal ligament, which is an extension of the ligamentum flavum. The fifth inferior articular processes project caudally and flank the sacral hiatus as sacral cornuae, connected to the coccygeal cornua by intercornual ligaments.

The sacral canal is formed by the sacral vertebral foramina and is triangular in shape. It is a continuation of the lumbar spinal canal. Each lateral wall presents four intervertebral foramina, through which the canal is contiguous with the pelvic and dorsal sacral foramina. The posterior sacral foramina are smaller than their anterior counterparts. The sacral canal contains the cauda equina (including the filum terminale) and the spinal meninges. Near its midlevel (typically the middle one third of S2, but varying from the midpoint of S1 to the midpoint of S3) the subarachnoid and subdural spaces cease to exist, and the lower sacral spinal roots and filum terminale pierce the arachnoid and dura maters.[3,4] The lowest margin of the filum terminale emerges at the sacral hiatus and traverses the dorsal surface of the fifth sacral vertebra and the sacrococcygeal joint to reach the coccyx. The fifth spinal nerves also emerge through the hiatus medial to the sacral cornua. The sacral canal contains the epidural venous plexus, which generally terminates at S4, but which may continue more caudally. Most of these vessels are concentrated in the anteriolateral portion of the canal. The remainder of the sacral canal is filled with adipose tissue, which is subject to an age-related decrease in its density. This change may be responsible for the transition from the predictable spread of local anesthetics administered for caudal anesthesia in children to the limited and unpredictable segmental spread seen in adults.[5]

Clinical Pearls

- Considerable variability occurs in sacral hiatus anatomy among individuals of seemingly similar backgrounds, race, and stature.
- With advancing age, the overlying ligaments and the cornua thicken; consequently identification of the hiatal margins become challenging.
- The practical problems related to caudal anesthesia are mainly attributable to wide anatomic variations in size, shape, and orientation of the sacrum.

Considerable variability occurs in sacral hiatus anatomy among individuals of seemingly similar backgrounds, race, and stature.[1] As individuals age, the overlying ligaments and the cornua thicken significantly. The hiatal margins often defy recognition by even skilled fingertips. The practical problems related to caudal anesthesia are mainly attributable to wide anatomic variations in size, shape, and orientation of the sacrum. Trotter[3] summarized the major anatomic variations of the sacrum. The sacral hiatus may be almost closed, asymmetrically open, or widely open secondary to anomalies in the pattern of fusion of the laminae of the sacral arches. Sacral spina bifida was noted in about 2% of males, and in 0.3% of females. The anteroposterior depth of the sacral canal may vary from less than 2 mm to greater than 1 cm. Individuals with sacral canals having anteroposterior diameters less than about 3 mm may not be able to accommodate anything larger than a 21-gauge needle (5% of the population).[1] Additionally, the lateral width of the sacral canal varies significantly. Since the depth and width of the canal may vary, the volume of the canal itself may also vary. Trotter found that sacral volumes varied between 12 and 65 mL, with a mean volume of 33 mL.[3] A magnetic resonance imaging (MRI) study in 37 adult patients found the volume (excluding the foramina and dural sac) to be 14.4 mL, with a range of 9.5 to 26.6 mL.[6] Patients with smaller capacities may not be able to accommodate the typical volumes of local anesthetics administered for epidural anesthesia via the caudal route. In a cadaver study of 53 specimens, the mean distance between the tip of the dural sac and the upper edge of the sacral hiatus as denoted by the sacrococcygeal membrane was 45 mm, with a range of 16 to 75 mm.[3] In the MRI study mentioned earlier, the mean distance was found to be 60.5 mm, with a range of 34 to 80 mm.[6] The sacrococcygeal membrane could not be identified in 10.8% of subjects using MRI.[6] A recent anatomic evaluation of 92 isolated sacra found that 42% of cases had both a hiatus and cornu; 4% of the cases showed an absent hiatus. The apex of the sacral hiatus, in that study, was noted in 64% of cases to exist at the S4 level. The hiatus was closed in 3% of cases.[7]

The sacral foramina afford anatomic passages that permit the spread of injected solutions such as local anesthetics and adjuvants (see Figure 15–1C and D). The posterior sacral foramina are essentially sealed by the multifidus and sacrospinalis muscles, but the anterior foramina are unobstructed by muscles and ligaments, permitting ready egress of solutions through them.[8] The sacral curvature also varies substantially.[9] This variability tends to be more pronounced in males than in females. The clinical significance of this finding is that a noncurving epidural needle will more likely pass easily into the canal of females than males. The angle between the axis of the lumbar canal and the sacral canal varies between 7 and 70 degrees in subjects with marked lordosis. The clinical implication of this finding is that the cephalad flow of caudally injected solutions may be more limited in lordotic patients with exaggerated lumbosacral angles than in those with flatter lumbosacral angles, in whom the axes of the lumbar and sacral canals are more closely aligned.

INDICATIONS FOR CAUDAL EPIDURAL BLOCK

The indications for caudal epidural block are essentially the same as those for lumbar epidural block, but its use may be preferred when sacral nerve spread of anesthetics and adjuvants is preferred over lumbar nerve spread. The unpredictability of ascertaining consistent cephalad spread of anesthetics administered through the caudal canal limits the usefulness of this technique when it is essential to provide lower thoracic and upper abdominal neuraxial blockade. Though this modality is described for perioperative use (diminishing role) and for managing chronic pain in adults (increasing role), it is essential to recognize that caudal block has an extremely wide range of applicability (Table 15–1).[10–13]

Clinical Pearls

- The indications for caudal epidural block are essentially the same as those for lumbar epidural block.
- Caudal may be preferred over lumbar epidural block when sacral nerve spread of anesthetics and adjuvants is preferred over lumbar nerve spread.
- The unpredictability of ascertaining consistent cephalad spread of anesthetics administered through the caudal canal limits the usefulness of this technique when it is essential to provide lower thoracic and upper abdominal neuraxial blockade.

Table 15–1.

Clinical Applications of Caudal Epidural Nerve Block

General Uses

Administration of anesthesia in infants, children, and adults, especially for surgery of the perineum, anus, and rectum; inguinal and femoral herniorrhaphy; cystoscopy and urethral surgery; hemorrhoidectomy; vaginal hysterectomy

Prognostic neural blockade to evaluate pelvic, bladder, perineal, genital, rectal, anal, and lower extremity pain

Provide sympathetic block for individuals suffering from acute vascular insufficiency of lower extremities secondary to vasospastic or vasocclusive disease, including frostbite and ergotamine toxicity

Relief of labor pain (mostly historical)

Conditions requiring epidural block where extensive segmental block is not important

Acute Pain Management

Management of pelvic and lower extremity pain secondary to trauma (without evidence of pelvic fracture)

Postoperative pain management

Temporizing measure for pain secondary to acute lumbar vertebral compression fractures

Chronic Pain Management

Injection of local anesthetics or medications for lumbar radiculopathy secondary to herniated disks and spinal stenosis

Approach to the epidural space in failed back surgery syndrome

Diabetic polyneuropathy

Postherpetic neuralgia

Complex regional pain syndromes

Orchalgia; pelvic pain syndromes

Percutaneous epidural neuroplasty

Cancer Pain Management

Chemotherapy-related peripheral neuropathy

Bony metastases to the pelvis

Injection therapy for pain secondary to pelvic, perineal, genital, or rectal malignancy

Prognostic indicator prior to performing neurodestructive sacral nerve ablation(s)

Injection of hyperbaric phenol solutions for management of sacral pain

Other newer indications in adults bear special mention and will be described later, including the performance of percutaneous epidural neuroplasty;[14,15] the use of caudal analgesia following lumbar spinal surgery;[16] caudal analgesia after emergency orthopedic lower extremity surgery;[17] administering local anesthetic adjuvants for postoperative analgesia;[18] and caudal block for performing neurolysis for intractable cancer pain.[19]

THE TECHNIQUE OF CAUDAL EPIDURAL BLOCK

The technique of caudal epidural block involves palpation, identification and puncture.[1] Patients are evaluated for any epidural block, and the indications and relative and absolute contraindications to its performance are identical. A full complement of noninvasive monitors is applied, and baseline vital signs are assessed. One must decide whether a continuous or single-shot technique will be employed. For continuous techniques, a Tuohy-type needle with a lateral facing orifice is preferred.

Patient Positioning

Several positions can be used in adults, compared with the lateral decubitus position in neonates and children. The lateral position is efficacious in pediatrics because it permits easy access to the airway when general anesthesia or heavy sedation has been administered prior to performing the block. In pediatric patients, blocks may be performed with the patient fully anesthetized; the same is not recommended for older children and adults. In adults, the prone position is the most frequently utilized, but the lateral decubitus position or the knee–chest (also known as knee–elbow) position may be employed. In the prone position, the procedure table or operating room table should be flexed, or a pillow may be placed beneath the symphysis pubis and iliac crests to produce slight flexion of the hips. This maneuver makes palpation of the caudal canal easier. The legs are separated with the heels rotated outward to smooth out the upper part of the anal cleft while relaxing the gluteal muscles. For placement of caudal epidural block in the parturient, the woman is in the lateral (Sim position) or in the knee–elbow position.

Anatomic Landmarks

A dry gauze swab is placed in the anal cleft to protect the anal area and genitalia from povidone-iodine (Betadine) or other disinfectants (especially alcohol) used to sterilize the skin. The skin folds of the buttocks are useful guides in locating the underlying sacral hiatus. Alternatively, a triangle may be marked on the skin over the sacrum, using the posterior superior iliac spines (PSIS) as the base, with the apex pointing inferiorly (caudally). Normally, this apex sits over or immediately adjacent to the sacral hiatus. The hiatus is marked and the tip of the index finger is placed on the tip of the coccyx in the natal cleft while the thumb of the same hand palpates the two sacral cornua located 3–4 cm more rostrally at the upper end of the natal cleft. The sacral cornua may be identified by gently moving the palpating index finger from side to side (Figure 15–2). The palpating thumb should sink into the hollow between the two cornua, as if between two knuckles of a fist.[1] A sterile skin preparation and draping of the entire region is performed in the usual fashion.

Technique

A small-gauge 1.5-in. needle is then utilized to infiltrate the skin over the sacral hiatus using 3–5 mL of 1–1.5% plain lidocaine HCl (Figures 15–3 through 15–5). If fluoroscopy is utilized, a lateral view is obtained to demonstrate the anatomic boundaries of the sacral canal. We routinely leave the local anesthetic infiltration needle in situ for this view, since it demonstrates whether the approach is at the appropriate level

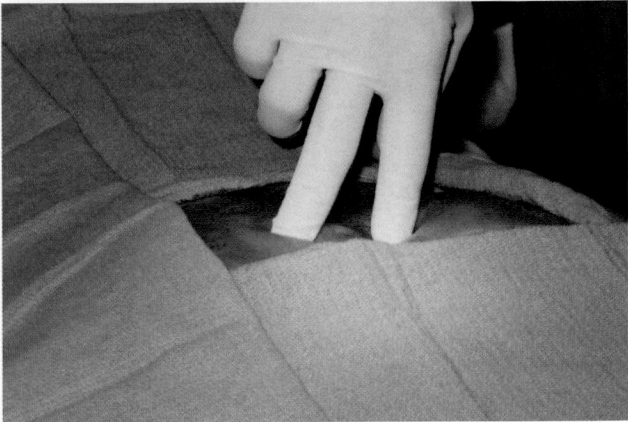

Figure 15–2. Technique of palpating the midline over the sacral hiatus. The palpating index and middle fingers are spread over the fifth sacral vertebral body. The sacrococcygeal ligament lies directly beneath the palpating fingers.

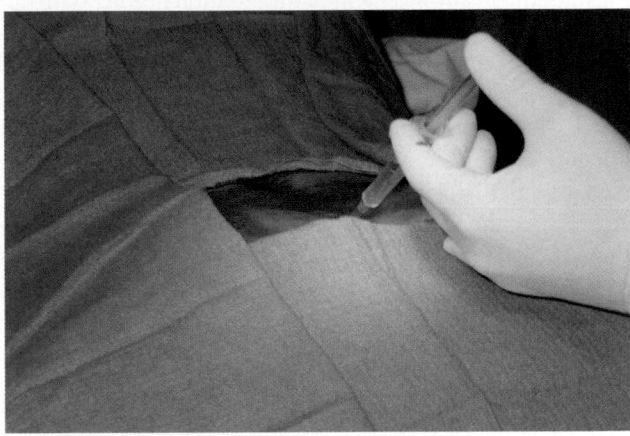

Figure 15–3. Technique of skin infiltration using a fine-bore needle and local anesthetic. The needle is inserted first above, and then into the substance of the sacrococcygeal ligament.

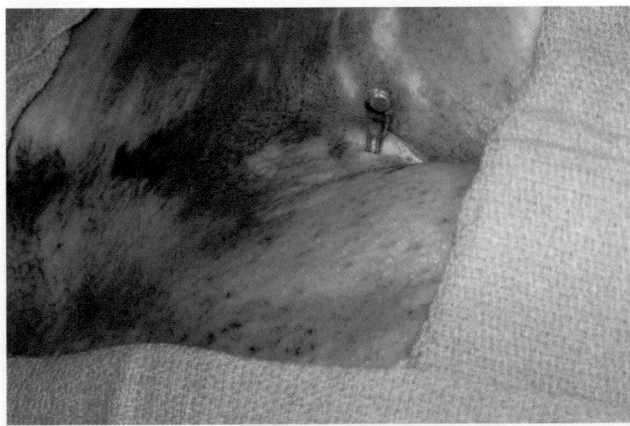

Figure 15–4. The fine-bore needle has been left in place, having engaged the sacrococcygeal ligament.

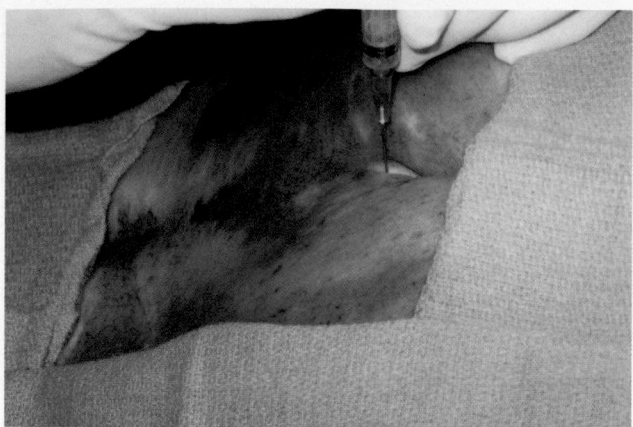

Figure 15–5. A longer, firmer infiltration needle for local anesthetic injection is now advanced through the sacrococcygeal ligament to anesthetize that structure and the overlying subcutaneous tissues.

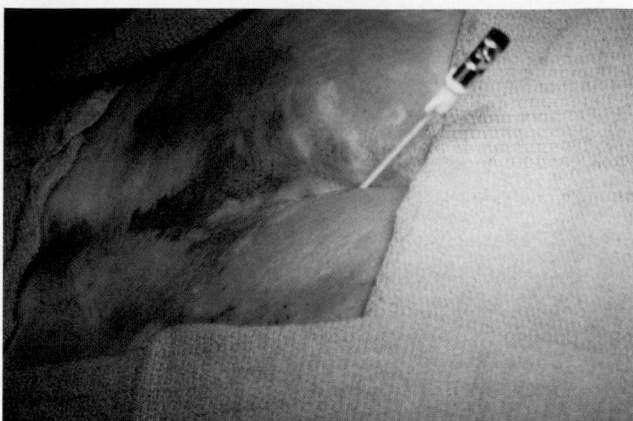

Figure 15–7. The 17-gauge needle has been advanced from the skin into the sacral hiatus through the sacrococcygeal ligament. Usually, when fluoroscopy is not available to verify correct needle placement, a syringe loaded with air or saline is attached to the needle and the loss-of-resistance technique is employed to identify the epidural space, as for conventional lumbar or cervical epidural injections.

for subsequent advancement of the epidural needle. With fluoroscopy, the caudal canal appears as a translucent layer posterior to the sacral segments (Figure 15–6). The median sacral crest is visualized as an opaque line posterior to the caudal canal. The sacral hiatus is usually visualized as a translucent opening at the base of the caudal canal. The coccyx may be seen articulating with the inferior surface of the sacrum.

Once the tissues overlying the hiatus have been anesthetized, a 17- or 18-gauge Tuohy-type needle is inserted either in the midline or, using a lateral approach, into the caudal canal (Figures 15–7 and 15–8). A feeling of a slight "snap" may be appreciated when the advancing needle pierces the sacrococcygeal ligament. Once the needle reaches the ventral wall of the sacral canal, it is slowly withdrawn and reoriented,

directing it more cranially (by depressing the hub and advancing) for further insertion into the canal (Figure 15–9). We utilize the anteroposterior view once the epidural needle is safely situated within the confines of the canal, and the epidural catheter is advanced cephalad. In this projection, the intermediate sacral crests appear as opaque vertical lines on either side of the midline. The sacral foramina are visualized as translucent and nearly circular areas lateral to the intermediate sacral crests. The presence of intestinal gas may obfuscate the recognition of these structures. A syringe loaded with either air or saline containing a small air bubble is attached to the needle, and the loss-of-resistance technique is used to establish entry into the epidural space.

Clinical Pearls

- The needle tip should stay below the S2 level to avoid tearing the dura.
- The needle should never be advanced in the space to the full length of the shaft.
- The skin corresponding to about 1 cm inferior to the PSIS indicates the S2 level (caudalmost extension of the dura mater).
- The dural sac extends lower in children than in adults, and epidural needles should be very carefully advanced no deeper than the S3 or S4 level in this patient population.

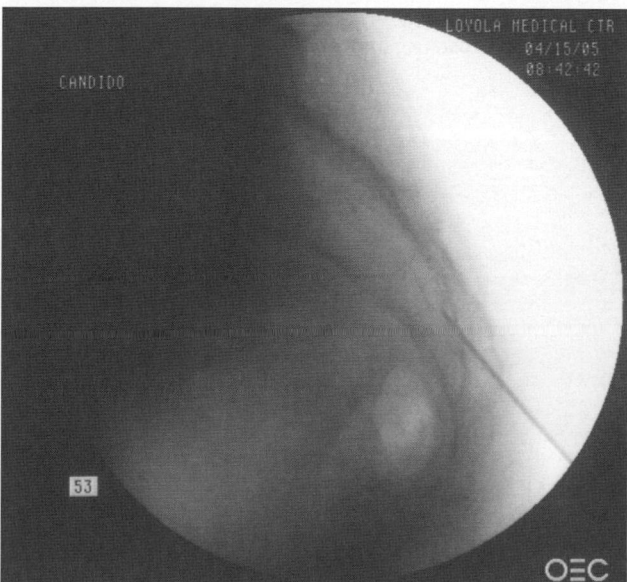

Figure 15–6. Lateral fluoroscopic image depicting the 17-gauge extracatheter device correctly seated in the caudal epidural space.

A "whoosh" test has been described for identifying correct needle placement in the caudal canal. This characteristic sound has been noted during auscultation of the thoracolumbar region during the injection of 2 to 3 mL of air into the caudal epidural space.[20] The test has been modified in pediatrics,

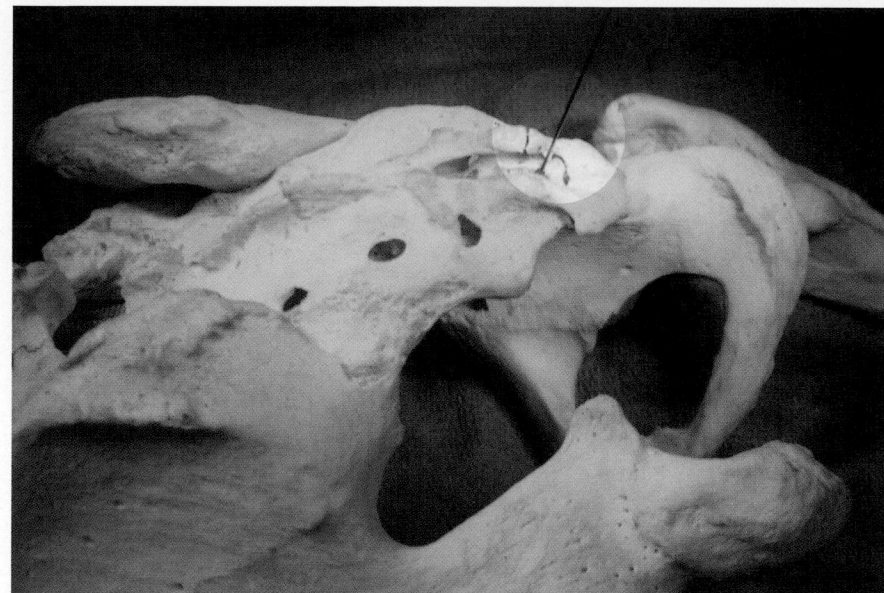

Figure 15–8. Skeletal specimen demonstrating the needle introducer from the 17-gauge extracatheter device situated correctly in the caudal epidural space, traversing the sacrococcygeal ligament (removed) and entering the sacral hiatus (lateral view).

wherein local anesthetic, and not air injection, is auscultated during the performance of the block. Of the 108 patients with a successful block in one study, 98 had a positive test, with no false-positive results.[21] Once the correct placement of the needle is confirmed, a catheter is inserted into the desired location (depth) (Figure 15–10), and its position confirmed fluoroscopically when desired (Figures 15–11 and 15–12).

Clinical Pearls

■ In pediatric patients, electrical stimulation has been used to ascertain correct needle placement in the caudal canal. Anal sphincter contraction (corresponding to stimulation of S2-S4) can be sought with a current of 1–10 mA.[22]

■ If the needle has been inserted correctly, it will swing easily from side to side at the hub while the shaft is held like a fulcrum at the sacrococcygeal membrane and the tip moves freely in the sacral canal.

■ If cerebrospinal fluid (CSF) is aspirated through the needle, it should be withdrawn and injection should not be undertaken.

■ If blood is aspirated, the needle should be withdrawn and reinserted until no blood is apparent at the hub.

■ When injection of air (or saline) for the loss-of-resistance technique results in a bulging over the sacrum, the needle tip most probably lies dorsal to the sacrum in the subcutaneous tissues.

■ If the needle tip is subperiosteal, the injection will meet with significant resistance, and the patient will find this to be a most unpleasant experience. The cortical layer of the sacral bone is often quite thin, particularly in infants and older subjects, and puncture of cancellous bone is relatively easy, especially if force is exerted while advancing the needle. The sensation of entering cancellous bone is not unlike penetrating the sacrococcygeal membrane; there is a feeling of resistance that is suddenly overcome and the needle advances more freely and subsequent injection is unhampered.

Injected solutions may be absorbed very rapidly by bone marrow and toxic drug reactions result. In this situation, pain is typically noted over the caudal part of the sacrum during the injection. If this occurs, the needle should be withdrawn slightly and rotated on its axis until it can be reinserted in a slightly different direction.[23–25]

If injection is made anterior to the sacrum (between the sacrum and coccyx), it is possible to perforate the rectum, or, in parturients, the baby's head may be injured. This limits the use of caudal block in laboring women once the presenting part has descended into the perineum. Inadvertent venous

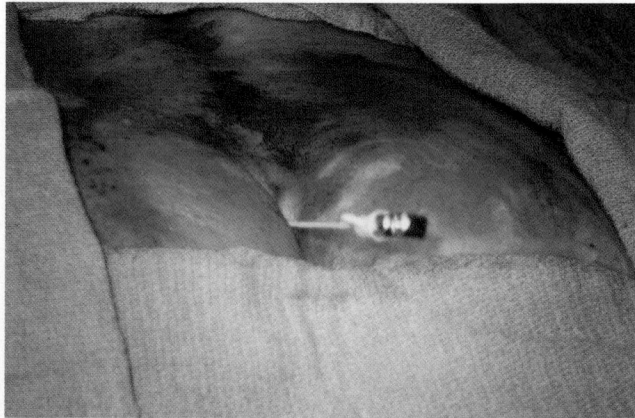

Figure 15–9. Caudocranial view of the 17-gauge extracatheter device situated correctly through the sacrococcygeal ligament into the sacral hiatus.

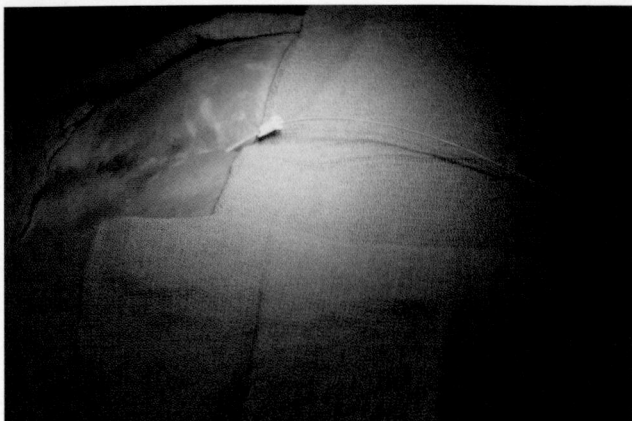

Figure 15–10. A continuous catheter with a stylet in place is shown. The catheter is advanced through either the short over-the-needle catheter that was left in situ (shown), or through a 17–18-gauge steel needle placed in the canal.

puncture also may occur, and the incidence of this has been reported to be about 0.6%.[26]

Caudal block may be used with a single-shot or continuous catheter technique. For continuous block, the catheter may be advanced anterogradely (conventionally) or retrogradely. Continuous caudal block may be performed in retrograde fashion using needle insertion into the lumbar epidural space, but directed inferiorly instead of superiorly. In one study of 10 patients, epidural catheters were advanced through 18-gauge Tuohy-type epidural needles in retrograde fashion from the L4-L5 interspace. This technique was associated with a 20% failure rate with the catheter going into the paravertebral or retrorectal spaces, despite easy epidural

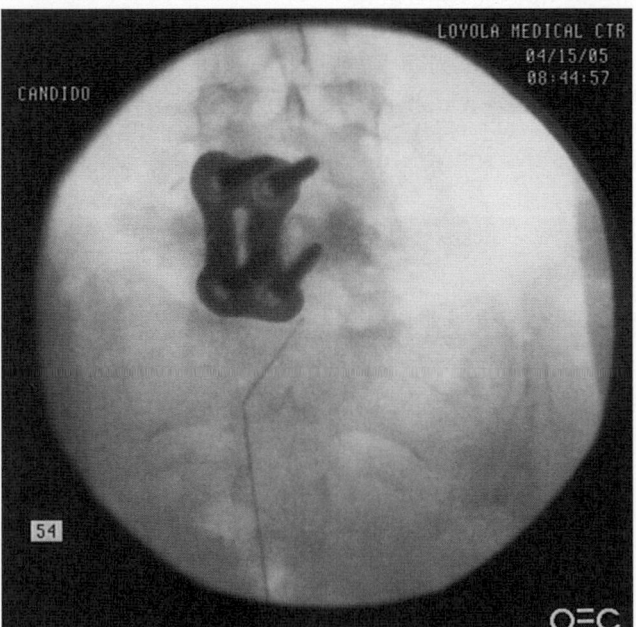

Figure 15–11. Anteroposterior fluoroscopic image depicting proper placement of the needle. The patient's hardware from previous fusion surgery is also seen.

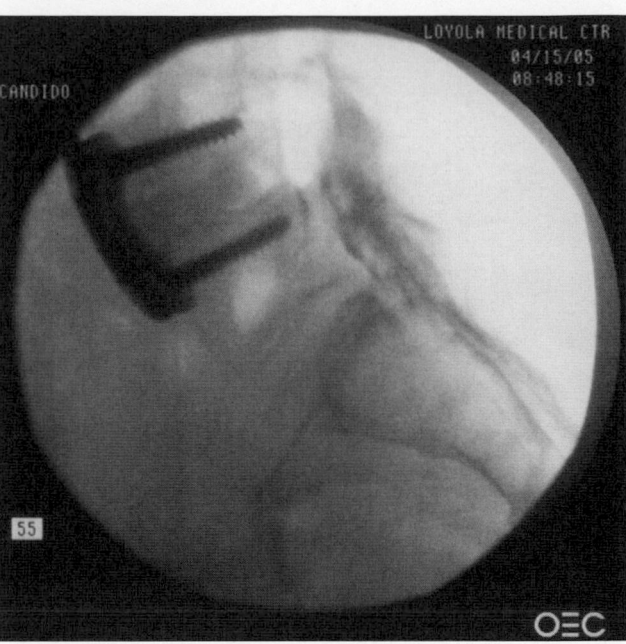

Figure 15–12. Lateral fluoroscopic image depicting radiopaque contrast medium in the caudal and lower lumbar epidural spaces. The image shows considerable spread, both anteriorly and posteriorly, following the injection of 2 mL of dye.

space entry.[27] Using the conventional approach, a Huber-tipped Tuohy needle is used as a conduit to pass the epidural catheter into the canal. This needle has a skilike tip that limits its being caught or snagged on the sacral periosteum. The needle is inserted with its shoulder facing anteriorly and its orifice dorsally. Alternatively, a standard 16- or 17-gauge catheter-over-needle assemblage (angiocatheter) may serve as the introducing needle for subsequent catheter placement. The catheter is advanced with fluoroscopic guidance, especially when it is performed for chronic pain management in failed back surgery syndrome. The catheters should be advanced gently, since there have been reports of dural puncture with rapid or aggressive advancement. The lateral and anteroposterior views should be obtained to demonstrate placement of the catheter in the epidural space (lateral view, see Figure 15–6) and to follow its path in a cephalad or cephalolateral direction (anteroposterior view, see Figure 15–11). When the desired level is attained, iodinated nonionic contrast media may be injected, followed by the injection of local anesthetics, corticosteroids or adjuncts (Figures 15–13 and 15–14). We usually do not advance the catheter higher than the level of the L4 vertebral body, although we have occasionally advanced it to the L1 or L2 level. Some authorities suggest avoiding advancement more than 8–12 cm cephaladly.

Clinical Pearl

Spread of local anesthetic solutions injected into the caudal epidural space is influenced by injected volume, speed of injection, and patient position.

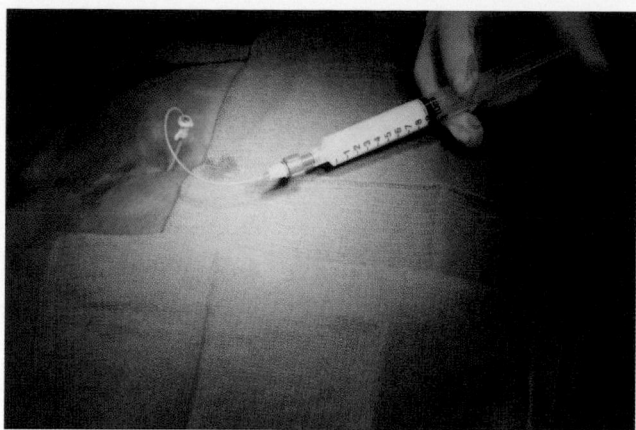

Figure 15–13. A syringe loaded with radiopaque contrast medium is attached to the continuous catheter or catheter system in place in the caudal epidural space. Injection of mixture of local anesthetic or corticosteroid medication (or both) into a continuous catheter placed into the caudal epidural space.

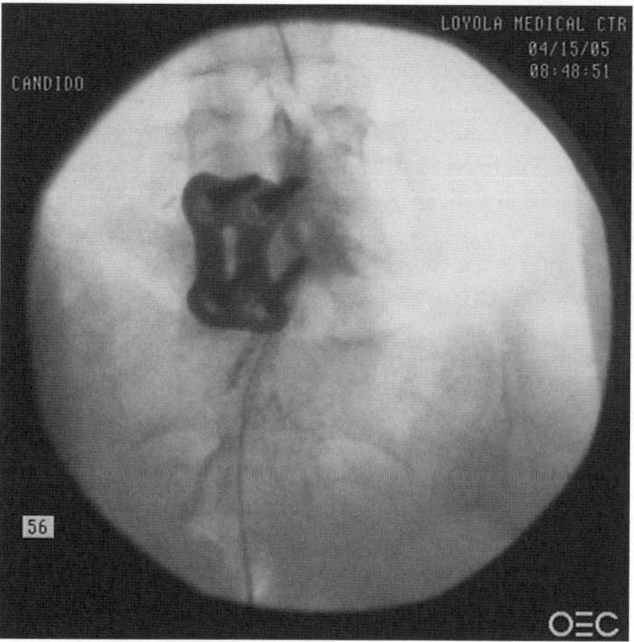

Figure 15–14. Anteroposterior fluoroscopic image depicting radiopaque contrast medium in the epidural space, beneath the patient's hardware from previous fusion surgery. In the face of previous spinal surgery, with or without hardware implantation, caudal epidural block may be significantly safer than conventional epidural block, since it obviates the need to penetrate the surgical scar.

CHARACTERISTICS & INDICATIONS OF CAUDAL EPIDURAL BLOCK IN ADULTS

Characteristics of the Blockade

Caudal epidural block results in sensory and motor block of the sacral roots and limited autonomic block. The sacral contribution of the parasympathetic nervous system is blocked, causing loss of visceromotor function of the bladder and intestines distal to the colonic splenic flexure. Sympathetic block, though limited compared with lumbar or thoracic epidural block, does occur. However, the sympathetic outflow from the spinal cord ends at the L2 level, and, therefore, caudal block should not routinely result in peripheral vasodilatation of the lower extremities to the degree witnessed with lumbar epidural blockade. Caudal epidural local anesthetic block in adults may be chosen for surgeries of the lower abdomen, perineum, or lower extremities. The local anesthetic mixtures and doses are similar to those for lumbar epidural block (Table 15–2).

Spread of the Local Anesthetic Solutions

The large capacity of the sacral canal accommodates correspondingly large volumes of solution; significant volumes may be lost through the wide anterior sacral foramina. Therefore, the caudal dose requirements of local anesthetics are significantly larger to effect the same segmental spread than are the corresponding lumbar doses. Roughly twice the lumbar epidural local anesthetic dose is needed for caudal blockade to attain similar levels of analgesia and anesthesia, and solutions injected in the caudal space take longer to spread (see Table 15–2). Bromage noted that age is not correlated with caudal segmental spread in adults and the upper level of analgesia resulting from 20-mL doses of local anesthetic solution varies widely between S2 and T8.[1] This unpredictability limits the usefulness of applying caudal anesthesia for surgical procedures that require cephalad analgesia levels above the pelvic level or the umbilicus. A recent study reconfirmed Bromage's findings. In 172 women undergoing minor gynecologic surgery using caudal anesthesia with 20 mL of 1.5% lidocaine, the highest sensory dermatome level reached was below T10.[28]

Clinical Pearls

- The sacral canal contains the cauda equina (including the filum terminale), the spinal meninges, adipose tissue, and the sacral venous plexus.
- The volume of the sacral canal averages 14.4 mL, but varies from 9.5 to 26.6 mL.
- The indications for performing caudal epidural block are essentially the same as for lumbar epidural block.
- Percutaneous epidural neuroplasty is a technique of administering local anesthetics, corticosteroids, hyaluronidase, and hypertonic saline through a caudal catheter for the purpose of lysing epidural adhesions.
- Adult patients are typically placed prone for the block, whereas the lateral decubitus position is preferred for pediatrics.
- Caudal blockade in pediatrics is used primarily for perioperative pain control, whereas in adults it is primarily for chronic pain management.

Table 15–2.

Local Anesthetics Commonly Used for Caudal Anesthesia in Adults[a,b]

AGENT	CONCENTRATION (%)	DOSE (mg)	SENSORY ONSET (4-segment spread) (min)	DURATION (2-segment regression) (min)
Lidocaine	1.5–2	300–600	10–20	90–150
Chloroprocaine	2–3	400–900	8–15	45–80
Mepivacaine	2	400–600	10–20	90–240
Ropivacaine	0.75–1	150–300	15–25	120–210
Bupivacaine/ Levobupivacaine	0.5–0.75	100–225	10–25	180–270

[a] *All solutions with epinephrine 1:200,000, except ropivacaine.*
[b] *All doses and times approximate.*

■ In adults, roughly twice the local anesthetic dose is required to attain the same segmental spread with caudal block compared with the dose used for lumbar epidural block.

Indications in Adults

Caudal block is indicated whenever the area of surgery involves the sacral and lower lumbar nerve roots. The technique is suitable for anal surgery (hemorrhoidectomy and anal dilatation), gynecologic procedures, surgery on the penis or scrotum, and lower limb surgeries. Using a catheter technique, it is possible to use caudal epidural block for vaginal hysterectomy and inguinal herniorrhaphy.

Caudal epidural block is used less frequently than lumbar or even thoracic epidural block for providing perioperative analgesia in adults. The pelvis enlarges markedly in puberty while the epidural fat in the lumbosacral region undergoes compaction and increased fibrous content. This hinders cephalad spread of solutions particularly when compared with the spread in children.

As an alternative to caudal epidural block in adults, one might consider a median approach to transsacral epidural block. In the original description of that technique, 87% of blocks were successful for transurethral resection of bladder tumors versus 100% success for sacral procedures. Anesthesia level, side effects, and hemodynamics were similar between the two groups studied in that initial report.[29]

■ CAUDAL BLOCK FOR LABOR ANALGESIA

The sacral canal shares in the general engorgement of extradural veins that occurs in late pregnancy, or in any clinical condition in which the inferior vena cava (IVC) is partially obstructed. Since the effective volume of the caudal canal is markedly diminished during the latter part of pregnancy, the caudal dosage should be reduced proportionately in women at term. The segmental spread of local anesthetics may increase substantially in pregnant women at term, necessitating a 28% to 33% decrease of dose requirement in this patient population.[1] The choice of a continuous catheter or a single-shot technique during active labor is limited by the relative lack of sterility at the sacral hiatus, which may be contaminated by feces and meconium.

Rare cases of Horner syndrome have been noted when large doses of local anesthetics are injected caudally during labor.[1] This is most likely to occur if injection is made with the patient on her back (engorgement of epidural venous plexus and IVC compression are maximal). The so-called dual technique (lumbar and caudal) of epidural block for labor is no longer widely used. Since the pain of uterine contractions is mediated by sympathetic nervous system fibers originating from T10 to L2, a lumbar epidural catheter suffices for both stage I and stage II of parturition, with dosage adjustments being made depending on the exact circumstances and requirements. Labor analgesia is discussed in greater detail in Chapter 53 (Regional Anesthesia for the Obstetric Patient).

■ CHARACTERISTICS & INDICATIONS OF CAUDAL EPIDURAL BLOCK IN CHILDREN

Characteristics of the Blockade

The sacral hiatus is usually very easy to palpate in infants and children, which makes this technique much easier and more predictable in children. Consequently, in many institutions with large numbers of pediatric patients, caudal epidural block is an integral part of the intra- and postoperative pain management for children undergoing a wide range of surgical procedures both below and above the diaphragm.

The technique is easily learned; one study demonstrated an 80% success rate in resident trainees after completing 32 procedures performed without fluoroscopic guidance.[30] In infants and small children, a 21-gauge short-beveled 1-in. needle may be used for single-injection techniques. For continuous blocks, a standard epidural catheter may be advanced through an 18-gauge angiocatheter or a thin walled 18-gauge epidural needle. It has been noted that by 4 or 5 years of age the sacral canal is usually large enough to accept such a needle for passage of a catheter.[1] The electrocardiogram has been used to verify appropriate thoracic catheter tip placement (epidural electrocardiography).[31]

Spread of the Local Anesthetic Solutions

Unlike in adults, the segmental spread of analgesia following caudal administration is more predictable in children up to about 12 years of age. Studies suggest that the cephalad spread of caudal solutions in children is not hampered by the same anatomic constraints that develop from puberty onward. Before puberty, anatomic impedance at the lumbosacral junction has not yet developed to a marked degree, and caudal solutions can flow freely upward into the higher recesses of the spinal canal. As a consequence, the rostral spread of caudal anesthesia is more extensive and more predictable in children than in adults.

Indications in Adults

In children, caudal block is usually combined with light general anesthesia with spontaneous ventilation. During lower abdominal and genitourinary surgery in children, caudal block with 0.25% bupivacaine (2 mg/kg) was shown to lower the metabolic and endocrine responses to stress, as measured by glucose concentrations, mean prolactin, insulin, and cortisol concentrations, as compared with general anesthesia alone.[32] Thoracic placement of catheters is possible in neonates and small children. However, one radiographic study of 115 infants found 10 caudally placed catheters to be in the high thoracic or low cervical region, when their intended site was in the lower thoracic segments.[33]

Clinical Pearls

- The following are the three groups of indications for caudal epidural block in children:
  1. Patients requiring sacral block (circumcision, anal surgery)
  2. Patients requiring lower thoracic block (inguinal herniorrhaphy)
  3. Patients requiring analgesia of the upper thoracic dermatomes (in some circumstances)

Pharmacologic Considerations for Caudal Epidural Anesthesia in Children

Caudal block with bupivacaine (4 mg/kg) and morphine (150 mcg/kg) was found to lower fentanyl requirements during cardiac surgery and shorten extubation times in a group of 30 pediatric patients randomized to receive general anesthesia alone or a combination of general and caudal block.[34]

Anesthetic dose requirements are about 0.1 mL/segment/year of age for 1% lidocaine or 0.25% bupivacaine.[1] The dose may also be calculated based on body weight. The relationship between age and dose requirements is strictly linear with a high degree of correlation up to 12 years old. Plasma bupivacaine concentrations in children receiving caudal block with 0.2% of the local anesthetic (2 mg/kg) were less than equivalent doses administered via ilioinguinal–iliohypogastric block for pain control following herniotomy or orchidopexy. Additionally, the times to peak plasma concentrations were faster in the peripheral nerve block group, indicating that caudal block is a safe alternative to local infiltration techniques in inguinal surgery.[35] In a study of children 1 to 6 years of age who underwent orchidopexy, a caudal block using larger volumes of dilute bupivacaine (0.2%) was shown to be more effective than a smaller volume of the standard (0.25%) concentration in blocking the peritoneal response to spermatic cord traction, with no change in the quality of postoperative analgesia. In that study the total bupivacaine dose was identical in both groups (20 mg).[36]

Ropivacaine 0.5% was shown to provide a significantly longer duration of analgesia following inguinal herniorrhaphy in children 1.5 to 7 years of age compared with 0.25% ropivacaine or 0.25% bupivacaine.[37] All children received 0.75 mL/kg of the local anesthetic. Unfortunately, however, the times to first voiding and to standing were significantly delayed in the group receiving 0.5% ropivacaine, and there was one case of motor block of the lower extremities. This demonstrates the tradeoff when one attempts to maximize analgesia by altering local anesthetic concentration or total dose.

Ropivacaine has also been used for caudal block for hypospadias repair in a double-blind, randomized study in 26 children. The minimal effective local anesthetic concentration of ropivacaine was found to be 0.11% under general anesthesia with a 0.5% monitored anesthesia care of enflurane.[38] Plasma concentrations of ropivacaine after caudal block in 20 children 1 to 8 years of age, using 2 mg/mL, 1 mL/kg, demonstrated free fractions to be 5%, clearance of 7.4 mL/min/kg, and terminal half-life of 3.2 h, well below those associated with toxic symptoms in adults.[39] Clonidine has been added to bupivacaine in 36 children undergoing elective surgery. A caudal catheter was placed using 1 mg/kg bupivacaine 0.125% with an equal volume of either clonidine (2 mcg/kg) or normal saline. No benefit of adding the clonidine was found, and, in addition, more children in the clonidine group vomited in the first 24 h postoperatively.[40]

The local anesthetics typically administered for single-shot caudal blocks in pediatric patients are listed in Table 15–3.

Table 15–3.

Typical Local Anesthetics for Caudal Block in Pediatric Patients (single–shot)

Agent	Concentration (%)	Dose	Onset (min)	Duration of Action (min)
Ropivacaine[50]	0.2	2 mg/kg	9	520
Bupivacaine[50]	0.25	2 mg/kg	12	253
Ropivacaine[51]	0.2	0.7 mg/kg	11.7	491
Bupivacaine[51]	0.25	0.7 mg/kg	13.1	457
Ropivacaine[52]	0.2	1 mL/kg	8.4	Not available
Levobupivacaine[52]	0.25	1 mL/kg	8.8	Not available
Bupivacaine[52]	0.25	1 mL/kg	8.8	Not available

Clinical Pearls

- The success of a caudal block in pediatric patients may be predicted from the laxity of the anal sphincter secondary to the reduction in sphincter tone from the local anesthetic block.

- This is fortuitous since most caudal blocks in children are performed while the child is anesthetized, and it is not possible to assess the effectiveness of the block by testing for sensory analgesia levels.

- One study demonstrated that the presence of a lax anal sphincter at the termination of surgery correlated with the reduced need to administer opioids perioperatively.[41]

Other Considerations for Use of Caudal Epidural Anesthesia in Children

Although caudal block is a mainstay of perioperative pain management in pediatric surgery and represents probably 60% of all regional anesthetic techniques in this patient population, not all studies demonstrated a marked benefit of caudal block for postoperative analgesia compared with other modalities. Following unilateral inguinal herniorrhaphy, caudal block was shown to provide effective, but not superior, pain management compared with local wound infiltration in 54 children. The side effects and rescue analgesia requirements did not differ between the two groups.[42]

Caudal epidural block in children may induce significant changes in descending aortic blood flow while maintaining heart rate and mean arterial blood pressure. In a study of 10 children 2 months to 5 years of age, a transesophageal Doppler probe was used to calculate hemodynamic variables after the injection of 1 mL/kg of 0.25% bupivacaine with epinephrine 5 mcg/mL. The aortic ejection volume increased, and aortic vascular resistance decreased by about 40%.[43] These data suggest that caudal block results in vasodilatation secondary to sympathetic nervous system blockade.

APPLICATIONS OF CAUDAL EPIDURAL BLOCK IN ACUTE & CHRONIC PAIN MANAGEMENT

Radiculopathy Refractory to Conventional Therapy

In cases of radiculopathy that is refractory to conventional therapies, caudal epidural treatment can significantly reduce the pain. Percutaneous epidural neuroplasty uses a caudal catheter left in place for up to 3 days to inject hypertonic solutions into the epidural space to treat radiculopathy with low back pain and epidural scarring, typically from previous lumbar spinal surgery. In addition to local anesthetics and corticosteroids, hypertonic saline and hyaluronidase are added to the injectate. The technique relies on fluoroscopic guidance and caudal epidurography, because the fluoroscopic findings of a filling defect of injected iodinated nonionic contrast medium correlates with the patient's reported level of pain.[15] Injection of solutions into the epidural space of a patient with adhesions may be quite painful because of distension of affected nerve roots.[14] Triamcinolone acetate, dexamethasone, or betamethasone have been recommended instead of methylprednisolone since particulate steroids can occlude an epidural catheter or possibly cause infarction of spinal tissue via vascular injection. Hypertonic saline is also used to prolong pain relief due to its local anesthetic effect and its ability to reduce edema in previously scarred or inflamed nerve roots.[14] The authors recommend a lateral needle placement into the caudal canal, directing the needle and catheter toward the affected side. Lateral placement tends to minimize the likelihood of penetrating the dural sac or subdural area.

When 5–10 mL of contrast medium is injected into the caudal canal through an epidural catheter, a "Christmas-tree" appearance develops as dye spreads into the perineural structures inside the bony canal and along the nerves as they exit the vertebral column.[14] Epidural adhesions prevent the spread of the dye so there is no outline of the involved nerve roots.

> ## Clinical Pearl
>
> - When the needle or catheter is inadvertently placed in the subarachnoid space, the fluoroscopic image will show the spread of the dye centrally and cephaladly to a level higher than that attained with epidural spread.

Once correct catheter placement in the epidural space is ensured, 1500 units of hyaluronidase in 10 mL of preservative-free saline is injected rapidly. This is followed by an injection of 10 mL of 0.2% ropivacaine and 40 mg of triamcinolone. Following these two injections, an additional injection of 9 mL of 10% hypertonic saline is infused over 20 to 30 min. On the second and third days, the local anesthetic (ropivacaine) injection is followed up by the hypertonic saline solution. Antibiotic coverage is provided to reduce the possibility of epidural abscess formation.

Postoperative Analgesia in Patients Undergoing Lumbar Spine Surgery

Another unique application of caudal block is to provide postoperative analgesia in patients undergoing lumbar spine surgeries. In one series, patients received 20 mL of 0.25% bupivacaine with 0.1 mg buprenorphine via the caudal epidural approach, performed prior to surgical incision. The patients underwent posterior interbody fusion and laminotomy for spinal stenosis, and postoperative pain control was compared in the caudal group with a group treated with conventional parenteral opioids. The caudal group required less rescue analgesic medication doses over the first 12 h following surgery.[16] A reduction in blood pressure in the caudal group patients undergoing laminotomy, but not fusion, was noted in the patients with a prolonged duration (24 h) of postoperative analgesia.

Other Applications

Caudal epidural block has also been compared with intramuscular opioids in the treatment of pain after emergency lower extremity orthopedic surgery. The caudal group received 20 mL of 0.5% bupivacaine and had 8 h of superior analgesia with a concomitant significant reduction in the need for rescue opioid medications.[17]

Caudal injection of clonidine, 75 mcg with 7 mL bupivacaine 0.5% and 7 mL lidocaine 2% with epinephrine 5 mcg/mL has been used for postoperative analgesia after elective hemorrhoidectomy. Thirty-two adults received the clonidine–local combination while a control group received local anesthetic alone. Analgesia averaged 12 hours in the clonidine group, compared to <5 h in the group receiving only local anesthetic. Bradycardia occurred in about 22% of patients in the clonidine group.[18] This contrasts with the results of an evaluation of clonidine used as an adjunct for pediatric caudal anesthesia as noted earlier.[40]

Caudal injections of alcohol or phenol have been used to treat intractable pain due to cancer. In a study of 67 blocks, it was found that the lower sacral roots were easily reached with the caudal injection, and that the S1 and S2 roots (contribution from the lumbosacral plexus) were spared.[19]

COMPLICATIONS ASSOCIATED WITH CAUDAL EPIDURAL BLOCK

The complications of caudal block are similar to those occurring following lumbar epidural block and include complications related to the technique itself and complications related to the injectate (local anesthetic or other injected substance). Fortunately, serious complications occur infrequently. The list of possibilities includes epidural abscess, meningitis, epidural hematoma, dural puncture and postdural puncture, headache, subdural injection, pneumocephalus and air embolism, back pain, and broken or knotted epidural catheters.

Systemic Toxicity of Local Anesthetics

The incidence of local anesthetic-induced seizures occurs more frequently following caudal epidural block than it does following lumbar or thoracic approaches. In a retrospective study of 25,697 patients who received brachial plexus blocks, caudal or lumbar epidural blocks from 1985 to 1992, Brown noted 26 seizures.[44] The frequency of seizures in adults was caudal > brachial plexus block > lumbar or thoracic epidural block. Nine overall seizures were attributed to local anesthetic injection in the caudal space, eight occurring with chloroprocaine and one occurring with lidocaine. There was a 70-fold increased incidence (0.69%) of local anesthetic toxic reactions with caudal epidural anesthesia than with lumbar or thoracic epidural anesthesia in adults.

> ## Clinical Pearls
>
> - The incidence of local anesthetic-induced seizures occurs more frequently following caudal epidural block than it does following lumbar or thoracic approaches.
> - The risk of local anesthetic toxicity follows this order: caudal > brachial plexus block > lumbar or thoracic epidural block.
> - Elevation of heart rate by >10 bpm or an increase in systolic blood pressure of >15 mm Hg after injection of epinephrine-containing local anesthetic is indicative of intravascular injection.

In children, however, one retrospective review identified only two toxic reactions (ie, local anesthetic-induced seizures) in 15,000 caudal blocks.[45] Dalens' group found that inadvertent intravascular injection occurs in up to 0.4% of pediatric caudal blocks,[46] demonstrating the importance of performing epinephrine-containing test dosing in this age group. It has been suggested that an elevation of heart rate by >10 bpm or an increase in systolic blood pressure of >15 mm Hg should be taken as indicative of systemic injection. T wave changes on the ECG occur earliest following intravascular injection, followed by heart rate changes, and lastly, by blood pressure changes. These changes may be delayed for up to 90 sec following the injection.[46]

Development of Spinal Anesthesia

Total spinal anesthesia can occur when the injected solution of local anesthetic gains access to the subarachnoid space. In the case report of an 18-month-old child weighing 10 kg who received a caudal block postoperatively after undergoing emergency repair of a recurrent diaphragmatic hernia 4 mL of 0.5% bupivacaine and 2.5 mcg/kg of buprenorphine were injected in a total volume of 10 mL. Eye opening and hand movement were delayed for 3 h following this complication.[47] In another infant undergoing revision of a fundoplication, a caudally placed catheter was inadvertently advanced to the cervical spinal region. Electrical stimulation of the catheter tip (Tsui test) resulted in phrenic nerve stimulation. On withdrawal and repositioning of the catheter further care was uncomplicated. This case report demonstrates the relative ease of passing the catheter to high vertebral levels in infants as opposed to adults.[48]

Infection

One case report documented the rare occurrence of distant discitis and vertebral osteomyelitis involving skip levels and without the development of epidural abscess formation in an elderly woman who received caudal epidural steroid and local anesthetic for degenerative spondylolisthesis. One month later she developed an L2-L3 and L4-L5 infective discitis, together with adjacent vertebral osteomyelitis. Cultures demonstrated *Pseudomonas aeruginosa* growth, which was treated with antibiotics.[49]

SUMMARY

Caudal epidural block is a technique of providing analgesia and anesthesia of the lumbosacral nerve roots that predates conventional lumbar approaches. The block has undergone several periods of acceptability and although it is infrequently applied to routine surgical cases in adults, it is the most commonly performed regional anesthetic technique in infants and children. Caudal block has enjoyed a resurgence lately, largely due to its easy access to the lumbar epidural space beneath scarring from spinal surgeries and for performing epiduroscopy. Clinicians who routinely utilize fluoroscopy will find that it has many applications, both for routine and complicated cases.

References

1. Bromage PR: *Epidural Analgesia.* WB Saunders, 1978, pp 258–282.
2. Racz G: Personal communication; October 12, 2003, American Society of Anesthesiologists Annual Meeting, San Francisco, Ca.
3. Trotter M: Variations of the sacral canal: Their significance in the administration of caudal analgesia. Anesth Analg 1947;26:192–202.
4. MacDonald A, Chatrath P, Spector T, et al: Level of termination of the spinal cord and the dural sac: A magnetic resonance study. Clin Anat 1999;12:149–152.
5. Igarashi T, Hirabayashi Y, Shimizu R, et al: The lumbar extradural structure changes with increasing age. Br J Anaesth 1997;78:149–152.
6. Crighton I, Barry B, Hobbs G: A study of the anatomy of the caudal space using magnetic resonance imaging. Br J Anaesth 1997;78:391–395.
7. Sekiguchi M, Yabuki S, Satoh K, et al: An anatomic study of the sacral hiatus: A basis for successful caudal epidural block. Clin J Pain 2004;20:51–54.
8. Bryce-Smith R: The spread of solutions in the extradural space. Anaesthesia 1954;9:201–205.
9. Brenner E: Sacral anesthesia. Ann Surg 1924;79:118–123.
10. Waldman S: Caudal epidural nerve block. In Waldman S (ed): *Interventional Pain Management,* 2nd ed. WB Saunders, 2001, p 520.
11. Winnie A, Candido KD: Differential neural blockade for the diagnosis of pain. In Waldman S (ed): *Interventional Pain Management,* 2nd ed. WB Saunders, 2001, pp 162–173.
12. Candido KD, Stevens RA: Intrathecal neurolytic blocks for the relief of cancer pain. Van Aken H. (ed). Best Pract Res Clin Anaesthesiol, 2003;17:407–428.
13. Lou L, Racz G, Heavner J: Percutaneous epidural neuroplasty. In Waldman S (ed): *Interventional Pain Management,* 2nd ed. WB Saunders, 2001, pp 434–445.
14. Heavner J, Racz G, Raj P: Percutaneous epidural neuroplasty: Prospective evaluation of 0.9% NaCl versus 10% NaCl with or without hyaluronidase. Reg Anesth Pain Med 1999;24:202–207.
15. Manchikanti L, Bakhit C, Pampati V: Role of epidurography in caudal neuroplasty. Pain Digest 1998;8:277–281.
16. Kakiuchi M, Abe K: Pre-incisional caudal epidural blockade and the relief of pain after lumbar spine operations. Int Orthop 1997;21:62–66.
17. McCrirrick A, Ramage D: Caudal blockade for postoperative analgesia: A useful adjunct to intramuscular opiates following emergency lower leg orthopaedic surgery. Anaesth Intensive Care 1991;19:551–554.
18. Van Elstraete A, Pastureau F, Lebrun T, et al: Caudal clonidine for postoperative analgesia in adults. Br J Anaesth 2000;84:401–402.
19. Porges P, Zdrahal F: Intrathecal alcohol neurolysis of the lower sacral roots in inoperable rectal cancer. (German) Anaesthetist 1985;34:627–629.
20. Chan S, Tay H, Thomas E: "Whoosh" test as a teaching aid in caudal block. Anaesth Intensive Care 1993;21:414–415.
21. Orme R, Berg S: The "swoosh" test—an evaluation of a modified "whoosh" test in children. Br J Anaesth 2003;91:157.
22. Tsui B, Tarkkila P, Gupta S, et al: Confirmation of caudal needle placement using nerve stimulation. Anesthesiology 1999;91:374–378.
23. Digiovanni A: Inadvertent interosseous injection—A hazard of caudal anesthesia. Anesthesiology 1971;34:92–94.
24. Lofstrom B: Caudal anaesthesia. In Ejnar Eriksson (ed): *Illustrated Handbook in Local Anaesthesia.* AB Astra, 1969, pp 129–134.
25. Caudal block. In Covino BG, Scott DB (eds): *Handbook of Epidural Anaesthesia and Analgesia.* Grune & Stratton, 1985, pp 104–108.
26. Dawkins C: An analysis of the complications of extradural and caudal block. Anaesthesia 1969;24:554–563.

27. Chung Y, Lin C, Pang W, et al: An alternative continuous caudal block with caudad catheterization via lower lumbar interspace in adult patients. Acta Anaesthesiol Scand 1998;36:221–227.

28. Wong S, Li J, Chen C, et al: Caudal epidural block for minor gynecologic procedures in outpatient surgery. Chang Gung Med J 2004;27:116–121.

29. Nishiyama T, Hanaoka K, Ochiai Y: The median approach to transsacral epidural block. Anesth Analg 2002;95:1067–1070.

30. Schuepfer G, Konrad C, Schmeck J, et al: Generating a learning curve for pediatric caudal epidural blocks: An empirical evaluation of technical skills in novice and experienced anesthesiologists. Reg Anesth Pain Med 2000;25:385–388.

31. Tsui B, Seal R, Koller J: Thoracic epidural catheter placement via the caudal approach in infants by using electrocardiographic guidance. Anesth Analg 2002;95:326–330.

32. Tuncer S, Yosunkaya A, Reisli R, et al: Effect of caudal block on stress response in children. Pediatr Int 2004;46:53–57.

33. Valairucha S, Seefelder C, Houck C: Thoracic epidural catheters placed by the caudal route in infants: The importance of radiographic confirmation. Paediatr Anaesth 2002;12:424–428.

34. Rojas-Perez E, Castillo-Zamora C, Nava-Ocampo A: A randomized trial of caudal block with bupivacaine 4 mg × kg-1 (1.8 mL × kg-1) plus morphine (150 micrograms × kg-1) vs general anaesthesia with fentanyl for cardiac surgery. Paediatr Anaesth 2003;13:311–317.

35. Stow P, Scott A, Phillips A, et al: Plasma bupivacaine concentrations during caudal analgesia and ilioinguinal-iliohypogastric nerve block in children. Anaesthesia 1988;43:650–653.

36. Verghese S, Hannallah R, Rice LJ, et al: Caudal anesthesia in children: Effect of volume versus concentration of bupivacaine on blocking spermatic cord traction response during orchidopexy. Anesth Analg 2002;95:1219–1223.

37. Koinig H, Krenn C, Glaser C, et al: The dose-response of caudal ropivacaine in children. Anesthesiology 1999;90:1339–1344.

38. Deng S, Xiao, W, Tang G, et al: The minimum local anesthetic concentration of ropivacaine for caudal analgesia in children. Anesth Analg 2002;94:1465–1468.

39. Lonnqvist P, Westrin P, Larsson B, et al: Ropivacaine pharmacokinetics after caudal block in 1–8 year old children. Br J Anaesth 2000;85:506–511.

40. Joshi W, Connelly R, Freeman K, et al: Analgesic effect of clonidine added to bupivacaine 0.125% in paediatric caudal blockade. Paediatr Anaesth 2004;14:483–486.

41. Verghese S, Mostello L, Patel R: Testing anal sphincter tone predicts the effectiveness of caudal analgesia in children. Anesth Analg 2002;94:1161–1164.

42. Schindler M, Swann M, Crawford M: A comparison of postoperative analgesia provided by wound infiltration or caudal analgesia. Anesth Intensive Care 1991;19:46–49.

43. Larousse E, Asehnoune K, Dartayet B, et al: The hemodynamic effects of pediatric caudal anesthesia assessed by esophageal Doppler. Anesth Analg 2002;94:1165–1168.

44. Brown D, Ransom D, Hall J, et al: Regional anesthesia and local anesthetic-induced systemic toxicity: Seizure frequency and accompanying cardiovascular changes. Anesth Analg 1995;81:321–328.

45. Giaufre E, Dalens B, Gombert A: Epidemiology and morbidity of regional anesthesia in children: A one-year prospective survey of the French-language Society of Pediatric Anesthesiologists. Anesth Analg 1996;83:904–912.

46. Dalens B, Hansanoui A: Caudal anesthesia in pediatric surgery: Success rate and adverse effects in 750 consecutive patients. Anesth Analg 1989;8:83–89.

47. Afshan G, Khan F: Total spinal anaesthesia following caudal block with bupivacaine and buprenorphine. Paediatr Anaesth 1996;6: 239–242.

48. Tsui B, Malherbe S: Inadvertent cervical epidural catheter placement via the caudal route using electrical stimulation. Anesth Analg 2004;99:259–261.

49. Yue W, Tan S: Distant skip level discitis and vertebral osteomyelitis after caudal epidural injection: A case report of a rare complication of epidural injections. Spine 2003;1:209–211.

50. Ivani G, Mereto N, Lampugnani E, et al: Ropivacaine in paediatric surgery: Preliminary results (abstr). Paediatr Anaesth 1998;8:127–129.

51. Ivani G, Lampugnani E, De Negri P, et al: Ropivacaine vs bupivacaine in major surgery in infants (abstr). Can J Anaesth 1999;46:467–469.

52. Ivani G, DeNegri P, Conio A, et al: Comparison of racemic bupivacaine, ropivacaine and levobupivacaine for pediatric caudal anesthesia. Effects on postoperative analgesia and motor blockade. Reg Anesth Pain Med 2002;27:157–161.

16

Combined Spinal–Epidural Anesthesia

J. Sudharma Ranasinghe, MD, FFARCSI • Elyad Davidson, MD • David J. Birnbach, MD

INTRODUCTION

In recent years, regional anesthesia techniques for surgery, obstetrics, and postoperative pain management have been used with increasing frequency.[1–3] The combined spinal–epidural (CSE) technique, a comparatively new anesthetic technique, includes an initial subarachnoid injection followed by epidural catheter placement and administration of epidural medications. This allows for almost immediate relief of pain or induction of regional anesthesia by the rapid onset of the spinal drugs, and subsequent administration of medications for prolonged anesthesia. In addition postoperative analgesia via the epidural catheter can be delivered for extended periods.

Clinical studies have demonstrated that the CSE technique provides excellent surgical conditions as quickly as the single-shot subarachnoid (SSS) block, and with advantages compared with the epidural block alone.[4–6] The introduction of CSE anesthesia offers benefits of both spinal and epidural anesthesia.

Although the CSE technique has become increasingly popular over the past two decades, it is a more complex technique that requires comprehensive understanding of epidural and spinal physiology and pharmacology.

This chapter discusses the technical aspects, advantages, potential complications, and limitations of the CSE technique for surgery and analgesia during labor.

CLINICAL USE OF CSE ANESTHESIA

The results of a recent survey demonstrate wide variation in CSE use and practice among experienced anesthesiologists,[7] reflecting concern over the frequency of CSE-related complications,[8,9] controversy over the technique,[10,11] and the potential for higher failure rates with CSE than with individual spinal or other anesthetic techniques.[12]

General Surgery

In the literature, the technique has been described for use in general, orthopedic, and trauma surgery of lower limb, as well as in urologic and gynecologic surgery. Clinical studies have demonstrated that the CSE technique provides excellent surgical conditions as quickly as with SSS block—conditions that are better than with epidural block alone.[4,13] With the CSE technique, surgical anesthesia is established rapidly, saving 15–20 min compared with epidural anesthesia. Furthermore, epidural catheterization provides the possibility of supplementing subarachnoid anesthesia, which may be insufficient when used alone. In a recent article it was also observed that various needles can be used in different combinations when performing CSE and may have different advantages and disadvantages for different patients and situations.[14] This will be discussed later in the chapter.

Labor Analgesia

The CSE technique is widely used in obstetric practice to provide optimal analgesia for parturients. It offers effective, rapid-onset analgesia with minimal risk of toxicity or motor block.[15] In addition, this technique provides the ability to prolong the duration of analgesia, as required, through the use of an epidural catheter. Furthermore, should an operative delivery become necessary, that same catheter can be used to provide operative anesthesia. The onset of spinal analgesia is almost immediate, and the duration is between 2 and 3 h, depending on which agent or agents are chosen. The duration of spinal analgesia, however, decreases when administered to a woman in advanced labor versus one in early labor.[16] Patients may have greater satisfaction

with CSE than with standard epidurals, perhaps because of a greater feeling of self-control.[17] The original description of spinal labor analgesia involved sufentanil or fentanyl,[18] but the addition of isobaric bupivacaine to the opioid produces a greater density of sensory blockade while still minimizing motor blockade.[19] Originally, 25 mcg of fentanyl or 10 mcg of sufentanil was advocated, but more recent studies have suggested using smaller doses of opioid combined with a local anesthetic.[20] For example, many clinicians are now routinely use 5 mcg of sufentanil or 15 mcg of intrathecal fentanyl. Recent studies have suggested that ropivacaine and levobupivacaine can be substituted for intrathecal bupivacaine to provide labor analgesia.[21,22] The CSE technique has also made ambulation possible for many women receiving neuraxial analgesia, although ambulation may be possible with other techniques. In addition to the advantage of rapid onset of pain relief, the CSE technique may reduce the incidence of several potential problems associated with the conventional epidural technique, including incomplete (patchy) blockade, motor block, and poor sacral spread. Another potential advantage of the CSE technique is that, as suggested by preliminary study, it may be associated with a significant reduction in the duration of the first stage of labor in primiparous parturients.[23,24]

Cesarean Delivery

The CSE technique, first reported as an option for cesarean section in 1984,[25] has recently increased dramatically in popularity. The advantage of this technique is that it provides rapid onset of dense surgical anesthesia while allowing the ability to prolong the block with an epidural catheter. In addition, because the block can be supplemented at any time, the CSE technique allows the use of smaller doses of spinal local anesthetics, which may in turn reduce the incidence of high spinal block or prolonged hypotension.[26] Potential problems of the CSE technique for cesarean delivery include an inability to test the catheter, the possibility of a failed epidural catheter after spinal injection, and the risk of enhanced spread of previously injected spinal drug after use of the epidural catheter.[27]

ADVANTAGES OF CSE

Compared with Conventional Epidural or Subarachnoid Anesthesia

When CSE block was compared with either epidural or subarachnoid block for hip or knee arthroplasty, CSE anesthesia was found to be superior to epidural anesthesia. With the CSE technique, surgical anesthesia was rapidly established, saving 15–20 min compared with epidural anesthesia. Furthermore, the epidural catheter provided the possibility of supplementing insufficient subarachnoid anesthesia.[4]

Patients who received the CSE technique had a more rapid onset of anesthesia and more intense motor blockade than those who received epidural anesthesia alone.

CSE has been reported to decrease the failure rate and incidence of adverse events of neuraxial analgesia.[28] In a retrospective analysis of 19,259 deliveries (75% neuraxial labor analgesia rate), the overall failure rate with this technique was 12%. The patients had adequate analgesia from initial placement, but 6.8% of patients had subsequent inadequate analgesia during labor and required epidural catheter replacement. Ultimately, 98.8% of all patients received adequate analgesia, even though 1.5% of patients had one or more replacements. However, when compared with epidural analgesia alone for labor, the incidence of overall failure, accidental intravascular placement of epidural catheters, accidental dural punctures, inadequate epidural analgesia, and catheter replacements were shown to be significantly lower in patients receiving CSE analgesia.[15,28,29]

Norris and coworkers. and Eappen and colleagues reported that CSE has higher success rate than the conventional epidural technique.[15,28] This difference may be due to the option to confirm questionable epidural location by successful spinal injection.

CSE enables low-dose spinal anesthesia for cesarean delivery.[30-34] When using SSS anesthesia for ambulatory surgery, many anesthesiologists tend to overdose because there is only one chance to ensure an effective spinal block. The presence of an epidural catheter as a "safety net" allows the anesthesiologist to use the lowest effective dose of local anesthetic. Urmey and coworkers used the CSE technique to investigate the appropriate dose of intrathecal isobaric lidocaine 2% for day-case arthroscopy.[35] The CSE technique provided excellent anesthesia for all 90 patients in his study. Patients receiving the smallest dose (40 mg) had a significantly shorter duration of anesthesia, which allowed quicker discharge than for the patients receiving 60 or 80 mg of intrathecal lidocaine.

Norris suggested the use of a CSE technique with intrathecal sufentanil alone for outpatient shock-wave lithotripsy, reserving the use of epidural catheter for patients with inadequate analgesia.[36]

Epidural volume extension (EVE) and enhancement of a small-dose intrathecal block by epidural saline infusion has been demonstrated via a CSE technique.[37] The advantage of this EVE technique is that a small-dose spinal block may provide an adequate level of anesthesia while allowing faster motor recovery of the lower limbs. In a prospective, randomized, double-blind study, the EVE technique was compared with SSS anesthesia with respect to its sensory and motor block profile and hemodynamic stability. Sixty-two patients scheduled for elective cesarean delivery were randomized to receive either spinal anesthesia with hyperbaric 0.5% bupivacaine (9 mg) and fentanyl (10 mcg) or CSE with intrathecal hyperbaric 0.5% bupivacaine (5 mg) with fentanyl (10 mcg), followed by 0.9% saline (6.0 mL) through the epidural catheter 5 min later. Both groups were comparable in terms of demographic data and duration of surgery. In the comparison of sensory block, both groups had similar peak sensory block height and VAS pain scores. The hemodynamic profile and ephedrine dose required were comparable between the two groups. Patients in the EVE group, however, demonstrated significantly faster motor recovery to modified Bromage score of 0 (73 ± 33 min versus 136 ± 32 min; $p < 0.05$). CSE with EVE provided adequate anesthesia with only 55% of the bupivacaine dose and allowed faster motor recovery of the lower limbs.

In another study, four different intrathecal doses of hyperbaric bupivacaine (2.5, 5, 7.5, and 10 mg) were compared in patients undergoing cesarean section under sequential CSE block, a technique that involves administration of a relatively small subarachnoid block that may be supplemented as needed by epidural local anesthetics. The authors demonstrated that 5 mg of intrathecal bupivacaine combined with an appropriate dose of epidural lidocaine provided adequate surgical analgesia while maintaining hemodynamic stability. Higher doses of intrathecal bupivacaine were associated with typical adverse effects of high subarachnoid block such as nausea, vomiting, and dyspnea.[38]

CSE for High-Risk Patients

The sequential CSE technique may be particularly advantageous in high-risk patients, such as those with cardiac disease, when slower onset of sympathetic blockade is desirable.[39] Most spinal anesthetics are administered as a single-injection procedure and rapid onset of sympathetic blockade may result in abrupt, severe hypotension. Traditionally, high-risk patients are treated with slow epidural anesthesia, which requires much higher total dosages of local anesthetic than is the case with sequential CSE. With careful positioning of the patient prior to induction of subarachnoid anesthetic, and by allowing titration with small incremental epidural doses to the precise level of anesthesia desired, the sequential CSE technique may enhance the safety of the neuraxial block.

In summary, CSE can reduce or eliminate many of the disadvantages of subarachnoid or epidural anesthesia alone while preserving their respective advantages. The CSE block offers the speed of onset, efficacy, and minimal toxicity of a subarachnoid block combined with the potential for improving an inadequate block or prolonging the duration of anesthesia with epidural supplements and extending the analgesia well into the postoperative period. Although the sequential CSE technique will take somewhat longer than the standard CSE technique, the use of minimal doses of local anesthetics has been shown to reduce the frequency and severity of hypotension when compared with epidural or spinal techniques.[40]

FUNCTIONAL ANATOMY RELATED TO CSE

When performing an epidural block, skin to epidural space distance (SED) and the posterior epidural space distance (PED) are measures that can help in reducing the inadvertent penetration of the dura and injury to neural structures.[41,42] The knowledge of these measures is also important in the success rate of epidural anesthesia. The PED, a measure of the epidural space depth, is particularly important with the CSE needle-through-needle (NTN) technique. Underestimation of this distance (short protrusion of the spinal needle through the epidural needle) will result in a higher incidence of spinal block failure. Any nonmidline approach also would increase the risk of not reaching the subarachnoid space because the dural sac has a triangular shape with the top pointing dorsally. Overestimation of PED will cause overprotrusion of the spinal needle that may increase the risk of neural damage.[43] These distances have been measured using various methods,[44] including MRI, CT, and measurement of CSE tip-to-tip distance or the amount of protrusion of the spinal needle beyond the Tuohy needle. The SED distance is most commonly 4 cm (50%) and is 4–6 cm in 80% of the population according to detailed records of 3200 cases.[44] The width of the PED varies with vertebral level, being the widest in the midlumbar region (5–6 mm) and decreasing toward the cervical vertebral column. In the midthoracic region, it is 3–5 mm in the midline and narrows laterally. In the lower cervical region, it is only 1.5–2 mm in the midline.[45] These spaces also correlate with the weight-to-height ratio and BMI.[46] Based on these measures, the present design of spinal needle protrusion varies between 10 and 15 mm beyond the epidural needle.

Epidural Space & Ligament Flavum

The thickness of the ligamentum flavum, distance to dura, and skin-to-dura distance vary with the area of vertebral canal (Table 16–1).

The two ligamenta flava are variably joined (fused) in the midline, and this fusion or lack of fusion of the ligamenta flavum occurs at different vertebral levels in individual patients. Lirk and coworkers investigated the incidence of midline gaps in the lumbar ligamentum flavum in embalmed cadavers.[47] Vertebral column specimens were obtained from

Table 16–1.

Characteristics of Ligamentum Flavum at Different Vertebral Levels

Site	Skin to Ligament (cm)	Thickness of Ligament (mm)
Cervical	—	1.5–3.0
Thoracic	—	3.0–5.0
Lumbar	3.0–8.0	5.0–6.0
Caudal	Variable	2.0–6.0

Data used, with permission, from Brown DL: Spinal, epidural, caudal anesthesia. In Miller RD (ed): Anesthesia, 6th ed. Churchill Livingstone, 2005, pp 1657.

45 human cadavers. The gaps in the lumbar ligamentum flavum are most frequent between L1 and L2 (22.2%) but are rare below this level (L2 through L3 = 11.4%, L3 through L4 = 11.1%, L4 through L5 = 9.3%, L5 through S1 = 0). Therefore, when using midline approach, one cannot rely on the ligamentum flavum to impede entering the epidural space in all patients.

TECHNIQUE

A number of recent reviews have discussed the technical factors related to performance and success of CSE.[48–50]

Although CSE is considered a new technique, Soresi in 1937 described the intentional injection of anesthetic agents outside and within the subarachnoid space.[51] Somewhat different from current practice, Soresi intentionally used a single needle. He first injected some local anesthetic into the epidural space and then advanced the needle and injected the rest of the medication to cause a subarachnoid block. Although this technique included both spinal and epidural anesthesia, no catheter was used. In 1979 Curelaru[52] reported the first CSE with an introduction of an epidural catheter through a Tuohy needle. Catheter insertion was followed by a test dose and then a traditional dural puncture, which was performed at a different interspace using a 26-gauge spinal needle. That same year, Brownridge suggested the use of CSE for obstetrics. He described successful use of CSE for elective cesarean section in 1981.[53,54] In 1982, the needle-through-needle (NTN) CSE technique was first described independently by Coates[55] and Mumtaz and colleagues,[56] and its use in obstetric practice was first published in 1984 by Carrie and O'Sullivan.[57]

Several approaches for initiation of CSE have been described in the recent literature.

Needle-Through-Needle Technique

In contrast to Serosi's description of CSE, in which a single needle was introduced into the epidural space and then

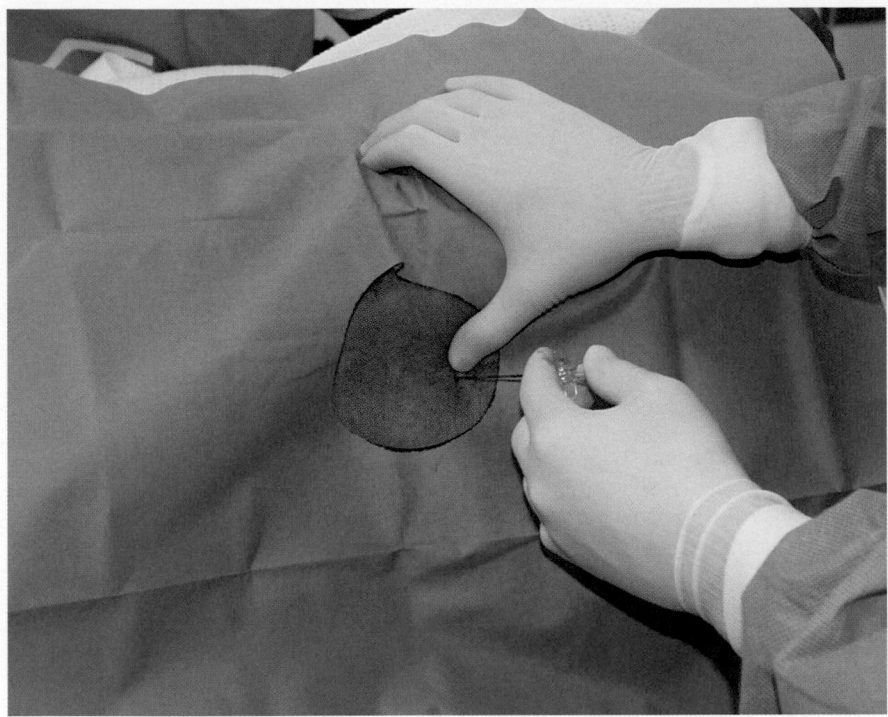

Figure 16–1. Epidural needle is placed in the epidural space indentically to the technique in epidural anesthesia.

advanced into the subarachnoid space, the needle-through-needle (NTN) technique includes use of separate epidural and spinal needles.

The epidural space is penetrated with a conventional epidural needle and technique, and then a long spinal needle is passed through the epidural needle until CSF appears in the hub of the spinal needle. Drug is administered into the subarachnoid space, the spinal needle is removed, and an epidural catheter is inserted into the epidural space (Figures 16–1 through 16–7). Although several different CSE techniques are used in clinical practice (including the two needle, two interspace technique), NTN is the most widely used CSE technique in the US.

Separate Needle Technique

CSE may be performed using two separate needles (separate needle technique; SNT), with spinal block and epidural

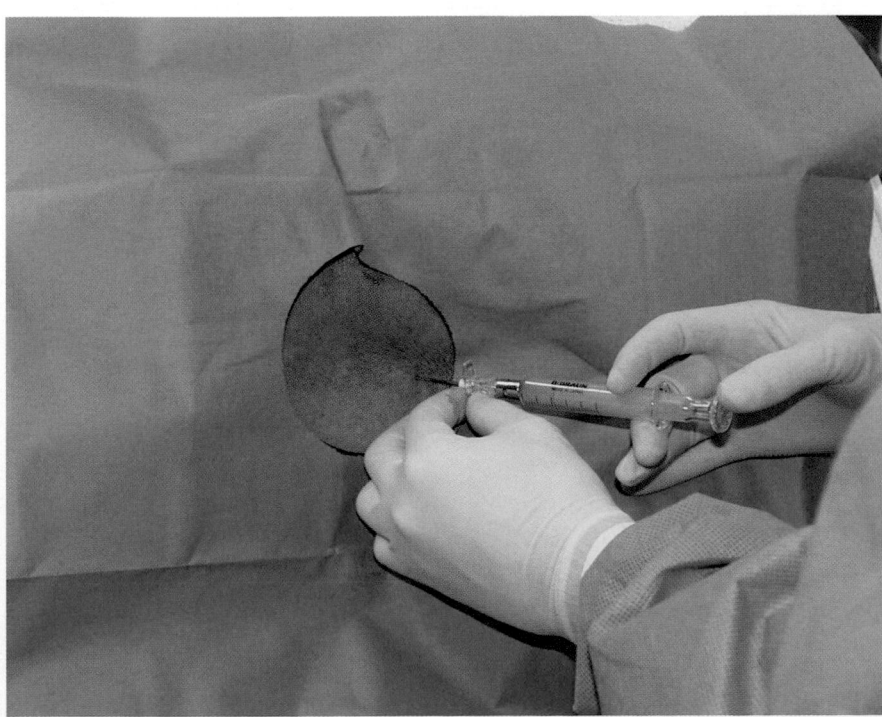

Figure 16–2. Figure 16–2. Entry of the needle into the epidural space is recognized by a sudden loss of resistance to injection of air.

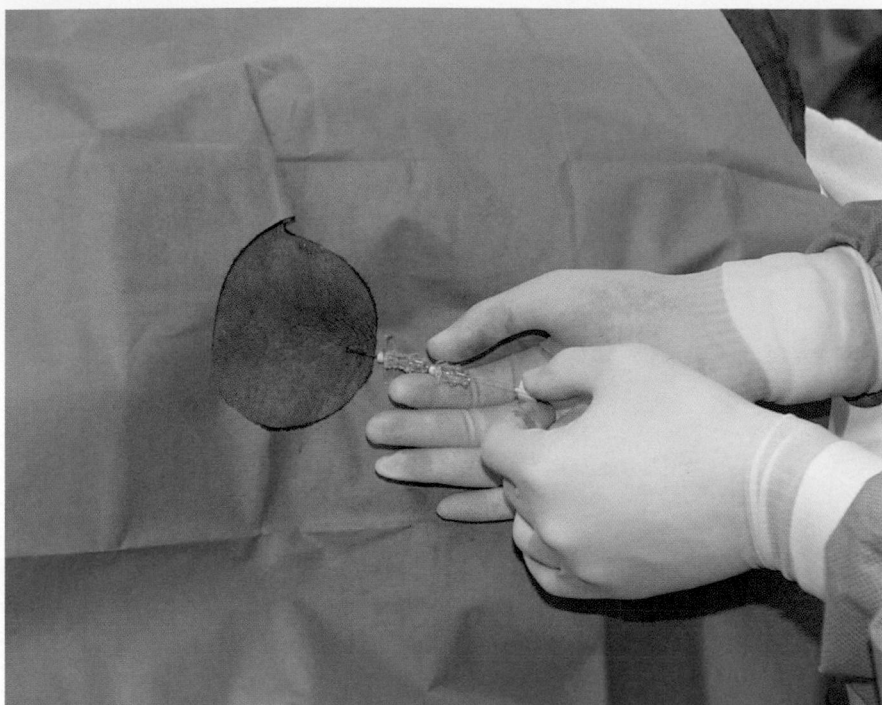

Figure 16–3. A small-bore spinal needle is placed through the epidural needle until CSF appears at the hub of the needle, indicating successful entrance of the spinal needle into the subarachnoid space. Typically, a loss of resistance is felt as the needle makes a slight bend to exit through the curved tip of the epidural needle and another as the spinal needle pierces the dura and enters the subarachnoid space.

catheter placement at either a single[58,59] or two different interspaces.[60–62] If the epidural catheter is placed first, proper placement can be tested before administration of spinal medications, potentially decreasing the risk of inadvertent intravascular or intrathecal catheter migration. Placing the epidural catheter first may also reduce the risk of neural damage, which may occur when the catheter is inserted after subarachnoid block, since paresthesia and other warning signs of improper needle placement may be absent

after administration of spinal medications. However, there is also a risk of striking the epidural catheter with the spinal needle.[63–65] Some authors consider this to be a purely hypothetical risk and have demonstrated that it is not possible to perforate an epidural catheter with commonly used spinal needles.[66,67]

Cook[68] recently reported a series of 201 consecutive CSEs performed with a novel separate-needle technique. The study was designed to avoid potential and actual problems

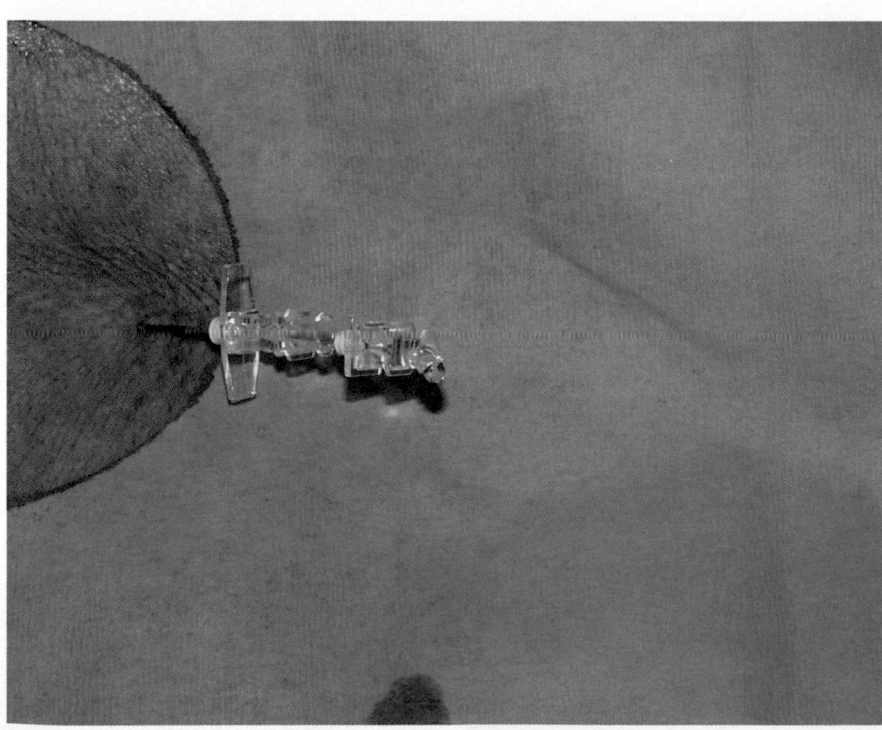

Figure 16–4. CSF appears in the hub of the spinal needle, indicating the subarachnoid placement of its tip.

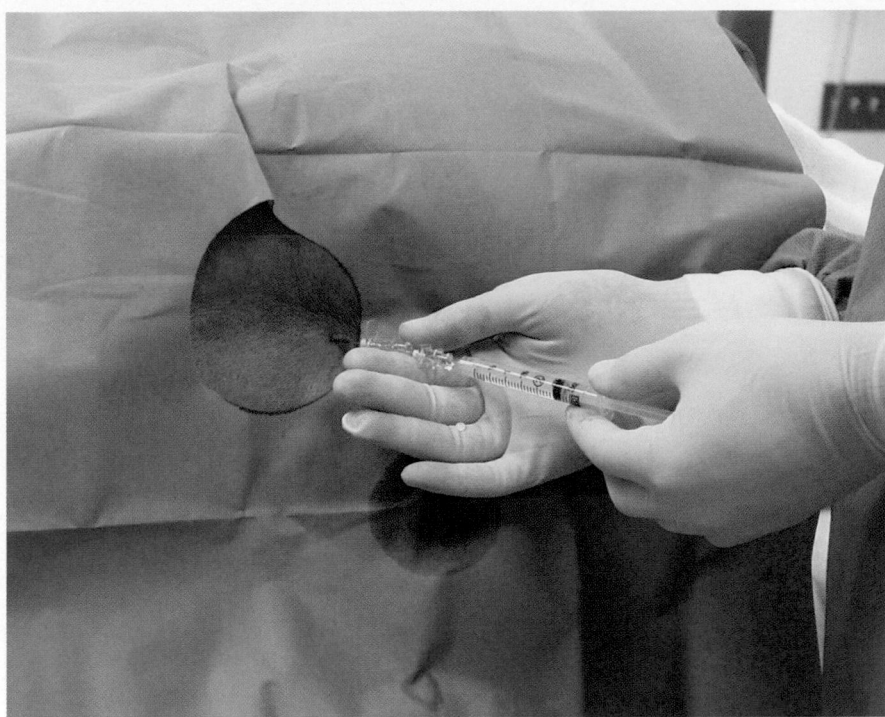

Figure 16–5. A desired dose of local anesthetic with or without additives is injected through the spinal needle.

associated with the CSE technique. Cook placed the spinal needle in the subarachnoid space and then replaced the spinal needle stylet to stop the CSF leak. He next placed the epidural catheter through a different interspace and returned to the spinal needle to inject the subarachnoid drug, thus avoiding epidural catheter insertion in an anesthetized patient. This method of CSE anesthesia, though more work, may be associated with high success and low complication rates.

Regardless of which component is performed first, the major disadvantage of the two-needle/two-interspace technique is that it takes longer to perform and requires two separate injections.

Comparison of Techniques

Comparison of NTN & SNT CSE Techniques

The SNT technique has a few theoretical advantages over the NTN technique. It enables placement of the epidural catheter prior to initiation of the spinal block. The SNT may thus theoretically reduce the risk for neurologic injury, since

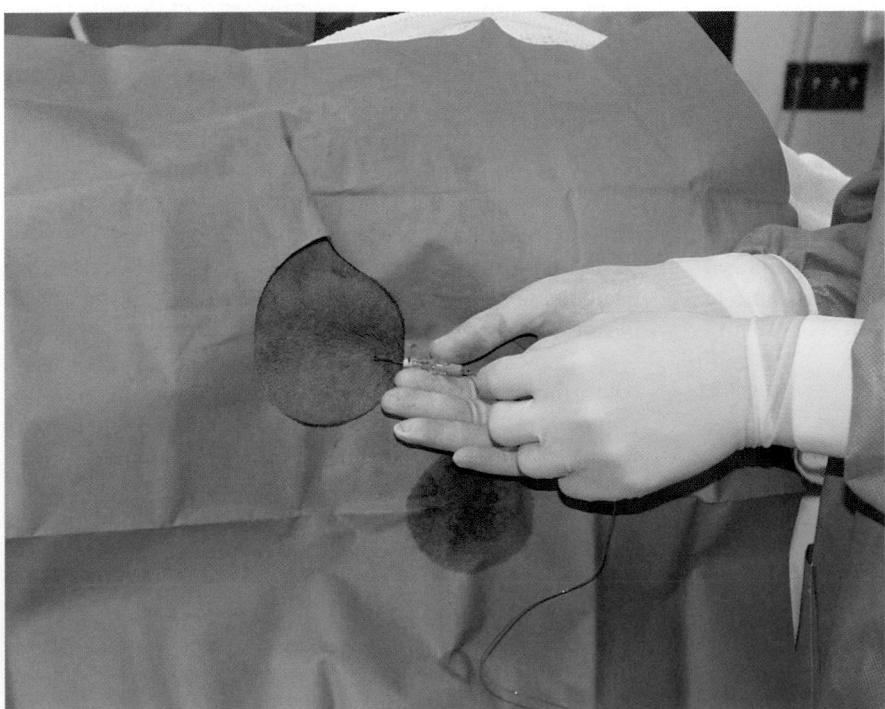

Figure 16–6. A flexible catheter is placed through the epidural needle and left about 5 cm in the epidural space.

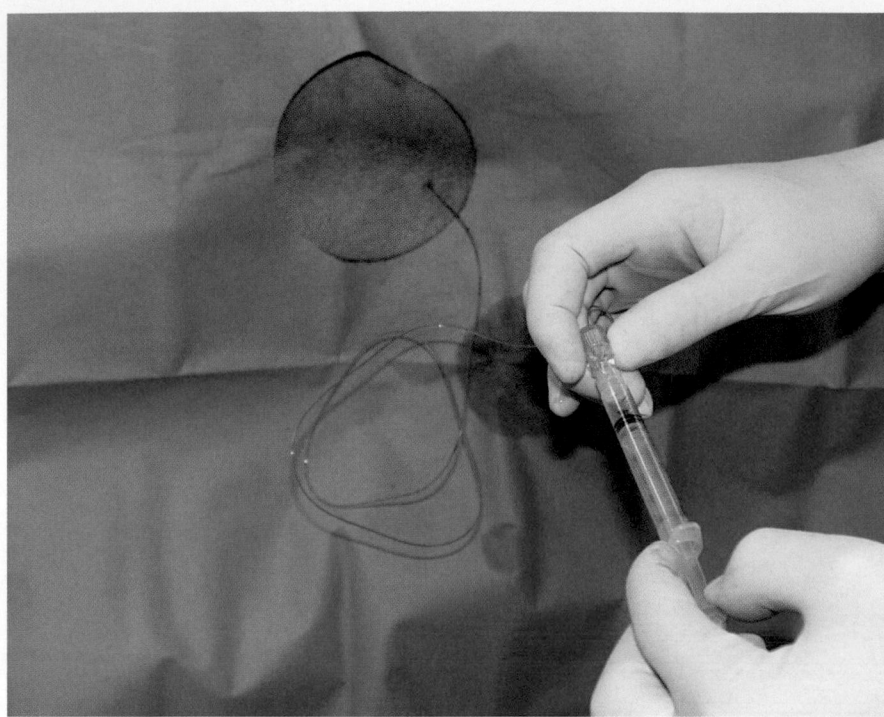

Figure 16–7. Epidural catheter is checked by the aspiration test to rule out its inadvertent intravascular (appearance of blood in the catheter) or intrathecal (appearance of CSF) placement.

paresthesia and other symptoms are not masked. Since the epidural catheter is placed early, problems that may occur due to delayed catheter placement (technical problems) after the injection of a hyperbaric spinal solution (such as unilateral, sacral, or low lumbar regional neuraxial block) are avoided.[69−71]

Several studies have compared NTN and SNT techniques.[72−75] Some have reported better success and lower failure rates with the SNT. However, these studies also report greater patient acceptance and less discomfort with the NTN technique. A recent prospective randomized study[76] compared the outcomes and techniques of NTN and SNT (double space) CSE in 200 patients receiving elective cesarean section. A successful block to the T5 level with the double–space and the NTN techniques were 80 vs 54, with an odds ratio of 0.29. SNT had a greater success rate than the NTN technique; the T5 dermatome was reached with fewer corrective manipulations (epidural augmentation or repeated blocks). Failure to enter the intrathecal space once the epidural space had been located occurred in 29 patients in the NTN group. Time to readiness for surgery was slightly increased with SNT (15 min with SNT vs 12.9 min with NTN).

Techniques to Improve Success & Safety of CSE

The success of CSE block depends heavily on accurate cannulation of the epidural space. The identification of the epidural space is traditionally achieved by a blind loss of resistance. With the blind handling of the needles, in which the feedback to the operator is merely tactile, deviation of the axis of the needle trajectory may occur. Because of the triangular

form of the dural sac, deviation from the midline of the spinal needle will cause the operator to miss the dural sac, leading to spinal component failure or unsuccessful dural puncture. Complications such as paresthesia, postdural puncture headache (PDPH) are also associated with the puncture technique.

Grau and coworkers performed real-time ultrasonic scanning of the lumbar spine to provide accurate reading of the location of the needle tip and to facilitate the performance of CSE anesthesia.[77] Their aim was to establish a less-invasive method to monitor the advancement of the needle in real time.

Thirty parturient patients scheduled for cesarean section were randomized to three equal groups. Ten control patients received conventional CSE anesthesia. Ten received ultrasonic scans by an offline technique. The remaining 10 received online imaging of the lumbar region during puncture. The Tuohy needle was inserted using the midline approach in all three groups. In the control group, CSE was performed using the single-space NTN technique with the standard loss of resistance to saline method.

In the offline group, ultrasound images were taken just before the puncture to improve needle trajectory. In the online group, ultrasonic images were taken to monitor and identify needle trajectory in real time.

They reported that in both ultrasound groups, a significant reduction in the number of necessary puncture attempts was found ($p < 0.036$); the number of interspaces necessary for puncture was reduced ($p < 0.036$); the number of spinal needle manipulations was significantly reduced ($p < 0.036$). Dural tenting was observed in 9 out of 10 in the online group (tenting length 2.4 mm). Asymmetric block was observed in 10% of those in the control group, but not in any of those in the ultrasound groups.

The authors concluded that the use of ultrasound imaging was obviously helpful in finding the ideal needle trajectory and to improve puncture conditions by demonstration of the relevant anatomy.

In the CSE NTN technique, there is no practical test to confirm correct epidural catheter placement. Tsui and colleagues proposed the use of nerve stimulators to confirm the proper placement of epidural catheter.[78] They studied 39 obstetric patients in labor who received epidural catheters (not CSE) for analgesia. A low-current (1–10 mA) electrical stimulation was used to confirm the correct placement of epidural catheter (19-gauge Arrow Flextip Plus). A positive motor response (truncal or limb) indicated that the catheter was in the epidural space. They reported that the sensitivity and specificity of this test was 100% and 100%, respectively, with 38 true-positive tests and 1 true-negative test. A case of intravascular epidural catheter migration was detected using this new test and was subsequently confirmed by a positive epinephrine test. If the motor response only occurs with larger currents (>10 mA) or does not respond at all (before receiving any local anesthetics), the catheter is outside the epidural space. If a positive response occurs at an unusually low milliamperage (<1 mA), intrathecal placement is likely. More detail on the electrical stimulation can be found in Chapter 5 (Electrophysiology of Nerve Stimulation).

The electrical stimulation test may not be applicable when the CSE technique is used for surgery in which anesthetic doses of local anesthetics are administered intrathecally prior to the placement of the epidural catheter. When using the CSE technique for labor analgesia, this test may be utilized as a simple and practical method for determining the epidural catheter placement. The standard test dose (3 mL of 1.5% lidocaine with 1:200,000 epinephrine) may help to identify vascular and intrathecal placement, but it does not verify appropriate epidural placement or function.

PHARMACOLOGIC CHOICES FOR CSE

Sufentanil and fentanyl, with or without local anesthetics, are most often administered intrathecally to provide analgesia for the laboring woman receiving CSE. The usual dosage of sufentanil is 2.5–10 mcg; however, most practitioners are now using 2.5 or 5 mcg. The ED_{50} and ED_{95} for laboring patients were found to be 2.6 mcg and 8.9 mcg, respectively.[79] The doses of fentanyl used are typically 10–25 mcg. The median effective dose (ED_{50}) and the effective dose for 95% of patients (ED_{95}) for laboring patients has been reported to be 5.5 and 17.4 mcg, respectively.[80] Although the original studies used much higher doses of intrathecal opioids (10 mcg sufentanil and 25–50 mcg of fentanyl), subsequent studies have suggested the use of smaller doses, with reduced side effects and similar analgesic effect.[81]

Morphine, a highly ionized, water-soluble opioid, produces analgesia of long duration, but with a slow onset (approximately 60 min between injection and onset). In addition it may be associated with an unacceptably high incidence of side effects such as nausea, vomiting, and pruritus, as well as the potential for delayed respiratory depression. These side effects, coupled with the slow onset of pain relief, limit the usefulness of intrathecal morphine for labor analgesia. Intrathecal meperidine (10 mg) may provide reliable analgesia in advanced labor,[82] but has been associated with a high incidence of nausea, vomiting, hypotension, and ephedrine requirement. In addition, it is the only opioid that has intrinsic local anesthetic properties at clinically used doses,[82] by blocking nerve conduction at the proximal end of the dorsal root[83] by a mechanism other than sodium channel blockade.[84] This nerve conduction blockade is not naloxone reversible.[83]

Clinical Pearl

- In many patients, a single intrathecal injection of a lipid-soluble opioid is insufficient to produce analgesia for the entire duration of labor.

In many patients, a single intrathecal injection of a lipid-soluble opioid is insufficient to produce analgesia for the entire duration of labor.

When the second stage of labor is imminent, the subarachnoid administration of local anesthetic plus opioid should be considered to achieve a greater depth of pain relief. The combination of 2.5 to 5 mcg sufentanil plus 2.5 mg bupivacaine provides rapid analgesia without motor block, alleviates the pain of the second stage of labor, and lasts longer than sufentanil alone.[85] Although the original reports[86] recommended the use of 10 mcg of sufentanil, Sia and colleagues showed that adequate relief of labor pain could be safely provided by administering half that dose of intrathecal sufentanil plus bupivacaine.[87]

New studies[88] have attempted to determine the ED_{50} for intrathecal bupivacaine, defined as the minimum local anesthetic dose (MLAD) and then use this to asses the effect of different doses of fentanyl. The MLAD of intrathecal bupivacaine has been found to be 1.99 mg, and the addition of 5 mcg of intrathecal fentanyl offered a similarly significant sparing effect to 15 or 25 mcg of fentanyl, resulting in less pruritus but with a shortening of duration of action.

Levin and coworkers compared a standard dose of intrathecal bupivacaine with sufentanil for CSE analgesia using two doses of ropivacaine (2 and 4 mg) with sufentanil and concluded that both local anesthetics provided similar duration of labor analgesia with equivalent side effects.[89] In addition, a recently published pilot study showed that intrathecal ropivacaine with or without sufentanil also provides effective analgesia and does not impair motor strength, which might facilitate ambulation during labor.[90]

COMPLICATIONS & CONCERNS OF CSE TECHNIQUE

Failure of the Spinal Component

The most common method of performing a CSE is the single-interspace NTN technique. In earlier reports, failure to achieve a spinal block with this technique has been reported in 10 to 15% of cases in the past.[91,92] However, more recent reports have demonstrated failure rates in the range of 2 to 5%.[93–95]

Clinical Pearls

Possible causes for failure include:

- The spinal needle is too short. The needle did not extend far enough beyond the epidural tip or tented the dura.[91] Hollway and Telford observed the distance from identification of the epidural space to penetration of the dura in 31 patients during the use of Tuohy needle to perform deliberate dural puncture for the insertion of lumbar drains.[96] Although many reference text books quote smaller distances from location of the epidural spaces to dural puncture, these authors found unexpectedly large distances of up to 2.25 cm in this study[97] and postulated that tenting of the dura by the blunt needle was the cause of this finding. Tenting is facilitated by the absence of a negative epidural space pressure when the needle opens the space to the atmosphere.

- The dura was not entered. This may occur with small-caliber needles that lack the rigidity to puncture the dura.[98] As postulated by Holloway and Telford,[96] the absence of negative epidural space pressure limits the transdural pressure gradient to the CSF pressure alone. Therefore, penetration of the dura (a relatively tough membrane) requires a substantial reactive force.[99]

- Divergence from the midline may cause the spinal needle to pass by the dura,[74,77] although the epidural space has been located.

- A long small-gauge spinal needle may penetrate the dura and then be advanced to the anterior epidural space due to the delay in the reflux of CSF.[100–102] Another potential problem may occur with the long, fine spinal needles currently in use. The spinal needle may be poorly anchored because it is located in the epidural needle and not in tissue. Therefore, the medication may be only partially administered to the subarachnoid space.[103–105] The ability to hold the spinal needle steady takes practice but is easily learned.

- After a subarachnoid drug has been administered, there can be a delay while placing the epidural catheter. This is usually brief and without consequences, but according to some authors[106,107] it may alter the final characteristics of the block. This complication is of greater clinical significance when performing CSE for cesarean delivery. However, should a delay occur and the block not reach optimum height, the epidural catheter can be used to supplement the block.

- Another concern with the NTN technique is that damage to either needle by friction between the two needles may lead to spread of metallic debris in to the neuraxial space or injury to proximal neural structures.[108]

Most current needle designs allow extension of the spinal needle 12–15 mm beyond the tip of the Tuohy needle. Excessively long needles, however, pose problems of handling and depth of placement. Deviation from midline will lengthen the epidural–dural distance and may also cause the spinal needle to miss the spinal space laterally (Figures 16–8 and 16–9). Saline used to identify the epidural space may enter the spinal needle and may be misinterpreted as CSF.

Spinal Migration of the Catheter or Intrathecal Administration of Epidural Drugs

Subarachnoid Placement of Intended Epidural Catheter

One of the concerns with the CSE technique is that the epidural catheter may inadvertently pass through the dural puncture hole into the subarachnoid space during CSE technique. This seems more likely with NTN CSE technique than with SNT or with epidural needles with back holes. Although this may seem a rare theoretical problem, several publications have reported its occurrence.[109–112]

Angle and coworkers[113] recently studied factors contributing to unintentional subarachnoid catheter passage after epidural placement with an in vitro model using human dural tissue. In that study, the dura was punctured with 25-gauge Whitacre spinal needles. The researchers compared the subarachnoid catheter passage of the intact dura with that of the dura with obvious epidural needle punctures, and single 25-gauge Whitacre spinal needle punctures after a CSE technique. Their conclusion was that the catheter passage intrathecally is unlikely in the presence of an intact dura or after an uncomplicated combined spinal–epidural technique.

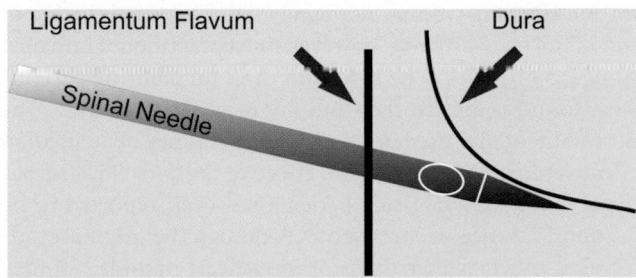

Figure 16–8. Successful entrance into the epidural space may not always guarantee successful subarachnoidal needle placement. This can particularly be the case with an odd angle of needle insertion or the use of excessively long needles that may bend during the advancement.

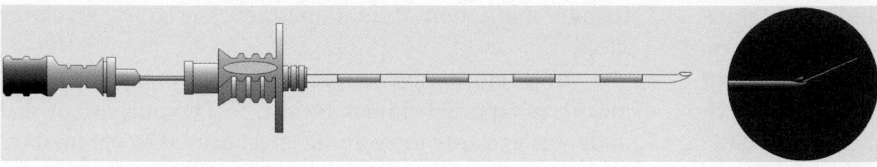

Figure 16–9. A CSE needle-through-needle design with the spinal needle exiting the epidural needle. The spinal needle is shown exiting at an angle that may cause it to miss the subarachnoid space.

Therefore, unintentional subarachnoid passage of the epidural catheter suggests dural damage with the epidural needle.

Holtz and colleagues investigated the possible passage of the epidural catheter into the subarachnoid space in an anatomic preparation.[114] In 10 series of experiments, the epidural compartment was entered with an 18-gauge Tuohy needle. The spinal puncture (27- or 29-gauge Quincke needle) was performed with the NTN technique. Subsequently, the internal side of the intrathecal compartment was examined endoscopically for penetration of the epidural catheter. In a similar way, the endoscope was inserted epidurally to visualize the movements of the epidural catheter in the epidural compartment. In this model of simulated physiologic intrathecal conditions, using a one-space NTN technique, they could not detect intrathecal passage of the epidural catheter.

Holmstrom and coworkers also reported, in a percutaneous epiduroscopy study using fresh cadavers that it was impossible to force an epidural catheter into the subarachnoid space after a single perforation of the dura with a small-gauge spinal needle. However, they found that the risk of intrathecal catheter migration increased to approximately 5% after multiple dural punctures with the spinal needle. Dural penetration of the epidural catheter after a dural puncture with a Tuohy needle was clearly demonstrated in the same study.[115]

Whether the incidence of an unintentional passage of the epidural catheter into the subarachnoid space is greater with CSE than with standard epidural technique alone is controversial. Therefore, regardless of the technique used, all epidural medications should be given in incremental doses.

Subarachnoid Spread of Epidurally Administered Drugs

Leighton and colleagues reported that following a CSE, a dose of epidural local anesthetic will produce a higher dermatomal level than expected, presumably due to subarachnoid flux of the drug. However, when used for labor analgesia, unless the dura is breached with the epidural needle[116] or large bolus volumes are administered,[117] flux should not be clinically significant. Suzuki and coworkers found that dural puncture using a 26-gauge Whitacre spinal needle before the epidural injection in nonpregnant patients increased caudal spread of analgesia induced by epidural local anesthetics with no change in the cephalad spread.[118]

Holst and coworkers investigated endoscopically the possible passage of the epidural catheter anesthetic through the dural puncture hole into the CSF compartment in an anatomic preparation.[114] Even 1 h after epidural administration of 20 mL of methylene blue-dyed local anesthetic (bupivacaine 0.5%, isobaric), no passage of local anesthetic into the intrathecal compartment could be detected under continuous endoscopic monitoring.

Clinical Pearls

- A dural puncture may allow dangerously large quantities of subsequently administered epidural drugs to reach the subarachnoid space.
- The magnitude of flux was a function of the diameter of the spinal needle. The risk may be decreased by using the smallest possible needle to puncture the meninges.

Theoretically, a dural puncture may allow dangerously large quantities of subsequently administered epidural drugs to reach the subarachnoid space. Bernard and colleagues investigated the risk of epidural drug reaching the subarachnoid space through the dural hole left by spinal needles and concluded that the magnitude of flux was a function of the diameter of the spinal needle. The risk may be decreased by using the smallest possible needle to puncture the meninges.[119]

However, the possibility of this hazard is supported by reports of high or total spinal block during epidural anesthesia administered following unintentional dural perforation with the epidural needle.[120,121] Eldor and coworkers reported a case of delayed respiratory arrest in the CSE anesthesia. They commented: "The event was likely due to morphine injected through the epidural catheter, unintentionally entering into the subarachnoid space through the hole in the dura that was made previously by the spinal needle in the needle-through-needle technique."[121] However, data from some clinical studies of the CSE technique have not indicated an increase in spread of sensory block due to subarachnoid leakage of epidurally administered medications.[114,122–124]

The administration of a test dose for spinal placement of an epidural catheter may be problematic and aspiration may fail, but test doses have been found to detect more intrathecal catheters than aspiration alone during labor analgesia.[125] Despite the studies that have reported that intrathecal migration is very rare and the flux should not produce clinically relevant complications, epidural drugs or catheters may migrate into the spinal space following CSE. Therefore, all epidural doses should be incremental and patients receiving continuous epidural infusions for analgesia should be checked every hour to rule out excessive motor or sensory block that may be indicative of intrathecal administration of drugs.

Hypotension

Does subarachnoid block induced by CSE (using loss of resistance to air) render a higher level of sensory anesthesia than single-shot spinal (SSS) when an identical mass of intrathecal anesthetic is injected?

Goy and Sia performed a prospective randomized study comparing CSE (using loss of resistance to air) vs SSS on 60 patients who were undergoing minor gynecologic procedures and concluded that subarachnoid block induced by CSE produces a greater sensorimotor anesthesia ($p < 0.01$) and prolonged recovery ($p < 0.05$) than SSS. They also found a more frequent incidence of hypotension and vasopressor use in the CSE group ($p < 0.05$), despite using identical doses of intrathecal medications.[126]

Another study reported similar findings when only 4 mL of air was used as part of the loss-of-resistance technique.[127] The objective of that study was to determine the ED_{50} of intrathecal hyperbaric bupivacaine for CSE and SSS by using the up–down sequential allocation technique. Sixty participants were separated into two groups in a double-blind, randomized, prospective study design. The researchers concluded, under similar clinical conditions, that the ED_{50} of intrathecal hyperbaric bupivacaine in CSE was 20% less than that in SSS. Although the mechanism that accounts for this finding is undetermined, the loss-of-resistance technique in CSE could introduce air pockets within the epidural space. MRI has demonstrated residual air pockets to extend up to three lumbar vertebral segments and compress the lumbar thecal sac dorsally and laterally.[128] This could result in a reduction of the lumbosacral CSF volume and enhance the extent of sensory anesthesia.[129]

Epidural administration of drugs seems to affect the thecal contents and therefore influences the spread of earlier induced subarachnoid block.[130,131] The magnitude of this effect depends on the time interval between the injections and the volume of the epidural injectate. Initially, the proposed mechanism for this effect was the subarachnoid leakage of epidurally administered medications.

In a retrospective study Klasen and colleagues examined whether the patients receiving spinal anesthesia as part of CSE experienced a more frequent incidence of relevant hypotension than patients receiving spinal anesthesia alone.[132] Anesthesia records from 1596 patients who received spinal anesthesia and 1023 patients who received CSE for elective surgery were reviewed. The investigators reported that the patients who had CSE had a significantly more frequent prevalence of arterial hypotension as a major risk factor. The level of sensory block after 10 min was higher with CSE than with spinal anesthesia alone. In this study after the typical loss of resistance, a volume of 5 to 10 mL of saline 0.9% was injected into the epidural space, followed by dural puncture and administration of intrathecal local anesthetic. They suggested that the increased volume in the lumbar epidural space with 5 to 10 mL of saline may lead to an enhanced cephalad spread of the local anesthetic in the subarachnoid space.

Blumgart and colleagues in a prospective, randomized study, demonstrated a similar increase in cephalad spread of subarachnoid block after either 10 mL of saline or 10 mL of local anesthetic solutions when injected epidurally after establishing a subarachnoid block.[133] Thus, they concluded that the mechanism of extension of spinal anesthesia by extradural injection of local anesthetics is largely a volume effect.

In a prospective randomized study Takiguchi and coworkers reported similar results.[134] The purpose of that study was to clarify the volume effect caused by epidural injection of saline after spinal anesthesia.[134] The participants were 20 patients undergoing cesarean delivery under CSE anesthesia whose analgesic levels did not reach the surgical regions 10 min after spinal medication. These patients were randomly assigned to two groups. The control group ($n = 10$) received no epidural saline, and the saline group received 10 mL of saline through the epidural catheter 10 min after spinal anesthesia. In the saline group, the levels of analgesia 15 and 20 min after spinal anesthesia were significantly higher than those in the control group ($p < 0.05$). Next, they examined the volume effect of epidural saline with myelography using two subjects. They reported that the diameter of the subarachnoid space diminished to less than 25% after injection of saline. Concurrently, the contrast medium injected into the lumbar subarachnoid space increased from L3 to L1 and from L2 to T12.

Hypotension can occur following the administration of intrathecal fentanyl or sufentanil, even if sympathetic blockade does not occur. However, the hemodynamic effects of intrathecal fentanyl are usually benign in nature and typically due to a decrease in catecholamines secondary to pain relief. Vasodilation due to sympathectomy, however, causes a decrease in preload, end-diastolic index, and in stroke index, as well as an increase in heart rate. Since the end-diastolic index and stroke index remained relatively stable and the heart rate decreased in a study by Mandell and colleagues, these authors concluded that the observed hypotension was not due to vasodilation.[135] The hypotensive episodes following administration of neuraxial opioids for labor are transient, easily treated, and not necessarily associated with adverse fetal heart rate changes.

Neurologic Injury

Neurologic complications directly related to spinal anesthesia may be caused by trauma, cord ischemia, infection, and neurotoxicity.

Needle Trauma

Needle- or catheter-induced trauma rarely results in permanent neurologic injury. However, Horlocker and coworkers, in a retrospective review of 4767 consecutive spinal anesthetics for CNS complications, concluded that the presence of a paresthesia during needle placement significantly increased the risk of persistent paresthesia ($p < 0.001$). In that review, paresthesia was elicited during needle placement in 298 (6.3%) cases. Six patients reported pain (persistent paresthesia) upon resolution of the spinal anesthetic; four of the cases resolved within 1 week, and the remaining two resolved in 18 to 24 months.[136] It is not known, however, how the report of the paresthesia by the patient can be used to avoid such complications from occurring.

The increase in the risk of neurologic sequelae following the CSE technique may have the following causes. In the single-space, NTN technique, the insertion of epidural needle and catheter after administration of spinal local anesthetics may prevent identification of paresthesias that may warn the anesthesiologist about needle misplacement. Higher incidence of paresthesia during CSE is a recognized factor. In accordance with the literature paresthesia is reported in 0.9 to 11% of patients undergoing CSE.[137] Browne and colleagues reported a 14% incidence of paresthesias with the Espocan needle (18-gauge Tuohy epidural needle with an extra lumen in the needle bevel) and a 42% incidence with the conventional Tuohy epidural needle.[14]

In a randomized prospective study, McAndrew and Harms reported that 37% (17 of 46) of women in the NTN group and only 9% (4 of 43) in the SSS group had paresthesia upon spinal needle insertion ($p < 0.05$). The equipment used was a 16-gauge/26-gauge CSE kit and a 26-gauge pencil point spinal needle with introducer (both Sims Portex, Australia). They postulated that the higher incidence of paresthesia may be related to deeper penetration of the subarachnoid space with CSE technique. However, in that study, none of the patients had persistent neurologic symptoms on examination at postoperative day 1.[138]

Holloway and coworkers conducted a pilot survey on anesthetists' experiences of neurologic sequelae following spinal and CSE anesthesia in obstetric units in the UK.[139] Because of the retrospective nature of the survey, many neurologic problems that were reported lacked detail. However, no obvious differences occurred in the incidence of problems associated with CSE vs the SSS techniques. Turner and Shaw suggested the possibility that painful insertion and subsequent root damage might be increased by the use of atraumatic pencil point spinal needles.[140] In that survey, problems were reported with both Whitacre and Sprotte needles, but none with Quincke needles. However, the numbers using Quincke needles were too small to permit statistical analysis. More dangerous than root damage is damage to the spinal cord, and in that survey[140] two cases of conus damage were reported: one with CSE and one with SSS. This complication is not a fault of atraumatic needles, but rather of the technique itself. In 19% of patients the spinal cord terminated below L1. In more than 50% of cases the chosen space is incorrectly identified.[141] Therefore, the L3-4 intervertebral space or below should be selected for CSE or SSS.

Risk of Metal Toxicity in CSE

It has been alleged that during the NTN technique, tiny metal particles abraded by the spinal needle from the inner edge of the Tuohy needle may be introduced into the epidural or spinal compartment.[108] In order to examine this concern, Holst and colleagues simulated the NTN technique in an in vitro model.[114] They used atomic absorption spectrography (AAS) to identify abraded metal particles. The needles were then examined under an electron microscope. They reported no increased alloy components detected in the rinse solution after either twofold or fivefold puncture compared with the control measurements. After five punctures, and handling the needle as in normal practice, no traces of use could be detected by electron microscopy on the inner ground edge of the Tuohy needle.[114]

Infectious Neurologic Complications

Although overall incidence of infections and their sequelae following placement of CSE is perceived to be extremely low, the relative risk compared with either a spinal or epidural alone is unknown.

In a classic study, Dripps and Vandem prospectively reported no cases of meningitis after 10,098 spinal anesthetics.[142] Phillips and coworkers also reported no cases after a prospective review of 10,440 such cases.[143] These studies included patients undergoing obstetric and urologic operations, which are known to be associated with perioperative bacteremia. However, case reports of meningitis following CSEs appear in the journals beginning mid-1990s.[144,145] Theoretically, CSE is thought to be associated with an increased risk of meningitis compared with epidural alone because the dura (protective barrier for the CNS) is punctured deliberately during CSE and then a foreign body, an epidural catheter, is placed nearby. The epidural catheter can lie close to the dural hole and is a potential focus of infection, especially following bacteremia.[146] Contamination of the subarachnoid space may occur from bleeding due to needle trauma in a bacteremic patient or from failure of aseptic technique.

Headache and neck pain or neck stiffness in a patient who recently received spinal anesthesia is often attributed to postdural puncture headache (PDPH). One case report highlighted the dangers associated with missed diagnosis of meningitis. The patient was misdiagnosed as having endometritis when she presented with headache, vomiting, and fever 2 days after uncomplicated epidural analgesia for labor. Her condition rapidly deteriorated, and meningitis was not considered as a diagnosis until it was too late. She died in intensive care a few weeks later.[147]

Several studies have shown that facemasks prevent forward dispersal of organisms from upper airway and downward dispersal during talking and head turning.[148,149] Despite this, in 1996 a postal survey of members of the Obstetric Anaesthetists Association found that over half those surveyed did not routinely wear facemasks when performing neuraxial anesthesia.[150] More discussion on the infectious complications of neuraxial techniques can be found in Chapter 72 (Infection Control in Regional Anesthesia).

Postdural Puncture Headache

The incidence of PDPH after CSE technique is controversial; some authors have reported decreased incidence when compared with epidural alone,[151] but others report an increased incidence.[152]

Norris and coworkers[15] reported that the patients who requested only epidural analgesia were more likely to suffer an accidental dural puncture (twofold increase; epidural vs CSE = 4.2%:1.7%). These investigators offered two possible explanations for this result. The first was that they usually choose CSE for women who are most often in early labor and reserved epidural analgesia for patients in the more painful active phase of labor. Therefore, the patients in the epidural group are more likely to move during the procedure, and thus cause a "wet tap." Secondly, during CSE if one is uncertain of the location of the epidural needle, the spinal needle can be inserted to look for CSF[153] or closeness to dura.

Other factors may decrease the incidence of PDPH following the CSE technique. Administration of intrathecal opioids has been shown to decrease the incidence of PDPH.[154] Subsequent infusion of an epidural local anesthetic increases the subarachnoid pressure and also may help to decrease the incidence of PDPH following CSE. Dunn and colleagues argued that the intentional dural puncture involved in the CSE technique would increase the risk of PDPH in obstetric patients compared with those receiving epidural analgesia alone.[152] The use of small-gauge atraumatic pencil point spinal needles (such as Whitacre, Pencan, Sprotte, and Gertie Marx) greatly reduce the incidence of PDPH in patients receiving CSE.[151,155]

Chan and Paech reported three cases of persistent CSF leak following uneventful CSE analgesia for labor.[156] Using β_2-transferrin immunofixation assay, they confirmed that the leaking fluid was CSF in two cases.[157] None of the patients developed PDPH or any other complications. Howes and Lenz also reported CSF cutaneous fistula in two patients following epidural anesthesia (not CSE) for postoperative pain relief. Both patients developed PDPH only after removal of the catheters and were treated successfully with an autologous blood patch.[158]

Complications Related to Labor Analgesia

Fetal Bradycardia

Reports in the literature suggest an increased frequency of nonreassuring fetal heart rate tracings and fetal bradycardia associated with CSE.[159–161] The cause of the fetal bradycardia after CSE remains elusive, but it may be related to an acute reduction in circulating maternal catecholamine levels after the quick onset of analgesia. In addition, it has been postulated that an imbalance between epinephrine and norepinephrine levels causes unopposed α-adrenoceptor effects on uterine tone and decreases uterine blood flow. However, preliminary reports suggest that there may be no alteration in uteroplacental blood flow.[102]

The resulting fetal bradycardia is usually short-lived and typically resolves within 5 to 8 min.[163] A retrospective study of 1240 patients who received regional labor analgesia (mostly CSE) and 1140 patient who received systemic medication or no analgesia demonstrated no significant difference in the rate of cesarean delivery, with rates of 1.3% and 1.4%, respectively. That study also reported that no emergency cesarean deliveries for acute fetal "distress" were necessary in the absence of obstetric indications up to 90 min after intrathecal sufentanil administration.[164]

EQUIPMENT

CSE technique has gained popularity and acceptance, especially in obstetrics. Special kits have been produced for CSE. (Example: B Braun Medical Ltd. comprising the standard 16-gauge, 8-cm Tuohy needle with a 26-gauge Quincke spinal needle). Various concerns of the CSE technique have led to some modification of the needles used.

The potential dangers of the single-level NTN kit include introduction of very fine metal particles abraded by the spinal needle as it is maneuvered through the tip of the Tuohy needle[108] and unintentional passage of epidural catheter through the dural hole caused by the spinal needle.[109] As previously mentioned, Holst and coworkers, using AAS, showed no contamination of the intrathecal space by metal particles after normal clinical use in the NTN technique.[114]

In order to direct the epidural catheter away from the dural puncture site, Rawal and colleagues recommended rotation of the epidural needle 180 degrees following dural puncture This maneuver directs the epidural catheter 2–2.5 mm away from the dural puncture site.[165] However, Meikljohn, using postmortem dura mater, demonstrated that rotation of the epidural needle significantly decreases the force required to puncture the dura.[99]

Recently, CSE kits designed with an orifice in the back curve (back hole) of the epidural needle for separate spinal needle passage have been made available[14] (Figure 16–10).

This needle is expected to reduce the likelihood of dural passage of the epidural catheter by directing the catheter away from the dural puncture site (Figure 16–11). However, the spinal needle may not always go through the spinal needle orifice and may exit through the Huber tip, thus losing the advantage of the back hole[14] Joshi and McCarroll suggested a technique to enhance the spinal needle exit through the spinal needle orifice.[91,166] The modified technique consisted of first aligning the bevel orifice of the spinal needle in the same direction as the Tuhoy bevel and then bending the spinal needle 10 degrees toward the Tuohy bevel while advancing through the Tuohy needle. This technique guides the spinal needle tip to exit through the back hole. In a prospective randomized study Pan evaluated the success rate of the spinal needle exiting through the spinal needle orifice, in two commonly

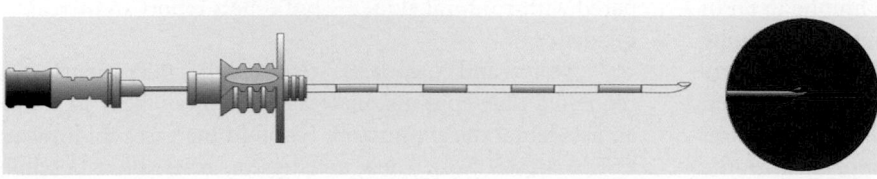

Figure 16–10. Epidural needle with a back hole (an exit on the back of the Tuohy tip) for introduction of the spinal needle.

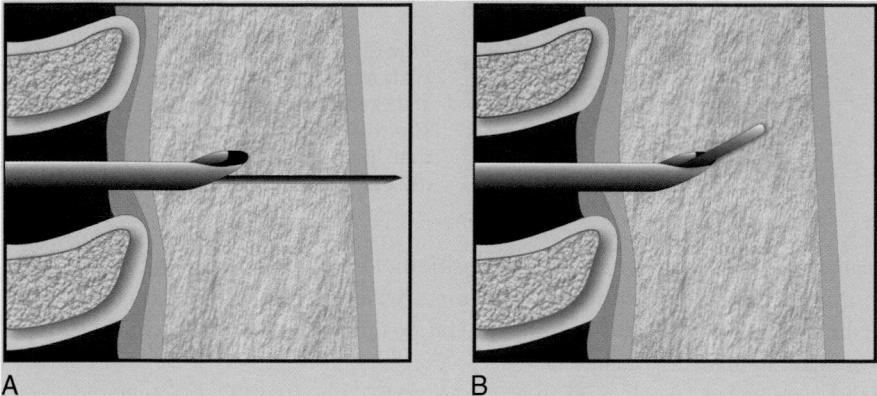

Figure 16–11. A specialized needle with an orifice in the back curve (back hole) of the epidural needle for separate spinal needle passage has been made available. **A:** The tip of the epidural needle is shown in the epidural space. A spinal needle is shown passing through the lumen of the epidural needle and entering the subarachnoid space. **B:** After the spinal anesthesia has been accomplished, the spinal needle is withdrawn and an epidural catheter is advanced into the epidural space.

available single-lumen, dual-orifice CSE needle kits.[167] The CSE kits studied were (1) Espocan CSE kit (Braun Medical Ltd.), which consists of a standard 18-gauge Tuohy needle with a 26-gauge sleeved Quincke spinal needle that extends 12 mm beyond the tip of the Tuohy needle through the back hole. The sleeve on the spinal needle was designed to guide the spinal needle to exit through the back hole. (2) Espocan CSE kit (Braun Medical Ltd.), which consists of the same epidural needle with a 27-gauge nonsleeved Sprotte spinal needle that extends 13 mm beyond the tip of the Tuohy needle through the back hole. This researcher performed 1600 attempts, which included modified technique described by Joshi and McCarroll. The modified technique improved the success rate of spinal needle exiting through the back hole from 67% to 94% for kit 1 and 50% to 81% for kit 2; cephalad orientation of the Tuohy needle bevel further improved the success rate to 96% and 91%, respectively. Overall, the sleeved spinal needle has a better success rate than the unsleeved spinal needle.

The failure of the spinal needle to exit through the back hole may also result in bending of the spinal needle and less protrusion beyond the tip of the Tuohy needle. This may contribute to the increased failure rate of dural puncture. The ideal length of spinal needle protrusion is reported to be at least 12–13 mm. In a prospective randomized study of 40 patients, Joshi and McCarroll reported a 15% failure rate of CSF return when the spinal needle protruded only 10 mm beyond the tip of the Tuohy needle, and 0% with 13 mm protrusion.[91] Riley and coworkers reported[168] similar results comparing 24-gauge Sorotte (9-mm protrusion past the tip of the Tuohy and 17% failure to obtain CSF) and Gertie Marx (protrusion 17 mm and 0% failure rate). The number of patients developing PDPH and requiring blood patch was greater with the Gertie Marx than the Sprotte needle. However, this difference was not statistically significant. It is possible that the longer spinal needle also punctures the anterior aspect of the dura and causes a greater CSF leak. Greater paresthesia was also noted (anecdotally) with the 127-mm needle, and the 124-mm Gertie Marx needle was suggested as an excellent compromise.

Herbstman and colleagues compared four pencil point spinal needles commonly used in the CSE technique and reported that longer spinal needles are associated with significantly more transient paresthesias (Gertie Marx 15-mm protrusion with 29% incidence; Whitacre 10-mm protrusion with 17% incidence). Success in obtaining CSF and the incidence of PDPH did not differ among the four needles.[169]

The conventional spinal needle in the CSE kit, which does not lock within the epidural needle, is difficult to handle and stabilize during injection of spinal medication. The displacement of the spinal needle during aspiration of the CSF and injection may result in failed anesthesia or may push the spinal needle deeper, leading to nerve damage or anterior dural perforation. To overcome this problem, Simsa suggested an external fixation device.[170] This device, however, is somewhat complicated to handle. Recently, spinal needles with an adjustable locking device have been introduced (CSEcure and Adjustble DursafeCSE needle). Studies on the lockable extensions reported that they provide safe and stable conditions during placement of the syringe and injection.[44,171] However, both studies reported frequent inability to feel dural perforation with the locking needles (15.3% with CSFcure and 25% with Adjustable Durasafe), the reason for which is unclear.

In a CSE technique, sometimes the epidural catheter cannot be threaded or threaded intravascularly after the intrathecal drugs has already been injected. To overcome this problem, a dual-lumen, dual-orifice CSE kit was developed, in which an epidural catheter can be inserted in place prior to inserting the spinal needle and mediation.[172,173] This is possible because the catheter and the spinal needle each have a separate lumen (Figure 16–12).

Recently, a dual-lumen CSE needle lumen has been commercialized in Europe (Epistar; Medimex, Germany).

CONTROVERSIAL ISSUES IN CSE TECHNIQUE

Test Dose

The issue of whether a test dose is needed when administering epidural analgesia for labor is controversial.[174,175] Because ultradilute solutions are commonly used and aspiration is often diagnostic, some authors believe that a test

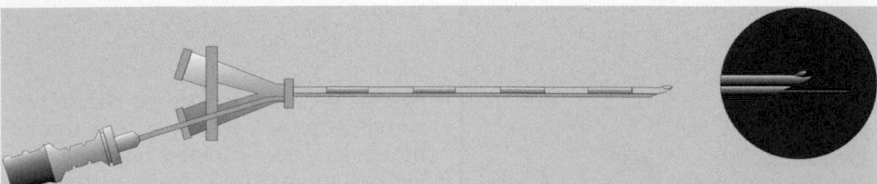

Figure 16–12. A dual-lumen CSE kit. This kit has two separate lumens: one for the catheter and another for the spinal needle. The theoretical advantage of this design is that the possibility of dural puncture with the epidural catheter is avoided.

dose is unnecessary.[176] However, because catheter aspiration is not always predictive (especially when using a single-orifice epidural catheter), others maintain the importance of a test dose to improve detection of intrathecal or intravascular placement of an epidural catheter.[177] Part of the controversy surrounding the testing of epidural catheters involves the use of epinephrine. Epinephrine has been shown to produce a reliable increase in heart rate in volunteers and surgical patients when the epidural has been sited in a blood vessel.[177] However, in a laboring patient, maternal heart rate variability from the pain of uterine contractions may confuse interpretation of the heart rate response, and intravenous epinephrine may have deleterious effects on uterine blood flow.[178] Means to improve the reliability of epinephrine include injecting the dose between uterine contractions and repeating the test dose when the response is equivocal. However, the lack of sensitivity and specificity of the test dose calls into question its usefulness as a diagnostic tool. Leighton and colleagues have described an alternative means of testing an epidural catheter for intravascular placement. They advocate the injection of 1 to 2 mL of air into the epidural catheter while listening over the precordium with the maternal external Doppler monitor for evidence of air.[179] With the recent reports of subarachnoid administration of chloroprocaine,[180] it is possible that in the future this agent will be utilized for testing epidural catheters. Before this happens, more information is essential.

If continuous infusion of dilute local anesthetic is administered and the patient remains comfortable without a motor block, proper epidural catheter placement is likely. If the epidural catheter is intravascular, the patient should have inadequate pain relief; if the catheter is subarachnoid, a solid motor block would develop. Although infusions of ultradilute local anesthetics do not pose a serious threat, such is not true of concentrated local anesthetics used for operative delivery. Some authors have suggested that a test dose is essential for any parturient receiving epidural anesthesia.[177] Regardless of the technique used, the safe practice of administering labor epidural analgesia dictates initial catheter aspiration, incremental injections, and continuous monitoring for evidence of local anesthetic toxicity.

Positioning for CSE

Neuraxial blocks are often performed with the patients in the sitting position, especially in obese individuals, because the midline is easily recognized. Sitting position has been shown to allow better spinal flexion in the parturients.[181] In addition, the SED was shown to be significantly greater when epidural puncture was performed in the lateral position than

in the sitting position. This change in distance may cause catheter dislodgment when the patient is turned from the sitting to the lateral position , with consequent inadequate analgesia.

Yun and coworkers compared the effects of induction of CSE anesthesia in the sitting vs lateral position in healthy women undergoing elective cesarean delivery.[182] The severity of hypotension, measured by the maximal percentage decrease in systolic blood pressure from control, as well as its duration, were significantly greater in the sitting group ($p < 0.05$). Patients in the sitting group required twice as much ephedrine to treat hypotension as those in the lateral recumbent group. The reason for the difference in the severity of hypotension is unclear. The authors postulated it to be related to a slower recovery from venous pooling in the lower extremities when assuming a supine position from an initial sitting position. These authors concluded that the position used for induction of CSE should be considered in cases associated with greater maternal or fetal risk from hypotension.

Traditional teaching is that the spread of hyperbaric intrathecal solutions follows gravity. Lewis and colleagues compared the development of spinal blocks in the left lateral position vs the supine wedge position, after performing the CSE in the sitting position.[183] The intrathecal medications consist of 2 mL of 0.5% hyperbaric bupivacaine with 15 mcg fentanyl. The left lateral position did not produce unilateral blockade. The left lateral position was associated with slower block onset ($p = 0.004$), but eventually produced a spinal block similar in characteristics to that obtained in the supine wedge position. The left lateral position is known to improve maternal cardiac output, and slower onset may be outweighed by the possible benefit to the fetus.

SUMMARY

Recent studies have shown that the CSE technique is gaining popularity[10,150] for various types of surgery and particularly in obstetrics. In our institution, CSE technique is the most commonly performed regional technique for labor analgesia (97%) as well as cesarean delivery (50%). Although it is not a perfect technique, it provides a method for administering optimal neuraxial anesthesia and analgesia in numerous clinical situations.

CSE technique offers the advantages of both spinal and epidural technique and therefore has a high success rate in providing regional anesthesia. CSE provides rapid onset and the ability to titrate a desired sensory level, control the duration of the block, and deliver postoperative analgesia. Another positive aspect of CSE is the ease with which the spinal needle enters the subarachnoid space. The Tuohy needle acts as a perfect introducer and guides the fine spinal needle almost to the subarachnoid space. When smaller gauge atraumatic spinal needles are used, PDPH is absent or very rare.[155]

On the other hand, the combined technique introduces potential side effects, such as PDPH, the increased risk of catheter migration into the subarachnoid space, and transient paresthesias from the spinal needle. Although the risk is extremely low, many technical adaptations have been suggested and developed to avoid penetration of the epidural catheter through the dural hole made by the spinal needle.

The ideal length of spinal needle protrusion beyond the tip of the epidural needle is reported to be at least 12–13 mm. Longer spinal needles were shown to be associated with significantly higher transient paresthesias. Inability to obtain CSF through the spinal needle may occur with shorter needles (<10 mm of protrusion) and result in failure of the spinal component of the technique. CSE failure is also related to a faulty puncture site or axis deviation during needle advancement. The risk of infection, hematoma, and neurologic damage increases with multiple attempts and multiple manipulations of the needles, but it is unclear if the CSE technique increases these risks. Noninvasive ultrasonic guidance has been proposed to enhance the safety and the success of the CSE technique.

References

1. Rodgers A, Walker N, Schug S, et al: Reduction of postoperative mortality and morbidity with epidural or spinal anaesthesia: Results from overview of randomised trials. BMJ 2000;321:1493–1504.
2. Buhre W, Rossaint R: Perioperative management and monitoring in anaesthesia. Lancet 2003;362:1839–1846.
3. Kehlet H, Wilmore DW: Multimodal strategies to improve surgical outcome. Am J Surg 2002;183:630–641.
4. Holmström B, Laugaland K, Rawal N, et al: Combined spinal epidural block versus spinal and epidural block for orthopaedic surgery. Can J Anesth 1993;40:601–606.
5. Stienstra R, Dahan A, Alhadi ZRB, et al: Mechanism of action of an epidural top-up in combined spinal epidural anaesthesia. Anesth Analg 1996;83:382–386.
6. Stienstra R, Dilrosun-Alhadi BZR, Dahan A, et al: The epidural top-up in combined spinal–epidural anaesthesia: The effect of volume versus dose. Anesth Analg 1999;88:810–814.
7. Blanshard HJ, Cook TM: Use of combined spinal–epidural by obstetric anaesthetists. Anaesthesia 2004;59(9):922–923.
8. Norris MC: Are combined spinal epidural catheters reliable? Int J Obstet Anaesth 2000;9:3–6.
9. Reynolds F: Damage to the conus medullaris following spinal anaesthesia. Anaesthesia 2001;56:238–247.
10. Cook TM: Combined spinal–epidural techniques. Anaesthesia 2000;55:42–64.
11. Hughes D, Simmons SW, Brown J, et al: Combined spinal–epidural versus epidural analgesia in labour. Cochrane Database Syst Rev 2003;(4):CD003401. Review.
12. Poulakka R, Pitkanen MT, Rosenberg PH: Comparison of technical and block characteristics of different combined spinal and epidural anesthesia techniques. Reg Anesth Pain Med 2001;26:17–23.
13. Cherng YG, Wang YP, Liu CC, et al: Combined spinal and epidural anesthesia for abdominal hysterectomy in a patient with myotonic dystrophy. Case report. Reg Anesth 1994;19(1):69–72.
14. Browne IM, Birnbach DJ, Stein DJ, et al: A comparison of Espocan and Tuohy needles for the combined spinal–epidural technique for labor analgesia. Anesth Analg 2005;101:535–540.
15. Norris M C, Grieco W M, Borkowski M, et al: Complications of labor analgesia: Epidural versus combined spinal epidural techniques. Anesth Analg 1994;79:529–537.
16. Viscomi CM, Rathmell JP, Pace NL: Duration of intrathecal labor analgesia. Early versus advanced labor. Anesth Analg 1997;84:1108–1112.
17. Collis RE, Davies DW, Aveling W: Randomised comparison of combined spinal epidural and standard epidural analgesia in labour. Lancet 1995;345:1413–1416.
18. Palmer CM, Randall CC, Hays R, et al: The dose-response relation of intrathecal fentanyl for labor analgesia. Anesthesiology 1998;88:355–361.
19. Campbell DC, Camann WR, Datta S, et al: The addition of bupivacaine to intrathecal sufentanil for labor analgesia. Anesth Analg 1995;81:305–309.
20. Sia AT, Chong JL, Chiu JW: Combination of intrathecal sufentanil 10 mcg plus bupivacaine 2.5 mg for labor analgesia. Is half the dose enough? Anesth Analg 1999;88:362–366.
21. Hughes D, Hill D, Fee JP: Intrathecal ropivacaine or bupivacaine with fentanyl for labour. Br J Anaesth 2001;87:733–737.
22. Vercauteren MP, Haus G, De Decker K, et al: Levobupivacaine combined with sufentanil for intrathecal labor analgesia: A comparison with racemic bupivacaine Anesth Analg 2001;93:996–1000.
23. Tsen L, Thue B, Datta S, et al: Is combined spinal–epidural analgesia associated with more rapid cervical dilation in nulliparous patients when compared with conventional epidural analgesia? Anesthesiology 1999;91:920–925.
24. Wong CA, Scavon BM, Peaceman AM, et al: The risk of cesarean delivery with neuraxial analgesia given early versus late in labor. N Engl J Med 2005;352(7):655–665.
25. Carrie LES, O'Sullivan GM: Subarachnoid bupivacaine 0.5% for cesarean section. Eur J Anaesthesiol 1984;1:275–283.
26. Crowhurst J, Birnbach DJ: Low dose neuraxial block. Heading towards the new millennium. Anesth Analg 2000;90:241–242.
27. Blumgart CH, Ryall D, Dennison B, et al: Mechanism of extension of spinal anaesthesia by extradural injection of local anesthetic. Br J Anaesth 1992;69:457.
28. Eappen S, Blinn A, Segal S: Incidence of epidural catheter replacement in parturients: A retrospective chart review. Int J Obstet Anesth 1998;7:220–225.
29. Pan PH, Bogard TD, Owen MD: Incidence and characteristics of failures in obstetric neuraxial analgesia and anesthesia: A retrospective analysis of 19,259 deliveries. Int J Obstet Anesth 2004;13(4):227–233.
30. Choi DH, Park YD: Comparison of combined spinal–epidural anaesthesia and spinal anaesthesia for Caesarean section. IMRAPT 2002;14:A129.
31. Reyes M, Pan PH: Very low-dose spinal anesthesia for cesarean section in a morbidly obese preeclamptic patient and its potential implications. Int J Obstet Anesth 2004;13(2):99–102.
32. Ranasinghe JS, Steadman J, Toyama T, et al: Combined spinal epidural anaesthesia is better than spinal or epidural alone for Caesarean delivery. Br J Anaesth 2003;91(2):299–300.
33. Lim Y, Loo CC, Goh E: Ultra low dose combined spinal and epidural anesthesia for cesarean section. Int J Obstet Anesth 2004;13(3):198–200.
34. Peng PW, Chan VW, Perks A: Minimum effective anaesthetic concentration of hyperbaric lidocaine for spinal anaesthesia. Can J Anesth 1998;45:122–129.
35. Urmey WF, Stanton J, Peterson M, et al: Combined spinal–epidural anaesthesia for outpatient surgery. Dose-response characteristics

of intrathecal isobaric lidocaine using a 27-gauge Whitacre needle. Anesthesiology 1995;83:528–534.

36. Norris MC: Combined spinal–epidural anaesthesia for urological and lower extremity vascular procedures. Tech Reg Anaesth Pain Manage 1997;1:131–136.

37. Lew E, Yeo SW, Thomas E: Combined spinal–epidural anesthesia using epidural volume extension leads to faster motor recovery after elective cesarean delivery: A prospective, randomized, double-blind study. Anesth Analg 2004;98(3):810–814.

38. Fan SZ, Suseti L, Wang YP, et al: Low dose of intrathecal hyperbaric bupivacaine combined with epidural lidocaine for Caesarean section—A balance block technique. Anesth Analg 1994;78:474–477.

39. Landau R, Giraud R, Morales M, et al: Sequential combined spinal–epidural anesthesia for cesarean section in a woman with a double-outlet right ventricle. Acta Anaesthesiol Scand 2004;48(7):922–926.

40. Thorén T, Holmström B, Rawal N, et al: Sequential combined spinal epidural block versus spinal block for Caesarean section: Effects on maternal hypotension and neurobehavioral function of the newborn. Anesth Analg 1994;78:1087–1092.

41. Hoffmann VL, Vercauteren MP, Vreugde JP, et al: Posterior epidural space depth: Safety of the loss of resistance and hanging drop techniques. Br J Anaesth 1999;83(5):807–809.

42. Han KR, Kim C, Park SK, et al: Distance to the adult cervical epidural space. Reg Anesth Pain Med 2003;28(2):95–97.

43. McAndrew CR, Harms P: Paraesthesiae during needle-through-needle combined spinal epidural versus single-shot spinal for elective caesarean section. Anaesth Intensive Care 2003;31(5):514–517.

44. Hoffmann VL, Vercauteren MP, Buczkowski PW, et al: A new combined spinal–epidural apparatus: Measurement of the distance to the epidural and subarachnoid spaces. Anaesthesia 1997;52(4):350–355.

45. Cousins MJ, Bridenbaugh PO: *Neural Blockade in Clinical Anesthesia and Management of Pain,* 3rd ed. Lippincott-Raven, 1998, pp 252–255.

46. Watts RW: The influence of obesity on the relationship between body mass index and the distance to the epidural space from the skin. Anesth Intensive Care 1993;21:309–310.

47. Lirk P, Moriggl B, Colvin J, et al: The incidence of lumbar Ligamentum flavum midline gaps. Anesth Analg 2004;98:1178–1180.

48. Cook TM: Combined spinal–epidural techniques. Anaesthesia 2000;55:42–64.

49. Landau R: Combined spinal–epidural analgesia for labor: Breakthrough or unjustified invasion? Semin Perinatol 2002;26(2):109–121. Review.

50. Rawal N, Holmstrom B: The combined spinal–epidural technique. Best Pract Res Clin Anaesthesiol 2003;17(3):347–364. Review.

51. Soresi AL: Episubdural anesthesia. Anesth Analg 1937;16:306–310.

52. Curelaru I: Long duration subarachnoid anesthesia with continuous epidural block. Prakt Anasth 1979;14:71–78.

53. Brownridge P: Central neural blockade and Cesarean Section, Part 1. Review and case series. Anaesth Intensive Care 1979;7:33–41.

54. Brownridge P: Epidural and subarachnoid analgesia for elective Cesarean section. Aneaesthesia 1981;36:70.

55. Coates MB: Combined subarachnoid and epidural techniques. Anaesthesia 1982;37:89–90.

56. Mumtaz MH, Daz M, Kuz M: Another single space technique for orthopaedic surgery. Anaesthesia 1982;37:90.

57. Carrie LES, O'Sullivan GM: Subarachnoid bupivacaine 0.5% for Cesarean section. Eur J Anaesthesiol 1984;1:275–283.

58. Turner MA, Reifenberg NA: Combined spinal epidural analgesia. The single space double-barrel technique. Int J Obstet Anesth 1995;55:158–160.

59. Cook TM: A new combined spinal–epidural technique. Int J Obstet Anesth 1999;55:3–6.

60. Brownridge P: Epidural and subarachnoid analgesia for elective Caesarean section. Anaesthesia 1981;55:70.

61. Carrie LES: Epidural versus combined spinal epidural block for Caesarean section. Acta Anaesth Scand 1988;55:595–596.

62. Morris GN, Kinsella M, Thomas TA: Pencil-point needles and combined spinal epidural block. Why needle through needle? Anaesthesia 1998;55:1132.

63. Kestin IG: Spinal anaesthesia in obstetrics. Br J Anaesth 1991;55:663.

64. Eldor J: Combined spinal–epidural anaesthesia through the Portex set. Anaesthesia 1993;55:836.

65. Soni AK, Sarna MC: Combined spinal epidural analgesia. The single space double-barrel technique. Int J Obstet Anesth 1996;55:206–207.

66. Sakuma N, Hori M, Suzuki H, et al: A sheared off and sequestered epidural catheter: A case report Masui 2004;53(2):198–200.

67. Roberts E, Brighouse D: Combined spinal–epidural anaesthesia for Caesarean section. Anaesthesia 1992;55:1006.

68. Cook TM: 201 combined spinal–epidurals for anaesthesia using a separate needle technique. Eur J Anaesthesiol 2004;21(9):679–683.

69. Levin A, Segal S, Datta S: Does combined spinalepidural analgesia alter the incidence of paraesthesia during epidural catheter insertion? Anesth Analg 1998;55:445–451.

70. Familton MJG, Morgan BM: 'Needle-through-needle' technique for combined spinal–extradural anaesthesia in obstetrics. Br J Anaesth 1992;55:327.

71. Patel M, Samsoon G, Swami A, et al: Posture and the spread of hyperbaric bupivacaine in parturients using the combined spinal epidural technique. Can J Anaesth 1993;55:943–946.

72. McAndrew CR, Harms P: Paraesthesiae during needle-through-needle combined spinal epidural versus single-shot spinal for elective caesarean section. Anaesth Intensive Care 2003;31(5):514–517.

73. Lyons G, Macdonald R, Mikl B: Combined epiduralspinal anaesthesia for Caesarean section. Through the needle or in separate spaces? Anaesthesia 1992;55:199–201.

74. Casati A, D'ambrosio A, De Negri P, et al: A clinical comparison between needle-through-needle and double segment techniques for combined spinal and epidural anesthesia. Reg Anesth Pain Med 1998;55:390–394.

75. Rawal N, Van Zundert A, Holmström B, et al: Combined spinalepidural technique. Reg Anesth 1997;55:406–423.

76. Backe SK, Sheikh Z, Wilson R, et al: Combined epidural/spinal anaesthesia: Needle-through-needle or separate spaces? Eur J Anaesthesiol 2004;21(11):854–857.

77. Grau T, Leipold RW, Fatehi S, et al: Real-time ultrasonic observation of combined spinal–epidural anaesthesia. Eur J Anaesthesiol 2004;21(1):25–31.

78. Tsui BC, Gupta S, Finucane B: Determination of epidural catheter placement using nerve stimulation in obstetric patients. Reg Anesth 1999;24:17–23.

79. Herman NL, Calicott R, Van Decar TK, et al: Determination of the dose-response relationship for intrathecal sufentanil in laboring patients. Anesth Analg 1997;84:1256–1261.

80. Herman NL, Choi KC, Affleck PJ, et al: Analgesia, pruritus, and ventilation exhibit in parturients receiving intrathecal fentanyl during labor. Anesth Analg 1999;89(2):378–383.

81. Palmer CM, Randall CC, Hays R, et al: The dose-response relation of intrathecal fentanyl for labor analgesia. Anesthesiology 1998;88:355–361.

82. Honet JE, Arkoosh VA, Norris MC, et al: Comparison among intrathecal fentanyl, meperidine, and sufentanil for labor analgesia. Anesth Analg 1992;75:734–739.

83. Jaffe RA, Rowe MA: Comparison of the local anesthetic effects of meperidine, fentanyl, and sufentanil on dorsal root axons. Anesth Analg 1996;83:776–781.

84. Flanagan MT, Walker FO, Butterworth J: Failure of meperidine to anesthetize human median nerve. A blinded comparison with lidocaine and saline. Reg Anesth 1997;22:73–79.

85. Abouleish A, Abouleish E, Camann W: Combined spinal–epidural analgesia in advanced labor. Can J Anaesth 1994;41:575–578.

86. Campbell DC, Camann WR, Datta S: The addition of bupivacaine to intrathecal sufentanil for labor analgesia. Anesth Analg 1995;81:305–309.

87. Sia ATH, Chong JL, Chiu JW: Combination of intrathecal sufentanil 10 mcg plus bupivacaine 2.5 mg for labor analgesia: Is half the dose enough? Anesth Analg 1999;88:362–366.

88. Stocks GM, Hallworth SP, Fernando R, et al: Minimum local analgesic dose of intrathecal bupivacaine in labor and the effect of intrathecal fentanyl. Anesthesiology 2001;94:593–598.

89. Levin A, Datta S, Camann W: Intrathecal ropivacaine for labor analgesia: A comparison with bupivacaine. Anesth Analg 1998;87:624–627.

90. Soni AK, Miller CG, Pratt SD, Hess PE, Oriol NE, Sarna MC: Low dose intrathecal ropivacaine with or without sufentanil provides effective analgesia and does not impair motor strength during labour: A pilot study. Can J Anaesth 2001;48(7):677–680.

91. Joshi GP, McCarroll SM: Evaluation of combined spinal–epidural anaesthesia using two different techniques. Reg Anaesth 1994;55:169–174.

92. Collis RE, Baxandall ML, Srikantharajah ID, et al: Combined spinal epidural analgesia with ability to walk throughout labour. Lancet 1993;55:76–78.

93. Hoffmann VLH, Vercauteran MP, Buczkowski PW, et al: A new combined spinal epidural apparatus: Measurement of the distance to the epidural and subarachnoid spaces. Anaesthesia 1997;55:350–355.

94. Westbrook JL, Donald F, Carrie LES: An evaluation of a combined spinal/epidural needle set utilising a 26-gauge pencil point spinal needle for Caesarean section. Anaesthesia 1992;55:990–992.

95. Randalls B, Broadway JW, Browne DA, et al: Comparison of four solutions in a needle-through-needle technique for elective Caesarean section. Br J Anaesth 1991;55:314–318.

96. Holloway TE, Telford RJ: Observations on deliberate dural puncture with a Touhy needle: depth measurement. Anesthesia 1991;46:722–724.

97. Cousins MJ, Bridenbaugh PO: *Neural Blockade in Clinical Anesthesia and Management of Pain*, 3rd ed. Lippincott-Raven, 1998, pp 255.

98. Brighouse D, Wilkins A: Failure of pencil-point spinal needles to enter the subarachnoid space. Anaesthesia 1994;55:176.

99. Meiklejohn BH: The effect of rotation of an epidural needle: an in vitro study. Anaesthesia 1987;42:1180–1182.

100. Husemeyer RP, White DC: Topography of the lumbar epidural space. Anaesthesia 1980;55:7–11.

101. Waldman SA, Liguori GA: Comparison of the flow rates of 27-gauge Whitacre and Sprotte needles for combined spinal and epidural anesthesia. Reg Anesth 1996;55:378–379.

102. Vandermeersch E: Combined spinal–epidural anaesthesia. Balliere's Clin Anaesth 1993;7:691–708.

103. Fukishige T, Sano T, Kano T: Lumbar dural sac deformation after epidural injection. Anesthesiology 1998;55:A870.

104. Norris MC, Grieco WM, Borkowski M, et al: Complications of labor analgesia: Epidural versus combined spinal epidural techniques. Anesthesia and Analgesia 1994;55:529–537.

105. Lesser P, Bembridge M, Lyons G, et al: An evaluation of a 30-gauge needle for spinal anaesthesia for Caesarean section. Anaesthesia 1990;55:76–78.

106. Dennison B: Combined subarachnoid and epidural block for Caesarean section. Can J Anaesth 1987;55:105.

107. Patel M, Swami M: Combined spinal–extradural anaesthesia for Caesarean section. Anaesthesia 1992;55:1005–1006.

108. Eldor J: Metallic fragments and the combined spinal–extradural technique. Br J Anaest 1992;69:663.

109. Robbins PM, Fernando R, Lim GH: Accidental intrathecal insertion of an extradural catheter during combined spinal extradural anaesthesia for Caesarean section. Br J Anaesth 1995;55:557.

110. Vucevic M, Russell IF: Spinal anaesthesia for Caesarean section: 0.125% plain bupivacaine 12 mL compared with 0.5% plain bupivacaine 3 mL. Br J Anaesth 1992;55:590–5.

111. Ferguson DJM: Dural puncture and epidural catheters. Anaesthesia 1992;55:272.

112. Muranaka K, Tsutsui T: Comparison of clinical usefulness of the two types of combined spinal epidural needles. Masui 1994;55:1714–1717.

113. Angle P, Kronberg JE, Thompson DE, et al: Epidural catheter penetration of human dura tissue: In vitro investigation. Anesthesiology 2004;100(6):141–46.

114. Holtz D, Mollman M, Schymroszcyk B, et al: No risk of metal toxicity in combined spinal–epidural anesthesia. Anesth Analg 1999;88(2):393–397.

115. Holmstrom B, Rawal N, Axelsson K, et al: Risk of catheter migration during combined spinal epidural block—percutaneous epiduroscopy study. Anesth Analg 1995;80:747–753.

116. Leighton BL, Arkoosh VA, Huffnagle S, et al: The dermatomal spread of epidural bupivacaine with and without prior intrathecal sufentanil. Anesth Analg 1996;83:526–529.

117. Stienstra R, Dilrosun-Alhadi BZ, Dahan A, et al: The epidural "top-up" in combined spinal-epidural anesthesia: The effect of volume versus dose. Anesth Analg 1999;88:810–814.

118. Suzuki N, Koganemaru M, Onizuka S, et al: Dural puncture with a 26G spinal needle affects spread of epidural anesthesia. Anesth Analg 1996;82:1040–1042.

119. Bernard CM, Kopacz DJ, Michel MZ: Effect of needle puncture on morphine and lidocaine flux through the spinal meninges of the monkey in vitro. Implications for combined spinal–epidural anaesthesia. Anesthesiology 1994;80:853–858.

120. Hodgkinson R: Total spinal block after epidural injection into an interspace adjacent to an inadvertent dural perforation. Anesthesiology 1981;55:593–595.

121. Eldor J, Guedj P, Levine S: Delayed respiratory arrest in combined spinal–epidural anesthesia. Case report. Reg Anesth 1994;19;418–422.

122. Leach A, Smith GB: Subarachnoid spread of epidural local anaesthetic following dural puncture. Anaesthesia 1988;43:671–674.

123. Gaiser RR, Lewin SB, Cheek TG, et al: Effects of immediately initiating an epidural infusion in the combined spinal and epidural technique in nulliparous parturients. Reg Anesth Pain Med 2000;25:223–227.

124. Beaubien G, Drolet P, Girard M, et al: Patient-controlled epidural analgesia with fentanyl-bupivacaine: Influence of prior dural puncture. Reg Anesth Pain Med 2000;25:254–258.

125. Kuczkowski KM, Birnbach DJ, O'Gorman DA, et al: Does a test dose increase the likelihood of identifying intrathecal placement of epidural catheters during labor analgesia? Abstract of Scientific Papers SOAP. Anesthesiology 2000; A26.

126. Goy RW, Sia AT: Sensorimotor anesthesia and hypotension after subarachnoid block: Combined spinal–epidural versus single-shot spinal technique. Anesth Analg 2004;98(2):491–496.

127. Goy RWL, Chee-Seng Y: The median effective dose of intrathecal hyperbaric bupivacaine is larger in the single-shot spinal as compared with the combined spinal–epidural technique. Anesth Analg 2005;100:1499–1502.

128. Gaur V, Gupta RK, Agarwal A, et al: Air or nitrous oxide for loss-of-resistance epidural technique? Can J Anaesth 2000;47:503–505.

129. Carpenter RL, Hogan QH, Liu SS, et al: Lumbosacral cerebrospinal fluid volume is the primary determinant of sensory block extent and duration during spinal anesthesia. Anesthesiology 1998;89:24–29.

130. Rawal N, Schollin J, Wesström G: Epidural versus combined spinal epidural block for Caesarean section. Acta Anaesthiol Scand 1988;32:61–66.

131. Kumar C: Combined subarachnoid and epidural block for Caesarean section. Can J Anaesth 1987;34:329–330.

132. Klasen J, Junger A, Hartmann B, et al: Differing incidences of relevant hypotension with combined spinal–epidural anesthesia and spinal anesthesia. Anesth Analg 2003;96:1491–1495.

133. Blumgart CH, Ryall D, Dennison B, et al: Mechanism of extension of spinal anaesthesia by extradural injection of local anaesthetic. Br J Anaesth 1992;69:457–460.

134. Takiguchi T, Okano T, Egawa H, et al: The effect of epidural saline injection on analgesic level during combined spinal and epidural anaesthesia assessed clinically and myelographically. Anesth Analg 1997;85:1097–1100.

135. Mandell GL, Jamnback L, Ramanathan S: Hemodynamic effects of subarachnoid fentanyl in laboring parturients. Reg Anesth 1995;21(2):103–111.

136. Horlocker TT, McGregor DG, Matsushige DK, et al: A retrospective review of 4767 consecutive spinal anesthetics: Central nervous system complications. Anesth Analg 1997;55:578–584.

137. Simsa J: Use of 29-G spinal needle s and a fixation device with combined spinal epidural technique. Acta Anaesthesiol Scand 1994;38:439–441.

138. McAndrew CR, Harms P: Paraesthesiae during needle-through-needle combined spinal epidural versus single-shot spinal for elective caesarean section. Anaesth Intensive Care 2003;31(5):514–517.

139. Holloway J, Seed PT, O'Sullivan G, et al: Paraesthesiae and nerve damage following combined spinal epidural and spinal anaesthesia: a pilot survey. Int J Obstet Anesth 2000;9(3):151–155.

140. Turner MA, Shaw M: Atraumatic spinal needles (letter). Anaesthesia 1993;48:452.

141. Broadbent CR, Maxwell WB, Ferrie R, et al:. Ability of anaesthetists to identify a marked lumbar interspace. Anaesthesia 2000;55:1106–1126.

142. Dripps Rd, Vandem LD: Long-term follow-up of patients who received 10.098 spinal anaesthetics. JAMA 1954;156:1486–1491.

143. Phillips OC, Ebner H, Melson AT, et al: Neurological complications following spinal anesthesia with lidocaine: A prospective review of 10,440 cases. Anesthesiology 1969;30:284–289.

144. Harding SA, Collis RE, Morgan BM:. Meningitis after combined spinal extradural anaesthesia in obstetrics. Br J Anaesth 1994;73:545–547.

145. Cascio M: Meningitis following a combined spinal–epidural technique in a labouring term parturient. Can J Anaesth 1996;43:399–402.

146. Pinder AJ, Dresner M: Meningococcal meningitis after combined spinal–epidural analgesia. Int J Obstet Anesth 2003;12:183–187.

147. Choy JC: Mortality from peripartum meningitis. Anaesth Intensive Care 2000;28:328–330.

148. McLure HA, Talboys CA, Yentis SM, et al: Surgical facemesks and downward dispersal of bacteria. Anaesthesia 1998;53:624–626.

149. Phillips BJ, Fergusson S, Armstrong P, et al: Surgical facemasks are effective in reducing bacterial contamination caused by dispersal from the upper airway. Br J Anaesth 1992;69:407–408.

150. Burnstein R, Buckland R, Pickett JA: A survey of epidural analgesia for labour in the United Kingdom. Anesthesia 1999;54:634–650.

151. Rawal N, Holmstrom B, Croehurst JA, et al: The combined spinal–epidural technique. Anaesthsiol Clin North Am 2000;18:267–295.

152. Dunn SM, Connelly NR, Parker RK: Postdural puncture headache (PDPH) and combined spinal anesthesia (CSE). Anesth Analg 2000;90:1249–1250.

153. Balestrieri PJ: The incidence of postdural puncture headache and combined spinal–epidural: Some thoughts. Int J Obstet Anesth 2003;12(4):305–306.

154. Brownridge P: Spinal anaesthesia in obstetrics. Br J Anaesth 1991;67:663–667.

155. Geurts JW, Haanschoten MC, Van Wijk RM, et al: Post-dural puncture headache in young patients. A comparative study between the use of 0.52 mm (25-gauge) and 0.33 mm (29-gauge) spinal needles. Acta Anaesthesiol Scand 1990;34:350–353.

156. Chan BO, Paech MJ: Persistent cerebrospinal fluid leak: A complication of the combined spinal–epidural technique. Anesth Analg 2004;98(3):828–830.

157. Reisinger PWM, Hochstrasser K: The diagnosis of CSF fistulae on the basis of detection of beta2-transferrin by polyacrylamide gel electrophoresis and immunoblotting. J Clin Chem Clin Biochem 1989;27:169–172.

158. Howes J, Lenz R: Cerebrospinal fluid cutaneous fistula—An unusual complication of epidural anaesthesia. Anaesthesia 1994;49:221–222.

159. Pan PH, Moore CH, Ross VH: Severe maternal bradycardia and asystole after combined spinal–epidural labor analgesia in a morbidly obese parturient. J Clin Anesth 2004;16(6):461–464.

160. Kuczkowski KM: Severe persistent fetal bradycardia following subarachnoid administration of fentanyl and bupivacaine for induction of a combined spinal–epidural analgesia for labor pain. J Clin Anesth 2004;16(1):78–79.

161. D'Angelo R, Eisenach JC: Severe maternal hypotension and fetal bradycardia after a CSE. Anesthesiology 1997;81:116–118.

162. O'Gorman D, Birnbach DJ, Kuczkowski KM, et al: Use of umbilical flow velocimetry in the assessment of the pathogenesis of fetal bradycardia following combined spinal epidural analgesia in parturients (Abs). Anesthesiology 2000;92:A2.

163. Clarke VT, Smiley RM, Finster M: Uterine hyperactivity after intrathecal injection of fentanyl for analgesia during labor: A cause of fetal bradycardia? Anesthesiology 1994;81:1083.

164. Albright GA, Forster RM: Does combined spinal–epidural analgesia with subarachnoid sufentanil increase the incidence of emergency cesarean delivery? Reg Anesth Pain Med 1997;22:400–405.

165. Rawal N, Schollin J, Wesstrom G: Epidural versus combined spinal epidural block for cesarean section. Acta Anaesthesiol Scand 1988;32:61–66.

166. Joshi GP, MaCarroll SM: Combined spinal—epidural anesthesia using needle-through-needle technique (Letter). Anesthesiology 1993;78:406–407.

167. Pan PH: Laboratory evaluation of single-lumen, dual-orifice combined spinal-epidural needles: Effects of bevel orientation and modified technique. J Clin Anesth 1998;10(4):286–290.

168. Riley ET, Hamilton CL, Ratner EF, et al: A comparison of the 24-gauge Sprotte and Gertie Marx spinal needles for combined spinal–epidural analgesia during labor. Anesthesiology 2002;97(3):574-577.

169. Herbstman CH, Jaffe JB, Tuman KJ, et al: An in vivo evaluation of four spinal needles used for the combined spinal–epidural technique. Anesth Analg 1998;86(3):520–522.

170. Simsa J: Needle fixation with combined spinalepidural anaesthesia. Acta Anaesthesiol Scand 1995;55:275.

171. Stocks GM, Hallworth SP, Fernando R: Evaluation of a spinal needle locking device for use with the combined spinal epidural technique. Anaesthesia 2000;55(12):1185–1188.

172. Eldor J, Chaimsky G: The Eldor combined spinal–epidural needle. Anesthesia 1993;48;173.

173. Torrieri A, Aldrete JA: Combined spinal–epidural needle. Acta Anaesthesio Belg 1998;39:65–66.

174. Birnbach DJ, Chestnut DH: The epidural test dose in obstetric practice: Has it outlived its usefulness? Anesth Analg 1999;88:971.

175. Steffek M, Owczuk R, Szlyk-Augustyn M, et al: Total spinal anaesthesia as a complication of local anaesthetic test-dose administration through an epidural catheter. Acta Anaesthesiol Scand 2004;48(9):1211–1213.

176. Norris MC, Ferrenbach D, Dalman H, et al: Does epinephrine improve the diagnostic accuracy of aspiration during labor epidural analgesia? Anesth Analg 1999;88;1073.

177. Moore DC, Batra MS: The components of an effective test dose prior to epidural block. Anesthesiology 1981;55:693.

178. Hood DD, Dewan DM, James FM III: Maternal and fetal effect of epinephrine in gravid ewes. Anesthesiology 1986;64:610.

179. Leighton BL, Norris MC, DeSimone CA, et al: The air test as a clinically useful indicator of intravenously placed epidural catheters. Anesthesiology 1990;73:610.

180. Kopacz DJ: Spinal 2-chloroprocaine: Minimum effective dose. Reg Anesth Pain Med 2005;30(1):36–42.

181. Hamza J, Smida M, Benhamou D, et al: Parturient's posture during epidural puncture affects the distance from skin to epidural space. J Clin Anesth 1995;7:1–4.

182. Yun EM, Marx GF, Santos AC: The effects of maternal position during induction of combined spinal–epidural anesthesia for Caesarean delivery. Anesth Analg 1998;87:614–618.

183. Lewis NL, Ritchie EL, Downer JP, et al: Left lateral vs. supine, wedged position for development of block after combined spinal–epidural anaesthesia for Caesarean section. Anaesthesia 2004;59:894–898.

17

Equipment for Peripheral Nerve Block

Ban C. H. Tsui, MD • Admir Hadzic, MD

INTRODUCTION

As in other areas of medicine, anesthesiologists increasingly rely on more sophisticated equipment in regional anesthesia. The advanced technology used to accomplish and increase the success rate of regional anesthesia techniques requires thorough understanding of the equipment. One of the most important advances in regional anesthesia was the introduction of the portable peripheral nerve stimulator in the late 1970s and early 1980s.[1] Since that time, many improvements in nerve stimulators were made, as well as to the needle and catheter designs. Over the last decade, ultrasound also developed into a promising method for nerve localization.[1-3] As technology continues to evolve, it will likely assume a more significant role in regional anesthesia. Nevertheless, the performance of regional anesthesia techniques still requires proper set-up, careful preparation, detailed planning, and continuous monitoring to provide safe and effective patient care.

INDUCTION & BLOCK ROOM

Clinical Pearl

- A designated area with proper equipment and monitoring devices is essential for providing effective and safe regional anesthesia.

Regional anesthesia should be performed only in a designated area with the proper equipment (Figure 17–1). This area could be the operating room or a separate area within the surgical suite. Regardless of where the actual procedure is performed, adequate space, proper equipment, and careful monitoring are essential to ensure time-efficient and safe care of the patient undergoing the peripheral nerve block.[4–6] To facilitate the successful implementation of a nerve block, all supplies, drugs, and other equipment must be readily available in the room. The designated area must be large enough to enable proper monitoring and resuscitation of patients. And it should have proper lighting, suction, and equipment for oxygen administration and emergency airway management, including positive-pressure ventilation.

MONITORING

Toxicity from an inadvertent intravascular injection or rapid absorption or channeling of local anesthetic into the systemic circulation is always a potential risk when administering

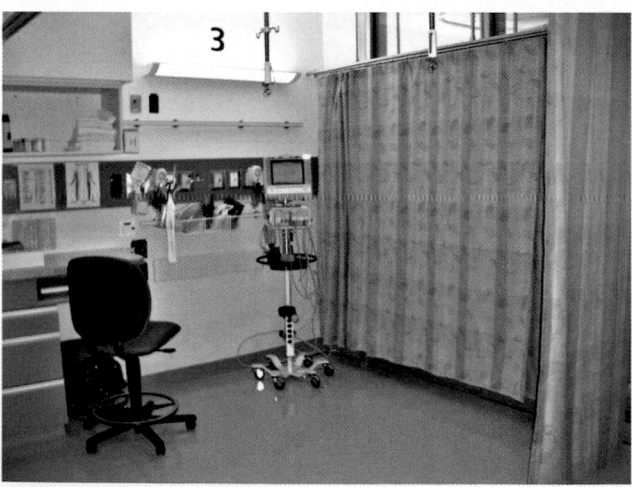

Figure 17–1. An example of room/area with basic monitoring equipment.

local anesthetic for any regional block. Vigilant monitoring is crucial for diagnosing and managing any potential complications that arise during or after a regional anesthesia or analgesia procedure.[4,7] Every patient should have vascular access secured prior to performing the procedure.

Clinical Pearls

- Patients having regional anesthesia should be monitored similarly to patients undergoing general anesthesia.
- Level of consciousness, pulse oximetry, vital signs (blood pressure and heart rate), electrocardiogram (ECG), and respiratory rate should be monitored and documented throughout the procedure.

The patient's baseline level of consciousness, pulse oximetry, vital signs (blood pressure and heart rate), ECG, and respiratory rate should be monitored throughout the procedure. After completion of the block, all patients should be monitored for at least 30 min for any signs of local anesthetic toxicity. It is important to keep in mind that although a toxic reaction typically occurs during or immediately following the injection of local anesthetic, it can also occur due to absorption. In the latter scenario, signs and symptoms of toxicity become apparent after the serum levels of local anesthetic peak (typically, 20 min following the injection).

Patients undergoing surgery under regional anesthesia should be cared for in the same way as patients having general anesthesia. Blood pressure, heart rate, respiratory rate, and ECG should be continuously monitored throughout the surgery. However, temperature monitoring is usually not necessary in minimally sedated and conversing patients.

REGIONAL ANESTHESIA EQUIPMENT STORAGE CART

Clinical Pearl

- An equipment cart should contain all the drugs, needles, and catheters necessary for regional anesthesia; it also should contain necessary emergency drugs and equipment.

A well-stocked and maintained regional anesthesia cart is essential for providing effective, time-efficient, and safe regional anesthesia (Figure 17–2). The cart should be organized logically to include all commonly used equipment, supplies, and local anesthetics. Supplies needed include draping and skin disinfecting supplies, nerve stimulators, and resuscitation drugs and equipment.[4,6] An atlas and textbook of regional anesthesia are invaluable resources and can be included in the cart. Finally, the cart should be organized and stocked

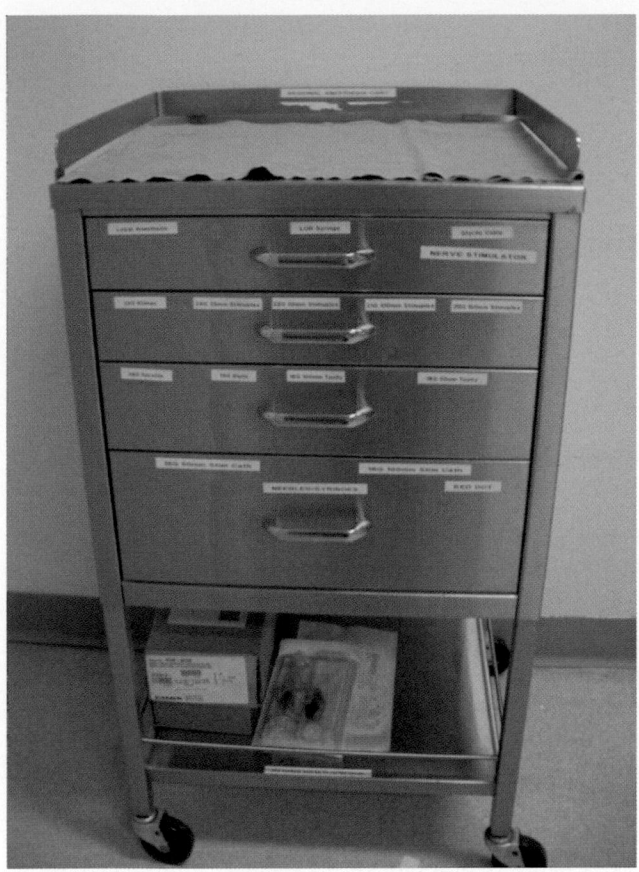

Figure 17–2. An example of regional anesthesia equipment storage chart.

in such a way that most regional blocks can be performed efficiently and without interruption in the designated area.

EMERGENCY DRUGS & EQUIPMENT

Although adverse effects and complications from peripheral nerve blocks are relatively rare, in the case of an untoward reaction or complication, immediate and timely intervention is necessary to prevent adverse outcomes.[4,6,7] Thus, all emergency drugs and airway equipment should be readily available in a neatly organized designated drawer in the regional block cart. Emergency drugs should include atropine, epinephrine, phenylephrine, ephedrine, propofol, and succinylcholine. In addition, laryngoscopic equipment with an assortment of commonly used blades, styletted endotracheal tubes and airways of various sizes, and a mask-valve ventilation device (Ambubag) with an oxygen source and a suction apparatus should be in the designated drawer.

PREMEDICATION

Sedation and analgesia is used commonly when preparing patients for regional anesthesia. Particular attention should be paid to the dosage and titration of these drugs in order to

Table 17–1.

Commonly Used Sedatives

Bolus	Infusion
Midazolam 1–2 mg (Titrated up to 0.07 mg/kg) Fentanyl 0.5 mcg/kg	Remifentanil 0.05 mcg/kg/min Propofol 12 mg/kg/h

obtain the maximum benefit with minimal side effects, especially in elderly patients.[8] Ideally, sedatives should be short-acting, easy to administer, and have a low side effect profile and a high safety margin. Effective sedation can be achieved with propofol, midazolam, fentanyl, remifentanil, or a combination of these drugs. The dosages of sedative and analgesic agents are titrated to achieve a level of sedation appropriate for a specific nerve block procedure and patient characteristics (Table 17–1).

SPECIALTY TRAYS

A commercially or institutionally prepared nerve block tray is useful for an efficient and successful nerve block. Ideally, such trays should be customized to contain all necessary equipment to perform the intended regional anesthesia procedure without interruption.[4–6,9] In practice, however, it is difficult to have a single set-up containing all desirable items, particularly with the extensive assortment of needles and catheters available. Instead, a basic regional anesthesia set-up that is suitable for most nerve blocks can be prepared or obtained commercially (Figure 17–3). Such a set-up should include

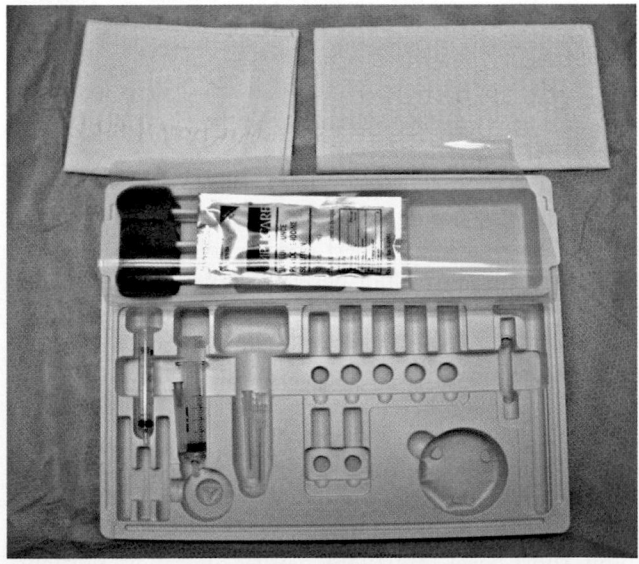

Figure 17–3. An example of a commercially available basic regional anesthesia tray.

items for sterile skin preparation and draping and needles and syringes for skin infiltration. The specific needle/catheter should then be selected and simply added to the tray for a specific block. Inclusion of a marking pen and ruler is helpful for outlining the patient's anatomy prior to performing the procedure. With proper preparation, the anesthesiologist can focus on performing the entire procedure without distraction.

REGIONAL BLOCK NEEDLES

Clinical Pearls

- For most single-shot peripheral nerve blocks, 21–25-gauge, short-bevel insulated needles are used.
- For continuous blocks, an 18-gauge, Tuohy tip needle with a stimulating catheter is becoming increasingly popular.

A wide variety of needles are available for peripheral nerve blocks. Depending on the block performed, the preference of the clinician, and the size of the patient, needles are chosen based on tip design, length, gauge, and the absence or presence of insulation.[4,6,7,9,10] Most anesthesiologists, however, now commonly use insulated needles for better block precision (see Chapter 5, Electrophysiology of Nerve Stimulation).

Needle Tip Design

Nerve injury following local anesthetic injection usually occurs from one of three mechanisms.[10,11] The first mechanism is from direct trauma to the nerve by the advancing needle. The second is from mechanical neural damage or ischemia to the nerve from a high-pressure intraneural injection of local anesthetic. Finally, nerve injury can occur as a result of a combination of the previous two mechanisms, with the possibility of toxic effects occurring from the local anesthetic or its preservative.

Currently, there is lack of clear evidence to suggest unequivocally that needle design is a significant factor in nerve injury; however, most expert anesthesiologists believe that pencil-point or short, blunt-bevel needle designs are less likely to cause injuries during nerve blockade. Intuitively, needles with short, blunt bevels or pencil points are much less likely to penetrate or cut nerves during needle advancement than are long- (cutting) bevel needles. Blunted, Tuohy-tip design needles recently were used with success for continuous peripheral nerve blocks.[12,13] The design of the needle tip can have a direct effect on an anesthesiologist's ability to appreciate the various tissue planes as it passes through them. Blunt, short-bevel, and Tuohy needles offer more resistance and thus give a better feel (with some techniques) as the needle traverses tissue layers than do sharper, long-bevel needles. In an in vitro study, anesthesiologists preferred needles that

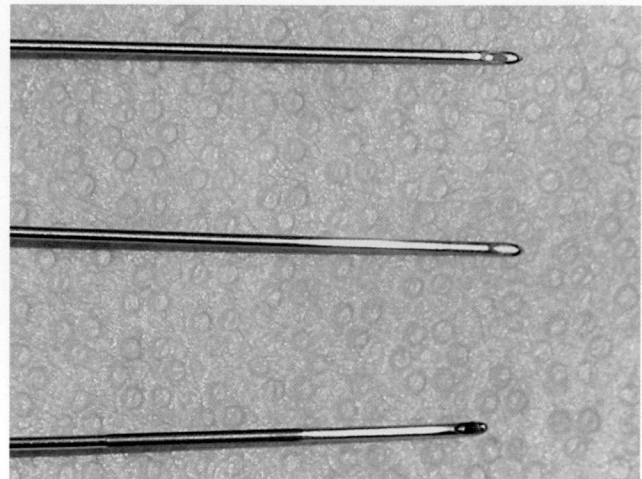

Figure 17–4. Various uninsulated single-shot needle tips. Top to bottom: Quincke, short-beveled, Tuohy.

offered moderate resistance and enhanced feel with the tissue penetration.[14] For a single-shot deep nerve or major plexus nerve block, most experts use short- and blunt-beveled needles with or without insulation (Figures 17–4 and 17–5). On the other hand, sharp and smaller gauge needles (eg, 25- and 26-gauge) are often used for transarterial axillary, superficial, and field blocks. If a block does not require nerve stimulation (eg, a paravertebral block), a 22-gauge, uninsulated Tuohy needle or Quincke spinal needle can be used. In the case of continuous blocks, short-bevel and Tuohy-style tips are used most commonly.

Needle Length

The appropriate length of a needle must be selected based on the block performed and the size of the patient. A needle that is too short will not reach its targeted depth. In contrast, excessively long needles carry a higher risk of causing serious complications, not only because they are more difficult

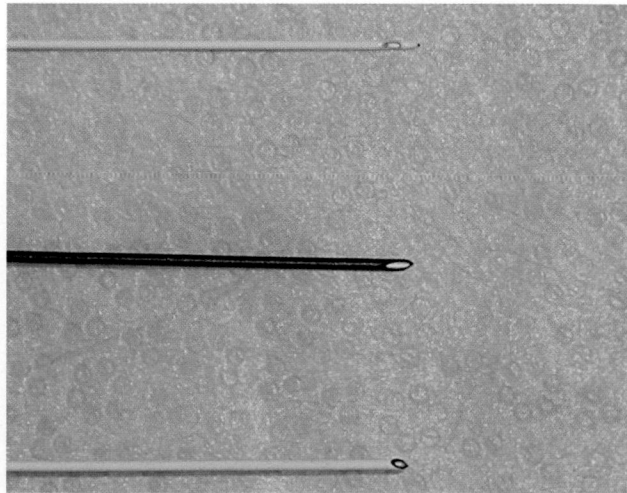

Figure 17–5. Various insulated single-shot needle designs. Top to bottom: Sprotte, Quincke, short-beveled.

Table 17–2.

Recommended Needle Length

Block Technique	Recommended Needle Length
Cervical plexus block	50 mm (2 in.)
Interscalene brachial plexus block	25 mm (1 in.) to 50 mm (2 in.)
Infraclavicular brachial plexus block	100 mm (4 in.)
Axillary brachial plexus block	25 (1 in.) to 50 mm (2 in.)
Thoracic paraverterbral block	90 mm (3.5–4 in.)
Lumbar paravertebral	100 mm (4 in.)
Lumbar plexus block	100 mm (4 in.)
Sciatic block–posterior approach	100 mm (4 in.)
Sciatic block–anterior approach	150 mm (6 in.)
Femoral block	50 mm (2 in.)
Popliteal block–posterior approach	50 mm (2 in.)
Popliteal block–lateral approach	100 mm (4 in.)

to manipulate but also because they tend to be inserted too deeply. The recommended needle lengths provided in this chapter are based on the authors' practice[4] and should be regarded as general guides only (Table 17–2).

Gauge

Choice of an appropriate gauge for a needle depends on whether the block will be a single-shot or a continuous catheter will be used. For a single-shot block, it is important to use a relatively small-gauge needle to reduce the risk of tissue trauma and undue discomfort. However, smaller gauge needles bend more easily, making it difficult to control the needle path. It is also more difficult to inject local anesthetics, assess injection pressure and resistance, and aspirate blood through the smaller gauge needles. In clinical practice, smaller gauge (eg, 25- and 26-gauge) needles are used for superficial and field blocks, whereas 22-gauge needles are commonly used for major conduction or deeper blocks. When using longer needles for deeper blocks, it may be necessary to use a larger gauge (eg, 21-gauge) to avoid bending the needle along its shaft and to retain control over the needle insertion path. For continuous blocks, the needle gauge must be large enough to allow the passage of a catheter. Currently, most clinicians use 18- or 19-gauge needles for continuous blocks (Figure 17–6). These needles usually are used with a 20-gauge catheter.

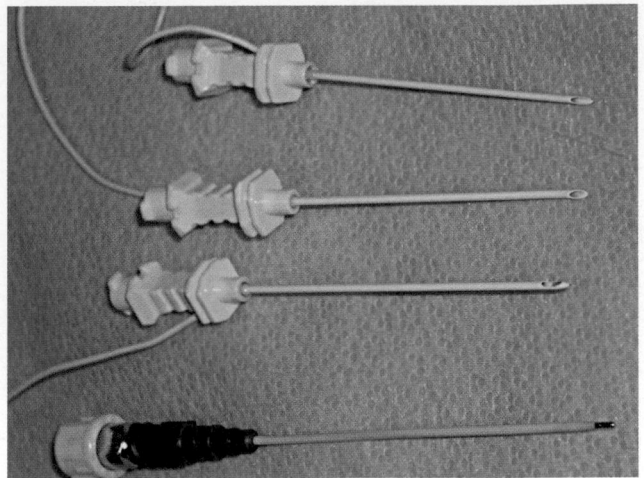

Figure 17–6. Various 18-gauge insulated needle for 20-gauge catheter. Top to bottom: Short-beveled, Tuohy, Sprotte, bullet-tipped.

Accessories

Extension tubing attached to the needle is useful in stabilizing the penetrating needle (immobile needle). With this tubing, the clinician or a helper is able to aspirate to test for intravascular needle placement and to change the syringe without moving the needle. Most commercial needles, therefore, have preattached extension tubing. Since greater force is required to initiate the injection, this technique may result in intraneural needle placement and it carries an increased risk of an intraneural injection.[15,16] A small pressure gauge can be used to objectively monitor and document the force of the injection (see Chapter 47, Injection & Current Delivery Monitoring).[4,11]

CONTINUOUS BLOCKS

When a continuous infusion is planned, a wide variety of special needle designs with larger diameters, catheters, and infusion pumps are available (see Chapter 48, Equipment for Continuous Peripheral Nerve Blocks). Some designs incorporate styletted catheters for increased ease and control of insertion; others designs have the ability to attach to a nerve stimulator.

Stimulating Catheters

The introduction of stimulating catheters (see Chapter 49, Stimulating Catheters) to facilitate optimal catheter positioning during placement (Figure 17–7)[17-19] gives the practitioner the ability to continuously stimulate a nerve during catheter advancement. This use is advantageous because the catheter greatly adds to the predictability of the procedure. Traditionally, normal saline is injected to dilate the perineural space to facilitate advancement of the stimulating catheter. However, the advantage of "real-time" stimulation is lost with the loss of the ability to elicit a motor response with a low current (<0.5 mA), which occurs often after dilating the perineural space with normal saline or local anesthetic.[1,18] The use of a nonconducting solution (eg, 5% dextrose in water,

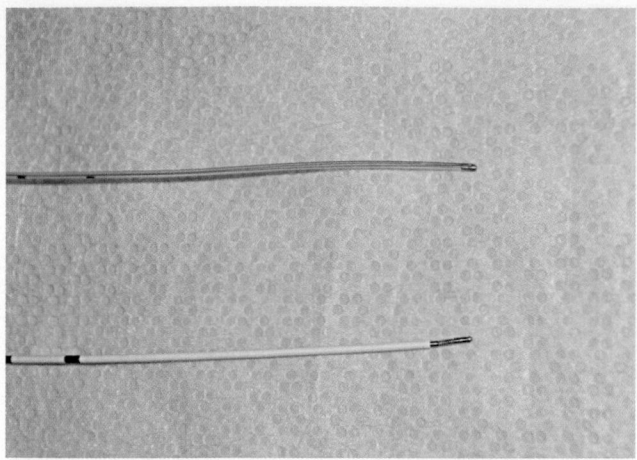

Figure 17–7. Examples of stimulating catheters. The two cathers vary in the insulation material and the length of the conducting surface at the tip of the catheter.

D_5W) instead of saline to dilate the perineural space helps to avoid misinterpretation of the catheter position.[20] The initial clinical experiences using D_5W to facilitate the placement of a stimulating catheter are very encouraging.[21,22] The ability to dilate the space while maintaining a motor response with a stimulating catheter allows for real-time monitoring of the catheter, an aid to successful catheter placement.[21]

Infusion Pumps

A number of infusion pump designs and systems for continuous peripheral nerve blocks recently were introduced for both inpatient- and outpatient-based local anesthetic infusion. These systems are mechanical, electrical spring, or elastic balloon-driven.[23–25] The accuracy of delivery rate varies significantly among the different type of pumps and between manufacturers. Factors such as infusion rate accuracy and consistency, infusion profile, temperature sensitivity, and battery life and source directly affect the actual drug dose delivered to patients. Thus, anesthesiologists must consider these factors when selecting a pump and infusion system, particularly if it is to be used in an unsupervised, ambulatory setting. For inpatient settings, with proper labeling, most epidural pumps also can be used for inpatients receiving continuous peripheral nerve blocks (Figure 17–8). The characteristics of infusion pumps are covered in more detail elsewhere in this text.

Accessories

Specialized connector holding or occlusive dressing is useful for securing the peripheral nerve catheter and avoiding accidental dislodgement (Figure 17–9). Extra care should be exercised to keep the site sterile and clean. It is important to clearly label the peripheral catheter and infusion tubing. In addition, the infusion tubing must be distinct from other intravenous tubing. To avoid accidental injection of other medications, infusion tubing should not have any injection ports.

NERVE STIMULATORS

Clinical Pearls

- A modern design, the constant-current stimulator should be used for nerve stimulation.
- Prior to using a nerve stimulator, clinicians should familiarize themselves with the machine and ensure that it is functioning properly.

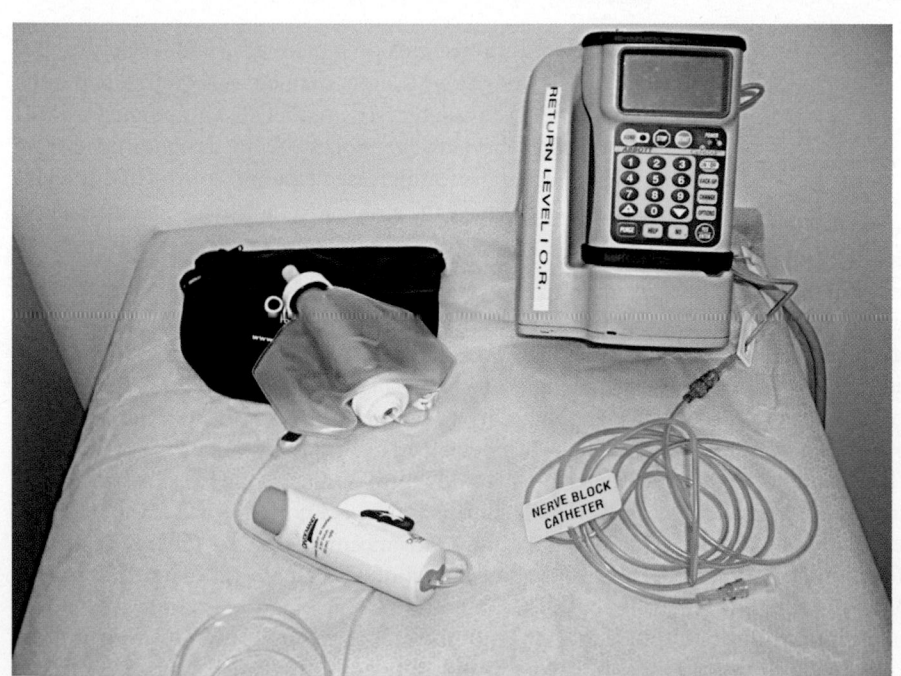

Figure 17–8. Examples of infusion pumps. (*Left*) Single-use, disposable, balloon-driven pump suitable for outpatient use. (*Right*) Standard epidural pump with proper labeling on the infusion tubing to indicate peripheral nerve catheter.

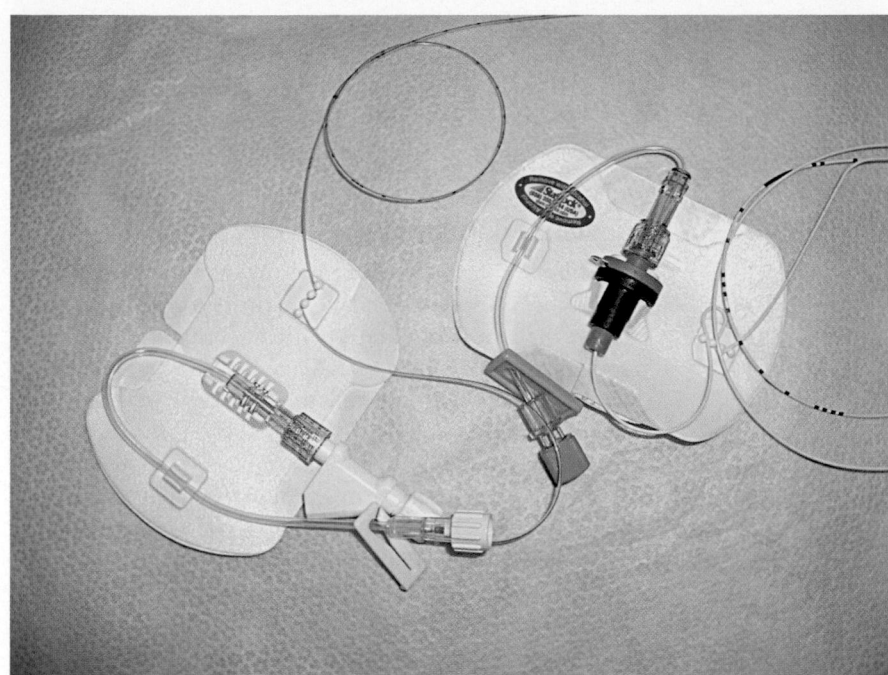

Figure 17–9. Examples of specialized connector holders for continuous catheters. The image shows two different ways of securing the injection port and catheters by using a clip-on mechanism on a self-adhesive apparatus.

A nerve stimulator is an extremely useful tool in regional anesthesia. The electrical properties of the nerve stimulators contribute to the successful localization of a peripheral nerve. Depending on the manufacturer and model of a nerve stimulator, the actual amount of current delivered during stimulation can vary significantly.[1,26] Thus, anesthesiologists should be familiar with the model of stimulator used in the institution before performing any peripheral nerve blocks.

Constant-Current Output & Display

Ideally, the current output of the nerve stimulator should remain unchanged during the advancement of a needle, regardless of the various resistances encountered from the tissue, needle, and connectors. In the past, most commercially produced nerve stimulators used a constant-voltage system (Figure 17–10). However, because the current and not the voltage stimulates the nerve, the amplitude of those nerve stimulators required constant adjustment to maintain a desirable current output. With the advances in technology, most modern models deliver a constant current, and the current output can be set in frequency, pulse width, and current milliamperes (mA) (Figure 17–11).[26] The primary advantage of a constant-current output nerve stimulator is its ability to deliver a stable current output in the presence of varied resistances.

The optimal current with which to begin nerve localization without discomfort and the current intensity to reliably indicate when a needle is positioned sufficiently close to the nerve for block success is unknown. In one study, the minimal

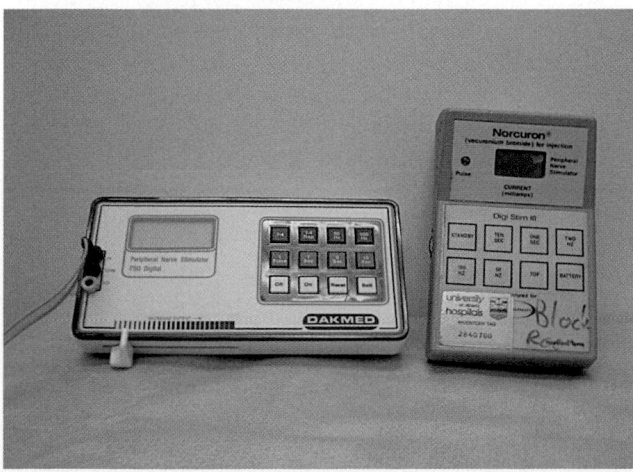

Figure 17–10. Examples of older model (constant-voltage) peripheral neural stimulators.

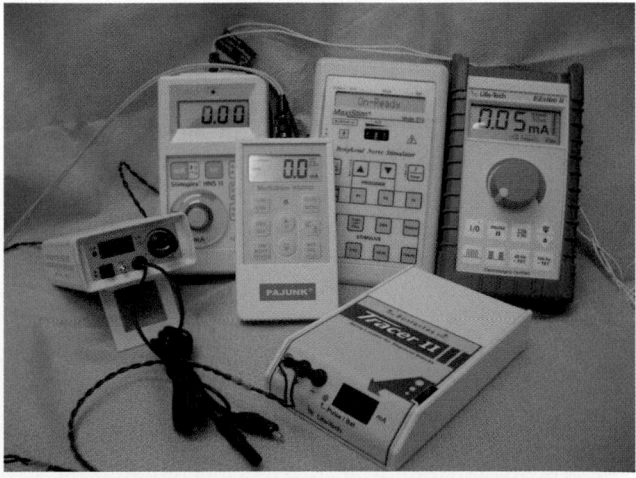

Figure 17–11. Examples of modern, constant-current nerve stimulators.

current required to obtain clearly seen motor response was 0.32 ± 0.05 (range 0.23–0.38 mA) for the brachial plexus and 0.29 ± 0.1 (range 0.15–0.4 mA) for the femoral nerve when the duration was 0.1 msec. This suggests that when performing interscalene brachial or femoral nerve blocks it is probably not necessary to continue searching for a nerve response with currents of less than 0.2 mA at a stimulus duration of 0.1 msec.[27]

Display

A clear digital display, especially in the lower range, is an important feature of the electrical nerve stimulator. This display must indicate the actual current delivered to the patient and not simply the target current setting. Some nerve stimulators are equipped with low (≤ 6 mA) and high output ranges (≤ 80 mA). The lower range is primarily for localizing peripheral nerves. The higher range is used mainly for monitoring neuromuscular blockade. Recently, higher ranges were used for percutaneous electrode guidance (2–5 mA) and the epidural stimulation test (1–10 mA). Although the majority of newer models with constant and linear output circuitry deliver current with greater accuracy and quality, it is advisable to have each machine periodically checked by a biomedical engineering department.[26] Future nerve stimulators may include externalized (remote) means of monitoring the nerve stimulator functionality with an LED mounted on the hub of the needle. Such designs will provide clinicians with a real-time indicator of current delivery (eg, the LED will flash with each successful delivery of the current), current intensity (eg, the LED will change color as the output current changes), and disconnect alarm (eg, the LED will not flash in case of a disconnect, poor electrical contact, or nerve stimulator malfunctions). Part IV of this textbook addresses these emerging technologies in more detail.

Variable Pulse Width

Most nerve stimulators deliver an electrical pulse width of 100 μs or 200 μs for stimulating motor nerves. The pulse width (duration) of the stimulation current is an important factor, not only for determining the amount of charge delivered, but also for selectivity stimulating different nerve fibers.[27] More sophisticated nerve stimulators also allow for variable pulse widths (from 50 μs to 1 μs), in an attempt to provide selective stimulation or increase the total charge delivered. The site of the cutaneous electrode is not critical when using a constant-current output nerve stimulator for nerve localization during interscalene brachial plexus and femoral nerve blockade.

The duration of current does not have an effect on the degree of discomfort during nerve stimulation.[27,28] This can be explained by the fact that the total energy delivered to the nerve(s) is greater with stimuli of longer duration as described by the equation E (energy; in nanocoulombs [nC]) = I (current intensity; in milliamperes [mA]) $\times$ t (duration of application; in microseconds [μsec]).[8] For example, when set

at a current of 1.0 mA, a stimulus duration of 1.0 msec will deliver 10 times more energy than a stimulus of 0.1 msec (1000 nC vs 100 nC). Consequently, the greater energy delivered to the nerve will result in a more forceful motor response, resulting in greater discomfort to the patient.

Specialized Polarity of the Electrodes

The cathode (black) is selected as the stimulating electrode because the "cathodal stimulation" is three to four times more effective than the anode at depolarizing the nerve membrane. A specialized male connector designed to fit in the female conducting portion of the stimulating needle is very common with newer nerve stimulators. Unfortunately, the receptacles for needle connection on various models of nerve stimulators are not compatible with various designs of stimulating needles. At the present time, there are no standards governing the stimulator-to-needle connection. Consequently, the use a nerve stimulator made by one manufacturer is best coupled with the needles of the same manufacturer to avoid the need for adapters to allow needle-to-stimulator connection.

A reversal of polarity may occur in clinical practice when the cables to the nerve stimulator are erroneously connected. A reversal of polarity from the usual negative to positive results in an almost threefold increase in the current required to elicit a motor response.[29]

Clinical Pearls

- The site of placement of the cutaneous electrode is not important during nerve localization for peripheral nerve blocks.

- The duration of the stimulus can significantly affect the intensity of current required to stimulate the nerve as well as the magnitude of the motor response obtained.

- Currents of greater intensity result in more pronounced motor responses and consequently may cause greater patient discomfort, regardless of current pulse duration. Selecting a current duration (0.05–1.0 msec) specifically to preferentially stimulate sensory or motor components of a mixed nerve does not appear to be important. Special attention must be paid to polarity because an erroneous connection of cables may lead to errors in estimating the needle–nerve relationship.

Variable Pulse Frequency

Most new stimulators have an option to change the frequency at which the electrical pulse is delivered. The optimal frequency of the electrical pulse is between 0.5 and 3 Hz. The slower stimulating frequency increases the specificity of the twitch response due to its slow repetition, whereas stimulating frequencies above 3 Hz lose specificity because such repetitive stimulation may be indistinguishable from patient tremor. As the best compromise between specificity and sensitivity, most

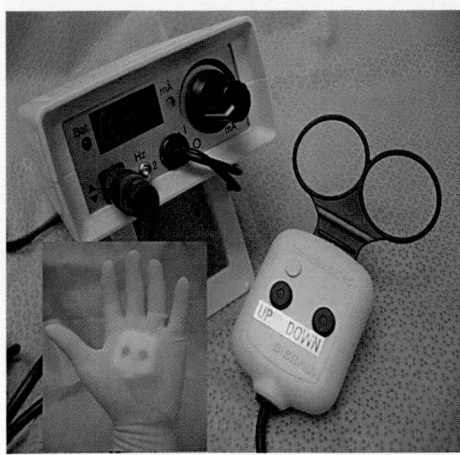
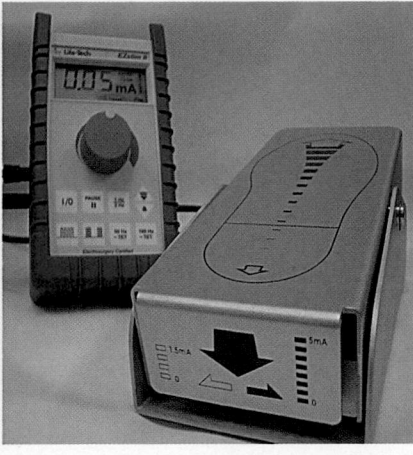

Figure 17–12. Examples of remote controllers. (*Left*) Hand controller (*Right*) Foot controller.

users select a frequency of 2 Hz. When using a lower frequency, such as 1 Hz (one stimulus per sec), the needle must be slowly advanced to avoid missing the nerve between stimulations.

Disconnection & Malfunction Indicators

The disconnection and malfunction of nerve stimulators should be a concern to anesthesiologists. Thus, stimulators should warn when the circuit is not complete and if the pulse is not being delivered. In addition, an indication of battery power is essential to prevent unnecessary needle insertions in search of a motor response when a disconnect of nerve stimulator malfunction occurs. As previously mentioned, future nerve stimulator designs may include an externalized (remote) means of monitoring the nerve stimulator functionality with an LED mounted on the hub of the needle. The LED will flash with the successful delivery of the current and will not flash when the stimulator is disconnected, has poor electrical contact, or malfunctions. Part IV of this textbook addresses these emerging technologies in more detail. More information on the circuitry of nerve stimulators and electrophysiologic principles of nerve stimulation can be found in Chapter 5 (Electrophysiology of Nerve Stimulation).

NEWER ACCESSORIES & TRENDS

In recent years a number of new, useful, or promising pieces of equipment and designs have been introduced to facilitate performance of nerve block or make their administration safer and more objective. A small remote hand control or foot pedal allows a single operator to adjust the current output of a nerve stimulator without an assistant (Figure 17–12). Recently, a commercially available probe was developed for performing percutaneous electrode guidance in surface nerve mapping (Figure 17–13). Finally, injection pressure monitors have recently been proposed to decrease the risk of mechanical injection injury to the nerve and facilitate objective documentation of the force exerted during nerve block performance (Figure 17–14). The reader should refer to Part IV of

this textbook for more information on emerging trends and equipment in regional anesthesia.[30,31]

DOPPLER ULTRASOUND

In the past, Doppler ultrasound was used to identify vascular structures and to indirectly estimate nerve location, based on the anatomy of a neurovascular relationship.

More recently, however, ultrasound was introduced in regional anesthesia to directly visualize the nerves (see Part V: Ultrasound-Guided Regional Anesthesia [Chapters 50–52]).[1,2,9] It is a noninvasive, real-time technique used to guide needles in the direction of target peripheral nerves. Promising results have been reported with ultrasound-guided interscalene, supraclavicular, infraclavicular, and axillary approaches to brachial plexus blocks, as well as femoral 3-in-1, lumbar plexus, and popliteal blocks.[3]

In recent years, the cost and the size of ultrasound machines decreased significantly, making this technology more affordable and portable (Figure 17–15). In clinical practice, one of the most important considerations when selecting an

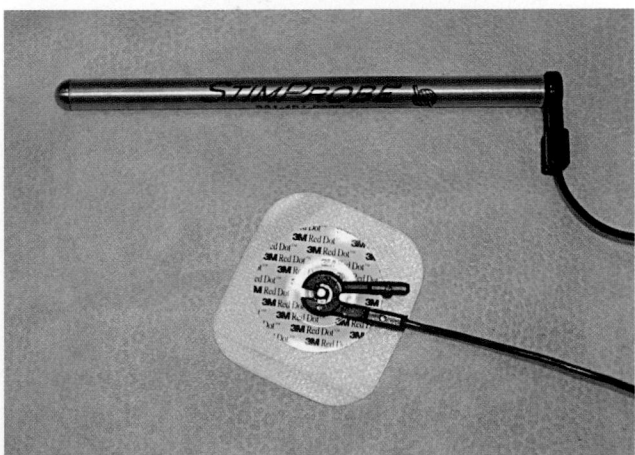

Figure 17–13. Example of probe for percutaneous electrode guidance.

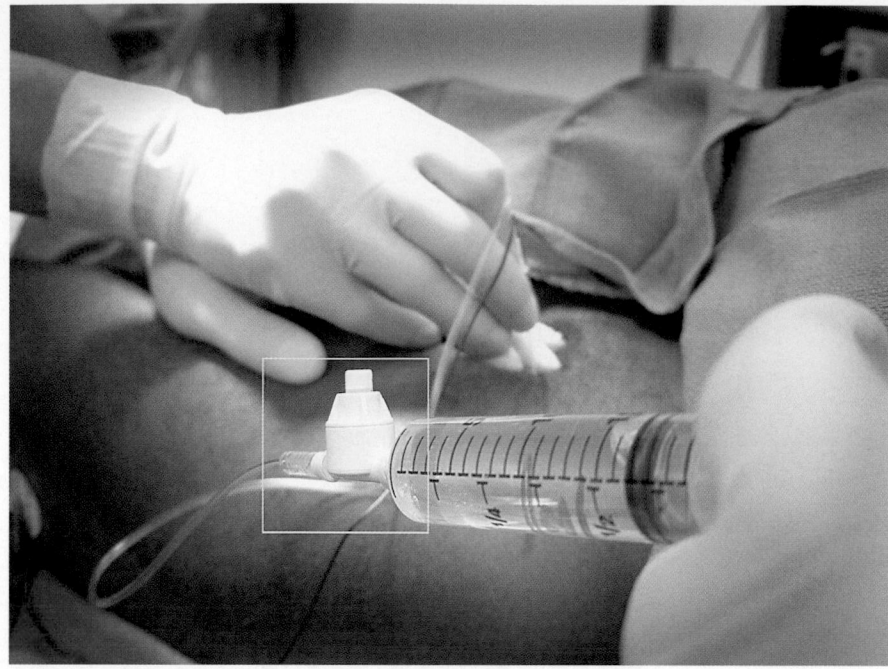

Figure 17–14. Injection pressure monitoring during administration of a (femoral) nerve block. The area of the detail shows a disposable, in-line pressure monitor with a movable piston indicating pressure throughout the injection.

ultrasound machine is the frequency of the transducer. In general, higher transducer frequencies (7.5–10 MHz) result in better image resolution, albeit with a reduced penetration of the tissue. Accordingly, the choice of a transducer must be based on a balance between resolution and penetration with respect to the expected depth of the nerve. In a transverse plane, peripheral nerves typically appear as multiple round or nodular, hypoechoic structures encircled by a relative hyperechoic background (Figure 17–16). The availability of a Doppler effect permits the confirmation of vascular structures to assist in the identification of nerves based on the anatomic relationship of the nerves to the vascular structures. Despite these features, optimal needle placement is often hindered by the limited imaging quality of the ultrasound machine. Inevitably, advances in imaging technology will continue to improve ultrasound technique and eventually lead to a more widespread use of ultrasound imaging as an aid in nerve localization, most likely in conjunction with peripheral nerve stimulation.

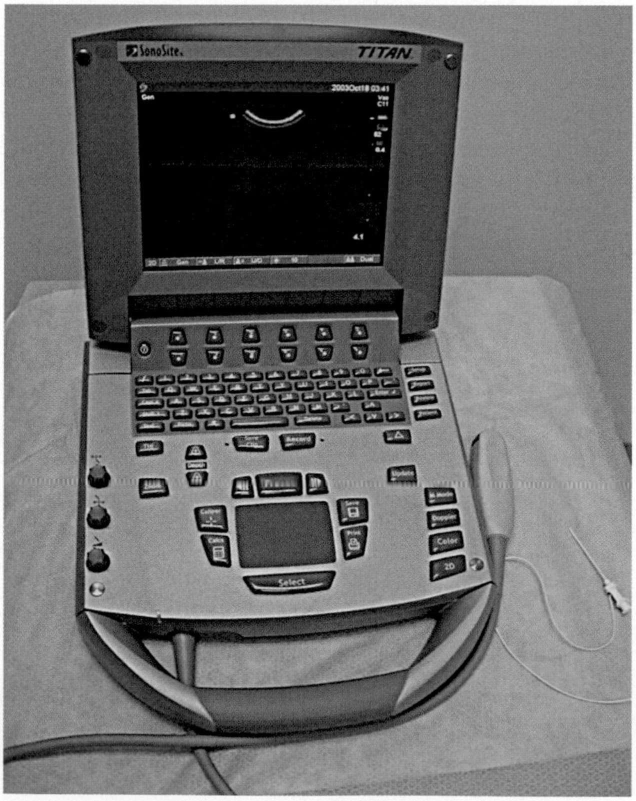

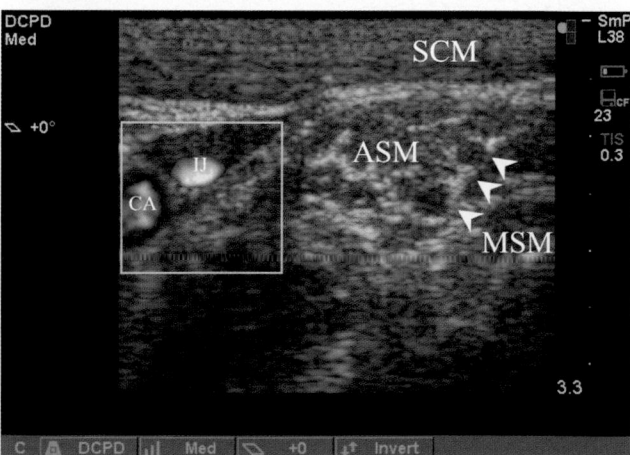

Figure 17–16. Ultrasound image of the interscalene groove. SCM = sternocleidomastoid muscle; ASM = anterior scalene muscle; MSM = middle scalene muscle; CA = carotid artery with Doppler flow; IJ = internal jugular vein with Doppler flow. Arrows indicate brachial plexus in the interscalene groove.

Figure 17–15. Portable ultrasound machine.

CONCLUSION

A well-maintained, designated area with proper equipment and set-up is essential to providing effective and safe regional anesthesia. In addition, patient monitoring and proper documentation of the peripheral nerve block are also important, not only for patient care and quality assurance but also for the purpose of research or legal issues. A useful standardized peripheral nerve procedure note form that can be easily adapted to regional anesthesia practice was recently developed (see Chapter 80, Documentation of Regional Anesthesia Procedures).[32]

As technology continues to evolve, more sophisticated equipment will likely assume a more significant role in regional anesthesia. At present, electrical stimulation to elicit motor response is used frequently to indicate that the probing needle is adjacent to the target nerve. Future research to improve electrical stimulation via the injection of nonconducting solutions is important, and current research is promising. Nevertheless, electrical stimulation relies on physiologic responses to an electric current to locate peripheral nerves, whereas ultrasound relies on anatomic images to visually guide needle placement. Individually, ultrasound and electrical stimulation have limitations, but together, these techniques may compensate for the other's weaknesses to assist with optimal needle placement.

References

1. Raj PP, de Andres J, Grossi P, et al: Aids to localization of peripheral nerves, in Raj PP (ed): *Textbook of Regional Anesthesia*. New York, Churchill Livingstone, 2002, pp 251–284.
2. Denny NM, Harrop-Griffiths W: Location, location, location! Ultrasound imaging in regional anaesthesia. Br J Anaesth 2005;94:1–3.
3. Marhofer P, Greher M, Kapral S: Ultrasound guidance in regional anaesthesia. Br J Anaesth 2005;94:7–17.
4. Hadzic A, Vloka JD: Equipment and patient monitoring in regional anesthesia. In Hadzic A, Vloka JD (eds): *Peripheral Nerve Blocks: Principles and Practice*. McGraw-Hill, 2004, pp 29–41.
5. Neal JM, McMahon DJ: Equipment. In Brown DL (eds): *Regional Anesthesia and Analgesia*, 1st ed. WB Saunders, 2005, pp 159–172.
6. Raj PP, Johnston M: Organization and function of the nerve block facility, in Raj PP (ed): *Textbook of Regional Anesthesia*. Churchill Livingstone, 2002, pp 147–156.
7. Plancarte RS, Mayer FJM: Monitoring in regional anesthesia, in Raj PP (ed): *Textbook of Regional Anesthesia*. Churchill Livingstone, 2002, pp 157–175.
8. Tsui BC, Wagner A, Finucane B: Regional anaesthesia in the elderly: A clinical guide. Drugs Aging 2004;21:895–910.
9. Barret JM, Harmon D, Loughnane F, et al: Peripheral nerve block materials. In Barret JM, Harmon D, Loughnane F, et al (eds): *Peripheral Nerve Blocks and Peri-operative Pain Relief*, Saunders, 2004, pp 43–48.
10. Raj PP: Guidelines for regional anesthetic technique. In Hahn MB, McQuillan PM, Sheplock GJ (eds): *Regional Anesthesia: An Atlas of Anatomy and Techniques*. Mosby, 1996, pp 21–38.
11. Hadzic A, Vloka JD: Neurologic complications of peripheral nerve blocks. In Hadzic A, Vloka JD (eds): *Peripheral Nerve Blocks: Principles and Practice*. McGraw-Hill, 2005, pp 67–77.
12. Grant SA, Nielsen KC, Greengrass RA, et al: Continuous peripheral nerve block for ambulatory surgery. Reg Anesth Pain Med 2001;26:209–214.
13. Steele SM, Klein SM, D'Ercole FJ, et al: A new continuous catheter delivery system. Anesth Analg 1998;87:228.
14. Sardesai AM, Denny NM, Herrick MJ, et al: A study of the characteristics of single-injection insulated block needles in a biologic model. Reg Anesth Pain Med 2004;29:476–479.
15. Claudio R, Hadzic A, Shih H, et al: Injection pressures by anesthesiologists during simulated peripheral nerve block. Reg Anesth Pain Med 2004;29:201–205.
16. Hadzic A, Dilberovic F, Shah S, et al: Combination of intraneural injection and high injection pressure leads to fascicular injury and neurologic deficits in dogs. Reg Anesth Pain Med 2004;29: 417–423.
17. Boezaart AP, De Beer JF, du TC, et al: A new technique of continuous interscalene nerve block. Can J Anaesth 1999;46:275–281.
18. Pham-Dang C, Kick O, Collet T, et al: Continuous peripheral nerve blocks with stimulating catheters. Reg Anesth Pain Med 2003;28:83–88.
19. Salinas FV: Location, location, location: Continuous peripheral nerve blocks and stimulating catheters. Reg Anesth Pain Med 2003;28:79–82.
20. Tsui BC, Wagner A, Finucane B: Electrophysiologic effect of injectates on peripheral nerve stimulation. Reg Anesth Pain Med 2004;29:189–193.
21. Tsui BC, Kropelin B, Ganapathy S, et al: Dextrose 5% in water: Fluid medium for maintaining electrical stimulation of peripheral nerves during stimulating catheter placement. Acta Anaesthesiol Scand 2005;49:1562–1545.
22. Tsui BC, Kropelin B: The electrophysiological effect of dextrose 5% in water on single-shot peripheral nerve stimulation. Anesth Analg 2005;100:1837–1839.
23. Ilfeld BM, Morey TE, Enneking FK: The delivery rate accuracy of portable infusion pumps used for continuous regional analgesia. Anesth Analg 2002;95:1331–1336.
24. Ilfeld BM, Morey TE, Enneking FK: Portable infusion pumps used for continuous regional analgesia: Delivery rate accuracy and consistency. Reg Anesth Pain Med 2003;28:424–432.
25. Ilfeld BM, Morey TE, Enneking FK: Delivery rate accuracy of portable, bolus-capable infusion pumps used for patient-controlled continuous regional analgesia. Reg Anesth Pain Med 2003;28: 17–23.
26. Hadzic A, Vloka J, Hadzic N, et al: Nerve stimulators used for peripheral nerve blocks vary in their electrical characteristics. Anesthesiology 2003;98:969–974.
27. Hadzic A, Vloka JD, Claudio RE, et al: Effects of surface electrode placement and duration of the stimulus on motor response. Anesthesiology 2004;100:1526–1530.
28. Kurc P, Hadzic A. Yufa M, et al: Painful paresthesiae are infrequent during brachial plexus localization using low-current peripheral nerve stimulation. Reg Anesth Pain Med 2003;28:380–383. This article is accompanied by an editorial.
29. Tulchinsky A, Weller RS, Rosenblum M, et al: Nerve stimulator polarity and brachial plexus block. Anesth Analg 1993;77:100–103.
30. Bosenberg AT, Raw R, Boezaart AP: Surface mapping of peripheral nerves in children with a nerve stimulator. Paediatr Anaesth 2002;12:398–403.
31. Urmey WF, Grossi P: Percutaneous electrode guidance: A noninvasive technique for prelocation of peripheral nerves to facilitate peripheral plexus or nerve block. Reg Anesth Pain Med 2002;27:261–267.
32. Gerancher JC, Viscusi ER, Liguori GA, et al: Development of a standardized peripheral nerve block procedure note form. Reg Anesth Pain Med 2005;30:67–71.

18

Nerve Blocks for the Head & Neck

James P. Rathmell, MD • Geoffrey J. Pollack, MD

INTRODUCTION

Regional anesthetic techniques have a well established role in head and neck surgery. Successful anesthesia and analgesia for a number of procedures can be accomplished with the proper application of these techniques. For example, regional blocks can be utilized during procedures such as endoscopic sinus surgery, facial plastic surgery, thyroidectomy, and parathyroidectomy surgery. Various ear nose and throat procedures are increasingly being performed in an office-based setting. These are often done using topical anesthesia of the airway or regional blockade. Because of the close proximity of many nerve and vascular structures in this region, practitioners should be familiar with possible complications of these techniques and means to prevent and treat them. This chapter will review the anatomy relevant to regional blocks of the head and neck and will highlight examples for use of each technique in current practice. Additional discussion on numerous regional anesthesia techniques and their application can be also found in Chapter 19 (Airway Blocks) and in Chapters 20 (Oral and Maxillofacial Regional Anesthesia) and 55 (Regional and Local Anesthesia in Pediatric General Dentistry). To avoid redundancy, this chapter will deal only with the anatomic and block techniques not covered in the aforementioned chapters.

TRIGEMINAL (GASSERIAN) GANGLION BLOCK

Indications

Gasserian ganglion block is used primarily for treatment of trigeminal neuralgia, a relatively rare but devastating form of neuropathic facial pain.[1-3] Patients with trigeminal neuralgia typically present with the spontaneous onset of pain in one or more divisions of the trigeminal nerve. The most common presentation involves both V_2 and V_3; however, any or all divisions may be involved. Patients report paroxysmal lancinating pain in the face that is often severe. The pain usually has a specific area of trigger—pressure on this trigger area elicits the pain.[4] Patients who present with new symptoms suggestive of trigeminal neuralgia should undergo a thorough neurologic evaluation, including imaging studies to rule out intracranial pathology. The majority of patients with trigeminal neuralgia will respond to oral neuropathic medications; carbamezapine remains the agent of choice.[4,5] Neural blockade is usually reserved for those with trigeminal neuralgia that do not respond to pharmacologic therapy.[1,6] Local anesthetic block of the trigeminal ganglion and its primary divisions is often used as a diagnostic test to predict response to neural blockade prior to proceeding with neurolysis.[7-9]

Clinical Pearls

- Neural blockade of the trigeminal ganglion is usually reserved for those with trigeminal neuralgia that do not respond to pharmacologic therapy.
- Local anesthetic block of the trigeminal ganglion and its primary divisions is often used as a diagnostic test to predict response to neural blockade prior to proceeding with neurolysis.

Anatomy

The trigeminal nerve, the fifth cranial nerve, supplies the majority of sensory innervation to the face (Figure 18–1). Preganglionic fibers exit the brainstem and travel anteriorly to synapse with second-order neurons within the trigeminal (gasserian) ganglion (Figure 18–2). The ganglion lies within the cranial vault at the base of the petrous portion of the temporal bone in a dural invagination containing cerebrospinal fluid known as Meckel's cave. Postganglionic fibers exit the

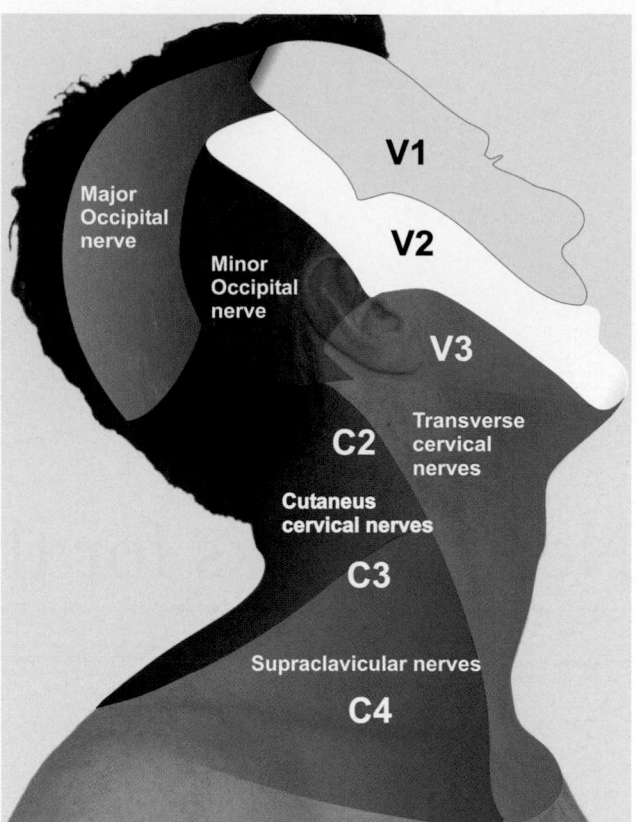

Figure 18–1. Cutaneous innervation of the head and neck.

ganglion to form the ophthalmic (V_1), maxillary (V_2), and mandubular (V_3) nerves (Figure 18–3). The three divisions of the trigeminal nerve and the functions they serve are detailed in Table 18–1. The first division, the ophthalmic nerve, is discussed in detail in Chapter 21 (Eye Blocks).

The second division of the trigeminal nerve, the maxillary nerve, exits the middle cranial fossa via the foramen rotundum. Outside the cranial vault, the maxillary nerve sends pterygopalatine branches to the pterygopalatine ganglion, zygomatic nerve, and the infraorbital nerve. The pterygopalatine branch supplies the pterygopalatine ganglion which, in turn, supplies sensory branches to the nasal septum, the lateral nasal wall, and the soft and hard palates. The zygomatic nerve supplies sensory innervation surrounding the zygomatic arch (zygomaticotemporal and zygomaticofacial nerves). The infraorbital nerve sends sensory branches to the upper teeth (superior alveolar nerves) and terminates in a small sensory branch over the maxillary prominence (infraorbital nerve; see Figure 18–3).

The third division of the trigeminal nerve, the mandibular nerve, exits the middle cranial fossa via the foramen ovale and divides into anterior and posterior divisions (Figure 18–4). The anterior division supplies motor innervation to the masseter muscle and other muscles involved in mastication and a small terminal sensory branch to the cheek (the buccal nerve). The posterior division divides into the auriculotemporal nerve (cutaneous sensation in front of the ear), the lingual nerve (sensation to the tongue), and the inferior alveolar nerve (sensation to the lower teeth). The

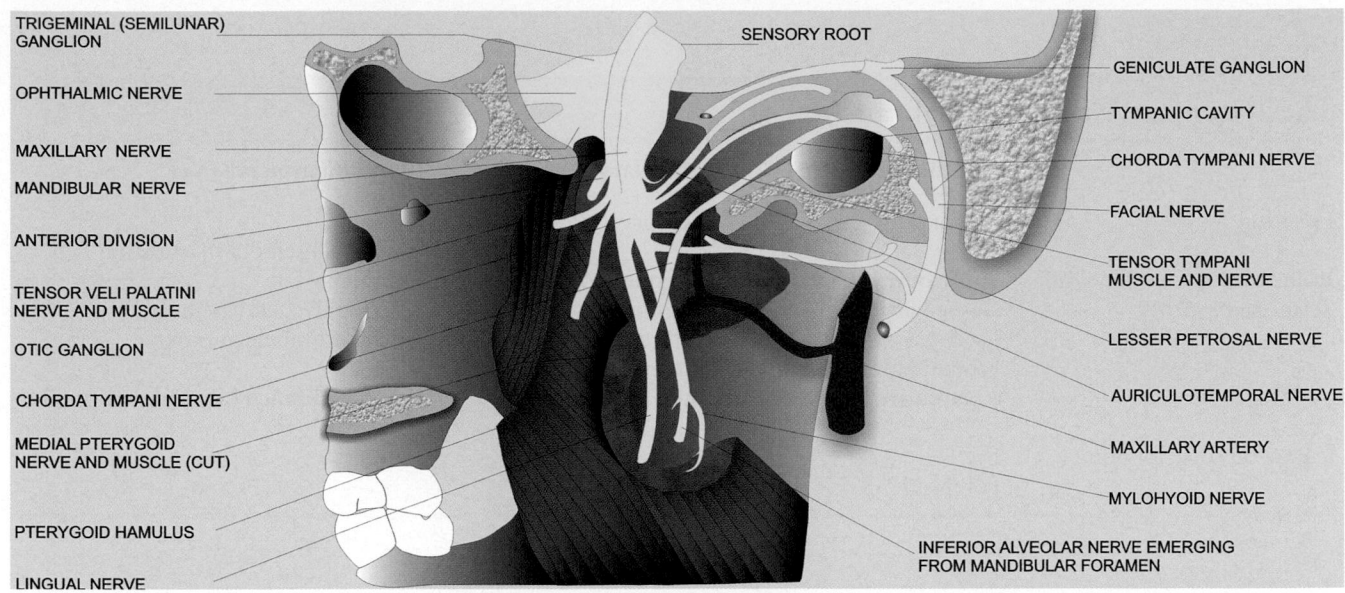

Figure 18–2. Trigeminal ganglion: organization and divisions.

inferior alveolar nerve terminates in a small cutaneous nerve supplying sensation to the chin (the mental nerve).

Block Technique

Block of the gasserian ganglion is performed with the patient in the supine position.[6] Location of the foramen ovale is facilitated by the use of fluoroscopic guidance. When fluoroscopy is used, the C-arm is angled so that the axis of the x-ray beam is aligned to reveal the foramen ovale (oblique and caudal angulation). A skin wheal of local anesthetic is raised 2–3 cm lateral to the corner of the mouth and a 22-gauge, 10-cm spinal needle is advanced upward toward the mandibular condyle in a plane in line with the pupil (Figure 18–5). The surface of the greater wing of the sphenoid bone is typically contacted at a depth of 4 to 6 cm, and the needle is withdrawn and redirected in a more posterior direction until the foramen ovale is entered. Once the needle enters the foramen, it is advanced an additional 1–1.5 cm. As the foramen is entered, a paresthesia in the mandible is usually elicited. As the advancement continues, paresthesia in the maxilla and orbit are also typically reported. Injection volume of 1.0 mL is usually sufficient to

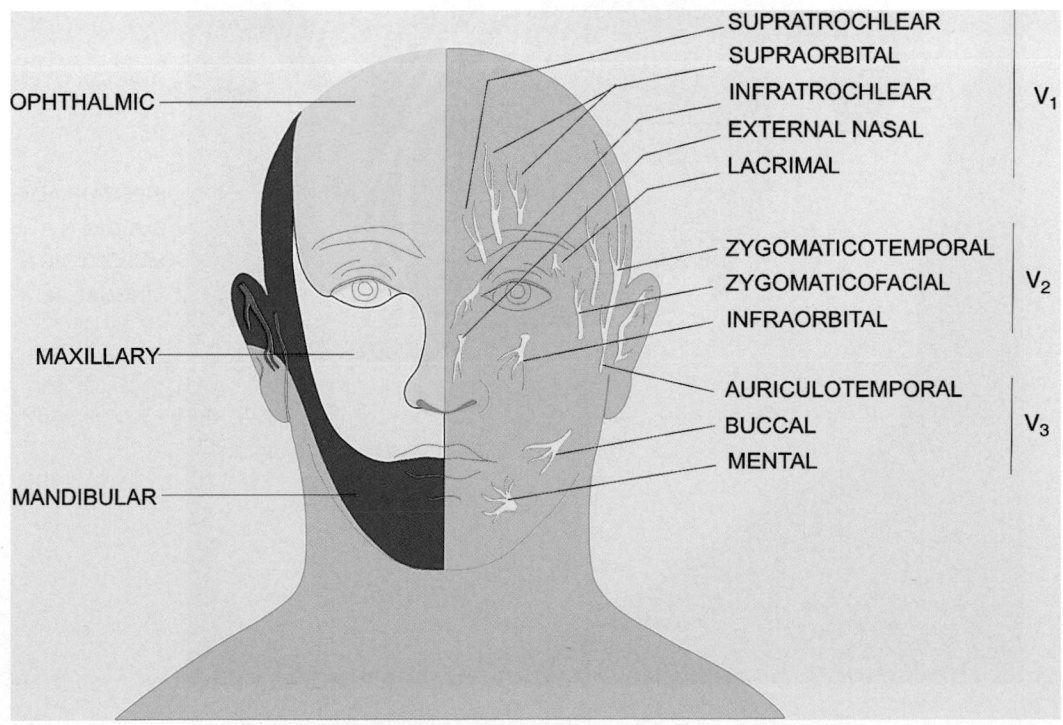

Figure 18–3. Cutaneous innervation of the face, anterior view.

Table 18–1.

The Trigeminal Nerve and Its Branches

	Ophthalmic nerve (V₁)	Maxillary nerve (V₂)	Mandibular nerve (V₃)
Function	Sensory	Sensory	Sensory Motor: Muscles of mastication
Route of exit from the skull	Superior orbital fissure	Foramen rotundum	Foramen ovale
Terminal branches	Nasociliary	Zygomatic	Inferior alveolar (mental)
	Lacrimal	Infraorbital	Anterior branch (motor)
	Frontal (supraorbital; supratrochlear)	Superior alveolar	Lingual
		Sphenopalatine	Posterior branch (auriculotemporal, buccal)
Cutaneous distribution	Eye	Midface	Lower jaw
	Forehead	Upper jaw	

produce dense analgesia. Paresthesia in the effected division is sought to guide needle placement prior to neurolysis.

Complications

Complications associated with local anesthetic block of the trigeminal ganglion include direct intravascular injection into the carotid artery, persistent paresthesia, and total spinal anesthesia due to local anesthetic deposition within the cerebrospinal fluid over the ventral surface of the brainstem. Complications associated with neurolysis are more common. Facial numbness occurs in nearly all patients and may be profound. Other complications include anesthesia

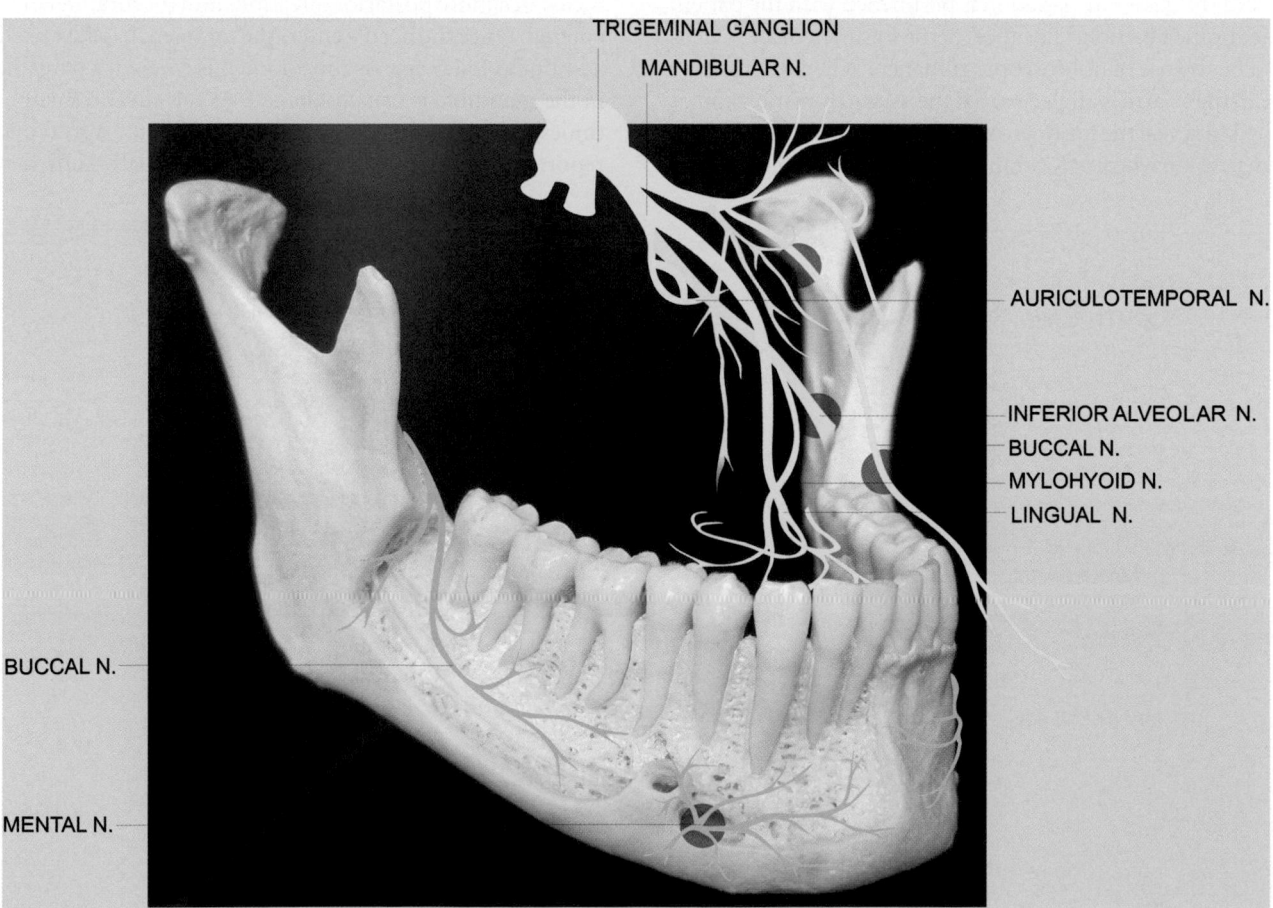

Figure 18–4. The mandibular nerve and its terminal branches. Shaded areas indicate typical sites for anesthetizing each branch.

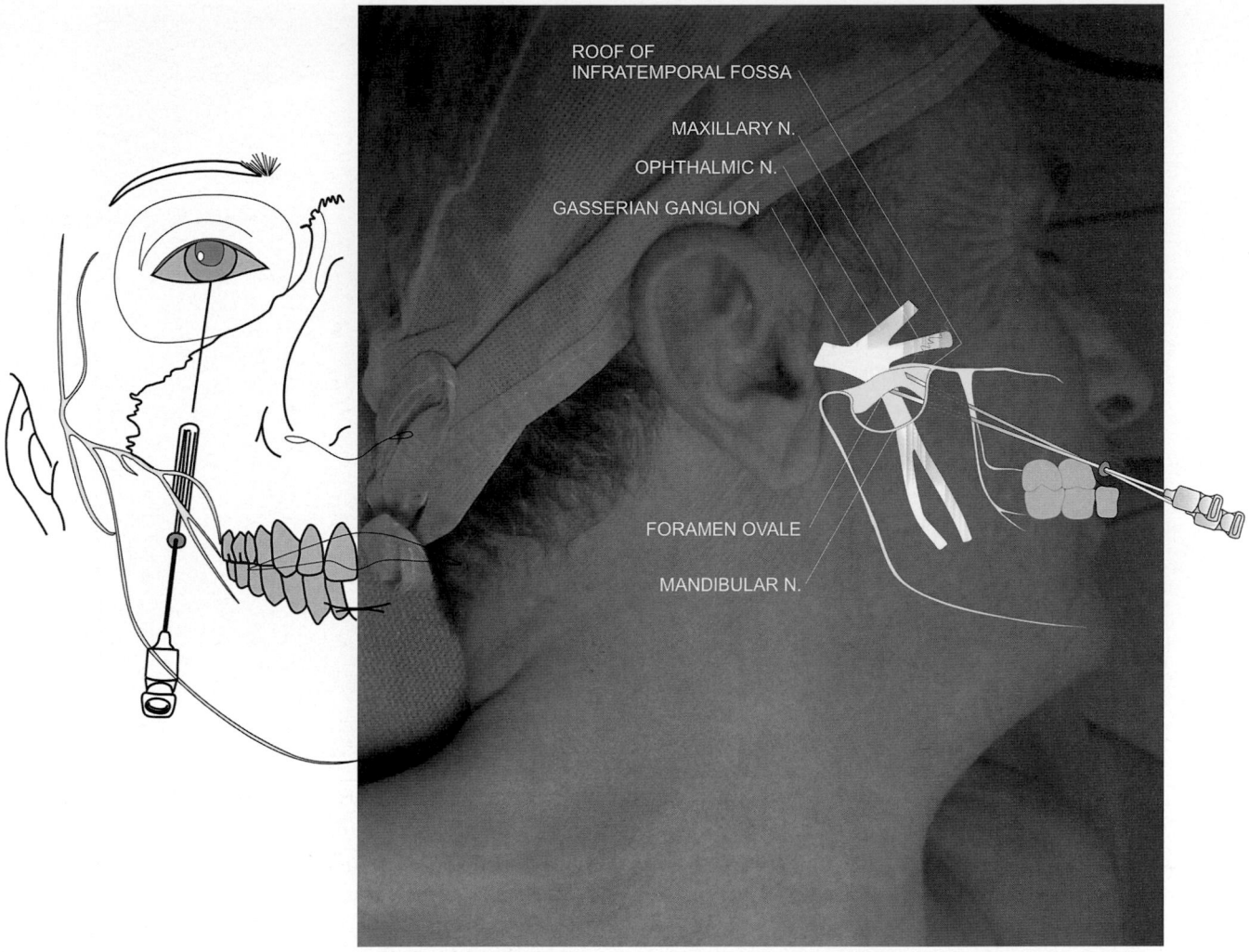

Figure 18–5. Trigeminal (gasserian) ganglion block. (1) The needle is placed through the skin 2–3 cm lateral to the lateral margin of the mouth and advanced toward the mandibular condyle and toward the ipsilateral pupil until bone is contacted. (2) The needle is then withdrawn and redirected more posteriorly until the foramen ovale is entered.

dolorosa (pain and numbness), reduced corneal reflex, abolition of the corneal reflex, keratitis, and masticatory weakness. Percutaneous trigeminal neurolysis (using either glycerol or radiofrequency lesioning) remains an effective, minimally invasive treatment for patients with trigeminal neuralgia.

Clinical Pearls

SPECIFIC COMPLICATIONS ASSOCIATED WITH HEAD AND NECK BLOCKS

- Subarachnoid or epidural placement of local anesthetic may lead to high-spinal and brainstem anesthesia.
- Generalized seizures may occur with the injection of even small intraarterial volumes of local anesthetic (0.5 mL or less) as the arterial blood flow continues directly from the arteries in the head and neck to the brain.
- Hematoma formation may lead to airway compromise.

- Respiratory distress may result from block of the phrenic or recurrent laryngeal nerves, pneumothorax, or loss of sensory or motor function of the nerves to the airway.
- Rapid and complete absorption of topical anesthetics from the oral mucosa can lead to unexpected systemic toxicity.

GREATER PALATINE BLOCK

Indications

Greater palatine block is useful for paranasal sinus anesthesia and vasoconstriction during endoscopic sinus surgery.

Technique

Via the oral cavity the greater palatine groove is finger palpated, and the needle is inserted into the groove and advanced

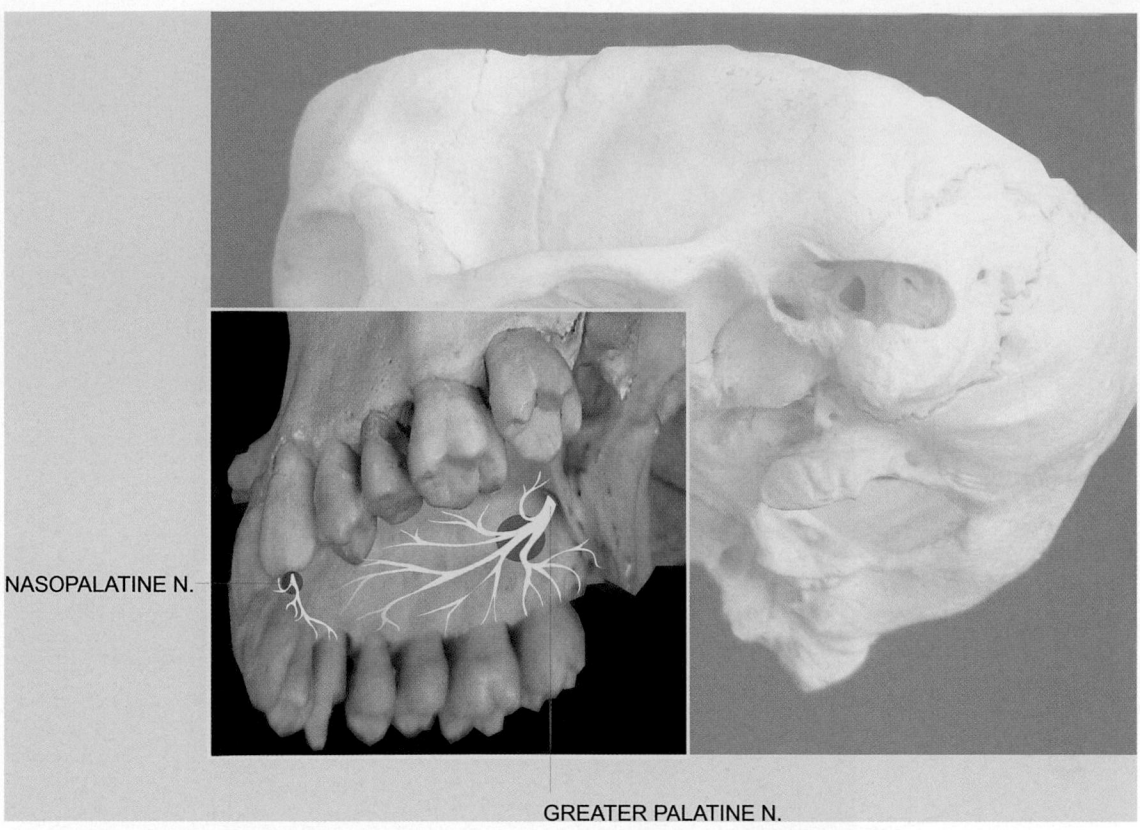

Figure 18–6. Location of the greater palatine and nasopalatine nerves and typical sites for the blockade.

to contact the bone at which point 2–3 mL of local anesthetic is injected (Figures 18–6 and 18–7).[6,10,11]

OCCIPITAL NERVE BLOCK

Indications

Occipital nerve block is most often used in the diagnosis and treatment of occipital neuralgia and cervicogenic headache. True occipital neuralgia typically follows blunt trauma to the nerves over the occiput and is characterized by pain in the distribution of the occipital nerves. Cervicogenic headache is more ill-defined, insidious in onset, and characterized by pain in the same distribution. Many patients with cervicogenic headaches have associated spondylosis of the cervical facet joints. When the pain is limited to the region overlying the occiput, occipital nerve blocks may be of some benefit in reducing the associated pain.

Anatomy

The greater occipital nerve arises from the posterior primary ramus of the second cervical nerve root (Figure 18–8). It travels deep to the cervical paraspinous musculature and becomes

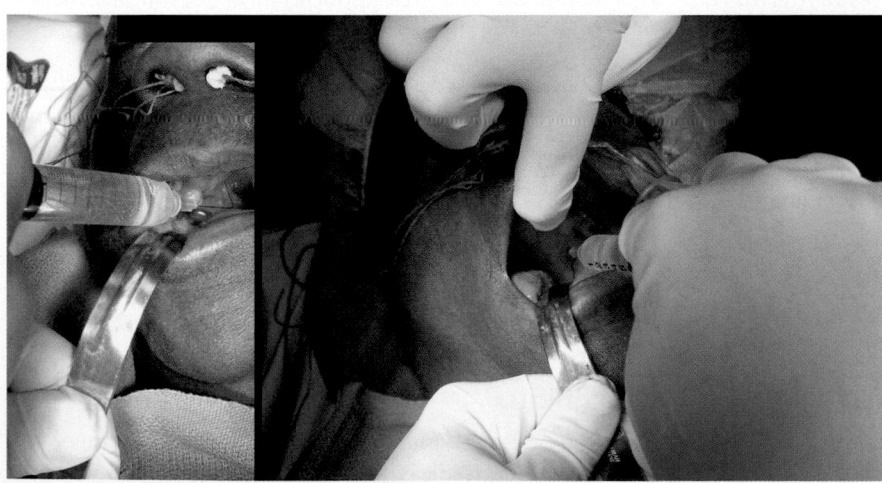

Figure 18–7. The greater palatine block. The greater palatine groove is finger palpated, and the needle is inserted into the groove and advanced to contact the bone at which point 2–3 mL of local anesthetic is injected.

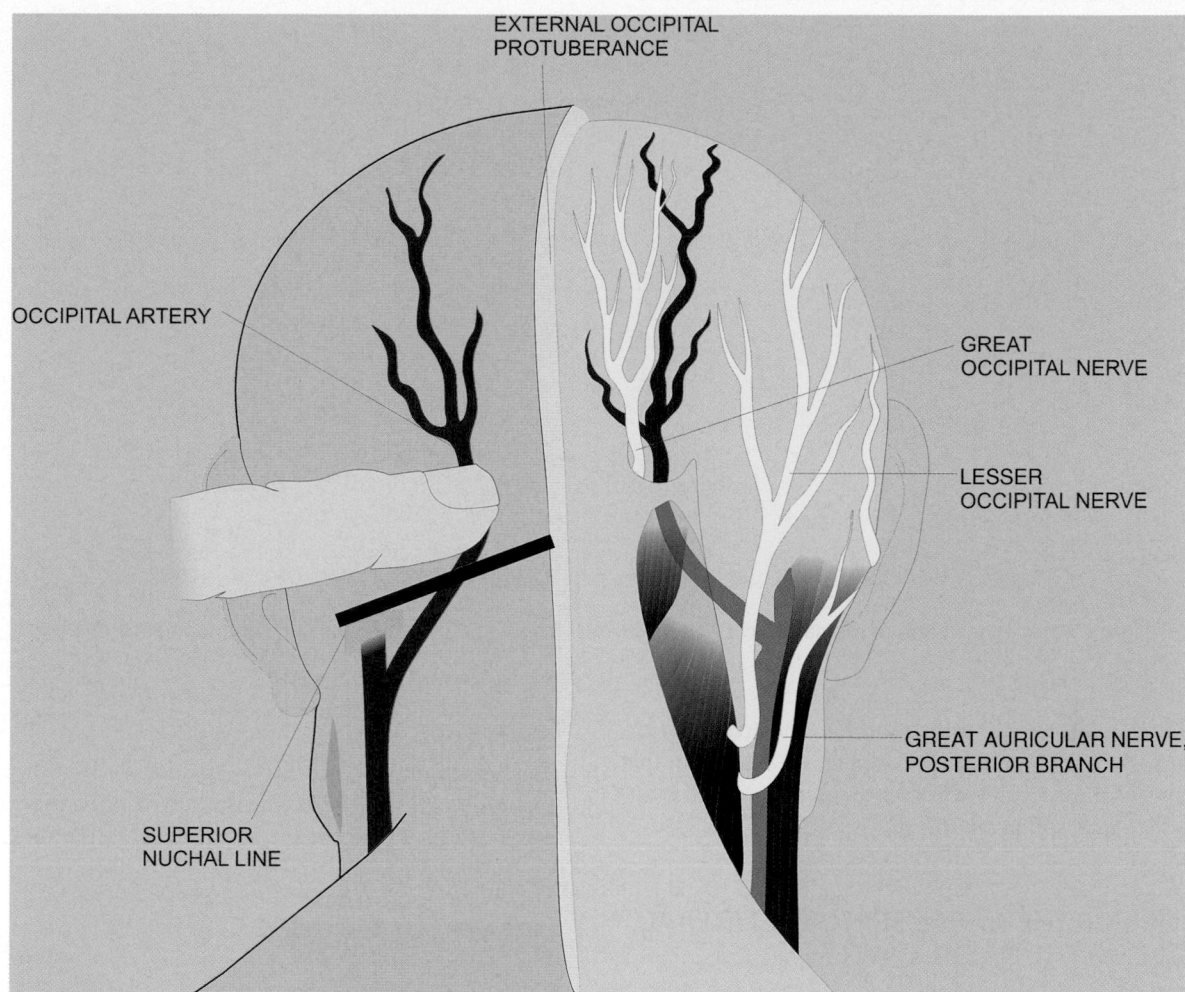

Figure 18–8. Localization of the occipital nerve. The greater occipital nerve is positioned medial to the pulse of the occipital artery; approximately one third of the distance from the occipital protuberance to the mastoid, whereas the lesser occipital nerve is more lateral, approximately two thirds of this distance.

superficial just inferior to the superior nuchal line and lateral to the occipital protuberance of the skull; at this point, the nerve is just lateral to the occipital artery. The lesser occipital nerve and great auricular nerve are terminal branches of the superficial cervical plexus. Both arise from the posterior primary ramus of the second and third cervical nerve roots, travel through the cervical paraspinous musculature, and become superficial over the inferior nuchal line of the skull, just superior and medial to the mastoid and just inferior to the tragus of the ear, respectively. The lateral section of the posterior scalp is supplied by the lesser occipital and great auricular nerves.

Technique

Occipital nerve block is typically performed with the patient in the sitting position with the head and neck held in the flexed position.[6,10,11] The occipital protuberance and mastoid process are identified, and an imaginary line connecting these two landmarks is made. The occipital artery is often palpable about a third of the distance from midline to the mastoid

process and is the site of greater occipital nerve block. The lesser occipital nerve is blocked at a distance two thirds of the way from the midline to the mastoid process along this imaginary line. The block can be carried out by using a single skin entry point midway between the mastoid process and the occipital protuberance. Three to 5 mL of local anesthetic is infiltrated medially and another 3–5 mL laterally, both along this line. An effective block can be achieved by using two separate skin entry sites one third and two thirds of the way along this line. The local anesthetic is deposited within the skin and subcutaneous tissues in a fanwise fashion to create a subcutaneous wall along the imaginary line. A 25- or 27-gague $1\frac{1}{2}$-in. needle is used.

Complications

Few complications are associated with occipital nerve blocks. The local anesthetic itself creates swelling of the scalp, and the patient should be warned that this is normal. Puncture of the occipital artery is not uncommon and can result in hematoma. Simple pressure by the patient may be applied.

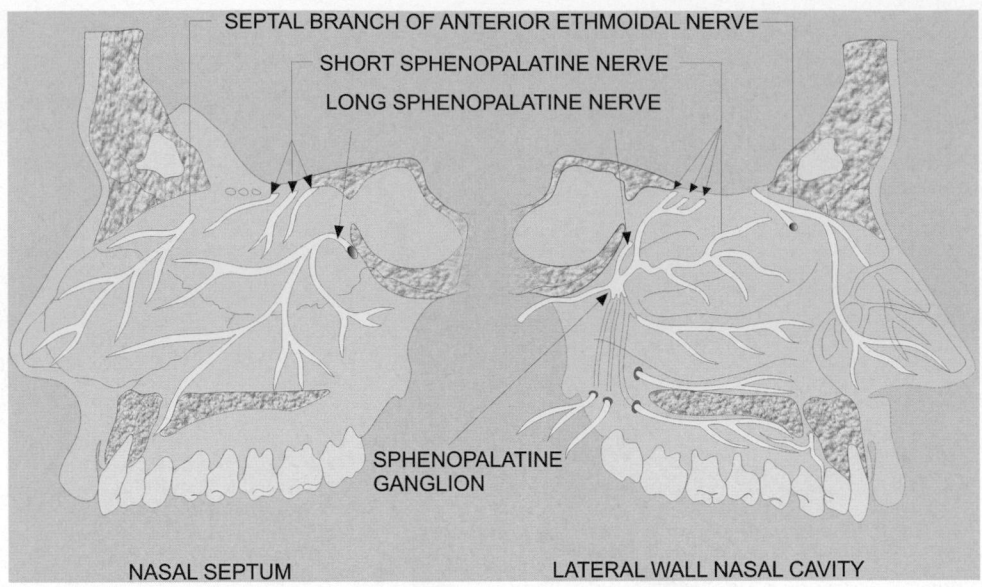

Figure 18–9. Innervation of the nasal cavity. Nasal cavity is innervated by ethmoidal and sphenopalatine nerves.

Patients with a history of blunt trauma to the area or prior posterior fossa intracranial surgery may have a defect in the bony cranium; in such cases, direct entry into the cranial vault may produce total spinal anesthesia.

BLOCK OF THE NASAL SEPTUM & LATERAL WALL OF THE NASAL CAVITY

Anesthesia of the nasal septum and the lateral wall of the nasal cavity facilitates nasotracheal intubation. Sensation to the superior portions of both the septum and lateral wall of the nasal cavity are supplied by the anterior ethmoidal nerve, a terminal branch of the ophthalmic division of the trigeminal nerve (Figure 18–9). The inferior and posterior portions of the septum and the lateral wall of the nasal cavity are innervated by branches arising from the sphenopalatine ganglion. These terminal branches lie superficially just beneath the nasal mucosa and can be anesthetized by direct topical application of local anesthetic (Figure 18–10).[12]

SUPRAORBITAL BLOCK

The supraorbital nerve emerges from the supraorbital foramen, which can be palpated along the upper border of the orbit, approximately 2.5 cm lateral to the midline of the face.[13] The supraorbital nerve exits along the upper border of the orbit, approximately 1 cm medial to the supraorbital foramen.

Indications

A supraorbital block is primarily used for the surgery on lower forehead and upper eyelid.

Technique

The supraorbital notch is palpated by the finger (Figure 18–11) and the needle is inserted along the upper orbital margin, approximately 1 cm medial to the supraorbital

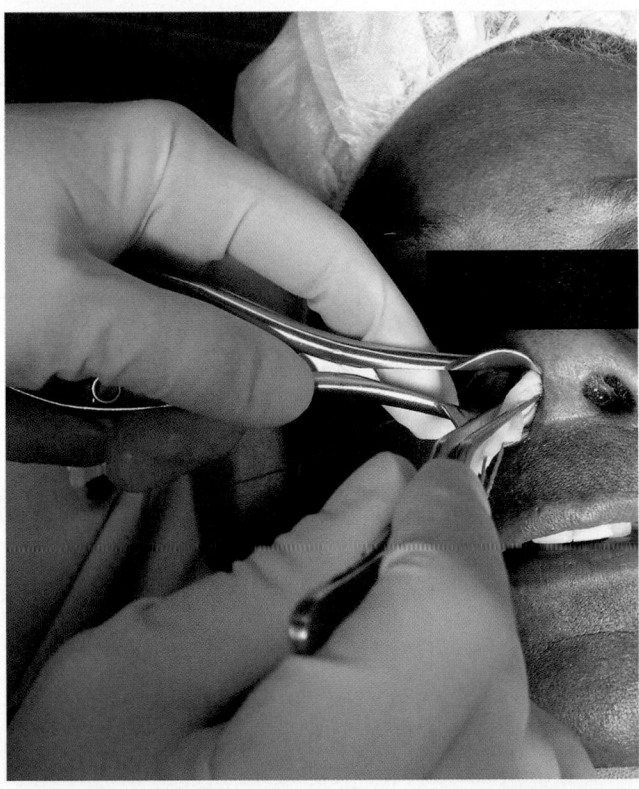

Figure 18–10. Application of the local anesthetic-soaked cotton packing to the nasal mucosae to accomplish anesthesia of the nasal cavity. The packing is left in position for several minutes to allow the topical anesthetic to penetrate the nasal mucosa.

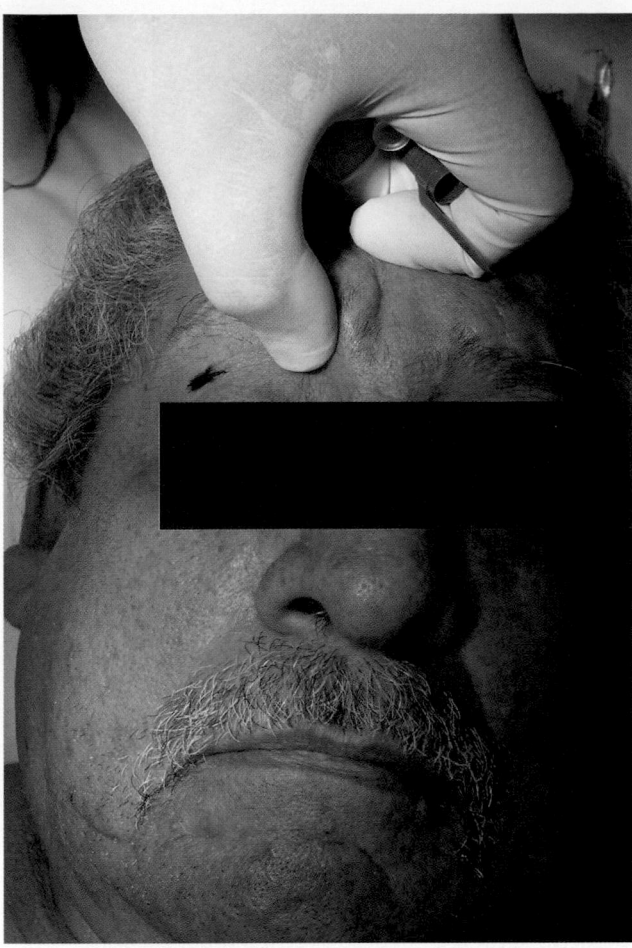

Figure 18–11. Palpation of the supraorbital notch.

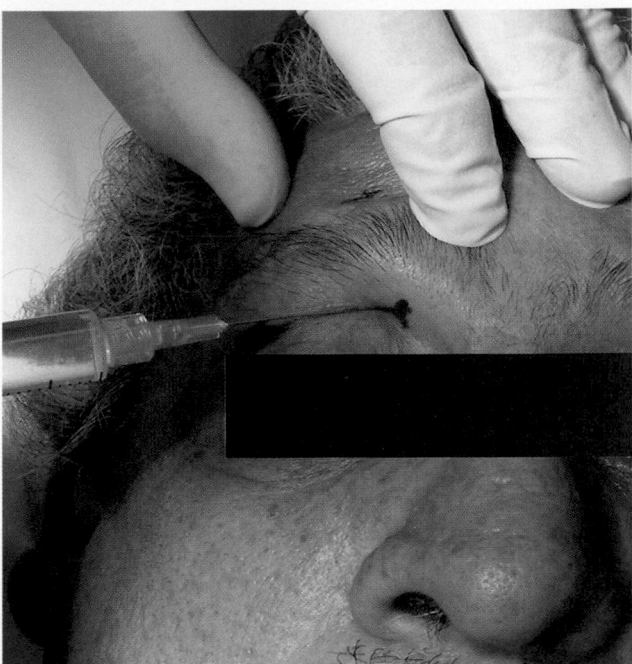

Figure 18–12. Supraorbital block.

foramen where 2–3 ml of local anesthetic is injected (Figure 18–12).

INFRAORBITAL NERVE BLOCK

An infraorbital block anesthetizes the anterior and middle maxillary alveolar nerves, inferior palpebral, lateral nasal, and superior labial nerves, resulting in anesthesia of the maxillary incisors, canines and premolars, including their vestibular osseous support and the soft tissues which cover them (Figure 18–13). In addition, mesiovestibular root of the maxillary first molar, part of the maxillary sinus, nose, superior labial, and inferior palpebral areas are also partly or completely anesthetized.

Anatomy

The second division of the trigeminal nerve, maxillary branch, exits the skull through the foramen rotundum, passes the pterygomaxillar fossa, enters the infraorbital canal, becomes the infraorbital nerve, and runs along the orbital floor (Figure 18–14). In other words, the infraorbital nerve is an extension of the maxillary nerve as it reaches the infraorbital fossa. The nerve emerges at the anterior side of the maxilla through the

infraorbital foramen, ending in three terminal branches: lateral nasal, superior labial, and inferior palpebral (see Figure 18–13). About 5 to 6 mm before the foramen, the infraorbital nerve supplies the anterior maxillary alveolar nerve, whose branches descend by narrow canals in the maxilla, running between the sinus mucosa and the bony wall, penetrating through the radicular apices, to innervate the pulp of maxillary incisors and canines. Its branches also go to the outer bone plate, periosteum, and other lining structures in the region of these teeth.

The middle superior alveolar nerve leaves the infraorbital nerve at the posterior part of the floor of the infraorbital canal and continues in a downward frontal direction until the premolar apices. At other times, it separates near the infraorbital foramen and descends by the anterior wall or the anterolateral maxillary sinus until the superior premolars, innervating the dental pulp, the external alveolar lamina, the periosteum and the mucosa.

Clinical Pearls

- The infraorbital nerve is the only sensory nerve. As the nerve exits the infraorbital foramen, it divides supplying the skin of the lower eyelid, nose, cheek, and upper lip.
- It is accompanied by the infraorbital artery and vein, which run parallel to the nerve.

Technique

The infraorbital foramen is located with a finger beneath the middle of the inferior margin of the orbit, just above the centered pupil.[14,15] The needle is inserted into the superior

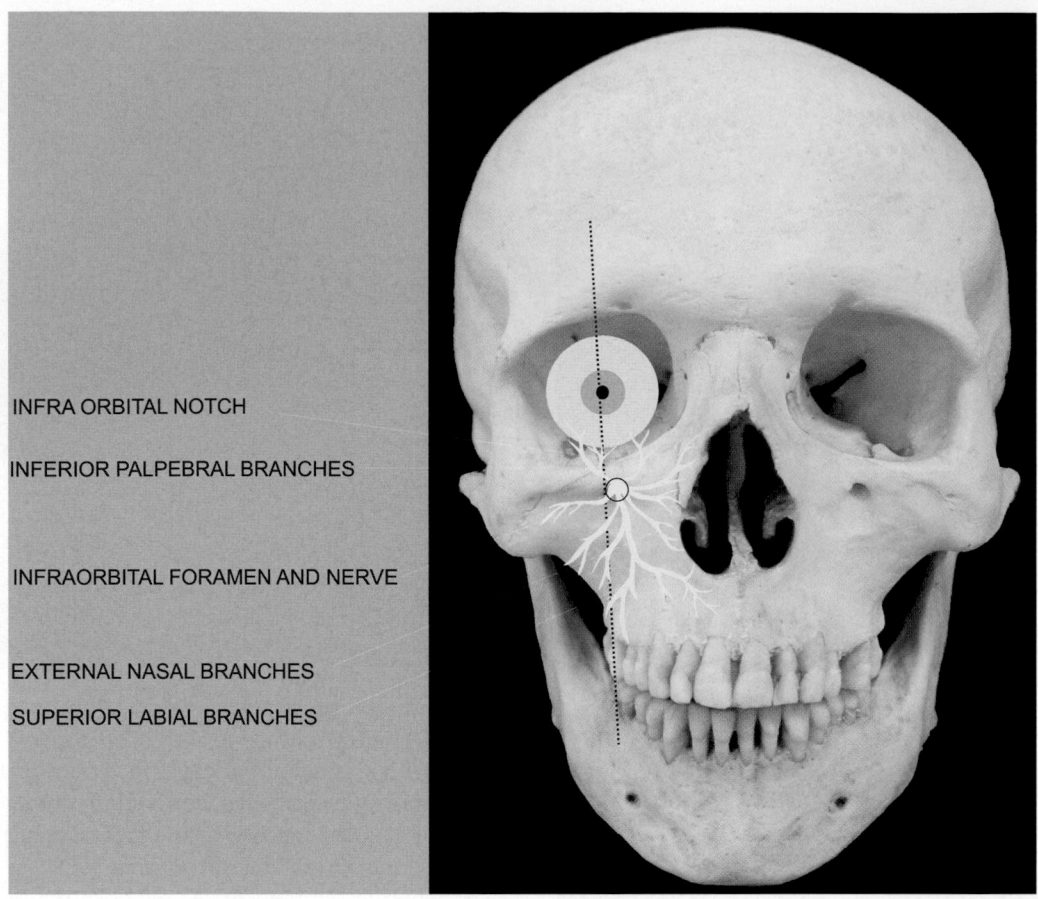

INFRA ORBITAL NOTCH

INFERIOR PALPEBRAL BRANCHES

INFRAORBITAL FORAMEN AND NERVE

EXTERNAL NASAL BRANCHES

SUPERIOR LABIAL BRANCHES

Figure 18–13. Infraorbital nerve and its branches. The infraorbital nerve can be anesthetized directly through the skin over where the infraorbital foramen is palpable along the inferior rim of the orbit. This nerve can also be anesthetized using a transoral approach or transnasal approach.

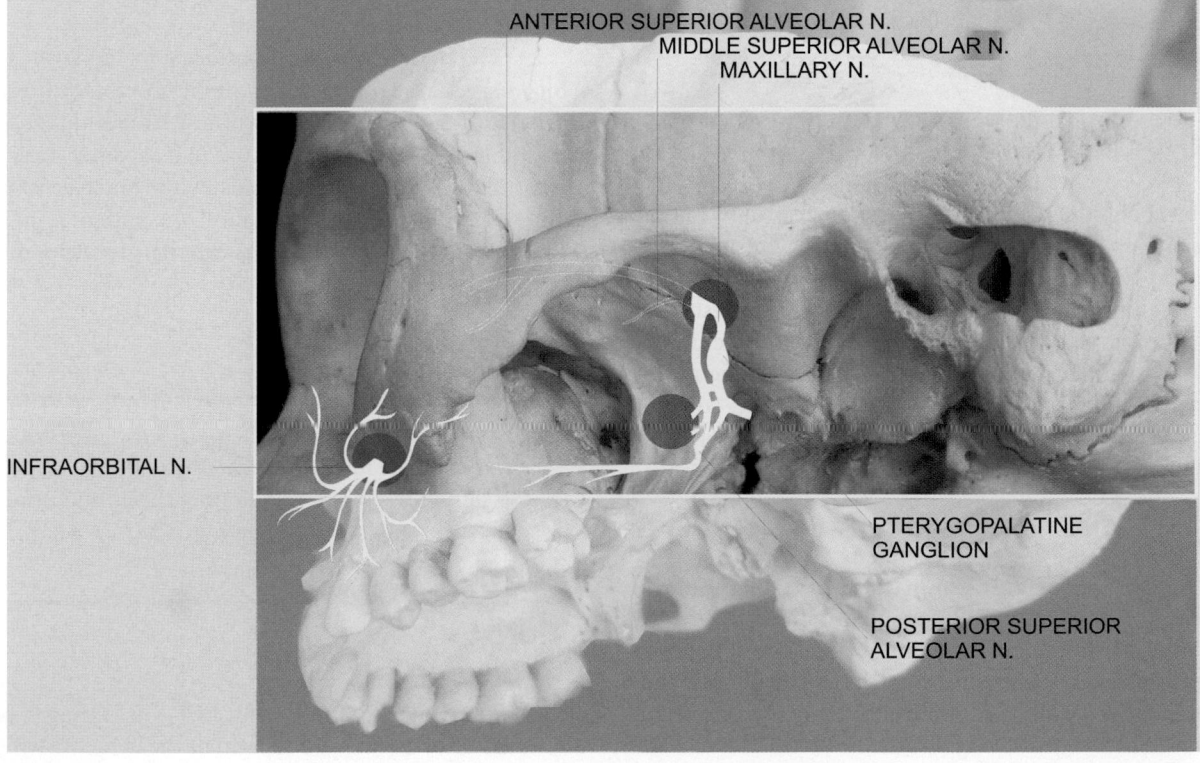

ANTERIOR SUPERIOR ALVEOLAR N.
MIDDLE SUPERIOR ALVEOLAR N.
MAXILLARY N.

INFRAORBITAL N.

PTERYGOPALATINE GANGLION

POSTERIOR SUPERIOR ALVEOLAR N.

Figure 18–14. Anatomy of the infraorbital nerve.

buccal groove and directed upward and outward, until contact with the finger, ie, injection site. A hypodermic needle (typically 25–27 gauge, 25 mm) is used. Lidocaine (1% or 2%), 0.25% bupivacaine, or 0.5% ropivacaine are all commonly used. In infants, 0.5–1 mL is used, 1–2 mL in children and 5 mL in adults.

For surgery on the upper lip, a bilateral infraorbital nerve block is always needed. For labiomaxillary fissure repair, this block should be combined with a nasopalatine nerve block.

Another technique of blocking the infraorbital nerve is by inserting the needle into the nasal vestibule and directing it lateral and superior in the direction of the infraorbital nerve. This is particularly useful for nasal work, such as nasal fractures.

SUMMARY

Several nerve block technique for head and neck applications can be used to provide successful anesthesia and analgesia for a variety of procedures performed on the head and neck. The same techniques are also used in the pain management practice either as diagnostic or therapeutic procedures. We suggest the reader consult Chapters 19-21 and 55 for more information on nerve block techniques for the head and neck surgery.

References

1. Perkin G: Trigeminal neuralgia. Curr Treat Options Neurol 1999;1: 458–465.
2. Green M, Selman J: Review article: The medical management of trigeminal neuralgia. Headache 1991;31:588–592.
3. Zakrewska J: Trigeminal neuralgia. Prim Dent Care 1997;1997: 17–9.
4. Sidebottom A, Maxwell A: The medical and surgical management of trigeminal neuralgia. J Clin Pharm Ther 1995;20:31–35.
5. Zakrewska J, Patsalos P: Drugs used in the management of trigeminal neuralgia. Oral Surg Oral Med Oral Pathol 1992;74:439–450.
6. Raj P, Pai U, Rawal N: *Techniques of Regional Anesthesia in Adults, Clinical Practice of Regional Anesthesia.* Churchill Livingston, 1991, p 271.
7. Han P, Shetter A, Smith K, et al: Gamma knife radiosurgery for trigeminal neuralgia: Experience at the Barrow Neurological Institute. Stereotact Funct Neurosurg 1999;73:131.
8. Zakrewska J: Surgical management of trigeminal neuralgia. Br Dent J 1991;170:61–62.
9. Kondziolka D, Lunsford L, Young R, et al: Stereotactic radiosurgery for trigeminal neuralgia: A multiinstitutional study using the gamma unit. J Neurosurg 1996;84:940–945.
10. Murphy T: Somatic blockade of head and neck. In Cousins M, Bridenbaugh P (eds): *Neural Blockade in Clinical Anesthesia and Management of Pain.* Lippincott-Raven, 1998, pp 489–514.
11. Tucker J, Flynn J: Head and neck regional blocks. In Brown D (ed): *Regional Anesthesia and Analgesia.* WB Saunders, 1996, pp 240–253.
12. Molliex S, Navez M, Baylor D, et al: Regional anaesthesia for outpatient nasal surgery. Br J Anaesth 1996;76:151–153.
13. Knize D: A study of the supraorbital nerve. Plant Reconstr Surg 1995;96:564–569.
14. Eaton J, Grekin R: Regional anaesthesia of the face. Derrnatol Surg 2001;27:1006–1009.
15. Lynch M, Syverud S, Schwab R, et al: Comparison of intraoral and percutaneous approaches for infraorbital nerve block. Acad Emerg Med 1994;1:514–519.

19

Regional & Topical Anesthesia for Endotracheal Intubation

Leroy Sutherland, MD • David Misita, MD

INTRODUCTION

Recent developments in regional anesthesia have resulted in a number of innovative and refined options to practitioners, often allowing regional techniques to be used for patients with presumed difficult airways. However, not every surgery can be performed under regional anesthesia. In addition, even in the hands of the most skilled regional anesthesiologist, blocks are subject to a certain rate of complications or failure.[1-4] In addition, there are many situations in which the anesthesiologist is called on to secure an airway in less than ideal circumstances. Expertise with regional anesthesia of the airway allows intubation in awake patients with suspected difficult intubation, upper airway trauma, or cervical spine fractures. Therefore,

it is essential that every regional anesthesiologist be skilled in the administration of general anesthesia and especially in the management of the difficult airway.

In recent years, there have been many advances in difficult airway management. The introduction of the laryngeal mask airway, and later the intubating laryngeal mask airway have changed the American Society of Anesthesiologists' difficult airway algorithm significantly.[5] Despite new devices and techniques being added to the arsenal daily, the mainstay of difficult airway management remains flexible fiberoptic laryngobronchoscopic intubation. Fiberoptic intubation can be performed under a variety of conditions. However, one major decision must be made with every procedure: Will the patient be intubated while under general anesthesia, or does the patient need to be awake during intubation?[6] Intubation under general anesthesia (even with inhalational induction and spontaneous respiration) carries the inherent risk of losing control of the difficult airway. For this reason, many anesthesiologists, on recognition of a difficult airway, elect to perform an awake intubation using either fiberoptic laryngobronchoscopy or awake direct laryngoscopy.

Direct laryngoscopy in an awake, unprepared patient can be extremely challenging. Excessive salivation and gag and cough reflexes can make intubation difficult, if not impossible, under awake conditions. In addition, the stress and discomfort may lead to undesirable elevations in the patient's sympathetic and parasympathetic outflow. Several highly effective topical and regional anesthesia techniques have been developed to subdue these reflexes and facilitate intubation. Each of these techniques has the common goal of reducing sensation over the specific regions that will be encountered by the fiberoptic bronchoscope and endotracheal tube.

Relevant Anatomy

To decide on a proper approach to an awake fiberoptic intubation, one must determine what structures need to be anesthetized along the two basic routes of intubation (oral or nasal) to facilitate optimal surgical conditions in the context of patient-specific anatomic considerations. Each of these routes has a well-defined pattern of innervation that can be specifically blocked to provide adequate anesthesia.

The nasal cavity is innervated by the **greater and lesser palatine nerves** and the **anterior ethmoidal nerve.** The palatine nerves arise from the trigeminal nerve via the pterygopalatine ganglion and innervate the nasal turbinates and most of the nasal septum. The pterygopalatine ganglion is located posterior to the middle turbinate in the pterygopalatine fossa. The anterior ethmoidal nerve arises from the olfactory nerve (CN I) and innervates the nares and the anterior third of the nasal septum.[7]

The oropharynx is innervated by branches of the **vagus, facial and glossopharyngeal nerves** (Figure 19–1). These

glossopharyngeal nerves travel anteriorly along the lateral surface of the pharynx, and the three branches provide sensory innervation to the posterior third of the tongue,[8] the vallecula, the anterior surface of the epiglottis (lingual branch), the walls of the pharynx (pharyngeal branch), and the tonsils (tonsillar branch). The sensory innervation of the anterior two thirds of the tongue is provided by the trigeminal nerve (lingual branch of the mandibular division).[8] Given that it is not a part of the reflex arcs controlling gag or cough, its blockade is not essential for comfort during fiberoptic intubation.

The **internal branch of the superior laryngeal nerve** is a branch of CN X (vagus nerve) (Figure 19–2). The superior laryngeal nerve provides sensory innervation to the base of the tongue, posterior epiglottis, aryepiglottic folds, and arytenoids.[7] This branch originates from the superior laryngeal nerve lateral to the greater cornu of the hyoid bone. The **recurrent laryngeal nerve** provides sensory innervation of the vocal folds and trachea and motor function of all intrinsic laryngeal muscles except the cricothyroid supplied by the external branch of the superior laryngeal nerve.[7]

Clinical Pearls

- Three major neural pathways supply sensation to airway structures (see Figure 19–1).
- Terminal branches of the ophthalmic and maxillary divisions of the trigeminal nerve supply the nasal cavity and turbinates.
- The oropharynx and posterior third of the tongue are supplied by the glossopharyngeal nerve.
- Branches of the vagus nerve innervate the posterior epiglottis and more distal airway structures.

TECHNIQUES FOR ANESTHETIZING THE AIRWAY

Preparation for Awake Intubation

The process of intubating an awake patient requires careful preparation. The anesthesiologist must evaluate each patient's needs on an individual basis. Nearly every patient experiences some degree of anxiety associated with the surgery, anesthesia, and perhaps outcome. For this reason, most patients require some degree of sedation and analgesia. For this purpose, it is best to use short-acting or reversible agents for sedation or agents that do not cause a considerable degree of respiratory depression. Some examples of commonly used medication for awake intubation include midazolam, alfentanil, and fentanyl. These sedatives/analgesics are particularly useful in this setting because of their easy titratability to effect easy reversal with flumazenil or naloxone. Similarly, dexmedetomidine does not cause respiratory depression and is suitable in this setting.[9]

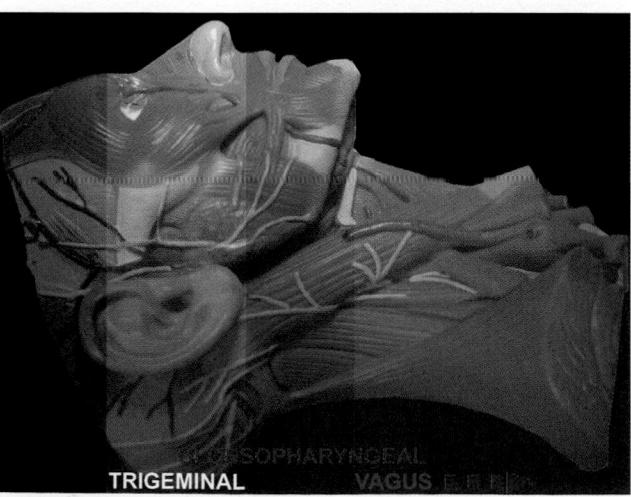

Figure 19–1. Innervation of the airway passages.

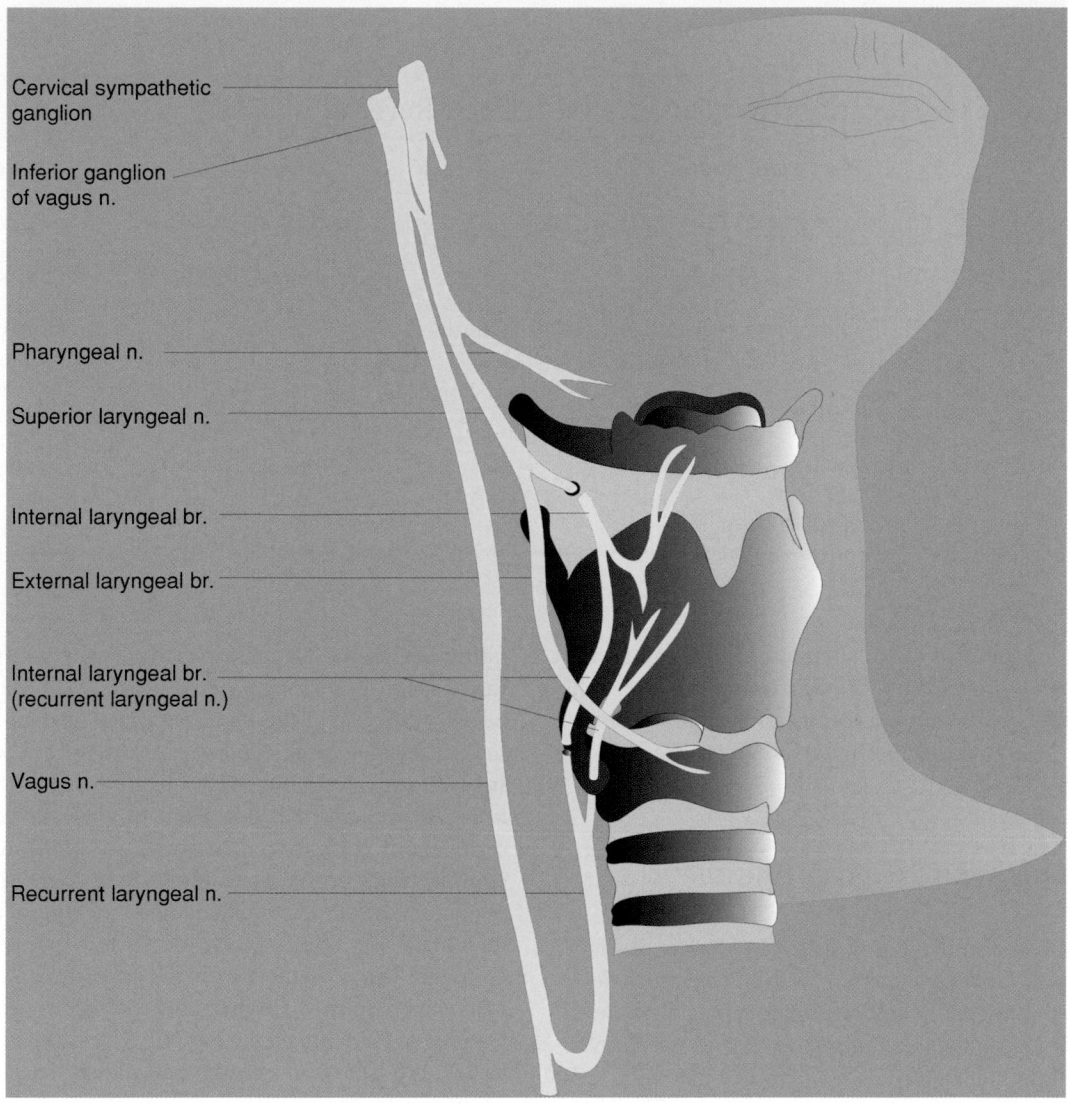

Figure 19–2. Innervation of the larynx.

Antisialogogues should be considered before any airway instrumentation. Oral secretions may make visualization via the fiberoptic equipment difficult and may serve as a barrier to effective penetration of local anesthetic into the mucosa. Glycopyrrolate 0.4 mg given intramuscularly or intravenously helps to diminish secretions.[10] Alternatively, atropine 0.5–1 mg may be used intramuscularly or intravenously to similar effect. Intramuscular administration is favored over intravenous administration to avoid undesired side effects such as tachycardia and, less commonly, psychosis (with atropine) (Table 19–1).

Topical Anesthesia of the Nose, Mouth, Tongue, & Pharynx

One way to achieve anesthesia for oral or nasal fiberoptic intubation is to topicalize the structures involved with a local anesthetic. **Topicalization** of the airway is the spreading of local anesthetic over a region of mucosa to achieve local uptake and neural blockade of that region.

By far, the simplest of these techniques involves the spraying or swishing of local anesthetic directly onto the mucosa of the mouth, pharynx, tongue, and/or nose. This can be accomplished with any of the many commercially available local anesthetics, particularly viscous lidocaine preparations and mixtures of benzocaine and tetracaine. One popular preparation, Cetacaine, is a pressurized solution of benzocaine, tetracaine, and butamben in a small canister, which delivers a spray via a long spray nozzle that is pointed in the desired direction (Figure 19–3). The anesthetic is delivered in an oily foam, which is absorbed rapidly into the mucosa and provides excellent topical anesthesia of the mucosa.

Alternatively, a 10-mL syringe can be filled with lidocaine 2–4% and sprayed via a small-bore single or multiperforated catheter or the working channel of the fiberoptic bronchoscope.[11] This arrangement produces a fine stream of local anesthetic liquid, which with sufficient aliquots directed

Table 19–1.

Commonly Used Medications and Dosages With Their Reversal Agents

Medication	Dosage and Route	Effect	Reversal Agent
Atropine	0.5–1 mg IV, IM	Antisialogogue	N/A
Glycopyrrolate	0.2–0.4 mg IV, IM	Antisialogogue	N/A
Dexmedetomidine	*Loading dose*: 1 mcg/kg/min over 10 min *Infusion*: 0.2–0.7 mcg/kg/min	Sedative	N/A
Midazolam	0.5–4 mg IV	Sedative	Flumazenil
Fentanyl	10–100 mcg IV	Opioid	Naloxone
Alfentanil	100–1000 mcg IV	Opioid	Naloxone

at the target mucosa achieves an adequate topical anesthetic effect. The safety and efficacy of both techniques are well established. Even with large amounts of swallowed anesthetic, plasma levels of local anesthetic should not reach toxic levels.[12,13]

Topicalization by Use of Local Anesthetic Reservoirs

Topicalization can also be accomplished by the use of local anesthetic-soaked cotton pledgets or swabs. These are soaked in either viscous or aqueous solutions of local anesthetic and then left for 5–15 minutes on the region of mucosa that re-

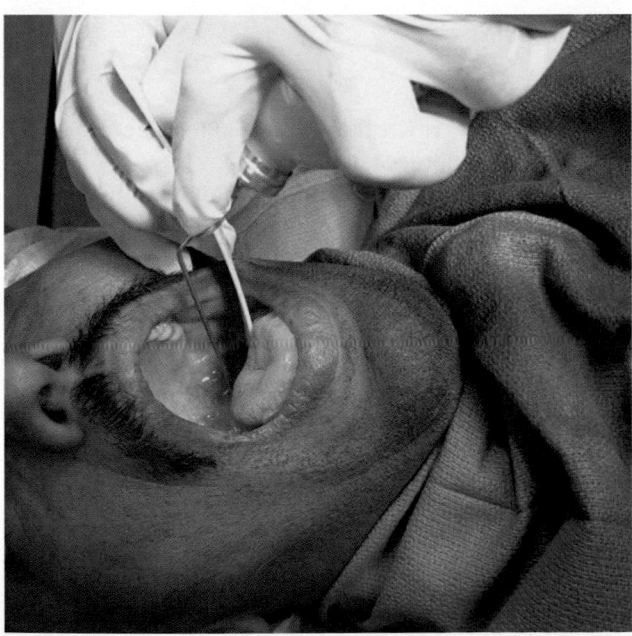

Figure 19–3. Topicalization of the mouth mucosa using a benzocaine spray.

quires anesthesia. The cotton acts as a reservoir for the anesthetic agent, producing a dense block. This technique is especially effective in the nasal passages. In the past, cocaine-soaked pledgets were used because they resulted both in a superb local anesthetic effect and in localized vasoconstriction. This practice has fallen out of favor, however, as concerns about cocaine toxicity grew. In addition, because of cocaine's high profile as an illicit drug, there are significant regulatory hurdles associated with stocking it in a hospital formulary (eg, DEA paperwork, theft, accurate accounting of usage). As a method of achieving similar results, most clinicians have used the technique of adding small concentrations of epinephrine (1:200,000 or less) or phenylephrine (0.05%) to lidocaine. Alternatively, a vasoconstricting nasal spray can be applied before application of the local anesthetic. This approach results in dry mucosa, which then can be more easily anesthetized with local anesthetic because the local anesthetic does not get diluted with nasal secretions or saliva. The resulting vasoconstriction is nearly as effective as that of cocaine and offsets lidocaine's powerful vasodilatation.

The application of highly concentrated local anesthetic-soaked cotton pledget reservoirs can be exploited to achieve highly specific nerve blocks as well. These methods are detailed later with the description of individual nerve blocks. More about topicalization can be found in Chapter 18.

Inhalation of Aerosolized (Atomized) Local Anesthetic

Inhalation of aerosolized local anesthetic is another simple technique to achieve oropharyngeal anesthesia (Figure 19–4). To perform this technique, local anesthetic is added to a standard nebulizer with a mouthpiece or face mask attached. The patient is then asked to inhale the local anesthetic vapor deeply. After a period of approximately 15–30 minutes, the patient should have inhaled a sufficient quantity

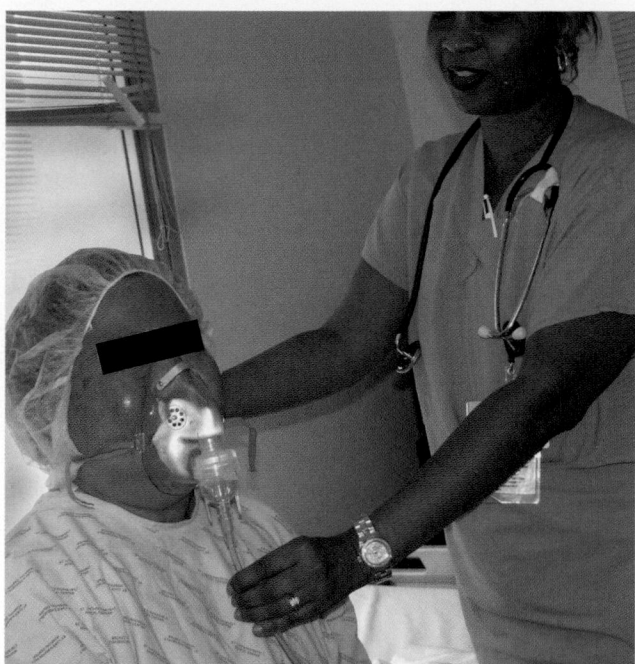

Figure 19–4. Anesthetizing airway using inhalation of aerosolized lidocaine.

of local anesthetic to achieve a reasonably good level of topical anesthesia throughout the oropharynx and trachea. Focused aerosolized local anesthetic from an atomizer is ideal for nasal intubation. A number of disposable commercially available syringe-powered atomizers are available but are deficient in achieving small particle size unless outfitted with a side-stream air/oxygen flow to enhance dispersion by virtue of the Venturi principle.

For these techniques, lidocaine in concentrations of 0.5%–4% has been suggested; quicker and denser blockade is achieved by using concentrations in the range of 2–4%. This technique has a proven clinical track record of safety; however, little data are available regarding the blood levels of local anesthetic that are achieved using these techniques or regarding metabolism of swallowed local anesthetics. Parkes et al.[14] showed plasma concentrations of 0.29–0.45 mg/L in healthy volunteers after inhalation of 10% lidocaine solution. Because these levels were well below the generally accepted 5 mg/L safe level, it can be inferred that inhaling a 2–4% lidocaine for 15–30 minutes should be safe in most patients, particularly as a stand-alone technique.[14]

The major advantage of this technique lies in its simplicity and lack of discomfort. In addition, very little working knowledge of the anatomy of the region is required for its successful implementation.

Although this technique may seem ideal, it does have some drawbacks that limit its usefulness. The main disadvantage is that the density of the anesthesia achieved throughout the airway is highly variable. Many patients still experience an intact cough reflex, which can make intubation technically challenging. The rate of onset of this technique is highly dependent on patient compliance. Many patients who need an awake intubation are incapable or unwilling to take deep breaths. Also, inhalation of local anesthetic vapors can lead to central nervous system depression in patients whose mental status may already be depressed owing to other disease processes.

Clinical Pearls

- Topicalization is the simplest method for anesthetizing the airway.
- Local anesthetic can be sprayed directly onto the desired mucosa.
- Nebulization of lidocaine 2–4% via face mask or oral nebulizer for 15–30 minutes can achieve highly effective anesthesia of the oral cavity and trachea for intubation.
- Atomization is ideal for airway topicalization during nasotracheal intubations.
- Density of anesthesia is variable and often requires supplementation to facilitate intubation.
- Anesthetic-soaked cotton can be applied to targeted mucosal surfaces for 5–15 minutes to effect selective blockade of underlying nerves.
- Vasoconstrictors such as epinephrine (1:200,000) or phenylephrine (0.05%) can be added to the solution to reduce mucosal bleeding.
- Adequate time allocation is needed to achieve optimal conditions.

TECHNIQUES FOR BLOCKING INDIVIDUAL NERVES OF THE AIRWAY

Blockade of the Glossopharyngeal Nerve

The oropharynx, soft palate, posterior portion of the tongue, and the pharyngeal surface of the epiglottis are innervated by the glossopharyngeal nerve. Blockade of the glossopharyngeal nerve facilitates endotracheal intubation by blocking the gag reflex associated with direct laryngoscopy as well as facilitating passage of a nasotracheal tube through the posterior pharynx. The glossopharyngeal nerve travels anterior along the lateral surface of the pharynx, and its three branches provide sensory innervation to the posterior third of the tongue, the vallecula, the anterior surface of the epiglottis (lingual branch), the walls of the pharynx (pharyngeal branch), and the tonsils (tonsillar branch). Logically, blockade of this nerve bilaterally would result in anesthesia of those structures.

The glossopharyngeal nerve can be anesthetized using either intraoral or extraoral (peristyloid) approaches. For the intraoral approach, the mouth is opened the overlying mucosa is anesthetized with topical anesthetic. A $3\frac{1}{3}$-in.,

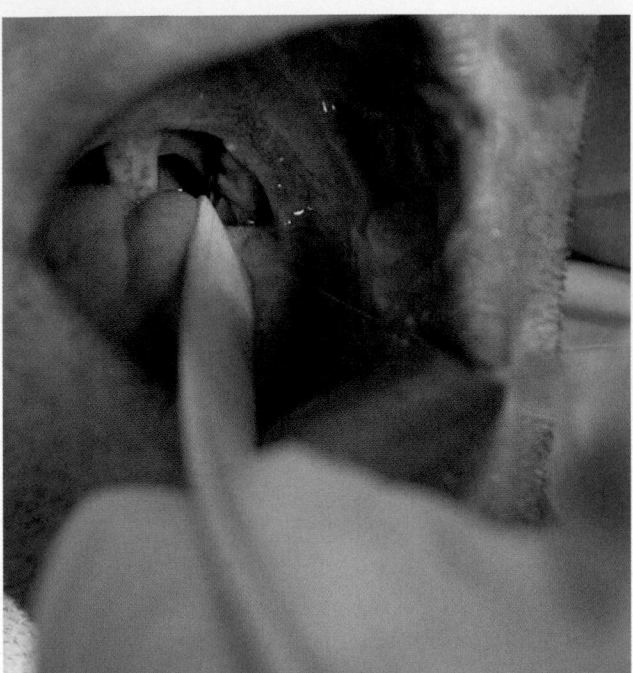

Figure 19–5. Glossopharyngeal block.

22-gauge needle is used to place 2–5 mL of local anesthetic solution submucosally at the base of the palatoglossal fold (Figure 19–5). To perform the peristyloid approach to the glossopharyngeal block, the patient is placed supine and a line is drawn between the angle of the mandible and the mastoid process. Using deep pressure, the styloid process is palpated just posterior to the angle of the jaw along this line, and a short, small-gauge needle is seated against the styloid process. The needle is then withdrawn slightly and directed posteriorly off the styloid process. As soon as bony contact is lost, 5–7 mL of local anesthetic solution are injected after careful aspiration for blood. Both approaches involve deposition of local anesthetic in close proximity to the carotid artery, and careful aspiration before injection is essential.

The applications of this block are limited by the specific anatomic regions that are innervated by the glossopharyngeal nerve. It is essential to ablate deep pressure symptoms from the tongue base during direct laryngoscopy. Blockade of the glossopharyngeal nerve is an integral part of effective block combinations, which is discussed later in the text.[5] Because of the high vascularity of the palatoglossal arch, accidental vascular injection is an ever-present risk. Careful aspiration helps to reduce this risk, but it cannot be avoided entirely. In addition, significant absorption of local anesthetic can be expected in this region. The addition of epinephrine to the local anesthetic solution helps to vasoconstrict the blood vessels in the region, reducing absorption as well as assisting in the diagnosis of intravascular injection by heart rate monitoring. As with any injection into a highly vascular region, this technique may be contraindicated in patients with coagulopathies or anticoagulation.

Clinical Pearls

- The glossopharyngeal nerve provides sensory innervation to the posterior third of the tongue, the vallecula, the anterior surface of the epiglottis (lingual branch), the walls of the pharynx (pharyngeal branch), and the tonsils (tonsillar branch).
- It is most easily blocked where it crosses the palatoglossal arch.
- It can be blocked using one of three methods: topical spray application, direct mucosal contact of soaked pledgets, or direct infiltration by injection.
- Glossopharyngeal nerve block is not adequate as a solo technique to facilitate intubation, but in combination with other techniques it is highly effective.

Superior Laryngeal Nerve Block

The internal branch of the superior laryngeal nerve (a branch of the vagus nerve) provides sensory innervation to the base of the tongue, posterior surface of the epiglottis, aryepiglottic fold, and the arytenoids. Blockade of the sensory input to this branch can often be accomplished by mucosal saturation with local anesthetic by the inhalational and direct topical application techniques described above. In some patients, however, this may not provide timely adequate anesthesia for a comfortable awake intubation. In these cases, a direct regional blockade of the superior laryngeal nerve is desired. Regional anesthesia of the superior laryngeal nerve can be accomplished by exploiting the anatomic course of the nerve as it arises from the vagus nerve and descends to the larynx. The internal branch originates from the superior laryngeal nerve lateral to the greater cornu of the hyoid bone. In most patients, the nerve should pass approximately 2–4 mm inferior to the greater cornu of the hyoid bone.[15] From here, it pierces the thyrohyoid membrane and travels under the mucosa in the pyriform recess.[16]

After topicalization, the most popular technique for superior laryngeal nerve block involves bilateral injections at the level of the greater cornu of the hyoid bone. The patient is placed supine with the head extended as much as possible. The patient's skin is cleaned with an appropriate antimicrobial solution (eg, betadine). The cornu of the hyoid bone is located below the angle of the mandible. It is easily identified (particularly in men) by palpating outward from the thyroid notch along the upper border of the thyroid cartilage until the greater cornu is encountered just superior to its posterolateral margin (Figure 19–6). The nondominant hand is used to displace the hyoid bone with contralateral pressure, bringing the ipsilateral cornu and the internal branch of the superior laryngeal nerve toward the anesthesiologist. The anesthesiologist can then appreciate the pulsation of the carotid artery being displaced deep to the palpating finger tip.

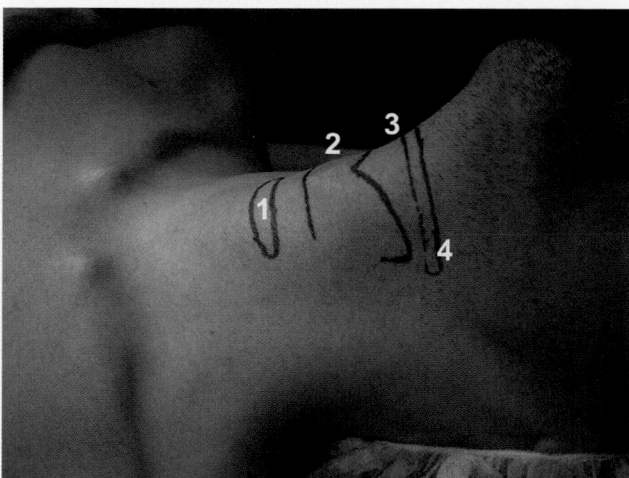

Figure 19–6. Surface anatomy of the larynx: (1) Cricoid cartilage; (2) thyroid cartilage; (3) hyoid bone; (4) cornu of the hyoid bone.

A $\frac{5}{8}$-in., 25-gauge needle is inserted in an anteroinferomedial direction until the lateral aspect of the greater cornu is contacted (Figure 19–7). If the needle is then walked downward toward the midline (1–2 mm) off the inferior border of the greater cornu, the thyrohyoid membrane is pierced and the internal branch alone is blocked. If the needle is retracted slightly after contacting the hyoid, both the internal and external branches of the superior laryngeal nerve are blocked. The syringe is then aspirated, and if aspiration is negative for air and blood, 2 mL of local anesthetic (2% lidocaine) with or without epinephrine (1:300,000) are then injected. If aspiration results in air, the needle tip is likely in the larynx and needs to be retracted. If blood is encountered, the needle may have encountered a blood vessel. Given the proximity of the carotid artery, it is advisable to withdraw the needle, reassess the landmarks, and reattempt the procedure.

Two milliliters of local anesthetic should reliably bathe the internal branch of the superior laryngeal nerve, given its proximity to the hyoid bone. If this volume is injected outside the thyrohyoid membrane, it is likely to block the external

branch of the superior laryngeal nerve as well. Isolated external superior laryngeal nerve branch blockade may result in cricothyroid muscle weakness, which eliminates its function as an airway dilator.[17] The motor input of the recurrent laryngeal nerve is spared, however, and therefore does not result in clinically significant change in laryngeal inlet diameters.[18]

The superior laryngeal nerve can also be approached in the pre-epiglottic space. The pre-epiglottic space is accessed at a point 2 cm lateral to the thyroid notch. The needle is advanced 1–1.5 cm superoposteriorly to pierce the thyrohyoid membrane, and the nerve can be blocked. Alternatively, using the thyroid cornu as a landmark and walking the needle superoanteromedially can accomplish this block.

Some patients may be unwilling or unable to undergo such injections. Common reasons include patient refusal, anticoagulation, and distorted anatomy due to tumors, arteriovenous malformations, surgical deformities, or reconstruction. In patients in whom injection is contraindicated or overly challenging, a less invasive technique for blocking the superior laryngeal nerve can be accomplished by using soaked pledgets. After topicalization, the patient is asked to stick the tongue out. The tongue is then grasped using a gauze pad. With a right-angled forceps (Jackson-Krause forceps) the anesthetic-soaked pledgets are placed in the pyriform fossae located on either side of the root of the tongue. After 5–10 minutes, a sufficient degree of anesthesia should be present for intubation.[19]

Clinical Pearls

- The superior laryngeal nerve innervates the base of the tongue, posterior surface of the epiglottis, aryepiglottic fold, and the arytenoids.
- Blockade is usually inadequate as a solo technique for intubation.
- Noninvasive blockade involves topicalization of the oral cavity, but this technique often proves inadequate.
- Direct infiltration is accomplished at the level of the thyrohyoid membrane inferior to the cornu of the hyoid bone. A reliable block with a definite endpoint is effected by retracting the needle marginally after contacting the greater cornu and injecting 2 mL of local anesthetic after negative aspiration.
- Less invasive blockade can be accomplished by placing anesthetic-soaked cotton pledgets into the pyriform fossae bilaterally.

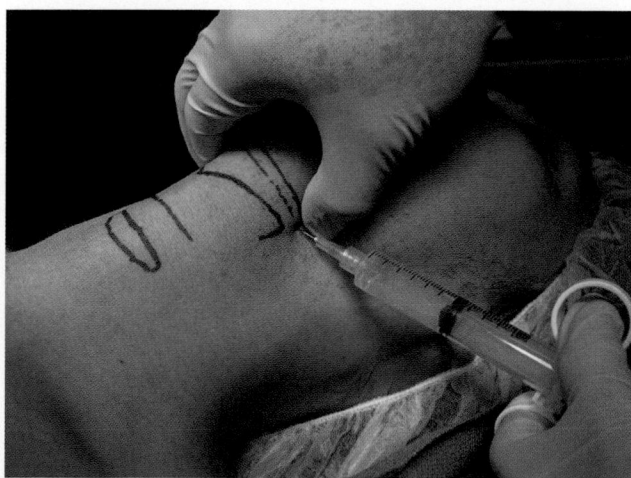

Figure 19–7. Superior laryngeal block.

Recurrent Laryngeal Nerve Block

The recurrent laryngeal nerve provides sensory innervation to the vocal folds and the trachea. Blockade of this nerve is necessary to provide comfort and prevent coughing while the endotracheal tube is being passed between the vocal cords. Sufficient blockade of the recurrent laryngeal nerve can often be accomplished using the inhalational technique previously

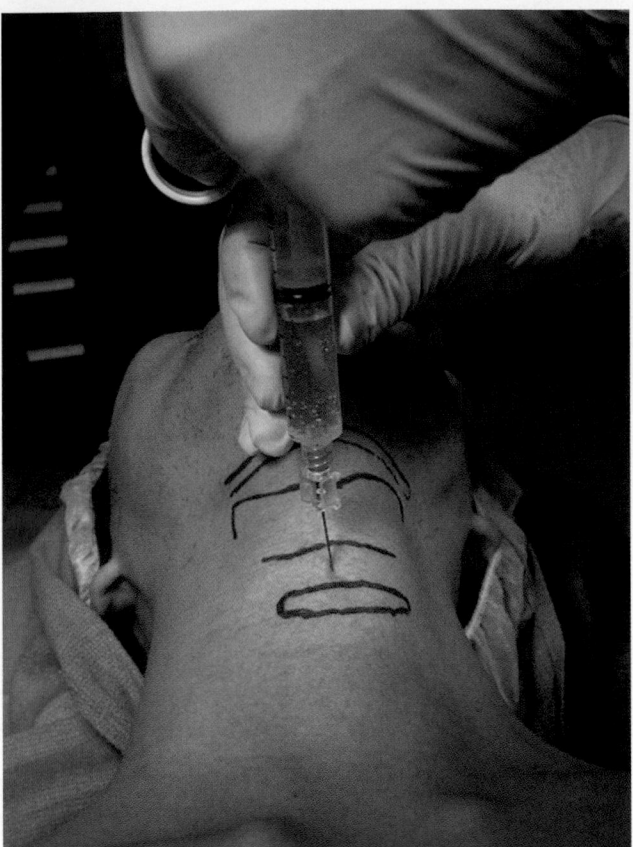

Figure 19–8. Transtracheal Block. The needle is inserted into the trachea transcutaneously.

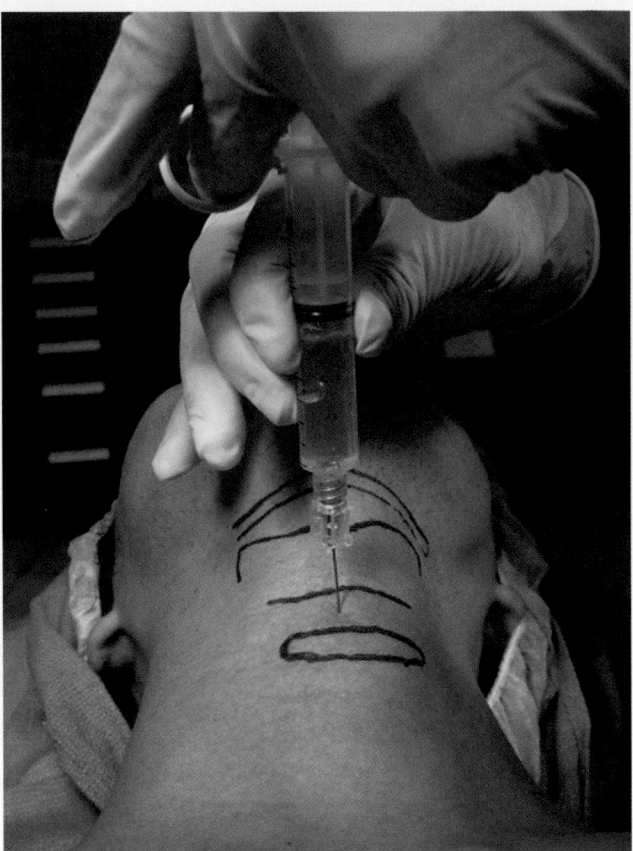

Figure 19–9. Transtracheal Block. Appearance of an air bubble in the syringe while the syringe is being aspirated during continuous advancement indicates intratracheal placement.

described. Again, some patients may not achieve a sufficient amount of anesthesia to facilitate intubation.

Another technique for blocking the sensory input of the recurrent laryngeal nerve is the **transtracheal block.** In this technique, the cricothyroid membrane is located in the midline of the neck. It can be located by palpating the thyroid prominence and proceeding in a caudad direction. The cricothyroid membrane is identified as the spongy fibro-muscular band between the thyroid and cricoid cartilages (Figure 19–8). After sterile skin preparation, the overlying skin is anesthetized by raising a small skin wheal of local anesthetic. Then a 22- or 20-gauge needle on a 10-mL syringe with 4 mL of 4% lidocaine is passed perpendicular to the axis of the trachea and pierces the membrane. (Alternatively, a 20-gauge angiocath can be passed.) While the needle is being advanced, the syringe is continuously aspirated. The needle is advanced until air is freely aspirated, signifying that the needle is now in the larynx (Figure 19–9). Instillation of local anesthetic at this point invariably results in coughing. Through coughing, the local anesthetic is dispersed, diffusely blocking the sensory nerve endings of the recurrent laryngeal nerve. Motor function remains completely unaffected. It is advisable to use a larger-gauge needle for this block. A more rapid delivery of local anesthetic reduces the risk of needle-induced trauma due to coughing.

Direct blockade of the recurrent laryngeal nerve is contraindicated. Bilateral blockade results in upper airway obstruction, since the recurrent laryngeal nerve provides motor

innervation for all the muscles of the larynx except the cricothyroid. In contrast, unilateral blockade typically manifests only as transient hoarseness.

Clinical Pearls

- Recurrent laryngeal nerve provides sensory innervation to the trachea and vocal folds. Blockade facilitates comfortable passing of the endotracheal tube into the trachea.
- This nerve can be blocked by using topicalization techniques described previously.
- Translaryngeal block of the recurrent laryngeal nerve is easily accomplished at the level of the cricothyroid membrane. A 10-mL syringe with a 22- or 20-gauge needle is advanced until air is aspirated into the syringe. Four milliliters of local anesthetic are then injected, inducing coughing that disperses the local anesthetic.
- The recurrent laryngeal nerve can also be blocked by spraying local anesthetic via the injection port of the fiberoptic bronchoscope.
- The block density diminishes rapidly in the distal tracheo-bronchial tree so special care should be taken to maintain the tip of the fiberoptic bronchoscope and endotracheal tube above the carina.

Blockade of the Palatine Nerves

To allow awake nasal fiberoptic intubation, one must also provide sensory blockade to the nasal passages. The greater and lesser palatine nerves innervate the nasal turbinates and the posterior two thirds of the nasal septum. The sensory input of these nerves can be blocked by topical application of the local anesthetic into nasal passages. If this proves inadequate, however, regional blockade of the palatine nerves can be accomplished by blocking the pterygopalatine ganglion from which both nerves arise. This can be accomplished noninvasively by taking a cotton-tipped applicator soaked in local anesthetic and passing it along the upper border of the middle turbinate to the posterior wall of the nasopharynx, where it is left for 5–10 minutes.[20]

An oral approach to the pterygopalatine ganglion is described with needle passage through the greater palatine foramen into the pterygopalatine fossa. A percutaneous approach via the mandibular notch is usual performed under fluoroscopic guidance for pain management. Because of technical difficulty and the high risk for vascular injury, these techniques are rarely needed or used for nasal-passage anesthesia during fiberoptic intubation. They are mentioned here only for the sake of completeness and academic discussion.

Clinical Pearls

- Nasal intubation requires blockade of the nasal passages.
- Blockade of the greater and lesser palatine nerves blocks sensation to the nasal turbinates and posterior two thirds of the nasal septum.
- Topicalization of these structures is typically effective for intubation.
- Alternatively, the pterygopalatine ganglion can be blocked by passing a local anesthetic-soaked cotton applicator along the upper border of the middle turbinate to the posterior wall of the nasopharynx, where it is left for 5–10 minutes.
- Transoral and percutaneous approaches to the pterygopalatine ganglion can be accomplished, but technical difficulty and an increased potential for complications preclude their routine use.

Blockade of the Anterior Ethmoid Nerve

The remaining portions of the nasal passages to be blocked are innervated by the anterior ethmoid nerve and is usually adequately blocked by inhalational or spray topicalization. This nerve can be selectively blocked by direct mucosal contact application with an anesthetic-soaked cotton applicator passed along the dorsal surface of the nose until the anterior cribriform plate is reached. The applicator is left in this position for 5–10 minutes.

Clinical Pearls

- The anterior ethmoid nerve innervates the remainder of the nasal passage.
- Anesthetic-soaked cotton applicator is passed along the dorsal surface of the nose until the anterior cribiform plate is reached to achieve selective blockade after 5–10 minutes.

Step-by-Step Method for Orotracheal Fiberoptic Intubation Using Topical Anesthesia Only

1. Administer antisialogogue (glycopyrrolate 0.2–0.4 mg + dyphenhydramine (Benadryl) 20 mg IM) at least 20–30 minutes before fiberoptic instrumentation.
2. Provide judicious sedation using appropriate doses of midazolam and fentanyl/alfentanil and/or dexmedetomidine.
3. Use benzocaine spray to anesthetize the oral cavity and pharynx.
4. Apply a generous amount of 2% lidocaine ointment on the Ovassapian airway, and insert the tip of the airway in the patient's mouth. As the lidocaine ointment is dissolved, it is carried deeper into the pharynx and swallowed by the patient. The airway is then advanced deeper as tolerated by the patient every 2–3 minutes. Eventually, the patient should be able to swallow the entire airway without discomfort.
5. Attach a 5-mL syringe containing a solution of 4% lidocaine to the insufflating port of the flexible bronchoscope.
6. Advance the bronchoscope until the epiglottis and vocal chords are seen and proceed as follows:
   - Inject 2 mL of local anesthetic over the epiglottis, wait 15 seconds, and advance the scope (anesthetizes the epiglottis and superior aspect of the cords).
   - Inject 1 mL of local anesthetic when the tip of the scope is just above the vocal cords; wait 15 seconds and advance the scope (anesthetizes cords).
   - Inject 2 mL of local anesthetic when the tip of the scope passes underneath the vocal cords (anesthetizes the trachea).
   - Advance the scope until the carina is seen.
   - Advance the endotracheal tube over the fiberoptic scope.
7. If unable to intubate using the above method, attempt appropriate blockade of individual nerves until the patient is able to tolerate intubation.

SUMMARY

An awake intubation often requires a combination of techniques to adequately anesthetize all the structures that will be encountered. The widest coverage is provided by the inhalational technique. This technique, however, does not always provide a dense enough level of anesthesia for all patients. Supplementation of this technique with any of the nerve specific blocks in this chapter is an excellent way to accomplish efficacious anesthesia for awake inubation.[21]

References

1. Faccenda KA, Finucane BT: Complications of regional anaesthesia: Incidence and prevention. Drug Saf 2001;24:413–442.
2. Auroy Y, Narchi P, Messiah A, et al: Serious complications related to regional anesthesia: Results of a prospective survey in France. Anesthesiology 1997;87:479–486.
3. Naguib M, Magboul MM, Samarkandi AH, Attia M: Adverse effects and drug interactions associated with local and regional anaesthesia. Drug Saf 1998;18:221–250.
4. Cotter JT, Nielsen KC, Guller U, et al: Increased body mass index and ASA physical status IV are risk factors for block failure in ambulatory surgery: An analysis of 9,342 blocks. Can J Anaesth 2004;51:810–816.
5. American Society of Anesthesiologists Task Force on Management of the Difficult Airway: Practice guidelines for management of the difficult airway: An updated report by the American Society of Anesthesiologists Task Force on management of the difficult airway. Anesthesiology 2003;98:1269–1277.
6. Rose DK, Cohen MM: The airway: Problems and predictions in 18,500 patients. Can J Anaesth 1994;41:372–383.
7. Netter F: *Atlas of Human Anatomy*. Ciba-Geigy Corporation, 1989, Plates 37–40.
8. Netter F: *Atlas of Human Anatomy*. Ciba-Geigy Corporation, 1989, Plate 56.
9. Avitsian R, Lin J, Lotto M, Ebrahim Z: Dexmedetomidine and awake fiberoptic intubation for possible cervical spine myelopathy: A clinical series. J Neurosurg Anesthesiol 2005;17:97–99.
10. Brookman CA, Teh HP, Morrison LM: Anticholinergics improve fibreoptic intubating conditions during general anaesthesia. Can J Anaesth 1997;44:165–167.
11. Vloka JD, Hadzic A, Kitain E: A simple adaptation to the Olympus LF1 and LF2 fiberoptic bronchoscopes for instillation of local anesthetic. Anesthesiology 1995;82:792.
12. Greenblatt DJ, Benjamin DM, Willis CR, et al: Lidocaine plasma concentrations following administration of intraoral lidocaine solution. Arch Otolaryngol 1985;111:298–300.
13. Nydahl PA, Axelsson K: Venous blood concentration of lidocaine after nasopharyngeal application of 2% lidocaine gel. Acta Anaesthesiol Scand 1988;32:135–139.
14. Parkes SB, Butler CS, Muller R: Plasma lignocaine concentration following nebulization for awake intubation. Anaesth Intensive Care 1997;25:369–371.
15. Furlan JC: Anatomical study applied to anesthetic block technique of the superior laryngeal nerve. Acta Anaesthesiol Scand 2002;46:199–202.
16. Netter F: *Atlas of Human Anatomy*. Ciba-Geigy Corporation, 1989, Plates 70, 71.
17. Wheatley JR, Brancatisano A, Engel LA: Respiratory-related activity of cricothyroid muscle in awake normal humans. J Appl Physiol 1991;70:2226–2232.
18. Woodson GE, Sant'Ambrogio F, Mathew O, Sant'Ambrogio G: Effects of cricothyroid muscle contraction on laryngeal resistance and glottic area. Ann Otol Rhinol Laryngol 1989;98:119–124.
19. Curran J, Hamilton C, Taylor T: Topical analgesia before tracheal intubation. Anaesthesia 1975;30:765–768.
20. Kundra P, Kutralam S, Ravishankar M: Local anaesthesia for awake fibreoptic nasotracheal intubation. Acta Anaesthesiol Scand 2000;44:511.
21. Reasoner DK, Warner DS, Todd MM, et al: A comparison of anesthetic techniques for awake intubation in neurosurgical patients. J Neurosurg Anesthesiol 1995;7:94–99.

20

Oral & Maxillofacial Regional Anesthesia

Benaifer D. Dubash, DMD • Adam T. Hershkin, DMD • Paul J. Seider, DMD •
Gregory M. Casey, DDS

INTRODUCTION

Oral surgical and dental procedures are routinely performed in an outpatient setting. Regional anesthesia is the most common method of anesthetizing the patient before office-based procedures. Many techniques can be used to achieve anesthesia of the dentition and surrounding hard and soft tissues of the maxilla and mandible. The type of procedure to be performed as well as the location of the procedure determines the technique of anesthesia to be used. Orofacial anesthetic techniques can be classified into three main categories: local infiltration, field block, and nerve block.

The local infiltration technique anesthetizes the terminal nerve endings of the dental plexus. This is indicated when an individual tooth or a specific, isolated area requires anesthesia. The procedure is performed in the direct vicinity of the site of infiltration.

The field block anesthetizes the terminal nerve branches in the area of treatment. Treatment can then be performed in an area slightly distal to the site of injection. The deposition of local anesthetic at the apex of a tooth for the purposes of achieving pulpal and soft tissue anesthesia is often used by many dental and maxillofacial professionals. Although this is commonly termed "local infiltration," it is important to note that this is a misnomer. Terminal nerve branches are anesthetized in this technique, and it is therefore correctly termed a **field block.**

A nerve block anesthetizes the main branch of a specific nerve, allowing treatment to be performed in the region innervated by the nerve.[1] This chapter reviews the essential anatomy of orofacial nerves and details the practical approach to performing nerve blocks and infiltrational anesthesia for a variety of surgical procedures in this region.

Anatomy of the Trigeminal Nerve

General Considerations

Anesthesia of the teeth and soft and hard tissues of the oral cavity cannot be achieved without knowledge of the trigeminal nerve (fifth cranial nerve) and its branches. Regional, field, and local anesthesia of the maxilla and mandible depend on the deposition of anesthetic solution near terminal nerve branches or a main nerve trunk of the trigeminal nerve.

The largest of all the cranial nerves, the trigeminal nerve gives rise to a small motor root originating in the motor nucleus within the pons and medulla oblongata, and a larger sensory root which finds its origin in the anterior aspect of the pons. The nerve travels forward from the posterior cranial fossa to the petrous portion of the temporal bone within the middle cranial fossa. Here, the sensory root forms the trigeminal (semilunar or gasserian) ganglion situated within Meckel's cavity on the anterior surface of the petrous portion of the temporal bone. The ganglia are paired, one innervating each side of the face. The sensory root of the trigeminal nerve gives rise to the ophthalmic division (V_1), the maxillary division (V_2), and the mandibular division (V_3) from the trigeminal ganglion (Figure 20–1).

The motor root travels from the brainstem along with but separate from the sensory root. It then leaves the middle cranial fossa through the foramen ovale after passing underneath the trigeminal ganglion in a lateral and inferior direction. The motor root exits the middle cranial fossa along with the third division of the sensory root; the mandibular nerve. It then unties with the mandibular nerve to form a single nerve trunk after exiting the skull. The motor fibers supply the muscles of mastication (masseter, temporalis, medial

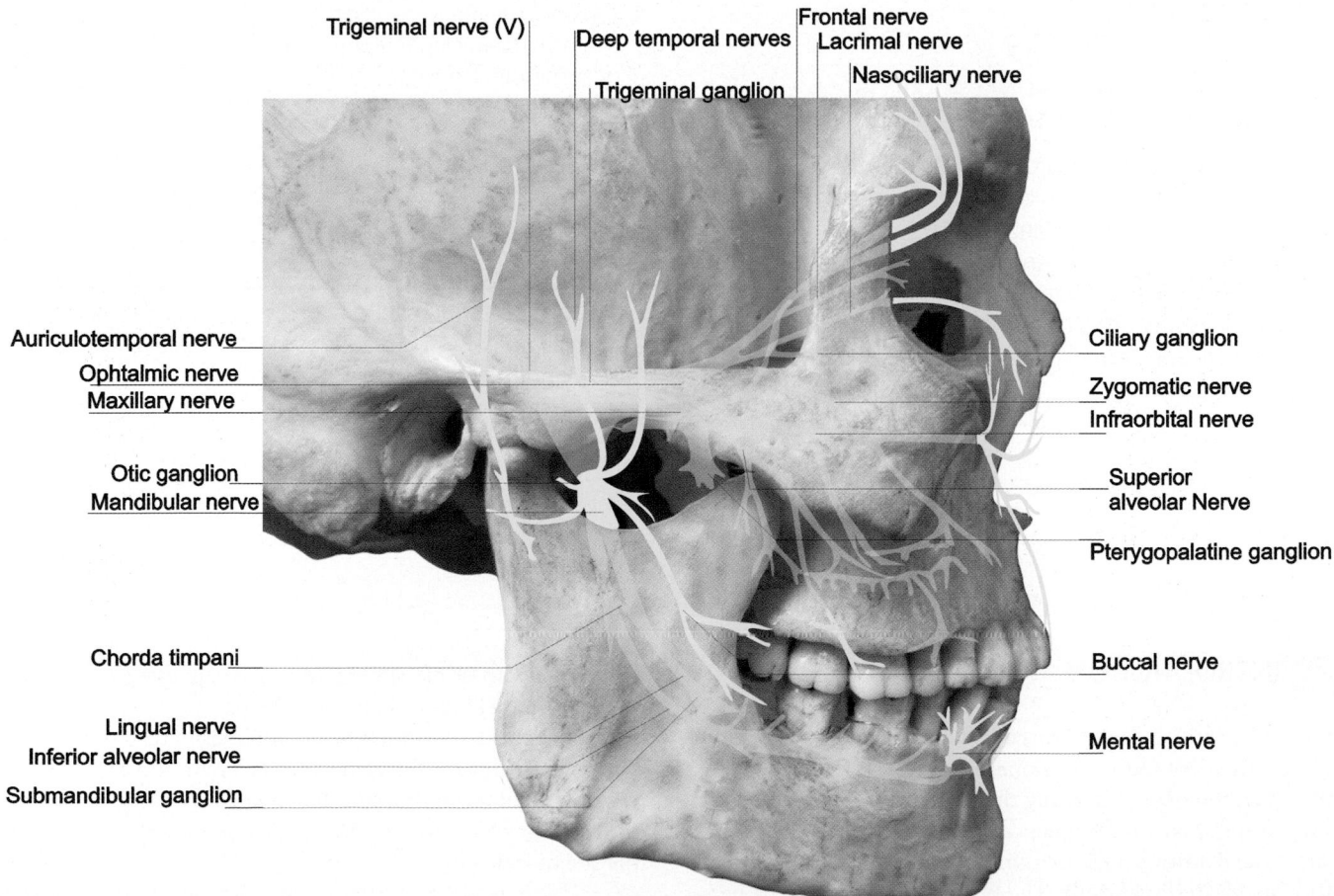

Figure 20–1. Anatomy of the trigeminal nerve The sensory root of the trigeminal nerve gives rise to the ophthalmic division (V_1), maxillary division (V_2), and the mandibular division (V_3) from the trigeminal ganglion.

pterygoid, and lateral pterygoid), mylohyoid, anterior belly of the digastric, tensor veli palatini and tensor tympani muscles.

Ophthalmic Division

The smallest of the three divisions, the ophthalmic division (V_1) is purely sensory and travels anteriorly in the lateral wall of the cavernous sinus in the middle cranial fossa to the medial part of the superior orbital fissure. Before its entrance into the orbit through the superior orbital fissure, the ophthalmic nerve divides into three branches: frontal, nasociliary, and lacrimal.

The **frontal nerve** is the largest branch of the ophthalmic division and travels anteriorly in the orbit, terminating as the supratrochlear and supraorbital nerves. The supratrochlear nerve lies medial to the supraorbital nerve and supplies the skin and conjunctiva of the medial portion of the upper eyelid and skin over the lower forehead close to the midline. The supraorbital nerve supplies the skin and conjunctiva of the central portion of the upper eyelid, the skin of the forehead, and the scalp as far back as the parietal bone and lambdoid suture.

The **nasociliary branch** travels along the medial aspect of the orbital roof, giving off various branches. The nasal cavity and the skin at the apex and ala of the nose are innervated by the anterior ethmoid and external nasal nerves. The mucous membrane of the anterior portion of the nasal septum and lateral wall of the nasal cavity are innervated by the internal nasal nerve. The skin of the lacrimal sac, lacrimal caruncle, and adjoining portion of the side of the nose are innervated by the infratrochlear branch. The ethmoid and sphenoid sinuses are supplied by the posterior ethmoidal nerve. The eyeball is innervated by the short and long ciliary nerves.

The **lacrimal nerve** supplies the skin and conjunctiva of the lateral portion of the upper eyelid and is the smallest branch of the ophthalmic division.

Maxillary Division

The maxillary division (V_2) of the trigeminal nerve is also a purely sensory division. Arising from the trigeminal ganglion in the middle cranial fossa, the maxillary nerve travels forward along the lateral wall of the cavernous sinus. Shortly after stemming from the trigeminal ganglion, the maxillary nerve gives off the only branch within the cranium; the middle meningeal nerve. It then leaves the cranium through the foramen rotundum, located in the greater wing of the sphenoid bone. After exiting the foramen rotundum, the nerve enters a space located behind and below the orbital cavity known as the pterygopalatine fossa. After giving off several branches within the fossa, the nerve enters the orbit through the inferior orbital fissure, at which point it becomes the infraorbital nerve. Coursing along the floor of the orbit in the infraorbital groove, the nerve enters the infraorbital canal and emerges onto the face through the infraorbital foramen.

The **middle meningeal nerve** is the only branch of the maxillary division within the cranium and provides sensory innervation to the dura mater in the middle cranial fossa.

Within the pterygopalatine fossa, several branches are given off, including the pterygopalatine, zygomatic, and posterior superior alveolar nerves. The **pterygopalatine nerves** are two short nerves that merge within the pterygopalatine ganglion and then give rise to several branches. They contain postganglionic parasympathetic fibers, which pass along the zygomatic nerve to the lacrimal nerve innervating the lacrimal gland, as well as sensory fibers to the orbit, nose, palate, and pharynx. The sensory fibers to the orbit innervate the orbital periosteum.

The posterior aspect of the nasal septum, mucous membrane of the superior and middle conchae, and the posterior ethmoid sinus are innervated by the nasal branches. The anterior nasal septum, floor of the nose, and premaxilla from canine to canine is innervated by a branch known as the nasopalatine nerve. The **nasopalatine nerve** courses downward and forward from the roof of the nasal cavity to the floor to enter the incisive canal. It then enters the oral cavity through the incisive foramen to supply the palatal mucosa of the premaxilla.

The hard and soft palate is innervated by the palatine branches: the greater (anterior) and lesser (middle and posterior) palatine nerves. After descending through the pterygopalatine canal, the greater palatine nerve exits the greater palatine foramen onto the hard palate. The nerve provides sensory innervation to the palatal mucosa and bone of the hard and soft palate. The lesser palatine nerves emerge from the lesser palatine foramen to innervate the soft palate and tonsillar region.

The pharyngeal branch leaves the pterygopalatine ganglion from its posterior aspect to innervate the nasopharynx.

The **zygomatic nerve** gives rise to two branches after passing anteriorly from the pterygopalatine fossa to the orbit. The nerve passes through the inferior orbital fissure and divides into the zygomaticofacial and zygomaticotemporal nerves supplying the skin over the malar prominence and skin over the side of the forehead, respectively. The zygomatic nerve also communicates with the ophthalmic division via the lacrimal nerve sending fibers to the lacrimal gland.

The **posterior superior alveolar (PSA) nerve** branches off within the pterygopalatine fossa before the maxillary nerve enters the orbit. The PSA travels downward along the posterior aspect of the maxilla to supply the maxillary molar dentition, including the periodontal ligament and pulpal tissues as well as the adjacent gingiva and alveolar process. The mucous membrane of the maxillary sinus is also innervated by the PSA. It is of clinical significance to note that the PSA does not always innervate the mesiobuccal root of the first molar.[1,2] Several dissection studies have been performed tracing the innervation of the first molar back to the parent trunk. These studies have demonstrated the variations in innervation patterns of the first molar and this is of clinical significance when anesthesia of this tooth is desired.

In a study by Loetscher and Walton,[3] 29 human maxillae were dissected to observe innervation patterns of the first molar. The study evaluated the innervation patterns by the

Table 20–1.

Branches of Three Major Divisions

Ophthalmic Division	Maxillary Division	Mandibular Division
1. Frontal • Supratrochlear • Supraorbital 2. Nasociliary • Anterior ethmoid • External nasal • Internal nasal • Infratrochlear • Posterior ethmoid • Short and long ciliary 3. Lacrimal	1. Middle meningeal 2. Pterygopalatine nerves • Sensory fibers to the orbit • Nasal branches • Nasopalatine nerve • Greater palatine nerve • Lesser palatine nerve • Pharyngeal branch 3. Zygomatic • Zygomaticofacial • Zygomaticotemporal 4. Posterior superior alveolar nerve block 5. Infraorbital • Middle superior alveolar • Anterior superior alveolar • Inferior palpebral • Lateral nasal • Superior labial	1. Main trunk • Nervous spinosus • Nerve to the pterygoid 2. Anterior division • Masseteric • Deep temporal • Lateral pterygoid • Buccal nerve 3. Posterior division • Auriculotemporal • Lingual • Inferior alveolar • Nerve to the mylohyoid

posterior, middle, and anterior superior alveolar nerves on the first molar. The posterior and anterior superior alveolar nerves were found to be present in 100% (29/29) of specimens. The middle superior alveolar (MSA) nerve was found to be present 72% of the time (21/29 specimens). Nerves were traced from the first molar to the parent branches in 18 of the specimens. The PSA nerve was found to provide innervation in 72% (13/18) of specimens. The MSA nerve provided innervation in 28% (5/18) specimens, whereas the anterior superior alveolar nerve did not provide innervation to the first molar in any of the specimens. In the absence of the MSA nerve, the PSA nerve may provide innervation to the premolar region. In a study by McDaniel,[4] 50 maxillae were decalcified and dissected to demonstrate the innervation patterns of maxillary teeth. The PSA was found to innervate the premolar region in 26% of dissections, when the MSA was not present. Table 20–1 lists the branches of the ophthalmic, maxillary, and mandibular divisions.

Within the infraorbital canal, the maxillary division is known as the **infraorbital nerve** and gives off the middle and anterior superior alveolar nerves. When present, the MSA nerve descends along the lateral wall of the maxillary sinus to innervate the first and second premolar teeth. It provides sensation to the periodontal ligament, pulpal tissues, gingival, and alveolar process of the premolar region as well as the mesiobuccal root of the first molar in some cases.[1,2] In a study by Heasman,[5] dissections of 19 human cadaver heads were performed and the MSA was found to be present in seven of the specimens. Loetscher and Walton[3] found that the mesial or distal position at which the MSA nerve joins the dental plexus (an anastomosis of the posterior, middle,

and anterior superior alveolar nerves described below) determines its contribution to the innervation of the first molar. Specimens in which the MSA joined the plexus mesial to the first molar were found to have innervation of the first molar by the PSA and the premolars by the MSA. Specimens in which the MSA joined the plexus distal to the first molar demonstrated innervation of the first molar by the MSA. In its absence, the premolar region derives its innervation from the PSA and anterior superior alveolar nerves.[4] The anterior superior alveolar nerve descends within the anterior wall of the maxillary sinus. A small terminal branch of the anterior superior alveolar communicates with the MSA to supply a small area of the lateral wall and floor of the nose. It also provides sensory innervation to the periodontal ligament, pulpal tissue, gingiva, and alveolar process of the central and lateral incisor and canine teeth. In the absence of the MSA, the anterior superior alveolar has been shown to provide innervation to the premolar teeth. In the previously mentioned study by McDaniel, the anterior superior alveolar was shown to provide innervation to the premolar region in 36% of specimens in which no MSA nerve was found.[4]

The three superior alveolar nerves anastomose to form a network known as the dental plexus, which comprises terminal branches coming off the larger nerve trunks. These terminal branches are known as the dental, interdental, and interradicular nerves. The dental nerves innervate each root of each individual tooth in the maxilla by entering the root through the apical foramen and supplying sensation to the pulp. Interdental and interradicular branches provide sensation to the periodontal ligaments, interdental papillae, and buccal gingiva of adjacent teeth.

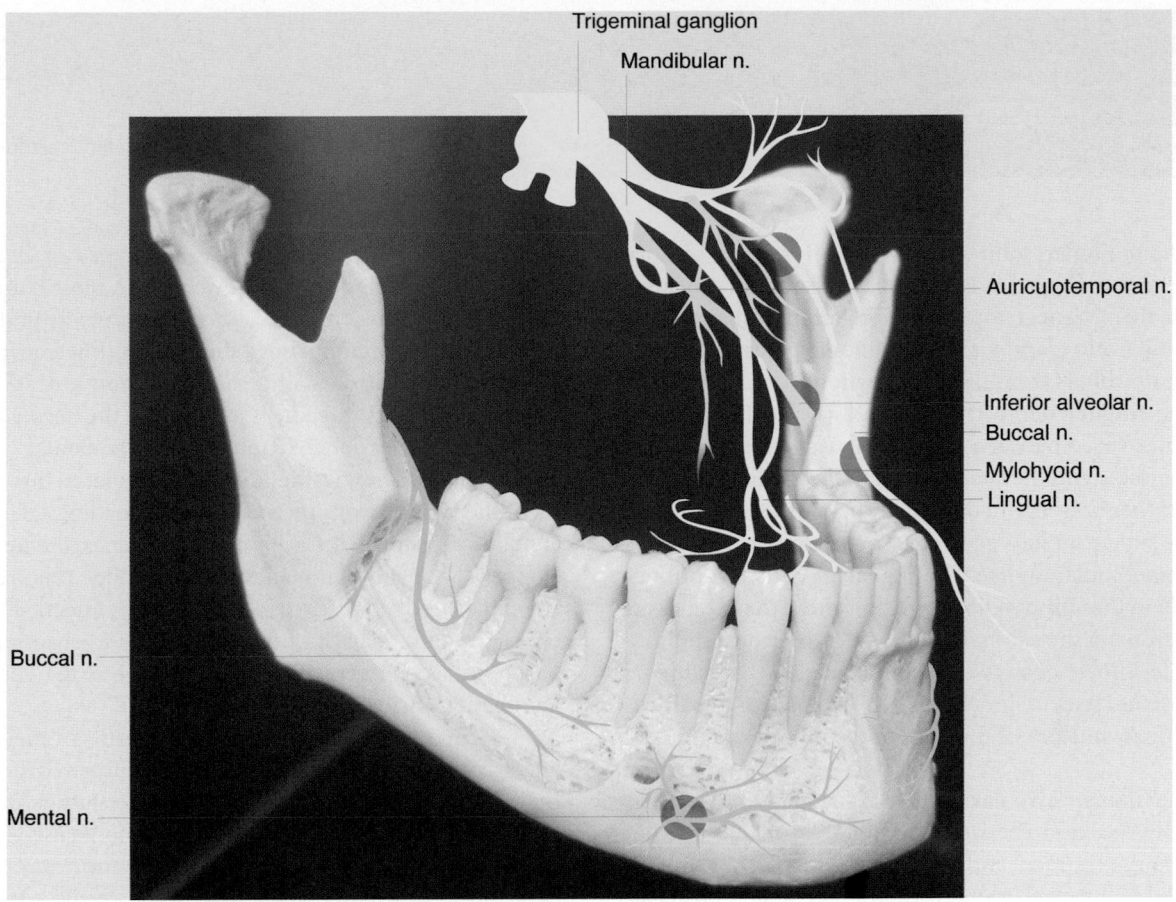

Figure 20–2. Anatomy of the mandibular nerve.

The infraorbital nerve divides into three terminal branches after emerging through the infraorbital foramen onto the face. The inferior palpebral, external nasal, and superior labial nerves supply sensory innervation to the skin of the lower eyelid, lateral aspect of the nose, and skin and mucous membranes of the upper lip, respectively.

Mandibular Division

The largest branch of the trigeminal nerve, the mandibular branch (V_3), is both sensory and motor (Figure 20–2). The sensory root arises from the trigeminal ganglion, whereas the motor root arises from the motor nucleus of the pons and medulla oblongata. The sensory root passes through the foramen ovale almost immediately after coming off the trigeminal ganglion. The motor root passes underneath the ganglion and through the foramen ovale to unite with the sensory root just outside the cranium, forming the main trunk of the mandibular nerve. The nerve then divides into anterior and posterior divisions. The mandibular nerve gives off branches from its main trunk as well as from the anterior and posterior divisions.

The main trunk gives off two branches known as the **nervus spinosus** (meningeal branch) and the **nerve to the medial pterygoid**. After branching off the main trunk, the nervus spinosus reenters the cranium along with the mid-

dle meningeal artery through the foramen spinosum. The nervus spinosus supplies the meninges of the middle cranial fossa as well as the mastoid air cells. The nerve to the medial pterygoid is a small motor branch that supplies the medial (internal) pterygoid muscle. It gives off two branches that supply the tensor tympani and tensor veli palatini muscles.

Three motor and one sensory branch are given off by the anterior division of the mandibular nerve. The **masseteric, deep temporal, and lateral pterygoid nerves** supply the masseter, temporalis, and lateral (external) pterygoid muscles, respectively. The sensory division known as the **buccal (buccinator or long buccal) nerve**, runs forward between the two heads of the lateral pterygoid muscle, along the inferior aspect of the temporalis muscle to the anterior border of the masseter muscle. Here, it passes anterolaterally to enter the buccinator muscle; however, *it does not innervate this muscle.* The buccinator muscle is innervated by the buccal branch of the facial nerve. The buccal nerve provides sensory innervation to the skin of the cheek, buccal mucosa, and buccal gingiva in the mandibular molar region.

The posterior division of the mandibular branch gives off two sensory branches (the auriculotemporal and lingual nerves) and one branch made up of both sensory and motor fibers (the inferior alveolar nerve).

The **auriculotemporal nerve** crosses the superior portion of the parotid gland, ascending behind the

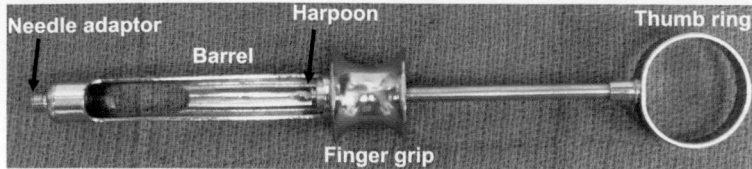

Figure 20-3. Breech-loading, metallic, cartridge-type, aspirating syringe.

temporomandibular joint and giving off several sensory branches to the skin of the auricle, external auditory meatus, tympanic membrane, temporal region, temporomandibular joint, and parotid gland via postganglionic parasympathetic secretomotor fibers from the otic ganglion.

The **lingual nerve** travels inferiorly in the pterygomandibular space between the medial aspect of the ramus of the mandible and the lateral aspect of the medial pterygoid muscle. It then travels anteromedially below the inferior border of the superior pharyngeal constrictor muscle deep to the pterygomandibular raphae. The lingual nerve then continues anteriorly in the submandibular region along the hyoglossus muscle, crossing the submandibular duct inferiorly and medially to terminate deep to the sublingual gland. The lingual nerve provides sensory innervation to the anterior two thirds of the tongue, mucosa of the floor of the mouth, and lingual gingiva.

The **inferior alveolar branch** of the mandibular nerve descends in the region between the lateral aspect of the sphenomandibular ligament and the medial aspect of the ramus of the mandible. It travels along with, but lateral and posterior to, the lingual nerve. While the lingual nerve continues to descend within the pterygomandibular space, the inferior alveolar nerve enters the mandibular canal through the mandibular foramen. Just before entering the mandibular canal, the inferior alveolar nerve gives off a motor branch known as the mylohyoid nerve (discussed below). The nerve accompanies the inferior alveolar artery and vein within the mandibular canal and divides into the mental and incisive nerve branches at the mental foramen. The inferior alveolar nerve provides sensation to the mandibular posterior teeth.

The **incisive nerve** is a branch of the inferior alveolar nerve that continues within the mandibular canal to provide sensory innervation to the mandibular anterior teeth.

The **mental nerve** emerges from the mental foramen to provide sensory innervation to the mucosa in the premolar/canine region as well as to the skin of the chin and lower lip.

The **mylohyoid nerve** branches off the inferior alveolar nerve before its entry into the mandibular canal. It travels within the mylohyoid groove and along the medial aspect of the body of the mandible to supply the mylohyoid muscle as well as the anterior belly of the digastric.[1,2]

EQUIPMENT FOR REGIONAL MAXILLARY & MANDIBULAR ANESTHESIA

Administration of regional anesthesia of the maxilla and mandible is achieved via the use of a dental syringe, nee-

dle, and anesthetic cartridge. Several types of dental syringes are available for use. However, the most common is the breech-loading, metallic, cartridge-type, aspirating syringe. The syringe comprises a thumb ring, finger grip, barrel containing the piston with a harpoon, and a needle adaptor (Figure 20-3). A needle is attached to the needle adaptor that engages the rubber diaphragm of the dental cartridge (Figure 20-4). The anesthetic cartridge is placed into the barrel of the syringe from the side (breech-loading). The barrel contains a piston with a harpoon that engages the rubber stopper at the end of the anesthetic cartridge (Figure 20-5). After the needle and cartridge have been attached, a brisk tap is given to the back of the thumb ring to ensure that the harpoon has engaged the rubber stopper at the end of the anesthetic cartridge (Figure 20-6).

Dental needles are referred to in terms of their gauge, which corresponds to the diameter of the lumen of the needle. Increasing gauge corresponds to a smaller lumen diameter. Needles of 25 and 25 gauge are most commonly used for maxillary and mandibular regional anesthesia and are available in long and short lengths. The length of the needle is measured from the tip of the needle to the hub. The conventional long needle is approximately 40 mm in length, whereas the short needle is approximately 25 mm. Variations in needle length do exist, depending on the manufacturer.

Anesthetic cartridges are prefilled, 1.8-mL glass cylinders with a rubber stopper at one end and an aluminum cap with a diaphragm at the other end (Figure 20-7). The contents of an anesthetic cartridge are the local anesthetic, vasoconstrictor (anesthetic without vasoconstrictor is also

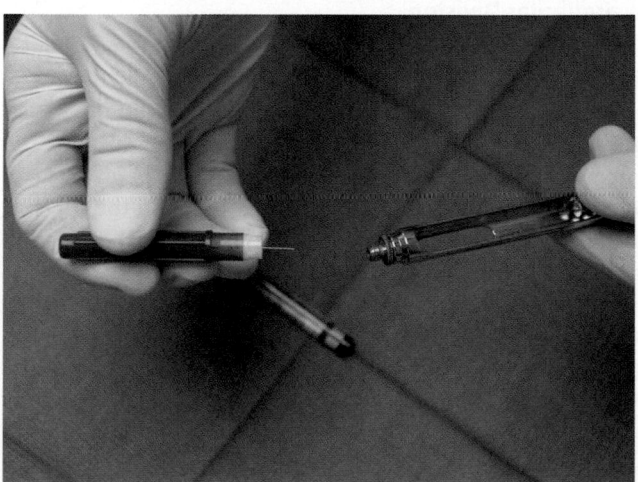

Figure 20-4. Needle-syringe assembling. A needle is attached to the needle adaptor.

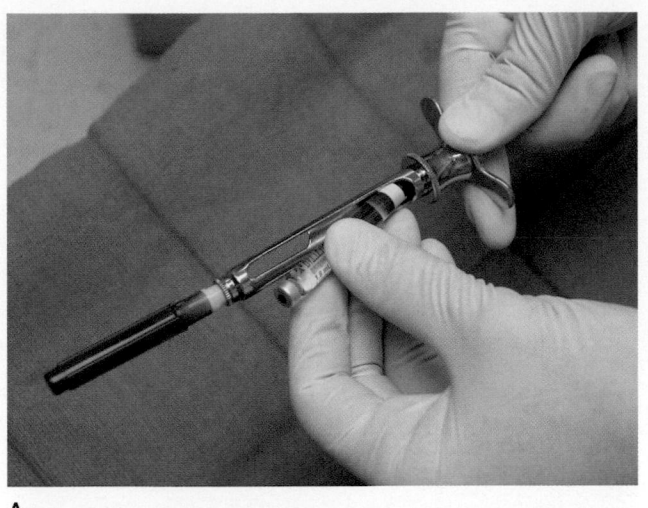

A

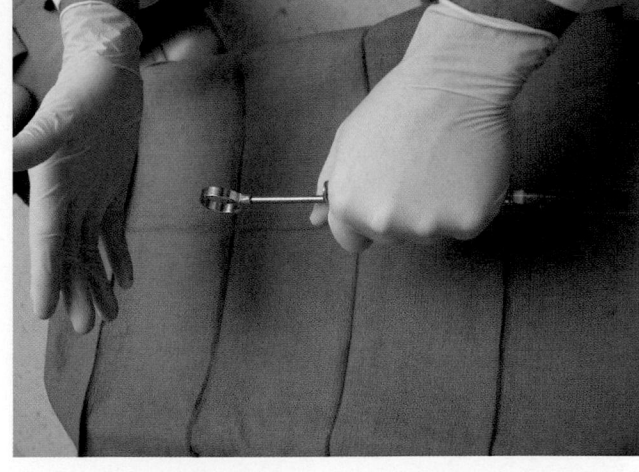

A

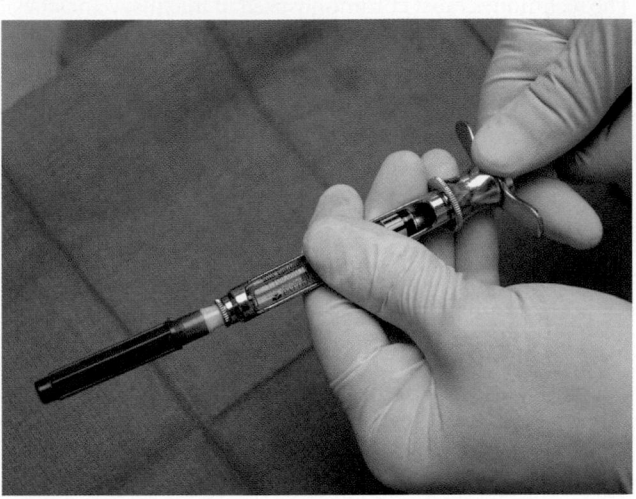

B

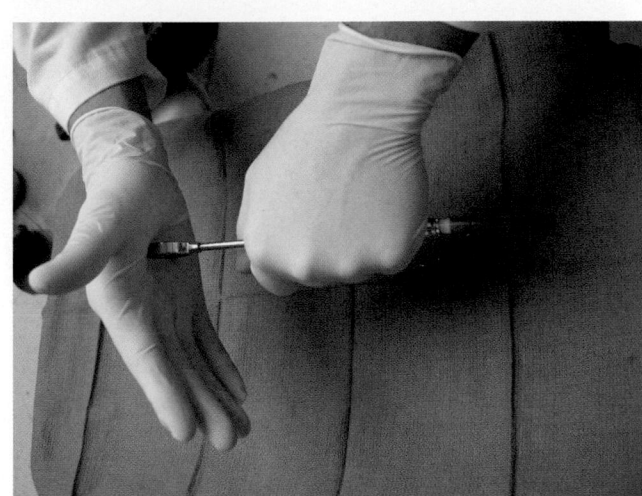

B

Figure 20–5. A: Needle–syringe assembling. The anesthetic cartridge is placed into the barrel of the syringe from the side (breech loading). **B:** A piston with a harpoon engages the rubber stopper at the end of the anesthetic cartridge while the needle adaptor engages the rubber diaphragm of the dental cartridge.

available), preservative for the vasoconstrictor (sodium bisulfite), sodium chloride, and distilled water. The most common anesthetics used in clinical practice are the amide anesthetics, lidocaine and mepivacaine. Other amide anesthetics available for use are prilocaine, articaine, bupivacaine, and etidocaine. Esther anesthetics are not as commonly used, but remain available. Procaine, procaine plus propoxycaine, chloroprocaine, and tetracaine are some common esther anesthetics.

Additional armamentaria include dry gauze, topical antiseptic, and anesthetic. The site of injection should be made dry with gauze, and a topical antiseptic should be used to clean the area. Topical anesthetic is applied to the area of injection to minimize discomfort during insertion of the needle into the mucous membrane (Figure 20–8). Common topical preparations include benzocaine, butacaine sulfate, cocaine hydrochloride, dyclonine hydrochloride, lidocaine, and tetracaine hydrochloride.

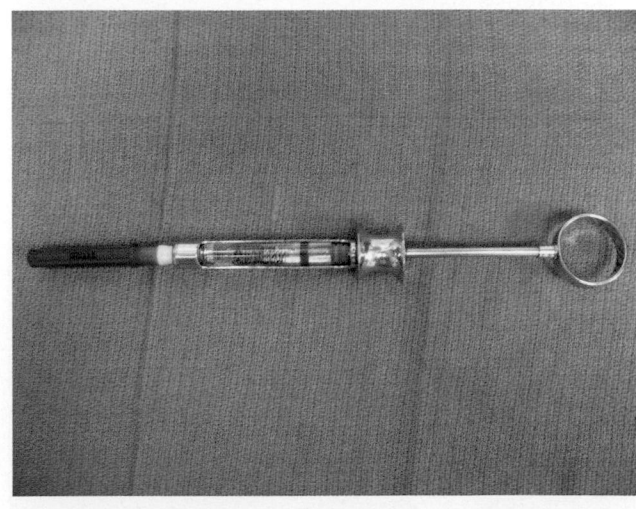

C

Figure 20–6. A and **B:** Needle–syringe assembling: A brisk tap is given to the back of the thumb ring to ensure that the harpoon has engaged the rubber stopper at the end of the anesthetic cartridge. **C:** A fully loaded anesthetic syringe.

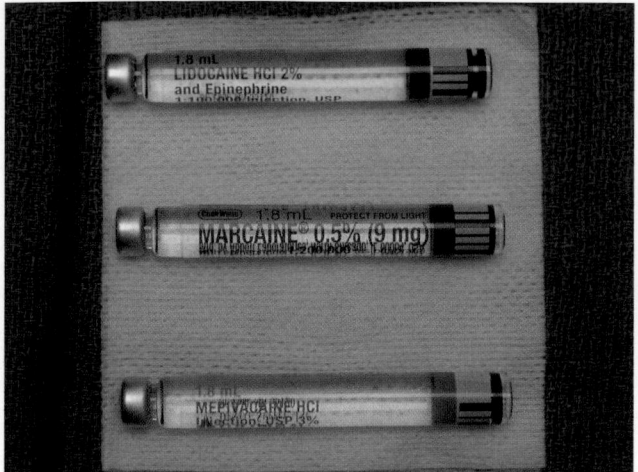

A

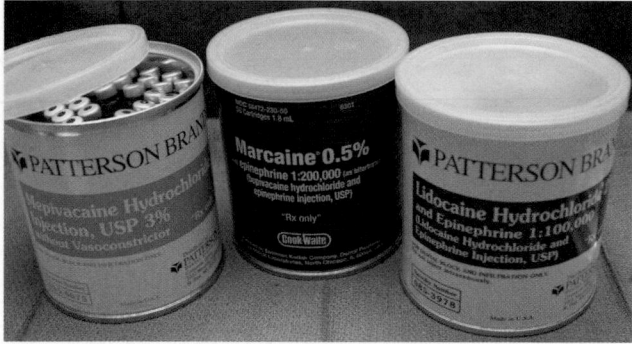

B

Figure 20–7. A: Dental cartridges. The rubber stopper is on the right end of the cartridge while the aluminum cap with the diaphragm is on the left end of the cartridge. **B:** Containers of dental anesthetic.

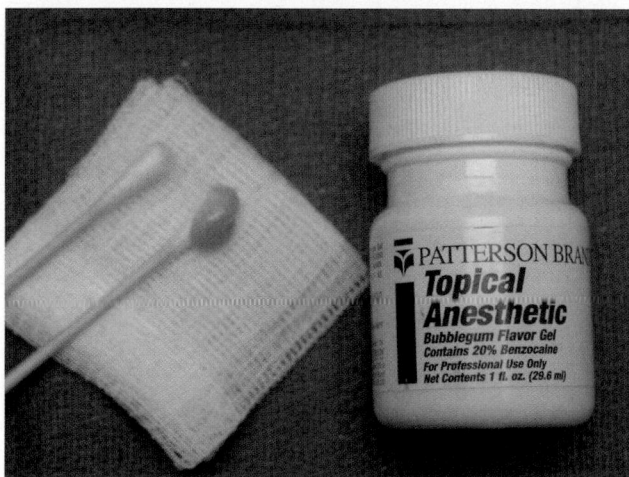

Figure 20–8. Topical anesthesia. Before injection, topical anesthetic can be applied on the mucosa in the area of an injection to minimize discomfort to the patient.

Universal precautions should always be observed by the clinician; these include the use of protective gloves, mask, and eye protection. After withdrawing the needle when a block has been completed, the needle should always be carefully recapped to avoid accidental needle stick injury to the operator.[1]

Retraction of the soft tissue for visualization of the injection site should be performed with the use of a dental mirror or retraction instrument. This is recommended for all maxillary and mandibular regional techniques discussed below. Use of an instrument rather than one's fingers helps to prevent accidental needle-stick injury to the operator.

TECHNIQUES OF REGIONAL MAXILLARY ANESTHESIA

The techniques most commonly used in maxillary anesthesia include supraperiosteal (local) infiltration, periodontal ligament (intraligamentary) injection, PSA (posterior superior alveolar) nerve block, MSA (middle superior alveolar) nerve block, anterior superior alveolar nerve block, greater palatine nerve block, nasopalatine nerve block, local infiltration of the palate, and intrapulpal injection (Table 20–2). Of less clinical application are the maxillary nerve block and intraseptal injection.

Supraperiosteal (Local) Infiltration

The supraperiosteal or local infiltration is one of the simplest and most commonly used techniques for achieving anesthesia of the maxillary dentition. This technique is indicated when any individual tooth or soft tissue in a localized area is to be treated. Contraindications to this technique are the need to anesthetize multiple teeth adjacent to one another (in which case a nerve block is the preferred technique), acute inflammation and infection in the area to be anesthetized, and, less significantly, the density of bone overlying the apices of the teeth. A 25- or 27-gauge short needle is preferred for this technique.

Table 20–2.

Techniques of Anesthesia for Treatment of a Localized Area or One or Two Teeth

Technique	Area Anesthetized
Supraperiosteal injection	Individual teeth and buccal soft tissue
Periodontal ligament injection	Individual teeth and buccal soft tissue
Intraseptal injection	Localized soft tissue
Intrapulpal injection	Individual tooth

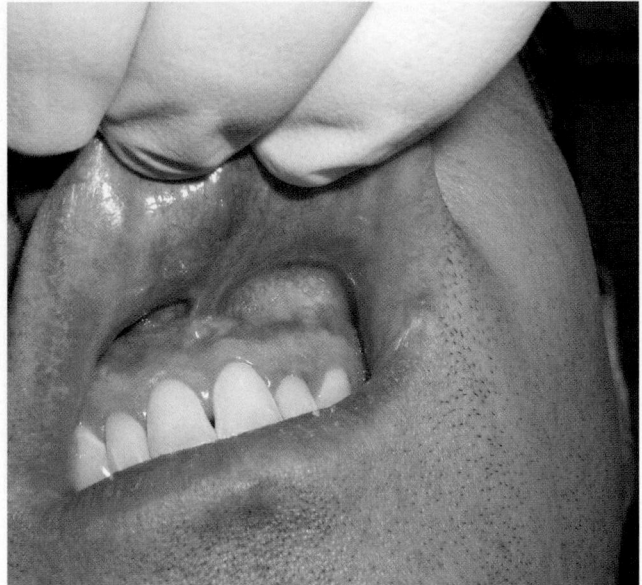

A

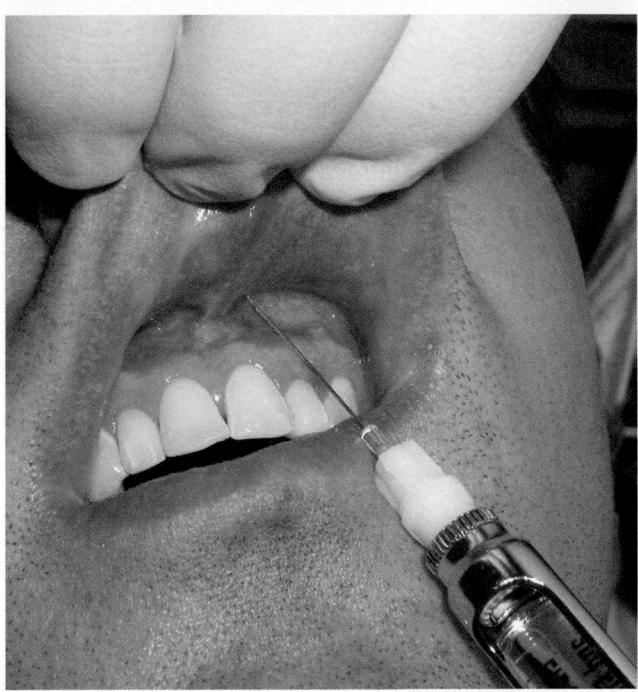

B

Figure 20–9. A: Locate the height of the mucobuccal fold over the tooth to be anesthetized. **B:** Clinical picture depicting a local infiltration of the maxillary left central incisor tooth. Note the penetration of the needle at the height of the mucobuccal fold above the maxillary left central incisor.

Procedure. Identify the tooth to be anesthetized and the height of the mucobuccal fold over the tooth. This will be the injection site. The right-handed operator should stand at the 9 o'clock to 10 o'clock position, whereas the left-handed operator should stand at the 2 o'clock to 3 o'clock position. Retract the lip and orient the syringe with the bevel toward bone. This prevents discomfort from the needle coming into

contact with the bone and minimizes the risk of tearing the periosteum with the needle tip. Insert the needle at the height of the mucobuccal fold above the tooth to a depth of no more than a few millimeters and aspirate (Figure 20–9). If aspiration is negative, slowly inject one third to one half (0.6–1.2 mL) of a cartridge of anesthetic solution, over the course of 30 seconds. Withdraw the syringe and recap the needle. Successful administration provides anesthesia to the tooth and associated soft tissue within 2–four minutes. If adequate anesthesia has not been achieved, repeat the procedure and deposit another one third to one half of the cartridge of anesthetic solution.[1]

Periodontal Ligament (Intraligamentary Injection)

The periodontal ligament or intraligamentary injection is a useful adjunct to the supraperiosteal injection or a nerve block. Often, it is used to supplement these techniques to achieve profound anesthesia of the area to be treated. Indications for the use of the intraligamentary injection technique are the need to anesthetize an individual tooth or teeth, need for soft tissue anesthesia in the immediate vicinity of a tooth, and partial anesthesia after a field block or nerve block. A 25- or 27-gauge short needle is preferred for this technique.

Procedure. Identify the tooth or area of soft tissue to be anesthetized. The sulcus between the gingiva and the tooth is the injection site for the periodontal ligament injection. Position the patient in the supine position. For the right-handed operator, retract the lip with a retraction instrument held in the left hand and stand where the tooth and gingiva are clearly visible. The same applies for the left-handed operator except that the retraction instrument is held in the right hand. Hold the syringe parallel with the long axis of the tooth on the mesial or distal aspect. Insert the needle (bevel facing the root) to the depth of the gingival sulcus (Figure 20–10). Advance the

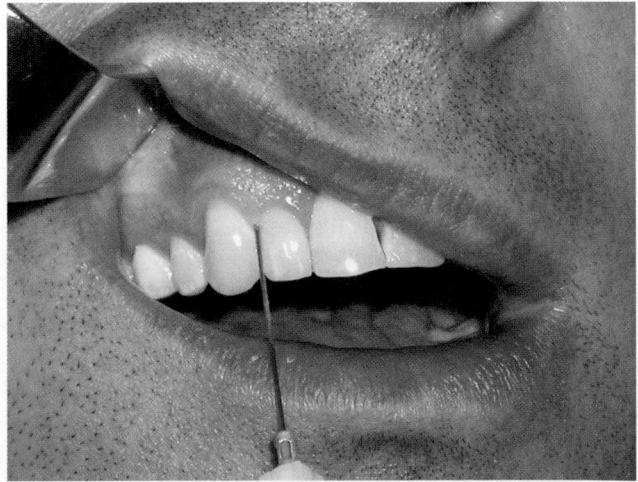

Figure 20–10. Clinical picture depicting a periodontal ligament injection. Note the position of the needle between the gingival sulcus and tooth with the needle parallel with the long axis of the tooth.

needle until resistance is met. A small amount of anesthetic (0.2 mL) is then administered slowly over the course of 20–30 seconds. It is normal to experience resistance to the flow of anesthetic. Successful execution of this technique provides pulpal and soft tissue anesthesia to the individual tooth or teeth to be treated.[1]

Posterior Superior Alveolar Nerve Block

The PSA nerve block, otherwise known as the tuberosity block or the zygomatic block, is used to achieve anesthesia of the maxillary molar teeth up to the first molar with the exception of its mesiobuccal root in some cases. A possible complication of this technique is the risk of hematoma formation from injection of anesthetic into the pterygoid plexus of veins or from accidental puncture of the maxillary artery. Aspiration before injection is indicated when the PSA block is given. The indications for this technique are the need to anesthetize multiple molar teeth. Anesthesia can be achieved with fewer needle penetrations, providing greater comfort to the patient than with the supraperiosteal technique. The PSA can be given to provide anesthesia of the maxillary molars when acute inflammation and infection are present. If inadequate anesthesia is achieved via the supraperiosteal technique, the PSA can be used to achieve more profound anesthesia of a longer duration. The PSA block also provides anesthesia to the premolar region in a certain percentage of patients in whom the MSA is absent.

Contraindications to the procedure are related to the risk of hematoma formation. In individuals with coagulation disorders, care must be taken to avoid injection into the pterygoid plexus or puncture of the maxillary artery. A short 25- or 27-gauge needle is preferred for this technique.

Procedure. Identify the height of the mucobuccal fold over the second molar. This is the injection site. The right-handed operator should stand at the 9 o'clock to 10 o'clock position, whereas the left-handed operator should stand at the 2 o'clock to 3 o'clock position. Retract the lip with a retraction instrument. Hold the syringe with the bevel toward the bone. Insert the needle at the height of the mucobuccal fold above the maxillary second molar at a 45-degree angle directed superiorly, medially, and posteriorly (one continuous movement). Advance the needle to a depth of three fourths of its total length (Figure 20–11). No resistance should be felt while advancing the needle through the soft tissue. If bone is contacted, the medial angulation is too great. Slowly retract the needle (without removing it) and bring the syringe barrel toward the occlusal plane. This allows the needle to be angulated slightly more lateral to the posterior aspect of the maxilla. Advance the needle, aspirate, and inject one cartridge of anesthetic solution slowly over the course of 1 minute, aspirating frequently during the administration. Before injecting, one should aspirate in two planes to avoid accidental injection into the pterygoid plexus. After the first aspiration, the needle should be rotated 1/4 turn. The operator should then re-aspirate. If positive aspiration occurs, slowly retract the needle 12 mL and re-aspirate in two planes. Successful injection technique results in anesthesia of the maxillary molars

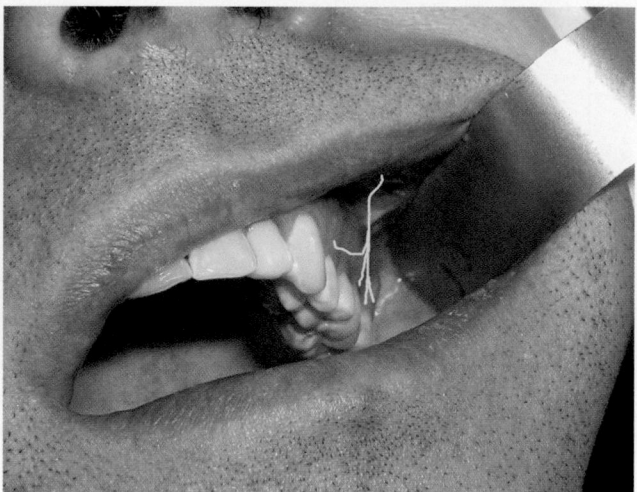

A

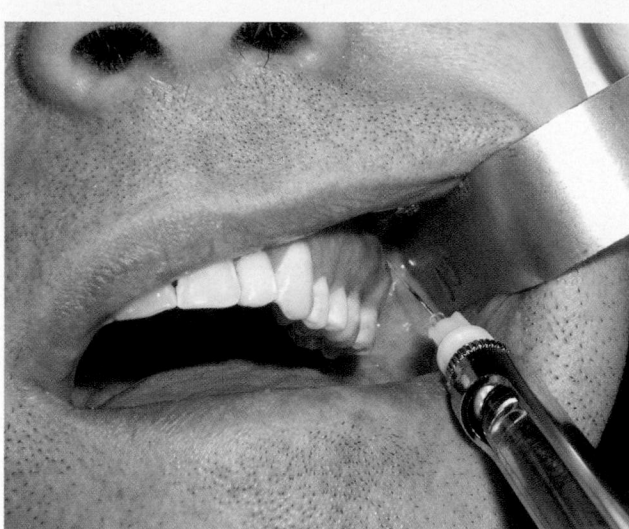

B

Figure 20–11. A: Location of the posterior superior alveolar (PSA) nerve. **B:** Position of the needle during the PSA nerve block. The needle is inserted at the height of the mucobuccal fold above the maxillary second molar at a 45-degree angle aimed superiorly, medially, and posteriorly.

(with the exception of the mesiobuccal root of the first molar in some cases) and associated soft tissue on the buccal aspect.[1]

Middle Superior Alveolar Nerve Block

The MSA nerve block is useful for procedures in which the maxillary premolar teeth or the mesiobuccal root of the first molar requires anesthesia. Although not always present, it is useful if the posterior or anterior superior alveolar nerve blocks or supraperiosteal infiltration fails to achieve adequate anesthesia. Individuals in whom the MSA nerve is absent, the PSA and anterior superior alveolar nerves provide innervation to the maxillary premolar teeth and the mesiobuccal root of the first molar.

Contraindications include acute inflammation and infection in the area of injection or a procedure involving one

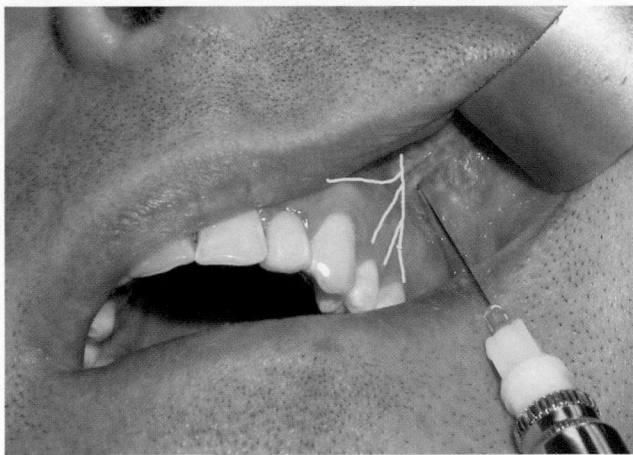

A

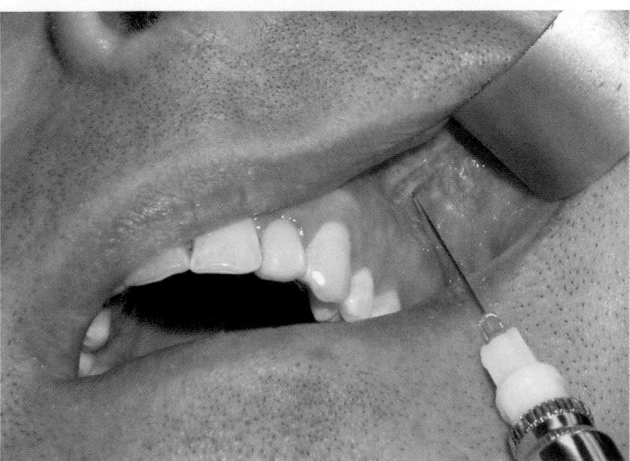

B

Figure 20–12. A: Location of the middle superior alveolar nerve. **B:** The needle is inserted at the height of the mucobuccal fold above the maxillary second premolar.

tooth in which local infiltration will be sufficient. A 25- or 27-gauge short needle is preferred for this technique.

Procedure. Identify the height of the mucobuccal fold above the maxillary second premolar. This is the injection site. The right-handed operator should stand at the 9 o'clock to 10 o'clock position, whereas the left-handed operator should stand at the 2 o'clock to 3 o'clock position. Retract the lip with a retraction instrument, and insert the needle until the tip is above the apex of the second premolar tooth (Figure 20–12). Aspirate and inject two thirds to one cartridge of anesthetic solution slowly over the course of 1 minute. Successful execution of this technique provides anesthesia to the pulp, surrounding soft tissue, and bone of the first and second premolar teeth and the mesiobuccal root of the first molar.[1]

Anterior Superior Alveolar Nerve Block/ Infraorbital Nerve Block

The anterior superior alveolar nerve block or infraorbital nerve block is a useful technique for achieving anesthesia of the maxillary central and lateral incisors and canine as well as

the surrounding soft tissue on the buccal aspect. In patients who do not have an MSA nerve, the anterior superior alveolar nerve may also innervate the premolar teeth and mesiobuccal root of the first molar. Indications for the use of this technique include procedures involving multiple teeth and inadequate anesthesia from the supraperiosteal technique. A 25-gauge long needle is preferred for this technique.

Procedure. Place the patient in the supine position. Identify the height of the mucobuccal fold above the maxillary first premolar. This is the injection site. The right-handed operator should stand at the 10 o'clock position, whereas the left-handed operator should stand at the 2 o'clock position. Identify the infraorbital notch on the inferior orbital rim (Figure 20–13A). The infraorbital foramen lies just inferior to the notch usually in line with the second premolar. Slight discomfort is felt by the patient when digital pressure is placed on the foramen. It is helpful but not necessary to mark the position

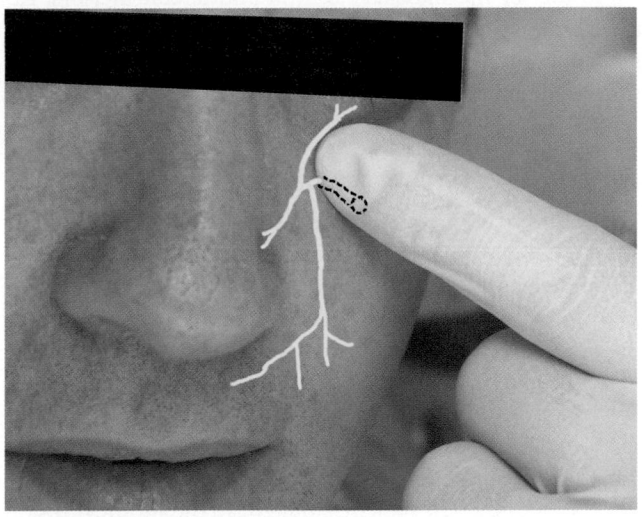

A

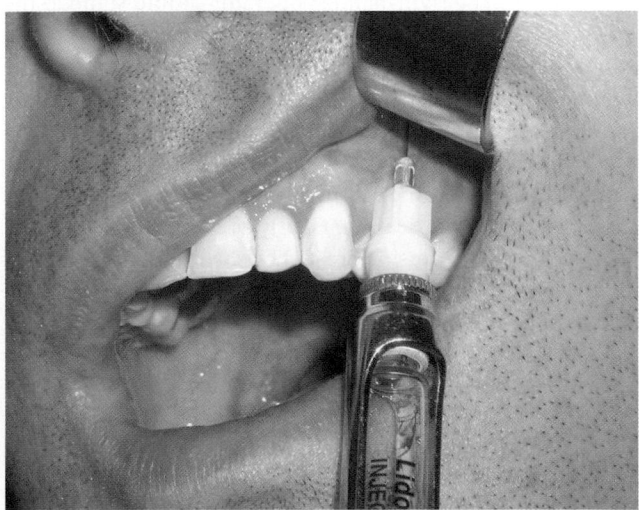

B

Figure 20–13. A: Location of the infraorbital nerve. **B:** The needle is kept parallel with the long axis of the maxillary first premolar and inserted at the height of the mucobuccal fold above the first premolar.

of the infraorbital foramen. Retract the lip with a retraction instrument while noting the location of the foramen. Orient the bevel of the needle toward bone and insert the needle at the height of the mucobuccal fold above the first premolar (Figure 20–13*B*).

The syringe should be angled toward the infraorbital foramen and kept parallel with the long axis of the first premolar to avoid hitting the maxillary bone prematurely. The needle is advanced into the soft tissue until the bone over the roof of the foramen is contacted. This is approximately half the length of the needle; however, this varies from individual to individual. After aspiration, approximately one half to two thirds (0.9–1.2 mL) of the anesthetic cartridge is deposited slowly over the course of 1 minute. It is recommended that pressure be kept over the site of injection to facilitate the diffusion of anesthetic solution into the foramen. Successful execution of this technique results in aesthesia of the lower eyelid, the lateral aspect of the nose, and the upper lip. Pulpal anesthesia of the maxillary central and lateral incisors, canine, buccal soft tissue, and bone is also achieved. In a certain percentage of people, the premolar teeth and the mesiobuccal root of the first molar is also anesthetized.[1]

Greater Palatine Nerve Block

The greater palatine nerve block is useful when treatment is necessary on the palatal aspect of the maxillary premolar and molar dentition. This technique targets the area just anterior to the greater palatine canal. The greater palatine nerve exits the canal and travels forward between the bone and soft tissue of the palate.

Contraindications to this technique are acute inflammation and infection at the injection site. A 25- or 27-gauge long needle is preferred for this technique.

Procedure. The patient should be in the supine position with the chin tilted upward for visibility of the area to be anesthetized. The right-handed operator should stand at the 8 o'clock position, whereas the left handed operator should stand at the 4 o'clock position. Using a cotton swab, locate the greater palatine foramen by placing it on the palatal tissue approximately 1 cm medial to the junction of the second and third molars (Figure 20–14). Although this is the usual position for the foramen, it may be located slightly anterior or posterior to this location. Gently press the swab into the tissue until the depression created by the foramen is felt.

Malamed and Trieger[6] found that the foramen is found medial to the anterior half of the third molar approximately 50% of the time, medial to the posterior half of the second molar approximately 39% of the time, and medial to the posterior half of the third molar approximately 9% of the time. The area approximately 1–2 mL anterior to the foramen is the target injection site. Using the cotton swab, apply pressure to the area of the foramen until the tissue blanches. Aim the syringe perpendicular to the injection site, which is 1–2 mL anterior to the foramen. While keeping pressure on the foramen, inject small volumes of anesthetic solution as the needle is advanced through the tissue until bone is con-

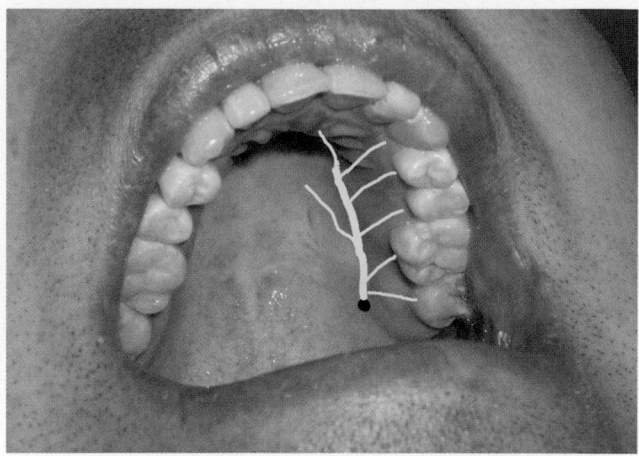

A

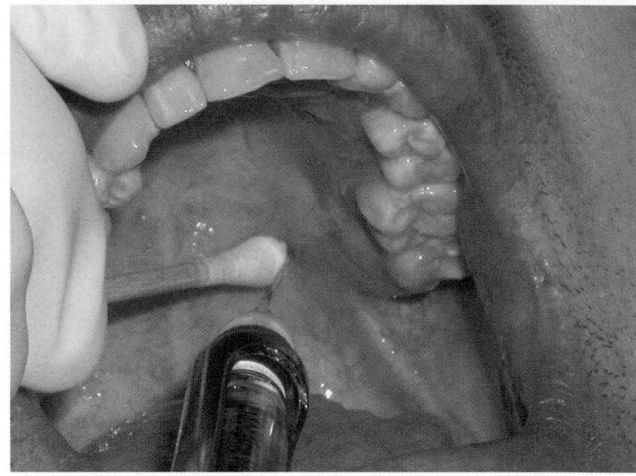

B

Figure 20–14. A: Location of the greater palatine nerve. **B:** Area of insertion for the greater palatine nerve block is 1 cm medial to the junction of the maxillary second and third molars.

tacted. The tissue will blanch in the area surrounding the injection site. Depth of penetration is usually no more than a few millimeters. Once bone is contacted, aspirate and inject approximately one fourth (0.45 mL) of the anesthetic solution. Resistance to deposition of anesthetic solution is normally felt by the operator. This technique provides anesthesia to the palatal mucosa and hard palate from the first premolar anteriorly to the posterior aspect of the hard palate and to the midline medially.[1,6]

Nasopalatine Nerve Block

The nasopalatine nerve block, otherwise known as the incisive nerve block and sphenopalatine nerve block, anesthetizes the nasopalatine nerves bilaterally. In this technique. anesthetic solution is deposited in the area of the incisive foramen. This technique is indicated when treatment requires anesthesia of the lingual aspect of multiple anterior teeth. A 25- or 27-gauge short needle is preferred for this technique.

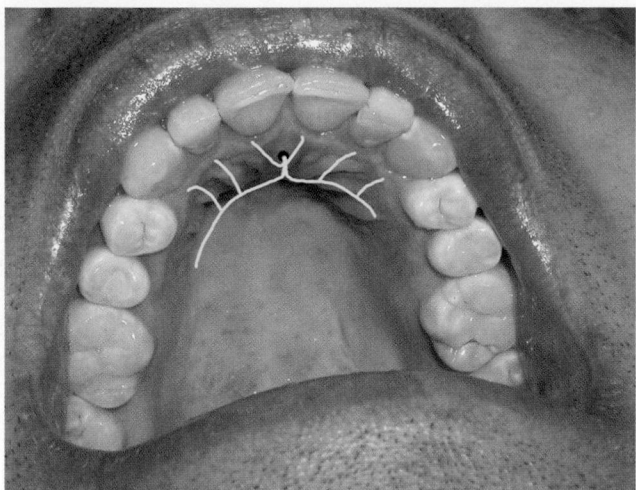

A

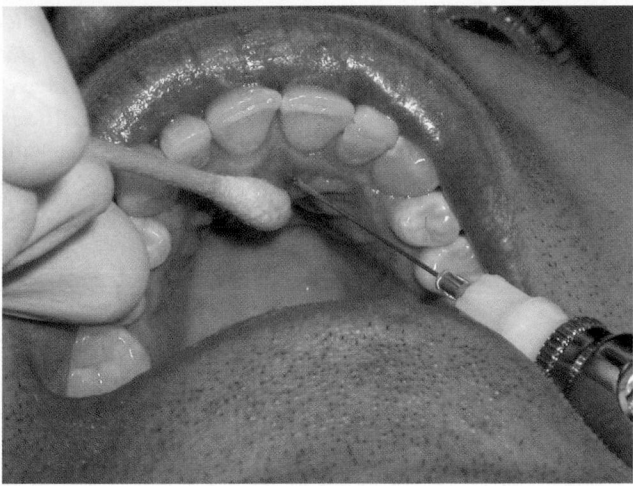
B

Figure 20–15. A: Location of the nasopalatine nerve. **B:** Insertion of the needle just lateral to the incisive papilla for the nasopalatine nerve block.

Procedure. The patient should be in the supine position with the chin tilted upward for visibility of the area to be anesthetized. The right-handed operator should be at the 9 o'clock position, whereas the left-handed operator should be at the 3 o'clock position. Identify the incisive papillae. The area directly lateral to the incisive papilla is the injection site. With a cotton swab, hold pressure over the incisive papilla. Insert the needle just lateral to the papilla with the bevel against the tissue (Figure 20–15). Advance the needle slowly toward the incisive foramen while depositing small volumes of anesthetic and maintaining pressure on the papilla. Once bone is contacted, retract the needle approximately 1 mm, aspirate, and inject one fourth (0.45 mL) of a cartridge of anesthetic solution over the course of 30 seconds. Blanching of surrounding tissues and resistance to the deposition of anesthetic solution are normal. Anesthesia is provided to the soft and hard tissue of the lingual aspect of the anterior teeth from the distal of the canine on one side to the distal of the canine on the opposite side.[1]

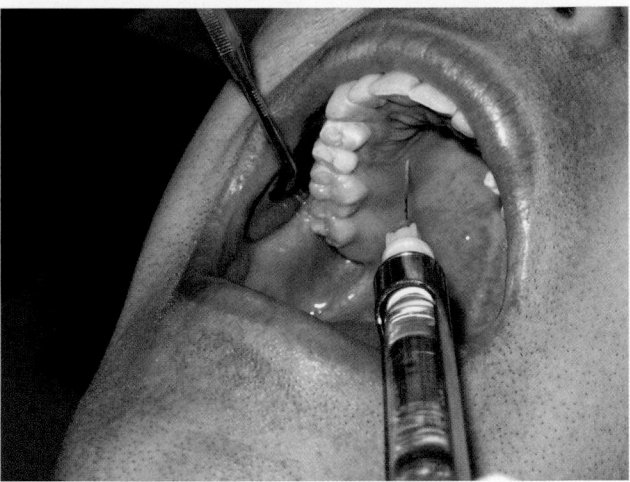

Figure 20–16. Local infiltration on the palatal aspect of the maxillary right first premolar. The needle is inserted approximately 5–10 mm palatal to the center of the crown.

Local Palatal Infiltration

The administration of local anesthetic for the palatal anesthesia of just one or two teeth is common in clinical practice. When a block is undesirable, local infiltration provides effective palatal anesthesia of the individual teeth to be treated. Contraindications include acute inflammation and infection over the area to be anesthetized. A 25- or 27-gauge short needle is preferred for this technique.

Procedure. The patient should be in the supine position with the chin tilted upward for visibility of the area to be anesthetized. Identify the area to be anesthetized. The right-handed operator should be at the 10 o'clock position, whereas the left-handed operator should be at the 2 o'clock position. The area of needle penetration is 5–10 mm palatal to the center of the crown. Apply pressure directly behind the injection site with a cotton swab. Insert the needle at a 45-degree angle to the injection site with the bevel angled toward the soft tissue (Figure 20–16). While maintaining pressure behind the injection site, advance the needle and slowly deposit anesthetic solution as the soft tissue is penetrated. Advance the needle until bone is contacted. Depth of penetration is usually no more than a few millimeters. The tissue is very firmly adherent to the underlying periosteum in this region, causing resistance to the deposition of local anesthetic. No more than 0.2–0.4 mL of anesthetic solution is necessary to provide adequate palatal anesthesia. Blanching of the tissue at the injection site immediately follows deposition of local anesthetic. Successful administration of anesthetic using this technique results in hemostasis and anesthesia of the palatal tissue in the area of injection.[1]

Intrapulpal Injection

Intrapulpal injection involves anesthesia of the nerve within the pulp canal of the individual tooth to be treated. When pain control cannot be achieved by any of the aforementioned methods, the intrapulpal method may be used once the pulp chamber is open. There are no contraindications to the use of this technique as it is at times the only effective method of pain control. A 25- or 27-gauge short needle is preferred for this technique.

Procedure. The patient should be in the supine position with the chin tilted upward for visibility of the area to be anesthetized. Identify the tooth to be anesthetized. The right-handed operator should be at the 10 o'clock position, whereas the left-handed operator should be at the 2 o'clock position. Assuming that the pulp chamber has been opened by an experienced dental professional, place the needle into the pulp chamber and deposit one drop of anesthetic. Advance the needle into the pulp canal and deposit another 0.2 mL of local anesthetic solution. It may be necessary to bend the needle in order to gain access to the chamber, especially with posterior teeth. The patient usually experiences a brief period of significant pain as the solution enters the canal, followed by immediate pain relief.[1]

Maxillary Nerve Block

Less often used in clinical practice, the maxillary nerve block (second division block) provides anesthesia of a hemimaxilla. This technique is useful for procedures that require anesthesia of multiple teeth and surrounding buccal and palatal soft tissue in one quadrant or when acute inflammation and infection preclude successful administration of anesthesia by the aforementioned methods. There are two techniques one can use to achieve the maxillary nerve block: the high tuberosity approach and the greater palatine canal approach.

The high tuberosity approach carries with it the risk of hematoma formation and is therefore contraindicated in patients with coagulation disorders. The maxillary artery is the vessel of primary concern with the high tuberosity approach. Both techniques are contraindicated when acute inflammation and infection are present over the injection site.

High Tuberosity Approach

A 25-gauge long needle is preferred for this technique.

The patient should be in the supine position with the chin tilted upward for visibility of the area to be anesthetized. Identify the area to be anesthetized. The right-handed operator should be at the 10 o'clock position, whereas the left-handed operator should be at the 2 o'clock position. This technique anesthetizes the maxillary nerve as it travels through the pterygopalatine fossa. Identify the height of the mucobuccal fold just distal to the maxillary second molar. This is the injection site. The needle should enter the tissue at a 45-degree angle aimed posteriorly, superiorly, and medially as in the PSA nerve block (see Figure 20–11B). The bevel should be oriented toward the bone. The needle is advanced to a depth of approximately 30 mm or a few millimeters shy of the hub. At this depth, the needle lies within the pterygopalatine fossa. The operator should then aspirate, rotate the needle one quarter turn, and aspirate again. After negative aspiration in two planes has been established, slowly inject one cartridge of anesthetic solution over the course of 1 minute. The needle is then slowly withdrawn and recapped.

Successful administration of anesthetic using the high tuberosity approach provides anesthesia to the entire hemimaxilla on the ipsilateral side of the block. This includes pulpal anesthesia to the maxillary teeth, buccal and palatal soft tissue as far medially as the midline, and the skin of the upper lip, lateral aspect of the nose, and lower eyelid.

Greater Palatine Canal Approach

A 25-gauge long needle is preferred for this technique.

Place the patient in the supine position. The right-handed operator should be at the 10 o'clock position, whereas the left-handed operator should be at the 2 o'clock position. Identify the greater palatine foramen as described in the technique for the greater palatine nerve block. The tissue directly over the greater palatine foramen is the target for injection. This technique anesthetizes the maxillary nerve as it travels through the pterygopalatine fossa via the greater palatine canal. Apply pressure to the area over the greater palatine foramen with a cotton-tipped applicator. Administer a greater palatine nerve block using the aforementioned technique (see Figure 20–14B). When adequate palatal anesthesia is achieved, gently probe for the greater palatine foramen with the tip of the needle. For this technique, the syringe should be held so that the needle is aimed posteriorly. It may be necessary to change the angulation of the needle to locate the foramen.

In a case study performed by Malamed and Trieger, the majority of canals were angled 45–50 degrees. Once the foramen has been located, advance the needle to a depth of 30 mm. If resistance is met, withdraw the needle a few millimeters and reenter at a different angle. Malamed and Trieger's study indicates that bony obstructions preventing passage of the needle were found in approximately 5–15% of canals. If resistance is met early and the operator is unable to advance the needle into the canal more than a few millimeters, the procedure should be aborted and the high tuberosity approach should be considered. If no resistance is met and

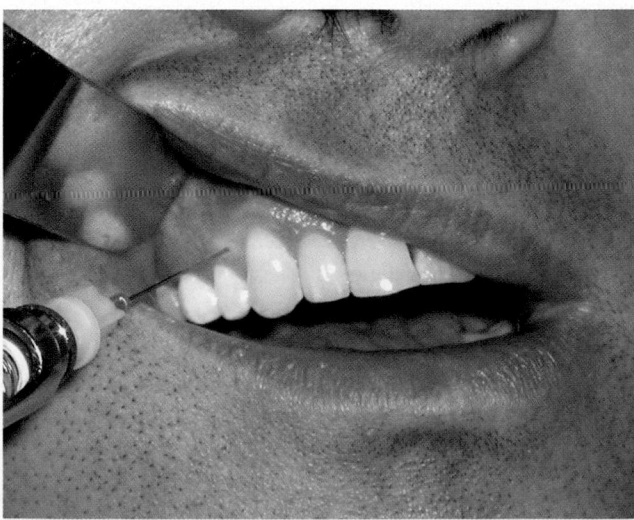

Figure 20–17. Note the position of the needle 3 mm apical to the apex of the papillary triangle for the intraseptal technique.

Table 20–3.

Techniques of Anesthesia for Treatment of a Quadrant or Multiple Teeth

Technique	Area Anesthetized
Maxillary	
Posterior superior alveolar nerve block	Maxillary molars (except the mesiobuccal root of maxillary first molar in some cases), hard and soft tissue on buccal aspect
Middle superior alveolar nerve block	Mesiobuccal root of maxillary first molar (in some cases), premolars, and surrounding hard and soft tissue on buccal aspect
Anterior superior alveolar nerve block/infraorbital nerve block	Maxillary central and lateral incisors and canine, surrounding hard and soft tissue on buccal aspect, mesiobuccal root of maxillary first molar (in some cases)
Greater palatine nerve block	Palatal mucosa and hard palate from first premolar anteriorly to posterior aspect of the hard palate, and to midline medially
Nasopalatine nerve block	Hard and soft tissue of lingual aspect of maxillary anterior teeth from distal of canine on one side to distal of canine on the contralateral side
Maxillary nerve block	Hemimaxilla on side of injection (teeth, hard and soft, buccal, and lingual tissue)
Mandibular	
Inferior alveolar nerve block	Mandibular teeth on side of injection, buccal and lingual hard and soft tissue, lower lip
Buccal nerve block	Buccal soft tissue of molar region
Gow-Gates mandibular nerve block	Mandibular teeth to midline, hard and soft tissue of buccal and lingual aspect, anterior $\frac{2}{3}$ of tongue, floor of mouth, skin over zygoma, posterior aspect of cheek, and temporal region on side of injection
Vazirani-Akinosi closed mouth	Mandibular teeth to midline, hard and soft tissue of buccal aspect, anterior $\frac{2}{3}$ of tongue, floor of mouth
Mental nerve block	Buccal soft tissue anterior to mental foramen, lower lip, chin
Incisive nerve block	Premolars, canine and incisors, lower lip, skin over chin, buccal soft tissue anterior to mental foramen

penetration of the canal is successful, aspirate in two planes as described in previous sections and slowly deposit one cartridge of local anesthetic solution. As with the high tuberosity approach, the hemimaxilla on the ipsilateral side as the injection becomes anesthetized with successful execution of this technique.[1,6,7]

Intraseptal Injection

The intraseptal technique is a useful adjunct to the aforementioned techniques (supraperiosteal, PSA, MSA, anterior superior alveolar). Although not used as often in clinical practice, the technique offers the added advantage of hemostasis in the area of injection. Terminal nerve endings in the surrounding hard and soft tissue of individual teeth are anesthetized with this technique. Contraindications to the procedure include acute inflammation and infection over the site of injection. A 27-gauge short needle is preferred for this technique.

Procedure. Place the patient in the supine position. The target area is the interdental palpillae 2–3 mm apical to the apex of the papillary triangle (Figure 20–17). The right-handed operator should be at the 10 o'clock position, whereas the left-handed operator should be at the 2 o'clock position. The operator may ask the patient to turn his or her head for optimum visibility. The syringe is held at a 45-degree angle to the long axis of the tooth with the bevel facing the apex of the root. The needle is inserted into the soft tissue and is advanced until bone is contacted. A few drops of anesthetic should be administered at this time. The needle is then advanced into the interdental septum, and 0.2 mL of anesthetic solution is deposited. Resistance to the flow of anesthetic solution is expected, and ischemia of the soft tissue surrounding the injection site ensues shortly after anesthetic solution is administered.[1]

Table 20–3 lists maxillary and mandibular techniques of anesthesia for treatment of a quadrant or multiple teeth.

TECHNIQUES OF MANDIBULAR REGIONAL ANESTHESIA

Techniques used in clinical practice for the anesthesia of the hard and soft tissues of the mandible include the supraperiosteal technique, periodontal ligament injection, intrapulpal anesthesia, intraseptal injection, inferior alveolar nerve block, long buccal nerve block, Gow-Gates technique, Vazirani-Akinosi closed-mouth mandibular block, mental nerve block, and incisive nerve block.

The supraperiosteal, periodontal ligament, intrapulpal, and intraseptal techniques are executed in the same manner as described for maxillary anesthesia. When anesthetizing the mandible, the patient should be in the semisupine or reclined position. The right-handed operator should stand at the 9 o'clock to 10 o'clock position, whereas the left-handed operator should stand at the 3 o'clock to 4 o'clock position.

Inferior Alveolar Nerve Block

The inferior alveolar nerve block is one of the most commonly used techniques in mandibular regional anesthesia. It is extremely useful when multiple teeth in one quadrant require treatment. While effective, this technique carries a high failure rate even when strict adherence to protocol is maintained. The target for this technique is the mandibular nerve as it travels along the medial aspect of the ramus before its entry into the mandibular foramen. The lingual, mental, and incisive nerves are also anesthetized. A 25-gauge long needle is preferred for this technique.

Procedure. The patient should be in the semisupine position. The right-handed operator should be in the 8 o'clock position, whereas the left-handed operator should be in the 4 o'clock position. With the patient's mouth open maximally, identify the coronoid notch and the pterygomandibular raphae. Three fourths of the anteroposterior distance between these two landmarks and approximately 6–10 mm above the occlusal plane is the injection site. Use a retraction instrument to retract the cheek and bring the needle to the injection site from the contralateral premolar region. As the needle passes through the soft tissue, deposit 1 or 2 drops of anesthetic solution. Advance the needle until bone is contacted. Once bone is contacted, withdraw the needle 1 mm, and redirect the needle posteriorly by bringing the barrel of the syringe toward the occlusal plane (Figure 20–18A and B). Advance the needle to three fourths of its depth, aspirate, and inject three fourths of a cartridge of anesthetic solution slowly over the course of 1 minute. As the needle is withdrawn, continue to deposit the remaining one fourth of anesthetic solution so as to anesthetize the lingual nerve (Figure 20–18C). Successful execution of this technique results in anesthesia of the mandibular teeth on the ipsilateral side to the midline, the associated buccal, and lingual soft tissue, the lateral aspect of the tongue on the ipsilateral side, and the lower lip on the ipsilateral side.[1]

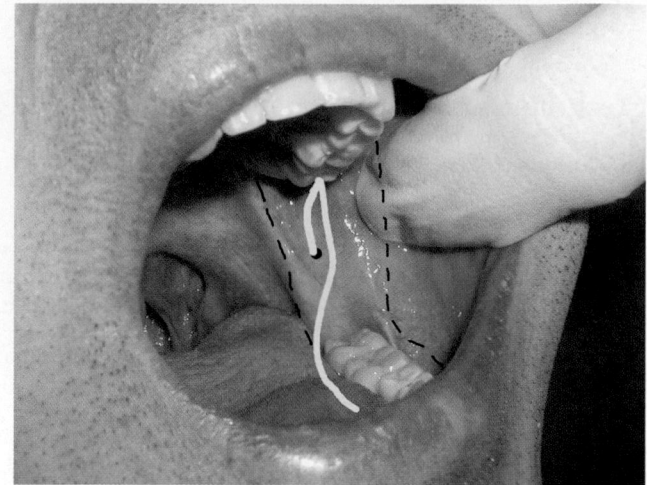

A

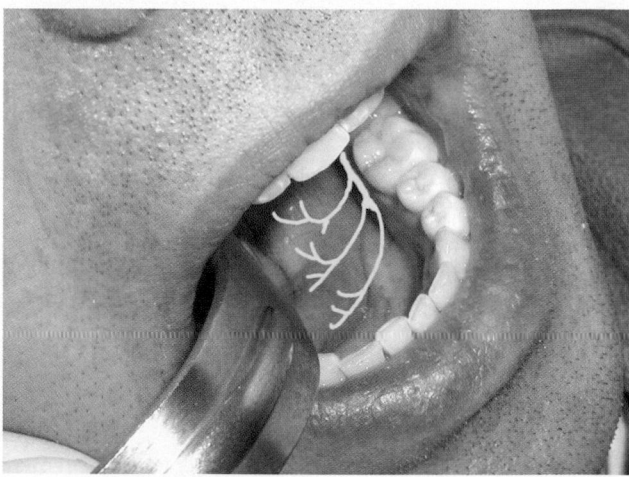

B

C

Figure 20–18. A: Location of the inferior alveolar nerve. **B:** After contacting bone, the needle is redirected posteriorly by bringing the barrel of the syringe toward the occlusal plane. The needle is then advanced to three fourths of its depth. **C:** Location of the lingual nerve, which is anesthetized during the administration of an inferior alveolar nerve block.

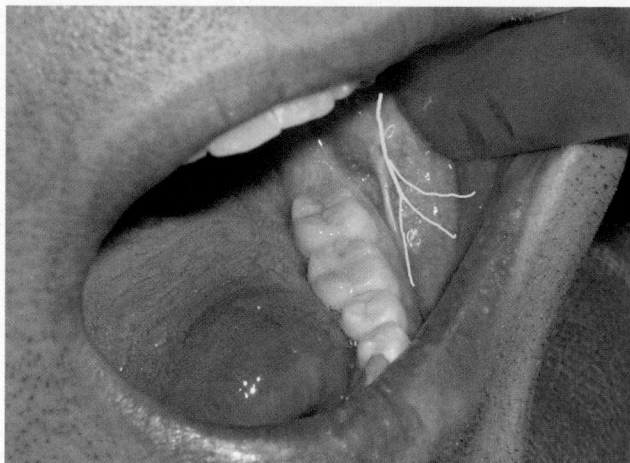

A

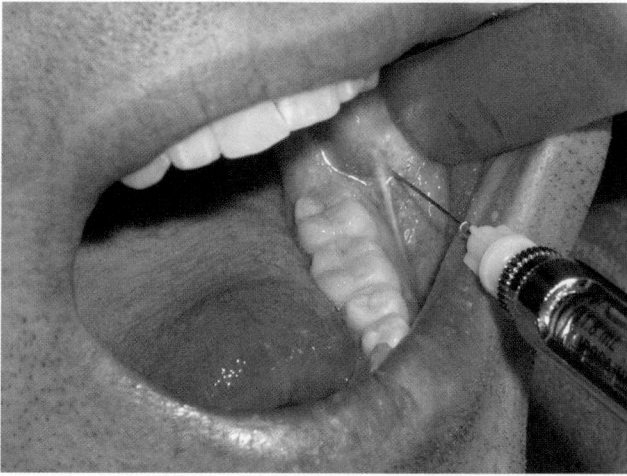

B

Figure 20–19. A: Location of the buccal nerve. **B:** The tissue just distal and buccal to the last molar tooth is the target area for injection.

Buccal Nerve Block

The buccal nerve block, otherwise known as the long buccal or buccinator block, is a useful adjunct to the inferior alveolar nerve block when manipulation of the buccal soft tissue in the mandibular molar region is indicated. The target for this technique is the buccal nerve as it passes over the anterior aspect of the ramus. Contraindications to the procedure include acute inflammation and infection over the site of injection. A 25-gauge long needle is preferred for this technique.

Procedure. The patient should be in the semisupine position. The right-handed operator should be in the 8 o'clock position, whereas the left-handed operator should be in the 4 o'clock position. Identify the most distal molar tooth on the side to be treated. The tissue just distal and buccal to the last molar tooth is the target area for injection (Figure 20–19). Use a retraction instrument to retract the cheek. The bevel of the needle should be toward bone and the syringe should be held parallel with the occlusal plane on the side of the injection. The needle is inserted into the soft tissue, and a few

drops of anesthetic solution are administered. The needle is advanced approximately 1 or 2 mm until bone is contacted. Once bone is contacted and aspiration is negative, 0.2 mL of local anesthetic solution is deposited. The needle is withdrawn and recapped. Successful execution of this technique results in anesthesia of the buccal soft tissue of the mandibular molar region.[1]

Gow-Gates Technique

The Gow-Gates technique or third division nerve block is useful alternative to the inferior alveolar nerve block and is often used when the latter fails to provide adequate anesthesia. Advantages of this technique compared with the inferior alveolar technique are its low failure rate and its low incidence of positive aspiration. The Gow-Gates technique anesthetizes the auriculotemporal, inferior alveolar, buccal, mental, incisive, mylohyoid, and lingual nerves. Contraindications include acute inflammation and infection over the site of injection and trismatic patients. A 25-gauge long needle is preferred for this technique.

Procedure. The patient should be in the semisupine position. The right-handed operator should be in the 8 o'clock position, whereas the left-handed operator should be in the 4 o'clock position. The target area for this technique is the neck of the condyle below the area of insertion of the lateral pterygoid muscle. A retraction instrument is used to retract the cheek. The patient is asked to open maximally and the mesiolingual cusp of the maxillary second molar on the side of desired anesthesia is identified. The insertion site of the needle should be just distal to the maxillary second molar at the level of the mesiolingual cusp. Bring the needle to the insertion site in a plane that is parallel with an imaginary line drawn from the intertragic notch to the corner of the mouth on the same side as the injection (Figure 20–20). The orientation of the bevel of the needle is not important in this technique. Advance the needle through soft tissue approximately 25 mm until bone is contacted. This is the neck of the condyle. Once bone is contacted, withdraw the needle 1 mm and aspirate. Redirect the needle superiorly and reaspirate. If aspiration in two planes is negative, slowly inject one cartridge of local anesthetic solution over the course of 1 minute. Successful execution of this technique provides anesthesia to the ipsilateral mandibular teeth up to the midline and the associated buccal and lingual hard and soft tissue. The anterior two thirds of the tongue, floor of the mouth, skin over the zygoma, posterior aspect of the cheek and temporal region on the ipsilateral side of injection are also anesthetized.[1,8]

Vazirani-Akinosi Closed-Mouth Mandibular Block

The Vazirani-Akinosi closed-mouth mandibular block is a useful technique for patients with limited opening due trismus or ankylosis of the temporomandibular joint. Limited mandibular opening precludes the administration of the inferior alveolar nerve block or use of the Gow-Gates technique,

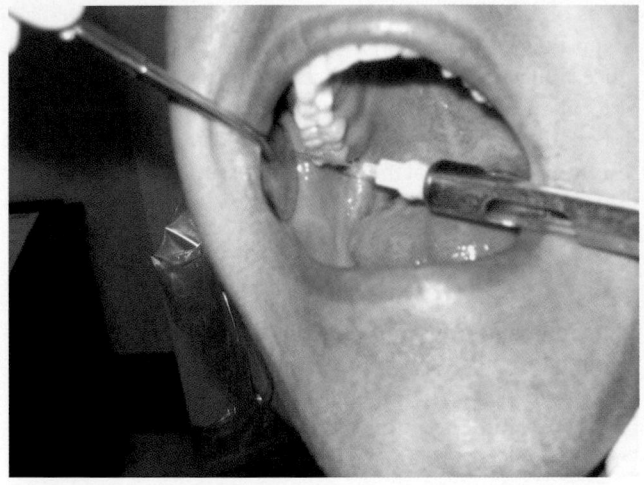

A

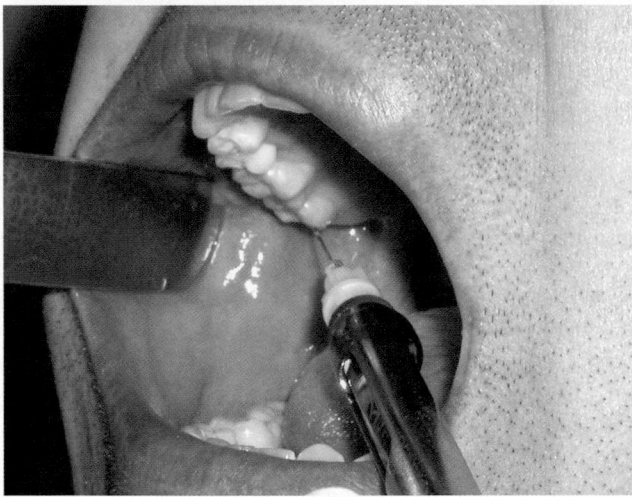

B

Figure 20–20. A: The patient is asked to open mouth maximally. The mesiolingual cusp of the maxillary second molar is the reference point for the height of the injection. **B:** The needle is then moved distally and is held parallel to an imaginary line drawn from the intertragic notch to the corner of the mouth.

both of which require the patient to be open maximally. Other advantages to this technique are the minimal risk of trauma to the inferior alveolar nerve, artery, vein, and pterygoid muscle, low complication rate, and minimal discomfort upon injection. Contraindications to this technique are acute inflammation and infection in the pterygomandibular space, deformity or tumor in the maxillary tuberosity region, and an inability to visualize the medial aspect of the ramus. A 25-gauge long needle is preferred for this technique.

Procedure. The patient should be in the semisupine position. The right-handed operator should be in the 8 o'clock position, whereas the left-handed operator should be in the 4 o'clock position. The gingival margin above the maxillary second and third molars and the pterygomandibular raphae serve as landmarks for this technique. A retraction instrument is used to stretch the cheek laterally. The patient should

occlude gently on the posterior teeth. The needle is held parallel with the occlusal plane at the level of the gingival margin of the maxillary second and third molars. The bevel is directed away from the bone facing the midline. The needle is advanced through the mucous membrane and buccinator muscle to enter the pterygomandibular space. The needle is inserted to approximately one half to three fourths of its length. At this point, the needle will be in the midsection of the ptyerygomandibular space. Aspirate and, if negative, one cartridge of local anesthetic solution is deposited over the course of 1 minute. Diffusion and gravitation of the local anesthetic solution anesthetizes the lingual and long buccal nerves in addition to the inferior alveolar nerve. Successful execution of this technique provides anesthesia of the ipsilateral mandibular teeth up to the midline and the associated buccal and lingual hard and soft tissue. The anterior two thirds of the tongue and floor of the mouth are also anesthetized.[9,10]

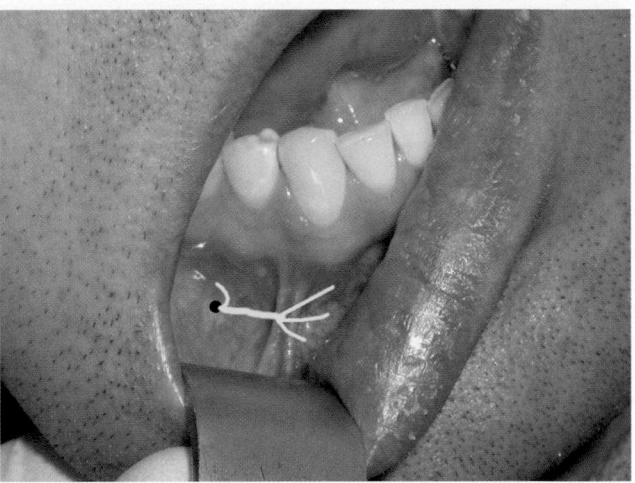

A

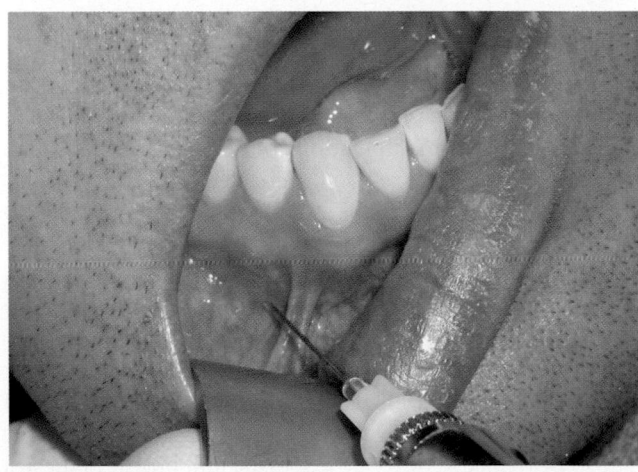

B

Figure 20–21. A: Location of the mental and incisive nerves. **B:** Block of the mental and incisive nerves. The needle is inserted at the height of the mucobuccal fold over the mental foramen for both the mental nerve block and the incisive nerve block.

Mental Nerve Block

The mental nerve block is indicated for procedures in which manipulation of buccal soft tissue anterior to the mental foramen is necessary. Contraindications to this technique are acute inflammation and infection over the injection site. A 25- or 27-gauge short needle is preferred for this technique.

Procedure. The patient should be in the semisupine position. The right-handed operator should be in the 8 o'clock position, whereas the left-handed operator should be in the 4 o'clock position. The target area is the height of the mucobuccal fold over the mental foramen (Figure 20–21*A* and *B*). The foramen can be manually palpated by applying gentle finger pressure to the body of the mandible in the area of the premolar apicies. The patient will feel slight discomfort upon palpation of the foramen. Use a retraction instrument to retract the soft tissue. The needle is directed toward the mental foramen with the bevel facing the bone. Penetrate the soft tissue to a depth of 5 mm, aspirate, and inject approximately 0.6 mL of anesthetic solution. Successful execution of this technique results in anesthesia of the buccal soft tissue anterior to the foramen, lower lip, and chin on the side of the injection.[1]

Incisive Nerve Block

The incisive nerve block is not as frequently used in clinical practice; however, it proves very useful when treatment is limited to mandibular anterior teeth and full quadrant anesthesia is not necessary. The technique is almost identical with the mental nerve block but with one additional step. Both the mental and incisive nerves are anesthetized using this technique. Contraindications to this technique are acute inflammation and infection at the site of injection. A 25- or 27-gauge short needle is preferred for this technique.

Procedure. The patient should be in the semisupine position. The right-handed operator should be in the 8 o'clock position, whereas the left-handed operator should be in the 4 o'clock position. The target area is the height of the mucobuccal fold over the mental foramen (see Figure 20–21*B*). Identify the mental foramen as previously described. Give the patient a mental nerve block as described above, and apply digital pressure at the site of injection during administration of anesthetic solution. Continue to apply digital pressure at the site of injection 2–3 minutes after the injection is complete to aid the anesthetic in diffusing into the foramen. Successful implementation of this technique provides anesthesia to the premolars, canine, incisor teeth, lower lip, skin of the chin, and buccal soft tissue anterior to the mental foramen.[1]

References

1. Malamed SF: *Handbook of Local Anesthesia,* 4th ed. Mosby-Year Book, 1997.
2. Snell RS: *Clinical Anatomy for Medical Students,* 5th ed. Little, Brown, 1995.
3. Loetscher CA, Walton RE: Patterns of innervation of the maxillary first molar: A dissection study oral surgery Oral Medicine. Oral Pathol 1988;65:86–90.
4. McDaniel WM: Variations in nerve distributions of the maxillary teeth. J Dent Res 1956;35:916–921.
5. Heasman PA: Clinical anatomy of the superior alveolar nerves. Br J Oral Maxillofacial Surg 1884;22:439–447.
6. Malamed SF, Trieger N: Intraoral maxillary nerve block: An anatomical and clinical study. Anesthesia Progr 1983;30:44–48.
7. Poore TE, Carney F. Maxillary nerve block: A useful technique. J Oral Surg 1973;31:749–755.
8. Gow-Gates GAE: Mandibular conduction anesthesia: A new technique using extraoral landmarks. Oral Surg 1973;36:321–328.
9. Akinosi JO: A new approach to the mandibular nerve block. Br J Oral Maxillofacial Surg 1977;15:83–87.
10. Vazirani SJ: Closed mouth mandibular nerve block: A new technique. Dent Digest 1960;66:10–13.

Local & Regional Anesthesia for Eye Surgery

Jacques Ripart, MD • Kenneth Merhige, MD • Robert Della Rocca, MD

INTRODUCTION

Ophthalmic surgery is one of the most frequent surgical procedures requiring anesthesia in developed countries.[1] Perioperative morbidity and mortality rates associated with eye (eg, cataract) surgery are low.[2,3] Nevertheless, because patients with cataracts tend to be older and to have serious comorbidities,[4–9] systematic preoperative evaluation should be performed to consider a patient eligible for surgery.[9] Anesthetic management may contribute to the success or failure of ophthalmic surgery. A closed-claims analysis by Gild and coworkers[10] found that 30% of eye injury claims associated with anesthesia were characterized by the patient moving during ophthalmic surgery. Clinical strategies to ensure patient immobility are essential, as blindness is the outcome in many cases of eye injury. Most problems occurred during general anesthesia. Quicker patient rehabilitation and fewer complications are the main reasons why many ophthalmic surgeons are choosing local (LA) over general anesthesia.[11–13]

In the past, regional anesthesia on the eye typically consisted of retrobulbar anesthesia (RBA), with the surgeon performing the block. Widespread use of the phacoemulsification technique, however, has changed the anesthesia requirements for this technique—total akinesia and lowered intraocular pressure are no longer necessary. Consequently, conventional RBA is used less frequently today, particularly since it carries a greater risk for complications than do the emerging techniques. The newer techniques do not provide akinesia of the globe paralleling that of the retrobulbar block; however, they are useful for anterior segment surgery, especially cataract surgery. Accurate knowledge of anatomy and of various anesthetic techniques are necessary to determine the appropriate block for specific clinical situations. This chapter will review the relevant anatomy of the eye, classic (retro and peribulbar) needle block techniques, emerging anesthesia techniques, and choice of LAs and adjuvant agents.

ANATOMY

The cavity of the orbit has a truncated pyramid shape, with a posterior apex, and a base corresponding to the anterior aperture. The orbit contains mainly adipose tissue, and the globe is suspended in the anterior part. The four rectus muscles of the eye insert anteriorly near the equator of the globe (Figure 21–1). Posteriorly, they insert together at the apex on the tendineus anulus communis of Zinn, through which the optic nerve enters the orbit. The four rectus muscles delineate the retrobulbar cone, which is not sealed by any intermuscular membrane.[14–17] Sensory innervation is supplied by the ophthalmic nerve (first branch of the trigeminal nerve [V]), which passes through the muscular cone (Figure 21–2). The

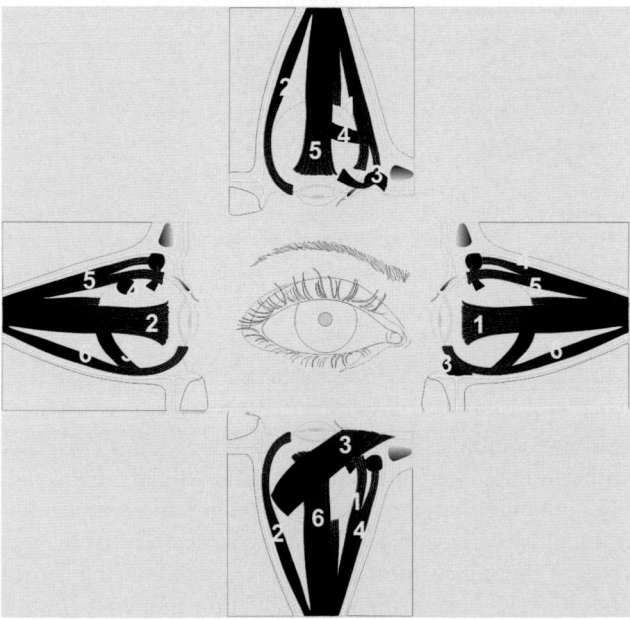

Figure 21–1. Insertion of the four rectus muscles of the eye and the two obliques. The muscles insert anteriorly near the equator of the globe. (1) Medial rectus, (2) Lateral rectus, (3) Inferior oblique, (4) Superior oblique, (5) Superior rectus, (6) Inferior rectus.

trochlear nerve (IV) provides motor control to the superior oblique muscles, the abducens nerve (VI) to the lateral rectus muscle, and the oculomotor nerve (III) to all other extraocular muscles. All but the trochlear nerve pass through the muscular conus. Injection of LA solution inside the cone will provide anesthesia and akinesia of the globe and the extraocular muscles. Only the motor nerve to the orbicularis muscle of the eyelids has an extraorbital course, coming from the superior branch of the facial nerve (VII). Many major structures are located within the muscular conus and are therefore at risk of needle and injection injury. These include the optic nerve with its meningeal coverings; blood vessels of the orbit; and the autonomic, sensory, and motor innervation of the globe. For this reason, some authors advise that introduction of the needle into the muscular cone be avoided and suggest that needle insertion be limited to the extraconal space.[18,19] However, posterior to the equator of the globe, the extraconal space is only a virtual space, because the rectus muscles are in contact with the bone walls of the orbit.

The scleral portion of the globe is surrounded by Tenon's capsule, a fibroelastic layer stretching from the corneal limbus anteriorly to the optic nerve posteriorly. Its proper anatomic name is the **facial sheath** of the eyeball. It delimits a potential space named the **episcleral space** (sub-Tenon's space). This is only a virtual space that expands when fluid is injected into it.

RETROBULBAR ANESTHESIA

Historically, RBA has been the gold standard for anesthesia of the eye and orbit. This technique generally consists of injecting a small volume of LA solution (3–5 mL) inside the muscular cone (Figure 21–3). A facial nerve block is occasionally required to prevent blinking. Because of its extraconal motor control, the superior oblique muscle may frequently remain functional, precluding total akinesia of the globe. The main hazard of RBA is risk of injury to the globe or to one of the anatomic structures in the muscular cone. Near the apex, these structures are packed in a very small space and are fixed by the tendon of Zinn, which prevents them from moving away from a needle.

Conventional Technique

Since its formal description by Atkinson toward the end of the nineteenth century,[20] conventional RBA has not changed for decades. The patient is asked to look in the "up-and-in" direction. The needle is introduced through the skin below the inferior lid at the junction between the lateral third and the medial two thirds of the inferior orbital edge (Figure 21–3). The needle is directed to the apex of the orbit (slightly medially and cephalad) and advanced to a depth of 25–35 mm. Two to 4 mL of LA solution is then injected. An additional facial nerve block is performed to prevent blinking; the technique most frequently used is the Van Lindt block.[21]

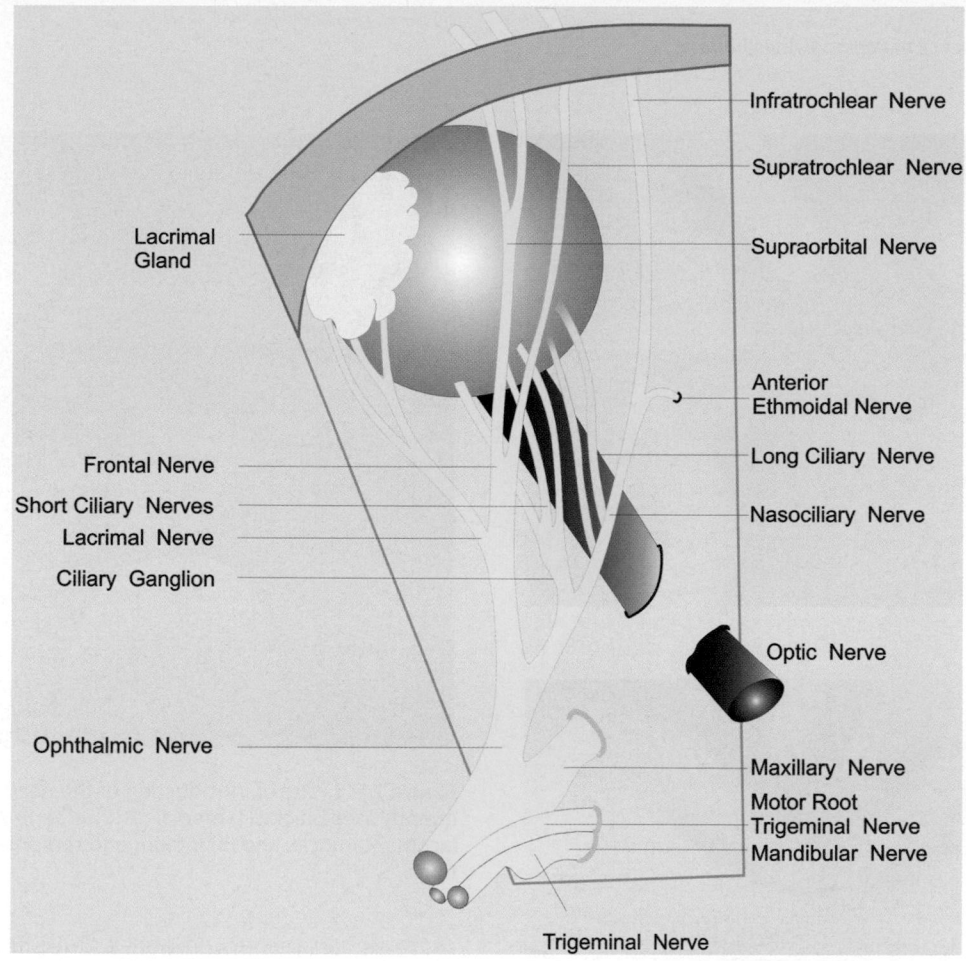

Figure 21–2. Sensory innervation of the eye and orbit is supplied by the ophthalmic nerve (first branch of the trigeminal nerve [V]), which passes through the muscular cone.

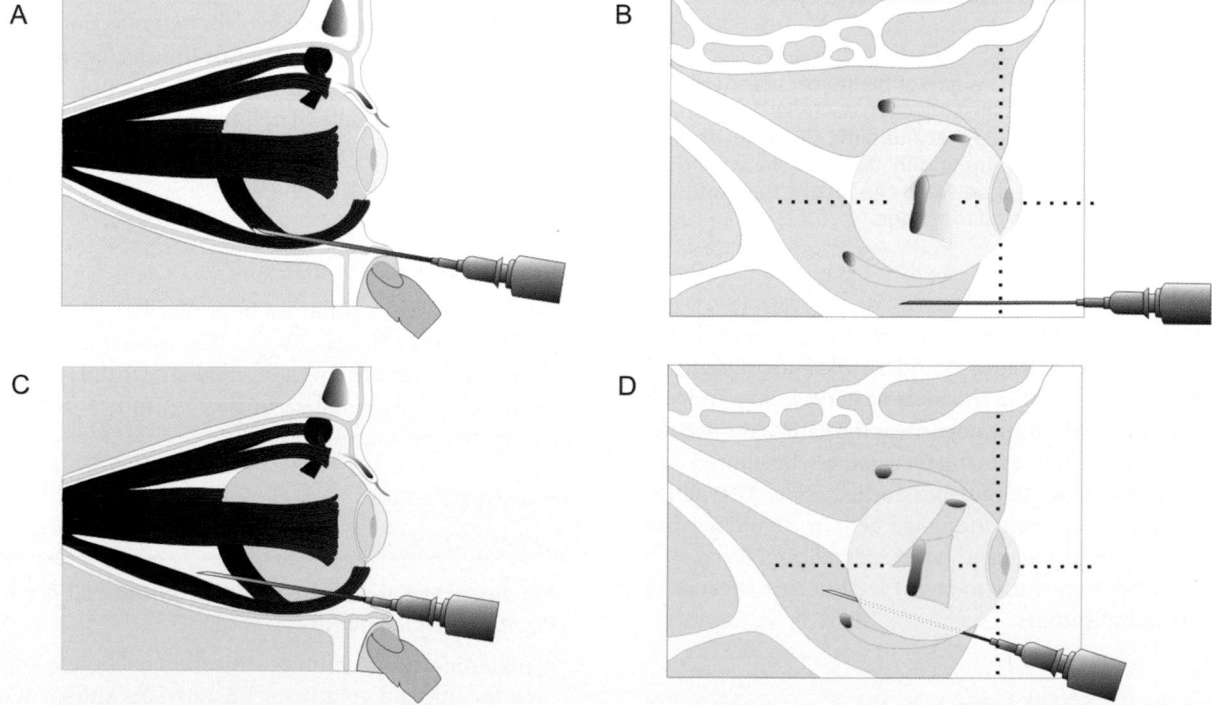

Figure 21–3. Retrobulbar anesthesia. The needle is introduced through the skin below the inferior lid at the junction between the lateral third and the medial two thirds of the inferior orbital edge.

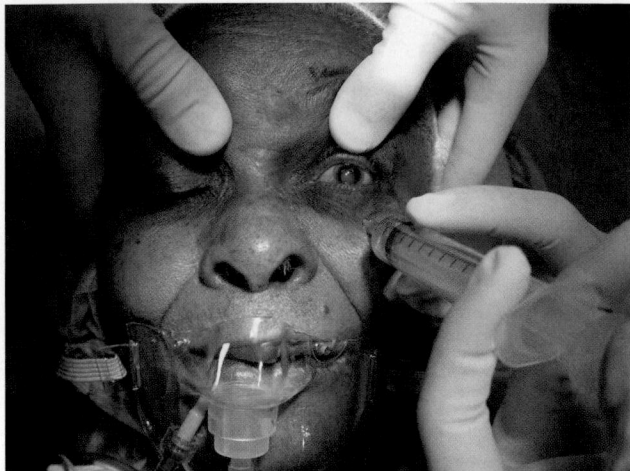

A

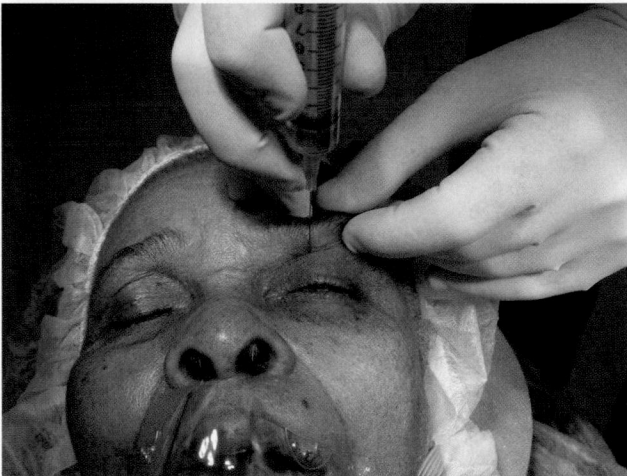

B

Figure 21–4. The classic technique of peribulbar anesthesia involves two injections. **A:** The first injection is inferior and temporal, the needle being introduced at the same site as for an RBA injection, but with a smaller "up-and-in" angle. **B:** The second injection is superior and nasal between the medial third and the lateral two thirds of the orbital roof edge.

Alternative Techniques

The Atkinson up-and-in position of the gaze was abandoned when Liu and colleagues[22] and Unsöld and colleagues[23] warned that it increases the risk of optic nerve injury. Indeed, this position places the optic nerve near the path of the needle. Moreover, the optic nerve is stretched and can be injured easily by the needle rather than being pushed aside. Alternative puncture sites and specially designed bent or curved needles have been proposed but have never gained popularity.[24–26] RBA is used less frequently today, at least in part because of its risks of complications.

■ PERIBULBAR ANESTHESIA

With peribulbar anesthesia, the needle is introduced into the extraconal space.[18,19,27,28] The injected volume of LA

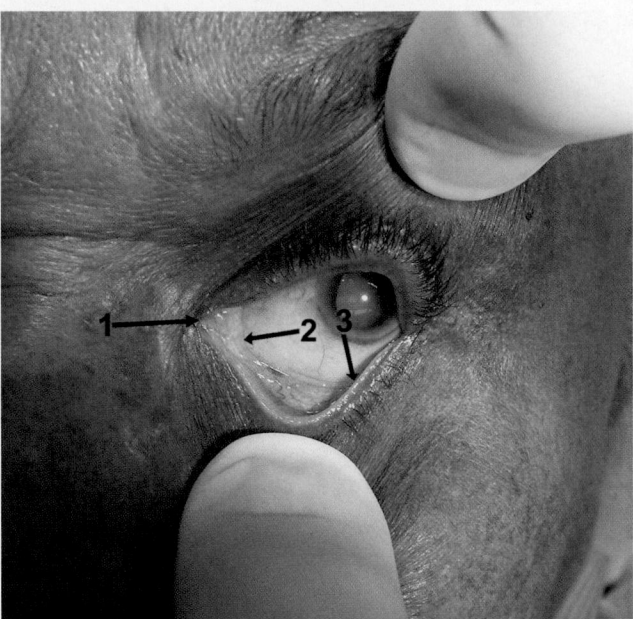

Figure 21–5. Site of introduction of the needle for the most frequently used blocks: (1) medial canthus peribulbar anesthesia, (2) lacrimal caruncle, and (3) inferior and temporal peribulbar injections.

(6–12 mL) is larger than that for a retrobulbar injection. This larger volume allows the LA to spread into the whole corpus adiposum of the orbit, including the intraconal space, where the nerves to be blocked are located. Additionally, such a large volume allows anterior spread of LA to the lids to provide a block of the orbicularis muscle and to avoid the need for additional lid block.

The classic technique involves two injections. The first injection is inferior and temporal, the needle being introduced at the same site as for an RBA injection, but with a smaller up-and-in angle. The second injection is superior and nasal between the medial third and the lateral two thirds of the orbital roof edge (Figure 21–4B).

Alternative Techniques

Several alternative techniques of peribulbar anesthesia have been described (Figure 21–5). The most common sites for needle insertion are (1) medial canthus peribulbar anesthesia,[29] (2) lacrimal caruncle,[30,31] and (3) inferior and temporal peribulbar injections.[18,19]

Clinical Pearls

Whichever technique of peribulbar anesthesia is chosen, several principles apply:

■ Single-injection vs multiple injection technique. Increasing the injected volume of LA provides sufficient anesthesia. Additional injections are not needed.[32] In addition, anatomic distortion following the first injection may increase the risk of complications associated with consecutive injections.[33] As a rule of thumb, a second injection should be performed only as a supplement when the first injection has failed to provide effective anesthesia.

- **Needle insertion sites.** Needle insertion through the superior nasal site should be avoided. At this level, the distance between the orbital roof and the globe is reduced, theoretically increasing the risk of globe perforation. Additionally, the superior oblique muscle may be injured by the needle. The inferior nasal puncture should be used instead. An alternative site of puncture for peribulbar anesthesia is the medial canthus (see Figure 21–5).[29] The needle is introduced at the medial junction of the lids, nasal to the lacrimal caruncle, in a strictly posterior direction to a depth of 15 mm or less. At this level, the space between the orbital wall and the globe is similar in size to that of the inferior and temporal approach and is free from blood vessels. Moreover, myopic staphyloma, an anatomic anomaly that represents a risk factor for perforation, is infrequently encountered on the nasal side of the globe.

- **Needle insertion depth.** Limit needle insertion depth to 25 mm. Posterior to the globe, the rectus muscles are in contact with the orbital walls, so that the extraconal space entirely disappears and becomes virtual. Increasing needle insertion depth would be expected to change a peribulbar to a retrobulbar injection.[34] Some "posterior peribulbar blocks" are in fact unintentional retrobulbar injections. This is a plausible explanation for optic nerve injury after an attempted peribulbar injection. Moreover, a long needle fully introduced into the orbit may reach the apex of the orbit, another hazardous area.[35] Inserting the needle to a depth of 40 mm has led to performing the injection directly through the optical foramen in 11% of cases.[36]

- Thin needles (25-gauge) are suggested for reducing pain on needle insertion. The use of short-beveled needles may be safer because they may enhance the tactile perception of resistance during needle insertion (intraneural or intramuscular placement). Indeed, on cadavers, more pressure is required with short-bevel needles to perforate the sclera.[37] Nevertheless, these are only theoretical considerations, since the complication rate with peribulbar blocks is low.

- Use compression to lower intraocular pressure, which increases after injection. Compression has not been shown to enhance the quality of the block. Applying a pressure of 30 mm Hg for 5 to 10 min is usually sufficient.

- In all cases, the spread of LA within the corpus adiposum of the orbit remains somewhat unpredictable, leading to the need for more anesthetic to prevent an imperfect block. Depending on the surgeon's preference for akinesia, additional anesthetic is required in up to half of all cases.[27,28] This poor reproducibility in block efficacy is the main disadvantage of peribulbar anesthesia.[19]

Retrobulbar Versus Peribulbar Blocks

Retrobulbar block has been traditionally assumed to be more effective than PBA. However, when a sufficient volume of LA is injected, both blocks have similar success rates.[38] There is a sound anatomic explanation for this: the absence of an intermuscular membrane to separate extra- from intraconal compartments results in a similar space for the spread of local anesthetic.[14–17] Therefore, if the effectiveness is similar, it would be logical to use the technique with less risk of complications. Because the retrobulbar block theoretically carries a higher risk of complications (optic nerve injury, brainstem anesthesia, retrobulbar hemorrhage), peribulbar block is deemed preferable to retrobulbar block.

MAJOR COMPLICATIONS OF EYE BLOCKS

The primary cause of serious complications is needle misplacement. Although patients' anatomic features may increase the risk of complications, the main risk factor is the lack of training and experience on the part of the physician. However, it should be noted that complications such as retrobulbar hemorrhage may occur with even the most experienced practitioners. Presenting signs, symptoms, and mechanism of common complications are summarized in Tables 21–1 and 21–2).

Central nervous system complications of eye blocks may occur by two different mechanisms:

1. An accidental intraarterial injection may reverse the blood flow in the ophthalmic artery up to the anterior cerebral or the internal carotid artery.[40] Consequently, injectate volume as small as 4 mL may produce seizures. Symptomatic treatment by maintaining patent airway; providing oxygenation; and abolishing seizure activity with small doses of benzodiazepam, propofol, or barbiturates, is usually adequate and results in a rapid recovery without sequelae.

2. An unintentional injection under the dura mater sheath of the optic nerve or directly through the optic foramen may result in subarachnoid spread of the LA. This causes partial or total brainstem anesthesia.[41–43] Katsev and coworkers[36] have shown that the apex of the orbit may be reached with a 40-mm needle in up to 11% of patients.[36] Depending on the dose and volume of LA spreading toward the brainstem, a bilateral block; cranial nerve palsy with sympathetic activation, confusion, and restlessness; or total spinal anesthesia with tetra paresis, arterial hypotension, bradycardia, and eventually respiratory arrest can occur. Symptomatic treatment (oxygen, vasopressors, and, if required, tracheal intubation and ventilation) should permit complete recovery after the spinal block wears off (a few hours).

Unintentional globe perforation and rupture is the most devastating complication of eye blocks. It has a poor prognosis, especially when the diagnosis is delayed. The

Table 21–1.

Signs, Symptoms and Mechanism of Complications of Retrobulbar Anesthesia

Complications	Signs and Symptoms	Mechanism
Ocular		
Perforation of globe	Ocular pain, intraocular hemorrhage, restlessness	Direct trauma: Myopic eye, posterior staphyloma, repeated injections
Retrobulbar hemorrhage	Subconjunctival or eyelid ecchymosis, increasing proptosis pain, and/or, increased intraocular pressure	Direct trauma (artery or vein)
Optic nerve damage	Visual loss, optic disc pallor	Direct injury to nerve or blood vessels, vascular occlusion
Systemic		
Intraarterial injection	Cardiopulmonary arrest, convulsions	Retrograde flow to internal carotid and access to midbrain structures
Optic nerve sheath injection	Agitation, ptosis, mydriasis dysphagia, dizziness, confusion, contralateral ophthalmoplegia, respiratory depression or cardiac arrest	Subdural or subarachnoid injection
Oculocardiac reflex	Bradycardia, other arrhythmias, asystole	Trigeminal nerve (afferent, arc) to floor of fourth ventricle with efferent arc via vagus nerve

incidence is between 1 in 350 and 7 in 50,000 cases.[44,45] Main risk factors include inadequate experience of the physician and a highly myopic eye (ie, long eyeball).[46] In a study of 50,000 cases, Edge and Navon[45] observed that myopic staphyloma was a significant risk factor. This suggests that isolated high myopia may not be a risk factor per se but acts as a confounding factor because myopic staphyloma occurs only in myopic eyes.[45] Vohra and Good[46] have observed with B-mode ultrasound that the probability of staphyloma is greater in highly myopic than in slightly myopic eyes. Moreover, staphyloma was more frequently located at the posterior pole of the globe (accounting for perforations after RBA) or in the inferior area of the globe (accounting for perforations after inferior and temporal punctures, both peri- and retrobulbar). As a result, at least in myopic patients and at best in all patients, ultrasound measurement of the axial length of the globe (biometry) should be available. In cases of high myopic eye (axial length greater than 26 mm), a needle block can carry an increased risk of globe perforation. In these cases, a sub-Tenon's or topical block may be preferable.

Injury to an extraocular muscle may cause diplopia and ptosis. Several mechanisms can be involved, including direct injury by the needle resulting in intramuscular hematoma, high pressure because of injection into the muscle sheath, or myotoxicity of the LA.[47] The injury may progress in three steps: first, the muscle is paralyzed; second, it seems to recover; and third, a retractile scar develops.

Clinical Pearls

- Retrobulbar hemorrhage is typically caused by an inadvertent arterial puncture. It may lead to a compressive hematoma, which can threaten retinal perfusion.

- At the time of hemorrhage, it is *imperative* to have an ophthalmologist present who can monitor intraocular pressure and take the appropriate steps to preserve central retinal artery perfusion. Lack of perfusion for even short periods of time can lead to permanent, devastating loss of vision.

- Surgical decompression may be required in severe cases, but in most cases surgery has only to be postponed.[48]

- Venous puncture may occur after both retrobulbar and peribulbar injection. It leads to noncompressive hematoma, the consequences of which are much less severe, so that in most cases surgery can be carried on.

- Patients who are on anticoagulants (even aspirin and similar medications) should probably undergo sub-Tenon's or topical anesthesia to minimize the risk of hemorrhage.

Direct optic nerve trauma by the needle is rare but may result in blindness. Computed tomography imaging usually shows optic nerve enlargement caused by intraneural hematoma.[35,49] Overall, there is a 1–3% chance of

Table 21–2.

Other, Minor Complications

Complication	Comment
Chemosis (subconjunctival edema)	Usually of minimal concern; disappears with pressure
Venous hemorrhage	Usually mild and while unsightly, it is easily controlled
Arterial hemorrhage	Can be dramatic, causing proptosis, extensive subconjunctival and lid hematoma, and a dramatic increase in intraocular pressure. It often necessitates postponement of surgery
Globe perforation	Probably more likely in long myopic eyes. A long eye has thinner sclera and may have an irregular outline (staphylomata). The needle should be inserted tangentially to the globe and should move freely in the orbital fat without rotating the globe
Damage to the optic nerve	A result from direct trauma, injection into nerve sheath, or the ischemic consequences of the pressure on injection
Decreased visual acuity	Resolves with resolution of the block
Myotoxicity	May follow the use of high concentrations of LA (eg, 4% lidocaine) or direct injection into a muscle and may result in muscle palsy[39]
Systemic complications:	Include potential for subarachnoid injection during retrobulbar block as a cause of respiratory arrest[30]
Grand mal seizures, loss of consciousness, and respiratory depression or cardiac arrest	These complications can result from systemic LA toxicity, injection of LA into the optic nerve sheath, or retrograde arterial flow
Pulmonary edema	Rare, the mechanism poorly understood[31]
Reaction to epinephrine	Often inappropriately referred to as "Epinephrine toxicity." In patients with hypertension, angina, or arrhythmias, the amount of epinephrine injected with the LA should be reduced
Oculocardiac reflex, vasovagal reaction	See text for presentation and management
Allergic reaction to LA	Extremely rare with amide-type local anesthetics

LA = local anesthetic

complications, often necessitating postponement of the planned surgery. Since some complications may be life-threatening if patients are not immediately resuscitated, it is recommended that an anesthesiologist be present and monitor the patient throughout the entire immediate perioperative period.[50]

Clinical Pearls

OCULOCARDIAC REFLEX: QUICK FACTS (FIGURE 21–6)

- Bradycardia occurs due to traction on the extraocular muscles, conjunctiva, orbital structures, pressure on the globe, retrobulbar block, ocular trauma, pressure on tissue remaining after enucleation.

- Pathways: trigeminal afferent, vagal efferent.
- Any arrhythmia including ventricular tachycardia and rarely asystole can occur.
- Incidence highest in children: up to 90% without pretreatment with atropine.
- Prophylaxis in children: 0.02 mg/kg or glycopyrolate. 0.01 mg/kg prior to surgery is indicated.
- Intramuscular atropine not useful: onset too slow.
- Prophylaxis in adults is usually not indicated.
- Treatment: removal of stimulus, anticholinergics, check depth of anesthesia (when general anesthesia is used).

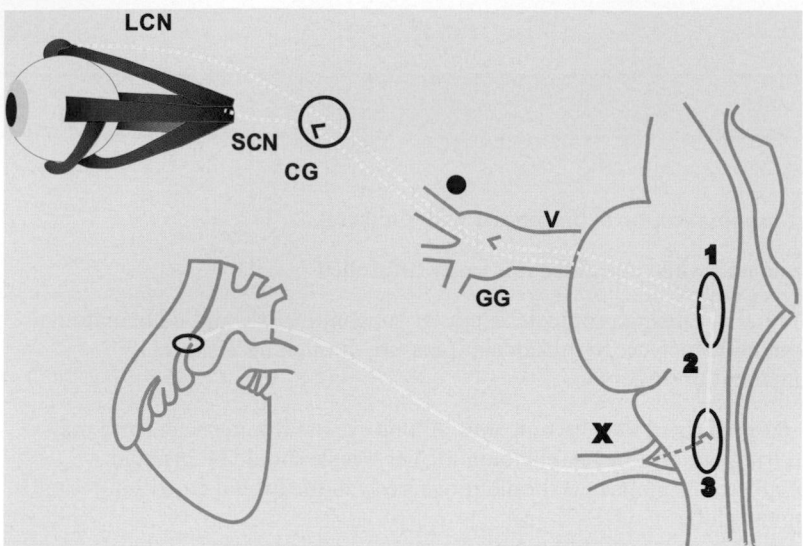

Figure 21–6. Oculocardiac reflex pathways. LCN = long ciliary nerve; SCN = short ciliary nerve; CG = ciliary ganglion; GG = geniculate ganglion; V = fifth cranial nerve; X = tenth cranial nerve; (1) main sensory nucleus of the trigeminal nerve; (2) short internuncial fibers in the reticular formation; (3) motor nucleus of the vagus nerve.

TOPICAL ANESTHESIA

Instillation of LA eye drops provides corneal anesthesia, thus allowing cataract surgery by phacoemulsification (Figure 21–7). It is quick and simple to perform and avoids the potential hazards of needle techniques. The technique is used in up to 50% of the cataract surgeries performed worldwide.[1] Some surgeons prefer topical anesthesia for routine phacoemulsification in more than 90% of their cases; however, the lack of akinesia and intraocular pressure control, along with its short duration, may make surgery hazardous.[51] Therefore, use of topical anesthesia is best limited to uncomplicated procedures performed by experienced surgeons in cooperative patients. Whenever phacoemulsification is not possible, total akinesia is still required and topical anesthesia may not be suitable. This may be the case in world areas in which phacoemulsification is not technically available

and in some specific indications.[52,53] Because anesthesia may be incomplete, patients randomly assigned to one technique for one eye and the other technique for the other eye prefer the retrobulbar to the topical technique (71% vs 10%).[54] Intraoperative comfort is more reproducibly obtained with retrobulbar[51,54,56] or sub-Tenon's[55] blocks than with topical anesthesia. Intracameral injection of LA has also been proposed to enhance analgesia.[57] It consists of injecting small amounts of LA (0.1 mL) in the anterior chamber at the beginning of, or during, surgery. Intracameral anesthetic should be preservative-free. Some concerns have been expressed about the toxicity effects of LA on corneal endothelium, which is unable to regenerate. The safety of intracameral injection seems acceptable in this regard,[58] but its analgesic benefit when compared with simple topical anesthesia has not been established.[56,59–62] The insertion of sponges soaked in LA into the conjunctival fornices has also been proposed.[63] The use of lidocaine jelly instead of eye drops seems to enhance the quality of analgesia of the anterior segment[55,62,64] and is becoming popular for improving the patient's comfort under topical anesthesia.

PERILIMBAL (SUBCONJUNCTIVAL) ANESTHESIA

Subconjunctival injection of LA may provide analgesia of the anterior segment without akinesia. This technique has not gained wide acceptance.

EPISCLERAL (SUB-TENON'S) BLOCKS

Common Principle

Episcleral (sub-Tenon's) anesthesia, also called **parabulbar anesthesia,** places the injection into the episcleral space. This

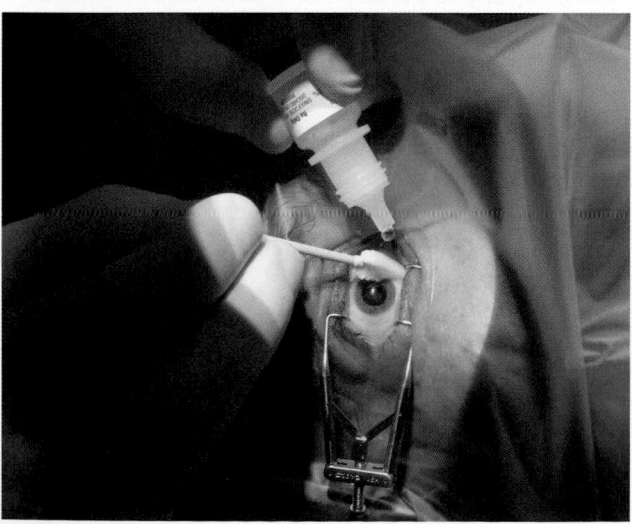

Figure 21–7. Application of topical anesthesia to the eye.

allows the LA to spread circularly around the scleral portion of the globe, ensuring high-quality analgesia of the entire globe with relatively low volumes of LA (usually 3–5 mL).[65,66] In addition, the use of a larger volume (up to 8–11 mL) causes the LA to spread to the extraocular muscle sheaths, ensuring effective and reproducible akinesia.[65–68] The occurrence of a chemosis (subconjunctival spread of the LA) is common after injecting such large volumes; it confirms the sub-Tenon's location of the injection and requires compression to resolve itself. Several approaches have been described, including needle and no-needle surgical approaches.

Needle Technique

The needle is introduced into the fornix between the semilunaris fold of the conjunctiva and the globe, tangentially to the globe (Figure 21–8).[65–67,69] After it has encroached the conjunctiva, the needle is slightly shifted medially and advanced strictly posteriorly, therefore attracting the globe and directing the gaze medially. After a small loss of resistance (click) is perceived, the globe comes back to its primary gaze position. This serves as a depth marker, thus indicating injection depth at 10 to 15 mm. The volume injected may be up to 10 mL, depending on the patient's anatomy and body size.

Using a large volume with this technique (6–11 mL) results in good globe and eye lid akinesia that is more reproducible than classic peribulbar anesthesia.[67] This technique is associated with a low risk of complications and it is simple to learn and use. In a series of 2000 cases no serious complications occurred.[69] However, as for all needle techniques, the risk of misplacement of the needle and its subsequent complications are always present and must be kept in mind.

Surgical Approach

This technique was first proposed as a supplement to (or rescue block) RBA.[70,71] After topical anesthesia, the bulbar conjunctiva is grasped with a small forceps in the inferior and nasal, superior and nasal, or superior and temporal quadrant, 5–10 mm from the limbus. Small scissors are used to open a small opening into the conjunctiva and Tenon's capsule to gain access to the episcleral space. A blunt cannula is then inserted into the episcleral space to allow the injection.[72,73] When a specialized cannula is not available, a short intravenous catheter (18- or 20-gauge) can also be used.

This technique is typically used with injection of low volumes of LA (3–5 mL). It provides good globe analgesia but only partial akinesia of the globe and lids.[74] The injection causes only a minor increase in intraocular pressure, so that preoperative compression of the globe is typically unnecessary. In a similar way, episcleral injection of a small volume of LA may be used in an open globe; it is the technique of choice as an intraoperative supplemental injection when anesthetic technique appears insufficient during surgery. Increasing the injected volume (eg, ≤11 mL) results in a good akinesia, allowing surgery of the posterior segment.[68] The main advantage of this technique is its safety as it avoids blind introduc-

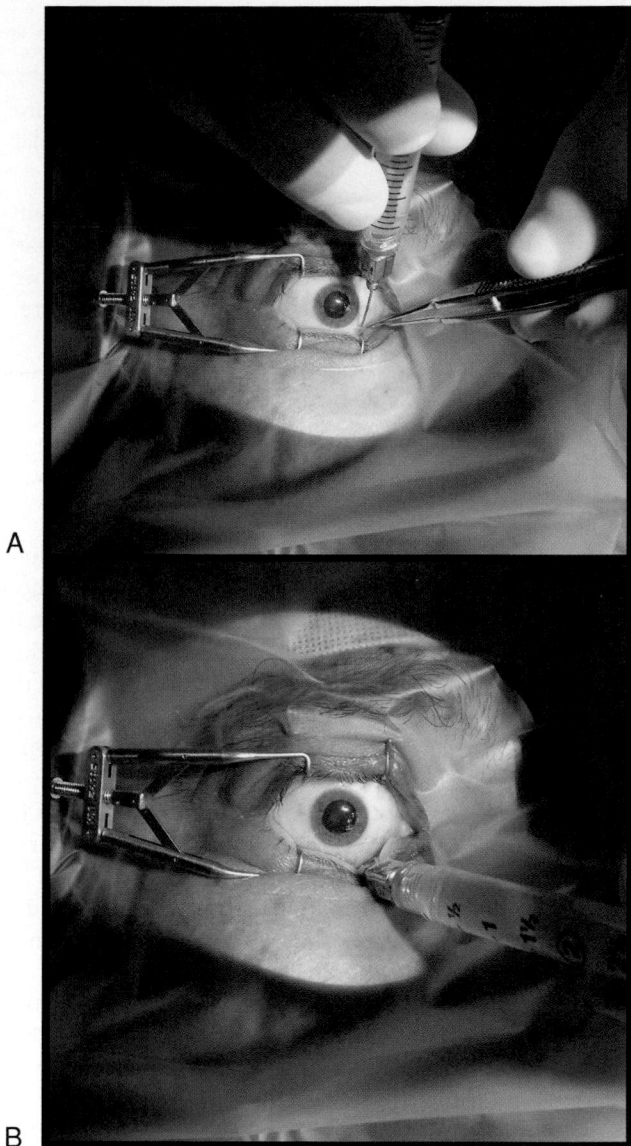

A

B

Figure 21–8. Sub-Tenon's (episcleral) block: The needle is introduced into the fornix between the semilunaris fold of the conjunctiva and the globe, tangentially to the globe.

tion of the needle into the orbit; in a series of 6000 cases, no serious complications were reported.[74] The blocks resulted in a 7% rate of subconjunctival hematoma without lasting consequences and a 6% rate of subconjunctival edema.[74] Surgery was cancelled because of subconjunctival hematoma in only 1 patient out of 6000.

USE OF EYE BLOCK FOR POSTOPERATIVE ANALGESIA

Regional anesthesia and especially sub-Tenon's block have been proposed as treatments for postoperative pain.[75] This is not required for anterior segment surgery, which usually results in minimal or no discomfort postoperatively.

Clinical Pearls

- Significant pain occurring after a cataract surgery is unusual and should raise suspicion for increased intraocular pressure or infection.

- Postoperative pain is more likely after posterior segment surgery. The use of an indwelling retrobulbar, peribulbar, or sub-Tenon's catheter has been proposed, to improve intraoperative anesthesia, to prolong postoperative regional analgesia, or to treat intractable eye pain.[76]

LOCAL ANESTHETICS & ADJUVANT AGENTS CONSIDERATIONS

All available LAs have been used for eye block, either alone or as a mixture of two different agents. The LAs used most often are lidocaine, bupivacaine, ropivacaine, mepivacaine, or a combination of two of these. The choice of LAs should be based on the pharmacologic properties and availability of the drugs, mainly depending on the requirement for a quick onset (lidocaine, mepivacaine), prolonged effect or postoperative residual block for analgesia (ropivacaine, bupivacaine), or akinesia (higher concentration). Because the amount of LA injected is usually small (3–11 mL), systemic toxicity is not a major concern.

Hyaluronidase is an enzyme that has been proposed to hasten the onset and increase the success rate of regional anesthesia for the eye. However, the literature is somewhat controversial about its benefit concerning akinesia.[77,78] Another possible benefit of hyaluronidase is in the lesser incidence of postoperative strabismus connected with its use, possibly by limiting LA myotoxicity owing to its faster spread.[79,80]

Clonidine enhances intra- and postoperative analgesia when added to the LA. At a dose of 1 mcg/kg, it does not increase the incidence of systemic adverse events such as hypotension or excessive sedation.[81] Moreover, it may help to prevent intraoperative arterial hypertension and lower intraocular pressure.

Epinephrine is sometimes used to increase the duration of eye block. However, the availability of long-acting LAs has decreased its value. Fear of vasospasm and subsequent retinal ischemia is probably not justified because the LA mixture does not spread inside the globe where retinal arteries are located.

Alkalinization of local anesthetic solutions has been proposed for decreasing pain during injection and accelerating the block onset; however, its efficacy remains unproven. Other adjuvant agents have been proposed but have not gained popularity. Small doses of a muscle relaxant may enhance akinesia, but concern has been expressed about their potential risk for systemic effects.[82] Opioids do not appear to be more efficient via a regional ophthalmic route than via systemic administration.[83] Warming the LA may decrease pain on injection and enhance block efficacy, but its benefit appears clinically negligible.[84]

Who Should Perform Eye Blocks

Since the 1980s, anesthesiologists have become increasingly involved in performing eye blocks that previously were performed only by surgeons. However, in some countries, anesthesiologists are not readily available, and surgeons have to manage the block themselves.[85] In other countries, anesthesiologists only provide sedation and monitoring, while the surgeon performs the block. In France and the United Kingdom however, anesthesiologists are often responsible for administering regional anesthesia. The available literature suggests that with proper training, anesthesiologists can perform eye blocks with the same degree of safety as for other regional anesthesia techniques.[24,29,69,74]

Perioperative Management

Eye surgery (eg, cataract surgery) carries a low risk of perioperative morbidity and mortality.[86–88] Eye block is associated with lower perioperative morbidity than is general anesthesia used for ophthalmic surgery, provided that heavy sedation is avoided.[87,88] Intraoperative monitoring should include basic monitoring (ie, electrocardiogram, pulse oximetry, and automated noninvasive blood pressure measurement). An intravascular access is often required. Older patients undergoing eye surgery frequently have coexisting diseases such as diabetes mellitus, hypertension, coronary artery disease, or cardiac insufficiency. A preoperative assessment should be routinely done to ensure that coexisting medical conditions are reasonably well controlled.

Anxiety and residual pain frequently occur during eye surgery under local or regional anesthesia. Patient immobility is required, and the presence of drapes over the head increases anxiety and impairs access to the airway. The patient should be positioned as comfortably as possible, with sufficient space to allow free breathing. Intraoperative sedation with judicious doses of sedatives may be used to limit anxiety and pain. However, exessive sedation may lead to restlessness, sleeping, snoring, or respiratory depression, which, in the absence of easy airway access, may pose a significant intraoperative challenge. Maintenance of meaningful patient contact is of paramount importance to avoid disasters that can occur with disoriented or combative patients while the surgery is underway.

SUMMARY

In summary, in developed countries, eye surgery is among the most frequently performed surgical procedures requiring anesthesia care. During the past 20 years, anesthesiologists have assumed an increasingly growing role in performing eye blocks. The requirement for a deep anesthetic block with total akinesia has been greatly lessened by use of phacoemulsification for cataract surgery, giving a more prominent role to topical anesthesia. Needle blocks carry a low but real risk of serious complications, mainly because of needle misplacement. Training and practice are required to prevent such problems.

The major patient risk factor is the presence of a myopic staphyloma. A surgical approach, sub-Tenon's block, lessens the risks of needle blocks but does not completely prevent complications. When akinesia and a dense block are required, the sub-Tenon's block appears to be the technique of choice.

References

1. Leaming DV: Practice styles and preferences of ASCRS members-2003 survey. J Cataract Refract Surg 2004;30:892–900.
2. Quigley HA: Mortality associated with ophthalmic surgery: A 20-year experience at the Wilmer Institute. Am J Ophthalmol 1974;77:517–524.
3. Breslin PP: Mortality in ophthalmic surgery. Int Ophthalmol Clin 1973;13:215–226.
4. McKibbin M: The pre-operative assessment and investigation of ophthalmic patients. Eye 1996;10:138–140.
5. Bass EB, Steinberg EP, Luthra R: Do ophthalmologists, anesthesiologists, and internists agree about preoperative testing in healthy patients undergoing cataract surgery? Arch Ophthalmol 1995;113:1248–1256.
6. Maltzman BA, Cinotti AA, Calderone JP Jr: Preadmission evaluation and elective cataract surgery. J Med Soc N J 1981;78:519–520.
7. Gilvarry A, Eustace P: The medical profile of cataract patients. Trans Ophthalmol Soc U K 1982;102:502–504.
8. Fisher SJ, Cunningham RD: The medical profile of cataract patients. Clin Geriatr Med 1985;1:339–344.
9. Hardesty DC: The Ophthalmic Surgical Patient, Medical Perioperative Management. Edited by Wolfsthal S. Appleton & Lange, 1989, pp 417–426.
10. Gild WM, Posner KL, Caplan RA, et al: Eye injuries associated with anesthesia. A closed claims analysis. Anesthesiology 1992;76:204–208.
11. Hodgkins P, Luff A, Morrell A: Current practice of cataract extraction and anaesthesia. Br J Ophthalmol 1992;76:323–326.
12. Hamilton R, Gimble H, Strunin L: Regional anaesthesia for 12,000 cataract extraction and intraocular lens implantation procedures. J Can Anaesth 1988;35:615–623.
13. Eke T, Thompson J: The national survey of local anaesthesia for ocular surgery. II. Survey methodology and current practice. Eye 1999;13:196–204.
14. Ropo A, Nikki P, Ruusuvaara P, et al: Comparison of retrobulbar and periocular injections of lignocaine by computerized tomography. Br J Ophthalmol 1991;75:417–420.
15. Koornneef L: The architecture of the musculo-fibrous apparatus in the human orbit. Acta Morphol Neerl Scand 1977;15:35–64.
16. Koornneef L: Details of the orbital connective tissue system in the adult. Acta Morphol Neerl Scand 1977;15:1–34.
17. Ripart J, Lefrant J, de La Coussaye J, et al: Peribulbar versus retrobulbar anesthesia for ophthalmic surgery. An anatomical comparison of extraconal and intraconal injections. Anesthesiology 2001;94:56–62.
18. Bloomberg L: Administration of periocular anesthesia. J Cataract Refract Surg 1986;12:677–679.
19. Davis D, Mandel M: Posterior peribulbar anesthesia: An alternative to retrobulbar anesthesia. J Cataract Refract Surg 1986;12:182–184.
20. Atkinson W: Retrobulbar injection of anesthetic within the muscular cone (cone injection). Arch Ophthalmol 1936;16:495–503.
21. Van Lindt M: Paralysie palpébrale transitoire provoquée dans l'opération de la cataracte. Ann Ocul 1914;151:420–424.
22. Liu C, Youl B, Moseley I: Magnetic resonance imaging of the optic nerve in the extremes of gaze. Implications for the positioning of the globe for retrobulbar anaesthesia. Br J Ophthalmol 1992;76:728–733.
23. Unsöld R, Stanley J, Degroot J: The C.T. topography of retrobulbar anesthesia. Anatomical correlation of implications and suggestion of a modified technique Albrecht Von Graefes. Arch Klin Exp Ophthalmol 1981;217:125–136.
24. Hamilton R, Loken R: Modified retrobulbar block. Can J Anaesth 1993;40:1219–1220.
25. Galindo A, Keilson L, Mondshine R, et al: Retro-peribulbar anesthesia: Special technique and needle design. Ophthalmol Clin North Am 1990;3:71–81.
26. Straus J: A new retrobulbar needle injection technique. Ophthalmic Surg 1988;19:134–139.
27. Bloomberg L: Anterior periocular anaesthesia: Five years experience. J Cataract Refract Surg 1991;17:508–511.
28. Davis D, Mandel M: Efficacy and complication rate of 16224 consecutive peribulbar blocks. A prospective multicenter study. J Cataract Refract Surg 1994;20:327–337.
29. Hustead R, Hamilton R, Loken R: Periocular local anesthesia: Medial orbital as an alternative to superior nasal injection. J Cataract Refract Surg 1994;20:197–201.
30. Wang BC, Bogart B, Hillman DE, et al: Subarachnoid injection—A potential complication of retrobulbar block. Anesthesiology 1989;71:845–857.
31. Kumar CM, Lawler PG: Pulmonary oedema after peribulbar block. Br J Anaesth 1999;82:777–779.
32. Demirok A, Simsek S, Cinal A, et al: Peribulbar anesthesia: One versus two injections Ophthalmic Surg Lasers 1997;28:998–1001.
33. Ball JL, Woon WH, Smith S: Globe perforation by the second peribulbar injection. Eye 2002;16:663–665.
34. Sarvela J, Nikki P: Comparison of two needle lengths in regional ophthalmic anesthesia with etidocaine and hyaluronidase. Ophthalmic Surg 1992;23:742–745.
35. Karampatakis V, Natsis K, Gigis P, Stangos N: The risk of optic nerve injury in retrobulbar anesthesia: A comparative study on 35 and 40 mm retrobulbar needles in 12 cadavers. Eur J Ophthalmol 1998;8:184–187.
36. Katsev D, Drews RC, Rose BT: Anatomic study of retrobulbar needle path length. Ophthalmology 1989;96:1221–1224.
37. Waller S, Taboada J, O'Connor P: Retrobulbar anesthesia risk: Do sharp needles really perforate the eye more easily than blunt needles? Ophthalmology 1993;100:506–510.
38. Demediuk O, Dhaliwal R, Papworth D, et al: A comparison of peribulbar and retrobulbar anesthesia for vitreoretinal surgical procedures. Arch Ophthalmol 1995;113:908–913.
39. Rainin EA, Carlson BM: Postoperative diplopia and ptosis. A clinical hypothesis based on the myotoxicity of local anesthetics. Arch Ophthalmol 1985;103:1337–1339.
40. Aldrete J, Romo-Salas F, Arora S, et al: Reverse arterial blood flow as a pathway for central nervous system toxic responses following injection of local anesthetics. Anesth Analg 1978;57:428–433.
41. Singer SB, Preston R, Hodge WG: Respiratory arrest following peribulbar anesthesia for cataract surgery: Case report and review of literature. Can J Ophthalmol 1997;32:450–454.
42. Loken R, Mervyn Kirker GE, Hamilton RC: Respiratory arrest following peribulbar anesthesia for cataract surgery: Case report and review of the literature. Can J Ophthalmol 1998;33:225–226.
43. Nicoll J, Acharya P, Ahlen K, et al: Central nervous system complication after 6000 retrobulbar blocks. Anesth Analg 1987;66:1298–1302.
44. Duker J, Belmont J, Benson W, et al: Inadvertent globe perforation during retrobulbar and peribulbar anesthesia. Ophthalmology 1991;98:519–526.
45. Edge R, Navon S: Scleral perforation during retrobulbar and peribulbar anesthesia: Risk factor and outcome in 50,000 consecutive injections. J Cataract Refract Surg 1999;25:1237–1244.
46. Vohra S, Good P: Altered globe dimensions of axial myopia as risk factors for penetrating ocular injury during peribulbar anaesthesia. Br J Anaesth 2000; 85: 242–245.
47. Carlson B, Rainin E: Rat extraocular muscle regeneration. Repair of local anesthetic-induced damage. Arch Ophthalmol 1985; 103: 1373–1377
48. Edge K, Nicoll M: Retrobulbar hemorrhage after 12,500 retrobulbar blocks. Anesth Analg 1993;76:1019–1022.

49. Hersch M, Baer G, Diecker JP, et al: Optic nerve enlargement and central retinal-artery occlusion secondary to retrobulbar anesthesia. Ann Ophthalmol 1989;21:195–197.

50. Rubin AP: Complications of local anaesthesia for ophthalmic surgery. Br J Anaesth 1995;75:93–96.

51. Rebolleda G, Munoz-Negrete FJ, Gutierrez-Ortiz C: Topical plus intracameral lidocaine versus retrobulbar anesthesia in phacotrabeculectomy: Prospective randomized study. J Cataract Refract Surg 2001;27:1214–1220.

52. Waddell KM, Reeves BC, Johnson GJ: A comparison of anterior and posterior chamber lenses after cataract extraction in rural Africa: A within patient randomized trial. Br J Ophthalmol 2004;88:734–739.

53. Bourne R, Minassian D, Dart J, et al: Effect of cataract surgery on the corneal endothelium: Modern phacoemulsification compared with extracapsular surgery. Ophthalmology 2004;11:679–685.

54. Boezaart A, Berry R, Nell M: Topical anesthesia versus retrobulbar block for cataract surgery: The patient's perspective. J Clin Anesth 2000;12:58–60.

55. Sekundo W, Dick HB, Schmidt JC: Lidocaine-assisted xylocaine jelly anesthesia versus one quadrant sub-Tenon infiltration for self-sealing sclero-corneal incision routine phacoemulsification. Eur J Ophthalmol 2004;14:111–116.

56. Pandey S, Werner L, Apple D, et al: No-anesthesia clear corneal phacoemulsification versus topical and topical plus intracameral anesthesia. Randomized clinical trial. J Cataract Refract Surg 2001;27:1643–1650.

57. Karp CL, Cox TA, Wagoner MD, et al: Intracameral anesthesia. A report by the American academy of ophthalmology. Ophthalmology 2001;108:1704–1710.

58. Heuerman T, Hartman C, Anders N: Long term endothelial cell loss after phacoemulsification: Peribulbar anesthesia versus intracameral lidocaine 1%. Prospective randomized study. J Cataract Refract Surg 2002;28:638–643.

59. Pang MP, Fujimoto DK, Wilkens LR: Pain, photophobia, and retinal and optic nerve function after phacoemulsification with intracameral lidocaine. Ophthalmology 2001;108:2018–2025.

60. Roberts T, Boytell K: A comparison of cataract surgery under topical anaesthesia with and without intracameral lignocaine. Clin Experiment Ophthalmol 2002;30:19–22.

61. Boulton J, Lopatazidis A, Luck J, et al: A randomized controlled trial of intracameral lidocaine during phacoemulsification under topical anesthesia. Ophthalmology 2000;107:68–71.

62. Bardocci A, Lofoco G, Perdicaro S, et al: Lidocaine 2% gel versus lidocaine 4% unpreserved drops for topical anesthesia in cataract surgery. A randomized controlled trial. Ophthalmology 2003;110:144–149.

63. Aziz ES: Deep topical fornix nerve block versus peribulbar block in one-step adjustable suture horizontal strabismus surgery. Br J Anaesth 2002;88:129–132.

64. Barequet IS, Soriano ES, Green WR, et al: Provision of anesthesia with single application of lidocaine gel. J Cataract Refract Surg 1999;25:626–631.

65. Ripart J, Prat-Pradal D, Charavel P, et al: Medial canthus single injection episcleral (sub-Tenon) anesthesia anatomic imaging. Clin Anat 1998;11:390–395.

66. Ripart J, Metge L, Prat-Pradal D, et al: Medial canthus single injection episcleral (sub-Tenon) anesthesia computed tomography imaging. Anesth Analg 1998;87:43–45.

67. Ripart J, Lefrant J, Vivien B, et al: Ophthalmic regional anesthesia: Canthus episcleral anesthesia is more efficient than peribulbar anesthesia. A double Blind Randomized study. J Anesthesiology 2000;92:1278–1285.

68. Li H, Abouleish A, Grady J, et al: Sub-Tenon's injection for local anesthesia in posterior segment surgery. Ophthalmology 2000;107:41–47.

69. Nouvellon E, L'Hermite J, Chaumeron A, et al: Medial canthus single injection sub-Tenon's anesthesia: A 2000 case experience. Anesthesiology 2004;100:370–374.

70. Mein C, Flynn HW: Augmentation of local anesthesia during retinal detachment surgery [letter]. Arch Ophthalmol 1989;107:1084.

71. Stevens JD: A new local anaesthesia technique for cataract extraction by one quadrant sub-Tenon's infiltration. Br J Ophthalmol 1992;76:670–674.

72. MacNeela BJ, Kumar CM: Sub-Tenon's block using ultrashort cannula. J Cataract Refract Surg 2004;30:858–862.

73. Kumar CM, Mac Neela BJ: Ultrasonic localization of anaesthetic fluids using sub Tenon's cannulae of three different lengths. Eye 2003;17:1–5.

74. Guise P: SubTenon's anesthesia: A prospective study of 6000 blocks. Anesthesiology 2003;98:964–968.

75. Duker J, Nielsen J, Vander J, et al: Retrobulbar bupivacaine irrigation for postoperative pain after scleral buckling surgery. Ophthalmology 1991;98:514–518.

76. Jonas JB, Jäger M, Hemmerling T: Continuous retrobulbar anesthesia for scleral buckling surgery using an ultra-fine spinal anesthesia catheter. Can J Anesth 2002;49:487–489.

77. Alwitryy A, Chaudhary S, Gopee K, et al: Effect of hyaluronidase on ocular motility in sub Tenon's anesthesia: Randomized controlled trial. J Cataract Refract Surg 2002;28:1420–1423.

78. Dempsey GA, Barrett PJ, Kirby IJ: Hyaluronidase and peribulbar block. Br J Anaesth 1997;78:671–674.

79. Brown S, Coats D, Collins MLZ, et al: Second cluster of strabismus cases after periocular anesthesia without hyaluronidase. J Cataract Refract Surg 2001;27:1872–1875.

80. Strouthidis NG, Sobba S, Lanigan L, et al: Vertical diplopia following peribulbar anesthesia: The role of hyaluronidase. J Pediatr Ophthalmol Starbismus 2004;41:25–30.

81. Bharti N, Madan R, Kaul HL, et al: Effect of addition of clonidine to local anaesthetic mixture for peribulbar block. Anaesth Intensive Care 2002;30:438–441.

82. Kücükyavuz Z, Arici MK: Effects of atracurium added to local anesthetics on akinesia in peribulbar block. Reg Anesth Pain Med 2002;27:487–490.

83. Hemmerling TM, Budde WM, Koppert W, et al: Retrobulbar versus systemic application of morphine during titratable regional anesthesia via retrobulbar catheter in intraocular surgery. Anesth Analg 2000;91:585–588.

84. Krause M, Weindler J, Ruprecht KW: Does warming of anesthetic solutions improve analgesia and akinesia in retrobulbar anesthesia? Ophthalmology 1997;104:429–432.

85. Hansen TE: Practice styles and preferences of Danish cataract surgeons-1995 survey. Acta Ophthalmol Scand 1996;74:56–59.

86. Eke T, Thompson JR: Eye: The national survey of local anesthesia for ocular surgery II. Safety profile of local anesthesia techniques. Eye 1999;13:196–204.

87. Glantz L, Drenger B, Gozal Y: Perioperative myocardial ischemia in cataract surgery patients: General vs local anesthesia. Anesth Analg 2000;91:1415–1419.

88. Katz J, Feldman MA, Bass EB, et al: Adverse intraoperative medical events and their association with anesthesia management strategies in cataract surgery. Ophthalmology 2001;108:1721–1726.

22

Functional Evaluation of Motor Responses for Upper Limb Blocks

André P. Boezaart, MD, PhD • Steven C. Borene, MD

INTRODUCTION

A nerve stimulator delivers a charge to a motor nerve fiber, which causes a flow of ions through the nerve membrane and initiates an action potential in the nerve fiber.[1] The larger the delivered charge, the more motor fibers in the motor nerve fascicle will fire and the stronger the resulting motor response until a maximal motor response is reached. Several factors influence the total charge delivered to a nerve fiber. The duration and intensity of the current are the main variables. The impedance of the tissue between the stimulating surface (needle or catheter) and the nerve further influence the current intensity. This is reduced as the distance from the stimulating surface to the nerve is reduced. In addition, the type of tissue between the stimulating surface and the nerve, the type of electrode used, and the polarity of the electrode affect the total impedance of the system and thus affect the motor response to stimulation. Muscle mass is also important, such that a stimulus in a frail 80-year-old woman differs substantially from a motor response from a similar electrical response delivered to a young muscular patient.[1]

Beyond exposure to regional anesthesia during training, an important aspect in developing confidence and proficiency in the placement of peripheral nerve blocks is through observing a well-defined motor response to neurostimulation. At the level of the roots, the brachial plexus originates from five separate nerve bundles, mainly divided into posterior sensory fibers and anterior motor fibers[2] (Figure 22–1). More distally, the five roots of the brachial plexus converge to form three trunks: the superior, middle, and inferior trunks. The brachial plexus then divides into the three cords, and finally the seven terminal branches are formed. The three cords are named according to their

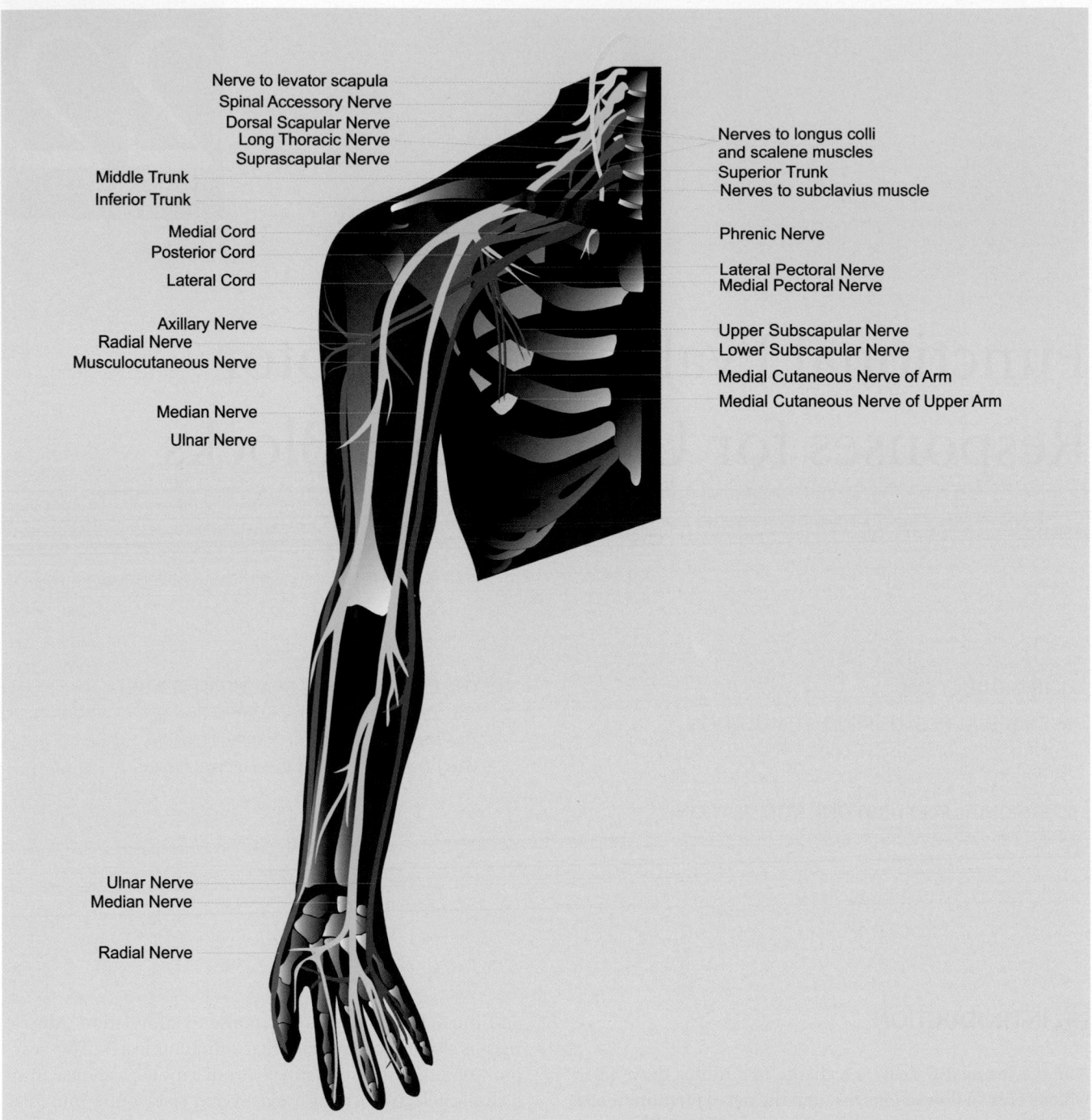

Nerve to levator scapula
Spinal Accessory Nerve
Dorsal Scapular Nerve
Long Thoracic Nerve
Suprascapular Nerve

Middle Trunk
Inferior Trunk

Medial Cord
Posterior Cord

Lateral Cord

Axillary Nerve
Radial Nerve
Musculocutaneous Nerve

Median Nerve

Ulnar Nerve

Nerves to longus colli
and scalene muscles
Superior Trunk
Nerves to subclavius muscle

Phrenic Nerve

Lateral Pectoral Nerve
Medial Pectoral Nerve

Upper Subscapular Nerve
Lower Subscapular Nerve
Medial Cutaneous Nerve of Arm
Medial Cutaneous Nerve of Upper Arm

Ulnar Nerve
Median Nerve

Radial Nerve

Figure 22–1. Schematic representation of the nerves of the brachial plexus and upper extremity.

relation to the axillary artery: posterior, lateral, and medial (see Figure 22–1).

Success with brachial plexus blockade requires the identification and block of the appropriate roots, trunks, cords, and peripheral nerves for the proposed surgery.[3] Accurately identifying the correct nerve bundles and avoiding injection of incorrect nerves may lead to higher success rates if the single stimulation technique of the infraclavicular block, for example, is followed,[4,5] or it may lead to shorter latency periods if the multiple stimulation technique[6] is chosen. In the case of blocks at the trunk level, it is also important to recognize false motor responses and avoid injecting local anesthetic when these are elicited.[7]

Whichever approach to blocks of the brachial plexus is chosen, elicitation of specific muscle twitches when each nerve bundle is stimulated is often confusing for trainees and experienced anesthesiologists alike. This chapter describes a simple and consistent way to teach and remember the motor responses elicited by electrical stimulation of the different nerve bundles.

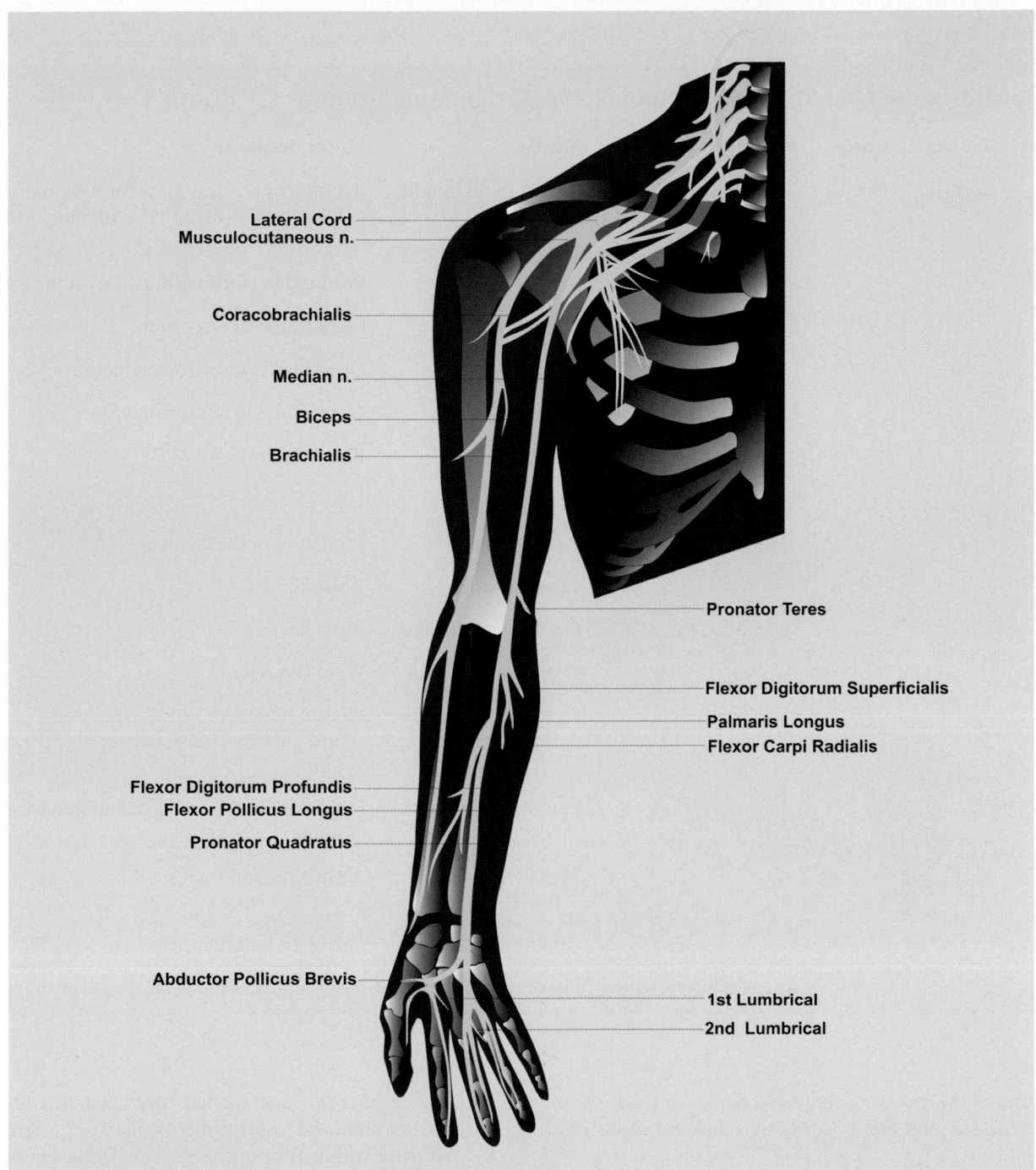

Figure 22–2. Schematic representation of the nerves derived from the lateral cord of the brachial plexus.

BRACHIAL PLEXUS ROOT STIMULATION

Fifth, Sixth, & Seventh Cervical Roots (C5, C6, & C7)

When studying Figure 22–1, it can be seen that the fifth cervical root (C5) and the superior parts of the sixth and seventh cervical roots (C6 and C7) form most of the superior and middle trunk and all of the lateral cord of the brachial plexus

(Figure 22–2). Fibers from the C5, C6, and C7 roots then terminate in the dorsal scapular nerve, suprascapular nerve, lateral pectoral nerve, musculocutaneous nerve, and part of the median nerve (Table 22–1). Electrical stimulation of only the C5 root, as with the cervical paravertebral block,[8,9] for example, therefore results in a motor response in any or all of the muscles supplied by the above nerves (rhomboid muscles, rotator cuff muscles, major pectoral muscle, biceps muscle,

Table 22–1.

Motor Response Due to Stimulation of Nerves Originating from the C5 Root

Roots	Trunks	Cords	Peripheral Nerves	Muscle	Motor Response
C5	Superior	Lateral	Nerve to scalene muscles	Anterior and middle scalene	Bending of cervical spine forward and ipsolaterally, with slight rotation to the other side
			Long thoracic	Serratus anterior	Protraction (forward drawing) of the scapula
			Suprascapular	Infraspinatus	Glenohumeral extension
				Supraspinatus	Glenohumeral vertical abduction
			Lateral pectoral	Pectoralis major	Glenohumeral adduction
			Musculocutaneous	Biceps brachii	Elbow flexion
				Brachialis	Elbow flexion
			Median	Pronator teres	Pronation of the forearm
				Palmaris longus	Wrist flexion
				Flexor carpi radialis	Wrist flexion
				Flexor carpi radialis	Wrist abduction
				Flexor digitorum superficialis	Flexion of fingers [metacarpal phalangeal and proximal interphalangeal (PIP) joints]
				Lumbrical I and II	Extension of PIP and distal interphalangeal joints
				Abductor pollicis brevis	Abduction and rotation thumb
				Opponens pollicis	Opposition of thumb
			Anterior interosseous	Flexor pollicis longus	Flexion of interphalangeal joint of thumb

pronators of the forearm, superficial flexors of the forearm, and first and second lumbricals of the hand and abductor of the thumb).

It is, however, almost never possible to achieve pure C5 stimulation. With cervical paravertebral block, the needle is aimed toward the C6 root.[8] Electrical stimulation of the C6 and C7 roots results in motor responses in the muscles supplied by nerves branching off the posterior cord (Figure 22–3), that is, the deltoid muscle (axillary nerve), extensors of the arm (radial nerve) (Table 22–2) and also any combination of the above muscles supplied by the nerves branching from the lateral cord (see Table 22–1).

Eighth Cervical & First Thoracic Root (C8 & T1)

The roots of C8 and T1 continue to form the inferior trunk (see Figure 22–1). Fibers coming from C8 continue to join the posterior and medial cords, whereas fibers of the T1 root continue to form the medial cord (Figure 22–4). Electrical stimulation of the inferior trunk causes contractions of all, or combinations of, the muscles supplied by nerves branching off the posterior cord (see Table 22–2), but mainly of the muscles supplied by the nerves coming from the medial cord (Table 22–3). These are the minor pectoral muscle (medial pectoral nerve) and muscles supplied by the ulnar nerve (flexor carpi ulnaris, flexor digitorum profundus, adductor pollicis, flexor pollicis, the interosseous muscles of the hand, the third and fourth lumbricals and flexors, and flexor and opponens digiti minimi (Table 22–3).

Sensory distribution of blocks performed at the level of root cover the total upper limb with the exception of the skin around the shoulder joint and clavicle, which is innervated by nerves from the superficial cervical plexus (Figure 22–5),

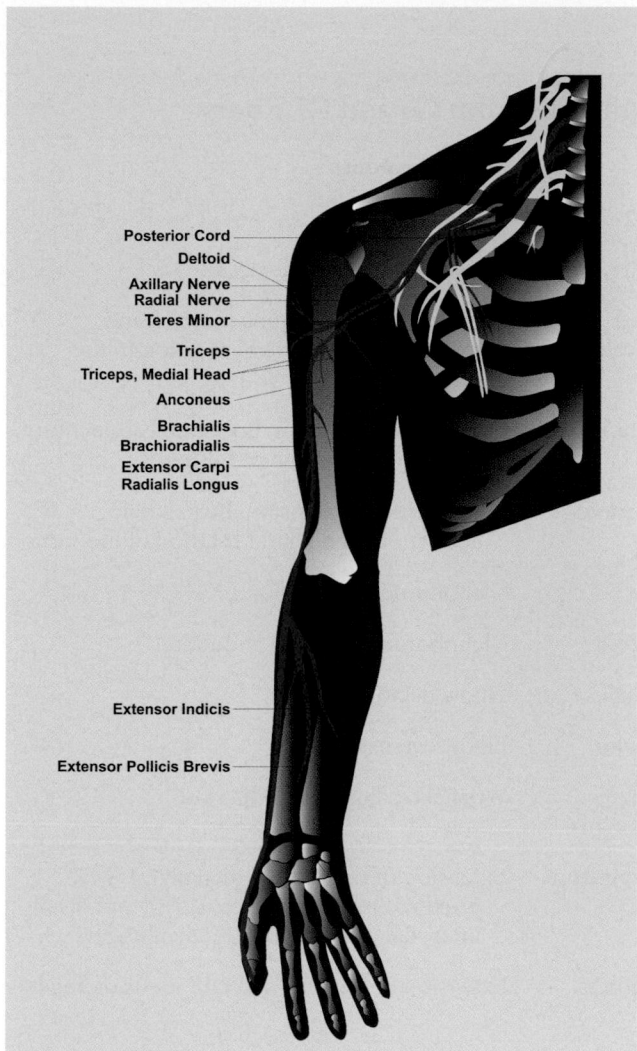

Figure 22–3. Schematic representation of the nerves derived from the posterior cord of the brachial plexus.

and the skin on the medial upper arm, just distal to the axilla, which is innervated by the intercostobrachial nerve.

Clinical Pearls

- Electrical stimulation of the superior three roots of the brachial plexus (C5, C6, and C7), as seen with cervical paravertebral block for shoulder surgery, results mainly in motor responses in the posterior and anterior shoulder girdle muscles and flexor and extensor muscles of the proximal arm.

- Electrical stimulation of the inferior two roots of the brachial plexus (C8 and T1), as seen with cervical paravertebral block for wrist surgery, results mainly in motor responses in the deep flexor muscles of the hand.

- The upper and lower limits of the current intensity for successful blocks at the level of the roots have not yet been established. For example, Wehling and colleagues[10] reported a case in which successful cervical paravertebral block was obtained without any untoward sequelae after stimulating through a catheter at a nerve stimulator current output of 0.05 mA and 300 μsec. On the other hand, in the original description of the continuous cervical paravertebral block currents of up to 3 mA were advocated.[8,9]

- Blocks at the level of the roots of the brachial plexus are ideal for continuous blocks for major surgery to all three large joints of the upper limb.

BRACHIAL PLEXUS TRUNK STIMULATION

Nerve conduction studies have demonstrated that electrical stimulation of the proximal aspects of all three brachial plexus trunks, as classically done during interscalene block, results in a motor response mainly of the muscles supplied by the radial nerve[11] (see Table 22–2). Moving the stimulating probe to the distal part of the superior trunk of the brachial plexus results in motor responses in the muscles supplied by the musculocutaneous nerve (flexion at the elbow due to biceps contraction) and axillary nerve (abduction of the arm due to deltoid contraction)[11] (see Table 22–1). If the inferior part of the inferior trunk is electrically stimulated, a flexor response can be observed in the hand resulting from a motor response in the muscles supplied by the median and ulnar nerves[11] (see Tables 22–1 and 22–3).

When attempting an interscalene block, it is equally important to know which motor responses are not acceptable. At the level at which the interscalene block is done, there are five other nerves that do not form part of the brachial plexus. Stimulating these nerves can lead to misleading motor responses, and if these "false" motor responses are incorrectly accepted, the confusion may ultimately lead to failed blocks.

From Figure 22–6, it can be seen that the phrenic nerve (1) is situated on the belly of the anterior scalene muscle. Stimulating this nerve results in a motor response of the diaphragm, which can clearly be seen as abdominal twitches. Phrenic nerve twitch should not be relied upon.

Approximately 1 cm posterior from the phrenic nerve between the anterior (2) and middle scalene muscles (4) are the trunks of the brachial plexus (3). Electrical nerve stimulation of the trunks here results in a triceps muscle motor response if stimulated proximally and in biceps and deltoid responses if stimulated distally on the superior trunk. A flexion hand motor response indicates that the inferior part of the inferior trunk is being stimulated, which means that the needle is deep to the superior and middle trunks and probably close to the dome of the lung.

Table 22–2.

Motor Response Due to Stimulation of Nerves Originating from C6 and C7 Roots

Roots	Trunks	Cords	Peripheral Nerves	Muscle	Motor Response
C6	Superior	Lateral	See Table 22–1	See Table 22–1	See Table 22–1
C7	Middle	Posterior	N. to longus colli	Longus colli	Forward flexion of the neck
			N. to scalene muscles	Anterior and middle scalene	Bending of cervical spine forward and ipsolaterally with slight rotation to the other side
			Axillary	Anterior deltoid	Glenohumeral flexion, horizontal abduction, and medial rotation of humerus
				Posterior deltoid	Glenohumeral extension, horizontal abduction, and lateral rotation of humerus
				Teres minor	Glenohumeral extension
				Middle deltoid	Glenohumeral vertical abduction
			Radial	Brachioradialis	Elbow flexion
				Triceps brachii	Elbow extension
				Extensor carpi radialis longus	Wrist extension and abduction
			Posterior interosseous	Extensor digitorum	Extension of metacarpal phalangeal (MP), proximal interphalangeal (PIP), and distal interphalangeal (DIP) joints of fingers
			Posterior interosseous	Extensor indices	Extension of MP, PIP, and DIP joints of fingers
			Posterior interosseous	Extensor digiti minimi	Extension of MP, PIP, and DIP of fifth finger
			Posterior interosseous	Extensor pollicis brevis	Extension of MP joint thumb
			Posterior interosseous	Extensor pollicis longus	Extension of interphalangeal joint of thumb
			Posterior interosseous	Abductor pollicis longus	Abduction of thumb

The dorsal scapular nerve (5), which originates from the C5 root, exits 1 cm farther posterior between the middle and posterior scalene muscles (see Figure 22–6). This nerve supplies the rhomboid muscles. Electrical stimulation results in medial and superior movements of the scapula. If the elbow is flexed and the hand of the patient rests on the abdomen, the elbow may be fixed on the bed and the medial movements of the scapula may be confused with abduction of the arm owing to deltoid contractions. This is a very common cause of confusion and failed block.

The suprascapular nerve (6) originates from the superior trunk and exits between the middle and posterior scalene muscles a few cm more lateral than the dorsal scapular nerve (see Figure 22–6). This nerve supplies mainly the muscles of the rotator cuff, which cause internal rotation of the humerus when the nerve is electrically stimulated. Like the dorsal scapular nerve, if the elbow is flexed and the hand of the patient is on the abdomen, rotation of the humerus can create an impression that the arm is abducting. This can mimic deltoid contractions. Electrical stimulation of this nerve, therefore, also frequently leads to confusion and failed block.

Farther posterior is the nerve to the levator scapulae muscle (7), which originates from the cervical plexus. Electrical stimulation of this nerve causes a motor response in

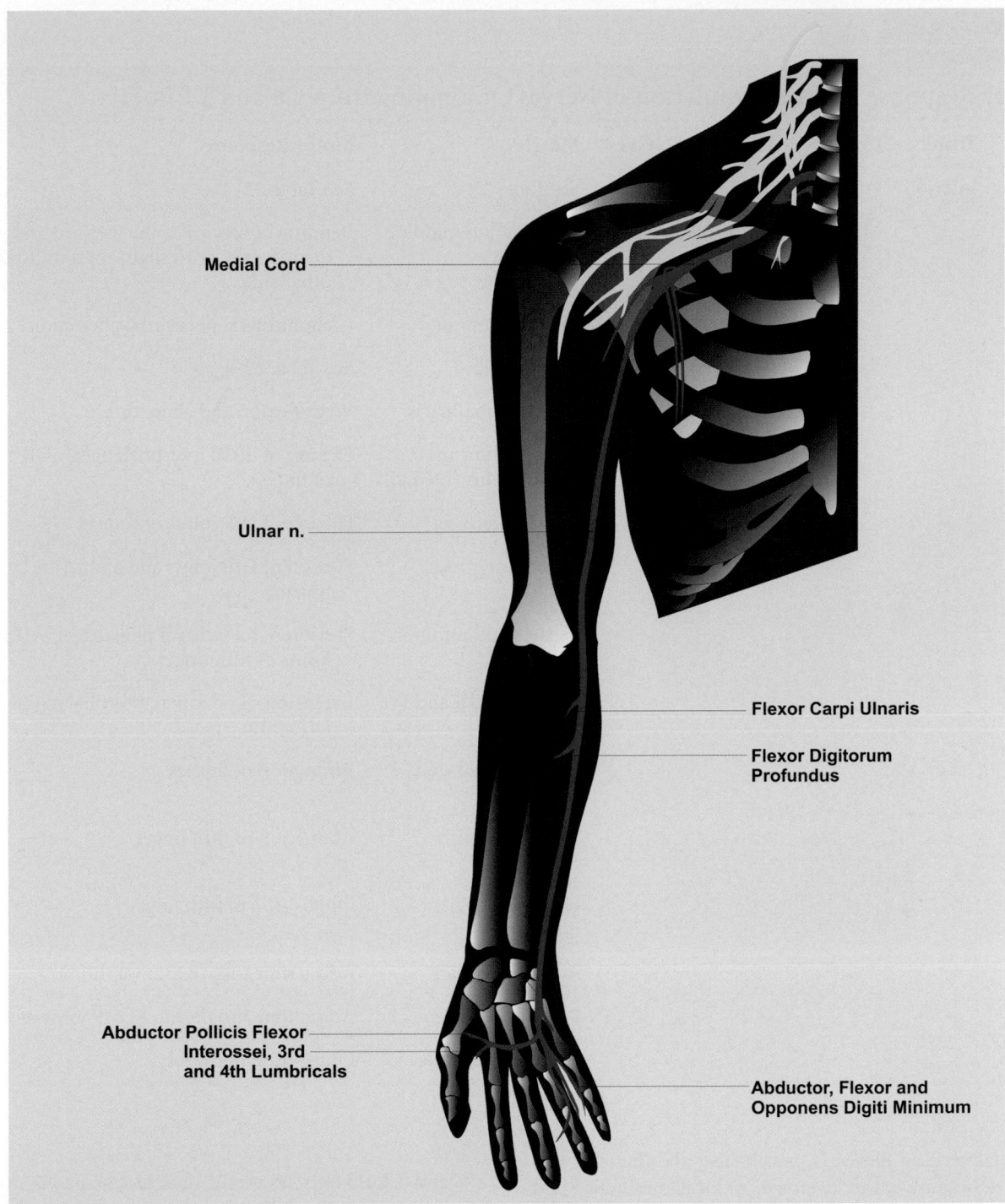

Figure 22–4. Schematic representation of the nerves derived from the medial cord of the brachial plexus.

the levator scapulae muscle and subsequent elevation of the scapula, which, like the dorsal scapular and suprascapular nerves, can cause confusion and failed block.

The accessory nerve (8), which is a cranial nerve, is farther posterior and superficial to the fascia, which forms the floor of the posterior triangle of the neck (see Figure 22–6). It runs parallel with the trapezius muscle, which it supplies. Electrical stimulation of this nerve causes a motor response on the trapezius muscle, which is elevation of the scapula. Like the other three nerves mentioned previously, electrical stimulation of the accessory nerve can result in failed block.

Sensory distribution of blocks done at the trunk level covers the lateral part of the upper limb if the superior and middle trunks are blocked. The skin around the shoulder joint and clavicle, which is innervated by nerves from the

Table 22–3.

Motor Response Due to Stimulation of Nerves Originating from C8 and T1 Roots

Roots	Trunks	Cords	Peripheral Nerves	Muscle	Motor Response
C8	Inferior	Posterior	See Table 22–2	See Table 22–2	See Table 22–2
T1		Medial	N. to scalene muscles	Anterior and middle scalene	Bending of cervical spine forward and ipsolaterally, with slight rotation to the other side
			Medial pectoral	Pectoralis minor	Glenohumeral horizontal abduction
			Median	See Table 22–1	See Table 22–1
			Ulnar	Flexor carpi ulnaris	Wrist flexion and abduction
				Flexor digitorum profundus (medial)	Flexion of distal interphalangeal (DIP) joints of fingers
				Dorsal interossei	Flexion of DIP joints of fingers
				Palmar interossei	Flexion of DIP joints and abduction of fingers
				Flexor digiti minimi brevis	Flexion of metacarpal phalangeal (MP) joints of fifth finger
				Lumbricals III and IV	Extension of proximal interphalangeal and DIP joints
				Dorsal interosseous muscles	Abduction of fingers
				Abductor digiti minimi	Abduction of fifth finger
				Opponens digiti minimi	Opposition of fifth finger
				Adductor pollicis	Adduction and rotation of thumb
				Palmar interosseous I	Adduction and flexion of MP joint of thumb
				Opponens pollicis	Opposition of thumb

superficial cervical plexus is usually also anesthetized with this block because of the "overflow" of local anesthetic agent to the superficial cervical plexus.

Clinical Pearls

- Electrical nerve stimulation of the proximal portion of all three trunks results in a triceps motor response *via* the radial nerve.
- Electrical nerve stimulation of the distal portion of the superior trunk results in a motor response of the biceps and deltoid muscles via the musculocutaneous and axillary nerves, respectively.

- Electrical stimulation of the inferior portion of the inferior trunk causes a flexor response of the hand.

- The phrenic nerve is on the belly of the anterior scalene muscle, and electrical stimulation of this nerve causes a motor response of the diaphragm.

- There are four nerves posterior to the brachial plexus at the trunk level that frequently cause confusion, leading to failed blocks (from anterior to posterior): the dorsal scapular nerve, which supplies the rhomboid muscles;

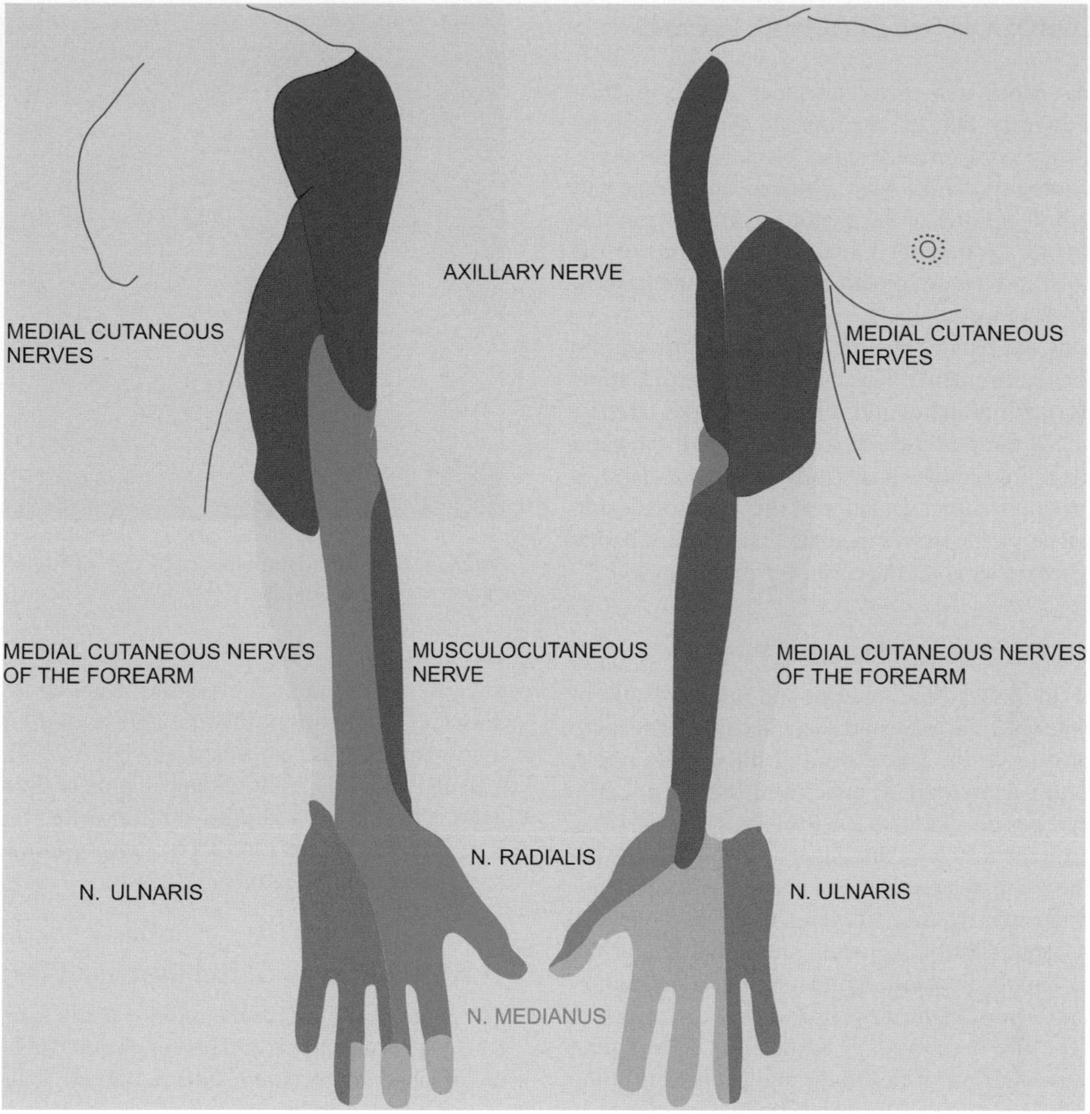

MEDIAL CUTANEOUS
NERVES

AXILLARY NERVE

MEDIAL CUTANEOUS
NERVES

MEDIAL CUTANEOUS NERVES
OF THE FOREARM

MUSCULOCUTANEOUS
NERVE

MEDIAL CUTANEOUS NERVES
OF THE FOREARM

N. RADIALIS

N. ULNARIS

N. ULNARIS

N. MEDIANUS

Figure 22–5. Sensory distribution of block of the brachial plexus.

the suprascapular nerve, which innervates the rotator cuff muscles; the nerve to the levator scapulae muscle, which elevates the scapula; and the accessory nerve, which is a cranial nerve and innervates the trapezius muscle.

- Blocks at the level of the trunks of the brachial plexus result in a dose- and volume-dependent sensory block of the lateral aspects of the arm and shoulder.

- Generally speaking, motor twitches anterior to the clavicle and in the arm result in successful interscalene block, whereas motor responses in muscles posterior to the clavicle result in failed blocks.

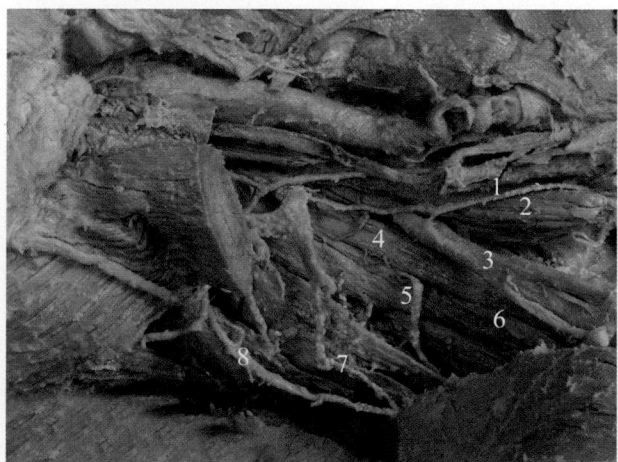

Figure 22–6. Anatomy of the lateral aspect of the neck (the nerve structures are labeled from anterior to posterior): (1) phrenic nerve; (2) anterior scalene muscle; (3) brachial plexus; (4) middle scalene muscle; (5) dorsal scapular nerve; (6) supraclavicular nerve; (7) nerve to levator scapulae; (8) accessory nerve.

THE CORDS OF THE BRACHIAL PLEXUS

Infraclavicular block is a cord-level block of the brachial plexus. It is essential that the appropriate cord or cords be blocked for successful infraclavicular block.[3] Anatomists[12] and anesthesiologists[13] alike have criticized this simple and practical method because of the anatomic variations in this region. There are 29 described anatomic variations of the brachial plexus, and it is not practical for anesthesiologists to remember all these variations.[14]

Basically, the pinkie, or fifth digit, moves toward the cord that is being stimulated. Thus, if the lateral cord is stimulated, the forearm pronates and the pinkie moves laterally (Figure 22–7). If the posterior cord is stimulated, the hand extends and the pinkie moves posteriorly. Finally, medial cord stimulation results in ulnar deviation at the wrist and flexion of the hand. The pinkie moves medially. Therefore, a handy acronym to remember is "at the cords, the pinkie towards."

The Lateral Cord of the Brachial Plexus

The anterior divisions of the superior and middle trunks of the brachial plexus unite to form the lateral cord.[15] The musculocutaneous nerve, the lateral head of the median nerve, and the lateral pectoral nerves arise from this cord.[16] The musculocutaneous nerve innervates the biceps brachii, coracobrachialis, all the flexors of the upper arm, and the medial portion of the brachialis muscle. The lateral head of the median nerve innervates the pronator teres, flexor carpi radialis, flexor pollicis longus, flexor digitorum profundus (lateral half to digits 2, 3), and the first and second lumbricals and abductor pollicis brevis muscles via the palmar digital and recurrent branches of the median nerve.[16–19] Stimulation of the lateral cord thus causes flexion of the elbow and pronation of the

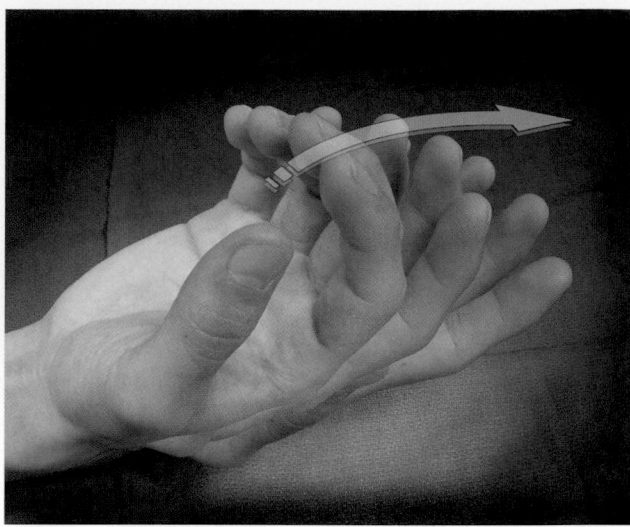

Figure 22–8. Neurostimulation of the posterior cord (pinkie moves mainly posteriorly).

forearm due to contractions of the biceps and pronator teres muscles.[16] In addition, the first and second lumbricals and thenar muscles also contract (see Figure 22–2). Overall, the fifth digit moves laterally with pronation of the forearm if the hand is held in the anatomic position when the lateral cord is stimulated (Figure 22–8). The sensory innervation of the lateral cord is outlined in Table 22–4.

The Medial Cord of the Brachial Plexus

The anterior division of the inferior trunk forms the medial cord.[15] The medial pectoral nerves, the medial brachial nerve, the antebrachial cutaneous nerve, the ulnar nerve, and the

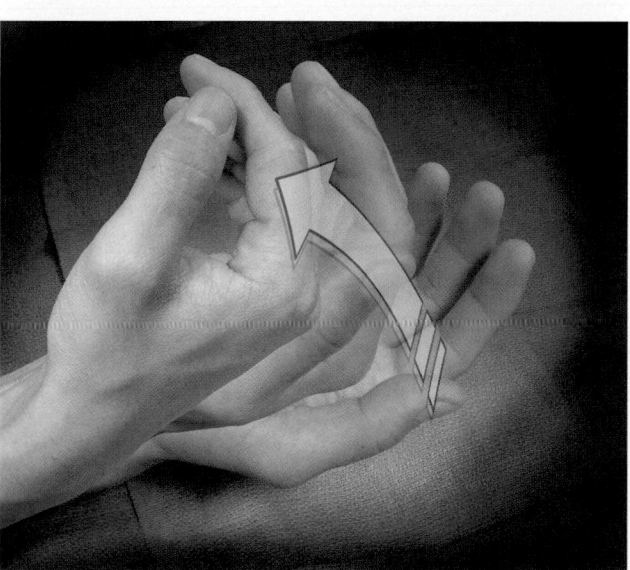

Figure 22–7. Neurostimulation of the lateral cord (pinkie moves mainly laterally).

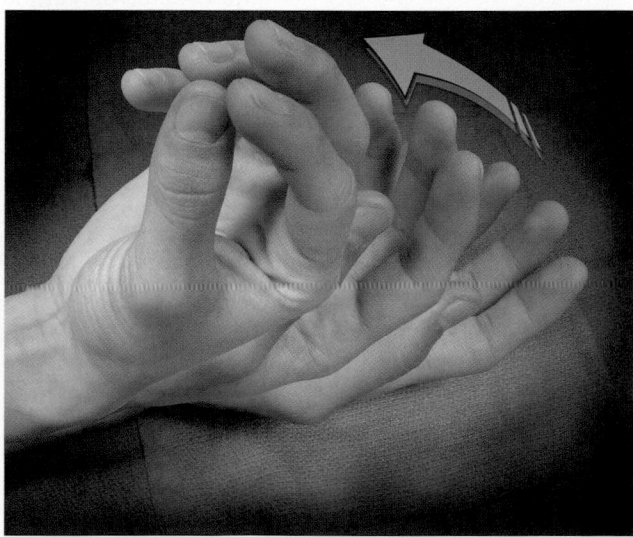

Figure 22–9. Neurostimulation of the medial cord (pinkie moves mainly medially).

Table 22–4.

Sensory Innervation of the Lateral Cord

Cord	Sensory Supply Area	Via Nerve
Lateral	Coracoclavicular ligaments, subacromial bursa, and acromioclavicular joint	Articular branch of lateral pectoral nerve (C6, 7) (also suprascapular nerve from superior trunk)
	Shoulder joint	Musculocutaneous nerve (C5, 6, 7)
	Preaxial border of the forearm as far distally as the ball of the thumb	Lateral cutaneous nerve of the forearm (terminal musculocutaneous nerve (C5, 6, 7)
	Anterior part of the capsule of the wrist joint and carpal joints	Anterior interosseous branch of the (lateral head) of median nerve (C6, 7)

medial head of the median nerve all arise from this cord.[16] The primary motor nerve of the medial cord is the ulnar nerve, which innervates flexor carpi ulnaris, palmaris brevis, flexor digitorum profundus (medial half to the fourth and fifth digits), and the palmar and dorsal interosseous muscles, the hypothenar muscles, and the third and fourth lumbrical muscles from the deep palmar branch.[17,18] Stimulation of the medial cord causes contraction of these deep flexors of the hand, as well as ulnar deviation of the wrist[16] (see Figure 22–4). Overall, it appears as if the fifth digit is moving medially if the hand is held in the anatomic position when the medial cord is stimulated (Figure 22–9). The sensory innervation of the medial cord is outlined in Table 22–5.

The Posterior Cord of the Brachial Plexus

The posterior divisions of all three trunks of the brachial plexus form the posterior cord.[15] The subscapular and tho-racodorsal nerves, axillary nerve, and radial nerve arise from this cord.[16] The subscapular nerve innervates the teres major muscle through the lower subscapular nerve and the subscapularis by the upper subscapular nerve. The thoracodorsal (middle subscapular) nerve innervates the latissimus dorsi. The axillary nerve innervates the deltoid muscle, as well as the teres minor muscle. The dominant posterior cord motor nerve is the radial nerve. It supplies all three heads of the triceps brachii muscle, the lateral portion of the brachialis muscle, and the entire extensor–supinator group of muscles.[19] Stimulation of the posterior cord causes muscle twitches of the extensor muscles of the forearm, hand, and fingers and contraction of the muscles of the rotator cuff and the deltoid muscle[16] (see Figure 22–3) Overall, the fifth digit moves posteriorly from the anatomic position with neurostimulation of the posterior cord (Figure 22–9). The sensory innervation of the posterior cord is outlined in Table 22–6.

Table 22–5.

Sensory Innervation of the Medial Cord

Cord	Sensory Supply Area	Via Nerve
Medial	Flexor surface and nails of $3\frac{1}{2}$ radial digits and a corresponding area of the palm	Medial head of median nerve (C8, T1)
	Skin on the front and medial sides of the upper arm	Medial cutaneous nerve of the arm (T1)
	Skin over medial side of the forearm	Medial cutaneous nerve of the forearm (C8, T1)
	Medial ligament of the elbow joint	Ulnar nerve (C7, 8, T1)
	Dorsum of the hand and dorsum of ulnar $1\frac{1}{2}$ fingers	Ulnar nerve (C7, 8, T1)
	Flexor surface of ulnar $1\frac{1}{2}$ fingers, including their nail beds	Ulnar nerve (C7, 8, T1) (Medial pectoral nerve apparently has no sensory function)

Table 22–6.

Sensory Innervation of the Posterior Cord

Cord	Sensory Supply Area	Via Nerve
Posterior	Glenohumeral (shoulder) joint	Axillary (circumflex)nerve (C5)
	Skin over lower half of deltoid muscle	Upper lateral cutaneous nerve (a branch of the axillary nerve)
	Skin over the center of deltoid muscle	Anterior branch of axillary nerve
	Skin along extensor surface of upper arm down to the elbow	Posterior cutaneous nerve of the arm (a branch of the radial nerve) (C5, 6, 7, 8, T-1)
	Skin over the lateral part of the upper arm	Lower lateral cutaneous nerve of the arm down to the elbow (a branch of the radial nerve) (C5, 6, 7, 8, T-1)
	Skin over extensor surface of the forearm to the wrist	Radial nerve (C5, 6, 7, 8, T-1)
	Interosseous membrane	Posterior interosseous nerve (a branch of the radial nerve) (C5, 6, 7, 8, T-1)
	Periosteum of the radius and ulna and wrist and extensor surfaces of carpal joints	Posterior interosseous nerve (a branch of the radial nerve) (C5, 6, 7, 8, T-1)
	Radial $3^{1}/_{2}$ digits (falling short of the nail beds) and corresponding area of the back of the hand	Radial nerve (C5, 6, 7, 8, T-1) (upper subscapular nerve [C6, 7], thoracodorsal nerve [C6, 7, 8], and lower subscapular nerve [C6, 7] apparently have no sensory function)

Clinical Pearls

- Ignoring all other associated arm movements, the fifth digit moves laterally (pronation of the forearm) when the lateral cord is stimulated, medially (flexion and ulnar deviation) when the medial cord is being stimulated, and posteriorly (extension) when the posterior cord is being stimulated. The pinkie thus always moves "toward" the cord that is stimulated.

- In using this method, remember not to look solely at the elicited motor response of the fifth digit. Rather, observe the overall change in space of the fifth digit (pinkie) at the time of neurostimulation.

References

1. Tsui B, Hopkins D: Electrical nerve stimulation for regional anesthesia. In: Boezaart AP (editor): *Orthopaedic Anesthesia.* McGraw-Hill, 2006.
2. Standring S (editor): *Gray's Anatomy: The Anatomical Basis of Clinical Practice,* 39th ed. Elsevier, 2001, pp. 801–942.
3. Borene SC, Edwards JN, Boezaart AP: At the cords, the pinkie towards: Interpreting infraclavicular motor response to neurostimulation. Reg Anesth Pain Med 2004;29:125–129.
4. Kapral S, Jandrasits O, Schabernig C, et al: Lateral infraclavicular plexus block vs. axillary block for hand and forearm surgery. Acta Anaesthesiol Scand 1999;43:1047–1052.
5. Jandard C, Gentili ME, Girard F, et al: Infraclavicular block with lateral approach and nerve stimulation: Extent of anesthesia and adverse effects. Reg Anesth Pain Med 2002;27:37–42.
6. Gaertner E, Estebe J-P, Zamfir A, et al: Infraclavicular plexus block: Multiple injections vs. single injection. Reg Anesth Pain Med 2002;27:590–594.
7. Boezaart AP, de Beer JF, du Toit C, van Rooyen K: A new technique of continuous interscalene block. Can J Anesth 1999;46:275–281.
8. Boezaart AP, Koorn R, Rosenquist RW: Paravertebral approach to the brachial plexus: An anatomic improvement in technique. Reg Anesth Pain Med 2003;28:241–244.
9. Boezaart AP, de Beer JF, Nell ML: Early experience with continuous cervical paravertebral block using a stimulating catheter. Reg Anesth Pain Med 2003;28:406–413.
10. Wehling MJ, Koorn R, Leddell C, Boezaart AP: Electrical nerve stimulation using a stimulating catheter: What is the lower limit? Reg Anesth Pain Med 2004;29:230–233.
11. Wilbourn AJ: Brachial plexus disorders. In: Dyck PJ, Thomas PK (eds): *Peripheral Neuropathy,* 3rd ed. WB Saunders, 1993, pp. 921–922.
12. Sala-Blanch X, Carrera A, Morro R, Llusa M: Interpreting infraclavicular motor response to neurostimulation of the brachial plexus: From anatomic complexity to clinical evaluation simplicity. Reg Anesth Pain Med 2004;29:618–621.
13. Groen GJ, Gielen MJ, Jack NJM, Knape JThA: At the cords, the pinkie towards: Interpreting infraclavicular motor response to neurostimulation. Reg Anesth Pain Med 2004;29:505–507.

14. Bergman R: *Illustrated Encyclopedia of Human Anatomical Variations.* http://www.vh.org/adult/provider/anatomy/AnatomicVariants/AnatomyHP.html.

15. Neal JM, Hebl JR, Gerancher JC, Hogan QH: Brachial plexus anesthesia: Essentials of our current understanding. Reg Anesth Pain Med 2002;27:402–428.

16. Wilbourn AJ: Brachial plexus disorders. In: Dyck PJ, Thomas PK (editors): *Peripheral Neuropathy,* 3rd ed. WB Saunders, 1993, pp. 911–950.

17. Gray H: Muscles of the hand. In: Pick TP, Howden R (eds): *Gray's Anatomy,* 15th ed. Barnes and Noble, 1995, p. 383.

18. Agur AMR: *Grant's Atlas of Anatomy,* 9th ed. Williams & Wilkins 1991, pp. 354–450.

19. Netter F: Upper limb. In: Colacino N (ed): *Atlas of Human Anatomy.* Ciba-Geigy Corporation, 1989, pp. 448–451.

20. Last RJ: *Anatomy: Regional and Applied,* 4th ed. J & A Churchill, 1970, pp. 131–133.

23

Cervical Plexus Block

Jerry D. Vloka, MD • Tony Tsai, MD • Admir Hadzic, MD

INTRODUCTION

Cervical plexus anesthesia was developed early in the twentieth century, and two main approaches were available to the early practitioners of regional anesthesia. In 1912, Kappis described a posterior approach to the brachial plexus while attempting to block spinal nerves at the point of emergence from the vertebral column.[1] The main reason for a posterior approach to blocking the cervical plexus is the relative position of the vertebral artery and vein anterior to the plexus.[2] However, the posterior approach is associated with discomfort during and after the blockade, most likely due to the puncture of the extensor muscles of the neck, and has been avoided by many practitioners. As a result, the posterior approach to the cervical plexus block has not been as popular as the lateral approach, although it has been utilized to block the brachial plexus either as a single-shot or continuous technique.[2–5]

In 1914 Heidenhein described the lateral approach, which has formed the basis for subsequent techniques of anesthetizing the cervical plexus.[6] Victor Pauchet described a lateral approach to blocking the cervical plexus in 1920 and mentioned the posterior approach; however, he advocated the use of the lateral approach.[7] Winnie revisited the lateral approach to the cervical plexus block in 1975, and it is currently the more used approach for the cervical plexus block.[8]

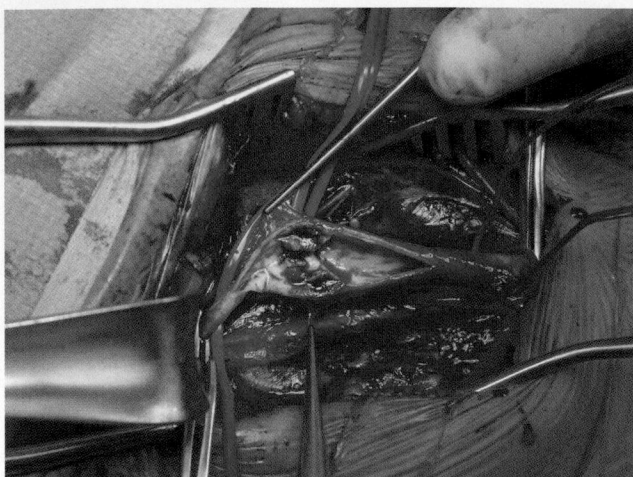

Figure 23–1. Carotid endarterectomy. The image shows open, cross-clamped carotid artery and a plaque inside its wall.

INDICATIONS & CONTRAINDICATIONS

Deep and superficial cervical plexus block can be used to provide anesthesia for a variety of surgical procedures, including superficial operations on the neck and shoulders, thyroid operations, and carotid endarterectomies in which awake neurologic monitoring is a simple and reliable method of neurologic assessment (Figure 23–1).[9,10] Eastcott described the first carotid endarterectomy in 1954, and the number of these surgeries performed in the United States grows each year.[11] Regional anesthesia is a viable anesthetic choice for carotid surgery, although debate continues about whether regional or general anesthesia is the better choice for carotid endarterectomy surgery. Most of the latest literature points to regional anesthesia as a better choice.[12–21] The outcome data from vascular surgery and neurosurgery literature shows that patients who undergo carotid endarterectomy under regional anesthesia may have better outcomes.[22–25]

The superficial cervical plexus block can be used for many superficial surgeries in the neck area, including lymph node dissection, excision of thyroglossal or branchial cleft cysts, carotid endarterectomy, and vascular access surgery.[26] If the superficial cervical plexus block is to be used alone for carotid endarterectomy, local anesthetic supplementation by the surgeon may be necessary.[27,28] Although both the deep and superficial cervical plexus blocks can be performed separately, they are most often performed in combination to provide anesthesia and postoperative analgesia for head and neck surgery.[29–31]

The main absolute contraindication to performing a cervical plexus block is patient refusal of regional anesthesia. Relative contraindications include infection at the site of injection, sepsis, preexisting central or peripheral nervous systems disorders, allergy to local anesthesia, and a long duration of surgery.

FUNCTIONAL ANATOMY OF DEEP CERVICAL PLEXUS BLOCKADE

The cervical plexus is formed by the anterior divisions of the four upper cervical nerves (Figure 23–2). The plexus is situated on the anterior surface of the four upper cervical vertebrae, resting on the levator anguli scapulae and scalenus medius muscles, and is covered by the sternocleidomastoid muscle. Their dorsal and ventral roots combine to form spinal nerves as they exit through the intervertebral foramen. The anterior rami of the second through fourth cervical nerves form the cervical plexus (the first cervical root is a primarily motor nerve and it is not blocked by this technique). The cervical plexus lies in the plane just behind the sternocleidomastoid muscle, giving off both superficial (superficial cervical plexus) and deep branches (deep cervical plexus). The branches of the superficial cervical plexus supply innervation to the skin and superficial structures of the head, neck, and shoulder (Figure 23–3). The deep branches of the cervical plexus innervate the deeper structures of the neck, including the muscles of the anterior neck and the diaphragm, which is innervated by the phrenic nerve. The third and fourth cervical nerves typically send a branch to the spinal accessory nerve, or directly into the deep surface of the trapezius to supply sensory fibers to this muscle. The fourth cervical nerve may send a branch downward to join the fifth cervical nerve and participate in the formation of the brachial plexus. The cutaneous innervation of both the deep and superficial cervical plexus blocks includes skin of the anterolateral neck and the ante- and retroauricular areas (Figure 23–4).

Anatomic Landmarks

The following three landmarks for a deep cervical plexus block are identified and marked (Figure 23–5):

1. Mastoid process
2. Chassaignac's tubercle (transverse process of the sixth cervical vertebra)
3. Posterior border of the sternocleidomastoid muscle

To estimate the line of needle insertion that overlies the transverse processes, the mastoid process (MP) and Chassaignac's tubercle, which is the transverse process of the sixth cervical vertebra (C6), are identified and marked (Figure 23–6). The transverse process of C6 is usually easily palpated behind the clavicular head of the sternocleidomastoid muscle at the level just below the cricoid cartilage (Figure 23–7). Next, a line is drawn connecting the MP to Chassaignac's tubercle. Position the palpating hand just behind the posterior border of the sternocleidomastoid muscle. Once this line is drawn, label the insertion sites over the C2, C3, and C4, which are respectively located on the MP–C6 line 2 cm, 4 cm, and 6 cm caudal to the mastoid process. It is also possible to perform a single injection at the C3 level, which is considered safe and effective.[32]

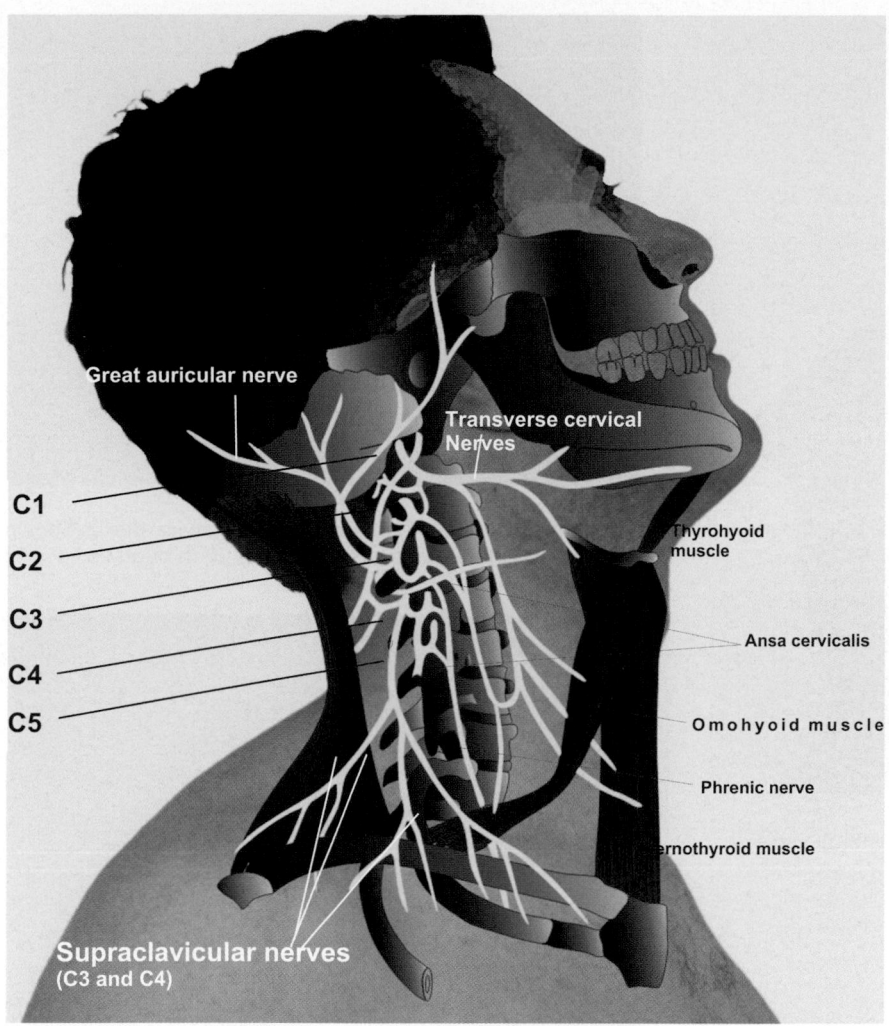

Figure 23–2. Anatomy of the cervical plexus.

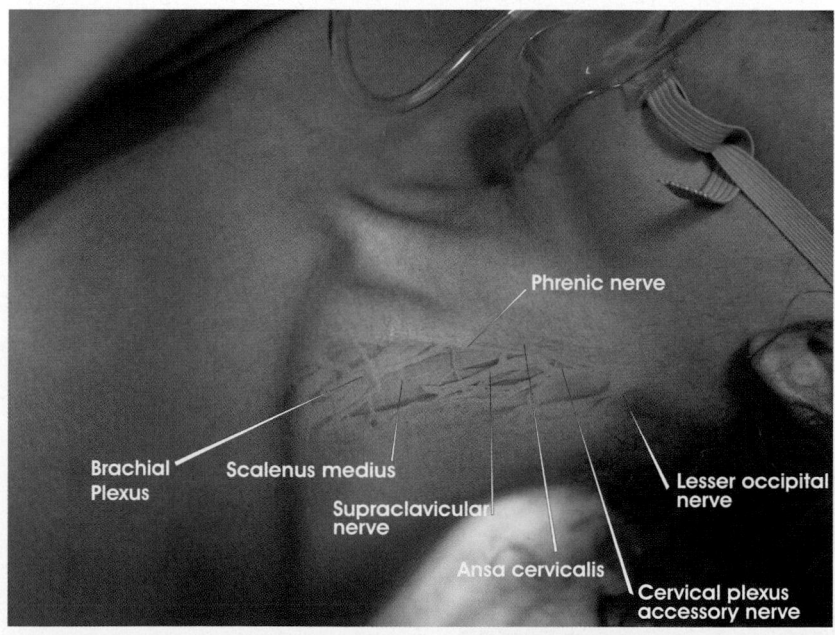

Figure 23–3. Topographic anatomy of the cervical plexus.

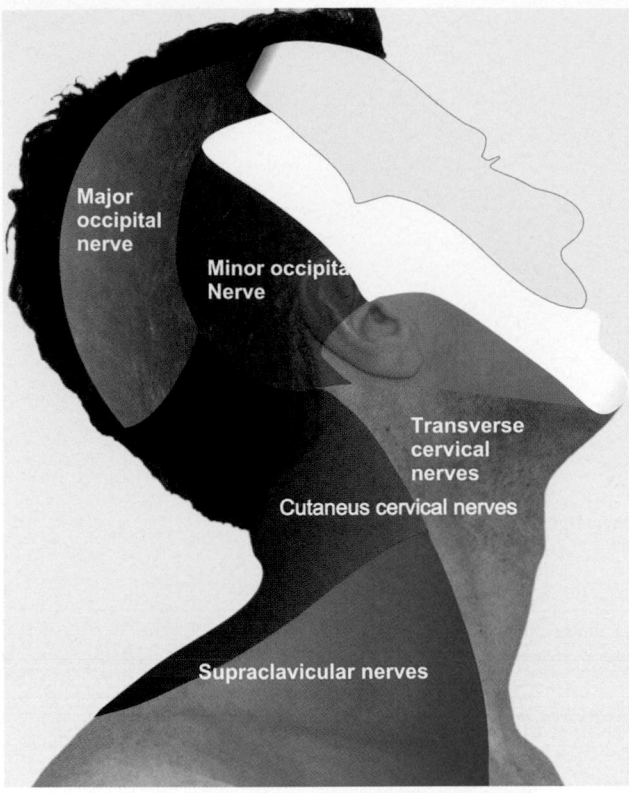

Figure 23–4. Cutaneous coverage of the cervical plexus.

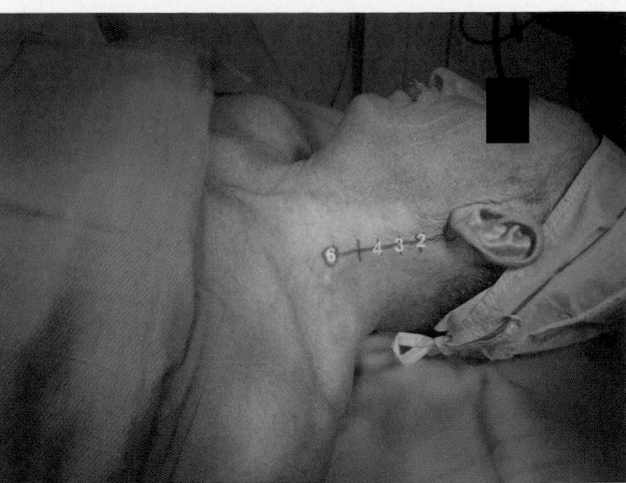

Figure 23–6. Anatomic landmarks for the cervical plexus. Shown are estimates of the transverse processes C2 through C6.

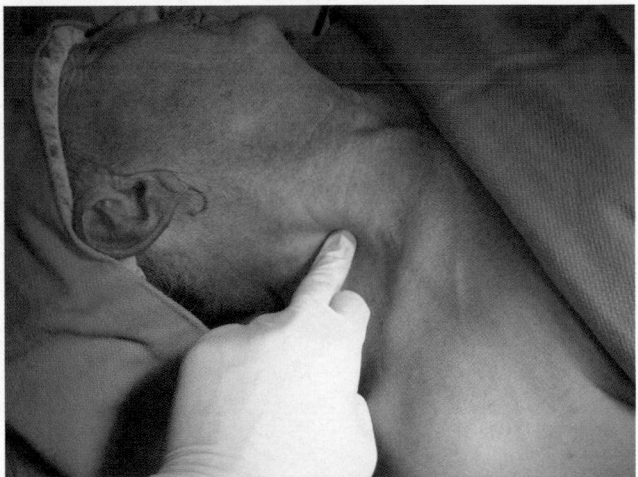

Figure 23–7. Palpation of the transverse process of C6.

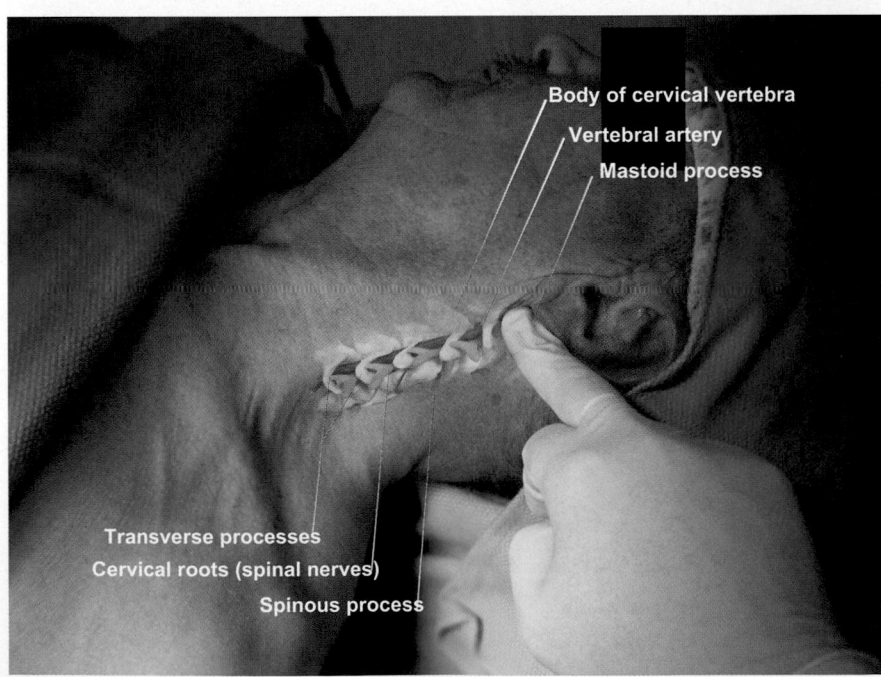

Figure 23–5. Anatomic landmarks for the cervical plexus block.

Choice of Local Anesthetic

A deep cervical plexus block requires 3–5 mL of local anesthetic per level to ensure reliable blockade. Except perhaps with patients with significant respiratory disease who rely on their phrenic nerve to adequately ventilate, most patients benefit from the use of a long-acting local anesthetic. Table 23–1 shows commonly used local anesthetics with onset and duration of anesthesia and analgesia for deep cervical plexus blocks. Ropivacaine is one option for deep cervical plexus block and 30–40 mL of the 0.5% concentration provides an excellent quality of block.[33] Ropivacaine has been shown to be a more suitable choice for carotid endarterectomy surgery.[34]

Equipment

A standard regional anesthesia tray is prepared with the following equipment:

- Sterile towels and 4- × 4-in. gauze pads
- 20-mL syringe(s) with local anesthetic
- Sterile gloves and marking pen

Table 23–1.

Commonly Used Local Anesthetics for Deep Cervical Plexus Blocks

	Onset (min)	Anesthesia (h)	Analgesia (h)
1.5% Mepivacaine ($+ HCO_3^- +$ epinephrine)	10–15	2.0–2.5	3–6
2% Lidocaine ($+ HCO_3^- +$ epinephrine)	10–15	2–3	3–6
0.5% Ropivacaine	10–20	3–4	4–10
0.25% Bupivacaine ($+$ epinephrine)	10–20	3–4	4–10

- One 1½-in., 25-gauge needle for skin infiltration
- A 1½-in.-long, 22-gauge, short-beveled needle

Technique

After cleaning the skin with an antiseptic solution, local anesthetic is infiltrated subcutaneously along the line over the transverse processes. The local anesthetic should be infiltrated over the entire length, rather than at the projected insertion sites to allow reinsertion of the needle slightly caudally or cranially when the transverse process is not contacted. This obviates the need to infiltrate the skin at a new insertion site.

The block needle is connected to a syringe with local anesthetic via flexible tubing. The needle is inserted between the palpating fingers and advanced at an angle perpendicular to the skin plane. The needle should never be oriented cephalad. A slight caudal orientation of the needle is the single best method for preventing the inadvertent insertion of the needle toward the cervical spinal cord. The needle is advanced slowly until the transverse process is contacted (Figure 23–8). At this point, the needle is withdrawn 1–2 mm and stabilized; then 4 mL of local anesthetic is injected after a negative aspiration test for blood. The block needle is then removed, and the entire procedure is repeated at the consecutive levels.

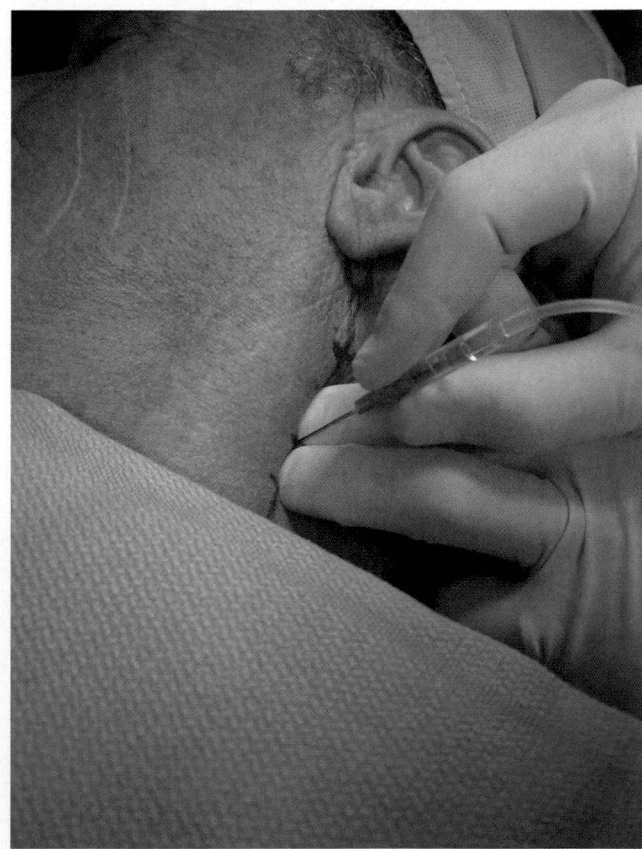

Figure 23–8. Needle insertion to block a single cervical level during deep cervical blockade.

The goal for the deep cervical plexus block is to contact the posterior tubercle of the transverse process because the spinal nerves at the individual levels are located just in front of the transverse process.

BLOCK DYNAMICS & PERIOPERATIVE MANAGEMENT

Although the placement of deep cervical block may be associated with moderate patient discomfort, avoid excessive sedation. During neck surgery, airway management may be difficult due to the need to share access to the head and neck with the surgeon. Surgeries like carotid endarterectomy require that the patient be fully conscious, oriented, and cooperative during the entire surgical procedure.[13] In addition, excessive sedation and the consequent lack of patient cooperation can result in restlessness and create difficulty for the surgeon. The onset time for this block is 10–15 min. The first sign of deep cervical plexus blockade is decreased sensation in the area of the distribution of the respective components of the cervical plexus. It should be noted that due to the complex arrangement of the neuronal coverage of the various layers in the neck area as well as the cross coverage from the contralateral side, the anesthesia achieved with cervical plexus block is rarely complete. Although this should not discourage the practitioner from using the deep cervical plexus block, its use does require an understanding surgeon who is willing to supplement the block with the local anesthetic as necessary.

FUNCTIONAL ANATOMY OF SUPERFICIAL CERVICAL PLEXUS BLOCKADE

The superficial cervical plexus supplies innervation to the skin of the anterolateral neck through anterior primary rami of the second through fourth cervical nerves (see Figure 23–4). The individual nerves emerge as four distinct nerves from the posterior border of the sternocleidomastoid muscle. The **lesser occipital nerve** usually is a direct branch from the main stem of the second cervical nerve. The larger remaining part of this stem then unites with a part of the third cervical nerve to form a trunk that arises as the **greater auricular** and the **transverse cervical nerves.** Another part of the third cervical nerve runs downward to unite with a major part of the fourth to form a supraclavicular trunk, which then divides into the three groups of **supraclavicular nerves.**

Anatomic Landmarks

A line extending from the mastoid to C6 is drawn (Figure 23–9). The site of needle insertion is marked at the midpoint of the line connecting the mastoid process with Chassaignac's tubercle of C6 transverse process (see Figure 23–9). This is the location of the branches of the superficial cervical plexus as they emerge behind the posterior border of the sternocleidomastoid muscle.

Choice of Local Anesthetic

A superficial cervical plexus block requires 10–15 mL of local anesthetic (3–5 mL per each redirection/injection). Most patients benefit from the use of a long-acting local anesthetic. Since motor block is not sought with this technique, some anesthesiologists suggest using a low concentration of local anesthetic (eg, 0.2–0.5% ropivacaine or 0.25% bupivacaine). Although a low concentration may suffice when the needle

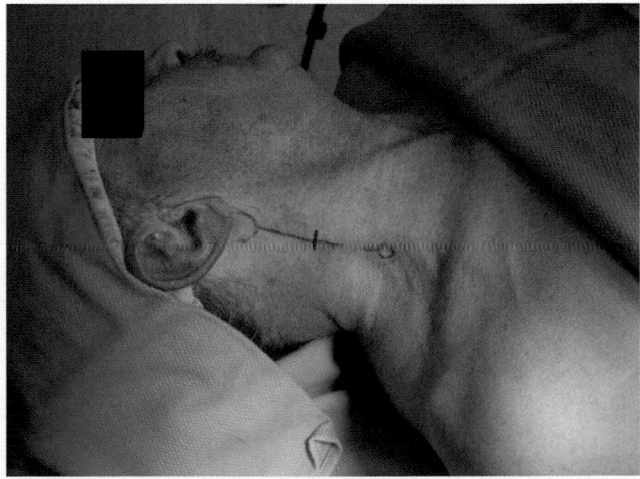

Figure 23–9. Landmarks for superficial cervical plexus block. The needle insertion site (horizontal line) is marked at the midpoint between mastoid process and transverse process of C6 behind the posterior border of the sternocleidomastoid muscle.

is ideally placed in the vicinity of the cervical plexus nerves, this is often not the case, and the higher concentration will result in both a higher success rate and a longer duration of blockade.[33] Table 23–1 shows choices of local anesthetic, with their onset time and duration of anesthesia and analgesia.

Equipment

A standard regional anesthesia tray is prepared with the following equipment:

- Sterile towels and 4- × 4-in. gauze pads
- 20-mL syringe with local anesthetic
- Sterile gloves, marking pen, and surface electrode
- A 1½-in., 25-gauge needle for block infiltration

Technique

After skin cleaning with an antiseptic solution, a skin wheal is raised at the site of needle insertion using a 25-gauge needle. Next, using a "fan" technique with superior–inferior needle redirections, the local anesthetic is injected alongside the posterior border of the sternocleidomastoid muscle 2–3 cm below and then above the needle insertion site. This injection technique should be adequate to achieve blockade of all four major branches of the superficial cervical plexus (Figure 23–10).

The goal of the injection is to infiltrate the local anesthetic subcutaneously and behind the sternocleidomastoid muscle. Deep needle insertion should be avoided (eg, >1–2 cm).

Block Dynamics & Perioperative Management

The superficial cervical plexus block is associated with minor patient discomfort. Small doses (1–2 mg) of midazolam for sedation and alfentanil (250–500 mcg) for analgesia just before needle insertion should produce a comfortable and cooperative patient during nerve localization. Similar to deep cervical plexus blockade, the sensory coverage of the neck is complex and a degree of cross-coverage from the cervical plexus branches from the opposite side of the neck should be expected. The onset time for this block is 10–15 min; the first sign of the blockade is decreased sensation in the area of the distribution of the respective components of the cervical plexus.

Clinical Pearls

- A subcutaneous midline injection of the local anesthetic extending from the thyroid cartilage distally to the suprasternal notch will block the nerve branches crossing from the opposite side.
- This "field" block is useful for preventing pain from surgical skin retractors on the medial aspect of the neck.

Complications & How to Avoid Them

Complications can occur with both deep and superficial cervical plexus block (Table 23–2). Infection, hematoma formation, phrenic nerve block, local anesthetic toxicity, nerve injury, and inadvertent subarachnoid or epidural anesthesia can all occur when performing these blocks.[35–39] In a large prospective study of 1000 blocks for carotid artery surgery, Davies and colleagues reported only 6 blocks (0.6%) showing evidence of intravascular injection.[13] Other possible complications include transient ischemic attacks either during surgery or in the postoperative period and recurrent laryngeal nerve blockade.[40–42] As with other nerve blockade procedures,

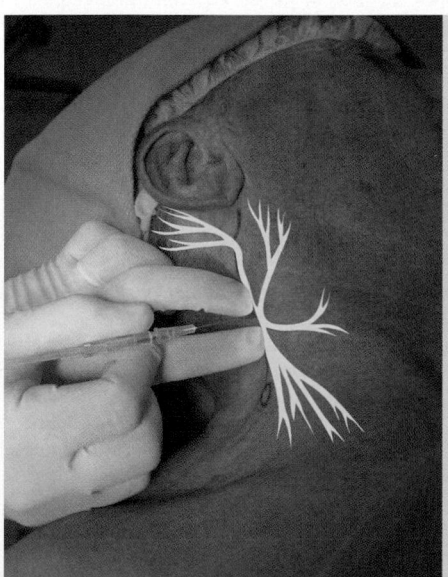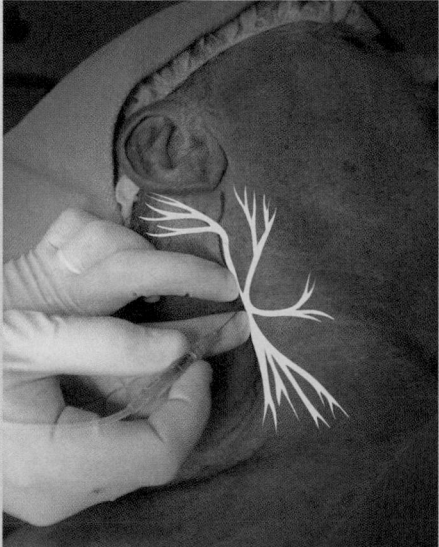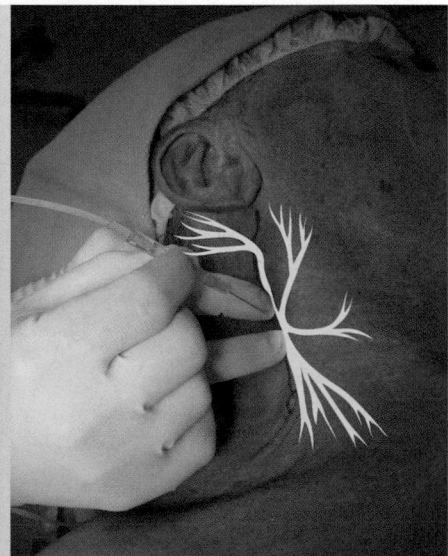

Figure 23–10. Technique of superficial cervical plexus block.

Table 23–2.

Complications of Cervical Plexus Block and Means to Avoid Them

Infection	• Low risk • A strict aseptic technique is used
Hematoma	• Avoid multiple needle insertions, particularly in anticoagulated patients • Keep five minutes of steady pressure on the site if the carotid artery is inadvertently punctured
Phrenic nerve blockade	• Phrenic nerve blockade (diaphragmatic paresis) invariably occurs with a deep cervical plexus block • A deep cervical block should be carefully considered in patients with significant respiratory disease • Bilateral deep cervical block in such patients may be contraindicated • Blockade of the phrenic nerve does not occur after superficial cervical plexus block
Local anesthetic toxicity	• Central nervous system toxicity is the most serious consequence of the cervical plexus block • This complication occurs because of the rich vascularity of the neck, including vertebral and carotid artery vessels and is usually caused by an inadvertent intravascular injection of local anesthetic rather than absorption • Careful and frequent aspiration should be performed during the injection
Nerve injury	• Local anesthetic should never be injected against resistance or when the patient complains of severe pain on injection
Spinal anesthesia	• This complication may occur with injection of a larger volume of local anesthetic inside the dural sleeve that accompanies the nerves of the cervical plexus • It should be noted that a negative aspiration test for CSF does not rule out the possibility of intrathecal spread of local anesthetic • Avoidance of high volume and excessive pressure during injection are the best measures to avoid this complication

CSF = cerebrospinal fluid.

if attention is paid to details, the risk of complications can be minimized when performing cervical plexus blocks and result in a safe and efficacious method of performing anesthesia that has high patient acceptance.[43–46]

SUMMARY

In summary, cervical plexus block has been in clinical use for nearly a century. Although modifications have been made to the approaches first described at the beginning of the twentieth century, the most common approach remains the lateral approach to deep cervical plexus block.

References

1. Kappis H: Über Leitunganaesthesie am Bauch, Brust, Arm, und Hals durch injection aus Foramen intervertebrale. Munchen Med Wschr 1912;59:794–796.
2. Boezaart AP, Koorn R, Rosenquist RW: Paravertebral approach to the brachial plexus: An anatomic improvement in technique. Reg Anesth Pain Med 2003;28:241–244.
3. Koorn R, Tenhundfel Fear KM, et al: The use of cervical paravertebral block as the sole anesthetic for shoulder surgery in a morbid patient: A case report. Reg Anesth Pain Med 2004;29:227–229.
4. Borene SC, Rosenquist RW, Koorn R, et al: An indication for continuous cervical paravertebral block (posterior approach to the interscalene space). Anesth Analg 2003;97:898–900.
5. Boezaart AP, Koorn R, Borene S, et al: Continuous brachial plexus block using the posterior approach. Reg Anesth Pain Med 2003;28:70–71.
6. Heidenhein L: Operations on the neck. In Braun H (ed): *Local Anesthesia, Its Scientific Basis and Practical Use.* Lea & Febiger, 1914, pp 268–269.
7. Sherwood-Dunn B: *Regional Anesthesia (Victor Pauchet's Technique).* FA Davis, 1920.
8. Winnie AP, Ramamurthy S, Durrani Z, et al: Interscalene cervical plexus block: A single-injection technique. Anesth Analg 1975;54:370–375.
9. Todesco J, Williams RT: Anaesthetic management of a patient with a large neck mass. Can J Anaesth 1994;41:157–160.
10. Kulkarni RS, Braverman LE, Patwardhan NA: Bilateral cervical plexus block for thyroidectomy and parathyroidectomy in healthy and high risk patients. J Endocrinol Invest 1996;19:714–718.
11. Eastcott HH, Pickering GW, Rob CG: Reconstruction of internal carotid artery in a patient with intermittent attacks of hemiplegia. Lancet 1954;267:994–996.
12. Stoneham MD, Knighton JD: Regional anaesthesia for carotid endarterectomy. Br J Anaesth 1999;82:910–919.
13. Davies MJ, Silbert BS, Scott DA, et al: Superficial and deep cervical plexus block for carotid artery surgery: A prospective study of 1000 blocks. Reg Anesth Pain Med 1997;22:442–446.

14. Stoneburner JM, Nishanian GP, Cukingnan RA, et al: Carotid endarterectomy using regional anesthesia: A benchmark for stenting. Am Surg 2002;68:1120–1123.

15. Harbaugh RE, Pikus HJ: Carotid endarterectomy with regional anesthesia. Neurosurgery 2001;49:642–645.

16. McCleary AJ, Maritati G, Gough MJ: Carotid endarterectomy; local or general anaesthesia? Eur J Vasc Endovasc Surg 2001;22:1–12.

17. Melliere D, Desgranges P, Becquemin JP, et al: Surgery of the internal carotid: Locoregional or general anesthesia? Ann Chir 2000;125:530–538.

18. Stone ME Jr, Kunjummen BJ, Moran JC, et al: Supervised training of general surgery residents in carotid endarterectomy performed on awake patients under regional block is safe and desirable. Am Surg 2000;66:781–786.

19. Knighton JD, Stoneham MD: Carotid endarterectomy. A survey of UK anaesthetic practice. Anaesthesia 2000;55:481–485.

20. Lehot JJ, Durand PG: Anesthesia for carotid endarterectomy. Rev Esp Anestesiol Reanim 2001;48:499–507.

21. Santamaria G, Britti RD, Tescione M, et al: Comparison between local and general anaesthesia for carotid endarterectomy. A retrospective analysis. Minerva Anestesiol 2004;70:771–778.

22. Bowyer MW, Zierold D, Loftus JP, et al: Carotid endarterectomy: A comparison of regional versus general anesthesia in 500 operations. Ann Vasc Surg 2000;14:145–151.

23. Papavasiliou AK, Magnadottir HB, Gonda T, et al: Clinical outcomes after carotid endarterectomy: Comparison of the use of regional and general anesthetics. J Neurosurg 2000;92:291–296.

24. Stoughton J, Nath RL, Abbott WM: Comparison of simultaneous electroencephalographic and mental status monitoring during carotid endarterectomy with regional anesthesia. J Vasc Surg 1998;28:1014–1021.

25. Bonalumi F, Vitiello R, Miglierina L, et al: Carotid endarterectomy under locoregional anesthesia. Ann Ital Chir 1997;68:453–461.

26. Brull SJ: Superficial cervical plexus block for pulmonary artery catheter insertion. Crit Care Med 1992;20:1362–1363.

27. Pandit JJ, Bree S, Dillon P, et al: A comparison of superficial versus combined (superficial and deep) cervical plexus block for carotid endarterectomy: A prospective, randomized study. Anesth Analg 2000;91:781–786.

28. Stoneham MD, Doyle AR, Knighton JD, et al: Prospective, randomized comparison of deep or superficial cervical plexus block for carotid endarterectomy surgery. Anesthesiology 1998;89:907–912.

29. Aunac S, Carlier M, Singelyn F, et al: The analgesic efficacy of bilateral combined superficial and deep cervical plexus block administered before thyroid surgery under general anesthesia. Anesth Analg 2002;95:746–750.

30. Masters RD, Castresana EJ, Castresana MR: Superficial and deep cervical plexus block: Technical considerations. AANA J 1995;63:235–243.

31. Dieudonne N, Gomola A, Bonnichon P, et al: Prevention of postoperative pain after thyroid surgery: A double-blind randomized study of bilateral superficial cervical plexus blocks. Anesth Analg 2001;92:1538–1542.

32. Gratz I, Deal E, Larijani GE, et al: The number of injections does not influence absorption of bupivacaine after cervical plexus block for carotid endarterectomy. J Clin Anesth 2005;17:263–266.

33. Umbrain VJ, van Gorp VL, Schmedding E, et al: Ropivacaine 3.75 mg/ml, 5 mg/ml, or 7.5 mg/ml for cervical plexus block during carotid endarterectomy. Reg Anesth Pain Med 2004;29:312–316.

34. Leoni A, Magrin S, Mascotto G, et al: Cervical plexus anesthesia for carotid endarterectomy: Comparison of ropivacaine and mepivacaine. Can J Anaesth 2000;47:185–187.

35. Pandit JJ, McLaren ID, Crider B: Efficacy and safety of the superficial cervical plexus block for carotid endarterectomy. Br J Anaesth 1999;83:970–972.

36. Carling A, Simmonds M: Complications from regional anaesthesia for carotid endarterectomy. Br J Anaesth 2000;84:797–800.

37. Emery G, Handley G, Davies MJ, et al: Incidence of phrenic nerve block and hypercapnia in patients undergoing carotid endarterectomy under cervical plexus block. Anaesth Intensive Care 1998;26:377–381.

38. Stoneham MD, Wakefield TW: Acute respiratory distress after deep cervical plexus block. J Cardiothorac Vasc Anesth 1998;12:197–198.

39. Castresana MR, Masters RD, Castresana EJ, et al: Incidence and clinical significance of hemidiaphragmatic paresis in patients undergoing carotid endarterectomy during cervical plexus block anesthesia. J Neurosurg Anesthesiol 1994;6:21–23.

40. Johnson TR: Transient ischaemic attack during deep cervical plexus block. Br J Anaesth 1999;83:965–967.

41. Lawrence PF, Alves JC, Jicha D, et al: Incidence, timing, and causes of cerebral ischemia during carotid endarterectomy with regional anesthesia. J Vasc Surg 1998;27:329–334.

42. Harris RJ, Benveniste G: Recurrent laryngeal nerve blockade in patients undergoing carotid endarterectomy under cervical plexus block. Anaesth Intensive Care 2000;28: 431–433.

43. Bergeron P, Benichou H, Dupont M, et al: Carotid surgery under cervical block anesthesia. A simple method of heart and brain protection in high risk patients. Int Angiol 1989;8:70–80.

44. Shah DM, Darling RC 3rd, Chang BB, et al: Carotid endarterectomy in awake patients: Its safety, acceptability, and outcome. J Vasc Surg 1994;19:1015–1019.

45. Lee KS, Davis CH Jr, McWhorter JM: Low morbidity and mortality of carotid endarterectomy performed with regional anesthesia. J Neurosurg 1988;69:483–487.

46. Love A, Hollyoak MA: Carotid endarterectomy and local anaesthesia: Reducing the disasters. Cardiovasc Surg 2000;8:429–435.

24

Cervical Paravertebral Block

André P. Boezaart, MD

INTRODUCTION

The cervical paravertebral approach to the brachial plexus results in a volume-dependent blockade of the roots of the brachial plexus. Cervical paravertebral block is indicated for anesthesia and postoperative analgesia in all major surgery on the upper extremity, including surgery on the shoulder, elbow, and wrist.[1] It is also suitable for patients in whom it is difficult to reach the brachial plexus trunks via the interscalene approach.[2] Because both the loss-of-resistance technique and nerve stimulation can be used for placement of this block, it is well suited to postoperative placement or for other patients (eg, patients with fractures of the arm) in whom motor activity due to nerve stimulation may be poorly tolerated.[1]

HISTORY

The technique described in this chapter is a modification of the single-injection block, originally described by Kappis in the 1920s[3] and modified by Pippa in 1990.[4] The original technique never gained popularity, probably because it was uncomfortable to patients due to penetration of the paraspinal extensor muscles of the neck. A modified technique, which does not penetrate these muscles, was described recently.[5,6] The modification is insertion of the needle in the V-shaped space between the levator scapulae and trapezius muscles at the level of the sixth cervical vertebra. By this method, penetration of the posterior paraspinal muscles is avoided, which minimizes the associated pain of this approach. Because all of the structures (eg, vertebral artery and vein, phrenic nerve, carotid and other major arteries, internal jugular vein, etc.) associated with complications from brachial plexus blockade are anterior to the nerve roots in the neck, where they exit the neuroforamina, Kappis' original argument that it is best to approach the roots from the posterior, where there are only muscles, remains valid. Furthermore, at the root level of the brachial plexus, which is the level at which this block is done,[5,6] the nerve fibers are arranged with sensory fibers posterior and motor fibers anterior. This probably explains the predominantly sensory block when approached from the posterior aspect of the neck.

SINGLE-INJECTION & CONTINUOUS BLOCK TECHNIQUE

Anatomy

The brachial plexus is situated between the anterior and middle scalene muscles (Figure 24–1). The phrenic nerve lies in front of the anterior scalene muscle. The vertebral artery and vein are situated anterior to the pars intervertebralis, or **articular column** of the vertebrae. The approach described in this section[1,2,5,6] avoids penetrating the extensor muscles of the neck by entering the neck through the "window" at the level of apex of the V formed by the trapezius and levator scapulae muscles (Figure 24–2).

Patient Positioning

Proper patient positioning is critical to the successful performance of this block. The patient is placed in the sitting or the lateral decubitus position (the levator scapulae muscle is usually easier to identify if the patient is in the sitting position). Elevating the head of the bed during the procedure facilitates venous drainage, and reduces venous oozing during the procedure. The patient's neck is flexed slightly forward and to the opposite side, and the anesthesiologist stands behind the patient.

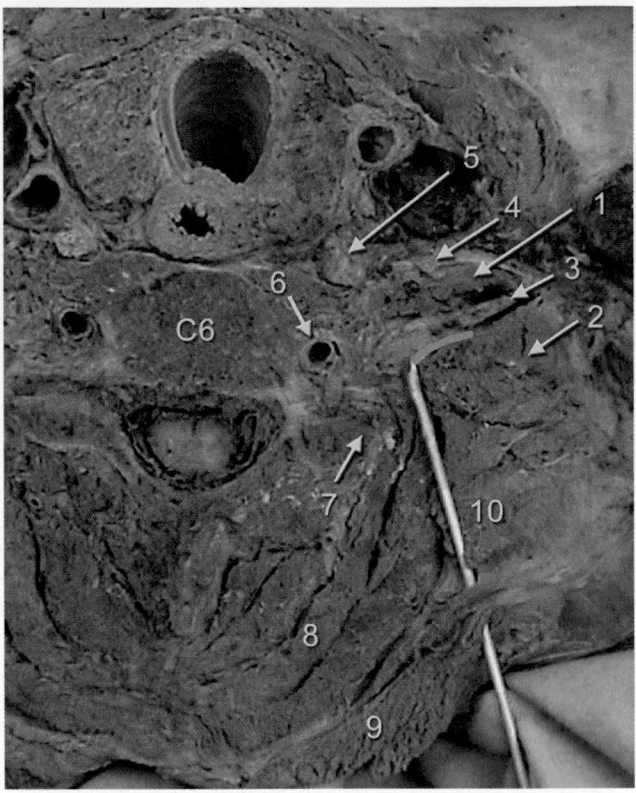

Figure 24–1. Anatomic considerations for cervical paravertebral block. 1 = Anterior scalene muscle; 2 = Middle scalene muscle; 3 = Brachial plexus; 4 = Phrenic nerve; 5 = Stellate ganglion; 6 = vertebral artery; 7 = Articular column of C6; 8 = Extensor muscles of the neck; 9 = Trapezius muscle; 10 = Levator scapulae muscle.

Needle Insertion

After preparing the skin with a disinfectant and placement of sterile drapes, local anesthetic is infiltrated into the skin and subcutaneous tissue to the level of the pars intervertebralis (**articular column**) and tunneling site for the catheter. Next, an insulated 17- or 18-gauge Tuohy needle is inserted at

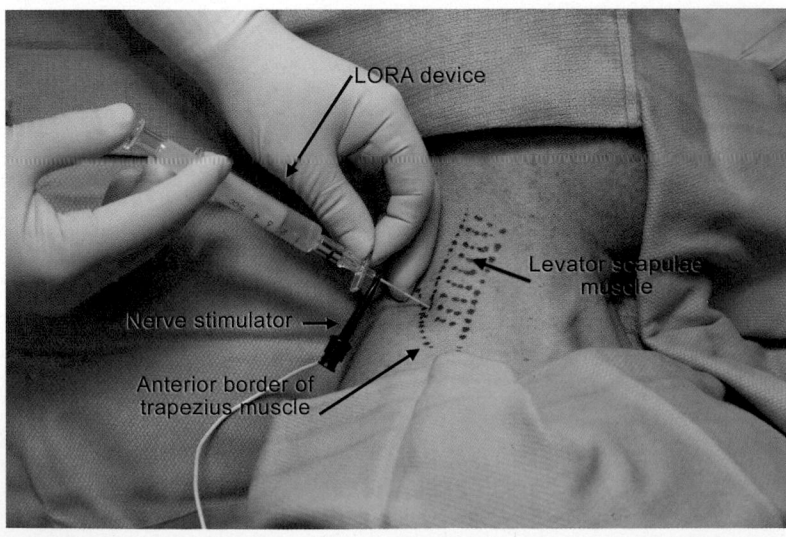

Figure 24–2. Cervical paravertebral block: needle insertion technique. The needle is inserted in the V-shaped region between the anterior border of the trapezius and levator scapulae muscles. LORA = loss of resistance to air.

the apex of the V formed by the trapezius and levator scapulae muscles at the level of the sixth cervical vertebrae (see Figure 24–2).

The nerve stimulator is set to deliver a current of 1 to 2 mA (frequency of 2 Hz and a pulse width of 100–300 μs) and its negative lead is attached to the needle. The needle is advanced anteromedially and approximately 30-degrees caudad, aiming toward the suprasternal notch or cricoid cartilage until the transverse process of C6 or the pars intervertebralis (articular column) of C6 is encountered. At this point, the stylet of the needle is removed, and a loss-of-resistance syringe is attached to the needle. While continuously testing for loss of resistance, the needle is *walked off* the bony structure (vertebra) by redirecting the needle laterally and then advancing it anteriorly. A distinct loss of resistance to air usually occurs simultaneously with contraction of the shoulder muscles when the cervical paravertebral space is entered (approximately 0.5–1 cm beyond the transverse process of the vertebra). At this level, the motor (anterior) and sensory (posterior) fibers have joined to form the roots of the brachial plexus, and typically, more current is required to elicit a motor response than with an anterior interscalene technique. If a single-injection technique is used, 20–40 mL of the local anesthetic is incrementally and slowly injected while monitoring the patient for the signs and symptoms of local anesthetic toxicity. The choice of type and concentration of local anesthetic depends on the desired degree of motor blockade and the desired duration of action. A catheter can also be inserted to allow prolongation of analgesia into the postoperative period. The onset of full surgical anesthesia with this technique typically requires 20 to 45 min. This somewhat slower block onset (compared to the interscalene block) is likely caused by thick dural sleeves, which continue along the nerve roots at this level.[1,2,5,6]

Clinical Pearls

- Occasionally, it is necessary to block the superficial cervical plexus to alleviate pain at skin incisions made for shoulder surgery or arthroscopy, especially the posterior portal for arthroscopic surgery or the incision for a posterior Bankart repair.
- Because the needle insertion site is relatively close to the patient's ipsilateral ear, the patient should be warned that a "crunching" sound may be heard when the Tuohy needle enters the skin and advances through the subcutaneous tissues.

Continuous Cervical Paravertebral Block

With continuous technique, when the tip of the needle approaches the roots of the brachial plexus, as indicated by a motor response, or the patient reporting sensory pulsation at a nerve stimulation output of approximately 0.5 mA, or loss of resistance to air is detected, the needle is held steady while the loss-of-resistance syringe is removed. If a nonstimulating technique is used for catheter placement, a bolus injection is given through the needle, and a standard epidural catheter is inserted. If a stimulating catheter technique is used, the nerve stimulator lead is attached to the proximal end of the 19- or 20-gauge stimulating catheter, and its distal end is inserted into the needle shaft. The nerve stimulator output is kept constant at a current that provides brisk muscle twitches of the shoulder or upper extremity muscles, and the catheter tip is advanced 5 cm beyond the tip of the needle. When the catheter is correctly placed, it is secured at a convenient position and covered with transparent dressing.

Clinical Pearls

- There is often slight resistance to catheter *advancement* beyond the tip of the needle. This is normal.
- Catheters usually do not follow the nerve root distally, but curl up at the root level; therefore, it is not necessary to insert the catheter deeper than 3–5 cm beyond the needle tip. Deeper insertion of the catheter may carry a risk of formation of a catheter knot around a nerve root.
- It is possible for the catheter to advance inappropriately and enter the epidural space. Stimulating the catheter before injections allows the operator to differentiate between plexus (stimulation possible at currents <1.0 mA) and epidural (stimulation requires current >1.0 mA) stimulation.
- A test dose of 2 mL of saline and 1/300,000 epinephrine should be used to rule out intravascular placement of the catheter.
- Catheter placement should be a strictly sterile procedure because an indwelling catheter will be left in situ.
- The catheter entry site should be covered with a transparent dressing to allow daily inspection of the catheter entry wound.
- Some patients experience discomfort at the catheter entry site; this discomfort can be treated with hot or cold compresses or oral analgesic medication. If this does not help, the catheter should be removed.

PERIOPERATIVE MANAGEMENT

An initial bolus of 20 to 40 mL of 0.5% bupivacaine, 0.5 to 0.75% ropivacaine, or 0.5% levobupivacaine may be used.[1,2,5,6] When used for postoperative analgesia, the bolus is followed by a continuous infusion of a lower concentration of the same drug; that is, 0.25% bupivacaine, 0.2% ropivacaine, or 0.2% levobupivacaine, at an infusion rate of 3 to 10 mL/h and patient-controlled boluses of 5 to 10 mL every 30 to 240 min.

COMPLICATIONS & SIDE EFFECTS

Horner syndrome can be expected in approximately 40% of patients.[1] However, this does not cause problems when patients are warned beforehand of this side effect. Due to phrenic nerve blockade, up to 8% of patients may complain of dyspnea in the recovery room. Dyspnea is usually experienced when both the phrenic and recurrent laryngeal nerves are blocked with oxygen supplementation, placing the patient in the Fowler's position and providing reassurance, this should not pose significant problems. Only 2% of patients continue to experience dyspnea after 6 h; no patients complained of dyspnea after 12 h.[1]

Infection at the catheter site is a potentially serious complication, especially after a major joint replacement (eg, shoulder, elbow, or wrist arthroplasty). In our study,[5] 5% (13 of 256 cases) of the catheter entry sites showed signs of localized infection. This was limited to redness of the skin at the catheter entry site ($n = 10$ of 13) and purulent discharge ($n = 3$ of 13). *Staphylococcus aureus* and *S. epidermidis* were cultured in 7 of the 13 cases. If infection is suspected, the cathe-ter should be removed and antibiotic therapy considered.

Posterior neck pain is a common complication seen with this block. In one report, 22% of the patients had some pain at the catheter insertion site.[1] Most of these patients were successfully treated with nonsteroidal antiinflammatory drugs, and it was not necessary to remove the catheters in the majority. This complication can largely be prevented by making sure that the catheter is inserted between the extensor muscles of the neck and not through them.

The subclavian artery, situated anterior to the brachial plexus, can be punctured by a posterior approach only if the plexus is penetrated. Puncture should not occur when the nerve stimulator is functioning properly.

Eleven of the 256 patients in this series (4%) experienced numbness in the fingers of the contralateral hand due to MRI-confirmed epidural spread of the local anesthetic agent. The numbness resolved in all the patients within 6 h without any respiratory or other sequelae.

CHOICE OF LOCAL ANESTHETIC & PRACTICAL MANAGEMENT FOR COMMON SURGICAL INDICATIONS

The choice of local anesthetic agent is not critical, except in situations when motor block is not desirable, such as "frozen shoulder." This author uses 0.5% ropivacaine as default agent; using bupivacaine or levobupivacaine in equipotent concentrations is equally suitable. Similar to other block procedure, a shorter acting local anesthetics can be used when desired.

Arthroscopic Subacromial Decompression

Arthroscopic subacromial decompression (ASAD) surgery typically does not result in significant postoperative pain,

and a continuous block is usually not indicated. A single-injection block provides analgesia for a few hours postoperatively. Brachial plexitis may well be the underlying cause of the shoulder pain in more patients than is commonly realized; therefore, blocks for this indication should be used with caution and carefully documented. If, however, a rotator cuff tear was found and repaired, a continuous cervical paravertebral block can be placed. Placement can be done in the operating room using resistance to air and before waking the patient or in the recovery room after the patient emerges from general anesthesia. The choice depends on the institutional protocol and the anesthesiologist's preference.

Shoulder, Elbow, & Wrist Arthroplasty; Shoulder Stabilization; & Rotator Cuff Repair

The continuous cervical paravertebral block is well suited for total or hemi- shoulder, elbow, and wrist arthroplasty. A relatively large volume of local anesthetic (20–40 mL) is injected as a bolus. These volumes usually block all the brachial plexus roots, which is ideal for the surgery since the innervation of the major joints of the upper limb is from the complete brachial plexus. Keep in mind that the onset of action is slower than in interscalene block, probably because of the dural sheath surrounding the roots. In placing the block, the needle tip is aimed more toward the lower roots (C7 through T1) for wrist arthroplasty and more toward the upper trunks (C5 and C6) for shoulder arthroplasty.

A continuous infusion of 5 mL/h of a lower concentration of the drug (eg, ropivacaine 0.2%) with patient-controlled regional analgesia (PCRA) boluses of 10 mL of the same drug at a lockout time of 1 h is used. Some investigators suggest that PCRA without continuous infusion is satisfactory.[7]

The motor block is denser in the proximal parts of the upper limb than in the distal parts, with a bolus injection of 30 mL of 0.5% ropivacaine and a continuous infusion of 0.2% ropivacaine at 0.1 mL/kg/h.[5] The distal motor block can also be expected to subside earlier than the proximal, and the sensory block outlasts the motor block. This feature makes the block suitable for shoulder surgery because it provides a dense sensory–motor block in the early postoperative period, while the motor function returns to the hand after approximately 36 h, and after 60 h in the shoulder area. The sensory block and analgesia are present for the duration of the surgery. The block virtually "tapers" itself as the need for motor block subsides over time.

Frozen Shoulder

Patients with **primary adhesive capsulitis,** or primary "frozen shoulder," require special considerations with regard to the use of the brachial plexus block. Frozen shoulder is a chronic fibrosing condition of the shoulder joint capsule.[8,9] Its histologic pathology is similar to Dupuytren's disease, and it shares a common biochemical pathway that leads to the contracture seen in Dupuytren's disease. The latter is, however, a progressive condition, whereas primary frozen shoulder is a self-limiting disorder that resolves with time. Primary frozen shoulder can have components of sympathetic dystrophy, having the characteristics of an algoneurodystrophic process similar to complex regional pain syndrome.[10] To rehabilitate primary frozen shoulder, it is essential that the patient be free from pain in the postoperative period. Motor blockade should be avoided so that the patient can participate in physical therapy. For these reasons, low concentrations (0.1%) of ropivacaine should be used. This author uses low infusion rates varying from 0 to 3 mL/h of 0.1% ropivacaine, and allows 5- to 10-mL PCRA boluses at a 60-min lockout time.

The block is probably not indicated for surgery of the clavicle because the clavicle receives its nerve supply from the entire brachial and cervical plexi. Similarly, this technique is not ideal for surgery on the acromioclavicular joint.

SUMMARY

The cervical paravertebral block is a newer technique for brachial plexus blockade. It presents an excellent alternative to continuous interscalene block for shoulder surgery and the continuous supra- and infraclavicular blocks for major elbow and wrist surgery. Experience with other approaches to brachial plexus block and strict adherence to the outlined precautions are necessary to ensure success and avoid complications.

References

1. Boezaart AP, De Beer JF, Nell ML: Early experience with continuous cervical paravertebral block using a stimulating catheter. Reg Anesth Pain Med 2003;28(5):406–413.

2. Borene SC, Rosenquist RW, Koorn R, et al: An indication for continuous cervical paravertebral block (posterior approach to the interscalene space). Anesth Analg 2003;97(3):898–903.

3. Kappis M: Weitere Erfahrungen mit der Sympathektomie. Kin Wchnschr 1923;2:1441.

4. Pippa P, Cominelli E, Marinelli C, et al: Brachial plexus block using the posterior approach. Eur J Anaesth 1990;7:411–420.

5. Boezaart AP: Continuous interscalene block for ambulatory shoulder surgery. Best Practice Res Clin Anaesthesiol 2002;16:295–310.

6. Boezaart AP, Koorn R, Rosenquist RW: Paravertebral approach to the brachial plexus: An anatomic improvement in technique. Reg Anesth Pain Med 2003;28(3):241–244.

7. Van de Putte P, van der Vorst M: Continuous interscalene block using a stimulating catheter: A review of technique. Acta Anaesthesiol Belg 2005;56:25–30.

8. Smith SP, Dvaraj VS, Bunker TD: The association between frozen shoulder and Dupuytren's disease. J Shoulder Elbow Surg 2001;10:149–151.

9. Bunker TD, Anthony PP: The pathology of frozen shoulder: A Dupuytren-like disease. J Bone Joint Surg [Br] 1995;77–B:677–683.

10. Müller LP, Müller LA, Happ J: Frozen shoulder: A sympathetic dystrophy? Arch Orthop Trauma Surg 2000;120:84–87.

25

Interscalene Brachial Plexus Block

Alain Borgeat, MD • Stephan Blumenthal, MD

INTRODUCTION

The first brachial plexus blocks were performed by Halsted, in 1885, at the Roosevelt Hospital in New York City. Later Crile, in 1902, described an "open approach" to expose the plexus to the direct application of cocaine. At the time, however, the clinical applicability of this approach was limited because of the need for surgical exposure of the brachial plexus. Percutaneous access to the brachial plexus was described in the early 1900s. In 1925, Etienne[1] reported the successful blockade of the brachial plexus by inserting a needle at the level of the cricothyroid membrane, halfway between the lateral border of the sternocleidomastoid and the anterior border of the trapezius muscle after a single injection through the area around the scalene muscles. This approach is most likely the first clinically useful interscalene block technique.

Different approaches were then tried until Winnie, in 1970,[2] described the percutaneous technique of injecting local anesthetic into the groove between the anterior and middle scalene muscles at the level of the cricoid cartilage. This approach was the first consistently effective and technically suitable technique, and it allowed wider applicability of interscalene brachial plexus block. Winnie's approach was further modified, in line with numerous developments in regional anesthesia, by the placement of a perineural catheter, for example.[3]

Indications

Interscalene block is well suited for surgical procedures involving the shoulder, including the lateral two thirds of the clavicle, proximal humerus, and shoulder joint. Interscalene block can be used in the setting of arm or forearm surgery, but incomplete blockade of the inferior trunk often results in insufficient analgesia in the ulnar distribution. The patient's positioning and comfort, the surgeon's preferences, and the duration of surgery sometimes necessitate a combined general anesthesia. The indications for single-shot and interscalene catheter are summarized in Table 25–1.

Table 25–1.

Single-Injection vs. the Choice of Technique: Interscalene Catheter According to Surgery.

Type of Surgery	Type of Block Single-Injection	Catheter
Open Surgery		
Arthroplasty	+	+
Rotator cuff repair	+	+
Arthrolysis	+	+
Acromioplasty	+	+
Bankart's repair	+	+
Latarjet	+	+
Proximal humerus osteosynthesis	+	±
Acromioclavicular resection	+	−
Shoulder luxation	+	−
Clavicle osteosynthesis	+ (± superficial cervical block)	−
Arthroscopic Surgery		
Rotator cuff repair	+	+
Arthrolysis	+	+
Bankart's repair	+	±
Acromioplasty	+	±

Skin infiltration of the posterior arthroscopic port insertion site with local anesthetics is often necessary despite a successful interscalene block.

Clinical Pearls

- Adequate control of pain is crucial after major open-shoulder surgery; early rehabilitation is necessary for improving success.
- A major characteristic of the pain after shoulder surgery is its dynamic component, which often interferes with rehabilitation.
- Up to 70% of patients report severe pain on movement after open major shoulder surgery, which is more than after hysterectomy (60%), gastrectomy, or thoracotomy (60%).[4]
- Major shoulder surgery entails massive nociceptive input from the richly innervated joint and periarticular tissues, which produce continuous deep somatic pain and reflex spasm of muscles.
- These structures are supplied by the same and adjacent spinal cord segments supplying the site of surgery[5]; moreover, periarticular structures exhibit not only C afferents, but also A-alpha and A-delta afferents, the latter being poorly blocked by opioids, which explains the relative inefficacy of opioids to control this type of postoperative pain.

Contraindications

Contraindications for interscalene brachial plexus block are rare. Absolute contraindications include patient's refusal, local infection, active bleeding in an anticoagulated patient, and proven allergy to local anesthetic. Relative contraindications include chronic obstructive airway disease, contralateral paresis of the phrenic or recurrent laryngeal nerves, and previous neurologic deficit of the involved arm. The risks and benefits of the chosen anesthetic technique should be discussed with the patient and the surgeon.

Anatomy

Understanding the relevant brachial plexus anatomy, ensuring precise needle location within the plexus diffusion space, and injection of appropriate volume and type of local anesthetic are fundamental for achieving high success rates with brachial plexus anesthesia. The plexus is formed by the ventral rami of the fifth to eighth cervical nerves and the greater part of the ventral ramus of the first thoracic nerve (Figure 25–1). In addition, small contributions may be made by the fourth cervical and the second thoracic nerves. The anatomy becomes complex because of the multiple connections to these ventral rami after they emerge from between the middle and the anterior scalene muscles until they end in the terminal nerves of the upper extremity. However, most of what happens to these roots on their way to becoming peripheral nerves is not clinically essential information to the anesthesiologist.

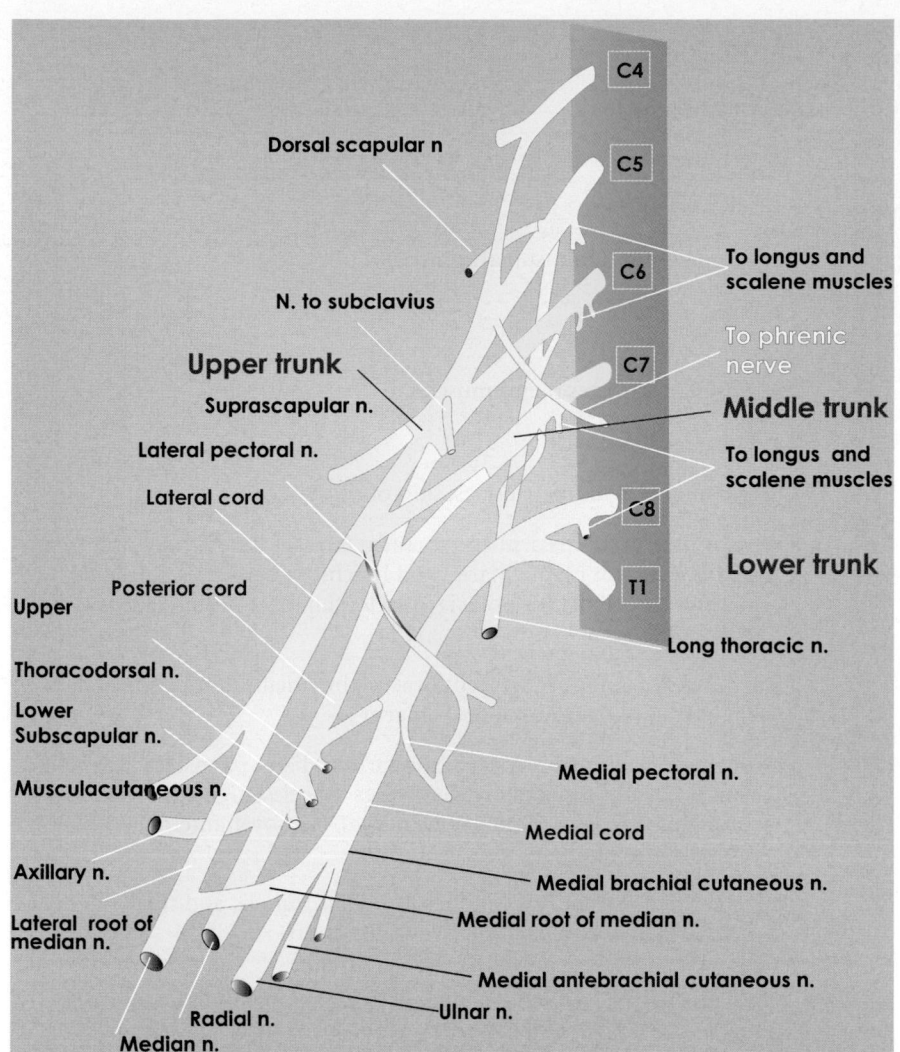

Figure 25–1. Organization of the brachial plexus.

Instead, broad concepts such as the spatial arrangement of the trunks (superior, middle, and inferior) and the muscular response elicited during electrostimulation can be helpful to clinicians (Table 25–2).

The brachial plexus supplies all the motor and most of the sensory functions of the shoulder except the cephalad cutaneous parts of the shoulder, which are innervated by the supraclavicular nerves originating from the lower part of the superficial cervical plexus (C3-4) (Figure 25–2). They supply sensation to the shoulder above the clavicle in addition to the first two intercostal spaces anteriorly. Furthermore, they supply sensation to the posterior cervical triangle and the upper thorax in this area as well as to the tip of the shoulder.[6]

Only three nerves of the brachial plexus have cutaneous representation in the shoulder. The most proximal of these is the upper lateral brachial cutaneous nerve, a branch of the axillary nerve that innervates the lateral side of the shoulder and the skin overlying the deltoid muscle. The upper medial side of the arm is innervated by both the medial brachial cutaneous and the intercostobrachial cutaneous nerves. In the anterior portion of the arm over the biceps muscle,

the skin is innervated by the medial antebrachial cutaneous nerve.[6]

Apart from the cutaneous nerve supply to the shoulder, the innervation of the joint deserves special consideration. In general, a nerve crossing a joint gives branches that innervate it. Therefore, the nerves supplying the ligaments, capsule, and synovial membrane of the shoulder are fibers from the axillary, suprascapular, subscapular, and musculocutaneous nerves.[7,8] The relative contributions of these nerves are variable, and the supply from the musculocutaneus nerve may be very small or completely absent. Anteriorly, the axillary nerve and suprascapular nerve provide most of the nerve supply to the capsule and glenohumeral joint (Figure 25–3). In some instances, the musculocutaneous nerve may innervate the anterosuperior portion of the joint. In addition, the anterior capsule may be supplied by either the subscapular nerves or the posterior cord of the brachial plexus after piercing the subscapularis muscle. Superiorly, primary contribution is from two branches of the suprascapular nerve, one branch supplying the acromioclavicular joint and proceeding anteriorly as far as the coracoid process and coracoacromial ligament and the other branch reaching the posterior aspect

Table 25–2.

Distribution of the Brachial Plexus

Nerve(s)	Spinal Segment(s)	Distribution
Subclavius nerve	C4 through C6	Subclavius muscle
Dorsal scapular nerve	C4-C5	Rhomboid muscles and levator scapulae muscle
Long thoracic nerve	C5 through C7	Serratus anterior muscle
Suprascapular nerve	C4, C5, C6	Supraspinatus and infraspinatus muscles
Pectoralis nerves (medial and lateral)	C5 through T1	Pectoralis muscles
Subscapular nerves	C5, C6	Subscapular and teres major muscles
Thoracodorsal nerve	C6 through C8	Latissimus dorsi muscle
Axillary nerve	C5 and C6	Deltoid and teres minor muscles; skin of shoulder
Radial nerve	C5 through T1	Extensor muscles of the arm and forearm (triceps brachii, extensor carpi radialis, extensor carpi ulnaris) and brachioradialis muscle; digital extension and abductor pollicis muscle; skin over posterolateral surface of the arm
Musculocutaneous nerve	C5 through C7	Flexor muscles of the arm (biceps brachii, brachialis, coracobrachialis); skin over lateral surface of the forearm
Median nerve	C6 through T1	Flexor muscles of the forearm (flexor carpi radialis, palmaris longus); pronator quadratus, and pronator teres muscles; digital flexors (through the palmar interosseous nerve); skin over anterolateral surface of the hand
Ulnar nerve	C8, T1	Flexor carpi ulnaris muscle, adductor pollicis muscle, and small digital muscles, skin over medial surface of the hand

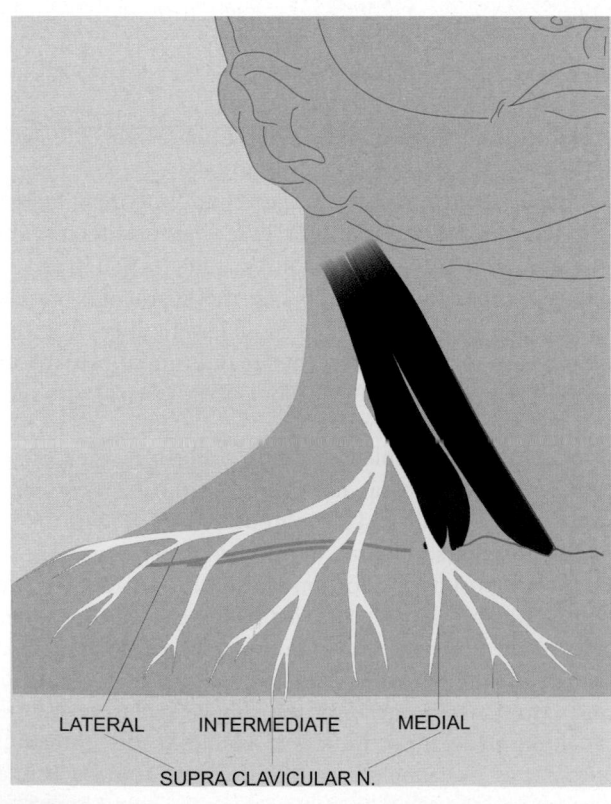

LATERAL   INTERMEDIATE   MEDIAL

SUPRA CLAVICULAR N.

Figure 25–2. The innervation of the skin over the shoulder and clavicle.

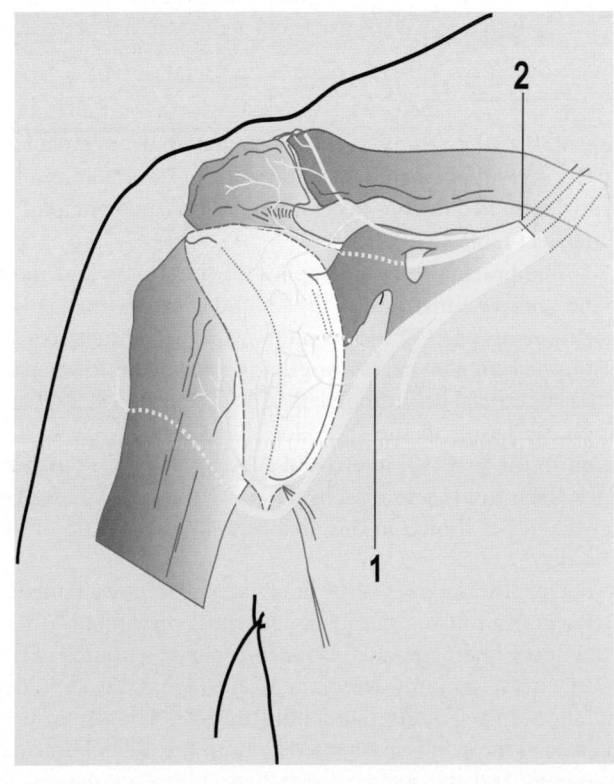

Figure 25–3. The innervation of the anterior portion of the shoulder. The axillary (1) and suprascapular (2) nerves form most of the nerve supply to the capsule and the glenohumeral joint.

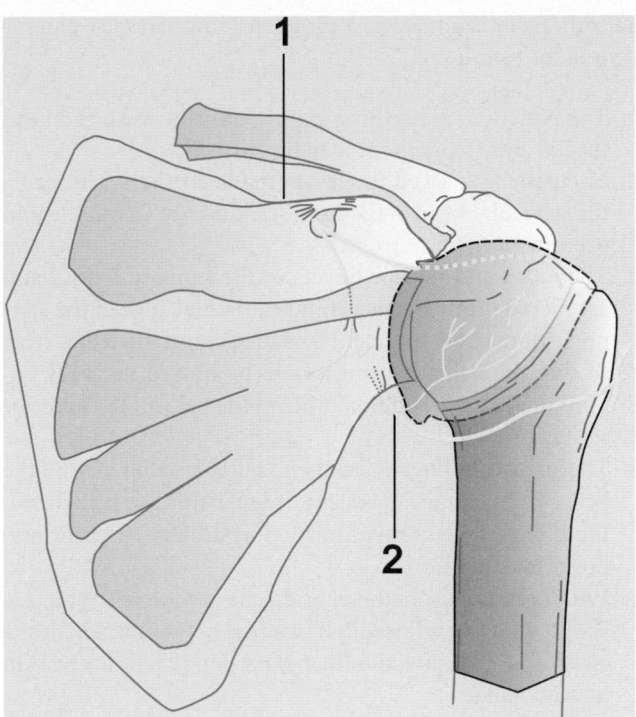

Figure 25–4. The posterior innervation of the shoulder joint. The primary nerves are the suprascapular (1) and the axillary (2).

of the joint. Other nerves contributing to this region of the joint are the axillary nerve and musculocutaneous nerve. Posteriorly, the main nerves are the suprascapular nerve in the upper region and the axillary nerve in the lower region (Figure 25–4).

Inferiorly, the anterior portion is primarily supplied by the axillary nerve, and the posterior portion is supplied by a combination of the axillary nerve and lower ramifications of the suprascapular nerve.

Clinical Pearls

■ The following nerves should be anesthetized to achieve anesthesia for arthroscopic surgery: supraclavicular, suprascapular, and axillary (radial) nerves.

■ For open shoulder surgery, knowledge of the surgical approach is useful because the surgical incision may also involve the territories of the median cutaneous, intercostobrachial, and the median antebrachial cutaneous nerves.

Landmarks

The following surface anatomy landmarks are necessary for identifying the interscalene groove:

1. Sternal head of the sternocleidomastoid muscle
2. Clavicular head of the sternocleidomastoid muscle
3. Upper border of the cricoid cartilage
4. Clavicle

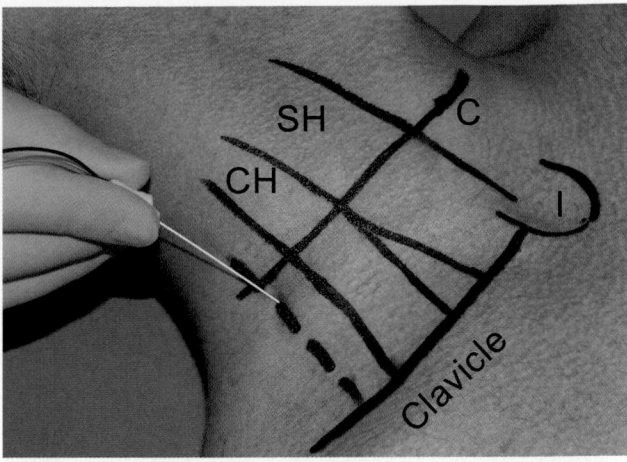

Figure 25–5. The lateral modified technique (Borgeat). The needle is inserted toward the plane of the interscalene space (*dashed line*) at an angle between 45 and 60 degrees. The needle is inserted approximately 0.5 cm under the level of the cricoid (C). SH, sternal head of the sternocleidomastoid muscle; CH, clavicular head of the sternocleidomastoid muscle. I, incisura jugularis sterni (sternal notch).

These landmarks should always be marked with a pen (Figure 25–5).

Equipment for Single-Shot Blockade

Standard regional anesthesia equipment for a single-shot blockade consists of the following items (Figure 25–6).

Marking pen, ruler
Sterile gloves
Peripheral nerve stimulator, surface electrode
Disinfection solution and sterile gauze packs

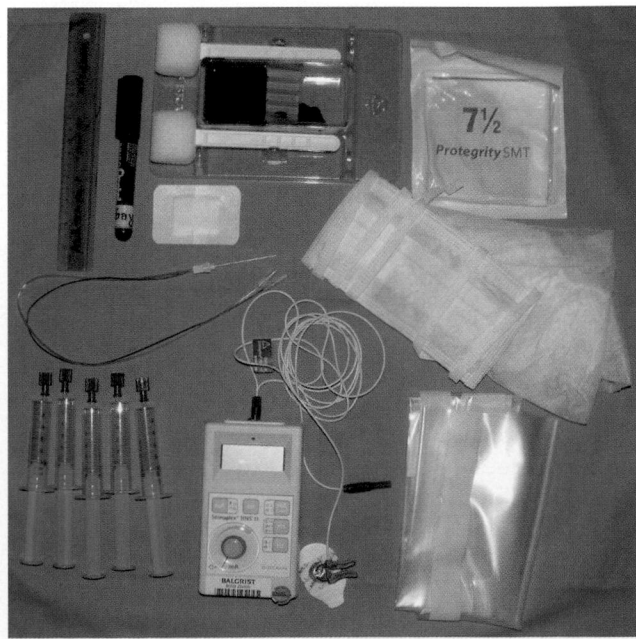

Figure 25–6. Equipment for single-injection interscalene block.

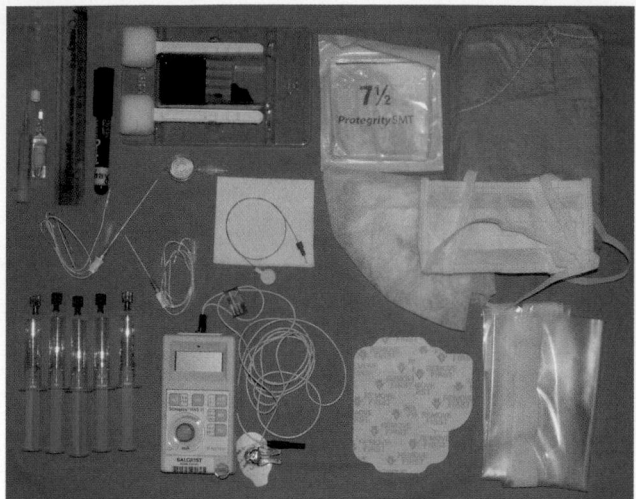

Figure 25–7. Equipment for continuous interscalene block.

2- to 5-cm, short-bevel, 22-gauge insulated stimulating needle

Syringes with local anesthetic

Equipment for Continuous Blockade

Standard regional anesthesia equipment for a continuous nerve block consists of the following items (Figure 25–7).

Marking pen, ruler

Peripheral nerve stimulator, surface electrode

Disinfection solution, sterile gauze packs

Sterile transparent drapes

Syringes with local anesthetic for skin infiltration and block injection

25-mm, 25-gauge needle for skin infiltration at puncture point and for tunneling

A set with stimulating needle for continuous nerve block and catheter

Adhesive transparent tapes for securing the catheter

Sterile gloves (cap, mask, and gown are optional)

APPROACHES TO & TECHNIQUES FOR BRACHIAL PLEXUS BLOCK AT THE LEVEL OF THE NECK

Several approaches for interscalene block are known; with all modern techniques, the use of a nerve stimulator is recommended to localize the brachial plexus. The common techniques are those of Winnie, Pippa, modified *lateral* techniques (Meier and Borgeat), and the *low interscalene* approach.

Classic Technique (Winnie)

The classic approach of Winnie[2] is performed at the level of the sixth cervical vertebra. Although Winnie originally used a

paresthesia technique, most clinicians nowadays use a nerve stimulator technique.

1. The patient is placed in a supine position with the head turned away from the side to be blocked.
2. The patient is asked to elevate the head slightly to bring the clavicular head of the sternocleidomastoid muscle into prominence.
3. The index and middle fingers of the nondominant hand are placed immediately behind the lateral edge of the sternocleidomastoid muscle. The patient is instructed to relax so that the palpating fingers can be moved medially behind this muscle and finally lie on the belly of the anterior scalene muscle.
4. The palpating fingers are then rolled laterally across the belly of the anterior scalene muscle until they fall into the interscalene groove (formed by scalene anterior and posterior muscles).
5. With both fingers in the interscalene groove, a $1\frac{1}{2}$ in., 22-gauge, short-bevel needle is inserted between them at the level of C6 in a direction that is perpendicular to the skin in every plane.
6. After a paresthesia (below the shoulder) is obtained, aspiration is carried out to rule out intravascular or intrathecal placement. While the patient is monitored closely for signs of local anaesthetic toxicity or inadvertent subarachnoid injection, 20–30 mL of local anesthetics are slowly injected.

Clinical Pearls

- In Winnie's original description, the needle is advanced slowly until a paresthesia is elicited or until the transverse process is encountered.
- Only a paresthesia below the level of the shoulder is acceptable because a paresthesia to the shoulder could result from stimulation of the suprascapular nerve inside or outside the interscalene space.
- If bone is contacted without producing a paresthesia, this is likely the transverse process and the needle should be gently "walked off" anteriorly millimeter by millimeter until a paresthesia is evoked.
- In modern practice, the paresthesia technique was replaced by the use of neurostimulation.

Reported complications with this technique included total spinal anesthesia,[9,10] epidural anesthesia,[11] cervical cord injection with resultant paraplegia, as well as injections into the vertebral artery and the cervical spinal cord.[12] Most of these complications are likely due to the perpendicular direction of the needle toward the cervical spine. Although an infrequent complication, pneumothorax can also occur with this technique. This technique is not well suited for the placement of an interscalene catheter because of the perpendicular approach to the trunks.

Posterior Approach (Pippa)

The posterior approach of Pippa[13] is performed using the loss of resistance technique.

Landmarks

The approach of Pippa requires the following surface landmarks to be drawn on the skin (see Chapter 24):

- *Point A*—Midpoint between the cutaneous projections of the spinal process of the sixth and the seventh cervical vertebrae.
- *Line B*—Cutaneous projection of the superoexternal edge of the trapezius muscle–aponeurotic line.
- The *point of needle insertion* is where the horizontal line through point A intersects with line B.
- The point of needle insertion lies approximately 3 cm lateral to the interspinous line C6 and C7 and corresponds to the upper edge of the transverse process of the seventh cervical vertebra.

Technique

After local infiltration of the skin at the point of needle insertion, a 9-cm, 21-gauge needle is inserted and directed perpendicular to the skin through the trapezius, splenius cervicis, and levator scapulae muscles as far as the transverse process of the seventh cervical vertebra. The patient is then asked to turn the head to the contralateral side, and the needle (attached to a 5-mL syringe filled with air) is passed over the transverse process and advanced slowly through the posterior and middle scalene muscle into the interscalene space, where a "loss of resistance" can be felt.

The patient is then asked to move the head back to the original position. After negative aspiration for blood and cerebrospinal fluid, the local anesthetic solution is injected. Apart from transient side effects, such as reduction of pulmonary function and Horner syndrome,[14,15] serious complications with Pippa's technique are not described. However, this technique represents a paravertebral approach to the brachial plexus and therefore can be associated with similar complications to those of Winnie's approach (eg, total spinal or epidural anesthesia; injections into the vertebral artery or the cervical spinal cord). This approach was recently modified by Boezaart.[16] It is described in greater detail in Chapter 24.

Modified Lateral Technique (Meier)

To reduce the risk of complications and to allow the placement of an interscalene catheter for postoperative analgesia, Meier and coworkers[17] modified Winnie's technique as follows.

- The same landmarks are identified as with Winnie's approach.
- The point of needle insertion is moved 2–3 cm cranial from the cricoid cartilage.
- In contrast to the technique of Winnie, the needle is not inserted perpendicularly, but at a 30-degree angle to the skin, and then directed toward the transition of the middle to the lateral third part of the clavicle.
- A nerve stimulator is used localize the brachial plexus in the interscalene groove.

This approach is also well designed for the placement of an interscalene catheter.

Modified Lateral Technique (Borgeat)

Similar to the technique described by Meier and coworkers,[17] this approach to the interscalene brachial plexus is a modification of the classic technique of Winnie. The positioning of the patient's head, the identification of the landmarks, and the palpation of the interscalene groove are carried out in a similar way. The palpation of the interscalene groove is crucial because it provides important information about its shape, depth, and course at the lateral neck and helps the anesthesiologist to gain a three-dimensional image of the interscalene space.[3]

Technique

- After palpation of the interscalene groove, a line is drawn along the interscalene groove (Figure 25–8).
- Similar to the Winnie's technique, the point of needle insertion on this line lies 3–5 mm below the level of the upper part of the cricoid cartilage.
- A 5-cm, 22-gauge, short-bevel needle is used.
- The needle is directed caudally and slightly laterally or medially, depending on the plane of the interscalene space (see Figure 25–5).
- Motor response to nerve stimulation is sought in the posterior and dorsal part of the superior or middle trunk of the brachial plexus (preferentially, a triceps or sometimes deltoid response [C5, C6]).
- The position of the needle is considered appropriate if twitches are still present with a current output between 0.2 and 0.4 mA (100 μsec).

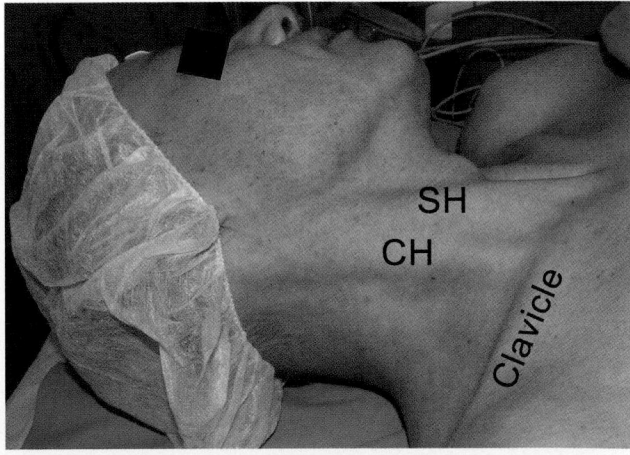

Figure 25–8. Surface landmarks for the interscalene groove are easier to recognize with the patient lifting his/her head off the table. CH, clavicular head; SH, sternal head.

This approach is equally suitable for single-shot inter-scalene anesthesia as well as for continuous interscalene anesthesia and analgesia through an interscalene catheter.

Low Interscalene Brachial Plexus Block

The low interscalene technique of brachial plexus block[18] differs in three important aspects from the classic approach and its modifications.

- Insertion of the needle is substantially below the cricoid cartilage and more lateral than with other approaches. This placement should reduce the risk of inadvertent insertion of the needle into the cervical cord as well as the risk of intraarterial injection into a vertebral artery.
- The brachial plexus is very superficial at this location; the skin to brachial plexus block distance is typically less than 1 cm and never deeper than 2 cm.
- The block can be considered anatomically and functionally a crossbreed between a classic interscalene block (the plexus is approached in the distal interscalene groove) and a supraclavicular block (the needle insertion is slightly above the clavicle).

In contrast to the other approaches, the low interscalene approach provides anesthesia for shoulder, elbow, and forearm surgeries alike.[19]

Landmarks

The landmarks for the low interscalene brachial plexus approach are as follows (Figure 25–9).

- Clavicle
- Posterior border of the clavicular head of the sternocleidomastoid muscle
- External jugular vein

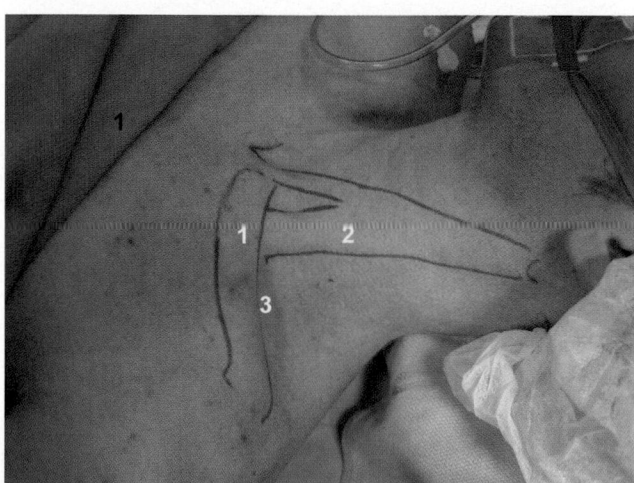

Figure 25–9. Landmarks for low interscalene approach to brachial plexus block: (1) Clavicle. (2) Posterior border of the sternocleidomastoid muscle. (3) External jugular vein.

Clinical Pearls

- The landmarks for the low interscalene approach to brachial plexus block can be accentuated by the following maneuver, which should be routinely performed:
  1. Ask the patient to face slightly away from the side to be blocked. This maneuver tenses the sternocleidomastoid muscles.
  2. Ask the patient to reach the ipsilateral knee on the side to be blocked or passively pull the wrist toward the knee. This maneuver flattens the skin of the neck and helps to identify both the scalene muscles and the external jugular vein.
  3. Ask the patient to lift the head off the table while facing away. This maneuver tenses the sternocleidomastoid muscles and helps to identify the posterior border of the clavicular head of the sternocleidomastoid muscle.

Technique

The fingers of the palpating hand should be gently but firmly pressed between the anterior and middle scalene muscles to shorten the skin to brachial plexus distance (Figure 25–10). The palpating hand should not be moved during the entire block placement procedure to allow for precise redirections of the angle of the needle insertion when necessary. A needle connected to the nerve stimulator is inserted between the palpating fingers and advanced at an angle almost perpendicular to the skin plane and in a slight caudad direction (Figure 25–11). The nerve stimulator should be initially set to deliver l mA (2 Hz, 100 μsec). The needle is advanced slowly until stimulation of the brachial plexus is obtained. Once any motor response of the brachial plexus is elicited, 35–40 mL of local anesthetic of choice is injected slowly, with intermittent aspiration.

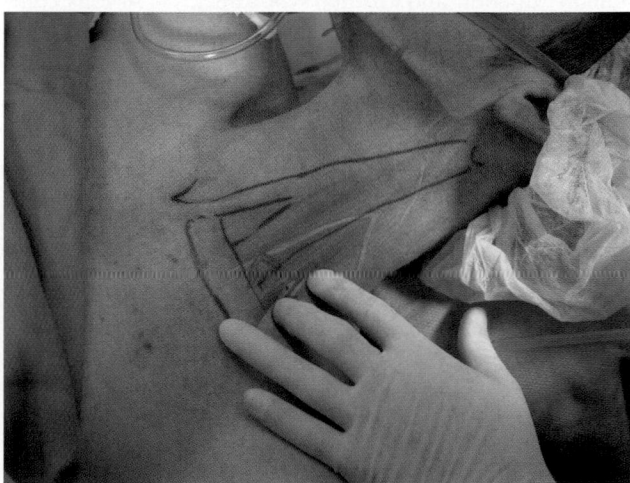

Figure 25–10. Fingers of the palpating hand are positioned in front of the external jugular vein and in the interscalene grove made up of anterior and middle scalene muscles. Interscalene groove is the widest and easiest to palpate in this position.

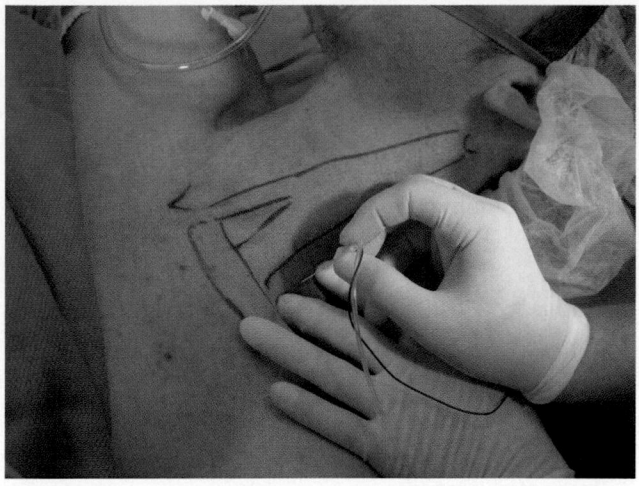

Figure 25–11. Low interscalene block. Proper angle of the needle direction is medial with a slight caudad angulation.

Clinical Pearls

Some common responses to nerve stimulation and the course of action to obtain the proper response are shown in Table 25–3. The following twitches all result from stimulation of the brachial plexus and can be accepted with a similar success rate:

- Pectoralis muscle
- Deltoid muscle
- Triceps muscles
- Any twitch of the hand or forearm (applicable only to low-interscalene approach)
- Biceps muscle

Table 25–3.

Guide to Troubleshooting Interscalene Block

Response Obtained	Interpretation	Problem	Action
Local twitch of the neck muscles	Direct stimulation of the anterior scalene *or* sternocleoidomastoid muscles	Needle pass is in the wrong plane; usually anterior and medial to the plexus	Withdraw the needle to the skin and reinsert 15-degrees posterior
Needle contacts bone at 1–2 cm depth; no twitches seen	The needle is stopped by the transverse process	The needle is inserted too posterior; the needle contacts anterior tubercles of the transverse process	Withdraw the needle to the skin and reinsert 15-degrees anterior
Twitches of the diaphragm	The result of stimulation of the phrenic nerve	The needle is inserted too anterior and medial	Withdraw the needle and reinsert 15 degrees posterior and lateral
Arterial blood noticed in the tubing	Puncture of the carotid artery (most likely)	The needle insertion and angulation are too anterior	Withdraw the needle and keep a steady pressure for 2–3 min; reinsert 1–2 cm posterior
Pectoralis muscle twitch	Brachial plexus stimulation (C4-5)		Accept and inject local anesthetic
Twitch of the scapula	Twitch of the serratus anterior muscle; stimulation of the thoracodorsal nerve	Needle position is posterior/deep to the brachial plexus	Withdraw the needle to the skin, and reinsert the needle anterior
Trapezius muscle twitches	Accessory nerve stimulation	Needle posterior to the brachial plexus	Withdraw the needle and insert more anteriorly
Twitch of pectorals, deltoid, triceps, biceps, forearm, and hand muscles	Stimulation of the brachial plexus	None	Accept and inject local anesthetic

Continuous Interscalene Brachial Plexus Block

The continuous interscalene brachial plexus blockade is an advanced regional anesthesia technique, and adequate experience with the single-shot technique is necessary. Paradoxically, although the single-shot interscalene block is one of the easiest intermediate techniques to perform and master, placement of the catheter in the interscalene groove may be one of the more challenging continuous block techniques. This discrepancy is mostly due to the shallow position of the brachial plexus and difficulties in stabilizing the needle during catheter advancement. In addition, there is a difference in stimulating characteristics between the smaller-caliber single-shot and larger-caliber (often) Tuohy-style tip needles. The technique is otherwise similar to the single-shot injection with the exception that the needle is inserted at a lower angle to allow for threading the catheter. This technique provides excellent analgesia in patients after shoulder, arm, and elbow surgery.

Technique

The patient is positioned in the same position as in the single-shot technique. The subcutaneous tissues at the projected site of needle insertion are anesthetized with local anesthetic. The needle is attached to the nerve stimulator (1.0 mA, 2 Hz, 100 μsec) and to a syringe with local anesthetic. With this technique, it is imperative that the palpating hand firmly stabilizes the skin to facilitate needle insertion and insertion of the catheter. A 5-cm block needle is inserted at a slightly caudal angle and advanced until the brachial plexus twitch is elicited at 0.2 to 0.5 mA (Figure 25–12). While paying meticulous attention to the position of the needle, the catheter is inserted some 2–3 cm beyond the tip of the needle (Figure 25–13). The catheter is secured using a benzoin skin preparation, followed by application of a clear dressing. Some clinicians prefer to tunnel the catheter to prevent its accidental withdrawal (Figure 25–14). The infusion port should be clearly marked as: "continuous interscalene block," and the catheter should be carefully checked for intravascular placement before ad-

ministering larger volumes or infusion of local anesthetics. Before initiating the infusion of local anesthetic, the catheter is first checked for patency, and intravascular placement is ruled out by administering a small volume (2–3 mL of 1% lidocaine with epinephrine 1:300,000). The management of the continuous infusion of local anesthetic is discussed in the section about intraoperative management.

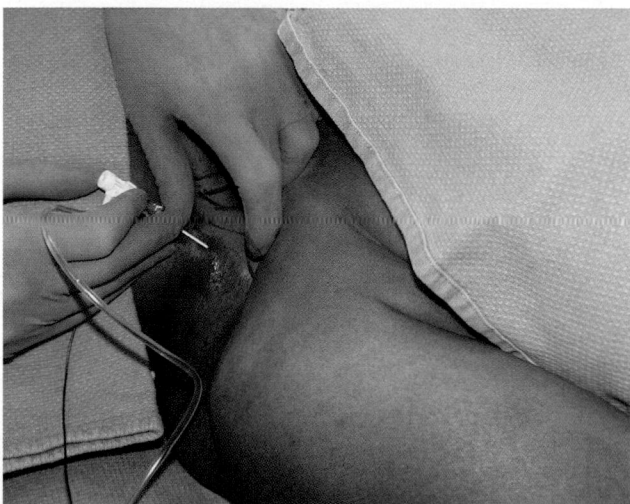

Figure 25–12. Continuous interscalene block. Note the low angle of needle insertion, which is necessary to facilitate insertion of the catheter.

Clinical Pearls

- Indeed, each patient has a different interscalene groove, which makes the block challenging in some patients because there are no bony or vascular landmarks.
- The following maneuvers help to precisely localize the interscalene groove:
  1. Ask the patient to turn the head away from the side to be blocked and then to lift the head off the table. This maneuver tenses the sternocleidomastoid muscle and helps to identify the lateral border of the clavicular head of the sternocleidomastoid muscle.
  2. In some patients, the clavicular head of the sternocleidomastoid and anterior scalene muscles are packed together. To help find out "what is what," the practitioner should ask the patient to take a deep breath as the practitioner places the fingers firmly on the muscles. With this maneuver, it is often possible to differentiate the two muscles; the part belonging to the anterior scalene muscle, contracting slightly before the clavicular part of the sternocleidomastoid muscle, is felt. Another tip is to look for the insertion of the muscle on the clavicle. The clavicular head of the sternocleidomastoid muscle inserts on the clavicle, whereas the anterior scalene muscle passes under the clavicle and is fixed on the first rib. This can be more or less easily palpated in each patient.
  3. It is important to make the difference between the anterior and the median and posterior scalene muscles. The anterior muscle is plump ("banana muscle"); the latter is flat. The feeling of the anterior scalene muscle is important to keep in mind.
  4. The supraclavicular nerve can be easily missed, particularly in patients with a short neck. It is also the only nerve to be blocked "in rescue," in case of incomplete interscalene block for shoulder surgery. The supraclavicular nerve can be easily blocked by injecting subcutaneously 6–8 mL of local anesthetics on the lateral–posterior side of the clavicular head of the sternocleidomastoid muscle.
  5. For certain surgeries (eg, Latarjet's procedure), the surgical incision goes below the lower part of the deltopectoral incision (usually performed). It may be useful to make a subcutaneous infiltration of local anesthetics in this area to block the cutaneous branches of the intercostobrachial nerve.

INTRAOPERATIVE MANAGEMENT OF AN INTERSCALENE BLOCK DURING SHOULDER SURGERY

Sedation is almost always necessary to improve patient's comfort and satisfaction and the quality of the anesthesia achieved with an interscalene block. In addition, most surgeons prefer

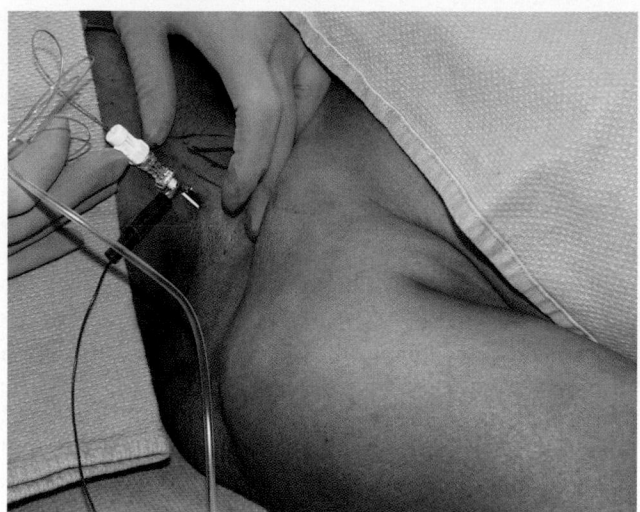

Figure 25–13. Continuous interscalene block. Insertion of the catheter.

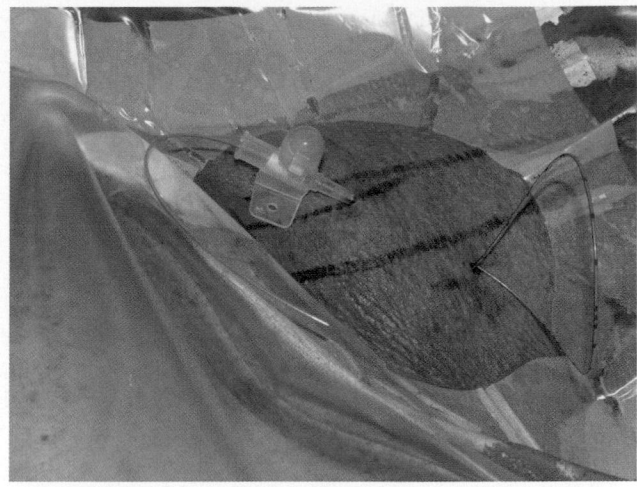

Figure 25–14. Subcutaneous tunneling of the interscalene catheter. The interscalene catheter is withdrawn retrogradely through the intravenous cannula.

patients to be lightly asleep during surgery. Similarly, most patients also prefer not to be "aware" of activities in the operating room. Drugs most commonly used to accomplish perioperative sedation are propofol, midazolam, and an intravenous opioid. A face mask with oxygen (4–6 L/min) is routinely applied. Because most operating rooms are kept cold, all patients undergoing surgery under interscalene block should be kept warm by using forced air or warm blankets. The onset of shivering can turn a successful regional anesthetic into a significant intraoperative challenge.

Intraoperative use of pneumatic equipment close to the patient's ear can result in noise levels over 100 dB and significant amount of sedation is often needed to mask this noise.[20] The use of earplugs, headphones with or without music, or blankets to cover the patient's ears and reduce the noise level can make a substantial difference in patient's comfort.

Hyperhydration should be avoided because the patients typically do not have or require urinary bladder catheterization. It is a good idea to ask patients to empty their bladders before administering any drugs.

Choice of Local Anesthetics

For single-shot techniques, a variety of local anesthetic mixtures can be used (Table 25–4), depending on the desired duration and density of blockade. This author prefers to use ropivacaine rather than bupivacaine and levobupivacaine because of the greater safety profile of ropivacaine.

The typical volume of local anesthetic used for interscalene blocks is 30–45 mL. The expected duration of the block varies between 3 and 5 hours with mepivacaine 1.5% or 2% and lidocaine 1.5%[21,22] and 8–12 hours with bupivacaine

Table 25–4.

Local Anesthetic Mixtures Used for Single-Injection Techniques

	Onset (min)	Anesthesia (h)	Analgesia (h)
3% 2-Chloroprocaine ($+$ HCO$_3$ $+$ epinephine)	5–10	1.5	2.0
1.5% Mepivacaine ($+$ HCO$_3$)	10–20	2–3	2–4
1.5% Mepivacaine ($+$ HCO$_3$ $+$ epinephrine)	5–15	2.5–4	3–6
2% Lidocaine ($+$ HCO$_3$)	10–20	2.5–3	2–5
2% Lidocaine ($+$ HCO$_3$ $+$ epinephrine)	5–15	3–6	5–8
0.5% Ropivacaine	15–20	6–8	8–12
0.75% Ropivacaine	5–15	8–10	12–18
0.5% Bupivacaine ($+$ epinephrine)	20–30	8–10	16–18

0.5% and ropivacaine 0.5 or 0.75%.[23,24] The duration of action is also proportional to the volume and dose administered. Clonidine,[25] but not opioids,[26,27] can prolong the duration of both anesthesia and analgesia with intermediate-acting local anesthetics.[25] The addition of epinephrine also prolongs the duration of action of most local anesthetics.[28] Results of studies that compared the outcome of interscalene block with that of general anesthesia in patients undergoing shoulder arthroscopy suggest that interscalene block provides a number of important advantages over general anesthesia in the outpatient setting.[21,29] The interscalene block provided excellent anesthesia and muscular relaxation, fewer postoperative side effects and hospital admissions, and a shorter hospital stay. It is important to note that complete recovery of the motor blockade is no longer a requirement before discharge home,[30] making the long-acting anesthetics more appropriate in this setting, even for day-case surgery.

Continuous infusion of local anesthetics through an interscalene catheter compared with traditional patient-controlled analgesia (PCA) with opioids provides significantly better control of pain, with a statistically significant lower incidence of side effects and greater patient satisfaction.[31,32] Catheters are typically left in place for 2–3 days. The use of a continuous infusion of 0.125% bupivacaine at a rate of 0.125 mL/kg per hour was shown to provide efficient pain relief, but at the cost of administrating a large volume of local anesthetics.[32] A better infusion protocol for perineural blocks would be to incorporate a PCA dose, which allows patients to affect the dynamic nature of the pain.

Clinical Pearls

- When compared with the continuous technique, a lower basal infusion of 5 mL/h bupivacaine 0.125% in addition to a small PCA bolus of 2.5 mL/30 min provides similar pain control, but reduces the consumption of local anesthetics by 37% and lowers the incidence of side effects, such as Horner syndrome and clinically apparent phrenic paresis.[31]

Either bupivacaine 0.15% or ropivacaine 0.2% as a primary agent at a rate of 5 mL/h plus a supplemental bolus of 4 mL/20 min was associated with better pain control; lower incidence of nausea, vomiting, and pruritus; and better patient satisfaction, compared with the classic PCA with opioids.[31,33]

Ropivacaine 0.2%, compared with interscalene PCA with bupivacaine 0.15%, was associated with better preservation of hand strength 24 and 48 hours after the beginning of the infusion, as well as 6 hours after the infusion was stopped.[34] Therefore, ropivacaine, compared with bupivacaine, may have better sensorimotor dissociation.[35,36]

SIDE EFFECTS & COMPLICATIONS & HOW TO AVOID THEM

Complications associated with the different techniques of interscalene block are summarized in (Table 25–5). The most common side effects encountered after interscalene block are hoarseness (10–20%) due to the blockade of the recurrent laryngeal nerve, which occurs more frequently on the right side. Claude-Bernard-Horner syndrome is characterized by ptosis, myosis, and enopthalmia due to the diffusion of the local anesthetic solution on the sympathetic cervical ganglion chain (including the stellatum ganglion) (Figure 25–15). The reason for this syndrome is the spread of the local anesthetic around the anterior scalene muscle behind the carotid artery and internal jugular vein toward the longus colli muscle (Figure 25–16). This results in blockade of the cervical ganglion (Horner syndrome) and phrenic nerve, which

Table 25–5.

Complications of Interscalene Block According to Approach

	Winnie	Posterior	Modified Lateral
Spinal injection	++	++	−
Epidural injection	++	++	−
Vertebral artery injection	+	(+)	−
Intravenous injection	+	+	+
Pneumothorax	+	+	+
Discomfort	(+)	++	(+)
Conditions for catheter placement	−	+	++

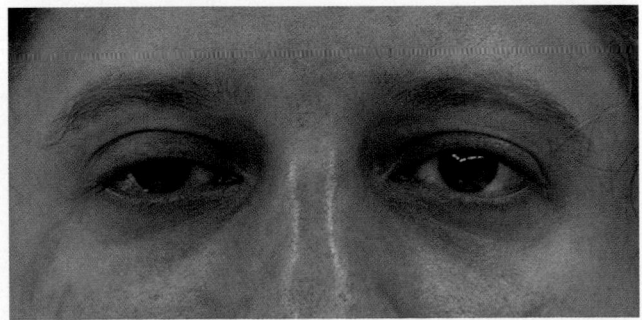

Figure 25–15. Horner syndrome is common after interscalene block and consists of ptosis, myosis, and enophthalmia (patient's right eye).

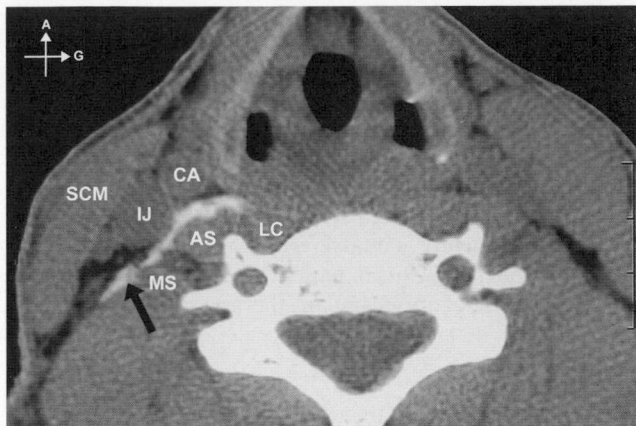

Figure 25–16. Spread of the local anesthetic (*arrow*) injectate in the interscalene block. Contrast medium is shown around anterior scalene muscle (AS), submerging in the space directly behind the carotid artery (CA) and internal jugular vein (IJ) and medially to the longus colli muscle (LC), where it results in blockade of the cervical ganglion (Horner syndrome) and phrenic nerve. Superior laryngeal nerve can be affected. MS, middle scalene muscle; SCM, sternocleidomastoid muscle.

rarely presents a problem clinically, and many patients are not even aware of it. The occurrence of the paradoxical Bezold-Jarisch reflex, that is, sudden bradycardia and hypotension (15–30%), is favored by the sitting position and can be often prevented by avoiding hypovolemia. It is easily treated by atropine and ephedrine administration.

Complications

Early complications (soon after block administration), such as epidural or spinal injection and intravertebral injection, are primarily related to the approach chosen (Table 25–5). Late complications include neuropathy, mechanical plexus injury, and infection.

Nerve injuries are a well-recognized complication of anesthesia.[38,39] It is generally believed that regional techniques are more prone to induce nerve damage because the aim of these techniques is to deposit the local anesthetic in close vicinity to the nerve. However, Kroll and coworkers[39] reported that 60% of the claims for nerve damage occurred after general anesthesia, with the reserve that more procedures were performed under general than under regional anesthesia. Postoperative brachial plexus plexopathy is well documented to occur regardless of the type of anesthesia administered. The American Society of Anesthesiologists, using the Closed Claims Database, performed a systematic analysis of nerve injury associated with anesthesia.[39] The results of this large study revealed that nerve damage represented 16% of the 4183 claims analyzed. The distribution of the nerve

are located in this area. In addition, superior laryngeal nerve can be affected. It occurs in 40–60% of patients and resolves with resolution of the block; patient reassurance is all that is needed for management. Ipsilateral hemidiaphragmatic paresis is a common finding and may be present in nearly 100% of patients[37] (Figure 25–17). This finding, however,

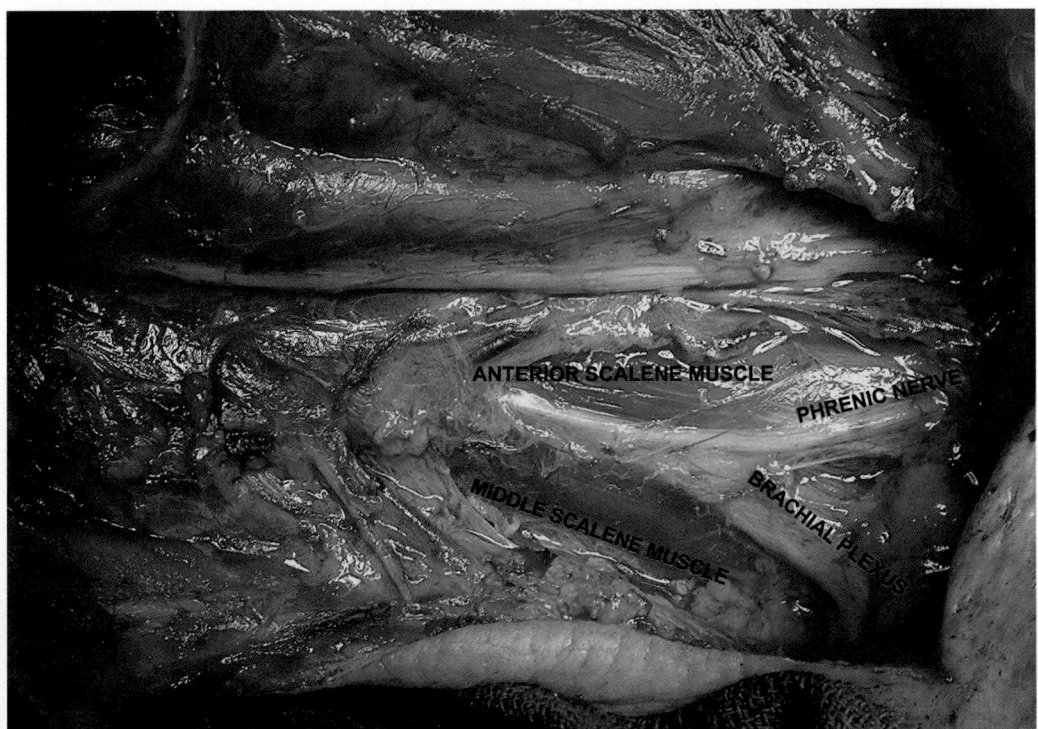

Figure 25–17. Neck dissection reveals the relation of the phrenic nerve, which leaves the brachial plexus anteriorly, and the rest of the brachial plexus, which remains sandwiched between the anterior and middle scalene muscles.

Table 25–6.	
Complications and How to Avoid Them	
Infection	• A strict aseptic technique is used
Hematoma	• Avoid multiple needle insertions, particularly in anticoagulated patients • Keep a 5-minute steady pressure when carotid artery is inadvertently punctured • Use a smaller gauge needle to localize the brachial plexus in patients with difficult anatomy • In the absence of spontaneous bleeding, the use of anticoagulant therapy should not be regarded as a contraindication for this block
Vascular puncture	• Vascular puncture is not common with this technique • Steady pressure of 5 minutes' duration should be maintained when the carotid artery is punctured (rare)
Local anesthetic toxicity	• Systemic toxicity due to absorption of local anesthetic after interscalene blockade is rare • Systemic toxicity most commonly occurs during or shortly after injection of local anesthetic; this is most commonly caused by an inadvertent intravascular injection or channeling of forcefully injected local anesthetic into small veins or lymphatic channels cut during needle manipulation • Large volumes of long-acting anesthetic should be reconsidered in older and frail patients. • Careful and frequent aspiration should be performed during the injection • Avoid forceful, fast injection of local anesthetic
Nerve injury	• Never inject local anesthetic when abnormal pressure on injection is encountered • Local anesthetic should never be injected when patient complains of severe pain or exhibits a withdrawal reaction on injection
Total spinal anesthesia	• When stimulation is obtained with current intensity of <0.2 mA, the needle should be pulled back to obtain the same response with current >0.2 mA before injecting local anesthetic to avoid injection into the dural sleeves and the consequent epidural or spinal spread • Never inject local anesthetic when abnormal resistance on injection is encountered
Horner syndrome	• Occurrence of ipsilateral ptosis, hyperemia of the conjunctiva, and nasal congestion is common, and it is dependent on the site of injection (less common with the low interscalene approach) and total volume of local anesthetic injected; patients should be instructed on the occurrence of this syndrome and reassured about its benign nature
Diaphragmatic paralysis	• Invariably present; avoid interscalene blockade or a large volume of local anesthetic in patients with severe, chronic respiratory disease, and use accessory respiratory muscles during breathing at rest

injury (670 cases) showed that the most common nerve injury involved the ulnar nerve (28%), immediately followed by the brachial plexus (20%). Among these, 78% and 22% occurred after general and regional anesthesia, respectively. Except for cases associated with spinal cord damage, no specific mechanism to explain these events was evident. However, in the cases of brachial plexus damage, factors related to patient position, such as the use of shoulder braces and the head position, malposition of the arms, and sustained neck extension were observed frequently. Little data are available on the rate of complication related to the use of the continuous interscalene catheters.[40,41] Table 25–6 lists reported complications of interscalene blocks and suggestions on how to avoid them.

SUMMARY

Interscalene nerve block is one of the most commonly used and most clinically applicable nerve block techniques. Modern techniques and equipment, when combined with appropriate training, result in a predictable success rate, excellent anesthesia, and superb postoperative analgesia. Recent studies affirmed the clinical impression that interscalene blocks offer several independent advantages over general anesthesia in outpatients undergoing shoulder surgery. Continuous interscalene block is a relatively new modality that can be used to extend the advantages of single-injection interscalene blocks well into the postoperative period.

References

1. Etienne J: Regional anesthesia: Its application in the surgical treatment of cancer of the breast [French], Faculté de Médecin de Paris, 1925.
2. Winnie AP: Interscalene brachial plexus block. Anesth Analg 1970;49:455–66.
3. Borgeat A, Ekatodramis G: Anaesthesia for shoulder surgery. Best Pract Res Clin Anaesthesiol 2002;16:211–25.
4. Bonica JJ: Anatomic and physiologic basis of nociception and pain, The Management of Pain, 2nd Edition. Edited by Bonica J. Philadelphia, Lea & Febiger, 1990, pp 28–94.
5. Bonica JJ: Postoperative pain, The Management of Pain, 2nd Edition. Edited by Bonica J. Philadephia, Lea & Febiger, 1990, pp 461–80.
6. Hollinshead WH: Anatomy for Surgeons, 3rd Edition. Philadelphia, Harper & Row, 1982.
7. DePalma AF: Surgery of the Shoulder, 3rd Edition. Philadelphia, JP Lippincott, 1983.
8. Gardner E: The innervation of the shoulder joint. The Anatomical Record 1948;102:1–18.
9. Dutton RP, Eckhardt WF 3rd, Sunder N: Total spinal anesthesia after interscalene blockade of the brachial plexus. Anesthesiology 1994;80:939–41.
10. Ross S, Scarborough CD: Total spinal anesthesia following brachial-plexus block. Anesthesiology 1973;39:458.
11. Scammell SJ: Case report: Inadvertent epidural anaesthesia as a complication of interscalene brachial plexus block. Anaesth Intensive Care 1979;7:56–7.
12. Benumof JL: Permanent loss of cervical cord function associated with interscalene block performed under general anesthesia. Anesthesiology 2000;93:151–4.
13. Pippa P, Cominelli E, Marinelli C, Aito S: Brachial plexus block using the posterior approach. Eur J Anaesthesiol 1990;7:411–20.
14. Dagli G, Guzeldemir ME, Volkan Acar H: The effects and side effects of interscalene brachial plexus block by posterior approach. Reg Anesth Pain Med 1998;23:87–91.
15. Rucci FS, Pippa P, Barbagli R, Doni L: How many interscalenic blocks are there? A comparison between the lateral and posterior approach. Eur J Anaesthesiol 1993;10:303–7.
16. Boezaart AP, De Beer JF, Nell ML: Early experience with continuous cervical paravertebral block using a stimulating catheter. Reg Anesth Pain Med 2003;28:406–13.
17. Meier G, Bauereis C, Heinrich C: [Interscalene brachial plexus catheter for anesthesia and postoperative pain therapy. Experience with a modified technique]. Anaesthesist 1997;46:715–9.
18. Hadzic A, Vloka JD: Interscalene brachial plexus block, Peripheral Nerve Blocks: Principles and Practice. Edited by Hadzic A, Vloka J. New York, McGraw-Hill, 2003, pp 1009–129.
19. Low interscalene abstract from ASRA 2005 presentation.
20. Dickerman D, Vloka JD, Koorn R, Hadzic A: Excessive noise levels during orthopedic surgery. Regional Anesthesia 1997;22:97.
21. Brown AR, Weiss R, Greenberg C, et al: Interscalene block for shoulder arthroscopy: Comparison with general anesthesia. Arthroscopy 1993;9:295–300.
22. Tetzlaff JE, Yoon HJ, O'Hara J, et al: Alkalinization of mepivacaine accelerates onset of interscalene block for shoulder surgery. Reg Anesth Pain Med 1990;15:242–244.
23. Klein SM, Greengrass RA, Steele SM, et al: A comparison of 0.5% bupivacaine, 0.5% ropivacaine, and 0.75% ropivacaine for interscalene brachial plexus block. Anesth Analg 1998;87:1316–1319.
24. Casati A, Borghi B, Fanelli G, et al: Interscalene brachial plexus anesthesia and analgesia for open shoulder surgery: A randomized, double-blinded comparison between levobupivacaine and ropivacaine. Anesth Analg 2003;96:253–259.
25. Singelyn FJ, Gouverneur JM, Robert A: A minimum dose of clonidine added to mepivacaine prolongs the duration of anesthesia and analgesia after axillary brachial plexus block. Anesth Analg 1996;83:1046–1050.
26. Picard PR, Tramer MR, McQuay HJ, Moore RA: Analgesic efficacy of peripheral opioids (all except intra-articular): A qualitative systematic review of randomised controlled trials. Pain 1997;72:309–318.
27. Bouaziz H, Kinirons BP, Macalou D, et al: Sufentanil does not prolong the duration of analgesia in a mepivacaine brachial plexus block: A dose response study. Anesth Analg 2000;90:383–387.
28. Tetzlaff JE, Yoon HJ, Brems J, Javorsky T: Alkalinization of mepivacaine improves the quality of motor block associated with interscalene brachial plexus anesthesia for shoulder surgery. Reg Anesth Pain Med 1995;20:128–132.
29. Hadzic A, Williams BA, Kraca PE, et al: For outpatient rotator cuff surgery, nerve block anesthesia provides superior same-day recovery over general anesthesia. Anesthesiology 2005;102:1001–1007.
30. Klein SM, Grant SA, Greengrass RA, et al: Interscalene brachial plexus block with a continuous catheter insertion system and a disposable infusion pump. Anesth Analg 2000;91:1473–1478.
31. Borgeat A, Schappi B, Biasca N, Gerber C: Patient-controlled analgesia after major shoulder surgery: Patient-controlled interscalene analgesia versus patient-controlled analgesia. Anesthesiology 1997;87:1343–1347.
32. Singelyn FJ, Seguy S, Gouverneur JM: Interscalene brachial plexus analgesia after open shoulder surgery: Continuous versus patient-controlled infusion. Anesth Analg 1999;89:1216–1220.
33. Borgeat A, Tewes E, Biasca N, Gerber C: Patient-controlled interscalene analgesia with ropivacaine after major shoulder surgery: PCIA vs PCA. Br J Anaesth 1998;81:603–605.
34. Borgeat A, Kalberer F, Jacob H, et al: Patient-controlled interscalene analgesia with ropivacaine 0.2% versus bupivacaine 0.15% after major open shoulder surgery: The effects on hand motor function. Anesth Analg 2001;92:218–223.
35. Rosenberg PH, Heinonen E: Differential sensitivity of A and C nerve fibres to long-acting amide local anaesthetics. Br J Anaesth 1983;55:163–167.
36. Wildsmith JA, Brown DT, Paul D, Johnson S: Structure-activity relationships in differential nerve block at high and low frequency stimulation. Br J Anaesth 1989;63:444–452.
37. Urmey WF, Talts KH, Shrarock NE: One hundred percent incidence of hemi-diaphragmatic paresis associated with interscalene brachial plexus anesthesia as diagnosed by ultrasonography. Anesth Analg 1991;72:498–503.
38. Todd MM, Brown DL: Regional anesthesia and postoperative pain management: Long-term benefits from a short-term intervention. Anesthesiology 1999;91:1–2.
39. Kroll DA, Caplan RA, Posner K, et al: Nerve injury associated with anesthesia. Anesthesiology 1990;73:202–207.
40. Borgeat A, Ekatodramis G, Kalberer F, Benz C: Acute and nonacute complications associated with interscalene block and shoulder surgery: A prospective study. Anesthesiology 2001;95:875–880.
41. Borgeat A, Dullenkopf A, Ekatodramis G, Nagy L: Evaluation of the lateral modified approach for continuous interscalene block after shoulder surgery. Anesthesiology 2003;99:436–442.

26

Supraclavicular Brachial Plexus Block

Carlo D. Franco, MD

INTRODUCTION

The supraclavicular block is one of several techniques used to anesthetize the plexus. The block is performed at the level of the brachial plexus trunks where almost the entire sensory, motor, and sympathetic innervation of the upper extremity is carried in just three nerve structures confined to a very small surface area. Consequently, typical features of this block include rapid onset, predictability, and dense anesthesia.[1-3] In 1911 Kulenkampff in Germany performed the first percutaneous supraclavicular approach, reportedly on himself, a few months after Hirschel described a surgical approach to the brachial plexus in the axilla. The technique was later published in the United States in 1928 by Kulenkampff and Persky.[4] As they described it, the technique was performed with the patient in the sitting position ("a regular chair will suffice") or in the supine position with a pillow between the shoulders if the patient could not adopt the sitting position. The operator sat on a stool at the side of the patient. The needle was inserted above the midpoint of the clavicle where the pulse of the subclavian artery could be felt and it was directed medially toward the spinous process of T2 or T3. Kulenkampff's familiarity with brachial plexus anatomy allowed him to recognize that "the best way to reach the trunks was in the neighborhood of the subclavian artery over the first rib." His technique was also simple; "all the branches of the plexus could be anesthetized through one injection." These two assertions are still valid today. Unfortunately his advice on needle direction carried an inherently high risk of pneumothorax. The popularity of the supraclavicular block remained high during the entire first half of the twentieth century until well after World War II. During this time the technique underwent several modifications, most of them intended to deal with the risk of pneumothorax.[1,5–8]

The introduction of axillary techniques by Accardo and Adriani[9] in 1949 and especially by Burnham[10] in 1958 marked the beginning of the decline in interest for supraclavicular block. The axillary block was particularly popularized after a publication in the journal *Anesthesiology* by De Jong in 1961.[11] The paper was based on cadaver dissections and included the now well-known calculation of 42 mL as the volume needed to fill a cylinder 6 cm long (axillary sheath). According to De Jong this dose "should be sufficient to completely bathe all branches of the brachial plexus." The article was also critical of the supraclavicular approach. Coincidentally the same journal published a paper by Brand and Papper[12] who compared axillary and supraclavicular techniques and managed to produce a 6.1% rate of pneumothorax. This uniquely high rate is frequently cited in the literature in reference to supraclavicular block.

More modern modifications of supraclavicular block include Winnie and Collins's subclavian perivascular technique[13] and the "plumb-bob" technique of Brown and collaborators.[14] The former is more a concept than a radically different technique, stating that plexus anesthesia is performed around a main vessel (perivascular) and within the confines of a sheath. Otherwise, their technique is similar to Murphey's,[7] who in 1944 described a single-injection technique performed just lateral to the anterior scalene muscle directing the needle caudad. The latter was published in 1993 by Brown and collaborators and is commonly known as plumb-bob approach.[14] It is based on cadaver dissections and magnetic resonance imaging performed on volunteers. In this technique the needle is introduced above the clavicle, just lateral to the sternocleidomastoid (SCM) muscle and advanced perpendicularly to the plexus in an anteroposterior direction (plumb bob). If the needle misses the plexus, the pleural dome could be penetrated.

Many authors perceive supraclavicular block technique as complex and as having a significant risk of pneumothorax. However, the advantages of a supraclavicular technique, namely its rapid onset, dense and predictable anesthesia, and its high success rate, make it a very useful approach, which Brown and collaborators[14] have promoted as "unrivaled" by other techniques. Indeed, in our practice the supraclavicular approach is the cornerstone of upper extremity regional anesthesia, and we use it extensively in all kinds of patients.[15]

INDICATIONS

The supraclavicular block is a technique that can be used to provide anesthesia for any surgery on the upper extremity that does not involve the shoulder. It is an excellent choice for elbow and hand surgery.

CONTRAINDICATIONS

General contraindications to the use of this technique are those that apply to any regional block, for instance, infection of the area, significant coagulation abnormalities, and personality disorders or mental illness that prevent the patient from lying still during surgery.

More specifically, this block is classically not attempted bilaterally because of the potential risk of respiratory emergency in case of pneumothorax or phrenic nerve block. Although this recommendation seems logical, the evidence is lacking in the literature.

ANATOMY OF THE BRACHIAL PLEXUS ABOVE THE CLAVICLE

The brachial plexus is usually formed by five roots originating from the ventral divisions of C5 through T1. The roots are sandwiched between the anterior and middle scalene muscles (Figure 26–1). The anterior scalene muscle originates in the anterior tubercles of the transverse processes of C3 through C6 and inserts on the scalene tubercle of the upper surface of the first rib. The middle scalene muscle originates in the posterior tubercles of the transverse processes of C2 through C7 and inserts on the upper surface of the first rib behind the subclavian groove. The five roots converge toward one another to form three trunks—upper, middle, and lower—which are stacked one on top of the other as they traverse the triangular interscalene space formed between the anterior and middle scalene muscles, commonly known as interscalene groove.

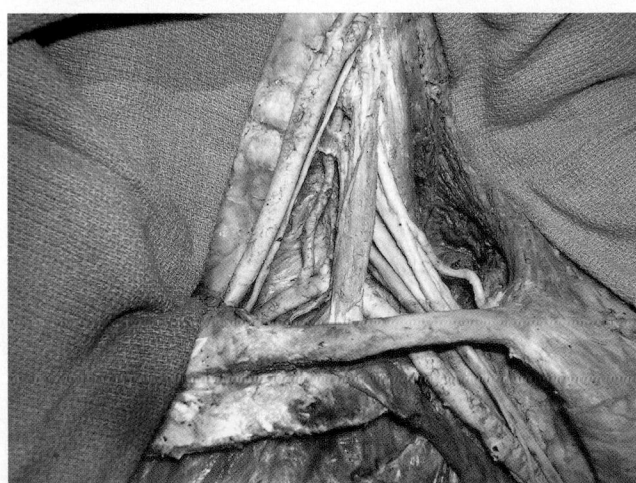

Figure 26–1. Cadaver dissection of left supraclavicular area. The SCM muscle has been removed. The roots and trunks of the plexus are visible lateral to the anterior scalene muscle. The trunks are all supraclavicular. The suprascapular nerve is seen arising from the upper trunk just proximal to the origin of the anterior and posterior divisions of this trunk. The phrenic nerve is visible in front of anterior scalene muscle. Medial to it, the origin of the vertebral artery can be seen, and more medially the common carotid artery and vagus nerve. The first intercostal space is visualized below the clavicle.

This space becomes wider in the anteroposterior plane as the muscles approach their insertion on the first rib. The subclavian artery accompanies the brachial plexus in the interscalene triangle anterior to the lower trunk. Although the roots of the plexus are long, the trunks are almost as short as they are wide, soon giving rise to anterior and posterior divisions as they reach the clavicle. Figure 26–1 shows the anatomy of the brachial plexus and surrounding structures in the supraclavicular area.

The pleura can potentially be violated in two places (the pleural dome and the first intercostal space) during a supraclavicular block, which can lead to pneumothorax. The pleural dome is the apex of the parietal pleura (inside lining of the rib cage), circumscribed by the first rib. Each first rib is a short, broad, and flattened bone structure with the shape of a letter C. They are located on each side of the upper chest with their concavities facing each other. This concavity, or medial border, forms the outer boundary of the pleural dome. The anterior scalene, by inserting in this border of the first rib, comes in contact medially with the pleural dome. There is no pleural dome lateral to the anterior scalene muscle. The first intercostal space on the other hand, is for the most part infraclavicular (see Figure 26–1) and consequently should not be reached when a supraclavicular block is properly performed, as will be explained later.

Clinical Pearls

- With the shoulder pulled down, the three trunks of the brachial plexus are located above the clavicle; therefore, the needle should never need to reach below the clavicle during a supraclavicular block.

- The first intercostal space is located below the clavicle, thus its penetration is unlikely during a properly performed supraclavicular block.

- The needle should never cross the parasagittal plane medial to the anterior scalene muscle because of risk of pneumothorax.

- The pulsatile effect of the subclavian artery exerted mainly against the lower trunk could explain why the C8 through T1 dermatome is often spared if the injection is not performed in the vicinity of the lower trunk.

- The SCM muscle inserts on the medial third of the clavicle, and the trapezius muscle on the lateral third of it, leaving the middle third for the neurovascular bundle. These proportions are maintained regardless of patient's size. Bigger muscle bulk resulting from exercise does not influence the size of the muscle insertion area.

- The brachial plexus crosses the clavicle at or near its midpoint. Because of the direction of the brachial plexus from medial to lateral as it descends, the higher in the supraclavicular area the more medial (closer to the SCM) the plexus is located.

LANDMARKS

The technique described in this chapter combines the simplicity of the original single-injection Kulenkampff technique with important anatomic principles, which should help make the technique safer than the original procedure. The main landmarks for this block are the lateral insertion of the SCM muscle in the clavicle, the clavicle itself, and the patient's midline. These three landmarks are easily identifiable in the majority of patients.

EQUIPMENT

- Gloves
- Antiseptic solution for skin disinfection
- Marking pen
- Sterile gauze
- Two 20-mL syringes for local anesthetic solution
- One 1-mL syringe with a 27-gauge needle for skin wheal
- One 5-cm, short-beveled, 22-gauge insulated needle
- Surface electrode
- Nerve stimulator

TECHNIQUE

Ideally the block is performed in a room dedicated to regional anesthesia. However, whether the block is performed inside or outside the operating room, the location must include American Society of Anesthesiologists standard monitors, an oxygen source, suctioning, and resuscitation equipment and drugs. A contingency plan for emergencies must be in place to safely and expeditiously treat any emergency that might arise.

If not contraindicated, this block is best performed after appropriate, light premedication (eg, midazolam 1 mg (IV) plus fentanyl 50 mcg IV for the average adult). In young and healthy patients this dose can be repeated as necessary. The patient is best kept sedated but cooperative.

A single-injection, nerve stimulator technique is preferred. The block is performed with the patient in a semisitting position with the head rotated to the opposite side as shown in Figure 26–2A. The semisitting position is more comfortable than the supine position both for the patient and the operator. Because patient positioning is very important in regional anesthesia, the operator should not try to recognize any landmarks until the patient has adopted the desired position. The patient is asked to lower the shoulder and flex the elbow, so the forearm rests on the lap. The wrist is supinated so the palm of the hand faces the patient's face as shown in Figure 26–2B. This maneuver allows for detection of any subtle finger movement produced by nerve stimulation. If the patient cannot turn the wrist on supination, a roll is placed under it so the fingers are free to move.

The operator usually stands on the side to be blocked, so for a left side block the palpation is done with the left hand and the needle is manipulated with the right (see Figure 26–2B). For a right-side block we teach exactly the opposite: the

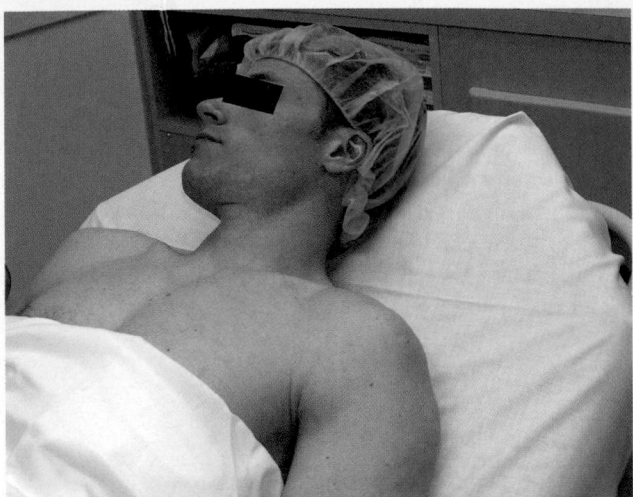

A

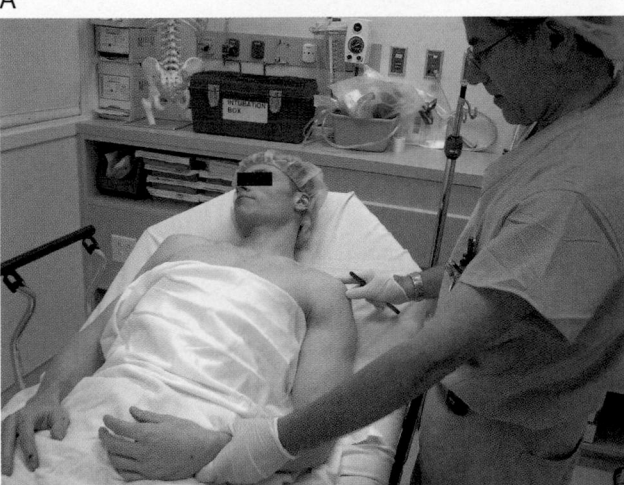

B

Figure 26–2. A: Patient positioning. The patient lies in a semisitting position with the head turned away from the side to be blocked. **B:** The shoulder is down, the elbow is flexed, and the palm of the hand rests on the patient's lap while it is turned toward his face.

operator manipulates the needle with the left hand and palpates with the right. Otherwise, the operator may choose to manipulate the needle always with his or her favored hand regardless of which side block is being performed. This is easily accomplished by standing on one side of the patient's head while reaching to the other side when necessary.

Point of Needle Entrance

With the patient in the described semisitting position and the shoulder down, the lateral (posterior) border of the SCM muscle is identified and followed distally to the point where it meets the clavicle. This particular point is marked on the skin over the clavicle, as shown in Figure 26–3. The lateral border of the SCM is usually clearly visible at the level where the external jugular vein crosses it. From this level the border can

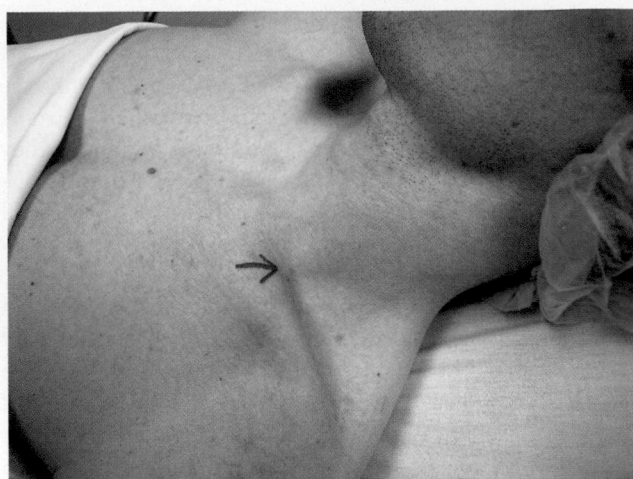

Figure 26–3. Landmarks. The lateral insertion of the SCM in the clavicle is marked (*arrow*).

be traced caudally to the point where it meets the clavicle. A parasagittal line (parallel to the midline) is imaginarily drawn at this level to recognize an area medial to it that is at risk for pneumothorax. The point of needle entrance is always lateral to this parasagittal plane, separated by a distance we call "margin of safety." This distance is about 1 in. (2.5 cm) lateral to the insertion of the SCM in the clavicle or one "thumb's breadth" lateral to the SCM as shown in Figure 26–4. The margin of safety can be alternatively established using a distance equal to the width of the clavicular head of the SCM at its insertion on the clavicle.[16] The palpating index finger is placed at this site as shown in Figure 26–5. We customarily draw two arrows at this location pointing to each other. The proximal arrow, above the finger, is used to localize the needle entrance point, the distal one shows the direction of the needle path.

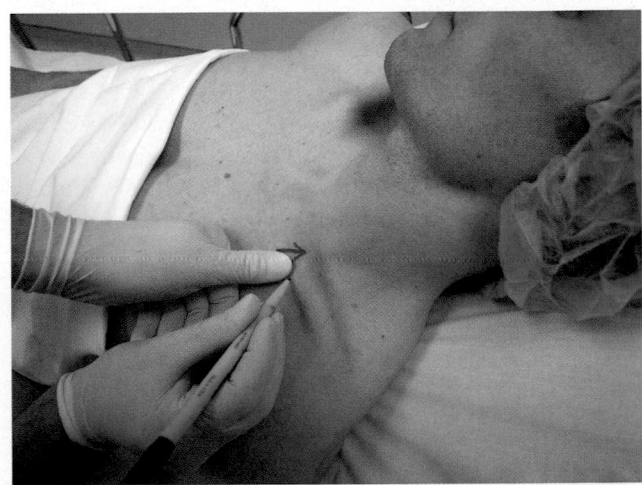

Figure 26–4. Margin of safety. A distance of approximately 1 in. (2.5 cm) is measured laterally from the SCM, away from the pleural dome.

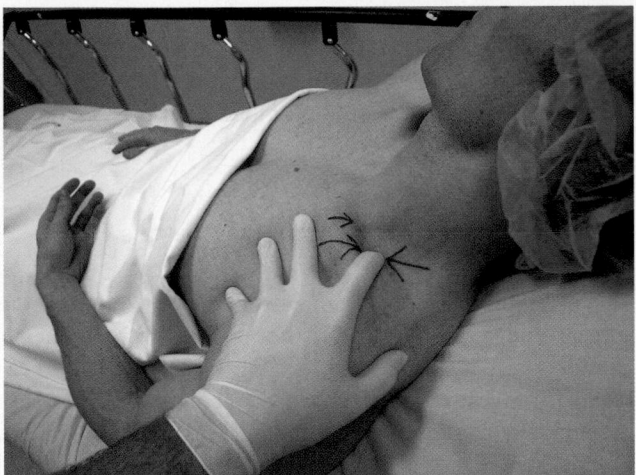

Figure 26–5. Point of needle entrance. The point of needle entrance is located just cephalad to the palpating finger and one fingerbreadth above the clavicle. The arrows on each side of the palpating finger help visualize the direction of the needle parallel to the midline.

The needle is inserted immediately cephalad to the palpating finger and advanced first perpendicularly to the skin for 2 to 5 mm (depending on the amount of the patient's subcutaneous tissue) and then turned caudally under the palpating finger to advance it in a direction that is parallel to the midline, as shown in Figure 26–6.

The block should take place above the clavicle, under the palpating finger. An isolated muscle twitch is elicited in all fingers either in flexion or extension, often mistakenly referred as "median nerve" and "radial nerve" responses, respectively (both nerves at this level are yet to be formed while their constituent fibers are traveling in all three trunks). Any other response carries a significantly lower success rate.

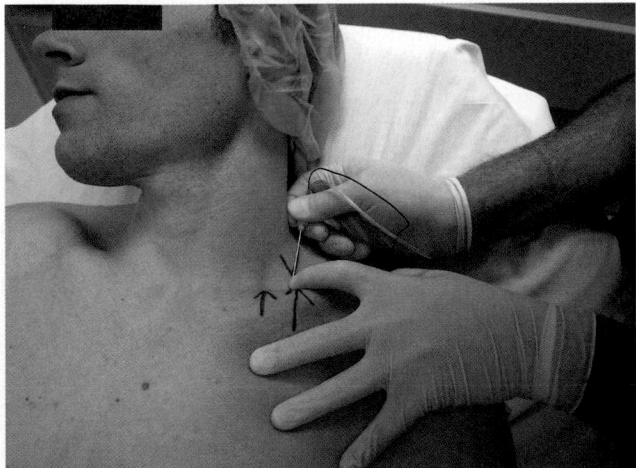

Figure 26–6. Needle direction. The needle is first introduced perpendicular to the skin and is then turned and advanced parallel to the midline in the direction of the two lateral arrows.

If reposition of the needle is necessary, the needle is withdrawn and the penetration angle is adjusted in the anteroposterior plane, either slightly more posterior or slightly more anterior, but always parallel to the midline.

Nerve Stimulator Settings

Modern nerve stimulators used in regional anesthesia are portable, accurate and easy to use. They should be checked periodically by the hospital engineering department to ensure proper function and be fitted with new batteries according to a schedule. The ground electrode should be fresh out of the package. If for any reason it needs to be relocated, it is better to use a new one to avoid the increase in impedance that comes with desiccation of the conductive gel. Its location in reference to the blocking site does not seem to have any significance. The negative electrode should be connected to the needle because less current is needed to produce a nerve response.[17] We always use a 5-cm, short-beveled, insulated needle to perform this technique.

We start the technique with a current of 0.8 mA and a pulse width of 100 μs. Once the desired response is obtained—ie, a muscle twitch of the fingers that is clearly visible—we start the injection without reducing the nerve stimulator current. This is a unique characteristic of the supraclavicular block. In a recent study, the onset, duration, and success rate with a supraclavicular block was unaffected by reducing the nerve stimulator to 0.5 mA or less.[18] Supraclavicular and lumbar plexus blocks are the only peripheral nerve blocks in which injecting at a higher current than 0.5 mA should be recommended.

Clinical Pearls

- To improve patient comfort, removal of a cast or splint prior to performing the block is not necessary as long as the fingers are visualized.
- The lateral border of the SCM muscle follows a straight line from the mastoid to the clavicle. Frequently a lateral deviation of this otherwise straight border can be seen in the proximity of the clavicle. This lateral extension should be disregarded because it usually represents the omohyoid muscle.
- The needle is inserted in a direction that is parallel to the midline. No other landmarks (eg, nipples) should be used to direct the needle, as their position is highly variable.
- Depending on the patient's weight, the palpating finger exerts different amounts of pressure on the deeper tissues. This maneuver helps bring the plexus closer to the skin and makes the trajectory of the needle shorter.
- The needle should never be inserted deeper than 1 in. (2.5 cm) if a twitch from the brachial plexus is not present.

- Because the trunks are contiguous, elicited twitches from one trunk follow the other without interruption. If the twitches instead disappear before reaching the lower trunk, the needle is withdrawn to the point of the previous twitch and advanced with a slight change in the anteroposterior angle of insertion.

- The margin of safety of about 1 in. (2.5 cm) lateral to the insertion of the SCM on the clavicle provides a safe distance lateral to the outer boundary of the pleural dome for the needle to travel. Because of the steep downward direction of the trunks, increasing this distance laterally may prevent the needle from contacting the plexus above the clavicle or miss the short trunks altogether.

- The risk of intraneural injection is minimized by using low injection pressures, meticulous technique, and possibly by avoiding blocks in heavily sedated or anesthetized patients.

- The injection is performed slowly with frequent aspirations while carefully observing the patient.

- If pain or abnormal pressure is felt at any point during injection, the needle should be withdrawn 1–2 mm, after which a new assessment is made.

CONTINUOUS TECHNIQUE

Traditionally the supraclavicular technique has not been considered an optimal choice for placement of catheters. The great mobility of the neck at this location carries a risk for catheter dislodgement. Tunnelization of the catheter to the infraclavicular level could help to make the catheter more stable; however; inadequate experience or data currently exist on this topic.

LOCAL ANESTHETIC CHOICES FOR SINGLE-SHOT & CATHETER TECHNIQUES

Most upper extremity surgeries performed under regional anesthesia last 1–3 h. Consequently, we most commonly use 35–40 mL of 1.5% mepivacaine with 1:400,000 epinephrine, which provides about 3–4 h of anesthesia. Most hand surgeries, including metacarpal and carpal fractures; radial and/or ulnar fractures; and tendons and digital nerve repairs can be performed using this combination. The same anesthetic solution without epinephrine provides about 2–3 h of anesthesia. Usually 2 mL of 8.4% sodium bicarbonate is added per every 20 mL of mepivacaine solution. Solutions of ropivacaine or bupivacaine provide longer acting anesthesia (5–12 h) when required. For continuous techniques, a bolus dose of about 10–15 mL of local anesthetic solution can be given, followed by an infusion rate of 8–10 mL/h. A solution of 0.2% levobupivacaine or ropivacaine can be used for this purpose. A patient-controlled analgesia (PCA) can be added to the system, thus allowing the patient to administer 3–5 mL every 30 min for breakthrough pain. If PCA is added, the basal infusion is decreased to around 5 mL/h. Breakthrough pain needs to be treated with a bolus of local anesthetic.

PERIOPERATIVE MANAGEMENT

The patient who receives single-shot blocks can undergo surgery under intravenous sedation titrated to the patient's comfort. The sedation requirements vary from patient to patient and range from small intermittent boluses of midazolam or fentanyl, to a propofol drip at 25–50 mcg/kg/min, to light general anesthesia.

COMPLICATIONS

Common side effects associated with this technique include phrenic nerve block with diaphragmatic paralysis and sympathetic nerve block with development of Horner's syndrome. They usually only require patient reassurance. Phrenic nerve block reportedly occurs about 50% of the time and is not associated with respiratory dysfunction in healthy volunteers.[19] Complications, such as intravascular injection with development of systemic local anesthetic toxicity and hematoma formation, are similar to those for other peripheral blocks. Neuropraxia and neurologic injury are similarly possible, but rarely reported.

The most feared complication of the supraclavicular block is pneumothorax, with rates quoted to be as high as 6.1%. As previously mentioned, this data was published by Brand and Papper in 1961.[12] The authors compared 230 consecutive supraclavicular blocks with 246 consecutive axillary blocks. However, the comparison was neither blinded nor randomized, and the study used several different techniques.[7] In contrast, this complication is rarely reported in the modern literature.[15] Our own experience with a large number of supraclavicular blocks is without any clinically manifested pneumothorax.

It is frequently mentioned also that the pneumothorax complicating a supraclavicular block has a delayed onset, making routine postoperative chest radiograph unjustifiable.[20,21] In fact the literature does include such cases.[1,22] However, most of the pneumothoraces published in relationship to supraclavicular block have usually been diagnosed within a few hours of the procedure and before the patient's discharge.

Based on the available literature it can be said that pneumothorax associated with supraclavicular block is an uncommon complication, often small, and it presents within a few hours following the procedure. Rarely, its presentation can be delayed up to 12 h. It is also important to emphasize that pneumothorax is a complication that for the most part is preventable with meticulous technique.

SUMMARY

Supraclavicular block is a reliable, fast-onset, and highly successful approach to brachial plexus anesthesia. The anatomy of the brachial plexus, with its three trunks confined to a much-reduced surface area, allows for a high success rate for achieving anesthesia in the upper extremity. The block should be performed with the shoulder down. This maneuver places the trunks above the clavicle, so the block can be truly supraclavicular and the risk of penetrating the first intercostal space is reduced. Inserting the needle at a distance lateral to the insertion of the SCM muscle in the clavicle and advancing it parallel to the patient's midline keeps it away (lateral) from the pleural dome. Performing the block under the palpating finger also confers a great degree of control. Supraclavicular block should not be performed without a thorough knowledge of the anatomy of not only the brachial plexus but also the important surrounding structures. Knowledge of anatomy, familiarity with simple landmarks, and meticulous technique are necessary to safely perform this highly efficacious technique of brachial plexus blockade.

References

1. Moore D: Supraclavicular approach for block of the brachial plexus. In Moore D (ed): *Regional Block. A Handbook for Use in the Clinical Practice of Medicine and Surgery,* 4th ed. Charles C Thomas Publisher, 1981, pp 221–242.

2. Lanz E, Theiss D, Jankovic D: The extent of blockade following various techniques of brachial plexus block. Anesth Analg 1983;62:55–58.

3. Urmey W: Upper extremity blocks. In Brown D (ed): *Regional Anesthesia and Analgesia.* WB Saunders Company, 1996; pp 254–278.

4. Kulenkampff D, Persky M: Brachial plexus anesthesia. Its indications, technique and dangers. Ann Surg 1928;87:883–891.

5. Labat G: *Regional Anesthesia. Its Technic and Clinical Application.* WB Saunders Company, 1922.

6. Patrick J: The technique of brachial plexus block anesthesia. Br J Surg 1940;27:734–739.

7. Murphey D: Brachial plexus block anesthesia: An improved technic. Ann Surg 1944;119:935–943.

8. Winnie A: *Plexus Anesthesia. Perivascular Techniques of Brachial Plexus Block.* WB Saunders Company, 1993.

9. Accardo N, Adriani J: Brachial plexus block: A simplified technic using the axillary route. South Med J 1949;42:920.

10. Burnham P: Regional anesthesia of the great nerves of the upper arm. Anesthesiology 1958;19:281–284.

11. De Jong R: Axillary block of the brachial plexus. Anesthesiology 1961;22:215–225.

12. Brand L, Papper E: A comparison of supraclavicular and axillary techniques for brachial plexus blocks. Anesthesiology 1961;22:226–229.

13. Winnie A, Collins V: The subclavian perivascular technique of brachial plexus anesthesia. Anesthesiology 1964;25:353–363.

14. Brown DL, Cahill D, Bridenbaugh D: Supraclavicular nerve block: Anatomic analysis of a method to prevent pneumothorax. Anesth Analg 1993;76:530–534.

15. Franco C, Vieira Z: 1,001 subclavian perivascular brachial plexus blocks: Success with a nerve stimulator. Reg Anesth Pain Med 2000;25:41–46.

16. Franco CD: The subclavian perivascular block. Tech Reg Anesth Pain Manag 1999;3:212–216.

17. Hadzic A, Vloka J: *Peripheral Nerve Blocks. Principles and Practice.* McGraw-Hill, 2004.

18. Franco C, Domashevich V, Voronov G, et al: The supraclavicular block with a nerve stimulator: To decrease or not to decrease, that is the question. Anesth Analg 2004;98:1167–1171.

19. Neal J, Moore J, Kopacz D, et al: Quantitative analysis of respiratory, motor, and sensory function after supraclavicular block. Anesth Analg 1998;86:1239–1244.

20. Greengrass R, Steele S, Moretti G, et al: Peripheral nerve blocks. In Raj P (ed): *Textbook of Regional Anesthesia.* Churchill Livingstone, 2002, pp 325–377.

21. Neal J, Hebl J, Gerancher J, et al: Brachial plexus anesthesia: Essentials of our current understanding. Reg Anesth Pain Med 2002;27:402–428.

22. Harley N, Gjessing J: A critical assessment of supraclavicular brachial plexus block. Anesthesia 1969;24:564–570.

27

Infraclavicular Brachial Plexus Block

Laura Lowrey Clark, MD

INTRODUCTION

The infraclavicular block is quick to perform and provides a complete block of the upper arm. Unlike the axillary approach, an infraclavicular block can be performed without abduction of the arm. Complications and contraindications are comparable to those for an axillary approach. It is conducive to placement of the continuous catheter by being more accessible and more comfortable for the patient than a catheter in the axilla. The infraclavicular area can be accessed by several approaches that permit flexibility, and the use of ultrasound guidance is also possible. The clinical application of this block has a short history and is continuing to evolve with modifications of the technique. Infraclavicular blockade is a useful alternative to the axillary approach and has the potential to be more popular than axillary block in the near future.

Hirschel in 1911 is considered to have performed the first percutaneous axillary block because he approached the plexus from the axilla.[1] His goal was to place the local anesthetic on top of the first rib via the axilla. He discovered after his own dissections of the plexus the reason for incompleteness of the axillary block and was the first to describe that the axillary and musculocutaneous nerves separated from the plexus much higher than in the axilla. However, the needles of the day were not long enough to reach this area to block those nerves.[2] To remedy this problem in 1911, Kulenkampff's supraclavicular description was soon to follow.[2] He felt his technique was safer and more accurate than Hirschel's, but after initial success the reports of complications of pneumothorax ensued.

In 1914, Bazy[3] described injecting below the clavicle just medial to the coracoid process along a line connecting with Chassaignac's tubercle. The needle trajectory was pointed away from the axilla, close to the clavicle and was felt to present little chance of pleural damage. A flurry of modifications came shortly after that during the next 8 years. Babitzsky[4] proposed an entry site where the clavicle and the second rib intersect, and Balog suggested actually impinging the second rib. It is also during this time period (in the early 1900s) that volumes were increased from the initial 5 mL to 20 mL. Also during this period an increased success rate was noted with increased volume.

Knowledge of the anatomy was at the forefront in this period as well. Babitzsky said that "to discuss the anatomical relationship and the technique more fully would be superfluous, as it is customary to familiarize oneself with the anatomy of the field in question on the cadaver any time one tends to use an unfamiliar technique."[2] The truth of this statement is still valid today.

Labat in 1922 essentially redescribed Bazy's technique in his textbook, *Regional Anesthesia,*[5] as did Dogliotti[6] in 1939. But the technique seemed to fade into obscurity. The technique was not included in Moore's *Regional Block*[7] in 1981 or Cousins and Bridenbaugh's *Neural Blockade.*[8] Raj[9] is credited with reintroducing the approach in 1973 with modification from the earlier descriptions. He described the initial entry point at the midpoint of the clavicle and directed the needle laterally toward the axilla using a nerve stimulator. This was thought to be the answer for the safe and complete block. His data supported that with this technique there was virtually no danger of pneumothorax. An additional advantage was that a more complete block was obtained, including the musculocutaneous, the intercostobrachial, and the ulnar nerves over the interscalene or axillary approaches.[9] This approach, however, did not become more popular than the axillary approach. A long trajectory passing thru the pectoralis major and minor muscles allowed more opportunity for individual error and created more discomfort for the patient. Many operators did not have the same success rate as Raj reported with the technique. Sims, in 1977, suggested a modification to attempt to increase the ability to approach the plexus more reliably and successfully from this approach.[10] His approach utilized a 1.5-in. needle rather than the 3.5-in. Raj suggested by moving the insertion point in the groove between the coracoid process and the clavicle. Identifying the depression of what is the deltopectoral groove is achieved by placing the operator's finger in the groove between the coracoid process and the clavicle. The finger is then advanced inferiorly and medially until the depression is felt. The needle was advanced inferiorly, laterally, and posteriorly toward

the apex of the axilla. He reports finding the plexus usually 2–3 cm from the insertion point because the plexus is much more superficial in this area.

Whiffler, in 1981, described what is commonly referred to today as the coracoid block. He, like his predecessors, did a dissection study to determine the feasibility of his technique. The injection site was very close to that detailed by Sims, but the technique was totally different. Whiffler felt that the shoulder should be depressed with the head turned to the opposite side and the arm abducted 45 degrees from the chest wall to make the plexus closer to the coracoid process. He described developing a three-dimensional view of the plexus to estimate the depth of the plexus to guide the placement of the needle. To estimate the depth of the plexus one identifies two points. One is the point past the midpoint of the clavicle where the subclavian pulse disappears. The second point is found by determining the highest pulse of the artery in the axilla and placing the thumb of the same hand on the anterior surface of the chest wall that corresponds to that point. Those points are connected, and the needle is then inserted inferior and medial to the coracoid process on that line to the depth that the plexus has been estimated to be. Whiffler did not use a nerve stimulator because he felt "this simpler approach does not require a nerve stimulator." Incremental injections were used, withdrawing the needle 1 cm one to two times. A total volume of 40 mL was injected.[11]

Understanding these earlier attempts gives new insight into performing the current techniques of today.

The infraclavicular block technique was not embraced by many anesthesiologists of the day because most seemed to prefer the axillary approach. In 1983, Winnie's book, *Plexus Anesthesia,* the chapter describing perivascular techniques of brachial plexus block relates the history of the infraclavicular block with the early evolution descriptions, and although including the technique of Raj (1973), Sims (1977), and Whiffler (1981), it does not devote a section to infraclavicular block. He states that "none of the infraclavicular techniques appears to offer significant advantages over the more established perivascular techniques . . . " and documents once again that the sheath can be entered at any level.[12]

Infraclavicular block reentered in the 1990s along with the upsurge in the popularity and applications of regional anesthesia in general and is rapidly regaining its place as a vital component in the armamentarium of the anesthesiologist who practices regional anesthesia.

The block as described by Raj underwent a modification after difficulties in reproducing his results. Klaastad in 1999 performed a magnetic resonance imaging (MRI) study and anatomically determined that if followed exactly as described, the MRI showed that the needle was not in close proximity to the cords. In a significant number of cases the cords were caudad and posterior to the target. Furthermore, the needle trajectory's shortest distance to the pleura was only 10 mm, and in one case hit the pleura. They concluded that a more lateral approach would make it more precise and provide less risk of complications. This was actually what Raj had found clinically and was suggesting in lectures but had not published. He had changed the point of needle insertion to be on a line between the pulsation of the subclavian and brachial artery and 2.5 cm from this line, crossing with the inferior border of the clavicle. This is what is commonly referred to as the modified Raj approach.[13]

Four approaches will be described in this chapter: (1) vertical infraclavicular block as described by Kilka and colleagues,[14] (2) the coracoid approach described by Whiffler[11] and modified by Wilson and coworkers,[15] (3) the modified Raj approach,[9] and (4) the lateral and sagittal approach described by Klaastad and associates often used for ultrasound.

INDICATIONS & CONTRAINDICATIONS

Clinical Pearls

- Distribution of anesthesia consists of the entire arm, including the hand, wrist, forearm, elbow, and most of the upper arm.
- Indications are similar to those for axillary block; hand, forearm, elbow and arteriovenous fistula surgery.
- Infraclavicular block provides greater coverage and obviates the need for special arm positioning (abduction).

Indications for infraclavicular block are similar to axillary blockade but expanded due to the advantages of reaching the plexus at a higher level. The approach is applicable for any surgery up to but *not* including the shoulder. Complete anesthesia of the arm is obtained from the lower shoulder to the hand. There have been reports of difficulty in blocking the medial cutaneous nerve, a branch of the medial cord innervating the upper inner aspect of the arm. Rodriquez and colleagues postulated that, this could be a result of the dominance of the intercostobrachial nerve (second thoracic root) in those patients.[16] Fortunately, tourniquet is well tolerated without supplementation of the intercostobrachial nerve; however if this area is involved in the surgery the medial upper arm should be specifically tested and the intercostobrachial nerve should be additionally blocked.

Not having to abduct the arm or include separate injections for the musculocutaneous or intercostobrachial nerve presents an advantage over the axillary approach. This is of significant value in patients whose injury precludes movement or for patients with arthritis or those whose shoulders cannot abduct for axillary block. Bilateral blocks can be carried out without fear of blocking the phrenic nerve. The coracoid process and clavicle landmarks are easily palpable even in obese patients. Infraclavicular access to the brachial plexus is also ideal for continuous catheter fixation and long-term infusion.

Other than an infection at or near the site or existing coagulopathy, there are no block-specific contraindications to infraclavicular block. Coagulopathy is relative and based on the risk-vs-benefit ratio. The primary concern is that should the artery be punctured, compression is difficult in this area. In patients with normal coagulation many punctures of the artery have been reported with no major problems occurring.

FUNCTIONAL ANATOMY

Clinical Pearls

- Block occurs at the cord level of the brachial plexus below the clavicle.
- Three cords surround the axillary artery.
- The organization of the brachial plexus is complex in this area and anatomic variability exists.
- Diagrams and the anatomic names of cords are often misleading; the relationship found clinically may differ.
- The lateral cord is the most superficial, the posterior cord is encountered next, the medial cord is the deepest and is below the axillary artery.
- The lateral cord and the medial cord both contribute fibers to the median nerve.
- The posterior cord contains all of the radial nerve.
- The musculocutaneous nerve is often outside but very close to the lateral cord.

The pertinent anatomy for this block begins at the level of brachial plexus divisions and extends to include transition to the cords of the brachial plexus (Figure 27–1). Divisions exist as the brachial plexus crosses the first rib into the infraclavicular area. They originate from the trunks and divide into anterior and posterior divisions, thus, the origin of the name division. Divisions are based on embryonic migration (see Chapter 2, Embryology) and locality. The anterior divisions usually supply flexor muscles (which are most often positioned anterior) and posterior divisions usually supply extensor muscles (which are generally posterior).

The brachial plexus makes most of its major changes in the infraclavicular area in just a few centimeters as it twists and turns from a parallel course in the neck to circumferentially surround the axillary artery in the infraclavicular area and progresses into the axilla as terminal nerves. Mixing of the nerves occurs, and although this is a great protective mechanism for the body its organization can be quite complex. In addition, the anatomic terms used to identify the nerves may be confusing to a nonanatomist.

Figure 27–2 is a fresh cadaveric tissue dissection showing the course of the brachial plexus from the interscalene to

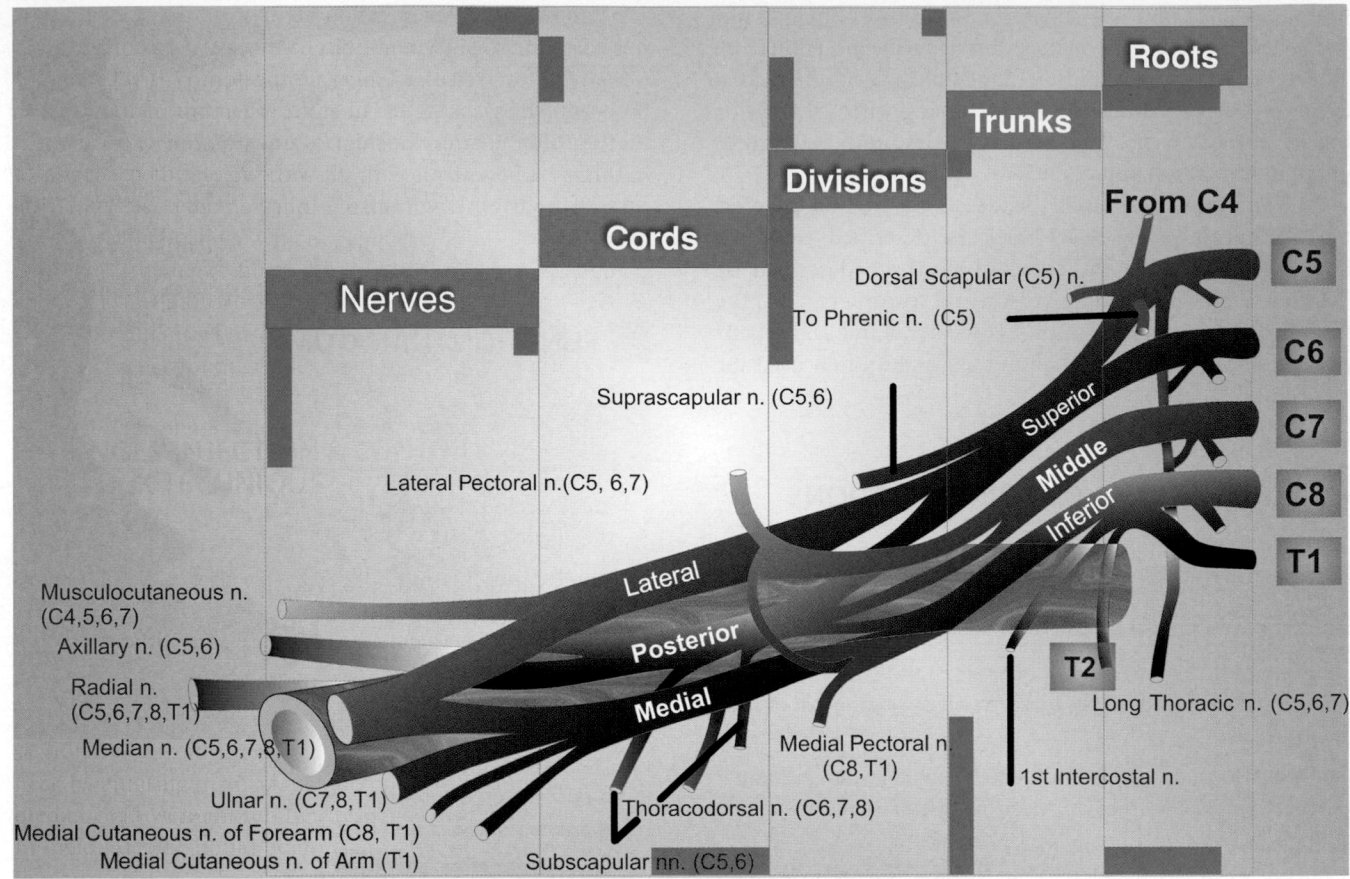

Figure 27–1. Organization of the brachial plexus.

the infraclavicular area. However, the anatomic descriptive terms for the cords are based with the body in anatomic position and relative to its center; this is not descriptive of how the brachial plexus is encountered clinically. Many textbooks feature two-dimensional rather than three-dimensional diagrams of the plexus in this area, which contributes to the confusion. However, a solid understanding of the three-dimensional organization of the plexus may be the most important factor in successful blockade.

Divisions, Branches, Cords, & Terminal Nerves

The anterior divisions of the upper (C5 and C6) and middle trunk (C7) unite to form the lateral cord, which lies lateral to the axillary artery and most superficial to the anterior chest skin. The anterior divisions of the lower trunk (C8 and T1) form the medial cord. It lies medial to the axillary artery and is the deepest. The posterior cord is formed from all of the posterior divisions (C5 through T1) and lies posterior to the artery just under the lateral cord. The cords end in terminal branches that are mixed nerves, which contain both sensory and motor components. They are the musculocutaneous, ulnar, median, axillary, and radial branches.

Other branches also exit the plexus prior to the formation of the terminal nerves. They are not mixed and are unique in that they are either sensory or motor nerves. These nerves are often not addressed but are important because the motor branches can be stimulated during performance of a block and knowing where they originate will help determine where to locate the tip of the needle. Tables 27–1 and 27–2 list the branches of the brachial plexus and their innervation.

Figure 27–2. Relationship of the brachial plexus, clavicle, and coracoid process.

Table 27–1.

Branches of Brachial Plexus

	Motor Innervation	Motion Observed	Sensory Innervation
Lateral			
Lateral pectoral nerve	Pectoralis major	Contraction of pectoralis	
Dorsal scapular nerve	Rhomboid major and minor; levator scapulae	Adducts and rotates shoulder, raises scapula	
Posterior			
Upper subscapular	Subscapularis (superomedial part)	Medial rotation or arm	
Thoracodorsal	Latissimus dorsi	Abduction of arm	
Lower subscapular	Subscapularis (lateral part), teres major	Internal rotation, adduction of shoulder	
Axillary	Deltoid, teres minor	Elevation of upper arm	Skin of upper lateral arm
Medial			
Medial pectoral	Pectoralis minor and major	Contraction of pectoralis	
Medial cutaneous nerve of arm			Skin of medial side or arm
Medial cutaneous nerve of forearm			Skin of medial side or forearm

Table 27–2.

Terminal Nerves of Brachial Plexus

	Motor Innervation	Motion Observed	Sensory Innervation
Lateral			
Musculocutaneous	Coracobrachialis, biceps brachii, brachialis	Flexion of elbow	Skin of lateral side of forearm
Median	Flexor digitorum superficialis—all, pronator teres, flexor carpi radialis palmaris longus	Flexion of first $3\frac{1}{2}$ fingers, opposition of thumb	Skin of radial half of palm and palmer side of radial $3\frac{1}{2}$ digits
Posterior			
Radial	Brachioradialis, abductor pollicis longus, extensor muscles of the wrist and fingers	Abduction of thumb, extension of wrist and fingers	Skin of posterior arm, forearm and hand
Medial			
Ulnar	Abductor pollicis interossei intrinsic muscles of the hand	Contraction of the 4th and 5th fingers and thumb abduction	Skin of medial side of wrist and hand and ulner $1\frac{1}{2}$ digits
Median	Flexor digitorum superficialis—all, pronator leres, flexor carpi radialis palmaris longus	Flexion of first $3\frac{1}{2}$ fingers, opposition of thumb	Skin of radial half of palm and palmer side of radial $3\frac{1}{2}$ digits

Note: *All branches from the medial cord carry C8 and T1 fibers, and that of the higher spinal segments in the brachial plexus (C5 through C6) tend to innnervate muscles more proximal on the upper extremity, whereas the lower segments (C8, T1) tend to innervate more distal muscles, such as those in the hand (T1). Anatomic variation and the comingling of fibers from both lateral and medial cords makes it impossible to tell with certainty which cord is being stimulated with distal median nerve response.*

CLINICAL ANATOMY

A simplified schematic diagram of the plexus is shown in Figure 27–1. This diagram depicts the plexus as it actually exists and a more clinical representation of how it is encountered when performing infraclavicular block. As shown, the posterior cord is not actually the most posterior cord but instead lies between the lateral and medial cords. The most helpful anatomic picture is in the sagittal plane as shown in Figure 27–3. This is a fresh cadaveric tissue dissection of the brachial plexus that was cut at the level of infraclavicular

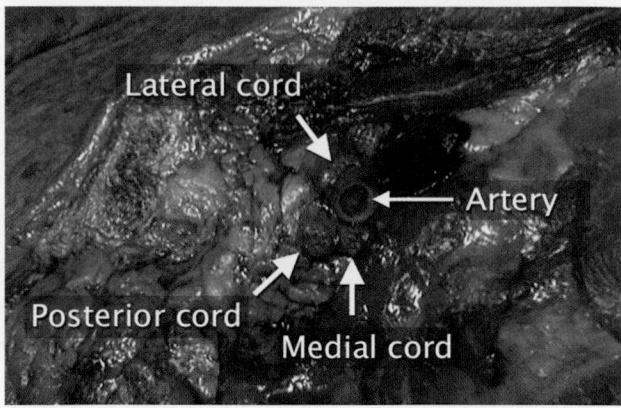

Figure 27–4. Close-up view of the relationship of the cords of the brachial plexus at the level of infraclavicular blockade to the subclavian/axillary artery.

blockade to show this relationship. The relationship shown in this picture is helpful for guiding needle placement while performing this block. The sagittal view shown in Figure 27–4 illustrates the cords in a close up view surrounding the artery. Once this relationship is learned, the ability to change the needle directions for correct positioning is based on anatomy, and the need for subsequent passes to achieve successful placement lessens.

The cord that is most often encountered first when performing the infraclavicular block is the lateral cord because it is the most superficial. Just beyond the lateral cord is the posterior cord, which is in close proximity but just a bit deeper than the lateral cord. The medial cord is actually caudal or below the axillary artery, as can be seen in the sagittal picture in Figure 27–4. The schematic diagram of the cord shown in Figure 27–5 demonstrates the 90-degree angle of needle insertion for the lateral and posterior cord. This picture also illustrates the proximity of the artery and the risk of puncturing the artery when attempting to encounter the medial cord.

The Lateral Cord

The lateral cord supplies the lateral half of the median nerve and the musculocutaneous and the pectoral nerve branches (see Tables 27–1 and 27–2). This lateral portion of the median nerve is the motor innervation to the flexor muscles in the

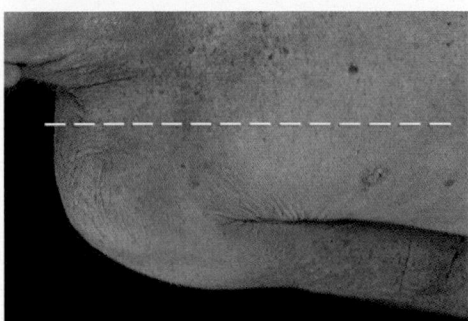
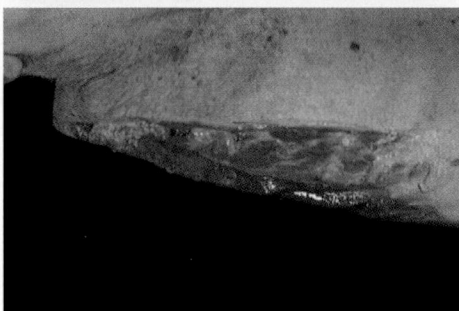
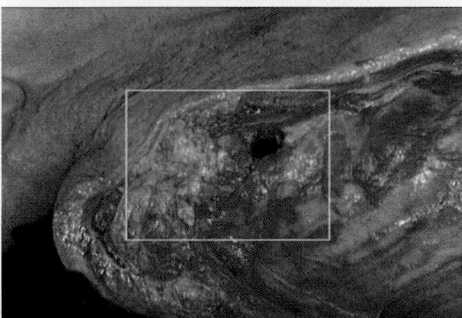
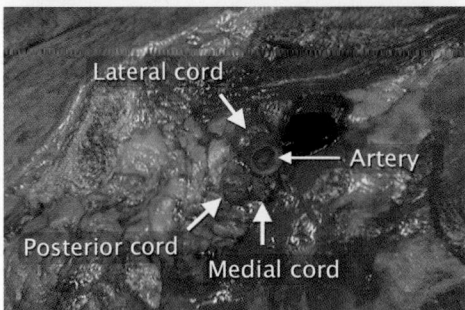

Figure 27–3. Relationship of the cords of the brachial plexus at the level of infraclavicular blockade to the subclavian/axillary artery.

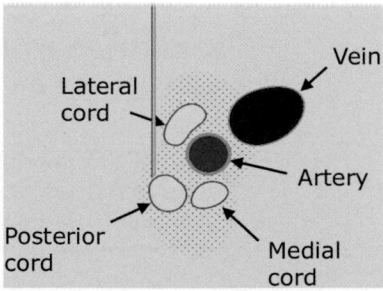

Figure 27–5. Schematic of the relationship of the cords of the brachial plexus to the subclavian/axillary artery.

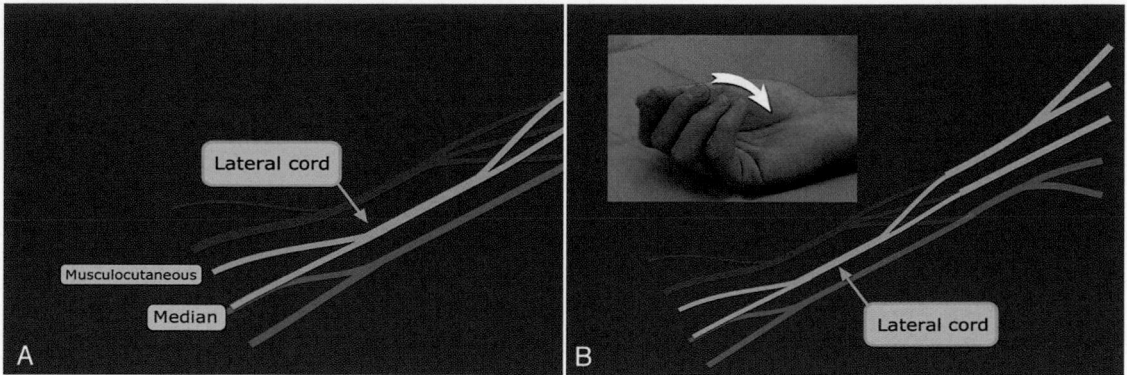

Figure 27–6. Organization (**A**) and motor response (**B**) of the lateral cord.

forearm, flexor carpi radialis, pronator teres (pronation of the forearm), and the thenar muscle of the thumb. It provides sensory innervation for the thumb to the lateral half of the fourth finger including the dorsal tips. The most distal motor response would be flexion of the fingers or flexion and opposition of the thumb.

The thumb has motor innervation from the ulnar nerve as well, which may be confusing if trying to interpret isolated thumb twitch. The ulnar nerve supplies the adductor pollicis, flexor pollicis brevis, and the first dorsal interosseous muscle. These muscles radially adduct the thumb. The flexor pollicis brevis assists in opposition of the thumb. The median nerve's innervation of the flexor pollicis longus, abductor pollicis brevis, and the opponens pollicis are the major flexors for opposition of the thumb.

The musculocutaneous nerve has only muscular branches above the elbow and is purely sensory below the elbow as it becomes the lateral antebrachial cutaneous nerve. The motor response is flexion of the elbow by contraction of the biceps and sensation to the middle to median part of the forearm.

The anatomic relationship of the musculocutaneous nerve to the cords and the coracoid process is pertinent to infraclavicular block. It could be considered a branch because it exits early but it is more like a terminal nerve because it has sensory and motor innervations. The musculocutaneous nerve is encountered commonly in infraclavicular blockade because it often is outside of the cord in this area. Variations in brachial plexus anatomy are common. Because the musculocutaneous nerve most often exits the lateral cord quite early, the stimulation of this nerve is felt to be an unreliable indicator of stimulation of the lateral cord.[17] This stimulation is not considered to be a distal response. It often overlies the lateral cord, which will be stimulated with deeper advancement of the needle as it passes the point of musculocutaneous nerve stimulation. Figure 27–6 depicts the lateral cord with its stimulated hand motor response.

The Posterior Cord

The posterior cord is just deep or inferior to the lateral cord. The axillary, the thoracodorsal, and upper and lower subscapular nerves are the branches from the posterior cord. They are involved in upper arm movement and shoulder movement and rotation as well as adduction of the shoulder and abduction of the arm. The branch most often encountered is the axillary nerve because it often has separated from the cord prior to the coracoid process. The axillary nerve to the deltoid elevates the upper arm. In addition to its branches, the posterior cord is responsible for the complete radial nerve. The distal responses from stimulation are abduction of the thumb and extension of the wrist and fingers (Figure 27–7). The

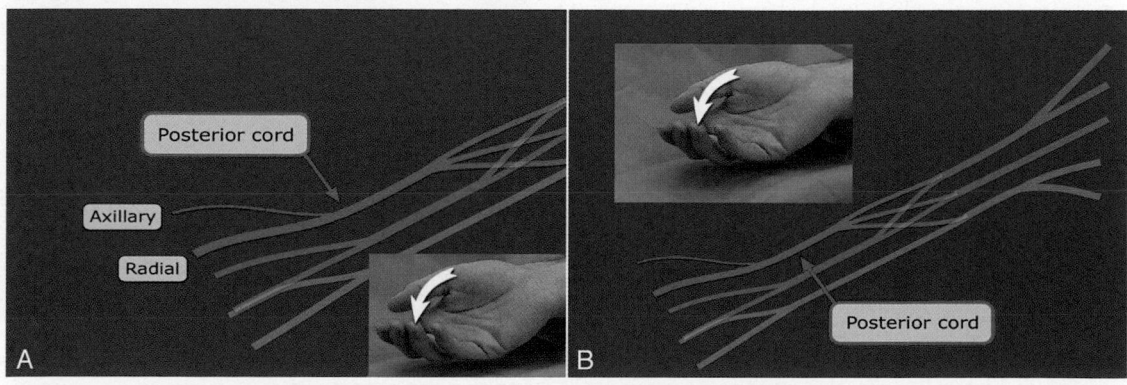

Figure 27–7. Organization (**A**) and motor response (**B**) of the posterior cord.

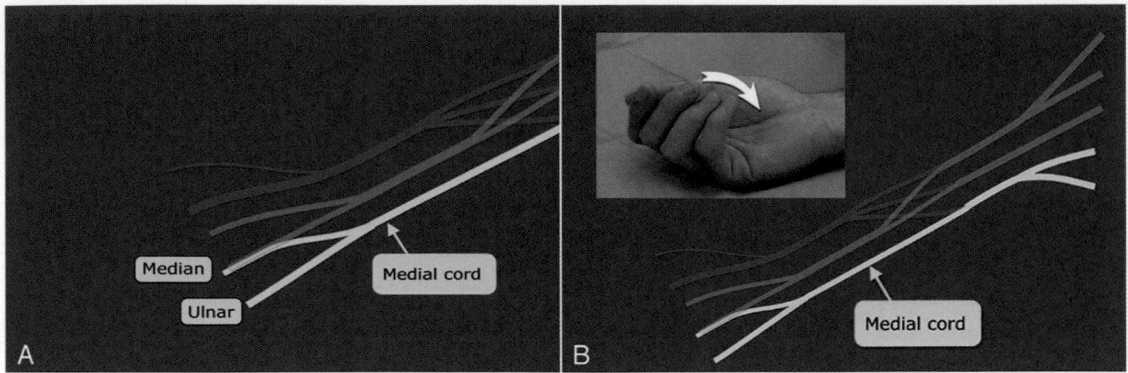

Figure 27–8. Organization (**A**) and motor response (**B**) of the medial cord.

brachioradialis muscle is innervated by the radial nerve and is classified as an extensor. Its stimulation should be characterized because it may be confused as a median nerve response because it actually flexes the elbow joint. Elbow flexion with radial deviation of the wrist represents stimulation of the brachioradialis muscle and a posterior cord response. The needle should be readjusted to obtain a more distal response of the radial nerve.

The Medial Cord

The medial cord branches into the ulnar nerve and the medial half of the median nerve. Branches include the medial pectoral, medial brachial cutaneous, and the medial antebrachial cutaneous nerves. These branches innervate the skin of the anterior and medial surfaces of the forearm to the wrist. The ulnar nerve innervates half of the fourth and the fifth fingers, the adductor pollicis, and all interossei, which results in contraction of the fourth and fifth fingers and thumb adduction. Median nerve stimulation results in flexion and sensation of the first three and one half fingers, opposition of the thumb, and sensation of the palm (Figure 27–8).

Unlike the axillary block, responses to stimulation of the median nerve during infraclavicular block could conceivably arise from either cord. Classic studies of fiber topography of the median nerve by Sunderland identified pronator teres fibers and flexor carpi radialis in the lateral root, along with nerves to the flexor digitorum profundus, flexor pollicis longus, and intrinsic thenar muscles in the median root.[18] Nerve injury studies also suggest that median fibers to the finger flexors are most likely found in the medial cord and medial root of the median nerve.[17] With the most commonly occurring plexus anatomy, finger flexion most likely identifies medial cord (or root) stimulation, but wrist flexion may result from either median or lateral cord (or root) stimulation.[19] Tables 27–1 and 27–2 summarize the cords, branches, terminal nerves, and their motor stimulus response. Because of anatomic variability and the mixing of the median nerve between the medial and lateral cords, the same responses are listed for both nerves. Except in rare variants the ulnar nerve is carried within the medial cord.

LANDMARKS & TECHNIQUE

Clinical Pearl

- The common approaches to infraclavicular block are the modified Raj, vertical infraclavicular, coracoid, lateral and sagittal.

General Guidelines

The bony landmarks used in most approaches are the clavicle, the jugular fossa or notch, the acromioclavicular joint, and the coracoid process, depicted in Figure 27–9. Bony landmarks and site of injection should be marked and the area

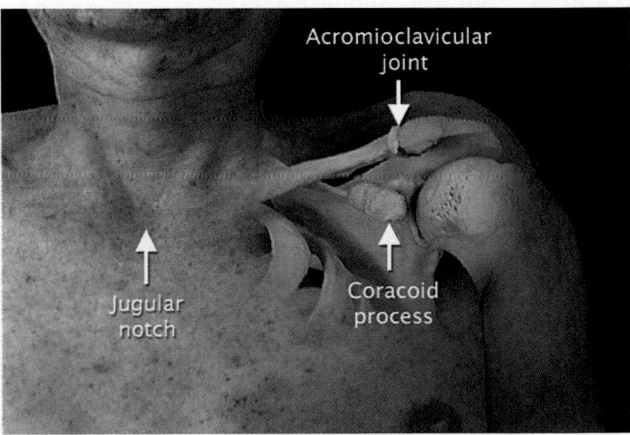

Figure 27–9. Relationship of the jugular (sternal) notch, clavicle and coracoid process.

Table 27–3.

Local Anesthetic Solutions for Infraclavicular Block

Duration	Anesthetic	
Short (1.5–3 h)	3% chloroprocaine 1.5% lidocaine 1–1.5% mepivacaine	
Intermediate (4–5 h)	2% lidocaine + epinephrine 1–1.5% mepivacaine	
Long-Lasting (10–14 h)	0.25–0.50% bupivacaine 0.50% ropivacaine	(0.0625–0.1% for infusion) 0.1–0.2% for infusion)

prepped with antiseptic solution. A small amount, approximately 5 mL, of local anesthetic is needed to anesthetize the skin and subcutaneous tissue. Care must be taken to avoid the pleura by never directing the needle in a medial direction. If the plexus is not encountered, the needle should be withdrawn and redirected sequentially by a factor of 10 degrees in either a cephalad or caudad direction. If those maneuvers are not successful, the landmarks should be reassessed before attempting another pass. Initial settings on the nerve stimulator are 1.5 mA, with an acceptable response occurring at less than 0.5 mA. The infraclavicular block is a large-volume block, and 30–40 mL of local anesthetic is necessary to accomplish block of the entire brachial plexus. Some commonly used local anesthetic solutions are listed in Tables 27–3 and 27–4.

MODIFIED RAJ APPROACH

Clinical Pearls

The relevant landmarks include:
- Line from the jugular fossa to the clavicular–acromial joint
- Middle point of that line—draw a perpendicular line 2.5–3 cm down for the insertion point
- 45- to 65-degree needle angle toward the axillay artery in the axilla
- 80- to 100-mm needle

The patient is in the dorsal recumbent position with the head turned to the side opposite the block. The subclavian artery is palpated where it dives under the clavicle, or the midpoint of the clavicle is marked. The brachial artery is palpated and marked at the lateral border of the pectoralis muscle. A line joining these two points is made with needle's insertion 2.5–3 cm below the midpoint of the clavicle at a 45-to 65-degree angle toward the axillary artery (Figure 27–10).

The practitioner stands on the opposite side to the site of block placement. Local anesthetic is infiltrated into the skin and the pectoralis muscle. The first two fingers of the palpating hand anchor the skin at the point of insertion, and the needle is advanced at a 45- to 65-degree angle toward the point of pulsation of the axillary artery (in axilla) or parallel to a line connecting the medial clavicular head with the coracoid process if the pulse cannot be felt (Figure 27–11).

If the plexus is not encountered, the needle should be withdrawn and redirected 10 degrees cephalad or caudad. At

Table 27–4.

Additives to Local Anesthetics

Drug	Dose	Notes
Epinephrine	Varies from zero 1:200,000–400,00 for vascular marking	Possible influence on duration and quality
Bicarbonate	Varied—1 mL/10 mL unless ropivacaine or upivacaine (1 mL/30 mL) is used	To speed onset of blockade
Clonidine		Small increase in pain relief post block. Possible sedation
Opioids		Most studies demonstrated no lasting effect
Buprenorphine	0.3 mg	Prolongs analgesia; greater duration of local anesthetic

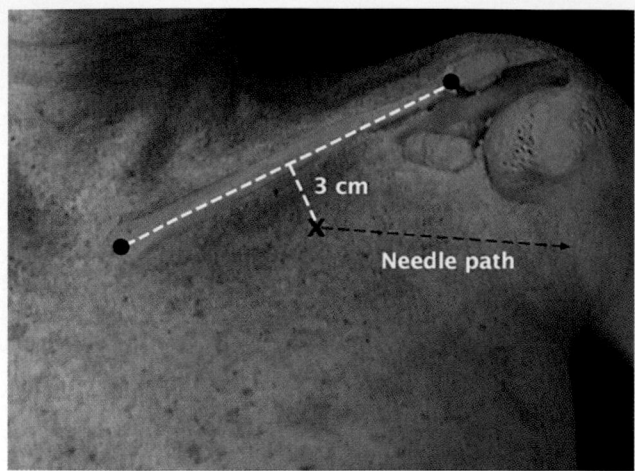

Figure 27–10. Raj approach: Landmarks and needle insertion plane.

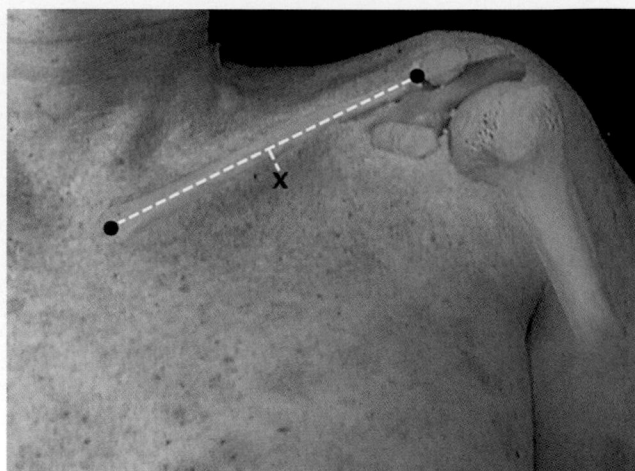

Figure 27–12. Vertical approach: Landmarks.

Clinical Pearls

- Needle insertion is at the midpoint of the line from the jugular fossa to the acromioclavicular joint. (Figure 27–12).
- Needle is inserted just under the clavicle.
- Needle assumes a 90-degree needle angle.
- A 50-mm needle is used.

A 50-mm needle is inserted close to the clavicle at an angle of 90 degrees (Figure 27–13). Local anesthetic is injected after a distal stimulus is obtained at or below 0.5 mA. This approach is popular in Europe and rapidly gaining in popularity in the United States.

If on the first pass the needle does not encounter the plexus, only the angle is changed while keeping the same plane by 10 degrees caudad or cephalad. The needle is never directed in a medial fashion.

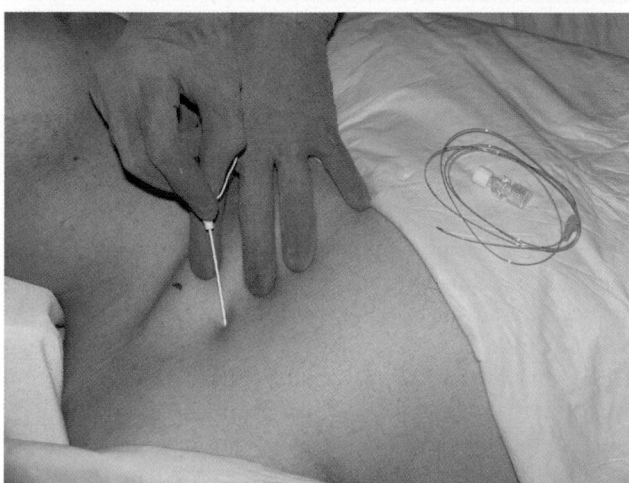

Figure 27–11. Raj approach: Needle insertion and orientation.

Clinical Pearls

The three most common errors that increase the risk of pneumothorax are:[20]
- Too medial insertion of the needle
- Depth of needle insertion >6 cm
- Medial direction of needle

no time should the needle be pointed medially or directed posteriorly (too steep of an angle) toward the lung.

VERTICAL INFRACLAVICULAR BLOCK

The vertical infraclavicular block was described by Kilka and coworkers in 1995.[14] The landmarks are the midpoint of a line from the middle of the fossa jugularis (jugular notch) and the ventral process of the acromion (Figure 27–12). The patient is lying in a supine position with the forearm relaxed on the chest with the head turned slightly to the side. The needle for most patients can be as short as 50 mm.

Adams reported improved success rate by moving the puncture site 1 cm laterally. The rate of unsuccessful block was reduced to 8.3%. Success was defined as not needing additional analgesics or sedation.[21] Using ultrasonographic assessment Greher and colleagues demonstrated topographic

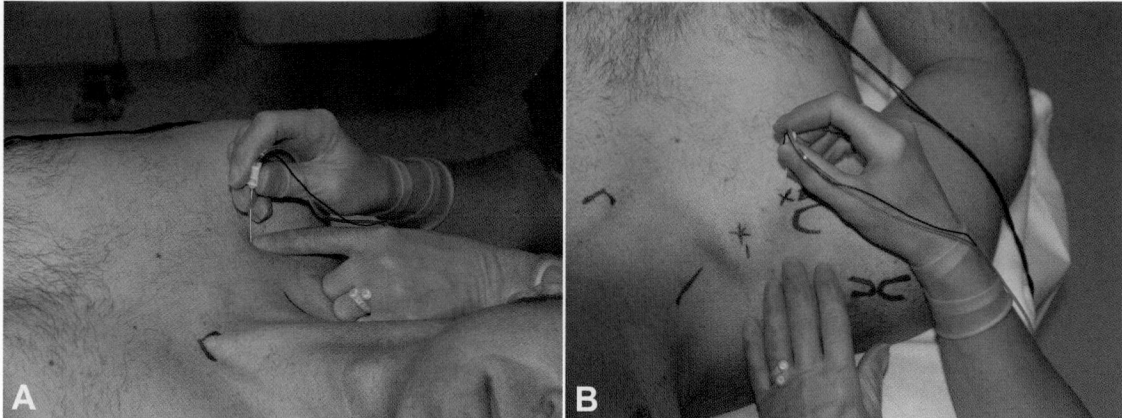

Figure 27–13. Vertical approach: Needle insertion (**A**) and orientation (**B**).

anatomy in volunteers and compared the classic approach to a puncture site determined by high-resolution ultrasound location of the plexus. A more lateral puncture site was suggested especially in women. They suggested that for every 1-cm decrease in the length of the distance of the line from the jugular fossa to the ventral process of the acromion from 22 to 22.5 cm, the puncture site should be moved 2 mm laterally from the center, and for every 1-cm increase, the puncture site moves 2 mm medially.[22]

CORACOID BLOCK

Clinical Pearls

- The needle insertion site is 2 cm inferior and 2 cm medial from the tip of the coracoid process.
- Needle assumes an angle of 90 degrees.
- An 80-mm needle is used.

The coracoid block as described by Whiffler[11] in 1981 has been revised from its original description. Whiffler's technique used a needle entry site that is most often inferior and medial to the coracoid process as determined by vascular landmarks, with the affected arm abducted and the shoulder depressed. In 1998 Wilson suggested that the insertion point should be 2 cm medial to the coracoid process and 2 cm caudad. At this skin entry site, direct posterior insertion of the needle makes contact with the cords at a mean range of 4.24 cm ± 1.49 (2.25–7.75 cm) in men and 4.01 ± 1.29 cm (2.25–6.5 cm) in women.[15] As shown in Figure 27–14, the lateral tip of the coracoid process (not the medial edge) is palpated. Kapral[20] in 1999 described a lateral approach with the patient in the same position. The point of needle insertion is lateral to the lateral point of the coracoid process. After identifying the coracoid process by touching the bone, the 7-cm needle is withdrawn 2–3 mm and redirected underneath the

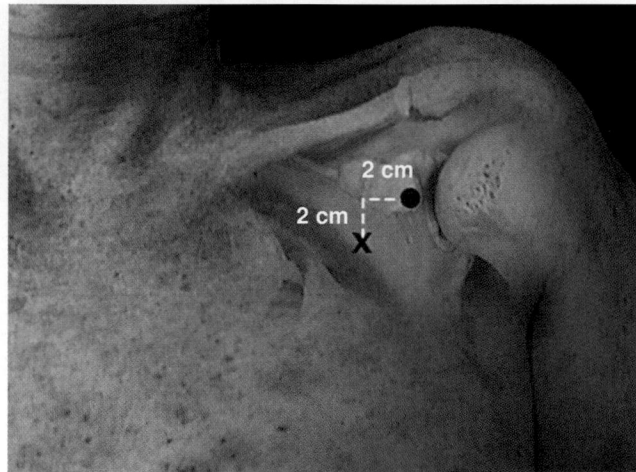

Figure 27–14. Coracoid approach: Landmarks.

coracoid process 2–3 cm until the brachial plexus is reached. The usual distance was 5.5–6.5 cm. Rodriguez described his series of coracoid blocks as closer to the coracoid process by making his puncture site 1 cm inferior and 1 cm medial to the coracoid process. He reported a similar success rate.[23,24]

THE LATERAL & SAGITTAL TECHNIQUE LANDMARKS

In 2004, Klaastad and coworkers described this technique and tested it in an MRI model.[25] The point of needle insertion is the intersection between the clavicle and the coracoid process (see Figure 27–2). The needle is advanced 15 degrees posterior, always strictly in the sagittal plane next to the coracoid process while abutting the anteroinferior edge of the clavicle. Unlike other approaches, the practitioner works from behind the shoulder of the patient. The coracoids' most medial palpable point close to the clavicle is determined. All needle directions in this method adhere strictly to the sagittal plane through this coracoid prominence. The posterior cord and

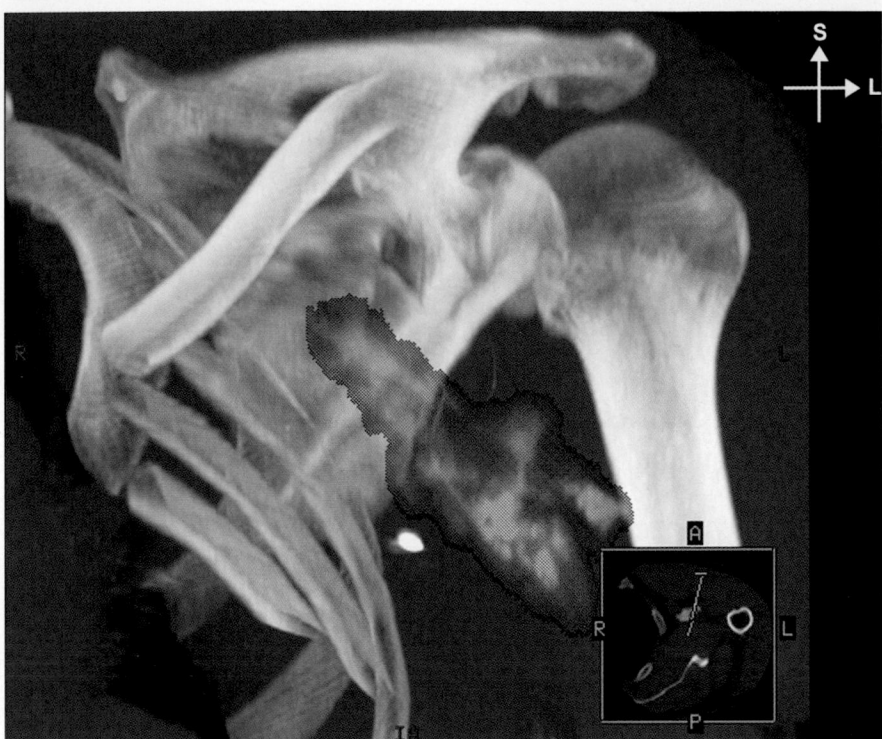

Figure 27–15. A contrast MRI image showing dispersion of the injectate after injection through an indwelling catheter.

medial cord were more often reached than the lateral cord. Insertion depth should be no greater than 6.5 cm. Although the cords are usually reached before the axillary artery and vein, puncture of these vessels as well as the cephalic vein is always a possibility.[26] Klaastad and coworkers reported occasionally needing to insert the needle more than 6.5 cm (their estimated maximal safe depth) to obtain satisfactory nerve contact and without a risk of pneumothorax.[27]

Although initially used with a nerve stimulator, this technique has become the preferred method for use with ultrasound localization of the brachial plexus cords.[14] Initial placement is adjacent (2 cm medial) to the coracoid process at the inferior border of the clavicle. The needle is advanced posteriorly with a 15-degree angle to the coronal plane to localize the cords. The cords are superior and posterior to the axillary artery, most commonly at a depth of 4 to 6 cm. Although it is always possible to puncture the artery, the trajectory of this approach appears to avoid puncture of the axillary vessels because the cords are encountered cephalad to the artery and 2–3 cm cephalad to the pleural cavity. Localization of the cords with the nerve stimulator is confirmed prior to injection. The use of ultrasound in combination with a nerve stimulator may improve block success and decrease morbidity.[28]

SINGLE INJECTION VS MULTIPLE INJECTION, & CONTINUOUS TECHNIQUE

Single stimulation has been reported to result in success rates from 82% to 100%.[20,26,29,30] Gaertner and colleagues compared single stimulation to stimulation of all three cords. Multistimulation took slightly longer (9 vs 7.5 min); however, 2 of the 40 patients in the multistimulation group were excluded because all three cords could not be localized within 15 min.[26] A distal response in the hand or wrist was considered adequate with 10 mL of local anesthetic injected at each site. In the single stimulation group, 30 mL of local anesthetic was injected after identifying a single response from any cord, (Figure 27–15). Their overall success rate was low for both techniques (40% for single stimulation and 72.5% for multiple stimulation) however, Gaertner and colleagues concluded that multiple stimulation was significantly more successful. The relatively low volume of local anesthetic (30 mL), could have contributed to the overall unusually low success rate. Most hand surgery can be performed with two or three of the nerves to the hand blocked if they are in the correct distribution of the surgery. However, Gaertner and colleagues felt more stringent criteria should be used. A complete motor and sensory block of all nerves was necessary for their criteria of success as compared with success defined as completing the procedure without supplementation or the need for general anesthesia.

An example of this criterion is demonstrated by Rodriguez and collaborators[23] in a random controlled trial comparing injection of 42 mL of mepivacaine using a single-, dual-, or triple-injection technique. A significantly less complete motor blockade was found with single injection versus the dual or triple injection. No significant difference was found in the dual- or triple-injection groups. However, musculocutaneous and axillary nerve responses were accepted as valid in their study. Seven patients in the single stimulation group (28%) had this proximal response considered a valid response. It is debatable whether this allows a direct comparison to the single technique. In another study,[24] comparing single and dual stimulation, 22% of the single stimulation group had a musculocutaneous or axillary response. The authors state that the recommendations for not accepting these responses is based on a published anecdotal report[31] on a noncoracoid approach. The authors demonstrated that triple injection offered no benefit over dual injection. Dual injection was described as the best balance between efficacy and comfort for patients and resulted in shorter block performance times and decreased vascular puncture rates compared with that for triple stimulation injection. To determine whether proximal or distal response was better, Rodriguez and collaborators devised a randomized, prospective, single-blind study comparing median versus musculocutaneous nerve response with a single injection infraclavicular block.[16] They concluded that elicitation of a median nerve response improved the effectiveness of blockade compared with a musculocutaneous nerve response. The median nerve response had a shorter time onset and a higher efficacy of brachial plexus anesthesia. However, complete blockade of the upper limb was low in both groups. They postulated that since the lateral cord is the shallowest and the medial cord is deeper, the musculocutaneous response is suggestive of a superficial injection of local anesthetic, whereas a median-type response corresponds to deposition of local anesthetic closer to the cords in a more "central" location.

An editorial categorizing the issue of multistimulation and acceptable response touts infraclavicular block as perhaps the ideal technique and delineates the debates of multistimulation versus single stimulation and the possible confusion that can exist in determining the exact cord that originates a distal response.[19] It is accepted that an axillary or musculocutaneous response is not a distal response. However, anatomic variability, multiple proximal branches, and dual-cord contribution all add to the possible difficulty in some cases of identifying with certainty and matching the correct cord stimulated with the demonstrated distal motor response. This must be taken in consideration with multiple cord stimulation.

Deluze and coworkers found a similar effective rate to triple stimulation by using 40 mL of 0.75% ropivacaine.[32] They compared infraclavicular block using a paracoracoid technique and accepted wrist or distal stimulation in the hand. A successful block was defined as abolition of cold and pinprick responses in all five nerve distributions distal to the elbow, (radial, ulnar, median, musculocutaneous, and medial antebrachial cutaneous) within 30 min. Successful blockade was achieved in 90%.

It remains to be seen if this dilemma could possibly be resolved by adjusting volume or an increase in anesthetic concentration without dealing with a toxicity issue. There are obvious advantages to obtaining a successful block with only one stimulation. This debate no doubt will continue for some time just as it has for axillary block.

Continuous Technique

The infraclavicular block has a particular advantage over the axillary approach for continuous pain management. With the infraclavicular approach, catheter management is simplified by its easy accessibility. The catheter is easier to care for and observe and there is less inherent movement than the axillary area, so there is less chance for dislodgement. Patient comfort is greater with an infraclavicular catheter rather than with a dressing in the axillary area. If the distribution of the pain is in the axillary nerve or musculocutaneous areas, the chance of sensory blockade of those areas and pain relief are greater.

All approaches have been utilized successfully with a continuous technique, and there is no overwhelming evidence that favors a particular approach.[20,27,33,34] One could postulate that the lateral sagittal approach or the modified Raj approach might offer an advantage because the catheter would not be required to make a 90-degree turn from the surface. Placement of the catheter should occur under sterile conditions, using, at a minimum, sterile gloves and sterile drapes.

Practical Management

The coracoid process can easily be found even in obese patients. The middle finger is placed just below the clavicle and the hand is moved laterally toward the shoulder. The first bony prominence that is felt by the index finger is the coracoid process. When a small circular pressure is applied to both the middle and index fingers, the middle finger should be in soft tissue, and the index finger will delineate the edges of the coracoid process. This can be confirmed by moving the arm because occasionally in a muscular or heavy individual the difference is not as great. As pressure is applied to it, the coracoid process will not move as the arm is raised. The patient should be positioned near the edge of the bed to allow enough room for stabilization of the operator's elbows. It is difficult to stabilize a needle if the operator's arm is "floating." The patient's arm can be extended at the side or flexed at the elbow, allowing the hand to rest on the abdomen.

The patient is often propped on the pillows with the shoulder in various positions. Pillows should be removed completely from the patient's head and back and if necessary used only for support of the lower arm. The head should be turned to the opposite side. Appropriate premedication will facilitate positioning.

SUMMARY

The infraclavicular block is a useful alternative to axillary block for surgery of the arm. Several approaches offer the anesthesiologist flexibility in achieving a successful block. The debate exists over single versus multistimulation and what is the optimal volume of local anesthetic. The infraclavicular block allows the anesthesiologist the advantages of providing complete blockade without having to abduct the arm or to individually block the musculocutaneous or intercostobrachial nerve. The block is reliable for surgery with comparable or decreased complications to other regional procedures. It is applicable to ultrasound technique and can be used for continuous as well as single-shot techniques.

References

1. Hirschel G: Die Anasthesierung des Plexus brachialis bei Operationen der oberen Extremitat. MMW Munch Med Wochenschr 1911;58:1555–1556.
2. Kulenkampff D: Anasthesie des Plexus brachialis. Zentralbl Chir 1911;8:1337–1350.
3. Bazy L, Pouchet V, Sourdat V, et al: J Anesth Reg 1917;222–225.
4. From Zentralbl Chir 45,1918. In Winnie AP: *Plexus Anesthesia.* WB Saunders, 1983, pp 215–217.
5. Labat's *Regional Anesthesia: Its Technique and Clinical Application,* WB Saunders, 1923, p 223.
6. Dogliotti AM: *Anesthesia: Narcosis, Local, Regional, Spinal.* SB Debour, 1939.
7. Moore DC: *Regional Block,* 4th ed. Charles C Thomas, 1981.
8. Cousins MJ, Bridenbaugh PO: *Neural Blockade in Clinical Anesthesia and Pain Management,* Lippincott, 1980.
9. Raj PP, Montgomery SJ, Nettles D, et al: Infraclaficular brachial plexus block—A new approach. Anesth Analg 1973;52:897–904.
10. Sims JK: A modification of landmarks for infraclavicular approach to brachial plexus block. Anesth Analg 1977;56:554–557.
11. Whiffler K: Coracoid block—A safe and easy technique. Br J Anaesth 1981;53:845.
12. Winnie AP: *Plexus Anesthesia.* WB Saunders, 1983.
13. Klaastad O, Lileas FG, Rotnes JS, et al: Magnetic resonance imaging demonstrates lack of precision in needle placement by the infraclavicular brachial plexus block described by Raj et al. Anesth Analg 1999;88:593–598.
14. Kilka HG, Geiger P, Mehrkens HH: Infraclavicular blockade. A new method for anesthesia of the upper extremity: An anatomical and clinical study. Anaesthesist 1995;44:339–344.
15. Wilson JL, Brown DL, Wongy GY: Infraclavicular brachial plexus block: Parasagittal anatomy important to the coracoid technique. Anesth Analg 1998;87:870–873.
16. Rodriguez J, Taboada-Muiz M, Barcena M, et al: Median versus musculocutaneous nerve response with single-injection infraclavicuar coracoid block. Reg Anesth Pain Med 2004:29:534–538.
17. Gelberman RH: Operative Nerve Repair and Reconstruction. Lippincott, 1991, p 1288.
18. Sunderland S: The intraneural topography of the radial, median, and ulnar nerves. Brain 1945;68(pt 4):243–299.
19. Weller RS, Gerancher JC: Brachial plexus block: "Best" approach and "best" evoked response—Where are we? Reg Anesth Pain Med 2004;29:520–523.
20. Kapral S, Jandrasits O, Schabernig C, et al: Lateral infraclavicular plexus block vs. axillary block for hand and forearm surgery. Acta Anaesthesiol Scand 1999;43:1047–1052.
21. Adam H, Hansel B: Vertical infraclavicular technique of brachial plexus block. Anaesthesiol Intensiv Med Notfallmed Schmerzther 2004;39(12):728–734.
22. Greher M, Retzl G, Niel P, et al: Ultrasound assessment of toporaphic anatomy in volunteers suggests a modification of the infraclavicular block. Br J Anaesth 2002;88:621–624.
23. Rodriguez J, Barcena M, Taboada-Muiz M, et al: A comparison of single versus multiple injections on the extent of anesthesia with coracoid infraclavicular brachial plexus block. Anesth Analg 2004;99:1225–1230.
24. Rodriguez J, Barcena M, Lagunilla J, et al: Increased success rate with infraclavicular brachial plexus block using a dual-injection technique. J Clin Anesthesia 2004;16:251–256.
25. Klaastad O, Smith HG, Smedby O, et al: A novel infraclavicular brachial plexus block: The lateral and sagittal technique, developed by magnetic resonance imaging studies. Anesth Analg 2004;98:252–256.
26. Gaertner E, Estebe JP, Zamfir A, et al: Infraclavicular plexus block: Multiple injection versus single injection. Reg Anesth Pain Med 2002;27:590–594.
27. Klaastad O, Smith H-J, Smedby O, et al: Response to letter to editor. Anesth Analg 2004;99:950–951.
28. Brull R, McCartney C, Chan V: A novel approach to the infraclavicular brachial plexus block: The ultrasound experience. Letter. Anesth Analg 2004;99:950.
29. Borgeat A, Ekatodramis G, Dumont C: An evaluation of the infraclavicular block via a modified approach of the Raj technique. Anesth Analg 2001;93:436–441.
30. Jandard C, Gentili ME, Girard F, et al: Infraclavicular block with lateral approach and nerve stimulation: Extent of anesthesia and adverse effects. Reg Anesth Pain Med 2002;27:37–42.
31. Fitzgibbon DR, Deps AD, Erjavec MK: Selective musculocutaneous nerve block and infraclavicular brachial plexus anesthesia. Reg Anesth 1995;20:239–241.
32. Deluze A, Gentili ME, et al: A comparison of a single-stimulation lateral infraclavicular plexus block with a triple stimulation axillary block. Reg Anesth Pain Med 2003;28:89–94.
33. Mehrkens HH, Geiger PK: Continuous brachial plexus blockade via the vertical infraclavicular approach. Anaesthesia 1998;53(Suppl 2):19–20.
34. Macaire P, Gaertner E, Capdevila X: Continuous post operative regional analgesia at home. Minerva Anestesiol 2001;67:109–116.

28

Axillary Brachial Plexus Block

Zbigniew Koscielniak-Nielsen, MD

INTRODUCTION

Brachial plexus block at the level of the axilla is typically chosen for anesthesia of the distal upper limb. Axillary block is a basic regional anesthesia technique and perhaps the most common approach to brachial plexus blockade. Low risk of serious complications, superficial location, and good analgesia of the upper arm muscles make this block suitable for ambulatory procedures of longer duration that require a tourniquet.

HISTORY

The surgical technique of this block was first described by Hall[1] in New York (Roosevelt Hospital) in 1884, and the percutaneous technique was described by Hirschel[2] in 1911. While dissecting the axilla in a child in 1958, Burnham,[3] recognized that filling the neurovascular sheath with local anesthetic could simplify the axillary block. He also described the characteristic fascial "click" felt on penetration by the needle. In 1961 while using the formula for a cylinder volume, De Jong[4] calculated that in an average adult, 42 mL of local anesthetic (LA) was necessary to fill the fascial compartment to the level of the cords and block all terminal nerves to the arm. A year later, Eriksson and Skarby,[5] in an effort to promote the proximal spread of LA, advocated wrapping a rubber tourniquet around the arm, distal to the needle. In 1979, Winnie and coworkers[6] found the tourniquet ineffective and painful and recommended firm distal digital pressure on the neurovascular sheath instead. In addition, they also recommended arm adduction after LA injection, thinking that the head of the abducted humerus compressed the neurovascular sheath. Both maneuvers were later proved to be clinically ineffective.[7–9] Thompson and Rorie,[10] in 1983, studied brachial plexus using computed tomograms and suggested that the median, ulnar, and radial nerves lie in separate fascial compartments within the neurovascular sheath; this finding provided a rational explanation for incomplete blocks. However, anatomic studies by Lassale and Ang[11] in 1984 and Vester-Andersen and coworkers[12] in 1986 did not confirm the existence of a true neurovascular sheath. The interfascial space they found contained the median and the ulnar nerves, infrequently the musculocutaneous, and occasionally the radial nerves. Moreover, the space was suggested to communicate proximally only with the medial cord of the plexus. In 1987 Partridge and coworkers[13] described the interneural septa, which were easily broken by injection of dyed latex. In 2002 Klaastad and coworkers[14] were the first to investigate the spread of the LA through the axillary catheter in studies using magnetic resonance imaging (MRI) scanning. They found that in most patients the spread of LA was uneven and the clinical effect inadequate.

Until the 1960s, the prevalent block techniques were double or multiple axillary injections. After the concept of the neurovascular sheath had been established by De Jong[4] in 1961, the single-injection technique, being the simplest, became standard. However, Vester-Andersen and coworkers[15,16] demonstrated in 1983 and 1984, that despite high volumes of LA, analgesia was often inconsistent ("patchy"). In the early 1990s, the double-injection, transarterial technique was popularized by Urban and Urquhart[17] and Stan and coworkers.[18] More recently, however, development of peripheral nerve stimulators and insulated atraumatic needles has allowed electrolocation and separate blockade of the individual terminal nerves (median, musculocutaneous, ulnar, and radial). This is known as the multiple-nerve stimulation technique. Baranowski and Pither[19] (in 1990), Lavoie and coworkers[20] (in 1992), Koscielniak-Nielsen and coworkers[21,22] (in 1997 and 1998), and Sia and coworkers[23,24] (in 2001 and 2002), independently showed that multiple-nerve stimulation was superior, both to the single- and the double-injection methods by increasing the success rate and shortening the block onset. A recent Cochrane review by Handoll and coworkers[25] validated these findings.

INDICATIONS & CONTRAINDICATIONS

The most common indications for axillary block include surgery of the forearm, wrist, or hand of moderate to long duration, with or without arm tourniquet. Relative contraindications to the use of this block are skin infection at the block site, axillary lymphadenopathy, and severe coagulopathy. In addition, this block is best avoided in patients with severe preexisting neurologic disease of the upper extremity because sensory assessments may be difficult.

PERTINENT ANATOMY

In the apex of the axilla, the three plexus cords (lateral, medial, and posterior) form the main terminal nerves of the upper extremity (axillary, musculocutaneous, median, ulnar, and radial). However, only the last three nerves accompany the blood vessels through the axilla where the blocks are performed (Figure 28–1), while the axillary and the musculocutaneous nerves leave the plexus approximately at the level of the coracoid process. The axillary nerve departs at a wider angle from the posterior cord, laterally and dorsally, and the musculocutaneous nerve, which originates from the lateral cord, runs obliquely laterally into the coracobrachial muscle and continues downward. The medial antebrachial and brachial cutaneous nerves run subcutaneously parallel to the axillary vessels, although the medial antebrachial cutaneous nerve often follows the median nerve within the neurovascular sheath. In the axilla, the median and musculocutaneous nerves lie superior to the artery, whereas the ulnar and radial nerves lie inferior to it. The depths at which the nerves are found vary. Typically, the median nerve is more superficial than the musculocutaneous, and the ulnar nerve is more superficial than the radial. Occasionally, the radial or the musculocutaneous nerves (or both) are found behind the artery. These two nerves progressively diverge from the neurovascular sheath, continuing down the upper arm, the musculocutaneous above (anterior) and the radial below (posterior) to the humerus, where they can be approached using the midhumeral approach.[26]

Landmarks

Surface landmarks for the axillary brachial plexus block include (Figure 28–2):

1. Pulse of the axillary artery
2. Coracobrachialis muscle
3. Pectoralis major muscle
4. Biceps muscle
5. Triceps muscle

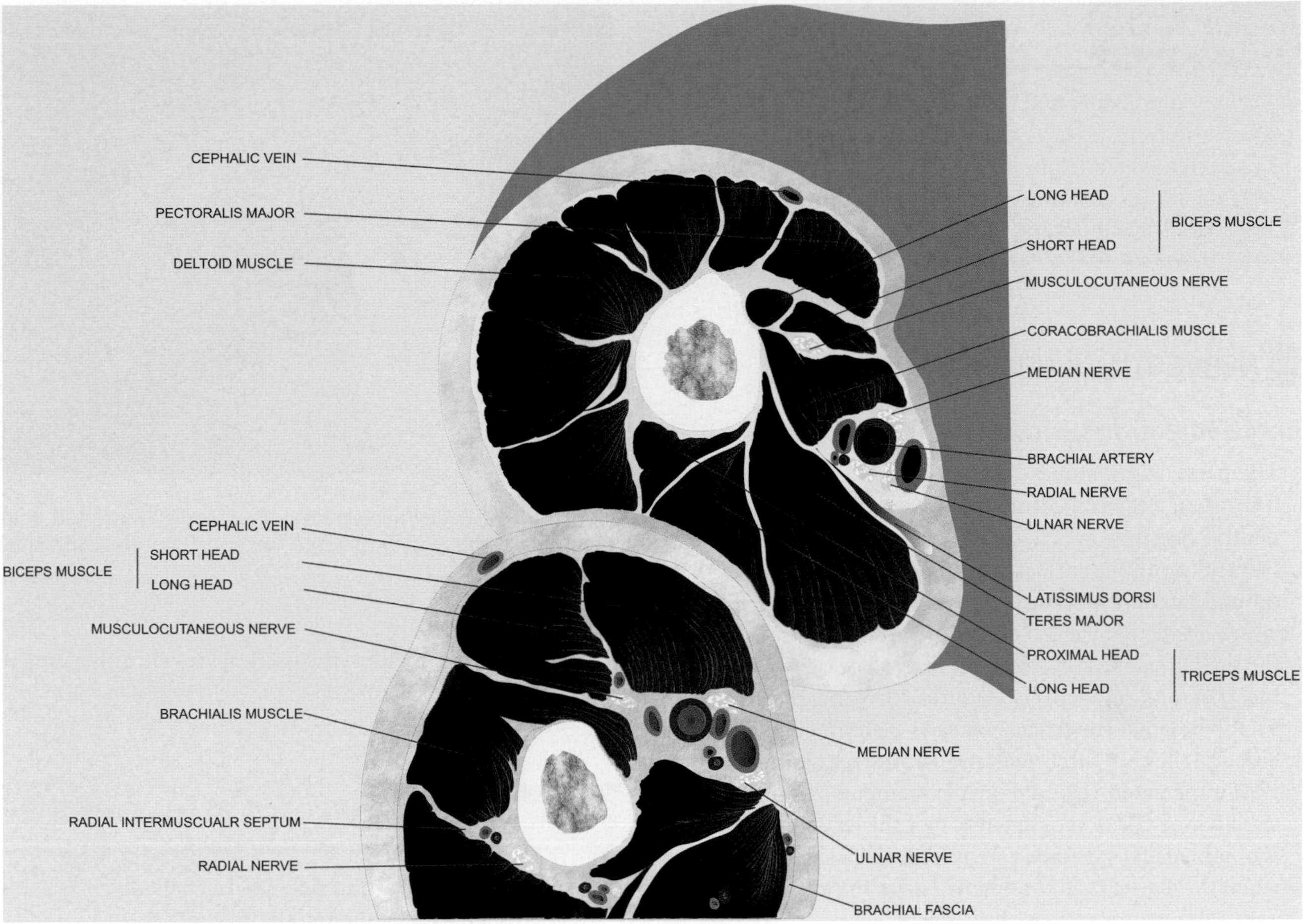

CEPHALIC VEIN

PECTORALIS MAJOR

DELTOID MUSCLE

LONG HEAD

SHORT HEAD

BICEPS MUSCLE

MUSCULOCUTANEOUS NERVE

CORACOBRACHIALIS MUSCLE

MEDIAN NERVE

BRACHIAL ARTERY

RADIAL NERVE

ULNAR NERVE

LATISSIMUS DORSI

TERES MAJOR

PROXIMAL HEAD

LONG HEAD

TRICEPS MUSCLE

CEPHALIC VEIN

SHORT HEAD

LONG HEAD

BICEPS MUSCLE

MUSCULOCUTANEOUS NERVE

BRACHIALIS MUSCLE

RADIAL INTERMUSCUALR SEPTUM

RADIAL NERVE

MEDIAN NERVE

ULNAR NERVE

BRACHIAL FASCIA

Figure 28–1. Anatomy of the brachial plexus at axilla and at the midhumeral level.

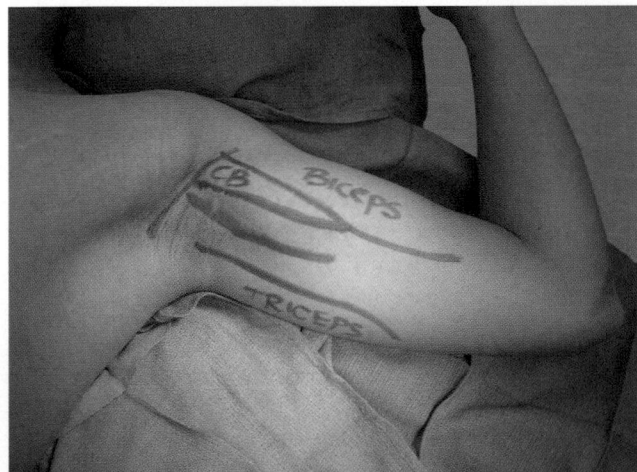

Figure 28–2. Landmarks for the classical approach to axillary brachial plexus block.

EQUIPMENT

- Sterile towels and 4-in. × 4-in. gauze packs
- Sterile gloves, marking pen, and a skin electrode
- 1-in., 25-gauge needle for skin infiltration
- 1- to 1.5-in. atraumatic, insulated stimulating needle
- 20-mL syringes containing LA of choice
- Peripheral nerve stimulator

INJECTION TECHNIQUES

Arm Position for the Block

The arm to be operated on is abducted approximately 90 degrees (see Figure 28–2). The elbow is flexed and the forearm rests comfortably, supported by a pillow. A skin electrode is typically placed on the patient's shoulder and connected to the positive electrode (anode) of the nerve stimulator. After scrubbing the axilla, the arterial pulse is palpated at the level of the major pectoral muscle, and the subcutaneous tissue overlying the artery is infiltrated with 4 to 5 mL of LA (to block the intercostobrachial and medial cutaneous nerves of the arm). Numerous techniques and approaches to the brachial plexus block at the level about the axilla have been described. Discussion of all the technique variations is beyond the scope of this text; we will describe some of the best studied and clinically useful techniques.

Clinical Pearl

- Various approaches and techniques described in the following sections all have their advantages and disadvantages. However, a triple-injection axillary block is probably the fastest and most efficient technique for axillary brachial plexus blockade.

NERVE STIMULATION TECHNIQUES

Single-Injection (Stimulation) Technique

1. The nerve stimulator is set to deliver 0.5–1.0 mA (2 Hz, 0.1 msec); electrical connections with the needle and the neutral electrode are checked.
2. Depending on the surgical site (palmar and medial or dorsal and lateral aspects of the hand/forearm), the stimulating needle is inserted above the arterial pulse (toward the median nerve) or below the arterial pulse (toward the radial nerve), respectively (Figures 28–3 and 28–4).
3. As the brachial superficial fascia is penetrated, a characteristic "click" is often felt, and the current amplitude is slowly increased (eg, at 1-mA increments) until the desired twitch (flexion or extension of the wrist and fingers) is obtained. This helps avoid painful electrical paresthesia when the elastic fascia suddenly "gives in" and the needle enters the neurovascular sheath.[27]
4. After the initial motor response is obtained, the needle is slowly advanced toward the stimulated nerve while reducing the amplitude.
5. Once the stimulation is obtained using a current intensity of 0.3 to 0.5 mA, the entire volume of LA is injected slowly, while intermittently aspirating to reduce the risk of accidental intravascular injection. This results in substantial

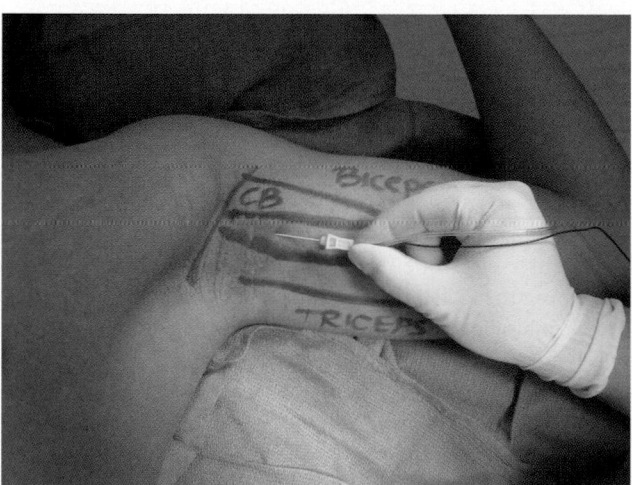

Figure 28–3. Median nerve block: The needle is inserted above the pulse of the axillary (brachial) artery. CB = coracobrachialis muscle.

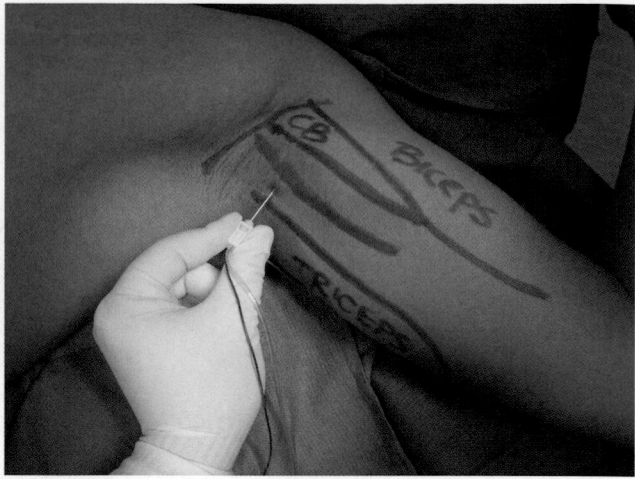

Figure 28–4. Radial nerve block: The needle is inserted below the pulse of the axillary (brachial) artery. CB = coracobrachialis muscle.

spread of the LA within the tissue layers encompassing the brachial plexus (Figure 28–5).

Clinical Pearls

- Arterial pulse palpation may prove challenging in some patients. In these patients, the first obtained motor response can be used to guide needle redirection to achieve the desired response.
- Elbow flexion (stimulation of the coracobrachialis muscle or the musculocutaneous nerve) indicates that the needle is outside the neurovascular sheath; the needle should be redirected downward and more superficially.
- Extension of the wrist and hand (radial nerve) indicates that the needle is below the artery.
- The more difficult differentiation is between the median and the ulnar nerves, which both result in wrist/finger flexion. In this scenario, the following method can be used to differentiate between the two nerves:
- When flexion is accompanied by forearm pronation, the stimulated nerve is the median (the needle is positioned above the artery).
- Another way to differentiate between these two nerves is by palpation of the flexor tendons at the wrist. Median nerve stimulation produces movements of the palmaris longus and the flexor carpi radialis tendons, which lie in the middle of the wrist, whereas ulnar nerve stimulation produces movement of the flexor carpi ulnaris tendon, which lies medially.
- Decreasing the intensity of the output current of the nerve stimulator helps facilitate differentiation between median and ulnar nerve stimulation.

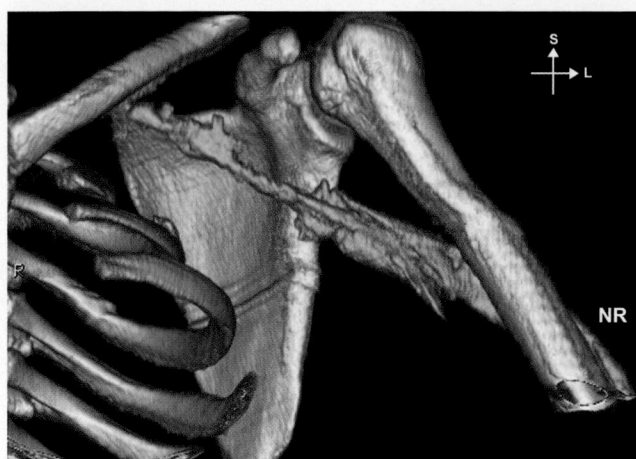

Figure 28–5. Distribution of local anesthetic injected during axillary brachial plexus blockade. NR = nervus radialis.

Double-Injection Technique

1. The stimulating needle is first inserted above the artery, below the coracobrachialis muscle (see Figure 28–3). After penetrating the fascia, the amplitude is increased until synchronous wrist flexion/pronation and flexion of the first three fingers are obtained (median nerve stimulation). The needle is advanced slowly toward this nerve while reducing the amplitude to 0.3 to 0.5 mA. At this point, half of the planned volume of LA is slowly injected with intermittent aspiration to rule out intravascular injection.
2. The needle is then withdrawn and inserted below the artery and above the triceps muscle (see Figure 28–4). The fascia is again penetrated and the amplitude slowly increased. The first response is usually either arm extension (muscular branches to the triceps) or thumb adduction and flexion of the last two fingers (ulnar nerve). However, these responses are ignored, and the needle is advanced deeper, often slightly upward, behind the artery (Figure 28–6) until wrist and finger extension is obtained (radial nerve). After stimulation is obtained using a current intensity lower than 0.5 mA, the remaining volume of LA is slowly injected with intermittent aspiration.

Multiple-Injection Technique

Needle insertion sites are identical to those for the double-injection technique

1. After electrolocation of the median nerve, 5–10 mL of the LA volume is injected (see Figure 28–3).
2. The needle is withdrawn subcutaneously and redirected obliquely, above and into the coracobrachialis muscle. After obtaining stimulation-synchronous elbow flexion, the amplitude is reduced to 0.3 to 0.5 mA and another 5–10 mL of LA is injected.

3. The needle is removed and inserted below the artery (see Figure 28–4). The first stimulated nerve is usually the ulnar, into which 5–10 mL of LA is injected.
4. The needle is advanced deeper until the radial nerve is found (see under Double-Injection Technique.)

Clinical Pearls

- Two recent studies by Sia and colleagues[23,28] suggest that two separate injections below the artery do not improve success rates, and therefore only one such injection is needed. This injection is made close to the radial nerve and should contain half of the planned LA volume.
- Electrolocation of multiple nerves may occasionally take some time. Because the first injection of the LA injection in the vicinity of the median nerve may partially block the ulnar nerve, the search for the nerves should be made expeditiously to minimize the risk of nerve injury by advancing needle or intraneural injection into an anesthetized nerve.
- For these reasons, this technique could be considered an advanced regional anesthesia technique. Careful assessment of resistance to injection by an experienced practitioner or objective monitoring of injection pressure should be used with each injection.

Transarterial Technique

The transarterial technique is perhaps most commonly used for axillary blockade. This relatively simple technique does not rely on a nerve stimulator; instead, placement of the needle within the neurovascular sheath is ensured by relying on the pulse of the axillary artery:

- The axillary artery is palpated and stabilized using a two-finger palpation technique.
- As the needle is advanced toward the pulse of the axillary artery, bright red arterial blood is aspirated. A thin, long-beveled needle (typically 1.5-in., 25-gauge) is used to minimize the risk of axillary hematoma.
- The needle is advanced deeper until blood cannot be aspirated (the tip of the needle has exited the artery) and half of the volume of the LA is injected behind the posterior wall. This should block the radial nerve.
- The needle is slowly withdrawn while aspirating. As the needle enters the axillary artery, bright red blood is again aspirated.
- The withdrawal of the needle is continued until blood can not be aspirated (the needle exits the artery and its tip is positioned superficial [medial] to the artery inside the neurovascular sheath).
- The remaining volume of LA is injected superficial to the anterior wall to block the median and the ulnar nerves.

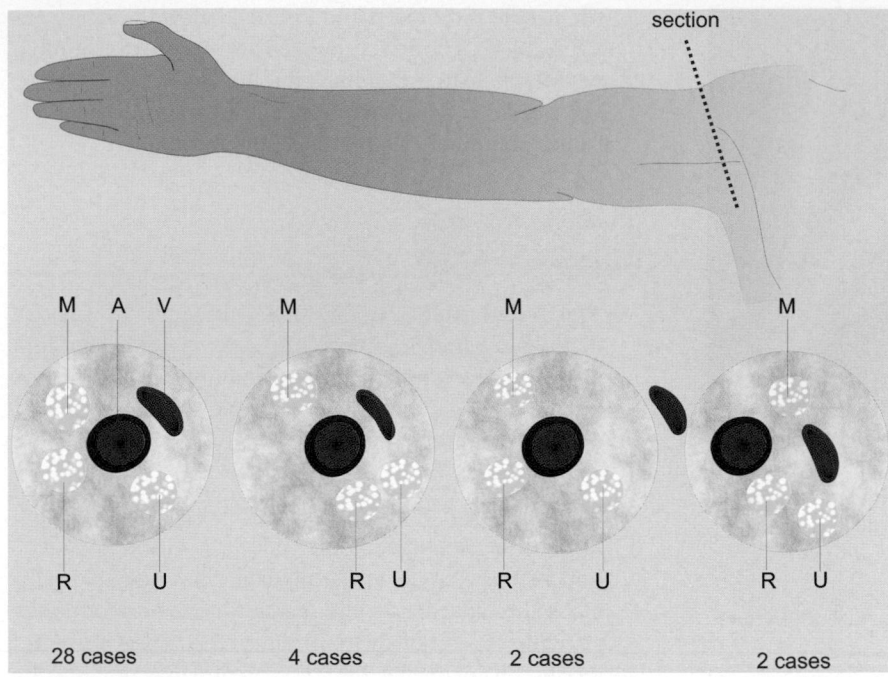

Figure 28–6. Spatial arrangement of the terminal nerves of the brachial plexus in the axilla. M = median nerve, A = artery, V = vein, R = radial nerve, U = ulnar nerve.

Clinical Pearl

- A transarterial injection is made as high up in the axilla as possible, and the needle should traverse the artery at an oblique angle. This reduces the risk of making the injection behind the artery intramuscularly and improves the spread of the LA to the plexus cords to block the musculocutaneous nerve.

Continuous Axillary Brachial Plexus Block Technique

Continuous axillary brachial plexus block is similar to the single-injection technique; nerve stimulator technique is typically used. The needle of choice is connected to the nerve stimulator, and the desired twitch response is sought. Once the stimulation is obtained with a current close to 0.5 mA, a catheter is advanced 5–8 cm cephalad into the neurovascular sheath. When a stimulating catheter is used, a nonconducting solution (eg, 5% dextrose[29]) can be injected through the catheter to dilate the sheath and facilitate insertion of the catheter. The catheter is secured using either a tunneling technique or application of a sterile clear dressing.

Clinical Pearl

- Strict aseptic precautions should be adhered to, just as with any other indwelling catheter technique.

MIDHUMERAL APPROACH (HUMERAL CANAL BLOCK)

The difference between the multiinjection axillary and the midhumeral (humeral canal) approaches is that in the latter, the two terminal nerves, the musculocutaneous and the radial, are blocked above and below the humeral bone, respectively (Figure 28–7). With any multistimulation technique, there is always a risk that an intraneural injection may be made into the already anesthetized nerves. For that reason, theoretically, the midhumeral approach may carry a lower risk of neurologic complications because the nerves are farther apart.

Although the four-injection midhumeral block has been found to be more effective than the double-injection axillary technique,[30] either block results in a high success rate when four injection techniques are used.[24] An advantage of the axillary approach is that incomplete axillary blocks can be supplemented with a midhumeral block.[31] The opposite is not possible, nor is it recommended because electrostimulation may be precluded by blockade distal to the site of nerve localization. An incomplete midhumeral block, on the other hand, can be supplemented at the elbow or the wrist.

Technique

The injection technique for the midhumeral block is similar to the four-injection axillary technique, except the injections are made more distally. In addition, the musculocutaneous and the radial nerves are sought at a deeper location than in the axillary approach (see Figure 28–7). Figure 28–8 demonstrates the spread of the injected local anesthetic in the midhumeral technique.

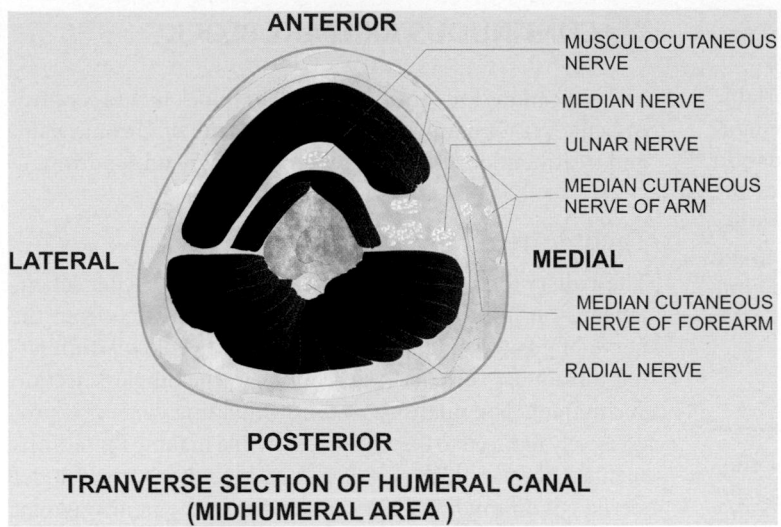

ANTERIOR

MUSCULOCUTANEOUS
NERVE

MEDIAN NERVE

ULNAR NERVE

MEDIAN CUTANEOUS
NERVE OF ARM

LATERAL   MEDIAL

MEDIAN CUTANEOUS
NERVE OF FOREARM

RADIAL NERVE

POSTERIOR

TRANVERSE SECTION OF HUMERAL CANAL
(MIDHUMERAL AREA)

Figure 28–7. Spatial arrangement of the terminal nerves of the brachial plexus at the midhumerus.

- The anesthesiologist's nondominant hand grips the biceps muscle while searching for the musculocutaneous nerve, and the stimulating needle is inserted below the muscle (to avoid direct stimulation).
- When the bone is contacted before eliciting the twitches, the needle is redirected upward, toward the belly of the biceps muscle.

- The triceps muscle is stabilized similarly while attempting stimulation of the radial nerve. It should be kept in mind that the radial nerve winds around the humeral shaft on its way downward, which makes electrolocation of this nerve challenging with distal approaches.

Clinical Pearl

- The technique's name, *midhumeral,* is a misnomer, as the block is typically performed between the upper and middle thirds of the arm.

CHOICE OF LOCAL ANESTHETIC

The choice of LA depends on the length of surgery and the desired density and duration of blockade. For single-injection blocks, short- and medium-acting LAs (prilocaine, 2-chloroprocaine, lidocaine, or mepivacaine) in concentrations of 1.5% to 2% (3% for 2-chloroprocaine), with or without epinephrine or sodium bicarbonate, will provide reliable sensory and motor block of rapid onset (10–20 min) and sufficient duration (3–4 h; 1.5–2 h for 2-chloroprocaine) for most common surgical procedures (wound debridement; closed fracture repositions; ligament-, tendon-, or nerve sutures; finger amputations; etc). For elective procedures of longer duration (arthrodeses, arthroplasties, osteosyntheses, extensive palmar fasciectomies, etc) ropivacaine 0.5–0.75% or bupivacaine 0.375–0.5%, with or without epinephrine, will provide analgesia of slightly slower onset (15–20 min) and longer duration (6–16 h). For specialized hand surgery that may last several hours—for example, multiple joint replacements or reimplantations of severed extremities—a continuous ropivacaine (0.2–0.375%) infusion via an axillary catheter is probably the best technique. Clonidine (0.5 mcg/kg) may be added to intermediate-acting LAs to prolong analgesia after single-shot blocks.[32]

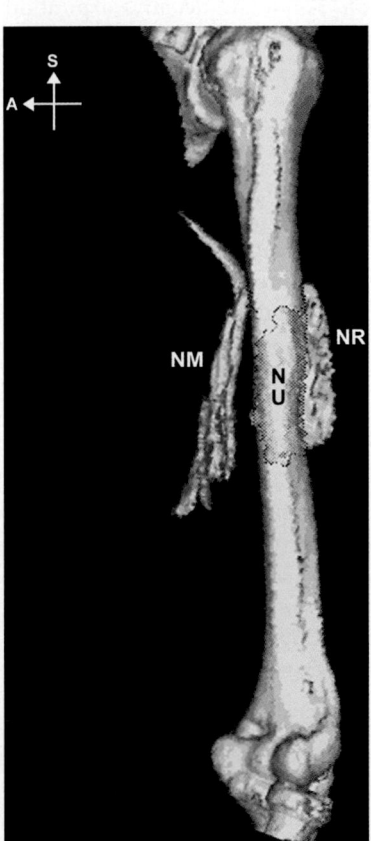

Figure 28–8. Distribution of injectates after midhumeral blockade. NM = nervus medialis, NU = nervus ulnaris, NR = nervus radialis.

PERIOPERATIVE MANAGEMENT

The multiple-nerve stimulation technique is uncomfortable to patients[27,33] and should be preceded by adequate premedication (eg, midazolam + sufentanil).[34] Adequate sedation and analgesia not only improve patients' acceptance of the block but also help relax the arm muscles. This makes precise needle manipulation as well as eliciting and interpreting the motor responses to nerve stimulation significantly easier for the practitioner and more acceptable to patients.

Clinical Pearls

- The first sign of a successful block is weakness of the upper arm muscles, which can be tested immediately after needle withdrawal. This can be done by asking the patient to place the hand on the abdomen or touch the practitioner's finger.

- Loss of coordination signifies that the mantle fascicles of the musculocutaneous and radial nerves, which supply flexors and extensors, are being blocked. Patients typically report an early loss of the position sense in the blocked extremity.

The onset and distribution of analgesia can be tested every 5 or 10 min after block administration in the sensory areas of the terminal nerves (Figure 28–9). Thirty minutes after block insertion, the unblocked nerves can be supplemented distal to the initial block site (eg, elbow blocks).

Clinical Pearls

- Most hand surgery (eg, palmar fasciectomies and nerve or tendon repair) is done on the volar aspect and theoretically can be performed with partial blocks (ie, without the radial or musculocutaneous nerves).

- Surgery on the thumb can also be performed without blocking the ulnar nerve. However, this is not advisable because patients are often very apprehensive about the preserved sensation in the nonanesthetized parts of the hand and demand heavy sedation. In addition, the surgeon may need to extend the operative site, encroaching on the sensory territory of the unblocked nerves. Hence, it is advisable to also ensure forearm, wrist, and hand anesthesia. Alternatively, the surgeon can supplement the block intraoperatively with injection of local anesthetic when necessary.

- For elbow surgery, an infraclavicular approach is a better choice then the axillary block.

- Tourniquet analgesia may be more related to the total injected dose of LA rather than to successful block of the medial cutaneous brachial nerves. Most of the injected LA is absorbed into the surrounding muscles, which are the main source of ischemic pain.[35]

CONTINUOUS AXILLARY BLOCK

The indications for continuous axillary block include control of acute postoperative pain, management of chronic pain, and treatment of vascular disease, (eg, Raynaud syndrome).

Technique

The axillary fossa is best shaved and disinfected. After subcutaneous LA infiltration, the specific muscle twitch from the nerve of greatest interest is elicited by a needle or stimulating introducer cannula (see section on the Single-Injection Technique). The intensity of the stimulating current is progressively reduced to 0.5 mA or less, while making fine adjustments to the cannula's position. A catheter is inserted (under sterile conditions) 5–8 cm cephalad into the neurovascular sheath and either sutured to the skin or tunneled. This helps maintain the catheter in place because the nerves are superficial and the arm sweat makes maintenance of an occlusive dressing difficult.

Clinical Pearl

- Difficulty with catheter insertion usually indicates that the introducer cannula is placed outside the neurovascular sheath. Following negative aspiration, 30–40 mL of LA (eg, ropivacaine 0.5%) is intermittently injected while closely observing the patient.

Maintenance

Diluted solutions of long-acting LAs (eg, 0.125% bupivacaine or 0.2% ropivacaine) are most often used for continuous infusions. Ropivacaine is preferable because of its relative sparing effect on the motor neurons and its lower cardiotoxicity.

Clinical Pearl

- Either electronic or elastomeric pumps may be used. The former are more expensive but allow for repeated adjustments, and they have alarms and data-storage capability. The latter are less expensive, simpler, and disposable, but may lack versatility and accuracy.

Different modes of LA administration may be employed: a continuous basal infusion, repeated boluses, and a combination of both (in which a bolus administration is patient-controlled). The first is limited by the size of pump's reservoir, for example, a 250-mL reservoir at 10 mL/h will last only 1 day. The combination of baseline infusion and boluses offers the advantage of adjusting the level of analgesia to individual needs and puts the patient "in charge" of pain control (which has an important psychological aspect). A typical infusion

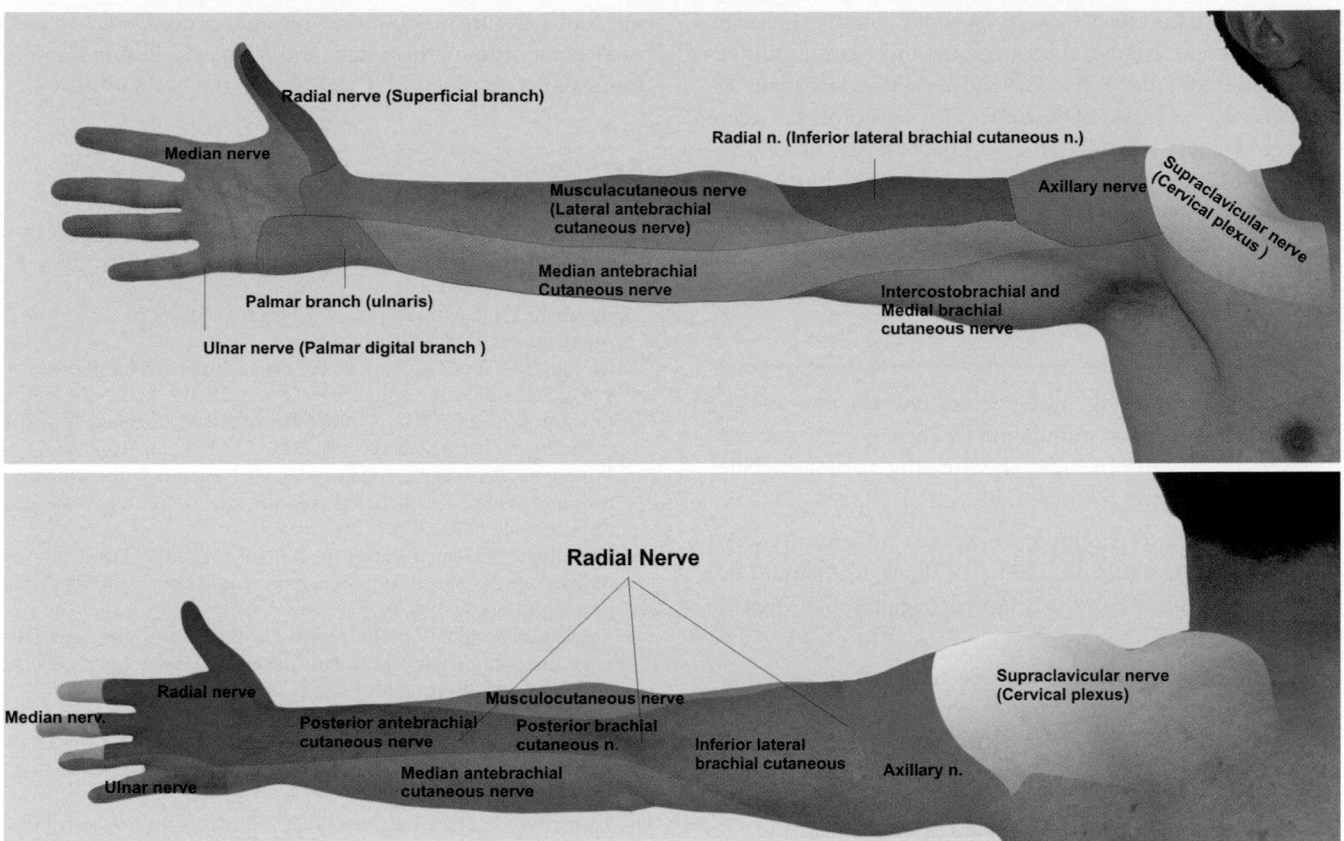

Figure 28–9. Sensory innervation of the upper extremity.

regimen for 0.2% ropivacaine is a basal rate of, for example, 0.1 mL/kg body weight per hour (minimum, 5 mL; maximum, 10 mL) and a 5 mL patient-controlled bolus with a lock-out time of 30 min. Such a regimen may be maintained for 2 to 3 days for the treatment of acute postoperative pain and as long as necessary in the chronic conditions.

Complications of Axillary Blocks
Acute

Vascular Puncture

Vascular puncture is frequent; however, intravascular injection usually can be avoided by repeated careful needle aspiration. However, venous puncture may go undetected when vigorous aspiration collapses the venous lumen.

Intravascular LA Injection

Intravascular LA injection (see earlier discussion) typically presents as lightheadedness and or tachycardia (ropivacaine- or epinephrine-containing solutions). Intraarterial injection produces hand paresthesia during injection, accompanied by sudden paleness, which may last a couple of minutes. Intravascular injection of a large LA dose may lead to loss of consciousness, seizures, and cardiac arrest. Slow injection with repeated needle aspirations is mandatory.

Hematoma

Hematoma may occur after arterial puncture, especially with large-bore blunt needles and in older patients. If the artery is punctured, firm, steady pressure should be applied over the puncture site for 5 to 10 min. For the transarterial technique, needles of smaller gauge should be used to minimize the risk of hematoma.

Toxicity Due to Absorption of LA

Toxicity due to absorption of LA (in contrast to the accidental intravascular injection, which becomes symptomatic during or immediately after the injection) usually becomes symptomatic 5–30 min after injection. The symptoms include lightheadedness, dizziness, tunnel vision, circumoral paresthesia, brady- or tachycardia, anxiousness (eventually progressing to unconsciousness), and seizures. Oxygen, a sedative/hypnotic in repeated, small doses, and airway support if necessary should be immediately administered.

Subacute & Chronic

Nerve Injury

Nerve injury may be caused by the advancing needle, intraneural injection, application of a tourniquet, or a combination of these. Intraneural injections are characterized by pain, extremity withdrawal, and resistance to injection. Needle and injection injuries typically manifest as neurologic deficit in the distribution of the affected nerve. Ischemic damage caused by prolonged application of the tourniquet more commonly results in a diffuse injury, affects several nerves, and is usually accompanied by soreness of the upper arm. Symptoms of nerve damage (sensory loss and persistent paresthesia) usually appear within a day or two after recovery from the block. Most nerve injuries are neurapraxia (functional damage), which carry a good prognosis and heal within a few weeks.

Clinical Pearls

- LA should probably not be injected when a motor response to nerve stimulation is seen with a current strength <0.2 mA (0.1 μsec) because the tip of the needle may be positioned intraneurally.

- When the motor response to nerve stimulation is seen with currents <0.2 mA, the tip of the needle should be slightly withdrawn or repositioned to maintain the twitch with 02 to 0.5 mA.

- LA should never be injected when abnormal resistance (high pressure) to injection is encountered. When this occurs, the needle should be pulled back slightly and the injection reattempted. If the resistance persists, the needle should be completely withdrawn and cleared; it should never be assumed that the cause of the resistance is related only to needle obstruction.

SUMMARY

For axillary brachial plexus block, a triple-injection nerve stimulator technique with electrolocation of median, musculocutaneous, and radial nerves is preferred. This technique is probably the best compromise with regard to block success rate, onset, and simplicity. A double-injection technique is the next best and may be used with or without a nerve stimulator. The midhumeral (a four-injection technique) is probably best suited for supplementing incomplete axillary blocks, although it can be used as a primary technique. For continuous blocks, a catheter should be placed close to the main nerve innervating the surgical site (eg, the median nerve for surgery of medial and volar surfaces; the radial nerve for surgery of lateral and dorsal surfaces). For more extensive surgery involving the entire circumference of the arm (eg, major trauma/amputation), an approach higher in the axilla or infraclavicular block may be better suited. An optimal perineural infusion technique is the basal rate with patient-controlled boluses; the suggested LA for this application is ropivacaine 0.2%. An accidental intravascular injection is the most common complication of axillary block. The risk of systemic toxicity of LA can be decreased by avoiding fast, forceful injection and using frequent aspiration to rule out intravascular injection. Pain, paresthesia, extremity withdrawal or high injection pressure may indicate intraneural needle placement; occurrence of any of these signs and symptoms should prompt immediate cessation of the injection and reevaluation.

References

1. Hall RJ: Hydrochlorate of cocaine. NY Med J 1884;40:643.
2. Hirschel G: Die Anästesierung der Plexus Brachialis bei die Operationen an der oberen Extremität. München Med Wochenschr 1911;58:1555–1556.
3. Burnham PJ: Regional block of the great nerves of the upper arm. Anesthesiology 1958;19:281–284.
4. De Jong RH: Axillary block of the brachial plexus. Anesthesiology 1961;22:215–225.
5. Eriksson E, Skarby HG: A simplified method of axillary brachial plexus block. Nord Med 1962;68:1325.
6. Winnie AP, Radonjic R, Akkineni SR, et al: Factors influencing distribution of local anesthetic injected into the brachial plexus sheath. Anesth Analg 1979;58:225–234.
7. Koscielniak-Nielsen ZJ, Horn A, Rotbøll-Nielsen P: Effect of arm position on the effectiveness of perivascular axillary nerve block. Br J Anaesth 1995;74:387–391.
8. Koscielniak-Nielsen ZJ, Quist Christensen L, Stens-Pedersen HL, et al: Effect of digital pressure on the effectiveness of perivascular axillary block. Br J Anaesth 1995;75:702–706.
9. Yamamoto K, Tsubokawa T, Ohmura S, et al: Effect of arm position on central spread of local anesthetics and on quality of the block with axillary brachial plexus block. Reg Anesth Pain Med 1999;24:36–42.
10. Thompson GE, Rorie DK: Functional anatomy of the brachial plexus sheaths. Anesthesiology 1983;59:117–122.
11. Lassale B, Ang ET: Particularités de l'organisation du tissu celluleux de la cavité axillaire. Bull Soc Anat Paris 1984;9:57–60.
12. Vester-Andersen T, Broby-Johansen U, Bro-Rasmussen F: Perivascular axillary block VI: The distribution of gelatine solutions injected into the axillary neurovascular sheath of cadavers. Acta Anaesthesiol Scand 1986;30:18–22.
13. Partrigde B, Katz J, Benirschke K: Functional anatomy of the brachial plexus sheath: Implications for anesthesia. Anesthesiology 1987;66:743–747.
14. Klaastad O, Smedby O, Thompson GE, et al: Distribution of local anesthetic in axillary brachial plexus block: A clinical and magnetic resonance imaging study. Anesthesiology 2002;96:1315–1324.
15. Vester-Andersen T, Christiansen C, Sørensen M, et al: Perivascular axillary block II: Influence of injected volume of local anaesthetic on neural blockade. Acta Anaesthesiol Scand 1983;27:95–98.
16. Vester-Andersen T, Husum B, Lindeburg T, et al: Perivascular axillary block IV: Blockade following 40, 50, or 60 mL mepivacaine 1% with adrenaline. Acta Anaesthesiol Scand 1984;28:99–105.
17. Urban MK, Urquhart B: Evaluation of brachial plexus anesthesia for upper extremity surgery. Reg Anesth Pain Med 1994;19:175–182.
18. Stan TC, Krantz MA, Solomon DL, et al: The incidence of neurovascular complications following axillary brachial plexus block using a transarterial approach. A prospective study of 1000 consecutive patients. Reg Anesth Pain Med 1995;20:486–492.
19. Baranowski AP, Pither CE: A comparison of three methods of axillary brachial plexus anaesthesia. Anaesthesia 1990;45:362–365.
20. Lavoie J, Martin R, Tétrault JP, et al: Axillary plexus block using a peripheral nerve stimulator: Single or multiple injections. Can J Anaesth 1992;39:583–586.
21. Koscielniak-Nielsen ZJ, Stens-Pedersen HL, Lippert Knudsen F: Readiness for surgery after axillary block: Single or multiple injection techniques. Eur J Anaesthesiol 1997;14:164–171.
22. Koscielniak-Nielsen ZJ, Hesselbjerg L, Fejlberg V: Comparison of transarterial and multiple nerve stimulation techniques for an initial

axillary block by 45 mL of mepivacaine 1% with adrenaline. Acta Anaesthesiol Scand 1998;42:570–575.

23. Sia S, Lepri A, Ponzecchi P: Axillary brachial plexus block using peripheral nerve stimulator: A comparison between double- and triple injection techniques. Reg Anesth Pain Med 2001;26:499–503.

24. Sia S, Lepri A, Campolo MC, et al: Four-injection brachial plexus block using peripheral nerve stimulator: A comparison between axillary and midhumeral approaches. Anesth Analg 2002;95:1075–1079.

25. Handoll HHG, Koscielniak-Nielsen ZJ. Single, double, or multiple injection techniques for axillary brachial plexus block for hand, wrist, or forearm surgery. Cochrane Database Syst Rev.2006 Jan 25(1):CD003842. Review.

26. Dupré LJ: Bloc du plexus brachial au canal huméral. Cah Anesth 1994;42:767–769.

27. Koscielniak-Nielsen ZJ, Rotbøll-Nielsen P, Rasmussen H: Patients' experiences with multiple stimulation axillary block for fast-track ambulatory hand surgery. Acta Anaesthesiol Scand 2002;46:789–793.

28. Sia S, Bartoli M: Selective ulnar nerve localization is not essential for axillary brachial plexus block using a multiple nerve stimulation technique. Reg Anesth Pain Med 2001;26:12–16.

29. Tsui BC, Wagner A, Finucane B: Electrophysiologic effect of injectates on peripheral nerve stimulation. Reg Anesth Pain Med 2004;29:189–193.

30. Bouaziz H, Narchi P, Mercier FJ, et al: The use of selective axillary nerve block for outpatient hand surgery. Anesth Analg 1998;86:746–748.

31. March X, Pardina B, Torres-Bahí S, et al: A comparison of triple-injection axillary brachial plexus block with the humeral approach. Reg Anesth Pain Med 2003;28:504–508.

32. Murphy DB, McCartney CJ, Chan VW: Novel analgesic adjuncts for brachial plexus block: A systematic review. Anesth Analg 2000;90:1122–1128.

33. Koscielniak-Nielsen ZJ, Rasmussen H, Nielsen PT: Patients' perception of pain during axillary and humeral blocks using multiple nerve stimulations. Reg Anesth Pain Med 2004;29:328–332.

34. Kinirons BP, Bouaziz H, Paqueron X, et al: Sedation with sufentanil and midazolam decreases pain in patients undergoing upper limb surgery under multiple nerve block. Anesth Analg 2000;90:1118–1121.

35. Koscielniak-Nielsen ZJ, Rotbøll Nielsen P, Sørensen T, et al: Low dose axillary block by targeted injections of the terminal nerves. Can J Anaesth 1999;46:658–664.

29

Wrist Block

Steven Glickel, MD • Paul Hobeika, MD • Douglas Unis, MD • Jerry D. Vloka, MD

INTRODUCTION

The wrist block is a technique for blocking branches of the ulnar, medial, and radial nerves at the level of the wrist. The wrist block is a basic peripheral nerve block technique that involves anesthesia of the median, ulnar, and radial nerves, as well as the dorsal sensory branch of the ulnar nerve. The wrist block is simple to perform, essentially devoid of systemic complications, and highly effective for a variety of procedures on the hand and fingers. As such, skill in performing a wrist block should be in the armamentarium of every anesthesiologist. Wrist blocks can be used in the outpatient setting and office setting along with the standard operating room setting, resulting in safe, effective, and cost-effective anesthesia that is well accepted by both surgeons and patients.[1–8] Wrist blocks are also useful in the emergency setting to provide anesthesia for repair of hand injuries in the emergency room because there is adequate anesthesia of the hand without motor blockade of the extrinsic hand muscles.[9]

INDICATIONS & CONTRAINDICATIONS

A wrist block is most commonly used for carpal tunnel and hand and finger surgery.[10,11] The most common hand surgery in the United States is carpal tunnel release. Paget described carpal tunnel syndrome in 1853.[1,12] Although Learmonth reported release of the carpal tunnel at the wrist in 1933, it was not until the 1950s that the surgery became popular through the efforts of Phalen.[13–15] Because of the ease of performing

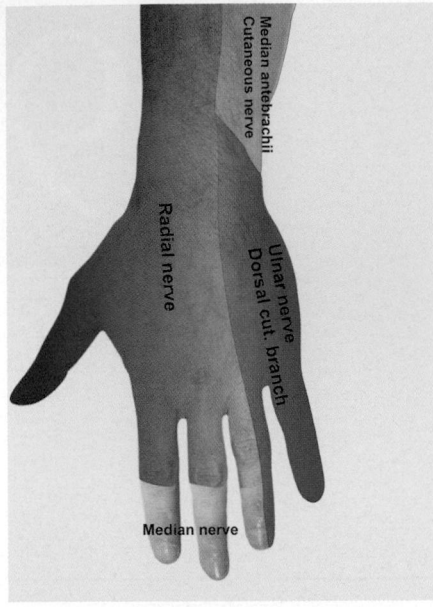
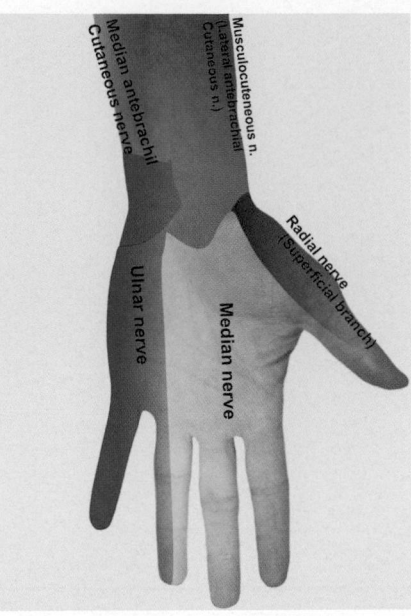

Figure 29–1. Innervation of the hand: Territorial distribution of nerves.

a wrist block, wrist blocks are used in a variety of settings including the emergency room, outpatient surgery centers, and office-based anesthesia practices. Hand surgeons also make use of the wrist block to perform minor procedures in their offices. A wrist block can be used in a patient with a full stomach requiring emergeny surgery, thereby obviating the need for general anesthesia and reducing the risk of aspiration.

The contraindications to wrist blocks are few, but include local infection at the sites of needle insertion, preexisting central or peripheral nervous systems disorders, and allergy to local anesthesia. Patients are usually able to tolerate a tourniquet on the arm without anesthesia for 20 min; a wrist tourniquet can be tolerated for about 120 min.

FUNCTIONAL ANATOMY OF WRIST BLOCK

Innervation of the hand is shared by the ulnar, median, and radial nerves (Figure 29–1). The ulnar nerve innervates more intrinsic muscles than the median nerve, which in turn innervates digital branches to the skin of the medial one and a half digits (Figure 29–2). A corresponding area of the palm is innervated by palmar branches that arise from the ulnar nerve in the forearm. The deep branch of the ulnar nerve accompanies the deep palmar arch and supplies innervation to the three hypothenar muscles, the medial two lumbrical muscles, all the interossei, and the adductor pollicis. The ulnar nerve also innervates the palmaris brevis muscle.

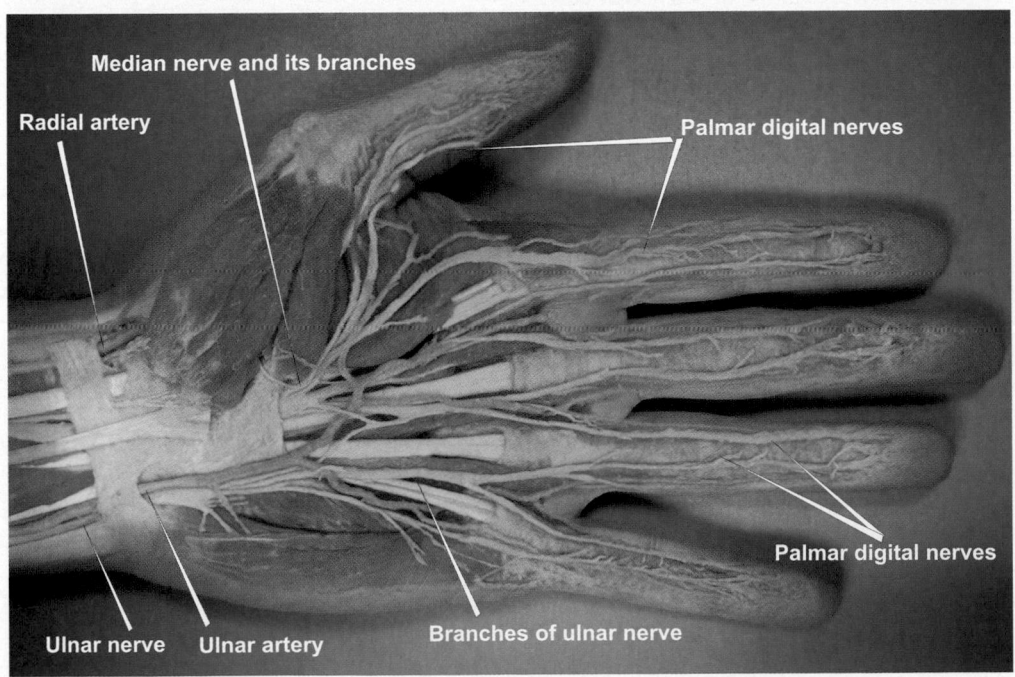

Figure 29–2. Innervation of the hand: The course of the terminal nerves.

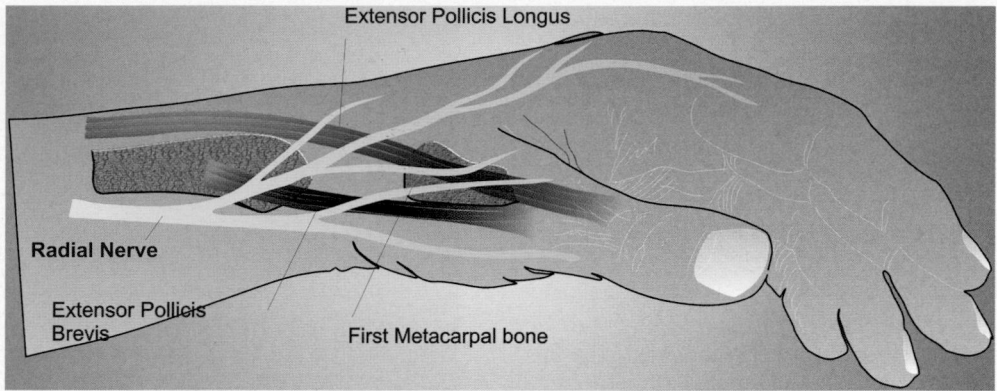

Figure 29–3. Position and course of the radial nerve at the wrist.

The median nerve traverses the carpal tunnel and terminates as digital and recurrent branches. The digital branches innervate the skin of the lateral three and a half digits and, usually, the lateral two lumbrical muscles. A corresponding area of the palm is innervated by palmar branches that arise from the median nerve in the forearm. The recurrent branch of the median nerve supplies the three thenar muscles. In the palm, the digital branches of the ulnar and median nerves lie deep in the superficial palmar arch, but in the fingers, they lie anterior to the digital arteries that arise from the superficial arch. Although the innervation of the ring and middle fingers may vary, the skin on the anterior surface of the thumb is always supplied by the median nerve and that of the little finger by the ulnar nerve. The palmar digital branches of the median and ulnar nerves also innervate the nail beds of their respective digits.

The radial nerve passes along the front of the radial side of the forearm. It arises first from the lateral side of the radial artery and beneath the supinator muscle. About 3 inches above the wrist, it leaves the artery, pierces the deep fascia, and divides into two branches (Figure 29–3). The superficial branch, the smaller of the two branches, supplies the skin of the radial side and base of the thumb, and joins the anterior branch of the musculocutaneous nerve. The deep branch of the radial nerve communicates with the posterior branch of the musculocutaneous nerve. On the dorsum of the hand, the deep branch of the radial nerve forms an arch with the dorsal cutaneous branch of the ulnar nerve.

ANATOMIC LANDMARKS

The superficial branch of the *radial nerve* runs along the medial aspect of the brachioradialis muscle (see Figure 29–3). It then passes between the tendon of the brachioradialis and radius to pierce the fascia on the dorsal aspect. Just above the styloid process of the radius (circle), it gives off digital branches for the dorsal skin of the thumb, index finger, and lateral half of the middle finger. Several of its branches pass superficially over the anatomic "snuff box."

The *median nerve* is located between the tendons of the palmaris longus and the flexor carpi radialis (see Figures 29–2 and 29–4). The palmaris longus tendon is usually the more

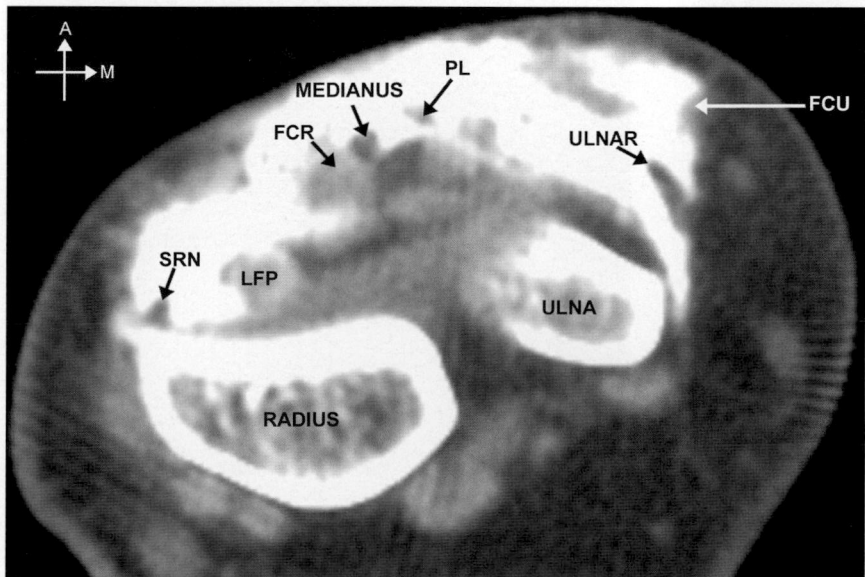

Figure 29–4. Cross-sectional anatomy of the wrist as shown on an MRI scan just above the carpal tunnel. A = anterior, FCR = flexor carpi radialis, FCU = tendon of the flexor carpi ulnaris, FPL = tendon of the flexor palmaris longus, M = medial, PL = tendon of the palmaris longus, SRN = superficial radial nerve.

prominent of the two tendons, and the median nerve passes just lateral to it.

The *ulnar nerve* passes between the ulnar artery and tendon of the flexor carpi ulnaris (see Figures 29–2 and 29–4. The tendon of the flexor carpi ulnaris is superficial to the ulnar nerve.

EQUIPMENT

A standard regional anesthesia tray is prepared with the following equipment:

- Sterile towels and 4 × 4-in. gauze pads
- 10-mL syringes with local anesthetic (LA)
- One 1½-in., 25-gauge needle

TECHNIQUE

The patient is in the supine position with the arm abducted. The wrist should be kept in a slight dorsiflexion.

Block of the Radial Nerve

The radial nerve is essentially a "field block" and requires a more extensive infiltration because of its less predictable anatomic location and division into multiple, smaller cutaneous branches. Five milliliters of LA is injected subcutaneously just above the radial styloid while advancing the needle medially (Figure 29–5). The infiltration is then extended laterally, using an additional 5 mL of LA.

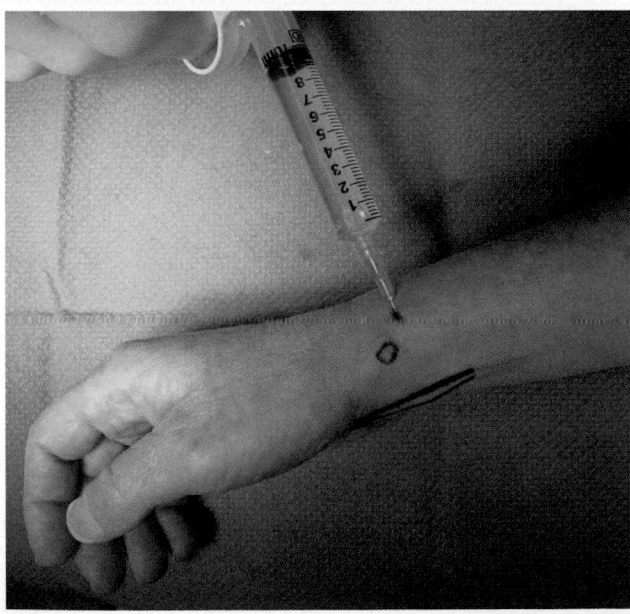

Figure 29–5. Block of the radial nerve above the head of the radius.

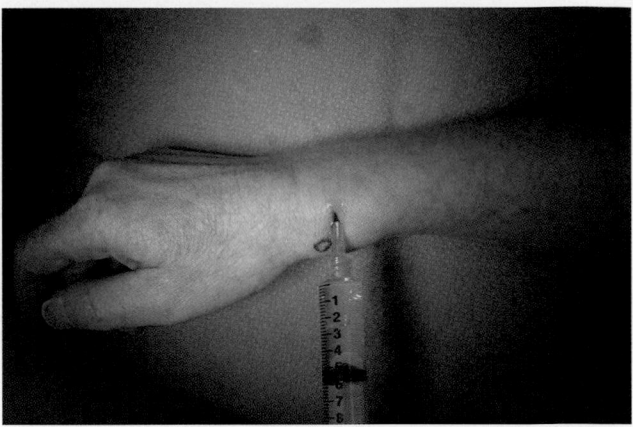

Figure 29–6. Block of the superficial radial nerve.

Block of the Dorsal Sensory Branch of the Radial Nerve

The dorsal sensory branch of the radial nerve is blocked by inserting the needle 1 cm proximal to the radial styloid, which is radial to the radial artery (Figure 29–6). This branch of the radial nerve exits from between the brachioradialis and extensor carpi radialis longus 5 to 8 cm proximal to the radial styloid. The needle is advanced to Lister's tubercle, and if there are no paresthesias, 5 mL of LA is injected subcutaneously throughout this area.

Block of the Ulnar Nerve

The ulnar nerve is anesthetized by inserting the needle under the tendon of the flexor carpi ulnaris muscle close to its distal attachment just above the styloid process of the ulna (Figures 29–4, 29–7 and 29–8). The needle is advanced 5 to 10 mm to just past the tendon of the flexor carpi ulnaris. Three to 5 mL of LA solution is injected. A subcutaneous injection of 2 to 3 mL of local anesthesia just above the tendon of the flexor carpi

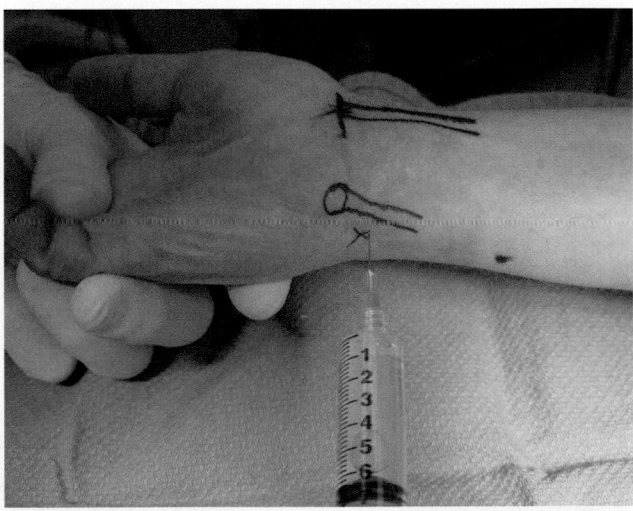

Figure 29–7. Block of the ulnar nerve. The needle is shown inserted just medial to the flexor carpi ulnaris.

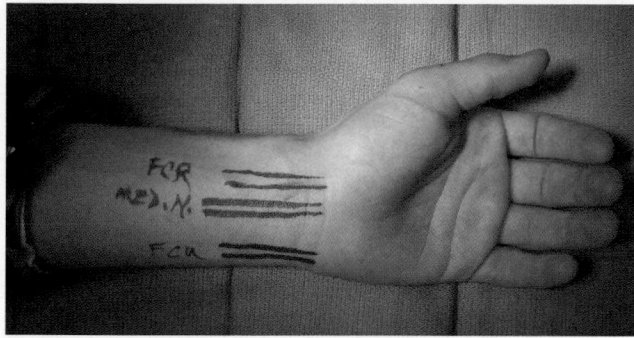

Figure 29–8. Tendons of the wrist flexors and position of the medianus nerve in relationship to the flexor tendons. FCR = flexor carpi radialis, FCU = flexor carpi ulnaris, Med. N = medianus nerve.

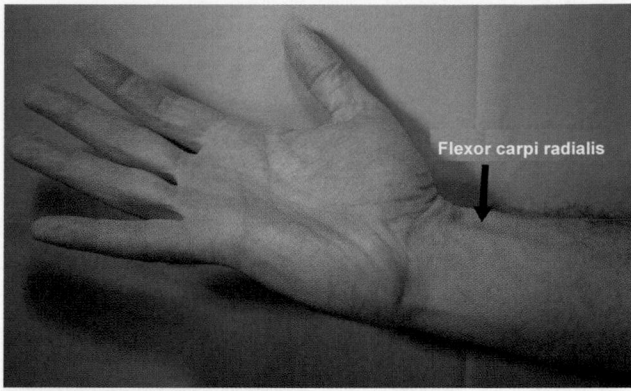

Figure 29–10. A maneuver to accentuate the tendon of the flexor carpi radialis.

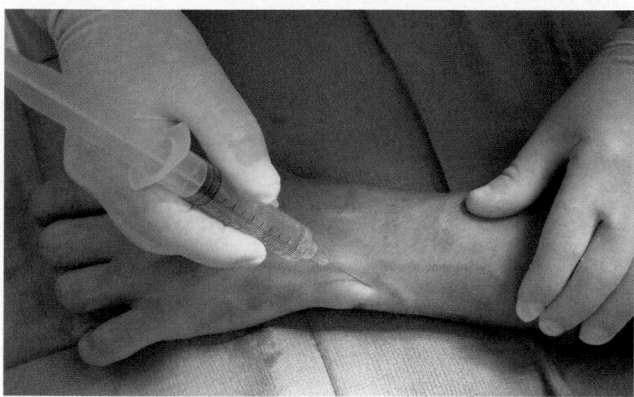

Figure 29–9. Block of the superficial branch of the ulnar nerve.

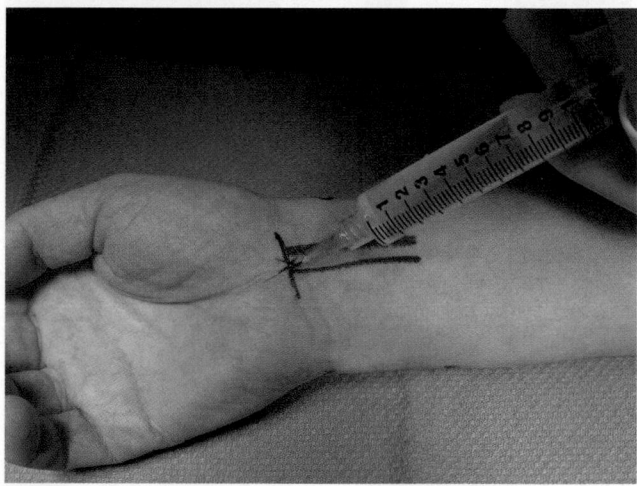

Figure 29–11. Block of the medianus nerve at the wrist. The needle is shown inserted just medial to the flexor carpi radialis.

ulnaris is also advisable in blocking the cutaneous branches of the ulnar nerve, which often extend to the hypothenar area.

Block of the Dorsal Sensory Branch of the Ulnar Nerve

The dorsal sensory branch of the ulnar nerve is blocked by inserting the needle at the level of the ulnar styloid because it travels from palmar to dorsal in the area of the ulnar styloid (Figure 29–9). Start the injection at the flexor carpi ulnaris and extend subcutaneously dorsally toward the distal radioulnar joint. Five mL of LA is injected subcutaneously throughout the area.

Block of the Median Nerve

The median nerve is anesthetized by inserting the needle between the tendons of the palmaris longus and flexor carpi radialis (Figures 29–8, 29–10 and 29–11). The needle is inserted until it pierces the deep fascia. Three to 5 mL of LA is injected. Although the piercing of the deep fascia has been described to result in a fascial "click," it is more reliable to simply insert the needle until it contacts the bone. At that point, the needle is withdrawn 2 to 3 mm and the LA is injected. Figure 29–12 demonstrates the spread of the LA after injection of 5 mL using the described technique.

Clinical Pearls

- A "fan" technique is recommended to increase the success rate of the median nerve block.
- After the initial injection, the needle is withdrawn back to the skin level, redirected 30 degrees laterally, and advanced again to contact the bone.
- After pulling back 1 to 2 mm off the bone, an additional 2 mL of LA is injected.
- A similar procedure is repeated with a medial redirection of the needle.

Nerve Stimulation Technique

Median and ulnar nerves can also be blocked at the wrist using a nerve stimulator. These blocks may be used for finger flexor tendon repairs, when the surgeon wishes to test their function intraoperatively (function of the forearm muscles

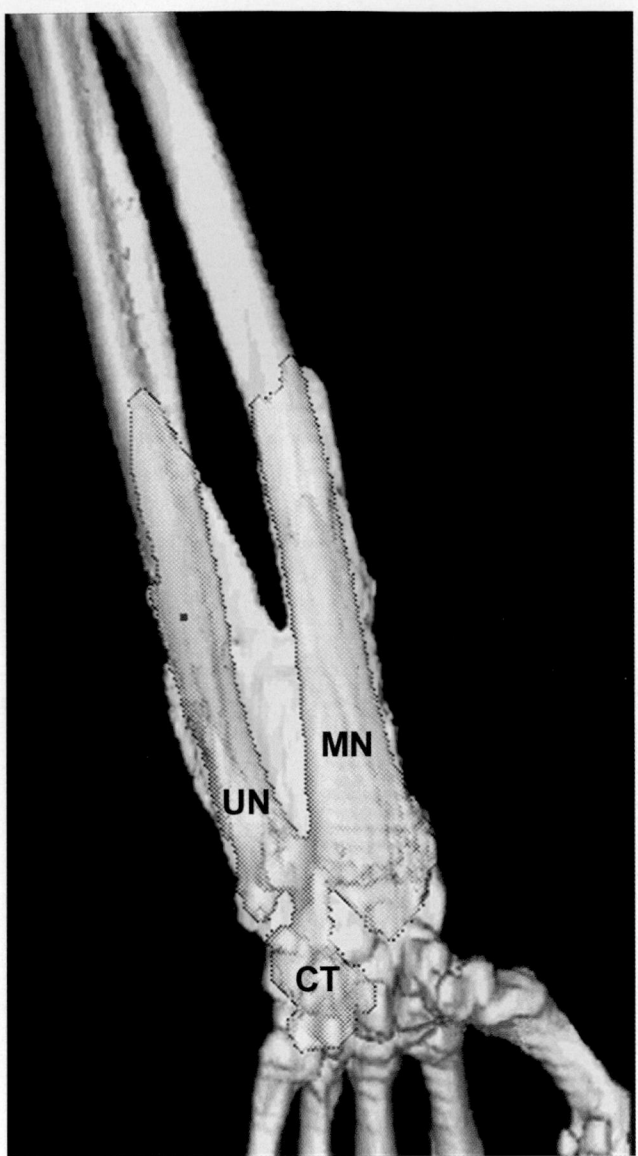

Figure 29–12. Distribution of the injectate, after wrist block. CT = carpal tunnel, MN = medianus nervus, UN = ulnaris nervus.

is not affected). The median nerve is found in the carpal tunnel between the palmaris longus and the flexor carpi radialis tendons, and the ulnar nerve is found between the flexor carpi ulnaris and the ulnar artery. Twitches are similar to elbow blocks except for the forearm pronation, which is missing. Two to 3 mL of LA is sufficient to block either nerve.

Clinical Pearl

- Both nerves lie quite superficially in tight compartments and cannot move readily away from the needle. Extra caution should therefore be used when advancing the needle and injecting LA.

Table 29–1.

Onset Times and Duration for Commonly Used Local Anesthetic Mixtures

	Onset (min)	Anesthesia (h)	Analgesia (h)
1.5% Mepivacaine (+ HCO$_3^-$)	15–20	2–3	3–5
2% Lidocaine (+ HCO$_3^-$)	10–20	2–5	3–8
0.5% Ropivacaine	15–30	4–8	5–12
0.75% Ropivacaine	10–15	5–10	6–24
0.5% Bupivacaine (or L-bupivacaine)	15–30	5–15	6–30

CHOICE OF LOCAL ANESTHETIC

The choice of the type and concentration of LA for wrist blockade is based on the desired duration. Lidocaine is the most used anesthetic for wrist block, but bupivacaine or ropivacaine can be used safely, also.[16] Table 29–1 provides onset times and duration for some commonly used LAs mixtures.

BLOCK DYNAMICS & PERIOPERATIVE MANAGEMENT

Wrist block is associated with moderate patient discomfort because multiple insertions and subcutaneous injections are required. Appropriate sedation and analgesia, midazolam (2–4 mg) and alfentanil (250–500 mcg), are required to ensure the patient's comfort. A typical onset time for a wrist block is 5 to 15 min, depending primarily on the concentration and volume of LA used. Sensory anesthesia of the skin develops faster than the motor block. Placement of an Esmarch latex-free bandage or a tourniquet at the level of the wrist is well tolerated and does not require additional blockade.

COMPLICATIONS & HOW TO AVOID THEM

Complications after wrist block are typically limited to residual paresthesias due to an inadvertent intraneural injection. Systemic toxicity is rare because of the distal location of the blockade and relatively small volumes (doses) of local anesthetic NMR required (Table 29–2).

Table 29–2.

Complications from Wrist Block

Infection	This should be very rare with the use of an aseptic technique.
Hematoma	Avoid multiple needle insertions for superficial blocks. Most superficial blocks can be accomplished with one or two needle insertions. Use 25-gauge needle and avoid puncturing superficial veins.
Vascular complications	Do not use epinephrine with wrist and finger blocks.
Nerve injury	Do not inject when the patient complains of pain or high pressure on injection is detected. Do not reinject the medianus and ulnaris nerves.
Other	Instruct the patient on the care of the insensate extremity.

References

1. Derkash RS, Weaver JK, Berkeley ME, et al: Office carpal tunnel release with wrist block and wrist tourniquet. Orthopedics 1996;19:589–590.
2. Gebhard RE, Al-Samsam T, Greger J, et al: Distal nerve blocks at the wrist for outpatient carpal tunnel surgery offer intraoperative cardiovascular stability and reduce discharge time. Anesth Analg 2002;95:351–355.
3. Martinotti R, Berlanda P, Zanlungo M, et al: Peripheral anesthesia techniques in surgery of the arm. Minerva Chir 1999;54:831–833.
4. Melone CP Jr, Isani A: Anesthesia for hand injuries. Emerg Med Clin North Am 1985;3:235–243.
5. Leversee JH, Bergman JJ: Wrist and digital nerve blocks. J Fam Pract 1981;13:415–421.
6. Dushoff IM: Hand surgery under wrist block and local infiltration anesthesia, using an upper arm tourniquet. Plast Reconstr Surg 1973;51:685–686.
7. Vatashsky E, Aronson HB, Wexler MR, et al: Anesthesia in a hand surgery unit. J Hand Surg [Am] 1980;5:495–497.
8. Klezl Z, Krejca M, Simcik J: Role of sensory innervation variations for wrist block anesthesia. Arch Med Res 2001;32:155–158.
9. Ferrera PC, Chandler R: Anesthesia in the emergency setting: Part I. Hand and foot injuries. Am Fam Physician 1994;50:569–573.
10. Delaunay L, Chelly JE: Blocks at the wrist provide effective anesthesia for carpal tunnel release. Can J Anaesth 2001;48:656–660.
11. Dupont C, Ciaburro H, Prevost Y, et al: Hand surgery under wrist block and local infiltration anesthesia, using an upper arm tourniquet. Plast Reconstr Surg 1972;50:532–533.
12. Paget J: *Lectures on Surgical Pathology.* Longman, Brown, Green, Langman, 1853.
13. Learmonth JR: The principle of decompression in the treatment of certain diseases of peripheral nerves. Surg Clin North Am 1933;13:905–913.
14. Dellon AL, Amadio PC: James R. Learmonth: The first peripheral nerve surgeon. J Reconstr Microsurg 2000;16:213–217.
15. Phalen GS: Spontaneous compression of the median nerve at the wrist. J Am Med Assoc 1951;145:1128–1133.
16. Nystrom A, Lindstrom G, Reiz S, et al: Bupivacaine: A safe local anesthetic for wrist blocks. J Hand Surg [Am] 1989;14:495–498.

30

Digital Block

Tagashige Iwata, MD • Louis Catalano, MD • Jerry D. Vloka, MD

INTRODUCTION

Strauss[1] provided the first description of the digital block in 1889 for the condition of an ingrown toenail, using 20% cocaine at the base and under the nail. In 1905, Braun reported the synergistic advantage of adding epinephrine to local anesthetics.[2,3] However, the use of epinephrine in digital block anesthesia has been avoided due to the theoretical risk of ischemia and possible gangrene. More recently, however, Wilhelmi and colleagues[4] demonstrated the safety and efficacy of epinephrine-containing local anesthetic for digital block, which made its use only more controversial. Digital block is one of the most common nerve block techniques, frequently used in the emergency department and primary care settings for various procedures such as lacerations of the finger or toe, nail removal, nail bed repair, paronychia drainage, removal of foreign bodies, and any other painful procedures on digits.

In 1990, approximately a century after the first publication of traditional digital block, Chiu[5] described a technique of digital block that produced complete finger anesthesia with a single injection into the flexor tendon sheath at the level of the distal palmar crease. In anatomic studies he showed that after injection of methylene blue into the flexor tendon sheath there was "complete staining of the entire flexor tendon sheath and centrifugal diffusion of the blue dye circumscribing the entire circumference of the proximal phalanx" (see section on Transthecal Digital Block). The advantages of this technique are (1) rapid onset of action, (2) only a small volume of anesthetic solution required, (3) only a single injection required, and (4) absence of risk of direct trauma to the neurovascular bundles.[6-8] Although Chevaleraud and coworkers[9] did not accomplish anesthesia of the dorsum of the finger in all cases, some authors consider the transthecal method to be as effective as a traditional digital nerve block.[10] Others have found that it results in anesthesia comparable to the newer single-injection subcutaneous digital blocks,[11] both in experimental and clinical situations.[12,13] Transthecal anesthesia appears to be safe and effective without a risk of any long-term damage to the tendon sheath.

A digital block is the technique of blocking the nerves of the digits to achieve anesthesia of the finger(s). This technique is simple to perform and essentially devoid of systemic complications. It is a commonly used and effective method of anesthesia for a wide variety of minor surgical procedures on the digits. As such, this block should be in the armamentarium of every anesthesiologist. Several different techniques of digital block and their modifications are available; in this chapter, we chose to describe the one that is most commonly used in our institution.

REGIONAL ANESTHESIA ANATOMY

The common digital nerves are branches of the median and ulnar nerves, which divide in the distal palm into the volar aspect, tip, and nail bed area (Figure 30–1). The main digital nerves, accompanied by digital vessels, run on the ventrolateral aspect of the finger immediately lateral to the flexor tendon sheath (Figure 30–2). Small dorsal digital nerves run on the dorsolateral aspect of the finger and supply innervation to the back of the fingers as far as the proximal joint.

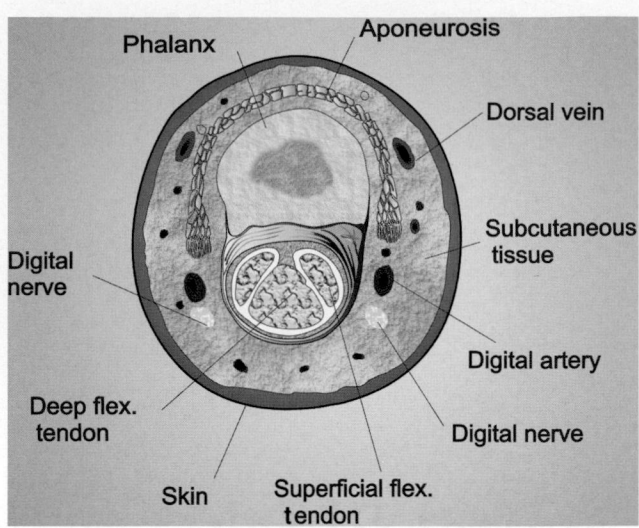

Figure 30–2. Cross-sectional view of the anatomy of the phalanx.

EQUIPMENT

A standard regional anesthesia tray is prepared with the following equipment:

- Sterile towels and 4-in. × 4-in. gauze pads
- A controlled, 10-mL syringe with local anesthetic
- One 1½-in., 25-gauge needle

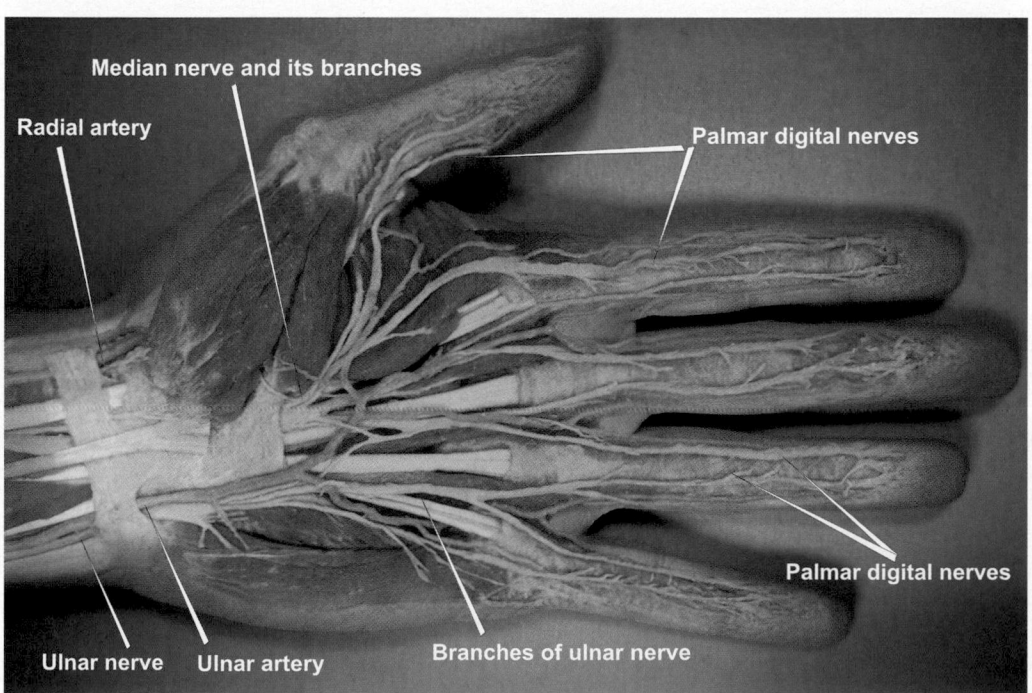

Figure 30–1. The origin and distribution of the digital nerves.

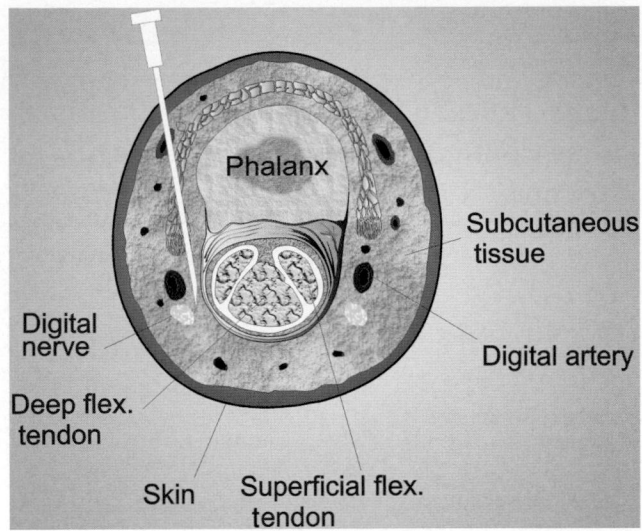

Figure 30–3. Angle and depth of needle insertion.

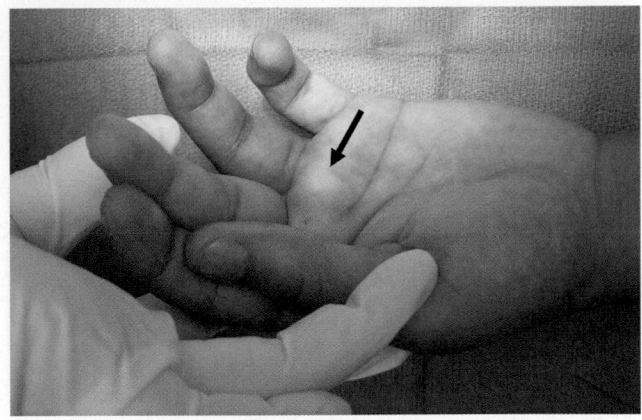

Figure 30–5. Advancement of the needle is stopped when the needle tip causes a skin bulge on the palmar side.

▮ TECHNIQUE

Block of Volar & Dorsal Digital Nerves at the Base of the Finger

A 25-gauge, 1½-in. needle is inserted at a point on the dorsolateral aspect of the base of the finger, and a small skin wheal is raised. The needle is then directed anteriorly toward the base of the phalanx (Figures 30–3 and 30–4). The needle is advanced adjacent to the phalanx, while the operator observes for any protrusion from the palmar dermis directly opposite the needle path (Figure 30–5). Two to three milliliters of solution is injected. An additional 1 mL is injected continuously as the needle is withdrawn back to the skin. The same procedure is repeated on each side of the base of the finger to achieve anesthesia of the entire finger (Figure 30–6).

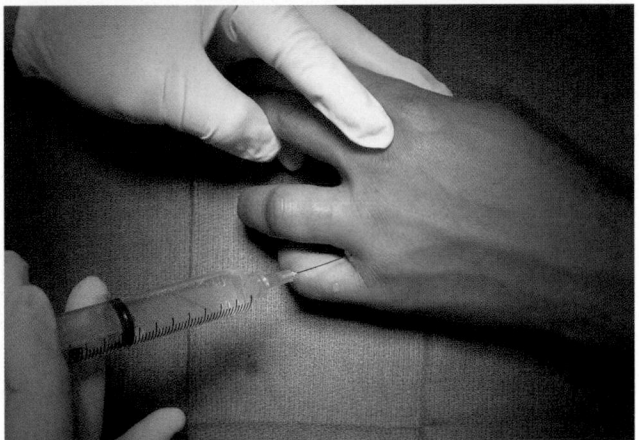

Figure 30–6. The identical procedure is repeated on the radial side of the proximal phalanx to block the ulnar branch of the digital nerve.

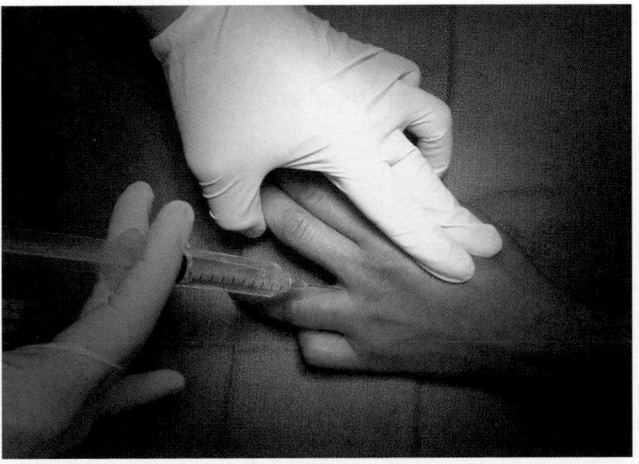

Figure 30–4. The needle is shown inserted at the base of the proximal phalanx to block the medial digital nerve.

Transthecal Digital Block

The transthecal digital block is placed by using the flexor tendon sheath for local anesthetic injection. In this technique, the patient's hand is supinated and the flexor tendon is located. Using a 25- to 27-gauge, 1-in. needle, 2–3 mL of local anesthetic is injected into the flexor tendon sheath at the level of the distal palmar crease (Figure 30–7). The needle should puncture the skin at a 45-degree angle. Resistance to the injection suggests that the needle tip is against the flexor tendon. Careful withdrawal of the needle results in the free flow of medication as the potential space between tendon and sheath is entered. Proximal pressure is applied to the volar surface during injection to promote diffusion of the medication within the synovial sheath.

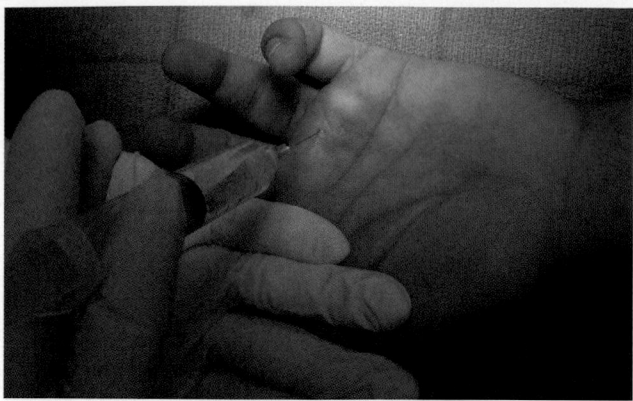

Figure 30–7. Transthecal digital block. The needle is placed into the flexor tendon sheath. To confirm the correct needle placement in the tendon sheath, the needle can be placed without the syringe, in which case the operator flexes and extends the finger. This should result in a free and substantial swinging of the needle as the tendon moves with this maneuver.

Table 30–1.

Onset Times and Duration of Anesthesia for Some Commonly Used Local Anesthetics Mixtures

	Onset (min)	Anesthesia (h)	Analgesia (h)
1.5% Mepivacaine (+ HCO_3^-)	15–20	2–3	3–5
2% Lidocame (+ HCO_3^-)	10–20	2–5	3–8
0.5% Ropivacaine	15–30	4–8	5–12
0.75% Ropivacaine	10–15	5–10	6–24
0.5% Bupivacaine (or L-bupivacaine)	15–30	5–15	6–30

Clinical Pearls

- The advantage of this approach is the provision of anesthesia to the entire digit with a single injection and a reportedly higher success rate.
- For more extensive surgery on the finger, it may be advantageous to combine both approaches discussed in this chapter for a greater success rate and more extensive distribution of anesthesia.

BLOCK DYNAMICS & PERIOPERATIVE MANAGEMENT

A skin wheal at the point of needle insertion significantly reduces the discomfort during the placement of the block. A digital block requires a small dose of a sedative or a narcotic during placement. Typical onset time for this block is approximately 5 min, depending on the concentration and volume of local anesthetic used.

Table 30–2.

Complications of Digital Blocks

Infection	This should be very rare with use of an aseptic technique.
Hematoma	Avoid multiple needle insertions. Use 25-gauge needle (or smaller) and avoid puncturing superficial veins.
Other	Instruct the patient on the care of the insensate finger.
Gangrene of the digit(s)	The use of epinephrine-containing solutions for this block is avoided by many; the safety of its use is controversial. Limit the injection volume to 3 mL on each side. The mechanical pressure effects of injecting solution into a potentially confined space should always be borne in mind, particularly in blocks at the base of the digit. In patients with small-vessel disease, perhaps an alternative method should be sought in addition to avoidance of digital tourniquet.
Nerve injury	Residual paresthesias are rare and may be due to an inadvertent intraneuronal injection. Systemic toxicity is rare because of the distal location of the blockade. Do not inject when the patient complains of pain or when high resistance to injection is encountered.

CHOICE OF LOCAL ANESTHETIC

The choice of the type and concentration of local anesthetic for a digital block is based on the desired duration of blockade (Table 30–1).

COMPLICATIONS & HOW TO AVOID THEM

One specific complication of digital blocks is vascular insufficiency and gangrene. This catastrophe is a result of digital artery occlusion, together with collateral circulation insufficiency. A series of causative factors is often involved to produce this rare, but serious complication (Table 30–2).

References

1. Strauss L: Über Gangran nach Lokalanasthesie. (Inaugural Dissertation.). Berlin, G. Schade, 1910.
2. Braun H: Zur Anwendung des Adrenalins bei anaethesierenden Gewebsinjektionen. Zentralbl Chir 1903;30:1025.
3. Geddes IC: A review of local anesthetics. Br J Anaesth 1954;26:208.
4. Wilhelmi BJ, Blackwell SJ, Miller JH, et al: Do not use epinephrine in digital blocks: Myth or truth? Plast Reconstr Surg 2001;107:393.
5. Chiu DTW: Transthecal digital block: Flexor tendon sheath used for anesthetic infusion. J Hand Surg 1990;15:471–473.
6. Morrison WG: Transthecal digital block. Arch Emerg Med 1993;10:35–38.
7. Morros C, Perez D, Raurell A, et al: Digital anaesthesia through the flexor tendon sheath at the palmar level. Int Orthop 1994;17:273–274.
8. Ramamurathy S Hickey, R: Anestheisa. In Green D (ed): Operative Hand Surgery, 3rd ed. Churchill Livingstone, 1993, p 41.
9. Chevaleraud E, Ragot JM, Brunelle E, et al: Anesthesie locale digitale par la gains des flechisseurs. [Local anaesthesia of the finger using the flexor tendon sheath.] Ann Fr Anesth Reanim 1993;12:237–240.
10. Hill RG , Patterson JW, Parker JC, et al: Comparison of transthecal digital block and traditional digital block for anesthesia of the finger. Ann Emerg Med 1995;25:604–607.
11. Whetzel TP, Mabourakh S, Barkhorder R: Modified transthecal digital block. J Hand Surg 1997;22A:361–363.
12. Low CK, Vartany A, Engstrom JW, et al: Comparison of transthecal and subcutaneous single-injection digital block techniques. J Hand Surg 1997a;22A:901–905.
13. Low CK, Wong HP, Low YP: Comparison between single injection transthecal and subcutaneous digital blocks. J Hand Surg 1997b;22B:582–584.

31

Cutaneous Blocks for the Upper Extremity

Joseph M. Neal, MD

INTRODUCTION

Although most upper extremity regional anesthesia is accomplished by means of various approaches to the brachial plexus, there are occasions when individual terminal nerves or their branches are blocked selectively. There are generally three instances in which the anesthesiologist desires to perform these selective nerve blocks. First, some surgical sites are partially innervated by sensory nerves that are not part of the brachial plexus or not consistently anesthetized with plexus blocks. This chapter describes how and when to anesthetize the most common of these nerves—the supraclavicular, the suprascapular, and the intercostobrachial. The second indication is when blocking the entire brachial plexus block is

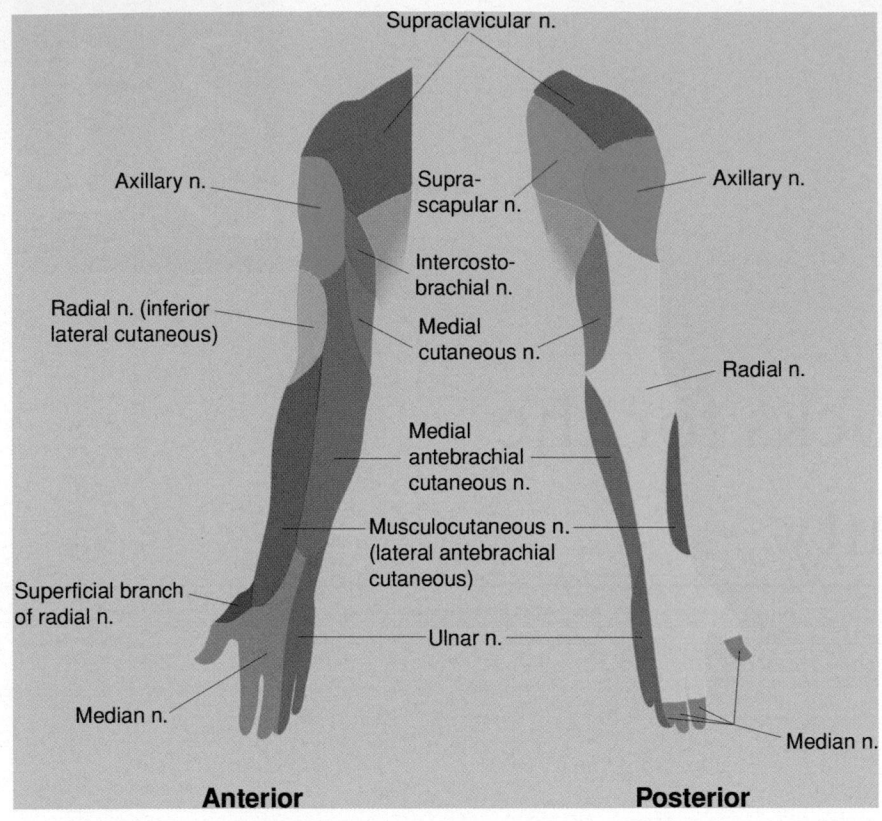

Figure 31–1. Cutaneous innervation of the upper extremity. Actual patients demonstrate large variation in the depicted pattern of innervation and have significant crossover between nerves.

not necessary for the planned procedure. In this case, selective upper extremity cutaneous anesthesia or analgesia may involve blocking terminal nerves (radial, median, or ulnar nerves) or their branches (lateral and medial antebrachial cutaneous nerves) distally at the elbow. A final and controversial indication for selective upper extremity nerve blocks is their use as a supplement to an incomplete brachial plexus block.

This chapter discusses individual nerve blocks as a means of furthering the reader's understanding of the indications and contraindications for selective upper extremity regional anesthesia. When considering the application of these various blocks, the reader is reminded that innervation of the upper extremity is often variable and overlapping.[1] Therefore, when faced with the choice of performing a single nerve block versus blocking several adjacent nerves, it is advisable to err on the side of multiple blocks, particularly in those adjacent cutaneous areas that represent potential crossover innervation (Figures 31–1 and 31–2). The relevant anatomy will be covered with specific nerve block description.

Local Anesthetic & Adjuvant Selection

Local anesthetics for individual upper extremity nerve blocks are selected for their desired duration of anesthesia and/or analgesia. If intermediate-acting local anesthetics are selected (lidocaine or mepivacaine), duration can be increased with either adjuvant epinephrine (2.5 mcg/mL) or clonidine

(0.5 mcg/kg). Neither adjuvant significantly increases duration when a long-acting local anesthetic such as bupivacaine or ropivacaine is chosen.[1]

SUPRACLAVICULAR NERVE BLOCK

Indications

The supraclavicular nerve provides sensory innervation to the "cape" of the shoulder (Figure 31–3). Commonly anesthetized as a component of cervical plexus block for carotid surgery, the supraclavicular nerve may also require blockade for surgery involving the shoulder or supraclavicular area. Local anesthetic spread in an interscalene approach to brachial plexus block is often adequate to block the supraclavicular nerve, but the nerve is frequently not anesthetized with a supraclavicular brachial plexus block. Particularly in patients undergoing supraclavicular or incomplete interscalene brachial plexus anesthesia without concomitant general anesthesia, the supraclavicular nerve can be blocked to accomplish more complete anesthesia for shoulder surgery.

Anatomy

The supraclavicular nerve is derived from the ventral rami of the third and fourth cervical nerve roots (C3-C4); it is thus separate from the brachial plexus. The nerve becomes

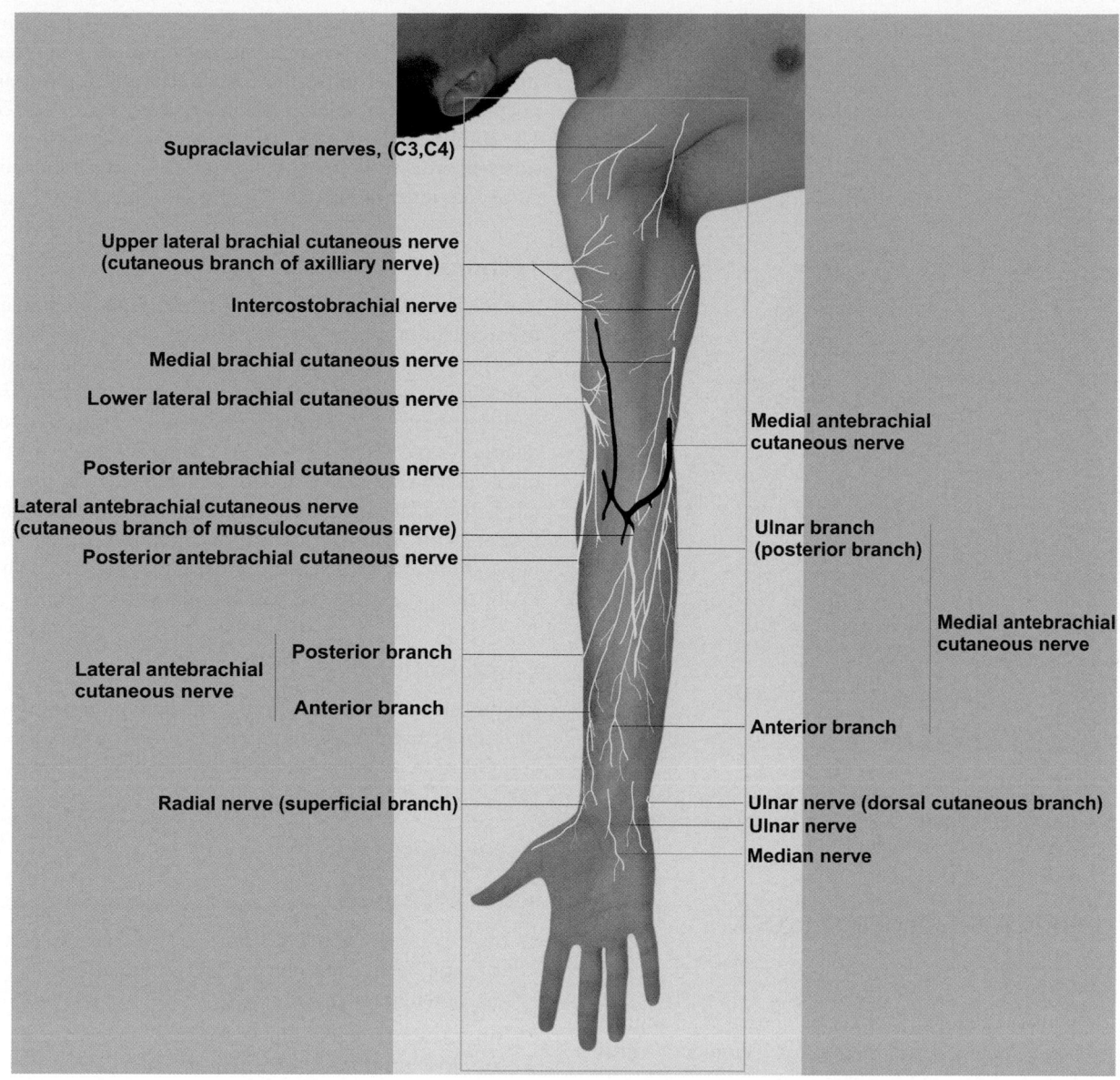

Figure 31–2. Idealized distribution of the cutaneous innervation of the upper arm and forearm.

superficial as it penetrates the mid-belly of the sternocleidomastoid muscle, thereafter forming three branches (Figure 31–3). These branches provide sensory innervation to the cape area, which spans from the midline to the deltoids, and from the second rib anteriorly to the top of the scapula posteriorly.

Technique

Blockade of the supraclavicular nerve is accomplished with 10 mL of an intermediate or long-acting local anesthetic, depending on analgesic requirements. Three milliliters are deposited with a 22- to 25-gauge sharp needle into the mid-belly of the sternocleidomastoid muscle. The remaining volume of local anesthetic is then injected subcutaneously in a cephalad

and caudad direction along the posterior border of the sternocleidomastoid (Figure 31–4).

Complications

Complications of the supraclavicular nerve block are minimal provided that aseptic technique is used and local anesthetic injection remains superficial. The external jugular vein should be avoided to prevent hematoma.

Clinical Pearl

- The supraclavicular nerve block should be used as a supplement to supraclavicular brachial plexus block for patients undergoing shoulder surgery.

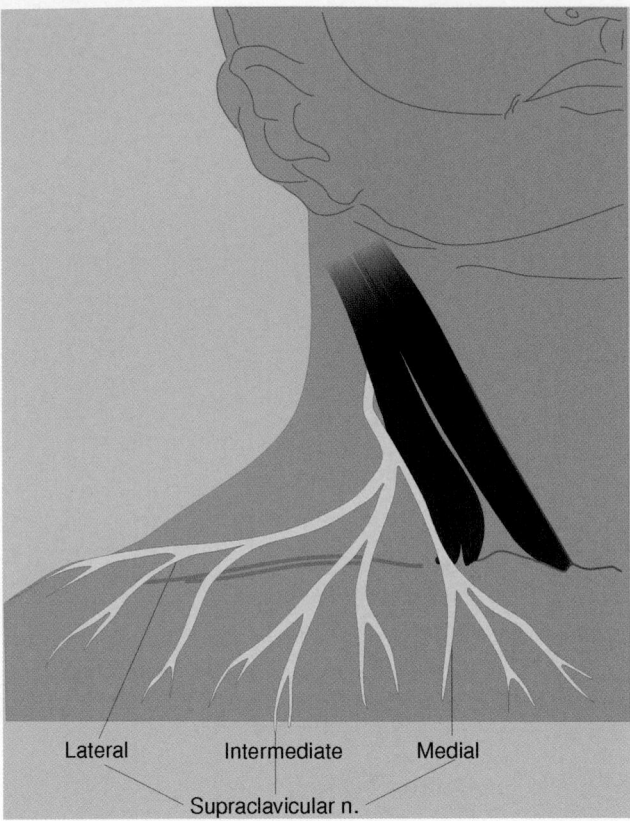

Figure 31–3. Supraclavicular nerve. This nerve is derived from C3-C4 nerve roots, is not part of the brachial plexus, and provides sensory innervation of the shoulder "cape."

SUPRASCAPULAR NERVE BLOCK

Indications

Suprascapular nerve block (SSNB) can be used as an adjunct to arthroscopic shoulder surgery and total shoulder arthroplasty. When combined with general anesthesia for shoulder arthroscopy, SSNB improves analgesia, reduces opioid-related side effects, and hastens hospital discharge,[2] although SSNB is not superior to interscalene block in this setting.[3] For anterior open shoulder surgery, supplemental SSNB does not affect outcome when combined with interscalene block.[4] Because it provides major sensory innervation to the shoulder joint, it can be used to block supplementally the suprascapular nerve for analgesia after total shoulder arthroplasty. Furthermore, because it may send branches to the anterior axilla, the suprascapular nerve may require supplementation to anesthetize the anterior arthroscopic port site in awake patients who receive an interscalene block as the sole anesthetic for surgery.

Anatomy

The suprascapular nerve (C4-C5) branches from the superior trunk of the brachial plexus and therefore is usually anesthetized by an interscalene block. It traverses the suprascapular notch and continues laterally along the superior border

of the scapular spine (Figure 31–5). The supraclavicular nerve provides sensory innervation to 70% of the posterior-superior shoulder joint, the acromioclavicular joint, and a portion of the anterior axilla in up to 10% of patients.[1] The suprascapular nerve provides motor innervation to the supraspinatus and infraspinatus muscles, but minimal if any cutaneous innervation over the scapula or posterior shoulder.

Technique

Surface landmarks are identified by drawing one line along the superior border of the scapular spine and then bisecting it with a second line drawn parallel with the vertebral spine. From where these two lines cross, the suprascapular notch underlies a point ~2–3 cm toward the middle of the upper/outer quadrant (see Figure 31–5). A 1.5-in. 22-gauge needle is placed at this entry mark and directed caudad in the parasagittal plane until it contacts the scapular spine, followed by injection of 10 mL of a long-acting local anesthetic. If a peripheral nerve stimulator is used, the suprascapular nerve is identified by the motor response of external shoulder rotation.

Complications

Pneumothorax can result from a needle that passes through the suprascapular notch and enters the pleural space. This complication is largely avoidable by directing the needle in a caudad, rather than anterior, direction.

Clinical Pearls

- Suprascapular nerve block is a valuable analgesic adjunct for shoulder arthroscopy performed with the patient under general anesthesia.

- Suprascapular nerve block does not add value to open shoulder procedures in which an interscalene block is the primary anesthetic.

- Suprascapular nerve block is probably a valuable supplement to interscalene block during total shoulder arthroplasty or in the occasional patient who experiences pain at the anterior arthroscopic port site.

INTERCOSTOBRACHIAL NERVE BLOCK

Indications

The intercostobrachial nerve block is indicated for surgery involving the medial/posterior upper arm and/or for anterior arthroscopic port placement. A secondary indication is to alleviate the sensation resulting from a pneumatic tourniquet applied to the upper arm. Despite a commonly held misperception, the intercostobrachial nerve block does not block the ischemic, compressive components that cause tourniquet pain. Rather, the intercostobrachial nerve block simply

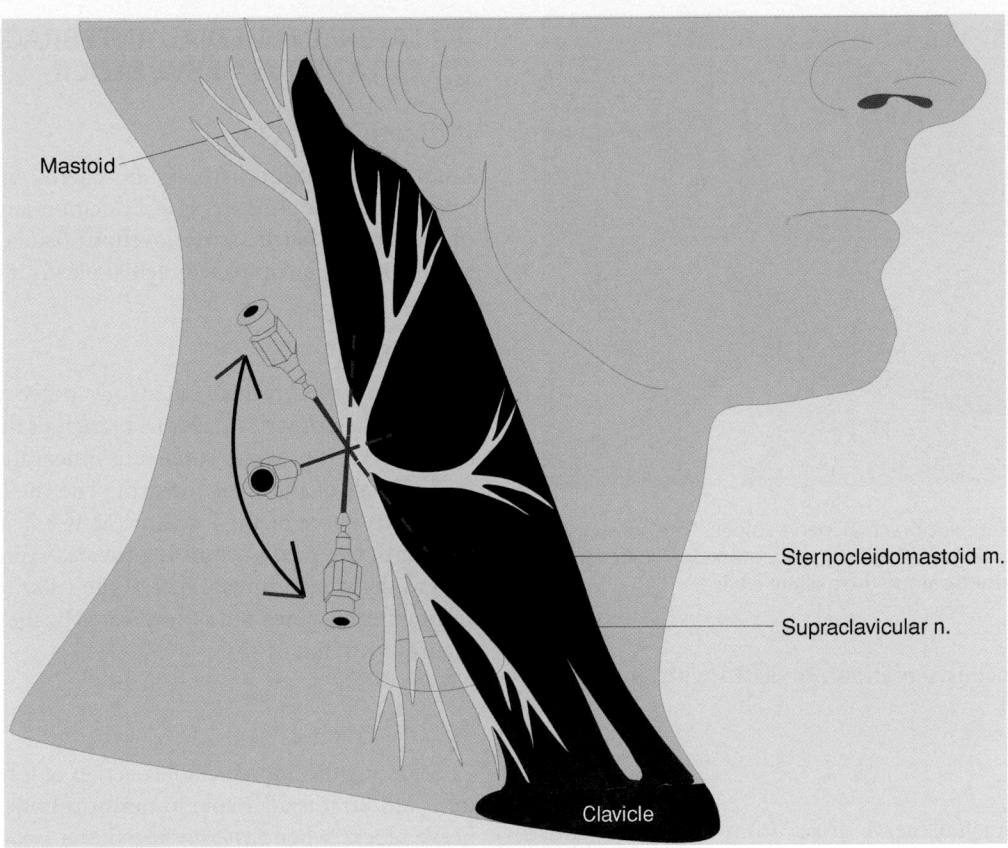

Figure 31–4. Supraclavicular nerve block. An initial injection of 3 mL local anesthetic is deposited at the midpoint of the sternocleidomastoid muscle, followed by 7 mL injected subcutaneously in a caudad and cephalad direction along the posterior border of the muscle.

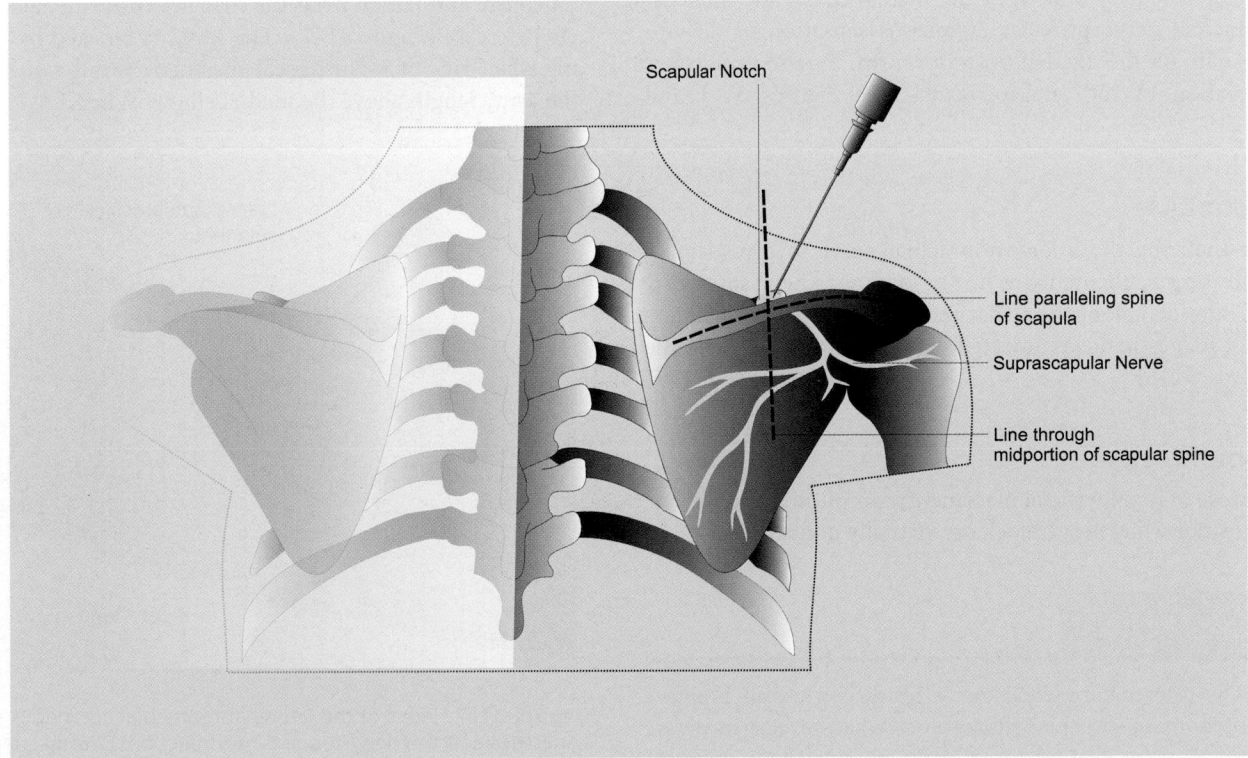

Figure 31–5. Suprascapular nerve block. The suprascapular nerve is blocked as it emerges from the suprascapular notch. Directing the needle caudally substantially reduces the risk of pneumothorax.

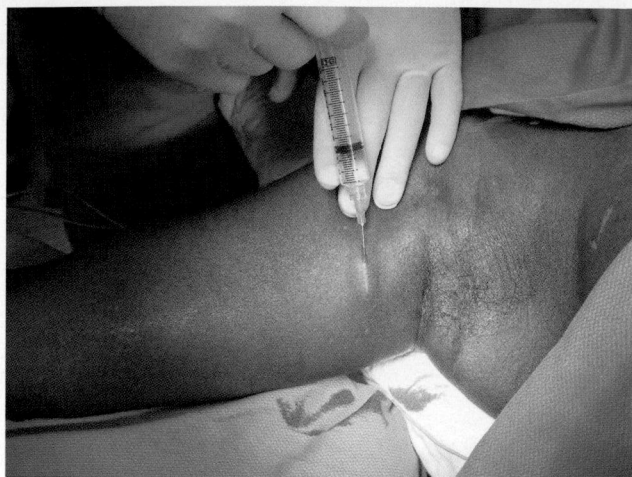

Figure 31–6. Intercostobrachial nerve block. The intercostobrachial nerve is anesthetized by subcutaneous injection of 3–5 mL local anesthetic along the axillary crease.

blocks the cutaneous sensation associated with tourniquet inflation.

Anatomy

The intercostobrachial nerve arises from the second thoracic (T2, and occasionally T1) nerve root (see Figure 31–2). As such, it is not a component of the brachial plexus and is therefore not anesthetized by any brachial plexus approach. Along with the medial cutaneous nerve of the arm (an intermediary branch of the medial cord), the intercostobrachial nerve provides cutaneous sensation to the upper half of the medial/posterior arm. It also innervates a portion of the anterior axilla (see Figures 31–1 and 31–2).

Technique

Anesthetizing the intercostobrachial nerve involves simply depositing a subcutaneous line of local anesthetic superiorly and inferiorly along the axillary crease. Three to five milliliters of local anesthetic are injected via a 1.5-in. 25-gauge needle (Figure 31–6).

Complications

Because of its superficial placement, complications of the intercostobrachial nerve block are virtually nonexistent.

Clinical Pearls

▪ The intercostobrachial nerve block is a useful supplement to any brachial plexus block when surgery involves the upper medial/posterior arm, a pneumatic tourniquet, and/or an anterior arthroscopic port.

LATERAL & MEDIAL ANTEBRACHIAL CUTANEOUS NERVE BLOCK

Indications

Local anesthetic blockade of the lateral and medial antebrachial cutaneous nerves is indicated for superficial surgery of the forearm, such as arteriovenous fistula surgery, or as a supplement to incomplete brachial plexus block.

Anatomy

The lateral antebrachial cutaneous nerve of the forearm (LAC) is the primary cutaneous branch of the musculocutaneous nerve. It provides cutaneous innervation to the lateral (radial) half of the volar forearm. The medial antebrachial cutaneous nerve of the forearm (MAC) is an intermediary branch of the medial cord. It provides cutaneous innervation to the medial (ulnar) half of the volar forearm, an area commonly misperceived as innervated by the ulnar nerve (see Figures 31–1 and 31–2).

Technique

Considering the unpredictable overlap of forearm cutaneous innervation, it is advisable to perform both LAC and MAC nerve blocks when forearm anesthesia is desired. Blocking the LAC is accomplished with two local anesthetic injections placed along the intercondylar line. The first 5 mL of local anesthetic are injected just deep to the lateral margin of the biceps tendon; the second 5 mL area injected subcutaneously and lateral from the first injection site, along the elbow crease (Figure 31–7). The MAC is blocked by injecting a half-ring of 5–7 mL local anesthetic about a quarter of the arm's length above the medial elbow. When LAC and/or

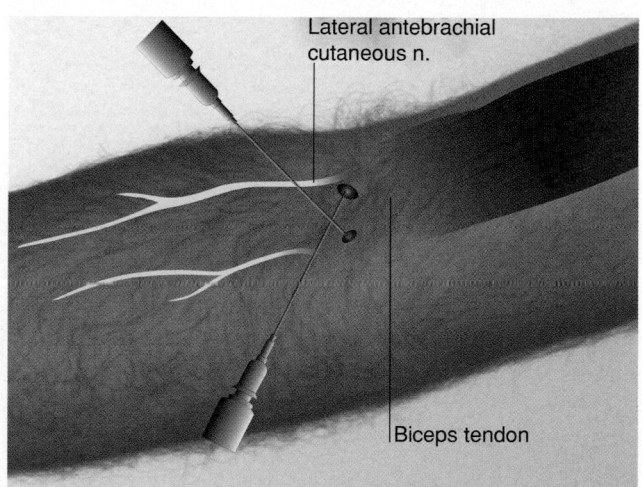

Lateral antebrachial cutaneous n.

Biceps tendon

Figure 31–7. Block of the lateral antebrachial cutaneous nerve. Anesthesia for this nerve requires two injections. The first deposits 5 mL local anesthetic just lateral to the border of the biceps tendon. A second 5 mL is then injected subcutaneously and lateral from the first injection site.

MAC nerve blocks are supplemental to a previous incomplete brachial plexus block, the additional 15–20 mL of local anesthetic should be well tolerated by patients if injected 20–30 minutes after the primary block.[5]

Complications

Techniques for anesthetizing the LAC and MAC nerves involve only superficial injection of local anesthetic; thus the risk of nerve injury is very low. For this reason, these blocks may be preferable to selective elbow or wrist blocks as a supplement to incomplete brachial plexus anesthesia involving the volar forearm cutaneous distribution.

Clinical Pearls

- Medial and lateral antebrachial cutaneous nerve blocks are useful techniques for superficial volar forearm procedures, such as creation of an arteriovenous fistula.

- These nerve blocks also represent a reasonable alternative for supplementation of anesthetic when proximal brachial plexus blocks are incomplete.

SELECTIVE NERVE BLOCKS AT THE ELBOW

Indications

Proximal techniques of brachial plexus block are often superior to selective nerve block at the elbow because the latter are more difficult to perform, are more time-consuming and uncomfortable, and potentially carry a greater risk of complications. For instance, the anesthesiologist who desires to provide selective analgesia strategies to specific terminal nerves may be better served by the midhumeral brachial plexus block, where selective application of clonidine[6] or low concentration of a long-acting local anesthetic[7] to the median and ulnar nerves prolongs analgesia without concomitant prolongation of motor block. Another reason to avoid selective elbow blocks is the commonly misunderstood cutaneous innervation of the forearm. For example, block of the musculocutaneous nerve must be performed in the axilla to render motor block of the biceps and brachioradialis muscles. But anesthetizing the cutaneous distribution of the musculocutaneous nerve is best accomplished with a LAC nerve block. Anesthetizing the skin of the medial forearm requires blockade of the MAC nerve, not the ulnar nerve at the elbow. A third issue is to avoid elbow blocks to supplement incomplete brachial plexus blocks because this practice theoretically increases the risk of anesthesia-related nerve injury. Indeed, the only indication for elbow approaches is to block forearm flexor and extensor muscles when the surgeon desires immobility of the fingers.

Radial Nerve block

Anatomy

The radial nerve supplies sensation to the dorsum of the forearm and hand (see Figures 31–1 and 31–2); it also innervates the musculature of the dorsal forearm. The radial nerve descends the posterior arm, traversing from the medial to the lateral side. At the epicondyles, the radial nerve lies relatively deep between the brachialis and brachioradialis muscles (Figure 31–8).

Technique

The patient is positioned supine for radial nerve block with the arm supinated and abducted. Selective block of the radial nerve is accomplished by placing a needle ∼1.5 cm lateral to the biceps tendon at the level of the epicondyles (see Figure 31–8). Three to five milliliters of local anesthetic are injected when a paresthesia to the hand is elicited. If using a peripheral nerve stimulator, one seeks the motor response of wrist extension.

Median Nerve Block

Anatomy

The median nerve provides sensation to the radial palm, the proximal fingers from the thumb to the long finger, and motor control to the forearm flexors (see Figures 31–1 and 31–2). It passes the elbow joint just medial to the brachial artery and in front of the brachialis muscle.

Technique

Median nerve block at the elbow is accomplished with a 1.5-in. needle that is placed just medial to the brachial artery at the level of the epicondyles (see Figure 31–8). Either a motor response that consists of wrist flexion and/or thumb opposition, or a paresthesia to the thumb or index finger, is sought before injecting 3–5 mL of local anesthetic.

Ulnar Nerve Block

Anatomy

The ulnar nerve at the elbow is located superficially in the ulnar groove (Figure 31–9). At this level, blockade of the ulnar nerve results in anesthesia of the little finger and motor block of the intrinsic muscles of the hand.

Technique

The patient is placed supine for ulnar nerve block and the forearm is flexed at the elbow (see Figure 31–9). After identification of the ulnar groove, a short needle is placed ∼1 cm proximal to the epicondyles and directed distally. The desired endpoint is paresthesia to the little finger or a motor response consisting of finger flexion, thumb adduction, and/or ulnar deviation of the wrist. It is suggested that only 2–3 mL of local anesthetic be injected to avoid excessive pressure within the tight fascial space of the ulnar groove and thereby lessen the possibility of compromising neural blood flow.

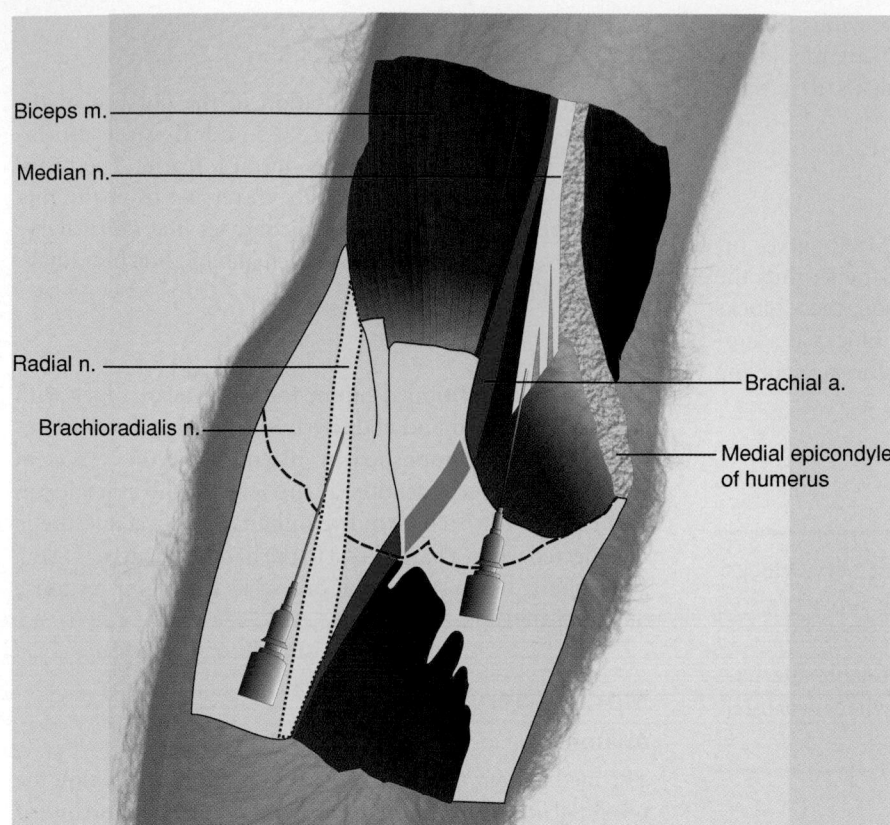

Figure 31–8. Radial and median nerve block at the elbow. Both nerves are approached at the level of the epicondyles. The radial nerve is found ~1.5 cm lateral to the biceps tendon. The median nerve is more superficial and identified by a needle placed just medial to the brachial artery.

Complications

Selective nerve blocks at the elbow may rarely cause hematoma. However, it is the potential for anesthesia-related nerve injury that adds risk when these blocks are used to supplement incomplete proximal brachial plexus block. This theoretical risk is based on the concept that needle placement in the vicinity of nerves that already have full or partial prox-

imal local anesthetic blockade may reduce the patient's ability to perceive a paresthesia or pain on injection. Although not conclusively proven, these fears are nevertheless based on reported perioperative nerve injuries that occurred in the setting of supplementation.[1] Conversely, supplemental injections placed within a brief time (≤5 minutes) from initial injection of local anesthetic may carry less risk.[8]

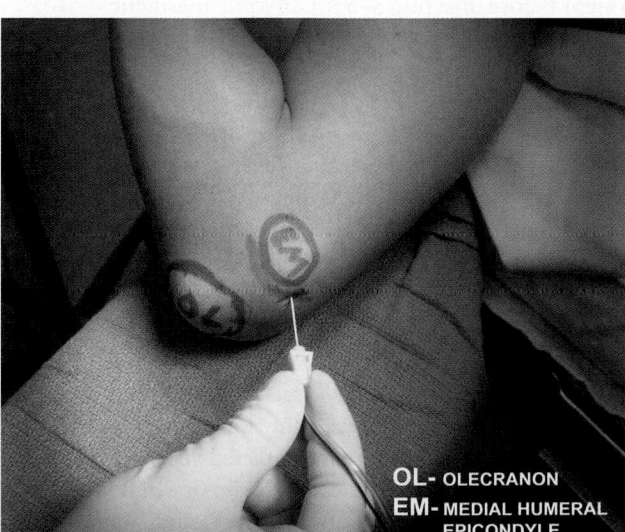

Figure 31–9. Ulnar nerve block at the elbow. The forearm is flexed, the ulnar groove identified, and a needle is placed 1 cm proximal to the epicondyles and directed distally.

Clinical Pearls

- Selective nerve blocks at the elbow can be recommended for hand surgery when forearm motor block is desired and motor block of the proximal brachial plexus block is not desired.
- Selective nerve blocks at the elbow to supplement incomplete proximal brachial plexus should be practiced with caution.

PERIOPERATIVE MANAGEMENT

Because cutaneous nerve blocks of the upper extremity require only small amounts of local anesthetic, which are typically injected subcutaneously and not proximate to major vessels, they can be placed with minimal monitoring and should require little postoperative observation. However, if these blocks are placed in conjunction with major plexus blocks, then full monitoring and recovery monitoring are required. Because most of the nerves considered in this chapter have insignificant motor innervation, prolonged motor block leading to positioning injuries is seldom a consideration. Nevertheless, outpatients should be warned to protect their insensate limbs from external pressure or temperature extremes.

SUMMARY

Selective upper extremity nerve blocks can be useful supplements to brachial plexus blocks. Supraclavicular, suprascapular, and superficial cutaneous nerve blocks are valuable adjuncts to the anesthesia and/or analgesia primarily provided by a plexus block or general anesthesia. The LAC and MAC nerve blocks can provide either primary anesthesia for superficial forearm operations or supplement an incomplete plexus block. Selective elbow blocks are inferior alternatives to brachial plexus blocks. Their use as a supplement to incomplete plexus blockade should be practiced with caution.

References

1. Neal JM, Hebl JR, Gerancher JC, Hogan QH: Brachial plexus anesthesia: Essentials of our current understanding. Reg Anesth Pain Med 2002;27:402–428.
2. Ritchie E, Tong D, Chung F, et al: Suprascapular nerve block for postoperative pain relief in arthroscopic shoulder surgery: A new modality? Anesth Analg 1997;84:1306–1312.
3. Singelyn RJ, Lhotel L, Fabre B: Pain relief after arthroscopic shoulder surgery: A comparison of intraarticular analgesia, suprascapular nerve block, and interscalene brachial plexus block. Anesth Analg 2004;99:589–592.
4. Neal JM, McDonald SB, Larkin KL, Polissar NL: Suprascapular nerve block prolongs analgesia after nonarthroscopic shoulder surgery, but does not improve outcome. Anesth Analg 2003;96:982–986.
5. Finucane BT, Yilling F: Safety of supplementing axillary plexus blocks. Anesthesiology 1989;70:401–403.
6. Iskandar H, Guillaume E, Dixmerias F, et al: The enhancement of sensory blockade by clonidine selectively added to mepivacaine after midhumeral block. Anesth Analg 2001;93:771–775.
7. Bouaziz H, Narchi P, Mercier FJ, et al: The use of selective axillary nerve block for outpatient hand surgery. Anesth Analg 1998;86:746–748.
8. Fanelli G, Casati A, Garancini P, Torri G: Nerve stimulator and multiple injection technique for upper and lower limb blockade: Failure rate, patient acceptance, and neurologic complications. Study Group on Regional Anesthesia. Anesth Analg 1999;88:847–852.

32

Clinical Assessment of Lower Extremity Nerve Blocks

Joseph M. Neal, MD

I. INTRODUCTION

II. SCIATIC NERVE ASSESSMENT

III. OBTURATOR NERVE ASSESSMENT

IV. LATERAL FEMORAL CUTANEOUS NERVE ASSESSMENT

V. FEMORAL NERVE ASSESSMENT

INTRODUCTION

The extent of anesthesia after selective blocks of the peripheral nerves originating from the lumbar and lumbosacral plexi is often assessed before surgery can begin. This assessment may be deceptively difficult if one has incomplete understanding of lower extremity innervation or if the evaluation is hindered by slow onset of sensory block. Conversely, timely evaluation of the block allows the anesthesiologist to identify inadequately anesthetized nerves, thus providing the opportunity to modify the block before incision.

A simple system for assessing the adequacy of upper extremity nerve block has been described and enjoys acceptance by anesthesiologists worldwide. The four P's (push, pull, pinch, punt) concept was likely developed during World War II as a straightforward method for medics to determine the extent of battlefield injury. The concept was later formalized and popularized by Thompson and Brown.[1] Herein is described a methodology for assessing lower extremity anesthesia that is a variation of the four P's concept. For lower extremity evaluation, the P's are modified slightly to become push, pull, pinch, punt.

Several minutes after depositing local anesthetic near a peripheral nerve, the following individual assessments are undertaken to determine blockade of the four major nerves of the lower extremity.

SCIATIC NERVE ASSESSMENT

The sciatic nerve is derived from the lumbosacral plexus and provides motor control to the posterior thigh and the entire lower leg and foot. Its sensory distribution includes the posterior thigh, the posterior knee joint, and all the lower leg except for the saphenous nerve distribution (medial lower leg and ankle). Because plantar flexion of the foot is controlled by the sciatic nerve, its function is evaluated by asking the patient to *push* the foot against the resistance of the examiner's hand or "step on the gas" (Figure 32–1). Anesthesia within the sciatic nerve distribution is indicated by weakness during

---

Portions of this text originally appeared in the following publication: Neal JM: Assessment of Lower Extremity Nerve Block: Reprise of the Four P's Acronym. Regional Anesthesia and Pain Medicine, vol 27: 618–620, 2002; copyright 2002 American Society of Regional Anesthesia and Pain Medicine, with permission.

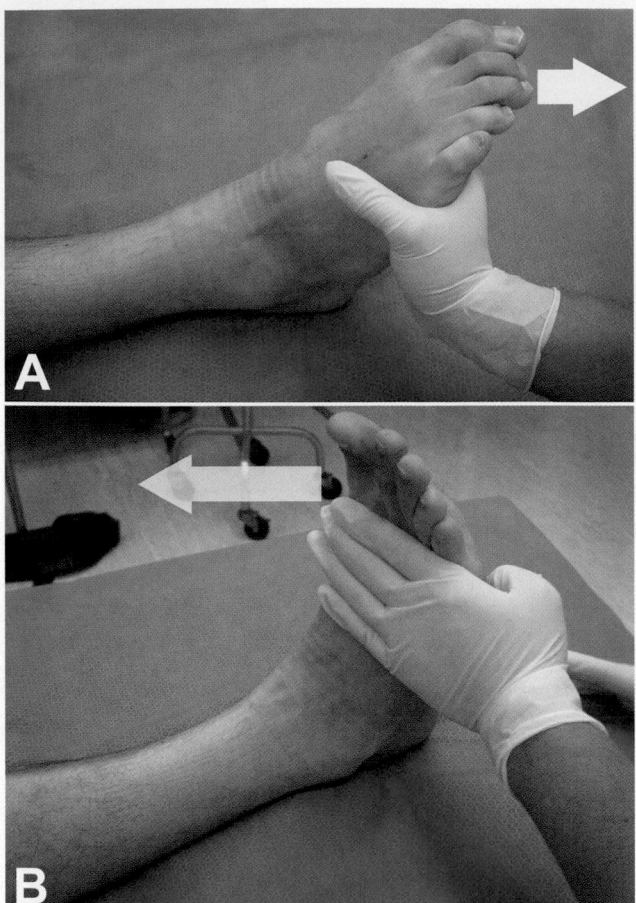

Figure 32–1. Push. Patients with successful sciatic or popliteal fossa block are unable to push the target with their foot. **A:** Tibial nerve or dorsiflex the foot; **B:** Common peroneal nerve.

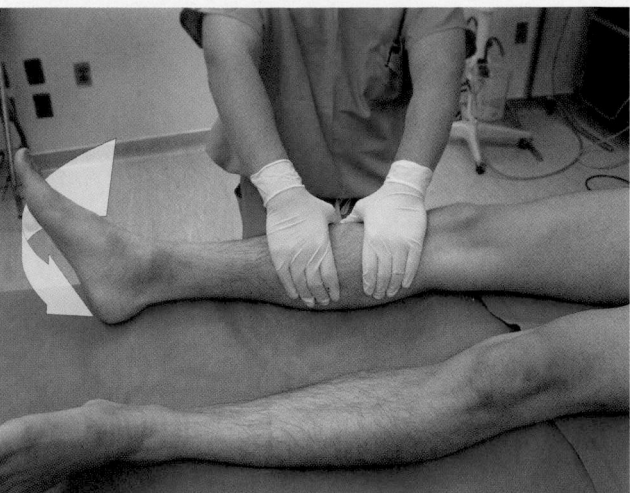

Figure 32–2. Pull. With obturator blockade, patients are unable to pull the blocked extremity toward midline.

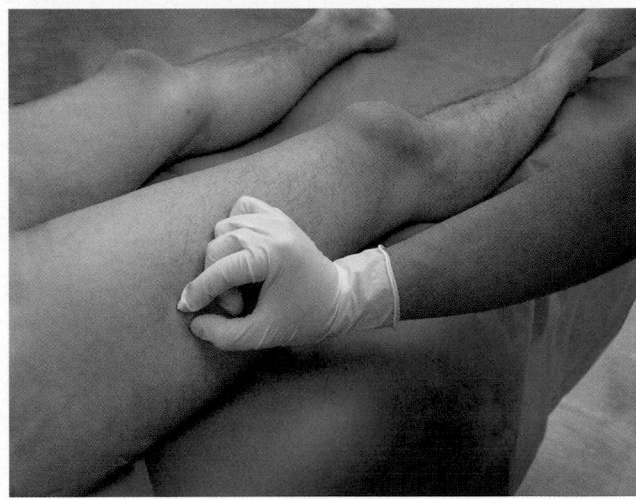

Figure 32–3. Pinch. With successful block of the lateral cutaneous nerve of the thigh, patients are unable to feel skin pinching on the lateral aspect of the thigh.

the performance of this maneuver. Because the evaluation is performed distally, it is applicable to all sciatic nerve block approaches, including the blocks at the popliteal fossa.

OBTURATOR NERVE ASSESSMENT

The obturator nerve, a component of the lumbar plexus, provides motor innervation to the adductors of the thigh and variable sensory innervation to the proximal medial thigh. It also has small branches to the knee and hip joints. To assess obturator nerve function, the anesthesiologist abducts the patient's leg and then requests that the patient *pull* the leg toward the midline against resistance (Figure 32–2). The obturator nerve has been successfully blocked if the patient exhibits adductor weakness during this task.

LATERAL FEMORAL CUTANEOUS NERVE ASSESSMENT

The lateral femoral cutaneous nerve, a part of the lumbar plexus, is the only purely sensory nerve of the four major lower

extremity nerves. The cutaneous innervation of this nerve includes the lateral buttock and the lateral thigh. Thus, the inability to detect a *pinch* on the proximal lateral thigh signals successful conduction block of the lateral femoral cutaneous nerve (Figure 32–3).

FEMORAL NERVE ASSESSMENT

The femoral nerve provides motor innervation to the quadriceps femoris and sartorius muscles. Its sensory distribution includes the anterior thigh, the saphenous nerve, and branches to the hip joint and the majority of the knee joint. To test femoral nerve function, the anesthesiologist supports the patient's knee by placing an arm under the popliteal fossa and slightly raising the knee off the bed. The patient is then

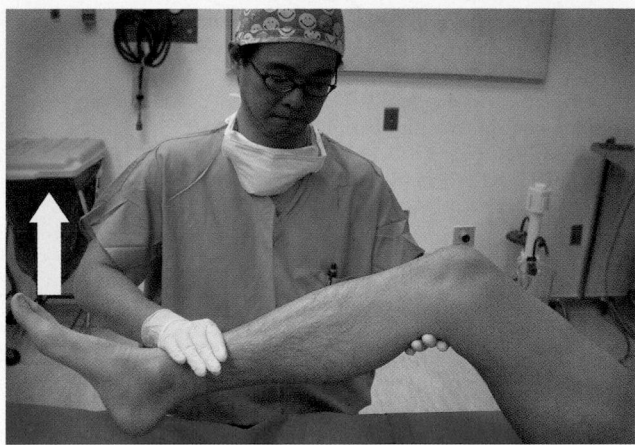

Figure 32–4. Punt. With successful femoral nerve block, patients are unable to extend the leg in the knee against resistance.

asked to *punt* an imaginary football against the resistance of the examiner's restraining hand (Figure 32–4). The inability to contract the quadriceps muscle and extend the lower leg at the knee indicates conduction block of the femoral nerve. If the leg is splinted, requesting the patient to contract the quadriceps muscle accomplishes the same purpose.

Clinical Pearls

- The earliest sign of femoral nerve block is the loss of temperature discrimination in the saphenous nerve territory (saphenous sign) (Figure 32–5).
- When this sign is present shortly after injection of local anesthetic, successful block of the femoral nerve is imminent.[2]

This chapter describes a simple and reliable method to verify lower extremity anesthesia after regional block techniques. By using push, pull, pinch, punt, the anesthesiologist can rapidly perform a qualitative assessment of conduction block of the sciatic, obturator, lateral femoral cutaneous, and femoral nerves, respectively.

Clinical Pearls

- The signs discussed in the previous text are present only when the block has full onset. However, surgery can be started before these signs are present as long as the patient shows early signs of onset shortly after injection of local anesthetic.
- Local anesthetic infiltration in the area of the surgical incision can be used to bridge the "time gap" until the block has full onset or to supplement incomplete dermatomal coverage.

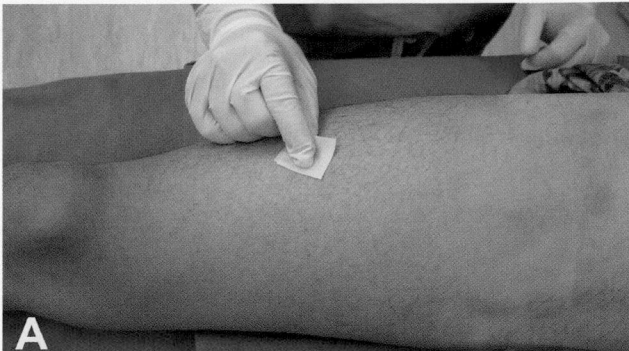

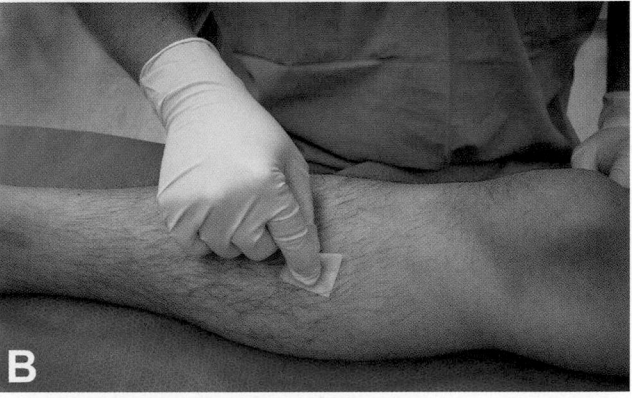

Figure 32–5. The first sign of onset of femoral nerve blockade is loss of temperature discrimination in the anterior thigh (**A**) and in the saphenous nerve territory below the knee (**B**).

Because cutaneous innervation of the lower extremity consists of multiple overlapping sensory fields, it can be difficult to accurately determine which specific peripheral nerve is inadequately anesthetized.[3,4] The four P's methodology takes advantage of the principle that peripheral nerves consist of an outer mantle layer surrounding an inner core layer. The mantle layer, which innervates the proximal extremity, is generally anesthetized first.[5] This arrangement causes proximal motor fibers to become anesthetized before distal sensory fibers.[6] Thus, motor function of the proximal lower extremity typically shows signs of conduction block before the more distal sensory fibers. For example, a patient may show early gastrocnemius weakness (*pushing* on the gas) before sensory changes in the foot. Furthermore, selecting motor or sensory function specific to an individual nerve will accurately show its functional integrity. Thus, adduction of the leg (pulling the leg toward the midline) is exclusively an obturator nerve function, whereas sensation of the proximal lateral thigh (*pinching*) is only within the lateral femoral cutaneous nerve's sensory field.

Because each described maneuver is specific to a peripheral nerve, early functional assessment facilitates selective supplementation of an inadequately anesthetized nerve well in advance of surgical incision. Therefore, the use of the four P's (push, pull, pinch, punt) is recommended as a simple, rapid, and reliable method for assessment of lower extremity nerve block.

References

1. Thompson G, Brown D: The common nerve blocks. In: Nunn J, Utting J, Brown B (editors): *General Anaesthesia*, 5th ed. Butterworths, 1989, pp. 1068–1069.

2. Hadzic A, Vloka JD: Femoral nerve block. In: *Peripheral Nerve Blocks: Principles and Practice.* McGraw-Hill, 2004, pp. 267–281.

3. Stopford J: The variation in distribution of the cutaneous nerves of the hand and digits. J Anat 1919;53:14–25.

4. Kirk E, Denny-Brown D: Functional variation in dermatomes in the macaque monkey following dorsal root lesions. J Comp Neurol 1970;139:307–320.

5. Kristerson L, Nordenram A, Nordqvist P: Penetration of radioactive local anaesthetic into peripheral nerve. Arch Int Pharmacodyn 1965;157:148–152.

6. Winnie A, Tay C-H, Patel K, et al: Pharmacokinetics of local anesthetics during plexus blocks. Anesth Analg 1977;56:852–861.

33

Lumbar Plexus Block

Christopher Robards, MD • Admir Hadzic, MD

INTRODUCTION

The use of lumbar or sacral plexus blockade for lower extremity surgeries has not been commonplace until recently. This is because these techniques were thought to be difficult to perform and resulted in frequent failure to accomplish surgical anesthesia.[1–3] Dogliotti[4] pointed out, "the nerve trunks of the lumbar plexus which run into the inferior extremity are at a great distance from each other, so much so that in order to produce anesthesia, multiple procedures are necessary with separate injections, for each nerve trunk." Hence, anesthesiologists preferred the quicker and more effective techniques of spinal or epidural anesthesia for most patients. Several variations of the original technique have been proposed, with the main differences being in the level of blockade and the distance from the midline for the needle insertion.[4–6] However, given the deep location of the lumbar plexus, various approaches often represent minuscule technical variations rather than clinically relevant modifications. For instance, Chayen's approach is thought to result in too high of an incidence of epidural blockade.[7] However, newly proposed techniques have also resulted in a 15% incidence of epidural blockade.[8] More recently, ultrasound-guided lumbar plexus block technique has been suggested; unfortunately this requires substantial ultrasonographic skill, and adequate images are difficult to obtain in many patients.[9] Regardless of which technique is followed, safety precautions must be used for successful and safe use of this technique.

Indications

Lumbar plexus block has been used for a number of lower extremity procedures. It has been shown to be particularly useful for femoral shaft and neck fractures, knee procedures, and procedures involving the anterior thigh.[1,10–12] Lumbar plexus block alone cannot provide adequate anesthesia for major surgery of the lower extremity because of the contributing innervation by the sciatic nerve. Even when combined lumbar plexus–sciatic blocks are used for anesthesia in patients undergoing total knee arthroplasty, conversion to general anesthesia may be required in up to 22% of the time.[13]

Regional Anesthesia Anatomy & Management

The lumbar plexus consists of six nerves on each side, the first of which emerges between the first and second lumbar vertebrae and the last between the last lumbar vertebra and the base of the sacrum. As soon as the L2, L3, and L4 roots of the lumbar plexus depart from their spinal nerves and emerge from the intervertebral foramina, they become embedded in the psoas major muscle[14] (Figure 33–1). This is because the psoas is attached to the lateral surfaces and transverse processes of the lumbar vertebrae. Within the muscle, these roots then split into anterior and posterior divisions, which reunite to form the individual branches (nerves) of the plexus.[15] The major branches of the lumbar plexus are the genitofemoral nerve, lateral femoral cutaneous nerve, femoral, and obturator nerves (Figure 33–2). Within the psoas major muscle, the lateral femoral cutaneous and femoral nerves are separated from the obturator nerve by a muscular fold in more than 50% of patients; anatomic variations are also common.[15,16]

The femoral nerve is formed by the posterior divisions of L2-4 and descends from the plexus lateral to the psoas

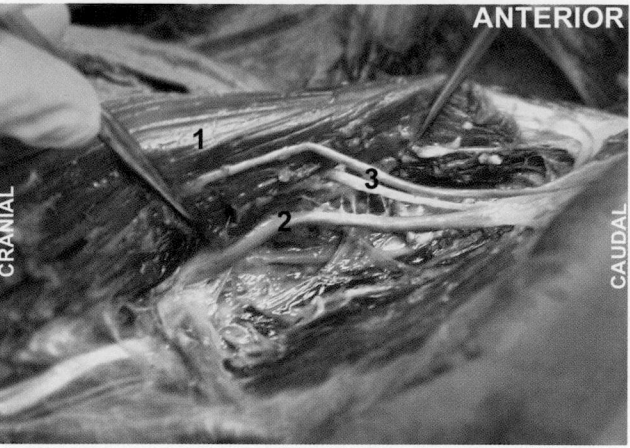

Figure 33–1. Psoas muscle (*1*) is shown exposed from within abdominal cavity with lumbar plexus branches (*2, 3*).

muscle. The anterior divisions of the same roots unite to form the other major branch of the lumbar plexus, the obturator nerve. The reader is referred to Chapter 3 for more in-depth discussions on anatomy.

Distribution of Anesthesia

Injection of local anesthetic during lumbar plexus block most commonly results in spread of the injectate within the body of the psoas muscle around the lumbar branches (L2-4), with cephalad spread to the lumbar nerve roots.[17]

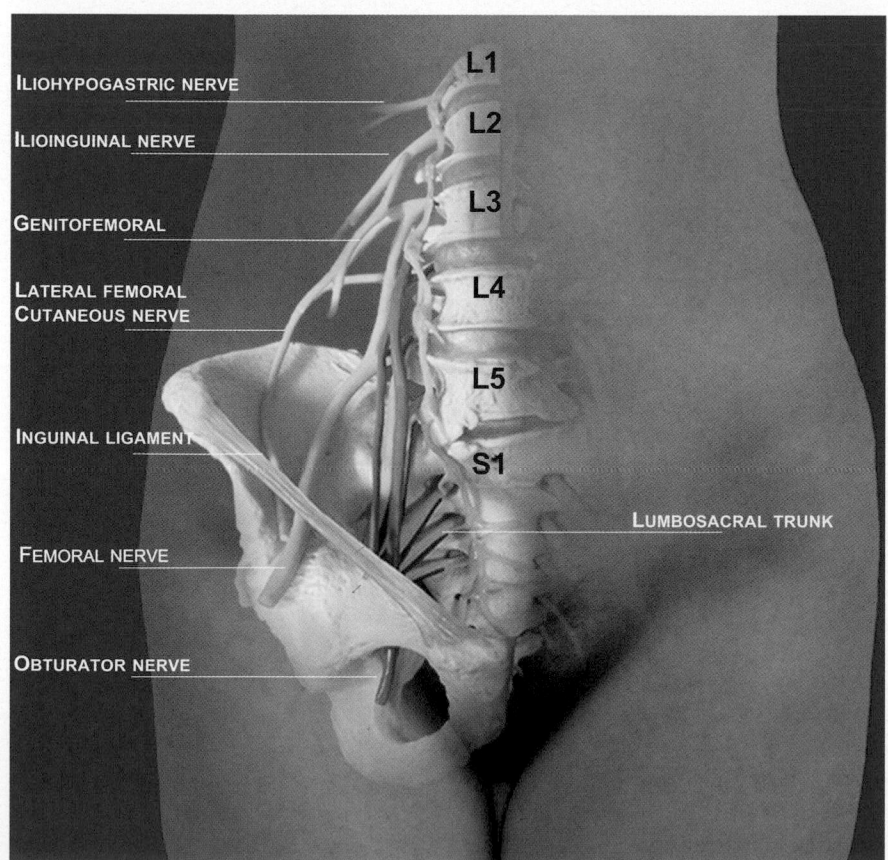

Figure 33–2. Lumbar plexus branches.

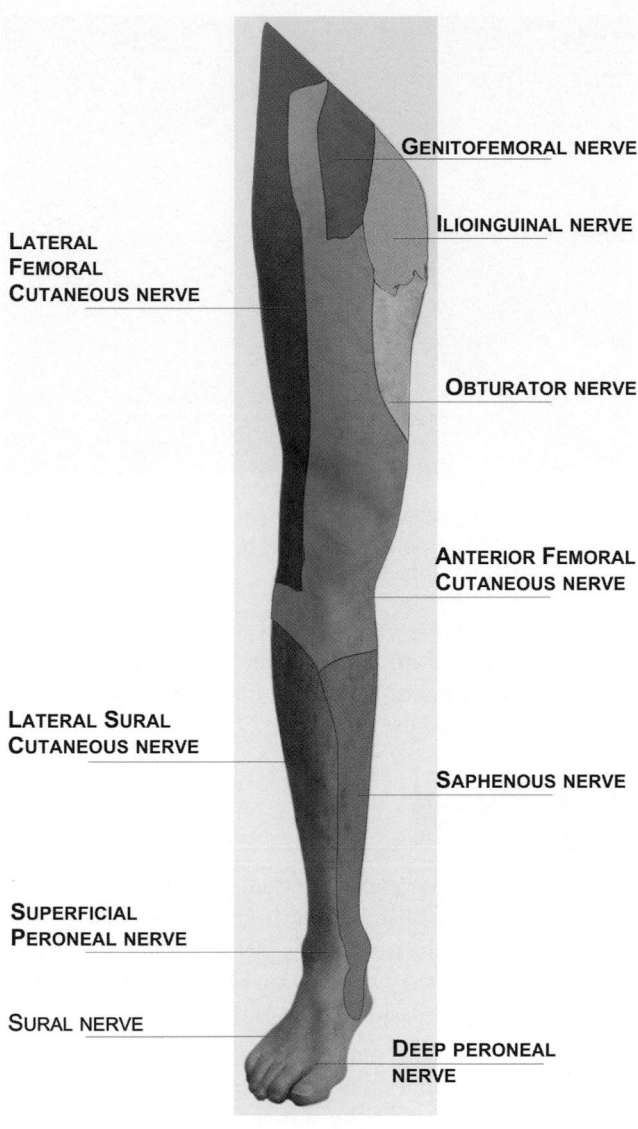

LATERAL
FEMORAL
CUTANEOUS NERVE

GENITOFEMORAL NERVE

ILIOINGUINAL NERVE

OBTURATOR NERVE

ANTERIOR FEMORAL
CUTANEOUS NERVE

LATERAL SURAL
CUTANEOUS NERVE

SAPHENOUS NERVE

SUPERFICIAL
PERONEAL NERVE

SURAL NERVE

DEEP PERONEAL
NERVE

ANTERIOR

Figure 33–3. Distribution of anesthesia and analgesia after a successful lumbar plexus block.

The femoral nerve supplies motor fibers to the quadriceps muscle (knee extension), the skin of the anteromedial thigh, and the medial aspect of the leg below the knee and foot. The obturator nerve sends motor branches to the adductors of the hip and a highly variable cutaneous area on the medial thigh or knee joint. The lateral femoral cutaneous and genitofemoral nerves are purely cutaneous nerves. Figure 33–3 illustrates the cutaneous innervation of the lumbar plexus.

Choice of Local Anesthetic

Lumbar plexus blockade requires a relatively large volume of local anesthetic to achieve anesthesia of the entire plexus. The choice of the type and concentration of local anesthetic should be based on whether the block is planned for surgical anesthesia or pain management. Because of the vascular nature of the area and the potential for inadvertent intravascular injection, rapid absorption from the deep mus-

Table 33–1.

Local Anesthetic Choices for Lumbar Plexus Block

	Onset (min)	Anesthesia (h)	Analgesia (h)
3% 2-Chloroprocaine (+ HCO₃; + epinephrine)	10–15	1.5	2.0
1.5% Mepivacaine (+ HCO₃)	10–15	2	2–4
1.5% Mepivacaine (+ HCO₃; + epinephrine)	10–15	2.5–3	2–5
2% Lidocaine (+ HCO₃)	10–20	2.5–3	2–5
2% Lidocaine (+ HCO₃ + epinephrine)	10–20	5–6	5–8
0.5% Ropivacaine	15–20	4–6	6–10

cle beds, and epidural spread, then rapid, forceful injections should be avoided. Epinephrine is almost routinely used as a vascular marker. The most commonly used local anesthetic for this block in our institution is alkalinized 2-chloroprocaine 3% 1:300,000 epinephrine in outpatients having knee arthroscopy.[18,19] Some common choices of local anesthetics for this block are listed in Table 33–1.

Technique

The patient is in the lateral decubitus position with a slight forward tilt (Figure 33–4). The foot on the side to be

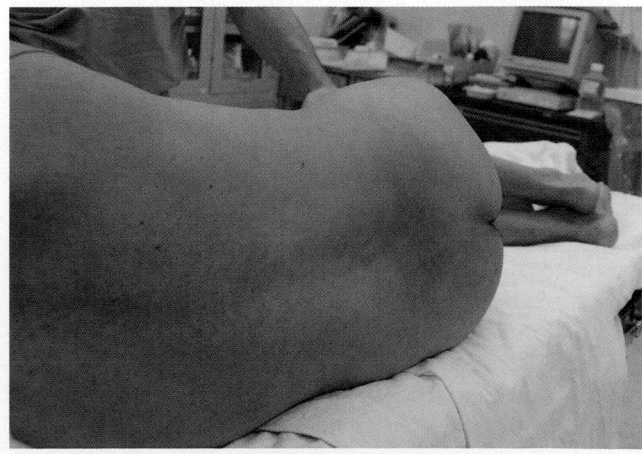

Figure 33–4. Patient position for lumbar plexus block.

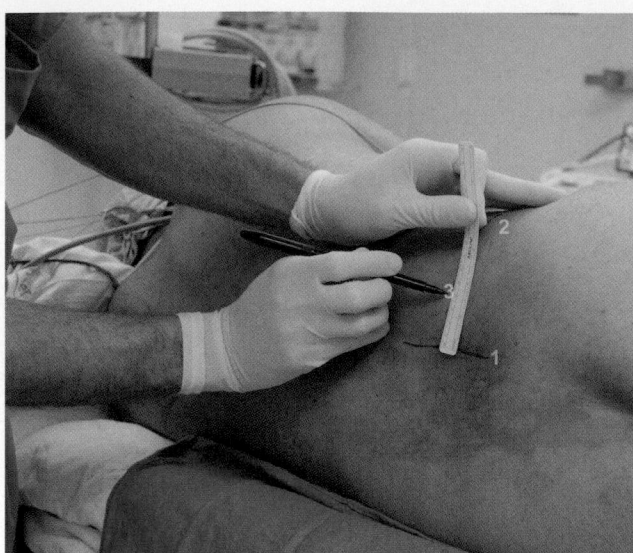

Figure 33–5. Landmarks for lumbar plexus block. *1*, Midline. *2*, Iliac crest. *3*, Needle insertion site is labeled 4 cm lateral to the midline.

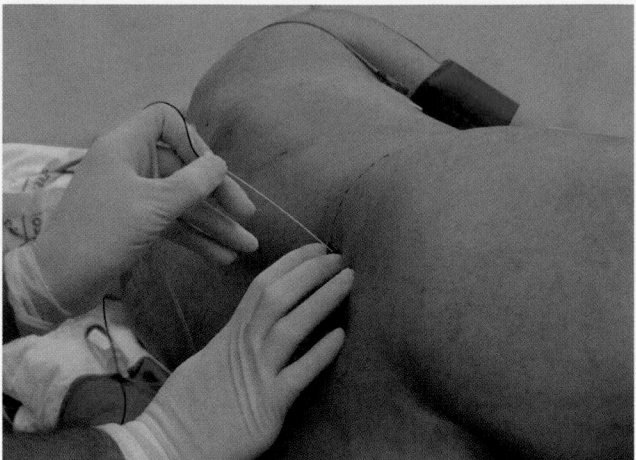

Figure 33–6. Needle insertion for the lumbar plexus block. The needle is inserted perpendicular to the body plane or with a slight medial orientation (shown).

At this point, 25–35 mL of local anesthetic is slowly injected with frequent aspiration to rule out inadvertent intravascular placement of the needle.

Clinical Pearls

- Successful lumbar plexus blockade depends on the dispersion of the local anesthetic in the fascial plane (psoas muscle) where the roots of the plexus are situated. Thus, the goal of the nerve stimulation is to identify this plane by eliciting stimulation of one of the roots.

- Stimulation at currents less than 0.5 mA should not be sought when using this technique. Dural sleeves thickly envelop the roots of the lumbar plexus. Motor stimulation with a low current may indicate placement of the needle inside a dural sleeve. An injection inside this sheath can result in tracking of the local anesthetic toward the epidural or subarachnoid space, with consequent epidural or spinal anesthesia.

blocked should be positioned over the dependent leg so that twitches of the quadriceps muscle and/or patella can be seen easily.

A standard regional anesthesia tray is prepared with the following equipment:

- Sterile towels and 4-in. × 4-in. gauze packs
- 20-mL syringes with local anesthetic
- Sterile gloves, marking pen, and surface electrode
- One 1½-in., 25-gauge needle for skin infiltration
- A 10-cm long, short-bevel, insulated stimulating needle
- Peripheral nerve stimulator

Landmarks for the lumbar plexus block include (Figure 33–5):

1. Midline (spinous processes)
2. Iliac crest
3. Needle insertion labeled 4-cm lateral to the intersection of landmarks 1 and 2

After a cleaning with an antiseptic solution, the skin is anesthetized by infiltrating local anesthetic subcutaneously at the determined needle insertion site.

The fingers of the palpating hand are firmly pressed against the paravertebral muscles to stabilize the landmark and decrease the skin–nerve distance. The needle is inserted at a perpendicular angle to the skin (Figure 33–6). The nerve stimulator should be initially set to deliver current intensity of 1.5 mA. As the needle is advanced, local twitches of the paravertebral muscles are obtained first at a depth of a few centimeters. The needle is then advanced further until twitches of the quadriceps muscle are obtained (usually at the depth of 6–8 cm). After the twitches are obtained, the current should be lowered to obtain stimulation between 0.5 mA and 1.0 mA.

When insertion of the needle does not result in quadriceps muscle stimulation, the maneuvers outlined in Table 33–2 should be followed.

Block Dynamics & Perioperative Management

A lumbar plexus block can be associated with significant patient discomfort during nerve localization owing to the needle passage through multiple muscle planes. Adequate sedation and analgesia are necessary to ensure a still and tranquil patient. Typically, we use midazolam 4–6 mg after the patient is positioned and alfentanil 500–750 mcg just before needle insertion. A typical onset time for this block is 15–25 minutes, depending on the type, concentration, and volume of local anesthetic and the level at which the needle is placed.

Table 33–2.

Troubleshooting Procedures During Lumbar Plexus Blocks

Response Obtained	Interpretation	Problem	Action
Local twitch of the paraspinal muscles	Direct stimulation of the paraspinal muscles	Too shallow placement of the needle	Continue advancing the needle
Needle contacts bone at 4–6 cm depth; no twitches are seen	The needle advancement is stopped by the transverse process	Indicates proper needle placement, but requires redirection of the needle	Withdraw the needle to the skin level, and redirect 5 degrees cranially or caudally
Twitches of hamstrings muscles are seen; needle inserted 6–8 cm	Result of stimulation of the roots of the sciatic plexus (sciatic nerve)	Needle inserted too far caudally	Withdraw the needle and reinsert 3–5 cm cranially
Flexion of thigh at the depth of >6–8 cm	This subtle and often missed response is caused by direct stimulation of the psoas muscle	Needle inserted too deep (missed the lumbar plexus roots); further advancement may place the needle intraperitoneally	Stop advancing the needle; withdraw the needle and reinsert using the protocol outlined in the technique description
Needle is placed deep (10 cm), but twitches were not elicited and bone is not contacted	Needle missed the transverse process and roots of the lumbar plexus	Needle placement too lateral	Withdraw the needle and reinsert with a slight medial angulation (5–10 degrees)

For example, although an almost immediate onset of anesthesia in the anterior thigh and knee can be achieved with an injection at the L3 level, additional time is required for local anesthetic to block the lateral thigh (L1) or obturator nerve (L5). The first sign of the onset of blockade is usually the loss of sensation in the saphenous nerve territory (medial skin below the knee).

CONTINUOUS LUMBAR PLEXUS BLOCK

Continuous lumbar plexus blockade is an advanced regional anesthesia technique, and adequate experience with the single-shot technique is a prerequisite to ensure its efficacy and safety. The technique is similar to the single-shot injection except that the Tuohy needle is preferable. The needle opening should be directed cephalad to facilitate threading of the catheter. This technique can be used for postoperative pain management in patients undergoing hip, femur, and knee surgery.[20] Because a large volume of local is required anesthetic to accomplish analgesia, continuous infusion requires intermittent boluses for success. Consequently, some feel that its advantages over continuous femoral block for postoperative analgesia are questionable at best and that continuous lumbar plexus block should not be in routine use for postoperative analgesia.[21]

Equipment

A standard regional anesthesia tray is prepared with the following equipment:

- Sterile towels and 4-in. × 4-in. gauze packs
- 20-mL syringe with local anesthetic
- Sterile gloves, marking pen, and surface electrode
- One 1½-in. 25-gauge needle for skin infiltration
- A 10-cm long, insulated stimulating needle (preferably Tuohy-style tip)
- Catheter
- Peripheral nerve stimulator

Technique

The skin and subcutanoues tissues are anesthetized with local anethetic. The needle is attached to the nerve stimulator (1.5 mA, 2 Hz, 100 μsec) and to a syringe with local anethetic. The palpating hand should be firmly pressed and anchored against the paraspinal muscles to facilitate the needle insertion and redirection of the needle when necessary. A 10-cm, Tuohy-style tip, continuous block needle is inserted at a perpendicular angle to the skin and advanced until the quadriceps twitch response is obtained at 0.5–1.0 mA current. At this point, the initial volume of local anesthetic is injected (eg, 15–25 mL), and the catheter is inserted approximately

8–10 cm beyond the needle tip. The needle is then withdrawn back to the skin level, while the catheter is simultaneously advanced. This method prevents inadvertent removal of the catheter and intravascular and intrathecal placement by negative aspiration test. Figure 33–7 shows dispersion of the dye within the sheath of the psoas muscle.

Clinical Pearls

- The opening of the needle tip should be oriented cephalad before threading the catheter.
- The skin in the lumber area is very movable; thus insertion of the catheter to a depth of 8–10 cm is necessary to help prevent its removal during patient repositioning, etc.

Continuous Infusion

Continuous infusion is always initiated after an initial bolus of dilute local anesthetic through the catheter. For this purpose, we routinely use ropivacaine 0.2% (15–20 mL). Diluted bupivacaine or l-bupivacaine is also suitable, but can result in more motor blockade. The infusion is maintained at 10 mL/h or 5 mL/h when a PCA dose is planned (5 mL/q30min). Figures 33–7 and 33–8 show the dispersion of 20 mL of a contrast solution within the psoas sheath.

Clinical Pearls

- Breakthrough pain in patients on continuous infusion is always managed by administering a bolus of local anesthetic.
- Simply increasing the rate of infusion is rarely adequate. With patients on the ward, a higher concentration of a shorter-acting local anesthetic (eg, 1% mepivacaine) is useful to both manage the pain and test the position of the catheter.

COMPLICATIONS & HOW TO AVOID THEM

The lumbar plexus block is an advanced technique with a significant clinical applicability but also with a potential for serious complications. The most common complications reported with lumbar plexus block are epidural spread with the potential for high neuraxial anesthesia,[22–25] hypotension, local anesthetic toxicity,[26–28] and iliopsoas or renal hematoma.[29–32] Plasma concentrations of local anesthetics are significantly higher after lumbar plexus block compared with other peripheral nerve block, and there is a potential for rapid absorption and intravascular channeling owing to the

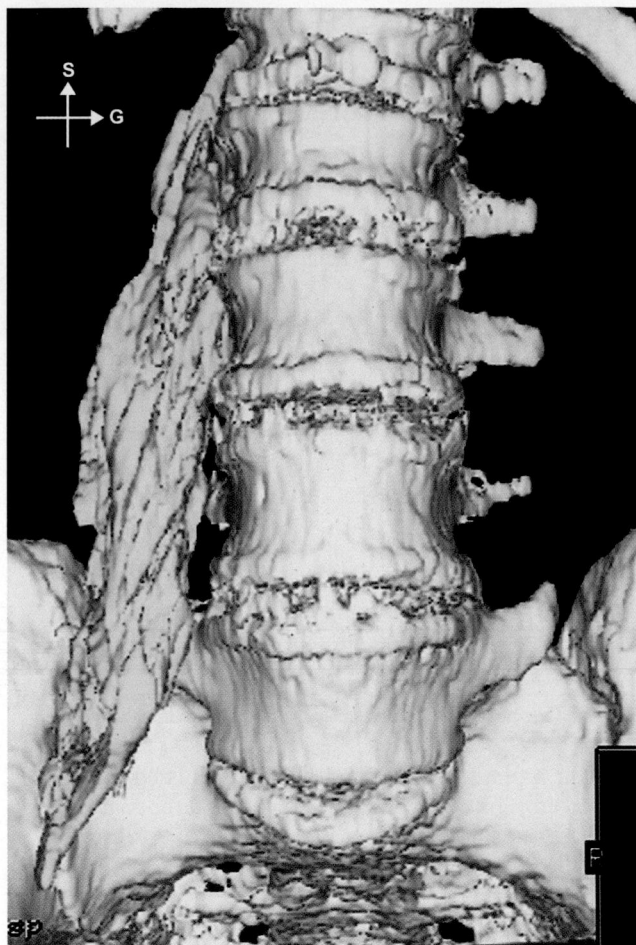

Figure 33–7. Distribution of 20 mL of injectate after lumbar plexus block. Shown is typical fusiform distribution within the psoas muscle.

large volumes required for this block and the intramuscular location of the needle.[33] This block is best avoided in anticoagulated patients.[31] Table 33–3 provides some general and

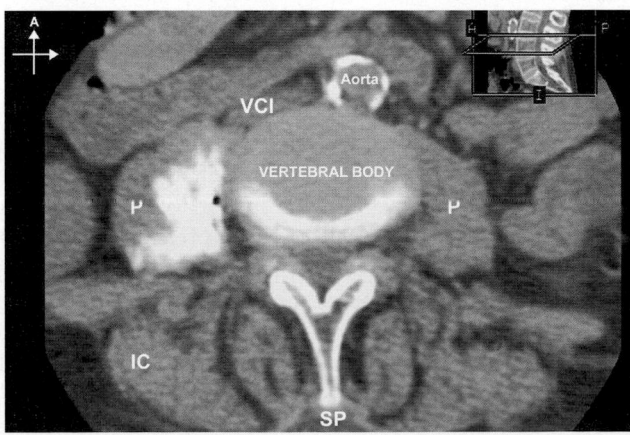

Figure 33–8. An MRI image demonstrating distribution of local anesthetic after lumbar plexus block. (A, anterior; I, inferior; IC, iliac crest; P (large), posterior; p, psoas muscle; S, spinous process; VCI, vena cava inferior.)

Table 33–3.	
Instructions on How to Avoid Complications	
Complication	**Instruction**
Infection	• A strict aseptic technique is used
Hematoma	• Avoid multiple needle insertions, particularly in anticoagulated patients • Avoid continuous lumbar plexus blocks in anticoagulated patients; however, once the catheter is placed, we use it even in patients on thromboembolic prophylaxis, such as low-molecular-weight and subcutaneous heparin therapy • Antiplatelet therapy is not a contraindication for lumbar plexus block in the absence of spontaneous bleeding
Vascular puncture	• Generally not common with this technique • Deep needle insertion should be avoided (vena cava, aorta)
Local anesthetic toxicity	• Systemic toxicity after sciatic blockade may be more common than with plexus blocks because of the location of the plexus in the proximity of large muscle beds • Higher volumes result in more solid, complete, and faster blockade, but they carry a higher risk of toxicity • Large volumes of long-acting anesthetic should be reconsidered in older and frail patients • Careful and frequent aspiration should be performed during the injection • Avoid forceful, fast injection of local anesthetic
Nerve injury	• Risk after lumbar plexus block is low • Local anesthetic should never be injected when the patient complains of pain or when abnormally high pressure on injection is noted • When stimulation is obtained with current intensity of <0.5 mA, the needle should be pulled back to obtain the same response with a current of 0.5 mA before injecting local anesthetic to avoid injection into the dural sleeves and the consequent epidural or spinal spread
Hemodynamic consequences	• Lumbar plexus blockade results in unilateral sympathectomy; as such, significant hypotension is rare • Spread of the local anesthetic to the epidural space may result in significant hypotension and occurs in up to 15% of patients • Every patient receiving a lumbar plexus block should be monitored to the same extent as patients receiving epidural anesthesia

specific instructions on possible complications and methods to avoid.

Summary

The main advantage of the lumbar plexus block over femoral nerve block is the ability to provide anesthesia or analgesia in the territories of the obturator nerve and lateral femoral cutaneous nerve of the thigh in addition to the block of the femoral nerve. However, this coverage requires a lare volume of local anesthetic or injections at two different spinal levels. Lumbar plexus block is an advanced regional anesthesia technique; experience with basic nerve block procedures is a prerequisite for its mastery and successful application in clinical practice. The proximity of the neuraxis requires astute monitoring to avoid the consequences of a high neuraxial block, which can occur even with a proper technique.

References

1. de Takats G: *Local Anesthesia.* WB Saunders, 1928.
2. Labat G: *Regional Anesthesia. In Its Technic and Clinical Application,* 2nd ed. WB Saunders, 1924.
3. Sherwood-Dunn B: *Regional Anesthesia.* FA Davis, 1920.
4. Dogliotti A: *Narcosis—Local-Regional-Spinal.* SB Debour, 1939.
5. Mannion S, O'Callaghan S, Walsh M, et al: In with the new, out with the old? Comparison of two approaches for psoas compartment block. Anesth Analg 2005;101:259–264.
6. Awad IT, Duggan EM: Posterior lumbar plexus block: Anatomy, approaches, and techniques. Reg Anesth Pain Med 2005;30:143–149.
7. Chayen D, Nathan H, Chayen M: The psoas compartment block. Anesthesiology 1976;45:95–99.
8. Molina Monleon I, Asensio Romero I, Barrio Mataix J, et al: [Epidural anesthesia after posterior lumbar plexus block]. Rev Esp Anestesiol Reanim 2005;52:55–56.

9. Kirchmair L, Entner T, Wissel J, et al: A study of the paravertebral anatomy for ultrasound-guided posterior lumbar plexus block. Anesth Analg 2001;93:477–478.

10. Capdevilla X, Macaire P, Dadure C, et al: Continuous psoas compartment blocks for postoperative analgesia after total hip arthroplasty: New landmarks, technical guidelines, and clinical evaluation. Anesth Analg 2002;94:1606–1613.

11. Indelli PF, Grant SA, Nielsen K, et al: Regional anesthesia in hip surgery. Clin Orthop Relat Res 2005;441:250–205.

12. Watson MW, Mitra D, McLintock TC, Grant SA: Continuous versus single-injection lumbar plexus blocks: Comparison of the effects on morphine use and early recovery after total knee arthroplasty. Reg Anesth Pain Med 2005;30:541–547.

13. Luber MJ, Greengrass R, Vail TP: Patient satisfaction and effectiveness of lumbar plexus and sciatic nerve block for total knee arthroplasty. J Arthroplasty 2001;16:17–21.

14. Di Benedetto P, Pinto G, Arcioni R, De Blasi RA, et al: Anatomy and imaging of lumbar plexus. Minerva Anestesiol 2005;71:549–554.

15. Sim IW, Webb T: Anatomy and anaesthesia of the lumbar somatic plexus. Anaesth Intensive Care 2004;32:178–187.

16. Farny J, Drolet P, Girard M: Anatomy of the posterior approach to the lumbar plexus block. Can J Anaesth 1994;41:480–485.

17. Mannion S, Barrett J, Kelly D, et al: A description of the spread of injectate after psoas compartment block using magnetic resonance imaging. Reg Anesth Pain Med 2005;30:567–571.

18. Khy V, Girard M: [The use of 2-chloroprocaine for a combined lumbar plexus and sciatic nerve block]. Can J Anaesth 1994;41:919–924.

19. Hadzic A, Karaca PE, Hobeika P, et al: Peripheral nerve blocks result in superior recovery profile compared with general anesthesia in outpatient knee arthroscopy. Anesth Analg 2005;100:976–981.

20. Chelly JE, Casati A, Al-Samsam T, et al: Continuous lumbar plexus block for acute postoperative pain management after open reduction and internal fixation of acetabular fractures. J Orthop Trauma 2003;17:362–367.

21. Bogoch ER, Henke M, Mackenzie T, et al: Lumbar paravertebral nerve block in the management of pain after total hip and knee arthroplasty: A randomized controlled clinical trial. J Arthroplasty 2002;17:398–401.

22. Litz RJ, Vicent O, Wiessner D, Heller AR: Misplacement of a psoas compartment catheter in the subarachnoid space. Reg Anesth Pain Med 2004;29:60–64.

23. Auroy Y, Benhamou D, Bargues L, et al: Major complications of regional anesthesia in France: The SOS Regional Anesthesia Hotline Service. Anesthesiology 2002;97:1274–1280.

24. Gentili M, Aveline C, Bonnet F: [Total spinal anesthesia after posterior lumbar plexus block]. Ann Fr Anesth Reanim 1998;17:740–742.

25. Farny J, Girard M, Drolet P: Posterior approach to the lumbar plexus combined with a sciatic nerve block using lidocaine. Can J Anaesth 1994;41:486–491.

26. Huet O, Eyrolle LJ, Mazoit JX, Ozier YM: Cardiac arrest after injection of ropivacaine for posterior lumbar plexus blockade. Anesthesiology 2003;99:1451–1453.

27. Mullanu CH, Gaillat F, Scemama F, et al: Acute toxicity of local anesthetic ropivacaine and mepivacaine during a combined lumbar plexus and sciatic block for hip surgery. Acta Anaesthesiol Belg 2002;53:221–223.

28. Pham-Dang C, Beaumont S, Floch H, et al: [Acute toxic accident following lumbar plexus block with bupivacaine]. Ann Fr Anesth Reanim 2000;19:356–359.

29. Hsu DT: Delayed retroperitoneal haematoma after failed lumbar plexus block. Br J Anaesth 2005;94:395.

30. Aveline C, Bonnet F: Delayed retroperitoneal haematoma after failed lumbar plexus block. Br J Anaesth 2004;93:589–591.

31. Klein SM, D'Ercole F, Greengrass RA, Warner DS: Enoxaparin associated with psoas hematoma and lumbar plexopathy after lumbar plexus block. Anesthesiology 1997;87:1576–1579.

32. Aida S, Takahashi H, Shimoji K: Renal subcapsular hematoma after lumbar plexus block. Anesthesiology 1996;84:452–455.

33. Blumenthal S, Ekatodramis G, Borgeat A: Ropivacaine plasma concentrations are similar during continuous lumbar plexus blockade using two techniques: Pharmacokinetics or pharmacodynamics? Can J Anaesth 2004;51:851.

34

Obturator Nerve Block

Hervé Bouaziz, MD • Vicente Roqués Escolar, MD • Xavier Sala-Blanch, MD

INTRODUCTION

Selective obturator nerve block was first described by Labat in 1922.[1] More interest in obturator nerve block emerged a few years later when Pauchet, Sourdat, and Labat stated, "obturator nerve block combined with blocks of the sciatic, femorocutaneous nerves, anesthetized the entire lower limb." However, a lack of clear anatomic landmarks, the block complexity, and inconsistent results were the reasons why this block had been used infrequently. Historically, Labat's classical technique remained forgotten until 1967, when it was modified by Parks.[2] In 1993, the interadductor approach was described by Wassef,[3] which was further modified by Pinnock in 1996.[4] In 1973, Winnie introduced the concept of the "3-in-1 block," an anterior approach to the lumbar plexus using a simple paravascular inguinal injection to anesthetize the femoral, lateral cutaneous nerve of the thigh and obturator nerves.[5] Since its

description however, many studies have refuted the ability of the 3-in-1 block to reliably block the obturator nerve with this technique. However, with the introduction of modern nerve stimulators, selective blockade of the obturator nerve has become more reliable and has seen a resurgence of interest in recent times.

Indications

Obturator nerve block is used to treat hip joint pain and is used in the relief of adductor muscle spasm associated with hemiplegia or paraplegia. Muscle spasticity is a relatively common problem among patients suffering from central neurologic problems, such as cerebrovascular pathology, medullar injuries, multiple sclerosis, and infantile cerebral palsy. Spasticity of the adductor muscle induced via the obturator nerve plays a major role in associated pain problems and makes patient grooming and mobilization very difficult. Obturator block, tenotomies, cryotherapy, botulin toxin infiltration, surgical neurolysis, and muscle interpositions all have been suggested to remedy this problem.[6-9] A number of diagnostic or therapeutic procedures on the knee and thigh can be performed by combining obturator nerve block with block of the sciatic, lateral cutaneous nerve and femoral nerves. Common clinical practice is to combine a sciatic nerve with the femoral nerve block for surgical procedures distal to the proximal third of the thigh. When deemed necessary, addition of a selective obturator nerve block may reduce intraoperative discomfort, improve tourniquet tolerance, and improve the quality of postoperative analgesia in these cases.

Obturator nerve block is also occasionally used in urologic surgery to suppress the obturator reflex during transurethral resection of the lateral bladder wall. Direct stimulation of the obturator nerve by the resector as it passes in close proximity to the bladder wall results in a sudden, violent adductor muscle spasm. This is not only distracting to the surgeon, but also potentially dangerous, increasing the risk of serious complications such as bladder wall perforation, vessel laceration, incomplete tumor resection, and obturator hematomas.[10,11] Prevention strategies include muscle relaxation, reduction in the intensity of the resector, the use of laser resectors, shifting to saline irrigation, peri-prostate infiltrations, and/or endoscopic transparietal blocks.[12-16] However, a selective obturator nerve block remains the safest and most effective alternative to this problem.[17-22]

Clinical Pearls

- The obturator reflex is not abolished by spinal anesthesia. It can be suppressed only by a selective obturator nerve block.

Neurolytic blockades with alcohol or phenol, performed with the help of a nerve stimulator and/or radioscopy, result in a cost-effective and effective reduction of muscle spasms.[3,9,23-26] The main drawback to neurolytic blockade is its temporal duration and the need to repeat the blockade when the previous block wears off. Selective obturator nerve block has also been used in the diagnosis and treatment of chronic pain states secondary to knee arthrosis or pelvic tumors resistant to conventional analgesic approaches.[27-31]

Contraindications

Patient refusal, inguinal lymphadenopathy, perineal infection, or hematoma at the needle insertion site are typical contraindications to obturator nerve blockade.

Preexisting obturator neuropathy, clinically manifested by groin pain, pain of the posteromedial aspect at the thigh and occasionally paresis of the adductor group of muscles, are relative contraindications to this block. Obturator nerve blocks should be avoided in the presence of a coagulopathy.

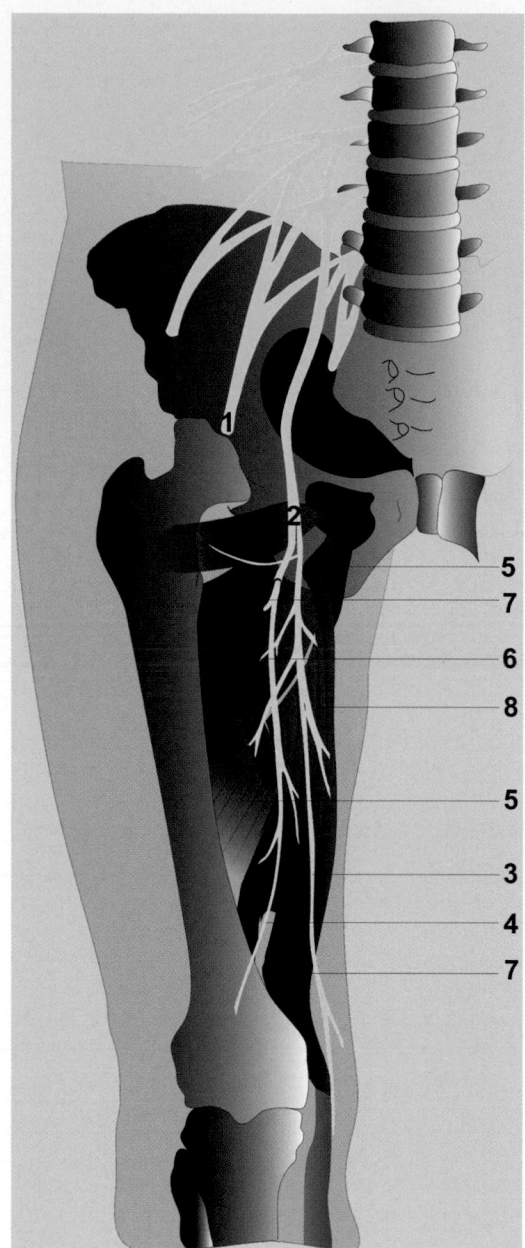

Figure 34–1. Anatomy of the obturator nerve. 1, Femoral nerve; 2, obturator nerve; 3, anterior branch; 4, posterior branch; 5, adductor longus; 6, adductor brevis; 7, adductor magnus; 8, gracilis.

Anatomy

The obturator nerve is a mixed nerve, which, in most cases, provides motor function to the adductor muscles and cutaneous sensation to a small area behind the knee. It is derived from the anterior primary rami of L2, L3 and L4 (Figure 34–1). On its initial course, it runs within the psoas major muscle. Taking a vertical course, it emerges from the inner border of the psoas, staying medial and posterior at the pelvis until it crosses at the level of the sacroiliac joint (L5) under the common iliac artery and vein and runs anterior/lateral to the ureter (Figure 34–2). At this level, it courses close to the wall of the bladder on its inferior/lateral portion

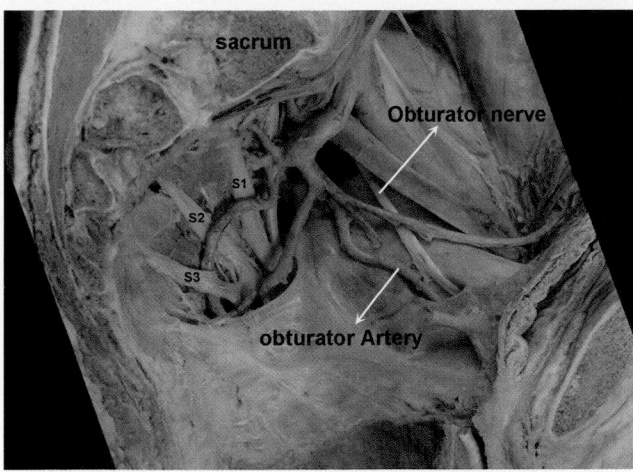

Figure 34–2. Intrapelvic trajectory of the obturator nerve. After crossing under the iliac vessels, the obturator nerve travels toward the obturator foramen via the lateral pelvic wall. During this course, the obturator artery and vein join the nerve, forming the obturator neurovascular bundle.

and then it takes place anterior to the obturator vessels within the superior part of the obturator foramen, exiting the pelvis below the pubic superior branch. In its intrapelvic course, the obturator nerve is separated from the femoral nerve by

the iliopsoas muscle and iliac fascia. It innervates the parietal peritoneum on the lateral pelvic wall and contributes collateral branches to the obturator externus muscle and the hip joint. It leaves the pelvis by passing through the obturator canal before entering the adductor region of the thigh (Figure 34–3). Here, 2.5–3.5 cm after leaving the obturator foramen, the obturator nerve divides into its two terminal branches, anterior and posterior, providing innervation to the hip adductor compartment (see Figure 34–3).[32]

The **anterior branch** descends behind the pectineus and adductor longus and in front of the obturator externus and adductor brevis. It gives muscular branches to the adductor longus, adductor brevis, gracilis, and occasionally the pectineus, and it terminates as a small nerve that innervates the femoral artery (Figure 34–4). In 20% of subjects, it contributes a branch, which anastamoses with branches of the femoral nerve and forms the subsartorial plexus, from which sensory branches emerge to supply sensation to posteromedial aspect of the inferior third of the thigh. The anterior branch contributes articular branches to anteromedial aspect of the hip joint capsule (Figure 34–5) but does not innervate the knee joint.

The **posterior branch** descends between the adductor brevis in front and the adductor magnus behind. It terminates by passing through the adductor hiatus to enter the popliteal

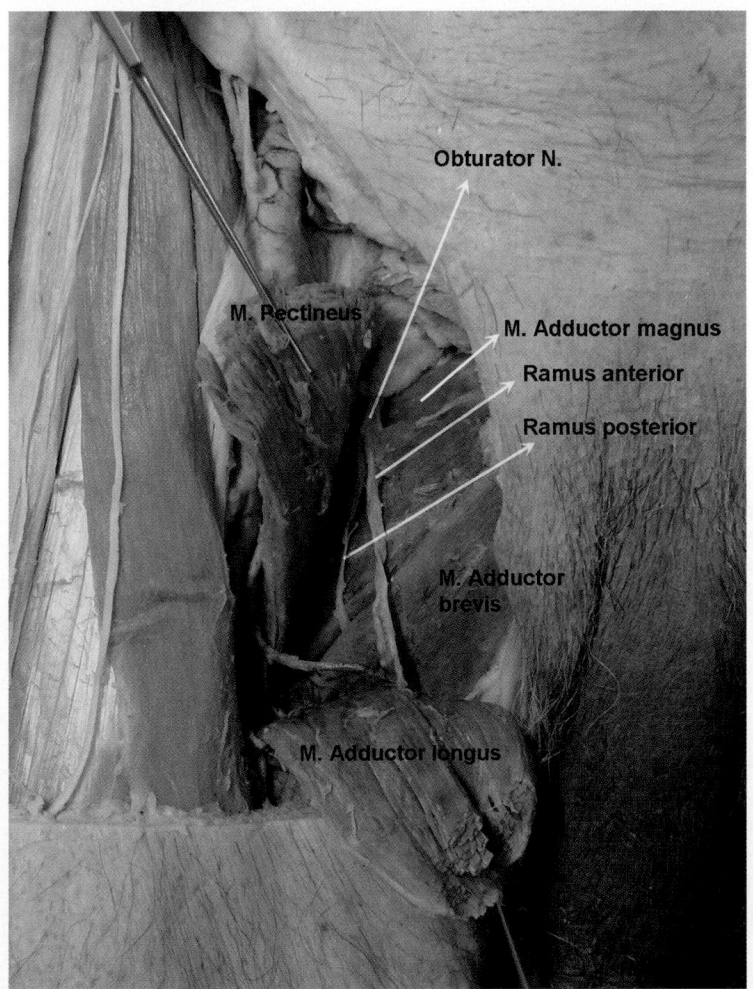

Figure 34–3. Distribution of the anterior and posterior divisions of the obturator nerve after exiting the obturator foramen.

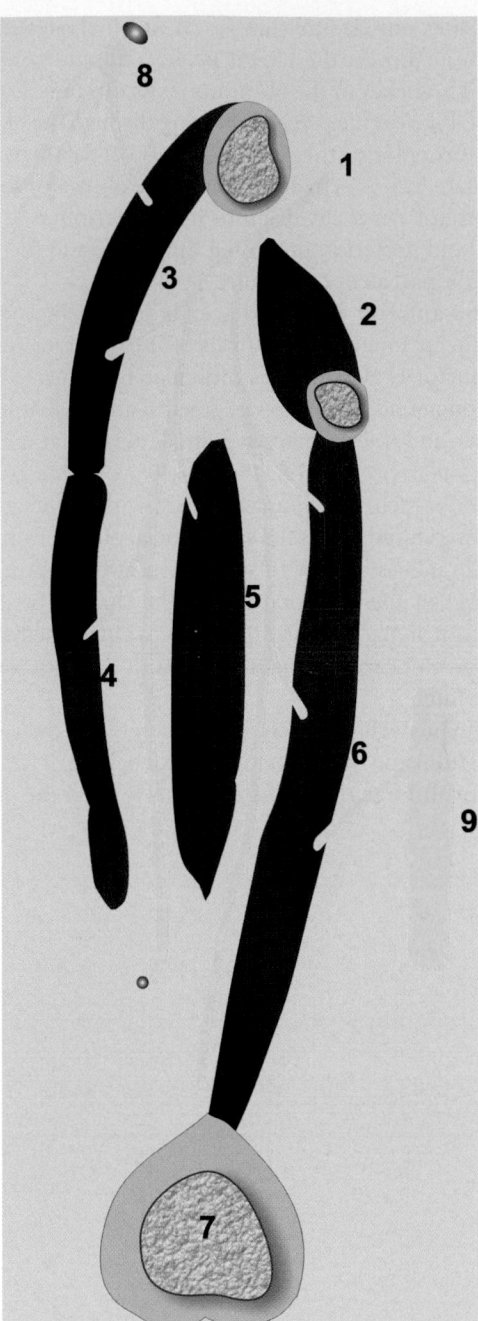

Figure 34–4. Sagittal section demonstrating the relationship of the obturator nerve to the adductor muscles. 1, Obturator nerve passing through the obturator canal; 2, obturator externus; 3, pectineus; 4, adductor longus, 5, adductor brevis; 6, adductor magnus; 7, medial femoral condyle; 8, femoral nerve; 9, sciatic nerve.

Clinical Pearls

- The functions of the muscles innervated by the obturator nerve are adduction of the thigh and assistance with hip flexion.
- The gracilis muscle assists knee flexion, and the obturator externus aids the lateral rotation of the thigh.
- Asking the patient to adduct the thigh therefore tests the function of the nerve. The patient should be supine with knees extended. The leg is then adducted against resistance while the examiner supports the contralateral leg.
- The paralysis (or block) of the nerve is characterized by a severe weakening of the adduction, although it is not completely lost as the adductor magnus (the most powerful adductor muscle) receives fibers from the sciatic nerve and eventually from the femoral nerve.

Anatomic Variants

Numerous variations to the formation, course, and distribution of the obturator nerve can have clinical implications. For instance, in 75% of cases, the obturator nerve divides into its two terminal branches as it passes through the obturator canal. In 10% of cases, this division occurs before the nerve reaches the obturator canal; in the remaining 15% of cases, after entering the thigh.

Occasionally, the anterior and posterior branches descend through the thigh behind the adductor brevis. Note that the sensory cutaneous branch of the obturator nerve is often absent.

Up to 20% of subjects possess an accessory obturator nerve that can be formed from variable combinations of the anterior rami L2-L4 or emanate directly from the trunk of the obturator nerve.[33] It accompanies the obturator nerve as it emerges from the medial border of the psoas but unlike the obturator, passes in front of the superior pubic ramus to supply a muscular branch, the pectineus. It contributes articular branches to the hip joint and terminates by anastomosing with the obturator nerve itself.

Equipment

To perform a block, the following equipment is required:

- Nerve stimulator
- Insulated stimulating needle (5–8 cm, depending on the approach chosen)
- Local anesthetic: 1% mepivacaine (onset of motor block 15 minutes, duration 3–4 hours) or 0.75% ropivacaine (onset of motor block 25 minutes, block duration 8–10 hours)
- Sterile fenestrated drape
- Marking pen
- Ruler
- A 10-mL syringe
- Disinfectant
- Sterile gloves

fossa, supplying the posterior aspect of the knee joint and the popliteal artery. During its course, the posterior branch sends muscular branches to the obturator externus, the adductor magnus, and occasionally the adductor brevis muscles (see Figure 34–4).

Cutaneous innervation by the obturator nerve varies according to the authors and is illustrated in Figure 34–6.

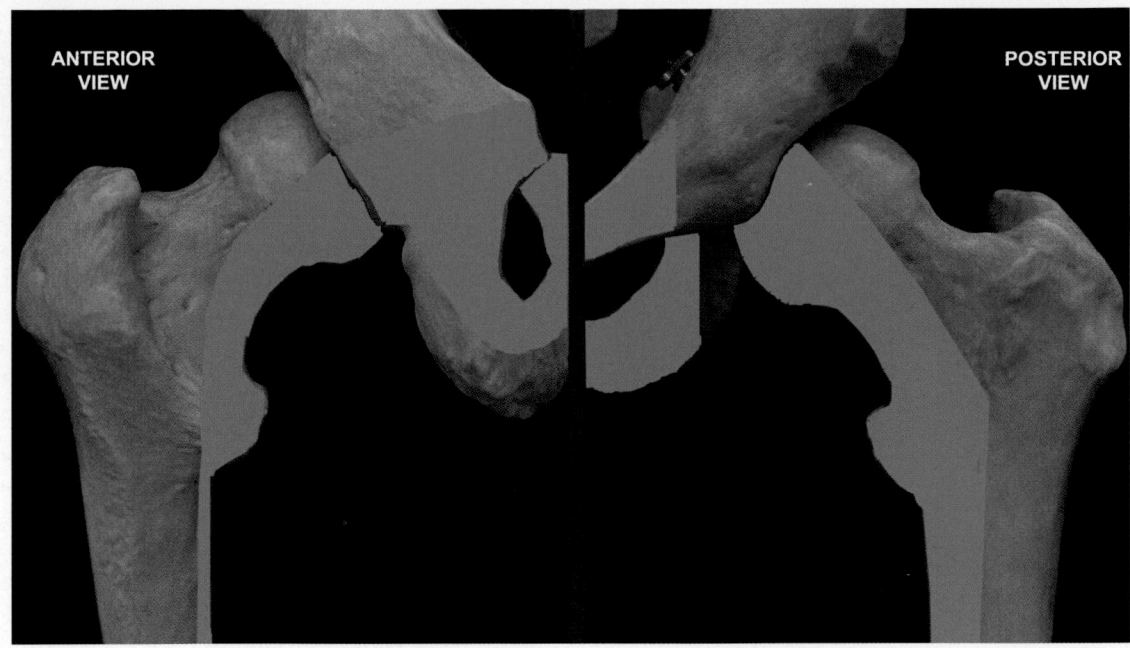

Figure 34–5. The role of the obturator nerve in the sensory innervation of the hip.

Landmarks

Anatomic landmarks vary depending on the chosen approach. The following landmarks are useful regardless of the approach chosen (Figure 34–7):

Bony landmarks: Anterior and superior iliac spine and pubic tubercle, inguinal ligament

Vascular landmarks: Femoral artery, femoral crease

Muscular landmarks: Tendon of the long abductor muscle

Techniques

Several methods can accomplish block of the obturator nerve. These approaches can be grouped into *plexus block techniques*

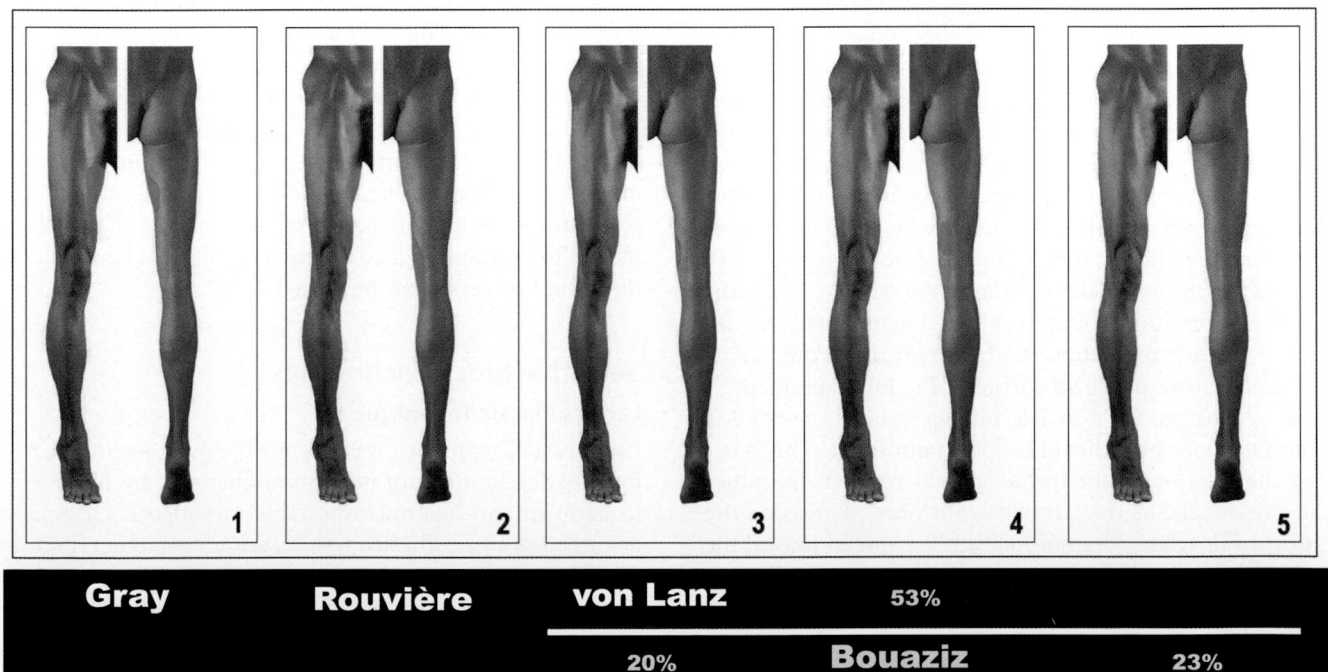

Figure 34–6. Skin innervation by obturator nerve according to different authors.

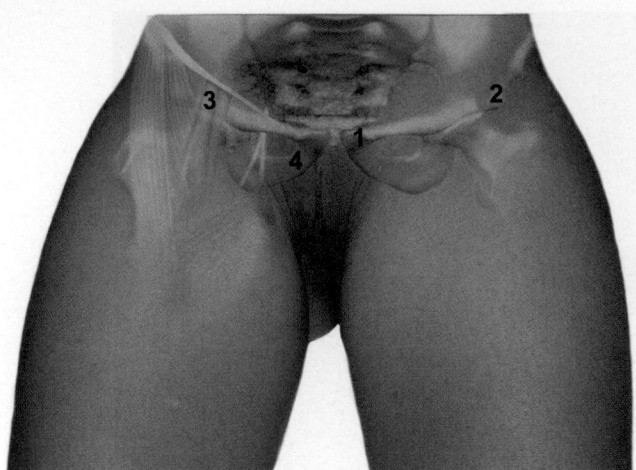

Figure 34–7. Anatomic landmarks for blockade of the obturator nerve. 1, Pubic tubercle; 2, anterosuperior iliac spine; 3, femoral artery; 4, tendon of the long adductor muscle.

where the obturator nerve is blocked along with other components of the lumbosacral plexus and *specific single-nerve block* techniques for the obturator nerve.

Plexus Block Techniques

Several approaches have been described; however, the lumbar plexus block via the posterior approach (in the psoas compartment) is the only technique that ensures an acceptable success rate of obturator nerve blockade.

3-in-1 Block Technique

Based on the theoretical existence of a suprainguinal compartment, in 1973 Winnie described the lumbar plexus block by an anterior approach or the 3 in 1.[5] According to the 3-in-1 concept, a large volume of local anesthetics is injected over the femoral nerve to spread underneath the fascia iliaca. When combined with distal compression, the local anesthetic spreads proximally reaching the lumbar plexus. Unfortunately, several studies have repeatedly failed to demonstrate the reliability of this technique to obtain a block of the lumbar plexus or the obturator nerve.[5,34–36] In addition, studies in human cadavers have documented the absence of a fluid-conducting compartment that would allow such an extensive proximal spread of the local anesthetic.[37] For these reasons, the 3-in-1 technique results in anesthesia of the cutaneous branches of the obturator nerve. This is because the local anesthetic spread laterally or medially, rather than proximally, as once thought. Of note, increasing the volume of injectate does not increase the spread toward the lumbar plexus; no differences were found when local anesthetic injection volumes of 20 or 40 mL were compared.[38] Theoretically, catheters inserted by an inguinal approach can ascend toward the psoas compartment, however, only a minor percentage (23%) of catheters can be reliably positioned.[39,40]

Iliofascial Block Technique

Dalens first described this approach in 1989 for use in pediatric patients.[41] Following Winnie's reasoning for the 3-in-1 block, he took a more lateral approach and reported a 100% success rate for femoral and femorocutaneous nerve blockade and 88% success rate for the obturator nerve. However, follow-up studies in adults did not confirm these results.[39,42] In adults, the iliofascial approach allows more successful blockade of the lateral femorocutaneous nerve when compared with the 3-in-1 technique. However, the obturator nerve remains spared.[42,43]

Psoas Compartment Block

Since Winnie's description of the posterior approach to the lumbar plexus in 1974 (psoas compartment block), numerous modifications of the technique have been described.[43,44–47] The obvious advantage is the ability to obtain a complete lumbar plexus block with a single injection. Indeed, studies have demonstrated femoral nerve block close to 100% plexus block with this technique, whereas femorocutaneous and obturator nerve blocks are anesthetized 88–93% of the time.[48,49]

Parasacral Sciatic Block

Mansour initially described this technique in 1993 with the objective of achieving a more complete sciatic nerve block.[50,51] Since this technique is a true plexus block, it provides more consistent anesthesia of all branches of the sciatic nerve. It successfully blocks the posterior cutaneous nerve of the thigh, the gluteal superior and inferior nerves, and the pudendal nerve. In addition, the splanchnic nerves, the inferior hypogastric plexus, the proximal portion of sympathetic trunks, and the obturator nerve are located close to the point of injection. Thus, a blockade of all these nervous structures would be theoretically achievable with a single injection. However, recent anatomic and clinical studies suggest that the parietal peritoneum and the pelvic fascia surrounding the sacral plexus are anatomically separated from the obturator nerve that runs along the medial border of the psoas. Consequently, although the parasacral approach to sciatic nerve block should result in a complete block of the sacral plexus, the obturator nerve may be spared.[52]

Selective Block Techniques

Labat's Classic Technique

Labat's classic approach was the most popular technique before the development of new approaches that are more easy to perform and less uncomfortable to patients. Originally described as a paresthesia method, the advent of nerve stimulation has increased the effectiveness and reduced patient discomfort, complications, and number of needle insertions. The procedure sequence consists of five phases, depicted in Figure 34–8.

Nerve stimulation is begun using a current intensity of 2–3 mA (2 Hz, 0.1–0.3 msec) and reduced to 0.3–0.5 mA

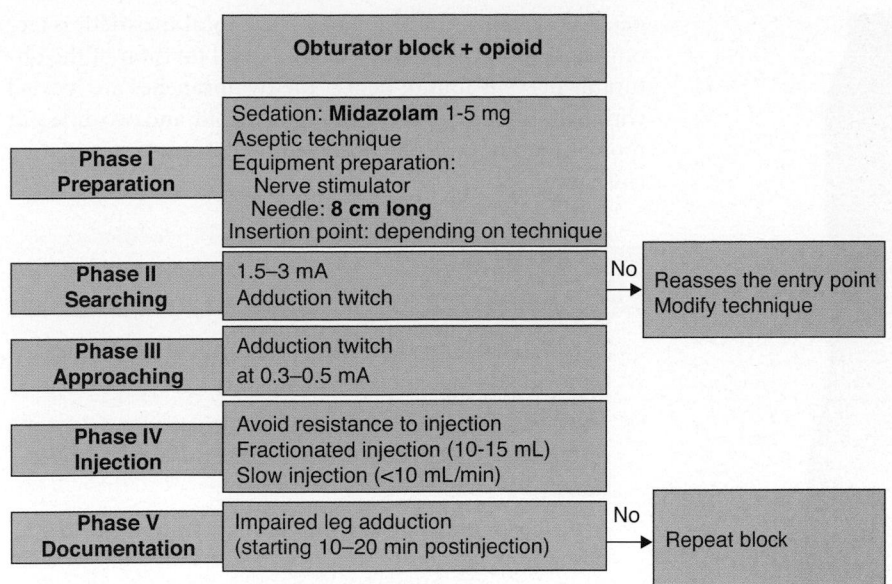

Figure 34–8. A practical algorithm to classical approach to obturator nerve block.

before injection of local anesthetic. The patient lies supine, with the limb to be blocked at 30 degrees abduction. The pubic tubercle is identified by palpation, and a 1.5-cm long line is drawn laterally and caudally; the injection insertion site is labeled at the tip of the end of the caudal line (Figure 34–9). The classical approach consists of carrying out three consecutive movements of the needle until the tip of the needle is placed over the top of the obturator foramen, where the nerve runs before splitting into its two terminal branches. With a 22-gauge, 8-cm long needle, the skin is penetrated perpendicularly and the needle is advanced until it makes contact with the inferior border of the superior pubic branch at a depth of 2–4 cm. During the second phase, the needle is slightly withdrawn and then slipped along the anterior pubic wall (another 2–4 cm). After this, it is redirected anteriorly/posteriorly. Finally, the needle is withdrawn again and slightly redirected (cephalically and laterally) at an angle of 45 degrees for another 2–3 cm until contractions of the thigh adductor muscles are observed.

This technique can be simplified by eliminating the second movement of the needle. Hence, after making contact with the pubic branch, the needle can be redirected 45 degrees laterally to the obturator foramen (see Figure 34–9).

Paravascular Selective Inguinal Block

This technique consists of a selective block of the two branches of the obturator nerve (anterior and posterior), performed at the inguinal level and slightly more caudad than the previously described techniques.[53] The femoral artery and the tendon of the long adductor muscle at the pubic tubercle are identified. For tendon identification, extreme leg abduction is required (Figure 34–10). A line is drawn over the inguinal fold from the pulse of the femoral artery to the tendon of the long adductor muscle. The needle is inserted at the mid-point of this line at an angle of 30 degrees anteriorly/posteriorly and cephalically (Figure 34–11). By following the needle a few centimeters in depth via the long adductor muscle, twitching

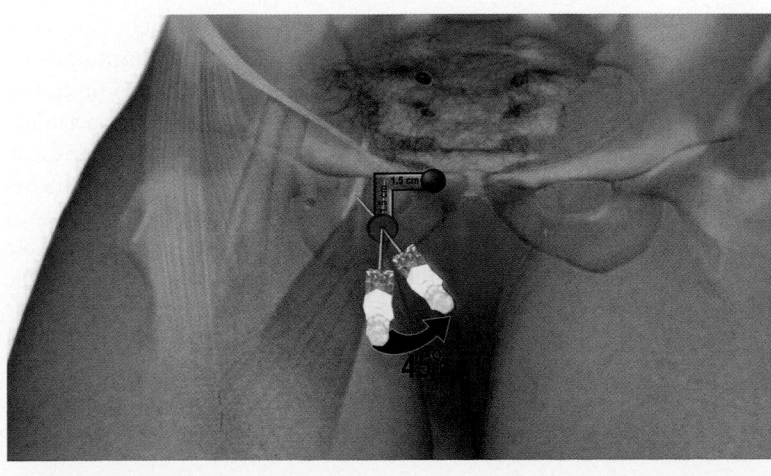

Figure 34–9. Obturator nerve block. Simplified Labat's classical technique.

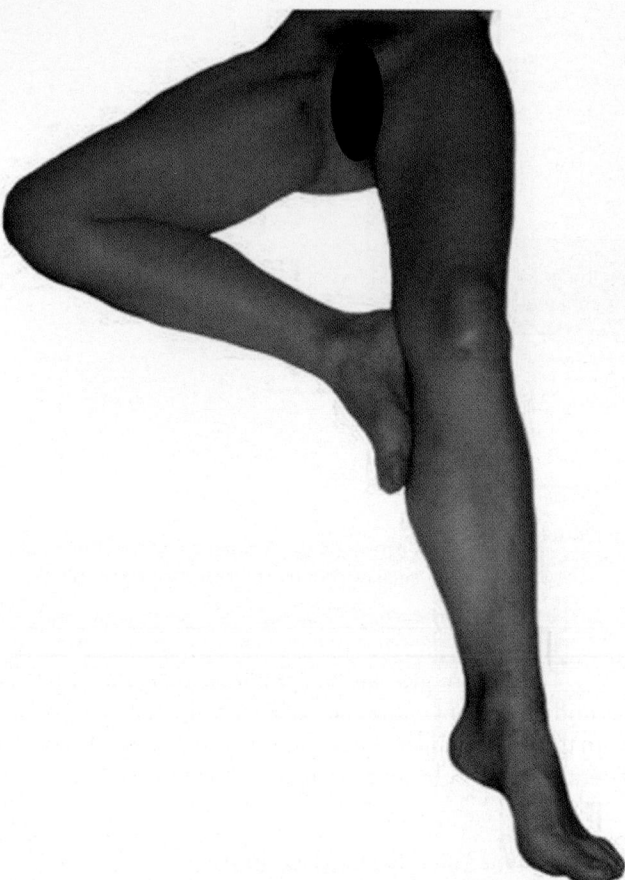

Figure 34–10. Paravascular selective inguinal approach to obturator nerve block. Leg abduction.

responses from the long adductor and gracilis muscles are easily detectable on the posterior and medial aspect of the thigh. Subsequently, the needle is inserted deeper (0.5–1.5 cm) and slightly laterally over the short adductor muscle until a response from the major adductor muscle is obtained and can be visualized on the posterior-medial aspect of the thigh. After

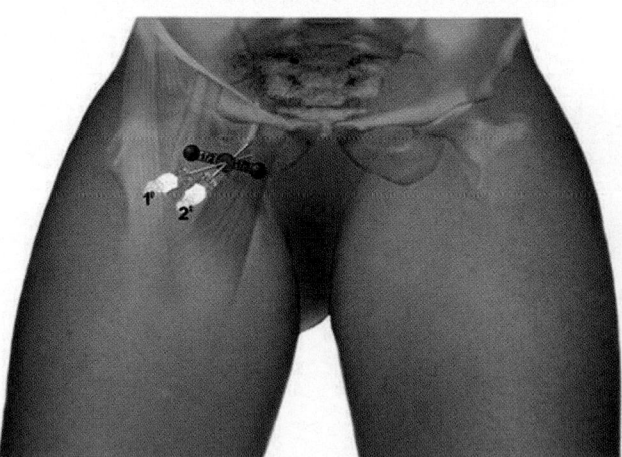

Figure 34–11. Paravascular selective inguinal approach to obturator nerve. Needle insertion and redirection.

needle insertion, infiltration of 5–7 mL local anesthetic is recommended. Occasionally, a more caudal division of the obturator nerve is found; hence, the two branches are located within the same location at the inguinal fold, and two different motor responses may be observed with a single stimulation (injection).

Clinical Pearls

- The inguinal approach to the obturator nerve is easier to perform and less uncomfortable to the patient.
- The needle insertion site with this approach is away from intrapelvic contents, resulting in lower risk of complications.
- Articular branches to the hip joint are not blocked with this approach

Choice of Local Anesthetic

Ten to 15 mL of local anesthetic are adequate in patients. The type and concentration of the local anesthetic depend on the indication for the block. For diagnostic–therapeutic blockades, highly concentrated neurolytic solutions are used to achieve long-lasting blocks. In the literature, combinations of phenol, ethanol, bupivacaine, levobupivacaine, and/or steroids are well reported.[3,9,23–26]

For lower limb surgeries, the recommended anesthetic technique consists of the administration of medium- to long-lasting local anesthetics that are associated with adequate postoperative analgesia, such as bupivacaine 0.25–0.5%; ropivacaine 0.25–0.75%, and levobupivacaine 0.25–0.5%. To avoid adductor muscle spasms during transurethral surgery, the use of medium to long local anesthetics is not required because the surgery does not last more than 2 hours. Therefore, mepivacaine 1–2% or lidocaine 1–2% should be adequate for this purpose.[17,54]

BLOCK EVALUATION

The onset of motor blockade is seen approximately 15 minutes after administration of 1% mepivacaine and 25 minutes after injection of 0.75% ropivacaine. Evaluation of an obturator block by sensory testing is unreliable due to the variability in its sensory distribution (see Figure 34–10). In some cases, the obturator nerve may not contain any sensory branches that can be clinically tested for adequacy of the blockade. In addition, even when a sensory branch is present, there is considerable overlap of cutaneous innervation from the obturator, femoral, and sciatic nerves. It is often erroneously thought that the skin of the medial aspect of the thigh is innervated by the obturator nerve; in fact, sensory branches of the femoral nerve contribute sensory innervation to this region.

Clinical Pearls

- Evaluation of an obturator block by sensory testing is difficult because of the variability in its sensory distribution.
- The most common sensory innervation of the obturator nerve is the skin in a small region located on the posteromedial aspect of the knee.
- A considerable overlap of cutaneous innervation exists among the obturator, femoral, and sciatic nerves.
- Reduction in adduction strength is the most reliable means of demonstrating successful obturator nerve blockade.

The area of skin most commonly regarded as having exclusive obturator nerve supply is a small region located on the posteromedial aspect of the knee. Also, the strength of the lower limb adductors relies 70% on the obturator nerve. Consequently, reduction in the strength of the adductors of the thigh is the most reliable sign of successful obturator nerve blockade. Adductor muscle strength can be objectively evaluated by comparing the maximal pressure exerted by the patient squeezing a sphygmomanometer that has been preinflated to 40 mm Hg and placed between the legs before and after block performance. Failure to demonstrate a reduction in adductor muscle strength from baseline is synonymous with block failure.

PERIOPERATIVE MANAGEMENT

Patients must be warned that ambulation may be impaired becauseof the blockade of the thigh adductors.

COMPLICATIONS

There are no reports of complications associated with obturator nerve block. The lack of reported complications, however, is more likely due to the infrequent use of this block rather than to its inherent safety. Needle orientation for the classical pubic approach of Labat is toward the pelvic cavity. Therefore, if advanced too far in a cephalad direction, the needle can pass over the superior pubic ramus and penetrate the pelvic cavity, perforating the bladder, rectum, and spermatic cord. Accidental puncture of the obturator vessels could result in unintentional intravasacular injection and hematoma formation. A retropubic anastamosis between the external iliac and obturator arteries (corona Mortis) is present in up to10% of patients: bleeding secondary to puncture of the corona Mortis can be difficult to control. Obturator neuropathy, secondary to needle trauma, intraneural injection, nerve ischemia, or local anaesthetic toxicity are also possible, as with other peripheral nerve block techniques.

References

1. Labat G: *Regional Anesthesia: Its Technique and Clinical Application.* WB Saunders, 1922.
2. Parks CR, Kennedy WF: Obturator nerve block: A simplified approach. Anesthesiology 1967;28:775–778.
3. Wassef M: Interadductor approach to obturator nerve blockade for spastic conditions of adductor thigh muscles. Reg Anesth 1993;18:13–17.
4. Pinnock CA, Fischer HBJ, Jones RP: *Peripheral Nerve Blockade.* Churchill Livingstone, 1996.
5. Winnie AP, Ramamurthy S, Durrani Z: The inguinal paravascular technic of lumbar plexus anaesthesia: The "3-in-1" block. Anesth Analg 1973;52:989–996.
6. Kim PS, Ferrante FM: Cryoanalgesia: A novel treatment for hip adductor spasticity and obturator neuralgia. Anesthesiology 1998;89:534–536.
7. Wheeler ME, Weinstein SL: Adductor tenotomy-obturator neurotomy. J Pediatr Orthop 1984;4:48–51.
8. Benzel EC, Barolat-Romana G, Larson SJ: Femoral obturator and sciatic neurectomy with iliacus and psoas muscle section for spasticity following spinal cord injury. Spine 1988;13:905–908.
9. Pelissier J: Chemical neurolysis using alcohol in the treatment of spasticity in the hemiplegic. Cah Anesthesiol 1993;41;139–143.
10. Akat T, Murakami J, Yoshinaga A: Life-threatening haemorrhage following obturator artery injury during transurethral bladder surgery: A sequel of an unsuccessful obturator nerve block. Acta Anaesthesiol Scand 1999;43:784–788.
11. Shulm MS: Simultaneous bilateral obturator nerve stimulation during transurethral electrovaporizacion of the prostate. J Clin Anesth 1998;10:518–521.
12. Prentiss RJ: Massive adductor muscle contraction in transurethral surgery: Cause and prevention; development of new electrical circuit. Trans Am Assoc Genitourin Surg 1964;56:64–72.
13. Shiozawa H: A new transurethral resection system: Operating in saline environment precludes obturator nerve reflex. J Urol 2002;168:2665–2657.
14. Biserte J: Treatment of superficial bladder tumors using the argon laser. Acta Urol Belg 1989;57:697–701.
15. Brunken C, Qiu H, Tauber R: Transurethral resection of bladder tumours in physiological saline. Urologe 2004;43:1101–1105.
16. Hobika JH, Clarke BG: Use of neuromuscular blocking drugs to counteract thigh-adductor spasm induced by electrical shocks of obturator nerve during transurethral resection of bladder tumors. J Urol 1961;85:295–296.
17. Atanassoff PG, Weiss BM, Brull SJ: Lidocaine plasma levels following two techniques of obturator nerve block. J Clin Anesth 1996;8:535–539.
18. Kakinohana M: Interadductor approach to obturator nerve block for transurethral resection procedure: Comparison with traditional approach. J Anesth 2002;16:123–126.
19. Deliveliotis C, Alexopoulou K, Picramenos D, et al: The contribution of the obturator nerve block in the transurethral resection of bladder tumor. Acta Urol Belg 1995;63:51–54.
20. Schwilick R, Wingartner K, Kissler GV, et al: Elimination of the obturator reflex as a specific indication for dilute solution of etidocaine. A study of the suitability of a local anesthetic for reflex elimination in the 3-in-1 block technic. Reg Anesth 1990;13:610.
21. Rubial M, Molins N, Rubio P, et al: Obturator nerve block in transurethral surgery. Actas Urol Esp 1989;13:79–81.
22. Gasparich JP, Mason JT, Berger RE: Use of nerve stimulator for simple and accurate obturator nerve block before transurethral resection. J Urol 1984;132:291–293.
23. Viel E, Pelissier J, Pellas F, et al: Alcohol neurolytic blocks for pain and muscle spasticity. Neurochirurgie 2003;49:256–262.
24. Viel E.J, Peennou D, Ripart J, et al: Neurolytic blockade of the obturator nerve for intractable spasticity of adductor thigh muscle. Eur J Pain 2002;6:97–104.

25. Kirazli Y, On AY, Kismali B, et al: Comparison of phenol block and botulinus toxin type A in the treatment of spastic foot aster stroke. A randomized double-blind trial. Am J Phys Med Rehabil 1998;77:510–515.

26. Loubser PG: Neurolytic interventions for upper extremity spasticity associated with head injury. Reg Anesth 1997;22:386–387.

27. Heywang-Kobrunner SH, Amaya B, Okoniewski M, et al: CT-guided obturator nerve block for diagnosis and treatment of painful conditions of the hip. Eur Radiol 2001;11:1047–1053.

28. Hong Y, O'Grady T, Lopresti D, et al: Diagnostic obturator nerve block for inguinal and back pain: A recovered opinion. Pain 1996;67:507–509.

29. Edmonds-Seal J, Turner A, Khodadadeh S, et al: Regional hip blockade in osteoarthrosis. Effects on pain perception. Anaesthesia 1982;37:147–151.

30. James CDT, Little TF: Regional hip blockade. A simplified technique for the relief of intractable osteoarthritic pain. Anaesthesia 1976;31:1060–1070.

31. Sunderland S: Obturator nerve. In: Sunderland S (editor): *Nerves and Nerve Injuries.* Livingstone, Ltd, 1968, pp. 1096–1109.

32. Whiteside JL, Walters MD: Anatomy of the obturator region: Relations to a trans-obturator sling. Int Urogynecol J Pelvic Floor Dysfunct 2004;15:223–226.

33. Falsenthal G: Nerve blocks in the lower extremities: Anatomic considerations. Arch Phys Med Rehabil 1974;55:504–507.

34. Parkinson SK, Mueller JB, Little WL, et al: Extend of blockade with various approaches to the lumbar plexus. Anesth Analg 1989;68:243–248.

35. Brindenbaugh PO, Wedel DJ. The lower extremity. Somatic blockade. In: Cousins MJ, Brindenbaugh PO (editors): *Neural Blockage in Clinical Anesthesia and Management of Pain.* Lippincott-Raven, 1998, pp. 373–394.

36. Atanassoff PG, Weiss BM, Brull SJ, et al: Electromyographic comparison of obturator nerve block to three-in-one block. Anesth Analg 1995;81:529–533.

37. Ritter JW: Femoral nerve "sheath" form inguinal paravascular plexus block is not found in human cadavers. J Clin Anesth 1995;7:470–473.

38. Seeberger MD, Urwyler A: Paravascular lumbar plexus extension after femoral nerve stimulation and injection of 20 vs 40 ml mepivacaine 10 mg/kg. Acta Anesthesia Scand 1995;39:769–813.

39. Singelyn FJ, Gouverneur JM, Gribomont BF: A high position of the catheter increases the success rate of continuous 3-in-1 block. Anesthesiology 1996;85:A723.

40. Capdevila X, Biboulet P, Morau D, et al: Continuous 3-in-1 block for postoperative pain after lower limb orthopedic surgery: Where did the catheter go? Anesth Analg 2002;94:1001–1006.

41. Dalens B, Vanneuville G, Tanguy A: Comparison of the fascia iliac block with the 3-in-1 block in children. Anesth Analg 1989;69:705–713.

42. Morau D, Lopez S, Biboulet P, et al: Comparison of continuous 3-in-1 and fascia iliaca compartment blocks for postoperative analgesia: Feasibility, catheter migration, distribution of sensory block, and analgesic efficacy. Reg Anesth Pain Med 2003;28:309–314.

43. Capdevila X, Biboulet P, Bouregba M, et al: Compartment of the 3-in-1 and fascia iliaca compartment block in adults: Clinical and radiographic analysis. Anesth Analg 1998;86:1039–1044.

44. Winnie AP, Ramamurthy S, Durrani Z, et al: Plexus blocks for lower extremity surgery. Anesthesiol Rev 1974;1:1–6.

45. Chayen D, Nathan H, Chayen M: The posterior compartment block. Anesthesiology 1976;45:95–99.

46. Hanna MH, Peat SJ, D'Costa F: Lumbar pexus block: An anatomical study. Anaesthesia 1993;48:675–678.

47. Schupfer G, Johr M: Psoas compartment block in children: Part I—Description of the technique. Pediatric Anesth 2005;15:461–464.

48. Pandin PC, Vandesteen A, d'Hollander AA: Lumbar plexus posterior approach: A catheter placement description using electrical nerve stimulation. Anesth Analg 2002;95:1428–1431.

49. Awad IT, Duggan EM: Posterior lumbar plexus block: Anatomy, Approaches, and Techniques. Reg Anesth Pain Med 2005;30:143–149.

50. Mansour NY: Reevaluating the sciatic nerve block: Another landmark for consideration. Reg Anesth 1993;18:322–323.

51. Morris GF, Lang SA, Dust WN, et al: The parasacral sciatic nerve block. Reg Anesth 1997;22:223–228.

52. Jochum D, Iohom G, Choquet, et al: Adding a selective obturator nerve block to the parasacral sciatic nerve block: An evaluation. Anesth Analg 2004;99:1544–1549.

53. Choquet O, Nazarian S, Manelli H. Bloc obturateur au pli inguinal: Étude anatomique. Ann Fr Anesth Réanim 2001;20:131s.

54. Fujita Y, Kimura K, Furukawa Y, et al: Plasma concentrations of lignocaine alter obturator nerve block combined with spinal anaesthesia in patient undergoing transurethral resection procedures. Br J Anaesth 1992;68:596–598.

Femoral Nerve Block

François J. Singelyn, MD

INTRODUCTION

The femoral nerve block is considered one of the basic nerve block techniques because it is relatively simple to perform, carries a low risk of complications, and results in a high success rate. When used alone, femoral nerve block is well suited for surgery on the anterior aspect of the thigh and for postoperative pain management after femur and knee surgery. However, when combined with a sciatic block, anesthesia of almost the entire lower limb from the mid-thigh level can be achieved.

Indications

Single-Dose Technique

When used alone, a femoral nerve block is well suited for surgery on the anterior aspect of the thigh and for superficial surgery on the medial aspect of the leg below the knee. Some examples include repair of the quadriceps tendon or quadriceps muscle biopsy, long saphenous vein stripping, and postoperative pain management after femur and knee surgery. Femoral nerve block significantly improves postoperative analgesia after knee surgery during the first 8–12 hours postoperatively.[1-5] However, when combined with a sciatic or popliteal block, femoral block provides anesthesia for entire lower leg or ankle surgery.

Continuous Technique

The primary indication of continuous femoral nerve block is pain management after major femur or knee surgery.[6-22] In addition, when compared with a single dose technique or placebo, continuous femoral nerve block significantly reduces postoperative morphine consumption in patients after total hip replacement.[23,24] For this application, the technique is as efficient as IV patient-controlled analgesia (PCA) with morphine or patient-controlled epidural analgesia, and it results in fewer technical problems and side effects.[13]

Continuous femoral nerve block provides excellent analgesia in patients with femoral shaft or femoral neck fractures.[14,15,21,25] Its relative simplicity makes it uniquely suitable for analgesia in the emergency room and facilitate physical and radiologic examinations as well as manipulations of the fractured femur or hip.

After major knee surgery, continuous femoral nerve block provides better pain relief than parenteral administration of opioids (IV PCA, intramuscular)[7,12,16,17,20] or intraarticular analgesia.[18,26] For knee surgery, continuous femoral block is as effective as continuous lumbar plexus block[27] or continuous epidural analgesia,[12,20] with fewer risks of complications. Because this technique results in faster postoperative knee rehabilitation than IV PCA with morphine and fewer side effects than epidural analgesia, continuous femoral nerve block is probably the analgesic technique of choice in patients after total knee arthroplasty.[7,12,20,28]

Contraindications

Relative contraindications for femoral nerve block may include previous ilioinguinal surgery (femoral vascular graft, kidney transplantation), large inguinal lymph nodes or tumor, local infection, peritoneal infection, and preexisting femoral neuropathy.

Anatomy

The femoral nerve is the largest nerve of the lumbar plexus. It is formed by the dorsal divisions of the anterior rami of the L2, L3, and L4 spinal nerves. It emerges from the lateral border of the psoas muscle, approximately at the junction of the middle and lower thirds of that muscle. Along its course to the thigh, it remains deep to fascia iliaca. It enters the thigh posterior to the inguinal ligament, where it is positioned immediately lateral and slightly posterior to the femoral artery (Figure 35–1). At this level, it is situated deep to fascia lata (Figure 35–2). As the nerve passes into the thigh, it divides into anterior and posterior branches (Figure 35–3). Located above the fascia iliaca, the anterior branches innervate the sartorius and pectineus muscles (Figure 35–4) and the skin of the anterior and medial aspects of the thigh.

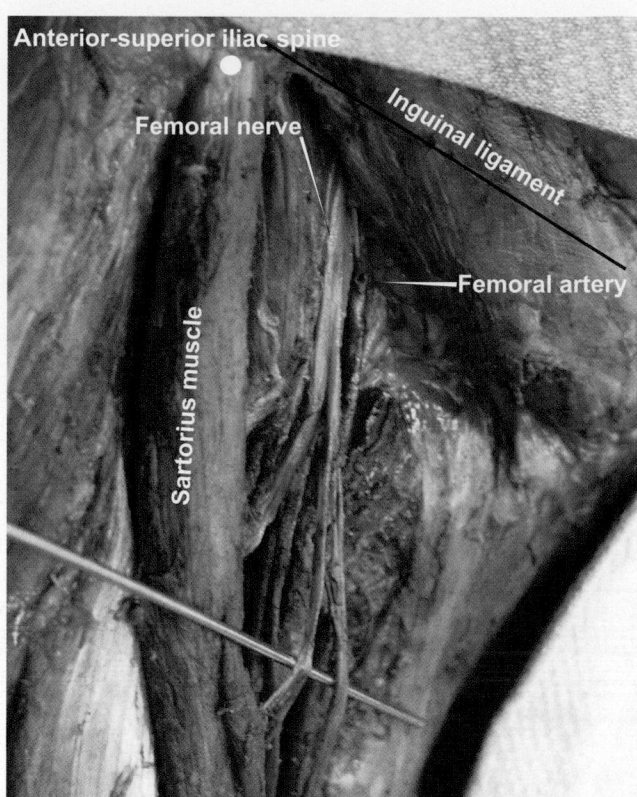

Figure 35–1. Anatomic relationship in the femoral triangle.

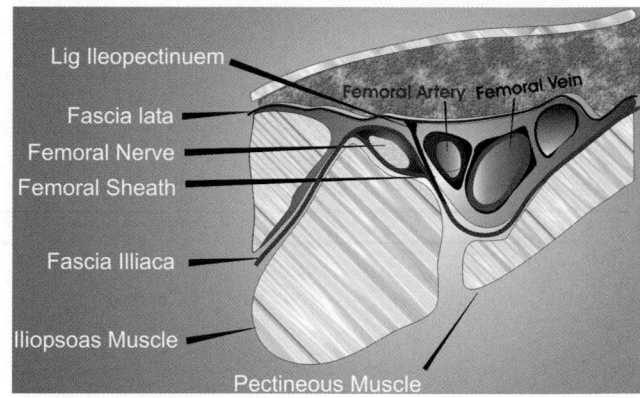

Figure 35–2. Tissue sheaths and femoral nerve. Femoral artery and vein relationships.

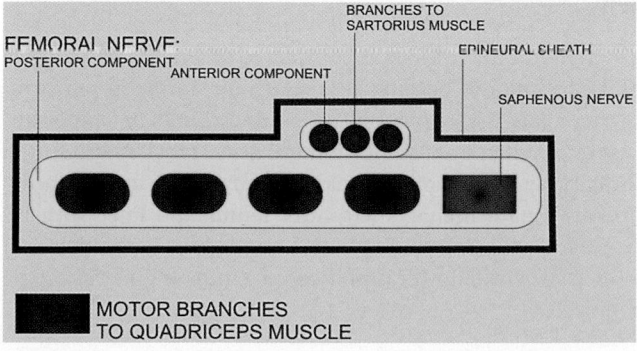

Figure 35–3. Composition of the femoral nerve at the level of blockade.

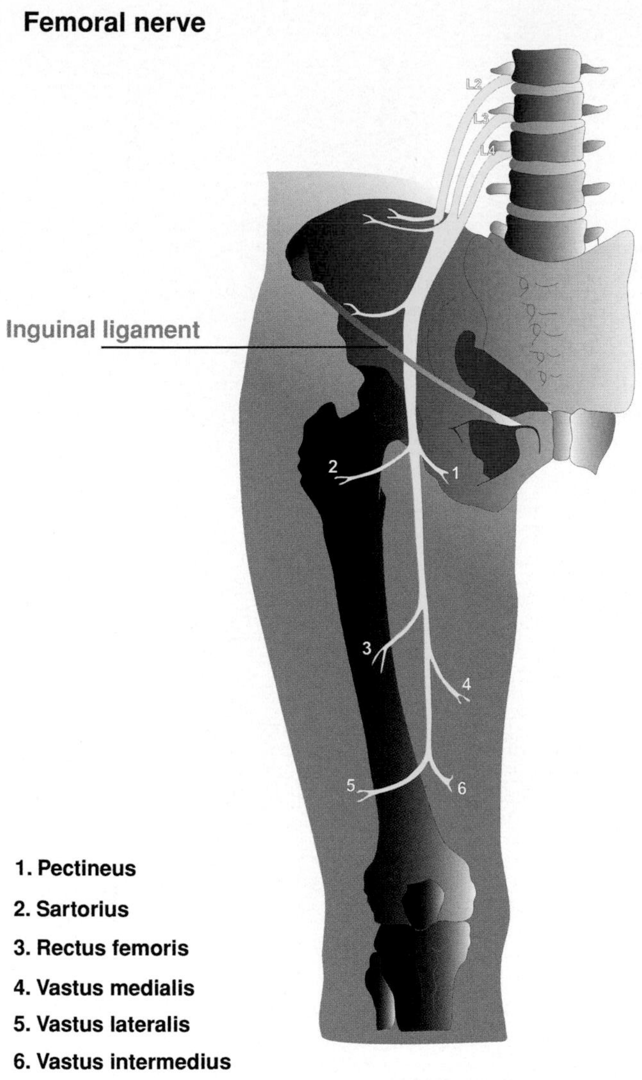

Femoral nerve

Inguinal ligament

1. Pectineus
2. Sartorius
3. Rectus femoris
4. Vastus medialis
5. Vastus lateralis
6. Vastus intermedius

Figure 35–4. Motor innervation of the femoral nerve.

Located under the fascia iliaca, the posterior branches innervate the quadriceps muscle and the knee joint and give off the saphenous nerve. The saphenous nerve supplies the skin of the medial aspect of the leg below the knee joint (Figure 35–5).

Clinical Pearls

- It is useful to think of the mnemonic NAVEL (nerve, artery, vein) going from lateral to medial when recalling the relationship of the femoral nerve to the vessels in the inguinal crease.

Landmarks

The following landmarks are used to determine the site of needle insertion: inguinal ligament, inguinal crease, femoral artery (Figure 35–6).

Clinical Pearl

- In obese patients, the identification of the inguinal crease can be facilitated by asking an assistant to retract the lower abdomen laterally (see Figure 36–7).

Equipment

A standard regional anesthesia tray is prepared with the following equipment:

- Sterile towers and gauze packs
- 20-mL Syringe with local anesthetic
- Sterile gloves, marking pen
- One 25-gauge, $1^{1}/_{2}$-in. needle for skin infiltration
- A 5-cm long, short-bevel, insulated stimulating needle
- A peripheral nerve stimulator and a surface electrode

BLOCK TECHNIQUE

Patient position. The patient lies in the supine position. The ipsilateral extremity is abducted 10–20 degrees.

Site of needle insertion. The site of needle insertion (see Figure 35–6) is located at the femoral crease but below the inguinal crease and immediately lateral (1 cm) to the pulse of the femoral artery.

Clinical Pearls

- Note that the description of the femoral nerve block technique provided here varies from the common description of this block, where the needle is inserted at the level of the inguinal ligament.[29]
- In fact, the femoral nerve is approached at the femoral crease, well below the inguinal ligament. This more distal needle insertion site prevents the possibility of insertion of the needle into the pelvis and allows insertion of the needle more tangentially.[30]
- This approach also facilitates insertion of the catheter when a continuous technique is performed.

Single-Injection Technique

After skin disinfection, local anesthetic is infiltrated subcutaneously. In obese patients, the lower abdomen is retracted laterally to allow access to the inguinal area (Figure 35–7). The needle is connected to a nerve stimulator set at a current intensity of 1.0 mA (0.1 msec/2 Hz) and introduced at 45-degree angle to the skin in a cephalad direction (Figure 35–8).

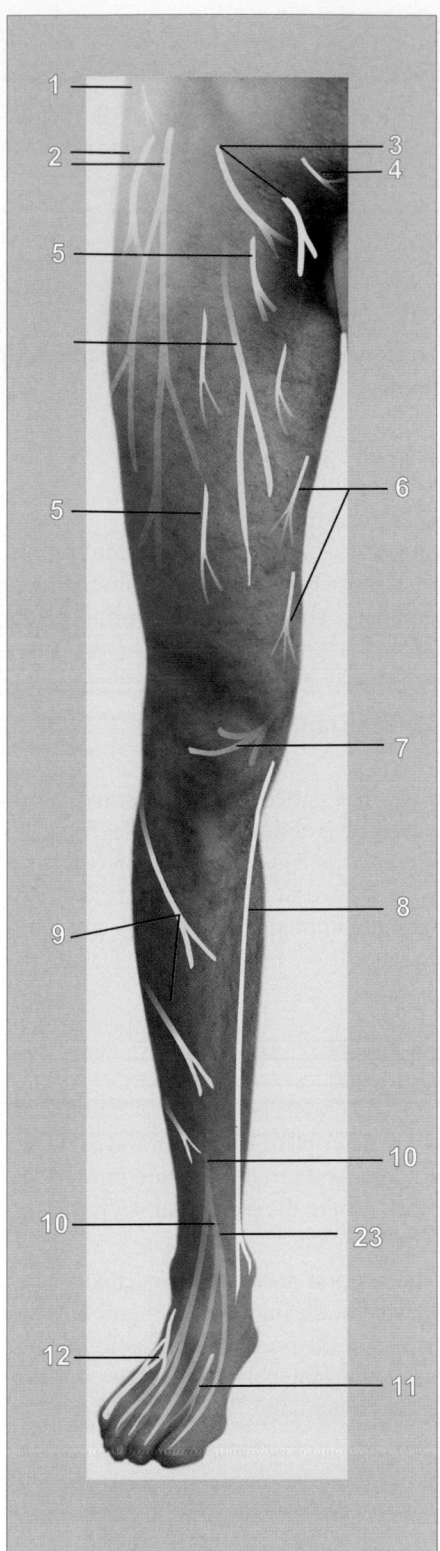

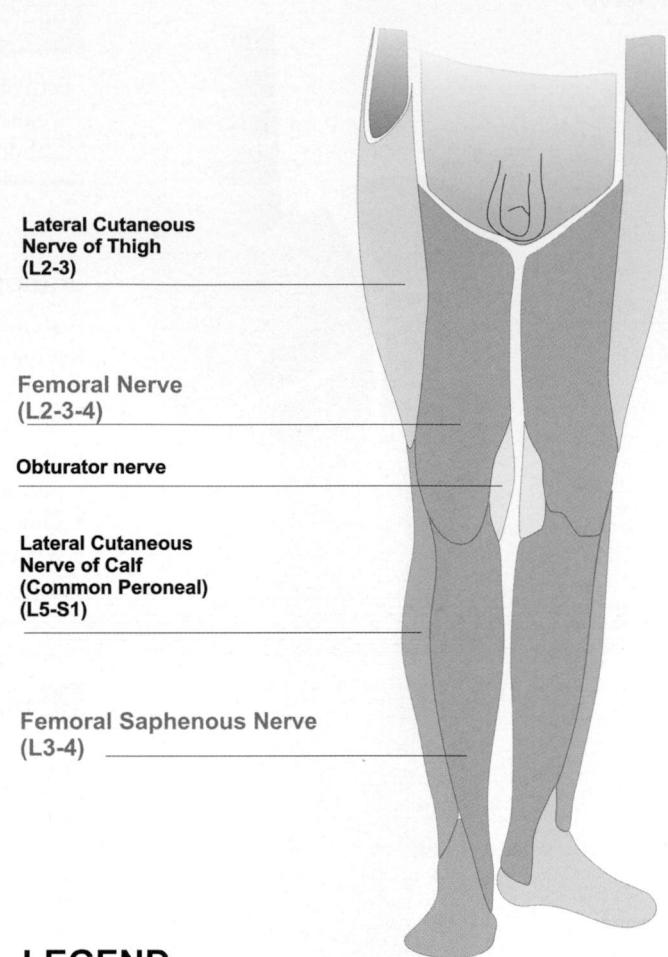

**Lateral Cutaneous
Nerve of Thigh
(L2-3)**

**Femoral Nerve
(L2-3-4)**

Obturator nerve

**Lateral Cutaneous
Nerve of Calf
(Common Peroneal)
(L5-S1)**

**Femoral Saphenous Nerve
(L3-4)**

LEGEND

1. Subcostal nerve (lateral cutaneous branch)

2. Lateral femoral cutaneous nerve

3. Femoral branch of the genitofemoral nerve

4. Genital branch of the genitofemoral nerve

5. Anterior femoral cutaneous nerve (from femoral nerve)

6. Cutaneous branches of the obturator nerve

7. Infrapatelar branch of the saphenous nerve

8. Saphenous nerve (terminal cutaneous branch of the femoral nerve)

9. Lateral sural cutaneous nerves (from common peroneal nerve)

10. Superficial peroneal nerve

11. Deep peroneal nerve

12. Lateral dorsal cutaneous nerve (branch of sural nerve)

Figure 35–5. Sensory innervation of the femoral nerve and distribution of anesthesia with femoral nerve block.

The needle is advanced through the fascia lata (a loss of resistance is often perceived, but not relied upon) until quadriceps muscle contractions (ie, patellar twitch) are obtained. The current output is then gradually decreased while the needle is advanced. The position of the needle is judged adequate when patellar twitches are elicited with current output between 0.2 and 0.5 mA. After a negative aspiration test for blood, 15–20 mL of local anesthetic is injected. Some

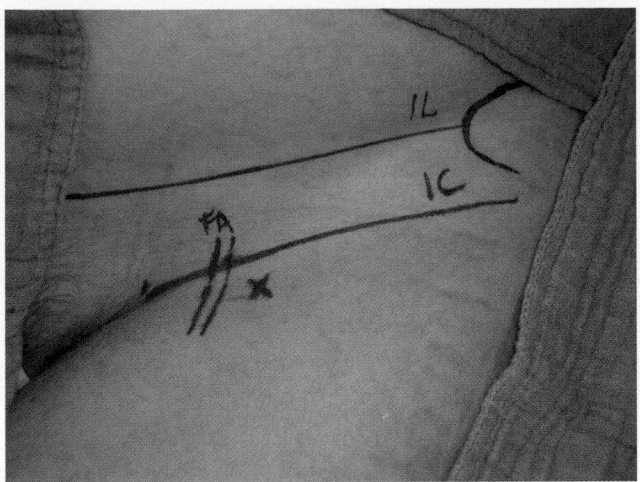

Figure 35–6. Anatomic landmarks for femoral nerve block. IL, Inguinal ligament; IC, inguinal crease; FA, femoral arterial pulse. The needle insertion site (*X*) is located just below the inguinal crease, 1–2 cm lateral to the pulse of the femoral artery.

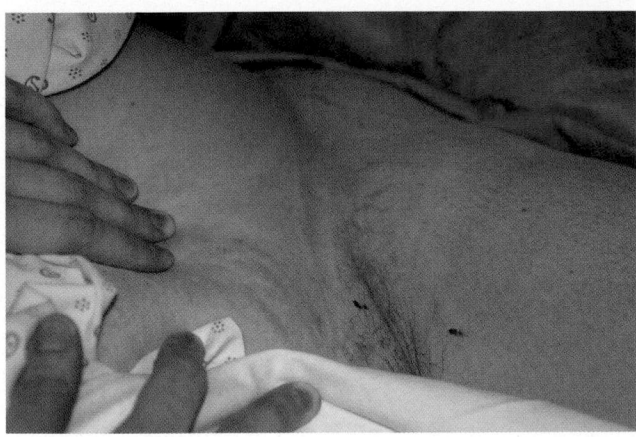

Figure 35–7. Maneuver to facilitate exposure of the anatomy during femoral nerve blockade: The lower abdomen in obese patients may obstruct the access to the femora/inguinal region. This can be remedied by simple retraction of the lower abdomen laterally throughout the procedure.

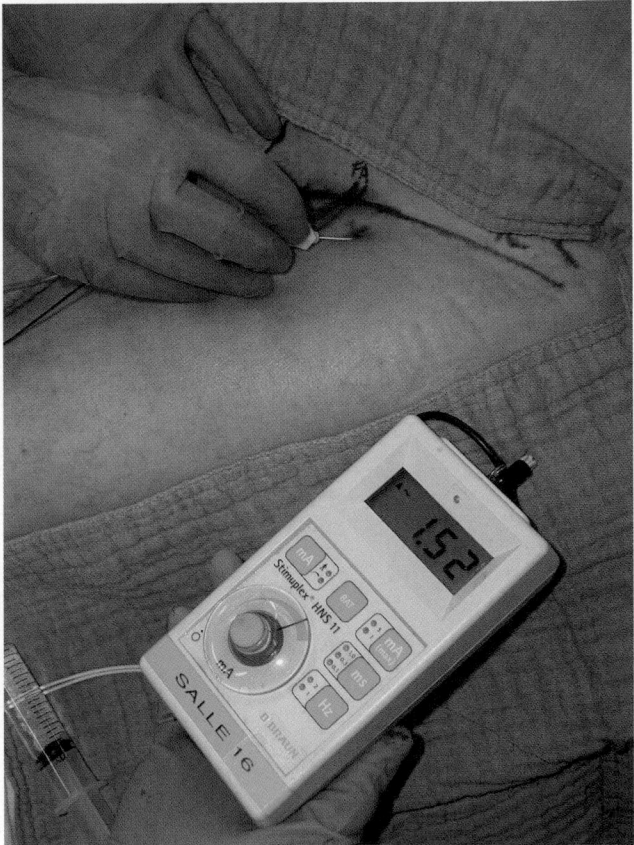

Figure 35–8. Needle insertion in femoral nerve blockade. The needle is connected to a nerve stimulator set at 1.05 mA current intensity and introduced at a 30- to 45-degree angle to the skin in a cephalad direction.

common responses to nerve stimulation and appropriate action to troubleshoot are featured in Table 35–1.

In an attempt to fasten the onset time and increase the safety of such block, a multiple injection technique, that is, elicitation of a vastus medialis, intermedius, and medialis twitch and separate injection of local anesthetic on each nerve branch, has been recently suggested.[31,32] When compared with a single injection, the volume of local anesthetic required to block the nerve and the onset time of anesthesia were significantly reduced. However, 14% of patients reported paresthesia, and 28% reported discomfort during block performance.[33] Therefore, more data and better injection monitoring techniques are necessary before this approach to femoral block can be widely recommended.

Clinical Pearls

- The sensation of "loss of resistance" may be better perceived when the bevel of the needle is oriented downward.
- The needle tip should be positioned below fascia lata and iliaca to obtain a complete femoral nerve block.
- Passage through the fascia iliaca may be difficult to perceive in some patients. In such circumstances, when patellar twitches are obtained, advance the needle deeper until it disappears. Increase the current output to 1 mA and withdraw the needle until the muscular twitches reappear. At this point, optimize the needle position.
- A volume of local anesthetic larger than 20 mL is frequently suggested in various texts. However, a larger volume is not necessary because it does not lead to better success rate.[34]
- A small dose (eg, 0.1 mL per 20 mL) of epinephrine to the initial bolus dose of local anesthetic solution may be added to rule out intravascular injection.

Table 35–1.

Common Responses to Nerve Stimulation and Action to Obtain Femoral Nerve Twitch

Response Obtained	Interpretation	Problem	Action
No response	The needle is inserted either too medially or to laterally	Femoral artery not properly localized or the palpating hand moved during the procedure	Follow the systematic lateral angulation and reinsertion of the needle as described in the technique
Bone contact	The needle contacts hip or superior ramus of the pubic bone	The needle is inserted too deep	Withdraw to the level of the skin and reinsert in another direction
Local twitch	Direct stimulation of the illiopsoas or pectineus muscle	Too deep insertion	Withdraw to the level of the skin and re-insert in another direction
Twitch of the sartorius muscle	Sartorius muscle twitch	The needle tip is slightly anterior and medial to the main trunk of the femoral nerve	Redirect the needle laterally and advance deeper 1–3 mm
Vascular puncture	Blood in the invariably indicates placement into the femoral artery	Too medial needle placement	Withdraw and reinsert laterally 1 cm
Patella twitch	Stimulation of the main trunk of the femoral nerve	None	Accept and inject local anesthetic

Continuous Technique

The continuous technique is similar to the single-injection technique. After passage through the fascia lata, the needle is advanced to elicit a patellar twitch using a current output between 0.2 and 0.5 mA (0.1 msec) (Figure 35–9). The catheter is then inserted 5–10 cm beyond the tip of the needle

or introducer. It is secured in place with a stitch tunnelling and/or a dressing. After a negative aspiration test for blood, a bolus dose of 20 mL of local anesthetic is injected and followed by a continuous infusion of dilute local anesthetic (Figure 35–10).

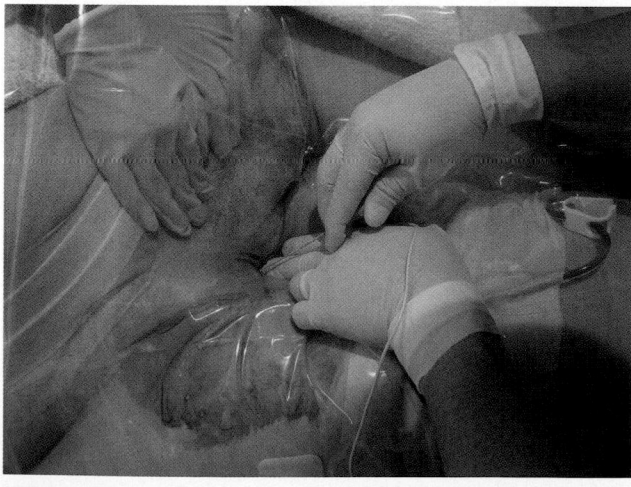

Figure 35–9. Continuous femoral nerve block: Needle insertion.

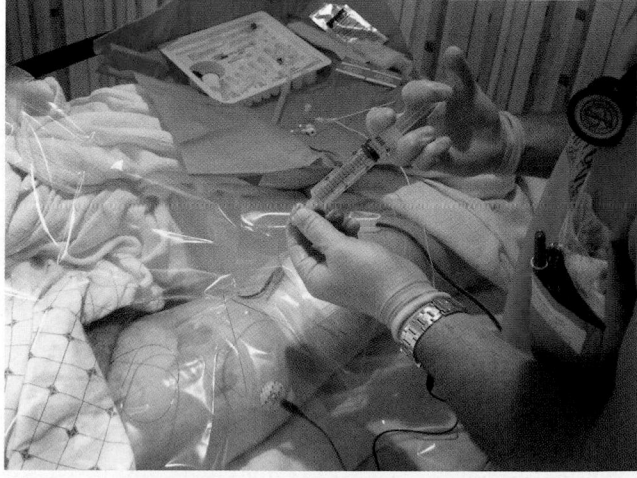

Figure 35–10. Testing the catheter for patency and accidental intravascular placement before initiation of continuous infusion of local anesthetic.

■ Catheter insertion should be without resistance. When this is not the case, the needle should be withdrawn to the skin and reinserted.

Block Assessment

Sensory blockade is assessed by cold or pin prick test on the anterior and medial aspect of the thigh (femoral nerve) and on the medial aspect of the leg (saphenous nerve). Motor blockade is evaluated by asking the patient to extend the knee (eg, to elevate the foot from the table).

CHOICE OF LOCAL ANESTHETIC

Single-Injection Technique

The choice of the type and concentration of local anesthetic should be based on whether the block is planned for surgical anesthesia or for pain management. Examples of onset times and mean duration of both anesthesia and analgesia with different types and concentrations of local anesthetic solution are presented in Table 35–2.

Table 35–2.

Onset and Duration of 20 mL of Local Anesthetic in Femoral Block

	Onset (min)	Anesthesia (h)	Analgesia (h)
3% 2-Chloroprocaine (+ HCO$_3$)	10–15	1	2
3% 2-Chloroprocaine (+ HCO$_3$ + epi)	10–15	1.5–2	2–3
1.5% Mepivacaine (+ HCO$_3$)	15–20	2–3	3–5
1.5% Mepivacaine (+ HCO$_3$ + epi)	15–20	2–5	3–8
2% Lidocaine (+ HCO$_3$ + epi)	10–20	2–5	3–8
0.5% Ropivacaine	15–30	4–8	5–12
0.75% Ropivacaine	10–15	5–10	6–24
0.5 Bupivacaine	15–30	5–15	8–30
(or L-bupivacaine)			

In our institution, when the technique is used to provide surgical anesthesia, 1% mepivacaine or 0.5% ropivacaine or levobupivacaine with epinephrine 1:300,000 is administered. When it is used only for postoperative analgesia, 0.25 ropivacaine or levobupivacaine with epinephrine 1:300,000 is injected.

■ The use of long-acting local anesthetics in outpatients who are expected to ambulate at home (eg, knee arthroscopy) should be avoided. The long-lasting motor block of the quadriceps muscle delays ambulation and carries a risk of falls at home.

Continuous Technique

Initial Bolus Dose

The choice of local anesthetic depends on the duration of surgery and whether the catheter is planned for surgical anesthesia or for postoperative analgesia alone. In our institution, when the technique is used to provide surgical anesthesia, 1% mepivacaine or 0.5% ropivacaine or levobupivacaine with epinephrine 1:300,000 is administered. When it is used only for postoperative analgesia, 0.2–0.25% ropivacaine or levobupivacaine with epinephrine 1:300,000 is injected. The spread of the local anesthetic after a bolus of 20 mL is shown in Figure 35–11.

Maintenance

The most suitable local anesthetic solution to maintain continuous femoral nerve block has not yet been determined. Most authors advocate the use of a dilute solution of long-acting local anesthetic such as 0.2% ropivacaine, 0.125% bupivacaine, or 0.125% levobupivacaine.[6–10,12,13,17,20,27,29] In our institution, we use 0.2% plain ropivacaine. Addition of clonidine to the local anesthetic infusion is not recommended

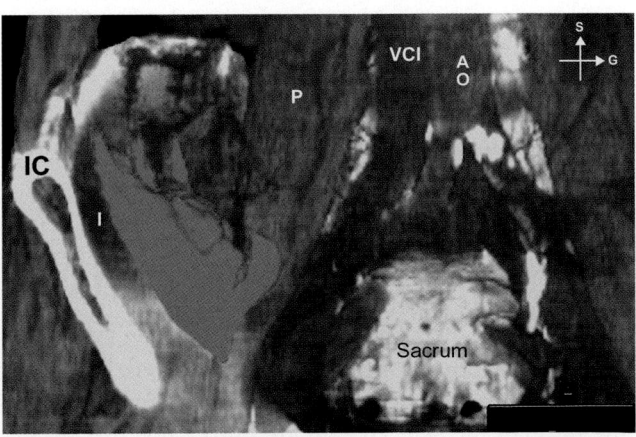

Figure 35–11. Distribution and spread of the injectate after femoral nerve block (20 mL). IC, Iliac crest; I, iliacus muscle; P, psoas muscle; VCI, vena cava inferior; AO, aorta; L, left side.

Table 35–3.	
Femoral Nerve Block: Complications	
Hematoma	• When the femoral artery or vein is punctured, the procedure should be stopped and pressure applied over the puncture site for 2–3 minutes.
Vascular puncture	• Maintain a palpating finger on the femoral pulse and insert the needle just lateral and parallel to the pulse. • Never redirect the needle medially.
Nerve injury	• Use a nerve stimulator. • Never seek paresthesia. Distinct paresthesia is almost never elicited with femoral nerve block and should not be sought or relied on to indicate an intraneural injection. However, should severe pain on injection is reported, abort the injection immediately. • Do not inject when high pressures on injection are encountered. • Use the minimal efficient volume and concentration of local anesthetic (eg, 20 mL 0.5%).
Catheter infection	• Use strict aseptic technique during catheter insertion. • Sterile drapes and generous application of antiseptic should be used with continuous techniques. • Remove the catheter after 48–72 hours (risk of infection increases with time).
Other	• Instruct patient on the inability to bear weight on the blocked extremity.

because it delays recovery of motor function without prolongation of analgesia.[35]

Several regimens of infusion through the femoral catheter have been recommended. Femoral perineural catheter can be managed by continuous infusion of a dilute local anesthetic solution (eg, 0.125% levobupivacaine, 0.2% ropivacaine) at the rate of approximately 8 mL/min.[6,7] A background infusion (eg, 5 mL/h) of 0.125% bupivacaine with small-volume (eg, 2.5 mL/30 min) PCA boluses provides excellent pain relief and a 32% reduction in the local anesthetic consumption.[8,36,37] The latter regimen also allows reinforcement of the block before a knee physiotherapy session. PCA boluses alone (eg, 10 mL/h^{-1}) achieved comparable results with a more significant reduction (58%) in the bupivacaine consumption. However, this regimen requires additional effort to educate the patients. Comparable results have been recently obtained when ropivacaine is used,[9] and also after total hip arthroplasty.[9] Thus, in most patients, a low basal infusion rate (eg 5 mL/h) associated with PCA boluses (eg, 2.5 mL–lockout: 30 minutes) could be recommended as the infusion regimen of choice to maintain continuous femoral nerve block.

PERIOPERATIVE MANAGEMENT OF FEMORAL NERVE BLOCKS

The performance of femoral nerve block is associated with minor patient discomfort because the needle passes only through the skin and adipose of the inguinal region. Regardless, patients should be premedicated to the level according to their own preferences. Femoral nerve block is associated with weakness of the quadriceps for the duration

of the blockade muscle. Knee extension and thus weight bearing on the blocked side are impaired. This must be clearly explained to the patient to prevent the risk of falls.

Complications & How to Avoid Them

Complications of femoral nerve block are relatively rare and may include[13] vascular puncture,[34] femoral nerve compression by a hematoma,[38] diffusion of the local anesthetic solution into the epidural space with resultant epidural block,[39] catheter shearing,[40] nerve injury and femoral dysesthesia (incidence of 0.25%).[13,41,42] With regard to continuous catheters, bacterial contamination of the catheter is common after 48 hours.[31,41,42] However, local or systemic infection remains rare, with the estimated risk of 0.13%.[43] Suggestions on how to decrease the risk of such complications is presented in Table 35–3.

SUMMARY

Femoral nerve block is easy to perform and associated with a low risk of complications. It is particularly suitable for catheter insertion. When used alone, it is well suited for surgery on the anterior aspect of the thigh and for postoperative pain management after femur and knee surgery. When combined with sciatic and/or obturator nerve blocks, anesthesia of almost the entire lower limb from the mid-thigh level can be achieved.

References

1. Fournier R, Van Gessel E, Gaggero G, et al: Postoperative analgesia with "3-in-1" femoral nerve block after prosthetic hip surgery. Can J Anaesth 1998;45:34–38.

2. Allen H, Liu S, Ware P, et al: Peripheral nerve blocks improve analgesia after total knee replacement surgery. Anesth Analg 1998;87:93–97.

3. Vloka JD, Hadzic A, Mulcare R, et al: Femoral nerve block versus spinal anesthesia for outpatients undergoing long saphenous vein stripping surgery. Anesth Analg 1997;84:749–752.

4. Yufa M, Kurc PE, Vloka JD, Hadzic A: Lower extremity blocks for analgesia. Reg Anesth Pain Med 2002;6:60–65.

5. Enneking FK, Chan V, Greger J, et al: Lower-extremity peripheral nerve blockade: Essentials of our current understanding. Reg Anesth Pain Med 2005;30:4–35.

6. Anker-Møller E, Spangsberg N, Dahl J, et al: Continuous blockade of the lumbar plexus after knee surgery: A comparison of the plasma concentrations and analgesic effect of bupivacaine 0.250% and 0.125%. Acta Anaesthesiol Scand 1990;34:468–472.

7. Ganapathy S, Wasserman R, Watson J, et al: Modified continuous femoral three-in-one block for postoperative pain after total knee arthroplasty. Anesth Analg 1999;89:1197–1202.

8. Singelyn F, Gouverneur JM: Extended "3-in-1" block after total knee arthroplasty: Continuous versus patient-controlled techniques. Anesth Analg 2000;91:176–180.

9. Eledjam JJ, Cuvillon P, Capdevila X, et al: Postoperative analgesia by femoral nerve block with ropivacaine 0.2% after major knee surgery: Continuous versus patient-controlled techniques. Reg Anesth Pain Med 2002;27:604–611.

10. Singelyn F, Vanderelst P, Gouverneur JM: Extended femoral nerve sheath block after total hip arthroplasty: Continuous vs patient-controlled techniques. Anesth Analg 2001;92:455–459.

11. Tetzlaff J, Andrish J, O'Hara J, et al: Effectiveness of bupivacaine administered via femoral nerve catheter for pain control after anterior cruciate ligament repair. J Clin Anesth 1997;9:542–545.

12. Capdevila X, Barthelet Y, Biboulet P, et al: Effects of perioperative analgesic technique on the surgical outcome and duration of rehabilitation after major knee surgery. Anesthesiology 1999;91:8–15.

13. Singelyn F, Gouverneur JM: Postoperative analgesia after total hip arthroplasty: IV PCA with morphine, patient-controlled epidural analgesia, or continuous "3-in-1" block? A prospective evaluation by our acute pain service in more than 1300 patients. J Clin Anesth 1999;11:550–554.

14. Ben-David B, Croituru M: Psoas block for surgical repair of hip fracture: A case report and description of a catheter technique. Anesth Analg 1990;71:298–301.

15. Capdevila X, Biboulet P, Bouregba M, et al: Bilateral continuous 3-in-1 nerve blockade for postoperative pain relief after bilateral femoral shaft surgery. J Clin Anesth 1998;10:606–609.

16. Serpell M, Millar F, Thomson M: Comparison of lumbar plexus block versus conventional opioid analgesia after total knee replacement. Anaesthesia 1991;46:275–277.

17. Dahl J, Christiansen C, Daugaard J, et al: Continuous blockade of the lumbar plexus after knee surgery – postoperative analgesia and bupivacaine plasma concentrations. Anaesthesia 1988;43:1015–1018.

18. De Andrés J, Bellver J, Barrera L, et al: A comparative study of analgesia after knee surgery with intraarticular bupivacaine, intraarticular morphine, and lumbar plexus block. Anesth Analg 1993;77:727–730.

19. Schultz P, Christensen E, Anker-Moller E, et al: Postoperative pain treatment after open knee surgery: Continuous lumbar plexus block with bupivacaine versus epidural morphine. Reg Anesth Pain Med 1991;16:34–37.

20. Singelyn F, Deyaert M, Joris D, et al: Effects of intravenous patient-controlled analgesia with morphine, continuous epidural analgesia, and continuous "3-in-1" block on postoperative pain and knee rehabilitation after unilateral total knee arthroplasty. Anesth Analg 1998;87:88–92.

21. Johnson C: Continuous femoral nerve blockade for analgesia in children with femoral fractures. Anaesth Intensive Care 1994;22:281–283.

22. Capdevila X, Biboulet P, Bouregba M, et al: Comparison of the three-in-one and fascia iliaca compartment blocks in adults: Clinical and radiographic analysis. Anesth Analg 1998;86:1039–1044.

23. Singelyn FJ, Ebongo F, Symens B, et al: Influence of the analgesic technique on postoperative rehabilitation after total hip replacement. Reg Anesth Pain Med 2001;26:39.

24. Boujlel S, Delbos A, Singelyn F: Continuous but not single-dose femoral nerve sheath block provides efficient pain relief after total hip replacement (THR). Reg Anesth Pain Med 2001;26:135.

25. Chudinov A, Berkenstadt H, Salai M, et al: Continuous psoas compartment block for anesthesia and perioperative analgesia in patients with hip fractures. Reg Anesth Pain Med 1999;24:563–568.

26. Dauri M, Polzoni M, Fabbi E, et al: Comparison of epidural, continuous femoral block and intraarticular analgesia after anterior cruciate ligament reconstruction. Acta Anaesthesiol Scand 2003;47:20–25.

27. Kaloul I, Guay J, Côté C, et al: The posterior lumbar plexus (psoas compartment) block and the three-in-one femoral nerve block provide similar postoperative analgesia after total knee replacement. Can J Anaesth 2004;51:45–51.

28. Chelly J, Greger J, Gebhard R, et al: Continuous femoral blocks improve recovery and outcome of patients undergoing total knee arthroplasty. J Arthroplasty 2001;16:436–445.

29. Winnie AP, Ramamurthy S, Durrani Z: The inguinal paravascular technic of lumbar plexus anesthesia. The "3-in-1 block." Anesth Analg 1973;52:989–996.

30. Vloka JD, Hadzic A, Drobnik L, et al Anatomical landmarks for femoral nerve block: A comparison of four needle insertion sites. Anesth Analg 1999;89:1467–1470.

31. Casati A, Fanelli G, Beccaria P, et al: The effects of single or multiple injections on the volume of 0.5% ropivacaine required for femoral nerve blockade. Anesth Analg 2001;93:183–186.

32. Casati A, Fanelli G, Beccaria P, et al: The effects of the single or multiple injection technique on the onset time of femoral nerve block with 0.75 % ropivacaine. Anesth Analg 2000;91:181–184.

33. Fanelli G, Casati A, Garancini P, et al: Nerve stimulator and multiple injection technique for upper and lower limb blockade: Failure rate, patient acceptance and neurologic complications. Anesth Analg 1999;88:847–852.

34. Seeberger M, Urwyler A: Paravascular lumbar plexus block: Block extension after femoral nerve stimulation and injection of 20 vs. 40 mL mepivacaine 10 mg/mL. Acta Anaesthesiol Scand 1995;39:769–773.

35. Casati A, Vinciguerra F, Cappelleri G, et al: Adding clonidine to the induction bolus and postoperative infusion during continuous femoral nerve block delays recovery of motor function after total knee arthroplasty. Anesth Analg 2005;100:866–872.

36. Esteve M, Veillette Y, Ecoffey C, et al: Continuous block of the femoral nerve after surgery of the knee: Pharmacokinetics of bupivacaine. Ann Fr Anesth Réanim 1990;9:322–325.

37. Kaloul I, Guay J, Cote C, et al: Ropivacaine plasma concentrations are similar during continuous lumbar plexus blockade using the anterior three-in-one and the posterior psoas compartment techniques. Can J Anaesth 2004;51:52–56.

38. Jöhr M: A complication of continuous femoral nerve block. Regional Anaesthesie 1987;10:37–38.

39. Singelyn F, Contreras V, Gouverneur JM: Epidural anesthesia complicating continuous 3-in-1 lumbar plexus blockade. Anesthesiolgy 1995;83:217–220.

40. Lee B, Goucke C: Shearing of a peripheral nerve catheter. Anesth Analg 2002;95:760–761.

41. Cuvillon P, Ripart J, Lalourcey L, et al: The continuous femoral nerve block catheter for postoperative analgesia: Bacterial colonization, infectious rate and adverse effects. Anesth Analg 2001;93:1045–1049.

42. Pirat P, Branchereau S, Bernard N, et al: Suivi prospectif descriptif des effets adverses non infectieux liés aux blocs nerveux périphériques continus: à propos de 1416 patients. Ann Fr Anesth Réanim 2002;21:R010.

43. Bernard N, Pirat P, Branchereau S, et al: Suivi multicentrique prospectif des effets adverses d'ordre infectieux sur 1416 blocs nerveux périphériques continus. Ann Fr Anesth Réanim 2002;21:R076.

36

Three-in-One Block

Peter Marhofer, MD • Stephan Kapral, MD • Xavier Sala-Blanch, MD

INTRODUCTION

The initial description of the 3-in-1 block was published by Winnie et al.[1] in 1973 involving a small number of patients. The authors postulated that a block of the entire lumbar plexus can be accomplished by a single perivascular injection slightly distal to the inguinal ligament. Consequently, a single injection should result in anesthesia of the femoral, the lateral femoral cutaneous, and obturator nerves. Winnie et al.[2,3] suggested that the underlying mechanism of this regional anesthetic technique should be a cephalad distribution of the local anesthetic along a fascial layer. This hypothesis, however, was never confirmed clinically. Moreover, an MRI study clarified the spread of local anesthetic after an inguinal injection of local anesthetic lateral to the femoral artery[4,5] and concluded that the distribution of local anes-

thetic follows a lateral and slightly medial direction, but never a cephalad direction. Figures 36–1 and 36–2 illustrate that the spread of local anesthetic does not follow a proximal direction.

One of the main proposed advantages of the 3-in-1 block was the ability to achieve block of the obturator nerve using this approach. However, most investigators have used clinical or electrophysiologic methods to analyze analgesia levels and involved nerves. In clinical practice, however, the obturator nerve has never been shown to be anesthetized effectively using this approach.[6,7] Cauhepe et al.[8] investigated the anesthetic route of the 3-in-1 blocks using standard pelvic radiography and computed tomography and reported two unexpected distributions of local anesthetic. The first type consisted of an internal distribution of local anesthetic toward the psoas major muscle. The second type was an external

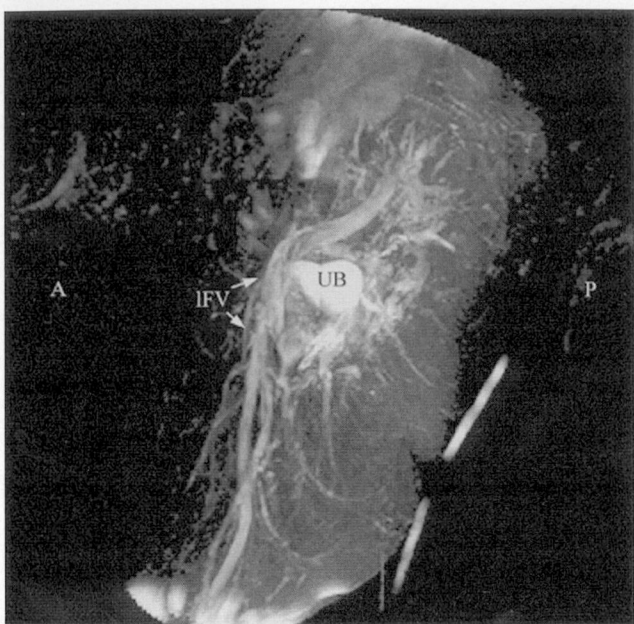

Figure 36–1. Relevant anatomy for the 3-in-1 block on sagittal T2-weighted MRI. (A, Anterior; P, posterior; lFV, left femoral vein; UB, urinary bladder.)

diffusion of local anesthetic in front of the iliac muscle. The main result of this study in human cadavers was that the local anesthetic never reached the obturator nerve. Capdevila et al.[9] reported that the local anesthetic used in 3-in-1 blocks spreads under the iliac fascia, but rarely to the lumbar plexus. Both techniques resulted in poor blocks of the obturator nerve.

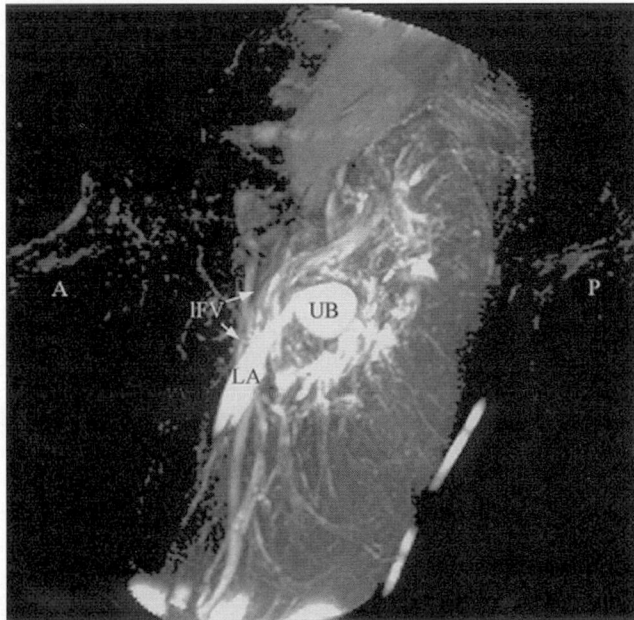

Figure 36–2. MRI image after administration of local anesthetic on sagittal T2-weighted MRI. (A, Anterior; P, posterior; lFV, left femoral vein; LA, local anesthetic; UB, urinary bladder.)

Indications & Contraindications

The following are indications for using 3-in-1 block:

- Surgical procedures in the sensory areas of the femoral, lateral femoral cutaneous, and anterior branches of the obturator nerves (eg, skin surgery, muscle biopsy)
- Patella surgery
- Perioperative pain therapy of hip fractures (additional block of the sciatic nerve is necessary)
- Perioperative pain therapy of femoral shaft fractures (additional block of the sciatic nerve is necessary for a complete analgesia)
- Perioperative pain therapy of knee surgery (popliteal area not involved—posterior branch of the obturator nerve)
- Together with a sciatic nerve block, all surgical procedures on the lower extremity
- Pain therapy and prevention of phantom limb pain following above-knee amputations (catheter technique)

The following are contraindications to 3-in-1 nerve block:

- General contraindications against peripheral nerve blocks (infection at the needle insertion site, severe blood coagulation abnormalities)
- Femoral–popliteal bypass graft (can be performed with ultrasound-guided technique)

Functional Anatomy

The femoral, lateral femoral cutaneous, and obturator nerves are formed by the ventral roots of the lumbar plexus from the 12th thoracic nerve (T12) to the 4th lumbar nerve (L4). The femoral nerve (L1/2-L4) is the largest of the three nerves from the lumbar plexus, and its position cephalad to the inguinal ligament is inside the greater psoas muscle and more distal between the greater psoas and the iliac muscles (Figure 36–3). The femoral nerve enters the thigh at the level of the inguinal ligament lateral to the femoral artery, where the iliopectineal arch (a deep layer of the inguinal ligament) and the fascia iliaca separate the two structures from each other (Figure 36–4). The femoral nerve divides slightly distal to the inguinal ligament in several branches, which is the rationale for the nerve block needle to be inserted close to the distal ligament when performing the 3-in-1 block. The femoral nerve supplies motor branches to the quadriceps femoris, sartorius, and pectineus muscles, and its sensory branch (saphenous nerve) innervates the anterior-medial side of the lower leg down to the medial ankle (Figures 36–5 and 36–6).

Both the obturator and the lateral femoral cutaneous nerves divide at variable levels from the femoral nerve. The obturator nerve enters through the craniomedial part of the obturator foramen on the medial side of the thigh and divides in an anterior branch, which lies between the adductor brevis, obturator externus, adductor longus, and pectineus muscles,

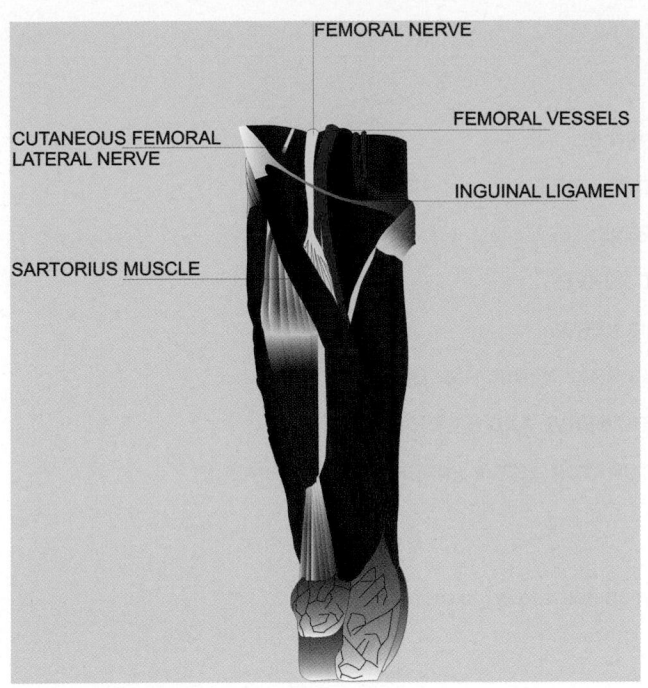

Figure 36–3. Anatomy of the inguinal region.

and a posterior branch, which pierces the obturator externus muscle and lies above the adductor magnus and brevis muscles. The obturator nerve supplies motor branches to all the mentioned muscles and also to the gracilis muscle. An accessory obturator nerve may divide from the lumbar plexus at the L3/4 level and supply a muscular branch of the pectineus muscle, then enter the hip joint.

The lateral femoral cutaneous nerve enters the thigh slightly medial to the anterior superior iliac spine and is a purely sensory nerve.

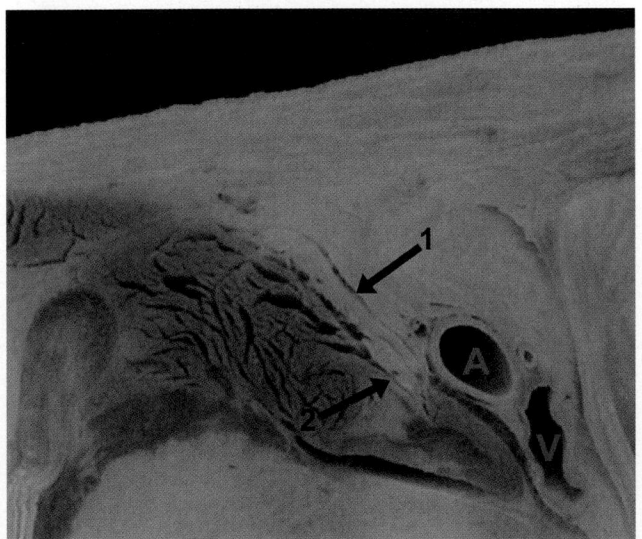

Figure 36–4. Anatomy of the inguinal region. Shown are the femoral artery (*A*) and vein (*V*), fascia lata (*1*), and femoral nerve (*2*).

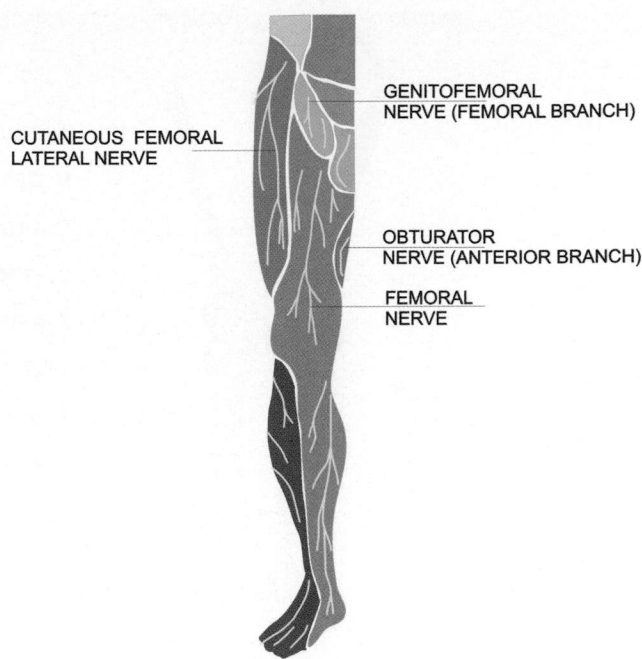

Figure 36–5. Sensory surface innervation of the lower extremity.

Distribution of Anesthesia

Figure 36–5 illustrates the anesthetic distribution of the femoral, lateral femoral cutaneous, and obturator nerves. It is important to notice that the sensory area of the anterior branch of the obturator nerve is inconsistent at the medial side of the thigh and that the posterior branch of the obturator nerve innervates a sensory area at the popliteal fold, which is never anesthetized by a 3-in-1 block. Also important to notice is that the most proximal parts of the thigh are sensory-innervated by nerves from the abdominal wall (femoral branch of the genitofemoral nerve) and therefore also not anesthetized by a 3-in-1 block. Innervation of the lower-extremity osteotomes are illustrated in Figure 36–6.

Landmarks

The landmarks for the 3-in-1 block are the anterior superior iliac spine, which is usually easy to palpate, and the inguinal ligament, an abdominal fascial layer fixed at the anterior superior iliac spine (Figure 36–7). In obese patients, identification of the inguinal ligament may be difficult. Below the inguinal ligament (or the femoral crease), the pulsation of the femoral artery is detectable, and the needle insertion site for the 3-in-1 block lies in the area between the inguinal ligament and lateral to the femoral artery (1–2 cm distal the ligament). In the inguinal area, it is useful to think of the mnemonic term NAVEL to remember the position of the femoral nerve and vascular components. From lateral to medial: **N** = femoral nerve; **A** = femoral artery; **V** = femoral nerve; **E** = empty space; **L** = lacunar ligament.

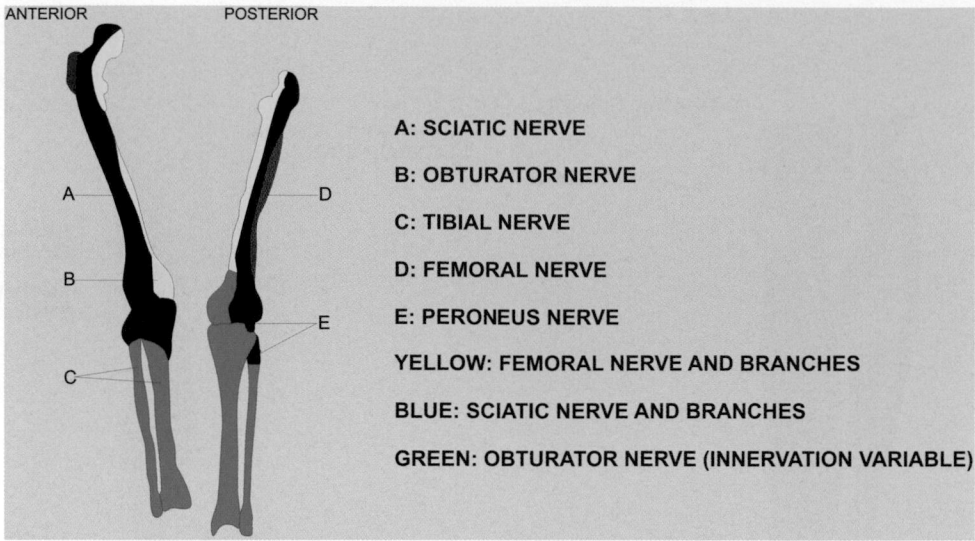

Figure 36–6. Osteotomal innervation of the lower extremity.

Equipment

The following items are used for 3-in-1 blockade:

Sterile prep solution

25-gauge needle, 2-mL syringe, and lidocaine 1% for skin infiltration

For continuous technique—peripheral nerve block catheter set of choice

20-mL syringe and the appropriate local anaesthetic

22-gauge, 40-mm insulated stimulation needle

Sterile gloves

Nerve stimulator and surface electrode *or*

Ultrasound machine with small parts software and a 5–12-MHz linear probe.

Techniques

Winnie described the paresthesia technique of the 3-in-1 block in 1973. Currently, only two techniques are used, the nerve stimulator and the ultrasonographic guidance techniques.

Nerve Stimulator–Guided Technique

The position of the patient is supine with both legs extended and the leg to be blocked with 15–30 degrees lateral rotation. After standard preparation (monitoring, intravenous access, sterile preparation of the needle insertion area, and skin anesthesia), the nerve stimulation needle is connected to a nerve stimulator. The needle insertion site is 1–2 cm distal to the inguinal ligament with an angle of 30–45 degrees and a cephalad direction (Figure 36–8). On the way to the femoral nerve, a twofold resistance loss can often be appreciated as the needle pierces the fascia lata and the fascia iliaca. Usually, the nerve is at a depth of 12 ± 4 mm. Once a distal motor response of the

quadriceps femoris muscle (patella twitch) at a current intensity of 0.3 mA (0.1 msec) or less is observed and a negative aspiration test is obtained, the local anesthetic may be injected according to Winnie's "immobile needle" technique.[10]

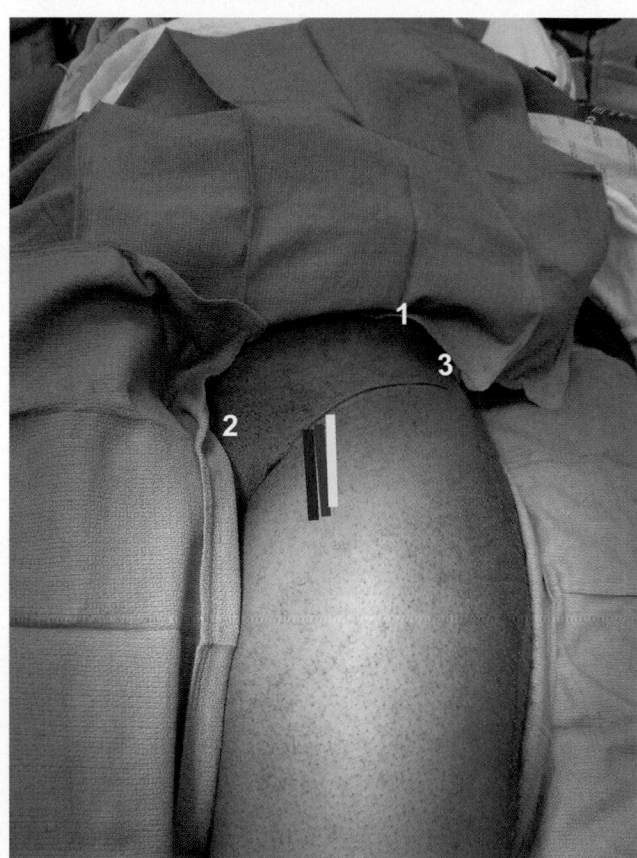

Figure 36–7. Landmarks for the 3-in-1 block. 1, Anterior superior iliac spine; 2, pubic bone; 3, femoral crease. Inguinal ligament stretches between 1 and 2. Femoral vein, artery, and nerve are represented as blue, red, and yellow lines, respectively.

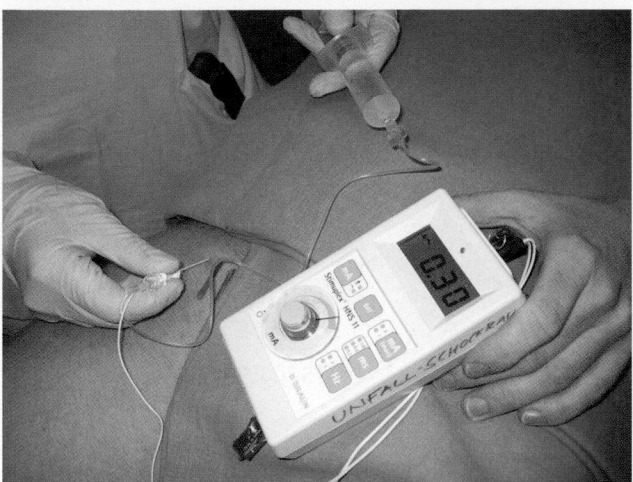

Figure 36–8. Nerve stimulator-guided 3-in-1 block technique.

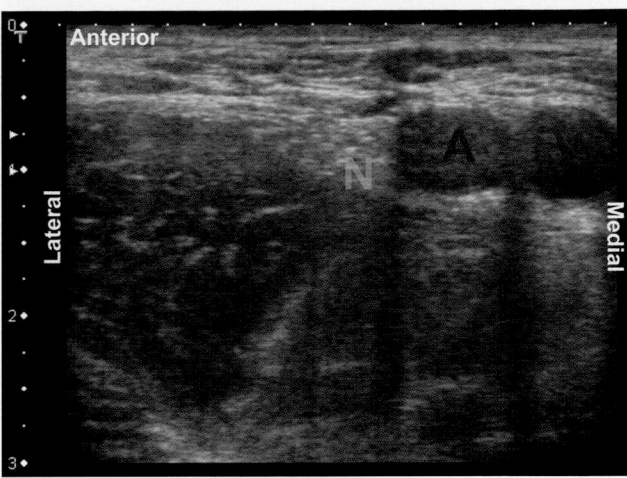

Figure 36–10. Cross-sectional ultrasonographic view of the inguinal region. Femoral vein, artery, and nerve are labeled as *VAN*, respectively.

Ultrasound-Guided Technique

Significantly faster sensory onset times and improved quality of blocks can be obtained with ultrasound guided technique when compared with the conventional nerve stimulator technique.[11] In addition, significantly reduced amount of local anesthetics can be used, illustrating that the quality of peripheral nerve blockade can be influenced by direct visualization of the spread of local anesthetic.[12] This can be particularly important in elderly patients and those with cardiovascular compromise, as well as in patients who require combined nerve blocks.[13]

Because of the superficial position of the femoral nerve, a high-frequency linear ultrasonographic probe can be used for the 3-in-1 block (Figure 36–9). Inguinal vessels are easily visualized (Figure 36–10); the femoral nerve can be imaged slightly distal to the inguinal ligament in a cross-sectional view (Figure 36–10) in which a 4-cm needle with a blunt tip is placed below the iliopectineal arch, and approximately 5 mL

(for a single femoral nerve block) or 20 mL (for a 3-in-1 block) of local anesthetic is injected. It is not necessary to visualize the lateral femoral cutaneous and obturator nerves by ultrasonography. Both nerves are small, and the anterior branch of the obturator nerve is particularly difficult to visualize by ultrasound because of its position between the adductor brevis and longus muscles. Similar technique can be used to insert a catheter for continuous blockade (Figure 36–11).

Volume & Choice of Local Anesthetics

Twenty milliliters is the adequate volume of local anesthetic for the 3-in-1 block, although much larger volumes are described in the literature. The appropriate technique significantly influences the success of the block.[12] A single femoral nerve block can be performed with as little as 5–10 mL local anesthesia.

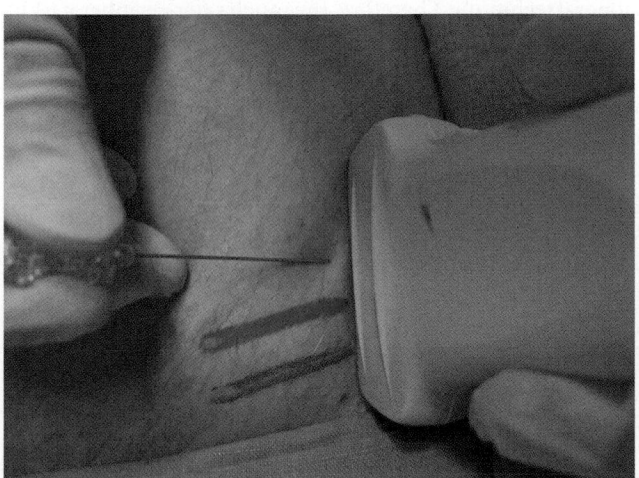

Figure 36–9. Ultrasound-guided 3-in-1 block technique with the linear probe relative to the stimulating needle to achieve a cross-sectional view.

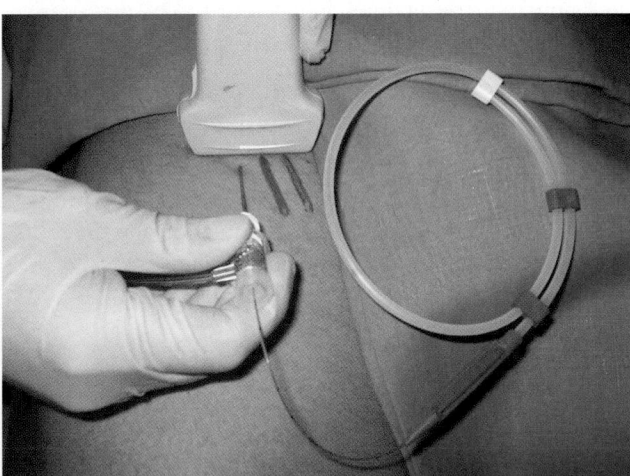

Figure 36–11. Ultrasound-guided placement of a 3-in-1 catheter.

Table 36–1.

Choice of Type, Volume, and Concentration of Local Anesthetics for Surgical Anesthesia and Pain Management for 3-in-1 Blocks

Technique	Local Anesthetic Regimen
3-in-1 Block Single-Shot Technique	
Surgical indication	20 mL Ropivacaine 0.75%
Analgesia	20 mL Ropivacaine 0.2%
Femoral Nerve Block Single-Shot Technique	
Surgical indication	5 mL Ropivacaine 0.75%
Analgesia	5 mL Ropivacaine 0.2%
3-in-1 Block Catheter Technique	
Surgical indication	2 × 20-mL bolus administration/day ropivacaine 0.75%
Analgesia	2 × 20-mL bolus administration/day ropivacaine 0.2%
Femoral Nerve Block Catheter Technique	
Surgical indication	5 mL/h Ropivacaine 0.75%
Analgesia	5 mL/h Ropivacaine 0.2%

Table 36–2.

Onset Time and Duration of Anesthesia and Analgesia of Common Local Anesthetics

	Onset (min)	Anesthesia (h)	Analgesia (h)
3% 2-Chloroprocaine ($+ HCO_3$)	10–15	1	2
3% 2-Chloroprocaine ($+ HCO_3 + $ epi)	10–15	1.5–2	2–3
1.5% Mepivacaine ($+ HCO_3$)	15–20	2–3	3–5
1.5% Mepivacaine ($+ HCO_3 + $ epi)	15–20	2–5	3–8
2% Lidocaine ($+ HCO_3 + $ epi)	10–20	2–5	3–8
0.5% Ropivacaine	15–30	4–8	5–12
0.75% Ropivacaine	10–15	5–10	6–24
0.5 Bupivacaine (or L-bupivacaine)	15–30	5–15	6–30

Ropivacaine is well investigated for the 3-in-1 block and shows similar onset times and quality of nerve blockade when compared with bupivacaine.[14] The exact duration of sensory and motor blocks with different concentrations of ropivacaine has not been investigated, but with 20 mL of ropivacaine 0.75%, a duration of nerve blockade of more than 24 hours was observed (Tables 36–1 and 36–2). For shorter blocks and faster onset times, mepivacaine 1–2% may be used. Levobupivacaine is also a valuable alternative.

Interpreting Responses to Nerve Stimulation

Ideally, obtain twitches of the distal quadriceps femoris muscle (patella twitch) at 0.2–0.5 mA current. Table 36–3 presents some common responses to nerve stimulation and the course of action to take to obtain the proper response.

PERIOPERATIVE MANAGEMENT

Usually, the 3-in-1 block should be performed (comparable to other regional anesthetic techniques) in the awake patient.

With the use of ultrasonography and direct visualization of the anatomic structures and the spread of local anesthetic, 3-in-1 block can be performed in anesthetized patients.

Nevertheless, in daily clinical practice most blocks are performed on awake patients.

Practical Management of Continuous Blocks

The first description of a 3-in-1 catheter was published by Rosenblatt in 1980.[15] In 1998, Singelyn et al.[16] compared epidural with 3-in-1 block catheters and systemic opioids after knee arthroplasty and found that the central regional anesthetic technique was equally as effective as with the peripheral technique. Therefore, the much safer peripheral technique was recommended.

The 3-in-1 technique itself is comparable to the single-injection technique. Figure 36–11 illustrates the performance of a continuous 3-in-1 block with ultrasonographic guidance and a catheter set specially designed for the ultrasound-guided technique (Nanoline peripheral catheter set, Pajunk, Geisingen, Germany). The catheter should be introduced only 2–5 cm above the tip of the stimulating needle to avoid a malposition of the tip of the catheter. In most cases, the catheter is not visible on the ultrasound; the main predictor of successful catheter placement is the distribution of the injected local anesthetic. Ultrasonography can also be used to troubleshoot a malfunctioning catheter.

To achieve a complete 3-in-1 block with a catheter, bolus administration of local anesthetic seems to be more successful than continuous administration of local anesthesia.[17] In cases in which only the femoral or saphenous nerve need to be blocked, continuous administration of local anesthesia

Table 36–3.

Responses to Nerve Stimulation and How to Obtain Appropriate Response

Response Obtained	Interpretation	Problem	Action
No response	Needle is inserted either too medially or too laterally	Femoral artery not properly localized or the palpating hand moved during the procedure	Follow the systematic lateral angulation and reinsertion of the needle as described in the technique.
Bone contact	Needle contacts hip or superior ramus of the pubic bone	Needle inserted too deep	Withdraw to the level of the skin, and reinsert in another direction.
Local twitch	Direct stimulation of the iliopsoas or pectineus muscle	Too deep insertion	Withdraw to the level of the skin, and reinsert in another direction.
Twitch of the sartorius muscle	Sartorius muscle twitch	Needle tip is slightly anterior and medial to main trunk of femoral nerve	Redirect the needle laterally and advance deeper 1–3 mm.
Vascular puncture	Blood in the syringe invariably indicates placement into the femoral artery	Too medial needle placement	Withdraw and reinsert laterally 1 cm.
Patella twitch	Stimulation of the main trunk of the femoral nerve	None	Accept and inject local anesthetic.

is appropriate. The rationale behind this recommendation is the fact that the 3-in-1 block is a volume block in which a sufficient lateral and medial distribution of local anesthetic is mandatory for a successful block.[5]

Complications & Measures to Avoid Them

The following are possible complications resulting from 3-in1-blockade:

> Direct stimulation of the sartorius muscle (failed block, tip of the needle is too superficial and/or too lateral)
>
> Intravascular injection of local anesthetic (aspiration before injection of local anesthesia is mandatory)
>
> Intraneuronal injection (pain during injection of local anesthesia in nonanesthetized patients may be present)[18]
>
> Complications after femoral 3-in-1 block are relatively rare. Table 36–4 provides some general as well as specific instructions on possible complications and how to avoid them.

SUMMARY

The 3-in-1 block is a useful regional anesthetic technique for a broad spectrum of indications. In light of the newer literature,

the 3-in-1 block could be more appropriately called a $2^{1}/_{2}$-in-1 block because the posterior branch of the obturator nerve is never blocked. There are alternatives to the 3-in-1 block. (1) The psoas compartment block has a greater spread but is more central and therefore may be associated with higher risk of complications. (2) The fascia iliaca compartment block is also often promoted; however, it is an inexact technique in which larger volumes of local anesthesia are needed for a hoped-for effect.[19] Nevertheless, both techniques have their spectrum of indications: The psoas compartment block is used when a complete block of the lumbar plexus is necessary, and the fascia iliaca compartment block is used when fast analgesia (eg, in a prehospital setting or for those who are inexperienced in regional anesthesia) is necessary.

The use of ultrasonographic guidance for the performance of 3-in-1 blocks is recommended. It is one of the simplest ultrasound-guided blocks to perform and results in improved quality of nerve blockade and possibly reduction in complications.

References

1. Winnie A, Ramamurthy S, Durrani Z: The inguinal paravascular technic of lumbar plexus anesthesia: The "3-in-1 block." Anesth Analg 1973;52:989–996.
2. Winnie A: Regional anesthesia. Surg Clin North Am 1975;55:861–892.

Table 36–4.

Possible Complications and How to Avoid Them

Infection	Use strict aseptic technique Catheters at this location are difficult to keep sterile and should be removed after 48 hours
Hematoma	Avoid advancement of the needle when the patient reports pain; this may indicate insertion of the needle through the iliopsoas or pectineus muscles When the femoral artery or vein is punctured, stop the procedure and apply firm and constant pressure over the femoral artery for 2–3 minutes before proceeding with block In a patient with difficult anatomy or severe peripheral vascular disease, use a single-shot smaller-gauge needle to localize the femoral nerve before proceeding with a larger-gauge needle for continuous technique
Vascular puncture	Never redirect the needle medially Needle is first inserted just lateral to the femoral artery, and the consequent insertions and redirections should all be progressively more lateral
Nerve injury	Use nerve stimulation and slow needle advancement or ultrasound guidance Distinct paresthesia is almost never elicited with femoral nerve block and should not be sought Do not inject when the patient complains of pain or when abnormal resistance or high pressures on injection are met
Other	Instruct the patient on the inability to bear weight on the blocked extremity

3. Winnie A, Ramamurthy S, Durrani Z, Radonjic R: Plexus blocks for lower extremity surgery. Anesthesiol Rev 1974;1:11–16.

4. Ritter J: Femoral nerve "sheath" for inguinal paravascular lumbar plexus block is not found in human cadavers. J Clin Anesth 1995;7:470–473.

5. Marhofer P, Nasel C, Sitzwohl C, Kapral S: Magnetic resonance imaging of the distribution of local anesthetic during the three-in-one block. Anesth Analg 2000;90:119–124.

6. Lang S, Yip R, Chang P, Gerard M: The femoral 3-in-1 block revisited. J Clin Anesth 1993;5:292–296.

7. Lang S: Electromyographic comparison of obturator nerve block to 3-in-1 block. Anesth Analg 1996;83:436–437.

8. Cauhepe C, Oliver M, Colombani R, Railhac N: The "3-in-1" block: myth or reality? Ann Fr Anesth Reanim 1989;8:376–378.

9. Capdevila X, Biboulet P, Bouregba M, et al: Comparison of the three-in-one and fascia iliaca compartment blocks in adults: Clinical and radiographic analysis. Anesth Analg 1998;86:1039–1044.

10. Winnie A: An "immobile needle" for nerve blocks. Anesthesiology 1969;31:577–578.

11. Marhofer P, Schrogendorfer K, Koinig H, et al: Ultrasonographic guidance improves sensory block and onset time of three in one blocks. Anesth Analg 1997;85:854–857.

12. Marhofer P, Schrogendorfer K, Wallner T, et al: Ultrasonographic guidance reduces the amount of local anesthetic for 3-in-1 blocks. Reg Anesth Pain Med 1998;23:584–588.

13. Marhofer P, Schrogendorfer K, Andel H, et al: Combined sciatic nerve—3-in-1 block in high risk patient. Anasthesiol Intensivmed Notfallmed Schmerzther 1998;33:399–401.

14. Marhofer P, Oismuller C, Faryniak B, et al: Three-in-one blocks with ropivacaine: Evaluation of sensory onset time and quality of sensory block. Anesth Analg 2000;90:125–128.

15. Rosenblatt R: Continuous femoral anesthesia for lower extremity surgery. Anesth Analg 1980;59:631.

16. Singelyn F, Deyaert M, Joris D, et al: Effects of intravenous patient-controlled analgesia with morphine, continuous epidural analgesia, and continuous three-in-one block on postoperative pain and knee rehabilitation after unilateral total knee arthroplasty. Anesth Analg 1998;87:88–92.

17. Singelyn F, Vanderelst P, Gouverneur J: Extended femoral nerve sheath block after total hip arthroplasty: Continuous versus patient-controlled techniques. Anesth Analg 2001;92:455–459.

18. Uhrbrand B, Jensen T: Success rate and complications of the 3-in-1 block method. Ugeskr Laeger 1988;150:928–929.

19. Paut O, Schreiber E, Lacroix F, et al: High plasma ropivacaine concentrations after fascia iliaca compartment block in children. Br J Anaesth 2004;92:416–418.

37

Sciatic Nerve Block

Elizabeth Gaertner, MD • Elisabeth Fouché, MD • Olivier Choquet, MD • Admir Hadzic, MD • Jerry D. Vloka, MD

INTRODUCTION

Victor Pauchet first described the sciatic nerve block in L'Anesthésie Régionale in 1920: "the site of needle insertion for blocking the sciatic nerve at the level of hip: 3 cm along the perpendicular that bisects a line drawn between the greater trochanter and the posterior superior iliac spine."[1] Although this technique is referred to as "The classic approach of Labat," it was in fact first described by Labat's teacher, Pauchet. Perhaps the reason for the name designation comes from the fact that the sciatic nerve block was first described in anesthesia literature in 1923 by Gaston Labat in his book, *Regional Anesthesia: Its Technic and Clinical Application*.[2] Of note, Labat in the same year founded the American Society of Regional Anesthesia (ASRA). Anecdotally, Labat intended to name the new group "the Labat Society" in his honor, but the name ASRA remains today as we know it. Labat's book went through several reprintings of the first edition and was one of the first English language anesthesia textbooks of regional anesthesia in the United States. Curiously, this book was similar to L'Anesthésie Régionale, written by Labat's tutor, Pauchet, from 1918 to 1920 in the University of Paris.

Alon Winnie eventually modified the Labat approach in 1975.[3] In 1963, Beck[4] described an anterior approach, and, in 1975, Raj proposed a lithotomy approach.[4,5] These alternative approaches were devised to allow the sciatic nerve to be blocked in the supine patient. Since its original description, a number of new approaches to sciatic nerve blocks were proposed, most of which include minor modifications of questionable clinical significance. Based on the clinical studies of various approaches, the most useful of these newer techniques appear to be the subgluteal and parasacral approaches introduced by di Benedetto and Mansour, respectively.[6–8] Discussion of all described techniques and approaches is beyond the scope of this chapter. Instead, this chapter focuses on the classic approach to sciatic nerve block, parasacral and subgluteal modifications, and the anterior approach.

Indications & Contraindications

Indications for sciatic nerve block include lower-limb surgery, often combined with a femoral or psoas compartment block.[8] For distal surgery of the lower extremity, however, more distal approaches such as ankle block or popliteal sciatic nerve block are preferable when feasible. Note that the sciatic nerve block almost always needs to be combined with supplemental block, which involves components of the lumbar plexus (femoral nerve).

Contraindications to sciatic nerve block are few, and may include local infection and bed sores at the site of insertion, coagulopathy, preexisting central or peripheral nervous systems disorders, and allergy to local anesthetics.

Functional Anatomy

The union of the lumbosacral trunk with the first three sacral nerves forms the sacral plexus (Figure 37–1). The lumbosacral trunk originates from the anastomosis of the last two lumbar nerves with the anterior branch of the first sacral nerve. This structure receives the anterior branches of the second and third sacral nerves, forming the sacral plexus. The sacral plexus is shaped like a triangle pointing toward the sciatic notch, with its base spanning across the anterior sacral foramina. It rests on the anterior aspect of the piriformis muscle and is covered by the pelvic fascia, which separates it from the hypogastric vessels and pelvic organs. Seven nerves stem from the sacral plexus: six collateral branches and one terminal branch—the sciatic nerve, the largest nerve of the plexus.

Strictly speaking, L4 through S3 nerve roots form the sacral plexus. These roots of the sacral plexus form on the anterior surface of the lateral sacrum and are assembled into the sciatic nerve on the ventral surface of the piriformis muscle[9] (Figure 37–2). The sciatic nerve is the largest peripheral nerve in the body and measures more than 1 cm in breadth at its origin. It exits the pelvis through the greater sciatic notch below the piriformis muscle, then descends between the greater trochanter of the femur and the ischial tuberosity. The nerve then runs along the posterior thigh to the lower third of the femur, where it diverges into two large branches, the tibial and

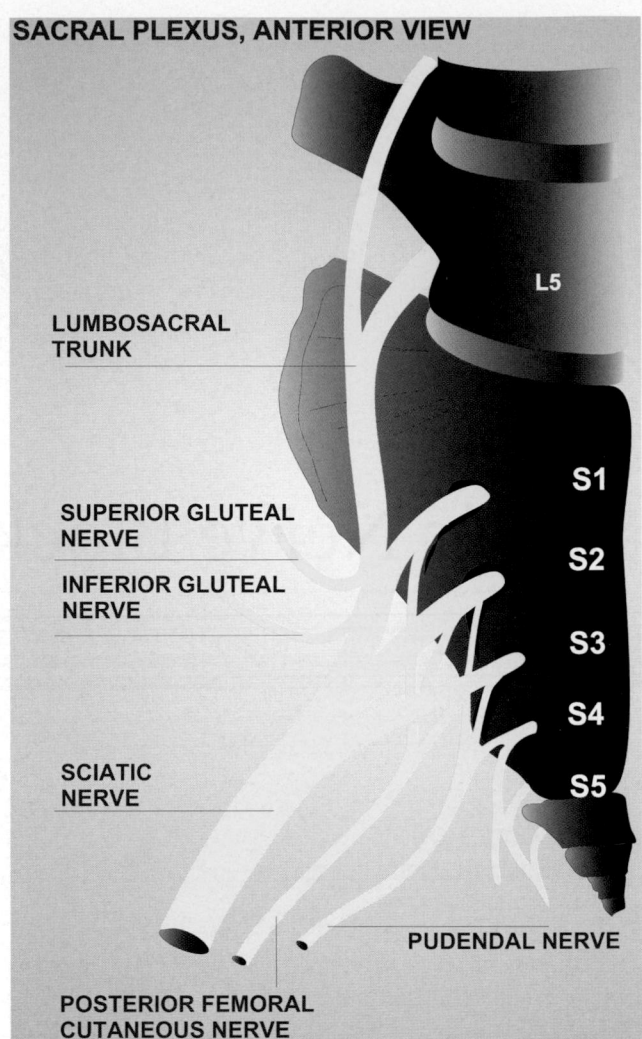

SACRAL PLEXUS, ANTERIOR VIEW

LUMBOSACRAL TRUNK

L5

SUPERIOR GLUTEAL NERVE

INFERIOR GLUTEAL NERVE

S1

S2

S3

S4

S5

SCIATIC NERVE

PUDENDAL NERVE

POSTERIOR FEMORAL CUTANEOUS NERVE

Figure 37–1. Formation of the sacral plexus.

common peroneal nerves. This division may occur at any level proximal to the lower third of the femur.[10,11] Fifteen percent of the time, the common peroneal and tibial nerves are separated from their onset at the sacral plexus; in this case, the common peroneal nerve typically pierces piriformis muscle. The course of the sciatic nerve can be estimated by drawing a line on the back of the thigh beginning from the apex of the popliteal fossa to the midpoint of the line joining the ischial tuberosity to the apex of the greater trochanter. From its onset, the sciatic nerve also gives off numerous articular (hip, knee) and muscular branches.

In the upper part of its course, the sciatic nerve lies deep in the gluteus maximus muscle and rests on the posterior surface of the ischium (Figures 37–3 and 37–4). The sciatic nerve crosses the external rotators, obturator internus, and gemelli muscles, then passes on to the quadratus femoris. The quadratus femoris separates the sciatic nerve from the obturator externus and the hip joint. Medially, the posterior cutaneous nerve of the thigh and the inferior gluteal plexus accompany the sciatic nerve, whereas more distally the sciatic nerve lies on the adductor magnus. The long head of

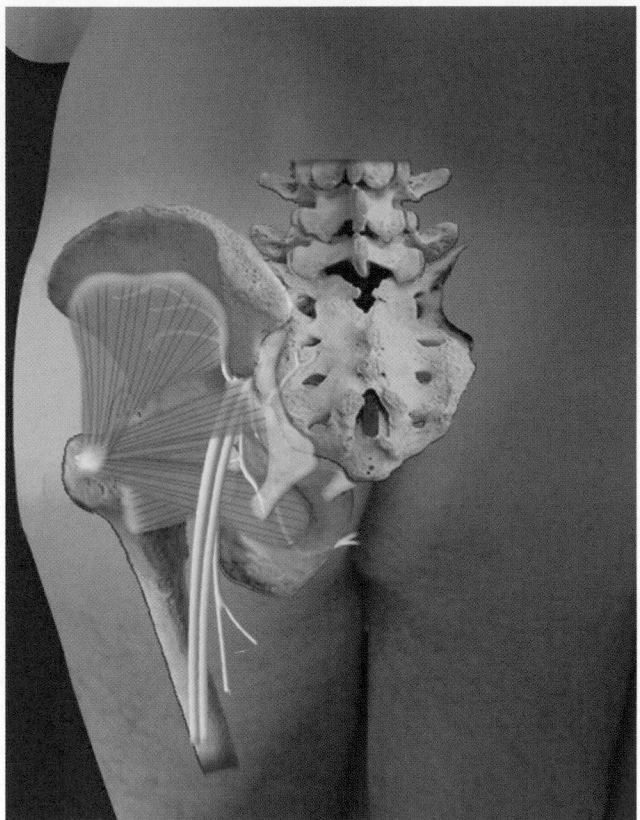

Figure 37–2. Course of the sciatic nerve at the exit from the pelvis. A posterior view.

the biceps femoris crosses the sciatic nerve obliquely. The *articular branches* of the sciatic nerve arise from the upper part of the nerve and supply the hip joint by perforating the posterior part of its capsule. However, the articular branches are sometimes derived directly from the sacral plexus. The

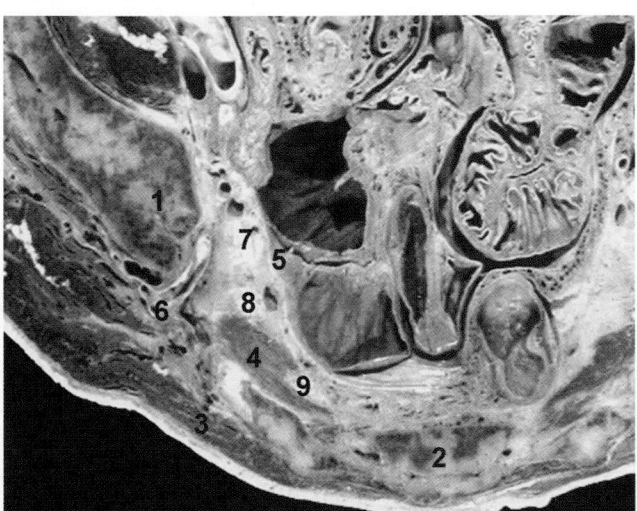

Figure 37–3. Parasacral area. Transversal coupe at the S3 level. 1, Iliac bone; 2, sacrum; 3, gluteal muscle; 4, piriformis muscle; 5, pelvic aponeurosis; 6, inferiorgluteal plexus; 7, lumbosacral trunk; 8, first sacral root; 9, second sacral root; muscle; (contributed by the Institute of Anatomy, Strasbourg, France).

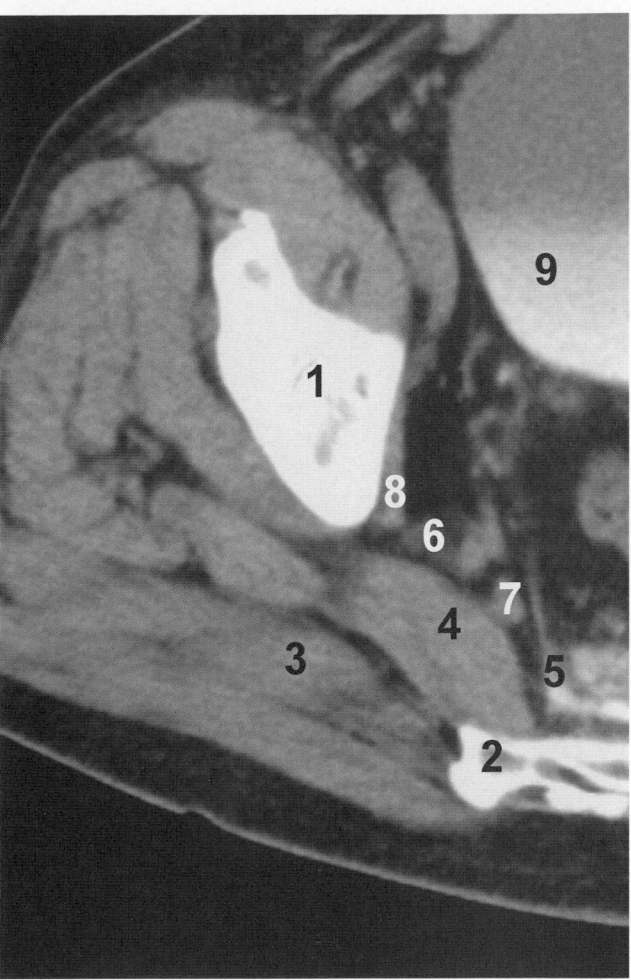

Figure 37–4. CT scan of the parasacral area, at the S3 level.1, Iliac bone; 2, sacrum; 3, gluteal muscle; 4, piriformis muscle; 5, pelvic aponeurosis; 6, first sacral root; 7, second sacral root; 8, obturator internis muscle; 9, bladder.

muscular branches of the sciatic nerve innervate the gluteus, the biceps femoris, the ischial head of the adductor magnus, the semitendinosus, and the semimembranosus muscles (Figure 37–5; Table 37–1). The branches of the ischial head of the adductor magnus and semimembranosus muscles arise from a common trunk. The nerve to the short head of the biceps femoris comes from the common peroneal division, whereas the other muscular branches arise from the tibial division of the sciatic nerve.

The parasacral area is delineated by the ventral aponeurosis of the piriformis muscle dorsally, by the pelvic aponeurosis medially, and by the aponeurosis of the obturator internis muscle laterally.[9] The common peroneal component passes through the piriformis muscle or above it, and only the tibial component passes below the muscle.

Choice of Local Anesthetic

Despite its large size, sciatic block requires a relatively low volume of local anesthetic to achieve anesthesia of the entire trunk of the nerve.[12] Generally, 20–25 mL of local anesthetic

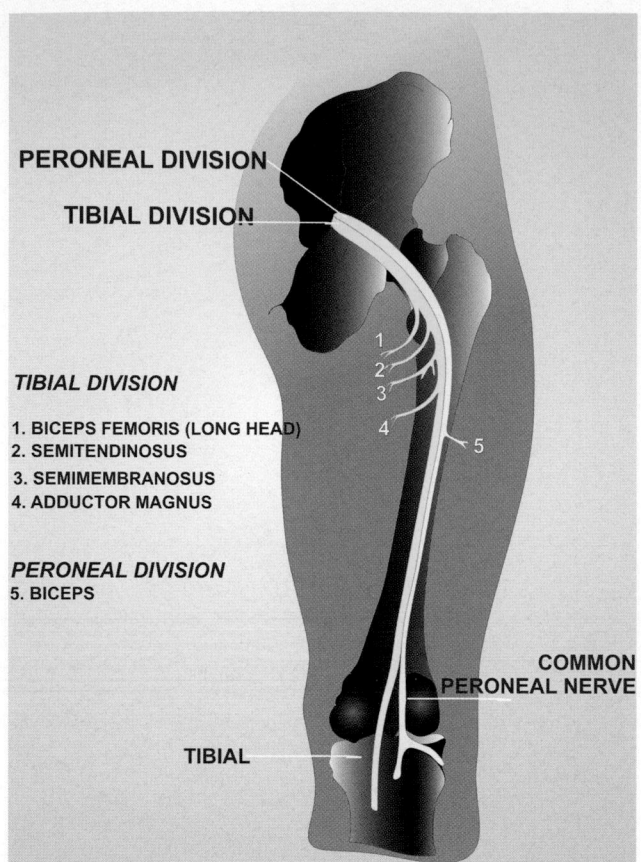

PERONEAL DIVISION

TIBIAL DIVISION

TIBIAL DIVISION

1. BICEPS FEMORIS (LONG HEAD)
2. SEMITENDINOSUS
3. SEMIMEMBRANOSUS
4. ADDUCTOR MAGNUS

PERONEAL DIVISION
5. BICEPS

COMMON PERONEAL NERVE

TIBIAL

Figure 37–5. Sciatic nerve. Downward course and motor branches to the hamstrings muscle.

Table 37–2.

Local Anesthetic Choices for Sciatic Nerve Block: Duration of Anesthesia and Analgesia

	Onset (min)	Anesthesia (h)	Analgesia (h)
3% 2-Chloroprocaine (+ HCO$_3$)	10–15	2	2.5
1.5% Mepivacaine (+ HCO$_3$)	10–15	4–5	5–8
2% Lidocaine (+ HCO$_3$)	10–20	5–6	5–8
0.5% Ropivacaine	15–20	6–12	6–24
0.75% Ropivacaine	10–15	8–12	8–24
0.5% Bupivacaine (or L-bupivacaine)	15–30	8–16	10–48

are sufficient. The choice of the type and concentration of local anesthetic should be based on whether the block is planned for surgical anesthesia or analgesia[13] (Table 37–2). When prolonged pain relief is desired long-acting local anesthetic may be more appropriate.[14,15] Epinephrine is not routinely used for sciatic nerve block because of the possibility of injury due to stretching or sitting on the anesthetized nerve with the long duration of block with epinephrine-containing local anesthetics. However, its use may be justified in patients undergoing above-knee amputation, in whom these issues are not pertinent and prolonged analgesia is always beneficial.

Equipment

All approaches to the sciatic nerve block necessitate assembly of a nerve block tray before placing the block. As with

Table 37–1.

Branches, Source, and Motor Innervation of the Sacral Plexus

Nerve	Source	Muscular Innervation
N. to obturator internus m.	Lumbosacral trunk and S1	Obturator internus
Superior gluteal n.	Lumbosacral trunk and S1	Gluteus medius Gluteus minimus Tensor fasciae lata
N. to piriformis muscle	S2	Piriformis
N. to biceps femoris superior	Anterior portion of plexus	Biceps femoris superior
N. to biceps femoris inferior and quadratus femoris	Anterior portion of plexus	Biceps femoris inferior Quadratus femoris Branch to coxofemoral articulation
Posterior femoral cutaneous nerve (lesser sciatic nerve)	Lumbosacral trunk, S1, S2	Inferior gluteal n. to gluteus maximus muscle Sensory branch to buttock, thigh, popliteal fossa, and lateral aspect of knee

Table 37–3.

Common Responses to Nerve Stimulation and Action to Take

Response Obtained	Interpretation	Problem	Action
Local twitch of the gluteus muscle	Direct stimulation of the gluteus muscle	Too shallow (superficial) placement of the needle	Continue advancing the needle
Needle contacts bone but local twitch of the gluteus muscle not elicited	Needle inserted close to the caudal aspect of the iliac bone or the lateral aspect of the sacrum	Too superior or too medial needle insertion	Slightly laterally and caudally redirect the needle
Needle encounters bone and sciatic twitches elicited	Needle missed the plane of the sciatic nerve and is stopped by the hip joint or ischial bone	Needle inserted too laterally (hip joint) or medially (ischial bone)	Withdraw the needle and redirect slightly medially or laterally (5–10 degrees)
Hamstring twitch	Stimulation of the main trunk of the sciatic nerve	None. These branches are within the sciatic nerve sheath at this level	Accept and inject local anesthetic
The needle placed deep (10 cm) but no twitches elicited and no bone contact	Needle has passed through the sciatic notch	Too inferior needle placement	Withdraw and redirect the needle slightly laterally, or cephalad
Paresthesia of the genital organs	Needle is stimulating the inferior roots of the sacral plexus (pudendal nerve)	Too inferior and too medial needle placement	Withdraw and redirect the needle slightly cephalad and laterally

all regional anesthesia techniques, the heart rate, blood pressure, and pulse oximeter are routinely monitored before performing the block. Resuscitation equipment and emergency medications must be immediately available and ready to use. Supplemental oxygen via face mask is routinely used before giving sedation. A standard regional anesthesia tray is prepared with the following equipment:

- Sterile towels and 4-in. × 4-in. gauze packs
- 20-mL syringe with local anesthetic
- Sterile gloves, marking pen, and surface electrode
- One $1\frac{1}{2}$-in., 25-gauge needle for skin infiltration
- A 10-cm long, short-bevel, insulated stimulating needle (15 cm for anterior approach)
- Peripheral nerve stimulator

Interpreting Responses to Nerve Stimulation

Twitches of the hamstrings, calf, foot, or toes at 0.2–0.5 mA current all can be used as signs of successful localization of the sciatic plexus (nerve). Table 37–3 presents common responses to nerve stimulation and the course of action to take to obtain the proper response.[16]

BLOCK DYNAMICS & PERIOPERATIVE MANAGEMENT

Sciatic nerve blockade technique may result in significant patient discomfort because the needle passes through the glu-

teus muscles. Adequate sedation and analgesia are important to ensure patient comfort. Midazolam 2–6 mg can be given for patient positioning, and alfentanil 500–750 mcg is given just before needle insertion. A typical onset time for this block is 10–25 minutes, depending on the type, concentration, and volume of local anesthetic used. The first signs of blockade onset are usually reported by the patient in the form of a feeling that the foot is "different" and/or that he or she cannot wiggle the toes.

Clinical Pearls

- Inadequate skin anesthesia despite an apparent timely onset of the blockade can occur.
- It can take up to 30 minutes for full sensory–motor anesthesia to develop.
- Local infiltration at the site of the incision by the surgeon is often all that is needed to allow the surgery to proceed.

POSTERIOR APPROACHES TO SCIATIC NERVE BLOCK

General Considerations

The posterior approach to sciatic blockade has wide clinical applicability for surgery and pain management of the lower

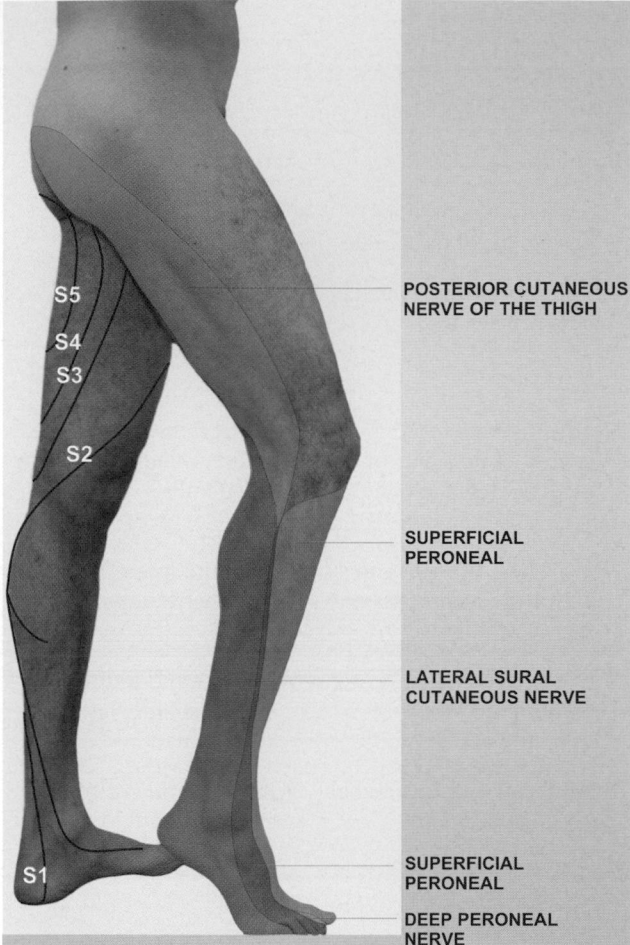

Figure 37–6. Sciatic nerve. Cutaneous innervation.

POSTERIOR CUTANEOUS NERVE OF THE THIGH

SUPERFICIAL PERONEAL

LATERAL SURAL CUTANEOUS NERVE

SUPERFICIAL PERONEAL

DEEP PERONEAL NERVE

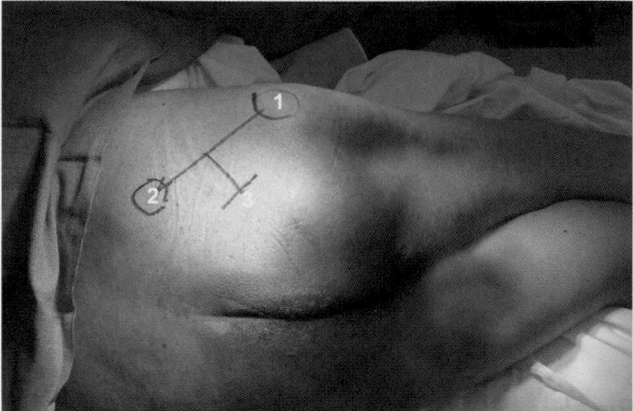

Figure 37–7. Sciatic nerve block, posterior approach. Landmarks: 1, Greater trochanter; 2, posterior–superior iliac spine; 3, point of needle insertion.

tion technique is of utmost importance because the adipose tissue over the gluteal area may obscure these bony prominences. The landmarks are outlined by a marking pen:

1. Greater trochanter
2. Posterior superior iliac spine
3. Needle insertion site 4 cm distal to the midpoint between the two landmarks

Technique

The patient is in the lateral decubitus position with a slight forward tilt. The foot on the side to be blocked should be positioned over the dependent leg so that twitches of the foot or toes can be easily noted. After cleaning with an antiseptic solution, local anesthetic is infiltrated subcutaneously at the determined needle insertion site. The anesthesiologist performing the block should assume an ergonomic position to allow precise needle maneuvering and monitoring of the responses to nerve stimulation.

Clinical Pearls

■ Raise the height of the bed enough to allow a comfortable and stable position for the patient during block placement and for observation of the muscle twitches obtained during nerve stimulation.

The fingers of the palpating hand should be firmly pressed on the gluteus muscle to decrease the skin–nerve distance (Figure 37–8). The skin below the index and middle finger is stretched for greater precision during block placement. The palpating hand should not be moved during block placement; even small movements of the palpating hand can substantially change the position of the needle insertion site because the skin and soft tissues in the gluteal region are highly movable. The needle is introduced at an angle perpendicular to the spherical skin plane (Figure 37–8). The

extremity. In contrast to common belief, this block is relatively easy to perform and is associated with a high success rate when properly performed.[17,18] It is particularly well suited for surgery on the knee, calf, Achilles tendon, ankle, and foot. It provides complete anesthesia of the leg below the knee with the exception of the medial strip of skin, which is innervated by the saphenous nerve (Figure 37–6). When combined with a femoral nerve or lumbar plexus block, anesthesia of almost the entire leg can be achieved.

Distribution of Anesthesia

Sciatic nerve blockade results in anesthesia of the skin of the posterior aspect of the thigh, hamstrings, and biceps muscles, part of the hip and knee joints, and the entire leg below the knee, with the exception of the skin of the medial aspect of the lower leg (see Figure 37–6). Depending on the level of surgery, the addition of a saphenous or femoral nerve block may be required.

Classic Posterior Approach

Anatomic Landmarks

Landmarks for the posterior approach to sciatic blockade are easily identified in most patients (Figure 37–7). Proper palpa-

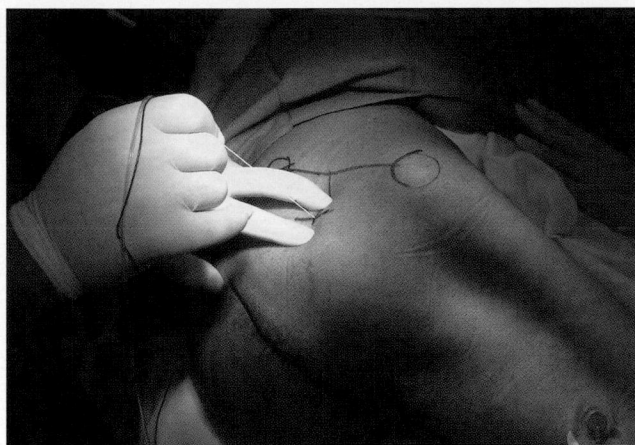

Figure 37–8. Sciatic nerve block, posterior approach. Needle insertion is in the perpendicular plane; the palpating hand is firmly pressed to decrease the skin–nerve distance and stabilize the anatomy.

nerve stimulator should be initially set to deliver 1.5 mA current (2 Hz, 100 μsec) to allow detection of twitches of the gluteal muscles and stimulation of the sciatic nerve.

As the needle is advanced, the first twitches observed are from the gluteal muscles. These twitches merely indicate that the needle position is still too shallow. The goal is to achieve visible or palpable twitches of the hamstrings, calf muscles, foot, or toes at 0.2–0.5 mA current. Twitches of the hamstrings are equally acceptable because this approach blocks the nerve proximal to the separation of the nerve branches to the hamstrings muscle. Once the gluteal twitches disappear, brisk response of the sciatic nerve to stimulation is observed (hamstrings, calf, foot, or toe twitches). After the initial stimulation of the sciatic nerve is obtained, the stimulating current is gradually decreased until twitches are still seen or felt at 0.2–0.5 mA current. This typically occurs at a depth of 5–8 cm.

After negative aspiration for blood, 15–25 mL of local anesthetic is injected (Figure 37–9). Any resistance to the

injection of local anesthetic should prompt needle withdrawal by 1 mm. The injection is then reattempted. Persistent resistance to injections should prompt complete needle withdrawal and flushing to ensure needle patency before reintroduction.

Clinical Pearls

- Since the level of the blockade with this approach is above the departure of the branches for hamstring muscles, twitch of any of the hamstring muscles can be accepted as a reliable sign of localization of the sciatic nerve.
- When the first needle pass does not result in nerve localization, do not regard it as a failure. Instead, use a systematic approach to troubleshooting:
  1. *Ascertain a functional nerve stimulator that is properly connected to the patient and needle and ensure that it is set to deliver the desired intensity of current.*
  2. *Mentally visualize the plane of the initial needle insertion, and redirect the needle in a slightly caudal direction (5–10 degrees) to the initial insertion plane.*
  3. *If the above maneuver fails, withdraw the needle to the skin and redirect it slightly cephalad (5–10 degrees) to the initial insertion plane.*
  4. *Failure to obtain foot response to nerve stimulation should prompt a reassessment of the landmarks and patient position.*

Continuous Block

The continuous sciatic nerve block is an advanced regional anesthesia technique, and experience with the single-shot technique is recommended to ensure its efficacy and safety. Continuous sciatic nerve block was described by Gross in 1956.[19] The current technique used is similar to the single-shot injection; however, slight angulation of the needle in the caudal direction is necessary to facilitate threading of the catheter. Securing and maintenance of the catheter are easy and convenient. This technique can be used for surgery and postoperative pain management in patients undergoing a wide variety of lower leg, foot, and ankle surgeries. Perhaps the single most important indication for use of this block is for amputation of the lower extremity.

Technique

The continuous sciatic block technique is similar to the single-shot technique. A standard regional anesthesia tray is prepared and an 8–10 cm long, insulated stimulating needle (preferably Tuohy-style tip) is used. Proper positioning at the outset and maintenance of the position during the continuous sciatic nerve block are crucially important to allow for precise catheter placement. A slight forward pelvic tilt prevents the "sag" of the soft tissues in the gluteal area and significantly facilitates block placement.

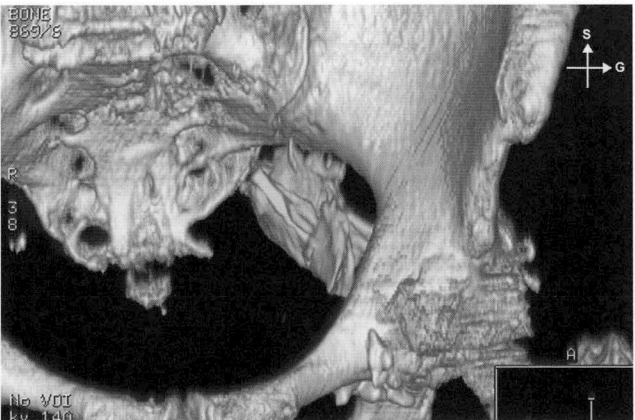

Figure 37–9. Sciatic nerve block, posterior approach. Dispersion of the local anesthetic after injection. The image represents an AP (anterior-posterior) view.

With the patient in the lateral decubitus position and a slight forward pelvic tilt, the landmarks are identified and marked with the pen. After a thorough skin cleaning with antiseptic solution, the skin at the needle insertion site is infiltrated with local anesthetic. A 10-cm long continuous-block needle is connected to the nerve stimulator (1.5 mA) and inserted at an angle perpendicular to the skin sphere. The opening of the needle should face distally (pointing toward the patient's foot) to facilitate catheter insertion. The initial intensity of the stimulating current should be 1.0–1.5 mA.

Clinical Pearl

- It is useful to inject some local anesthetic intramuscularly to prevent pain on advancement of larger-gauge and blunt-tipped needles typically used for this block.

As the needle is advanced, the first twitches obtained are from the gluteus muscle. Deeper needle advancement results in stimulation of the sciatic nerve. The principles of nerve stimulation and needle redirection are identical with those in the single-shot technique. After obtaining the appropriate twitches, manipulate the needle until the desired response is seen or felt using a current of 0.2–0.5 mA. At this point, a bolus of local anesthetic is injected (20 mL) after negative aspiration for blood. This is followed by insertion of the catheter 5–10 cm beyond the needle tip (Figure 37–10).

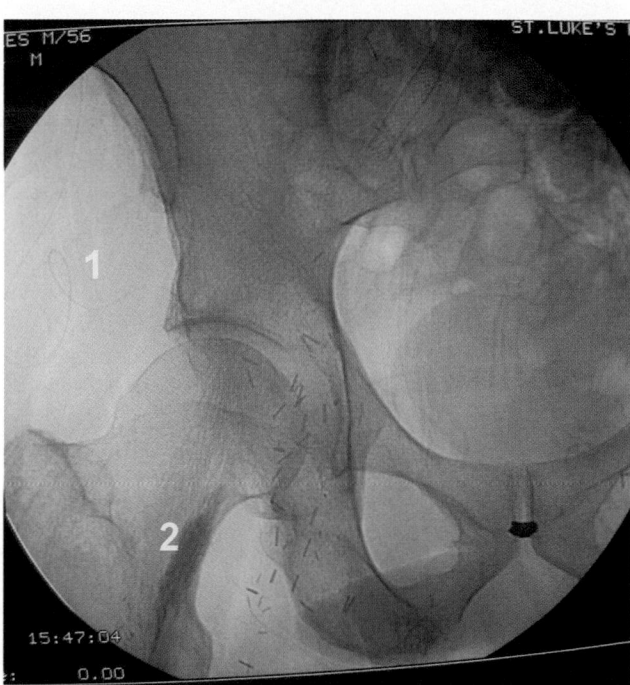

Figure 37–10. Continuous sciatic nerve block, posterior approach. Shown is the course of the catheter (*1*) and the fusiform-shaped contrast area indicating the spread of the local anesthetic in the sheath of the sciatic nerve (*2*). In this example, a mere 2 mL of the local anesthetic is injected.

Before administering local anesthesia, the catheter is checked for inadvertent intravascular placement by a negative test for blood.

Clinical Pearl

- When insertion of the catheter proves difficult, lowering the angle of the needle can be helpful.

A number of techniques to secure the catheter to the skin have been proposed. A benzoin skin preparation, followed by application of a clear dressing and a cloth tape is a simple and often sufices. The infusion port should be clearly marked as "continuous sciatic block."

Continuous Infusion

Continuous infusion is initiated after an initial bolus of dilute local anesthetic through the catheter. Ropivacaine 0.2% is commonly used for this purpose (15–20 mL). Diluted solutions of bupivacaine or L-bupivacaine are also suitable, but can result in undesirably greater motor blockade. The infusion is initiated at 10 mL/h or 5 mL/h when a patient-controlled analgesia (PCA) dose is planned (5 mL).[20,21]

Clinical Pearls

- Always manage breakthrough pain in patients on continuous infusion by administering a bolus of local anesthetic.
- Increasing the rate of infusion is never adequate alone in treating breakthrough pain.
- With patients on the ward, a higher concentration of a shorter-acting local anesthetic (eg, 1% lidocaine) is useful to both quickly treat the pain and test the position of the catheter.
- When the bolus injection through the catheter fails to result in blockade after 30 minutes, the catheter should be considered dislodged and should be removed.
- Patients receiving a sciatic nerve block infusion should be prescribed an immediately available alternative pain management protocol because incomplete analgesia and catheter dislodgment can occur.
- For inpatients, this is probably best done using a back-up IV PCA.

Parasacral Approach

Described by Mansour in 1993, the parasacral sciatic nerve block features relatively simple landmarks, and it is well suited for continuous infusion of local anesthetic.[8,22−27] In addition, the extension of the sciatic nerve block has characteristics of a plexus block. As such, there is a high success rate, anesthesia of the entire sacral plexus, and motor blockade of the obturator nerve.[23,24,28] Ripart[25] reports a 94% success rate in his series of 400 parasacral sciatic nerve block cases.

The parasacral approach to sciatic blockade has a wide clinical applicability for surgery and analgesia of the lower extremity, particularly when combined with a femoral or psoas compartment block.[23,28] The technique is associated with a high success rate and is particularly well suited for surgery on the popliteal fossa and the knee.[23]

Distribution of Anesthesia

Parasacral sciatic nerve blockade results in anesthesia of the skin of the posterior thigh, hamstrings, and biceps muscles; part of the hip and knee joint; and the entire leg below the knee except the medial cutaneous skin of the lower leg (see Figure 37–6). Morris[23] demonstrated extension of anesthesia to the obturator nerve after sciatic nerve block, as tested by the presence of adductor muscle weakness on a numeric scale. However, Jochum[29] suggested that the obturator nerve is only occasionally blocked by the parasacral sciatic nerve block. These conflicting data may be due to the fact that the parasacral plexus could be responsible for one third of adductor muscle strength. Depending on the level of surgery, the addition of a psoas compartment or femoral nerve block may be required.

Anatomic Landmarks

Landmarks for the parasacral approach to sciatic blockade are easily identified in most patients (Figure 37–11). Proper palpation technique is of the utmost importance because the adipose tissue over the gluteal area may obscure these bony

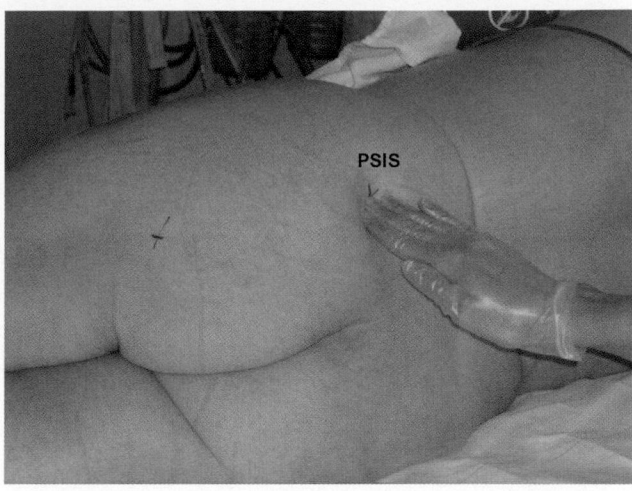

Figure 37–12. Parasacral sciatic nerve block. Proper palpation technique to identify the posterior superior iliac spine (PSIS).

prominences (Figures 37–12 and 37–13). The following landmarks are outlined by a marking pen:

- Posterior–superior iliac spine (PSIS)
- Ischial tuberosity (IT)
- A line between the PSIS and the IT is drawn. The needle insertion point lies 6 cm caudad to the PSIS on this line. The insulated needle is inserted at this point and advanced in a sagittal plane.

Technique

The patient is positioned in a lateral decubitus position, similar to the position required for the classic posterior approach to sciatic block (Figure 37–13). The dependent limb at the knee and hip is kept straight, and the limb to be blocked is flexed at both the hip and knee. Appropriate sedation and analgesia are mandatory to ensure the patient's comfort throughout the procedure. After cleaning with an antiseptic

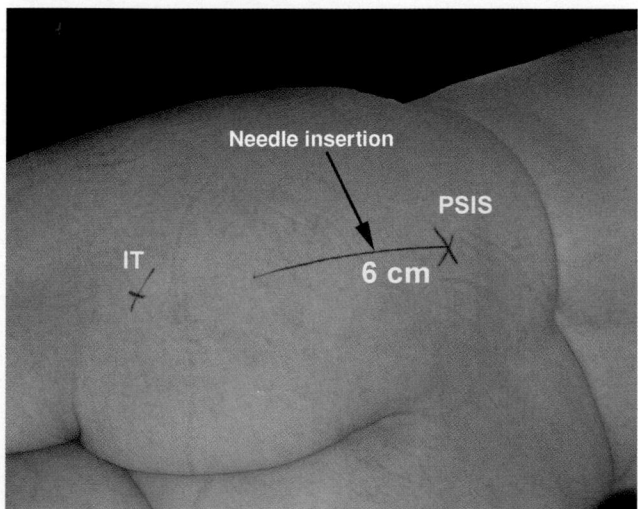

Figure 37–11. Parasacral approach to sciatic nerve block. Shown are the posterior superior iliac spine (*PSIS*) and the ischial tuberosity (*IT*). The needle insertion site is marked as 6 cm caudad to the PSIS on the line connecting PSIS with IT.

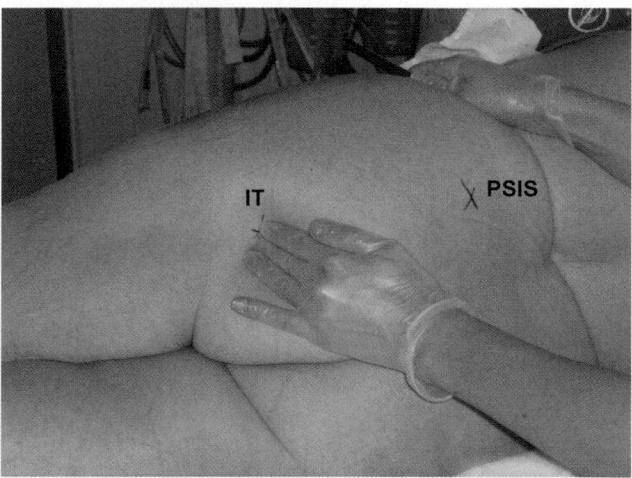

Figure 37–13. Parasacral sciatic nerve block. Proper palpation technique to identify ischial spine. (IT, ischial tuberosity; PSIS, posterior superior iliac spine.)

solution, local anesthetic is infiltrated subcutaneously at the determined needle insertion site. The practitioner performing the block should assume an ergonomic position to allow precise needle maneuvering and monitoring of the responses to nerve stimulation.

Clinical Pearl

- The height of the bed is adjusted to allow a comfortable and stable position for the patient during block placement and for observation of the motor responses obtained during nerve stimulation.

The needle is inserted perpendicular to the skin and advanced slowly (Figure 37–14). The motor response of the sciatic plexus is usually obtained at a depth between 6 and 8 cm. The goal is to achieve visible or palpable twitches of the hamstrings, calf muscles, foot, or toes at the current intensity of 0.2–0.5 mA. Twitches of the hamstrings are equally acceptable because this approach blocks the sciatic nerve proximal to the separation of the nerve branches to the hamstring muscles. The distal motor response may be either a tibial or a peroneal response with equal success of sciatic nerve blockade (Figure 37–15). Extension or flexion of the toes (responses of the common peroneal nerve and tibial nerve, respectively) rarely occur deeper than 8 cm. It is not necessary to stimulate both the common peroneal nerve and the tibial nerve; either response is adequate.[30,31]

Clinical Pearls

- Contact with the bone usually indicates the needle contact with the wings of the sacrum or the iliac bone, superior to and near the greater sciatic notch.
- In this case, the needle is withdrawn and redirected slightly caudally and laterally.
- Contact with the bone can be used as a depth test. The needle depth is noted; the needle should not be advanced more than 2 cm beyond this depth. At this site, the sciatic nerve is approached at the top of the greater sciatic foramen while leaving the pelvis. Advancing the needle deeper may expose pelvic viscera and vessels to risk of injury.

Once the aforementioned distal motor response is obtained with low-intensity stimulation (<0.5 mA), the local anesthetic solution is injected slowly while performing frequent aspiration tests. Twenty to 25 mL of local anesthesia is sufficient to produce sciatic nerve blockade (Figure 37–16).

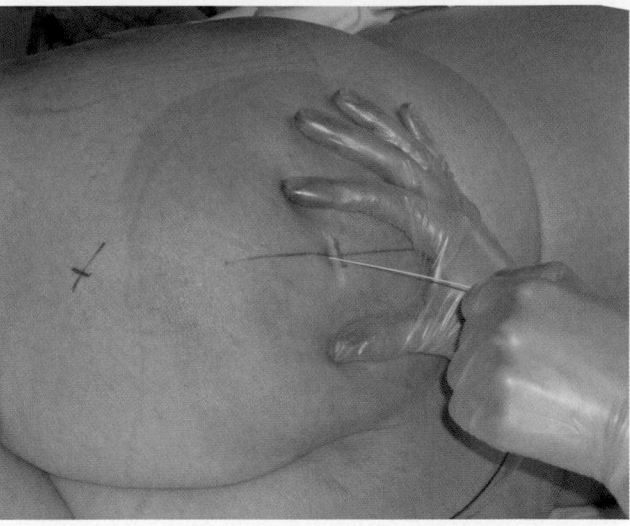

Figure 37–14. Parasacral sciatic nerve block. Needle insertion is perpendicular to the horizontal plane.

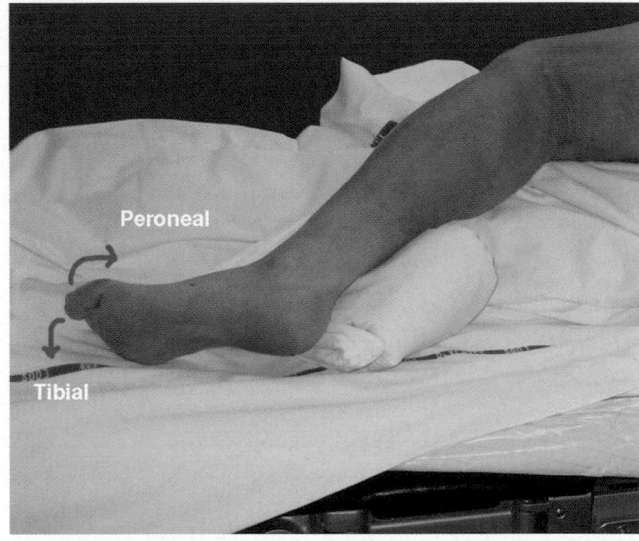

Figure 37–15. Sciatic nerve stimulation: motor response of the common peroneal or tibial nerves indicate proper localization of the sciatic nerve.

Cuvillon et al.[7] compared the parasacral sciatic nerve block with Winnie's approach, eliciting one or two stimulations. Winnie's approach with double-injection technique required more time to perform the block compared to Winnie's single-injection technique and the parasacral method. Although the onset of sensory and motor blocks were significantly faster with the double-injection method, the additional time needed to perform the double-injection block eliminated the advantage of the faster onset.

Continuous Parasacral Sciatic Nerve Block

The continuous parasacral sciatic nerve block is similar to the single-shot injection; however, slight caudad angulation

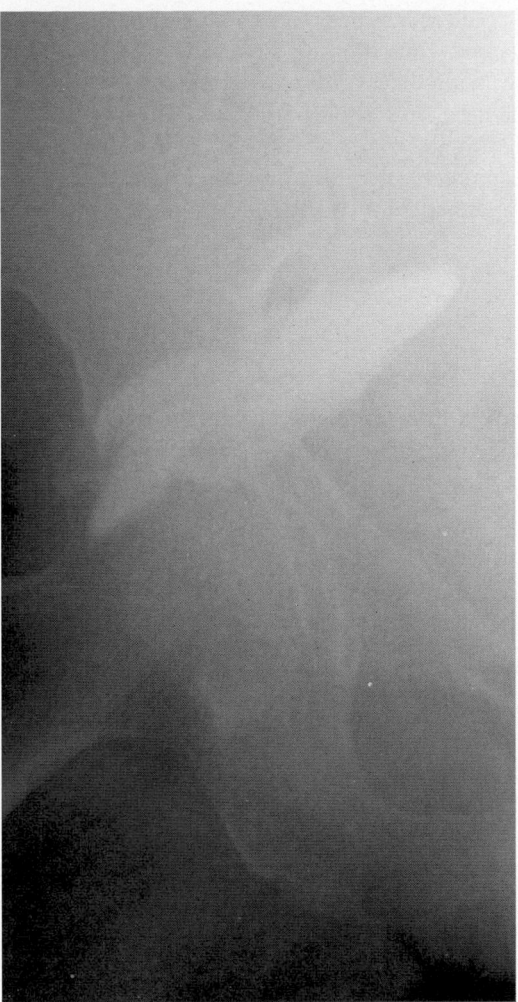

Figure 37–16. Parasacral nerve block: Dispersion of the contrast after injection, the "negative" contrast sign, and a typical fusiform distribution of the injectate.

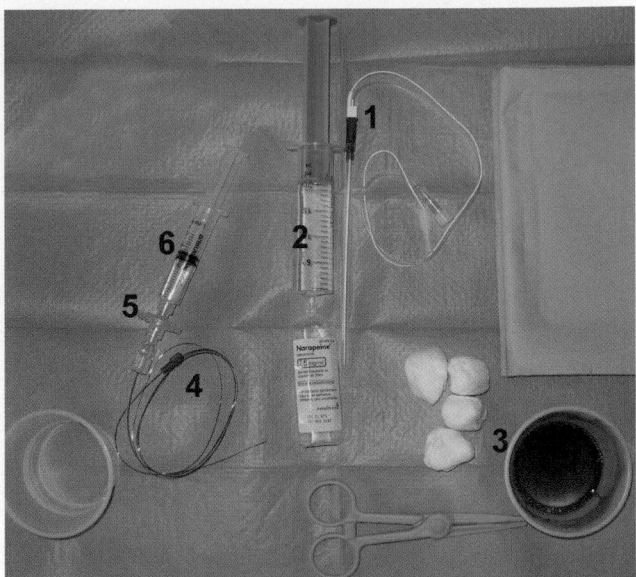

Figure 37–17. Equipment for continuous sciatic block. 1, Insulated needle; 2, syringe; 3, prep solution; 4, catheter; 5, filter; 6, syringe for test dose.

catheter insertion.[33] The initial intensity of the stimulating current should be 1.0–1.5 mA.

Clinical Pearls

- It is useful to inject some local anesthetic intramuscularly to prevent pain on advancement of larger-gauge and blunt-tipped needles typically used for this block.

of the needle is necessary to facilitate threading of the catheter. Securing and maintenance of the catheter are easy and convenient.[32] This technique can be used for surgery and postoperative pain management in patients undergoing a wide variety of knee, lower leg, foot, and ankle surgeries. Perhaps the single most important indication for use of this block is for cancer surgery of the lower extremity and for knee surgery.

Several kits for catheter insertion are currently commercially available. An ideal kit should include an insulated needle with a short bevel, a stimulating needle for catheter insertion, a catheter, an electrical wire connection, and an antibacterial filter (Figure 37–17). With the patient in the lateral decubitus position, the landmarks are identified and marked with a pen. After a thorough skin cleaning with an antiseptic solution, the skin is infiltrated with local anesthetic at the needle insertion site. A continuous-block needle is connected to the nerve stimulator and inserted at an angle perpendicular to the skin sphere. The opening of the needle should face distally (pointing toward the patient's foot) to facilitate

As the needle is advanced, twitches of the gluteus muscle are obtained first. Deeper needle advancement results in stimulation of the piriformis muscle first, then the sciatic nerve. The principles of nerve stimulation and needle redirection are identical with those of the single-shot technique. After obtaining the appropriate twitches, manipulate the needle until the desired response is seen or felt using a current of 0.2–0.5 mA. At this point, a bolus of local anesthetic is injected (20 mL) after negative aspiration for blood (Figure 37–18). This is followed by insertion of the catheter tip. Before administering the local anesthetic, the catheter is checked for inadvertent intravascular placement. If confirmation of catheter placement is desired, contrast media can be injected through the catheter and radiographic images can be studied.[31] The presence of a spindle 2–3 cm in length with an oblique orientation crossing the sciatic notch on the anteroposterior radiograph and/or shadowing of the sacral roots are considered to indicate injection into the correct plane and adequate placement of the catheter (Figure 37–16). For continuous infusion, ropivacaine 0.2% is maintained at 5 mL/h and a PCA dose is often planned (5 mL, lock-out time 30–45 minutes).

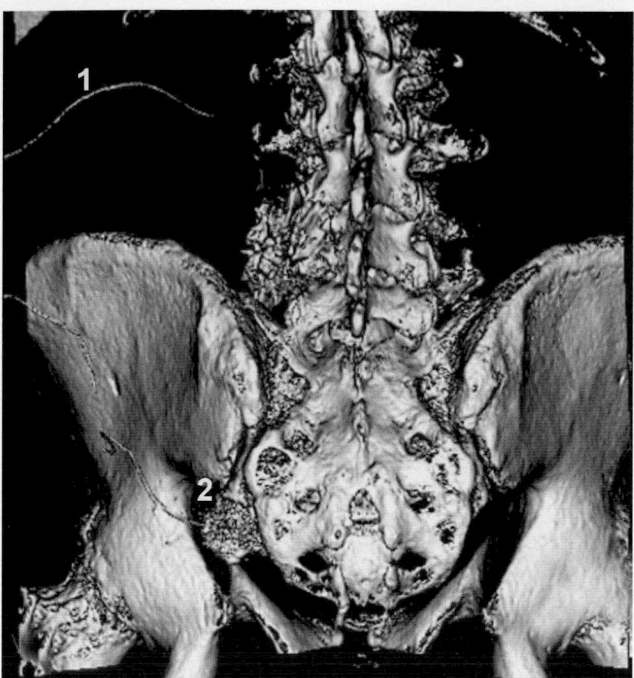

Figure 37–18. Parasacral sciatic block: Shown is the course of the catheter (1) This image is a PA (posterior-anterior) view and visualization of the injectate around the sciatic nerve (2).

ALTERNATIVE POSTERIOR APPROACHES

Di Benedetto[34] recently described a *subgluteal approach* to the sciatic nerve block. The study by di Benedetto suggested that the sciatic nerve is easily approachable through the posterior subgluteal approach. This technique is also a good alternative to the more proximal approaches to the sciatic nerve, with the potential for reducing the discomfort experienced by the patient during block placement. The landmarks with the subgluteal approach are the greater trochanter of the femur, the ischial tuberosity, and a line between the two with the midpoint marked. From the midpoint, another line is drawn perpendicularly and extended 4 cm in the caudad direction to identify the needle insertion point. A 20-gauge, 10-cm needle and nerve stimulator, are used and 20 mL of local anesthetic is injected when twitches of the sciatic nerve are obtained at ≤0.5 mA current.

Traditional approaches to the sciatic nerve at the pelvic level require identification of pelvic bone structures. Although the size of the buttocks is variable among different individuals and in the same individual at different stages of adult life, the relation of the sciatic nerve to the pelvis is constant throughout life. Using this premise, Franco[35] has suggested a more simplified approach to the sciatic nerve block that does not require palpation of deep bony structures. The landmarks in this approach are the intergluteal sulcus, the midline of the intergluteal sulcus, and a point 10 cm lateral to the midline of the intergluteal sulcus where the

block needle will be inserted. The curvature of the buttocks is disregarded when locating the needle insertion point. However, it is important not to stretch the skin when measuring the needle insertion point; this can distort the anatomy and lead to difficulties with localizing the sciatic nerve. The equipment, nerve stimulation and required volume of local anesthetic are comparable to those of the traditional approaches.

Complications & Strategies in Posterior Approaches & How to Avoid Them

Table 37–4 lists some general and specific instructions on possible complications of sciatic nerve blockage and methods to avoid them.

ANTERIOR APPROACH

General Considerations

The anterior approach to sciatic block is an advanced nerve block technique. The block is suited for surgery on the leg below the knee, particularly on the ankle and foot. It provides complete anesthesia of the leg below the knee with the exception of the medial strip of skin innervated by the saphenous nerve (Figure 37–19). When combined with the femoral nerve block, anesthesia of the entire knee and leg below the knee level is achieved.[36] The anterior approach is much less clinically desirable compared with the posterior approach. This is because the distribution of anesthesia is more limited and a much higher level of skill is required to achieve reliable anesthesia and avoid multiple needle insertions. In addition, this technique is not suitable for catheter insertion because of the deep location and perpendicular angle of insertion required to reach the sciatic nerve. Consequently, this block is best reserved for patients who cannot be repositioned into the lateral position needed for the posterior approach. The block has been suggested to be useful to manage postoperative pain in children in whom the anterior approach allows block placement in the supine position.[37,38] This obviously presents an advantage over other approaches to the sciatic block because these children are typically anesthetized for surgery using general anesthesia and the anterior approach does not require patient repositioning.

Since the original description by Beck,[4] several investigators have suggested modifications with more reliable landmarks for this block. However, all described approaches derive the needle insertion site at nearly identical points regardless of whether they use bony prominences, soft tissue, or femoral artery as landmarks.[36,39–43] In addition, even if these different approaches varied slightly in the site of needle insertion, the long path by the needle required to reach the sciatic nerve (8–12 cm) and the tendency of long, blunt-tipped needles

Table 37–4.	
Complications and How to Avoid Them	
Infection	Use strict aseptic technique
Hematoma	Avoid multiple needle insertions, particularly in anticoagulated patients Do not perform the sciatic nerve block in anticoagulated patients
Vascular puncture	Vascular puncture is not common with the sciatic nerve block technique Avoid deep needle insertion (pelvic vessels)
Local anesthetic toxicity	Systemic toxicity after sciatic blockade is not common Avoid using large volumes and doses of local anesthetic owing to the proximity of the large vessels and the potential for rapid absorption Injection of local anesthetic should be carried out slowly and with frequent aspiration to rule out intravascular injection
Nerve injury	Sciatic block has a unique predisposition for mechanical and pressure injury Use nerve stimulation and slow needle advancement Never inject local anesthesia when the patient complains of pain or when abnormally high pressure on injection is noted Never assume that the needle is obstructed with tissue debris when resistance to injection is met Take the needle out and check it for patency (flush) before reinsertion When stimulation is obtained with a current intensity of <0.2 mA, withdraw the needle slightly to obtain the same response with a current intensity of >0.2 mA before injecting local anesthesia
Nerve injury	Advance the needle slowly when twitches of the gluteus muscle cease to avoid impaling the sciatic nerve on a rapidly advancing needle
Other	Instruct the patient and nursing staff on the care of the insensate extremity Explain the need for frequent body repositioning to avoid stretching and prolonged ischemia (sitting) on the anesthetized sciatic nerve Advise heel padding during prolonged bed rest or sleep
Perforation of pelvic organs	Directing the needle medially should be exercised with this complication in mind
Anesthesia of the pudendal nerve	The pudendal nerve, a branch of the sacral plexus, may be anesthetized by the parasacral nerve block owing to diffusion of the injected local anesthesia Inform patients that this problem is transient
Tourniquet	Avoid the use of a tourniquet when possible Injection of the local anesthetic within the sciatic nerve sheath, epinephrine, and a tourniquet over the site of injection all can combine to cause ischemia of the sciatic nerve

to bend on insertion through the tissues make any proposed advantages questionable at best.

Equipment

A standard regional anesthesia tray is prepared with the following equipment:

Sterile towels and 4-in. × 4-in. gauze packs
20-mL syringes with local anesthetic
Sterile gloves, marking pen, and surface electrode
One 1½-in., 25-gauge needle for skin infiltration
A 15-cm long, short-bevel, insulated stimulating needle
Peripheral nerve stimulator

Anatomic Landmarks

The following landmarks should routinely be outlined using a marking pen (Figure 37–20):

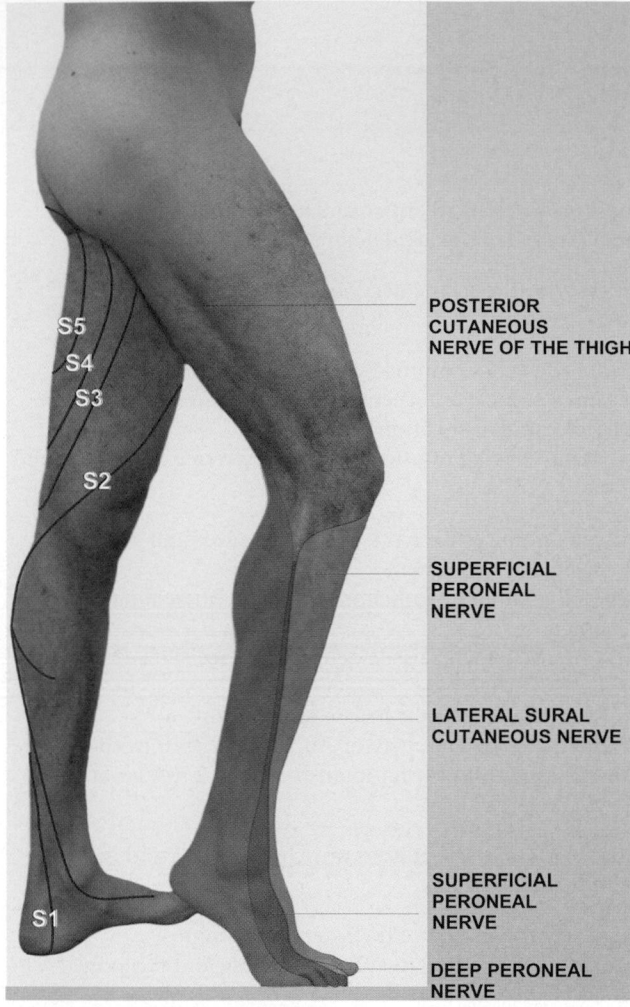

Figure 37–19. Distribution of anesthesia with anterior approach to sciatic nerve block.

1. Femoral crease
2. Femoral artery pulse
3. Needle insertion point is marked 4–5 cm distally on the line passing through the pulse of the femoral artery and perpendicular to the femoral crease

Technique

The leg to be blocked is fully extended on the table with the patient in the supine position. After cleaning the area with an antiseptic solution, local anesthetic is infiltrated subcutaneously at the determined needle insertion site. The fingers of the palpating hand should be firmly pressed against the quadriceps muscle to decrease the skin–nerve distance, and a needle connected to a nerve stimulator (1.5 mA) is introduced at a perpendicular angle to the skin plane (Figure 37–21). Motor response of the sciatic nerve (foot twitch) is typically obtained at a depth of 8–12 cm (visible or palpable twitches of the calf muscles, foot, or toes at a current of 0.2–0.5 mA). After negative aspiration for blood, 20 mL of local anesthetic is slowly injected. Any resistance to injection of local anesthetic

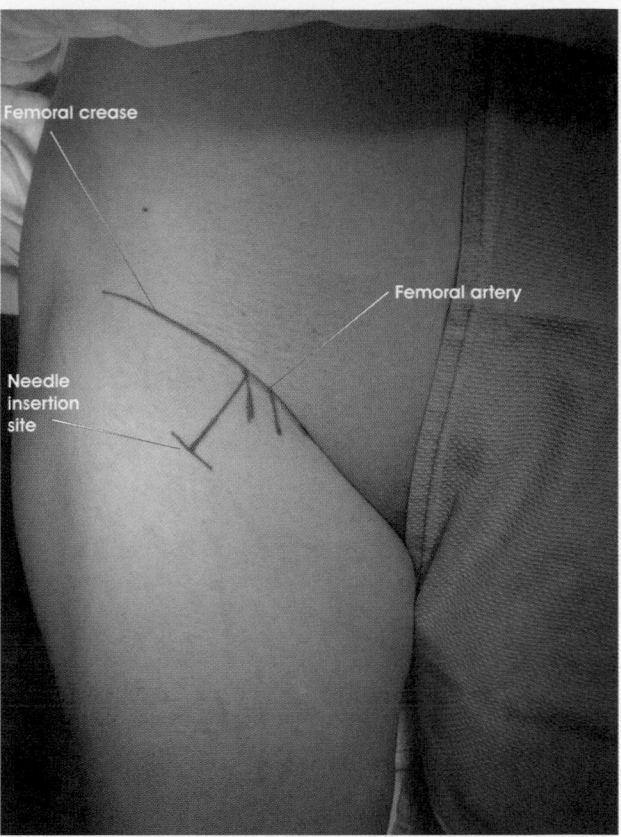

Figure 37–20. Sciatic nerve block through the anterior approach. Landmarks.

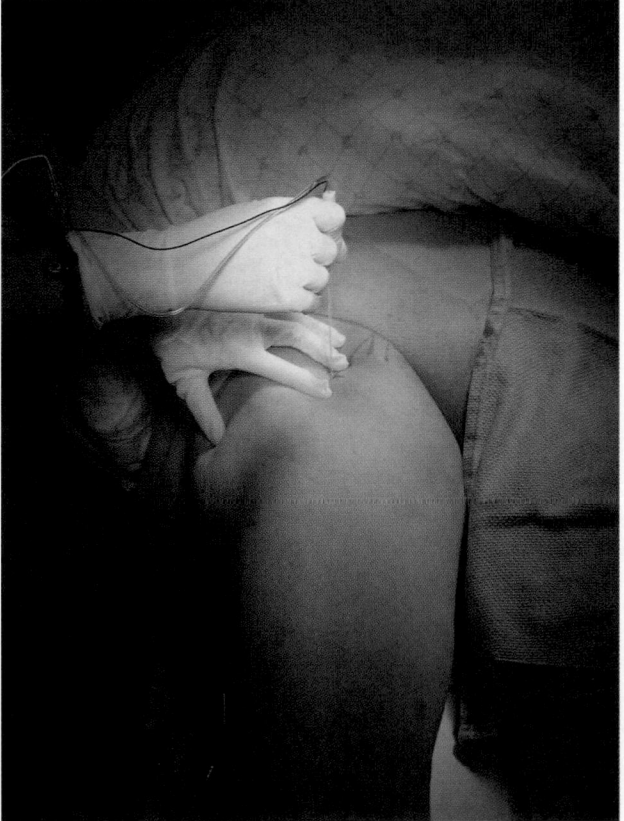

Figure 37–21. Sciatic nerve block through the anterior approach. Needle insertion.

Table 37–5.			
Interpreting Responses to Nerve Stimulation			
Response Obtained	**Interpretation**	**Problem**	**Action**
Twitch of the quadriceps muscle (patella twitch)	Common; stimulation of the branches of the femoral nerve	Too shallow (superficial) placement of needle	Continue advancing the needle
Local twitch at the femoral crease area	Direct stimulation of the iliopsoas or pectineus muscles	Too superior insertion of needle	Stop the procedure and reassess the landmarks
Hamstring twitch	Needle may be stimulating branch(es) of the sciatic nerve to the hamstring muscle; direct stimulation of the hamstrings with higher current is also possible	Unreliable-difficult to determine whether the needle is in the proximity of the sciatic nerve	Withdraw the needle and redirect slightly medially or laterally (5–10 degrees)
The needle is placed deep (12–15 cm) but twitches were not elicited and bone is not contacted	The needle is likely too medial		Withdraw and redirect slightly laterally
Twitches of the calf, foot, or toes	Stimulation of the sciatic nerve	None	Accept and inject local anesthetic

should prompt cessation of the attempts to inject and needle withdrawal by 1 mm. The injection is then reattempted. Persistent resistance to injection should prompt complete needle withdrawal and flushing before reintroduction of the needle.

Clinical Pearls

- Local twitches of the quadriceps muscle are often elicited during needle advancement. The needle should be advanced past these twitches.
- Although there is a concern of femoral nerve injury with further needle advancement, this concern is theoretical. At this level, the femoral nerve is divided into smaller terminal branches that are movable and unlikely to be penetrated by a slowly advancing, blunt-tipped needle.
- Resting the patient's heel on the bed surface may prevent the foot from twitching even when the sciatic nerve is stimulated. This can be prevented by placing the ankle on a foot rest or by having an assistant continuously palpate the calf or Achilles tendon.
- Because branches to the hamstring muscle may depart the main trunk of the sciatic nerve at the level of needle insertion, twitches of the hamstrings should not be accepted as a reliable sign of sciatic nerve localization with this approach.

Bone contact is frequently encountered during needle advancement. This indicates that the needle has contacted the

femur (usually lesser trochanter). In this case, the foot is first rotated laterally, which should swing the minor trochanter out of the path of the needle and allow deeper advancement of the needle and nerve localization. If this maneuver fails, the needle is redirected or reinserted more medially. Table 37–5 lists some common responses to nerve stimulation and the course of action to take to obtain the proper response during the anterior sciatic blockade.

SUMMARY

Although the sciatic nerve block was described long ago, many practitioners avoided this block because of the perceived technical complexity. However, practice and knowledge of anatomy, high success rates can be achieved. Many approaches have been proposed to blocking the sciatic nerve posteriorly, and some of the most relevant have been presented in this chapter. Sciatic nerve block is an important technique for the regional anesthesiologist to master, because the combination of this block and a femoral nerve block or lumbar plexus block can anesthetize almost the entire leg.

References

1. Sherwood-Dunn B: *Regional Anesthesia: (Victor Pauchet's Technique).* FA Davis, 1921.
2. Labat G: *Regional Anesthesia: Its Technic and Clinical Application.* WB Saunders, 1924.
3. Winnie AP: Regional anesthesia. Surg Clin North Am 1975;55:861–892.

4. Beck GP: Anterior approach to sciatic nerve block. Anesthesiology 1963;24:222–224.

5. Raj PP, Parks RI, Watson TD, Jenkins MT: A new single-position supine approach to sciatic-femoral nerve block. Anesth Analg 1975;54:489–493.

6. Di Benedetto P, Bertini L, Casati A, et al: A new posterior approach to the sciatic nerve block: A prospective, randomized comparison with the classic posterior approach. Anesth Analg 2001;93:1040–1044.

7. Cuvillon P, Ripart J, Jeannes P, et al: Comparison of the parasacral approach and the posterior approach, with single- and double-injection techniques, to block the sciatic nerve. Anesthesiology 2003;98:1436–1441.

8. Mansour NY, Bennetts FE: An observational study of combined continuous lumbar plexus and single-shot sciatic nerve blocks for post-knee surgery analgesia. Reg Anesth 1996;21:287–291.

9. Agur AMR, Lee MJ: *Grant's Atlas of Anatomy,* 10th ed. Lippincott Williams & Wilkins, 1999.

10. Babinski MA, Machado FA, Costa WS: A rare variation in the high division of the sciatic nerve surrounding the superior gemellus muscle. Eur J Morphol 2003;41:41–42.

11. Vloka JD, Hadzic A, April EW, et al: Division of the sciatic nerve in the popliteal fossa and its possible implications in the popliteal nerve blockade. Anesth Analg 2001;92:215–217.

12. Smith BE, Siggins D: Low volume, high concentration block of the sciatic nerve. Anaesthesia 1988;43:8–11.

13. Sinnott CJ, Strichartz GR: Levobupivacaine versus ropivacaine for sciatic nerve block in the rat. Reg Anesth Pain Med 2003;28:294–303.

14. Eledjam JJ, Ripart J, Viel E: Clinical application of ropivacaine for the lower extremity. Curr Top Med Chem 2001;1:227–231.

15. Casati A, Fanelli G, Borghi B, Torri G: Ropivacaine or 2% mepivacaine for lower limb peripheral nerve blocks. Study Group on Orthopedic Anesthesia of the Italian Society of Anesthesia, Analgesia, and Intensive Care. Anesthesiology 1999;90:1047–152.

16. Hadzic A, Vloka J: *Peripheral Nerve Blocks: Principles and Practice.* McGraw-Hill, 2004.

17. Bruelle P, Muller L, Bassoul B, Eledjam JJ: Block of the sciatic nerve. Cah Anesthesiol 1994;42:785–791.

18. Dalens B, Tanguy A, Vanneuville G: Sciatic nerve blocks in children: Comparison of the posterior, anterior, and lateral approaches in 180 pediatric patients. Anesth Analg 1990;70:131–137.

19. Gross G: Continuous sciatic nerve block. Br J Anaesth 1956;28:373–376.

20. Ilfeld BM, Thannikary LJ, Morey TE, et al: Popliteal sciatic perineural local anesthetic infusion: A comparison of three dosing regimens for postoperative analgesia. Anesthesiology 2004;101:970–977.

21. di Benedetto P, Casati A, Bertini L: Continuous subgluteus sciatic nerve block after orthopedic foot and ankle surgery: Comparison of two infusion techniques. Reg Anesth Pain Med 2002;27:168–172.

22. Mansour NY: Reevaluating the sciatic nerve block: Another landmark for consideration. Reg Anesth 1993;18:322–323.

23. Morris GF, Lang SA: Continuous parasacral sciatic nerve block: Two case reports. Reg Anesth 1997;22:469–472.

24. Morris GF, Lang SA, Dust WN, Van der Wal M: The parasacral sciatic nerve block. Reg Anesth 1997;22:223–228.

25. Ripart J, Cuvillon P, Nouvellon E, et al: Parasacral approach to block the sciatic nerve: A 400-case survey. Reg Anesth Pain Med 2005;30:193–197.

26. Bertini L, Borghi B, Grossi P, et al: Continuous peripheral block in foot surgery. Minerva Anestesiol 2001;67:103–108.

27. di Benedetto P, Borghi B, Ricci A, van Oven H: Loco-regional anaesthesia of the lower limbs. Minerva Anestesiol 2001;67:56–64.

28. Ho AM, Karmakar MK: Combined paravertebral lumbar plexus and parasacral sciatic nerve block for reduction of hip fracture in a patient with severe aortic stenosis. Can J Anaesth 2002;49:946–950.

29. Jochum D, Iohom G, Choquet O, et al: Adding a selective obturator nerve block to the parasacral sciatic nerve block: An evaluation. Anesth Analg 2004;99:1544–1549.

30. Bailey SL, Parkinson SK, Little WL, Simmerman SR: Sciatic nerve block. A comparison of single versus double injection technique. Reg Anesth 1994;19:9–13.

31. Gaertner E, Lascurain P, Venet C, et al: Continuous parasacral sciatic block: A radiographic study. Anesth Analg 2004;98:831–834.

32. Souron V, Eyrolle L, Rosencher N: The Mansour's sacral plexus block: An effective technique for continuous block. Reg Anesth Pain Med 2000;25:208–209.

33. Chelly J, Fanelli G, Casati A (editors): *Continuous Peripheral Nerve Blocks: An Illustrated Guide.* CV Mosby, 2001.

34. di Benedetto P, Casati A, Bertini L, Fanelli G: Posterior subgluteal approach to block the sciatic nerve: Description of the technique and initial clinical experiences. Eur J Anaesthesiol 2002;19:682–686.

35. Franco CD: Posterior approach to the sciatic nerve in adults: Is euclidean geometry still necessary? Anesthesiology 2003;98:723–728.

36. Magora F, Pessachovitch B, Shoham I: Sciatic nerve block by the anterior approach for operations on the lower extremity. Br J Anaesth 1974;46:121–123.

37. McNicol LR: Anterior approach to sciatic nerve block in children: Loss of resistance or nerve stimulator for identifying the neurovascular compartment. Anesth Analg 1987;66:1199–1200.

38. McNicol LR: Sciatic nerve block for children. Sciatic nerve block by the anterior approach for postoperative pain relief. Anaesthesia 1985;40:410–414.

39. Mansour NY: Anterior approach revisited and another new sciatic nerve block in the supine position. Reg Anesth 1993;18:265–266.

40. Chelly JE, Delaunay L: A new anterior approach to the sciatic nerve block. Anesthesiology 1999;91:1655–1660.

41. Vloka JD, Hadzic A, April E, Thys DM: Anterior approach to the sciatic nerve block: The effects of leg rotation. Anesth Analg 2001;92:460–462.

42. Van Elstraete AC, Poey C, Lebrun T, Pastureau F: New landmarks for the anterior approach to the sciatic nerve block: Imaging and clinical study. Anesth Analg 2002;95:214–218.

43. Hadzic A, Vloka JD: Anterior approach to sciatic nerve block. In: Hadzic A, Vloka J (editors): *Peripheral Nerve Blocks.* McGraw-Hill, 2003.

38

Block of the Sciatic Nerve in the Popliteal Fossa

Jerry D. Vloka, MD • Admir Hadzic, MD

INTRODUCTION

Distal sciatic nerve block (popliteal fossa block) is a relatively simple technique that results in reliable surgical anesthesia of the calf, tibia, fibula, ankle, and foot.[1,2] Consequently, this technique is used primarily for anesthesia or analgesia for foot, ankle, and lower-leg surgery.[3] The sciatic nerve can be approached from either the posterior approach described by Rorie,[3] or the lateral approach, which eliminates the need to reposition patients in the supine position.[1] With the lateral popliteal fossa block, patients remain supine for the block and catheter placement, rather than being prone and then turning supine after the block is placed. Both approaches provide equivalent surgical anesthesia after nerve blockade.[1] With both approaches, catheters can be inserted to provide prolonged postoperative analgesia; catheters, however, are more easily secured in the lateral position. Because of the slower resolution of neural blockade in the lower extremity, popliteal fossa block performed with long-acting local anesthetics such as ropivacaine can provide 12–24 hours of analgesia after foot surgery. The remarkable safety of the block has been demonstrated in numerous studies.[3,4]

Analgesia with lower-extremity blocks typically lasts longer than analgesia with ankle block. For instance, McLeod found that lateral popliteal fossa block with 0.5% bupivacaine lasted 18 hours when compared with ankle block, which lasted only 6.2 hours.[5] Popliteal fossa block has also been used as an effective analgesic technique in children.[6] In a study of the efficacy of the popliteal sciatic nerve blockade (0.75 mL/kg of ropivacaine 0.2%) after foot and ankle surgery, 19 of 20 children required no analgesic agents during the first 8–12 hours postoperatively. Blocking the sciatic nerve in the popliteal fossa is an excellent choice for foot and ankle surgery.[1] When used as a sole technique in outpatients, popliteal fossa block provides excellent anesthesia and postoperative analgesia, allows use of a calf tourniquet, and is devoid of disadvantages of neuraxial blockade.[7]

Indications & Contraindications

The popliteal block is one of the most commonly used regional anesthesia techniques in regional anesthesia practice. Common indications include corrective foot surgery, foot debridement, short saphenous vein stripping, repair of the Achilles tendon, and others.[8] As opposed to the more proximal block of the sciatic nerve, popliteal fossa block anesthetizes the leg distal to the hamstring muscles, allowing patients to retain knee flexion.[9,10]

Functional Anatomy

The **sciatic nerve** is a nerve bundle consisting of two separate nerve trunks, the tibial and common peroneal nerves. A common epineural sheath envelops these two nerves at their outset in the pelvis.[11] As the sciatic nerve descends toward the knee, the two components eventually diverge in the popliteal fossa, giving rise to tibial and common peroneal nerves (Figure 38–1). This division of the sciatic nerve occurs usually between 50 and 120 mm proximal to the popliteal fossa crease.[12,13] From

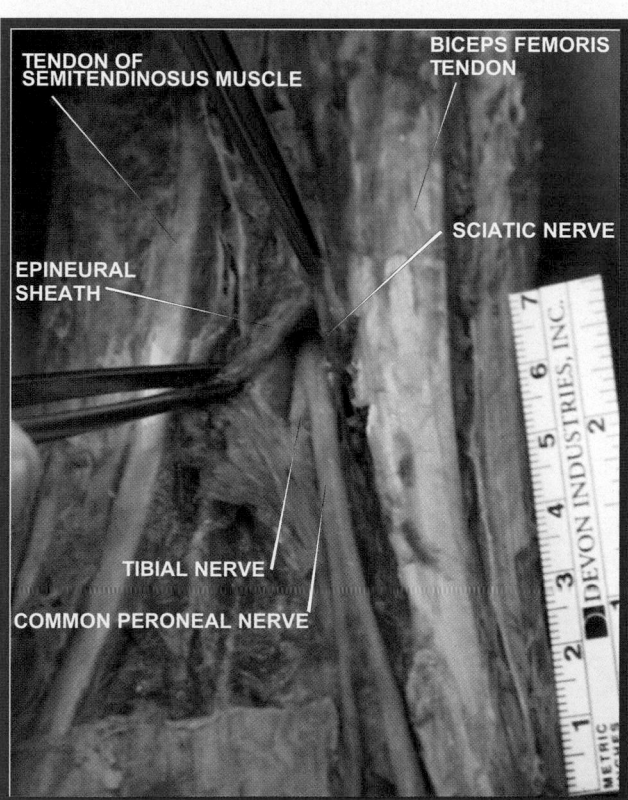

Figure 38–1. Anatomy of the distal sciatic nerve. The sciatic nerve descends between the hamstring muscles and diverges as tibial and common peroneal nerves approximately at or below 7–8 cm above the popliteal fossa crease. A common epineural sheath that serves as a conduit for injected local anesthetic is shown dissected.

its divergence from the sciatic nerve, the **common peroneal nerve** continues its path downward and descends along the head and neck of the fibula. Its major branches in this region are branches to the knee joint and cutaneous branches that form the sural nerve. Its terminal branches are superficial and deep peroneal nerves. The **tibial nerve** is the larger of the two divisions of the sciatic nerve and continues its path vertically through the popliteal fossa. Its terminal branches are the medial and lateral plantar nerves. Its collateral branches give rise to the cutaneous sural nerves, muscular branches to the muscles to the calf, and articular branches to the ankle joint. The tibial nerve is enveloped by a well-defined epineural sheath; consequently, single injection of a large volume of local anesthetic into the sheath of the tibial nerve may carry a higher success rate than injection into the sheath of the common peroneal nerve.[11] Note that in contrast to the common assumption, the sciatic nerve and popliteal vessels are *not* enveloped by the same tissue sheath; consequently, the concepts of the neurovascular sheath are not applicable to this block.[11] Instead, in the popliteal fossa the sciatic nerve components are lateral and superficial to the popliteal artery and vein. This anatomic characteristic is important in understanding why vascular punctures and systemic toxicity are so rare after popliteal blockade.

Distribution of Anesthesia

Popliteal blockade results in anesthesia of the entire distal two thirds of the lower extremity, with the exception of the medial aspect of the leg)[14] (Figure 38–2). Cutaneous innervation of the medial leg below the knee, however, is provided by the saphenous nerve, a superficial terminal extension of the femoral nerve. Depending on the level of surgery, the addition of saphenous nerve block may be required for surgery. Popliteal block alone is typically sufficient as anesthesia for the tourniquet pain, because this pain is the result of the pressure and ischemia of the deep muscle beds.

Choice of Local Anesthetic

Popliteal blockade requires a larger volume of local anesthetic (35–45 mL) to achieve anesthesia of both divisions of the nerve.[7] The choice of type, volume, and concentration of local anesthetic should be based on the patient's size and general condition and whether the block is planned for surgical anesthesia or pain management. The type and concentration of local anesthetics and the choice of additives to local anesthetic influence the onset and, particularly, the duration of the blockade (Table 38–1).

TECHNIQUES

Intertendinous (Posterior) Approach

The patient is in the prone position.[15] The foot on the side to be blocked should be positioned so that even the slightest movement of the foot or toes can be easily observed. This is best achieved by allowing the foot to protrude off the bed.

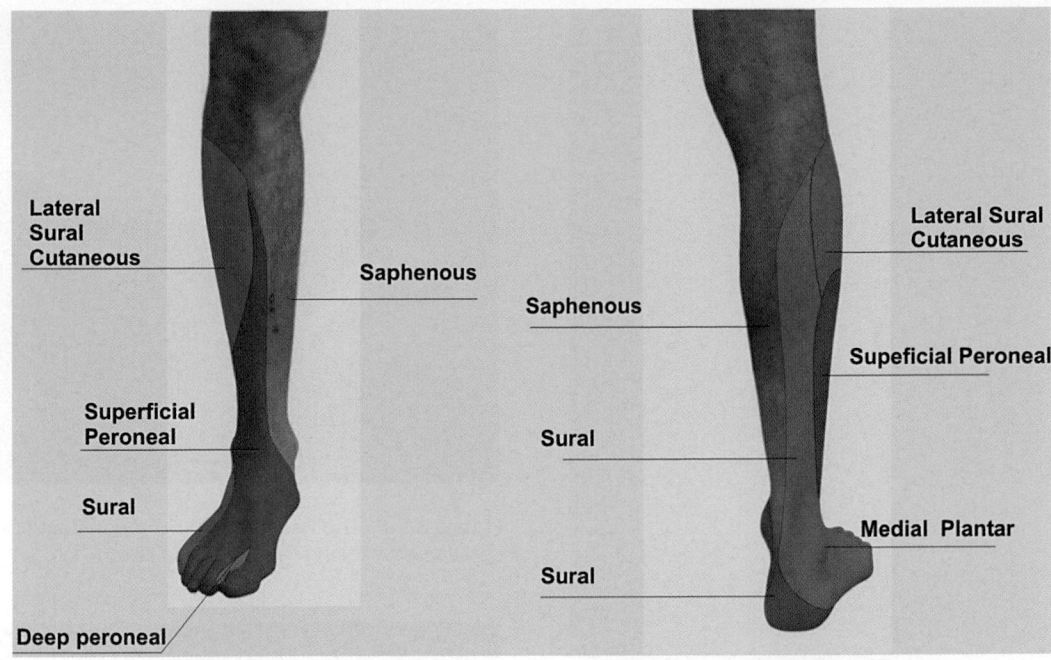

Figure 38–2. Sensory distribution of anesthesia after popliteal blockade.

Equipment

A standard regional anesthesia tray is prepared with the following equipment:

> Sterile towels and 4-in. × 4-in. gauze packs
> Three 20-mL syringes with local anesthetic

Table 38–1.

Local Anesthetics Choice for Popliteal Block

	Onset (min)	Anesthesia (h)	Analgesia (h)
3% 2-Chloroprocaine (+ HCO₃)	10–15	1	2
3% 2-Chloroprocaine (+ HCO₃ + epinephrine)	10–15	1.5–2	2–3
1.5% Mepivacaine (+ HCO₃)	15–20	2–3	3–5
1.5% Mepivacaine (+ HCO₃ + epinephrine)	15–20	2–5	3–8
2% Lidocaine (+ HCO₃ + epinephrine)	10–20	2–5	3–8
0.5% Ropivacaine	15–30	4–8	5–12
0.75% Ropivacaine	10–15	5–10	6–24
0.5 Bupivacaine (or L-bupivacaine)	15–30	5–15	6–30

> Sterile gloves, marking pen, and surface electrode
> One 1½-in., 25-gauge needle for skin infiltration
> A 5-cm long, short-bevel, insulated stimulating needle
> Peripheral nerve stimulator

Anatomic Landmarks

Landmarks for the intertendinous approach to popliteal block are easily recognizable even in obese patients (Figure 38–3). The landmarks should be routinely outlined by a marking pen: (1) popliteal fossa crease, (2) tendon of biceps femoris (laterally), and (3) tendons of semitendinosus and semimembranosus (medially).

The needle insertion point is marked at 7 above the popliteal fossa crease at the midpoint between the tendons. This point is just above the sciatic nerve in the popliteal fossa in nearly two thirds of patients (Figure 38–4).

Clinical Pearls

■ Relying on tendons rather than on subjective interpretation of the "popliteal fossa triangle" gives a much more precise and consistent localization of the popliteal nerve.

■ When not immediately apparent visually, these landmarks can be accentuated by asking the patient to flex the leg in the knee joint (Figure 38–5). This maneuver tightens the hamstring muscles and allows an easy and accurate palpation of the tendons.

Technique

After application of an antiseptic solution, local anesthetic is infiltrated subcutaneously at the site of the block needle

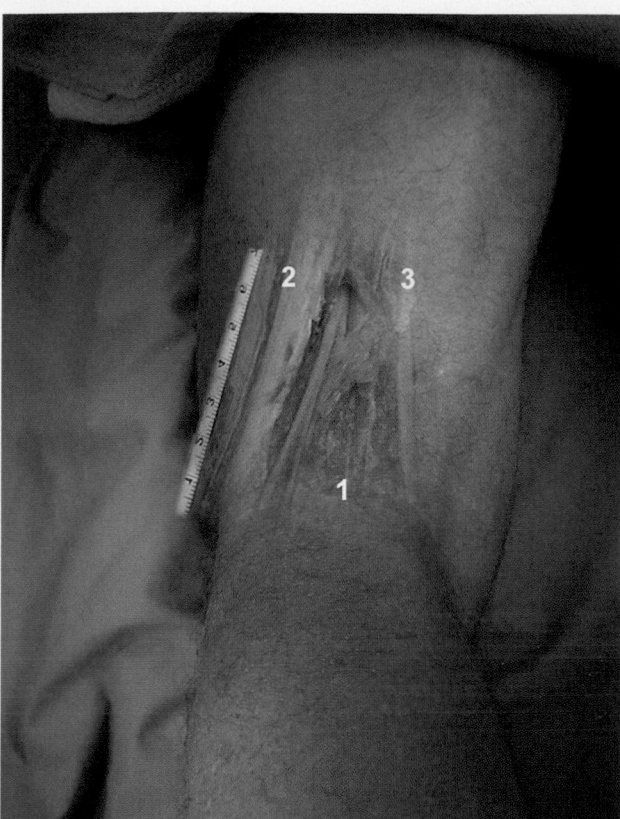

Figure 38–3. Popliteal block. Landmarks for the intertendinous approach. Seven centimeters above the popliteal fossa crease (1) the sciatic nerve is shown positioned between the tendons of the biceps femoris (2) and semitendinosus (3) muscles.

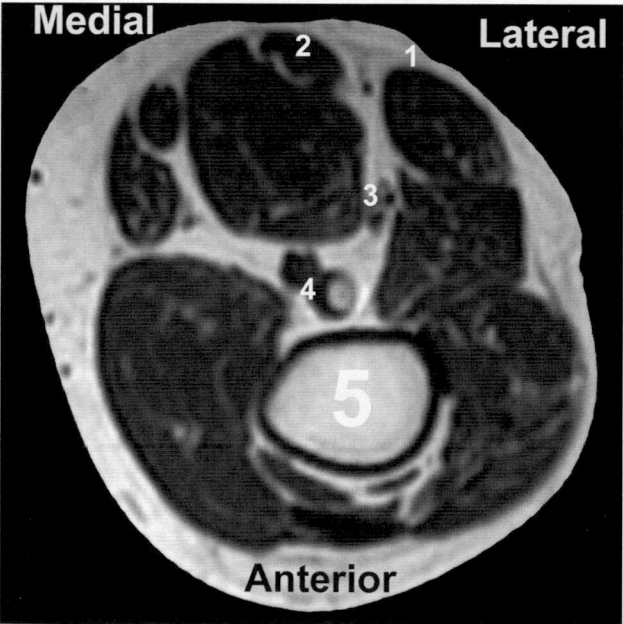

Figure 38–4. MRI of the popliteal fossa 7 cm above the popliteal fossa crease. 1, Tendon of the biceps femoris muscle; 2, tendon of the semitendinosus muscle; 3, sciatic nerve in the popliteal fossa (shown are both components: the tibial nerve is positioned more anteriorly and medially, whereas the common peroneal nerve is more posterior and lateral); 4, popliteal artery and vein; 5, femur.

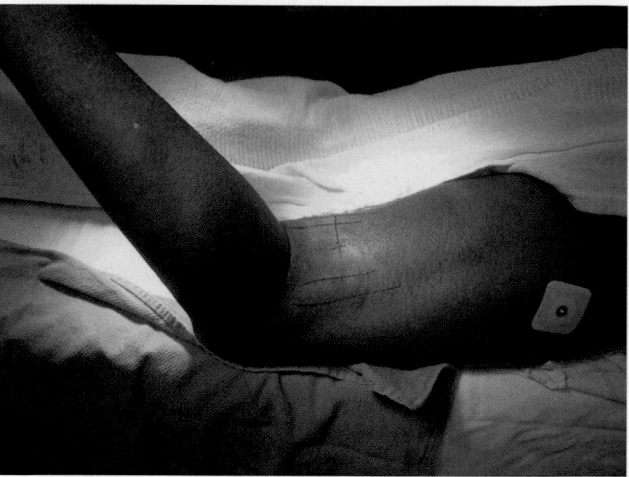

Figure 38–5. The landmarks for the popliteal block can be accentuated by asking the patient to flex the leg.

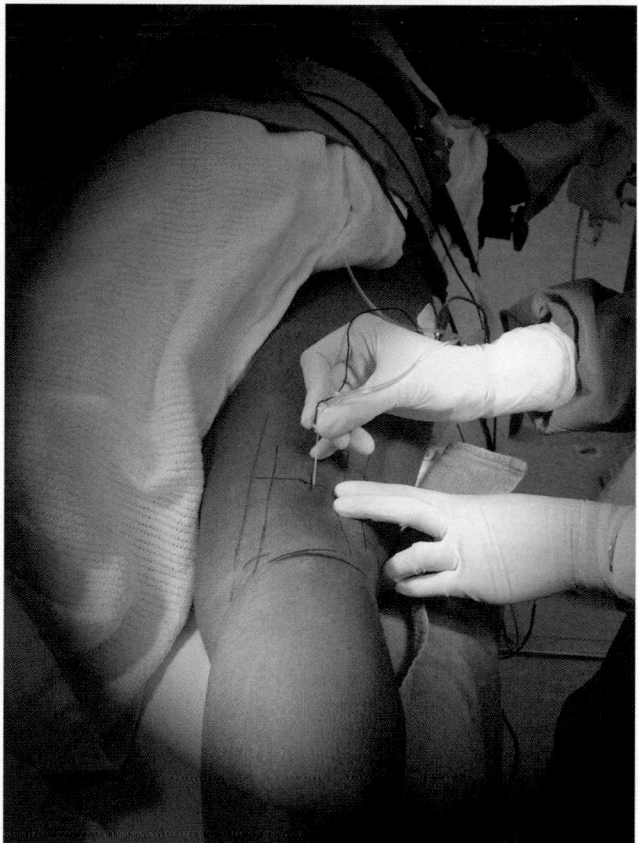

Figure 38–6. Popliteal block, intertendinous approach. The needle is inserted between tendons of the biceps femoris and semitendinosus muscles.

entry. The practitioner is best positioned on the side of the patient with the palpating hand on the biceps femoris muscle while observing the motor response of the foot and toes (Figure 38–6). The needle is introduced at the midpoint between the tendons. The nerve stimulator should be initially set to deliver 1.5 mA current (2 Hz, 100 μsec). When the needle is inserted in a correct plane, advancement of the needle should not result in local muscular twitches; the first response to nerve stimulation is typically that of the sciatic nerve (foot twitch). After the initial stimulation of the sciatic nerve is obtained, the stimulating current is gradually decreased until twitches are still seen or felt at 0.2–0.5 mA. This typically occurs at a depth of 3–5 cm from the skin. After negative aspiration for blood, 35–45 mL of local anesthetic is slowly injected.

Clinical Pearls

- Stimulation using current intensity of less than 0.5 mA may not be possible in some patients. This is occasionally (but not frequently) the case in patients with long-standing diabetes mellitus, peripheral neuropathy, sepsis, or severe peripheral vascular disease. In these cases, stimulating currents up to 1.0 mA should be accepted as long as a specific motor response is clearly seen or felt.

- When a rather small change in the needle position (eg, 1 mm) results in a change of the motor response from that of the popliteal nerve (plantar flexion of the foot) to that of the common peroneal nerve (dorsiflexion of the foot), the needle tip is stimulating the sciatic nerve at the level above its divergence into tibial and common peroneal nerve.

There are two basic types of motor responses that can be elicited with sciatic nerve stimulation at the level of the popliteal fossa. Stimulation of the common peroneal nerve results in dorsiflexion and eversion of the foot, whereas stimulation of the tibial nerve results in plantar flexion and inversion (Figure 38–7). As the stimulating current is being decreased, the twitch of the great toe often remains the only motor response seen with currents of <0.5 mA. Either response is adequate when the response is still present with current intensity of 0.2–0.4 mA (0.1 msec) as long as a large volume of local anesthetic is used. However, when the stimulation can not be accomplished with current <0.5 mA, stimulation of the tibial nerve may result in a higher success rate. Some common responses to nerve stimulation and the course of action to obtain the proper response are shown in Table 38–2.[16]

Block Dynamics and Perioperative Management

The intertendinous approach to popliteal block is associated with relatively minor patient discomfort because the needle passes only through the adipose tissue of the popliteal fossa. Regardless, adequate sedation and analgesia are always important to ensure a still and tranquil patient. Midazolam 1–2 mg after the patient is positioned and alfentanil 250–500 mcg just before block placement suffices for most patients. A typical onset time for this block is 10–25 minutes, depending on the type, concentration, and volume of local anesthetic used. The first signs of the onset of blockade are usually spontaneously reported by the patient who reports that the foot "feels different" or that he or she is unable to wiggle the toes. Sensory anes-

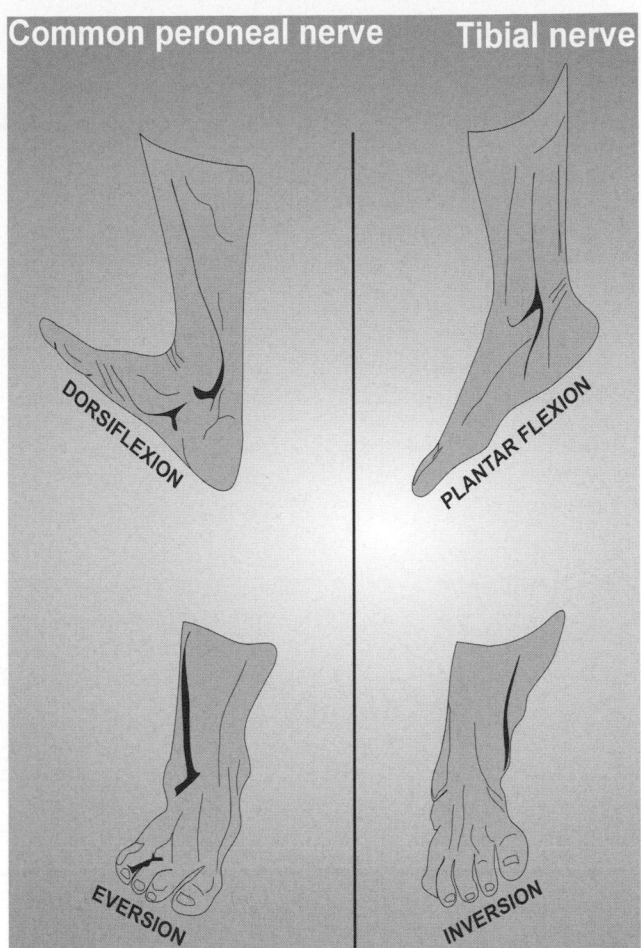

Figure 38–7. Motor responses obtained on stimulation of the sciatic nerve in the popliteal fossa.

thesia of the skin with this block is often the last to develop. Inadequate skin anesthesia despite the apparent timely onset of the blockade is common because it may take up to 30 minutes for full blockade to develop. However, local infiltration at the site of the incision by the surgeon is often all that is needed to allow the surgery to proceed until the block fully sets in.

Continuous Popliteal Block

Continuous popliteal block is an advanced regional anesthesia technique, and adequate experience with the single-shot technique is necessary to ensure its efficacy. The technique is similar to the single-shot injection; however, slight angulation of the needle cephalad is necessary to facilitate insertion of the catheter. Securing and maintaining of the catheter are easy and convenient. This technique can be used for surgery and postoperative pain management in patients undergoing a wide variety of lower leg, foot, and ankle surgeries.

Catheters may be inserted through a variety of approaches and equipment/infusion-specific techniques. There are also a variety of infusion systems, such as simple elastomeric pumps, which are easy for the patient to use. These infusion systems are disposable, deliver a fixed rate, and are generally inexpensive. Mechanical, battery-operated pumps

Table 38–2.

Intertendinous Popliteal Block: Troubleshooting

Response Obtained	Interpretation	Problem	Corrective Action
Local twitch of the biceps muscle	Direct stimulation of the biceps femoris muscle	Too lateral placement of the needle	Withdraw the needle and redirect slightly medially (5–10 degrees)
Local twitch of the semitendinosus/ membranosus muscles	Direct stimulation of the semitendinosus/ membranosus muscles	Too medial placement of the needle	Withdraw the needle and redirect slightly laterally (5–10 degrees)
Twitch of the calf muscles without foot or toe movement	Stimulation of the muscular branches of the sciatic nerve	These small branches are often outside the sciatic sheath	Disregard and continue advancing the needle until the foot/toes twitches are obtained
Vascular puncture	Blood in the syringe most commonly indicates placement into the popliteal artery or vein	Too medial needle placement	Withdraw and redirect laterally
Bone contact	The needle encounters the femur	Too deep needle insertion—either the nerve was missed or motor response was not appreciated	Withdraw the needle slowly and look for the foot twitch; if twitches are not seen, reinsert in another direction

The reader should also refer to Figure 38–4 for better understanding.

offer more flexibility of programming and bolus dosing, but tend to be more costly.[10] Souron et al.[17] reported the use of the continuous catheter technique to provide high-quality postoperative analgesia after oncologic orthopedic surgery of the leg.

Ilfeld[9] reported excellent postoperative analgesia using a continuous catheter in the popliteal fossa and a portable infusion pump for outpatients having moderately painful, lower extremity orthopedic surgery. Eighty percent of patients receiving ropivacaine infusion did not require oral opioid therapy and reported an average resting pain score of less than 1 (on a verbal pain score scale of zero to 10). Seven percent of patients who received placebo delayed their first dose of oral opioid until after infusion discontinuation, with an average resting pain score of 3–4 (out of 10). Breakthrough pain resulted in the worst resting pain score, with the difference between treatment and control groups being even more pronounced. The patients who received ropivacaine experienced a significant decrease in sleep disturbances, oral opioid use, and opioid-related adverse effects. These benefits were attained for ambulatory patients with the use of a portable, programmable, patient-controlled infusion pump. The degree of analgesia and the relative simplicity of the catheter pump system led to a very high rate of satisfaction for all subjects receiving ropivacaine.

Klein et al.[18] examined the efficacy and complications of long-acting popliteal nerve block after discharge home.

This prospective study included 1791 patients who had received an upper- or lower-extremity nerve block with 0.5% ropivacaine and were discharged the day of surgery. In all, 2382 blocks were placed: 1119 upper-extremity blocks and 1263 lower-extremity blocks. There were 733 interscalene, 193 supraclavicular, 193 axillary, 338 lumbar plexus, 263 femoral, and 662 sciatic blocks. Block efficacy was demonstrated by a low rate of conversion to general anesthesia (1–6%) and a low percentage of opioid use in the postanesthesia care unit (8–11%). The results showed that long-acting popliteal nerve block may be used in the ambulatory setting with a high degree of efficacy, safety, and satisfaction. Chelly et al.[19] documented the benefits of a continuous lateral popliteal sciatic nerve block infusion technique for postoperative analgesia in patients who had undergone open reduction and internal fixation of the ankle. Continuous infusion of ropivacaine 0.2% was associated with a significant reduction of morphine consumption by 29% and 62% during postoperative days 1 and 2, respectively.

Equipment

A standard regional anesthesia tray is prepared with the following equipment:

Sterile towels and 4-in. × 4-in. gauze packs

Three 20-mL syringes with local anesthetic

Sterile gloves, marking pen, and surface electrode

One $1\frac{1}{2}$-in., 25-gauge needle for skin infiltration

A 5-cm long, insulated stimulating needle

Catheter

Peripheral nerve stimulator

The needle insertion site is marked at 7 cm proximal to the popliteal fossa crease and between the tendons of the biceps femoris and semitendinosus muscles.

Technique

The continuous popliteal block technique is similar to the single-shot technique. With the patient in the prone position, the skin is infiltrated with local anesthetic using a 25-gauge needle at the injection site 7 cm above the popliteal fossa crease and between the tendons of biceps femoris and semitendinosus muscles. A 5- to 10-cm needle connected to the nerve stimulator (1.5 mA current) is inserted at the midpoint between the tendons of the biceps femoris and semitendinosus muscles (Figure 38–8). The block needle is advanced slowly with a slight cranial direction while seeking a plantar or dorsiflexion of the foot or toes. After obtaining appropriate motor response, the needle is manipulated until the desired response is seen or felt using a current of approximately 0.5 mA. The catheter should be advanced some 5 cm beyond the needle tip (see Figure 38–8). The needle is then withdrawn back to the skin while simultaneously advancing the catheter to prevent its inadvertent removal. Before activating, the catheter is checked for inadvertent intravascular placement by negative aspiration test for blood.

Continuous Infusion

Continuous infusion is initiated after an initial bolus of local anesthetic through the catheter. For this purpose, we routinely use ropivacaine 0.2% (15–20 mL). Diluted bupivacaine or L-bupivacaine is also suitable, but may result in more motor blockade. The infusion is maintained at 10 mL/h or 5 mL/h when a patient-controlled analgesia (PCA) dose is planned (5 mL). The dosing interval for the PCA dose is 20–60 minutes.

Clinical Pearls

- Breakthrough pain in patients on continuous infusion is always managed by administering a bolus of local anesthetic. Increasing only the rate of infusion is never adequate.

- Patients receiving continuous nerve block infusion should also be prescribed an alternative pain management protocol because incomplete analgesia and catheter dislodgment can occur. For inpatients, this is probably best done using a back-up IV PCA.

Popliteal (Lateral) Approach

The main advantage of the lateral approach to the popliteal block is that the patient does not need to be positioned in the prone position as with all posterior approaches.[5,16,20]

Regional Anesthesia Anatomy

The sciatic nerve is positioned between the biceps and semitendinosus muscles (see Figure 38–4). During block performance, stimulation of the common peroneal nerve is usually obtained first (65%) because this nerve is positioned lateral and more superficial than the tibial nerve.

Patient Positioning

The patient is in the supine position. The foot on the side to be blocked should be positioned so that even the slightest movement of the foot or toes can be easily observed. This is best achieved by placing the foot on a foot rest. Attention should be paid so that the Achilles tendon is also protruding off the foot rest. This positioning allows easy visualization of any foot movement during nerve stimulation.

Equipment

The equipment is identical with that for the posterior intertendinous approach except that a 10-cm stimulating needle is used.

Anatomic Landmarks

Landmarks for the lateral approach to popliteal block include popliteal fossa crease, vastus lateralis muscle, and biceps femoris muscle (Figure 38–9). The needle insertion site is marked in the groove between the vastus lateralis and biceps femoris muscles (Figure 38–10).

Technique

The operator should be seated, facing the side to be blocked. The height of the bed with the patient is adjusted to allow for an ergonomic position and a greater precision during

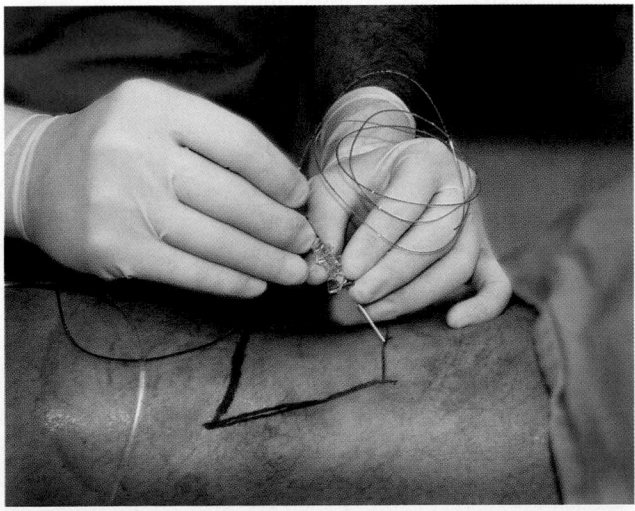

Figure 38–8. Popliteal block, intertendinous approach. Catheter insertion.

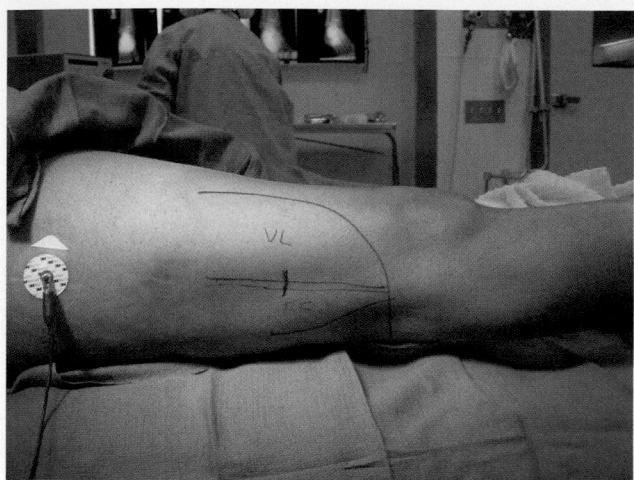

Figure 38–9. Popliteal block, lateral approach. Landmarks for this technique include vastus lateralis (VL), biceps femoris (BF) and popliteal fossa crease. The needle insertion site is marked 8 cm above the popliteal fossa crease (*thick vertical line*).

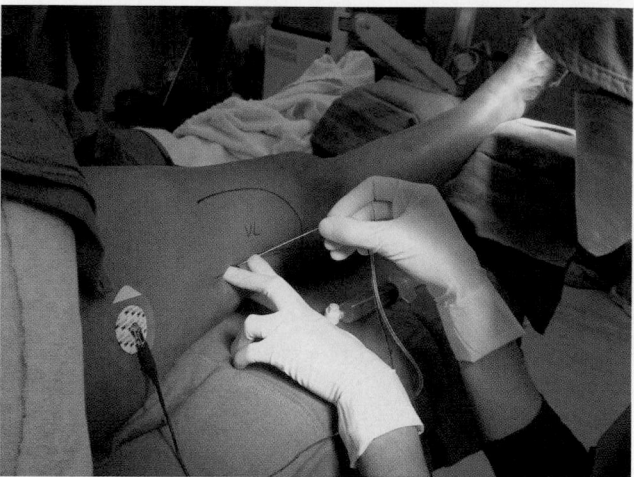

Figure 38–11. After the femur is contacted, the needle is redirected 30 degrees posterior to the plane in which the femur was contacted. VL, vastus lateralis.

block placement. This position also allows the performer to simultaneously monitor both the patient and the responses to nerve stimulation. The site of needle insertion is cleaned with an antiseptic solution and infiltrated with local anesthetic at the site of estimated needle insertion using a 1½-in., 25-gauge needle.

A 10-cm, 22-gauge needle is connected to a nerve stimulator, inserted in a horizontal plane between the vastus lateralis and biceps femoris muscles, and advanced to contact the femur (see Figure 38–10). The contact with the femur is important because it provides information on the depth of the nerve (typically 1–2 cm beyond the skin–femur distance) as well as on the angle at which the needle will need to be redirected posterior to stimulate the nerve. The current intensity is initially set at 1.5 mA. Keeping the fingers of the palpating hands firmly pressed and immobile in the groove, the needle

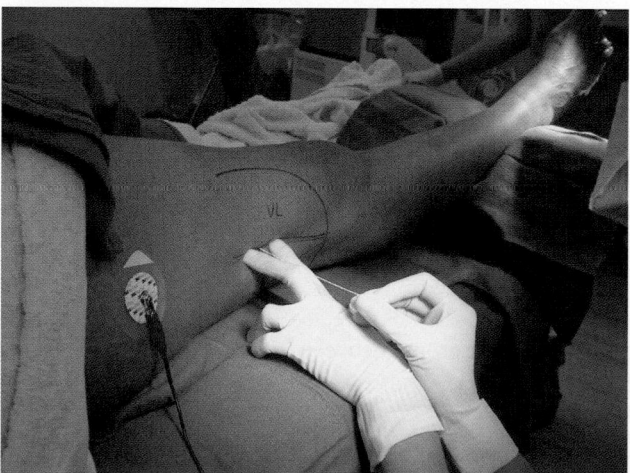

Figure 38–10. Popliteal block, lateral approach. The needle is inserted between vastus lateralis and biceps femoris in the horizontal plane to contact the femur. VL, vastus lateralis.

is then withdrawn to the skin, redirected 30 degrees posterior to the angle at which the femur was contacted, and advanced toward the nerve (Figure 38–11).

When the sciatic nerve is not localized on the first needle pass, the needle is withdrawn to the skin level and the following procedure is followed:

1. Make sure that the nerve stimulator is functional and properly connected to the patient and to the needle and that it is set to deliver current of desired intensity.
2. Make sure that the leg is not externally rotated in the hip joint and that the foot forms a 90-degree angle to the horizontal plane of the table. Any deviation from this angle changes the relationship of the sciatic nerve to the femur and biceps femoris muscle.
3. Mentally visualize the plane of the initial needle insertion and redirect the needle in a slightly posterior direction (5–10 degrees posterior angulation).
4. If the above maneuver fails, withdraw the needle and reinsert with an additional 5–10 degrees posterior redirection.
5. If the above maneuvers fail, withdraw the needle to the skin and reinsert 1 cm inferior to the initial insertion site; then repeat the above steps.
6. Failure to obtain foot response to nerve stimulation should prompt reassessment of the landmarks and arm position. In addition, the stimulating current should be increased to 2 mA.

After the initial stimulation of the sciatic nerve is obtained, the stimulating current is gradually decreased until motor response of the foot or toes is still seen or felt at 0.2–0.5 mA. This typically occurs at a depth of 5–7 cm. At this point, the needle should be stabilized, and after negative aspiration for blood, 35–45 mL of local anesthetic are slowly injected. The hands should be kept as immobile as possible to prevent injection outside the sheath of the sciatic nerve.

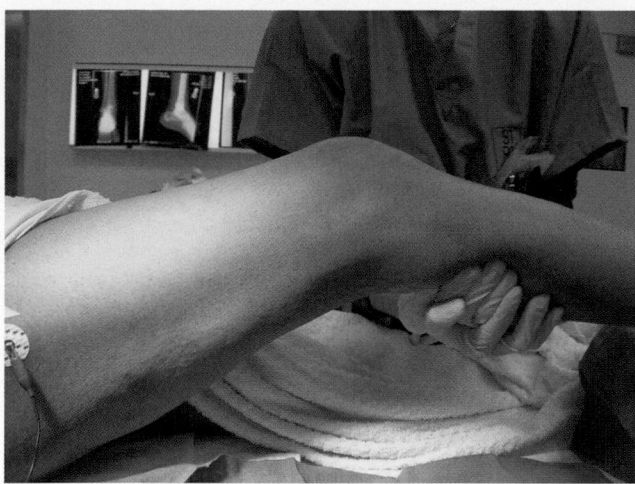

Figure 38–12. Popliteal block, lateral approach. Asking the patient to flex the leg in the knee joint facilitates identification of the landmarks (popliteal fossa crease, vastus lateralis, and biceps femoris).

Clinical Pearls

- In some patients, the biceps muscle may be atrophic and the iliotibial aponeurosis may be more prominent. In such cases, the needle insertion site is labeled in the groove between the vastus lateralis and the iliotibial tract.
- Flexing the patient's leg in the knee helps with identification of the popliteal fossa crease and the biceps and vastus lateralis muscles (Figure 38–12).

Some common responses during block placement using a nerve stimulator and the course of proper action to obtain twitches of the foot (Table 38–3).

Continuous Popliteal Block Through the Lateral Approach

The continuous popliteal block technique through the lateral approach is similar to the single-injection technique. With the patient in the prone position, the skin is infiltrated with local anesthetic at the injection site 8 cm above the popliteal fossa crease and in the groove between the biceps femoris and vastus lateralis muscles using a 25-gauge needle. A 10-cm Tuohy-style tip needle for continuous nerve block is connected to the nerve stimulator (at 1.5 mA current intensity) and inserted to contact the femur. Once the femur is contacted, the needle is withdrawn to the skin and redirected in a slight cranial and posterior direction relative to the plane in which the femur was contacted (usually 30 degrees to the horizontal plane) (Figure 38–13).

The needle is advanced slowly while seeking a plantar flexion or dorsiflexion of the foot or toes. After obtaining appropriate twitches, the needle is manipulated until the desired response is seen or felt using a current of 0.5 mA. The catheter should be advanced some 5–7 cm beyond the tip of the needle. The management of the catheter is similar to that of the intertendinous technique.

COMPLICATIONS & HOW TO AVOID THEM

Complications after a popliteal block are uncommon. Table 38–4 provides specific instructions on possible complications and how to avoid them.

SUMMARY

Popliteal sciatic block is an extremely useful technique to accomplish anesthesia or analgesia after ankle and foot surgery.

Table 38–3.

Lateral Popliteal Block: Troubleshooting

Response Obtained	Interpretation	Problem	Corrective Action
Local twitch of the biceps muscle	Direct stimulation of the biceps femoris muscle	Too shallow placement of the needle	Advance the needle deeper
Local twitch of the vastus lateralis muscle	Direct stimulation of the vastus lateralis muscles	Too anterior placement of the needle	Withdraw the needle and reinsert posterior
Twitch of the calf muscles without foot or toe movement	Stimulation of the muscular branches of the sciatic nerve	These small branches are often outside the sciatic sheath	Disregard and continue advancing the needle until the foot/toes twitches are obtained
Vascular puncture	Blood in the syringe most commonly indicates placement into the popliteal artery or vein	Too deep and anterior placement of the needle placement	Withdraw and redirect laterally
Twitches of the foot or toes	Stimulation of the sciatic nerve	None	Accept and inject local anesthetic

Table 38–4.

Complications of Popliteal Block and Measures to Prevent Them

Infection	• Use strict aseptic technique
Hematoma	• Avoid multiple needle passes with a continuous block needle; the larger needle diameter and/or Tuohy design may result in a hematoma of the biceps femoris or vastus lateralis muscles • When the nerve is not localized on first two or three needle passes, localize the nerve using a smaller gauge, single-shot needle first and then reinsert the continuous needle using the same angle; this technique is essentially similar to the localization of the internal jugular vein with a "localization needle" before inserting a large needle for canalization
Vascular puncture	• Avoid too deep insertion of needle because the vascular sheath is positioned medially and deeper to the sciatic nerve • When the nerve is not localized within 2 cm after the local twitches of the biceps muscle cease, the needle should be withdrawn and reinserted at a different angle, rather than advanced deeper
Nerve injury	• Uncommon; use nerve stimulation and slow needle advancement; do not inject when patient complains of pain or high pressures on injection are met; do not inject when stimulation is obtained at <0.2 mA current (100 μsec) • Avoid a combination of epinephrine in local anesthetic and application of a tourniquet over injection site to decrease risk of prolonged ischemia of the nerve
Pressure necrosis of the heel	• Instruct patient on the care of the insensate extremity • Use heel padding and frequent repositioning

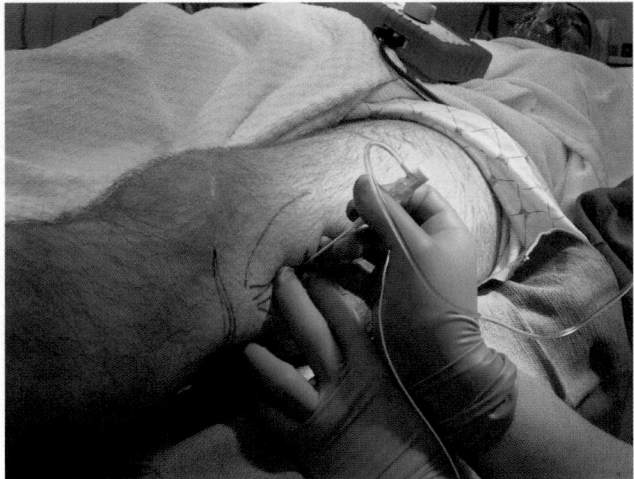

Figure 38–13. Popliteal block, lateral approach. Continuous technique is similar to the single-injection method except that a larger needle is used. The needle opening should be directed cephalad, and a slight cephalad needle angulation is used after localization of the sciatic nerve; these maneuvers facilitate insertion of the catheter.

Posterior and lateral approaches are both highly effective and applicable in numerous clinical scenarios.

References

1. Hadzic A, Vloka JD: A comparison of the posterior versus lateral approaches to the block of the sciatic nerve in the popliteal fossa. Anesthesiology 1998;88:1480–1486.

2. Rongstad K, Mann RA, Prieskorn D, et al: Popliteal sciatic nerve block for postoperative analgesia. Foot Ankle Int 1996;17:378–382.

3. Rorie DK, Byer DK, Nelson DO, et al: Assessment of block of the sciatic nerve in the popliteal fossa. Anesth Analg 1980;59:371–376.

4. Singelyn FJ, Gouverneur JM, Gribomont BF: Politeal sciatic nerve block aided by a nerve stimulator : A reliable technique for foot and ankle surgery. Reg Anesth 1991;16:278–281.

5. McLeod DH, Wong DH, Claridge RJ, Merrick PM: Lateral popliteal sciatic nerve block compared with subcutaneous infiltration for analgesia following foot surgery. Can J Anaesth 1994;41:673–676.

6. Tobias JD, Mencio GA: Popliteal fossa block for postoperative analgesia after foot surgery in infants and children. J Pediatr Orthop 1999;19:511–514.

7. Hansen E, Eshelman MR, Cracchiolo A: Popliteal fossa neural blockade as the sole anesthetic technique for outpatient foot and ankle surgery. Foot Ankle Int 2000;21:38–44.

8. Vloka JD, Hadzic A, Mulcare R, et al: Combined blocks of the sciatic nerve at the popliteal fossa and posterior cutaneous nerve of the thigh for short saphenous vein stripping in outpatients: An alternative to spinal anesthesia. J Clin Anesth 1997;9:618–622.

9. Ilfeld BM, Morey TE, Wang DR, Enneking F K: Continuous popliteal sciatic nerve block for postoperative pain control at home: A randomized, double-blinded, placebo-controlled study. Anesthesiology 2002;97:959–965.

10. Mulroy MF, McDonald SB: Regional anesthesia for outpatient surgery. Anesthesiol Clin North Am 2003;21:289–303.

11. Vloka JD, Hadzic A, Lesser JB, et al: A common epineural sheath for the nerves in the popliteal fossa and its possible implications for sciatic nerve block. Anesth Analg 1997;84:387–390.

12. Sunderland S: The sciatic nerve and its tibial and common peroneal divisions. Anatomical features. In: Sunderland S (editor): *Nerves and Nerve Injuries.* E & S Livingstone, 1968, pp. 1012–1095.

13. Vloka JD, Hadzic A, April EW, et al: Division of the sciatic nerve in the popliteal fossa and its possible implications in the popliteal nerve blockade. Anesth Analg 2001;92:215–217.

14. Benzon HT, Kim C, Benzon HP, et al: Correlation between evoked motor response of the sciatic nerve and sensory blockade. Anesthesiology 1997;87:548–552.

15. Vloka JD, Hadzic A, Koorn R, Thys D: Supine approach to the sciatic nerve in the popliteal fossa. Can J Anaesth 1996;43:964–967.

16. Hadzic A, Vloka JD: Popliteal block. In: Hadzic A, Vloka J (editors): *Peripheral Nerve Blocks: Principles and Practice.* McGraw-Hill, 2004.

17. Souron V, Eyrolle L, Rosencher N: The Mansour's sacral plexus block: An effective technique for continuous block. Reg Anesth Pain Med 2000;25:208–209.

18. Klein SM, Nielsen KC, Greengrass RA: Ambulatory discharge after long-acting peripheral nerve blockade: 2382 blocks with ropivacaine. Anesth Analg 2002;94:65–70.

19. Chelly JE, Greger J, Casati A: Continuous lateral sciatic blocks for acute postoperative pain management after major ankle and foot surgery. Foot Ankle Int 2002;23:749–752.

20. Zetlaoui PJ, Bouaziz H: Lateral approach to the sciatic nerve in the popliteal fossa. Anesth Analg 1998;87:79–82.

39

Ankle Block

Joseph Kay, MD • Rick J. Delmonte, DPM • Paul M. Greenberg, DPM

INTRODUCTION

Foot anesthesia is readily accomplished by blocking the five peripheral nerves that innervate the area by means of local anesthetic deposition either slightly proximal or distal to the malleoli.[1-5] This technique is easily learned and simple to perform, using straightforward visual and palpable anatomic landmarks. It does not require special equipment, paresthesia elicitation, nerve stimulation, special positioning, or patient cooperation.[1-5]

Ankle block can be used for all types of foot surgery and is safe and reliable, with success rates of 89–100%.[2,3,5-9] Because it does not cause motor blockade of the leg, patients are able to ambulate with crutches immediately after surgery and can be discharged home without recovery.[4] With the use of long-acting local anesthetics such as bupivacaine or ropivacaine, prolonged postoperative analgesia of up to 17 hours or longer may be accomplished.[6,9]

Indications & Contraindications

All types of foot surgery can be carried out with the patient under ankle block, including hallux valgus repair, forefoot reconstruction, arthroplasty, osteotomy, and amputation.[1-10] Ankle block can also provide analgesia for fracture and soft tissue injuries[11] and gouty arthritis.[12] Moreover, it can be used for diagnostic and therapeutic purposes with spastic talipes equinovarus[13] and sympathetically mediated pain.[14] Because motor block of the leg is avoided, ankle block may be preferable to sciatic/femoral (saphenous) nerve block for outpatient forefoot surgery.[15]

Ankle block should be avoided whenever there is infection, edema, burn, soft tissue trauma, or distorted anatomy with scarring in the area of block placement. Ankle block should also be avoided in a patient with vascular compromise due to compartment syndrome. In patients with severe coagulopathy, the risk of hematoma is increased, and if ankle block is performed, a more distal approach such as the mid-tarsal approach, in which blood vessels are more superficial and compressible, may be preferable.

Clinical Pearls

- Ankle block an excellent choice for ambulatory foot surgery.
- In extremely ill patients requiring foot surgery, general, neuraxial, or regional anesthesia with large volumes of local anesthetic can be avoided by using an ankle block.

Pertinent Anatomy

The foot is supplied by five nerves (Figures 39–1 and 39–2). The medial aspect is innervated by the *saphenous nerve,* a terminal branch of the femoral nerve (Figure 39–3). The rest of the foot is innervated by branches of the sciatic nerve:

- The lateral aspect is innervated by the *sural nerve* arising from the tibial and communicating superficial peroneal branches (Figure 39–4).
- The deep plantar structures, muscles and sole of the foot are innervated by the *posterior tibial nerve,* arising from the tibial branch (Figure 39–5).
- The dorsum of the foot is innervated by the *superficial peroneal nerve,* arising from the common peroneal branch (Figure 39–6).

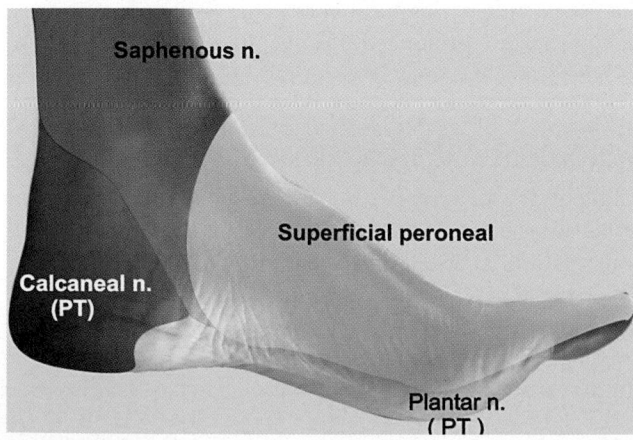

Figure 39–1. Sensory innervation of the foot.

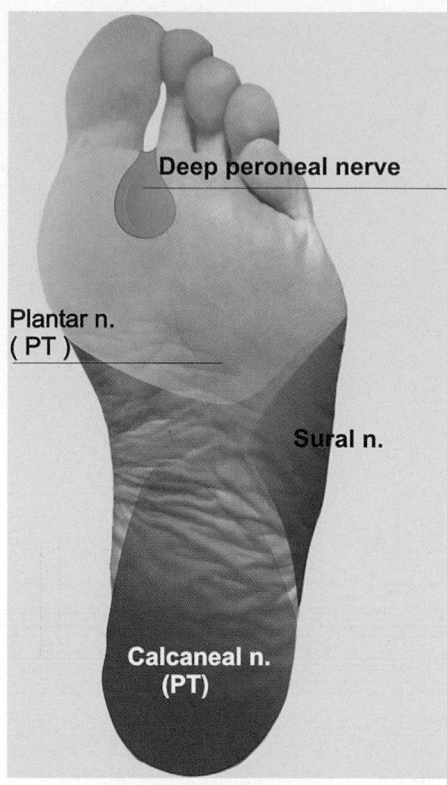

Figure 39–2. Sensory innervation of the sole of the foot.

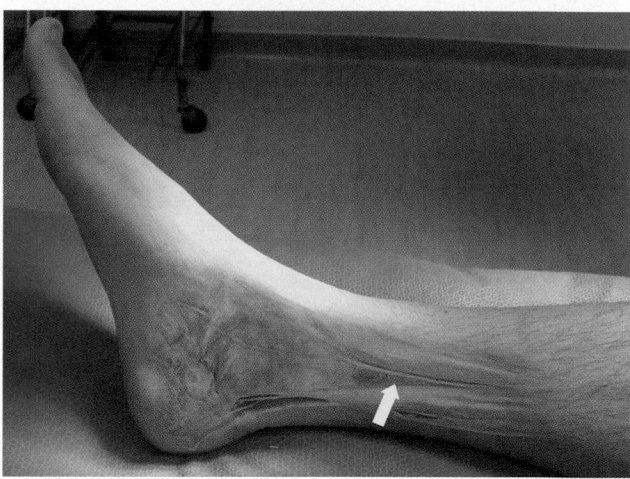

Figure 39–3. Saphenous nerve at the level of the ankle (*white arrow*).

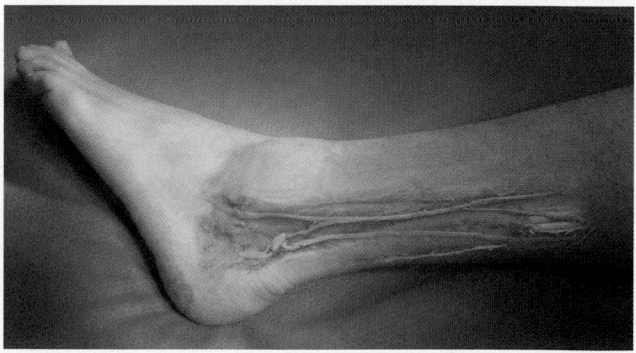

Figure 39–4. Sural nerve at the level of the ankle.

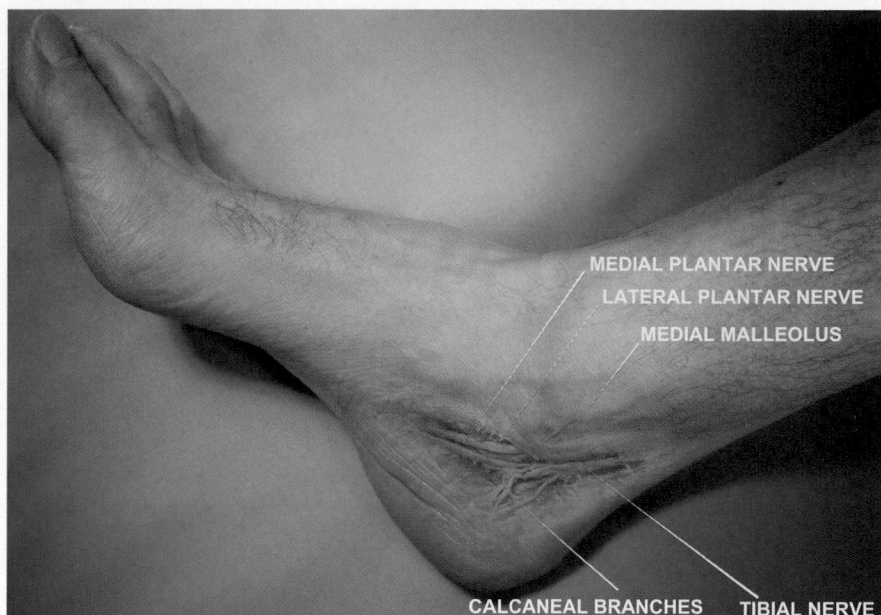

Figure 39–5. Posterior tibial nerve at the level of the medial malleolus.

MEDIAL PLANTAR NERVE
LATERAL PLANTAR NERVE
MEDIAL MALLEOLUS
CALCANEAL BRANCHES
TIBIAL NERVE

- The deep dorsal structures and web space between the first and second toes are innervated by the *deep peroneal nerve* (see Figure 39–2).[16,17]

At the level of the malleoli, the saphenous, superficial peroneal, and sural nerves are relatively superficial and subcutaneous. The posterior tibial and deep peroneal nerves are deep to the flexor and extensor retinaculi, respectively, and are more difficult to locate.

The posterior tibial nerve passes with the artery posterior to the medial malleolus deep to the flexor retinaculum, giving off a medial calcaneal branch to supply the lower and posterior surface of the heel.[18] The nerve and artery then become superficial and more accessible as they curve behind and underneath the sustentaculum tali, a bony ridge on the calcaneus about 2 to 3 cm below the medial malleolus. The nerve then divides into medial and lateral plantar nerves.[2]

The deep peroneal nerve passes lateral to the anterior tibial artery, extensor hallucis longus, and tibialis anterior tendons, and medial to the extensor digitorum longus tendon deep to the extensor retinaculum. It becomes more superficial to travel with the dorsalis pedis artery on the dorsum of the foot, where it is easily accessible.

Sensory innervation of the foot is highly variable. For example, in a study of 100 patients, 40% had the sural nerve extend medially to involve the fourth toe, and 10% had the saphenous nerve extend distally to involve the first metatarsophalangeal joint and occasionally the great toe.[18]

Because the deep structures of the foot are supplied by the deep peroneal and posterior tibial nerves and because cutaneous innervation is variable, all five nerves should be blocked for any foot surgery, especially if a tourniquet is used.[19] The one exception would be purely cutaneous surgery without tourniquet in the distribution of the sural, saphenous, or superficial peroneal nerves.[20] Selective versus complete ankle block for forefoot surgery under ankle tourniquet demonstrated that 43 versus 89% of patients were completely pain-free during surgery, suggesting that complete ankle block is preferable under these conditions.[8]

Clinical Pearls

- Always block all five nerves for any foot surgery under tourniquet.
- Block the deep peroneal and posterior tibial nerves distally where they are more superficial, whenever possible.

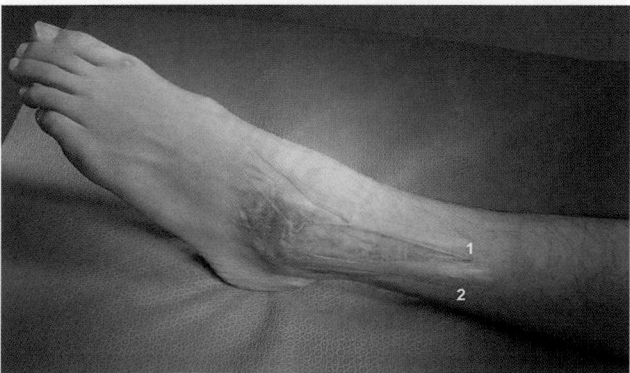

Figure 39–6. Superficial peroneal nerve. Shown is the emergence of the superficial nerve and its distribution on the dorsum of the foot. 1, Superficial peroneal nerve; 2, sural nerve.

Landmarks

The landmarks for ankle block are the medial and lateral malleoli, the Achilles tendon, extensor hallucis longus tendon (identified by having the patient extend the great toe)

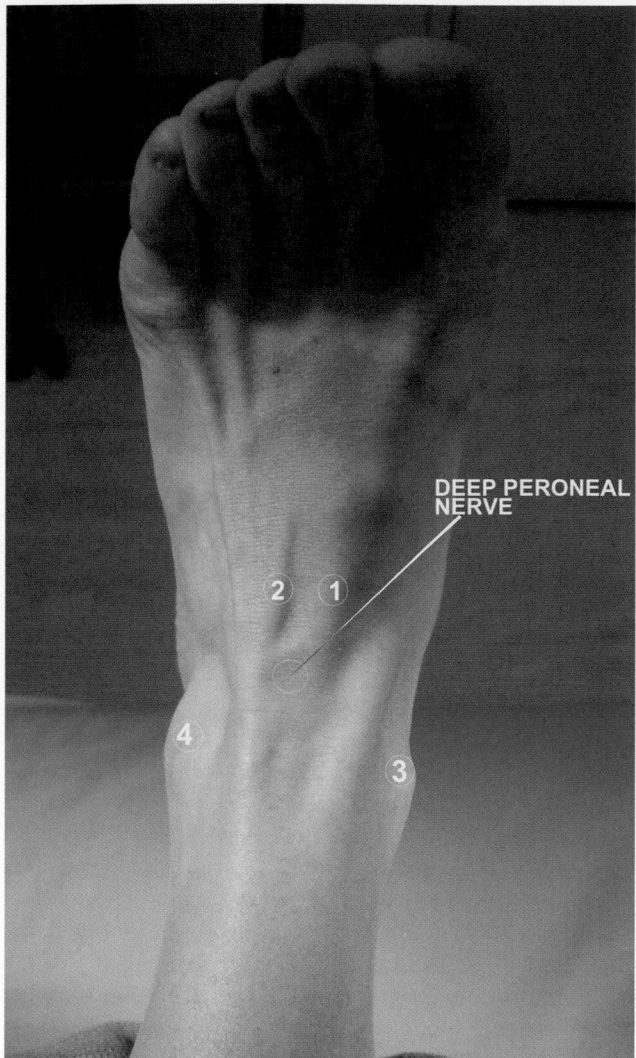

Figure 39–7. Maneuver to accentuate the landmarks for the deep peroneal nerve block (extensor hallucis longus). 1, Extensor hallucis longus; 2, extensor digitorum longus; 3, medial malleolus; 4, lateral malleolus.

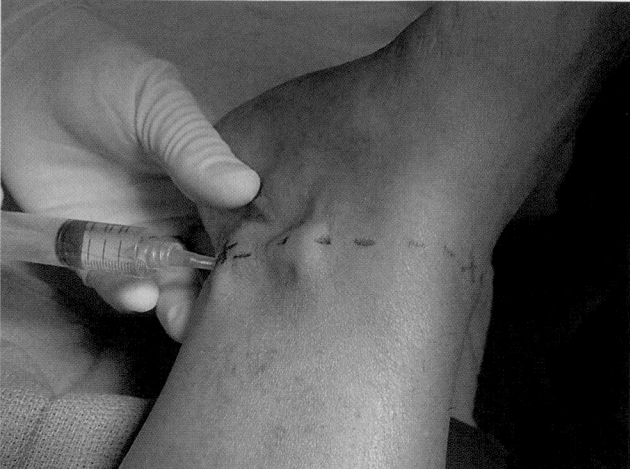

Figure 39–8. Saphenous nerve block is accomplished by injection of 5–8 mL of local anesthetic subcutaneously at the level of the medial malleolus.

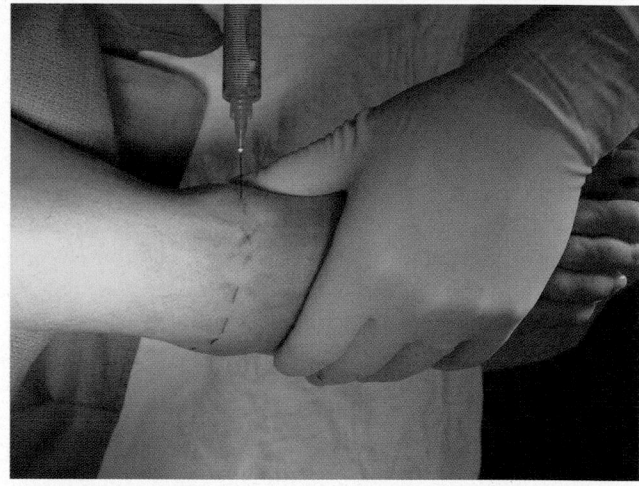

Figure 39–9. Superficial peroneal block.

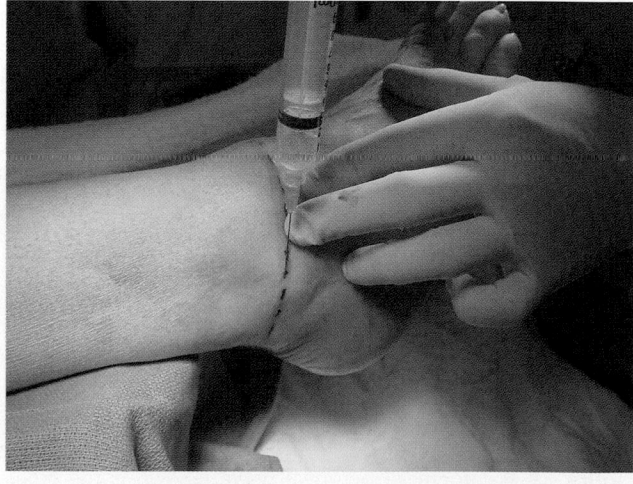

Figure 39–10. Block of the sural nerve.

(Figure 39–7), the posterior tibial and dorsalis pedis arteries, and the sustentaculum tali (a bony medial calcaneal ridge 2 to 3 cm below the malleolus).

For blockade at the level of the malleoli, the saphenous, sural, and superficial peroneal nerves are blocked with a circumferential subcutaneous injection of 10–15 mL of local anesthetic along a line just proximal to the malleoli and anterior from the Achilles tendon medially to laterally (Figures 39–8 through 39–10). The deep peroneal nerve is blocked by injection of 5–8 mL of local anesthetic just lateral to the extensor hallucis longus tendon deep to the retinaculum along the same circumferential line (Figure 39–11). The posterior tibial nerve is blocked by injection of the same volume of local anesthetic just posterior to the posterior tibial artery if palpable, or midway between the Achilles tendon and medial malleolus deep to the retinaculum (Figure 39–12).

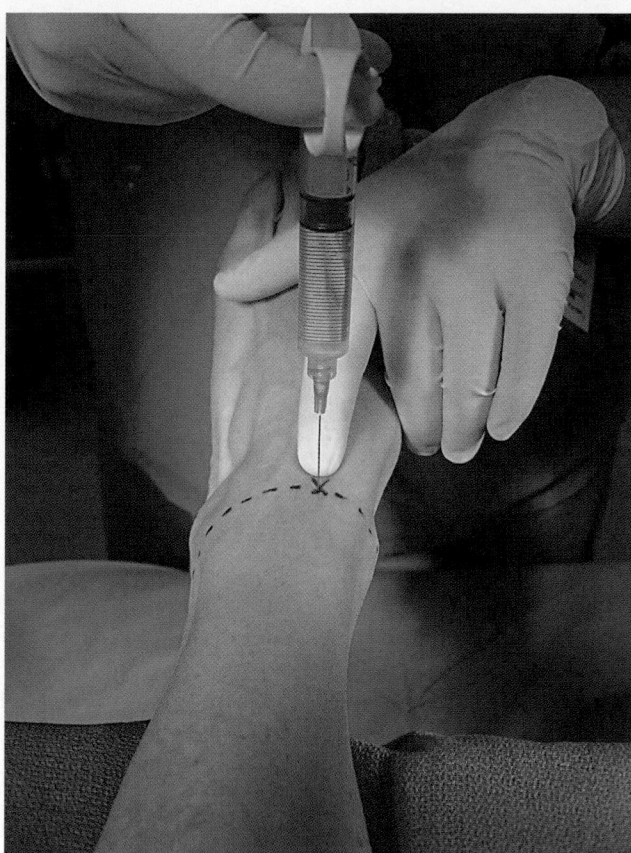

Figure 39–11. Block of the deep peroneal nerve.

For block at the *midtarsal level,* the saphenous, sural, and superficial peroneal nerves are blocked with a circumferential subcutaneous injection of 10–15 mL of local anesthetic along a line distal to the malleoli from the Achilles tendon medially to laterally. The deep peroneal nerve is blocked just lateral to the extensor hallucis longus tendon and medial to the dorsalis pedis artery. The posterior tibial nerve is blocked on the calcaneus on either side of the posterior tibial artery (if palpable) or posterior and inferior to the ridge of the sustentaculum tali.

Equipment

No special equipment other than disinfectant, gauze, and 10-mL syringes with $1\frac{1}{2}$-in., 25-gauge needles is required for ankle block. Although nerve stimulation is not necessary for distal approaches, it has been described for the proximal approach to the posterior tibial nerve.[21] Although there are no data regarding the use of ultrasound for ankle block, this modality can identify nerves, visualize needles and the spread of local anesthetic around the nerves, and may be useful for proximal approaches to the deep peroneal and posterior tibial nerves.

If a tourniquet is required for surgery, a pneumatic ankle tourniquet should be used rather than an Esmarch bandage, because pressures with the latter are variable, are unknown, and may be extremely high, up to 380 mm Hg.[22,23] Tourniquet pressures just above the malleoli between 200 and 250 mm Hg should ensure a bloodless field and maximize safety.[24,25] Ankle tourniquets are tolerated better than those placed at the midcalf or thigh, with less pain and no increase in neurologic complications.[26–30] An audit of 1000 cases of ankle block revealed that with proper tourniquet application and the option of sedation, only 3.1% of patients complained of tourniquet pain. Risk factors for tourniquet pain were age over 70 and tourniquet times greater than 30 minutes.[30]

Clinical Pearl

- Always ensure that when a tourniquet is required, a padded ankle tourniquet is used to maximize patient comfort, minimize sedation, and prevent general anesthesia.

Sterile disposable tourniquets are available if the surgery requires a more proximal operative area.

Alternative Techniques

There are several techniques for performing ankle block; they can be classified as perimalleolar or inframalleolar (midtarsal) block. The location of the block determines the procedures that can be done. With midtarsal block, forefoot surgery is easily accomplished. For midfoot and more proximal foot surgery, perimalleolar block is required. Because success rates are higher with inframalleolar technique, in which the deep

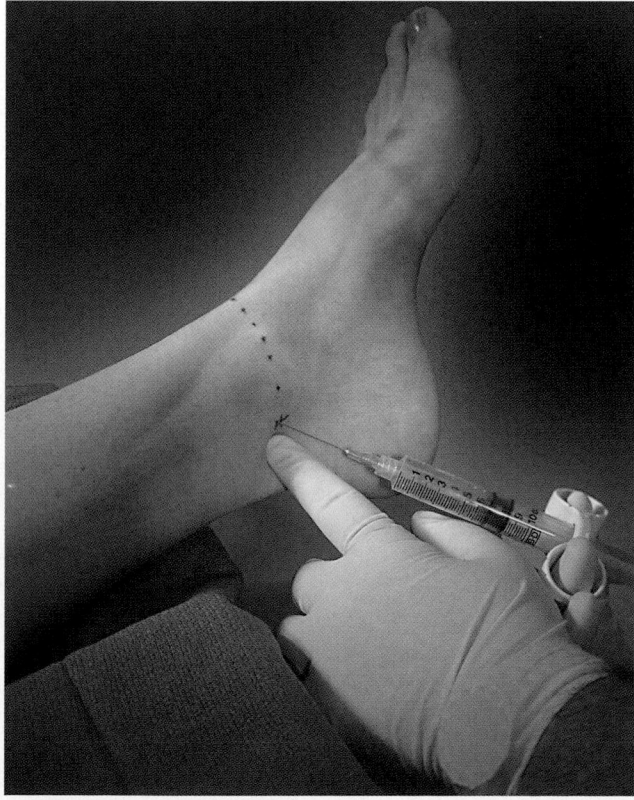

Figure 39–12. Block of the posterior tibial nerve.

peroneal and posterior tibial nerves are more superficial, this technique is preferable for forefoot surgery.[2,3]

For all approaches, the patient can be supine, with a pillow under the calf of the leg to be blocked to facilitate access. The anesthesiologist can sit on a stool at the foot of the bed, if desired.

Saphenous, Superficial Peroneal, and Sural Nerve Blocks

The saphenous, superficial peroneal, and sural nerves are already subcutaneous just proximal to the malleoli, and all can be blocked by a subcutaneous ring of local anesthetic at this location from just anterior to the Achilles tendon medially to laterally (see Figures 39–8 through 39–10). The advantage of blocking these nerves here is that the area under an ankle tourniquet will be anesthetized and tourniquet pain is less likely. By injecting slowly and continuously advancing a $1\frac{1}{2}$-in., 25-gauge needle into the previously injected area, the number of injections and discomfort from them can be minimized. This subcutaneous ring of local anesthetic can also be performed distal to the malleoli for a midtarsal block.

Deep Peroneal Nerve Blocks

For the perimalleolar approach, the patient is asked to extend the great toe, which will tense and identify the extensor hallucis tendon (see Figure 39–7). A $1\frac{1}{2}$-in., 25-gauge needle is inserted immediately lateral to the tendon, perpendicular to the tibia, and is advanced until it contacts bone (see Figure 39–11). The needle is then withdrawn a few millimeters, and after negative aspiration, 8 mL of local anesthetic are injected. For the inframalleolar or midtarsal approach, the extensor hallucis tendon is identified as previously mentioned above, but more distally, and the pulse of the dorsalis pedis artery is identified on the top of the foot as well. A $1\frac{1}{2}$-in., 25-gauge needle is inserted immediately lateral to the tendon and medial to the artery, and after negative aspiration, 5 mL of local anesthetic are injected.

Posterior Tibial Nerve Block

For the retrotibial approach, a $1\frac{1}{2}$-in., 25-gauge needle is inserted just posterior to the pulse of the posterior tibial artery behind the medial malleolus, or if it cannot be palpated, midway between the Achilles tendon and the posterior aspect of the medial malleolus (see Figure 39–12). The needle is directed toward the tibia at a 45-degree angle to contact bone. The needle is then withdrawn a few millimeters, and after negative aspiration, 8 mL of local anesthetic are injected.

For the midtarsal, there are two approaches. Either the posterior tibial artery is identified below and distal to the medial malleolus on the calcaneus, or the sustentaculum tali is identified. The needle is directed toward the calcaneus, slightly under the bony shelf of the sustentaculum tali, or on either side of the tibial artery. After contact with bone, the needle is withdrawn 2 mm, and 8 mL of local anesthetic are injected.

Clinical Pearl

■ Because the posterior tibial artery is not palpable in all individuals, the sustentaculum tali is a more consistent, easily palpable landmark for posterior tibial nerve block.

Block of the saphenous, sural, and superficial peroneal nerves by circumferential subcutaneous injection can always be performed proximal to the malleoli even when the deep peroneal and posterior tibial nerve blocks are done more distally. This may help with tourniquet tolerance.

MAYO BLOCK

Anatomic Facts

The Mayo block is a combination of the nerve block and a field block that involves the infiltration of local anesthesia through the tissues proximal to a surgical site in a ring shape around the first metatarsal (most commonly) or a lesser metatarsal base.[29] When the Mayo block is used around the first metatarsal base, the nerves that are anesthetized include the medial dorsal cutaneous nerve and the deep peroneal nerve on the dorsal aspect. The first and second branches of the common plantar digital nerves, which are superficial branches of the medial plantar nerve, provide sensation to the plantar aspect of the first metatarsal.

Indications

The Mayo block is commonly used in podiatric office surgery to anesthetize the area before performing bunion or hallux surgery. The injection can be used with or without epinephrine because it is not being injected into the toe.

Technique

The Mayo block consists of three or four separate injections. The block is performed by raising a wheal of local anesthesia proximally and dorsally in the first intermetatarsal space and advancing the needle in the plantar direction while injecting 3–5 mL of local anesthetic (Figure 39–13). The needle is then withdrawn partially and redirected medially, raising a subcutaneous wheal along its course (3–5 mL) (Figure 39–14). The needle is then removed and re-entered and directed laterally to raise a subcutaneous wheal along the course (3–5 mL) (Figure 39–15). Finally, the needle is removed and directed plantarmedially to the metatarsal and injected from medial to lateral underneath the metatarsal bone (3–5 mL) (Figure 39–16). The block encircles the entire metatarsal bone.

Choice of Local Anesthetic

The decision regarding which local anesthetic solution to use depends on the anticipated duration of surgery and the degree

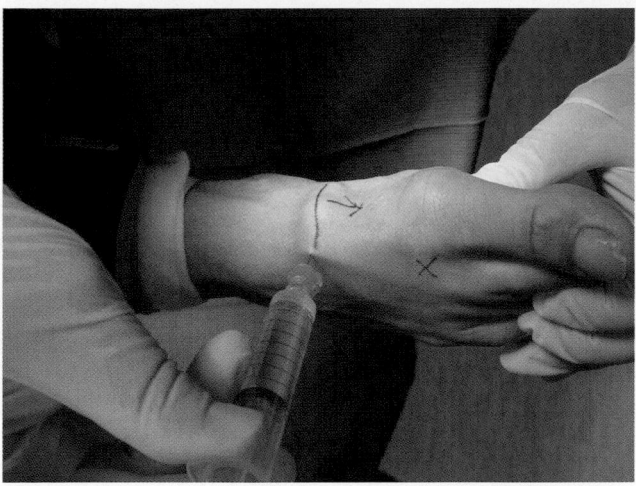

Figure 39–13. Mayo block, step 1. After a wheal of local anesthesia is raised at the level of the first intermetatarsal space, the needle is advanced in the plantar direction and 3–5 mL of local anesthetic is injected. (X, First metatarsal space; arrow, first metatarsal bone.)

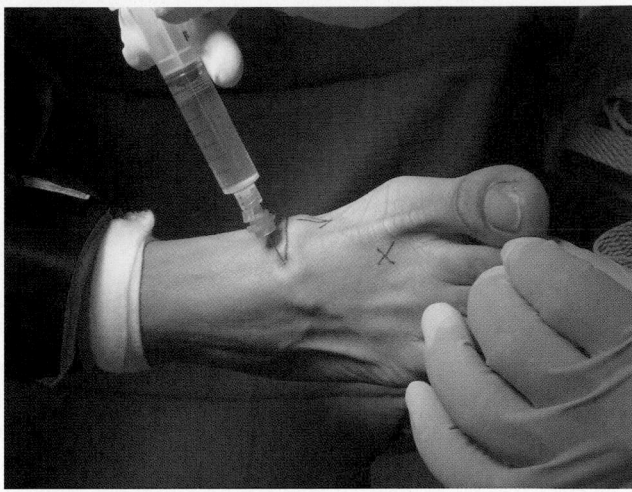

Figure 39–15. Mayo block, step 3. The needle is directed medial to lateral subcutaneously and 3–5 mL is injected. (X, First metatarsal space; arrow, first metarsal bone.)

of postoperative pain. The most commonly used local anesthetics are lidocaine 0.5–2%,[1–3] mepivacaine 1%,[8,30] bupivacaine 0.5–0.75%,[3,4] and ropivacaine 0.75%.[7] For example, removal of a superficial foreign body would require only a short-acting local anesthetic such as lidocaine, which provides a minimum of 1 hour of surgical anesthesia. However, long-acting anesthetics such as ropivacaine 0.75% and bupivacaine 0.75%, which give a mean duration of 14 or 17 hours of analgesia, respectively, after ankle block would be more beneficial after a longer surgery such as a complex forefoot reconstruction with severe postoperative pain.[6,9] When 20–25 mL of 0.5% bupivacaine are used, onset time is 15–20 minutes with a duration of anesthesia from 10–25 hours.[5] Mepivacaine 1% is a good choice for intermediate-length procedures.

Combinations of short- and long-acting local anesthetics have been used to speed onset but provide longer postoperative analgesia. A combination of 2% lidocaine and 0.5% bupivacaine in equal parts provides a minimum of 3 hours of anesthesia with an onset time of 10 ± 3 minutes.[32] Mixtures of 1.5% lidocaine and 0.75% ropivacaine in equal parts have been reported to have an intermediate mean duration of analgesia of 8 hours.[6]

Various additives to local anesthetic solutions have been used to prolong the duration of postoperative analgesia. Adding clonidine 1 mcg/kg to 0.75% ropivacaine increases the duration of analgesia from 14 to 17 hours.[6] Another study found a duration of 15.9 hours.[7] Similarly, the addition of clonidine 10 mcg/mL to lidocaine improves the quality and duration of postoperative analgesia.[36]

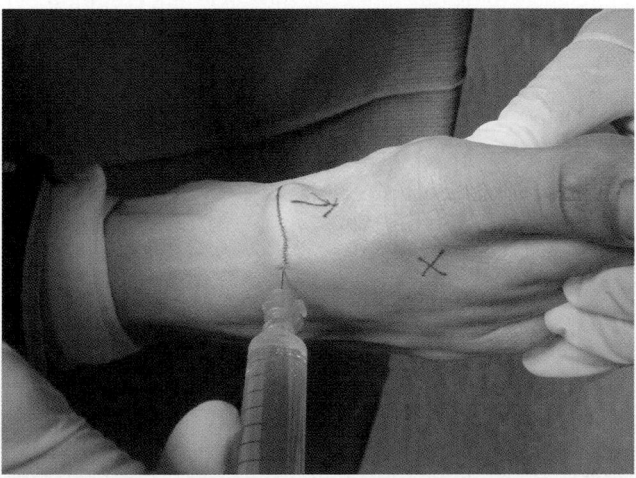

Figure 39–14. Mayo block, step 2. The needle is entered subcutaneously dorsomedially raising a wheal along the course. (X, First metatarsal space; arrow, first metarsal bone.)

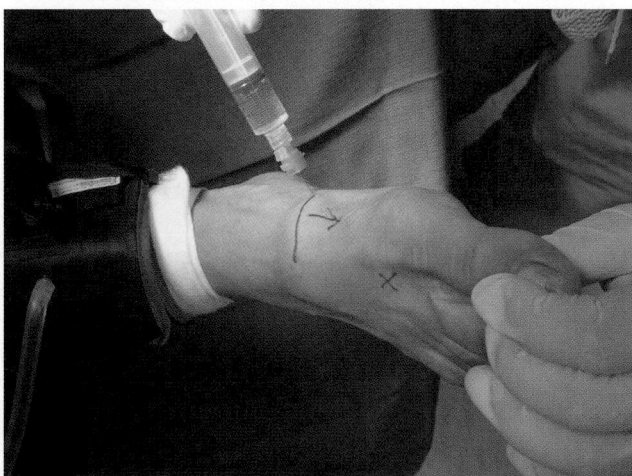

Figure 39–16. Mayo block, step 4. The needle is directed medial to lateral and plantar underneath the metatarsal bone while injecting 3–5 mL of local anesthetic. (X, First metatarsal space; arrow, first metarsal bone.)

Blood levels of plain local anesthetic are well below toxic levels, even when large amounts are used. Bilateral midtarsal blocks performed with up to 30 mL of plain 0.75% bupivacaine resulted in peak venous blood levels of 0.5 mcg/mL, whereas 13 mL of 2% lidocaine for unilateral block resulted in 1.1 mcg/mL.[9] No adverse local anesthetic effects were reported in a series of 66 patients receiving bilateral ankle blocks with mixtures of plain lidocaine and ropivacaine 0.75%, ropivacaine 0.75% or ropivacaine 0.75% with clonidine 1 mcg/kg.[6] The addition of epinephrine with ankle block remains controversial. The preponderance of the literature suggests that epinephrine should not be used in distal extremity local anesthesia.[33,34] However, low concentrations of epinephrine in local anesthetic solutions have been used with remarkable safety.[35] The overall incidence of severe vascular complications after injection of epinephrine-containing local anesthetics has been estimated to be 1 per 132,000 injections. Note that the use of 1:000,000 solutions of epinephrine has a 2.5 greater risk of complications compared with 1:200,000, suggesting that when epinephrine is indicated, it should be used only as dilute concentrations (ie, 1:300,000 or less). Regardless, epinephrine is probably best avoided altogether in patients with peripheral vascular disease or compromised circulation.

The high-efficacy, prolonged postoperative analgesia and safety of plain bupivacaine and ropivacaine suggest that these drugs should be the choice for surgery in which postoperative pain is expected. However, blocks should be performed 30 minutes before surgery (minimum of 20 minutes) when using bupivacaine or ropivacaine to maximize the success rate. In a prospective analysis of 1000 patients, the failure rate was significantly lower after waiting 20 minutes after the injection, with the lowest failure rates occurring after 50 minutes.[7]

Clinical Pearl

- When using ropivacaine or bupivacaine, perform the block at least 30 minutes before surgery to ensure maximal effect.

PERIOPERATIVE MANAGEMENT

Before block placement, consideration should be given to loading the patient preoperatively with nonopioid analgesics such as acetaminophen, celecoxib, or a nonsteroidal anti-inflammatory drug (NSAID), and gabapentin.

Because performing an ankle block requires more than one injection and requires subcutaneous infiltration, it can cause more discomfort than single-injection blocks. Apart from gentle, slow injection and infiltration, patients usually benefit from anxiolysis and analgesia with midazolam 1–4 mg and fentanyl 25–100 mcg. Before starting surgery, the block should be checked in all five nerve distributions, and supplemental local anesthetic can be injected if necessary.

Many patients benefit from continuing sedation during the procedure. Tourniquets should have a soft lining or padding and should be placed just above the malleoli. Sterile tourniquets are available for use if the surgeon requires a larger exposed field. Midcalf or thigh tourniquets should be avoided because they cause more discomfort. Discomfort from an ankle tourniquet may occur rarely, and more sedation may be required. Supplementation by the surgeon intraoperatively may rescue an incomplete block.

Postoperatively, acetaminophen and an NSAID can be continued routinely. Depending on the extent and type of surgery, small doses of a long-acting opioid such as controlled-release oxycodone may provide a smooth transition from block to postoperative analgesia and may facilitate rehabilitation. Ambulation is possible right after surgery. Elevation of the leg, when not ambulating, may decrease pain.

COMPLICATIONS & HOW TO AVOID THEM

Complications may occur from injection or from application of the tourniquet. Because most surgery is done under tourniquet, it is difficult to differentiate the cause of neurologic complications. In a retrospective study of 3027 patients with pneumatic ankle tourniquet at relatively high pressures of 325 mm Hg, there were three cases (0.1%) of posttourniquet syndrome.[28] Ankle tourniquets have been used routinely with as little as 200 mm Hg pressure,[5] although a bloodless surgical field may require 218.6 ± 34.6 mm Hg, with younger normotensive patients requiring only 203.9 ± 22.3 mm Hg.[25] Thus, no more than 250 mm Hg pressure is necessary, and more pressure may be harmful.

The incidence of complications after ankle block is low and is usually from transient paresthesias, which almost always resolve. The incidence is usually less than 1%, although it ranges from 0 to 10%, depending on the source of the data. In a prospective survey of 284 patients with posterior tibial, sural, and saphenous blocks at the ankle and common peroneal block at the knee, no patient developed postanesthetic neuralgia or other complications.[31] In three other studies with a total of 120 patients who received ankle blocks, no patients developed complications.[2,5,10] After midtarsal ankle block in 71 out of 100 patients available for follow-up, one patient developed transient posterior tibial paresthesias, which resolved in 4 weeks.[3] In another study of 40 patients, one developed paresthesias lasting 6 weeks, which resolved.[1] In a retrospective study of 1373 patients who received ankle block followed by a posterior tibial nerve catheter for postoperative analgesia, five patients had transient paresthesias, with one patient developing neurolysis (probably related to the catheter insertion) but with complete recovery.[21] In a prospective randomized trial of 32 patients (40 total feet) undergoing forefoot surgery under ankle tourniquet (inflation pressure 100 mm Hg over systolic) under complete or selective ankle block of which 26 patients (33 total feet) were available for follow-up between 16 and 80 weeks, one patient had paresthesias related to injection or tourniquet, one had ankle pain, and one had cold toes.[8]

Local anesthetic toxicity would be expected to be rare, given the low blood levels after injection. In the retrospective series of 1373 patients previously mentioned, one patient had a convulsion, thought to be secondary to an intravascular injection.[21] In another series of 1295 patients who received standard and modified ankle blocks as well as digital nerve blocks, three patients had vasovagal reactions and one had an episode of hypotension and supraventricular tachycardia, thought by the authors to be from lidocaine toxicity. No other complications were seen in this series.[4]

There are single case reports of injection-related complications such as an Achilles tendon avulsion from tibial nerve block in a patient with spastic talipes equinovarus,[13] and acute compartment syndrome from ankle block in a patient with previous scarring from forefoot arthroplasty.[37] Both of these patients had an altered anatomy, which may have predisposed them to the complication.

Clinical Pearls

- Ensure that the patient's anatomy is normal before injection and avoid injecting in scarred or swollen areas. Avoid injection of large volumes; most ankle blocks can be performed with less than 30 mL of local anesthetic.
- There should be no resistance to injection at any time. If there is, stop the injection and reposition the needle.

References

1. Schurman DJ: Ankle block anesthesia for foot surgery. Anesthesiology 1976;44:348–352.
2. Wassef MR: Posterior tibial nerve block. A new approach using the bony landmark of the sustentaculum tali. Anaesthesia 1991;46:841–844.
3. Sharrock NE, Waller JF, Fierro LE: Midtarsal block for surgery of the forefoot. Br J Anaesthesia 1986;58:37–40.
4. Myerson MS, Ruland CM, Allon SM: Regional anesthesia for foot and ankle surgery. Foot Ankle 1992;13:282–288.
5. Sarrafian SK, Ibrahim IN, Breihan JH: Ankle-foot peripheral nerve block for mid- and forefoot surgery. Foot Ankle 1993;4:86–90.
6. Rudkin GE, Rudkin AK, Dracopoulos GC: Bilateral ankle blocks: A prospective audit. ANZ Surg 2005;75:39–42.
7. Rudkin GE, Rudkin AK, Dracopoulos GC: Ankle block success rate: A prospective analysis of 1,000 patients. Can J Anesth 2005;52:209–210.
8. Delgado-Martinez AD, Marchal JM, Molina M, et al: Forefoot surgery with ankle tourniquet: Complete or selective ankle block? Reg Anesth Pain Med 2001;26:184–186.
9. Mineo R, Sharrock NE: Venous levels of lidocaine and bupivacaine after mid-tarsal ankle block. Reg Anesth Pain Med 1992;17:47–49.
10. Needoff M, Radford P, Costigan P: Local anesthesia for postoperative pain relief after foot surgery: A prospective clinical trial. Foot Ankle Int 1995;16:11–13.
11. Winiecke DG, Louis JM: Local anesthetic nerve blocks in the treatment of foot fractures. J Am Podiatr Med Assoc 1977;67:87–90.
12. Haber GR, Johnson DR, Nashel DJ, et al: Lidocaine regional block in the treatment of gouty arthritis of the foot. J Am Podiatr Med Assoc 1985;75:492–493.
13. Deltombe T, Nisolle JF, De Cloedt P, et al: Tibial nerve block with anesthetics resulting in Achilles tendon avulsion. Am J Phys Rehabil 2004;83:331–334.
14. Harvey CK: Dilute lidocaine ankle blocks in the diagnosis of sympathetically mediated pain. J Am Podiatr Med Assoc 1997;87:473–477.
15. McLeod DH, Wong DHW, Vaghadia H, et al: Lateral popliteal sciatic nerve block compared with ankle block for analgesia following foot surgery. Can J Anaesth 1995;42:765–769.
16. Agur AMR, Lee MJ: Grant's Atlas of Anatomy, 9th ed. Williams & Wilkins, 1991, pp. 255–352.
17. Clemente CD: Anatomy: A Regional Atlas of the Human Body, 4th ed. Williams & Wilkins, 1997, pp. 309–402.
18. McCutcheon R: Regional anaesthesia for the foot. Can Anesth Soc J 1965;12:465–474.
19. Hoerster W: Blocks in the area of the ankle. In: Zenz M, Panhans C, Niesel H (ed): Regional Anesthesia. Year Book Medical Publishers, 1988, p. 88.
20. Cohen SJ, Roenigk RK: Nerve blocks for cutaneous surgery on the foot. J Dermatol Surg Oncol 1991;17:527–534.
21. Frederic A, Bouchon Y: Analgesia in surgery of the foot. Can Anesthesiol 1996;44:115–118.
22. Biehl WC, Morgan JM, Wagner FW, et al: The safety of the Esmarch tourniquet. Foot Ankle 1993;14:278–283.
23. Finsen V, Kasseth AM: Tourniquets in forefoot surgery. Less pain when placed at the ankle. J Bone Jt Surg Br 1997;79B:99–101.
24. Pauers RS, Carocci MA: Low pressure pneumatic tourniquets: Effectiveness at minimum recommended inflation pressures. J Foot Ankle Surg 1994;33:605–609.
25. Diamond EL, Sherman M, Lenet M: A quantitative method of determining the pneumatic ankle tourniquet setting. J Foot Surg 1985;24:330–334.
26. Lichtenfeld NS: The pneumatic ankle tourniquet with ankle block anesthesia for foot surgery. Foot Ankle 1992;13:344–349.
27. Chu J, Fox I, Jassen M: Pneumatic ankle tourniquet: Clinical and electrophysiologic study. Arch Phys Med Rehabil 1981;62:570–575.
28. Derner R, Buckholz J: Surgical hemostasis by pneumatic ankle tourniquet during 3027 podiatric operations. J Foot Ankle Surg 1995;34:236–246.
29. McGlamry DE, Banks AS, Downey M: Ankle block. In: McGlamry DE, Banks AS, Downey M (eds): Comprehensive Textbook of Foot Surgery, 2nd ed. Williams & Wilkins, 1992, pp. 243–244.
30. Rudkin AK, Rudkin GE, Dracopoulos GC: Acceptability of ankle tourniquet use in midfoot and forefoot surgery: Audit of 1000 cases. Foot Ankle Int 2004;25:788–794.
31. Reinhart DJ, Wang W, Stagg KS, et al: Postoperative analgesia after peripheral nerve block for podiatric surgery: Clinical efficacy and chemical stability of lidocaine alone versus lidocaine plus clonidine. Anesth Analg 1996;83:760–765.
32. Kofoed H: Peripheral nerve blocks at the knee and ankle in operations for common foot disorders. Clin Orthop 1982;168:97–101.
33. Wylie WD: A Practice of Anesthesia. Year Book Medical Publishers, 1972, pp. 1166–1172.
34. Hardy JD: Rhoads Textbook of Surgery Principles and Practice, 5th ed. JB Lippincott, 1973, pp. 2310–2315.
35. Roth RD: Utilization of epinephrine-containing anesthetic solutions in the toes. J Am Podiatr Med Assoc 1981;71:189–199.
36. Hui Bon Hoa S, O'Bryne P, Messai EL: Peripheral foot block at the ankle: An additional landmark for localizing the tibial nerve. A study of 71 patients. Ann Fr Anesth Reanim 1989;8:371–375.
37. Noorpuri BS, Shahane SA, Getty CJ: Acute compartment syndrome following revisional arthroplasty of the forefoot: The dangers of ankle block. Foot Ankle Int 2000;21:680–687.

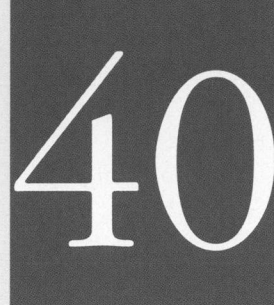

Cutaneous Nerve Blocks of the Lower Extremity

Anna Barczewska-Hillel, MD • Jerry D. Vloka, MD

INTRODUCTION

Blocks of the lateral femoral cutaneous, posterior femoral cutaneous, saphenous, sural, and superficial peroneal nerves are useful anesthetic techniques for a variety of superficial surgical procedures. These blocks are simple to learn and perform. They are essentially devoid of complications and can nicely complement major conduction blocks of the

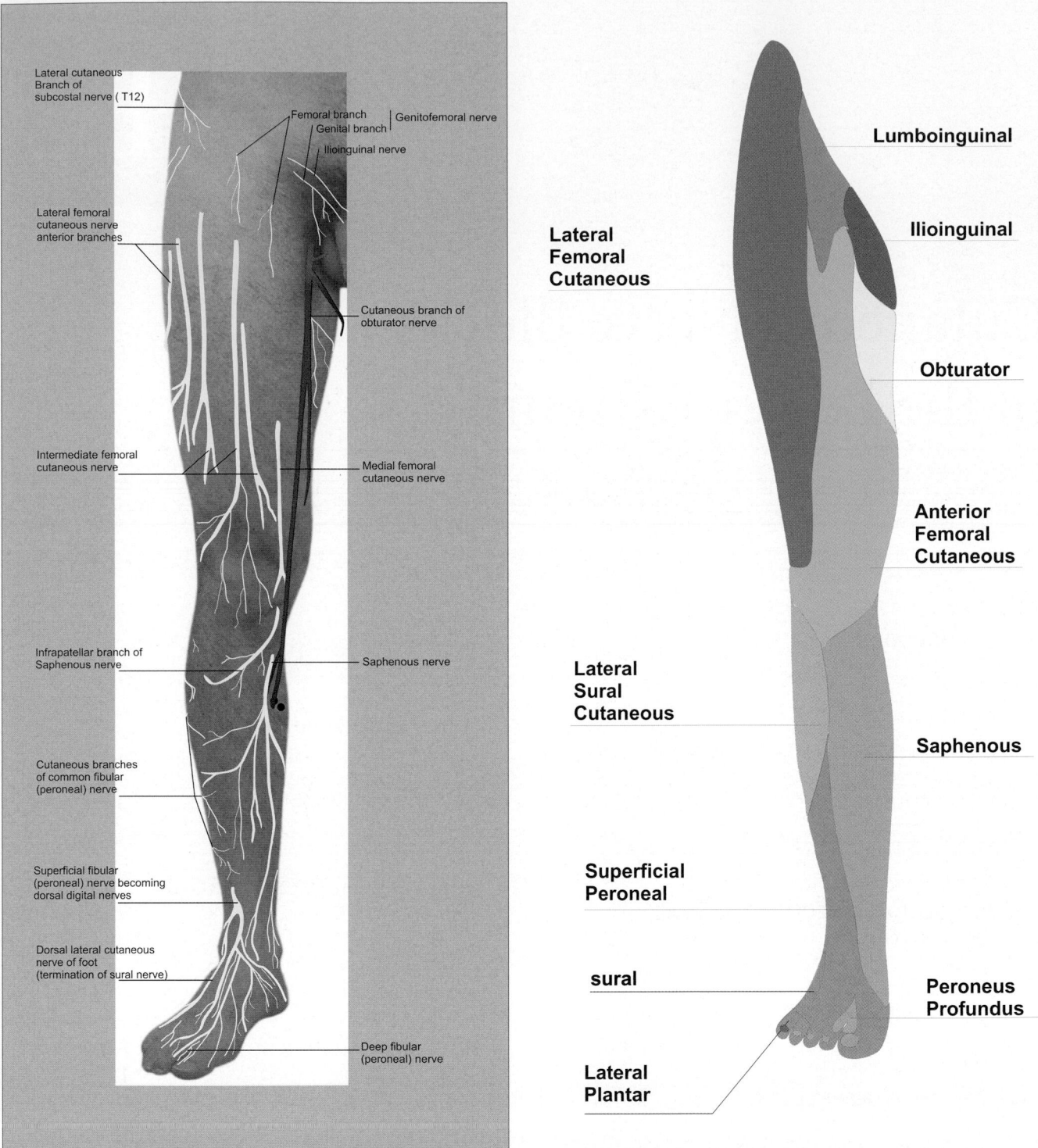

Figure 40–1. Cutaneous innervation of the lower extremity, anterior view.

lower extremity.[1,2] The combination of their applicability and simplicity mandate that these blocks should be in the armamentarium of every anesthesiologist.

Indications & Contraindications

Cutaneous nerve blocks of the lower extremity can be used to anesthetize patients for a variety of surgical procedures.

The lateral femoral cutaneous nerve block has been used to provide anesthesia for pediatric patients undergoing muscle biopsy[3] and to provide analgesia after femoral neck surgery in older patients.[4,5] The posterior femoral cutaneous nerve block is used for any surgical procedure performed on the posterior aspect of the thigh.[6] The saphenous, sural, and superficial peroneal nerve blocks can be used as part of an ankle block to provide complete anesthesia to the foot and ankle, or

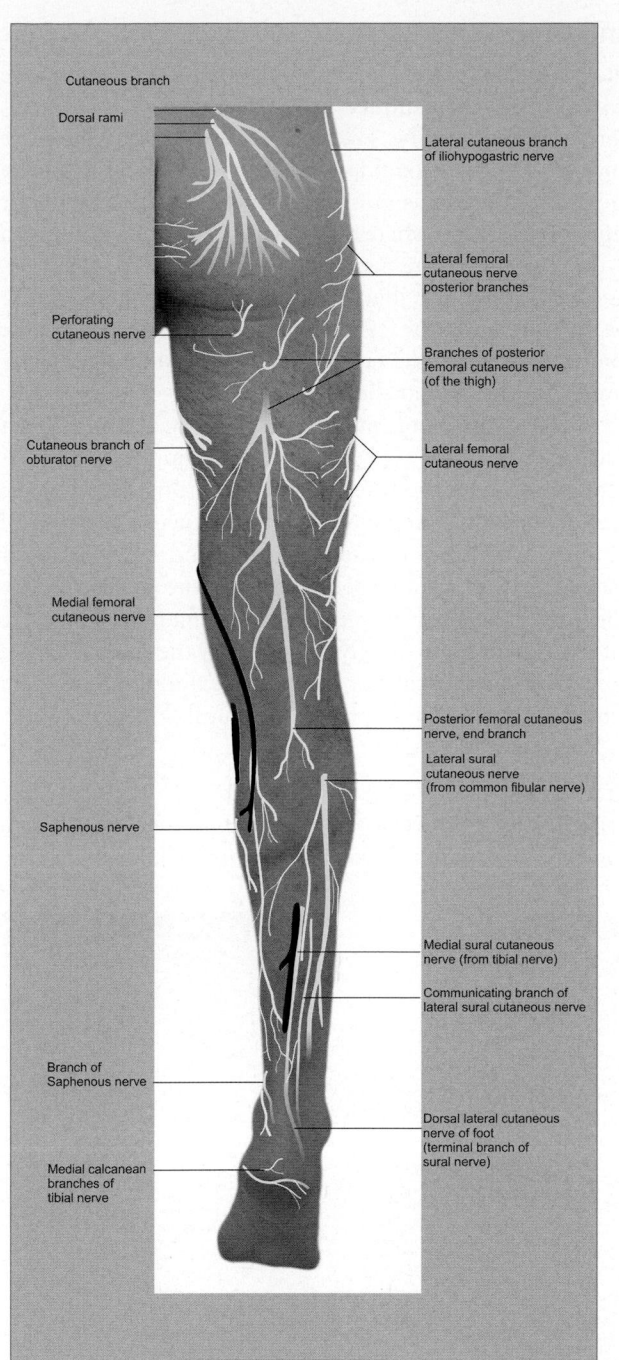

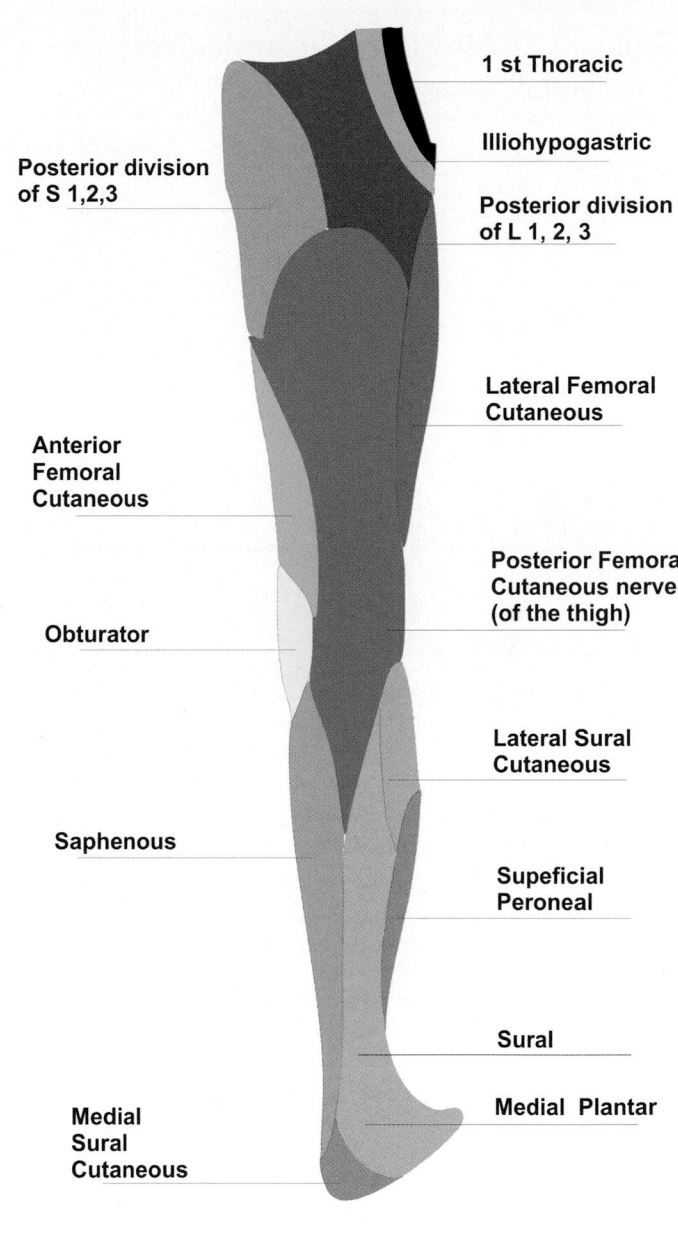

Figure 40–2. Cutaneous innervation of the lower extremity, posterior view.

they can be used separately to provide anesthesia to specific portions of the foot and ankle. These blocks can be used for a variety of foot and ankle procedures.

The contraindications to performing cutaneous nerve blocks of the lower extremity are few, but include local infection at the sites of needle insertion, preexisting central or peripheral nervous systems disorders, and allergy to local anesthetic.

Functional Anatomy

The cutaneous nerves of the extremities are blocked by injection of local anesthetic in the subcutaneous layers above the muscle fascia. The subcutaneous tissue contains a variable amount of fat, superficial nerves, and vessels. Deep into this area lies a tough membranous layer, deep fascia of the lower extremity enclosing muscles of the leg. Deep fascia is penetrated by numerous superficial nerves and vessels.

The cutaneous innervation of the lower extremity is accomplished by nerves that are part of the lumbar and sciatic plexuses (Figures 40–1 and 40–2). The largest cutaneous nerves are the lateral femoral cutaneous nerve, the posterior femoral cutaneous nerve, the saphenous nerve, the sural nerve, and the superficial peroneal nerve. A more detailed review of the relevant anatomy is provided with a description of the individual block procedures and in Chapter 3.

Table 40–1.

Choice of Anesthetic for Cutaneous Nerve Block of the Lower Extremity

	Onset (min)	Anesthesia (h)	Analgesia (h)
1.5% Mepivacaine (+ HCO₃)	15–20	2–3	3–5
2% Lidocaine (+ HCO₃)	10–20	2–5	3–8
0.5% Ropivacaine	15–30	4–8	5–12
0.75% Ropivacaine	10–15	5–10	6–24
0.5% Bupivacaine (or L-bupivacaine)	15–30	5–15	6–30

Choice of Local Anesthetic

Any local anesthetic can be used for cutaneous blocks of the lower extremity. The choice of local anesthetic is based primarily on the desired duration of the blockade. Because these blocks do not result in motor blockade, longer-acting local anesthetics are most commonly chosen (eg, 0.2–0.5% ropivacaine and 0.5% bupivacaine). When performing blocks in the ankle area, it is always prudent to avoid using epinephrine owing to the risk of decreasing blood flow to the toes. Onset time for the block depends on the local anesthetic used[7] (Table 40–1).

LATERAL FEMORAL CUTANEOUS NERVE BLOCK

General Considerations

Lateral femoral cutaneous nerve block can be used to provide complete anesthesia in patients undergoing small skin grafts on the lateral aspect of the thigh, or it can be combined with femoral block[8–10] or sciatic block to complement them and extend sensory coverage for tourniquet pain. Its use has also been reported as a diagnostic tool for meralgia paresthetica, neuralgia of the lateral femoral cutaneous nerve of the thigh.

Distribution of Anesthesia

The lateral femoral cutaneous nerve provides sensation to the anterolateral aspect of the thigh (see Figure 40–1).

Patient Positioning

The patient is in a supine position with the anesthesiologist at the patient's side. The anterior superior iliac spine is palpated and marked.

Anatomic Landmarks

The main landmark for lateral femoral cutaneous nerve blockade is easily identified in most patients; it is the anterior superior iliac spine. The lateral femoral cutaneous nerve emerges from the lateral border of the psoas major muscle and crosses the iliacus muscle obliquely toward the anterior superior iliac spine, where it supplies the parietal peritoneum of the iliac fossa. The nerve then passes into the thigh behind or through the inguinal ligament, variably medial to the anterior iliac spine (typically about 1 cm) or through the tendinous origin of the sartorius muscle, dividing into anterior and posterior branches.

The anterior branch becomes superficial about 10 cm distal to the anterior superior iliac spine supplying innervation to the skin of the anterior and lateral thigh as far as the knee. It connects terminally with the cutaneous branches of the anterior division of the femoral nerve and the infrapatellar branch of the saphenous nerve, forming the patellar plexus. The posterior branch pierces the fascia lata higher than the anterior, dividing to supply the skin on the lateral surface from the greater trochanter to about the middle of the thigh and occasionally also supplying the gluteal skin.

Technique

A 4-cm, 22-gauge needle is inserted 2 cm medial and 2 cm caudal to the anterior superior iliac spine (Figure 40–3). The

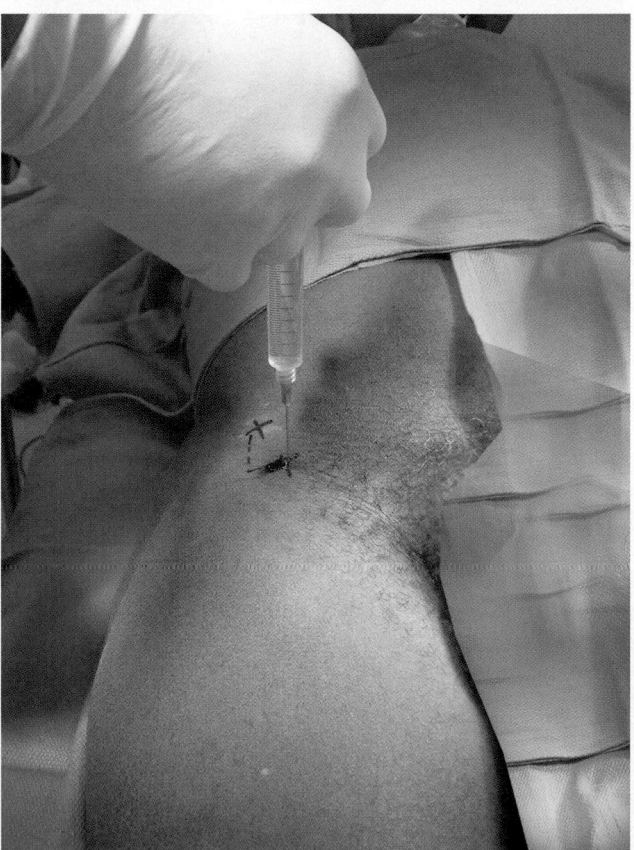

Figure 40–3. Lateral femoral cutaneous nerve block. The landmark for this block is the anterior superior iliac spine.

needle is advanced until a loss of resistance is felt as the needle passes through the fascia lata. A short-bevel needle is suggested to exaggerate the loss of resistance as the needle passes through the fascia. Because this fascia "give" is not consistent and its perception may vary among performers, local anesthetic is injected in a fanwise fashion both above and below the fascia lata from medial to lateral direction. A volume of 10 mL of local anesthetic is injected for this block. Although the lateral femoral cutaneous nerve is a sensory nerve, relatively higher concentrations of long-acting local anesthetic are useful to increase the success rate (0.5% ropivacaine or bupivacaine) because this is essentially a "blind" technique.

When used to provide anesthesia for a skin graft harvest site on the lateral thigh, the peripheral innervation of the lateral femoral cutaneous nerve in specific patients is outlined before beginning skin harvesting.

Because no larger vascular structures or other organs are nearby, blockade of the lateral femoral cutaneous nerve carries a minimal risk of systemic toxicity due to an inadvertent intravascular injection.

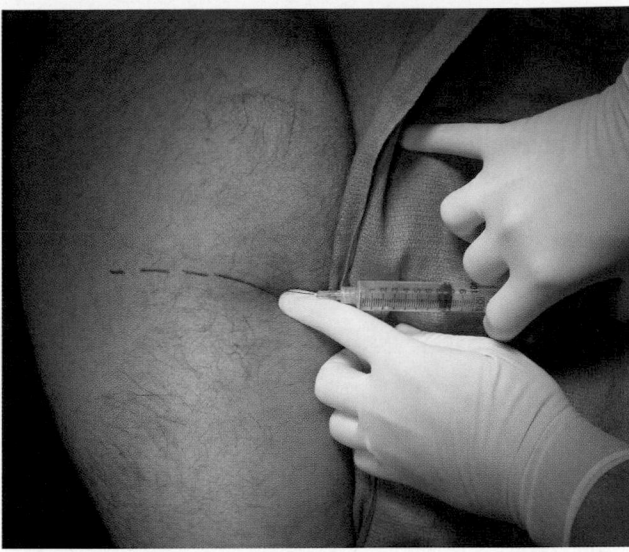

Figure 40–4. Posterior cutaneous nerve of the thigh block, subgluteal approach.

POSTERIOR CUTANEOUS NERVE BLOCK OF THE THIGH

General Considerations

The posterior cutaneous thigh nerve block has been used in burn patients for donor skin grafting taken from the posterior thigh or as part of a popliteal/posterior femoral cutaneous nerve block in short saphenous vein stripping.[11]

Distribution of Anesthesia

The posterior cutaneous nerve of the thigh innervates the skin over the posterior thigh between the lateral femoral cutaneous and anterior femoral cutaneous nerves (see Figure 40–2).

Patient Positioning

The patient can be positioned prone, in the lateral decubitus position (shown in Figures 40–4 and 40–5), or supine with the leg elevated 90 degrees.

Anatomic Landmarks

The posterior femoral cutaneous nerve originates from the dorsal branches of the first and second and from the ventral branches of the second and third sacral rami. It runs through the greater sciatic foramen below the piriformis and descends under the gluteus maximus muscle with the inferior gluteal vessels, posterior or medial to the sciatic nerve. The nerve then descends in the back of the thigh deep to the fascia lata. Its branches are all cutaneous and are distributed to the gluteal region, the perineum, and the flexor aspect of the thigh and leg.

Technique

The gluteal fold is identified and 10 mL of local anesthetic are injected subcutaneously to raise a skin wheal (Figure 40–4). In addition, at the midpoint of the gluteal crease, 5 mL of local anesthetic are injected at a deeper level, using a fan technique

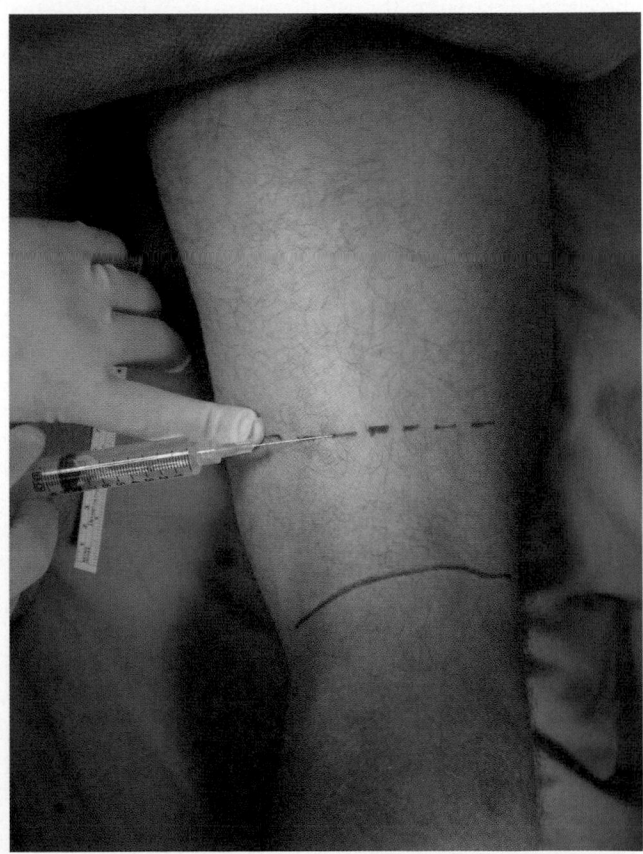

Figure 40–5. Posterior cutaneous nerve of the thigh block, midthigh approach.

to reach the nerve that has not emerged through the deep fascia.

To block the posterior cutaneous nerve of the thigh above the knee level, as for short saphenous vein stripping (as a complement to popliteal block),[11] 10 mL of local anesthetic are injected subcutaneously along a line 5 cm above and parallel with the popliteal crease (Figure 40–5). The patient is in the prone position for both blocks.

SAPHENOUS NERVE BLOCK

General Considerations

The saphenous nerve block is most commonly used in combination with a sciatic nerve block or popliteal block to complement anesthesia of the lower leg for various vascular, orthopedic, and podiatry procedures. The saphenous nerve is a terminal cutaneous branch of the femoral nerve. Its course is in the subcutaneous tissue of the skin on the medial aspect of the ankle and foot. All cutaneous nerves of the foot should be thought of as a neuronal network rather than single strings of nerves with a well-defined and consistent anatomic position.

Distribution of Anesthesia

The saphenous nerve innervates the skin over the medial, anteromedial, and posteromedial aspect of the lower leg from above the knee (part of the patellar plexus) to as low as the first metatarsophalangeal joint in some instances (Figures 40–1 and 40–6).

Patient Positioning

The patient is placed supine with the leg to be blocked supported by a footrest.

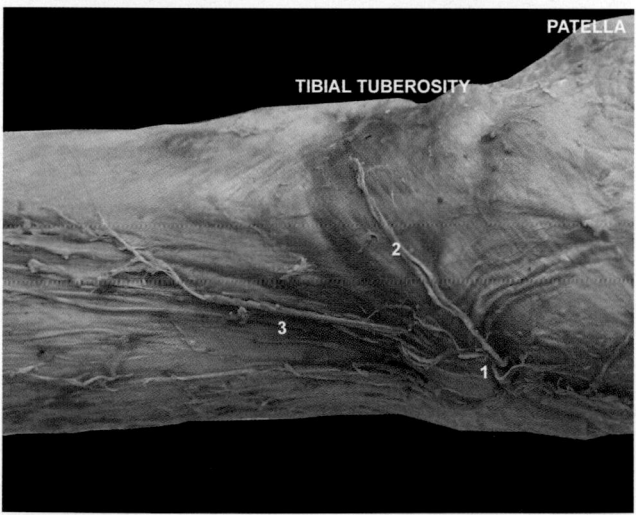

Figure 40–6. Saphenous nerve anatomy. Saphenous nerve pierces through the sartorius muscle (1), subpatellar branch (2), saphenous nerve in its descent on the medial aspect of the thigh (3).

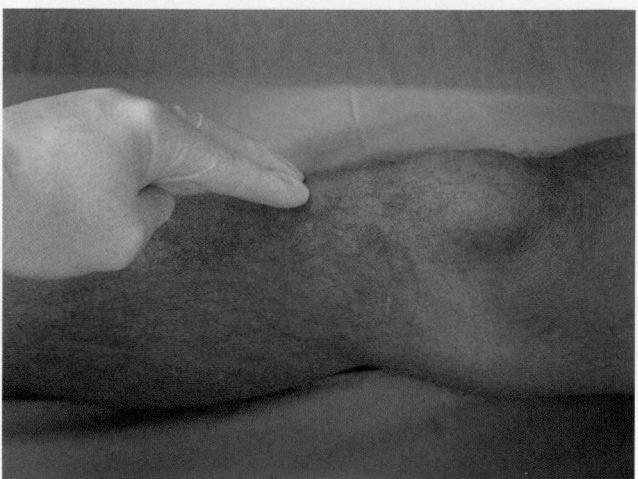

Figure 40–7. Tibial tuberosity. Palpation of the landmark for the saphenous nerve block.

Anatomic Landmarks

The main landmark for this block is the tibial tuberosity, an easily recognizable and easily felt bony prominence on the anterior aspect of the tibia a few centimeters distal from the patella (Figure 40–7). The saphenous nerve is the largest cutaneous branch of the femoral nerve. It descends laterally to the femoral artery into the adductor canal, where it crosses anteriorly to become medial to the artery. It proceeds vertically along the medial side of the knee behind the sartorius, pierces the fascia lata between the tendons of the sartorius and gracilis, and then becomes subcutaneous. From here, it descends on the medial side of the leg with the long saphenous vein along the medial tibial border. Note that the saphenous nerve branches into numerous small branches as it enters the subcutaneous space, and, as such, it is often difficult to achieve blockade of the entire extensive saphenous nerve network. For this reason, it is always preferable to block the saphenous nerve as distally as possible. For instance, to achieve anesthesia of the foot, the saphenous nerve is best approached at the level of the ankle, which is identical with the technique for performing an ankle block.

Techniques

The below-knee field block is performed with the patient in supine position. Five to 10 mL of local anesthetic are injected as a ring deeply subcutaneously, starting at the medial surface of the tibial condyle and ending at the dorsomedial aspect of the upper calf (Figure 40–8).

The paravenous technique has also been described, which is based on the close relation of the saphenous vein and nerve, to achieve a higher success rate. First, the saphenous vein is identified using a tourniquet around the leg in dependent position. The technique involves injection of 5 mL of local anesthetic in a fan-like fashion around the vein on the medial side of the leg just distal from the patella.[12] This technique, however, carries a small risk of creating a hematoma when the saphenous vein is punctured.

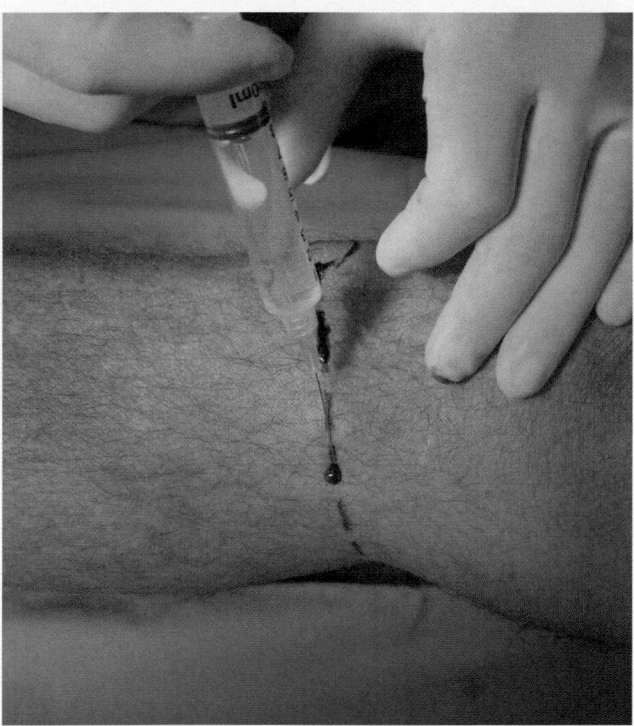

Figure 40–8. Saphenous nerve block. Shown is a subcutaneous injection of 10 mL of local anesthetic in a circumferential fashion on the medial aspect of the leg at the level of the tibial tuberosity.

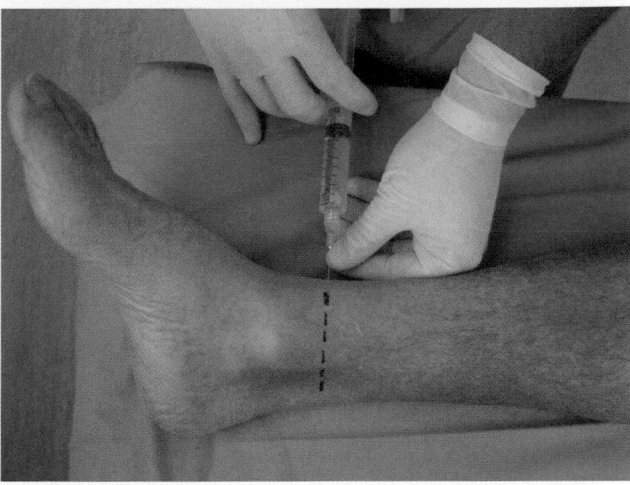

Figure 40–9. Saphenous nerve block, distal approach above the medial malleolus.

In the transsartorial approach, with the patient in the supine position, a skin wheal is raised over the sartorius muscle belly. The sartorius muscle can be palpated just above the knee with the leg extended and actively elevated. The needle is inserted at one finger-width above the patella slightly posterior to the coronal plane and slightly caudad through the muscle belly of the sartorius until a loss of resistance identifies the subsartorial adipose tissue. The depth of insertion is typically between 1.5 and 3 cm. After negative aspiration for blood, 10 mL of local anesthetic are injected.

For surgery on the foot, the saphenous nerve is best blocked just above the medial malleolus, similar to the technique in ankle block (Figure 40–9). Using a 1½-in. needle, 6–8 mL of local anesthetic are injected subcutaneously immediately above the medial malleolus in a ring-like fashion. The most commonly reported complication of this block is a painless hematoma of the saphenous vein at the injection site.

The saphenous nerve can also be blocked by using a nerve stimulator technique and performing a low-volume femoral nerve block. Injection of 10 mL of local anesthetic after obtaining either a medial muscle response, signified by contraction of the vastus medialis muscle, or an anterior muscle response, signified by contraction of the rectus femoris muscle and elevation of the patella, results in a high rate of block success.[13,14] Neurostimulation of the medial compartment of the femoral nerve requires even less volume of local anesthetic, compared with that of a standard femoral block.[115]

Clinical Pearls

- The most effective method of blocking the saphenous nerve is a low-volume femoral nerve block.
- Injection of a mere 10 mL of local anesthetic upon obtaining twitches of the patella or vastus medialis muscle results in a high success rate.

In a recent comparison of the different approaches to saphenous nerve block, the transsartorial, perifemoral, below-knee field block, and block at the medial femoral condyle were evaluated for efficacy. The transsartorial approach resulted in 100% sensory blockade of the medial aspect of the leg, whereas the perifemoral and the below-knee field block resulted in 70%. The medial femoral condyle block resulted in 40% of the patients having sensory blockade of the medial aspect of the leg with only 25% having complete anesthesia at the medial malleolus.[16] This supported the findings of a previous study in which 94% of patients had complete anesthesia of the medial malleolus after a transsartorial saphenous nerve block.[17] However, both of these studies have limited numbers of patients, and more research needs to be conducted.

SURAL NERVE BLOCK

General Considerations

The sural nerve block is used for superficial surgery on the lateral aspect of the ankle and foot and in conjunction with ankle block for foot and toe surgery.

Distribution of Anesthesia

The sural nerve innervates the posterior and lateral skin of the distal third of the leg along the lateral side of the foot and little toe (see Figure 40–1).

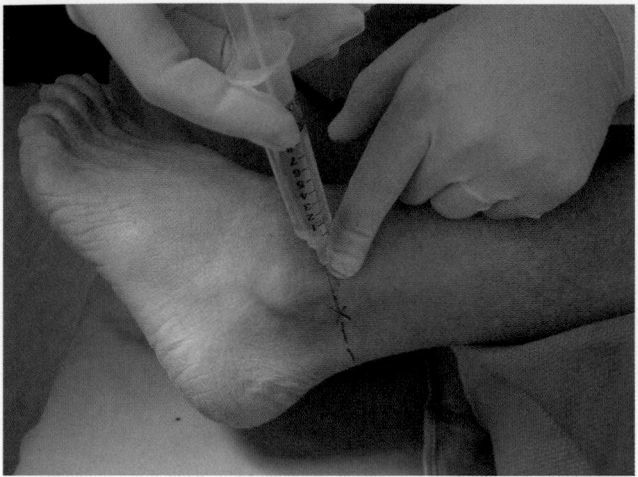

Figure 40–10. Sural nerve block.

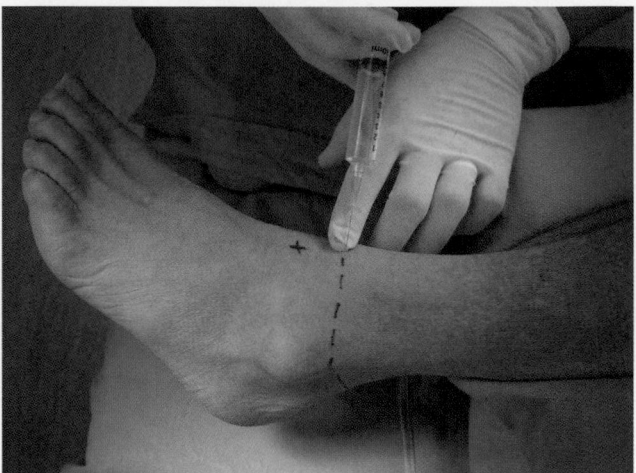

Figure 40–11. Superficial peroneal block.

Patient Positioning

For the block procedure, the patient can be positioned prone or supine with the ankle supported by a footrest.

Anatomic Landmarks

The sural nerve, a branch of the tibial nerve, pierces the deep fascia proximally in the leg and is joined by a branch of the common peroneal nerve. It descends near the lesser saphenous vein and between the lateral malleolus and the calcaneus.

Technique

Using a 1½-in., 25-gauge needle, a skin wheal is raised lateral to the Achilles tendon and just above the lateral malleolus (Figure 40–10). The needle is then inserted through the wheal and advanced toward the fibula while injecting 6–8 mL of local anesthetic.

■ SUPERFICIAL PERONEAL BLOCK

General Considerations

A superficial peroneal block is used alone or in combination with other blocks for foot surgery or ascending venography.[18,19]

Distribution of Anesthesia

The superficial peroneal branches supply innervation to the dorsal skin of all the toes except that of the lateral side of the fifth and adjoining sides of the first and second toes (see Figures 40–1 and 40–2).

Patient Positioning

For the block procedure, the patient can be positioned supine with the ankle supported by a footrest.

Anatomic Landmarks

The superficial peroneal nerve begins at the common peroneal bifurcation. It pierces the deep fascia in the distal third of the leg. It descends the leg adjacent to the extensor digitorum longus muscle, where it divides into terminal branches above the ankle.

Technique

The superficial peroneal nerve is blocked immediately above and medial to the lateral malleolus by injecting local anesthetic to form a subcutaneous wheal of 5–10 mL of local anesthetic from the site of insertion of the needle for the deep peroneal nerve to the anterior surface of the lateral malleolus (Figure 40–11).

Table 40–2.

Possible Complications From Cutaneous Nerve Blocks of the Lower Extremity

Systemic toxicity of local anesthetic	• Risk is small and may be of concern only when higher volumes are used in conjunction with other high-volume major conduction blocks
Hematoma	• Avoid multiple needle insertions and insertion of the needle through superficial veins
Nerve injury	• Usually manifested as transient paresthesias or dysesthesias and is the result of an inadvertent intraneuronal injection • Avoid injecting when high pressures on injection are felt or when the patient reports pain in the distribution of the nerve

COMPLICATIONS & HOW TO AVOID THEM

Few complications result from performing cutaneous nerve blocks of the lower extremity (Table 40–2).

SUMMARY

There are many uses for cutaneous nerve blocks of the lower extremity in everyday anesthetic practice. These blocks are easy to perform and have very few complications associated with them. As such, anesthesiologists are encouraged to learn how to perform cutaneous nerve blocks and incorporate them into their anesthetic plan.

References

1. Hopkins P, Ellis F, Halsall P: Evaluation of local anaesthetic blockade of the lateral femoral cutaneous nerve. Anaesthesia 1991;46:95–96.
2. Coad N: Post-operative analgesia following femoral-neck surgery: A comparison between 3 in 1 femoral nerve block and lateral cutaneous nerve block. Eur J Anaesthesiol 1991;8:287–290.
3. Maccani R, Wedel D, Melton A, Gronert G: Femoral and lateral femoral cutaneous nerve block for muscle biopsies in children. Paediatr Anaesth 1995;5:223–227.
4. Jones S, White A: Analgesia following femoral neck surgery. Lateral cutaneous nerve block as an alternative to narcotics in the elderly. Anaesthesia 1985;40:682–685.
5. Hood G, Edbrooke D, Gerrish S: Postoperative analgesia after triple nerve block for fractured neck of femur. Anaesthesia 1991;46:138–140.
6. Hughes P, Brown T: An approach to posterior femoral cutaneous nerve block. Anaesth Intensive Care 1986;14:350–351.
7. Elmas C, Elmas Y, Gautschi P, Uehlinger P: Combined sciatic 3-in-1 block. Application in lower limb orthopedic surgery. Anaesthetist 1992;41:639–643.
8. McNicol L: Lower limb blocks for children. Lateral cutaneous and femoral nerve blocks for postoperative pain relief in paediatric practice. Anaesthesia 1986;41:27–31.
9. Wardrop P, Nishikawa H: Lateral cutaneous nerve of the thigh blockade as primary anaesthesia for harvesting skin grafts. Br J Plast Surg 1995;48:597–600.
10. Brown T, Dickens D: A new approach to lateral cutaneous nerve of thigh block. Anaesth Intensive Care 1986;14:126–127.
11. Vloka J, Hadzic A, Mulcare R, et al: Combined popliteal and posterior cutaneous nerve of the thigh blocks for short saphenous vein stripping in outpatients: An alternative to spinal anesthesia. J Clin Anesth 1997;9:618–622.
12. De Mey J, Deruyck L, Cammu G, et al: A paravenous approach for the saphenous nerve block. Reg Anesth Pain Med 2001;26:504–506.
13. Comfort V, Lang S, Yip R: Saphenous nerve anaesthesia: A nerve stimulator technique. Can J Anaesth 1996;43:852–857.
14. Mansour N: Sub-sartorial saphenous nerve block with the aid of nerve stimulator. Reg Anesth Pain Med 1993;18:266–268.
15. Chassery C, Gilbert M, Minville V, et al: Neurostimulation does not increase the success rate of saphenous nerve blocks. Can J Anaesth 2005;52:269–275.
16. Benzon H, Sharma S, Calimaran A: Comparison of the different approaches to saphenous nerve block. Anesthesiology 2005;102:633–638.
17. van der Wal M, Lang S, Yip R: Transsartorial approach for saphenous nerve block. Can J Anaesth 1993;40:542–546.
18. Mussurakis S: Combined superficial peroneal and saphenous nerve block for ascending venography. Eur J Radiol 1992;14:56–59.
19. Lieberman R, Kaplan P: Superficial peroneal nerve block for leg venography. Radiology 1987;165:578–579.

Intravenous Regional Block for Upper & Lower Extremity Surgery

Kenneth D. Candido, MD • Alon P. Winnie, MD

INTRODUCTION

The technique of intravenous regional anesthesia (IVRA) was first introduced by August Bier in 1908.[1] Bier block essentially consists of injecting local anesthetic solutions into the venous system of an upper or lower extremity that has been exsanguinated by compression or gravity and that has been isolated by means of a tourniquet from the central circulation. In Dr. Bier's original technique, the local anesthetic procaine in concentrations of 0.25% to 0.5% was injected through an intravenous cannula, which had been placed between two Esmarch bandages utilized as tourniquets to divide the arm into proximal and distal compartments.[2–4] After injecting the local anesthetic, Dr. Bier noted two distinct types of anesthesia; an almost immediate onset of "direct" anesthesia between the two tourniquets, and then, after a delay of 5 to 7 min, an "indirect" anesthesia distal to the distally placed tourniquet. By performing dissections of the venous system of the upper extremity in cadavers after injecting methylene blue, Bier was able to determine that the direct anesthesia was the result of local anesthesia bathing bare nerve endings in the tissues, whereas the indirect anesthesia was most probably due to local

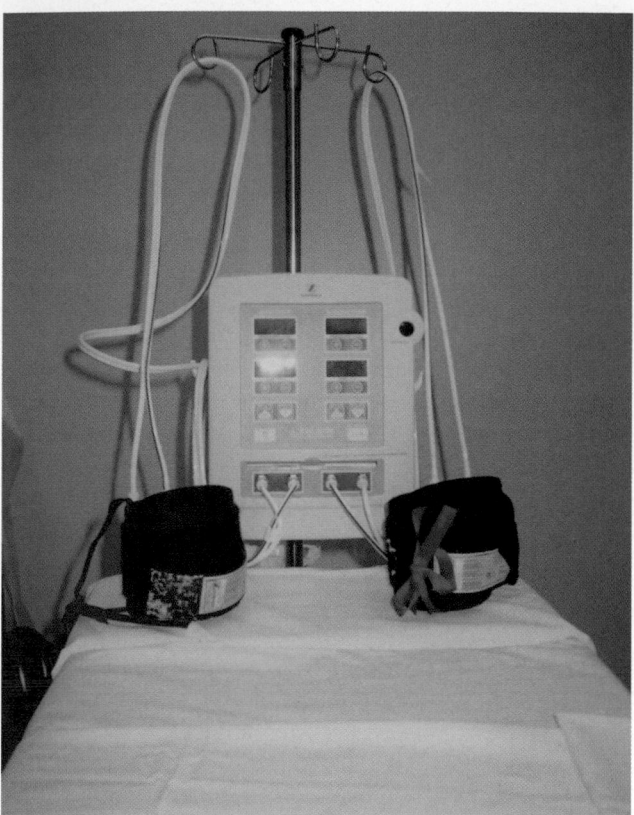

Figure 41–1. Double pneumatic tourniquet system for use in IV regional anesthesia of the upper or lower extremity.

anesthesia being transported to the substance of the nerves via the vasa nervorum, where a typical conduction block occurs. Dr. Bier's conclusion was that two mechanisms of anesthesia were associated with his technique: peripheral infiltration block and conduction block. The technique, as originally described by Dr. Bier, remains essentially unchanged in modern practice for the past 95 years, except for the introduction of the double-tourniquet preparation used in current clinical practice[5–7] (Figure 41–1).

Bier block can be used for brief surgical procedures or manipulations of the upper or lower extremity. However, the technique found its greatest acceptance for use for the upper extremity because tourniquet problems and other safety issues seem to arise more frequently when IVRA is used on the lower extremities. Bier block is also a procedure that has found utility as a treatment adjunct for patients suffering from complex regional pain syndromes (CRPS) (formerly know as reflex sympathetic dystrophy, or sympathetically maintained pain) as an alternative to repeated sympathetic blocks. In this regard, IVRA has been shown to decrease neurogenic inflammation, a phenomenon possibly associated with CRPS, with little impairment of sensory function, at least when mepivacaine is the local anesthetic chosen for the block. Sensibility to cold is significantly decreased 10 and 30 min after the block, even with a reduction in the skin temperature on the blocked side.[8] Chemical sympathectomy using IVRA with agents such as guanethidine or bretylium may last up to 5 days,

as compared with local anesthetic blocks, which typically provide analgesia lasting only several hours. Quantitative sensory testing before and after such blocks has demonstrated that it is possible to predict which patients will have long-lasting pain alleviation using IVRA guanethidine blocks following traumatic injury or surgery.[9]

Although IVRA is a safe and effective method of administering local anesthetics for extremity block both for surgery and for pain control, one recent large survey noted that most third-year (CA-3) anesthesia residents had performed fewer than 10 such blocks during the entire course of their training.[10]

ANATOMY

The only relevant anatomy is the location and distribution of the veins of the hand, antecubital fossa, and of the foot and ankle region.

INDICATIONS

Upper Extremity

IVRA is appropriate for surgeries and manipulations of the extremities requiring anesthesia of up to an hour's duration. It is most suited for peripheral, soft-tissue operations such as ganglionectomies, carpal tunnel release, Dupuytren's contractures, or reduction of fractures. However, the necessity of exsanguinating the extremity using an Esmarch bandage, a potentially painful maneuver, may preclude certain procedures from being undertaken with this technique (see Figures 41–5, 41–6, and 41–10). Likewise, manipulations of the ulnar, median, or radial nerves may cause paresthesias, which may require the use of analgesics or sedatives. A novel use of IVRA is for anesthetizing the hand prior to injecting botulinum toxin A (BTX-A) for the treatment of hyperhidrosis. BTX-A significantly reduces sweat production, as measured by Minor's test and as quantified by corneometer analysis, but the injection is painful unless the hand is anesthetized beforehand; IVRA has been found to be very suitable for this purpose.[11] IVRA of the upper extremity has been occasionally utilized for prolonged analgesia/anesthesia, with a mandatory tourniquet deflation period of at least 1 min prior to reestablishing the anesthetized state.[12]

Lower Extremity

IVRA may be used for brief surgical interventions of the lower extremity in a manner analogous to that described earlier for upper extremity surgery. Surgical procedures that may be completed using this approach include excision of a mass, digital nerve repair, phalangeal fracture/dislocation surgery, and accessory navicular excision. Any foot, ankle, or distal lower extremity orthopedic procedure requiring approximately 45 min or less may be amenable to this modality. Although IVRA has been associated with an increased incidence of compartment syndrome when treating tibial shaft fractures, and has therefore been deemed contraindicated in such cases, a recent study in volunteers showed no significant difference in tissue pressures before and after tourniquet inflation regardless of the volume of saline used (≤1.5 mL/kg) or as a function of time following saline injection during tourniquet inflation. The authors concluded that in the normal atraumatic limb, simulated IVRA using normal saline (NS) does not increase tissue pressure within the anterior compartment of the leg.[13]

Clinical Pearls

- ▪ IVRA for the lower extremity has been associated with an increased incidence of compartment syndrome when treating tibial shaft fractures. Although not proven, it is suggested that IVRA be used with caution in these patients.

- ▪ Some patients, especially with painful fractures of the extremities, may not be able to tolerate the placement of the Esmarch bandage with subsequent exsanguination of the leg (or arm). If simply elevating the extremity is not sufficient to effect this process, and IVRA is still considered the technique of choice, then exsanguination may be painlessly but effectively accomplished using a zippered pneumatic splint.[14] The leg (or arm) is placed on the open splint, after which the splint zipper is closed. The splint is then inflated to a pressure well above arterial pressure, after which time the proximal cuff is inflated, and the splint is deflated and removed. Whereas applying an Esmarch bandage to a painful fracture produces excessive pain, as the pressure is increased gradually in the pneumatic splint, the fracture usually becomes more comfortable, and this, of course improves the likelihood of the patient accepting the technique and hence enhances the chance for success with IVRA.

Pediatrics

IVRA has been an acceptable choice in selected pediatric patients for the reduction of fractures of the upper extremity. One large study of 470 children ages 2–19 years found that IVRA was adequate for fracture reduction in 99% (467 total). No complications were noted. The technique was only aborted in three children due to failure to gain peripheral venous access.[15] However, the technique of IVRA was found not to be superior to administration of nitrous oxide for the same purpose in a smaller sample of 28 children. Additionally, the nitrous oxide use was more rapidly applicable and dissipated more readily.[16]

CONTRAINDICATIONS

The only absolute contraindication to IVRA is patient refusal. Relative contraindications include:

- • Crush injuries of an extremity
- • Inability to locate peripheral veins
- • Local skin infections
- • Cellulitis
- • Compound fractures
- • Patients with convincing history of allergy to local anesthetics
- • Patients with severe vascular injuries to the extremity
- • Preexisting vascular arteriovenous shunts and patients in whom a tourniquet is unsuitable (ie, patients with severe peripheral vascular disease)

Clinical Pearls

- ▪ Bier block is an acceptable form of regional anesthesia in the anticoagulated patient.

- ▪ The feasibility of using a pneumatic tourniquet in those diagnosed with sickle cell disease must be balanced against the need for performing this type of anesthesia. Tourniquet use in this instance may induce localized stasis of blood, acidosis, and hypoxemia, with the subsequent formation of sickle cells. On the other hand, for lower extremity procedures in which regional block is considered preferable in the sickle cell patient, spinal or epidural block may result in compensatory vasoconstriction and a decreased Pao_2 in the nonblocked areas, making these areas possible sites for infarction. Under these circumstances, IVRA may actually be less offending than central neuraxial block.

EQUIPMENT

(Figures 41–1 through 41–11)

1. Local anesthetic agents: Lidocaine HCl, 0.25–0.5% (alternative is prilocaine, 0.5%)

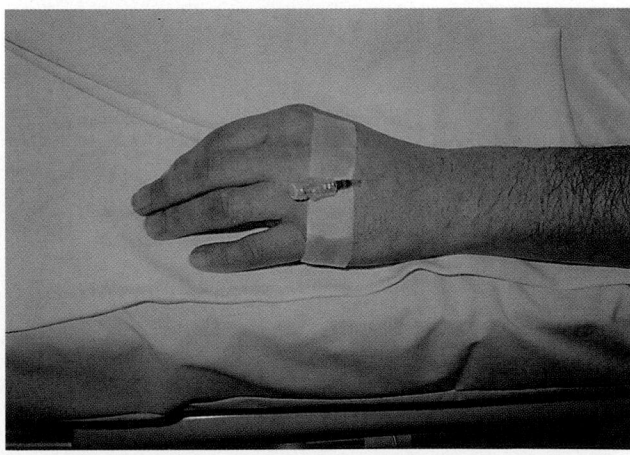

Figure 41–2. Intravenous cannula and Hep-Lock placed in a distal vein of the hand in preparation for IVRA.

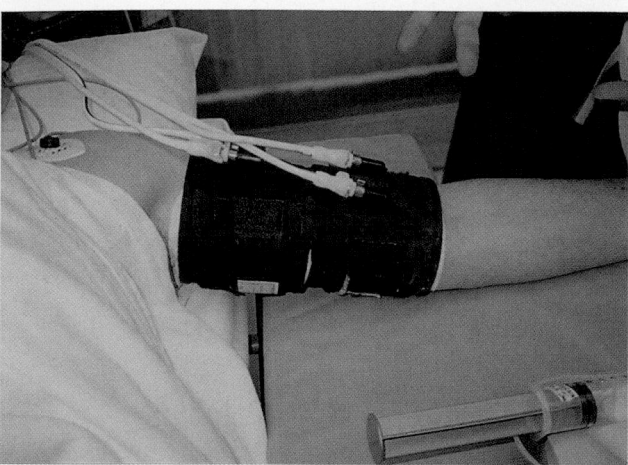

Figure 41–3. Placement of a proximal and distal tourniquet of the double pneumatic tourniquet system on the left upper extremity in preparation for IVRA.

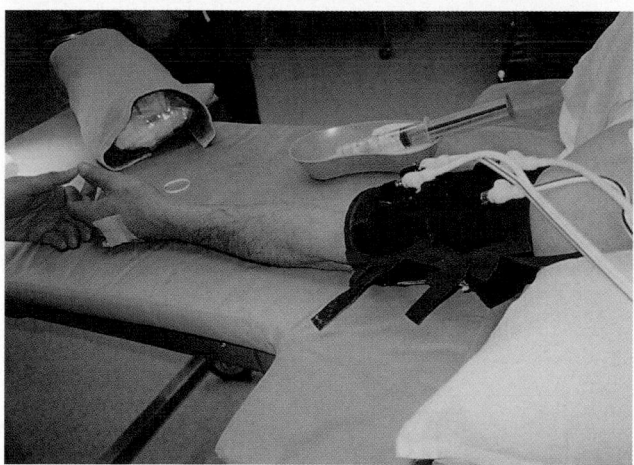

Figure 41–4. Double pneumatic tourniquet system on the left upper extremity; IV access port on the left hand; 50-mL syringe loaded with local anesthetic.

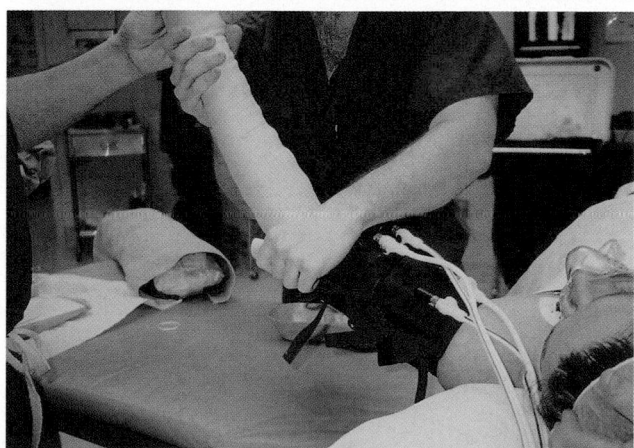

Figure 41–5. Beginning of the exsanguination process of the left upper extremity using a tightly wrapped Esmarch bandage from the distal hand to the proximal upper extremity at the base of the distal tourniquet.

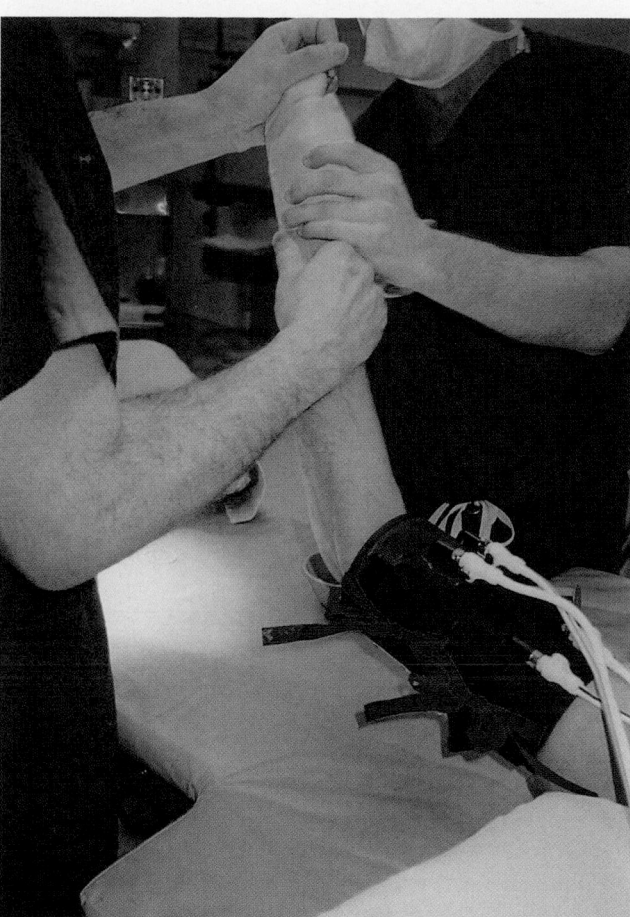

Figure 41–6. Completion of the exsanguination process of the left upper extremity with demonstration of the Esmarch bandage wrapped from distal to proximal.

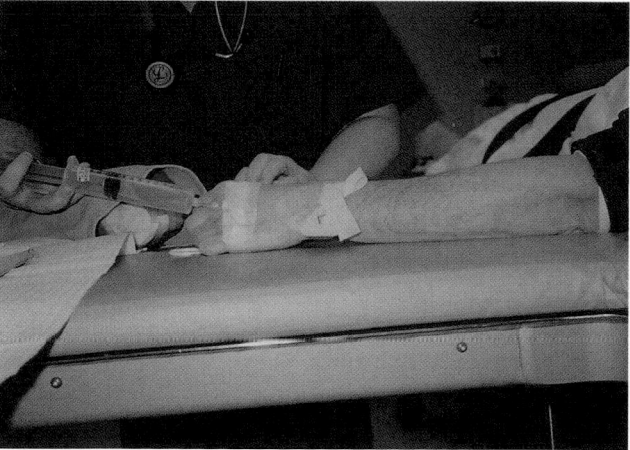

Figure 41–7. Injection of the local anesthetic through the left hand intravenous access port. Note the peripherally placed elastic tourniquet used to encourage distal and minimize proximal flow of the local anesthetic.

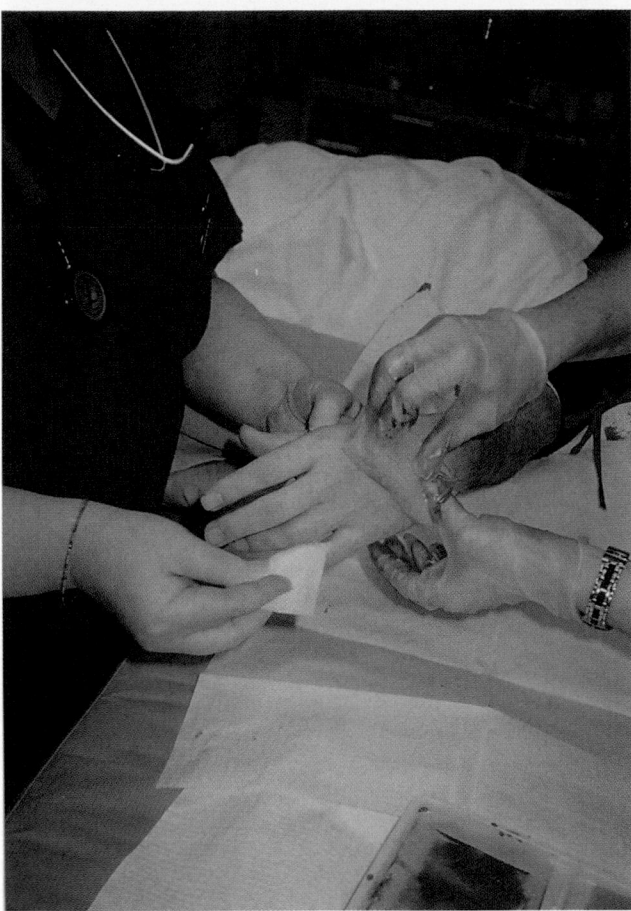

Figure 41–8. Removal of the left hand IV access port and application of Betadine-soaked sponge pad.

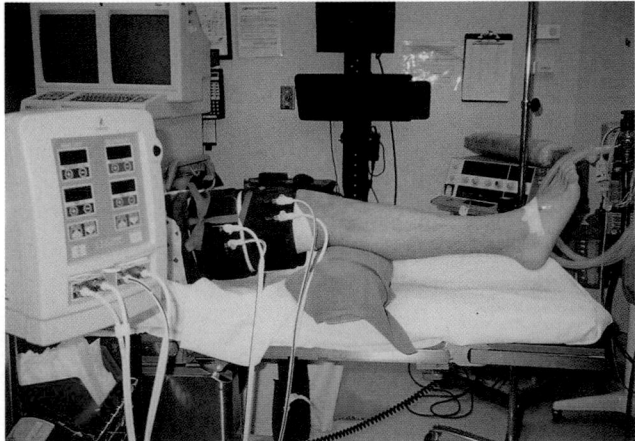

Figure 41–9. The right lower extremity prepared for IVRA. The double pneumatic tourniquets are in place, the leg is elevated on a bolster, and the IV access port is visible on the distal foot.

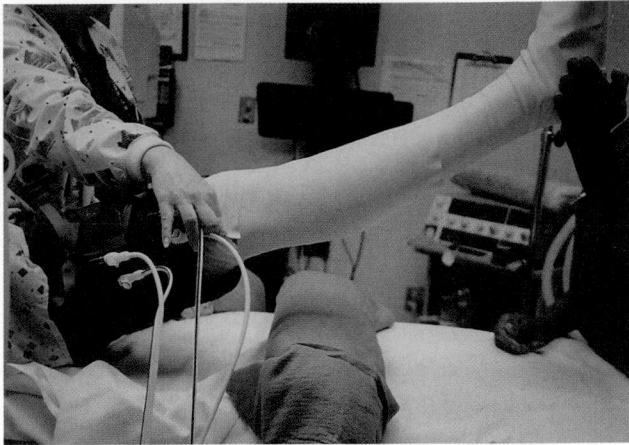

Figure 41–10. The right lower extremity is wrapped with a tightly wound Esmarch bandage in preparation for exsanguination by the proximal tourniquet.

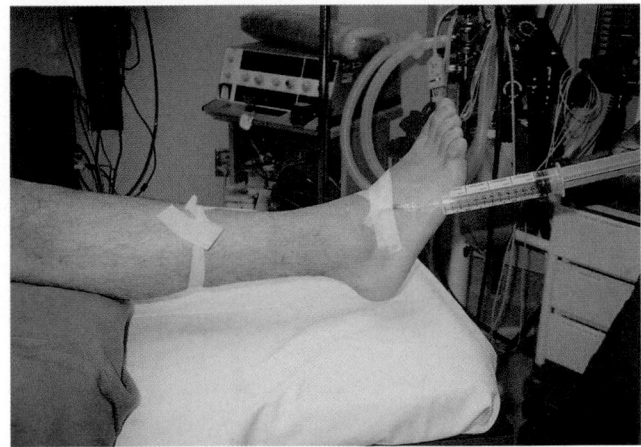

Figure 41–11. Injection of the local anesthetic through a distally placed peripheral IV access port on the dorsum of the right foot. Note the placement of the distal elastic tourniquet to promote distal and minimize proximal spread of the local anesthetic.

4. One 500-mL or 1-L bag of IV solution connected to an infusion set (vs a Hep-Lock) to be connected to the IV cannula to maintain its patency until the anesthetic solution is injected in the isolated extremity (may substitute a saline-flushed IV port instead)

5. Standard American Society of Anesthesiologists (ASA) monitors (electrocardiograph, blood pressure, pulse oximeter)

6. Resuscitation equipment (IV catheter, crystalloid solution, and infusion set for the contralateral upper extremity) (for upper extremity IVRA)

7. A functional IV catheter, crystalloid solution, and infusion set for the contralateral upper extremity

8. Two pneumatic tourniquets of appropriate size for the selected extremity (see Figures 41–1, 41–3 through 41–6, 41–9, and 41–10)

9. One Esmarch bandage 60 in. in length (152 cm) and 4 in. wide (10 cm) for exsanguinating the arm (see Figures 41–5, 41–6, and 41–10)

2. One rubber tourniquet (Penrose drain) 12–18 in. in length (30–45 cm) and $\frac{7}{8}$ in. wide (2.3 cm) for use prior to placing the intravenous cannula (see Figures 41–7 and 41–11)

3. One 18- or 20-gauge intravenous (IV) extracatheter (catheter-over-needle) (see Figures 41–2 and 41–11)

10. Sterile skin preparatory set
11. Fifty-milliliter Luer-Lok syringe (see Figures 41–7 and 41–11)
12. One graduated measuring cup for the mixing of solution, preferably with a 100-mL capacity
13. Adhesive tape; various sizes

Clinical Pearl

▪ Adjuvants to local anesthetics: There is some evidence suggesting that ketorolac, clonidine, and certain muscle relaxants may have efficacy as adjuvants. These include fentanyl citrate, pancuronium bromide, rocuronium, D-tubocurarine, ketorolac, sodium bicarbonate, and clonidine.

PATIENT PREPARATION

The patient lies in the dorsal recumbent position or in any other position as long as the vein selected for placement is readily accessible. The resuscitative equipment is checked, and the pneumatic tourniquets are tested and prepared for use. For surgery on the elbow, the needle will be placed in the forearm or antecubital fossa. For procedures on the hand or forearm, a vein on the dorsum of the hand is best selected (see Figure 41–2).

Clinical Pearls

▪ Some authors have demonstrated excellent results for hand surgery when placing the IV port either on the distal forearm[17] or in the antecubital fossa.[18] Therefore, when a patient having surgery on the distal extremity presents with difficult venous access on the hand, using a vein in the antecubital fossa should be considered instead.

For lower extremity procedures, a vein in the foot, ankle, or lower leg is chosen (see Figure 41–11). After obtaining intravenous access in a nonoperated extremity (alternatively, a central venous access may be secured), a full complement of ASA monitors is applied and baseline vital signs are assessed. If the patient is in severe pain, small aliquots of IV analgesics may now be administered (ie, fentanyl 1–2 mcg/kg) to facilitate the exsanguination process. Since total patient cooperation is not essential to be successful, small doses of a water-soluble benzodiazepine (ie, midazolam 15–25 mcg/kg) may alternatively be administered for anxiolysis. An important benefit to choosing a benzodiazepine is the suppression of the convulsant response associated with local anesthetic toxicity, a valid concern in the patient undergoing IVRA due to the large volume of agent being directly administered into the vascular system.

TECHNIQUE

Upper Extremity IVRA

The following is the technique of IVRA for upper extremity procedures as previously taught at Cook County Hospital by Alon P. Winnie, MD.

1. A double pneumatic tourniquet is placed on the proximal cuff high on the upper arm (see Figures 41–3 through 41–6)
2. An indwelling plastic extracatheter is inserted into a peripheral vein as far distally as feasible.
3. The entire arm is elevated, and a rubber Esmarch bandage is wound around the arm spirally from the hand to the distal cuff of the double tourniquet to exsanguinate the arm (see Figures 41–5 and 41–6).
4. The axillary artery is digitally occluded, and while pressure is maintained on it, the proximal pneumatic cuff is inflated to 50–100 mm Hg above the systolic arterial blood pressure, after which time the Esmarch bandage is removed.
5. Following inflation of the proximal cuff and removal of the Esmarch bandage, 30–50 mL of 0.5% lidocaine HCl is injected via the indwelling plastic catheter, the volume depending on the size of the arm being anesthetized (see Figure 41–7).
6. After injection of the local anesthetic, the arm is brought down to the level of the procedure table, the IV cannula in the surgical extremity is withdrawn, and pressure is quickly applied over the site using sterile povidone–iodine (Betadine)-soaked sponges (see Figure 41–8).
7. About 25–30 min after the onset of anesthesia or when a patient complains of tourniquet pain, the distal cuff is inflated and the proximal cuff is deflated, to minimize the development of tourniquet pain.

Clinical Pearls

▪ Compression of the axillary artery both before and during inflation of the pneumatic tourniquet is important, since as the pressure in the tourniquet rises, venous outflow is prevented before arterial inflow; and therefore, without occlusion of arterial inflow, exsanguination of the extremity may be incomplete. In fact, one study showed that arm elevation and arterial compression alone (ie, vs an Esmarch bandage or pneumatic vinyl splint for exsanguination) was sufficient in preventing maximum venous pressure (MVP), an indicator of leakage under the tourniquet. Nevertheless, using an Esmarch bandage, in that study, was associated with the most effective exsanguination of the limb, when compared with the use of vinyl splint or arm elevation/arterial compression alone.[19]

▪ For patients with painful fractures of the upper arm, it may be completely appropriate to forego the Esmarch bandage, and instead, simply elevate the arm (while occluding the artery) for a minimum of 5 min to effect the requisite venous drainage of the extremity.

- The usual dose of lidocaine (without epinephrine) administered is approximately 3 mg/kg, which is a relatively large dose in terms of systemic toxicity. Systemic toxic reactions can and do occur due to leakage past the tourniquet, sudden accidental deflation of the tourniquet during the procedure, or intentional deflation following brief surgical procedures.[20,21]

- Block can be also accomplished using a smaller volume of more concentrated local anesthetic (eg, 12–15 mL of lidocaine 2%).

Lower Extremity IVRA

The only significant difference is that the IVRA technique for the lower extremity requires relatively larger volume of local anesthetic. This is necessary to more completely fill the larger vascular compartment of the lower extremity from the distally placed IV cannula to the proximal tourniquet (100 mL vs 50 mL) (see Figures 41–9 through 41–11).

PHARMACOLOGIC CONSIDERATIONS

Clinical Pearls

- Lidocaine is the prototypical local anesthetic used for IVRA in the United States.
- Most authors use one of the following mixtures of preservative-free lidocaine for IVRA:

Upper extremity:
　　30–50 mL of 0.5% lidocaine or
　　12–15 mL of 2% lidocaine

Lower extremity:
　　50–100 mL of 0.5% lidocaine or
　　15–30 mL of 2% lidocaine

Local Anesthetic Considerations

Lidocaine is the prototypical local anesthetic used for IVRA in the United States. In Europe, however, prilocaine has been the subject of most clinical trials to date. Attempts have been made to maximize the efficacy of lidocaine, while minimizing side effects or toxicity of the agent. Alkalinization of 0.5% lidocaine (using 1.4% sodium bicarbonate) for IVRA was studied in 31 patients. The authors found no clinical advantage to the

practice of alkalinization of lidocaine with respect to sensory block, motor block, or the appearance of postoperative pain.[22] When lidocaine was compared with alkalinized and nonalkalinized 2-chloroprocaine, both used as 0.5% concentrations and used for hand surgery, alkalinized chloroprocaine behaved similarly to lidocaine, but plain chloroprocaine offered no benefit and produced more minor side effects than seen with lidocaine.[23] Lidocaine has been compared with ropivacaine for upper extremity IVRA in two separate studies. Two doses of ropivacaine (1.2 and 1.8 mg/kg) were compared with one dose of lidocaine (3.0 mg/kg) in 15 volunteers. Recovery of sensory and motor block after tourniquet release was slowest with the high-dose ropivacaine group. More patients in the lidocaine group (5 out of 5) experienced light-headedness following tourniquet release, vs only 1 in the high-dose ropivacaine group.[24] In the second study, 51 patients were randomized to receive either ropivacaine 0.375% or lidocaine 0.5% in a volume of 0.4 mL/kg up to 25 mL. Postoperative analgesia as measured by first request for analgesics was superior in the ropivacaine group.[25]

Prilocaine has been compared with lidocaine, as well as with other local anesthetics used for IVRA. Forty milliliters of 0.5% prilocaine (100 mg) was compared with the same volume and same concentration of chloroprocaine in 10 volunteers undergoing IVRA, while evaluating onset of sensory and motor block. Motor block onset did not differ between groups, and sensation recovered almost equally well. However, recovery of motor function was shorter in the prilocaine group, and more chloroprocaine patients demonstrated signs of venous irritation or antecubital urticaria for 30–45 min after tourniquet deflation. Heart rate changes were also more notable in the chloroprocaine group.[26] The same group of investigators expanded their study to include 60 patients; 30 in each of the two respective groups detailed earlier. Now, the investigators found that complete recovery of sensory block was faster in the prilocaine group (7.1 vs 9.8 min). Otherwise, the incidence of side effects remained higher in the chloroprocaine group.[27] Next, these investigators compared 0.5% prilocaine with the same concentration of articaine (a newer amino amide–type local anesthetic that contains thiophene and that is pharmacologically similar to mepivacaine) for upper extremity IVRA. Articaine, a potent local anesthetic with a low degree of toxicity by virtue of its rapid metabolism with esterases, was felt to be a suitable alternative to prilocaine. Ten volunteers participated in this double-blinded, crossover comparison of the two agents. They found no significant difference between the two with respect to onset of anesthesia or motor block, or in recovery of sensory or motor function. However, 80% of the subjects experienced skin rashes after receiving articaine, vs 20% in the prilocaine group.[28] When 0.5% prilocaine was compared with the same concentrations of articaine or lidocaine in three groups of 10 patients each for IVRA, it was found that the onset of sensory block was significantly shorter in the articaine group, which also had the lowest peak plasma concentrations of local anesthetic following tourniquet release.[29] Plain prilocaine 1% has been compared with the same local anesthetic combined with four different additives for IVRA; bupivacaine 0.25%, clonidine 150 mcg, sufentanil 25 mcg, or tenoxicam 20 mg. The sufentanil-added group demonstrated the most rapid onset of sensory block; postoperative pain scores were improved by adding either clonidine or tenoxicam. Otherwise, there were no significant differences among the five groups with respect to onset and duration of sensory and motor block.[30] Unlike the situation noted for lidocaine with the addition of bicarbonate as an adjuvant, the addition of bicarbonate to prilocaine does seem to shorten onset time and prolong the duration of anesthesia.[31,32]

The use of mepivacaine for IVRA has been studied. Sixteen patients were evaluated using 1.4 mg/kg in 40 mL for IVRA vs saline IVRA blocks performed in the same individuals on the contralateral arm. Arterial occlusion was maintained for 20 min. Reactive hyperemia was attenuated in the mepivacaine-treated arm for the 60-min evaluation period, indicating that mepivacaine is a potent vasoconstrictor of long duration of action. This finding has implications for the use of mepivacaine in individuals with either compromised upper extremity blood flow, or in those suffering from CRPS, wherein it probably should not be considered the local anesthetic of choice.[33] The same study group evaluated the effects of mepivacaine IVRA on intracutaneous capsaicin-induced burning pain and on microvascular skin blood flow as measured by Doppler perfusion imaging. The reactive hyperemia was less in the mepivacaine-treated arm 10 min after tourniquet release, and the area of the flare was smaller after capsaicin in the mepivacaine-treated arms. The authors concluded that mepivacaine IVRA had no effect on post-IVRA sensory function of thin afferents, but differentially decreased the spread of capsaicin-induced flare.[34]

Adjuncts to Local Anesthetics for IVRA

A systematic review of the literature was undertaken to evaluate the use of adjuncts to local anesthetics for IVRA. Twenty-nine studies met the criteria of being randomized, double-blinded, and controlled. Data on 1217 study subjects were reviewed, and the agents studied included opioids (fentanyl, sufentanil, meperidine, morphine), clonidine, muscle relaxants (atracurium, pancuronium, mivacurium), tramadol, nonsteroidal antiinflammatory agents (NSAIDs) (ketorolac, tenoxicam, acetylsalicylate), alkalinization using sodium bicarbonate, and the addition of potassium, and temperature alterations. The authors found solid evidence supporting the use of NSAIDs in general, and ketorolac in particular, for improving postoperative analgesia. Clonidine 1 mcg/kg also appeared to improve postoperative analgesia and prolong tourniquet tolerance. Opioids fared poorly when used for IVRA, with only meperidine in doses of ≥30 mg showing substantial postoperative benefit at the expense of postdeflation nausea, vomiting, and dizziness. Muscle relaxants improved postoperative motor block and were beneficial in fracture reduction in which muscular relaxation is imperative for good results.[35]

Alpha₂-Agonists (Clonidine and Dexmedetomidine)

Clonidine has been added to both prilocaine and lidocaine as an adjunct to IVRA, both for surgery and for the management of CRPS. When 2 mcg/kg was added to prilocaine 0.5% in a randomized, double-blind fashion in 56 patients undergoing upper extremity surgery, there was no difference between groups regarding sensory or motor block onset or duration. The patients who had clonidine added had a significant reduction in arterial blood pressure after tourniquet release (24–48%), while heart rate remained unchanged. The authors concluded that clonidine was of limited benefit as an adjunct to IVRA local anesthetics.[36] When a dose of 1 mcg/kg in a total volume of 50 mL of 0.5% lidocaine was used for lower extremity IVRA for patients suffering from CRPS, five of seven subjects obtained complete pain relief after four to six blocks. The remaining two study patients derived partial benefit from the blocks. There were no cases of significant hypotension, bradycardia, hypoxemia, or excessive sedation.[37] The addition of clonidine to prilocaine did dramatically suppress tourniquet pain, but it did not alter postoperative pain following tourniquet deflation.[38] Dexmedetomidine is approximately eight times more selective toward the α₂-adrenoreceptors than is clonidine. As such, it has been used in IVRA to determine if it might advance some of the beneficial findings noted with the latter agent. Thirty patients undergoing hand surgery under IVRA received 0.5% lidocaine alone or lidocaine plus dexmedetomidine 0.5 mcg/kg. The dexmedetomidine group showed a more rapid onset of sensory and motor block, a prolonged sensory and motor block recovery, prolonged tolerance for the tourniquet, and improved quality of analgesia compared with the group that received local anesthetic only.[39]

Opioids

Since opiate receptors were discovered to exist in the peripheral nervous system[40,41] and with the demonstration that opioids may produce effective, long-lasting analgesia when injected in conjunction with local anesthetics for brachial plexus block,[42–46] several investigators have attempted to decrease the potential for toxicity from local-anesthetic-only IVRA by adding opioids to reduce the concentration of lidocaine. Although it has not been proven that the addition of fentanyl to lidocaine for IVRA results in improved analgesia while reducing the risks,[47,48] the addition of fentanyl in 200-mcg doses to prilocaine 0.5% did result in more complete anesthesia than in patients who had 100 mcg added, or when plain prilocaine was used for IVRA. Postoperative nausea and central nervous system side effects were higher in the fentanyl-added groups vs those who received local anesthetic alone.[49] Two other studies, however, found that the addition of opioids to prilocaine did not improve success with the technique.[50,51] More research on the effects of the addition of opioids to prilocaine for IVRA may ultimately resolve this apparent discrepancy.

Some investigators have found that adding opioid and muscle relaxants to 0.25% lidocaine provides the same analgesia and muscular relaxation as that provided by 0.5% lidocaine alone, while reducing the likelihood of systemic toxicity. Adjuvants added to lidocaine have included fentanyl 50 mcg plus pancuronium 0.5 mg,[52,53] fentanyl plus rocuronium,[54] and fentanyl plus D-tubocurarine.[55] In each case, the authors reported outstanding operating conditions, and since the lidocaine concentration was able to be reduced to 0.20%, the potential for systemic toxicity was at least halved.

When meperidine 0.25%, 40 mL (100 mg), was used as a solitary agent for IVRA, complete motor block was produced, just as effective as that produced by lidocaine. Motor block onset was as rapid or more rapid than sensory block onset in each of the 15 patients in this study group. However, when compared with plain lidocaine in this study, there was a higher incidence of dizziness, nausea, and pain at the injection site.[56]

Tramadol

Tramadol has been evaluated for use in IVRA of the upper extremity. Sixty volunteers divided into four groups of 15 patients each received IVRA with 40 mL of tramadol 0.25% (100 mg), 0.9% NS, lidocaine 0.5%, or lidocaine plus tramadol 0.25%. The onset and recovery of sensory and motor block was similar between the tramadol and NS-only groups. However, the addition of tramadol to lidocaine resulted in faster onset of sensory block at the expense of an increase in skin rash development and painful burning sensations at the injection site. The conclusion of the authors was that tramadol alone does not possess local anesthetic effects, but might modify the effect if added to a local anesthetic like lidocaine.[57] In another study comparing 0.5% lidocaine with and without 50 mg of tramadol for upper extremity IVRA, the tramadol-added group experienced less tourniquet pain than the local-only group, but, as in the study mentioned earlier, there were several cases of skin urticaria in the tramadol group, but not in the lidocaine-only group.[58] Tramadol (100 mg) added to lidocaine for IVRA for upper extremity anesthesia acted similarly to sufentanil (25 mcg) or clonidine (1 mcg/kg) added to the local anesthesia with respect to intraoperative hemodynamic data, time to recovery of sensory block, onset and recovery of motor block, sedation scores, and postoperative pain.[59] In summary, tramadol is ineffective as a solo agent for IVRA, but may confer some advantage when added to lidocaine. This advantage, however, may be offset by the significant incidence of dermatologic side effects of tramadol given intravenously in an exsanguinated extremity.

Muscle Relaxants

A small dose of nondepolarizing muscle relaxant may be chosen as an adjunct to the local anesthetic administered for IVRA; however, since D-tubocurarine releases histamine even in judicious doses, it is probably best to avoid this agent altogether. Atracurium has been added to lidocaine in an effort to improve muscular relaxation during IVRA, particularly during the reduction of upper extremity fractures and dislocations. Adding 3 mg of atracurium to lidocaine for IVRA resulted in a decrease in the onset time of analgesia in the

hand, but not at the tourniquet site. There was no added benefit to adding this agent, or adding alfentanil to lidocaine in the same study.[60] A prior study using 2 mg of atracurium added to 40 mL of 0.5% lidocaine for IVRA for hand surgery in 40 patients randomized to one of two groups found that the addition of the atracurium provided a greater degree of muscular relaxation, easier reduction of fractures, and better operating conditions, as well as less pain after surgery.[61]

Neostigmine

Neostigmine has been suggested as a co-analgesic when used for epidural and intrathecal analgesia and anesthesia, but evidence of its benefit in the peripheral nervous system is controversial. In two studies, one using neostigmine added to lidocaine, and the other using the adjuvant added to prilocaine, there have been conflicting findings. When neostigmine (1 mg) was added to 0.5% lidocaine for IVRA in a study of 54 volunteers randomized into one of three study groups, it was found that the addition of the adjuvant provided no benefit in terms of analgesia or anesthesia compared with controls.[62] When one-half the dose of neostigmine (0.5 mg) was added to prilocaine (3 mg/kg) for IVRA in 30 patients randomized to one of two treatment groups, it was found that the adjuvant group demonstrated shortened sensory and motor block onset times, prolonged sensory and motor block recovery times, improved quality of anesthesia, and prolonged time to first analgesic requirement vs the plain prilocaine group.[63] It appears that these conflicting findings with neostigmine added to two distinct local anesthetics for IVRA will need to be confirmed by additional work incorporating larger patient sample sizes to resolve the apparent discrepancy in the two small studies mentioned earlier.

Nonsteroidal Antiinflammatory Agents

Other attempts to improve IVRA with lidocaine have included using NSAIDs like ketorolac[64] to suppress tourniquet pain while enhancing postoperative analgesia. Although ketorolac has shown some efficacy, other NSAIDs have not fared as favorably. Ketorolac has been added to lidocaine for IVRA for the treatment of sympathetically mediated pain syndromes. In a retrospective review of 61 patients referred to a university pain center with a diagnosis of reflex sympathetic dystrophy (RSD) who all underwent IVRA with the combination of ketorolac-lidocaine, 26% (16/61) had a complete analgesic response to the block(s). Forty-three percent (26/61) had a partial response, and 31% had no response. The authors stated that the only symptom predicting failure was the presence of allodynia. However, allodynia is the hallmark of RSD, so one must wonder whether the clinicians correctly categorized the patients as being afflicted with RSD, vs an alternative diagnosis.[65] When used for upper extremity surgery, ketorolac added to lidocaine for IVRA was shown to be safe and effective, and furthermore, using a forearm tourniquet instead of an upper arm tourniquet in this study demonstrated that the dose of both agents could be reduced by 50%, while also providing for prolonged sensory block and prolonged postoperative analgesia. Twenty milligrams of ketorolac was added to lidocaine 0.5% for the upper arm tourniquet group, and half the dose of both agents (by virtue of halving the volume administered of an equipotent concentration of both drugs) was used in the forearm tourniquet group.[66]

Another NSAID, tenoxicam, was added to prilocaine in one study of 45 total patients. A 20-mg dose of the NSAID was used in patients undergoing IVRA for reduction of Colles' fractures, with patients divided into three groups. One group received local anesthetic only, one received local plus tenoxicam, and one group had IVRA with local anesthetic only plus IV NSAID. In this last group, the tenoxicam (20 mg) was injected into the contralateral arm, opposite the IVRA procedure arm. The group receiving the NSAID added to the local had superior analgesia and lower pain scores than either of the other two groups of patients.[67]

Other Specific Agents: Corticosteroids

The antiinflammatory properties of steroids have been evaluated when these agents have been added to local anesthetics for IVRA in patients with rheumatoid arthritis (RA). In a randomized, double-blind, crossover, placebo-controlled study, 20 RA patients received either 50 mg methylprednisolone in mepivacaine 0.25% or mepivacaine plain for upper extremity IVRA. The other extremity received the opposite treatment. One week later, the same medications were injected into the contralateral extremities, respectively. Fifty percent of patients reported subjective improvement at 1 and 6 weeks; objective parameters like grip strength did not change until the 6-week evaluation, at which time a significant increase was noted, as was the reduction in grip diastasis and movement-invoked pain. This report suggests that corticosteroids administered by IVRA may provide sustained analgesia in certain RA sufferers.[68] Steroid IVRA has also been used as adjunctive treatment of CRPS type I. Methylprednisolone (40 mg) was added to lidocaine for IVRA in a randomized, double-blinded, placebo-controlled fashion in 22 patients. Treatments were applied once per week, for up to three sessions of blocks. The investigators found no benefit in adding the steroid to the local with regard to improvement in pain severity or shortening the course of the disease.[69]

Specific IVRA Treatments for CRPS

Adrenergic blocking agents or antagonists, particularly those effective at the alpha receptor, have shown promise in the treatment of CRPS, particularly when these agents are used for IVRA. Other adrenergic adjuvants release and then subsequently prevent the reuptake of norepinephrine at the neurovascular junction. Their use in CRPS is intuitive, since the pathophysiology of the disease is suspected to include the alpha receptor and to be mediated by norepinephrine. However, there is significant controversy regarding this topic, particularly when current research is compared with the findings of studies conducted almost 40 years ago. Guanethidine, reserpine, and bretylium have all been evaluated for IVRA for CRPS. When 15 mg guanethidine was added to

0.5% prilocaine in a group of 57 patients with CRPS of the upper extremity and hand, the guanethidine was found not to be more effective than NS in treating allodynia and burning pain of CRPS, following distal radius fractures.[70] These findings corroborated work done in a double-blind, randomized, multicenter study 7 years earlier. Sixty patients with RSD/causalgia received four IVRA blocks at 4-day intervals with either guanethidine or placebo in 0.5% lidocaine. Long-term, there was no difference noted between the placebo group and the guanethidine group, and only 35% of patients overall in all groups had a resolution of their pain problem.[71] Bretylium has been used as well in CRPS. In a randomized, controlled trial, 0.5% lidocaine was compared with the same local anesthetic to which bretylium 1.5 mg/kg was added. A decrease in pain of $\geq 30\%$ was considered significant. The bretylium-local group had pain relief for 20 ± 17.5 days, as opposed to the lidocaine-only group, wherein analgesia persisted for only 2.7 ± 3.7 days. The bretylium was far superior to the local anesthetic alone in treating CRPS in this study.[72] IVRA with bretylium was utilized to demonstrate that a reduction in sympathetic tone to exercising forearm muscles would increase blood flow, reduce muscle acidosis, and attenuate reflex responses. IVRA with bretylium increased blood flow as well as oxygen consumption in the exercising forearm, although both venous potassium and hydrogen ion content were elevated during the exercise phase, implying that reflex effects are unaffected by bretylium block.[73]

COMPLICATIONS

Complications due to IV regional anesthesia may be classified either as drug- or equipment- (ie, tourniquet) related. Drug-related complications depend on the agents being administered directly into the vascular system, including local anesthetics and adjuvants. Equipment-related complications include all devices and techniques used to isolate the vascular space from the systemic circulation. Inadvertent deflation of the cuff, cuff failure, a sudden increase in venous pressure within the occluded tissue to a level higher than cuff pressure, and an intact interosseous circulation may all contribute to complications due to IVRA. Lidocaine is the most commonly utilized local anesthetic for IVRA and is therefore the agent about which most complications have been reported. Fortunately, lidocaine does not accumulate to any great extent at sodium channels at therapeutic plasma concentrations, and since it both rapidly binds to and dissociates from the channel, toxic accumulations of the drug at the channel is atypical.[74,75] Excessive plasma concentrations of lidocaine, as are associated with IV boluses of large doses with a faulty tourniquet system, result in peripheral vasodilatation and diminished cardiac contractility, usually seen clinically as hypotension. The usual onset of IVRA using lidocaine in 0.5% concentrations is rapid (about 4.5 ± 0.3 min) and the termination of anesthesia once the tourniquet has been deflated is also quite rapid $(5.8 \pm 0.5 \text{ min}).$[76] Usually, there are no signs or symptoms of cardiovascular or central nervous system toxicity if the tourniquet is deflated at least 30 min after the drug is injected into the venous system, although tinnitus has been noted at the 20- and 27-s postdeflation periods following standard inflation times.[77] Although about 70% of the administered lidocaine dose remains within the tissues of the isolated limb after tourniquet deflation, the remaining 30% enters the systemic circulation during the ensuing 45 min.[75] Much more drug is released from the tissues of the isolated limb into the circulation after tourniquet deflation if the limb is inadvertently exercised, emphasizing the importance of maintaining the previously anesthetized extremity quiescent for some time immediately following tourniquet deflation. The other commonly utilized local anesthetic used for IVRA, prilocaine, is associated with the formation of methemoglobin, which occurs about 4 to 8 h after its administration.[74] Fortunately, significant methemoglobinemia has not been reported when prilocaine has been used for IVRA. Prilocaine (0.5%) administered for IVRA has an onset of analgesia of about 11 min ($\pm$6.8 min) and termination of analgesia following tourniquet deflation averages 7.2 min ($\pm$4.6 min).[26] The use of this agent for IVRA appears to be extraordinarily safe. Indeed, in one survey of 45,000 prilocaine IVRA blocks, there were no serious side effects and no deaths from using this drug via this technique.[78] In terms of effectiveness, prilocaine seems to be equivalent to lidocaine when used for IVRA.

When opioids are administered in combination with local anesthetics for IVRA in an attempt to prolong analgesia following cuff deflation, occasional side effects typically attributed to opioids administered systemically may be noted following cuff deflation. These include nausea, vomiting, and mild sedation.[47,50] When neuromuscular blocking drugs are administered in conjunction with local anesthetics to improve surgical conditions in patients undergoing fracture reduction, there have been no reports of complications from these adjuvants.

Clinical Pearls

- An intact tourniquet system is absolutely essential for the successful and safe performance of IVRA.

- Unintentional deflation of the tourniquet or the presence of a vascular communication even with an intact, functioning tourniquet may result in serious toxic sequelae due to IVRA.

- Intermittent cuff deflation may effectively prolong the time to achieve peak arterial concentrations of the local anesthetic, but may not be entirely reliable in minimizing toxicity due to release of local anesthetic into the circulation.[79]

- The tourniquet should not be deflated until at least 30 min has elapsed from the time the local anesthetic (and adjuvants, if used) is injected into the isolated venous system.

Additionally, the tourniquet itself may be a source of complications since it may cause ischemic pain and discomfort. Systemic hypertension may result from prolonged tourniquet inflation that is sustained or prolonged. Equipment misuse or malfunction is an important, and avoidable, source of complications due to this technique. Even an intact, fully functional tourniquet may be associated with leakage of administered drugs from a supposedly isolated extremity into the systemic circulation.[80,81] Lower limb IVRA has an almost 100% incidence of local anesthetic leakage from beneath the tourniquet, versus about a 25% incidence for upper extremity block.[82] As a corollary to this leakage phenomenon, the use of IVRA for lower extremity analgesia has an associated high incidence of poor-quality block (almost 40% in one prospective study).[83] Drug may leak past an apparently fully functioning cuff and gain access to the systemic circulation via the interosseous circulation, which is not affected by the occlusion of muscles, soft-tissues, and the accompanying vascular channels included therein. This factor has been recognized for almost 40 years, yet it does not appear to be significant in the production of complications due to IVRA.[84] Tourniquet deflation after IVRA is associated with signs and symptoms of systemic local anesthetic toxicity, ranging from mild CNS-related events such as tinnitus and perioral numbness, to seizures, and finally, to devastating cardiovascular collapse. These correlate with local anesthetic concentrations in arterial blood, and not to venous concentrations.[79,85] Another complication due to IVRA is tourniquet pain, which not uncommonly occurs if a double-pneumatic device is not utilized[81] (see Figures 41–1 and 41–2). We recommend the use of such a tourniquet for any procedure performed using IVRA that is expected to last longer than 30 min. Even when such guidelines are followed, however, some investigators have reported untoward events occurring following tourniquet deflation after a "safe" time interval. A 47-year-old patient with a history of CRPS type I underwent an IVRA block with a combination of lidocaine and clonidine. The tourniquet was deflated after 60 min and within the ensuing 10 min, he developed partial complex seizures that were persistent.[86]

Very rare, isolated reports of neurologic complications, including damage to the median, ulnar, and musculocutaneous nerves, are associated with IVRA.[87] The cause of such complications appears to be direct pressure of the tourniquet applied to these nerves, which subsequently exhibit histologic changes resembling crush injuries. It is recommended that tourniquet time not exceed 2 h, to reduce the likelihood of capillary and muscle damage secondary to tissue acidosis.[87,88] Compartment syndrome may occur rarely following IVRA, especially when IVRA is used for reduction of long bone lower extremity fractures, and may be due both to the large volume of anesthetic injected to effect analgesia as well as to inadequate or incomplete exsanguination of the limb prior to performing the block.[89,90] There is also a case report of this complication following inadvertent injection of hypertonic saline solution when local anesthetic was intended to be injected.[91] A 33-year-old pregnant patient undergoing

IVRA for endoscopic carpal tunnel release experienced a severe episode of phantom limb sensation after the injection of the local anesthetic. The symptoms resolved on dissipation of the IVRA.[92] There is one report of the devastating necessity for amputation of the arm in a 28-year-old patient whose radial and ulnar arteries thrombosed following IVRA after a brief tourniquet occlusion time.[93] Whether this resulted from unsuspected intraarterial injection of drug, a drug administration error, or perhaps an idiosyncratic drug reaction is purely speculative.

Local Anesthetic Toxicity

Although lidocaine is the most commonly utilized local anesthetic agent for IVRA in the United States, in Europe prilocaine 0.5% is more routinely chosen. Prilocaine, however, is metabolized to orthotoluidine, an oxidizing compound capable of converting hemoglobin to methemoglobin. This is usually only of concern when the dose of prilocaine exceeds 600 mg, which, even for lower extremity IVRA in which volumes as large as 100 mL are utilized, should not be attained (ie, 100 mL × 0.5% prilocaine = 500 mg). Deflation of the tourniquet after surgery is a critical step to minimizing the possibility of toxicity associated with IVRA. First, it is absolutely mandatory that the tourniquet not be deflated unless at least 30[34] min has elapsed since the injection of the local anesthetic, even if the duration of surgery or of the manipulation has been very brief. If the surgery is very brief, and the patient needs to recover in a postanesthesia care unit (PACU), it is acceptable to clamp off the distal tourniquet while it is inflated, remove the patient from the operating area (with the tourniquet inflated), and transfer the patient to a monitored care setting. At no time should anyone remove the clamped tourniquet, however, until the 30-min period commencing with the injection of local anesthetic solution has elapsed. At such time, the patient should be continually monitored for at least 15 min following tourniquet unclamping in the PACU. At least one case of cardiac arrest has been reported when the tourniquet was released soon after the injection of local, where the duration of surgery was extremely short.[94] Second, it is absolutely essential that the deflation of the tourniquet be accomplished in a "cyclical" fashion as follows: the cuff is deflated (after a minimum of 30 min) and is immediately reinflated. The patient is observed or questioned carefully for the occurrence of symptoms associated with local anesthetic toxicity, such as tinnitus, light-headedness, metallic taste in the mouth, etc. Obviously, signs of stimulation of the CNS may also represent local anesthetic toxicity and must be sought. If there are no such signs or symptoms after about 1 min, the cuff is once again deflated, and once again immediately reinflated for a period of about 1 to 2 min, with the patient being observed and queried for systemic local anesthetic toxicity. If none appear by this time, the tourniquet may be safely deflated and removed from the extremity. The safety of such cycled deflating/reinflating is that with each deflation, only a small fraction of the administered (and unbound) local anesthetic is allowed to enter the systemic circulation, minimizing the possibility of a sudden, sustained increase in the blood level of the local anesthetic.[79]

SUMMARY

IVRA is a valuable adjunct to the armamentarium of clinicians in any specialty dealing with the acutely injured patient. The simplicity of the technique and the relative safety (if strict adherence to the previously listed protocol is maintained) make it an attractive alternative to brachial plexus block (for upper extremity surgery or manipulation) and spinal or epidural block (for lower extremity surgery or manipulation). Simply being able to identify and access a peripheral vein and apply a pneumatic tourniquet make this one of the most "user-friendly" regional block modalities in clinical practice. One of the only potential disadvantages associated with IVRA is the very finite duration of anesthesia/analgesia associated with its use. A relative inability to prolong analgesia long into the postprocedure period detracts from its utility. For those occasions, continuous catheter insertion and maintenance by way of plexus anesthesia surely offers an attractive alternative.

References

1. Bier A: Über einen neun weg localanaesthesia an den gliedmassen zu erzeugen. Arch Klin Chir 1908;86:1007–1016.
2. Bier A: On a new method of local anesthesia. Muench Med Wschir 1909;56:589.
3. Bier A: Concerning venous anesthesia. Berl Klin Wschr 1909;46:477–489.
4. Bier A: On local anesthesia with special reference to vein anesthesia. Edinburgh Med J 19105:103–123.
5. Morrison J: Intravenous local anesthesia. Brit J Surg 1930–1931;18:641–647.
6. Herreros L: Regional anesthesia by the intravenous route. Anesthesiology 1946;7:558–60.
7. Holmes CMcK: Intravenous regional analgesia. Lancet 1963;1:245–247.
8. Kalman S, Svensson H, Lisander B, et al: Quantitative sensory changes in humans after intravenous regional block with mepivacaine. Reg Anesth Pain Med 1999;24:236–241.
9. Wahren L, Torebjork E, Nystrom B: Quantitative sensory testing before and after regional guanethidine block in patients with neuralgia in the hand. Pain 1991;46:23–30.
10. Smith M, Sprung J, Zura A, et al: A survey of exposure to regional anesthesia techniques in American anesthesia residency training programs. Reg Anesth Pain Med 1999;24:11–16.
11. Blaheta H, Vollert B, Zuder D, et al: Intravenous regional anesthesia (Bier's block) for botulinum toxin therapy of palmar hyperhidrosis is safe and effective. Dermatol Surg 2002;28:666–671.
12. Glickman L, Mackinnon S, Rao T, et al: Continuous intravenous regional anesthesia. J Hand Surg 1992;17:82–86.
13. Mabee J, Shean C, Orlinsky M, et al: The effects of simulated Bier block IVRA on intracompartmental tissue pressure. Acta Anaesthesiol Scand 1997;41:208–213.
14. Winnie A, Ramamurthy S: Pneumatic exsanguination for intravenous regional anesthesia. Anesthesiology 1970;33:664–665.
15. Blasier R, White R: Intravenous regional anesthesia for management of children's extremity fractures in the emergency department. Pediatr Emerg Care 1996;12:404–406.
16. Gregory P, Sullivan J: Nitrous oxide compared with intravenous regional anesthesia in pediatric forearm fracture manipulation. J Pediatr Orthop 1996;16:187–191.

17. Karalezli N, Karalezli K, Iltar S, et al: Results of intravenous regional anaesthesia with distal forearm application. Acta Orthop Belg 2004;70:401–405.

18. Blyth M, Kinninmonth A, Asante D: Bier's block: A change of injection site. J Trauma 1995;39:726–728.

19. Mabee J, Orlinsky M: Bier block exsanguinations: A volumetric comparison and venous pressure study. Acad Emerg Med 2000;7:105–113.

20. Brown E, McGill J, Malinowski R: Intravenous regional anesthesia (Bier block): A review of 20 years' experience. Can J Anaesth 1989;36:307–310.

21. Mazze R, Dunbar R: Intravenous regional anesthesia—Report of 497 cases with a toxicity study. Acta Anaesthesiol Scand 1969;36: 27–34.

22. Benlabed M, Jullien P, Guelmi K, et al: Alkalinization of 0.5% lidocaine for intravenous regional anesthesia. Reg Anesth 1990;15: 59–60.

23. Lavin P, Henderson C, Vaghadia H: Non-alkalinized and alkalinized 2-chloroprocaine vs lidocaine for intravenous regional anesthesia during outpatient hand surgery. Can J Anaesth 1999;46:939–945.

24. Chan V, Weisbrod M, Kaszas Z, et al: Comparison of ropivacaine and lidocaine for intravenous regional anesthesia in volunteers: A preliminary study on anesthetic efficacy and blood level. Anesthesiology 1999;90:1602–1608.

25. Peng P, Coleman M, McCartney C, et al: Comparison of anesthetic effect between 0.375% ropivacaine versus 0.5% lidocaine in forearm intravenous regional anesthesia. Reg Anesth Pain Med 2002;27:595–599.

26. Pitkanen M, Suzuki N, Rosenberg P: Intravenous regional anaesthesia with 0.5% prilocaine or 0.5% chloroprocaine. A double-blind comparison in volunteers. Anaesthesia 1992;47:618–619.

27. Pitkanen M, Kytta J, Rosenberg P: Comparison of 2-chloroprocaine and prilocaine for intravenous regional anaesthesia of the arm: A clinical study. Anaesthesia 1993;48:1091–1093.

28. Pitkanen P, Xu M, Haasio J, et al: Comparison of 0.5% articaine with 0.5% prilocaine in intravenous regional anesthesia of the arm: A cross-over study in volunteers. Reg Anesth Pain Med 1999;24:131–135.

29. Simon M, Gielen M, Alberink N, et al: Intravenous regional anesthesia with 0.5% articaine, 0.5% lidocaine, or 0.5% prilocaine. A double-blind randomized clinical study. Reg Anesth 1997;22:29–34.

30. Hoffman V, Vercauteren M, Van Steenberge A, et al: Intravenous regional anesthesia. Evaluation of 4 different additives to prilocaine. Acta Anaesthesiol Belg 1997;48:71–76.

31. Armstrong P, Brockway M, Wildsmith J: Alkalinization of prilocaine for intravenous regional anesthesia. Anaesthesia 1990;45:11–13.

32. Solak M, Akturk G, Erciyes N, et al: The addition of sodium bicarbonate to prilocaine solution during I.V. regional anesthesia. Acta Anaesthesiol Scand 1991;35:572–574.

33. Kalman S, Bjorhn K, Tholen E, et al: Mepivacaine as an intravenous regional block interferes with reactive hyperemia and decreases steady-state blood flow. Reg Anesth 1997;22:552–556.

34. Kalman S, Liderfalk C, Wardell K, et al: Differential effect on vasodilatation and pain after intradermal capsaicin in humans during decay of intravenous regional anesthesia with mepivacaine. Reg Anesth Pain Med 1998;23:402–408.

35. Choyce A, Peng P: A systematic review of adjuncts for intravenous regional anesthesia for surgical procedures. Can J Anaesth 2002;49:32–45.

36. Kleinschmidt S, Stockl W, Wilhelm W, et al: The addition of clonidine to prilocaine for intravenous regional anaesthesia. Eur J Anaesthesiol 1997;14:40–46.

37. Reuben S, Skair J: Intravenous regional anesthesia with clonidine in the management of complex regional pain syndrome of the knee. J Clin Anesth 2002;14:87–91.

38. Cucchia G, Chasot-Di Dio V, et al: Effect of addition of clonidine to local anesthetic during the Bier block on the pre- and postoperative analgesia. Br J Anaesth 1997;78(suppl 1):78–79.

39. Memis D, Turan A, Karamanlioglu B, et al: Adding dexmedetomidine to lidocaine for intravenous regional anesthesia. Anesth Analg 2004;98:835–840.

40. Fields H, Emson P, Leigh B, et al: Multiple opiate receptor sites on primary afferent fibers. Nature 1980;284:351–353.

41. Young W, Wamsley J, Zarbin M, et al: Opioid receptors undergo axonal flow. Science 1980;210:76–78.

42. Boogaerts J, Balatoni E, Lafont N, et al: Utilisation des morphiniques dans les blocs nerveux peripheriques. Congres Ser Ars Medicina 1985;3:143–150.

43. Gobeaux D, Landais A: Utilisation de deux morphiniques dans les blocs du plexus brachial. J Can Anesth 1988;36:437–440.

44. Gobeux D, Landais A, Bexon G, et al: Adjonction de fentanyl la lidocaine adrenaline pour le blocage du plexus brachial. J Can Anesth 1987;35:195–199.

45. Viel E, Eledjam J, de la Coussaye J, et al: Brachial plexus block with opioids for postoperative pain relief: Comparison between buprenorphine and morphine. Reg Anesth 1989;14:274–278.

46. Candido K, Khan M, Raja D, et al: Brachial plexus block with buprenorphine for postoperative pain relief. Reg Anesth 2000;25:23.

47. Arthur J, Mian T, Heavner J, et al: Fentanyl and lidocaine versus lidocaine for Bier block. Reg Anesth 1992;17:223–227.

48. Bobart V, Hartmannsgruber M, Atanassoff P, et al: Analgesia/anesthesia after fentanyl plus lidocaine vs. plain lidocaine for intravenous regional anesthesia. Anesth Analg 1998;86:S-3.

49. Pitkanen M, Rosenberg P, Pere P, et al: Fentanyl-prilocaine mixture for intravenous regional anaesthesia in patients undergoing surgery. Anaesthesia 1992;47:395–398.

50. Armstrong P, Power I, Wildsmith J: Addition of fentanyl to prilocaine for intravenous regional anaesthesia. Anaesthesia 1991;46:278–280.

51. Gupta A, Begntsson M, Bjornsson A, et al: Lack of peripheral analgesic effect of low-dose morphine during intravenous regional anesthesia. Reg Anesth 1993;18:250–253.

52. Abdulla W, Fadhil N: A new approach to intravenous regional anesthesia. Anesth Analg 1992;75:597–601.

53. Sztark F, Thicoipe M, Favarel-Garriques J, et al: The use of 0.25% lidocaine with fentanyl and pancuronium for intravenous regional anesthesia. Anesth Analg 1997;84:777–779.

54. Subxedar D, Gevirtz C, Malik V, et al: Intravenous regional anesthesia: Prospective evaluation of 0.25% lidocaine with fentanyl and rocuronium. Reg Anesth 1997;22:41.

55. Thapar P, Skerman J: Evaluation of 0.2% lidocaine with fentanyl and D-tubocurarine for intravenous regional anesthesia. Reg Anesth 1997;84:S342.

56. Acalovschi I, Cristea T: Intravenous regional anesthesia with meperidine. Anesth Analg 1995;81:539–543.

57. Acalovschi I, Cristea T, Margarit S, et al: Tramadol added to lidocaine for intravenous regional anesthesia. Anesth Analg 2001;92:209–214.

58. Tan S, Pay L, Chan S: Intravenous regional anesthesia using lignocaine and tramadol. Ann Acad Med Singapore 2001;30:516–519.

59. Alayurt S, Memis D, Pamukcu Z: The addition of sufentanil, tramadol or clonidine to lignocaine for intravenous regional anaesthesia. Anaesth Intensive Care 2004;32:22–27.

60. Kurt N, Kurt I, Aygunes B, et al: Effects of adding alfentanil or atracurium to lidocaine solution for intravenous regional anesthesia. Eur J Anaesthesiol 2002;19:522–525.

61. Elhakim M, Sadek R: Addition of atracurium to lidocaine for intravenous regional anaesthesia. Acta Anaesthesiol Scand 1994;38:542–544.

62. McCartney C, Brill S, Rawson R, et al: No anesthetic or analgesic benefit of neostigmine 1 mg added to intravenous regional anesthesia with lidocaine 0.5% for hand surgery. Reg Anesth Pain Med 2003;28:414–417.

63. Turan A, Karamanlyoglu B, Memis D, et al: Intravenous regional anesthesia using prilocaine and neostigmine. Anesth Analg 2002;95:1419–1422.

64. Reuben S, Steinberg R, Kreitzer J, et al: Intravenous regional anesthesia using lidocaine and ketorolac. Anesth Analg 1995;81:110–113.

65. Connelly N, Reuben S, Brull S: Intravenous regional anesthesia with ketorolac-lidocaine for the management of sympathetically-mediated pain. Yale J Biol Med 1995;68:95–99.

66. Reuben S, Steinberg R, Maciolek H, et al: An evaluation of the analgesic efficacy of intravenous regional anesthesia with lidocaine and ketorolac using a forearm versus upper arm tourniquet. Anesth Analg 2002;95:457–460.

67. Jones N, Pugh S: The addition of tenoxicam to prilocaine for intravenous regional anaesthesia. Anaesthesia 1996;51:446–448.

68. Bengtsson A, Bengtsson M, Nilsson I, et al: Effects of intravenous regional administration of methylprednisolone plus mepivacaine in rheumatoid arthritis. Scand J Rheumatol 1998;27:277–280.

69. Taskaynatan M, Ozgul A, Tan A, et al: Bier block with methylprednisolone and lidocaine in CRPS type I: A randomized, double-blinded, placebo-controlled study. Reg Anesth Pain Med 2004;29:408–412.

70. Livingstone J, Atkins R: Intravenous regional guanethidine blockade in the treatment of posttraumatic complex regional pain syndrome 1 (algodystrophy) of the hand. J Bone Joint Surg Br 2002;84:380–386.

71. Ramamurthy S, Hoffman J: Intravenous regional guanethidine in the treatment of reflex sympathetic dystrophy/causalgia: A randomized, double-blind study. Guanethidine Study Group. Anesth Analg 1995;81:718–723.

72. Hord A, Rooks M, Stephens B, et al: Intravenous regional bretylium and lidocaine for treatment of reflex sympathetic dystrophy: A randomized, double-blind study. Anesth Analg 1992;74:818–821.

73. Lee F, Shoemaker J, McQuillan P, et al: Effects of forearm Bier block with bretylium on the hemodynamic and metabolic responses to handgrip. Am J Physiol Heart Circ Physiol 2000;279:H586–593.

74. Bader A, Concepcion M, Hurley R, et al: Comparison of lidocaine and prilocaine for intravenous regional anesthesia. Anesthesiology 1988;69:409–412.

75. Tucker G, Boas R: Pharmacokinetic aspects of intravenous anesthesia. Anesthesiology 1971;34:538–549.

76. Ware R: Intravenous regional anesthesia using bupivacaine. A double blind comparison with lignocaine. Anaesthesia 1979;34:231–235.

77. Smith C, Steinhaus J, Haynes C: The safety and effectiveness of intravenous regional anesthesia. South Med J 1968;61:1057–1060.

78. Bartholomew K, Sloan J: Prilocaine for Bier's block: How safe is safe? Arch Emerg Med 1990;7:189–195.

79. Sukhani R, Garcia C, Munhall R, et al: Lidocaine disposition following intravenous regional anesthesia with different deflation technics. Anesth Analg 1989;68:633–637.

80. Mazze R, Dunbar R: Plasma lidocaine concentrations after caudal, lumbar epidural, axillary block and intravenous regional anesthesia. Anesthesiology 1966;27:574–579.

81. Dunbar R, Mazze R: Intravenous regional anesthesia: Experience with 779 cases. Anesth Analg 1967;46:806–813.

82. Davies J, Walford A: Intravenous regional anaesthesia for foot surgery. Acta Anaesthesiol Scand 1986;30:145–147.

83. Kim D, Shuman C, Sadr B: Intravenous regional anesthesia for outpatient foot and ankle surgery: A prospective study. Orthopedics 1993;16:1109–1113.

84. Cotev S, Robin G: Experimental studies on intravenous regional anaesthesia using radioactive lignocaine. Br J Anaesth 1966;38:936–940.

85. Hargrove R, Hoyle J, Parker J: Blood lidocaine levels following intravenous regional analgesia. Anaesthesia 1966;21:37–41.

86. Ahmed S, Vallejo R, Hord E: Seizures after a Bier block with clonidine and lidocaine. Anesth Analg 2004;99:593–594.

87. Larsen U, Hommelgaard P: Pneumatic tourniquet paralysis following intravenous regional analgesia. Anaesthesia 1987;42:526–528.

88. Shaw-Wilgis E: Observations on the effects of tourniquet ischaemia. J Bone Joint Surg 1971;1104:190.

89. Mabee J, Bostwick T, Burke M: Iatrogenic compartment syndrome from hypertonic saline injection in Bier block. J Emerg Med 1994;12:473–476.

90. Quigley J, Popich G, Lanz U: Compartment syndrome of the forearm and hand: A case report. Clin Orthop 1981;161:247–251.

91. Hastings H 2nd, Misamore G: Compartment syndrome resulting from intravenous regional anesthesia. J Hand Surg 1987;12:559–562.

92. Dominguez E: Distressing upper extremity phantom limb sensation during intravenous regional anesthesia. Reg Anesth Pain Med 2001;26:72–74.

93. Luce E, Mangubat E: Loss of hand and forearm following Bier block: A case report. J Hand Surg 1983;8:280–283.

94. Kennedy B, Duthie A, Parbrook G, Carr T: Intravenous regional anesthesia: An appraisal. Br Med J 1965;5440:954–957.

42

Ilioinguinal & Iliohypogastric Blocks

Roy A. Greengrass, MD

INTRODUCTION

"Almost all cases of hernia, with the possible exception of those in young children, could undoubtedly be subjected to the radical operation under local anesthesia." This quote by Harvey Cushing reported in the *Annals of Surgery* in 1900 illustrates that over 100 years ago the attributes of regional anesthesia for lower abdominal and inguinal surgery were appreciated. Ilioinguinal and iliohypogastric blocks are among the most frequently used regional blocks performed for these surgical procedures. Postherniorrhaphy pain is moderate to severe and often poorly controlled with opioids as single modal therapy.[1] Ilioinguinal and iliohypogastric blocks have been shown to significantly reduce pain associated with herniorrhaphy, regardless of whether the blocks are used as the primary anesthetic[2] or for pain control after general[3,4] or spinal[5] anesthesia.

Anatomy

Both the iliohypogastric and ilioinguinal nerves emanate from the first lumbar spinal root. Superomedial to the anterior superior iliac spine, the iliohypogastric and ilioinguinal nerves pierce the transversus abdominis to lie between it and the internal oblique muscles. After traveling a short distance inferomedially, their ventral rami pierce the internal oblique to lie between the internal and external oblique muscles before giving off branches, which pierce the external oblique to provide cutaneous sensation. The iliohypogastric nerve supplies the skin over the inguinal region. The ilioinguinal nerve

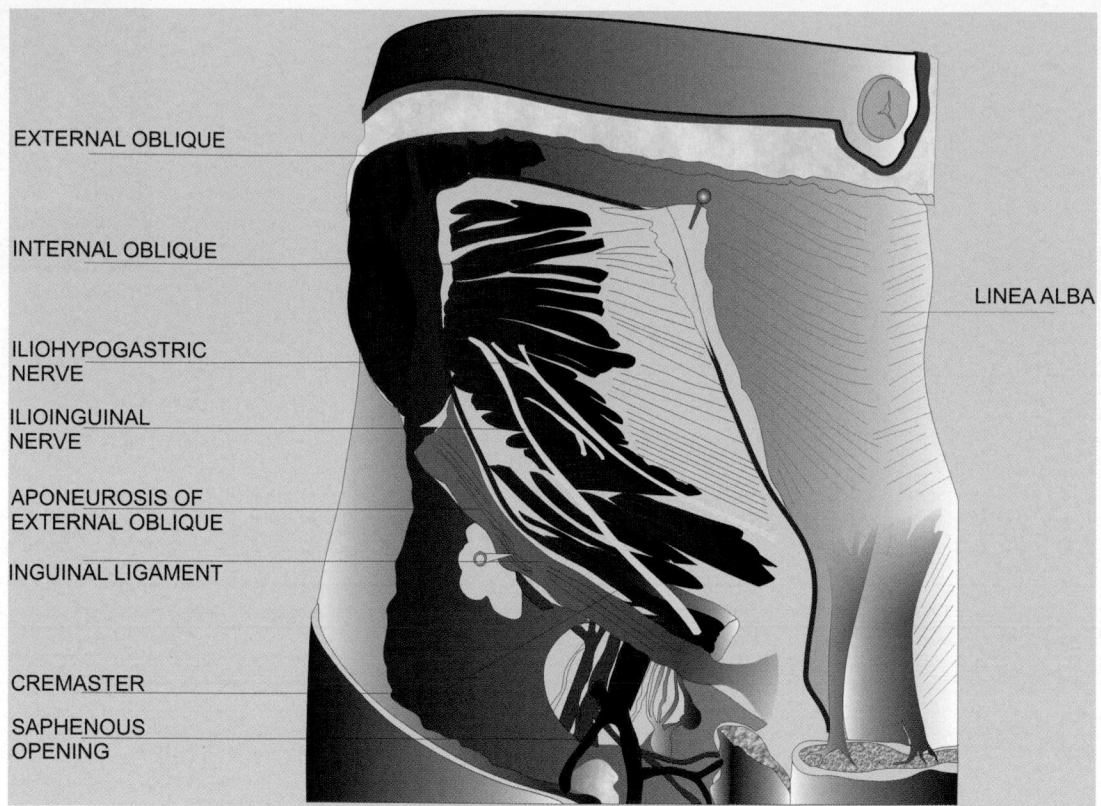

Figure 42–1. Anatomic relationship of the ilioinguinal and iliohypogastric nerves.

runs anteroinferiorly to the superficial inguinal ring, where it emerges to supply the skin on the superomedial aspect of the thigh (Figure 42–1).

Of note, the ventral rami of the lower intercostal nerves (T11 and T12) also pierce the transversus abdominis muscle to lie between it and the internal oblique. These latter nerves also supply sensation to the inferior abdominal wall, and block of these nerves as well as the iliohypogastric and ilioinguinal nerves is essential to provide anesthesia for procedures involving the lower abdominal wall.

METHOD OF BLOCK

Using the anatomic knowledge previously described, one needs to provide a method of block that allows accurate placement of local anesthetic between the internal oblique and external oblique muscles.

Methods of local anesthetic administration that do not accurately define placement between these muscular layers provide inconsistent anesthesia and analgesia of the abdominal wall and inguinal region. Unfortunately, this may result in the reporting of inadequate analgesia for a procedure that is more a problem of technique than of the block itself.[6] Accurate block techniques must define the specific muscular layers of the abdominal wall. The only way to facilitate this is to use loss of resistance techniques that define fascial layers.

Initially, the anterior superior iliac spine is palpated and a mark made 2 cm medial and 2 cm superior from it (Figure 42–2). After skin preparation and infiltration with local anesthetic, a small puncture is made in the skin with a sharp needle to allow subsequent insertion of a blunt needle. The needle is inserted through the skin puncture site perpendicular to the skin. Increased resistance is met as the needle encounters the external oblique muscle. A loss of resistance

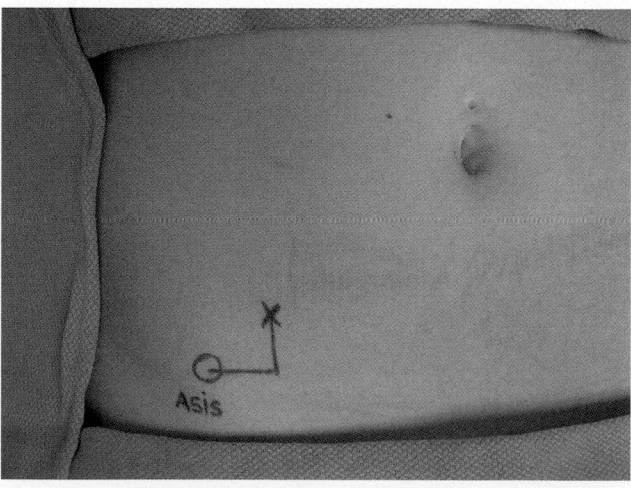

Figure 42–2. Surface landmarks for ilioinguinal block. The point of needle insertion is marked 2 cm medial and 2 cm superior from the anterior superior iliac spine (ASIS).

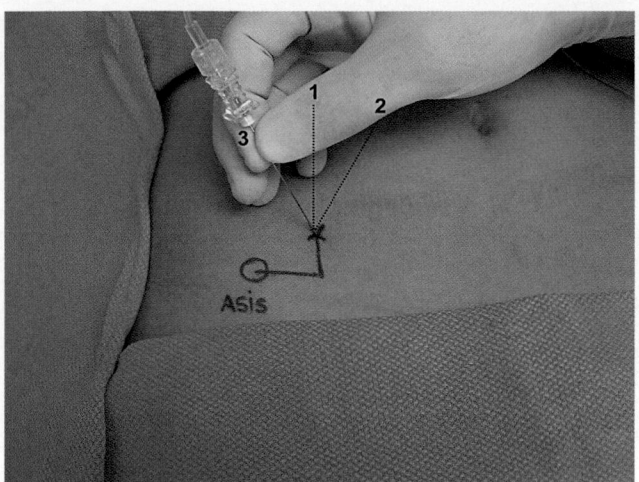

Figure 42–3. Needle maneuvers to block the iliohypogastric and ilioinguinal nerves. Shown is perpendicular needle insertion (1), lateral (2), and medial (3) redirections (fan technique).

is appreciated as the needle passes through the muscle to lie between it and the internal oblique. After the initial loss of resistance and negative needle aspiration for blood, 3 mL of local anesthetic is injected.

The needle is then withdrawn to skin and redirected at a 45-degree angle medially to again pierce the external oblique muscle (Figure 42–3). After loss of resistance, 3 mL of local anesthetic is again administered. The needle is then returned to skin and inserted 45 degrees laterally, and the procedure is repeated. Thus, a total of 9 mL of local anesthetic is placed in a fan-like distribution between the external and internal oblique muscles.

After completion of the block, the skin of the lower abdominal wall or inguinal region is tested for anesthesia.

Equipment

Any atraumatic needle blunt enough to appreciate a loss of resistance is used for this block. Examples are 22-gauge Whitacre, Sprotte, 18-gauge Tuohy-type(which can also be used to place catheters), 21-gauge Stimuplex needles, etc.

INDICATIONS & CONTRAINDICATIONS

Indications for ilioinguinal/iliohypogastric blocks include anesthesia for any somatic procedure involving the lower abdominal wall/inguinal region such as inguinal herniorrhaphy[2–5] and for analgesia after surgical procedures using a Pfannenstiel incision as for cesarean section[7] and abdominal hysterectomy.[8] These blocks do not provide visceral anesthesia and thus cannot be used as the sole anesthetic for procedures such as lower intraabdominal surgery. When used for inguinal herniorrhaphy, the sac (containing peritoneum) must be infiltrated with local anesthetic by the surgeon to complete anesthesia for the procedure.

There are no specific contraindications for these blocks apart from the generic contraindications to performance of any regional block such as infection at the procedure site, allergy to local anesthetics, indeterminate neuropathy, and so on.

CHOICE OF LOCAL ANESTHETIC

Unless unusual circumstances occur requiring immediate anesthesia (thus requiring an intermediate-acting agent), a long-acting local anesthetic agent is used to provide the benefits of prolonged postoperative analgesia. We currently use ropivacaine in concentrations of 0.5–1% without adjuvants for ilioinguinal/iliohypogastric blocks (less than 1% concentrations when bilateral block such as Pfannenstiel incisions or bilateral herniorrhaphy are scheduled). For continuous infusions, ropivacaine in concentrations of 0.2–0.5% is used.

COMPLICATIONS & HOW TO AVOID THEM

Because proper performance of ilioinguinal/iliohypogastric blocks requires multiple small volume injections the possibility of local anesthetic toxicity is remote. Pharmacokinetic studies of 3 mg/kg of 0.5% plain ropivacaine in children revealed peak plasma concentrations of ropivacaine well below the toxic level.[9] A similar study in adults receiving 60–70 mL of 0.5% ropivacaine again revealed low peak plasma concentrations.[10]

Because the block is limited to the lower abdominal wall and inguinal region, any hemodynamic changes would be unusual. As with other blocks, the patient is advised to protect the anesthetized area from trauma.

Proper performance of ilioinguinal/iliohypogastric blocks places the injection medial and superior to the anterior superior iliac spine. Some texts advocate performing the block from a point medial and inferior to the anterior superior iliac spine, which essentially places the injection within or inferior to the inguinal ligament. This may result in lateral femoral cutaneous or femoral block with little or no ilioinguinal/iliohypogastric anesthesia. However, even properly performed ilioinguinal/iliohypogastric blocks can result in transient femoral anesthesia with a reported incidence of 3.7–5%.[11,12] The mechanism of femoral anesthesia with these methods is tracking of local anesthetic along the fascia iliaca.[13] In the event of femoral anesthesia associated with ilioinguinal/iliohypogastric blocks, the surgeon is notified and the patient is advised to protect the lower extremity until the block recedes.

Perforation of both the small[14] and large[15] bowels and creation of a pelvic hematoma[16] have been reported after ilioinguinal/iliohypogastric blocks. This illustrates the importance of using blunt needles to appreciate the loss of resistance as the needle traverses the layers of the abdominal wall.

CONTINUOUS ILIOINGUINAL/ ILIOHYPOGASTRIC BLOCKS

Prolonged postoperative analgesia for procedures using a Pfannenstiel incision has been successfully produced using bilateral catheters. Such catheters are an excellent alternative to epidural analgesia by allowing unlimited ambulation without the need for urinary catheterization. Control of visceral pain with NSAIDS or other agents is necessary to complete analgesia.

Method

From a point 2 cm medial and 2 cm cephalad from the anterior superior iliac spine, an 18-gauge Tuohy-type needle is inserted in a slightly medial and caudal orientation to the skin to pierce the external oblique muscle (see Figure 42–2). After loss of resistance, a multilumen catheter is inserted and directed medially for 5 cm and secured to skin. The procedure is repeated on the other side. The catheters are either infused using separate pumps or a single pump with flow-restrictor catheters that allow accurate individual catheter flow are used. Individual catheter flow rates of 4 mL/h (0.2% ropivacaine) have been used.

SUMMARY

Regional anesthesia for surgical procedures involving the lower abdomen and inguinal region can be safely and successfully performed using ilioinguinal and iliohypogastric blocks. These techniques accord excellent postoperative analgesia, obviating the need for large-dose opioids and thus facilitating early ambulation and discharge.

References

1. Salet G: Patient survey after inguinal hernia repair in ambulatory surgery. Ambulatory Surg 1993;1:194–196.
2. Ding Y, White PF: Post-herniorrhaphy pain in outpatients after preincision ilioinguinal-hypogastric nerve block during monitored anaesthesia care. Can J Anaesth 1995;42:12–15.
3. Harrison CA, Morris S, Harvey JS: Effect of ilioinguinal and iliohypogastric nerve block and wound infiltration with 0.5% bupivacaine on postoperative pain after hernia repair. Br J Anaesth 1994;72:691–693.
4. Bugedo GJ, Carcamo CR, Mertens RA, et al: Preoperative percutaneous ilioinguinal and iliohypogastric nerve block with 0.5% bupivacaine for post-herniorrhaphy pain management in adults. Reg Anesth 1990;15:130–133.
5. Toivonen J, Permi J, Rosenberg PH: Effect of preincisional ilioinguinal and iliohypogastric nerve block on postoperative analgesic requirement in day-surgery patients undergoing herniorrhaphy under spinal anaesthesia. Acta Anaesthesiol Scand 2001;45:603–607.
6. Huffnagle HJ, Norris MC, Leighton BL, Arkoosh VA: Ilioinguinal iliohypogastric nerve blocks—before or after cesarean delivery under spinal anesthesia? Anesth Analg 1996;82(1):8–12.
7. Bell EA, Jones BP, Olufolabi AJ, et al: Women's Anesthesia Research Group. Iliohypogastric-ilioinguinal peripheral nerve block for post-Cesarean delivery analgesia decreases morphine use but not opioid-related side effects [English, French]. Can J Anaesth 2002;49(7):694–700.
8. Kelly MC, Beers HT, Huss BK, Gilliland HM: Bilateral ilioinguinal nerve blocks for analgesia after total abdominal hysterectomy. Anaesthesia 1996;51(4):406.
9. Dalens B, Ecoffey C, Joly A, et al: Pharmacokinetics and analgesic effect of ropivacaine following ilioinguinal/iliohypogastric nerve block in children. Paediatr Anaesth 2001;11:415–420.
10. Wulf H, Behnke H, Vogel I, Schroder J: Clinical usefulness, safety, and plasma concentration of ropivacaine 0.5% for inguinal hernia repair in regional anesthesia. Reg Anesth Pain Med 2001;26(4):348–351.
11. Shandling B, Steward DJ: Regional analgesia for post-operative pain in pediatric outpatient surgery. J Pediatr Surg 1980;15:477–480.
12. Ghani KR, McMillan R, Paterson-Brown S: Transient femoral nerve palsy following ilio-inguinal nerve blockade for day case inguinal hernia repair. J R Coll Surg Edinb 2002;47:626–629.
13. Rosario DJ, Jacob S, Luntley J, et al: Mechanism of femoral nerve palsy complicating percutaneous ilioinguinal field block. Br J Anaesth 1997;78(3):314–316.
14. Amory C, Mariscal A, Guyot E, et al: Is ilioinguinal/iliohypogastric nerve block always totally safe in children? Paediatric Anaesth 2003;13:164–166.
15. Johr M, Sossai R: Colonic puncture during ilioinguinal nerve block in a child. Anesth Analg 1999;88:1051–1052.
16. Vaisman, J: Pelvic hematoma after an ilioinguinal nerve block for orchialgia. Anesth Analg 2001;92:1048–1049.

43

Thoracic & Lumbar Paravertebral Block

Manoj K. Karmakar, MD • Anthony M-H. Ho, MD

THORACIC PARAVERTEBRAL BLOCK

Thoracic paravertebral block (TPVB) is the technique of injecting local anesthetic alongside the thoracic vertebra close to where the spinal nerves emerge from the intervertebral foramen.[1,2] This produces unilateral, segmental, somatic, and sympathetic nerve blockade,[3] which is effective for anesthesia and in treating acute and chronic pain of unilateral origin from the chest and abdomen.[1] Hugo Sellheim of Leipzig (1871–1936) is believed to have pioneered TPVB in 1905.[1,2] Kappis, in 1919, developed the technique of paravertebral injection, which is comparable to the one in present-day use. Although paravertebral block was fairly popular in the early 1900s, it seemed to have fallen into disfavor during the mid and later part of the century, the reason for which is not known. In 1979 Eason and Wyatt rekindled interest by describing a technique of paravertebral catheter placement.[4] Our understanding of the safety and efficacy of TPVB has improved significantly in the last 25 years, and there has been a gradual renewal of interest in this technique. Currently it is used not only for analgesia but also for surgical anesthesia,[5–7] and its application has been extended to children.[8–10]

Anatomy

The thoracic paravertebral space (TPVS) is a wedge-shaped space located on either side of the vertebral column (Figure 43–1). The parietal pleura forms the anterolateral boundary. The base is formed by the vertebral body, intervertebral disc, and the intervertebral foramen with its contents. The transverse process and the superior costotransverse ligament form the posterior boundary. Lying in between the parietal pleura anteriorly and the superior costotransverse ligament posteriorly is a fibroelastic structure, the **endothoracic fascia,** which is the deep fascia of the thorax (Figure 43–1 through 43–3).[1,11–15] Medially the endothoracic

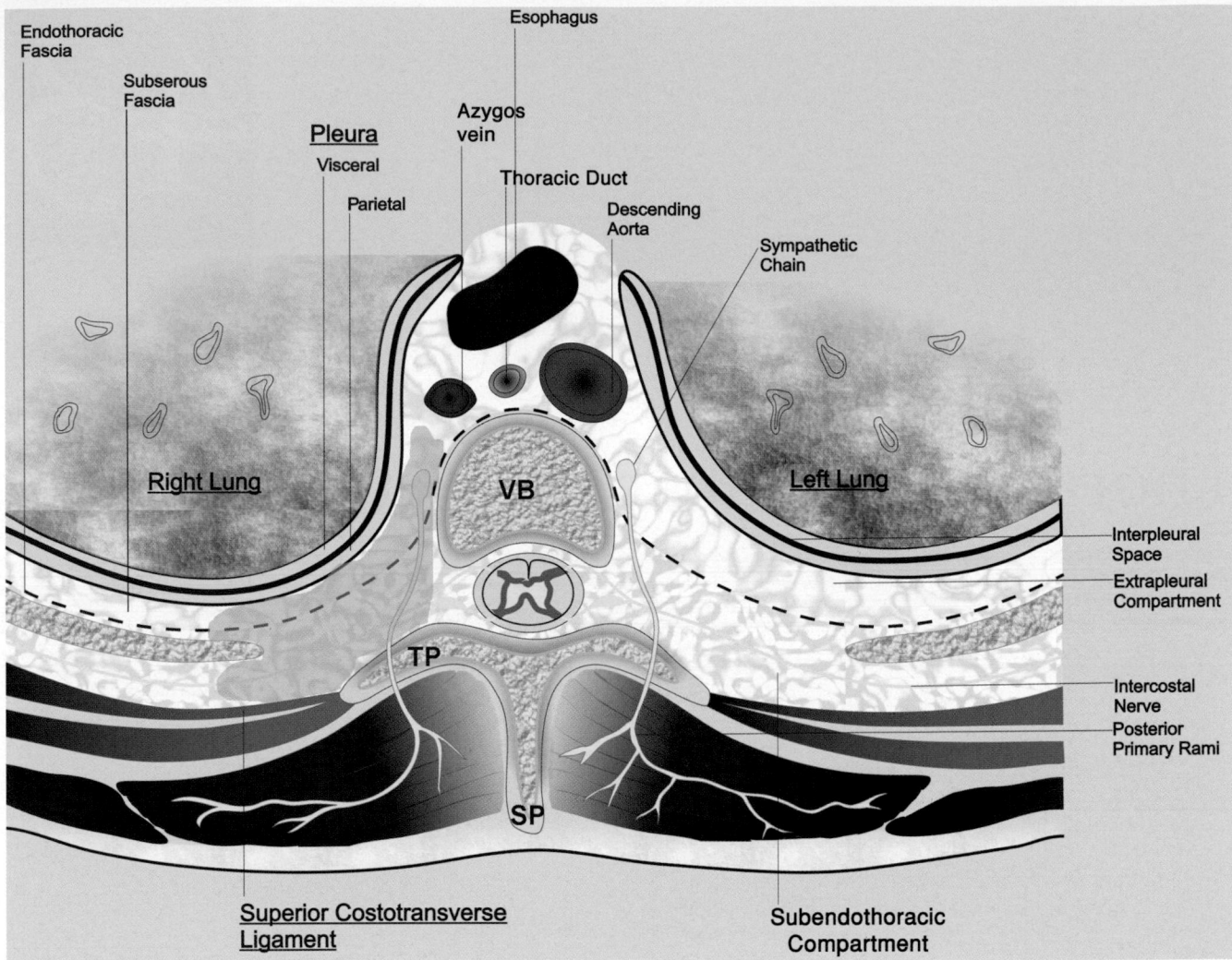

Figure 43–1. Anatomy of the thoracic paravertebral space. SP, spinous process; TP, transverse process; VB, vertebral body. The blue shaded area represents the paravertebral space.

fascia is attached to the periosteum of the vertebral body. A layer of loose areolar connective tissue, the **subserous fascia,** lies between the parietal pleura and the endothoracic fascia. Therefore there are two potential fascial compartments in the TPVS: the anterior **extrapleural paravertebral compartment** and the posterior **subendothoracic paravertebral compartment** (see Figures 43–1 and 43–2). The TPVS contains adipose tissue within which lie the intercostal (spinal) nerve, the dorsal ramus, intercostal vessels, rami communicantes, and anteriorly the sympathetic chain. The spinal nerves are segmented into small bundles and lie freely in the adipose tissue of the TPVS, which make them accessible to local anesthetic solutions injected into the TPVS.[16]

The TPVS communicates with the epidural space medially[17,18] and with the intercostal space laterally. The TPVS on either side of the thoracic vertebra also communicate with each other through the epidural and prevertebral space.[1,12,15] The cranial extension of the TPVS is challenging to define and may significantly vary; however, we have observed direct paravertebral spread of radiopaque contrast medium from the thoracic to the cervical paravertebral space, indicating a direct anatomic continuity. The TPVS

also communicates caudally through the medial and lateral arcuate ligaments with the retroperitoneal space behind the fascia transversalis, where the lumbar spinal nerves are located.[13,19–21]

Mechanism of Block & Distribution of Anesthesia

TPVB produces ipsilateral somatic and sympathetic nerve blockade (Figure 43–4) due to a direct effect of the local anesthetic on the somatic and sympathetic nerves in the TPVS, extension into the intercostal space laterally, and the epidural space medially. The overall contribution of epidural spread to the dermatomal distribution of anesthesia following a TPVB is not well defined. However, some degree of ipsilateral spread of local anesthetic toward the epidural space probably occurs in the majority of patients, resulting in a greater distribution of anesthesia than occurs with paravertebral spread alone.[18] The dermatomal distribution of anesthesia following a single injection of a large volume (eg, injection of 15–25 mL of local anesthetic at one level) varies and is often unpredictable.[1,3,22] However, the injected solutions routinely

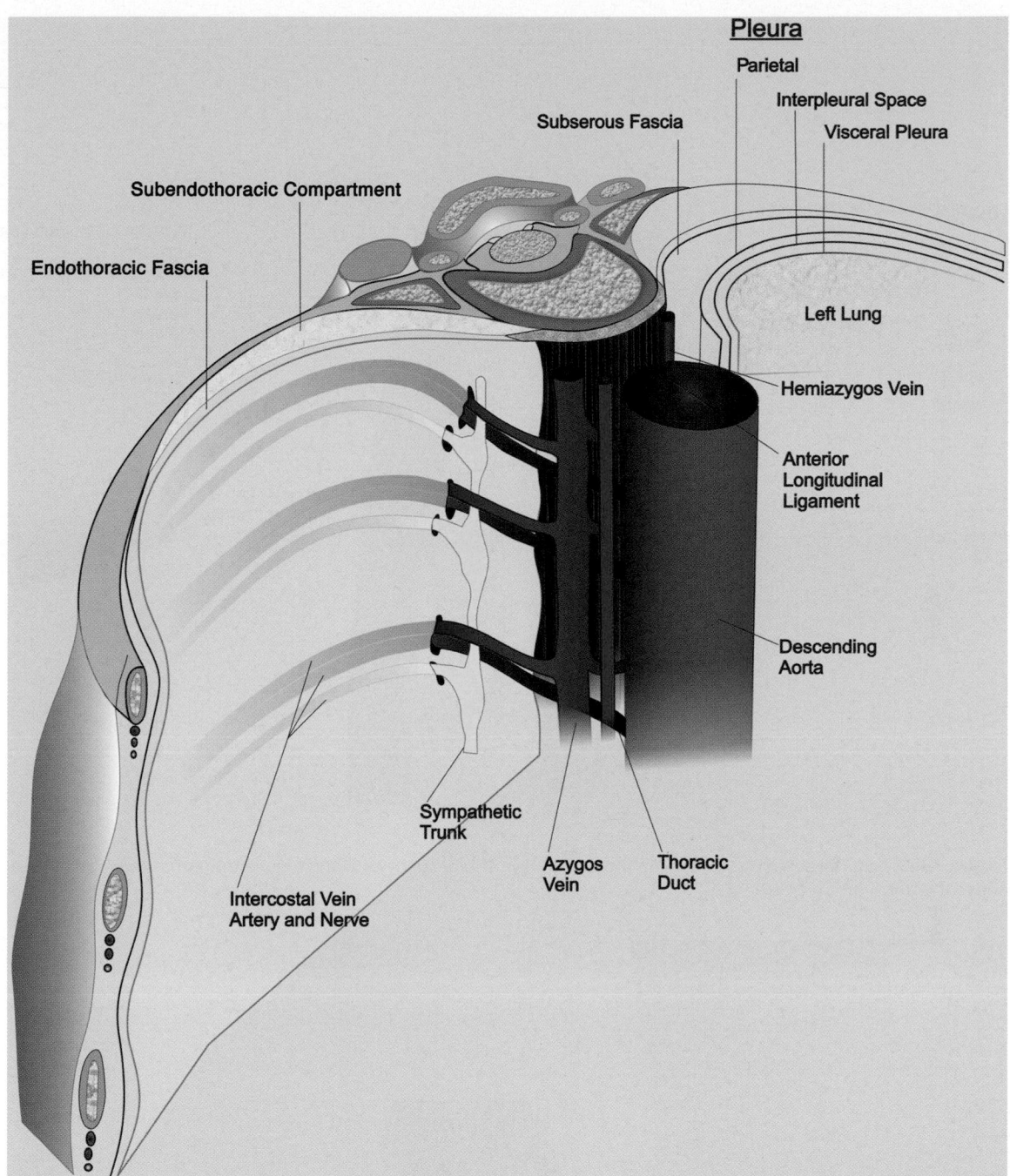

Figure 43–2. The endothoracic fascia and its anatomic relation to the structures in the thoracic paravertebral space. Note the fascial compartments and the location of the neurovascular structures in relation to the endothoracic fascia.

spread both cephalad and caudad to the site of injection to some extent (Figure 43–5). Nevertheless, the multiple-injection technique, where small volumes (3–4 mL) of local anesthetic are injected at several contiguous thoracic levels, is preferable over single, large-volume injection. This is particularly important when reliable anesthesia over several ipsilateral thoracic dermatomes is desired, such as when TPVB is used for anesthesia during breast surgery.

Segmental contralateral anesthesia, adjacent to the site of injection, occurs in approximately 10% of patients after single-injection TPVB and may be due to epidural or pre-

vertebral spread. Bilateral symmetrical anesthesia due to extensive epidural spread or unintentional intrathecal injection into a dural sleeve may occur, particularly when the needle is directed medially or when a larger volume of local anesthetic (>25 mL) is used. For this reason, during placement of TPVB, patients should be monitored using the same vigilance and methods as those employed for injection using the large-volume, single-injection epidural technique. The ipsilateral ilioinguinal and iliohypogastric nerves may also occasionally be involved after lower thoracic paravertebral injections. This is either due to epidural spread or extended

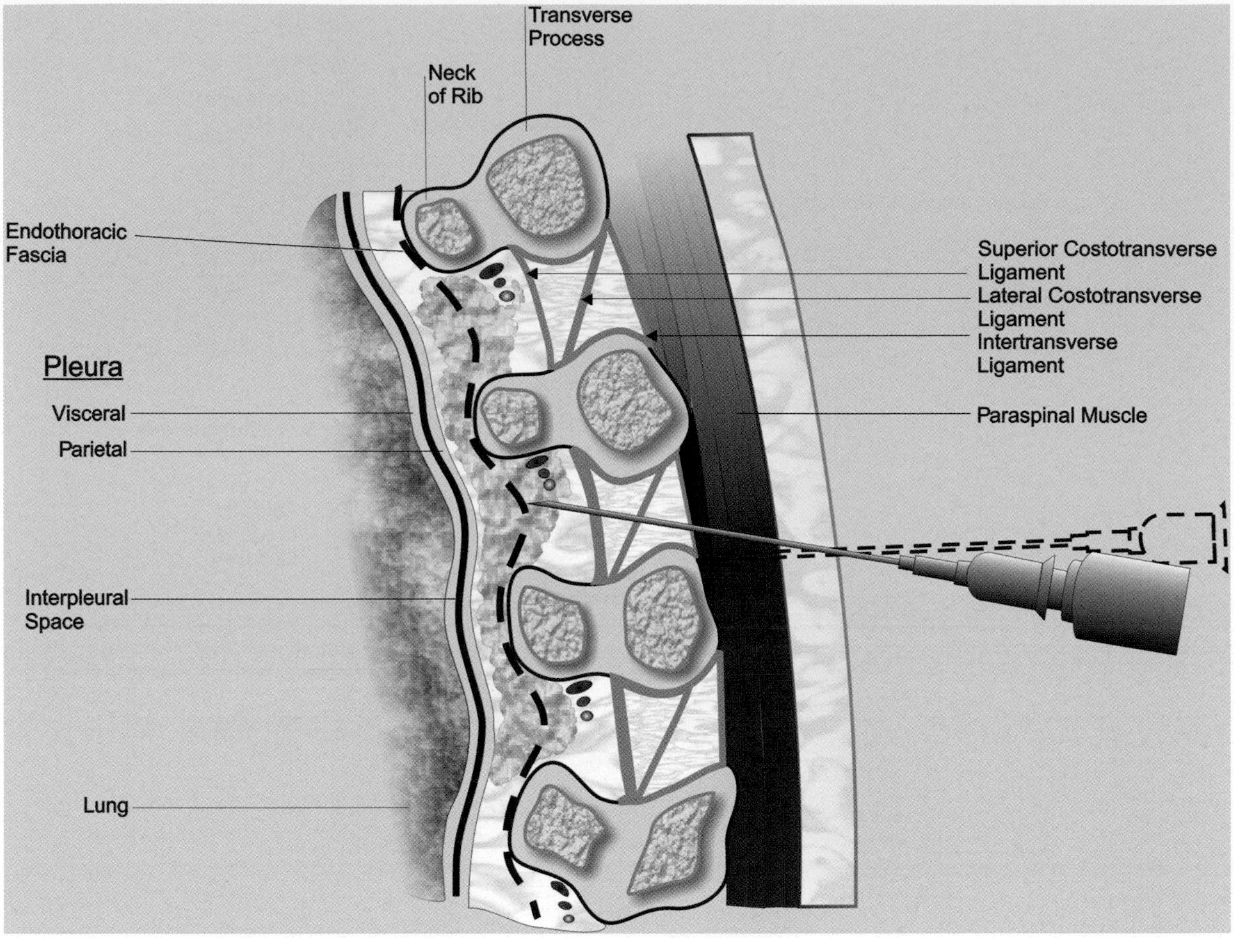

Transverse Process
Neck of Rib
Endothoracic Fascia
Pleura
Visceral
Parietal
Interpleural Space
Lung
Superior Costotransverse Ligament
Lateral Costotransverse Ligament
Intertransverse Ligament
Paraspinal Muscle

Figure 43–3. Sagittal section through the thoracic paravertebral space showing a needle that has been advanced above the transverse process.

C8
C8
C3
C5
C5
C4
C6
C7
T1
T2
T3
T4
T5
T6
T7
T8
T9
C8
C3
C4
C5
C6
C7
T1
T2
T3
T4
T5
T6
T7
T8

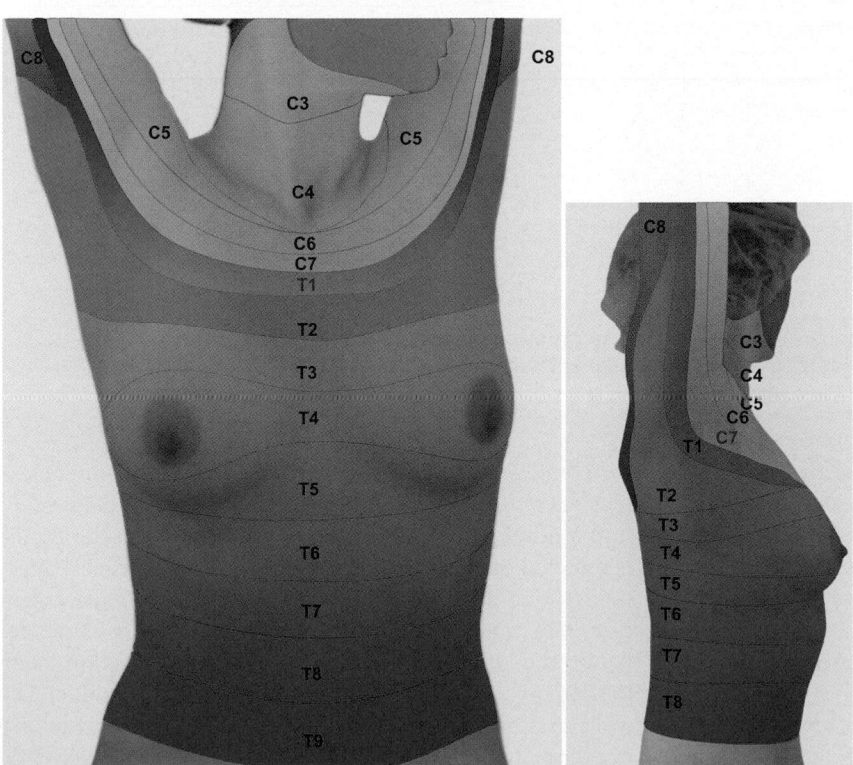

Figure 43–4. Segmental thoracic anesthesia achieved with paravertebral blocks.

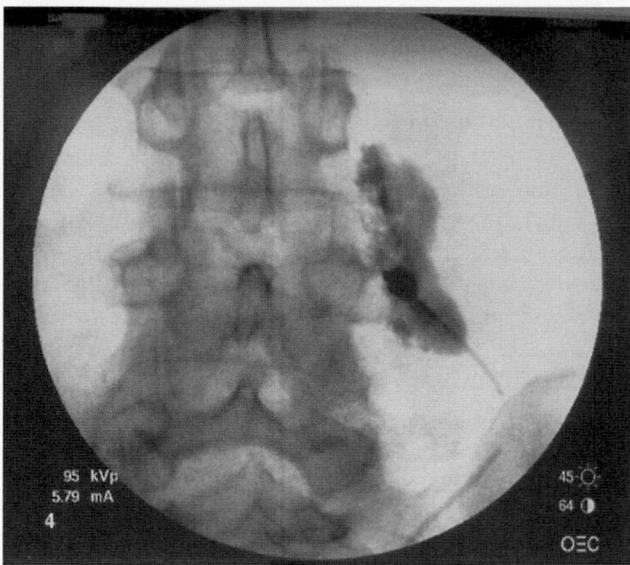

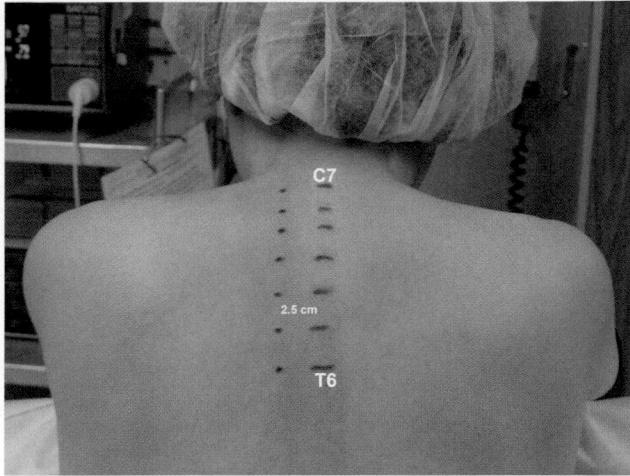

Figure 43–6. Surface landmarks for thoracic paravertebral blocks.

identified and marked with a skin marker before block placement (Figure 43–6). Skin markings are also made 2.5 cm lateral to the midline at the thoracic levels that are to be blocked. These markings indicate the needle insertion sites and should lie over the transverse process of the vertebra (Figure 43–7).

A standard regional anesthesia tray is prepared, and strict asepsis should be maintained during block placement. A 22-gauge Tuohy- or Quincke-tip spinal needle is used for a single- or multiple-injection TPVB (Figure 43–8). If the needle does not have depth markings on its shaft, a depth guard (see Figure 43–8) is recommended. An epidural set is used if insertion of a catheter into the TPVS is planned. Multiple injections during TPVB are uncomfortable and require a proper premedication (eg, midazolam 2–3 mg plus fentanyl

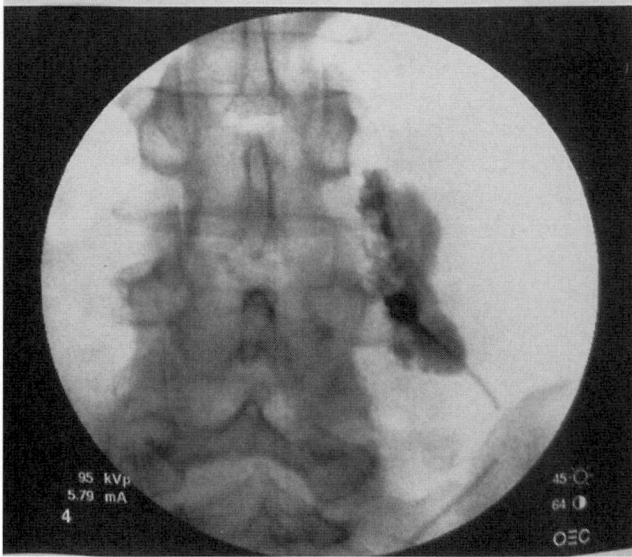

Figure 43–5. Radiopaque contrast imaging shows spread of the injectate (3 mL) cephalad and caudad to the tip of the catheter placed in the paravertebral space.

subendothoracic fascial spread to the retroperitoneal space where the lumbar spinal nerves are located. The effect of gravity on the dermatomal spread of anesthesia after TPVB is unknown, but there may be a tendency for preferential pooling of injected solution toward the dependent levels.[3,23,24]

Technique

It is preferable to perform TPVB with the patient in the sitting position because the surface anatomy is better visualized and patients are often more comfortable. However, when this is not possible or practical, TPVB can also be performed with the patient in the sitting, lateral, or prone position. The number and level of injections are selected according to the desired spread of local anesthesia. In this example, description of the TPVB for breast surgery is described. Surface landmarks are

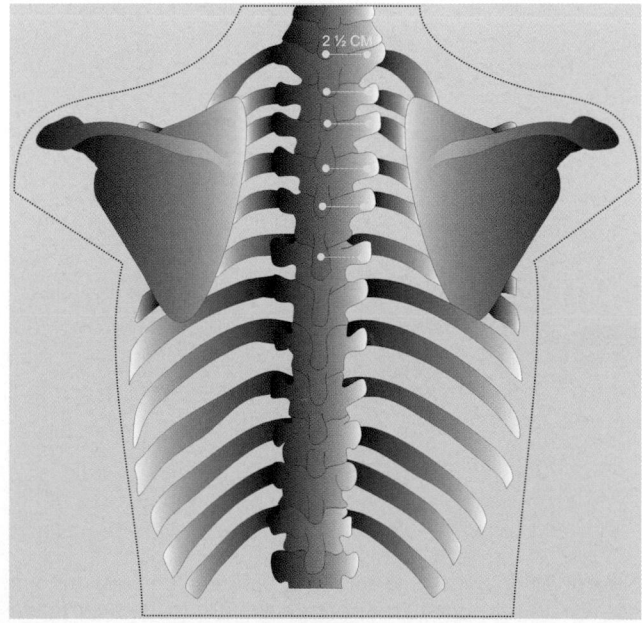

Figure 43–7. Relationship between spinous and transverse processes.

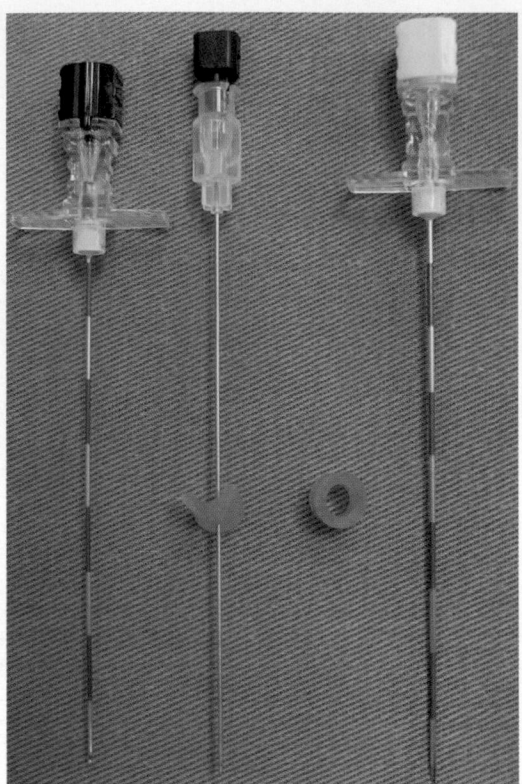

Figure 43–8. Needles commonly used for a single- or multiple-injection thoracic paravertebral block. Note the depth guard that is attached to the Quincke-tip spinal needle (*middle*).

50–100 mcg) to ensure patient acceptance and comfort during the block placement.

Loss-of-Resistance Technique

There are several different techniques of TPVB. The classical technique involves eliciting loss of resistance. The skin and underlying tissue is infiltrated with lidocaine 1%, and the block needle is inserted perpendicular to the skin in all planes to contact the transverse process of the vertebra. Note that due to the acute angulation of the thoracic spines in the midthoracic region, the transverse process that is contacted is the one from the lower vertebra (Figures 43–9 and 43–10).

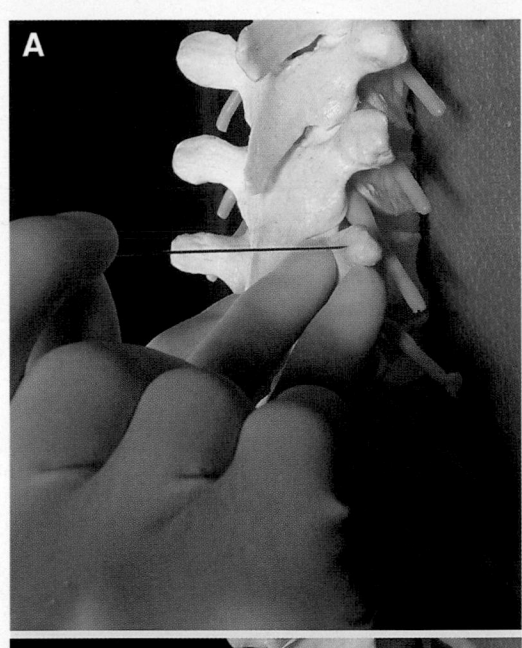

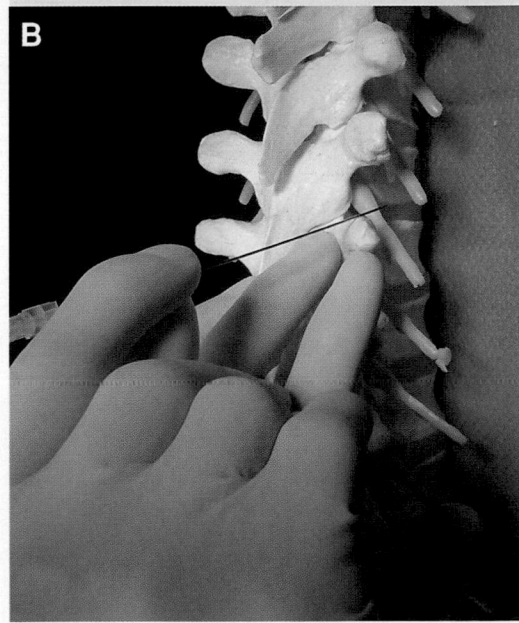

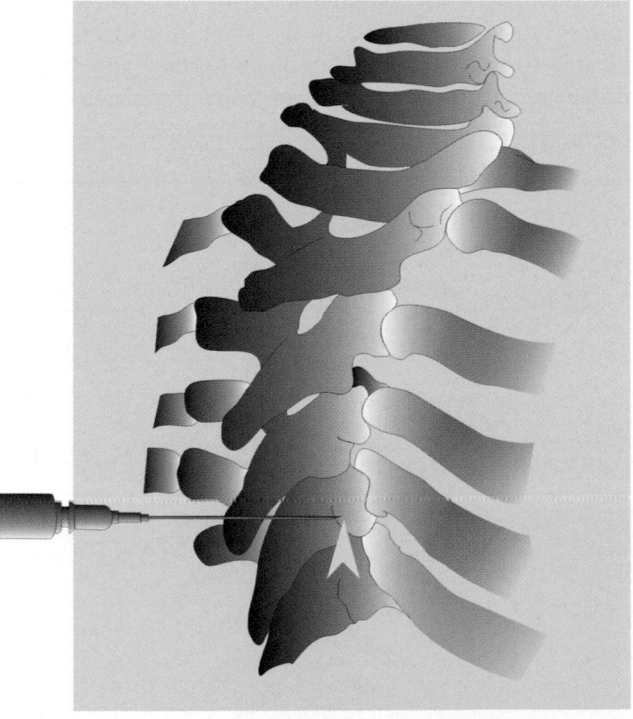

Figure 43–9. Special relationship between the spinous and transverse processes at the thoracic level. Due to the steep downward angulation of the spinous processes at the thoracic levels, the needle inserted at the level of the spinous process contacts the transverse process that belongs to the vertebra below it.

Figure 43–10. Technique of "walking off" the transverse process. **A:** The needle is shown contacting the transverse process. **B:** The needle is shown walking off the superior aspect of the transverse process.

The depth at which the transverse process is contacted varies (3–4 cm) and depends on the build of the individual and the level at which the needle is inserted. The depth is deeper at the cervical and lumbar spine level and shallower at the thoracic levels. During needle insertion it is possible to miss the transverse process and inadvertently puncture the pleura. Therefore it is imperative to search and make contact with the transverse process before advancing the needle too deep and risking pleural puncture. To minimize this complication, the block needle should initially be inserted only to a maximum depth of 4 cm at the thoracic and 5 cm at the cervical and lumbar levels. If bone is not contacted it should be assumed that the needle is in between two adjacent transverse processes. The needle should be withdrawn to the subcutaneous tissue and reinserted with a cephalad or caudad direction to the same depth (4 cm) until bone is contacted. If bone is still not encountered, the needle is advanced a further centimeter and the above procedure repeated until the transverse process is identified. The needle is then walked above (these authors' preference) or below the transverse process and gradually advanced until a loss of resistance is elicited as the needle traverses the superior costotransverse ligament into the TPVS (Figures 43–3 and 43–11). This usually occurs within 1 to 1.5 cm from the superior edge of the transverse process (see Figure 43–3). Although a subtle "pop" or "give" may be appreciated as the needle traverses the superior costotransverse ligament, this should not be entirely relied on. Instead, the depth of the needle placement should be guided by the initial bone contact (skin–transverse process plus 1 to 1.5 cm). Unlike localization of the epidural space, in which the loss of resistance is typically unequivocal, loss of resistance elicited during TPVB is very subtle and takes time to appreciate and master. The use of a glass syringe may facilitate recognition of the loss of resistance when this method is used.

Predetermined Distance Technique

TPVB can also be performed by advancing the needle by a fixed predetermined distance (1 cm) once the needle is walked off the transverse process, without eliciting loss of resistance (Figure 43–12).[5–7,23] Proponents of this technique have used it very successfully with low risk of pneumothorax. The use of a depth marker is recommended to avoid inadvertent pleural or pulmonary puncture.

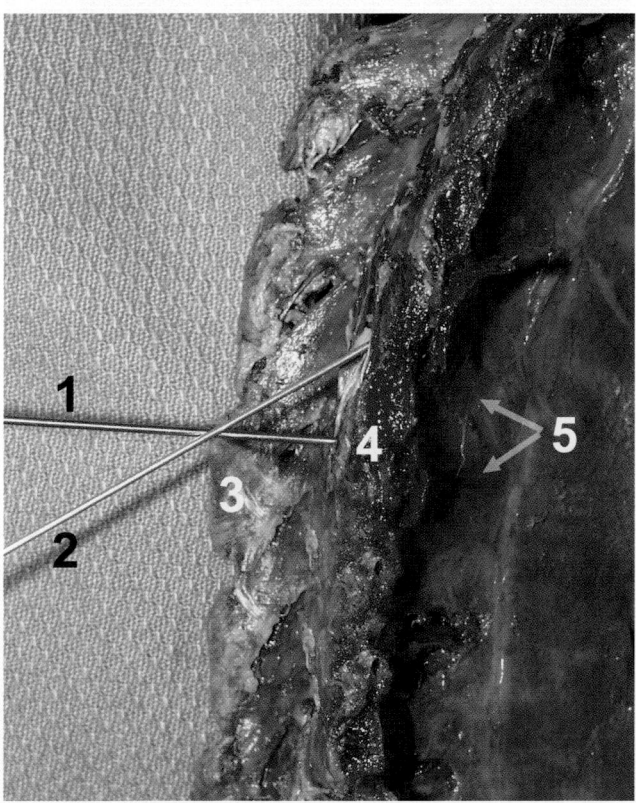

Figure 43–11. Paravertebral block technique. The needle (1) is first advanced to contact the transverse process (4), then redirected cephalad (2) or caudad to walk off the transverse process and enter the paravertebral space. Other structures shown are spinous process (3) and the dispersion of the dye in the paravertebral space and intercostal sulcus (5).

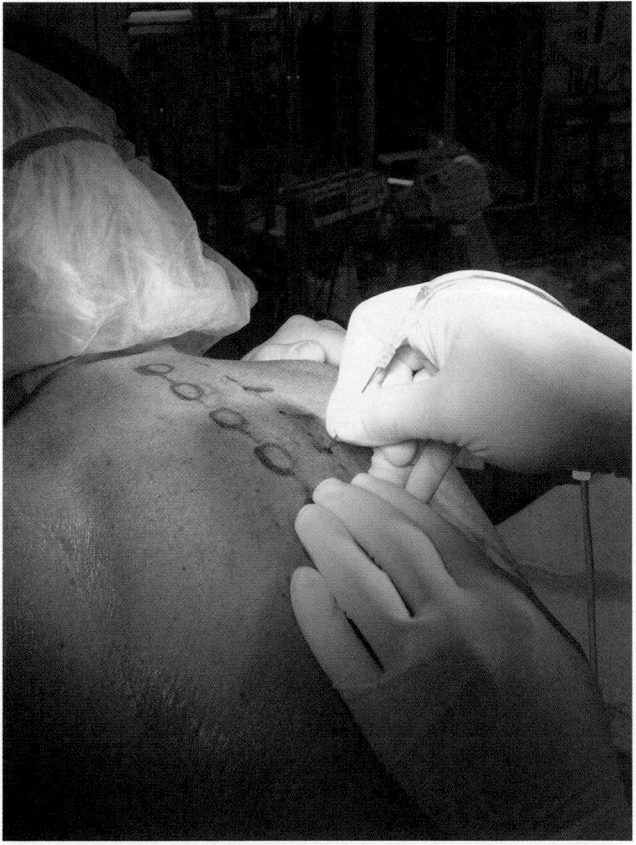

Figure 43–12. Paraverterbral block—the image shows needle advancement at the predetermined level. The fingers of the advancing hand are preventing insertion of the needle too deep.

Clinical Pearls

- Perform TPVB with the patient in the sitting position.
- Surface landmarks should always be identified and marked with a skin marker.
- Since TPVB produces unilateral anesthesia/analgesia, one must ensure that the surface markings for the injections are made on the indicated (correct) side.
- Use needles with depth markings to facilitate estimation of the depth of insertion.
- It is imperative to search and make contact with the transverse process before advancing the needle any further.
- The depth at which the transverse process is contacted varies in the same patient at different thoracic levels. It is deepest in the cervical, upper and lower thoracic, and shallowest in the midthoracic region.
- The loss of resistance is subtle and best appreciated using a 5-mL glass syringe.
- The needle should not be advanced more than 1.5 cm beyond the contact with the transverse process.
- Avoid directing the needle medially to prevent inadvertent epidural or intrathecal injection.

Placement of Thoracic Paravertebral Catheter

If a continuous TPVB (CTPVB) is planned, a catheter is inserted through a Tuohy needle into the TPVS.[4,22] Unlike epidural catheterization, certain resistance is commonly encountered during insertion of the paravertebral catheter. This can be overcome by manipulating (rotating or angling) the needle or injecting 5–10 mL of saline to create a space before catheter insertion. An unusually seamless passage of catheter should arouse the suspicion of interpleural placement.

Perhaps the safest and simplest method of placing a catheter into the TPVS is to place it under direct vision from within the open chest cavity.[8,25] Obviously, this requires an open thorax and is therefore done exclusively in patients undergoing a thoracotomy. This technique involves reflecting the parietal pleura from the posterior wound margin onto the vertebral bodies over several thoracic segments, thereby creating an extrapleural paravertebral pocket (Figure 43–13) into which a percutaneously inserted catheter is placed against the angles of the exposed ribs. The pleura is reapposed to the chest wall, and the thorax is closed. This method can be combined very effectively with a preincisional, single-shot, percutaneous thoracic paravertebral injection to provide perioperative analgesia during thoracic surgery.[26]

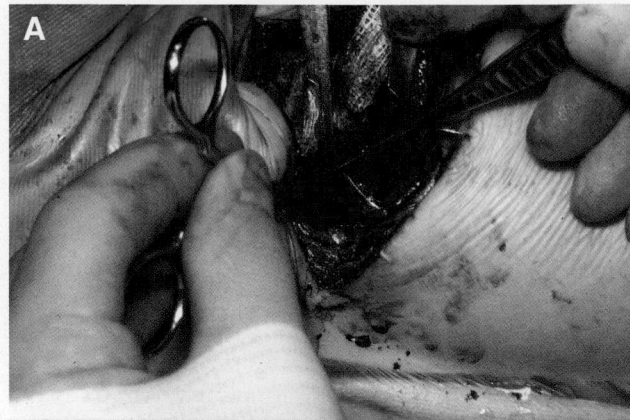

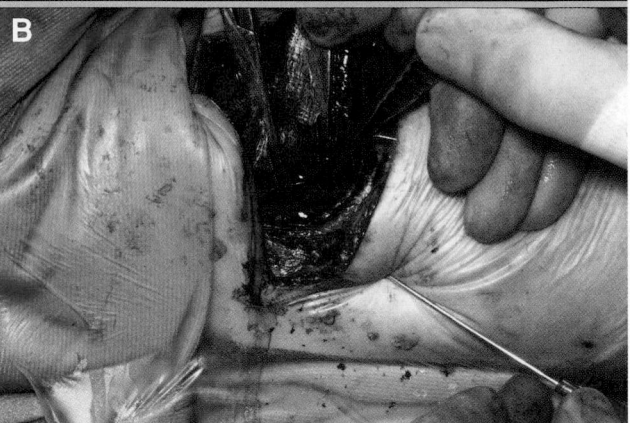

Figure 43–13. A: Extrapleural paravertebral catheter placement under direct vision in an infant. Figure shows a curved artery forceps that has been inserted into the extrapleural paravertebral pocket that was created by reflecting the parietal pleura from the posterior wound margin onto the vertebral bodies over several thoracic dermatomes. **B:** Extrapleural paravertebral catheter placement under direct vision in an infant. The figure shows a Tuohy needle that has been inserted from the lower intercostal space into the thoracic paravertebral space, ie, the extrapleural paravertebral pocket previously created. A catheter is then inserted through the Tuohy needle and secured in place against the angles of the exposed ribs, after which the pleura is reapposed and the chest is closed.

Clinical Pearls

- Injecting saline or the bolus dose of the local anesthetic before catheter insertion makes it easier to insert a catheter.
- Very easy passage of catheter (>6 cm) suggests intrapleural placement.

Indications

TPVB is indicated for anesthesia and analgesia for unilateral surgical procedures in the chest and abdomen. Commonly reported indications are listed in Table 43–1. The use of bilateral TPVB has also been reported.

Table 43–1.

Indications for Thoracic Paravertebral Block

Anesthesia

Breast surgery
Herniorrhaphy (thoracolumbar anesthesia)
Chest wound exploration

Postoperative Analgesia (as part of a balanced analgesic regimen)

Thoracotomy
Thoracoabdominal esophageal surgery
Video-assisted thoracoscopic surgery
Cholecystectomy
Renal surgery
Breast surgery
Herniorrhaphy
Liver resection
Appendicectomy
Minimally invasive cardiac surgery
Conventional cardiac surgery (bilateral TPVB)

Chronic Pain Management

Benign and malignant neuralgia

Miscellaneous

Postherpetic neuralgia
Relief of pleuritic chest pain
Multiple fractured ribs
Treatment of hyperhydrosis
Liver capsule pain after blunt abdominal trauma

TPVB = thoracic paravertebral block.

Contraindications

There are very few absolute contraindications for TPVB. These include infection at the site of injection, allergy to local anesthetic drug, empyema, and a neoplastic mass occupying the paravertebral space. Coagulopathy, bleeding disorders, or patients receiving anticoagulant drugs are relative contraindications for TPVB. One must exercise caution in patients with kyphoscoliosis or deformed spines and those who have had previous thoracic surgery. The chest deformity in the former may predispose to inadvertent thecal or pleural puncture, and the altered paravertebral anatomy due to fibrotic obliteration of the paravertebral space or adhesions of the lung to the chest wall in the latter may predispose to pulmonary puncture.

Choice of Local Anesthetic

Since TPVB does not result in motor weakness of the extremities, long-lasting analgesia is nearly always desirable with TPVB. Consequently, long-acting local anesthetic drugs are typically used. These include bupivacaine or levobupivacaine 0.5% and ropivacaine 0.5–0.75%. For single-injection TPVB, 20–25 mL of local anesthetic is injected in aliquots, whereas

for multiple-injection TPVB, 4–5 mL of local anesthetic is injected at each level planned. Higher concentrations of local anesthetic (eg, ropivacaine 0.75%) may reduce the onset time and prolong the duration of anesthesia and analgesia. The maximum dose of local anesthetic must be adjusted in the elderly, poorly nourished, and frail patients. The TPVS is well vascularized, leading to relatively rapid absorption of local anesthetic into the systemic circulation. Consequently, peak plasma concentration of the local anesthetic agent is attained quickly. Epinephrine (2.5–5 mcg/mL) containing local anesthetic solutions may be used during the initial injection because it reduces systemic absorption and thereby reduces the potential for toxicity. Epinephrine also helps in increasing the maximum allowable dose of local anesthetic. The duration of anesthesia after TPVB ranges from 3 to 4 h, but analgesia often lasts much longer (8–18 h). If CTPVB is planned, eg, for postoperative analgesia after thoracotomy or continuous pain relief for multiple fractured ribs, then an infusion of bupivacaine or levobupivacaine 0.25% or ropivacaine 0.2% at 0.1 to 0.2 mL/kg/h is started after the initial bolus injection and continued for 3 to 4 days or as indicated. It is our experience that using a higher concentration of local anesthetic (eg, bupivacaine 0.5% instead of 0.25%) for the CTPVB does not result in better quality of analgesia, and it may increase the potential for local anesthetic toxicity.

Clinical Pearls

- Consider using lidocaine or chloroprocaine for skin and subcutaneous infiltration during a multiple-injection TPVB to reduce the total dose of the more toxic long-acting local anesthetic.
- Use an epinephrine-containing (eg, 1:200 000 or 1:400 000) long-acting local anesthetic for the initial bolus injection because it reduces systemic absorption and therefore the potential for systemic toxicity.
- Local anesthetic dosage must be adjusted in the elderly and those with impairment of hepatic and renal function as they are more prone for systemic accumulation and local anesthetic toxicity.
- Increasing the dose of the local anesthetic infused during a continuous thoracic paravertebral block may not always improve pain management. Adjunct analgesics [eg, a nonsteroidal antiinflammatory drug (NSAID), as part of a multimodal analgesic regimen] may be more effective.
- Catheter dislodgement is not uncommon and must be excluded whenever patients complain of breakthrough pain that is not easily controlled.
- Exclude local anesthetic toxicity whenever a patient becomes confused while on a continuous thoracic paravertebral infusion.

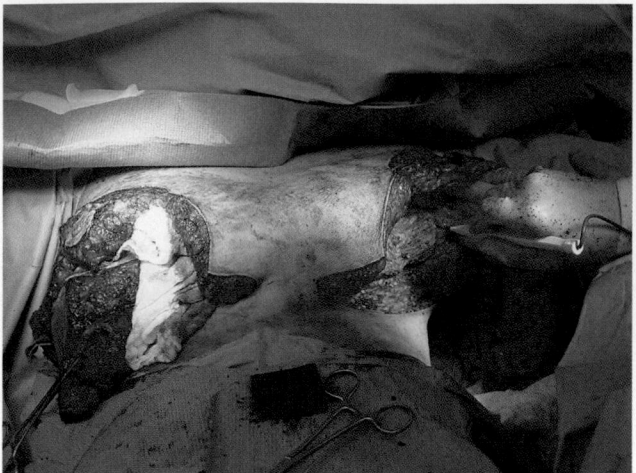

A

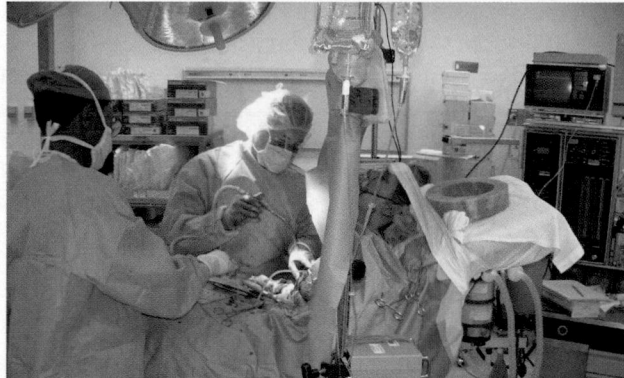

B

Figure 43–14. A: Extensive breast reconstruction surgery being performed under paravertebral block. **B:** The patient is sedated using propofol infusion. The images demonstrate how potent paravertebral blocks can be both as anesthetic and analgesic techniques.

Practical Management of Thoracic Paravertebral Block

Breast Surgery

Thoracic paravertebral injection of local anesthetic at multiple levels (C7 through T6) in conjunction with intravenous sedation is effective for surgical anesthesia during major breast surgery (Figure 43–14).[5,6,27] The C7 spinous process is the most prominent cervical spinous process; the inferior border of the scapula corresponds to T7. Compared with patients who receive only general anesthesia (GA), patients who receive a multiple-injection TPVB for major breast surgery have less postoperative pain, require fewer analgesics, and have less nausea and vomiting after surgery. However, to effectively use the multiple-injection TPVB technique for anesthesia during breast surgery, one must understand the complex innervation of the breast. The anterior and lateral chest wall receives

sensory innervation from the anterior and lateral cutaneous branches of the intercostal nerves (T2 through T6), the axilla (T1 to T2), the infraclavicular region from the supraclavicular nerves (C4 to C5), and the pectoral muscles from the lateral (C5 to C6) and medial (C7 to C8) pectoral nerves. There also may be overlapping sensory innervation from the contralateral side of the chest. This complex innervation of the breast from the C4 to T6 spinal segments explains why TPVB may not provide complete anesthesia for dissection over the pectoral muscle or the infraclavicular region. However, this can be overcome with proper sedation during surgery as well as by injections of local anesthetic by the surgeon intraoperatively into the sensitive areas. Injection of a local anesthetic subcutaneously along the inferior border of the clavicle or to perform an ipsilateral superficial cervical plexus block, in order to anaesthetize the supraclavicular nerves (C4 to C5) will minimize discomfort and sedative and analgesic requirements during surgery. A combination of midazolam, or propofol infusion, or IV opioid can be used to provide comfort to the patients intraoperatively. Dexmedetomidine, a highly selective α_2-adrenoceptor agonist, with its sedative, analgesic, and minimal or no respiratory depression properties is a useful alternative for sedation during breast surgery under TPVB.

When combined with general anesthesia, a single-injection TPVB with ropivacaine (2 mg/kg diluted to 20 mL with 0.9% saline) with 1:200,000 epinephrine, performed prior to the induction of GA can be used. This provides excellent postoperative analgesia, reduces postoperative analgesic requirement, reduces postoperative vomiting, facilitates the earlier resumption of oral fluid intake, reduces the postoperative decline in respiratory function, and augments the recovery of postoperative respiratory mechanics.

Postthoracotomy Pain Relief

CTPVB is an effective method of providing analgesia after thoracotomy (Figure 43–15). Ideally, TPVB should be established before the thoracotomy incision, via a catheter that is inserted percutaneously, and continued for 4 to 5 days after surgery. However, if an extrapleural paravertebral catheter is being placed under direct vision from within the chest during surgery, then a single-injection TPVB can be performed at the level of the thoracotomy incision before the surgical incision, and a continuous infusion of local anesthetic is commenced after the catheter placement. Either method provides effective perioperative analgesia.

It is important to note that CTPVB is inadequate on its own for complete pain relief after a thoracotomy and must be combined with an opioid [best as intravenous patient-controlled analgesia (IVPCA)] and a NSAID to provide optimal analgesia.[26] Analgesia achieved by CTPVB is comparable to epidural analgesia but with less hypotension, urinary retention, and the side effects commonly seen with epidural opioid administration.[1,26,28,29] The opioid requirement with such an approach is significantly reduced by the CTPVB, and analgesia is superior to IVPCA alone.[1,30]

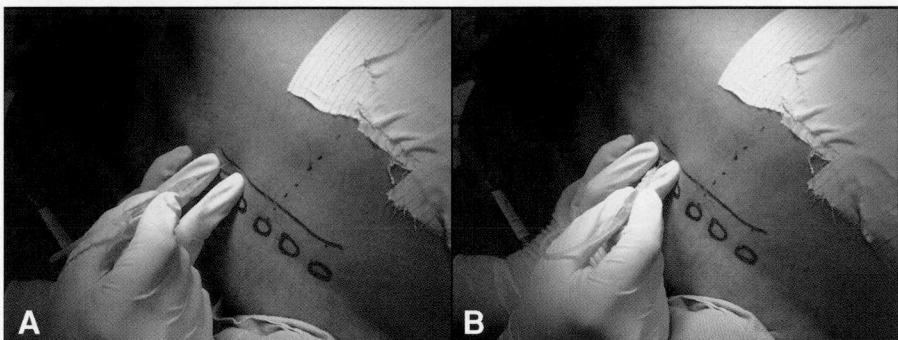

Figure 43–15. Thoracic paravertebral block after thoracotomy. A typical sequence of touching the transverse process (**A**) and walking off 1 cm deeper to the transverse process superiorly or inferiorly (**B**).

Multiple Fractured Ribs

TPVB is an effective method of providing pain relief in patients with unilateral multiple fractured ribs.[1,22,23] A single thoracic paravertebral injection of 25 (SD 5) mL of bupivacaine 0.5% produces pain relief for a mean duration of 9.9 (SD 1.2) h and improves respiratory function and arterial blood gases.[1,23] To avoid recurrence of pain and deterioration in respiratory function, a thoracic paravertebral catheter can be inserted midway between the highest and the lowest fractured rib, and a CTPVB can be commenced after administration of the initial bolus injection. CTPVB in combination with a NSAID provides continuous pain relief and produces a sustained improvement in respiratory parameters and arterial oxygenation.[22] Since TPVB does not cause urinary retention or affect lower limb motor function, it is useful in patients with multiple fractured ribs who also have concomitant lumbar spinal trauma since it also allows continuous neurologic assessment for signs of spinal cord compression.[31]

Pharmacokinetic Considerations

Relatively large doses of local anesthetics are commonly used during CTPVB. Therefore there is the potential for local anesthetic toxicity, and patients should be closely monitored during CTPVB and the infusion stopped if signs develop. During a prolonged thoracic paravertebral infusion there is progressive accumulation of local anesthetic in the plasma, and the plasma concentration of the drug may exceed the threshold for central nervous system toxicity (eg, 2–4.5 mcg/mL for bupivacaine). Despite the systemic accumulation, local anesthetic toxicity is rare. This may be the case because, although the total plasma concentration of the local anesthetic increases postoperatively, the free fraction of the drug remains unchanged[32] and may be due to the postoperative increase in α_1-acid glycoprotein concentration,[32] the protein that binds to local anesthetic drugs. There is also a greater increase in the *S*-bupivacaine enantiomer,[33,34] which is associated with lower toxicity, than the *R*-enantiomer. Due to concerns of systemic accumulation and local anesthetic toxicity with prolonged paravertebral infusion, it is preferable to use a local anesthetic with lower potential for toxicity, such as ropivacaine. One must also exercise caution in the elderly and frail

patients as well as in patients with impaired hepatic and renal function.

Complications & How to Avoid Them

Based on published data the incidence of complications after TPVB is relatively low and varies from 2.6 to 5%.[1,5,35,36] These include vascular puncture (3.8%), hypotension (4.6%), pleural puncture (1.1%), and pneumothorax (0.5%).[35] Unlike with thoracic epidural anesthesia, hypotension is rare in normovolemic patients after TPVB because the sympathetic blockade is unilateral. However TPVB may unmask hypovolemia and result in hypotension. Therefore TPVB should be used with caution in patients who are hypovolemic or hemodynamically labile. Nevertheless, hypotension is rare even after bilateral TPVB, probably owing to the segmental nature of the bilateral sympathetic blockade.

Pleural puncture and pneumothorax are two complications that often dissuade anesthesiologists from performing a TPVB. Inadvertent pleural puncture is uncommon after TPVB and may or may not result in a pneumothorax, which is usually minor and can be managed conservatively. Clues that suggest pleural puncture during a TPVB are a gritty pleural pop sensation, irritating cough, onset of sharp chest or shoulder pain, or sudden hyperventilation. Contrary to common belief, air cannot be aspirated through the needle unless the lung is also inadvertently punctured or air that may have entered the pleural cavity during removal of the stylet is aspirated. Such patients should be closely monitored for the possible development of a pneumothorax. It should be kept in mind that pneumothorax may be delayed in onset and a chest radiograph taken too early to exclude a pneumothorax may not be conclusive. Even a radiologic contrast study using a chest radiograph may be difficult to interpret because the intrapleural contrast disperses rapidly, does not define any specific anatomic plane, and tends to spread to the diaphragmatic angles or horizontal fissure.

Systemic local anesthetic toxicity can occur due to inadvertent intravascular injection or from using an excessive dose of local anesthetic. The local anesthetic solution must be injected in aliquots, and the dosage must be adjusted in the elderly and frail patient. An epinephrine-containing local anesthetic solution is suggested to enable the recognition of intravascular injection and reduce the systemic absorption of the local anesthetic.

Inadvertent epidural, subdural, or intrathecal injection and spinal anesthesia can also occur. Published data suggest that these complications are more frequent when the needle is directed medially but may also occur with a normally positioned needle due to the close proximity of the needle to the dural cuff and intervertebral foramen. Therefore the needle must never be directed medially, and care must be taken to exclude intrathecal injection by routinely performing an aspiration test before injection. Transient ipsilateral Horner syndrome can occasionally develop after TPVB. This is due to cephalad spread of the local anesthetic to the stellate ganglion or to the preganglionic fibers of the first few segments of the thoracic spinal cord. Bilateral Horner syndrome has also been reported and may be due to epidural spread or prevertebral spread to the contralateral stellate ganglion. Sensory changes in the arm and lower extremity may also occur after a TPVB. The former is due to spread of local anesthetic to the lower components of the ipsilateral brachial plexus (C8 and T1), and the latter is due to extended subendothoracic fascial spread to the ipsilateral retroperitoneal space where the lumbar spinal nerves are located (discussed earlier), but epidural spread as a cause cannot be excluded. Motor blockade or bilateral symmetrical anesthesia involving the lower extremity is rare. It generally suggests significant epidural spread and may be more common if large volumes of local anesthetic (>25–30 mL) are injected at a single level. Therefore if a wide segmental spread of anesthesia is desired, it is preferable to perform the multiple-injection technique or inject a smaller volume of local anesthetic at several levels a few dermatomes apart.

LUMBAR PARAVERTEBRAL BLOCK

Lumbar paravertebral block (LPVB) is technically similar to a TPVB but due to differences in anatomy between the thoracic and lumbar paravertebral spaces the two paravertebral techniques are described separately. LPVB is technically simple to perform and used most commonly in combination with a TPVB, as a thoracolumbar paravertebral block, for surgical anesthesia during inguinal herniorrhaphy.

Anatomy

The lumbar paravertebral space (LPVS) is limited anterolaterally by the psoas major muscle; medially by the vertebral bodies, the intervertebral disks, and the intervertebral foramen with its contents; and posteriorly by the transverse process and the ligaments that are interposed between the adjoining transverse processes. Unlike the TPVS, which contains adipose tissue, the LPVS is occupied primarily by the psoas major muscle. The psoas major muscle is made up of a fleshy anterior part that forms the main bulk of the muscle, and a thin accessory posterior part.[37] The main bulk origi-

nates from the anterolateral surface of the vertebral bodies and the accessory part originates from the anterior surface of the transverse process.[37] The two parts fuse to form the psoas major muscle except near the vertebral bodies where the two parts are separated by a thin fascia within which lie the lumbar spinal nerve roots and the ascending lumbar veins.[37] The ventral rami of the lumbar spinal nerve roots extend laterally in this intramuscular plane formed by the two parts of the psoas major muscle and form the lumbar plexus within the substance of the psoas major muscle.[37] The psoas muscle is enveloped by a fibrous sheath, "the psoas sheath," which continues laterally as the fascia covering the quadratus lumborum muscle. During a LPVB the local anesthetic is injected anterior to the transverse process into a triangular space between the two parts of the psoas major muscle containing the lumbar spinal nerve root.

The LPVS communicates medially with the epidural space. A series of tendinous arches extends across the constricted parts of the lumbar vertebral bodies, which are traversed by the lumbar arteries and veins and sympathetic fibers. These tendinous arches may provide a pathway for the spread of local anesthetic from the LPVS to the anterolateral surface of the vertebral body, the prevertebral space, and the contralateral side and may be the pathway through which the ipsilateral lumbar sympathetic chain may occasionally be involved.

Mechanism of Block & Distribution of Anesthesia

A lumbar paravertebral injection produces ipsilateral dermatomal anesthesia (Figure 43–16) by a direct effect of the local anesthetic on the lumbar spinal nerves and by medial extension into the epidural space via the intervertebral foramen. The contribution of epidural spread to the overall distribution of anesthesia after a LPVB is unknown but probably occurs in the majority of patients and depends on the volume of local anesthetic injected at a given level. Ipsilateral sympathetic blockade may also occur due to epidural spread or spread of local anesthetic anteriorly via the tendinous arches to the rami communicantes or the lumbar sympathetic chain.

Technique

Lumbar paravertebral block can be performed with the patient in the sitting, lateral, or prone position. Surface landmarks must be identified and marked with a skin marker before block placement. The spinous process of the vertebra at the levels to be blocked represents the midline, the iliac crest corresponds to the L3-4 interspace, and the tip of the scapula corresponds to the T7 spinous process. Skin markings are also made 2.5 cm lateral to the midline at the levels that are to be blocked (Figure 43–17) or one can draw a line 2.5 cm lateral to the midline and perform the injections along this line. A standard regional anesthesia tray is prepared; strict asepsis should be maintained during block placement. An 8-cm, 22-gauge, Tuohy or Quincke tip spinal needle (see Figure 43–8) is used

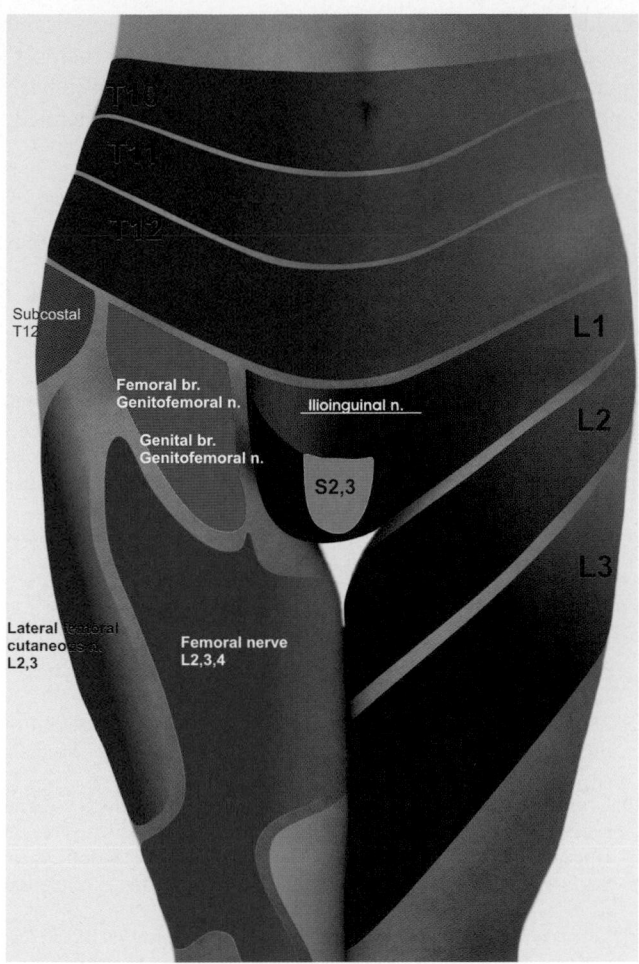

Figure 43–16. Segmental distribution of anesthesia with lumbar paravertebral levels.

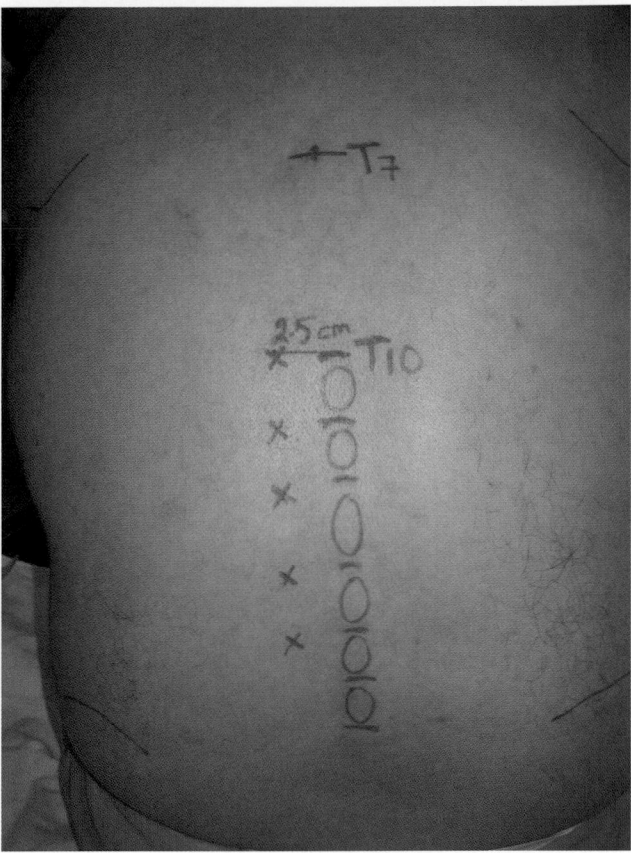

Figure 43–17. Surface landmarks and needle insertion sites for low thoracic/lumbar paravertebral block.

for LPVB. Similarly to the recommendations for TPVB, the use of needles with depth markings on the shaft of the needle or a guard indicating the depth (see Figure 43–8) is recommended.

Advancing the needle by a fixed predetermined distance (1 cm) beyond the transverse process, without eliciting paresthesia, is the method most commonly used to perform LPVB. The block needle is inserted perpendicular to the skin until the transverse process is contacted. The depth at which the transverse process is contacted is variable (4–6 cm) and depends on the build of the patient. Once the transverse process is identified, the marking on the needle is noted or the depth marker is adjusted so that it is 1 cm beyond the skin–transverse process depth. The needle is then withdrawn to the subcutaneous tissue and reinserted at a 10- to 15-degree superior or inferior angle so that it slides off the superior or inferior edge of the transverse process, similarly to the technique in thoracic paravertebral block (see Figure 43–11). The needle is advanced by a further 1 cm beyond the point at which it made contact with the transverse process or until the depth marker is reached. After negative aspiration for blood or CSF, the local anesthetic is injected. Since spread of local anesthetic after a single large-volume lumbar paravertebral injection is unpredictable, the multiple-injection technique in which 4–5 mL of local anesthetic is injected at each level is more commonly used.

Choice of Local Anesthetic

As for TPVB, long-acting local anesthetic agents such as bupivacaine 0.5%, ropivacaine 0.5–0.75%, or levobupivacaine 0.5% are commonly used for LPVB. During a multiple-injection LPVB, 4–5 mL of the local anesthetic is injected at each level. Anesthesia develops in about 15–30 min and lasts for 3 to 6 h. Analgesia is also long-lasting (12–18 h) and generally outlasts the duration of anesthesia. There are no data on the pharmacokinetics of local anesthetic after LPVB. Nevertheless, the addition of epinephrine (2.5–5 mcg/mL) to the local anesthetic may reduce systemic absorption and reduce the potential for toxicity.

Indications & Contraindications

The indications for LPVB are limited. Published data suggest that it is most commonly used in combination with TPVB (T10 through L2) for surgical anesthesia during inguinal herniorrhaphy. It can also be used for diagnostic purpose during evaluation of groin or genital pain, such as that following nerve entrapment syndrome after inguinal herniorrhaphy. Contraindications for LPVB are similar to TPVB, but one must exercise caution in patients who are anticoagulated or are receiving prophylactic anticoagulants since psoas hematoma with lumbar plexopathy has been reported.

Complications & How to Avoid Them

Published data suggest that complication is rare after LPVB.[38,39] Nevertheless, it is possible to inadvertently inject local anesthetic into the intravascular, epidural, or intrathecal spaces during LPVB and may be more common if the needle is directed medially. Therefore the direction of the block needle should be maintained perpendicular to the skin during insertion, and medial angulation should be avoided. Intraperitoneal injection or visceral injury (renal) may also occur, although this can occur only as a result of gross technical error. Motor weakness involving the ipsilateral quadriceps muscle may result if the L2 spinal nerve is blocked (femoral nerve L2 to L4).

Clinical Pearls

- Needles with depth markings are suggested to facilitate monitoring of the depth of needle insertion.

- The transverse process should always be contacted to avoid a needle insertion that is too deep. In addition, the success of the technique of LPVB depends on the transverse process/paravertebral space relationship; advancing the needle 1 cm beyond the transverse process is the best means of reducing the risk of complication and achieving successful blockade.

- Avoid medial orientation of the needle as it may predispose to inadvertent epidural or intrathecal injection.

- The size of the lumbar transverse process varies at each level. The transverse process of the L3 vertebra is the longest, and the transverse processes of the L4 and L5 vertebrae are much shorter. Therefore the block needle has to be inserted slightly more medially (2 cm lateral to the midline) in the lower lumbar region.

SUMMARY

Paravertebral block is conceptually a simple technique with few contraindications. Proper training is necessary to acquire stereotactic skills required to ensure a high success rate. Thoracic paravertebral block produces unilateral somatic and sympathetic nerve blockade that is adequate for surgical anesthesia during breast surgery and for analgesia when pain is of unilateral origin from the chest or abdomen. Lumbar paravertebral block is less commonly used in clinical practice. As a thoracolumbar paravertebral block it is effective for surgical anesthesia during inguinal herniorrhaphy. Hemodynamic stability is usually maintained after a paravertebral block due to the unilateral nature of sympathetic blockade.

Bladder and lower limb motor function is also preserved, and no additional nursing vigilance is required during the postoperative period. Bilateral paravertebral block has also been reported, but its role in clinical practice is still to be defined.

References

1. Karmakar MK: Thoracic paravertebral block. Anesthesiology 2001;95:771–780.
2. Richardson J, Lonnqvist PA: Thoracic paravertebral block. Br J Anaesth 1998;81:230–238.
3. Cheema SP, Ilsley D, Richardson J, et al: A thermographic study of paravertebral analgesia. Anesthesia 1995;50:118–121.
4. Eason MJ, Wyatt R: Paravertebral thoracic block—A reappraisal. Anesthesia 1979;34:638–642.
5. Coveney E, Weltz CR, Greengrass R, et al: Use of paravertebral block anesthesia in the surgical management of breast cancer: Experience in 156 cases. Ann Surg 1998;227:496–501.
6. Greengrass R, O'Brien F, Lyerly K, et al: Paravertebral block for breast cancer surgery. Can J Anaesth 1996;43:858–861.
7. Klein SM, Bergh A, Steele SM, et al: Thoracic paravertebral block for breast surgery. Anesth Analg 2000;90:1402–1405.
8. Karmakar MK, Booker PD, Franks R, et al: Continuous extrapleural paravertebral infusion of bupivacaine for post-thoracotomy analgesia in young infants. Br J Anaesth 1996;76:811–815.
9. Lonnquist PA, Hesser U: Radiological and clinical distribution of thoracic paravertebral blockade in infants and children. Paediatr Anaesth 1993;3:83–87.
10. Lonnqvist PA: Continuous paravertebral block in children. Initial experience. Anesthesia 1992;47:607–609.
11. Dugan DJ, Samson PC: Surgical significance of the endothoracic fascia. The anatomic basis for empyemectomy and other extrapleural technics. Am J Surg 1975;130:151–158.
12. Karmakar MK, Kwok WH, Kew J: Thoracic paravertebral block: Radiological evidence of contralateral spread anterior to the vertebral bodies. Br J Anaesth 2000;84:263–265.
13. Karmakar MK, Chung DC: Variability of a thoracic paravertebral block. Are we ignoring the endothoracic fascia? [letter]. Reg Anesth Pain Med 2000;25:325–327.
14. Moore DC, Bush WH, Scurlock JE: Intercostal nerve block: A roentgenographic anatomic study of technique and absorption in humans. Anesth Analg 1980;59:815–825.
15. Tenicela R, Pollan SB: Paravertebral-peridural block technique: A unilateral thoracic block. Clin J Pain 1990;6:227–234.
16. Nunn JF, Slavin G: Posterior intercostal nerve block for pain relief after cholecystectomy. Anatomical basis and efficacy. Br J Anaesth 1980;52:253–260.
17. Conacher ID: Resin injection of thoracic paravertebral spaces. Br J Anaesth 1988;61:657–661.
18. Purcell-Jones G, Pither CE, Justins DM: Paravertebral somatic nerve block: A clinical, radiographic, and computed tomographic study in chronic pain patients. Anesth Analg 1989;68:32–39.
19. Karmakar MK, Gin T, Ho AM: Ipsilateral thoraco-lumbar anesthesia and paravertebral spread after low thoracic paravertebral injection. Br J Anaesth 2001;87:312–316.
20. Saito T, Gallagher ET, Cutler S, et al: Extended unilateral anesthesia. New technique or paravertebral anesthesia? Reg Anesth 1996;21:304–307.
21. Saito T, Den S, Tanuma K, et al: Anatomical bases for paravertebral anesthetic block: Fluid communication between the thoracic and lumbar paravertebral regions. Surg Radiol Anat 1999;21:359–363.
22. Karmakar MK, Critchley LA, Ho AM, et al: Continuous thoracic paravertebral infusion of bupivacaine for pain management in patients with multiple fractured ribs. Chest 2003;123:424–431.
23. Gilbert J, Hultman J: Thoracic paravertebral block: A method of pain control. Acta Anaesthesiol Scand 1989;33:142–145.

24. Richardson J, Jones J, Atkinson R: The effect of thoracic paravertebral blockade on intercostal somatosensory evoked potentials. Anesth Analg 1998;87:373–376.

25. Sabanathan S, Smith PJ, Pradhan GN, et al: Continuous intercostal nerve block for pain relief after thoracotomy. Ann Thorac Surg 1988; 46:425–426.

26. Richardson J, Sabanathan S, Jones J, et al: A prospective, randomized comparison of preoperative and continuous balanced epidural or paravertebral bupivacaine on post-thoracotomy pain, pulmonary function and stress responses. Br J Anaesth 1999;83:387–392.

27. Weltz CR, Greengrass RA, Lyerly HK: Ambulatory surgical management of breast carcinoma using paravertebral block. Ann Surg 1995;222:19–26.

28. Sabanathan S, Mearns AJ, Bickford SP, et al: Efficacy of continuous extrapleural intercostal nerve block on post-thoracotomy pain and pulmonary mechanics. Br J Surg 1990;77:221–225.

29. Matthews PJ, Govenden V: Comparison of continuous paravertebral and extradural infusions of bupivacaine for pain relief after thoracotomy. Br J Anaesth 1989;62:204–205.

30. Carabine UA, Gilliland H, Johnston JR, et al: Pain relief for thoracotomy. Comparison of morphine requirements using an extrapleural infusion of bupivacaine. Reg Anesth 1995;20:412–417.

31. Karmakar MK, Chui PT, Joynt GM, et al: Thoracic paravertebral block for management of pain associated with multiple fractured ribs in patients with concomitant lumbar spinal trauma. Reg Anesth Pain Med 2001;26:169–173.

32. Dauphin A, Gupta RN, Young JE, et al: Serum bupivacaine concentrations during continuous extrapleural infusion. Can J Anaesth 1997;44:367–370.

33. Berrisford RG, Sabanathan S, Mearns AJ, et al: Plasma concentrations of bupivacaine and its enantiomers during continuous extrapleural intercostal nerve block. Br J Anaesth 1993;70:201–204.

34. Clark BJ, Hamdi A, Berrisford RG, et al: Reversed-phase and chiral high-performance liquid chromatographic assay of bupivacaine and its enantiomers in clinical samples after continuous extraplural infusion. J Chromatogr 1991;553:383–390.

35. Lonnqvist PA, MacKenzie J, Soni AK, et al: Paravertebral blockade. Failure rate and complications. Anesthesia 1995;50:813–815.

36. Richardson J, Sabanathan S: Thoracic paravertebral analgesia. Acta Anaesthesiol Scand 1995;39:1005–1015.

37. Farny J, Drolet P, Girard M: Anatomy of the posterior approach to the lumbar plexus block. Can J Anaesth 1994;41:480–485.

38. Klein SM, Greengrass RA, Weltz C, et al: Paravertebral somatic nerve block for outpatient inguinal herniorrhaphy: An expanded case report of 22 patients. Reg Anesth Pain Med 1998;23:306–310.

39. Wassef MR, Randazzo T, Ward W: The paravertebral nerve root block for inguinal herniorrhaphy—A comparison with the field block approach. Reg Anesth Pain Med 1998;23:451–456.

44

Intercostal Nerve Block

Anthony M-H. Ho, MD • Manoj K. Karmakar, MD

INTRODUCTION

The intercostal nerves (ICNs) innervate the major parts of the skin and musculature of the chest and abdominal wall. The block of these nerves was first described by Braun in 1907, in the textbook *Die Lokalanästesie*.[1] In the 1940s, clinicians noticed that intercostal nerve blocks (ICNBs) could favorably effect a reduction in pulmonary complications and in narcotic requirements after upper abdominal surgery.[1] In 1981, continuous ICNB was introduced to overcome the problems associated with repeated multiple injections.[1] Today, ICNB is used in a great variety of acute and chronic pain conditions affecting the thorax and upper abdomen. Less commonly, it is also used for breast and minor chest wall surgery and, in combination with celiac plexus blockade, abdominal operations, usually with light sedation or general anesthesia. As with many other regional techniques, the advantages of ICNBs include superior analgesia, opioid-sparing effect, improved pulmonary mechanics, reduced central nervous system depression, and avoidance of urinary retention. It should be noted, however, that supplemental systemic analgesia is also almost always needed. The disadvantages of the technique include the requirement for technical expertise, risks of pneumothorax, and local anesthetic toxicity with multiple levels of blockade.

INDICATIONS

ICNB provides excellent analgesia for chest trauma such as rib fractures[2,3] and for postsurgical pain after chest and upper abdominal surgery such as thoracotomy, thoracostomy, mastectomy, gastrostomy, and cholecystectomy.[4] Respiratory parameters typically improve with relief of pain.[2,3] Blockade of the two dermatomes above and the two below the level of surgical incision is required. ICNB does not block visceral abdominal pain, for which a celiac plexus block is required. It is inadequate for renal surgery since a block from T5 to L3 is required. In itself, ICNB alone does not provide adequate intraoperative anesthesia, and supplemental analgesics or sedatives are usually required except for minor body surface surgery. Neurolytic ICNB may be used to manage chronic pain conditions such as postmastectomy pain (T2) and post-thoracotomy pain.

CONTRAINDICATIONS

1. When pneumothorax would be a disaster. ICNBs may help a patient tethering on the brink of respiratory decompensation, but if an unintended pneumothorax could have serious consequences, an alternative block should be considered unless a chest tube is in place.
2. Coagulation abormalities. This contraindication is not as strong as in central neuraxial blocks but may become absolute if severe.
3. Local infection, lack of expertise and resuscitating equipment, and lack of any short-term plan to wean from the ventilator should also discourage the use of this block.

FUNCTIONAL ANATOMY

As thoracic nerves T1 to T12 emerge from their respective intervertebral foramina, they divide into the following rami (Figure 44–1):

1. The paired gray and white anterior rami communicantes, which pass anteriorly to the sympathetic ganglion and chain
2. The posterior cutaneous ramus, supplying skin and muscle in the paravertebral region
3. The ventral ramus (ICN, the main focus of this chapter)

    T1 and T2 send nerve fibers to the upper limbs and the upper thorax, T3 through T6 supply the thorax, T7 through T11 supply the lower thorax and abdomen, and T12 innervates the abdominal wall and the skin of the front part of the gluteal region (Figure 44–2). Carrying both sensory and motor fibers, the ICN pierces the posterior intercostal membrane about 3 cm (in adults) distal to the intervertebral foramen to enter the subcostal grove where it, for the most part, continues to run parallel to the rib although branches may often be found anywhere between adjacent ribs. Its course within the

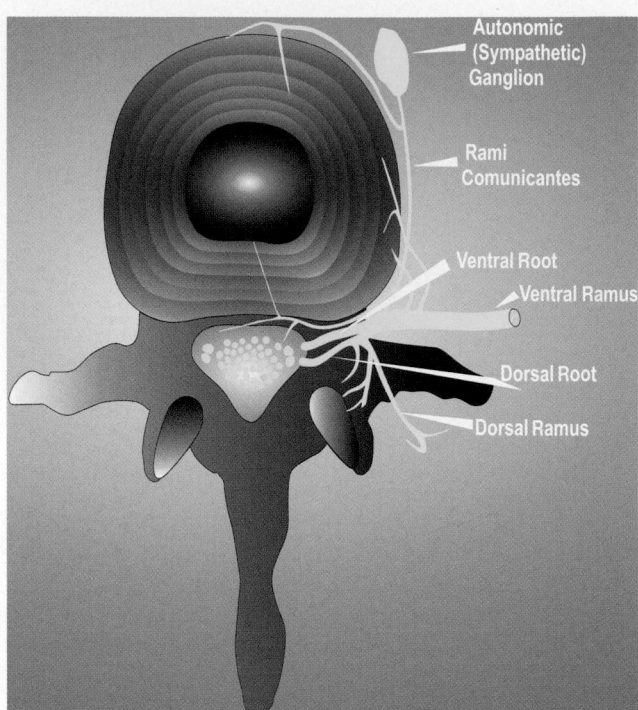

Figure 44–1. Anatomy of the spinal nerve.

thorax is sandwiched between the parietal pleura and innermost intercostal (also called the intercostalis intimus) muscles (inwardly) and the external and internal intercostal muscles (outwardly) (Figures 44–3 and 44–4). Just anterior to the midaxillary line, it gives off the lateral cutaneous branch. As the ICN approaches the midline, it turns anteriorly and pierces the overlying muscles and skin to terminate as the anterior cutaneous. There are notable variations. The first thoracic nerve (T1) has no anterior cutaneous branch, usually has no lateral cutaneous branch, and most of its fibers leave the intercostal space by crossing the neck of the first rib to join those from C8, while a smaller bundle continues on a genuine intercostal course to supply the muscles of the intercostal space. Some fibers of T2 and T3 give rise to the intercostobrachial nerve, which innervates the axilla and the skin of the medial aspect of the upper arm as far distal as the elbow. In addition, the ventral ramus of T12 is similar to the other ICNs but is called a subcostal nerve because it is not positioned between two ribs.

Lateral Cutaneous Branch

From their origins just anterior to the midaxillary line, the lateral cutaneous branches of T2 through T11 pierce the internal and external intercostal muscles obliquely before dividing into the anterior and posterior branches (see Figure 44–4). These branches supply the muscles and skin of the lateral torso. The anterior branches supply of T7 to T11 innervate the skin as far forward as the lateral edge of the rectus abdominis. The posterior branches of T7 to T11 supply the skin overlying the latissimus dorsi. The lateral cutaneous branch of T12 does not divide. Most of the ventral ramus of T12 joins

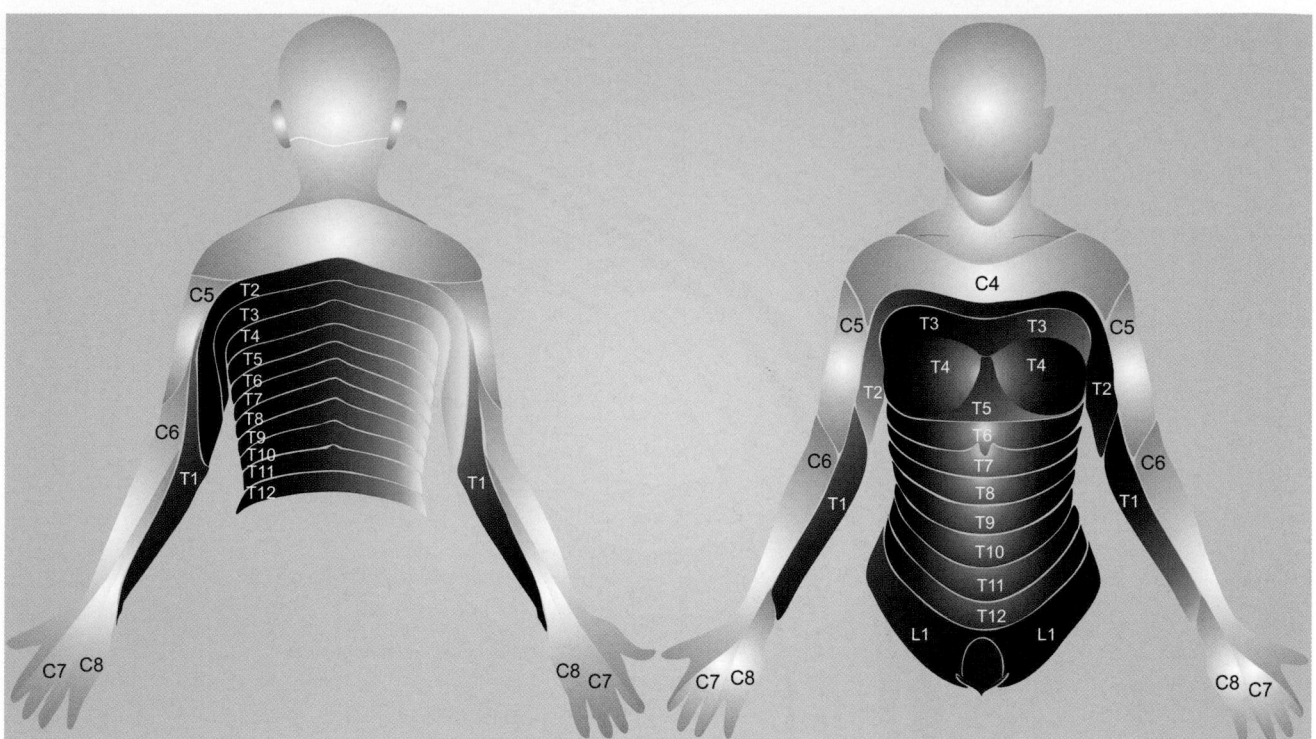

Figure 44–2. Dermatomal distribution of the intercostal nerves.

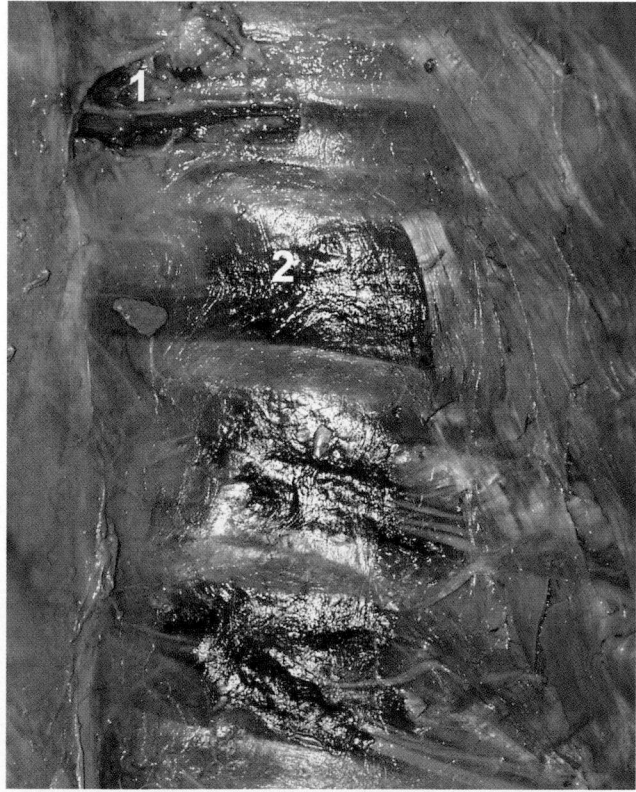

Figure 44–3. Intercostal nerves (accompanied by intercostal artery and vein) shown in the intercostal sulcus as seen from within the open chest cavity in a cadaver. The red dye illustrates spread of solutions injected into the intercostal sulcus during intercostal block. 1. Intercostal nerve. 2. Distribution of the dye after injection into the intracostal sulcus.

that of L1 to form the iliohypogastric, ilioinguinal, and genitofemoral nerves; the remaining part pierces the transverse abdominal muscle to lie between it and the internal oblique muscle.

Anterior Cutaneous Branch

The anterior cutaneous branches of T2 through T6 pierce the external intercostals and pectoralis major muscles to enter the superficial fascia near the lateral border of the sternum to supply the skin of the anterior part of the thorax near the midline and slightly beyond (see Figure 44–4). Smaller branches (T1 through T6) exist to supply the intercostal muscles and parietal pleura, and these branches may cross to adjoining intercostal spaces. The anterior cutaneous branches of T7 through T12 pierce the posterior rectus sheath to supply motor nerves to the rectus muscle and sensory fibers to the skin of the anterior abdominal wall. Some final branches of T7 through T12 continue anteriorly and, together with L1, innervate the parietal peritoneum of the abdominal wall. Their anterior course continues and becomes superficial near the linea alba to provide cutaneous innervation to the midline of the abdomen and a couple of centimeters beyond.

MECHANISM OF BLOCK & DISTRIBUTION OF ANESTHESIA

ICNB blocks the ipsilateral sensory and motor fibers of the ICNs by a direct effect of the local anesthetic. Three milliters of solution injected through a needle spreads easily for some

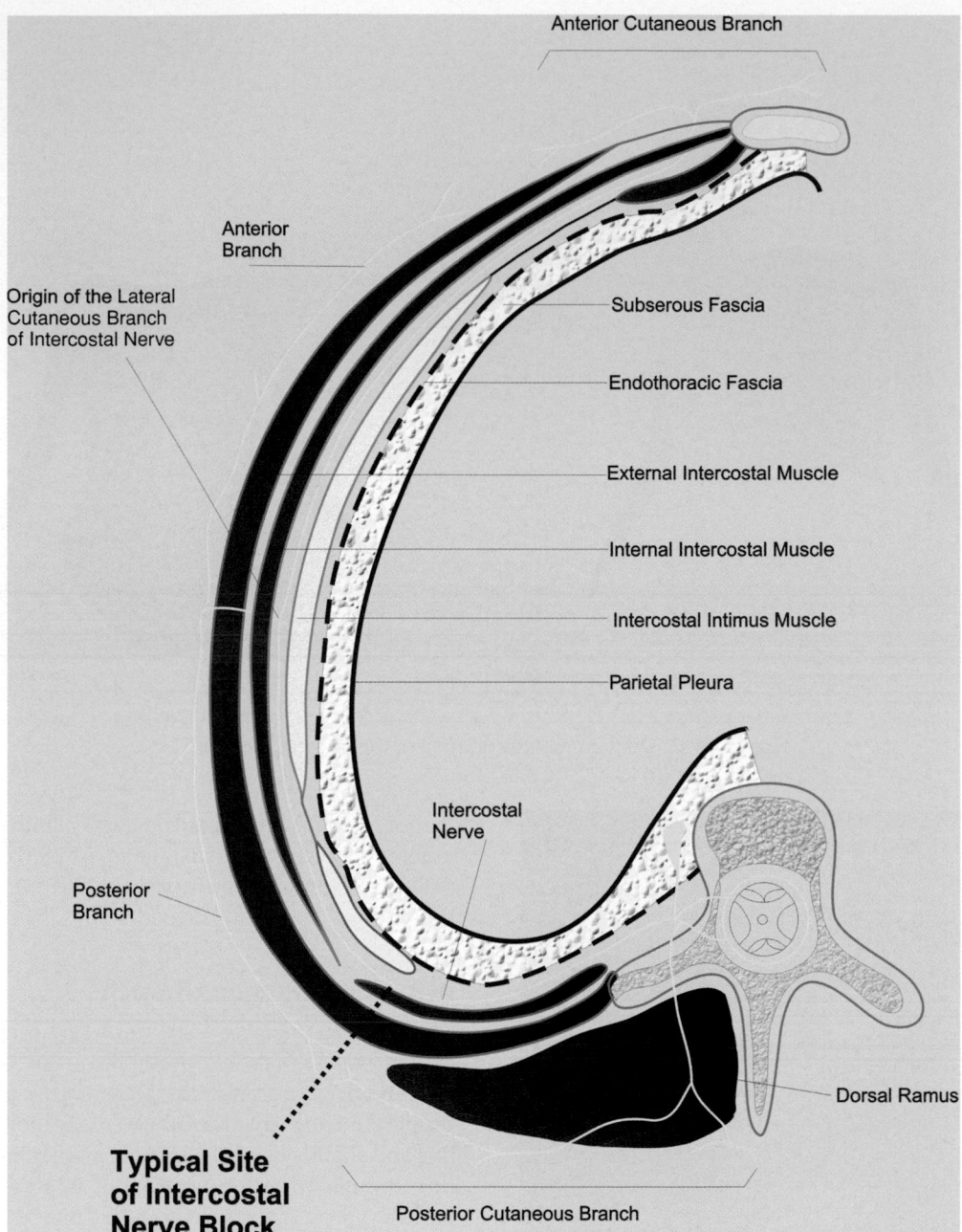

Figure 44–4. Anatomy of the intercostal nerve.

4–6 cm along that single subcostal groove distally and proximally (see Figure 44–3). If a catheter is inserted at the angle of the rib and directed medially 2–3 cm, the tip of the catheter will lie medial to the medial border of the intercostalis intimus muscle; 20 mL of solution can spread to the paravertebral space to contact 3–5 ICNs.

◼ TECHNIQUE

As with any regional block, some basic safety rules apply. The patient's airway and breathing must first be assessed and monitored. An intravenous line should be established, and resuscitation drugs should be readily available. Sedation and analgesia may be used in selected cases. Supplemental oxygen may be required. During the block, the clinician's hand controlling the needle should be firmly in contact with the patient's body. ICNB may be performed in an anesthetized patient, although spinal anesthesia has been reported in patients when ICNB was performed under general anesthesia,[4] and there is a concern that the risk of pneumothorax may be increased in a patient under positive pressure ventilation. After the block, the patient should be monitored for potential complications. In the case of ICNB, they include pneumothorax, local anesthetic toxicity, hematoma, nerve damage, infection, and, rarely, spinal anesthesia.

The ICN can be blocked anywhere proximal to the mid-axillary line, where the lateral cutaneous branch originates. In children, the block is commonly carried out at the posterior axillary line or, alternatively, just lateral to the paraspinal muscles, at the angle of the rib. In adults, the most popular site for ICNB is at the angle of the rib (6–8 cm from the spinous processes, Figures 44–5). Blocking the ICN at this location is relatively easy, is unlikely to result in direct injection into the dural sheath, and ensures that the tissues innervated by the lateral cutaneous nerve are blocked. At the angle of the rib, the rib is relatively superficial and easy to palpate, and the subcostal groove is the widest, theoretically reducing the probability of pleural puncture. Within this groove, the nerve is inferior to the posterior intercostal artery, which is inferior to the intercostal vein (Figures 44–6 and 44–3) (Mnemonic: VAN (vein/artery/nerve). They are surrounded mainly by adipose tissue and are sandwiched between the internal intercostal and the innermost intercostal (intercostalis intimus) muscles. The nerve often runs as three or four separate bundles, without an enclosing endoneural sheath, making it easily accessible to blockade. Blockade medial to the angle of the rib is not recommended because the nerve lies deep to the posterior intercostal membrane with very little tissue between it and the parietal pleura, and the overlying sacrospinalis muscle makes rib palpation difficult. Blockade distal to the anterior axillary line is more difficult because the nerve has left the subcostal groove, reentered the intercostal space and lies in the substance of the internal intercostal muscle.

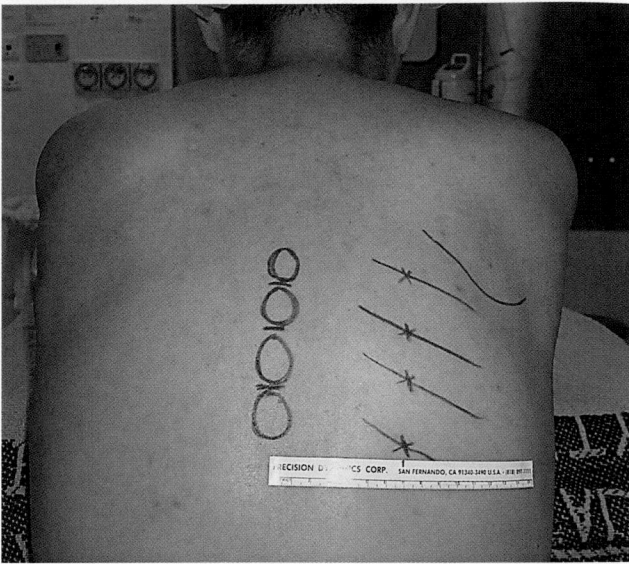

Figure 44–5. The sitting patient should lean slightly forward and be supported. The arms should pull the scapulae laterally to facilitate access to the posterior rib angles above T7. The inferior edges of the ribs to be blocked are marked just lateral to the lateral border of the sacrospinalis (paraspinous) muscle group, corresponding to the angles of the ribs. Points of needle entry are marked at 6–8 cm from the midline in most adults.

ICNB can be performed with the patient in the prone, sitting, or lateral position (block side up), with due considerations given to age, mental, physical, and ventilatory

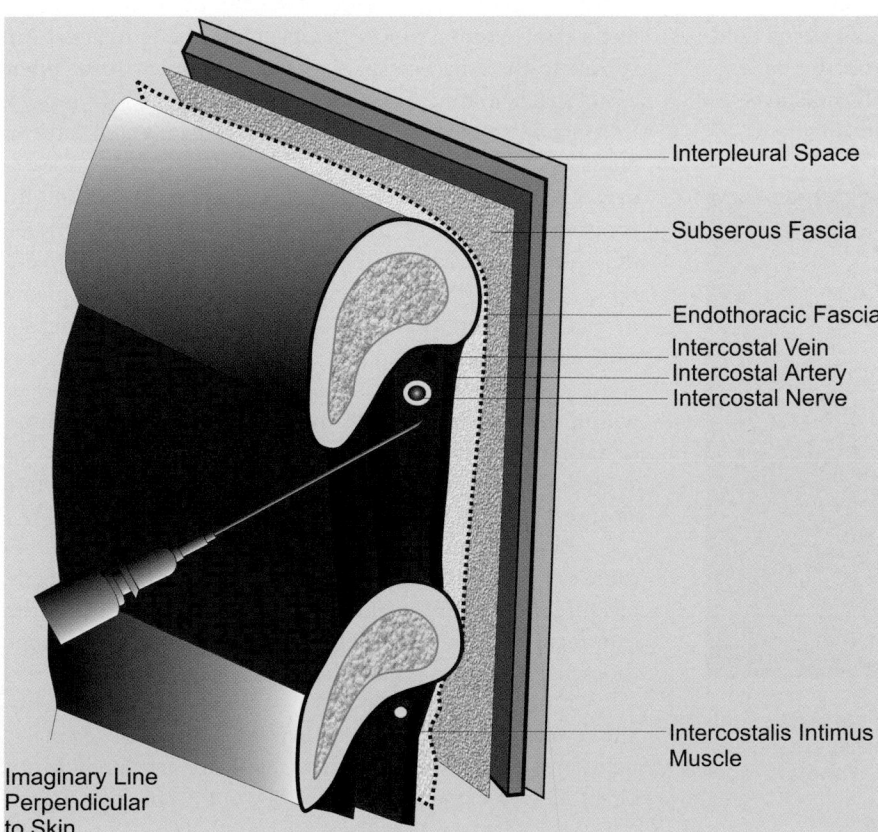

Interpleural Space

Subserous Fascia

Endothoracic Fascia
Intercostal Vein
Intercostal Artery
Intercostal Nerve

Intercostalis Intimus Muscle

Imaginary Line Perpendicular to Skin

Figure 44–6. Needle angle required to enter intercostal sulcus. Note the relationship of the intercostal vessels to the nerve (Superior-to-inferior, VAN: V = vein, A = artery, N = nerve).

status, along with any other concomitant blocks contemplated. For the prone position, a pillow should be placed under the patient's upper abdomen, and the arms are allowed to hang off the sides. The sitting patient should lean slightly forward holding a pillow and be supported. The arms should be forward. The position of the arm in either position is to pull the scapulae laterally and facilitate access to the posterior rib angles above T7 (see Figure 44–5).

Under aseptic conditions, the block sites are identified. Rib counting, if required, can be achieved by starting from the twelfth rib, or from the seventh rib, which is the lowest rib covered by the inferior tip of the scapula. The inferior edges of the ribs to be blocked are marked just lateral to the lateral border of the sacrospinalis (paraspinous) muscle group (usually 6–8 cm from the midline at the lower ribs and 4–7 cm from the midline at the upper ribs), corresponding to the angles of the ribs. Next, palpate the inferior borders of the ribs to be blocked and mark them, (see Figure 44–5).

The sites of skin entry are infiltrated with a small volume of lidocaine 1–2%. A site of entry is well-placed when a needle introduced through it at 20 degrees cephalad (sagittal plane; see Figure 44–6) just scrapes underneath the inferior border of the rib and reaches the subcostal groove. The skin is first drawn cephalad with the palpating hand by about 1 cm, and a 4- to 5-cm, 22- to 24-gauge (for single-shot injection), short-beveled needle is introduced through the chosen entry site at a 20-degree cephalad angle with the bevel facing cephalad. The needle is advanced until it contacts the rib (at a depth of less than 1 cm in most patients). A small amount of local anesthetic may be injected to anesthetize the periosteum. With the palpating hand holding the needle firmly and resting securely on the patient's back, the injecting hand gently walks the needle caudally while the skin is allowed to move back over the rib (Figure 44–7).

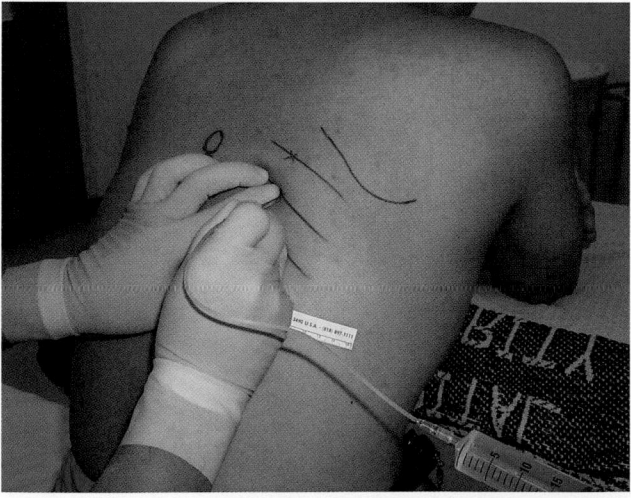

Figure 44–7. With the palpating hand holding the needle firmly and resting securely on the patient's back, the injecting hand gently walks the needle caudally while the skin is allowed to move back over the rib.

The needle is now advanced 3 mm, still maintaining the 20-degree tilt angle cephalad (even a slight caudad-pointing angle by the needle greatly reduces the chance of success). A subtle "give" or "pop" of the fascia of the internal intercostal muscle may be felt, especially if a short-beveled needle is used. As the average distance from the posterior aspect of the rib to the pleura averages 8 mm, advancement of the needle much beyond 3 mm increases the risk of pneumothorax.[5]

Paresthesia, although not actively sought, confirms needle placement. Radiologic guidance is advised for neurolytic blocks. At this point, on negative aspiration for blood, 3–5 mL of local anesthetic is injected. For a single ICNB, it is desirable to block at least one ICN cephalad and one caudad because some degree of overlapping innervation from adjacent ICNs is common. To ensure that the tip of the needle remains in the optimal location, unaffected by hand and chest movement, some clinicians prefer to connect an extension tubing between the needle and the syringe and have an assistant perform the aspiration and injection.

When repeated injections at multiple levels are desired, patient comfort, the increased risk of complications and convenience become important issues, and a continuous ICNB should be considered. The technique is the same as for a single-injection block except that a Tuohy 17- or 18-gauge needle (in adults) is used to facilitate the placement of a catheter. The site of entry should be the intercostal space midway between the dermatomes to be blocked. By orientating the bevel of the Tuohy needle medially or laterally, the epidural catheter is directed medially or laterally, respectively. A catheter tip threaded medially by 3 cm would effect a paravertebral block; the local anesthetic injected can spread to the adjacent spaces involving three to five intercostal spaces in total if sufficient volume (eg, 20 mL) is used. In contrast, solution injected via a laterally directed catheter tends to stay mainly in the same intercostal groove. A lesser degree of spread may be possible because the intercostalis intimus muscle is flimsy, and local anesthetic can pass between the separate fascicles of that muscle to reach the subpleural space, from where it can spread between ribs and pleura to reach adjacent ICNs.[5] It is usually difficult to thread a catheter much beyond 3 cm. Ability to pass a catheter beyond several centimeters suggests that the catheter may be within the pleura. It is also common for continuous intercostal block catheters to be placed under direct vision by surgeons at the end of a thoracotomy and before wound closure.[6]

Blockade of T1 through T7 is made more difficult because of the scapulae and the rhomboid muscles. Fortunately, few surgeries require blockade above T7. We prefer to perform a thoracic paravertebral block or an epidural blocks when high thoracic blockade is required.

ICNB, either single-shots or continuous, may actually result in injection of local anesthetic or catheter placement into the interpleural space or pulmonary parenchyma. Great ease of catheter insertion beyond 3 cm may suggest interpleural placement. Although analgesia may be provided with interpleural analgesia, it will not be the case with intraparenchymal injection.

EQUIPMENT

Needle: Single-shot: 20- to 22-gauge short-beveled 4- to 5-cm needle (adults)

Catheter placement: 18-to 20- gauge Tuohy needle (adults)

Syringe and needle for local infiltration

Syringe with extension tubing

Sterilizing and resuscitation equipment and drugs, drapes, marking pen, pillow, portable fluoroscope (for neurolytic blocks)

CHOICE OF LOCAL ANESTHETIC

The choice of local anesthetic for single-shot ICNB includes bupivacaine 0.25–0.5%, lidocaine 1–2% with epinephrine 1/200,000–1/400,000, and ropivacaine 0.5–0.75%. Three to 5 mL of local anesthetic is injected at each level during a multiple-injection ICNB. The duration of action is usually 12 ± 6 h. Addition of epinephrine to bupivacaine or ropivacaine does not significantly prolong the duration of block, but may slow the systemic absorption and increase the maximum allowable dose with a single shot by 30%.[4] Maximum bupivacaine dose is 2 (for plain solution) to 3 (with epinephrine) mg/kg/injection (total at one time)[7] and 7–10 mg/kg/day. Maximum lidocaine dose is up to 5 (for plain solution) and 7 (with epinephrine) mg/kg/single injection[7] and 20 mg/kg/day. Volunteers have been found to tolerate 30% more ropivacaine than bupivacaine before neurologic symptoms develop.[8] The maximum single injection dose for ropivacaine is 2.5 mg/kg (for plane solution) and 4 mg/kg (with epinephrine),[7] and the daily dose should probably be <9–12 mg/kg/24 h. The maximum single injection of epinephrine in stable patients is 4 mcg/kg. Depending on the volume of local anesthetic required, a 1/400,000 instead of 1/200,000 concentration of epinephrine may be chosen. Richly supplied areas favor rapid local anesthetic absorption, and the blood levels of local anesthetics after ICNB are higher than for any other regional anesthetic procedure. As such, it is advisable to leave a safety margin between the doses given and the maximum recommended dosages, especially in young children, the elderly, debilitated patients, and those with underlying cardiac, hepatic, or renal impairment. For continuous infusion, patients can usually tolerate a gradual build-up of the plasma local anesthetic level better than acute rises. An apparently safe regimen is a loading dose of 0.3 mL/kg followed by an infusion of 0.1 mL/kg/h of either bupivacaine 0.25% or lidocaine 1%.[5]

Clinical Pearls

- A relatively easy site for ICNB is the angle of the rib, about 7 cm lateral to midline in adults.

- The ideal angle of entry into the subcostal groove is about 20 degrees cephalad.

- A continuous catheter may be better tolerated in cases that require repeated blocks at multiple levels.

- ICNB provides excellent analgesia but is seldom adequate for intraoperative anesthesia.

- Supplemental analgesia may be required in continuous ICNB especially if the area of pain is wide.

- Epidural block should be considered as a better alternative to bilateral ICNBs because of the risk of bilateral pneumothorax and the potential for local anesthetic toxicity due the increased amount of local anesthetic required.

- Absorption of local anesthetic from the intercostal space is rapid and toxicity is usually an important concern.

- ICNB above T7 may be difficult because of the scapulae, and an alternative technique such as paravertebral or epidural block should be considered.

COMPLICATIONS

The foremost concern in a patient without an ipsilateral tube thoracostomy is pneumothorax, the rate of occurrence of which, as detected by chest radiograph and not necessarily accompanied by signs and symptoms, is well below 1%. Tension pneumothorax and the subsequent need for tube thoracostomy is rare. The risks of pneumothorax and lung injury, however, are increased in patients who have had previous chest surgery. If an asymptomatic pneumothorax is detected, the best management is observation, reassurance, and, if necessary, supplemental oxygen.

The peritoneum and abdominal viscera are at risk of penetration when lower ICNs are blocked, and the incidence should not be greatly different from that for pneumothorax.

Absorption of local anesthetic from the intercostal space is rapid. Peak arterial plasma concentration develops in less than 5 to 10 min, and peak venous plasma concentration peaks several minutes later. Because of this, toxicity is always a concern with multiple or continuous intercostal injections. Sometimes the dilemma comes when a frail elderly patient has multiple fractured ribs. The concern over systemic anesthetic toxicity may at times necessitate the use of a different regional technique.

Finally, as the dural sheath can extend up to 8 cm laterally, there is a slight risk of spinal anesthesia after an ICNB.

Clinical Pearls

- ICNB is indicated for management of acute and chronic pain involving the thorax and upper abdomen.

- ICNB by itself is inadequate for most intraoperative anesthesia except for minor body surface surgery.

- ICNB is contraindicated when pneumothorax would spell disaster, in the presence of severe hemostatic deficiencies, and when there are better alternatives.

- In the presence of minor hemostatic abnormalities, ICNB may be an attractive alternative to neuraxial blocks. Serious hemostatic deficiencies contraindicate all nerve blocks.

- General anesthesia is not a contraindication to ICNB.

SUMMARY

ICNB is a very satisfying block for both the clinician and patient because it is technically easy to perform and effective in the controlling pain involving the thorax and upper abdomen. It avoids many of the problems associated with central neuraxial blocks. Although there is the risk of pneumothorax and local anesthetic toxicity, these can be reduced with good technique and due consideration given to the maximum allowable drug dose and the patient's clinical condition. The proper use of this technique includes balancing its advantages and disadvantages against those of alternative techniques such as epidural and thoracic paravertebral block.

References

1. Strømskag KE, Kleiven S: Continuous intercostals and interpleural nerve blockades. Tech Reg Anesth Pain Manage 1998;2:79–89.
2. Karmakar MK, Ho AMH: Acute pain management of patients with multiple fractured ribs. J Trauma 2003;54:612–615.
3. Karmakar MK, Critchley LAH, Ho AMH, et al: Continuous thoracic paravertebral infusion of bupivacaine for pain management in patients with multiple fractured ribs. Chest 2003;123:424–431.
4. Kopacz DJ, Thompson GE: Intercostal blocks for thoracic and abdominal surgery. Tech Reg Anesth Pain Manage 1998;2:25–29.
5. Nunn JF, Slavin G: Posterior intercostal nerve block for pain relief after cholecystectomy. Anatomical basis and efficacy. Br J Anaesth 1980;52:253–60.
6. Barron DJ, Tolan MJ, Lea RE: A randomized controlled trial of continuous extra-pleural analgesia post-thoracotomy: Efficacy and choice of local anaesthetic. Eur J Anaesthesiol 1999;16:236–245.
7. Lagan G, McLure HA: Review of local anaesthetic agents. Curr Anaesth Crit Care 2004;15:247–254.
8. Scott DB, Lee A, Fagan D, et al: Acute toxicity of ropivacaine compared with that of bupivacaine. Anesth Analg 1989;69:563–569.

New & Emerging Concepts in Peripheral Nerve Blocks: Equipment & Practice

45

Percutaneous Nerve Localization

William F. Urmey, MD

INTRODUCTION

Conventional methods for peripheral nerve or plexus blockade have involved the identification of surface anatomic landmarks. Such landmarks serve as an approximate starting point for a search for the targeted nerve or nerves by needle exploration. The objective of needle exploration is to reach a finite endpoint that indicates the tip of the needle is sufficiently close to the targeted nerve or nerve plexuses. Two distinct types of endpoint exist:

1. An **anatomic** endpoint based on encountering anatomic relations to the targeted nerve or nerves. Examples of blocks that make use of anatomic endpoints include field block, transarterial techniques, or ultrasonographic guidance.

2. A **functional** endpoint based on a nerve response to mechanical or electrical stimulation. The main types of functional endpoints used clinically are either sensory response to mechanical stimulation of the nerve (mechanical paresthesia) or a motor response to electrical stimulation.

Designated anatomic landmarks are limited because they vary from patient to patient and do not always correlate with the location of the underlying nerve or plexus. In addition, traditional landmark measurements are sometimes complicated, requiring linear measurements with a ruler, bisecting lines, and they are not always normalized to patient size or body habitus. For many blocks, accepted descriptions of the technique include insertion of the block needle at a certain distance from a designated palpable landmark, without regard to patient size. Consequently, with many techniques, dexterity and delicate proprioception are often required for successful block performance.

Techniques such as ultrasonography or other imaging techniques or percutaneous localization utilizing transcutaneous electrical stimulation help to decrease needle exploration. Transcutaneous electrical stimulation, in contrast to an imaging technique such as ultrasonography, utilizes a functional neural response, either motor or sensory. Prelocalization of the nerve prior to needle insertion serves to decrease the amount of invasive search with the needle, increasing patient comfort while decreasing the potential for complications. The purpose of this chapter is to discuss how transcutaneous electrical stimulation helps to localize the underlying nerve or plexus through the skin, in a noninvasive manner before the needle is introduced transcutaneously. The chapter will necessarily discuss basic elements of nerve stimulation; however, for more in-depth coverage of principles of nerve stimulation and nerve stimulators, the reader is referred to Chapters 5 (Electrophysiology of Nerve Stimulation) and 17 (Equipment for Peripheral Nerve Blocks).

CLINICAL EXAMPLES

Elicitation of a paresthesia is an all-or-nothing phenomenon, ie, the needle either contacts the nerve or it does not. By contrast, use of electrical nerve stimulation yields graded information, which may be useful at a distance from the targeted nerve. Furthermore, visual cues of motor responses from untargeted nerves allow for redirection of the needle. This concept has been extended to the use of transcutaneous electrical stimulation to yield visual cues and motor responses, noninvasively, through the intact overlying skin.

Transcutaneous electrical stimulation to elicit a motor response has been used to assist in determining the optimal entry point for needle insertion, thereby narrowing the invasive search for the nerve with the needle. Ganta and colleagues[1] reported on the use of a modified electrocardiographic electrode 0.5 cm in diameter with adherent coupling gel to assist in the performance of interscalene block. The electrode was coupled to a nerve stimulator and was "passed along the skin" to locate the optimal entry point for needle insertion. More recently, an exploring skin electrode was proposed to help find the interscalene groove in patients with difficult anatomy.[2]

Transcutaneous stimulation to elicit a sensory response (electrical paresthesia) to nerve stimulation of a purely sensory nerve (eg, lateral femoral cutaneous nerve) was described by Shannon and coworkers.[3] These investigators used a small handheld electrical nerve stimulator equipped with 0.5-cm diameter metal electrodes to elicit sensory paresthesias of the lateral femoral cutaneous nerve. Following this, they made measurements to determine the approximate location of the nerve. Based on these measurements, injection of local anesthetic was made to block the nerve.

SCIENCE OF ELECTRICAL NERVE STIMULATION

The objective of peripheral nerve location by electrical stimulation is to elicit a targeted motor response by a block needle coupled to a (square-wave) current generator (ie, nerve stimulator). The stimulator provides a stream of square-wave pulses, typically at a frequency (f) of 1 to 2 Hz. Ability to elicit designated motor responses below threshold current levels that have been empirically associated with high success rates indicates immediate proximity to the nerve.

Electrical Variables

The ability to electrically stimulate a peripheral nerve or neural plexus depends on:

1. Electric current amplitude (I), ie, the amperage applied to the stimulator electrode or needle
2. Pulse duration or width of the square wave of current generated by the pulse oximeter

And is inversely proportional to:

3. The distance between the stimulating electrode and the nerve
4. Tissue electrical impedance (mostly resistance) of the tissues that lie between and around the electrode and the targeted nerve or nerves

Current Amplitude (Amperage)

Use of higher amperage (eg, 2–5 mA) to stimulate peripheral nerves allows one to elicit a motor response at a greater distance from the nerve. As an electrode (the needle) approaches the nerve, motor response to electrical stimulation can be achieved at lower amperage (Figure 45–1). This is governed by Coulomb's law equation,

$$E = K(Q/r^2) \qquad (45.1)$$

where E = required stimulating current, K = constant, Q = minimal required stimulation current, and r = distance between electrode and nerve.

Empirically, motor response to stimulation with current below 0.5 mA with pulse duration of 0.1 ms signifies that the needle's tip is sufficiently close to the nerve to translate to a high block success rate.

Clinical Pearl

- According to Coulomb's law, if a motor response can be elicited at very low amperage (<0.5 mA), then the stimulating electrode must be very close to the nerve. Stimulation at very low amperage maximizes specificity.

According to Coulomb's law, if a motor response can be elicited at very low amperage (<0.5 mp), then the stimulating

A $E = K(Q/r^2) + C$

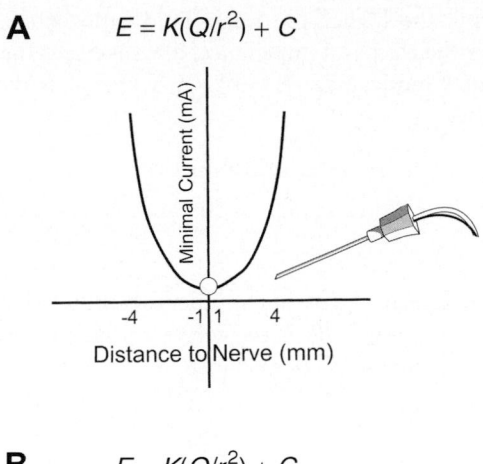

B $E = K(Q/r^2) + C$

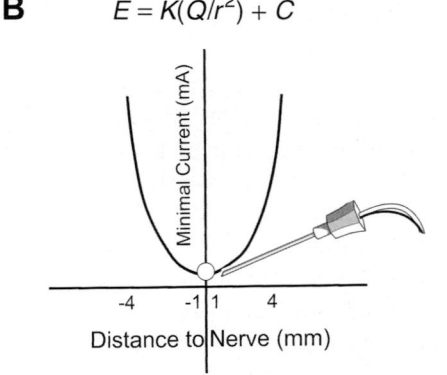

Figure 45–1. Electrical current from the stimulating microelectrode tip dissipates quickly, to the inverse square to the distance from the nerve. **A:** Needle tip position within 1 mm of nerve at minimal current amplitude (amperage) required for stimulation. **B:** Movement of needle tip to position just 4 mm from nerve results in a 16-fold increase in the amount of current required for stimulation.

electrode must be very close to the nerve. Stimulation at very low amperage maximizes specificity. In contrast, using a higher amperage (eg, 2–5 mA), maximizes sensitivity. This principle is used when monitoring the neuromuscular function by cutaneous electrodes and comparably very high (≈50 mA) currents during general anesthesia. Here, specificity of electrode location relative to the nerve is of less importance. For peripheral nerve location, 2- to 5-mA currents increase sensitivity, providing clues at a distance, but ultimate specificity is achieved by successful stimulation at very low current (<0.5 mA). However, it should be noted that using current of high intensity has practical disadvantages in that (1) it is associated with patient discomfort and (2). higher current intensity (eg, >1.0 mA) is sufficient to elicit direct muscle stimulation, which may produce confusing twitches of the local muscles. For these reasons, many nerve localization procedures are best initiated using relatively lower initial stimulating current (eg, <1.5 mA).

The surface area of the conductive electrode and its conductance are very important in nerve stimulation according to Ohm's law: $I = V/R$, where I = current flow (amperage), V = potential difference (voltage), and R = resistance (ohms).

The nerve stimulator varies current flow by altering the voltage. Most modern nerve stimulators are constant-current generators that automatically adjust the voltage output to maintain the set current flow despite changes in tissue resistance (within a certain range specified by the electrical design of the nerve stimulator).

Resistance, on the other hand, is related to the conductive area of the electrode by the equation $R = \rho L/A$, where R = electrical resistance, ρ = tissue resistivity, and A = conductive area. An example of the clinical importance of this principle is the use of defibrillating paddles. Defibrillation paddles are characterized by a large surface area to minimize impedance or resistance. By contrast, the microelectrode tip of a shielded block needle serves to maximize resistance outside of the microconductive area. This ensures that the electrode tip must be very close to the nerve if a motor response is to be elicited, thereby enhancing specificity.

Clinical Pearl

- If a motor response can be elicited at (1) very low amperage and by Ohm's law, with a (2) microelectrode (small conductive area), then the stimulator electrode must be very close to the nerve.

If a motor response can be elicited at (1) very low amperage and, by Ohm's law, with a (2) microelectrode (small conductive area), then the stimulator electrode must be very close to the nerve. This phenomenon has led to the clinical use of needles with electrically insulated shafts to ensure specificity of location to the microelectrode (needle's tip) relative to the targeted nerve. Bashein and colleagues[4] looked at the difference in the relative dispersion of current between electrically shielded and unshielded needles. Indeed, the ability to elicit a motor response to electrical stimulation following the initial elicitation of a mechanical paresthesia differs from 40%, using noninsulated needles, to 10% with insulated needles.[5] The 30% increase in the ability to cause motor nerve stimulation with a noninsulated needle compared with an insulated needle can be explained by the difference in current dispersion between the two needles (see Chapter 5, Electrophysiology of Nerve Stimulation, for more information).

Electrical Pulse Duration

Electrical pulse duration refers to the duration of the periodic pulsed square wave generated by the nerve stimulator. For the purpose of nerve localization, short pulse duration ranging between 0.05 and 1 ms is typically used in clinical practice, with 0.1 ms being most common. Increasing electrical pulse duration increases the total flow of electrons (electrical energy) proportional to the calculated area under the curve (Figure 45–2). Increasing the duration of the electrical pulse therefore results in increased ability to stimulate the nerve without changing other variables. Similar to current flow

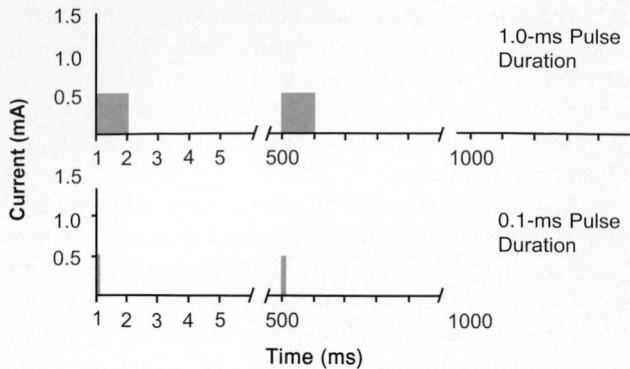

Figure 45–2. Graph of current in milliamperes (*y*-axis) versus time in milliseconds (*x*-axis). Increasing pulse duration from 0.1 to 1.0 ms at the same amperage (0.5 mA in this example) results in a larger area under the curve and a larger pulse of electrons, increasing the ability to stimulate the nerve transcutaneously without patient discomfort.

(amperage), higher pulse durations of 0.3 to 1.0 ms also result in enhanced sensitivity for transcutaneous or initial invasive prelocation of the nerve. By contrast, by using a lower pulse duration, specificity is maximized. This principle has been demonstrated clinically when higher current amplitude (amperage) was needed to elicit a motor response at lower pulse duration (Figure 45–3).[6]

Tissue Electrical Impedance

Clinical Pearl

- Condensing the tissues by indenting the overlying skin, adipose, etc toward the nerve serves to decrease electrical impedance, increasing conductance.

Tissue impedance is a function of electrical resistance, capacitance, and inductance of the biologic tissue. In general, the higher the water–lipid ratio of the tissue, the lower the electrical impedance, or conversely, the higher the tissue conductance, $R = \rho L/A$, where ρ is the tissue resistivity.

$$\text{Most conductive} \rightarrow \text{Least conductive}$$
$$\text{Nerves} > \text{Blood Vessels} > \text{Muscle} > \text{Skin} > \text{Fat} > \text{Bone}$$
$$(45.2)$$

Condensing the tissues by indenting the overlying skin, adipose, etc toward the nerve serves to decrease electrical impedance, increasing conductance.

Electrical Pulse Frequency

The frequency (f) of the square-wave electrical pulse generated by the nerve stimulator is typically set at 1 or 2 Hz. Increasing frequency to 2 Hz gives more rapid feedback with little added discomfort to the patient. Frequency must be sufficiently low so as to allow time for the relaxation phase period following depolarization. For example, frequency of 50 Hz causes sustained tetanus and is extremely painful and is therefore unacceptable for locating peripheral nerves for regional blockade. In addition, stimulation at frequencies greater than 3 Hz results in a loss of specificity; ie, motor response may be indistinguishable from a muscle fasciculations.

PERCUTANEOUS ELECTRODE GUIDANCE OF THE BLOCK NEEDLE

Percutaneous electrode guidance (PEG) of a block needle for peripheral nerve or plexus blockade is a recently proposed technique to assist with nerve location for regional anesthesia. PEG makes use of transcutaneous electrical stimulation to prelocate the nerve or plexus prior to needle insertion and exploration. The underlying motivation for the development of PEG was to devise a method to facilitate prelocation of the

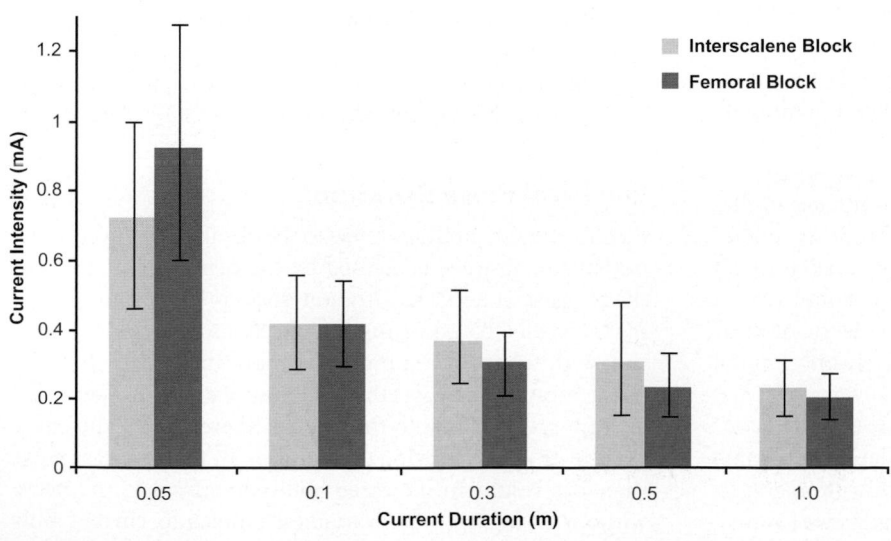

Figure 45–3. Increasing pulse durations in milliseconds (*x*-axis) resulted in lower required minimal stimulating current flow (intensity, *y*-axis) during interscalene or femoral nerve block. (Reprinted, with permission, from Hadzic A, Vloka JD, Claudio RE, et al: Electrical nerve localization: Effects of cutaneous electrode placement and duration of the stimulus on motor response. Anesthesiology 2004;100:1526–1530.)

targeted nerve in order to minimize dependence on anatomic landmarks and measurements and to simplify the process of nerve location, particularly for the trainees.

Multiple Injection Peripheral Nerve/Plexus Blockade via PEG

PEG allows for noninvasive, rapid identification of multiple superficial peripheral nerves. For example, all four nerves in the axillary brachial plexus (median, ulnar, radial, and musculocutaneous) can be located by stimulation and blocked (Figure 45–4).[7] Multiple–injection techniques may result in a higher success rate with smaller volumes of local anesthetic. This is especially true in certain areas of a peripheral nerve plexus, eg, the axillary brachial plexus, where high compliance may lead to incomplete spread of anesthetic.[8] For instance, Fanelli and coworkers studied multiple small-volume injection techniques for femoral–sciatic, axillary, or interscalene blocks in almost 4000 patients.[9] Nerve stimulator–assisted separate identification and injection resulted in excellent (93–94%) success rates with low total local anesthetic volumes (22.6–28.1 mL). With axillary block, these investigators separately identified and injected the radial, median, ulnar, and musculocutaneous nerves. Interscalene block was performed following separate identification of supraclavicular, radial, and musculocutaneous nerves. Similarly, femoral nerve block followed separate elicited motor responses of the vastus medialis, intermedius, and lateralis components of the quadriceps muscles. Sciatic block was performed following separate motor responses of foot flexion, extension, and biceps femoris contractions. Percutaneous electrical guidance is a promising technology for noninvasively prelocating and aiding in these multiple injection techniques.

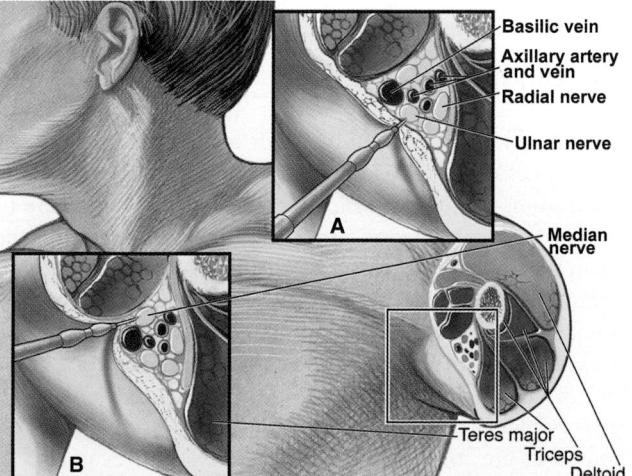

Figure 45–4. Cross-section illustration of percutaneous electrical stimulation (PEG) at the anatomic level of the axilla. Ulnar nerve indentation (**A**) is followed by median nerve stimulation (**B**). (Reprinted, with permission, from Urmey W: Percutaneous electrode guidance of the block needle for peripheral or plexus nerve blockade. Tech Reg Anesth Pain Manage 2002;6:145–149.)

Initial Experience with PEG

In the initial report, a cylindrical electrically shielded cutaneous electrode with a 1-mm diameter metallic conductive tip was used.[7] The probe was positioned over the skin overlying the nerve. Maximal motor response at minimal cutaneous probe amperage (2 Hz, 0.2 ms) was taken as evidence that the probe was directly above the nerve. A standard commercial nerve stimulator needle was then physically guided by the probe to the nerve. Block characteristics are shown in Table 45–1. Since nerves were prelocated by cutaneous probe, needle insertion in all but one case was made with a small current intensity of 0.5 mA. The milliamperage of a minimal transcutaneous stimulation current correlated directly with measured needle depth (beyond the probe tip) when minimal stimulating needle current occurred. Following the original publication of the PEG technique, a significant progress in improving the probe and simplifying the technique was made.[10]

Clinical Pearls

- Although electrical coupling gel is not necessary for percutaneous localization, transcutaneous conduction of electricity is enhanced by cleaning and removing oil from the skin with alcohol or another antiseptic. Ensure that if body lotion has been applied, none remains prior to cutaneous electrode stimulation.

- Indentation of the skin with a stimulating probe facilitates nerve stimulation by (1) decreasing the distance to the nerve, (2) decreasing resistance by condensing underlying subcutaneous tissues and directing subcutaneous adipose laterally, and (3) by minimizing the sphere of current diffusion. This improves accuracy of the relationship of the electrode's tip to the underlying nerve.

- Pure or predominantly sensory nerves such as the lateral femoral cutaneous or saphenous nerves can be localized percutaneously by elicitation of sensory paresthesias to electrical stimulation.

- Percutaneous localization of the brachial plexus at the interscalene block level is usually achieved by stimulation of the most superficial nerve roots, C5 and C6. This is manifested by contraction of the deltoid, biceps, or brachioradialis muscles. It is usually not possible, at normal nerve stimulator settings, to stimulate C7, C8, or T1 nerve roots. If stimulation of the phrenic nerve occurs, manifested by ipsilateral abdominal motion, the electrode lies anterior to the brachial plexus.

Capdevila and colleagues[11] published a larger study in which the needle tip itself was used to transcutaneously and noninvasively locate the nerves of the axillary brachial plexus. This was accomplished at nerve stimulator settings between 5 mA and 0.5 mA (0.2-ms pulse duration) prior to needle

Table 45–1.

Block Characteristics

Patient No.	Nerve Block	Minimal Electrode Current (mA)	Electrode Motor Response	Minimal Needle Current (mA)	Needle Motor Response	Needle Depth (cm)
1	Interscalene block	2.3	Deltoid, biceps	0.21	Deltoid, biceps	0.4
2	Interscalene block	2.8	Deltoid, biceps, brachioradialis	0.70	Biceps, biceps	0.6
3	Interscalene block	2.8	Biceps, brachioradialis	0.25	Biceps,* brachioradialis	0.6
4	A. Midhumeral median nerve block	2.3	Hand median distribution	0.21	Hand median distribution	0.4
	B. Axillary block	1.3	Hand ulnar distribution	0.31	Hand ulnar distribution	0.4
5	A. Axillary block (median nerve—conventional)	2.0	Hand median distribution	0.29	Hand median distribution	0.5
	B. Axillary block (median nerve transcoracobrachialis)	3.0	Hand median distribution	0.29	Hand median distribution	1.0
6	Femoral nerve block	8.2	Quadriceps, patellar motion	0.20	Quadriceps, patellar motion	1.1
7	A. Femoral nerve block	3.4	Quadriceps, patellar motion	0.44	Quadriceps, patellar motion	0.8
	B. Popliteal fossa peroneal	4.7	Foot dorsiflexion	0.50	Foot dorsiflexion	2.0

* *Patient noted simultaneous paresthesia to shoulder.*

† *Transmuscular approach.*

Reprinted, with permission, from Urmey W, Grossi P: Percutaneous electrode guidance (PEG): A noninvasive technique for pre-location of peripheral nerves to facilitate nerve block. Reg Anesth Pain Med 2002; 27:261–267.

insertion. These investigators, however, found a linear relationship between the needle depth at final location and minimal transcutaneous stimulating current (in milliamperes) (Figure 45–5). Subsequently, a report of PEG to perform femoral nerve block in obese patients without palpable arterial pulse was published by Pham Dang and coworkers.[12] These authors used a metallic probe to indent the skin and stimulate the nerve (which required up to 8 mA, 0.5-ms pulse duration). The skin was marked, and the standard block needle advanced using the skin markings as a guide. Although this method does not entirely represent PEG in that the needle was not physically guided by the transcutaneous stimulating electrode, it exemplifies the value of the concept. The technique used by Pham Dang and coworkers would be more correctly termed transcutaneous prelocation using a cutaneous electrode and is useful in determining the site of needle insertion.

SUMMARY

In summary, conventional methods for peripheral nerve or plexus blocks have relied on anatomic landmarks and needle exploration. Percutaneous localization allows prelocation of nerves by transcutaneous stimulation before invasive needle exploration. Electrical variables that include current flow or amplitude, pulse duration, and tissue impedance can be manipulated to enhance sensitivity and specificity for optimal transcutaneous nerve location. Percutaneous electrode guidance of the block needle can be used to facilitate superficial nerve or plexus blockade, or when more traditional palpable landmarks are absent. Percutaneous localization can also be used for teaching blockade techniques to the novice and has been successfully used to demonstrate nerve or plexus blocks in a workshop setting.

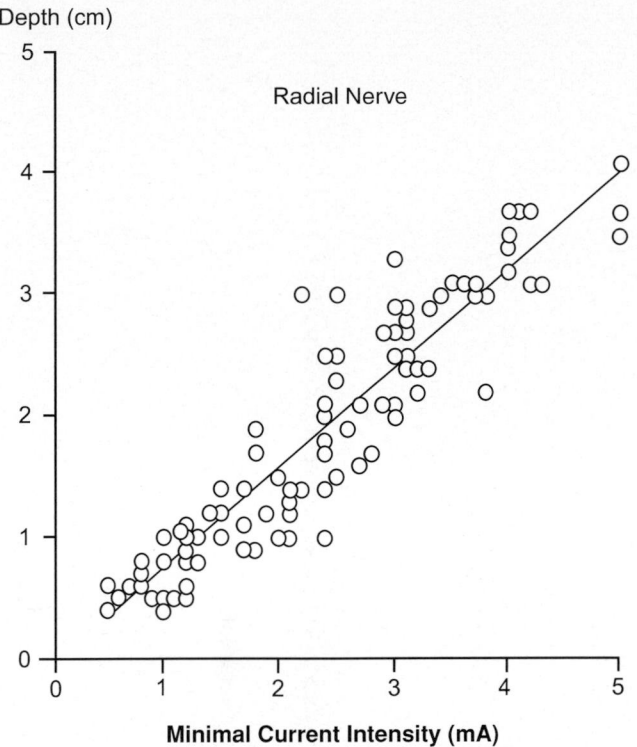

Figure 45–5. Needle depths for radial nerve are displayed on the y-axis as a function of minimal percutaneous electrode currents on the x-axis. (Reprinted, with permission, from Capdevila X, Lopez S, Bernard N, et al: Percutaneous electrode guidance using the insulated needle for prelocation of peripheral nerves during axillary plexus blocks. Reg Anesth Pain Med 2004;29: 206–211.)

References

1. Ganta R, Cajee R, Henthorn R: Use of a transcutaneous nerve stimulation to assist interscalene block. Anesth Analg 1993;76:914–915.
2. Urmey W: Upper extremity blocks. In Brown D (ed): *Regional Anesthesia and Analgesia.* WB Saunders, 1996, pp 254–278.
3. Shannon J, Lang S, Yip R: Lateral femoral nerve block revisited: A nerve stimulator technique. Reg Anesth 1995;20:100–104.
4. Bashein G, Haschke RH, Ready LB: Electrical nerve location: Numerical and electrophoretic comparison of insulated vs uninsulated needles. Anesth Analg 1984;63:919–924.
5. Urmey W, Stanton J: Inability to consistently elicit a motor response following sensory paresthesia during interscalene block administration. Anesthesiology 2002;96:552–554.
6. Hadzic A, Vloka JD, Claudio RE, et al: Electrical nerve localization: Effects of cutaneous electrode placement and duration of the stimulus on motor response. Anesthesiology 2004;100:1526–1530.
7. Urmey W, Grossi P: Percutaneous electrode guidance (PEG): A noninvasive technique for pre-location of peripheral nerves to facilitate nerve block. Reg Anesth Pain Med 2002;27:261–267.
8. Klaastad O, Smedby O, Thompson G, et al: Distribution of local anesthetic in axillary brachial plexus block: A clinical and magnetic resonance imaging study. Anesthesiology 2002;96:1315–1324.
9. Fanelli G, Casati A, Garancini P, et al: Nerve stimulator and multiple injection technique for upper and lower limb blockade: Failure rate, patient acceptance, and neurologic complications. Study Group on Regional Anesthesia. Anesth Analg 1999;88:847–852.
10. Urmey W, Grossi P: Percutaneous electrode guidance (PEG) and subcutaneous stimulating electrode guidance (SSEG): Modifications of the original technique. Letter to the Editor. Reg Anesth Pain Med 2003;28:253–255.
11. Capdevila X, Lopez S, Bernard N, et al: Percutaneous electrode guidance using the insulated needle for prelocation of peripheral nerves during axillary plexus blocks. Reg Anesth Pain Med 2004;29:206–211.
12. Pham Dang C, Kick, Pinaud M, Malinge M: Percutaneous electrode guidance for femoral nerve block in case of unperceivable artery pulsation (abstract). Reg Anesth Pain Med 2005;30:A40.

46

Multistimulation Techniques for Peripheral Nerve Blocks

Andrea Casati, MD • Marta Putzu, MD

INTRODUCTION

Contrary to common, oversimplified representations by medical illustrators, the arrangement of peripheral nerves and plexuses is quite complex. Various tissue compartments contain connective tissue and fat; terminal branches of plexuses and nerves divide and separate frequently, and the different branches may run at some distance from one another. Accordingly, once injected at a particular site, the local anesthetic molecules have to diffuse through several barriers before reaching the nerves, the first barrier being the distance between the injection site and each branch.

In regional anesthesia, the most frequently used strategy for overcoming this "spatial dispersion" of nerve branches is to place the needle somewhere close to the nerves and then inject a volume of local anesthetic large enough to spread toward desired different branches. This practice has been traditionally taught and clinically used for decades throughout the development of regional anesthesia. However, with the advent of modern nerve stimulators and nerve-stimulating techniques, electrolocation can be utilized to augment selectivity in nerve location, increase the success rate, and minimize the amount of local anesthetic required to accomplish a nerve block.

This chapter will discuss general principles of multistimulation for the commonly used peripheral nerve block procedures. For more discussions on anatomy and techniques, the reader is referred to the respective technique and detailed description of the anatomy elsewhere in this book.

PRINCIPLES OF MULTISTIMULATION

The use of a nerve stimulator makes it possible to readily identify different muscular twitches during block placement, by simply redirecting the stimulating needle according to the anatomic topography of each nerve block considered, using the so-called multiple injection technique. The rationale of the multiple-injection technique is to specifically and separately localize and block each major nerve required for surgical anesthesia using a small volume of local anesthetic solution.

Clinical Pearl

- The rationale of the multiple-injection technique is to specifically and separately localize and block each major nerve required for surgical anesthesia using a small volume of local anesthetic solution.

The needle is inserted as usual based on classical anatomic landmarks, with the nerve stimulator set at 1- to 1.5-mA intensity until the initial motor response is obtained. Thereafter, the intensity of the stimulating current is progressively reduced to less than 0.5 mA while maintaining the twitch response, at which point an injection of 5 to 7 mL of local anesthetic solution is made. When the desired component (nerve) is blocked, the current intensity of the nerve stimulator is again increased to 1 to 1.5 mA, and the needle is redirected according to the anatomic relationship among the individual components of the nerve being blocked. When the twitch of another component of the nerve is accomplished, an additional 5–7 mL of local anesthetic is injected. This maneuver is then repeated for all the main branches of the nerve required for surgery.

CLINICAL ADVANTAGES

Several clinical studies have demonstrated the advantages of the multiple-injection technique. The first report was by Lavoie and coworkers in 1992, who demonstrated that when performing an axillary block with the help of a nerve stimulator, stimulating three or four of the terminal nerves of the brachial plexus resulted in a higher success rate than a single injection of a larger volume of local anesthetic.[1] Subsequently, several authors reported on the improved quality and shorter onset time of the nerve block when using a multiple-injection rather than a single-injection technique.[2–5] And recent meta-analytic studies supported the evidence that, at least for axillary brachial plexus, the multiple injection should be always used. Similar results have also been reported with lower limb nerve blocks, including sciatic and femoral nerve blocks.[6,7] Of note, multiple-injection techniques also allowed a reduction (30–40%) in the volume of local anesthetic solution required to produce

an effective nerve block.[8,9] This may help minimize the risk of systemic local anesthetic toxicity, especially when multiple nerve blocks are used, such as for lower limb surgery.

Clinical Pearl

- Multiple-injection techniques typically allow a reduction in the volume of local anesthetic solution required to produce an effective nerve block

One disadvantage and possible problem with the multiple-injection technique is the increase in discomfort to the patient and in time for block placement. Several reports indicated that seeking multiple twitches resulted in a prolongation of the time required to place the block. However, the latency of the nerve block is also shorter, which helps offset this delay; consequently, the readiness for surgery of the multiple- and single-injection techniques remains similar.[4–7]

MULTIPLE STIMULATION & THE RISK OF NERVE INJURY

The use of multiple injections theoretically may increase the risk of nerve injury, because the additional needle manipulation and injections are made after some volume of local anesthetic has already been injected. In other words, the needle can be inserted into an anesthetized nerve, and the pain or paresthesia symptoms of intraneural injection may be missed when present. However, a certain time is required to achieve anesthesia with peripheral nerve blockade. This time typically ranges from 10 to 30 min according to the type, volume, and concentration of local anesthetic used; longer times may be required after injection of small volumes (5–7 mL) of local anesthetic. In contrast, the time required to electrolocalize two or three neural components of a nerve or plexus is typically a few minutes in experienced hands. For these reasons, the multiple-stimulation technique should be considered an advanced technique, with adequate training and experience with single-injection blocks required for effective and safe use. Regardless, in a large observational investigation involving nearly 4000 peripheral nerve blocks performed with the multiple-injection technique, the withdrawal and redirection of the stimulating needle was not associated with an increased incidence of neurologic complications. An incidence of 2.5/1000 of persistent nerve injury (resolving after more than 6 months), was reported, similar to that reported using a conventional immobile needle technique.[10,11] When electrolocating components of the nerve or plexus, increasing the intensity of the stimulating current to 1.5 to 2 mA may be helpful in increasing sensitivity and recruiting partially blocked or inner mantle nerve fibers. In the near future, objective monitoring of injection pressure to avoid intraneural injection may make these techniques safer even in the hands of those with less experience in multiinjection techniques.

CLINICAL EXAMPLES

Brachial Plexus Block

The brachial plexus can be blocked at several different levels from the interscalene groove to the axilla, or even more distally. Consequently, a number of approaches can be used to produce a block of the brachial plexus. However, because of the specific anatomic characteristics of the brachial plexus, the multiple-injection technique is not recommended for all approaches. For instance, the multiple-injection technique is suitable in the interscalene, axillary, and midhumeral approaches, but is not recommended for a supraclavicular brachial plexus block. This is due to the increased risk for complications related to the greater number of needle passes in the proximity of the pleural cavity and large blood vessels in this area. Multistimulation with the infraclavicular brachial plexus has been reported,[12,13] but it is the preference of this author that this technique should be reserved for those with significant experience. In this chapter, we will discuss the use of the multiple-injection technique for the interscalene, axillary, and midhumeral approaches to the brachial plexus block.

Interscalene Brachial Plexus Block

To perform an interscalene block using a multiple-stimulation technique, three different muscular twitches should be considered:

1. Contractions of the deltoid muscle, induced by stimulation of C4 and C5 roots.
2. Contractions of the biceps muscle with flexion of the forearm, induced by stimulation of the C6 root.
3. Contractions of the triceps muscle with extension of the forearm, induced by stimulation of the C7 root.

The patient is placed in a supine position with the head slightly turned away from the side to be blocked, similar to the single-injection technique. The interscalene groove formed by the anterior and middle scalene muscles is palpated at the level of the cricoid cartilage (C6). The nerve stimulator is set at 1 mA, 2 Hz, and 0.1 ms, and a 22- to 25-gauge, 3.75- to 5-cm needle is introduced at a 45-degree angle, with a slight caudal and posterior direction. The needle is advanced slowly until obtaining a specific motor response. The first motor response usually observed is contraction of the deltoid muscle. The position of the needle is then adjusted to maintain the same motor response with a current of 0.2 to 0.5 mA. After negative blood aspiration to rule out an intravascular needle placement, 8 mL of local anesthetic solution is slowly injected. Next, the insulated needle is withdrawn to the level of the skin, and the intensity of the current is increased to 1 to 1.5 mA. The needle is then introduced through the same skin insertion site in a more caudal direction on the same plane, identifying the projection of the brachial plexus between the two scalene muscles and running toward the midpoint of the clavicle and the sulcus between the pectoralis major and deltoid muscles, in order to elicit the second motor response

(contraction of the biceps muscle with flexion of the forearm). After obtaining the biceps muscle twitch at 0.2 to 0.5 mA, 6–8 mL of local anesthetic is injected after a careful aspiration test. Afterward, the insulated needle is withdrawn again to the level of the skin with the intensity of the current set at 1 to 1.5 mA and then introduced in a more caudal direction on the same plane identifying the pathway of the brachial plexus to elicit contractions of the triceps muscle with extension of the forearm. After the same twitch is elicited with a current ≤0.5 mA, another 6 mL of local anesthetic is injected slowly after a careful aspiration test.

Clinical Pearls

- The first motor response determines how the needle must be reoriented to look for the next motor response.
- Occasionally, it may be difficult to feel the interscalene groove at the C6 level; in these cases the groove can be more easily palpated at the level of the clavicle, where it is larger; from there, the groove can be followed cranially to the C6 level.

Axillary Brachial Plexus Block

The multiple-injection technique in the axillary brachial plexus block is based on eliciting motor responses from three or even four terminal nerves (the median, ulnar, radial, and musculocutaneous nerves). Accordingly, the muscular twitches that need to be elicited are:

1. Median nerve: Flexion of the wrist and fingers.
2. Radial nerve: Extension of the forearm or wrist and fingers, induced by the stimulation of the radial nerve.
3. Ulnar nerve: Flexion of the fourth and fifth fingers with adduction of the wrist or opposition of the first finger.
4. Musculocutaneous nerve: Contraction of the biceps muscle with flexion of the forearm.

At the level of the axilla, the trunks of the brachial plexus are already divided into their posterior and anterior divisions originating in the lateral, medial, and posterior cords. The axillary artery is surrounded by the nerves within the sheath, whereas at the level of the distal axilla the artery is surrounded by the terminal branches of the plexus: the radial, ulnar, and median nerves. The musculocutaneous nerve leaves the axilla more proximally, often as proximal as the coracoid process, entering the coracobrachialis muscle. The radial nerve is usually found posterior to the artery, the ulnar nerve lies on the inferior or posterior border of the artery, and the median nerve lies on the superior surface of the artery.

The patient is placed in the supine position with the arm to be blocked abducted and forming an angle of about 90 degrees, while the head is slightly turned toward the contralateral side. The landmarks are represented by the axillary artery, the inferior border of the pectoralis major muscle, and the coracobrachialis muscle. The nerve stimulator is set to deliver a stimulating current of 1- to 1.5-mA intensity, 0.1-ms duration, and 2-Hz frequency. A 3- to 5-cm, 22-gauge needle is usually inserted first above the axillary artery and as proximally as possible at the level of insertion of the long head of the biceps muscle to stimulate the musculocutaneous nerve. The position of the needle is then adjusted to maintain the same motor response with a current ≤0.5 mA; then, after negative aspiration, 5 mL of the anesthetic solution is slowly injected. The intensity of the stimulating current is then set again to 1 to 1.5 mA, and the needle is withdrawn to the skin and redirected to elicit the next twitch. Since the musculocutaneous nerve exits early from the brachial plexus, if the first twitch elicited is flexion of the forearm, the needle must be redirected more caudally and superficially, closer to the artery, in order to stimulate the median nerve; if the first nerve stimulated is the median nerve, the needle must be oriented more cranially toward the coracobrachialis muscle to stimulate the musculocutaneous nerve. Then the intensity is again decreased to 0.2 to 0.5 mA, and 5 mL of local anesthetic solution is injected. Since the ulnar and radial nerves run below and behind the axillary artery, stimulation of these nerves can be accomplished by redirecting the needle behind the axillary artery, or better yet, removing the needle and inserting it again through a second skin puncture performed below the axillary artery. The needle is then redirected behind the axillary artery looking for elicitation of extension of the arm, wrist, and fingers (stimulation of the radial nerve). After proper needle positioning with a stimulating intensity of 0.2 to 0.5 mA, and a negative aspiration test, 5 mL of local anesthetic solution is slowly injected. Then the needle is withdrawn to the skin, and the stimulating current increased to 1 to 1.5 mA, while the needle is reoriented looking for stimulation of the ulnar nerve (flexion of fourth and fifth fingers with the opposition of the first finger or adduction of the wrist). After the desired twitch is observed, the intensity of the stimulating current is progressively reduced to 0.2 to 0.5 mA; then, after a negative aspiration test, 5 mL of the local anesthetic solution is injected.

Clinical Pearls

- For multistimulation, one must have a clear three-dimensional idea of the paths of the nerves sought.
- When contractions of the biceps muscle are observed as the first muscular twitch, the next redirection of the stimulating needle (after the injection has been made) should be toward the artery to enter the brachial plexus sheath, since the musculocutaneous nerve exits early from the brachial plexus sheath.
- Elicitation of three of the four terminal nerves is enough to significantly improve the quality of the nerve block compared with that for the single-injection technique.
- Selective block of the ulnar nerve is not necessary if surgery does not directly involve the ulnar nerve territories.

Midhumeral Brachial Plexus Block

The terminal nerves reaching the upper limb exit from the axilla still surrounding the humeral artery, and then as they go toward the elbow, they progressively separate. The median nerve is usually felt superficially above the humeral artery in the proximal one-third of the arm, and the musculocutaneous nerve is located in the coracobrachialis muscle above the artery. In contrast, the ulnar and radial nerves are located below the artery, the ulnar nerve more superficial and the radial nerve deeper and close to the humerus. All of these nerves can be reached with the help of a nerve stimulator and blocked through a single skin puncture by moving and redirecting the stimulating needle.

The patient is placed supine with the arm abducted at 90 degrees. If possible, the forearm is also flexed at 90 degrees. The humeral artery is palpated in the proximal one-third of the humerus, and then the stimulating needle is inserted perpendicular to the skin above the artery with a stimulation frequency of 2 Hz and a stimulating current intensity of 1 mA. The needle is advanced approximately 1 to 2 cm under the skin until the flexion of wrist and fingers is elicited due to the stimulation of the median nerve. After a good contraction is elicited with an intensity ≤0.5 mA and after negative aspiration, 5–8 mL of local anesthetic solution is injected. Then the needle is withdrawn to the skin and reintroduced with an intensity of 1 to 1.5 mA at an angle of approximately 10 degrees more cranial toward the coracobrachialis muscle until biceps muscle contraction is elicited (stimulation of musculocutaneous nerve). Then, after aspiration and Raj tests, another 5 mL of the same anesthetic solution is injected. The needle is then withdrawn to the skin and redirected below the artery at an angle of 45 degrees with an intensity of 1 to 1.5 mA. It is advanced to a depth of approximately 2 cm until elicitation of opposition of the first finger and adduction of the wrist due to stimulation of the ulnar nerve with a stimulating intensity of 0.2 to 0.5 mA. Then, another 5–8 mL of the anesthetic solution is injected. The stimulating needle is then further advanced in the same direction with a 1- to 1.5-mA intensity until an extension of the wrist and fingers is elicited due to stimulation of the radial nerve. Once the muscular twitch is elicited with an intensity of 0.2 to 0.5 mA, another 5–8 mL of the same anesthetic solution is injected.

Femoral Nerve Block

To perform a femoral nerve block using the multiple-stimulation technique, three different muscular stimulations should be elicited: (1) contraction of the vastus medialis, induced by stimulation of the vastus medialis/saphenous nerve; (2) contraction of the rectus femoris muscle with movements of the patella, induced by the stimulation of the vastus intermedius nerve; and (3) contraction of the vastus lateralis muscle, induced by stimulation of the vastus lateralis nerve.

The patient is placed in a supine position. The needle is inserted just lateral to the femoral artery at the level of the inguinal crease and advanced perpendicularly to the skin. Usually the contraction of the vastus medialis is the first to be elicited. The needle position is then adjusted to maintain the same motor response with a stimulating current intensity of 0.2 to 0.5 mA. After negative aspiration, 5–6 mL of local anesthetic is slowly injected. Then the intensity of the stimulating current is increased to 1.5 mA, and the needle is oriented slightly laterally and introduced again in search of contraction of the rectus femoris with movement of the patella. Again, the needle position is adjusted to maintain the motor response with a stimulating current intensity of 0.2 to 0.5 mA. After negative aspiration, another 5–6 mL of the same anesthetic solution is injected. Finally, the insulated needle is withdrawn at the level of the skin, and the intensity of the stimulating current is increased to 1.5 mA. The needle is redirected more laterally by increasing the angle by another 2–3 degrees and then reintroducing it in search of contraction of the vastus lateralis muscle. Again, the needle position is then adjusted to maintain the motor response with an intensity of 0.2 to 0.5 mA. After negative aspiration, an additional 5–6 mL of local anesthetic solution is injected.

Clinical Pearls

- To minimize the risk of arterial puncture, the initial insertion of the needle should be in a sagittal plane; individual branches of the femoral nerve are best localized by redirecting the needle laterally (away from the artery).

- The contraction of the vastus lateralis muscle is often associated with residual movements of the patella and sometimes can only be seen distally at the level of the knee.

- Often contraction of the vastus lateralis is preceded by contraction of the sartorious muscle; to obtain the desired motor response, the needle needs to be introduced slightly deeper, maintaining the same direction.

- Contrary to the 3-in-1 block, a multiple-injection femoral nerve block does not result in block of the lateral femoral cutaneous and obturator nerves; if these blocks are required they need to be performed individually, or the injected volume must be significantly increased.

Sciatic Nerve Block

Stimulation of the sciatic nerve produces motor responses that vary according to the level at which the nerve is stimulated. At a high level (parasacral, posterior, and subgluteal), three types of responses are elicited:

1. Dorsiflexion or eversion of the foot, induced by stimulation of the common peroneal branch of the sciatic nerve.
2. Plantar flexion of the foot and toes produced by the stimulation of the tibial branch of the sciatic nerve.
3. Contraction of the biceps femoris induced by stimulation of the branches innervating the hamstring muscles. Above the knee (lateral sciatic and posterior popliteal), only contractions of the foot and toe muscles are observed. Although the sciatic nerve branches divide into the common peroneal and tibial nerves above or at the level of the popliteal fossa, the two branches can be clearly identified from their origin.

High Sciatic Approaches

Labat's Approach

NEEDLE SIZE. A 10- to 12-cm (sometimes 15-cm for very obese patients) insulated needle.

LANDMARKS. A line is drawn from the posterior superior iliac spine to the midpoint of the greater trochanter. A perpendicular line is drawn bisecting this line and intersecting a second line drawn from the greater trochanter to the sacral hiatus. The intersection of these two lines indicates the point of needle entry.

Subgluteal Approach

NEEDLE SIZE. A 5- to 8-cm insulated needle.

LANDMARKS. The patient is placed in the lateral decubitus position, with the leg to be blocked up with the knee flexed at 90 degrees (Sim position). A line is drawn from the greater trocanter to the ischial tuberosity. From the midpoint of this line a second line is drawn perpendicularly and extending caudally for 4 cm. At this level a skin depression is palpated, representing the groove between the biceps femoris and the lateral border of the quadriceps muscle. This point represents the needle entry.

TECHNIQUE. The patient is placed in the Sim position. The needle is introduced perpendicularly to the skin and advanced slowly until a stimulation of either the common peroneal or the tibial nerve is elicited. The position of the needle is then adjusted to maintain the same motor response with a stimulating current of 0.2 to 0.5 mA. After negative aspiration, 6–10 mL of the local anesthetic solution is injected. The stimulating needle is withdrawn to the level of the skin with a stimulating current set at 1 to 1.5 mA and then redirected slightly either laterally (if the tibial nerve was first stimulated) or medially (if the common peroneal nerve was first stimulated) and advanced until the appropriate motor response is elicited. The position of the needle is then adjusted to maintain the same motor response with a stimulating current of 0.2 to 0.5 mA. After negative blood aspiration, 8–10 mL of local anesthetic solution is injected.

Clinical Pearls

- Considering the length of the stimulating needle and the depth of the sciatic nerve, the changes in the angle direction should be very minor.
- Avoid flexing the stimulating needle; keeping the shaft of the needle straight markedly improves the predictability of the needle tip location.
- The depth at which the first motor response is obtained is a reliable clue as to how deeply the needle must be inserted to block the consecutive nerves (branches).

Popliteal Approaches

At the level of the popliteal fossa the two branches of the sciatic nerve divide, and the more caudally the nerve is approached, the more distant the two branches are from one another. The spatial distribution of common peroneal and tibial nerves must also be considered. The tibial nerve lies closer to the bone and more medial, and thus it is slightly more anterior and deeper than the common peroneal nerve when we approach it from the lateral side of the thigh. In contrast, the common peroneal nerve is more lateral and superficial and exits the popliteal fossa just above the head of the fibula. To perform a multiple-stimulation sciatic nerve block at the popliteal fossa, a proximal approach is usually recommended.

Posterior Popliteal Sciatic Nerve Block

NEEDLE SIZE.   A 22-gauge, 5- to 8-cm insulated needle.

LANDMARKS AND TECHNIQUE.   The popliteal fossa is a triangle defined by the tendon of the biceps femoris muscle laterally, the semitendinosus and semimembranosus muscles medially, and the popliteal crease caudally. At the lower part of the popliteal fossa, the sciatic nerve comes into proximity of the popliteal artery and vein. The tibial and common peroneal nerves are medial to the tendon of the biceps femoris 4–6 cm deep to the skin. The patient is placed in a prone position. The site of introduction of the needle is 7 cm from the popliteal crease and 1 cm lateral to middle. The needle is introduced perpendicular to the skin in search of a motor response related to either the stimulation of the common peroneal or tibial nerve (usually the common peroneal nerve). The needle position is adjusted to maintain the same motor response with a stimulating current ≤0.5 mA. After negative aspiration for blood, 10 mL of local anesthetic solution is injected. As with all approaches to the sciatic nerve, the first motor response determines how the needle is oriented when searching for the next motor response. If the first motor response elicited is dorsiflexion of the foot (common peroneal nerve), the needle will be directed more medially and slightly deeper in search of stimulation of the tib-

ial nerve (plantar flexion with flexion of the toes); if the first motor response is plantar flexion of the foot (tibial nerve), the stimulating needle will be redirected more laterally.

Lateral Popliteal Sciatic Nerve Block

NEEDLE SIZE.   A 22-gauge, 10-cm insulated needle.

LANDMARKS AND TECHNIQUE.   The patient is placed in the supine position with a pillow under the leg. A vertical line is drawn at the level of the superior border of the patella. The site of introduction of the needle is represented by the intersection of this line and the line drawn at the level of the groove between the biceps femoris and the sartorius muscles. The needle is inserted with an angle of 20 to 30 degrees posterior to the horizontal plane with a slight caudal direction, and advanced slowly in search usually of the common peroneal nerve, which produces either a dorsiflexion or an eversion of the foot. The needle position is then adjusted to maintain the same motor response with a stimulating current intensity of 0.2 to 0.5 mA. After negative aspiration, 8–10 mL of local anesthetic solution is injected. Next the needle is withdrawn to the skin and oriented at 45 degrees.

The tibial nerve is located more medially and slightly deeper than the common peroneal nerve. Its stimulation produces plantar flexion and flexion of the toes. The needle position is then adjusted to maintain the same motor response with a stimulating current intensity of 0.2 to 0.5 mA. After negative aspiration, 8–10 mL of local anesthetic solution is injected.

SUMMARY

In summary, multistimulation techniques for peripheral nerve blocks have been introduced relatively recently to clinical practice. Multiple injection of smaller volumes of local anesthetic after localization of major components of the peripheral nerve or more commonly, plexuses, are logically expected to result in a faster onset, higher success rate, and reduced volume of local anesthetic necessary to achieve clinically satisfactory blockade. Initial clinical experience with multistimulation techniques suggests that multiple injection is not associated with significantly higher risk of neurologic complications. However, more research is necessary before this can be extrapolated to general practice because the currently available reports emanated from a few select institutions and authors with unique expertise in peripheral nerve blocks. As the multistimulation techniques are continually refined, better methods to localize nerves (ultrasound) and avoid excessive injection force and intraneural injection become available in a near future, multistimulation may become the preferred method to many currently practiced peripheral nerve block techniques.

References

1. Lavoie J, Martin R, Tetrault JP, et al: Axillary plexus block using peripheral nerve stimulator: Single or multiple injections. Can J Anaesth 1992;39:583–586.

2. Koscielniak-Nielsen ZJ, Rotboll Nielsen P, Sorensen T, et al: Low dose axillary block by targeted injections of the terminal nerves. Can J Anaesth 1999;46:658–664.

3. Sia S, Bartoli M: Selective ulnar nerve localization is not essential for axillary brachial plexus block using a multiple nerve stimulation technique. Reg Anesth Pain Med 2001;26:12–6.

4. Koscielniak-Nielsen ZJ, Stens-Pedersen HL, Lippert FK: Readiness for surgery after axillary block: Single or multiple injection techniques. Eur J Anaesth 1997;14:164–171.

5. Fanelli G, Casati A, Beccaria P, et al: Interscalene brachial plexus anaesthesia with small volumes of ropivacaine 0.75%: Effects of the injection technique on the onset time of nerve blockade. Eur J Anaesthesiol 2001;18:54–58.

6. Paqueron X, Bouaziz H, Macalou D, et al: The lateral approach to the sciatic nerve at the popliteal fossa: One or two injections? Anesth Analg 1999;89:1221–1225.

7. Casati A, Fanelli G, Beccaria P, et al: The effects of the single or multiple injection technique on the onset time of femoral nerve blocks with 0.75% ropivacaine. Anesth Analg 2000;91:181–184.

8. Casati A, Fanelli G, Beccaria P, et al: The effects of single or multiple injections on the volume of 0.5% ropivacaine required for femoral nerve blockade. Anesth Analg 2001;93:183–186.

9. Serradell A, Herrero R, Villanueva JA, et al: Comparison of three different volumes of mepivacaine in axillary plexus block using multiple nerve stimulation. Br J Anaesth 2003;91:519–524.

10. Fanelli G, Casati A, Garancini P, et al: Nerve stimulator and multiple injection technique for upper and lower limb blockade: Failure rate, patient acceptance, and neurologic complications. Anesth Analg 1999;88:847–852.

11. Auroy Y, Benhamou D, Bargues L, et al: Major complications of regional anesthesia in France: The SOS Regional Anesthesia Hotline Service. Anesthesiology 2002;97:1274–1280.

12. Gaertner E, Estebe JP, Zamfir A, et al: Infraclavicular plexus block: Multiple injection versus single injection. Reg Anesth Pain Med 2002;27:590–594.

13. Rodriguez J, Barcena M, Taboada-Muniz M, et al: A comparison of single versus multiple injections on the extent of anesthesia with coracoid infraclavicular brachial plexus block. Anesth Analg 2004;99:1225–1230.

47

Injection & Current Delivery Monitoring

Christopher Robards, MD • Admir Hadzic, MD

I. GENERAL CONSIDERATIONS
  Monitoring the Depth of Needle Insertion
  Current Delivery & Disconnect Monitoring
  Resistance to Injection

II. NERVE PRELOCALIZATION USING SURFACE STIMULATION

 GENERAL CONSIDERATIONS

Only in the past decade or so has research on functional regional anesthesia anatomy, outcome, and equipment slowly begun to transform regional anesthesia into a modern discipline. However, in many ways the equipment used for peripheral nerve block remains in its infancy. The sophistication and functionality of the equipment used for peripheral nerve blocks (PNBs) are, at best, rudimentary and lag far behind those of general anesthesia, as depicted in the following examples.

Monitoring the Depth of Needle Insertion

Spinal cord injury after interscalene block is perhaps the most serious complication of a PNB. This devastating complication, however, can occur only with an excessively deep needle insertion (ie, >2.5 cm).[1] Monitoring the depth of the needle insertion is substantially important to avoid a too-deep insertion (eg, spinal cord or chest cavity with interscalene block). In fact, the recently suggested standardized block documentation procedure requires clinicians to document the depth at which the needle is inserted. Nevertheless, most commercially available needles still do not have depth markings for such objective documentation.[2] Despite that fact, there is much work underway to remedy this deficiency, and it is inevitable that all needles used in regional anesthesia will eventually incorporate depth markings on their shafts.

Current Delivery & Disconnect Monitoring

Nerve stimulator–assisted nerve localization has become a standard technique in PNB. In contrast to paresthesia techniques, nerve stimulation provides a more objective assessment of the needle position in relation to the nerve, does not require patient cooperation, and permits the use of sedatives and analgesics for patient comfort during a nerve block procedure. The basic premise of the nerve stimulator–assisted nerve blocks is that the electrical current ("field") in front of the advancing needle should elicit a motor response before the tip of the needle enters the nerve. In many nerve block techniques, a functioning nerve stimulator is essential to decrease the risk of inadvertent placement of the needle intraneurally or intravascularly. For instance, because of the close proximity of the subclavian artery anterior and inferior to the brachial plexus during cervical paravertebral block, the functionality of the nerve stimulator is of paramount importance to avoid vascular complications.[3] With a functioning nerve stimulator, a motor response of the shoulder muscle is seen when the brachial plexus is stimulated, which should occur before the subclavian artery is punctured by the advancing needle. In the case series on continuous paravertebral blocks using a stimulating catheter reported by Boezaart et al.,[3] vascular complications consisting of large-vessel puncture with a 17-gauge needle occurred only in patients in whom the nerve stimulators were found to be malfunctional.

Consequently, the ability of the nerve stimulator to deliver accurate current output and integrity of the stimulator-needle-return (skin) electrode circuit is of utmost importance for both the block success and the safety of the procedure. Problems with the reliability and accuracy of nerve stimulators have long been recognized but have been addressed only within the past few years by introduction of modern, constant-current, PNB-specific nerve stimulators.[4,5] However, the contemporary nerve stimulators still do not incorporate a convenient means of continuously monitoring current delivery by the operator to allow detection of a nerve stimulator malfunction that could lead to complications.[3]

The following case summaries describe several scenarios in which malfunction of the nerve stimulators or electrical connection was not detected owing to the absence of a convenient means of monitoring current delivery.

Example 1: A 90-year-old, 4-ft 10-in., 112-pound woman presented to the operating room with an infected right arm after open reduction and internal fixation of a fracture of her right humerus. She was scheduled to undergo incision and drainage of her right arm under interscalene brachial plexus block. After application of standard ASA (American Society of Anesthesiologists) monitors, the patient was premedicated with midazolam 2 mg IV, and the equipment, consisting of a Stimuplex-DIG nerve stimulator (B. Braun Medical, Inc.) and an insulated 22-gauge × 2-in. needle (Stimuplex A2250) was prepared. The return electrode (ECG electrode, Cleartrace, CONMED, Utica, NY) was placed on the right forearm. Interscalene technique through the classic approach was attempted with the nerve stimulator current set at 1.0 mA. Although the patient had easily identifiable landmarks, nerve stimulation could not be obtained despite multiple needle passes and changes of the needle entry site. During the attempts, the LCD (liquid crystal display) on the nerve stimulator did not indicate a problem with the patency of the electrical circuit. After the anesthesia team empirically switched to another nerve stimulator (the same model), nerve stimulation was promptly accomplished. A defective nerve stimulator was determined to be responsible for the many unsuccessful attempts at nerve localization, yet the operator was unaware of the equipment malfunction.

Example 2: A 31-year-old, 5-ft 2-in., 135-lb man with a history of end-stage renal disease was scheduled to undergo creation of an A-V fistula in the left arm. Interscalene brachial plexus block was planned as the anesthesia technique. After premedication with midazolam 2 mg IV and identification of the anatomic landmarks, a block was attempted using a Stimuplex DIG nerve stimulator and Stimuplex 22-gauge, 2–in. insulated needle. Several attempts to localize the brachial plexus using the initial current of 1.5 mA did not produce a twitch response. Several more attempts using another nerve stimulator (the same model) evoked no motor response. At this point, it was noticed that when the current setting was raised above 0.5 mA, the nerve stimulator indicated that the set current was not being delivered. It is possible that both stimulators indicated disconnect, but this could have been overlooked while the anesthesia team was preoccupied with the block technique. Careful inspection of the electrical connections led to detection of the defect in the connecting cable–needle assembly. Changing the stimulating needle, while paying close attention to the wire connection between the needle and the nerve stimulator, quickly led to a prompt motor response at 0.35 mA and a successful block for surgery.

Example 3: A 61-year-old, 5-ft 2-in., 169-lb woman with a history of mild asthma was scheduled to undergo repair of her left shoulder rotator cuff under interscalene brachial plexus block. Midazolam 4 mg was given intravenously, anatomic landmarks were identified, and the area was cleaned using povidone-iodine solution. Interscalene block was then attempted with a Stimuplex nerve stimulator and the 22-gauge × 2-in. insulated needle. With the return ECG electrode (3M) placed on the arm and the stimulator set to deliver 1.0 mA, several attempts to localize the brachial plexus were made without success. At this point, it was noted that the LCD on the stimulator indicated that the electrical circuit was incomplete. Checking all wire connections, changing several needles, and using multiple nerve stimulators were all unsuccessful in fixing the problem. As the last resort, the return ECG electrode was taken off the patient's arm and connected to the tip of the needle, at which point the LCD disconnect alert stopped blinking, indicating that the electrical circuit was completed. However, when a new ECG (3M) electrode was applied to the skin, the LCD again indicated that the set current was not being delivered. Firm pressure on the ECG electrode against the patient's skin resulted in the disappearance of the disconnect signal on the LCD. It became apparent that the "problem" was with the skin electrodes. Indeed, on careful inspection, the ECG electrodes were found to be desiccated and lacked their original conductive properties.

When measured with an ohmmeter, the electrical resistance ranged between several kiloOhms and several megaOhms (normal resistance is very low and typically does not exceed a few ohms). Changing the ECG electrode to an ECG electrode from a freshly opened stock resulted in the disappearance of the disconnect alarm and allowed nerve localization to be accomplished.

These case summaries emphasize the importance of ensuring proper functionality of the nerve stimulator and detection of abnormal circuit impedance (desiccated, poorly conducting skin electrode, circuit disconnect, or stimulator failure) or electric disconnect to successfully localize a peripheral nerve, achieve reliable blockade, and avoid needle trauma to the nerve. Unfortunately, there are no manufacturing standards when it comes to alarms, which can indicate a problem with the delivery of the current. Although older models of nerve stimulators did not incorporate a disconnect indicator at all, most new models of nerve stimulators incorporate a disconnect indicator. However, the indicators of the functionality are located on the nerve stimulator (thus, remotely from the operator) and vary substantially in how they display the information when there is a problem with the circuit connections, nerve stimulator, or return electrode–skin contact.

Some stimulators deliver an audible signal only when the current *is* successfully delivered; some emit an audible signal when the current is *not* delivered; others do not have any indicators. In a typical clinical setting, it may be rather challenging for the operator to concentrate on the block technique, observe the motor response, communicate with the patient, and monitor the information provided by a small-sized and difficult-to-read LCD indicator of the nerve stimulator on the current setting and occurrence of a disconnect.

The functionality of the nerve stimulator and the integrity of the circuit can and should be checked *before* the block procedure; however, many problems with the current delivery occur *during* the actual block procedure, such as electrical disconnect, nerve stimulator battery failure, and skin–electrode disconnect. For this reason, whenever nerve localization proves challenging, clinicians should often suspect a problem with the equipment (peripheral nerve stimulator) or electrical circuit as another variable in addition to the possible anatomic difficulties (ie, insertion of the needle in a wrong plane or a wrong anatomic position).

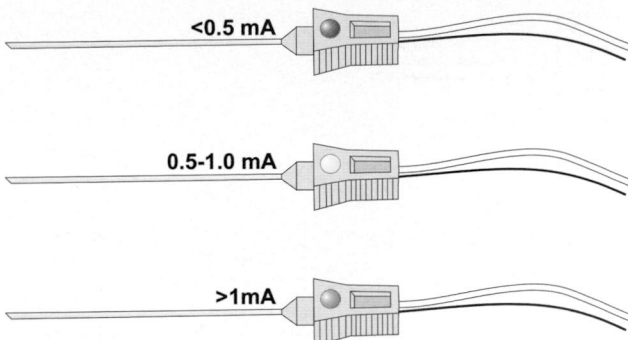

Figure 47–1. A needle with a current delivery monitor mounted on the hub of the needle. An LCD (liquid crystal display) flashes only when the current is reliably delivered. The color of the light indicates the current intensity (eg, green >1.0 mA, yellow 0.5–1.0 mA, red < 0.5 mA). Such a design allows the clinician to have real-time, continuous information on the current intensity, circuit integrity, and nerve stimulator functionality. Similar designs may incorporate a digital display with a similar information.

a design would allow continuous monitoring of the current delivery by the clinician performing the block, as well an immediate detection of the circuit disconnect or other electrical problems (eg, stimulator failure).

Resistance to Injection

Assessing resistance to injection during PNB is a common practice.[2] This practice is similar to the loss of resistance to injection of air or saline using a "syringe feel" during administration of epidural, paravertebral, or lumbar plexus blocks (Figure 47–2). Assessing tissue compliance has long been used as an additional means of estimating the anatomic location

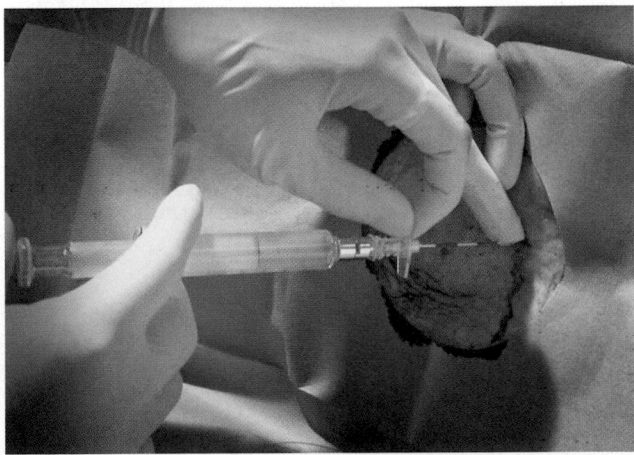

Figure 47–2. Resistance to injection of air or saline is routinely used in epidural anesthesia techniques to identify the epidural space. Because tissue layers vary in their compliance to injection of solutions, change of the resistance to injection as the needle exits the ligament (high resistance) and enters the epidural space (low resistance) helps to determine the location of the tip of the epidural needle. Similar concepts can be used to avoid intraneural injections or injection into tight compartments containing nerves to decrease the risk of mechanical/pressure injury to the nerves.

Clinical Pearls

The following steps should be taken before attempting a nerve stimulator–assisted nerve localization:

1. Clinicians should be familiar with how the nerve stimulator indicates proper current delivery and failure to deliver the set stimulus (disconnect alarm).

2. Only high-quality skin electrodes should be used for nerve localization.

3. Before application, the skin electrode should be visually and palpably inspected to ensure that the conducting gel is present and not desiccated.

4. Clinicians should verify the absence of the disconnect alarm as soon as the needle is inserted into skin and should periodically check the LCD indicator during the procedure to ensure that the set current is being delivered.

Inevitably, equipment designed in the future should incorporate a remote indicator of current delivery, which would be best mounted on the hub of the needle (Figure 47–1). Such

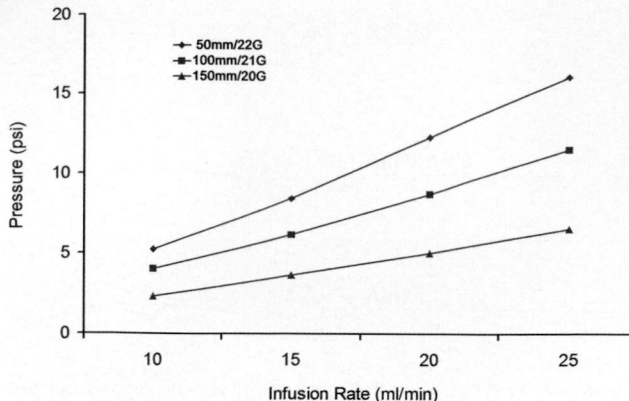

Figure 47–3. Resistance to injection of solutions significantly varies among needle designs and depends on injection speed. These factors combine to make subjective assessment of what constitutes normal or abnormal resistance to injection unreliable.

of the needle tip during application of a PNB. For this, clinicians typically use a "syringe feel" to estimate what may be an abnormal resistance to nerve block injection to reduce the risk of intraneural injection.[6–8] However, this practice has significant inherent limitations because of the subjective nature of the assessment and the inherent variability in the feel.[9] In addition, the resistance to injection is greater with smaller needles, adding to the confusion as to what constitutes normal or abnormal resistance (Figure 47–3). In contrast to loss of resistance in an epidural injection, there is no baseline pressure information or change in tissue compliance during nerve block injection, which means that with nerve block injection, there is no change in pressure that can be relied on. In a study by Claudio and colleagues,[9] all anesthesiologists detected a *change* in pressure of as little as 0.5 psi during a simulated nerve block injection. However, when gauging the absolute pressure, clinicians substantially varied (by as much

as 40 psi) in their perceptions of what constituted an appropriate resistance to injection. In addition, no information has been available on what constitutes normal and abnormal injection pressure during nerve block performance (Figure 47–4).

When asked to inject local anesthetic for a colleague performing a simulated interscalene block in a mannequin, the studied anesthesiologists significantly varied in their perception of what constituted normal versus abnormal resistance (pressure) to injection. A substantial number of injections resulted in pressures higher than 20 psi. If needles were indeed inserted intraneurally, such injection pressures would allow an intraneural administration of local anesthetic and consequent neurologic injury.

To explain the mechanisms responsible for the development of neuraxial anesthesia after an interscalene block,[10,11] Selander and coworkers[12] injected solutions of local anesthetic into rabbit sciatic nerves and traced the spread of the anesthetic along the nerve sheath. They postulated that an intraneural injection results in significant intraneural spread of local anesthetic. In their model, the investigators noticed that intraneural injections often resulted in much higher injection pressures than those required for perineural injections. Injection into a nerve fascicle resulted in rupture of the perineurium and histologic evidence of disruption of the fascicular anatomy. Researchers in this study, however, used a small animal model, microinjections (10–200 μL), miniature needles, clinically irrelevant injection rates (100–300 μL/min), and did not study neurologic consequences after intraneural injections. For these reasons, their foretelling of results on the possible association of injection pressure with intrafascicular injection did not generate the deserved interest among researchers and clinicians.

More recent studies used more clinically applicable injection speeds and volumes of local anesthetic in a large animal model.[5] The results of these studies suggest that

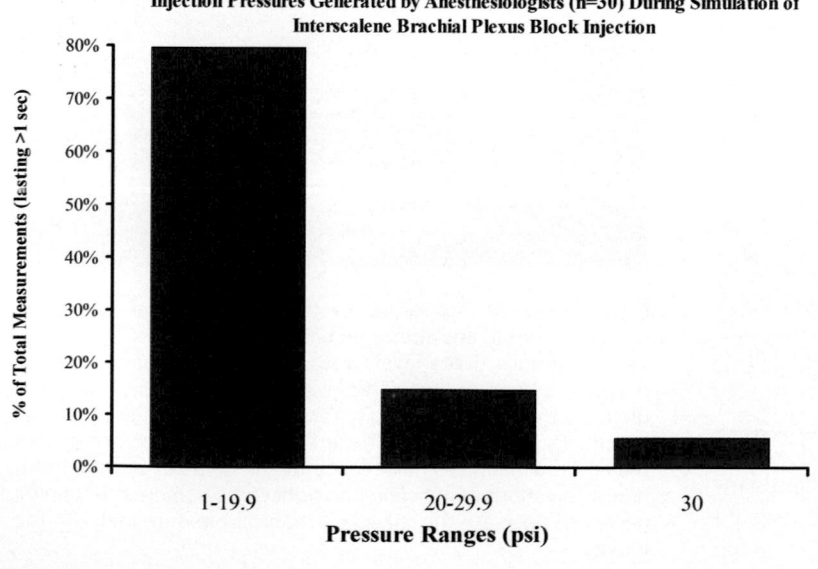

Figure 47–4. Subjective assessment of the resistance to injection significantly varies among anesthesiologists. In a simulation of the interscalene brachial plexus block, tested anesthesiologists often used excessive force (pressure) to inject local anesthetic (>20 psi). Had this occurred in actual patients and the needle was lodged intraneurally, a neurologic complication could have occurred.

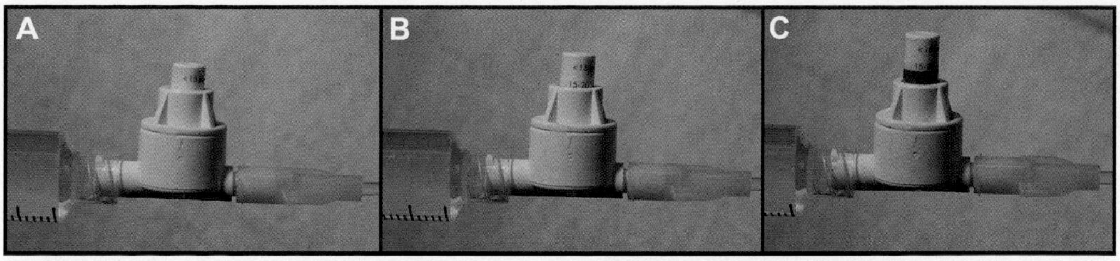

Figure 47–5. An example of an in-line injection pressure monitor. **A:** As the injection begins, the piston engages and raises to indicate the injection pressure. **B:** Normal injection pressures range from 5 to 20 psi using typical injection speed of 10–20 mL/min. **C:** When the injection pressure reaches 20 psi, the piston turns red, indicating that the pressure required to inject intrafascicularly has been reached. Similar designs may incorporate digital displays with similar information.

perineural injections are associated with low-injection pressures (<15–20 psi). In contrast, high-injection pressures (>20 psi) are associated with intrafascicular injections and as such carry a risk of neurologic injury.[5] In the dog model of intraneural injury, only intraneural injections resulting in pressures greater than 20 psi were associated with clinically detectable neurologic deficits as well as histologic evidence of injury to nerve fascicles.[13]

Note that current evidence suggests that neurologic injury does not always develop after an intraneural injection.[14] In fact, injection after an intraneural needle placement is more likely to result in deposition of the local anesthetic between and not into the fascicles.[5] Intraneural, but *extrafascicular* (interfascicular) injection, probably occurs more commonly than thought in clinical practice.[14] Such an injection results in a block of fast onset and long duration rather than in a neurologic injury.[13] This is because an intraneural but extrafascicular injection leads to intimate exposure of nerve fascicles to high concentration of local anesthetics. In this scenario, permanent neurologic injury does not develop because the local anesthetic is deposited *outside* the fascicles and the block slowly resolves after the injection without evidence of histologic derangement. However, intraneural *intrafascicular* needle placement results in high injection pressures and leads to neurologic injury.

For these reasons, subjective estimation of resistance to injection is at least as inaccurate as, perhaps, estimating blood pressure by palpating radial artery pulse. Objective means of assessing resistance to injection should be far superior in standardizing injection force and pressure. The future needle–syringe designs for use in PNBs will inevitably incorporate a simple, unobtrusive, and inexpensive in-line pressure monitor to allow clinicians to avoid injection force (pressure) consistent with intraneural injection. Figure 47–5 is an example of such a system.

NERVE PRELOCALIZATION USING SURFACE STIMULATION

Administration of PNBs relies on localization of a peripheral nerve using a percutaneously placed needle aimed at the nerve

to be blocked. Electrical current used for the purpose of nerve localization with PNBs is of a relatively low intensity (typically 0.2 mA–2 mA). Astute knowledge of anatomy is essential to avoid multiple needle insertions during attempts at nerve localization. However, a current of higher intensity (5–20 mA) can be used to transcutaneously stimulate and prelocalize nerves before needle insertion.

It is interesting that this practice is relatively new in peripheral nerve blockade despite the fact that the equipment has been available for decades and that the same principle is used on a daily basis in general anesthesia. For instance, stimulation of a motor nerve and evaluation of the resultant motor response constitute standard monitoring of the neuromuscular junction after the administration of muscle relaxants. The principle behind neuromuscular monitoring is that an electrical stimulus applied using a cutaneous electrode over a nerve should result in depolarization of the nerve and a consequent certain degree of motor response distal to the stimulation. Neuromuscular monitoring constitutes the nerve stimulator and stimulating electrodes (typically pre-gelled surface electrodes). Electrical current is applied using a peripheral nerve stimulator designed to deliver current intensity up to 80 mA (up to 700 volts in some units).[4]

Similar to monitoring of the function of the neuromuscular junction, surface prelocation of the peripheral nerves is possible, primarily with nerves and plexi that are superficial (eg, interscalene, axillary, femoral nerves). This is because the electrical current flows in all directions from the electrode and not necessarily toward the nerve or a plexus. Consequently, the intensity of the current reaching the nerve is inadequate to depolarize nerve(s) that are deeper below the skin surface.

Figure 47–6 demonstrates the apparatus and the procedure. In short, the electrode sites are prepared with a degreasing agent (eg, alcohol) to decrease the skin resistance and increase the loss of the stimulus at the electrode–skin interface. The stimulation is usually begun with a current of 5 mA when a stimulus of longer duration is used (eg, 1 ms) or up to 20 mA when a stimulus of shorter duration is used (eg, 0.1 ms). Once a distal motor response specific to the nerve under localization is elicited, the current is lowered to the minimal intensity at which this response is still seen or felt.

re-angling is often necessary to needle-electrolocalize (percutaneous) the nerve.

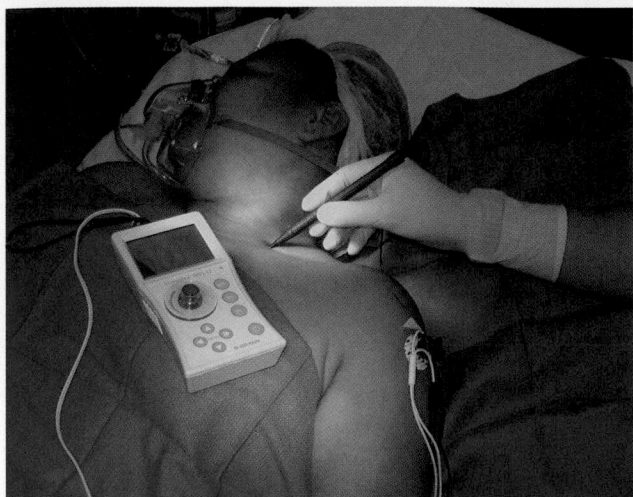

Figure 47–6. Transcutaneous stimulation of the brachial plexus in the axilla for the purpose of nerve prelocalization. For this purpose, electrical charge significantly greater than that used for needle nerve localization is used. This can be accomplished using a 5-mA, 1-ms setting on the nerve stimulator or using a higher-current output stimulator, such as units used for monitoring of neuromuscular blockade (10–20 mA). Once the motor response is obtained using current of minimal intensity, the needle entry point is marked on the skin and a stimulating needle connected to a low-output nerve stimulator is inserted.

The point on the skin at which the stimulation is elicited with the minimal possible current is labeled as the approximate position of the nerve (plexus). During the localization, the electrode is continuously and firmly pressed against the skin to shorten the skin–nerve distance and decrease the resistance of the skin–electrode interface (Figure 47–6).

In some patients, stimulation with a current of significantly greater intensity than 5 mA may be necessary to evoke a motor response. In these patients, a higher output nerve stimulator (ie, a unit used for neuromuscular monitoring) can be used. The current is set at 15–20 mA and applied via an alligator clip; the current is decreased as the motor response is established. It is important to realize, however, that surface nerve prelocation provides only a rough estimate of the location of the nerve or a plexus, and needle repositioning and

References

1. Benumof J: Permanent loss of cervical spinal cord function associated with interscalene block performed under general anesthesia. Anesthesiology 2000;93:1541–1544.
2. Gerancher J, Viscusi E, Liguori G, et al: Development of a standardized peripheral nerve block procedure note form. Reg Anesth Pain Med 2005;30:67–71.
3. Boezaart A, De Beer J, Nell M: Early experience with continuous cervical paravertebral block using a stimulating catheter. Reg Anesth Pain Med 2003;28:406–413.
4. Hadzic A, Vloka J, Hadzic H, et al: Nerve stimulators used for peripheral nerve blocks vary in their electrical characteristics. Anesthesiology 2003;98:969–974.
5. Vloka J, Hadzic A, Mulcare R, et al: Combined popliteal and posterior cutaneous nerve of the thigh blocks for short saphenous vein stripping in outpatients: An alternative to spinal anesthesia. J Clin Anesth 1997;9:618–622.
6. Weaver M, Tandatnick C, Hahn M: Peripheral nerve blockade. In: Raj P (editor): *Regional Anesthesia.* Churchill Livingstone, 2002, pp. 857–870.
7. Selander D: Peripheral nerve injury after regional anesthesia. In: Finucane B (editor): *Complications of Regional Anesthesia.* Churchill Livingstone, 1999, pp. 105–115.
8. Jankovic D, Wells C: Brachial plexus. In: Jankovic D, Wells C (editors): *Regional Nerve Blocks,* 2nd ed. Blackwell Science Berlin, 2001, pp. 58–86.
9. Claudio RE, Hadzic A, Shih H, et al: Injection pressures by anesthesiologists during simulated peripheral nerve block. Reg Anesth Pain Med 2004;29:201–205.
10. Passannante AN: Spinal anesthesia and permanent neurologic deficit after interscalene block. Anesth Analg 1996;82:873–874.
11. Dutton RP, Eckhardt WF III, Sunder N: Total spinal anesthesia after interscalene blockade of the brachial plexus. Anesthesiology 1994;80:939–941.
12. Selander D, Sjostrand J: Longitudinal spread of intraneurally injected local anesthetics. An experimental study of the initial neural distribution following intraneural injections. Acta Anesth Scand 1978;22:622–634.
13. Hadzic A, Dilberovic F, Shah S, et al: Combination of intraneural injection and high injection pressure leads to severe fascicular injury and neurologic deficits in dogs. Reg Anesth Pain Med 2004;29:417–423.
14. Sala-Blanch X, Pomes J, Matute P, et al: Intraneural injection during anterior approach for sciatic nerve block. Anesthesiology 2004;101:1027–1030.

48

Equipment for Continuous Peripheral Nerve Blocks

Holly Evans, MD • Karen C. Nielsen, MD • Roy A. Greengrass, MD • Susan M. Steele, MD

I. INTRODUCTION

II. HISTORICAL PERSPECTIVE

III. CURRENTLY AVAILABLE EQUIPMENT

IV. FUTURE DIRECTIONS

INTRODUCTION

Continuous peripheral nerve blocks (CPNBs) provide many advantages in the perioperative period.[1] These techniques provide the flexibility to prolong intraoperative anesthesia while avoiding the risks and side effects of general anesthesia. After surgery, CPNBs offer extended postoperative analgesia. When compared with parenteral opioid analgesia, CPNBs are associated with superior analgesia, reduced opioid consumption, and decreased opioid-related side effects such as postoperative nausea and vomiting, sedation, and respiratory depression.[2–12] Analgesia results are of a quality similar to epidural anesthesia results; however, CPNBs are associated with less hypotension, urinary retention, pruritus, and mobility restrictions than epidural analgesia.[8,13–15] There is also evidence supporting the beneficial effect of CPNBs on postoperative sleep patterns and cognitive function[16,17] as well as early rehabilitation.[8,9] Concurrent sympathectomy is ideal after microvascular surgery, reimplantation, and free-flap surgery[18,19] as well as for treatment of accidental intraarterial drug injection.[20–22] Extended analgesia can also be provided for chronic pain patients[23] and those requiring palliation of terminal illness.[24]

Despite these benefits, CPNBs have historically been relatively underused techniques. These reasons for the underutilization were multifactorial; however, inadequate CPNB equipment likely contributed. Until recently, there had been few commercially available equipment items dedicated for CPNBs. A number of relatively new advances in the area of CPNB needles and catheters have been essential for the safe use and advancement of these regional anesthesia techniques. This chapter summarizes the chronology of the development of CPNB equipment, outlines currently available equipment, and theorizes about possible future directions.

HISTORICAL PERSPECTIVE

The earliest report of CPNB is attributed to Ansbro[25] in 1946 (Figure 48–1). He attached a malleable blunt needle to injection tubing and a syringe. The needle was placed in the

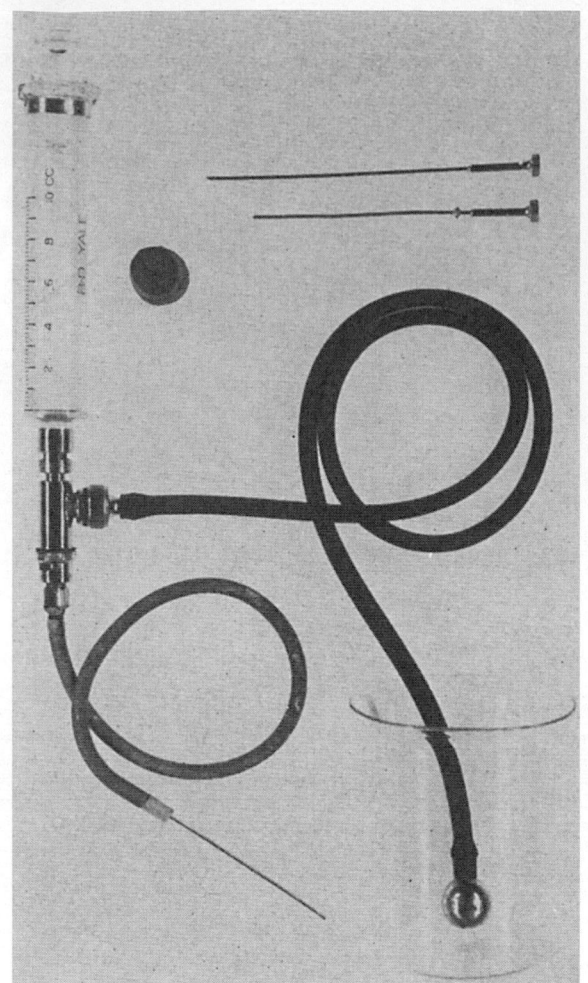

A

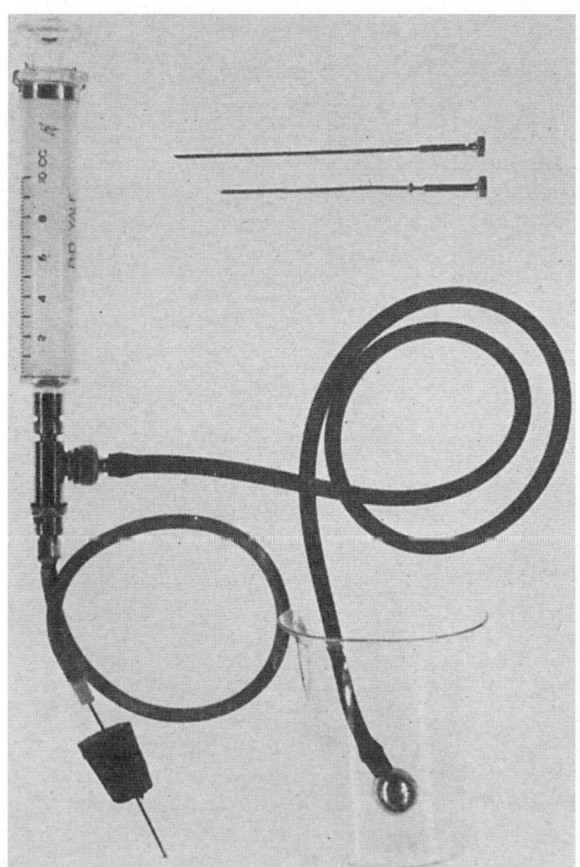

B

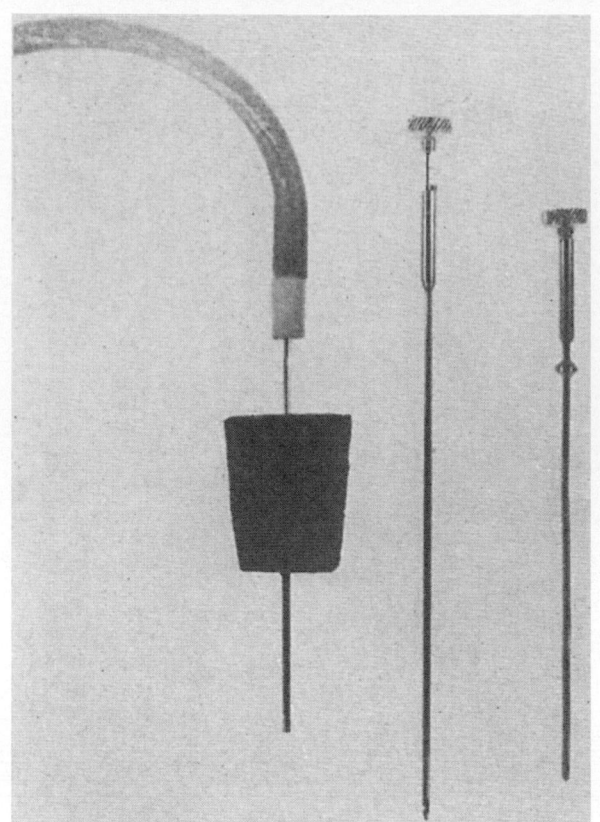

C

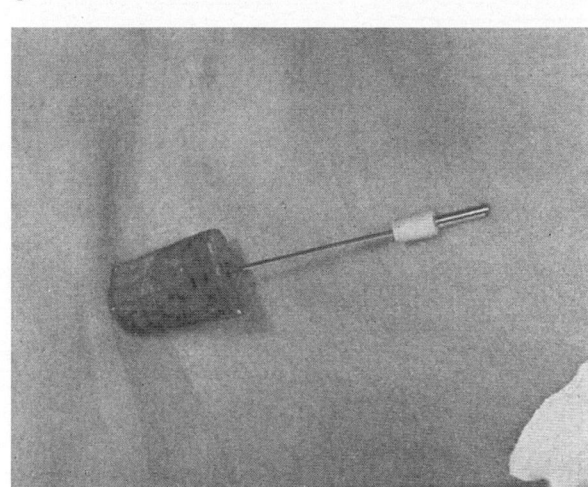

D

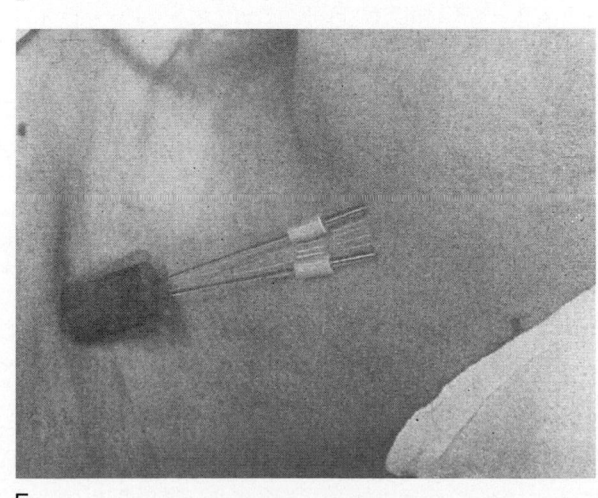

E

Figure 48–1. (continued)

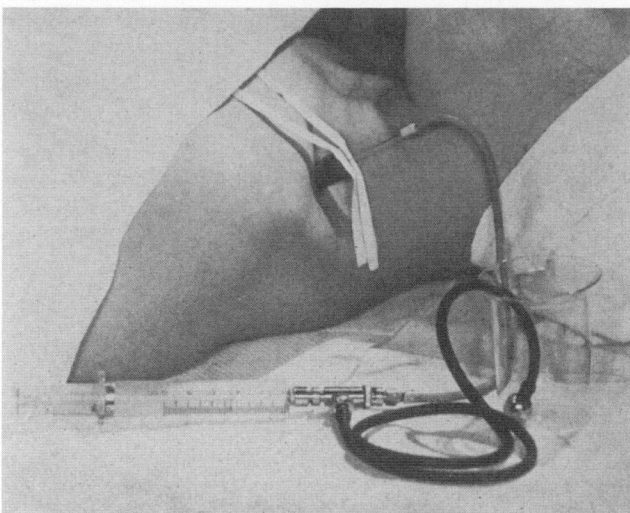

F

Figure 48–1. A: Apparatus consists of a 10-mL Luer-lock syringe and the two-way valve as used in the Hingson-Edwards continuous caudal method. The tubing can be of any desired length (18 inches is sufficient). A malleable needle (Becton-Dickinson & Company) is used, which has been filed to a blunt end to prevent perforation of blood vessels. A cork stopper from an ether can completes the apparatus. **B:** Apparatus with needle through the cork, usually 4–6 cm. **C:** Close view of blunted needle through the cork guard. The cork, when placed flush with the skin in the supraclavicular area, prevents the needle from going in deeper. **D:** Needle in place in the supraclavicular area. The cork prevents displacement inward and holds it upright. **E:** Pulsation of the needle, indicating its close apposition to the subclavian artery. If the needle is placed lateral to the artery and on top of the first rib, it is of necessity in close proximity to the plexus. Injection of 30–40 mL of 1% procaine induces anesthesia within 15 minutes. **F:** Apparatus in place and ready for fractional injections. The adhesive strapping over the cork keeps the needle in place and prevents its outward displacement. The cork firmly holding the needle prevents its inward displacement. (Reprinted, with permission, from Ansbro FP: A method of continuous brachial plexus block. Am J Surg 1946;71:716–722.)

supraclavicular area lateral to the pulsations of the subclavian artery and approximately 1 cm cephalad to the midpoint of the clavicle. A cork stopper from an ether can was used to secure the needle in place. Intermittent injections of procaine were given to 27 patients to extend the duration of intraoperative anesthesia for up to 4 hours and 20 minutes.

In 1951, Sarnoff and Sarnoff[26] published one of the first reports involving the use of a flexible indwelling catheter for CPNB. They performed continuous phrenic nerve blocks on patients with intractable hiccups. They used a 2-in., 18-gauge needle to locate the nerve and subsequently threaded a 9-in. piece of polyethylene tubing (inner diameter 0.023 in.; outer diameter 0.038 in.) with an inner stylet. A blunt 23-gauge needle was fit into the proximal end of the tubing and attached to a needle stopper to occlude the opening between local anesthetic injections. It is interesting to note that in their early trials these investigators used Vinylite tubing for the indwelling catheter but discovered that it became brittle and

less pliable over time. They presumed that this was due to the material's inherent solubility in animal fat and so abandoned it in favor of polyethylene.

The next report occurred almost a quarter century later when DeKrey et al.[27] described their experience using continuous subclavian perivascular blocks intraoperatively for upper extremity surgery of long duration. They used a 15- to 18-gauge Rochester-type plastic needle. After elicitation of paresthesia, they advanced the overlying plastic part of the needle (cannula) into the brachial plexus sheath and removed the inner metal stylet. A total of 25 patients received intermittent local anesthesia boluses for up to 9 hours. Shortly thereafter, Winnie[28] outlined continuous interscalene block using similar equipment. He described using a small "extra-cath" intravenous-type needle and cannula set. After identification of the brachial plexus with the paresthesia technique, the inner metal needle was removed while the outer plastic cannula was advanced. The cannula was subsequently used for repeated doses of local anesthesia. Selander[29] published one of the first reports of continuous axillary brachial plexus blocks in a series of 137 patients having hand surgery. He used an intravenous needle (external diameter 0.65 mm) and cannula (external diameter 1 mm; length 47 mm) and identified the axillary sheath with the fascial pop method (Figure 48–2). The cannula was threaded off the needle and into the sheath to provide a more secure attachment for a syringe containing local anesthesia and, consequently, to minimize the risk of block failure due to needle movements. The catheter was dosed with intermittent boluses of mepivacaine and left in place for up to 24 hours.

Although these early accounts primarily involved "cannula-over-needle" devices, subsequent descriptions also included "catheter-through-needle" equipment. In the earliest report of a continuous lower extremity block, Brands and Callahan[30] provided details of a series of 21 patients who received continuous lumbar plexus blocks for 72 to 96 hours after femoral neck fractures. An intravenous cannula had insufficient length for this block and would likely have been too susceptible to kinking when inserted at 90 degrees to the course of the plexus. Consequently, these authors used a 15-cm, 18-gauge needle and the loss-of-resistance method to identify the lumbar plexus psoas compartment. They subsequently threaded an epidural catheter through the needle. Rosenblatt[31] described another technique to facilitate catheter placement when the block needle approaches the neural structures perpendicularly. They reported using a Seldinger technique for a continuous interscalene brachial plexus block. After using a 25-gauge single-injection needle to identify the brachial plexus, an 8.9-cm, 18-gauge epidural needle was inserted. After injection of local anesthesia, a 0.53 mm diameter, 35-cm long spring guidewire was threaded through the needle and into the sheath about 4 cm. The epidural needle was subsequently removed and a 5-cm, 18-gauge diameter catheter was threaded over the guidewire into place. The guidewire was then removed and bupivacaine 0.25% was given as a continuous infusion at 10 mL/h to provide 24 hours of analgesia.

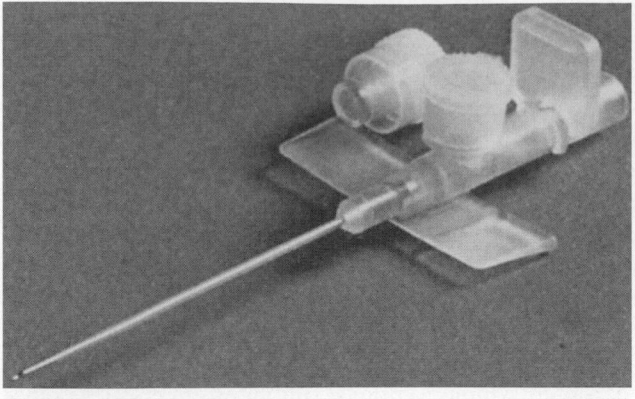

A

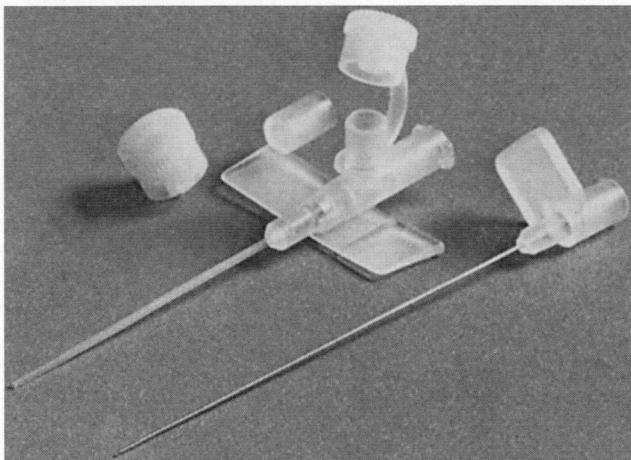

B

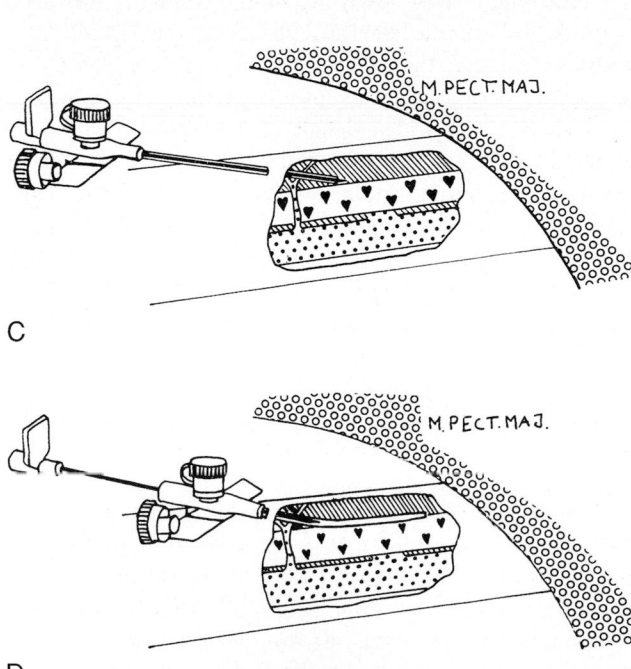

C

D

Figure 48–2. A and **B:** The Venflon cannula. **C** and **D:** Schematic views of the introduction of the Venflon catheter into the axillary neurovascular sheath. (Reprinted, with permission, from Selander D: Catheter technique in axillary plexus block. Presentation of a new method. Acta Anaesthesiol Scand 1977;21[4]:324–329.)

The identification of important neuroanatomic features occurred concurrently with the description of these early CPNBs and was instrumental in the further understanding of plexus anatomy and the development of continuous regional anesthesia techniques. Landmark papers were published by Winnie[28] as well as Thompson and Rorie[32] outlining the existence of a brachial plexus sheath and suggesting the potential for continuous plexus anesthesia. Tuominen et al.[33] provided early evidence of the safety of continuous plexus infusions of local anesthesia when they studied blood levels of bupivacaine during continuous axillary brachial plexus infusion.

Reflecting the popularity of the paresthesia, fascial pop and loss-of-resistance techniques from the 1970s through the early 1990s, most subsequent reports of CPNBs also involved the use of intravenous-type needles and cannula ("cannula-over-needle" devices)[33–38] as well as epidural-type needles and catheters ("catheter-through-needle" equipment).[3,4,39–42] In the late 1970s, however, concern surfaced in the regional anesthesia literature over the association between long-bevel needles used for peripheral nerve blocks and the occurrence of neurologic complications.[43] Consequently, the use of short-bevel needles was suggested to decrease the risk of intraneural injections. For example, Buttner et al.[44] described a modification of intravenous-type equipment to include an inner metal stylet with a 45-degree or short-bevel needle.

Concerns over neurologic injury from the elicitation of paresthesia[45] together with the introduction of nerve stimulator techniques[46] led to a decline in the popularity of the paresthesia method in favor of identification of neural structures by electrolocation. Although uninsulated needles could be used with nerve stimulators, insulated needles were found to provide more focused current output and consequently more accurate localization of neural structures.[47] As nerve stimulator techniques came into more widespread use in the 1990s, commercially insulated single-injection needles became available, but the design of CPNB needles and catheters was unsuitable. To circumvent this obstacle, regional anesthesia practitioners assembled intravenous access and spinal and epidural equipment to create their own CPNB apparatus.

There are numerous reports of various adaptations used for connecting an intravenous needle and cannula to a current source to enable nerve stimulation. Smith et al.[1] provided one of the first descriptions of a CPNB using an "insulated needle" and a nerve stimulator. They connected the metal trocar of a 16-gauge intravenous needle—catheter assembly (Medicut) to a low-powered nerve stimulator. On appropriate sciatic nerve stimulation, the trocar was removed and local anesthesia injected through the cannula. A 16-gauge epidural catheter (Simms-Portex, UK) was threaded through the cannula, and the cannula was subsequently removed. Anker-Moller et al.[48] used a similar system that consisted of a 14-gauge intravenous needle and cannula set (Viggo). After identification of the femoral nerve with a nerve stimulator, the inner needle was removed and a 16-gauge epidural catheter (Portex) inserted through the

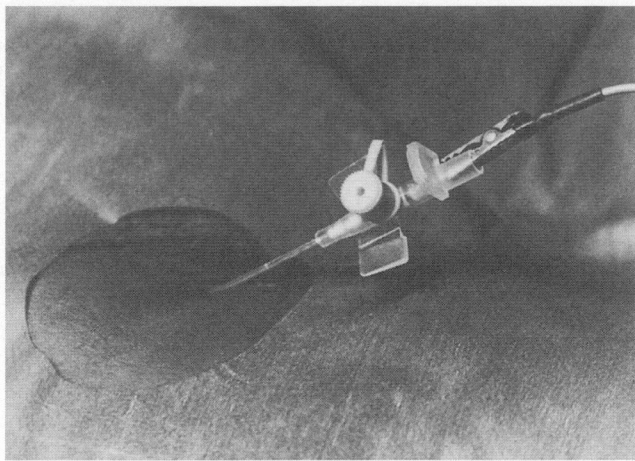

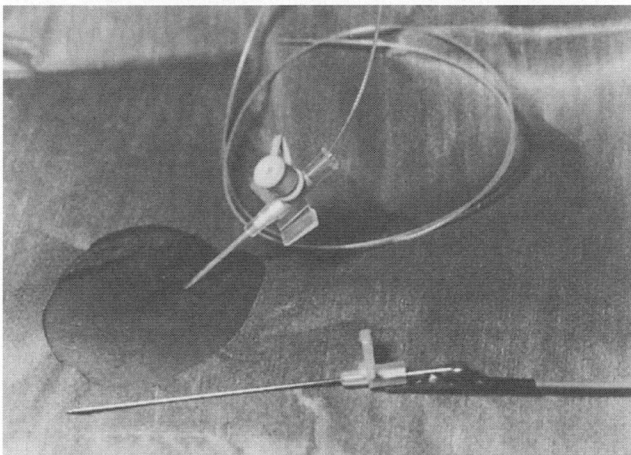

Figure 48–3. A: Placement of the infusion cannula. Nerve stimulator attached to the trocar (lateral view). **B:** The catheter is inserted through the infusion cannula (lateral view). (Reprinted, with permission, from Anker-Moller E, et al: Continuous blockade of the lumbar plexus after knee surgery: A comparison of the plasma concentrations and analgesic effect of bupivacaine 0.250% and 0.125%. Acta Anaesthesiol Scand 1990;34[6]: 468–472.)

intravenous cannula (Figure 48–3). In a unique adaptation of intravenous equipment, Ben-David et al.[49] inserted the metal needle of a 20-gauge intravenous catheter (Venflon, Viggo) inside the proximal end of a 16-gauge central venous pressure needle (Secalon, Viggo). They attached the negative electrode of the nerve stimulator to the exposed metal needle of the 20-gauge intravenous catheter and obtained appropriate stimulation during lumbar plexus block. The over-the-needle central venous cannula was then advanced beyond the tip of the needle and used for continuous lumbar plexus block (Figure 48–4). Using an innovative design, Concepcion[50] described wrapping the stylet of a 26-gauge spinal needle around the metal introducer of a typical intravenous over-the-needle cannula. An alligator clip was then attached to the stylet to allow electrical stimulation using a nerve stimulator (Figure 48–5).

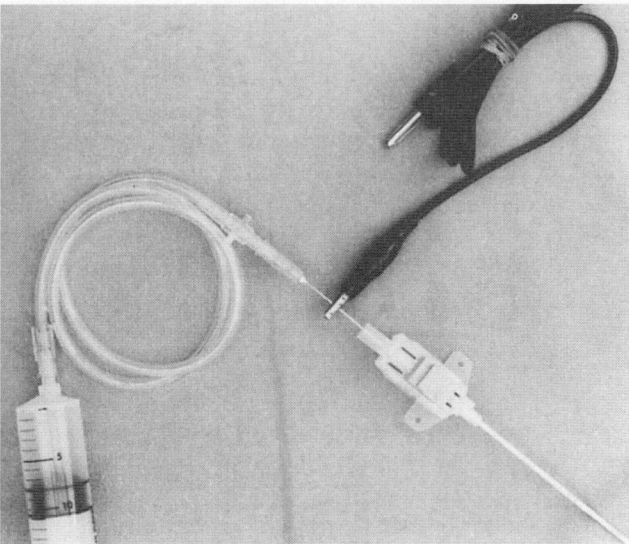

Figure 48–4. Assembly shows a 21-gauge needle inserted into the proximal end of the 16-gauge Secalon (Viggo) central venous pressure catheter. Metal contact of the smaller needle inside the larger needle allows an electrical impulse to be conveyed to the Secalon needle tip. An alligator clip from the electrical stimulator is attached to the shaft of the 21-gauge needle. Intravenous extension tubing inserts into the hub of the 21-gauge needle. (Reprinted, with permission, from Ben-David B, Lee E, Croitoru M: Psoas block for surgical repair of hip fracture: A case report and description of a catheter technique. Anesth Analg 1990;71[3]:298–301.)

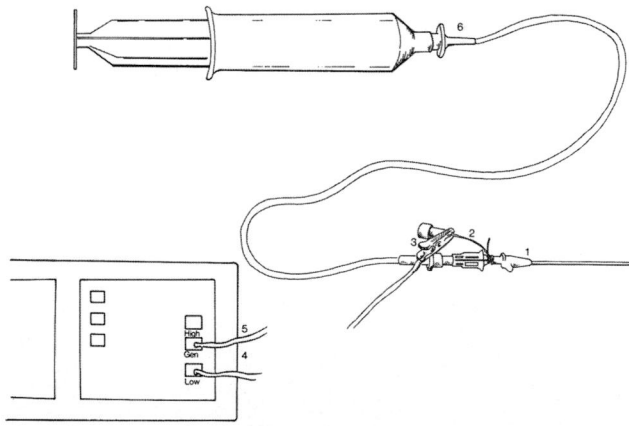

Figure 48–5. Assembly of needle and nerve stimulator for continuous brachial plexus blockade using an over-the-needle intravenous catheter: (1) intravenous over-the-needle catheter, (2) stylet from 26-gauge spinal needle, (3) alligator clip attached to the stylet and to the low-output terminal of a nerve stimulator, (4) nerve stimulator, (5) ground wire attached to the common port of the nerve stimulator (marked as "Gen" in the diagram) and to the patient, and (6) extension set and syringe for "immobile needle technique." (Reprinted, with permission, from Concepcion M: Continuous brachial plexus techniques. In: Ferrante FM, VadeBoncoeur TR [editors]: *Postoperative Pain Management*. Churchill Livingstone, 1993.)

Spinal and epidural equipment has similarly been adapted for CPNBs performed with nerve stimulators. Several groups[2,51] have placed an 18-gauge intravenous cannula over a 22-gauge spinal needle to provide insulation to the distal part of the needle. A current source was then attached to the bare proximal metal needle, and local anesthesia was injected upon identification of neural structures. The cannula was then threaded off the spinal needle into the perineural space and used for continuous infusion of local anesthesia for up to two days. Similarly, our group has placed an intravenous cannula over an epidural needle to insulate the distal part of the needle and has attached a current source to the proximal needle. Upon identification of neural structures, a catheter was threaded through the epidural needle into place. Alternatively, spinal needles and microcatheters have been used. The spinal microcatheters, however, were of such small size that injection was difficult and they were prone to kinking. This equipment was eventually withdrawn from the market because of neurotoxicity associated with continuous spinal anesthesia.

Prosser[52] devised yet another method to provide nerve stimulation during CPNBs for pediatric patients. This author connected a jackplug electrode into the hub of an intravenous cannula (Abbocath-T Venisystems) to make an electrical contact between the nerve stimulator and the central metal needle of the intravenous set (Figure 48–6). The surrounding Teflon-coated sheath insulated all but the tip of the cannula. This adaptation was successful with 20-, 22- and 24-gauge intravenous catheters and consequently was nearly ideal for the pediatric population.

Further advancing pediatric regional anesthesia, Tan et al.[53] used a radial artery catheterization set (#RA-04120;

Arrow, Reading, PA) with a 20-gauge cannula over a 22-gauge, thin-walled, short-bevel needle for continuous axillary brachial plexus block. The set had a 0.018-in. integral spring wire that this group connected via an alligator clip to the negative pole of a nerve stimulator to enable electrolocation of the brachial plexus. Using the Seldinger technique, the guidewire was then advanced and used to direct the cannula into the brachial plexus sheath.

Although these designs allowed nerve stimulation through an insulated needle, a number of drawbacks still existed. Several steps were required between identification of the nerve and threading of the catheter. This increased the risk of catheter misplacement and the likelihood of committing a breach in sterility. Despite the insulation provided by an intravenous-type cannula over a metal needle, the uninsulated area of the distal needle tip was of significant size and could adversely affect the accuracy of nerve location. Unfortunately, in these self-assembled systems, the cannula rarely provided a snug fit over the needle. In addition, there was continued concern about the risk of neurologic complications from long-bevel intravenous-type needles. Finally, the shape of the needle tip did not facilitate catheter threading in directions other than parallel with the course of the needle.

Increased effort into the development of CPNB equipment and the introduction of the safer long-acting local anesthesia ropivacaine (Astra, Westborough, MA) in the 1990s further stimulated the expansion of CPNB techniques. The original Contiplex A system (B. Braun-Melsungen AG, Germany) involved a cannula over a short-bevel needle and an accompanying catheter. The advantages of this equipment consisted of components that were designed to fit together, a theoretically less traumatic short-bevel needle (32-degree tip), and a catheter of compatible size (Figure 48–7). Although similar to the early equipment individually assembled and used by many regional anesthesiologists, this became one of the first commercially available CPNB products. This system was subsequently modified to create the Contiplex D model,

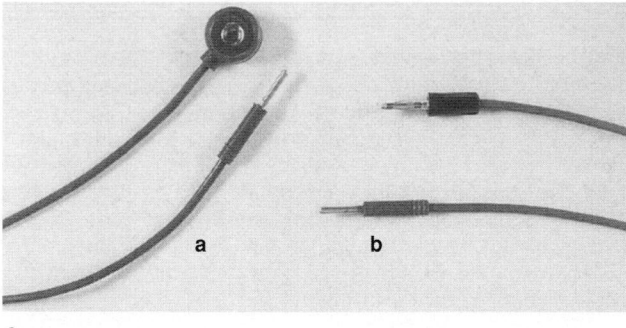

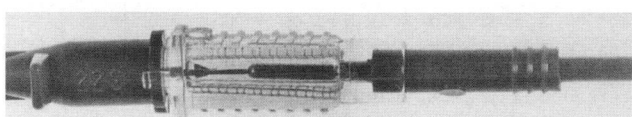

Figure 48–6. A: Peripheral nerve stimulator lead fitted with standard press stud and jackplug connectors (a); modified connectors, press stud replaced with second jackplug (b). **B:** Electrical contact between the Abbocath's central metal cannula and original jackplug from the lead. (Reprinted, with permission, from Prosser DP: Adaptation of an intravenous cannula for paediatric regional anaesthesia. Anaesthesia 1996;51[5]:510.)

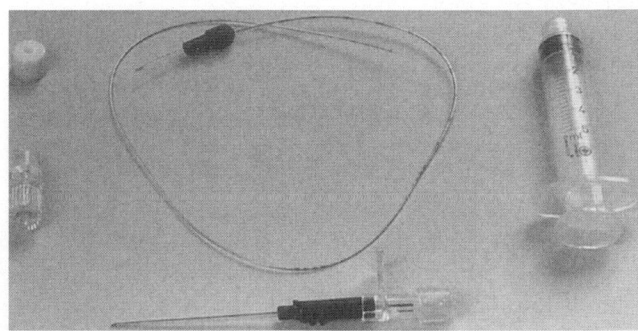

Figure 48–7. Brachial plexus infusion kit as used in this study (Contiplex, B. Braun Australia Pty, Ltd). The introducing cannula is 18-gauge, with a 0.85-mm diameter catheter, which is threaded into the axillary brachial plexus sheath. The needle within the cannula is a short-bevel type (30 degrees). (Reprinted, with permission, from Mezzatesta JP, et al: Continuous axillary brachial plexus block for postoperative pain relief. Intermittent bolus versus continuous infusion. Reg Anesth 1997;22[4]:357–362.)

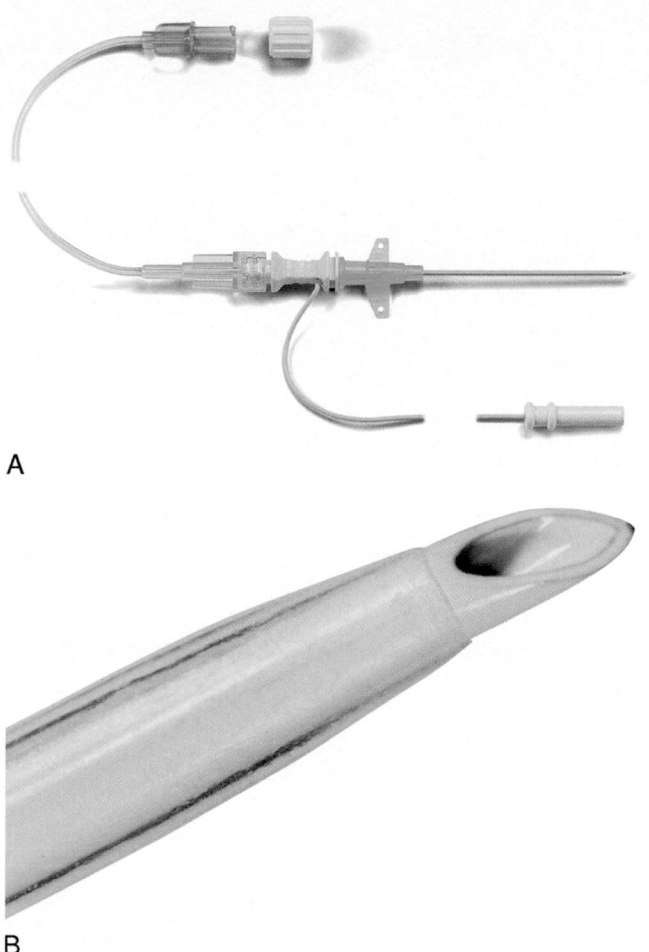

A

B

Figure 48–8. A: Pajunk MiniSet consisting of a cannula-over-needle design and integrated stimulating cable and extension tubing. **B:** Pajunk MiniSet distal short-bevel needle tip and cannula. (Photographs used with permission from Pajunk, Geisengen, Germany.)

which included an integrated wire for nerve stimulation and connection tubing for concurrent aspiration and injection. The use of both the Contiplex A and D became popular throughout the 1990s.[5,7,54–65] Other manufacturers subsequently developed similar systems. Notable among these is the MiniSet (Pajunk, Geisengen, Germany) (Figure 48–8). This system offers the choice of 21- or 24-gauge needles with either Sprotte or Facet tip. These alternatives enhanced the usefulness of this system and made it appealing for use in pediatrics.

In the late 1990s, a bullet-tip needle (Brachial Plexus Set #BP-01200, Arrow) was introduced and its use was described in the literature[66,67] (Figure 48–9). The theoretical advantage of this system consisted of an enhanced sensation of fascial penetration and a theoretical reduction in neurologic injury thought to occur in association with long-bevel needles. The extreme bluntness of the needle, however, required skin nicking and significant force on advancement of the needle, which made it difficult to control the path of the needle. In addition, the opening of the needle was in a 90-degree angle to the needle shaft causing difficulties when

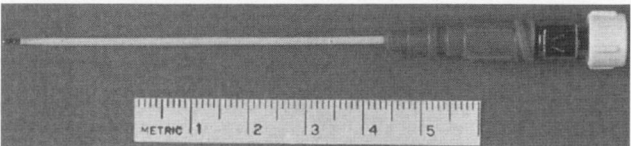

Figure 48–9. Arrow single-shot or continuous brachial plexus catheter. (Reprinted, with permission, from Longo SR, Williams DP: Bilateral fascia iliaca catheters for postoperative pain control after bilateral total knee arthroplasty: A case report and description of a catheter technique. Reg Anesth 1997;22[4]:372–377.)

threading a catheter. The difficulties in advancing the needle and controlling its path as well as the absence of a port conducive to catheter threading made this needle unpopular for peripheral nerve blocks.

The development of this equipment was important, but the weaknesses of these systems were evident. Even these commercially available devices required multiple manipulations for catheter insertion, thereby increasing the risk of contamination and improper catheter placement. In addition, few of the early systems allowed for concurrent nerve stimulation, aspiration for blood, and injection of local anesthesia. To address these concerns, to provide a system that would allow single-operator use and to develop a product that would have applicability at multiple anatomic sites, the modern Contiplex Tuohy system (B. Braun Medical, Bethlehem, PA) was created.[68] This apparatus involves an 18-gauge Tuohy-type needle insulated with polytetrafluroroethylene coating along its length with the exception of a pinpoint area at the most distal tip of the Tuohy bevel.

The Tuohy needle was designed with a Huber tip to facilitate placement of a catheter in a direction parallel with the nerve(s) in question. An adapter with a Luer-lock head and a hemostatic valve is fitted to the proximal end of the needle. It incorporates a side arm connected to 50 cm of extension tubing, which allows for continuous aspiration for blood and injection of local anesthesia by an assistant and which facilitates an immobile needle technique. The adapter also has a central diaphragm that allows passage of a catheter through a port separate from where aspiration and injection occur. This eliminates the need for equipment disconnection and minimizes the likelihood of needle movement, catheter misplacement, and secondary block failure.

The early prototype of the Tuohy system included a wire with an alligator clip on one end and a plug for a nerve stimulator on the other end (Figure 48–10). In the subsequent model, the 40-cm stimulating wire is permanently affixed to the metal needle and serves as a connector to a nerve stimulator (Figure 48–11). This wire also serves as a marker for the open face of the needle bevel distally. Various needle lengths are manufactured, allowing CPNB of nerves of varying depths. A 20-gauge multi-orificed epidural catheter and connector are included in the needle packaging. The ease of use and reliability of this apparatus have repeatedly been documented.[11,16,69–76] Subsequently, other manufacturers have developed comparable systems. The Plexolong system

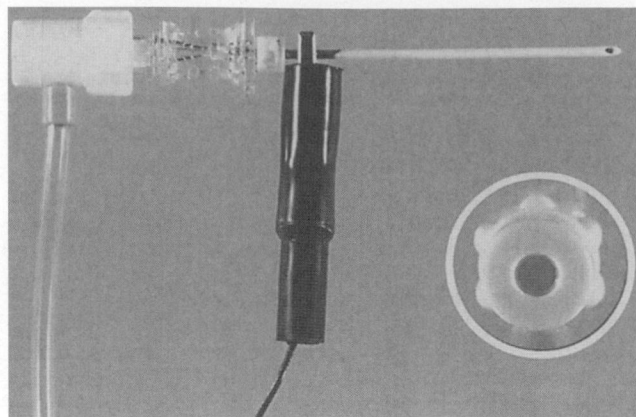

Figure 48–10. An 18-gauge, insulated Tuohy system (B. Braun, Contiplex; B. Braun Medical, Bethlehem, PA). Inset shows a Luer-lock head with central diaphragm at the proximal end of the needle. (Reprinted, with permission, from Klein SM, Grant SA, Greengrass RA, et al: Interscalene brachial plexus block with a continuous catheter insertion system and a disposable infusion pump. Anesth Analg 2000;91(6):1473–1478.)

(Pajunk, Geisengen, Germany) incorporates an insulated needle, a styletted epidural catheter coiled in a thread-assist device, an integrated stimulating wire, and detachable injection tubing[77-80] (Figure 48–12). Various needle diameters (18 and 19.5 gauge), lengths, and needle tip configurations (Tuohy, Sprotte, Facet with 30- or 45-degree bevel) are available. These options enable catheter threading at various needle angle approaches to neural structures. The catheter stylet imparts additional rigidity and enables catheter advancement; however, an interesting case report documents catheter shearing when

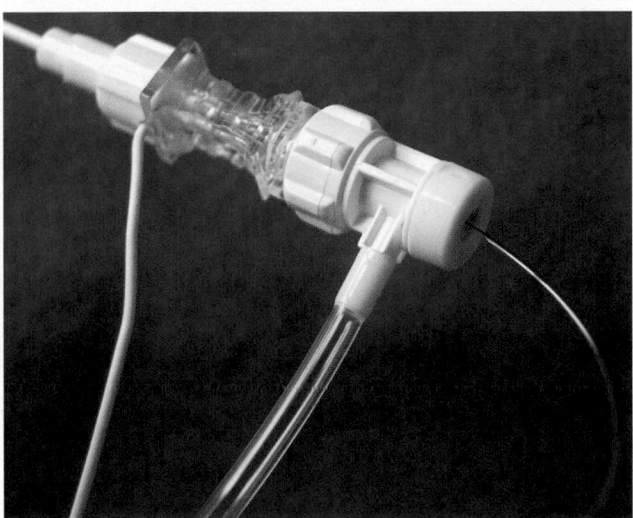

Figure 48–11. The Contiplex Tuohy (B. Braun, Melsungen AG, Germany) consists of an insulated Tuohy needle with a pinpoint uninsulated tip, an integrated stimulating wire, extension tubing, and a connector with a hemostatic valve, allowing the insertion of a catheter. This design enables simultaneous nerve stimulation, aspiration, and injection and allows for an immobile needle during catheter insertion.(Photograph provided for use by Dr. H. Evans.)

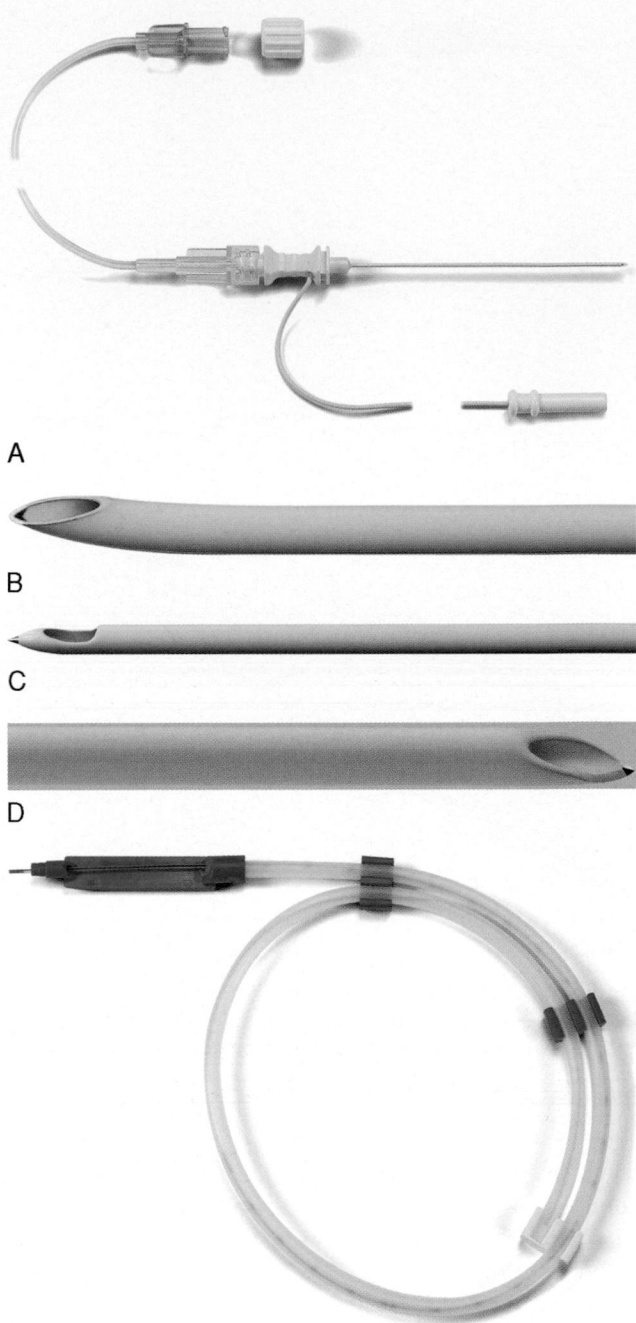

Figure 48–12. A: The Plexolong system (Pajunk, Geisengen, Germany) incorporates an insulated needle, integrated stimulating wire, and extension tubing. **B:** The Plexolong Tuohy tip. **C:** The Plexolong Sprotte tip. **D:** The Plexolong Facet (or short-bevel) tip. **E:** The Plexolong catheter with thread-assist device. (Photographs used with permission from Pajunk, Geisengen, Germany.)

the catheter stylet was removed before needle removal.[81] Further increasing the range of use of this system, a pediatric kit is available and consists of a 21-gauge Sprotte needle of 30 or 50 mm length and a 25-gauge catheter. Other manufacturers have developed similar products (see Table 48–2 later in this chapter).

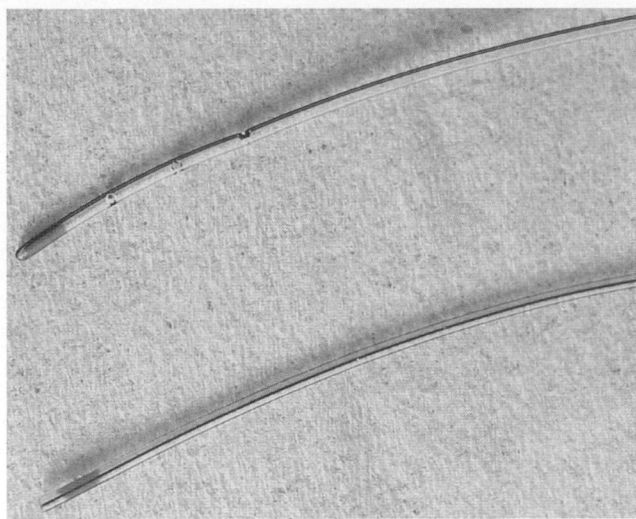

Figure 48–13. A closed-tip multi-orificed catheter (*above*) and an open-tip single-orifice catheter (*below*). (Photograph provided by Dr. H. Evans.)

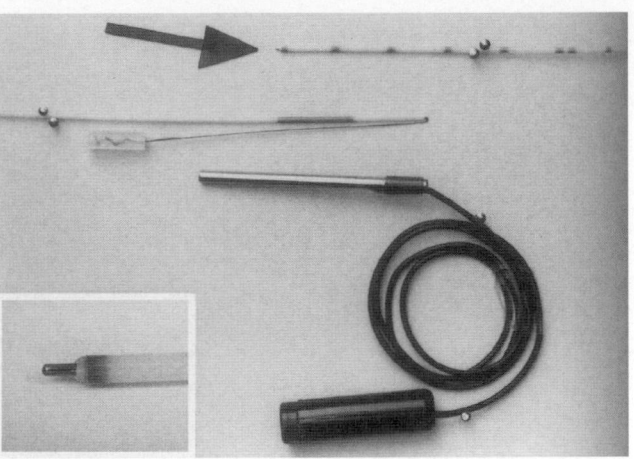

Figure 48–14. Shortened catheter with stylet just protruding from the distal end (*inset*) and folded over to maintain the position at the proximal end. Electrical connection is made by sliding a firmly fitting metal tube over the proximal end of the catheter. (Reprinted, with permission, from Sutherland ID: Continuous sciatic nerve infusion: Expanded case report describing a new approach. Reg Anesth Pain Med 1998;23[5]:496–501.)

Catheters initially manufactured for epidural use have been adapted for CPNBs. They are well suited for this application because they are nonirritating and flexible and generate minimal friction on passage through needles. Graduated markings provide an indicator of insertion depth, and radiopacity provides an additional method to confirm placement location. Some advocate the use of styletted catheters, believing that they are easier to advance; however, use of these catheters may result in greater tissue or blood vessel trauma. Multi-orificed catheters have a closed distal tip and three distal openings 0.5, 1.0, and 1.5 cm from the tip. Single-orificed catheters have a single opening at the distal end of the catheter (Figure 48–13).

The most recent advance in CPNB equipment involves the development of stimulating catheters. These catheters provide the ability to conduct current to their distal end and so may be used to confirm appropriate perineural catheter placement. In one of the first published reports, Sutherland[82] used a 1.0-mm outer-diameter ureteral catheter (Portex-Boots, Kent, UK) with a metal stylet. This author adapted the catheter by removing 50 mm from its distal tip and by rethreading the metal stylet so that it just protruded from the distal end (Figure 48–14). The proximal part of the stylet was folded over the proximal end of the catheter to maintain correct length and to facilitate an electrical connection to the nerve stimulator. This equipment was used successfully for continuous sciatic nerve block after foot surgery.

Boezaart et al.[83] subsequently described their adaptation of a wire-reinforced epidural catheter for use as a stimulating catheter. They used a polyurethane (Tecothane) thermoplastic catheter with an inner steel spring reinforcement and a nonferromagnetic stainless-steel stylet (Arrow Theracath, Arrow International) and removed part of the outer catheter to provide a 5-mm unsheathed metal tip. These authors describe removing the inner stylet from an uninsulated 17-gauge Tuohy needle and advancing the epidural catheter

through the needle so that the metal tip of the catheter did not make contact with the metal needle. This effectively allowed electrolocation during needle and catheter placement for continuous interscalene brachial plexus block. A later modification involved the addition of an insulated needle with an inner metal stylet to the set (StimuCath, Arrow International)[84,85] (Figure 48–15).

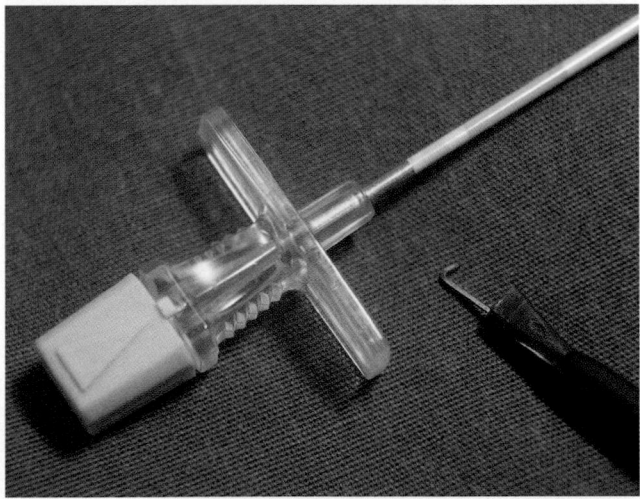

A

Figure 48–15. A: An alligator clip connects to an uninsulated segment on the proximal needle shaft of the StimuCath system (Arrow International, Reading, PA). **B:** The StimuCath system consists of an insulated Tuohy-tip needle, a stimulating catheter, and an alligator clip connector. **C:** The alligator clip is removed from the needle and attached to the catheter's proximal end. This provides current output to the catheter's distal tip. **D:** The Tuohy needle tip with a 5-mm long uninsulated segment is seen with the distal tip of the StimuCath stimulating catheter. (Photographs provided by Dr. H. Evans.)

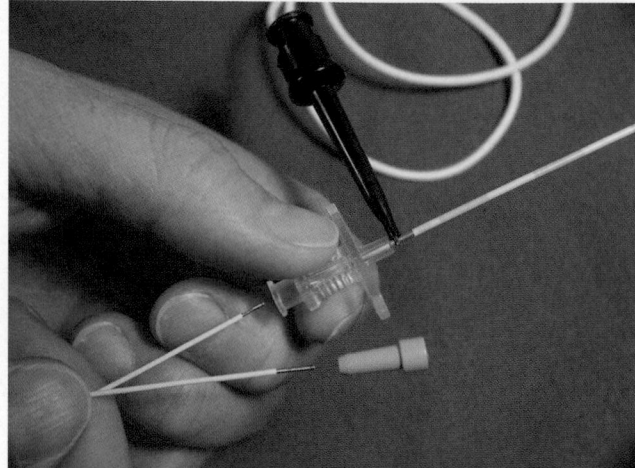

B

C

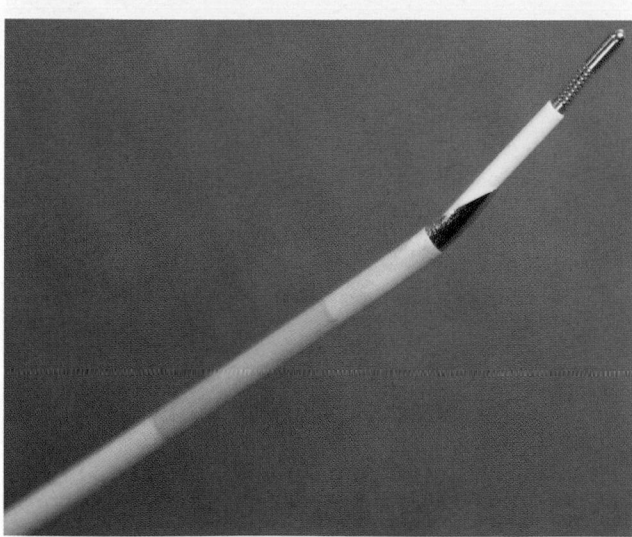

D

Figure 48–15. *(continued)*

Further revisions resulted in the addition of an alligator clip to allow direct connection to a nerve stimulator and, more recently, the addition of an integrated stimulating wire attached to the needle. Various sizes are available and initial clinical use has been successful.[86,87] Shortly after Boezaart's original description, Kick et al.[88] described another unique stimulating catheter (Stimulong Catheter Set; Pajunk, Geisengen, Germany) and reported its reliability in a series of 10 supraclavicular brachial plexus blocks. It consisted of a 20-gauge, single-hole, 400-mm polyamide catheter with a 405-mm indwelling removable conducting stylet. The metal wire stylet was insulated with Teflon coating along its length with the exception of the distal 0.3 mm. The proximal end had a plug to allow connection to a nerve stimulator. Subsequent modification involved incorporation of an integrated wire within the catheter (Stimulong Plus, Pajunk)[89] (Figure 48–16). Subsequently, other manufacturers have developed similar systems[90] (see Table 48–3; Figures 48–17 and 48–18). At the time of publication, the stimulating catheter remains a relatively new and novel device. Studies are underway to determine its safety and potential benefit compared with nonstimulating continuous catheter techniques. In addition, the stimulating characteristics of these catheters need to be elucidated and compared with those of insulated needles.[89,91]

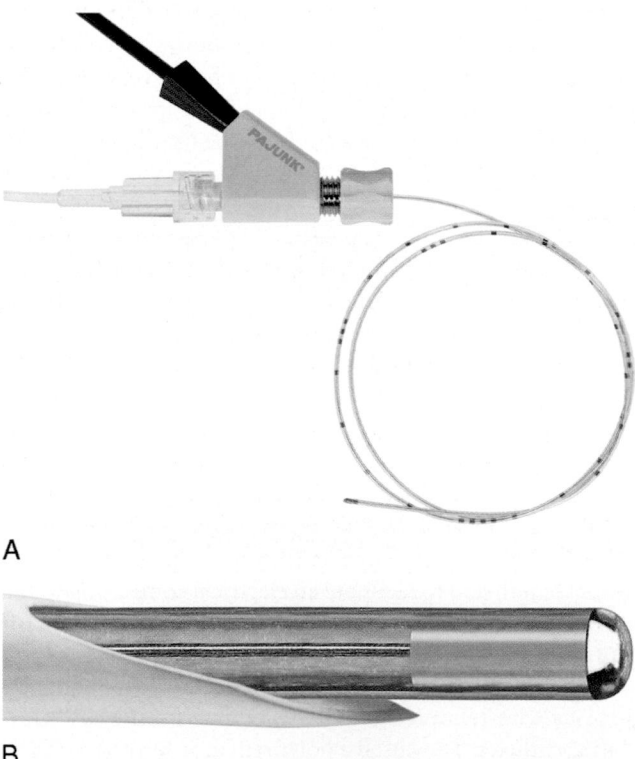

A

B

Figure 48–16. A: The stimulating catheter with integrated wire, Stimulong Plus (Pajunk, Geisengen, Germany), is shown with its screw connector. The connector accepts an electric cable and extension tubing. **B:** The tip of the Stimulong Plus stimulating catheter is shown with its conductive golden tip. (Photographs used with permission from Pajunk, Geisengen, Germany.)

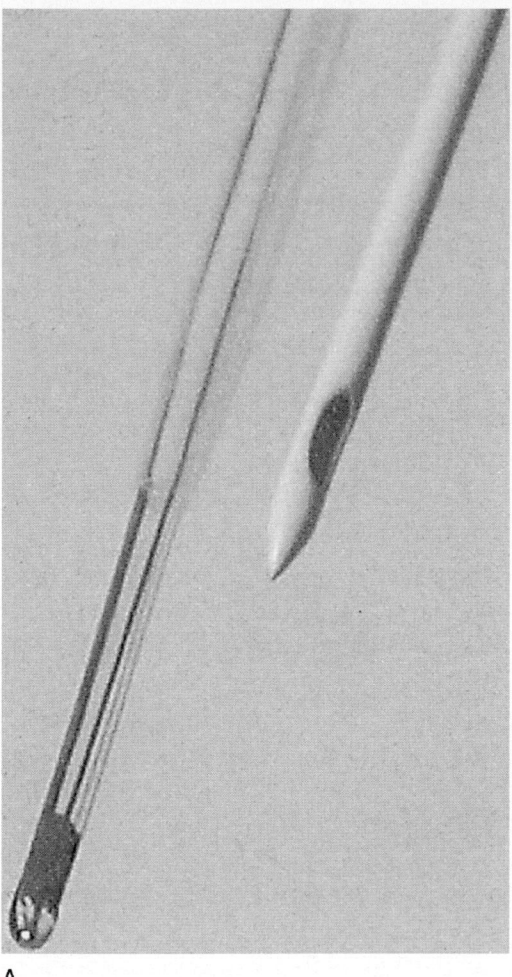

A

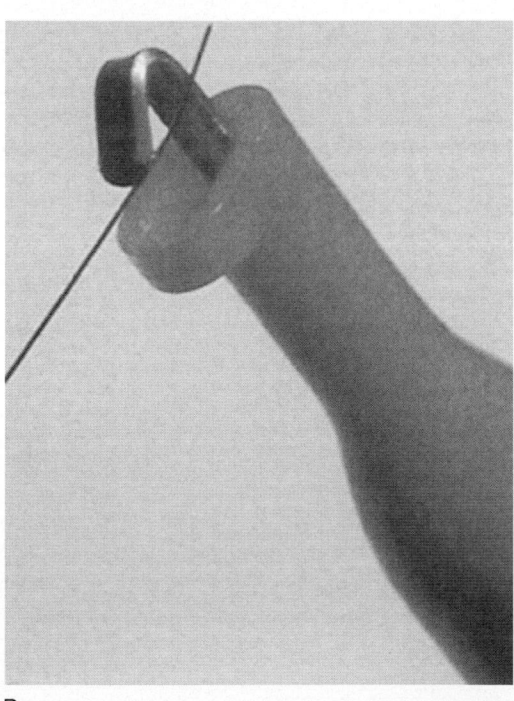

B

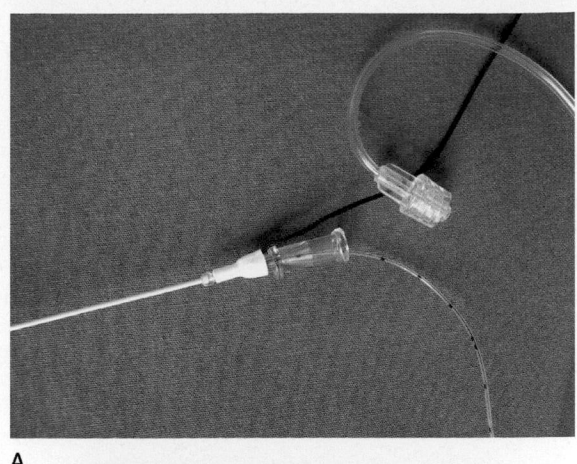

A

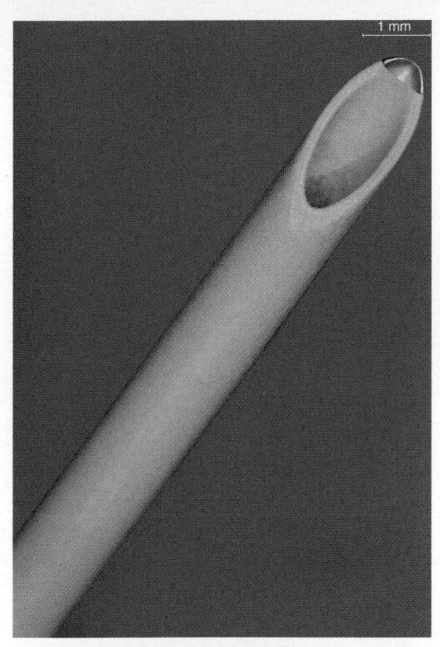

B

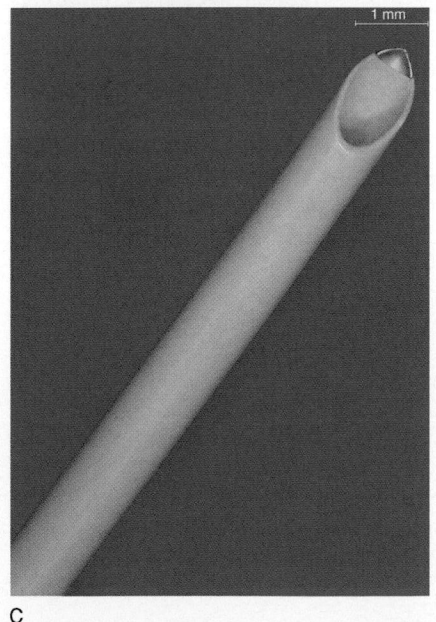

C

Figure 48–17. A: Distal end (*left*) of Polyplex stimulating catheter with integral wire visible. Distal tip (*right*) of Polyplex insulated pencil-point needle. **B:** Spring-closure stimulating catheter clip and stimulating catheter wire. (Reprinted, with permission, from Copeland SJ, Laxton MA: A new stimulating catheter for continuous peripheral nerve blocks. Reg Anesth Pain Med 21(6):589–590;2001.)

Figure 48–18. A: The Prolong system (Life-Tech, Stafford, TX). The extension tubing attached to the needle must be removed before threading the catheter. **B:** The Prolong needle with a Tuohy-type bevel. **C:** The Prolong needle with a 30-degree bevel. (Photographs used with permission from Life-Tech, Stafford, TX.)

Table 48–1.

Cannula-Over-Needle Systems

System	Needle Features	Cannula Features	Catheter Features	Additional Features
B. Braun, Contiplex A (Figure 48–7)	20-gauge needle Short-bevel: 32 degrees Length: 5.4 cm	Cannula-over-needle design 18-gauge Uninsulated area of needle tip 2 mm	20-gauge diameter 40 cm long Open tip with single distal orifice Centimeter gradations up to 20 cm Translucent Tungsten strip but not highly radiopaque	No integrated stimulating cable No integrated extension tubing Cost: $11
B. Braun, Contiplex D	20-gauge needle, 54 mm long with 15- or 30-degree bevel 18-gauge cannula 20-gauge catheter, 40 cm long *or* 20-gauge needle, 110 mm long with 15-degree bevel 18-gauge cannula 20-gauge catheter, 90 cm long *or* 22-gauge needle, 33 or 55 mm long with 15-degree bevel 20-gauge cannula 24-gauge catheter, 40 cm long exposed at tip	Cannula-over-needle design Cannula made of fluroroethylene propylene Needle fully coated with PTFE coating except for micropoint electrode	Open tip with single distal orifice Centimeter gradations up to 20 cm (for 40 cm long catheter) and 25 cm (for 90 cm long catheter) Translucent Catheter has tungsten strip but not highly radiopaque Inner metal stylet in 24-gauge catheter only	Integrated stimulating cable 36 cm long Integrated extension tubing 31 cm long Cost: $19–$35
Pajunk MiniSet (Figure 48–8)	*Sprott tip:* 21-gauge needle, 64 mm long 20-gauge cannula, 50 mm long 20-gauge catheter, 50 cm long *or* 24-gauge needle, 64 mm long 20-gauge cannula, 50 mm long 25-gauge catheter, 40 cm long *Facet tip:* 21-gauge needle, 64 or 88 mm long 18-gauge cannula, 50 or 75 mm long 20-gauge catheter, 50 cm long *or* 24-gauge needle, 64 mm long 18-gauge cannula, 50 mm long 25-gauge catheter, 40 cm long	Cannula-over-needle design Special tapered cannula tip to prevent rollback or buckling	Catheter size corresponds to cannula size	Integrated stimulating cable Detachable 40 cm extension tubing

Information obtained from manufacturers.
PTFE, polytetrafluroroethylene.

CURRENTLY AVAILABLE EQUIPMENT

Refer to Tables 48–1, 48–2, and 48–3 for currently available equipment that can be used for CPNBs.

FUTURE DIRECTIONS

The entire field of CPNBs is still in its infancy; consequently, many areas are available for future investigation. For instance,

Table 48–2.

Catheter-Through-Needle Systems

System	Needle Features	Catheter Features	Additional Features
B. Braun Contiplex Tuohy (Figure 48–11)	18-gauge Tuohy needle Huber-type atraumatic bevel Available lengths: 38.1 mm, 50.1 mm, 102 mm, 152 mm Insulated with PTFE Micropoint-uninsulated electrode on leading edge of needle-tip bevel No cm gradations on needle (this feature is expected 2006)	Catheter-through-needle design 20-gauge catheter Length: 100 cm Polyamide nylon catheter Centimeter gradations up to 20 cm Three distal orifices with closed tip Translucent Tungsten filament but not highly radiopaque No catheter stylet Small catheter threading–assist device	Integrated stimulating cable (40 cm) Detachable sideport with 50-cm extension tubing Luer-lock head with hemostasis valve and diaphragm for catheter insertion Cost: $24–$35
Pajunk, Plexolong (Figure 48–12)	*Tuohy tip:* 18-gauge needle Available lengths: 30 mm, 50 mm, 100 mm, 150 mm long *Sprott tip:* 19.5-gauge needle Available lengths: 60 mm, 120 mm *45-degree Facet tip:* 19.5-gauge needle Available lengths: 30 mm, 50 mm, 100 mm, 150 mm *30 degree Facet tip:* 19.5-gauge needle Available lengths: 30 mm, 50 mm, 100 mm, 150 mm Needles insulated with Teflon Small uninsulated part of needle tip 0.5 mm long All needles at least 40 mm long have centimeter gradations	Catheter-through-needle design 20-gauge catheter Length is either 50 or 90 cm Centimeter gradations up to 40 cm Translucent Radiopaque Styletted catheter Larger catheter threading–assist device keeps catheter in sterile coil	Integrated stimulating cable 40 cm long Detachable 40 cm extension tubing Cost: $17–$22 Pediatric set available and consists of: 21-gauge needle 30 or 50 mm long 25-gauge catheter
Life-Tech, Prolong (Figure 48–18)	*Tuohy tip:* 18-gauge needle Available lengths: 40 mm, 50 mm, 100 mm, 150 mm *Short-bevel tip (30-degree B bevel):* 19-gauge needle Available lengths: 40 mm, 50 mm, 100 mm, 150 mm Needles insulated with fluorocarbon coating Uninsulated tip area ~0.2 mm^2 No centimeter gradations on needle	Catheter-through-needle design 21-gauge catheter Length: 91.44 cm Centimeter gradations up to 25 cm Three distal orifices with closed tip Translucent Radiopaque No catheter stylet Small catheter threading–assist device	Integrated stimulating cable 61 cm Integrated extension tubing 45.7 cm Metal ball on needle shaft indicates needle diameter Cost: $25–$40

Information obtained from manufacturers.
PTFE, polytetrafluroroethylene.

little objective data are available to define the best needle-tip configuration that would facilitate catheter insertion and minimize the risk of neural injury. In addition, the ideal design and magnitude of the uninsulated portion of the needle tip have not been studied nor has the effect of varying the type of insulation material used. There have been few if any comparisons of the ease of use and clinical effectiveness of the various CPNB systems that are available. Moreover, although a number of large series document the safety of CPNBs, further evidence of the long-term safety of this technique

Table 48–3.

Stimulating Catheter Systems

System	Needle Features	Catheter Features	Additional Features
Pajunk, Stimulong Plus (Figure 48–16)	Any Pajunk Plexolong needle of sufficient diameter to accommodate a 20-gauge catheter can be used	Catheter-through-needle design 20-gauge stimulating catheter Available lengths: 50 cm, 90 cm Catheter covered with Teflon coating Distal 0.5 cm of tip of catheter uninsulated Centimeter gradations up to 40 cm Single distal orifice Catheter is radiopaque Catheter comes with threading device	Catheter has plug to allow connection of stimulating stylet to nerve stimulator Associated 40-cm extension tubing
Arrow International, StimuCath (Figure 48–15)	17- or 18-gauge Tuohy needle Available lengths: 40 mm, 80 mm, 110 mm, 140 mm Needles insulated with thin wall of polyester 5 mm long uninsulated segment at distal tip One option: uninsulated segment at proximal end that allows connection to nerve stimulator via alligator clip Another option: an integrated stimulating wire on the needle Winged hub Metal stylet Centimeter gradations	Catheter-through-needle design 19-gauge stimulating catheter (for 17-gauge Tuohy) 20-gauge stimulating catheter (for 18-gauge Tuohy) Stimulating wire-reinforced catheter with bullet tip Available length: 60 cm Catheter material is polyurethane with stainless steel Distal 5 mm of catheter uninsulated with exposed metal wire (19-gauge catheter) Distal 6 mm of catheter uninsulated with exposed metal wire (20-gauge catheter) Segment of uninsulated wire coil at proximal end Safety ribbon runs internally over the entire length of the needle Centimeter gradations up to 20 cm Single distal orifice termed "Omniport" 19-gauge catheter is white; 20-gauge catheter is blue Radiopaque Catheter comes with stylet to provide stiffness during catheter advancement No accompanying threading device	In early version, detachable stimulating cable with alligator clip could be connected to needle, proximal catheter or Snap lock catheter connector Later version has integrated stimulating cable on needle Integrated detachable extension tubing either 6 or 18 inches long Cost: $55–$85
Te Me Na SAS Polyplex. Distributed by Avid Medical (Figure 48–17)	*Polyplex T (Tuohy tip):* 18-gauge needle Available lengths 50 mm, 90 mm, 120 mm, 150 mm Uninsulated tip 0.05 mm *Polyplex N (Pencil point tip):* 21-gauge needle Available lengths: 30 mm, 50 mm, 90 mm 18-gauge cannula over needle	Catheter-through-needle design with Polyplex T and CK Cannula-over needle design with Polyplex N, M, C 20-gauge stimulating catheter 90 cm in length Overlying PTFE sleeve Uninsulated tip 0.1 mm Centimeter gradations Closed tip with 3 distal orifices	Integrated stimulating wire attached to needle Integrated stimulating wire *or* alligator clip added to stimulating catheter Integrated extension tubing attached to needle (20-cm length) Cost: ~$40

(continued)

Table 48–3.			
Stimulating Catheter Systems (*Continued*)			
System	**Needle Features**	**Catheter Features**	**Additional Features**

	Uninsulated tip is 0.5–0.7 cm
	*Polyplex M (short-bevel tip,
	    45 degrees):*
	21-gauge needle
	Available length: 50 mm
	18-gauge cannula over needle
	Uninsulated tip 0.5–0.7 cm
	Polyplex C (long-bevel tip, 20 degrees):
	21-gauge needle
	Available lengths: 30 mm, 50 mm,
	    90 mm
	18-gauge cannula over needle
	Uninsulated tip 0.5–0.7 cm
	*Polyplex CK (long-bevel tip,
	    20 degrees):*
	18-gauge diameter
	Available lengths: 30 mm, 50 mm,
	    70 mm, 90 mm, 120 mm, 150 mm
	Uninsulated tip 0.05 mm
	Insulated with polyester mix
	All needles ≥50 mm have cm
	    gradation
		Translucent
		Radiopaque
		Stylet
		Threading device included	

Information obtained from manufacturers.
PTFE, polytetrafluroroethylene.

is warranted. The literature supports the analgesic efficacy of CPNBs; however, more outcome studies are required to show their effects on postoperative cognitive function, sleep, fatigue, and other measures of quality of life in addition to their effects on rehabilitation, hemostasis, systemic stress response, and immune function.

The recent application of CPNBs for use in outpatients is an additional area requiring further evaluation. It is hoped that regional anesthesiologists will continue to work with equipment manufacturers to further advance the field. For instance, questions remain about the ideal magnitude and design of the uninsulated distal catheter tip, the acceptable stimulating current during electrolocation, and the risk of neural injury from some currently available systems. Consequently, some investigators accept higher current output from stimulating catheters than from insulated needles,[89] whereas others have observed that a lower stimulating current can be achieved owing to a high current density at the tip of the stimulating catheter.[87]

Despite the well-known advantages of CPNBs, relatively few clinicians are adequately trained to introduce these techniques into their practice. Efforts aimed at physician education are underway and a number of quality workshops, and training sessions are available throughout the United States. Similar educational efforts have been underway in Europe for several years. In this technologic era, virtual reality or simulation training may prove to be an excellent alternative to clinical training. In addition, education of patients and surgeons about the benefits of CPNBs may be instrumental to the further advancement of regional anesthesia. Future studies documenting physiologic outcome advantages from CPNBs may provide further impetus for the use of these techniques. It remains to be seen whether the use of ultrasound guidance will facilitate placement of CPNBs. Finally, it is not known how the introduction of ultralong-acting encapsulated local anesthesia solutions will impact the development and clinical use of CPNB equipment and techniques.

References

1. Smith BE, Fischer HB, Scott PV: Continuous sciatic nerve block. Anaesthesia 1984;39(2):155–157.
2. Serpell MG, Millar FA, Thomson MF: Comparison of lumbar plexus block versus conventional opioid analgesia after total knee replacement. Anaesthesia 1991;46(4):275–277.
3. Edwards ND, Wright EM: Continuous low-dose 3-in-1 nerve blockade for postoperative pain relief after total knee replacement. Anesth Analg 1992;75(2):265–267.
4. Matheny JM, Hanks GA, Rung GW, et al: A. A comparison of patient-controlled analgesia and continuous lumbar plexus block after anterior cruciate ligament reconstruction. Arthroscopy 1993;9(1):87–90.
5. Borgeat A, Schappi B, Biasca N, Gerber C: Patient-controlled analgesia after major shoulder surgery: Patient-controlled interscalene analgesia versus patient-controlled analgesia. Anesthesiology 1997;87(6):1343–1347.

6. Singelyn FJ, Aye F, Gouverneur JM: Continuous popliteal sciatic nerve block: An original technique to provide postoperative analgesia after foot surgery. Anesth Analg 1997;84(2):383–386.

7. Borgeat A, Tewes E, Biasca N, Gerber C: Patient-controlled interscalene analgesia with ropivacaine after major shoulder surgery: PCIA vs PCA. Br J Anaesth 1998;81(4):603–605.

8. Singelyn FJ, Deyaert M, Joris D, et al: Effects of intravenous patient-controlled analgesia with morphine, continuous epidural analgesia, and continuous three-in-one block on postoperative pain and knee rehabilitation after unilateral total knee arthroplasty. Anesth Analg 1998;87(1):88–92.

9. Capdevila X, Barthelet Y, Biboulet P, et al: Effects of perioperative analgesic technique on the surgical outcome and duration of rehabilitation after major knee surgery. Anesthesiology 1999;91(1): 8–15.

10. Lehtipalo S, Koskinen LO, Johansson G, et al: Continuous interscalene brachial plexus block for postoperative analgesia following shoulder surgery. Acta Anaesthesiol Scand 1999;43(3):258–264.

11. Chelly JE, Greger J, Gebhard R, et al: Continuous femoral blocks improve recovery and outcome of patients undergoing total knee arthroplasty. J Arthroplasty 2001;16(4):436–445.

12. White PF, Issioui T, Skrivanek GD, et al: The use of a continuous popliteal sciatic nerve block after surgery involving the foot and ankle: Does it improve the quality of recovery? Anesth Analg 2003;97(5):1303–1309.

13. Matthews PJ, Govenden V: Comparison of continuous paravertebral and extradural infusions of bupivacaine for pain relief after thoracotomy. Br J Anaesth 1989;62(2):204–205.

14. Schultz P, Anker-Moller E, Dahl JB, et al: Postoperative pain treatment after open knee surgery: Continuous lumbar plexus block with bupivacaine versus epidural morphine. Reg Anesth 1991;16(1):34–37.

15. Turker G, Uckunkaya N, Yavascaoglu B, et al: Comparison of the catheter-technique psoas compartment block and the epidural block for analgesia in partial hip replacement surgery. Acta Anaesthesiol Scand 2003;47(1):30–36.

16. Nielsen KC, Greengrass RA, Pietrobon R, et al: Continuous interscalene brachial plexus blockade provides good analgesia at home after major shoulder surgery–report of four cases. Can J Anaesth 2003;50(1):57–61.

17. Zaric D, Boysen K, Christiansen J, et al: Continuous popliteal sciatic nerve block for outpatient foot surgery–a randomized, controlled trial. Acta Anaesthesiol Scand 2004;48(3):337–341.

18. Buettner J, Klose R, Hoppe U, Wresch P: Serum levels of mepivacaine-HCl during continuous axillary brachial plexus block. Reg Anesth 1989;14(3):124–127.

19. van den Berg B, Berger A, van den Berg E, et al: Continuous plexus anesthesia to improve circulation in peripheral microvascular interventions. Handchir Mikrochir Plast hir 1983;15(2):101–104.

20. Camprubi Sociats I, Garcia Huete L, Sabate Pes A, et al: Use of axillary perivascular blockage of the brachial plexus with a catheter as treatment in accidental intra-arterial injection of drugs. Rev Esp Anestesiol Reanim 1989;36(3):167–170.

21. Haynsworth RF, Heavner JE, Racz GB: Continuous brachial plexus blockade using an axillary catheter for treatment of accidental intra-arterial injections. Reg Anesth 1985;10:187.

22. Berger JL, Nimier M, Desmonts JM: Continuous axillary plexus block in the treatment of accidental intraarterial injection of cocaine. N Engl J Med 1988;318(14):930.

23. Aguilar JL, Domingo V, Samper D, et al: Long-term brachial plexus anesthesia using a subcutaneous implantable injection system. Case report. Reg Anesth 1995;20(3):242–245.

24. Fischer HB, Peters TM, Fleming IM, Else TA: Peripheral nerve catheterization in the management of terminal cancer pain. Reg Anesth 1996;21(5):482–485.

25. Ansbro FP: A method of continuous brachial plexus block. Am J Surg 1946;71:716–722.

26. Sarnoff SJ, Sarnoff LC: Prolonged peripheral nerve block by means of indwelling plastic catheter. Treatment of hiccup. Anesthesiology 1951;12(3):270–275.

27. DeKrey JA, Schroeder CF, Buechel DR: Continuous brachial plexus block. Anesthesiology 1969;30(3):332.

28. Winnie AP: Interscalene brachial plexus block. Anesth Analg 1970;49(3):455–466.

29. Selander D: Catheter technique in axillary plexus block. Presentation of a new method. Acta Anaesthesiol Scand 1977;21(4):324–329.

30. Brands E, Callanan VI: Continuous lumbar plexus block—analgesia for femoral neck fractures. Anaesth Intensive Care 1978;6(3):256–258.

31. Rosenblatt RM: Modified Seldinger technique for continuous interscalene brachial plexus block. Reg Anesth 1981;6:82.

32. Thompson GE, Rorie DK: Functional anatomy of the brachial plexus sheaths. Anesthesiology 1983;59(2):117–122.

33. Tuominen M, Rosenberg PH, Kalso E: Blood levels of bupivacaine after single dose, supplementary dose and during continuous infusion in axillary plexus block. Acta Anaesthesiol Scand 1983;27(4):303–306.

34. Manriquez RG, Pallares V: Continuous brachial plexus block for prolonged sympathectomy and control of pain. Anesth Analg 1978;57(1):128–130.

35. Economacos G, Skountzos V: Nerve blocking of the sciatic and femoral nerves. Continual block with vein catheter on 44 patients. Acta Anaesthesiol Belg 1980;31(Suppl):223–228.

36. Vatashsky E, Aronson HB: Continuous interscalene brachial plexus block for surgical operations on the hand. Anesthesiology 1980;53(4):356.

37. Sada T, Kobayashi T, Murakami S: Continuous axillary brachial plexus block. Can Anaesth Soc J 1983;30(2):201–205.

38. Neimkin RJ, May JW Jr, Roberts J, Sunder N: Continuous axillary block through an indwelling Teflon catheter. J Hand Surg (Am) 1984;9(6):830–833.

39. Conacher ID, Kokri M: Postoperative paravertebral blocks for thoracic surgery. A radiological appraisal. Br J Anaesth 1987;59(2):155–161.

40. Lonnqvist PA: Continuous paravertebral block in children. Initial experience. Anaesthesia 1992;47(7):607–609.

41. Vaghadia H, Kapnoudhis P, Jenkins LC, Taylor D: Continuous lumbosacral block using a Tuohy needle and catheter technique.[see comment] Can J Anaesth 1992;39(1):75–78.

42. Chan V, Ferrante FM. Continuous thoracic paravertebral block. In: Ferrante FM, VadeBoncouer TR (eds): *Postoperative Pain Management.* Churchill Livingstone, 1993.

43. Selander D, Dhuner KG, Lundborg G: Peripheral nerve injury due to injection needles used for regional anesthesia. An experimental study of the acute effects of needle point trauma. Acta Anaesthesiol Scand 1977;21(3):182–188.

44. Buttner J, Kemmer A, Argo A, et al: Axillary blockade of the brachial plexus. A prospective evaluation of 1133 cases of plexus catheter anesthesia. Reg Anaesth 1988;11(1):7–11.

45. Selander D, Edshage S, Wolff T: Paresthesiae or no paresthesiae? Nerve lesions after axillary blocks. Acta Anaesthesiol Scand 1979;23(1):27–33.

46. Montgomery SJ, Raj PP, Nettles D, Jenkins MT: The use of the nerve stimulator with standard unsheathed needles in nerve blockade. Anesth Analg 1973;52(5):827–831.

47. Ford DJ, Pither C, Raj PP: Comparison of insulated and uninsulated needles for locating peripheral nerves with a peripheral nerve stimulator. Anesth Analg 1984;63(10):925–928.

48. Anker-Moller E, Spangsberg N, Dahl JB, et al: Continuous blockade of the lumbar plexus after knee surgery: A comparison of the plasma concentrations and analgesic effect of bupivacaine 0.250% and 0.125%. Acta Anaesthesiol Scand 1990;34(6):468–472.

49. Ben-David B, Lee E, Croitoru M: Psoas block for surgical repair of hip fracture: A case report and description of a catheter technique. Anesth Analg 1990;71(3):298–301.

50. Concepcion M: Continuous brachial plexus techniques. In: Ferrante FM, VadeBoncoeur TR (eds): *Postoperative Pain Management.* Churchill Livingstone, 1993.

51. Rosenblatt R, Pepitone-Rockwell F, McKillop MJ: Continuous axillary analgesia for traumatic hand injury. Anesthesiology 1979;51(6):565–566.

52. Prosser DP: Adaptation of an intravenous cannula for paediatric regional anaesthesia. Anaesthesia 1996;51(5):510.

53. Tan TS, Watcha MF, Safavi F, et al: Cannulation of the axillary brachial sheath in children. Anesth Analg 1995;80(3):640–641.

54. Thomson S: Long-term indwelling catheter for intermittent axillary plexus blocks with bupivacaine.[comment]. Anaesth Intensive Care 1990;18(2):276–277.

55. Pere P, Tuominen M, Rosenberg PH: Cumulation of bupivacaine, desbutylbupivacaine and 4-hydroxybupivacaine during and after continuous interscalene brachial plexus block. Acta Anaesthesiol Scand 1991;35(7):647–650.

56. Tuominen MK, Pere P, Rosenberg PH: Unintentional arterial catheterization and bupivacaine toxicity associated with continuous interscalene brachial plexus block. Anesthesiology 1991;75(2):356–358.

57. Pere P, Pitkanen M, Rosenberg PH, et al: Effect of continuous interscalene brachial plexus block on diaphragm motion and on ventilatory function. Acta Anaesthesiol Scand 1992;36(1):53–57.

58. De Andres J, Bellver J, Barrera L, et al: A comparative study of analgesia after knee surgery with intraarticular bupivacaine, intraarticular morphine, and lumbar plexus block. Anesth Analg 1993;77(4):727–730.

59. Pere P: The effect of continuous interscalene brachial plexus block with 0.125% bupivacaine plus fentanyl on diaphragmatic motility and ventilatory function. Reg Anesth 1993;18(2):93–97.

60. Guzeldemir ME, Ustunsoz B: Ultrasonographic guidance in placing a catheter for continuous axillary brachial plexus block. Anesth Analg 1995;81(4):882–883.

61. Larsen VH, Treschow M: Venous blood gas analysis for evaluation of blood circulation of the hand during continuous axillary block. Acta Anaesthesiol Scand 1995;39(5):554–556.

62. Pham-Dang C, Meunier JF, Poirier P, et al: A new axillary approach for continuous brachial plexus block. A clinical and anatomic study. Anesth Analg 1995;81(4):686–693.

63. Lucas MA, Harrop-Griffiths AW: Interscalene patient-controlled analgesia. Anaesthesia 1997;52(3):263–264.

64. Mezzatesta JP, Scott DA, Schweitzer SA, Selander DE: Continuous axillary brachial plexus block for postoperative pain relief. Intermittent bolus versus continuous infusion. Reg Anesth 1997;22(4):357–362.

65. Iskandar H, Rakotondriamihary S, Dixmerias F, et al: Analgesia using continuous axillary block after surgery of severe hand injuries: Self-administration versus continuous injection. Ann Fr Anesth Reanim 1998;17(9):1099–1103.

66. Longo SR, Williams DP: Bilateral fascia iliaca catheters for postoperative pain control after bilateral total knee arthroplasty: A case report and description of a catheter technique. Reg Anesth 1997;22(4):372–377.

67. Ganapathy S, Wasserman RA, Watson JT, et al: Modified continuous femoral three-in-one block for postoperative pain after total knee arthroplasty.[see comment] Anesth Analg 1999;89(5):1197–1202.

68. Steele SM, Klein SM, D'Ercole FJ, et al: A new continuous catheter delivery system. Anesth Analg 1998;87(1):228.

69. Klein SM, Greengrass RA, Gleason DH, et al: Major ambulatory surgery with continuous regional anesthesia and a disposable infusion pump. Anesthesiology 1999;91(2):563–565.

70. Klein SM, Grant SA, Greengrass RA, et al: Interscalene brachial plexus block with a continuous catheter insertion system and a disposable infusion pump. Anesth Analg 2000;91(6):1473–1478.

71. Grant SA, Nielsen KC, Greengrass RA, et al: Continuous peripheral nerve block for ambulatory surgery. Reg Anesth Pain Med 2001;26(3):209–214.

72. Klein SM, Greengrass RA, Grant SA, et al: Ambulatory surgery for multi-ligament knee reconstruction with continuous dual catheter peripheral nerve blockade. Can J Anaesth 2001;48(4):375–378.

73. Horlocker TT, Hebl JR, Kinney MA, Cabanela ME. Opioid-free analgesia following total knee arthroplasty–a multimodal approach using continuous lumbar plexus (psoas compartment) block, acetaminophen, and ketorolac. Reg Anesth Pain Med 2002;27(1):105–108.

74. Denny NM, Barber N, Sildown DJ: Evaluation of an insulated Tuohy needle system for the placement of interscalene brachial plexus catheters. Anaesthesia 2003;58(6):554–557.

75. Kaloul I, Guay J, Cote C, et al: Ropivacaine plasma concentrations are similar during continuous lumbar plexus blockade using the anterior three-in-one and the posterior psoas compartment techniques. Can J Anaesth 2004;51(1):52–56.

76. Kaloul I, Guay J, Cote C, Fallaha M: The posterior lumbar plexus (psoas compartment) block and the three-in-one femoral nerve block provide similar postoperative analgesia after total knee replacement. Can J Anaesth 2004;51(1):45–51.

77. di Benedetto P, Casati A, Bertini L: Continuous subgluteus sciatic nerve block after orthopedic foot and ankle surgery: Comparison of two infusion techniques. Reg Anesth Pain Med 2002;27(2):168–172.

78. Casati A, Borghi B, Fanelli G, et al: Interscalene brachial plexus anesthesia and analgesia for open shoulder surgery: A randomized, double-blinded comparison between levobupivacaine and ropivacaine. Anesth Analg 2003;96(1):253–259.

79. Casati A, Vinciguerra F, Scarioni M, et al: Lidocaine versus ropivacaine for continuous interscalene brachial plexus block after open shoulder surgery. Acta Anaesthesiol Scand 2003;47(3):355–360.

80. Dadure C, Raux O, Gaudard P, et al: Continuous psoas compartment blocks after major orthopedic surgery in children: A prospective computed tomographic scan and clinical studies. Anesth Analg 2004;98:623–628.

81. Lee BH, Goucke CR: Shearing of a peripheral nerve catheter. Anesth Analg 2002;95(3):760–761.

82. Sutherland ID: Continuous sciatic nerve infusion: Expanded case report describing a new approach. Reg Anesth Pain Med 1998;23(5):496–501.

83. Boezaart AP, de Beer JF, du Toit C, van Rooyen K: A new technique of continuous interscalene nerve block. Can J Anaesth 1999;46(3):275–281.

84. Boezaart AP, De Beer JF, Nell ML: Early experience with continuous cervical paravertebral block using a stimulating catheter. Reg Anesth Pain Med 2003;28(5):406–413.

85. Borene SC, Rosenquist RW, Koorn R, et al: An indication for continuous cervical paravertebral block (posterior approach to the interscalene space). Anesth Analg 2003;97(3):898–900.

86. Ilfeld BM, Morey TE, Enneking FK: Infraclavicular perineural local anesthetic infusion: A comparison of three dosing regimens for postoperative analgesia. Anesthesiology 2004;100(2):395–402.

87. Wehling MJ, Koorn R, Leddell C, Boezaart AP: Electrical nerve stimulation using a stimulating catheter: What is the lower limit? Reg Anesth Pain Med 2004;29(3):230–233.

88. Kick O, Blanche E, Pham-Dang C, et al: A new stimulating stylet for immediate control of catheter tip position in continuous peripheral nerve blocks. Anesth Analg 1999;89(2):533–534.

89. Pham-Dang C, Kick O, Collet T, et al: Continuous peripheral nerve blocks with stimulating catheters. Reg Anesth Pain Med 2003;28(2):83–88.

90. Copeland SJ, Laxton MA: A new stimulating catheter for continuous peripheral nerve blocks. Reg Anesth Pain Med 2001;26(6):589–590.

91. Salinas FV: Location, location, location: Continuous peripheral nerve blocks and stimulating catheters. Reg Anesth Pain Med 2003;28(2):79–82.

Stimulating Catheters

André P. Boezaart, MD

INTRODUCTION

It has been well established that peripheral nerve blocks and neuraxial blocks provide superior analgesia for the treatment of acute pain, especially postoperative pain. The main limitation of these modalities is that acute postoperative pain usually outlasts the relief afforded by single-injection techniques. As a result, continuous peripheral nerve blocks have been developed to overcome these limitations, to extend analgesia beyond duration of a single-injection method, and to allow for greater ability to titrate sensory–motor differentiation of the blockade. Unlike the case for single-injection techniques, continuous nerve block via a perineural catheter, can be discontinued or the infusion changed if unwanted side effects occur. The main emphasis during the past decade has been to develop catheters and techniques that allow relatively simple, accurate, and noninvasive catheter placement to ensure effectiveness and to reduce secondary block failure. These aims

have been largely accomplished in the past decade; the current efforts seek to define indications and infusion strategies for continuous peripheral nerve blocks, especially in the setting of outpatient surgery.

Two techniques are currently used to place perineural catheters: the nonstimulating catheter technique described by Steele and colleagues[1] and the stimulating catheter technique.[2] With a nonstimulating technique, an insulated needle (usually a Tuohy needle) is inserted near a nerve with the aid of a nerve stimulator. Saline or a local anesthetic agent is then injected through the needle to "expand" the perineural space, and a catheter (usually an epidural, multiorifice catheter) is inserted. This technique is relatively simple to perform and provides a reliable primary block (local anesthetic agent injected through the needle). However, because the catheter is placed without confirmation of the tip position, the success rate of the secondary block (infusion through the catheter) may be lower than for the primary block.

With the stimulating catheter technique, an insulated needle (typically a Tuohy needle) is inserted close to a nerve, and a nerve stimulator is used, similar to the procedure for a nonstimulating technique (Figure 49–1). Once the nerve or plexus is electrolocalized, a catheter with an electrically conductive connection to the tip of the catheter (a spring wire[2] or a steel stylet[3]) is then inserted through the needle (Figure 49.2). This allows stimulation of the nerve via the catheter to ensure accurate positioning. With this technique, both the bolus dose and continuous infusion of local anesthetic are injected through the catheter. This technique requires a few extra steps; however, the confirmation of the needle tip position logically should provide a lower risk of secondary block failure due to more accurate catheter placement.[4]

HISTORICAL OVERVIEW AND FUTURE TRENDS

F. Paul Ansbro[5] is credited with the first use of a continuous nerve block in 1946, although he did not use a perineural catheter. Instead, he inserted a blunt needle lateral to the subclavian artery in contact with the first rib after eliciting paresthesia in the patient's arm (Chapter 48). He then secured the needle by inserting it through a cork and strapping the cork to the skin with adhesive tape. The needle was connected with a rubber tube to a 10-mL Luer-Lok syringe for repeated injections of a local anesthetic agent. The objective of the continuous nerve block was to increase the duration of action of the 1% procaine that was used. The author presented 27 cases in which the average duration of the anesthesia was 2 h, ranging from 90 min to 4 h and 20 min. This was a significant improvement over the usual 15-min duration obtained with a single injection of 1% procaine.

Interestingly, the earliest recorded uses of electrical nerve stimulation for peripheral nerve block[3] and neuraxial block[6] were in 1951 and 1949, respectively, to assist in accurate placement of catheters for continuous block and not for needle placement (Chapters 5 and 17). Stanley and Lili-Charlotte Sarnoff pioneered the use of nerve stimulation for continuous peripheral perineural and subarachnoid block for the accurate placement of catheters. In the midst of the polio epidemic of the late 1940s and early 1950s, the Sarnoffs worked on the development of the "Electrophrenic Respirator" at the Harvard School of Public Health.[7] This device was capable of eliciting breathing by stimulating the phrenic nerve transcutaneously in cases of bulbar polio in which respiration could not be established by the iron lung. At the time, the couple's daughter, Daniela, was stricken by bulbar polio and saved by this method. This event made worldwide news under the headline "The Device (that) Cheats Death."

Armed with this knowledge and previous experience of precise placing of intrathecal catheters with nerve stimulation,[6] Stanley Sarnoff was confronted with a patient suffering from intractable hiccups.[3] He placed a "prolonged peripheral nerve block" catheter to continuously and accurately block the patient's phrenic nerve by stimulating it

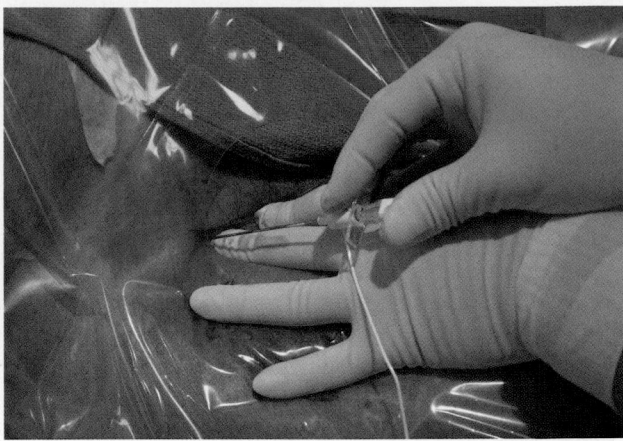

Figure 49–1. The first step is nerve localization techniques identical to those with nonstimulating catheters. Shown here is the needle insertion for femoral nerve block.

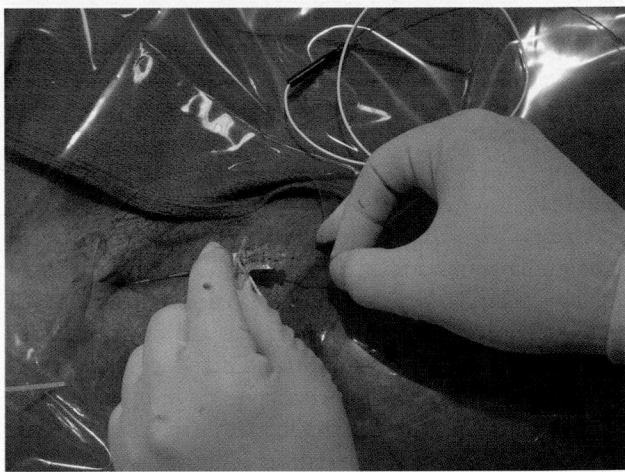

Figure 49–2. Once the nerve is localized using stimulation with the needle, the needle is disconnected from the nerve stimulator and the motor response ceases. The stimulating *catheter* is now connected to the nerve stimulator and inserted through the needle, which brings back the motor response.

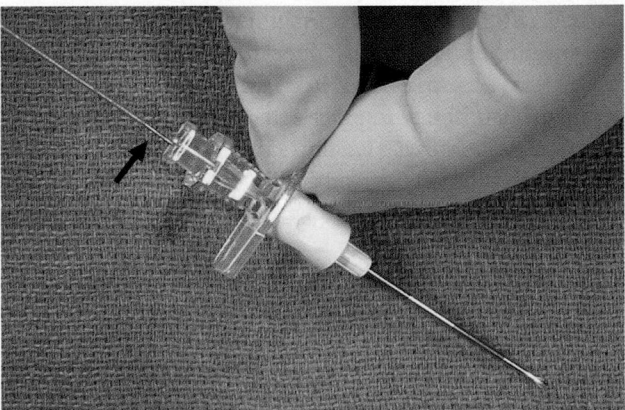

Figure 49–3. As the stimulating catheter is inserted through the needle, the exposed tip (*arrow*) of the catheter makes electrical contact with the inner metal lining of the needle and again enables stimulation with the needle until the tip of the catheter exits the needle.

via the catheter. In his description of the technique he stated that

> "The accurate placement of the tip of the needle and catheter is important to the success of the procedure . . . we adapted a previously described method of electrical localization of catheters to the purpose . . . by applying an electrical potential to the tip of the catheter by way of its stylet in the subarachnoid space. The same principle was used in localizing the tip of the needle in relation to the phrenic nerve in this study."

Indeed, early on nerve stimulation in nerve block was used to accurately place catheters for continuous blockade of a motor nerve—the phrenic nerve. Paradoxically, the nonstimulating catheter technique is often referred to as the "classical technique," when in fact the stimulating technique was the technique that was described first.

It was only decades later after the use of nerve stimulators for single-injection blocks of peripheral nerves became more popular that the technique of placing catheters for continuous peripheral nerve blocks by stimulating the nerve via both the needle and the catheter was "reinvented."[2,8] In the 30 years after the first descriptions by Sarnoff and Sarnoff, the main focus in the development of continuous peripheral nerve blocks was on the upper extremity, and mainly to improve blood flow by sympathetic block for reimplantations of traumatic amputated parts of the upper limb. Most authors used variations of the axillary perivascular technique in the 1970s and 1980s.[9–12] For example, during the Angola Civil War in 1975 the present author, acting as anesthesiologist for the Number 1 Forward Surgical Unit, used a cutdown technique and under direct vision, placed central line catheters in the perivascular space to manage the pain due to severe battlefield injuries of the hand and arm.[13] Of note, the main indication for continuous blocks in the 1970s and 1980s was to achieve sympathetic block and improve blood flow; at that time analgesia was considered merely, as an additional "bonus" and did not become the primary goal until the early 1990s.

During the 1990s the emphasis shifted toward the use of continuous nerve blocks to manage acute postoperative pain. This was, among other factors, driven by the quest for cost-effective ambulatory surgery following the exponential escalation of health-care costs in the mid- to late 1980s. Because of the efficiency and relative safety of neuraxial nerve blocks, the lower extremity received little attention during the early development of the technique, and the main focus was on continuous blocks for the upper extremity.[14–17] During this era, only the nonstimulating catheter technique was used by most investigators in postoperative treatment of patients undergoing a variety of major surgical procedures on the upper and lower extremities. Francois Singelyn and coworkers[18] were the first to demonstrate that continuous femoral nerve block in patients having total knee replacement provides superior pain control to intravenous morphine and epidural analgesia. This report was followed by others also documenting excellent analgesic potential, fewer complications, and faster rehabilitation with continuous nerve blocks.[19,20]

The secondary failure of continuous nerve block catheters, however, represents a significant obstacle to the ability to reproduce results cited in these and other reports.[21–25] Ganapathy and coworkers[26] and Klein and colleagues[27] alerted practitioners to the importance of ensuring the functionality of the catheters before discharging patients home. Discharging patients from the hospital with continuous nerve blocks that malfunction after the primary block wears off can increase the costs of postoperative management if a patient has to be readmitted to the hospital to treat resulting acute pain.[27] It is for these reasons that the concept of the stimulating catheter (or the Sarnoff technique) was revisited in the mid- to late 1990s.[2,8]

THE STIMULATING CATHETER TECHNIQUE

The technique described here is a general description of the stimulator technique applicable to most peripheral nerve blocks; the specifics of the techniques, however, vary somewhat for individual nerve block procedures. Figures 49–1 through 49–7 illustrate maneuvers specific to the stimulating catheter placement.

Stimulation Through the Needle

- Nerve stimulator is attached to an insulated 17- to 20-gauge needle (eg, StimuCath, Arrow International, Reading PA, USA) and set to deliver 1–1.5 mA (see Figure 49–1).
- The needle is advanced until a brisk motor response of the desired muscle group(s) is elicited with a current output of 0.3 to 0.5 mA (100–300 μsec; frequency 1–2 Hz).
- The needle is then held steady in the stimulating position; no local anesthetic or saline is injected through the needle.
- The nerve stimulator is now disconnected from the needle and attached to the proximal end of the stimulating catheter (see Figure 49–2).

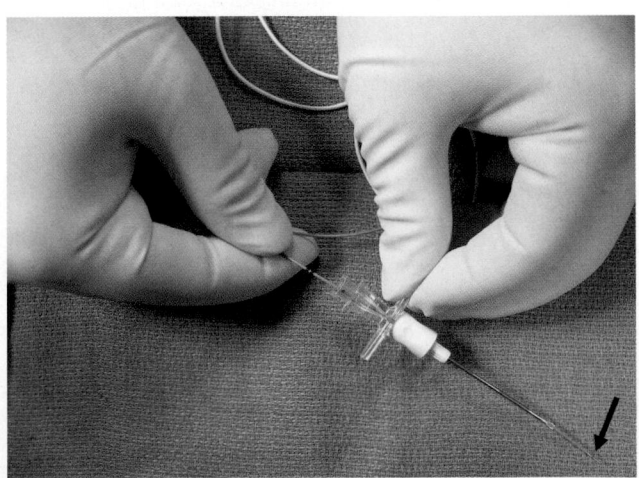

Figure 49–4. As the catheter is advanced through the needle, the tip of the catheter (*arrow*) eventually exits the needle, resulting in transition of the electrical stimulation through the *needle* into stimulation through the tip of the *catheter*.

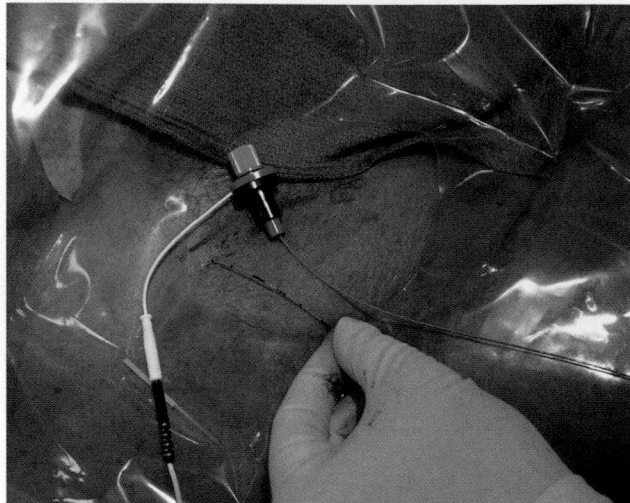

Figure 49–5. Once the catheter is successfully placed, the depth markings are used to position the catheter to the desired depth.

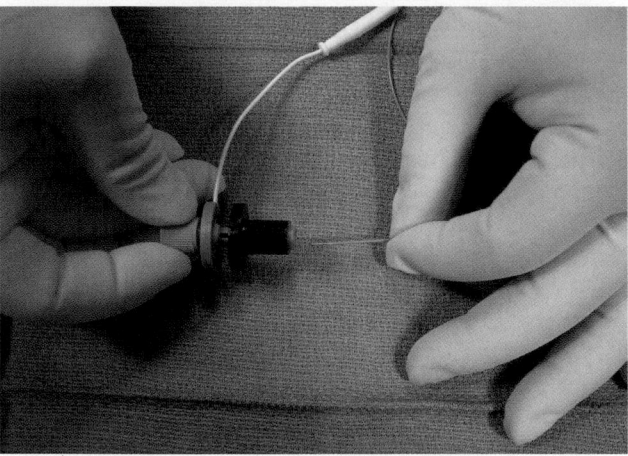

Figure 49–6. Similarly to its tip, the injection end of the catheter has an exposed conducting surface. This end is attached to an injection port, which allows for both electrical connection (neurostimulation) and fluid path (injection or infusion of local anesthetic).

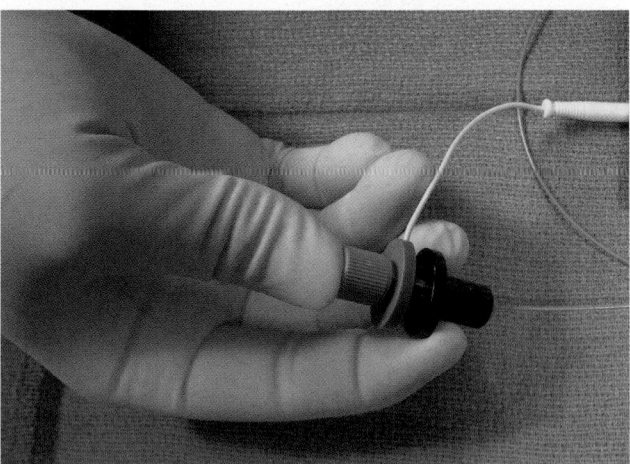

Figure 49–7. Shown is the maneuver required to lock the end of the catheter being secured to the injection/electrostimulation port.

Stimulation Through the Catheter

- The catheter is advanced through the needle to elicit a motor response similar to that elicited by stimulating via the needle (see Figures 49–2 through 49–4).
- The catheter is advanced beyond the distal end of the needle while maintaining the desired motor response (the motor response should remain qualitatively similar).
- The depth markings on the catheter should be observed throughout the procedure. One should be familiar with how these depth markings relate to the shaft of the needle (see Figure 49–5). In other words, the operator should always know the depth of the catheter placement (and whether the catheter tip is inside the needle or exited the needle tip).
- The catheter is then connected to an infusio-stimulation port (Figures 49–6 and 49–7).

Clinical Pearl

CATHETER INSERTION AND TROUBLESHOOTING

- When the motor response disappears or changes to an undesired quality with advancement of the catheter, the catheter is carefully (to prevent shearing off the catheter) withdrawn to inside the shaft of the needle.

- With the catheter in the needle (which converts stimulation from the catheter to the stimulation through the needle) the needle is manipulated slightly by rotating clockwise or counterclockwise or by moving it a few millimeters inward or outward, while maintaining the desired motor response. It is not necessary to reconnect the needle to the stimulator because the tip of the catheter maintains the electrical contact with the inner wall of the needle.

- Once the needle is repositioned, and desired stimulation obtained, the catheter is advanced again. This process is repeated by making small changes to the needle after careful catheter withdrawal until the desired motor response is elicited when the catheter is advanced. The catheter is then advanced 3 to 5 cm along the appropriate nerve.

Catheter-Securing Techniques

Various catheter-securing techniques have been described to prevent dislodgment of the catheters. The catheter can be tunneled subcutaneously to significantly decrease the chance of dislodgment. There are basically two approaches to tunneling the catheter: (1) tunneling without and (2) tunneling with a "skin bridge." Leaving a skin bridge makes catheter removal easier and is normally used for a short-term (1 to 7 days) catheterization, whereas tunneling without a skin bridge is typically used for long-term infusion (>7 days) catheterization and has the potential advantage of preventing infection. The first method may be associated with more leakage at the skin–bridge area, whereas the latter method may make catheter removal more difficult.

With a commonly used technique, the inner steel stylet of the Tuohy needle is used as a guide. If a skin bridge is planned, the needle enters the skin 2 to 3 cm from the catheter exit site, but through the catheter exit site (taking special care not to damage the catheter) if a skin bridge is not wanted. The stylet is then advanced subcutaneously for approximately 8 to 10 cm. The Tuohy needle is then "railroaded" back over the stylet, the stylet is removed, and the distal end of the catheter advanced retrogradely through the needle. The needle is then removed, and the catheter is tunneled. If a skin bridge is left, a small piece of plastic or silicone tubing can be inserted to protect the skin under the skin bridge. Various adhesive materials and methods have been used with success (eg, medical adhesive spray, Steri-Strips, and transparent occlusive dressings).[25]

SUMMARY

The development of the stimulating catheter technique has significantly improved the precision with which catheters are placed near the peripheral nerves and plexuses. More research is needed to clarify optimal surgical indications and infusion strategies for continuous nerve block techniques.

References

1. Steele SM, Klein SM, D'Ercole FJ, et al: A new continuous catheter delivery system (Letter). Anesth Analg 1998; 87(1):28.
2. Boezaart AP, de Beer JF: Accurate placement of a catheter for selective continuous interscalene brachial plexus nerve block (abstract). World Congress of Anesthesiologists, 1996, Sydney, Australia, Abstract number V14.
3. Sarnoff SJ, Sarnoff LC: Prolonged peripheral nerve block by means of indwelling plastic catheter. Treatment of hiccup. Anesthesiology 1951;12(3):270–277.
4. Salinas FV, Neal JM, Sueda LA, et al: Prospective comparison of continuous femoral nerve block with nonstimulating catheter placement versus stimulating catheter-guided perineural placement in volunteers. Reg Anesth Pain Med 2004;29(3):212–220.
5. Ansbro FP: A method of continuous brachial plexus block. Am J Surg 1946;71(6):716–722.
6. Sarnoff SJ: Functional localization of intraspinal catheters. Anesthesiology 1950;11:360–366.
7. Sarnoff, SJ, Hardenbergh E, Whittenberger JL: Electrophrenic Respiration. Science 1948;108:482.
8. Boezaart AP, de Beer JF, Du Toit C, et al: A new technique of continuous interscalene nerve block. Can J Anaesth 1999;46(3):275–281.
9. Selander D: Catheter technique in axillary plexus block. Acta Anaesthesiol Scand 1977;21:324–329.
10. Manriquez RG, Pallares V: Continuous brachial plexus block for prolonged sympathectomy and control of pain. Anesth Analg 1978;57:128–130.
11. Sada T, Kobayashi T, Murakami S: Continuous axillary brachial plexus block. Can Anaesth Soc J 1983;30(2):201–205.
12. Ang ET, Lassale B, Goldfarb G: Continuous axillary brachial plexus block—A clinical and anatomical study. Anesth Analg 1984;63:680–684.
13. Buckenmaier CC III: Battlefield Orthopaedic Injuries. In: Boezaart AP (ed): *Anesthesia and Orthopaedic Surgery.* McGraw-Hill, 2006 (in press).
14. Haasio J, Tuominen M, Rosenberg PH: Continuous interscalene brachial plexus block during and after shoulder surgery. Ann Chir Gynaecol Suppl 1990;79:103–107.
15. Rosenberg PH, Pere P, Hekali R, et al: Plasma concentrations of bupivacaine and two of its metabolites during continuous interscalene brachial plexus block. Br J Anaesth 1991;66:25–30.
16. Pere P, Tuominen M, Rosenberg PH: Cumulation of bupivacaine, desbutylbupivacaine and 4-hydroxybupivacaine during and after continuous interscalene brachial plexus block. Acta Anaesthesiol Scand 1991;35:647–650.
17. Koh DLH, Lim BH: Postoperative continuous interscalene brachial plexus blockade for hand surgery. Ann Acad Med Singapore 1995;24(4)(Suppl):3S–7S.
18. Singelyn FJ, Deyaert M, Joris D, et al: Effects of intravenous patient-controlled analgesia with morphine, continuous epidural analgesia, and continuous three-in-one block on postoperative pain and knee rehabilitation after unilateral total knee arthroplasty. Anesth Analg 1998;87:88–92.
19. Capdevila X, Barthelet Y, Biboulet P, et al: Effects of perioperative analgesic technique on the surgical outcome and duration of rehabilitation after major knee surgery. Anesthesiology 1999;19(1):8–15.
20. Chelly JE, Greger J, Gebhard R, et al: Continuous femoral blocks improve recovery and outcome of patients undergoing total knee arthroplasty. J Arthroplasty 2001;16(4):436–445.
21. Borgeat A, Schäppi B, Biasca N, et al: Patient-controlled analgesia after major shoulder surgery. Anesthesiology 1997;87(6):1343–1347.
22. Ilfeld BM, Morey TE, Wright TW, et al: Interscalene perineural ropivacaine infusion: A comparison of two dosing regimens for postoperative analgesia. Reg Anesth Pain Med 2004;29(1):1–3.
23. Ilfeld BM, Morey TE, Enneking FK: Infraclavicular perineural local anesthetic infusion: A comparison of three dosing regimens for postoperative analgesia. Anesthesiology 2004;100(2):395–402.
24. Ilfeld BM, Thannikary LJ, Morey TE, et al: Popliteal sciatic perineural local anesthetic infusion: A comparison of three dosing regimens for postoperative analgesia. Anesthesiology 2004;101(4):970–977.
25. Grant SA, Nielsen KC, Greengrass RA, et al: Continuous peripheral nerve block for ambulatory surgery. Reg Anesth Pain Med 2001;26(3):209–214.
26. Ganapathy S, Wasserman RA, Watson JT, et al: Modified continuous femoral three-in-one block for postoperative pain after total knee arthroplasty. Anesth Analg 1999;89:1197–1202.
27. Klein SM, Steele SM, Nielsen KC, et al: The difficulties of ambulatory interscalene and intra-articular infusions for rotator cuff surgery: A preliminary report. Can J Anesth 2003;50(3):265–269.

Ultrasound-Guided Regional Anesthesia

50

Introduction to Ultrasound-Assisted Regional Anesthesia Techniques

Andrew T. Gray, MD, PhD

I. ULTRASOUND IMAGING

II. DOPPLER

III. NERVE IDENTIFICATION WITH ULTRASOUND

IV. BLOCK NEEDLE TIP VISIBILITY

V. APPROACHES TO REGIONAL BLOCK WITH ULTRASOUND

VI. LIMITATIONS OF ULTRASOUND IMAGING

VII. TRAINING AND SAFETY

ULTRASOUND IMAGING

Ultrasound imaging utilizes high-frequency sound waves (3–17 MHz). Because the speed of sound in soft tissue is fairly constant (1540 m/sec), the position of objects can be inferred from the time of flight of their received echoes. The product of wavelength and frequency is the speed of sound, so high-frequency sound waves have shorter wavelengths, and therefore provide better axial resolution. Attenuation of sound waves is frequency-dependent (approximately 0.75 dB/cm/MHz), so penetration of high-frequency sound waves into deep tissue is limited. For interventional guidance, one of the biggest advantages of ultrasound over other imaging modalities is the real-time acquisition of images. Frame rates of 30 Hz or higher are common in clinical practice.

Theoretically, ultrasound imaging can cause warming of tissue through absorption of sound waves (quantified by the thermal index). Transmission of sound waves also can cause cavitation (gas body formation, quantified by the mechanical index). However, no adverse biological effects have been confirmed for diagnostic ultrasound. Nevertheless, it is prudent to limit scanning to that necessary for clinical care and related education.

The most common artifact associated with ultrasound imaging is contact artifact. **Contact artifact** is defined as loss of acoustic coupling between transducer and skin. Scanning gel is normally applied to exclude air from the transducer–skin interface. This interface can be disrupted simply because the transducer does not touch the skin. Another common cause is trapping of air bubbles under the sterile cover of the transducer. If the block needle is inserted too close to the transducer, the skin contact will be disturbed. Firm, even pressure with the transducer (like holding a mask to ventilate an anesthetized patient) is required to produce optimal scans. Manual compression exerted with the transducer is usually optimal for regional block when sufficient to just cause coaptation of the walls of superficial veins within the field of imaging.

Throughout this chapter I will use the American Institute of Ultrasound in Medicine (AIUM) standard nomenclature for transducer manipulation: tilting, rocking, sliding, compression, and rotation.[1]

DOPPLER

In 1842 Christian Johann Doppler described the frequency shift that occurs when a wave source or receiver moves. Doppler's stellar observation has been applied to estimate the velocity of moving reflectors in the body (typically red blood cells) by measuring the frequency shift of sound waves. Modern color Doppler velocity imaging maps the mean velocity to a color scale. Specifically, color flow mapping systems overlay a pseudocolor velocity map on a gray-scale, two-dimensional image.[2]

Recently a new color Doppler technology has been developed.[3] Rather than estimate the mean Doppler frequency shift, these new technologies are based on estimating the integrated Doppler power spectrum. The advantage of power Doppler is that it is more sensitive at detecting blood flow than velocity imaging (by a factor of 3 to 5 in some cases). In addition, the integrated power Doppler signal is almost independent of the angle between the vessel and the transducer beam. Finally, power Doppler is not subject to aliasing artifacts.[4] The disadvantages of power Doppler are the high motion sensitivity (flash artifact) and the lack of directional information.

When performing regional blocks it is important to distinguish small arteries from small monofascicular nerves because these two anatomic structures often run together. For the reasons cited earlier, power Doppler is the best tool for this purpose. In addition, visible pulsations with probe compression also can be useful in identifying small arteries.

Nerve vasculature can be demonstrated with color Doppler in some normal subjects. Longitudinal vessels within the epineurium or microvasculature within nerves can occasionally be detected,[5,6] However, a robust Doppler signal clearly distinguishes small arteries from nerves (Figure 50–1).

NERVE IDENTIFICATION WITH ULTRASOUND

Peripheral nerves have a fascicular echotexture (Figure 50–2). This means that when viewed on a transverse scan (short-axis view) peripheral nerves have a "honey-comb" appearance.[7] When questions regarding nerve identification arise it is often useful to trace the known course and divisions of the nerve. Transverse scanning by sliding a broad linear transducer is the preferred method for following a nerve along its course. Long-axis slides are useful for panoramic views of the nerve course but are difficult and time-consuming to construct.[8]

Nerves can change shape along the nerve path depending on the surrounding tissues. Nerve paths also can be curved and even change with extremity motion. However, in the absence of major branching the cross-sectional area of nerves is relatively constant along the nerve path and can be used as a discriminating feature. Using these techniques monofascicular nerves as small as 1 mm in diameter have been imaged with high-resolution ultrasound.[9]

Peripheral nerves exhibit anisotropy.[10,11] This implies the amplitude of the received echoes will vary with the angle of insonation. Angle changes as small as 10 degrees away from perpendicular to the axis of the nerve will substantially reduce its echogenicity. Tendons are even more highly ordered than nerves, so anisotropic effects are seen with angle changes as small as 2 degrees. Transducer manipulation plays a major role in optimizing nerve imaging. Trained clinicians will naturally

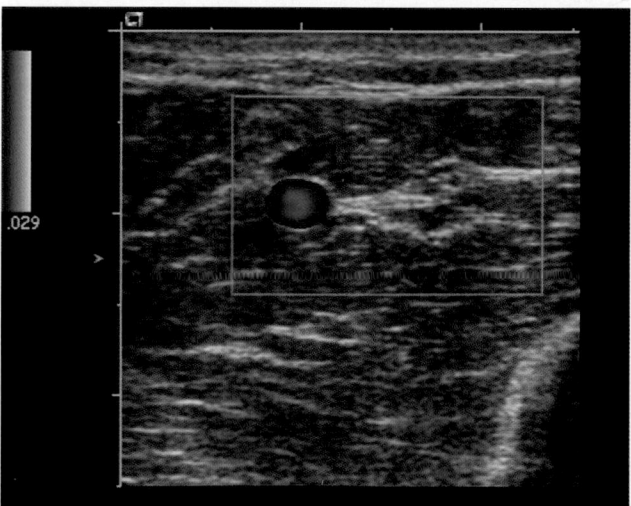

Figure 50–1. Color power Doppler imaging. In this forearm sonogram the ulnar artery and ulnar nerve are seen in transverse (short-axis) view. The robust color power Doppler signal clearly distinguishes the ulnar artery from the adjacent ulnar nerve.

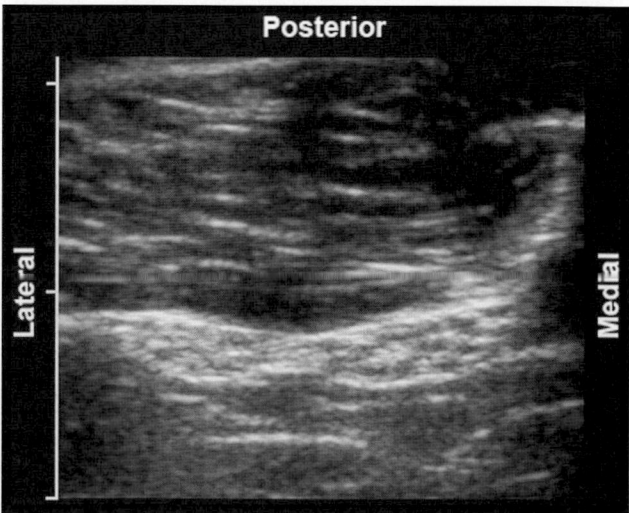

Figure 50–2. Fascicular echotexture of peripheral nerves. In this sonogram obtained from the thigh the fasciculated echotextures of the common peroneal (lateral) and tibial (medial) nerves are seen.

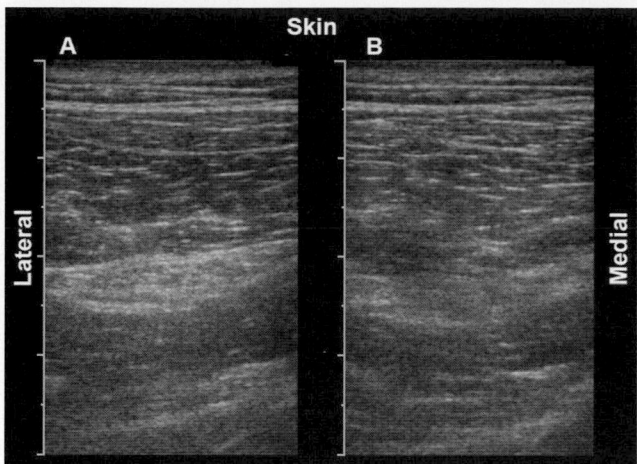

Figure 50–3. Anisotropy of peripheral nerves. In these side-by-side sonograms the sciatic nerve is seen in transverse (short-axis) view. Tilting the transducer from neutral position (**A**) to approximately 10 degrees (**B**) markedly reduces the received echoes from the nerve.

adjust the transducer to fill in the received echoes from the nerve (Figure 50–3).

Nerve motion can be revealed by dynamic ultrasound imaging.[12] With this method nerves are imaged with extremity movement. This best example of nerve motion is in the popliteal fossa. Foot movement will result in a characteristic "seesaw" pattern of nerve motion that can be used to identify the common peroneal, tibial, and common sciatic nerves.

BLOCK NEEDLE TIP VISIBILITY

A number of factors influence needle tip visibility,[13] one of the most important of which is the angle of the block needle with respect to the ultrasound beam. Strong specular reflections occur from beam angles perpendicular to the needle, even when the needle is slightly out of the scan plane.[14] Studies of needle tip echo have found a linear correlation between angle of incidence and mean brightness.[15]

One recent strategy to improve needle tip visibility is to use spatial compound imaging (beam steering to differing angles to produce overlapping scans that will form a composite image). Although spatial compounding has been found to reduce the effect of angle on needle tip echo when compared with single-line imaging, decreases in needle visibility still occur.[16] The needle tip is best visualized when the bevel is oriented either directly toward or away from the transducer.[17,18] As expected, increasing needle diameter improves visualization of the needle tip echo.

Needle visibility is more difficult during deeper blocks for a number of reasons. At steep angles only backscatter from the needle is received by the transducer rather than a strong specular reflection. The beam also attenuates and widens past the focal zone. Visualization of the needle tip can be problematic, particularly within echo-rich tissues such as adipose tissue. It may be necessary to slowly advance or withdraw the needle (a moving echo confirms needle tip identification). An alternative is to slowly turn the needle to change the bevel orientation.

APPROACHES TO REGIONAL BLOCK WITH ULTRASOUND

Two basic approaches to needle placement with ultrasound guidance are in common use. With the out-of-plane approach the needle crosses the plane of imaging as an echogenic dot. The target is typically placed in the center of the field of view. The first pass of the needle is usually made shallow to the target. The transducer can be manipulated using sliding and tilting to follow the needle tip as the needle is advanced. For the out-of-plane technique it is important to distinguish the needle tip echo from the shaft echo. This can usually be confirmed by slightly withdrawing the needle to move the needle tip back away from the plane of imaging.

With the in-plane approach the full needle tip and shaft are visualized along the axis of the needle. The target is positioned on the opposite side of the imaging field (away from the side of approaching needle). It is essential to establish needle tip visibility before advancing the needle. Detection of partial lineups of the needle with the plane of imaging is critical.

This overall scheme is a simplification (the sound beam resembles the shape of an hour glass more than a plane). Although there would seem to be an obvious advantage in visualizing the approaching needle, limitations regarding needle tip visibility in clinical practice make the comparison less clear. We use both out-of-plane and in-plane approaches at our institution and have observed similar rates of paresthesias, vascular punctures, and overall block success. These results need to be confirmed with controlled studies. Furthermore, the results may not apply to all blocks because the consequences of needle misplacement vary with anatomic location. Nevertheless, operator training and skill are probably more important than the approach to regional block per se. With either approach the needle tip is aimed at the edge of the nerve (not directly at the nerve itself).

The target nerve can be viewed in short axis (SAX) or in long axis (LAX). SAX views of the target have dominated regional blocks because the views are stable and provide assessment of circumferential distribution of the injected local anesthetic. LAX views of large, straight vessels are sometimes used for vascular access procedures because if the vessel and needle are both maintained in the plane of imaging the needle is constrained to enter the vessel.

LIMITATIONS OF ULTRASOUND IMAGING

As ultrasound technology improves so will the quality of nerve imaging. However, there are clearly some limitations today for imaging smaller and deeper nerves. Direct imaging of the lumbar plexus has only proved feasible in children who weigh 30 kg or less.[19] Although ultrasound imaging of the sciatic nerve was uniformly successful, imaging of its division in the popliteal fossa failed in 21 of 74 adult patients (28%).[20] In this latter study the only correlate of lack of visibility was the extremity size.

In the context of the current obesity epidemic, it is important to discuss difficult-to-image patients. For some regional blocks vascular surrogate landmarks are appropriate rather than relying on direct nerve imaging. This may be the underlying reason why the infraclavicular block (with three arterial wall-hugging cords of the brachial plexus) and axillary block (with three arterial wall-hugging branches of the brachial plexus) have become so popular with ultrasound imaging. Another alternative is to use ultrasound imaging combining nerve stimulation as a functional assay of nerve location.

Ultrasound is currently limited in its ability to determine the endpoints for local anesthetic injection. Although a volume-sparing effect has been shown for ultrasound guidance for regional block,[21–23] the lower limits and sonographic signs that predict local anesthetic blockade of peripheral nerves have yet to be firmly established.

TRAINING AND SAFETY

Ultrasound imaging plays a key role in our clinical practice for transesophageal echocardiography, line placement, and blocks. There is probably considerable cross training among these skills.

Several steps are critical in achieving proficiency with ultrasound imaging for regional block.[24,25] The first step is scanning skills (the ability to obtain images and recognize nerves). Scanning practice and review of teaching files are critical. In this process it is important to develop image quality control presets, so that the number of adjustments is minimal when actually performing blocks. Learn with the highest quality imaging available before "graduating" to another machine (some people start on the low end and experience frustration). Regarding the art and practice of neural imaging, it is best to begin with nerves that are easier to visualize (ulnar and median in the forearm, tibial nerve near the popliteal crease) before working up to the more difficult ones (brachial plexus in the interscalene groove or infraclavicular region). Of course, some people are difficult to image, but transducer manipulation skills can help a great deal in such cases.

The second step is the phantom skills (the use of tissue equivalent material for simulation of probe and needle manipulation). Purchase of a phantom (or construction of a home-made one) is a worthwhile investment, especially at a teaching institution.[26–28] The physical setup for performance of blocks also can be critical to success. The ideal place for an ultrasound machine is a block room or block bay where there is sufficient space and the lights can be dimmed.

Despite good practice, serious complications can occur during ultrasound-guided interventions.[29] However, there is considerable evidence that ultrasound guidance reduces (but does not eliminate) complications associated with internal jugular vein catheterization.[30] It is likely that we will have parallel findings for ultrasound guidance for regional block. Because of the low incidence of serious complications, examining the overall safety of ultrasound-guided regional anesthesia will require controlled clinical trials with careful patient follow-up.

References

1. AIUM technical bulletin: Transducer manipulation. American Institute of Ultrasound in Medicine. J Ultrasound Med 1999;18:169–175.
2. Ferrara K, DeAngelis G: Color flow mapping. Ultrasound Med Biol 1997;23:321–345.
3. Bude RO, Rubin JM: Power Doppler sonography. Radiology 1996;200:21–23.
4. Chen JF, Fowlkes JB, Carson PL, et al: Autocorrelation of integrated power Doppler signals and its application. Ultrasound Med Biol 1996;22:1053–1057.
5. Martinoli C, Bianchi S, Derchi LE: Tendon and nerve sonography. Radiol Clin North Am 1999;37:691–711, viii.
6. Gassner EM, Schocke M, Peer S, et al: Persistent median artery in the carpal tunnel: Color Doppler ultrasonographic findings. J Ultrasound Med 2002;21:455–461.
7. Martinoli C, Bianchi S, Derchi LE: Ultrasonography of peripheral nerves. Semin Ultrasound CT MR 2000;21:205–213.
8. Peer S, Bodner G: *High-Resolution Sonography of the Peripheral Nervous System.* Springer-Verlag, 2003.
9. Bodner G, Harpf C, Gardetto A, et al: Ultrasonography of the accessory nerve: Normal and pathologic findings in cadavers and patients with iatrogenic accessory nerve palsy. J Ultrasound Med 2002;21:1159–1163.
10. Grechenig W, Clement HG, Peicha G, et al: [Ultrasound anatomy of the sciatic nerve of the thigh] Biomed Tech (Berl) 2000;45:298–303. German.
11. Soong J, Schafhalter-Zoppoth I, Gray AT: The importance of transducer angle to ultrasound visibility of the femoral nerve. Reg Anesth Pain Med 2005;30:505.
12. Schafhalter-Zoppoth I, Younger SJ, Collins AB, et al: The "seesaw" sign: Improved sonographic identification of the sciatic nerve. Anesthesiology 2004;101:808–809.
13. Schafhalter-Zoppoth I, McCulloch CE, Gray AT: Ultrasound visibility of needles used for regional nerve block: An in vitro study. Reg Anesth Pain Med 2004;29:480–488.
14. Cheung S, Rohling R: Enhancement of needle visibility in ultrasound-guided percutaneous procedures. Ultrasound Med Biol 2004;30:617–624.
15. Bondestam S, Kreula J: Needle tip echogenicity. A study with real time ultrasound. Invest Radiol 1989;24:555–560.
16. Cohnen M, Saleh A, Luthen R, et al: Improvement of sonographic needle visibility in cirrhotic livers during transjugular intrahepatic portosystemic stent-shunt procedures with use of real-time compound imaging. J Vasc Interv Radiol 2003;14:103–106.
17. Bradley MJ. An in-vitro study to understand successful free-hand ultrasound guided intervention. Clin Radiol 2001;56:495–498.
18. Hopkins RE, Bradley M: In-vitro visualization of biopsy needles with ultrasound: A comparative study of standard and echogenic needles using an ultrasound phantom. Clin Radiol 2001;56:499–502.
19. Kirchmair L, Enna B, Mitterschiffthaler G, et al: Lumbar plexus in children. A sonographic study and its relevance to pediatric regional anesthesia. Anesthesiology 2004;101:445–450.
20. Schwemmer U, Markus CK, Greim CA, et al: Sonographic imaging of the sciatic nerve division in the popliteal fossa. Ultraschall Med 2005;26:496–500.

21. Marhofer P, Schrogendorfer K, Wallner T, et al: Ultrasonographic guidance reduces the amount of local anesthetic for 3-in-1 blocks. Reg Anesth Pain Med 1998;23:584–588.

22. Sandhu NS, Maharlouei B, Patel B, et al: Simultaneous bilateral infraclavicular brachial plexus blocks with low-dose lidocaine using ultrasound guidance. Anesthesiology 2006;104:199–201.

23. Sandhu NS, Bahniwal CS, Capan LM: Feasibility of an infraclavicular block with a reduced volume of lidocaine with sonographic guidance. J Ultrasound Med 2006;25:51–56.

24. Grau T, Bartusseck E, Conradi R, et al: Ultrasound imaging improves learning curves in obstetric epidural anesthesia: A preliminary study. Can J Anaesth 2003;50:1047–1050.

25. Sites BD, Gallagher JD, Cravero J, et al: The learning curve associated with a simulated ultrasound-guided interventional task by inexperienced anesthesia residents. Reg Anesth Pain Med 2004;29:544–548.

26. Fornage BD: A simple phantom for training in ultrasound-guided needle biopsy using the freehand technique. J Ultrasound Med 1989;8:701–3.

27. Xu D, Abbas S, Chan VW: Ultrasound phantom for hands-on practice. Reg Anesth Pain Med 2005;30:593–594.

28. Chapman GA, Johnson D, Bodenham AR: Visualisation of needle position using ultrasonography. Anaesthesia 2006;61:148–158.

29. Nolsoe C, Nielsen L, Torp-Pedersen S, et al: Major complications and deaths due to interventional ultrasonography: A review of 8000 cases. J Clin Ultrasound 1990;18:179–184.

30. Randolph AG, Cook DJ, Gonzales CA, et al: Ultrasound guidance for placement of central venous catheters: A meta-analysis of the literature. Crit Care Med 1996;24:2053–2058.

51

Ultrasound-Assisted Nerve Blocks in Adults

Anahi Perlas, MD • Vincent Chan, MD

RATIONALE

In recent years interest has been growing in the practice of regional anesthesia and, in particular, in peripheral nerve blocks for surgical anesthesia and postoperative analgesia. Peripheral nerve blocks have been found to be superior to general anesthesia[1] because they provide effective analgesia with few side effects[2] and can hasten patient recovery.[3] Unfortunately, the practice of regional anesthesia does not enjoy widespread endorsement because of inconsistent success, varying from one anesthesiologist to another. Current methods of nerve localization (eg, paresthesia and nerve stimulation) are es-

sentially "blind" procedures, since they both rely on indirect evidence of needle-to-nerve contact.[4,5] Seeking nerves by trial and error and random needle movement can cause complications. Although uncommon, complications such as intravascular local anesthetic injection resulting in systemic toxicity, inadvertent spinal cord injury following interscalene block, pneumothorax following supraclavicular block, and nerve injury have all been reported.[6,7]

Imaging guidance for nerve localization holds the promise of improving block success and decreasing complications. Among imaging modalities currently available, ultrasonography seems to be the one most suitable for regional anesthesia. Perhaps the most significant advantage of ultrasound technology is the ability to provide anatomic examination of the area of interest in real time.[8] Ultrasound imaging allows one to visualize neural structures (plexus and peripheral nerves) and the surrounding structures (eg, blood vessels and pleura), navigate the needle toward the target nerves, and visualize the pattern of local anesthetic spread.[9]

ULTRASOUND PRINCIPLES

An ultrasound probe (transducer) has dual functions. It emits and receives sound waves, thus functioning both as a speaker and a microphone. As the name implies, ultrasound waves are high-frequency sound waves ($\geq$20,000 cycles/sec, 20 kHz) that are not audible to the human ear. Ultrasound frequencies useful in clinical medicine are in the megahertz (MHz) range.[10] When an electric current is applied to an array of piezoelectric crystals (quartz) within the ultrasound transducer, mechanical energy, in the form of vibration, is generated, resulting in ultrasound waves. As the ultrasound waves move through body tissues of different acoustic impedances, they are attenuated (lose amplitude with depth), reflected, or scattered. Waves reflected to the transducer are then transformed back into an electrical signal that is then processed by the ultrasound machine to generate an image on the screen.

Depending on the amount of wave returned, anatomic structures take on different degrees of echogenicity. Structures with high water content, such as blood vessels and cysts, appear hypoechoic (black or dark) because ultrasound waves are transmitted through the structures easily with little reflection. On the other hand, bone and tendons block ultrasound wave transmission, and the strong signal returned to the transducer gives these structures a hyperechoic appearance (bright, white) on the screen. Structures of intermediate density and acoustic impedance, such as the liver parenchyma or the thyroid gland, appear gray on the screen. Knowing the speed of sound in tissue (1540 m/sec on average) and the time of echo return, the distance between the probe and the target structure (depth) is calculated.

ULTRASOUND IN REGIONAL ANESTHESIA

Ultrasound Equipment

Ultrasonography has many applications in clinical anesthesia. With appropriate probes, vascular imaging, echocardiography, and nerve imaging can be performed with the same unit. Compound imaging is an advanced feature in some of the cart-based units. The resolution of nerve images is enhanced with compound imaging when multiple lines of crystals on the transducer (as opposed to a single line) emit and receive ultrasound in multiple planes before final display of the image that is electronically reconstructed. Color Doppler is another useful feature that differentiates vascular from nonvascular structures (eg, nerves). Compact portable units currently available with many of these sophisticated features are also suitable for peripheral nerve imaging.

Transducers (Probes)

Ultrasound scanning of deep abdominal organs, such as liver, gallbladder, and kidneys, requires low-frequency probes (3–5 MHz). Scanning superficial structures such as the brachial plexus, on the other hand, requires high-frequency probes (10–15 MHz) that provide high axial resolution; however, beam penetration is limited to 3 to 4 cm. A lower frequency probe (4–7 MHz) is suited for scanning deeper structures, such as the brachial plexus in the infraclavicular region and the sciatic nerve in adults.

PERIPHERAL NERVE IMAGING

Probe Orientation

It is advisable to follow the tradition of pointing the premarked end of the probe toward the head when scanning in a sagittal or parasagittal plane, and pointing toward the patient's right when scanning in an axial plane, so that saved images will be correctly interpreted at a later time.

Scanning Technique

Patient positioning for each block is essentially the same as that used for standard, non-image–guided peripheral nerve blocks. Sterile technique should be followed, especially when a continuous catheter technique is performed, in which case a long sterile sheath covering the probe and the cord and sterile transmission gel are recommended.

Transverse and longitudinal views are most commonly used for nerve imaging. When the probe is perpendicular to the long axis of the nerve, the transverse (short axis, cross-sectional) view shows nerves in round to oval shape with internal hypoechoic nerve fascicles surrounded by the hyperechoic epineurium. When the probe is parallel to the long axis, nerves in longitudinal view appear tubular with linear hypoechoic fascicular components mixed with hyperechoic bands corresponding to the interfascicular epineurium.[11,12] Nerves have different degrees of echogenicity. For example, nerve roots and trunks of the brachial plexus in the interscalene and supraclavicular regions appear mostly hypoechoic, whereas peripheral branches of the brachial plexus and the sciatic nerve are largely hyperechoic.

IMAGING OF THE BRACHIAL PLEXUS

High-frequency linear probes, in the range of 10 to 15 MHz, are best suited for imaging the brachial plexus in most locations, except perhaps the infraclavicular region, where the cords may be more deeply located and thus probes in the 4- to 7-MHz range may be required.

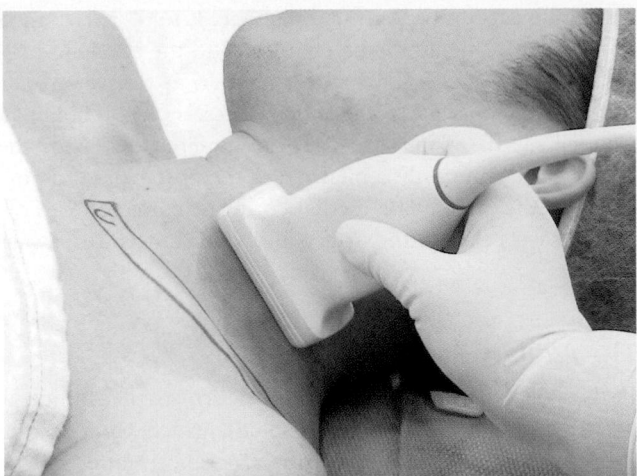

The Supraclavicular Region

In the supravlavicular region, the brachial plexus is best scanned with a linear probe in a coronal oblique plane (Figure 51–2A).[14] The subclavian artery is the most prominent landmark identified immediately superior to the first rib (Figure 51–2B). The trunks, or divisions, of the plexus in this region are tightly arranged within what seems to be a single sheath, immediately lateral and cephalad to the subclavian artery. The anterior and middle scalene muscles can be identified as they insert on the first rib. The pleura can be seen immediately deep to the first rib.

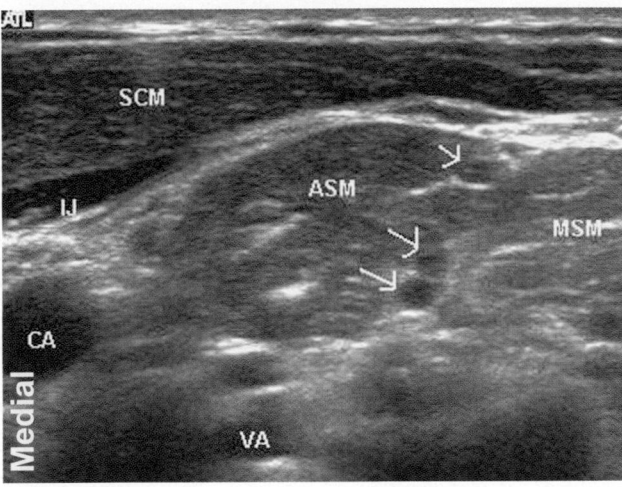

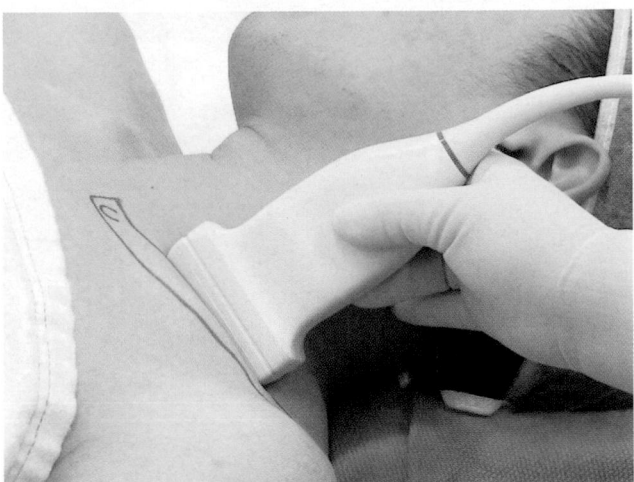

Figure 51–1. A: Ultrasound probe position to obtain a transverse view of the brachial plexus in the interscalene area. **B:** Ultrasound image of the brachial plexus in the interscalene area. SCM = sternocleidomastoid muscle, ASM = anterior scalene muscle, MSM = middle scalene muscle, IJ = internal jugular vein, CA = carotid artery, VA = vertebral artery. Arrows mark brachial plexus roots in the interscalene groove.

The Interscalene Region

In the interscalene region, the cervical roots forming the plexus are located between the anterior and middle scalene muscles. They are best visualized when scanned in the lateral aspect of the neck in an axial oblique plane (Figure 51–1A). In this manner, the sternocleidomastoid muscle can be identified superficially. Deep to it are the anterior and middle scalene muscles where one or more roots are visualized in the interscalene groove.[13] They appear mostly hypoechoic, with few internal punctuate echoes (Figure 51–1B). Deeper to this plane, the vertebral artery and vein are seen next to the vertebral transverse process. The carotid artery and internal jugular vein can be identified medially.

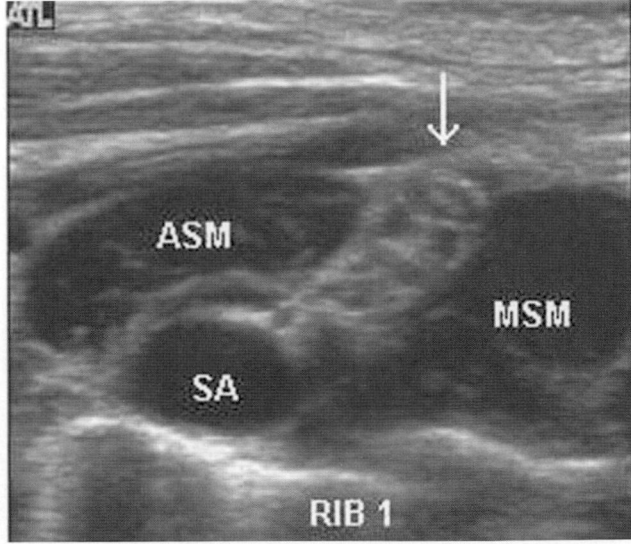

Figure 51–2. A: Ultrasound probe position for imaging the brachial plexus in the supraclavicular area. **B:** Ultrasound image of the brachial plexus in the supraclavicular area. ASM = anterior scalene muscle, MSM = middle scalene muscle, SA = subclavian artery, RIB 1 = first rib. The arrow signals the brachial plexus located in the most distal part of the interscalene space, just cephalad and lateral to the subclavian artery.

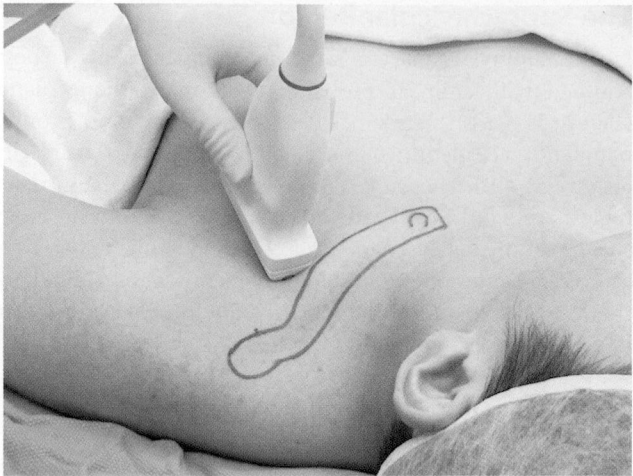

A

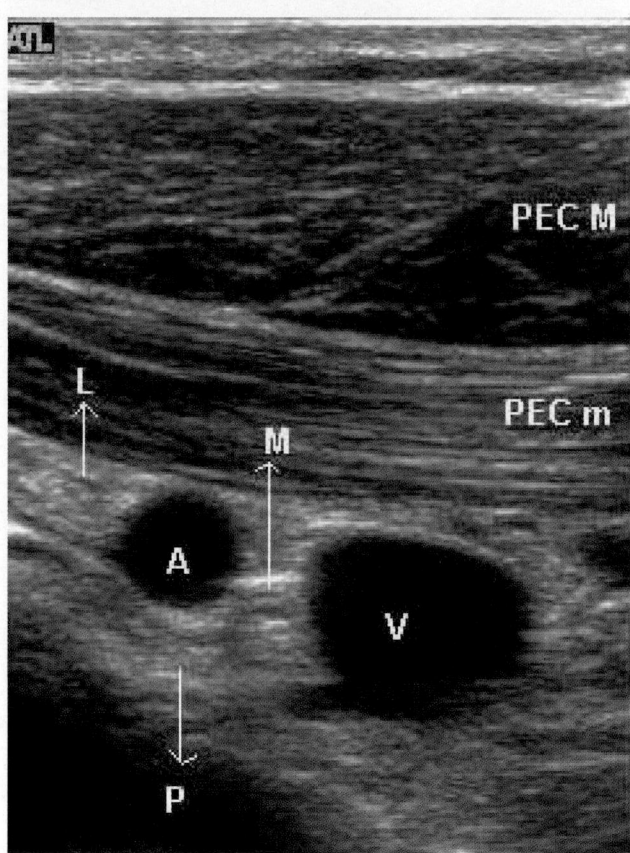

B

Figure 51–3. A: Ultrasound probe position for imaging the brachial plexus in the infraclavicular area.(Drawing on the patient with a "C" indicates the clavicle.) **B:** Ultrasound image of the brachial plexus in the infraclavicular area. PEC M = pectoralis major muscle, PEC m = pectoralis minor muscle, A = axillary artery, V = axillary vein, L = lateral cord, M = medial cord, P = posterior cord.

The Infraclavicular Region

In the infraclavicular region next to the coracoid process, the cords of the plexus lie deep to the pectoralis major and pectoralis minor muscles. They can be best imaged

with a linear probe in the range of 4 to 7 MHz, in a parasagittal plane, immediately medial to the coracoid process (Figure 51–3A).[15,16] In this manner, a transverse view of the cords adjacent to the axillary vessels can be obtained (Figure 51–3B). The cords appear hyperechoic, with the lateral cord commonly cephalad and the posterior cord posterior to the artery. The medial cord in this region can often be seen between the artery and vein, but is not always visible.

The Axillary Region

In the axilla and the upper arm, the neurovascular bundle is located in the internal bicipital sulcus, which separates the flexor muscle compartment of the arm (biceps and coracobrachialis muscles) from the extensor compartment (triceps). At this level, terminal braches of the brachial plexus, such as the musculocutaneous, median, ulnar, and radial nerves, are located superficially, usually within 1 to 2 cm of the skin. A linear 10- to 15-MHz probe is therefore recommended. To obtain a transverse view of the neurovascular bundle with the arm abducted at 90 degrees and the forearm flexed, the probe is positioned perpendicular to the long axis of the arm, as close to the axilla as possible (Figure 51–4A). The round pulsatile axillary artery is easily identified in the bicipital sulcus and is distinguished from the axillary veins that are readily compressed. Nerves in the axilla are round to oval-shaped and hypoechoic with internal hyperechoic areas, presumably the epineurium. In the axillary region, the median and ulnar nerves are usually lateral and medial to the artery, respectively (Figure 51–4B). The radial nerve is often posterior or posteromedial to the artery, but nerve location is highly variable.[17] The musculocutaneous nerve often branches off more proximally and can be seen as a hyperechoic structure. It can be found between the biceps and coracobrachialis muscles for a short distance before entering the body of the coracobrachialis muscle (see Figure 51–4B). When performing an axillary block, it is best to inject local anesthetic around each nerve individually to achieve consistent success. Local anesthetic spread within the sheath compartment may be presumably restricted by the septa when observed under ultrasound.[18]

LUMBOSACRAL PLEXUS

The lumbar plexus (L1 to L5) and the sacral plexus (S1 to S4) provide innervation to the lower extremity. Unlike the brachial plexus, the lumbosacral plexus and its proximal branches are quite deep. Sonographic imaging can be more challenging except for the distal peripheral branches.

Paravertebral Anatomy & Lumbar Plexus Blocks

Ultrasound imaging of the lumbar plexus in the paravertebral region in adults is technically difficult because of its deep

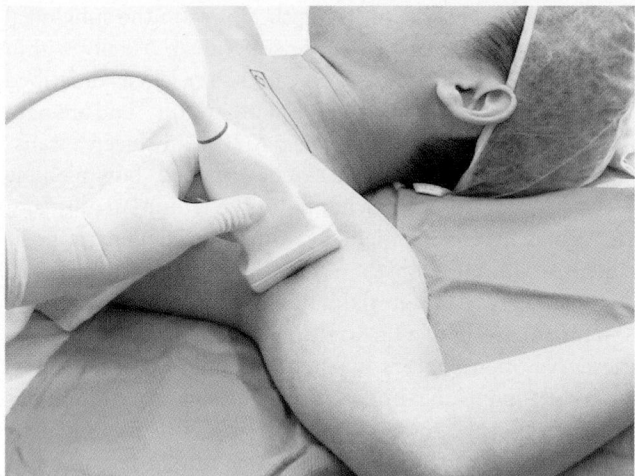

A

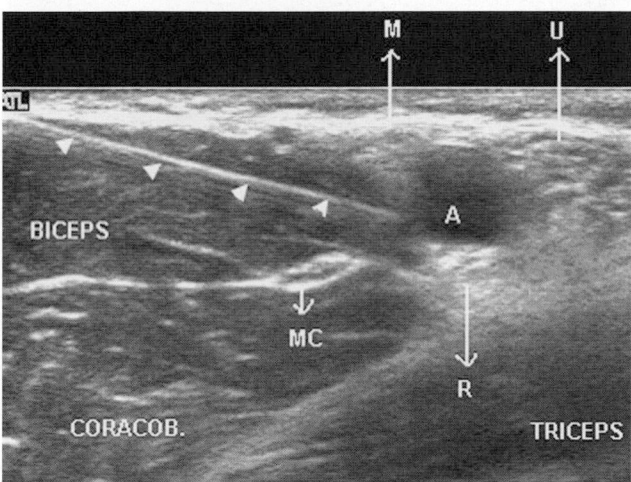

B

Figure 51–4. A: Ultrasound probe position for imaging the brachial plexus in the axillary area. **D.** Ultrasound image of the brachial plexus in the axillary area. A = axillary artery, M = median nerve, U = ulnar nerve, R = radial nerve, MC = musculocutaneous nerve. CORACOB = coracobrachialis muscle, arrowheads signal the needle shaft.

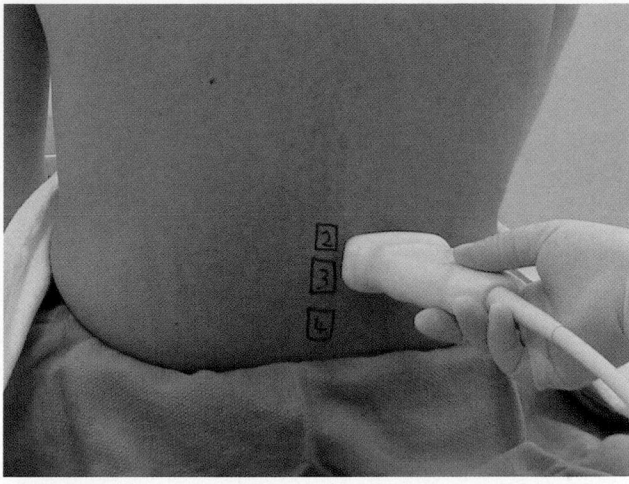

A

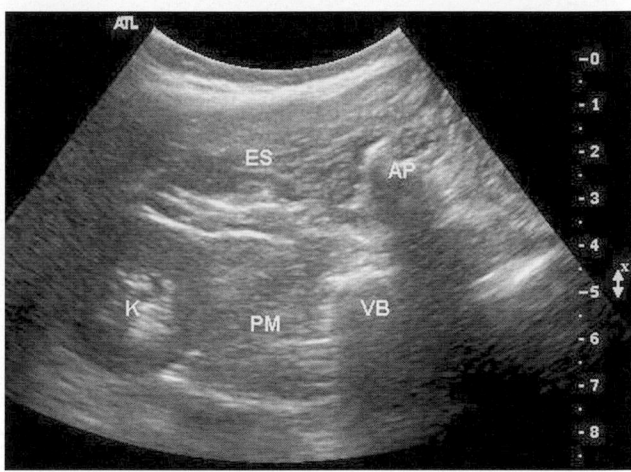

B

Figure 51–5. A: Ultrasound probe position for imaging the paravertebral anatomy relevant to performing lumbar plexus block. **B:** Ultrasound image of the paravertebral anatomy at the L2 to L3 level. AP = articular process, VB = vertebral body, ES = erector spinae muscle, PM = psoas muscle, K = kidney. The actual lumbar plexus roots are not seen in this image. They traverse the posterior third of the psoas muscle and are difficult to identify due to the depth and similar echogenicity of surrounding muscle tissue.

location. Using curved 4- to 5-MHz transducers, Kirchmair and associates identified the lumbar plexus within the psoas muscle and correlated ultrasound images with anatomic specimens.[19] Scanning is performed with the patient either prone with a pillow under the abdomen to reduce lumbar lordosis or in the sitting position. The transducer is placed longitudinally, in a parasagittal plane, approximately 3 cm from the midline to determine the location of the lumbar transverse processes. Once accomplished, the transducer is turned 90 degrees to the transverse axial plane and positioned between two transverse processes so that bony interference to ultrasound beam penetration is minimized (Figure 51–5A). In the axial image, two muscles are identified deep to the subcutaneous plane: the erector spinae muscle immediately lateral to the spinous process and the smaller quadratus lumborum more laterally. The psoas muscle lies deep (anterior)

to these two muscles and is adjacent to the vertebral bodies and intervertebral discs (Figure 51–5B). Previous anatomic studies demonstrate that the lumbar plexus most often lies between the posterior third and anterior two thirds of the psoas muscle; the average skin-to-plexus distance is 5–6 cm.[20] For this reason it has been recommended that local anesthetic be administered in the posterior one third of the muscle. Ultrasound also identifies the inferior pole of the kidney (as low as the L3 to L4 level) and can potentially avoid renal hematoma due to inadvertent needle trauma.[21]

Femoral Nerve

The three main terminal branches of the lumbar plexus are the femoral, obturator, and lateral femoral cutaneous nerves. The

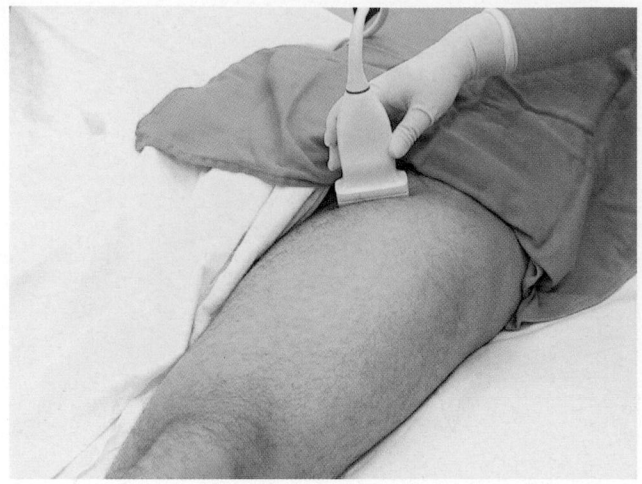

A

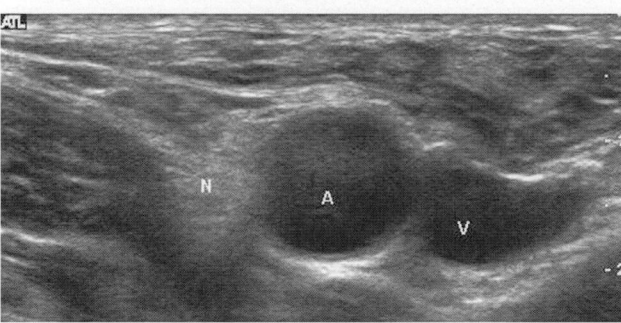

B

Figure 51–6. A: Ultrasound probe position for imaging the femoral nerve in the inguinal area. **B:** Ultrasound image of the femoral nerve in the inguinal area. V = femoral vein, A = femoral artery, N = femoral nerve.

femoral nerve derived from L2 to L4 is the largest branch and can be easily imaged in the inguinal region using a linear 8–12 MHz transducer (Figure 51–6A).[22] The probe placed over the inguinal crease in the transverse axial plane shows the femoral nerve immediately lateral to the femoral vessels, often appearing oval or triangular in shape (Figure 51–6B). It lies deep to the ileopectineal arch and overlying the groove between the iliac and psoas muscles. The femoral nerve can be imaged further distally for a short distance until it divides into small terminal branches that become indistinguishable from the surrounding tissue. It is possible to image the saphenous nerve, which is next to the femoral vessels in the mid to distal third of the thigh.

Sciatic Nerve

The sciatic nerve also originates from the lumbosacral plexus (L4 through S3) and enters the gluteal region through the greater sciatic foramen, between two muscle planes. The anterior muscle plane is formed by the obturator internus and inferior gemellus muscles, and the posterior, more superficial muscle plane by the gluteus maximus muscle. In the gluteal region the sciatic nerve is not easily identified by ul-

trasonography because of its depth. Lower in the subgluteal region, the sciatic nerve is more superficial, usually within 5 cm from the skin surface, and can be blocked as described by Raj and coworkers[23] and later by Sutherland[24] and Sukhani and associates.[25] With a curved 5–7 MHz transducer, a transverse view of the sciatic nerve can be obtained showing bony landmarks, the greater trochanter of the femur laterally, and the ischial tuberosity medially, when the patient is positioned semiprone with the limb to be blocked uppermost (Figure 51–7A). The approximate location of the sciatic nerve is in the midpoint of a line uniting both landmarks. The sciatic nerve often appears hyperechoic and elliptical deep to the distal gluteus maximus muscle and lateral to the biceps femoris muscle (Figure 51–7B).[26] It is usually surrounded by a well-defined border, presumably the aponeurosis of the surrounding muscles.

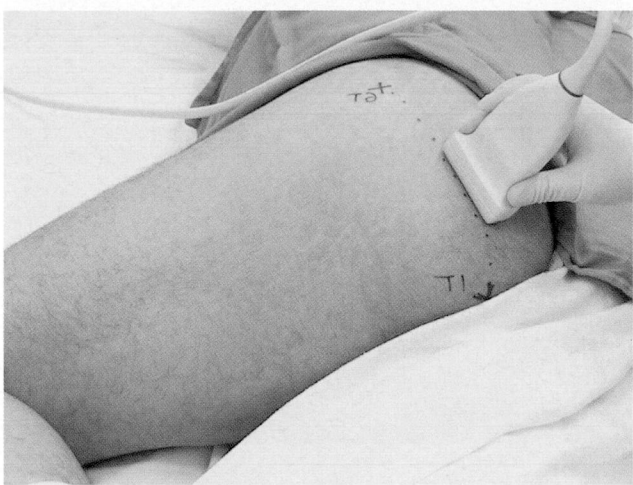

A

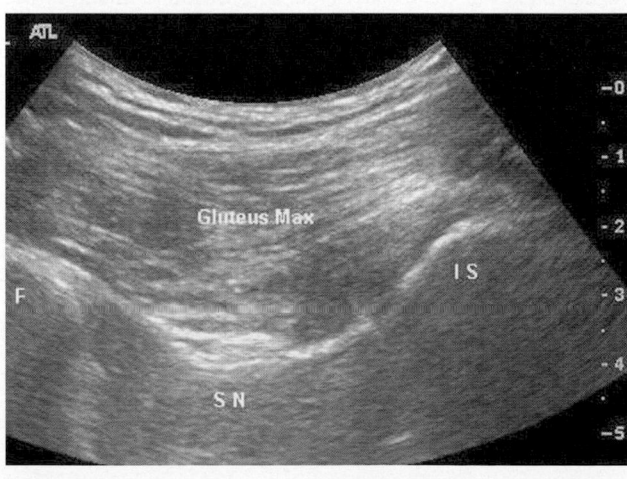

B

Figure 51–7. A: Ultrasound probe position for imaging the sciatic nerve in the gluteal area. (Markings on the patient: GT = greater trochanter, IT = ischial tuberosity). **B:** Ultrasound image of the sciatic nerve in the gluteal area using a curved probe: IS = ischial tuberosity, F = femur, Gluteus max = gluteus maximus muscle, SN = sciatic nerve.

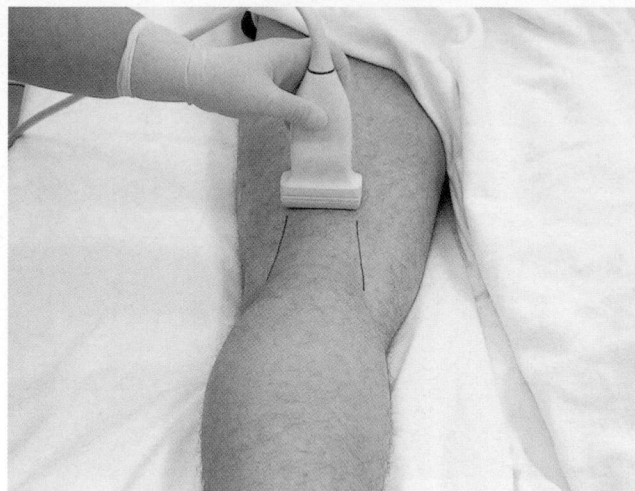

A

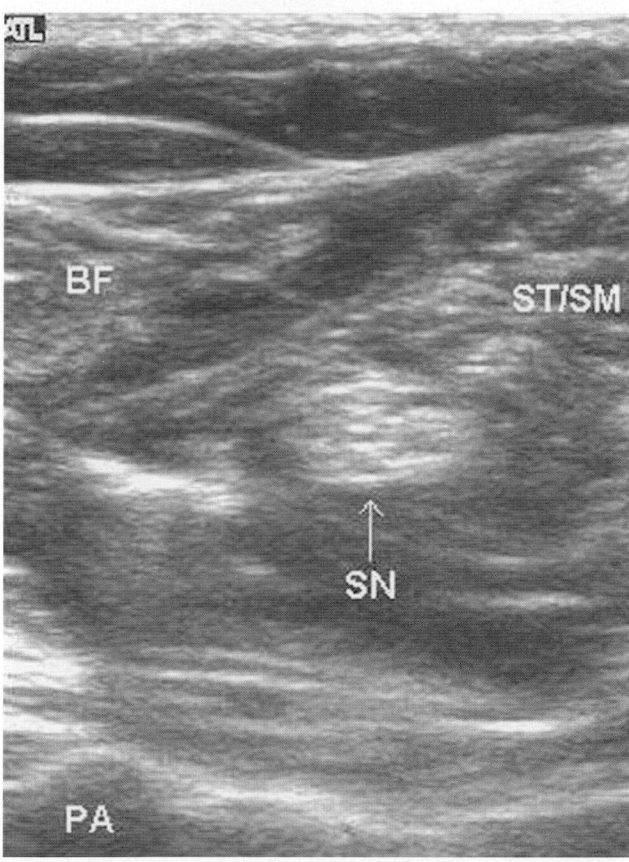

B

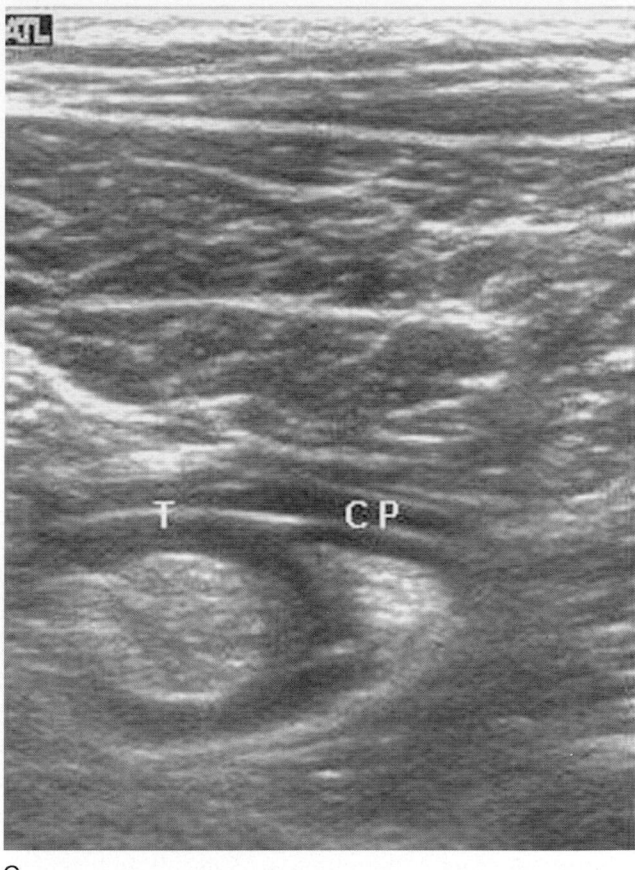

C

Figure 51–8. (*Continued*)

Figure 51–8. A: Ultrasound probe position for imaging the sciatic nerve in the popliteal area. **B:** Ultrasound image of the sciatic nerve in the popliteal area. BF = biceps femoris, ST/SM = semimembranous/semitendinous muscle, PA = popliteal artery, SN = sciatic nerve. **C:** Ultrasound image of the sciatic nerve in the popliteal area after local anesthetic injection. Notice the division of the sciatic nerve into two branches. T = tibial nerve, CP = common peroneal. The local anesthetic solution appears as a hypoechoic (black) space surrounding both nerve branches.

Moving caudally, the sciatic nerve can be imaged using a 7-MHz probe up to the popliteal fossa, where it divides into the peroneal and tibial nerves (Figure 51–8A). Here, the sciatic nerve often appears round and hyperechoic and is located posterior to the femur, lateral to the popliteal artery, and deep (anterior) to the semitendinous and semimembranous muscles medially and the biceps femoris muscle laterally (Figure 51–8B and 51–8C). More distally, the peroneal nerve may be followed as far laterally as the head of the fibula.

GENERAL PRINCIPLES OF ULTRASOUND-GUIDED NERVE BLOCK TECHNIQUES

Ultrasound-guided blocks for peripheral nerves follow several general principles.

1. The quality of ultrasonographic nerve images captured depends on the quality of the ultrasound machine and transducers, proper transducer selection (eg, frequency) for each nerve location, the anesthesiologist's familiarity and interpretation of sonographic anatomy pertinent to the block, and good eye-to-hand coordination to track needle movement during advancement.

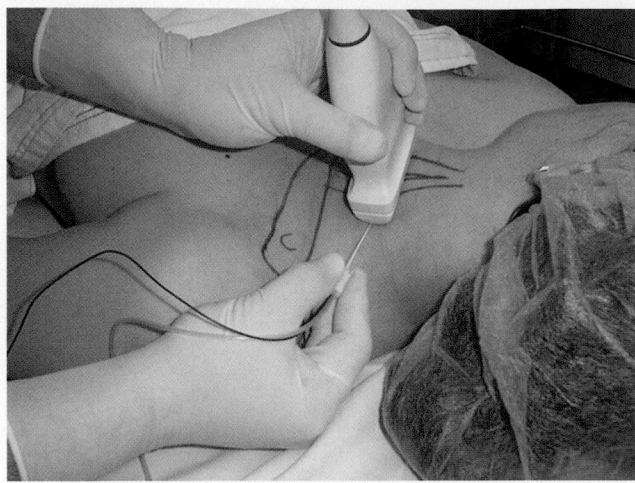

Figure 51–9. Probe and needle alignment during performance of an interscalene block. Notice the relative position of the needle in line with the probe, which allows visualization of the entire needle trajectory.

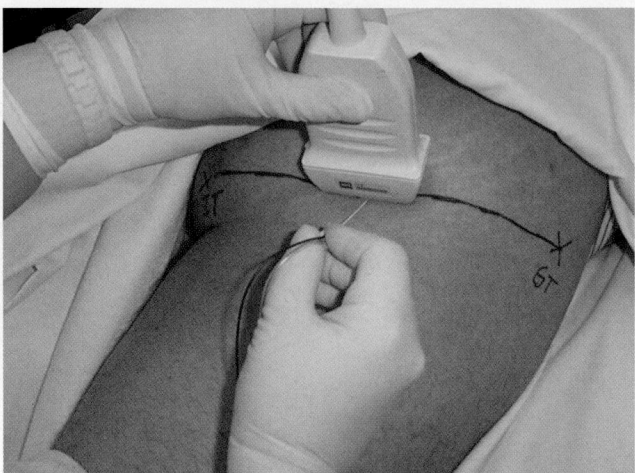

Figure 51–10. Probe and needle alignment during performance of a subgluteal sciatic nerve block. Notice the relative position of the needle perpendicular, or "out of plane" with the probe.

2. Optimal patient positioning and sterile technique are encouraged. This is particularly important for the continuous catheter technique, for which it is necessary to use sterile transmission gel and a sterile plastic sheath to fully cover the entire transducer.

3. Nerve localization by ultrasound can be combined with nerve stimulation. Both tools are valuable and complementary, not mutually exclusive. Ultrasonography provides anatomic information, while a motor response to nerve stimulation provides functional information about the nerve in question.

4. Observing local anesthetic spread is another valuable feature of ultrasound in addition to real-time visual guidance to navigate the needle toward the target nerve.

5. Two approaches are generally available to block peripheral nerves. The first approach aims to align and move the block needle in line with the long axis of the ultrasound transducer, so the needle stays within the path of the ultrasound beam (Figure 51–9). In this manner, the needle shaft and tip can be clearly visualized. This approach is preferred when it is important to track the needle tip at all times (eg, during supraclavicular block to minimize inadvertent pleural puncture). The second approach places the needle perpendicular to the probe (Figure 51–10). In this case, the ultrasound image captures a transverse view of the needle, which is shown as a hyperechoic "dot" on the screen. Accurate moment-to-moment tracking of the needle tip location can be difficult, and needle tip position is often inferred indirectly by tissue movement. This approach, however, is particularly useful for continuous catheter placement along the long axis of the nerve.

Outcome Studies

Ultrasound-guided techniques may improve the accuracy, success, and safety of regional anesthesia. However, few prospective randomized outcome studies have been conducted and published so far. Williams and coworkers suggested that the addition of ultrasound guidance improves the quality of supraclavicular block[27] when compared with neurostimulator guidance alone. Marhofer and associates also suggest that ultrasound guidance speeds the onset, improves the quality, and reduces the incidence of vascular puncture during three-in-one blocks.[28] No study to date, however, has examined the effect of ultrasound on nerve injury. In summary, although preliminary experience has been encouraging, more outcome data are required to define the success and safety profile of ultrasound-guided peripheral nerve blocks.

ULTRASONOGRAPHY & NEURAXIAL BLOCKS

Neuraxial anesthetic techniques can be challenging because of anatomic variability among patients[29] and imprecise determination of the level of the vertebral interspace by physical examination alone (inaccurate 70–80% of the time).[30,31] Spinal needle insertion and local anesthetic injection at the wrong lumbar interspace (ie, too cephalad) may have been implicated in previously reported injuries to the conus medullaris.[32] Potentially, imaging guidance may improve accuracy and safety of needle placement during neuraxial blocks.

Over two decades ago, attempts were made to image the ligamentum flavum using ultrasonography.[33] Because the epidural and subarachoid spaces are surrounded by bones, anatomic assessment in this region is difficult since the majority of the ultrasound beam is reflected on contacting the bony spinous processes. With a linear or curved 4- to 7-MHz probe, limited ultrasound beam passage is possible only through the interspinous space (Figure 51–11A), especially in the paramedian region. The ligamentum flavum and the dura mater are dense tissues that appear hyperechoic on ultrasound, whereas

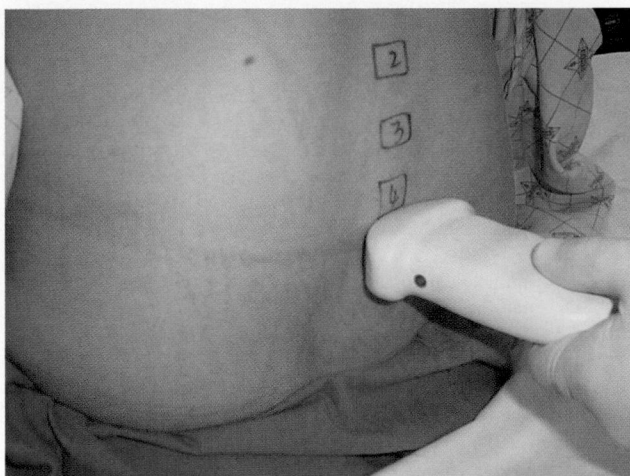

A

B

Figure 51–11. A: Ultrasound probe position to obtain an axial view of the neuraxial structures at the L4-5 interspace. **B:** Ultrasound image if the neuraxial structures at the L4-5 interspace, in an axial plane. TP = transverse process, VB = vertebral body, IT = intrathecal space, IL = interspinous ligament.

the low-density epidural space and the cerebrospinal fluid in the intrathecal space appear hypoechoic (Figure 51–11B).

Ultrasound determination of the spinal level is more accurate than clinical examination. This has been confirmed in two recent studies showing accurate ultrasound determi-

nation in over 70% of patients when compared with MRI examination.[31,34] The markers were always placed within one interspace of the intended level. Ultrasonography can also determine the depth of needle penetration to reach the epidural space[35] and can help reduce the number of needle puncture attempts. The paramedian region has been suggested by some to be the optimal window for ultrasound imaging, especially in the thoracic spine[36] because of a higher soft tissue to bone ratio.[37] In contrast to peripheral nerve blocks, real-time, image-guided neuraxial techniques have not been reported. Ultrasonography has been used primarily to help define the anatomy, depth, and angle of needle penetration immediately prior to performing the technique.

References

1. Mulroy M, Larkin K, Batra M, et al: Femoral nerve block with 0.25% or 0.5% bupivacaine improves post-operative analgesia following outpatient arthroscopic anterior cruciate ligament repair. Reg Anesth Pain Med 2001;26(1):24–29.
2. Chan VW, Peng PW, Kaszas Z, et al: A comparative study of general anesthesia, intravenous regional anesthesia, and axillary block for outpatient hand surgery: Clinical outcome and cost analysis. Anesth Analg 2001;93:1181–1184.
3. Pavlin DJ, Rapp SE, Polissar NL, et al: Factors affecting discharge time in adult outpatients. Anesth Analg 1998;87:816–826.
4. Choyce A, Chan V, Middleton W, et al: What is the relationship between paresthesia and nerve stimulation for axillary brachial plexus block? Reg Anesth Pain Med 2001;26:100–104.
5. Urmey W, Stanton J: Inability to consistently elicit a motor response following sensory paresthesia during interscalene block administration. Anesthesiology 2002;96:552–554.
6. Fortuna A, Fortuna Ade O: Bupivacaine induced cardiac arrest. Anesth Analg 1990;71:561–562.
7. Durrani Z, Winnie AP: Brainstem toxicity with reversible locked–in syndrome after interscalene brachial plexus block. Anesth Analg 1991;72(2):251–252.
8. Perlas A, Chan VWS, Simons M: Brachial plexus examination and localization using ultrasound and electrical stimulation—A volunteer study. Anesthesiology 2003;99:429–435.
9. Chan VWS, Perlas A, Rawson R, et al: Ultrasound guided supraclavicular brachial plexus block. Anesth Analg 2003;97:1514–1517.
10. Kossoff G: Basic physics and imaging characteristics of ultrasound. World J Surg 2000;24:134–142.
11. Peer S, Kovacs P, Harpf C, et al: High resolution sonography of lower extremity peripheral nerves: Anatomic correlation and spectrum of disease. J Ultrasound Med 2002;21:315–322.
12. Silvestri E, Martinoli C, Derchi LE, et al: Echotexture of peripheral nerves: Correlation between ultrasound and histologic findings and criteria to differentiate tendons. Radiology 1995;197:291–296.
13. Chan VWS: Applying ultrasound imaging to interscalene brachial plexus block. Reg Anesth Pain Med 2003;28(4):340–343.
14. Perlas A, Chan VWS: Ultrasound guided interscalene brachial plexus block. Tech Reg Anesth Pain Manage 2004;8(4):143–148.
15. Ootaki C, Hayashi H, Amano M: Ultrasound guided infraclavicular brachial plexus block: An alternative technique to anatomical landmark-guided approaches. Reg Anesth Pain Med 2000;25:600–604.
16. Sandhu NS, Capan LM: Ultrasound guided infraclavicular brachial plexus block. BJA 2002;89(2):254–259.
17. Retzl G, Kapral S, Greher M, et al: Ultrasonographic findings of the axillary part of the brachial plexus. Anesth Analg 2001;92:1271–1275.
18. Partridge BL, Benirschke K: Functional anatomy of the brachial plexus sheath: Implications for anesthesia. Anesthesiology 1987;66:743.

19. Kirchmair L, Entner T, Wissel J, et al: A study of the paravertebral anatomy for ultrasound-guided posterior lumber plexus block. Anesth Analg 2001;93:477–481.

20. Farny J, Drolet P, Girard M: Anatomy of the posterior approach to the lumbar plexus block. Can J Anesth 1994;41:480–485.

21. Aida S, Takahashi H, Shimoji K: Renal subcapsular hematoma after lumbar plexus block. Anesthesiology 1996;84:452–455.

22. Gruber H, Peer S, Kovacs P, et al: The ultrasonographic appearance of the femoral nerve and cases of iatrogenic impairment. J Ultrasound Med 2003;22:163–172.

23. Raj PP, Parks RI, Watson TD, et al: A new single position supine approach to the sciatic-femoral nerve block. Anesth Analg 1975;54:489–493.

24. Sutherland ID: Continuous sciatic nerve infusion: Expanded case report describing a new approach. Reg Anesth Pain Med 1998;23:496–501.

25. Sukhani R, Candido KD, Doty R, et al: Infragluteal parabiceps sciatic nerve block: an evaluation of a novel approach using a single injection technique. Anesth Analg 2003;96:868–873.

26. Gray AT, Collins A, Schafhalter-Zoppoth I: Sciatic nerve block in a child: A sonographic approach. Anesth Analg 2003;97:1300–1302.

27. Williams SR, Chouinard P, Arcand G, et al: Ultrasound guidance speeds the execution and improves the quality of supraclavicular block. Anesth Analg 2003;97:1518–1523.

28. Marhofer P, Schrogendorfer K, Koining H, et al: Ultrasonographic guidance improves sensory block and onset time of three-in-one blocks. Anesth Analg 1997;85:854–857.

29. Reimann AF, Anson BJ: Vertebral level of termination of the spinal cord with report of a case of sacral cord. Anat Rec 1944;88:127–138.

30. Broadbent CR, Maxwell WB, Ferrie R, et al: Ability of Anesthetists to identify a marked lumbar interspace. Anesthesia 2000;55:1122–1126.

31. Furness G, Reilly MP, Kuchi S: An evaluation of ultrasound imaging for identification of lumbar intervertebral level. Anesthesia 2002;57:277–280.

32. Reynolds F: Damage to the conus medularis following spinal anesthesia. Anaesthesia 2001;56:238–247.

33. Cork RC, Kryc JJ, Vaughan RW: Ultrasonic localization of the lumbar epidural space. Anesthesiology 1980;52:513–516.

34. Watson MJ, Evans S, Thorp JM: Could ultrasonography be used by an anesthetist to identify a specified lumbar interspace before spinal anesthesia? BJA 2001;90(4):509–511.

35. Grau T, Leipold RW, Conradi R, et al: Ultrasound imaging facilitates localization of the epidural space during combined spinal and epidural anesthesia. Reg Anesth Pain Med 2001;26(1):64–67.

36. Grau T, Leipold R, Delorme S, et al: Ultrasound imaging of the thoracic epidural space. Reg Anesth and Pain Med 2001;27(2);200–206.

37. Grau T, Leipold R, Horter J, et al: Paramedian access to the epidural space: The optimum window for ultrasound imaging. J Clin Anesth 2001;13:213–217.

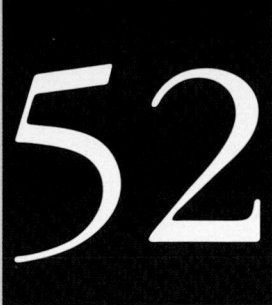

Ultrasound-Guided Peripheral Nerve Blocks in Children

Peter Marhofer, MD • Stephan Kapral, MD

INTRODUCTION

Modern pediatric anesthesia would not be conceivable without the use of regional anesthetic techniques. For instance, regional anesthesia decreases the need for mechanical ventilation following major thoracic or abdominal surgery. In addition, the need for intraoperative and postoperative opioids decreases accordingly. Perhaps most importantly, the entire perioperative experience is less stressful for children whose perioperative pain is adequately managed. Most of the advantages of perioperative regional anesthesia are demonstrated in central neuraxial blocks, specifically for caudal continuous lumbar or thoracic epidural blocks.

In contrast to central blocks, peripheral nerve blocks (PNBs) have not been studied extensively in children. A Medline search in April 2005 yielded 42 reports for *pediatric anesthesia & epidural* and only 17 for *pediatric anesthesia & peripheral nerve block*. This finding suggests that peripheral nerve blockade in children is used less frequently in clinical practice than in adults. This is compounded by the fact that some pediatric anesthesiologists are still reluctant to use the nerve stimulator, the accepted standard tool for locating nerves in adults. "Blind" methods, such as those used for blockade of the ilioinguinal/iliohypogastric nerves, continue to be the most prevalent approach in pediatric anesthesia. Even techniques that today are used exclusively in conjunction with nerve stimulators in adults, are frequently performed "blind" in children by using anatomic landmarks as the sole reference or by relying on fascial click techniques. Giaufré and coworkers[1] reported in a much-quoted overview article on a study performed under the auspices of the French Language Society of Pediatric Anesthesiologists (ADARPEF). In that study, a total of 24,409 regional anesthetic procedures were performed in children over a 1-year period, 15,013 (>60%) of them being central blocks. By comparison, only 38% of these were peripheral blocks. In this large series, no complications were reported, suggesting that PNBs in children can be used with remarkable safety. However, it is possible that some complications were minor or went clinically undetected. For example, complications during blockade of the ilioinguinal/iliohypogastric nerves were not observed in that study. It is unlikely that complications were virtually nonexistent, since the conventional techniques described are well known to carry a risk of peritoneal puncture.

Ultrasound-guided nerve blocks are rapidly becoming popular in adults. The smaller body size of children, allows the use of high-frequency, high-resolution probes, making ultrasound particularly suitable to the practice of PNBs in the pediatric patient. The reader should be advised that at the time of the publication of this book, this area of regional anesthesia is still in its infancy and scientific data on the true efficacy and safety of ultrasound-guided nerve blocks in children are limited. Consequently, some views expressed in this chapter necessarily reflect our own bias and clinical experience. Finally, because of our group's specific interest in anesthesia for pediatric trauma, most discussion in this chapter focuses on blocks in pediatric patients with traumatic injury of the upper and lower extremities.

Technical & Practical Details

Most blocks can be performed with 5- to 10-MHz linear ultrasound transducers. In addition, small probes are required due to the narrow anatomic relationships in children. "Hockey-stick" probes, with a surface length of 25 mm, are particularly well suited for this purpose. Also, higher frequency transducers are available for portable ultrasound units. Theoretically, superficial nerve structures can be better visualized using these higher frequencies. The discussion of techniques in the following sections, however, is based on ultrasound probes working at somewhat lower frequencies. Lower frequencies are preferable for deeper blocks, such as psoas compartment blocks in larger children, because the nerve structures to be

visualized are located deeper in this situation. Therefore, we use 2- to 4-MHz sector transducers for this specific indication.

The term *anisotropy* indicates the degree to which peripheral nerves can be optimally visualized only if the sonographic signals are oriented perpendicular to the nerve. Different nerves are characterized by different degrees of anisotropy. In general, the nerves of the upper limbs, for example, are characterized by high anisotropy. However, even minute deviations from the optimal angulation of the probe can greatly reduce the quality of visualization. In this situation, the chances of effectively blocking the sciatic nerve under ultrasound guidance are limited. The phenomenon of different nerves having different anisotropic properties is still poorly understood. Presumably, however, the degree of anisotropy has to do with the inner architecture of the neuronal structures involved and can vary among subjects.

It is important to note that some of the images shown in the discussion that follows were obtained with high-end, costly ultrasound units, which allow anatomic structures to be visualized in greater detail: This was done with didactic considerations in mind. Regardless, we challenge the widespread view that ultrasound-guided regional anesthesia is a technique reserved for "rich" institutions, where such high-end equipment is available. In contrast, all techniques described in the chapter can be carried out with portable systems, which can be acquired for a fraction of the price typically expended for anesthesia machines.

In accordance with the *immobile needle* concept, we use short-beveled needles with flexible injection tubing for most PNB techniques. We feel that the short-beveled needle design optimizes the precision of needle guidance inside the tissue. The surgical instrument industry is making major efforts to develop more suitable needles and catheters for better ultrasound visualization. The future will show whether it will be possible to strike a meaningful balance between sonographic visualization of the cannula and the appearance of artifacts.

Nerve Block Techniques

Techniques of nerve blockade fall into two major groups depending on the position of the needle relative to the ultrasound transducer: the *cross-sectional* and the *in-line* technique.

Cross-Sectional Technique

With the cross-sectional technique (Figures 52–1 and 52–2), the needle is positioned transverse to the ultrasound probe, such that visualization in the ultrasound image is confined to the needle tip of a small needle cross-section. The angle of needle insertion must be selected in such a way that the needle tip can be advanced precisely to the depth of the target structure. In addition to direct visualization, the needle is identified in the ultrasound image both by tissue displacement and by an acoustic shadow emerging dorsally at its tip. Attention must be paid when injecting the local anesthetic to visualize the spread of the

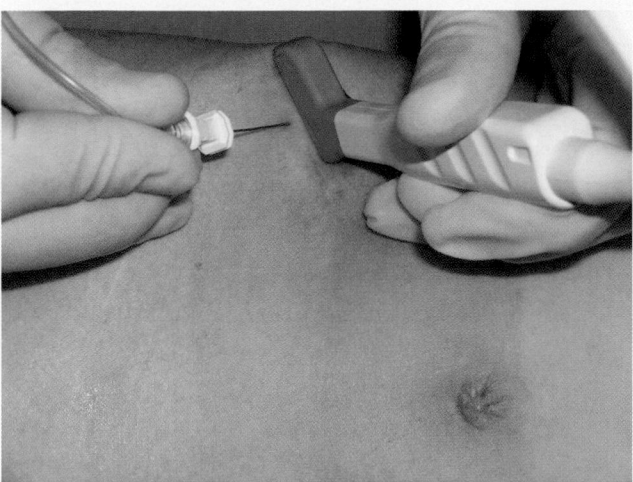

Figure 52–1. Needle position relative to the ultrasound probe (cross-sectional technique).

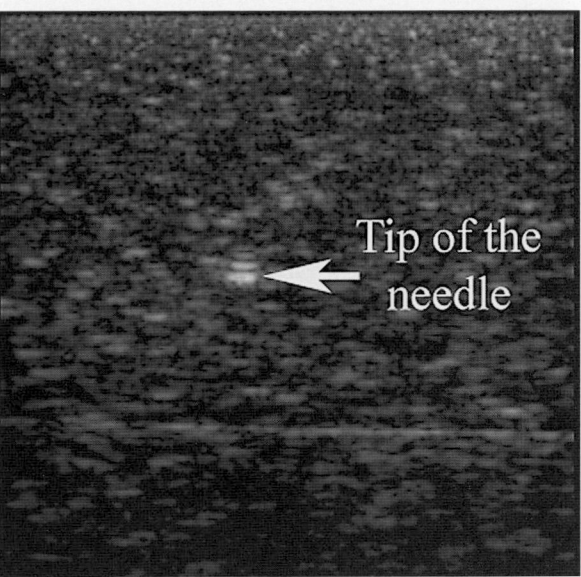

Figure 52–2. Sonographic visualization of the needle using the cross-sectional technique (in gel cushion). There is only one hyperechoic area (*center*), representing the needle tip.

anesthetic. Failure to visualize the local anesthetic in the ultrasound image during injection indirectly indicates that the needle tip is located outside of the ultrasound window as the needle tip is not always visualized. The described technique is used for most nerve blocks described in this chapter.

Clinical Pearls

- The most reliable way to obtain ultrasound-assisted nerve blockade is by using a cross-sectional approach and the transverse needle insertion.

- The needle-to-nerve distance is shorter with the cross-sectional than with the in-line technique; the shorter distance is associated with less tissue trauma and less patient discomfort.

- Precise location of the needle tip in the ultrasound image is not a prerequisite for successful blockade; always remember:
    1. *Nerves are blocked not by the needle but by the local anesthetic!*
    2. *Discernment of the location of the needle on ultrasound is helped by identifying both tissue displacement and an acoustic shadow, which emerges posterior to its tip.*

In-Line Technique

With the in-line technique (Figures 52–3 and 52–4), the needle is advanced longitudinally to the ultrasound probe. The advantage of this technique is that visualization is not confined to the tip but also extends to the shaft of the needle. This result can only be achieved, however, if the needle is located strictly within the range of the emitted ultrasound signals. Therefore, the requirements of positioning the probe relative to the needle are even more exacting. In case of transversal deviations as small as 1–2 mm, the needle will disappear from

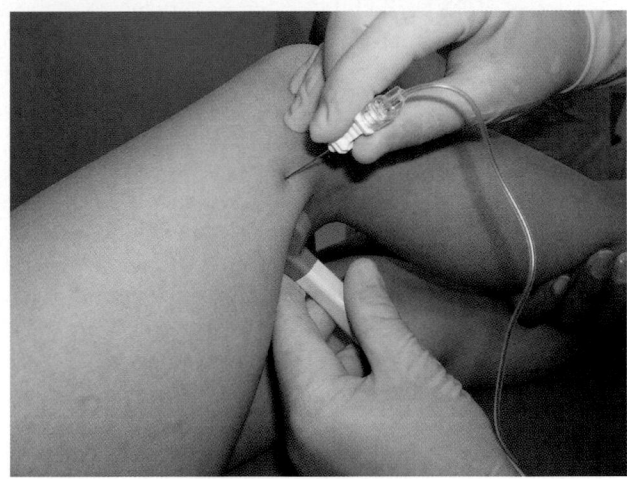

Figure 52–3. Needle position relative to the ultrasound probe (in-line technique).

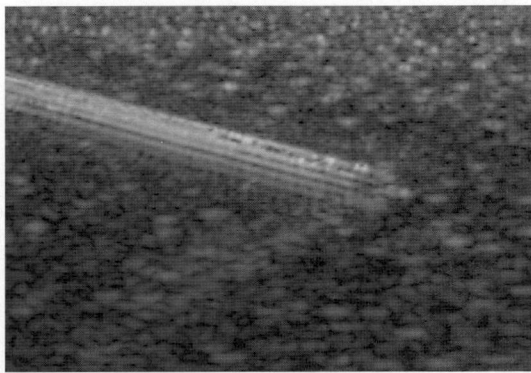

Figure 52–4. Sonographic visualization of the needle using the in-line technique (in gel cushion). Due to reverberation artifacts, the needle shaft emerging from the left margin of the image appears thicker than it really is.

the image. In practice, this technique remains confined to a few specific applications.

Infection Precautions

The approach to pediatric regional anesthesia with regard to infection control is essentially the same as in adults. For single punctures, a surface disinfectant is used on the transducer, making sure that the disinfectant selected is compatible with the manufacturer's recommendations regarding probe cleaning. Subsequently, the area for needle insertion is disinfected, and a sterile ultrasound gel is applied. A *no-touch technique* is then followed; contact between the needle and the transducer or any other objects is avoided.

For perineural catheter insertion, sterile draping is used, and the ultrasound probe is enclosed in sterile wrapping. For this purpose, an ultrasound gel is filled into a sterile plastic pouch or glove, and the sterile gel is again applied to the pouch or glove.

Special Considerations

The success of PNBs in children can be difficult to evaluate because pain or postoperative anxiety in children depend on numerous criteria and need to be evaluated on an individual basis. There is no consensus on using *"smiley face scales"* or other modes of evaluating perioperative pain in a uniform manner. However, information on pain and well-being of children is fundamental, since these patients enable us to evaluate the efficacy of our therapeutic interventions.

Assessment of postoperative pain versus anxiety in children is age-dependent and makes it difficult to accurately assess the efficacy of pain blocks.[2] Currently only limited data are available on the efficacy of the landmark-oriented techniques, nerve stimulator-guided blocks, and surface nerve-mapping techniques.[3] For these reasons alone, children in particular may benefit from the more exacting, ultrasound-guided techniques. In addition, more precise ultrasound-guided techniques may allow for reduction of the dose of the local anesthetic.[4,5] Although systemic toxicity of local anesthetic in pediatric regional anesthesia is rare, it is very likely that such events are underreported. Local anesthetics are mainly bound by acidic α_1-glycoprotein and albumin, which are not sufficiently produced in younger children, making the pediatric population at particular risk for systemic toxicity from local anesthetics.[6]

Additional advantages of ultrasound-based nerve block techniques are that anatomic structures can be visualized, the spread of the local anesthetic monitored, and intravascular or intraneuronal punctures are less likely to occur. However, adequacy of the clinician's training in ultrasound-guided nerve blocks deserves special consideration. Such training is currently offered only through specialized workshops and self-study methods. A more extended period of training, best done under the supervision of a regional anesthesiologist with experience in ultrasound-guided blocks until adequate expertise is achieved, is indispensable.

Finally, adequate technical specifications, proper selection of ultrasound probes, and proper adjustment of the ultrasound unit are all important for the success and safety of PNBs. This knowledge can be acquired in specialized workshops. The technical potential of these systems to optimize imaging must be fully utilized precisely because anatomic structures are highly condensed in children.

Clinical Pearl

- The pediatric nerve block techniques described in this chapter can be greatly simplified if the ultrasound unit is correctly adjusted. In fact, expertise in optimizing images is what sets "ultrasound professionals" apart.

Adjustment of the Ultrasound Unit

The ultrasound machine must be properly configured and adjusted to make it suitable for use in ultrasound-guided nerve blocks in children. The following list of steps delineates the important parameters of that adjustment:

1. *Image Depth.* It is necessary to strike a balance between overview and detail, considering that the quality of the ultrasound image gets significantly reduced at large magnifications as the individual pixels become visible.
2. *Gain.* Care must be taken to select an optimal gain relative to the image depth. Most modern ultrasound machines feature selection of independent gain in different sections of the image (TGF = time gain compensation). Other systems offer only a coarse type of depth gain adjustment (surface/ depth gain).
3. *Focus.* Given the dense vertical structures in children, the focus of the ultrasound image has to be adjusted so that the level of the target structures is optimally visible. With high-end systems, different focal zones can be defined. Here, the zone of optimal resolution becomes smaller as the focal zones decrease. As a rule, two or three focal zones are selected.

Nerve Block Preparation Strategies

The success of PNBs in children is not only a function of the blocking procedure itself but also requires an appropriate general strategy. Particularly when "novel" techniques are used, the environment and concomitant measures must be selected with great care, since first impressions by the surgeons, colleague anesthesiologists, parents, and other involved caregivers are very important to the success of the new techniques. Once a poor general impression is created, it often takes heroic efforts to improve it.

Whether a child is best kept sedated or alert during the block procedure depends on the individual clinical circumstances. Although it is possible in an occasional child to conduct the block procedure without premedication, as a general rule, however, sedation or general anesthesia is beneficial and preferred in most instances. The selection of the medications is left to the anesthesiologist's discretion and experience. One sedation regimen commonly used in our institution consists of midazolam (0.1 mg/kg) and ketamine (0.5–1.5 mg/kg), with or without a bolus of a hypnotic, such as propofol (0.5–1 mg/kg). Always bear in mind, however, that acutely injured children are rarely hospitalized with an empty stomach.[7] Appropriate intubation equipment and medications must be present and ready for use. When deeper levels of sedation are necessary to perform a nerve block procedure or comfort the child intraoperatively, general anesthesia with protection of the airway may often be a safer alternative to mask ventilation.

Presence of the parents prior to administration of sedatives and often during the block placement is invaluable. Experience in regional anesthesia and ultrasound-guided nerve block procedures is essential. In our institution, anesthesiologists must have adequate training to be allowed to perform ultrasound-guided nerve blocks.

SPECIFIC PERIPHERAL NERVE BLOCK TECHNIQUES

The following sections are dedicated to the various types of peripheral nerve blockade. We place special emphasis on the implications of ultrasound guidance and not on extensive review of the anatomy; anatomic structures are only discussed if they are clearly relevant to the execution of specific block types. For in-depth treatment of anatomic details, the reader is referred to the numerous textbooks available on the subject.

Clinical Pearl

- The block needle/syringe system must be completely purged of air because even minute amounts of air can cause artifacts in the ultrasound image.

Prior to conducting the block procedure, the equipment must be properly prepared and checked—including an ultrasound unit, an appropriate ultrasound probe, sterile ultrasound gel, a needle, and, of course, an appropriate local anesthetic. Other accessories required for all types of block procedures include disinfectant swabs, a 2-mL syringe, and a small-gauge hypodermic needle to anesthetize the skin prior to the needle insertion. The block needle/syringe system must be completely purged of air because even a minute quantity of air can result in artifacts in the ultrasound image.

In our pediatric regional anesthesia practice, we primarily use newer amide local anesthetics such as levobupivacaine or ropivacaine because of their decreased cardiotoxicity potential. By selecting the appropriate concentration (levobupivacaine: 0.125, 0.25, or 0.5%; ropivacaine: 0.2%, 0.475%, or 0.75%), differential (sympathetic, sensory, motor) nerve blockade of desired density and duration can be achieved.

NERVE BLOCKS OF THE UPPER LIMB

Although nearly all surgical interventions on upper limbs can be conducted under regional anesthesia, the reports on the use of these blocks in children are limited. Lack of training in regional anesthesia, and pediatric regional anesthesia in particular, is likely the main reason for the dearth of data. However, at the Department of Anesthesia and Intensive Care at the Medical University of Vienna, anesthetic management of upper-limb injuries in children is routinely performed using brachial plexus blockade and conscious sedation.

Clinical Pearls

- In adults and children alike, any approach to the brachial plexus is possible.
- The most useful brachial plexus blocks in children are supraclavicular, infraclavicular, and axillary blocks.
- Axillary blocks can be conducted for all procedures below the elbow; infraclavicular or supraclavicular blocks are better suited for procedures above the elbow.

Interscalene Approaches to Brachial Plexus Block

Interscalene block is the most proximal approach to the brachial plexus.[8] Shoulder surgery is the main indication for scalene blocks in adults. However, these procedures are relatively infrequently performed in children. One specific concern with interscalene blocks in children is the difficulty in achieving blockade of the roots of C8 and T1. Using a perpendicular needle orientation, these roots are not blocked at all or require very large amounts of local anesthetic. Use of a tangential route under guidance of a nerve stimulator carries a high risk of pleural injury. Ultrasound guidance is advantageous in this situation, as it allows direct visualization and blockade of both roots C8 and T1.

Tobias reported on the technique of interscalene brachial plexus blockade using a *perpendicular* (90-degree) needle insertion plane relative to the skin.[9] This approach, however, is not well suited for application in children. The narrow anatomic relationships in the neck areas of children pose a special risk of an inadvertent puncture of the vertebral artery or the epidural/subarachnoidal space. Instead, Büttner and Meier used a *tangential* insertion in adults,[10] which also may be a safer alternative in pediatric patients. Dalens and colleagues reported on a technique of parascalene brachial plexus blockade for pediatric shoulder surgery that uses an exaggerated, retroflexed head position and a needle insertion site between the lower and middle thirds of the line extending from the clavicle center to the C6 transverse process (Chassaignac's tubercle).[11] The rationale for this technique was to decrease the risk of puncturing the vertebral artery and pleura. Unfortunately, the success of the blockade depends on the use of large volumes of local anesthetic (1 mL/kg).

Clinical Pearls

- To visualize the anatomic structures of a child's neck, linear ultrasound probes working at frequencies as high as possible should be used.
- The exposure is facilitated by slightly turning the child's head to the contralateral side.
- The ultrasound probe should be oriented from the medial to the lateral aspect.

To visualize the anatomic structures of a child's neck, linear ultrasound probes working at frequencies as high as possible should be used. The exposure is facilitated by slightly turning the child's head to the contralateral side. The probe should be oriented from the medial to the lateral aspect. Medially, the thyroid gland and the major vessels in the neck area (carotid artery and internal jugular vein) are easily identified (Figure 52–5). Then, the probe is moved along the sternocleidomastoid muscle until its lateral border is reached. At the same time, the transducer is descended in a caudal direction such that the posterior scalene gap and the upper anterior roots (C5 to C7) of the brachial plexus become visible between the anterior and medial scalene muscles. In very small children, all roots of the brachial plexus (C5 to T1) can be visualized simultaneously (Figure 52–6). Special care must be exercised to place the needle accurately, due to the narrow spatial relationship between the plexus and the neck vessels. It should be noted that in children, the interscalene groove is not always

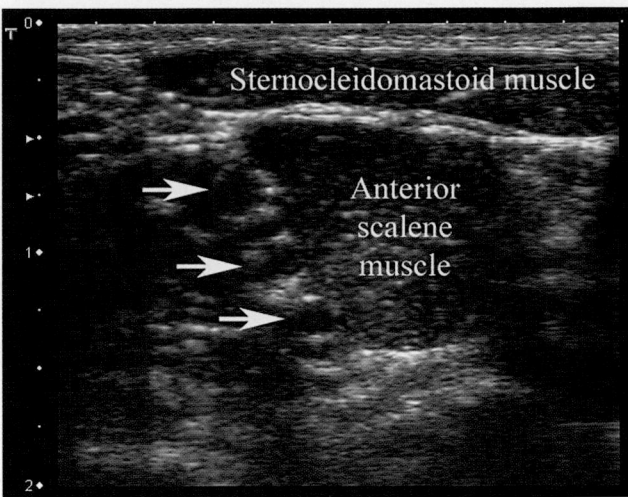

Figure 52–6. Sonographic visualization of the brachial plexus inside the posterior scalene gap (arrows indicate the roots of the brachial plexus; left side = lateral; SonoSite TITAN ultrasound unit with a 10 MHz linear probe).

located exactly at the lateral border of the sternocleidomastoid muscle; it is often situated away either medially or laterally.

The needle is inserted in a tangential direction relative to the neck above the transducer (Figure 52–7). The C5 root will be encountered only a few millimeters deep. As a rule, the needle should be lateral to the C7 root, which will ensure that the neck vessels remain at an adequate distance. Once the local anesthetic is injected, it will invariably spread toward the C5 root, which can be observed in the ultrasound image (Figure 52–8). Depending on the blockade required, the needle can be advanced to a deeper level for injection after the deep roots (C8 and T1) are visualized. In the majority of cases, the local anesthetic will spread medially, even when the needle is in a lateral position. However, if the local anesthetic fails to spread adequately in a medial direction, the needle is withdrawn to the subcutaneous level and repositioned on the medial side

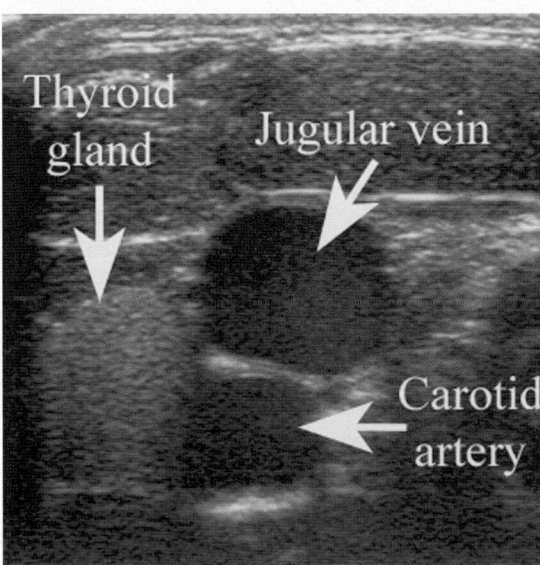

Figure 52–5. Sonographic visualization of anatomical structures in the medial neck area (left side = medial; Toshiba Aplio ultrasound unit with a 14-MHz linear probe).

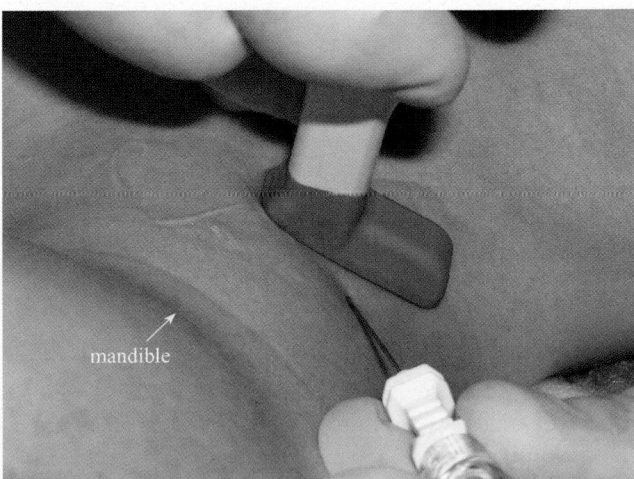

Figure 52–7. Needle position relative to the ultrasound probe during interscalene brachial plexus blockade.

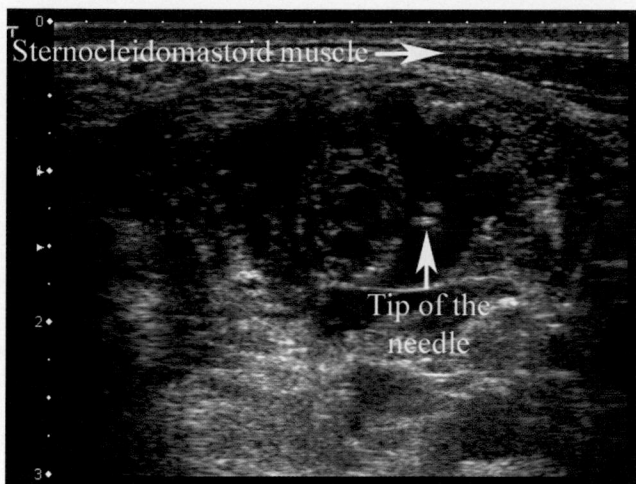

Figure 52–8. C5 to C7 roots covered by 4 mL of local anesthetic. The tip of the needle is placed on the medial side of the nerve roots (left side = lateral; Toshiba Aplio ultrasound unit with a 14-MHz linear probe).

to the posterior scalene gap in the area of the C7 root. Rather than using a specific, arbitrary volume, the injected volume of local anesthetic should be adequate to cover the root surfaces. In general, complete blockade of the brachial plexus in the interscalene groove can be accomplished with approximately 0.15–0.25 mL/kg of local anesthetic.

    Interscalene blocks are almost always best performed under general anesthesia because the patient needs to be immobile to avoid puncture-related complications due to the narrow anatomic relationships in the neck region. The posterior scalene gap is especially well suited for catheter techniques, since a catheter can be conveniently positioned and easily secured in place. Based on the current knowledge, however, catheters or single punctures through a scalene approach are rarely indicated in children.

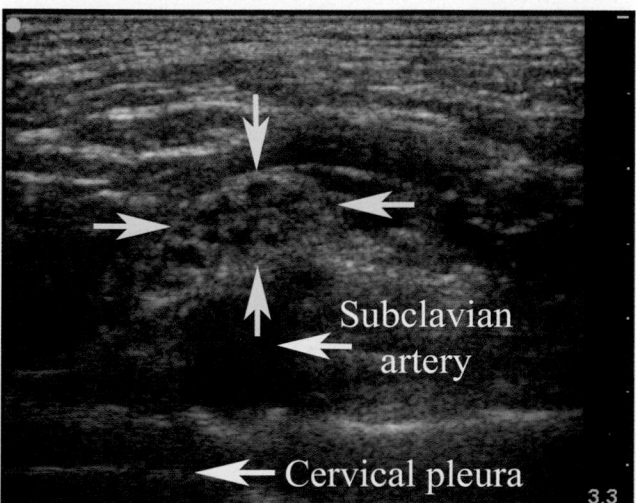

Figure 52–9. Ultrasound visualization of the brachial plexus (between the colored arrows) at the supraclavicular level, which is seated directly on top of the cervical pleura (SonoSite MicroMaxx ultrasound unit with a 6-13-MHz linear probe).

Supraclavicular Approaches to Brachial Plexus Blockade

Pediatric applications for supraclavicular brachial plexus blockade have been previously described.[12] Because of the anatomic proximity of the cervical pleura and the consequent risk of pneumothorax, we use this approach only with ultrasound guidance and in the few cases where infraclavicular visualization in the ultrasound image is inadequate. The brachial plexus is located close to the surface in this area, and it can be visualized readily. However, adequate experience is mandatory for this access route because the risk of puncturing the cervical pleura can be unacceptably high in inexperienced hands.

Clinical Pearls

- The proximity of the cervical pleura poses a specific risk of pneumothorax with supraclavicular block.
- We use this approach only as an ultrasound-guided technique and when infraclavicular visualization is inadequate.
- Adequate experience is mandatory to decrease the risk of injuring the pleura.

Anatomically, in the supraclavicular region, the brachial plexus is approached at the region where the trunks become divisions or cords. It is, therefore, difficult to identify the neuronal structures visible in the ultrasound image with any certainty. However, the brachial plexus, including the musculocutaneous and axillary nerves, remains located in a medial position to the artery (Figure 52–9). The suprascapular nerve, however, occasionally may leave the upper trunk at a more cranial level.

    Using a high-frequency, linear ultrasound probe with a small array surface (preferably a hockey-stick probe), the brachial plexus is approached lateral to the subclavian artery and above the level of the lateral clavicle. The needle is inserted according to the in-line technique, that is, parallel to the long axis of the ultrasound probe (Figure 52–10). In this way, the shaft of the needle can be visualized as well, such that the needle can be positioned very accurately between the artery and plexus. This approach offers complete nerve blockade at doses of local anesthetic as low as 0.15–0.2 mL/kg.

    At our institution, the supraclavicular approach is the preferred method for catheter techniques. Although catheters are more challenging to place using the infraclavicular route and difficult to maintain in a stable position using the axillary approach, supraclavicular catheters can be placed and stabilized readily, when a supraclavicular access is used. The technique, as such, is similar to the single-puncture technique, although the needle insertion site is selected so that it offers maximum immobility. The catheter is advanced once an appropriate volume of local anesthetic (see previous discussion) is injected. Today, suitable catheter kits, which feature a

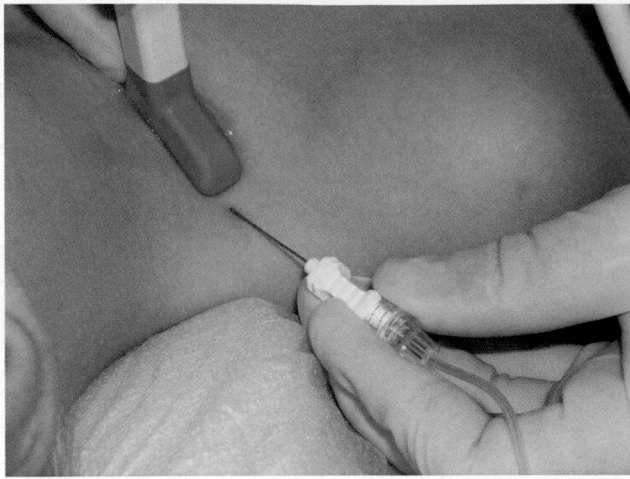

Figure 52–10. In-line puncture technique for supraclavicular plexus blockade using a hockey-stick probe (array surface: 25 mm).

- A 5- to 10-MHz linear ultrasound probe is positioned close to the subclavian artery in the infraclavicular area.
- Visualization of the artery as a round structure is essential in this technique because the brachial plexus is located lateral to the artery.
- Individual cords are difficult to identify in the infraclavicular technique.

hemostatic valve, are available, thus enabling the anesthesiologist to administer the local anesthetic and subsequently place the catheter without having to manipulate the cannula. Even though the catheter can be visualized directly if the ultrasound technique is handled correctly, the best way to verify its position is by visualizing the distribution of the local anesthetic.

Infraclavicular Approaches to Brachial Plexus Blockade

Although infraclavicular blockade with the help of a nerve stimulator is reported to be safe and effective in children,[13,14] the vertical approach to infraclavicular plexus blockade is not recommended because any puncture halfway between the jugular incisure and the acromion carries a risk of injuring the pleura.[15] Fleischmann and coworkers used a lateral approach below the level of the coracoid process under nerve stimulation and thereby achieved a more effective sensory blockade of the musculocutaneous, axillary, and medial brachial cutaneous nerves, as well as better motor blockade of the musculocutaneous and axillary nerves, than through the axillary route.[13] Based on Vester-Andersen's criteria, 100% of these infraclavicular blocks, as compared with 80% of axillary blocks, were successful. This technique of lateral infraclavicular blockade is relatively simple. A 40-mm needle attached to a nerve stimulator is inserted 0.5–1 cm below the coracoid process in the sagittal plane. The local anesthetic is injected after peripheral muscle stimulation is accomplished. It is often necessary to slightly reposition the needle in a cranial or caudal direction.

Ultrasound-guided block may result in shorter sensory–motor onset times than a nerve stimulator-guided technique (mean difference: 9 vs 15 min) as well as significantly longer block durations (mean difference: 1 h).[16] Additionally, the block placement in awake, sedated children resulted in less discomfort using ultrasound-guided nerve blocks than with nerve stimulation.

The ultrasound-guided technique consists of advancing a 5- to 10-MHz linear ultrasound probe into the subclavian artery in the infraclavicular area. It is essential to visualize the artery as a round structure because the brachial plexus is located lateral to the artery. Individual cords are difficult to identify. The lateral cord, being the most ventral and medial cord relative to the posterior cord in this area, is usually identified first. As the structures are tracked further in a lateral direction to the medial border of the coracoid process, the brachial plexus will descend, and the distance to the pleura will increase. At the same time, however, the quality of neural structure imaging will deteriorate as overlapping muscle structures (major and minor pectoral muscles) impose limitation on the high-frequency ultrasound spectrum. The area where the ultrasound image offers the best view of all anatomic structures is selected as a needle insertion site (Figure 52–11). The needle is inserted along the short axis either below (Figure 52–12) or above the transducer and advanced to a point around the lateral or medial cords where the needle tip is located lateral to the subclavian artery. Since the clavicle is located above the transducer, it is easier to insert the needle below the

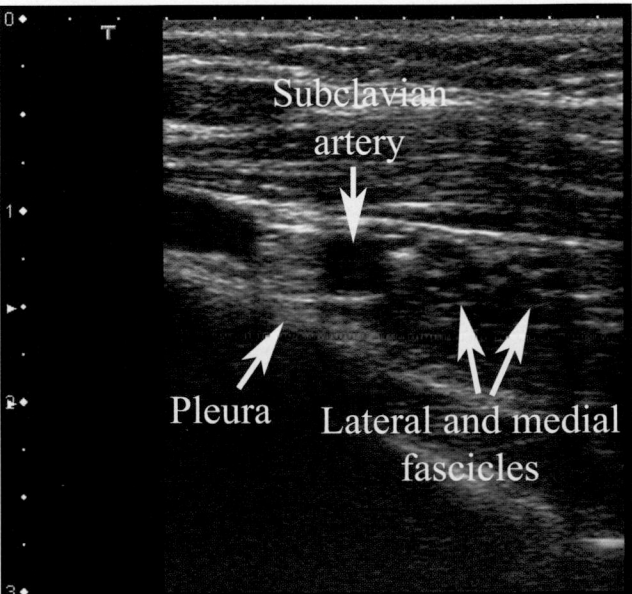

Figure 52–11. Sonographic visualization of the puncture area during lateral infraclavicular blockade of the brachial plexus (left side = medial; Toshiba Aplio ultrasound unit with a 12-MHz linear probe).

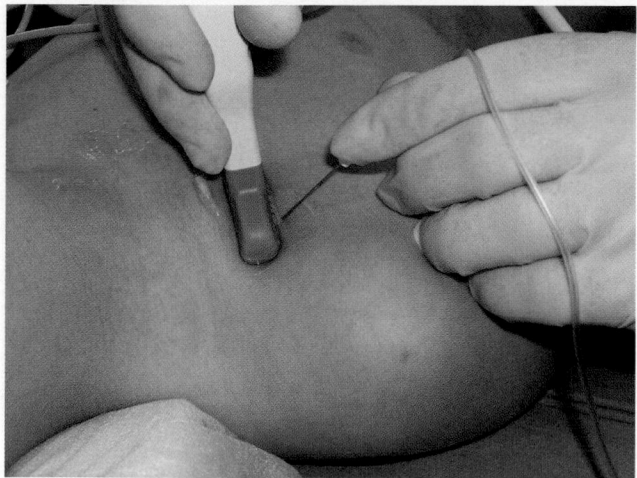

Figure 52–12. Puncture technique below the ultrasound probe during lateral infraclavicular blockade of the brachial plexus.

transducer. In this case, the needle is advanced toward the pleura, a maneuver that requires great care and tactile sensitivity to obtain correct positioning. Therefore, it should be noted that the technique is not "vertical" in a strict sense. In very small children, the brachial plexus may be close to the pleura even when the lateral infraclavicular approach is selected.

Clinical Pearls

- With the infraclavicular block, the needle has to pass through several muscle and fascia layers to reach the plexus; therefore, the local anesthetic may not spread correctly at the first injection attempt.
- Injection into the wrong tissue layer is easily recognized on ultrasound at the beginning of the injection.
- This mistake is easily corrected by advancing the needle to a deeper layer.

Because the local anesthetic will normally spread so that it encircles the artery, there is no need to reposition the needle. In contrast to the axillary approach, this method is essentially a single-shot technique. However, since the needle has to pass through several muscle and fascia layers to reach the plexus, there is always a chance that the local anesthetic may not spread correctly at the first injection attempt. Such maldistribution usually occurs cranial to the plexus as the needle tip is located within a wrong layer. However, this mistake is recognized on the initiation of the injection and easily corrected by advancing the needle to a deeper layer. Since the fascial layers are very elastic in children, accurate needle positioning occasionally may be difficult to achieve; in many cases, practical experience is required to implement the nerve blockade quickly and safely.

Although the published report on this ultrasound-guided block technique was based on a volume of local anesthetic of 0.5 mL/kg,[16] we currently use as little as 0.3–0.4 mL/kg. In contrast to other techniques in which an optimal volume is administered depending on how much volume is needed to fully cover the surface of the targeted nerve structures, the infraclavicular block technique requires the use of a defined volume of local anesthetic. This requirement arises from the fact that not all cords in the infraclavicular area can be visualized in a single ultrasound section, so that the distribution of the local anesthetic cannot be readily visualized in its entirety. Rather, the local anesthetic has to be discretely repositioned during injection to visualize the exact distribution pattern, including the posterior and medial fascicles.

Axillary Approaches to Brachial Plexus Blockade

The axillary route is the most common approach to the brachial plexus. It is indicated for surgical procedures below the level of the cubital fossa. The reasons are that most anesthesiologists are familiar with this technique and the potential for serious complications is significantly lower. These advantages are, however, offset by frequently incomplete blockade or the need for arm positioning required for the block, which may be painful in cases of arm fracture.

Fisher and coworkers used a tangential route to advance the needle to the neurovascular sheath very close to the chest area, using a fascial click to verify that the needle is in its correct position.[17] The mean volume of local anesthetic in this report was relatively large (0.55 mL/kg), and additional perioperative analgesics had to be administered in 46% of the children. Blind perivascular injection of 0.75 mL/kg of local anesthetic also was recommended in the text by Jöhr, which is popular in parts of Europe.[18] This recommendation referred to children younger than 8 years old; in larger children, the author favored the use of a nerve stimulator. He also indicated additional signs of appropriate cannula positioning when the blind technique was used, such as pulsation of the needle and a spindle/sausage-like distribution pattern of local anesthetic.

Carre and colleagues compared the success rate between single and multiple injections for axial plexus anesthesia by advancing the needle with the help of a nerve stimulator and injecting on stimulation of one or two nerves (0.5 mL/kg of local anesthetic).[19] Although a better success rate was reported with the multiple-injection technique, the nerve sensory–motor blockade was still incomplete in 54% of multiple-injection blocks.

Clinical Pearls

- The ultrasound probe must be perpendicular to the axis of the body when the axillary technique is used.
- Nerve structures must be followed in a distal direction to be identified properly.
- The median nerve always remains close to the artery.
- The ulnar nerve is located near the surface on its path to the ulnar nerve sulcus.
- The radial nerve becomes deeper on its descent toward the radial sulcus.

When ultrasound is used, the various neuronal structures involved (radial, median, ulnar, and musculocutaneous nerves) should be identified in the ultrasound image prior to injection, which rarely succeeds at the first attempt. Usually, the nerve structures must be followed in a distal direction to be properly identified. The median nerve always remains close to the artery, while the ulnar nerve is located near the surface on its path to the ulnar nerve sulcus, and the radial nerve quickly becomes deeper on its path to the radial sulcus. The ultrasound probe must be perpendicular to the axis of the body when the axillary technique is used therefore, if the upper arm is in 90-degree abduction, which is the optimal arm position for this type of blockade. Figures 52–13 and 52–14 illustrate the direction of needle insertion and the needle position relative to the ultrasound probe. The needle insertion should be in the lower third, near the distal border of the ultrasound probe. In this way, all targeted nerves are accessible while the

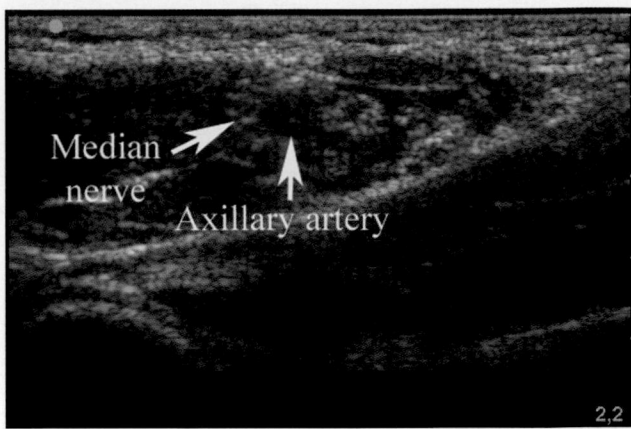

Figure 52–15. Sonographic visualization of the median nerve cranial to the axillary artery. The nerve is surrounded by a thin layer of local anesthetic 0.8 mL (SonoSite MicroMaxx ultrasound unit with a 13-MHz probe).

vessels remain protected. The pressure exerted by the probe itself should be very light to avoid compression of the venous vessels on the ultrasound image. Excessive pressure by the probe may change the relative position of the nerves, as well as the relationship of the nerves to the vessels.

The radial nerve, which can be easily located dorsal to the axillary artery, is routinely blocked first. Depending on the distribution of the local anesthetic, the needle is repositioned such that the ulnar and median nerves are blocked; these are invariably located superficially to the axillary artery (Figure 52–15). The musculocutaneous nerve, which branches off the lateral fascicle and is most commonly located between the short head of the biceps muscle and the coracobrachial muscle, has to be blocked separately (Figure 52–16). In very small (and some larger) children, the musculocutaneous nerve may be located close to the median nerve. In these cases, the amount of local anesthetic injected to block the median nerve may be sufficient to block the musculocutaneous nerve as

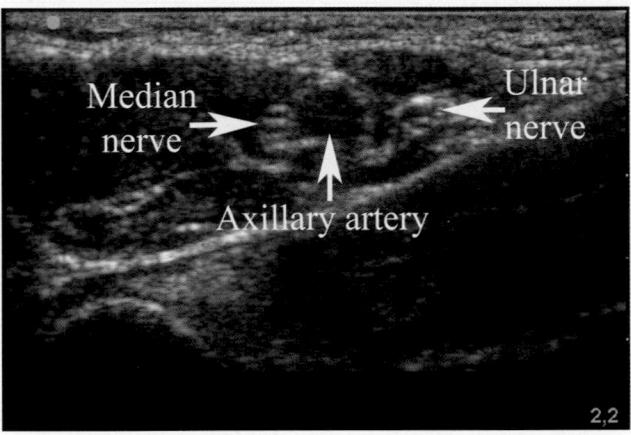

Figure 52–13. Sonographic visualization of the median and ulnar nerves (both surrounded by local anesthetic) at the axillary level. The radial nerve is in a position below the artery and therefore not visible from this view (left side = cranial; SonoSite MicroMaxx ultrasound unit with a 13-MHz probe).

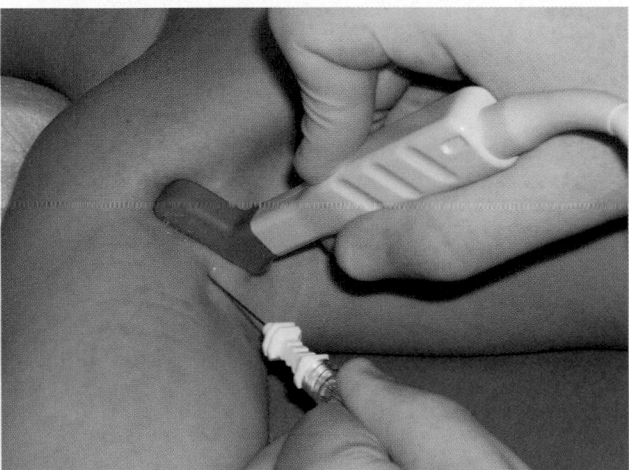

Figure 52–14. Puncture technique for axillary plexus blockade close to the chest region from the lower margin immediately distal to the ultrasound probe, with the upper arm in 90-degree abduction.

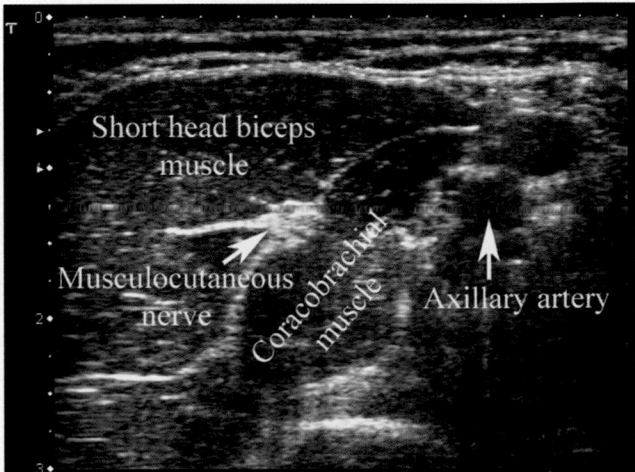

Figure 52–16. Sonographic visualization of the musculocutaneous nerve cranial the axillary artery between the short head of the biceps muscle and the coracobrachial muscle (left side = cranial; Toshiba Aplio ultrasound unit with a 14-MHz linear probe).

well. In addition, separate blockade of the brachial cutaneous and medial antebrachial nerves (branching off the medial fascicle) is recommended. These nerves are located within a fascial layer above the other segments of the brachial plexus and often cannot be well imaged. Occasionally, however, the nerves in this area may be seen after insertion of the needle underneath the fascia and an injection of as little as 0.5 mL of local anesthetic. In very small children, however, the local anesthetic will diffuse into this fascial space. Furthermore, the axillary nerve can be visualized close to the humeral circumflex artery on the medial side of the humerus. However, patients in whom blockade of the axillary nerve is required should normally receive regional anesthesia through a supraclavicular or infraclavicular approach. Therefore, this nerve is virtually never blocked with the axillary brachial plexus techniques.

As in other ultrasound-guided PNBs, we use the minimum amount of local anesthetic required for effective brachial plexus blockade. As a general rule, 0.2–0.3 mL/kg is sufficient.

The axillary route is also technically very suitable for catheter insertion. The bigger problem, however, is maintaining the catheter in a stable position; the catheters often dislodge, especially in very small children. For this reason, we prefer to use the supraclavicular route for catheters in children (see previous discussion).

RESCUE BLOCKS OF THE UPPER EXTREMITY

Specific blocks of the upper limb nerves have been used in children to compensate for incomplete brachial plexus blockade through the axillary route. The higher success rate of axillary blockade using nerve stimulation, multiple stimulation, and ultrasound techniques made specific distal nerve blockade largely obsolete. Consequently, indications for these procedures are narrowed down to localized surgical procedures in the sensory regions supplied by the individual nerves.

Although the nerves discussed as follows essentially can be blocked at any location visible in the ultrasound image, the cubital area is generally preferable. Distal blocks in the wrist area are challenging because the targeted nerves are located very close to the surface—which requires the use of very high ultrasound frequencies—and are firmly embedded in surrounding structures, including tendons, muscles, and connective tissue. Consequently, there is a theoretic risk of nerve damage due to the pressure increase caused by injection of the local anesthetic. In general, it is advisable to avoid nerve block injections in anatomic locations with limited space for the nerves to escape the increase in the compartmental pressure. Alternatively, injections may be made but the injection pressure and postinjection compartmental pressure should be monitored. For the same reasons, blocks should be avoided in the vicinity of bone structures or the ulnar nerve sulcus.

All three nerve blocks discussed require a high-frequency probe (at least 10 MHz). They also require insertion of the needle along the short axis with a 40-mm faceted needle. The amount of local anesthetic should be minimized such

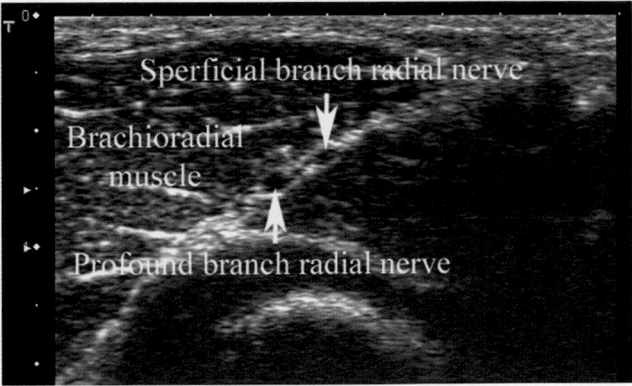

Figure 52–17. Sonographic visualization of the radial nerve (superficial and deep branches) in the cubital area (Toshiba Aplio ultrasound unit with a 14-MHz linear probe).

that the nerve is only covered by a thin film of the injected substance.

Radial Nerve

The radial nerve starts at the posterior fascicle and is located along the cubital fossa between the biceps tendon and the brachioradial muscle. In most cases, the superficial and deep segments are already distinguishable in this area, although both rami are still embedded in the same fascial sheath. Therefore, both nerves can be blocked from the same needle position at the same time (Figure 52–17). Figure 52–18 illustrates the position of the ultrasound probe relative to the puncture needle. In the majority of cases, the needle can be placed successfully between the two rami of the radial nerve, such that both are reached by the local anesthetic.

Ulnar Nerve

The ulnar nerve can be blocked either above or below the ulnar nerve sulcus. The level selected will depend mainly on the quality of visualization in the ultrasound image. The ulnar nerve is formed from the medial fascicle and remains at

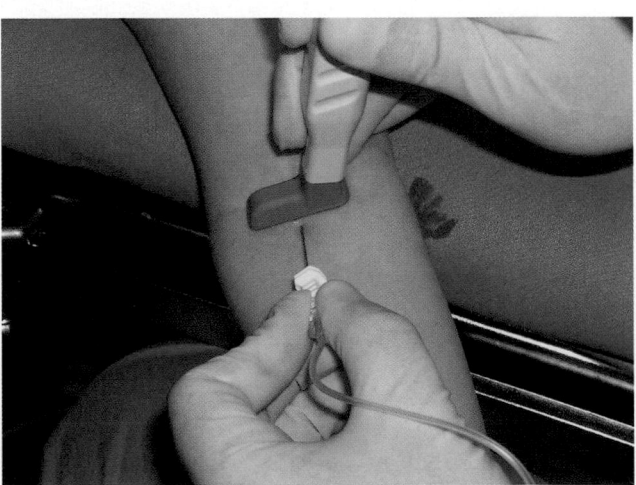

Figure 52–18. Puncture technique for radial nerve blockade inside the cubita.

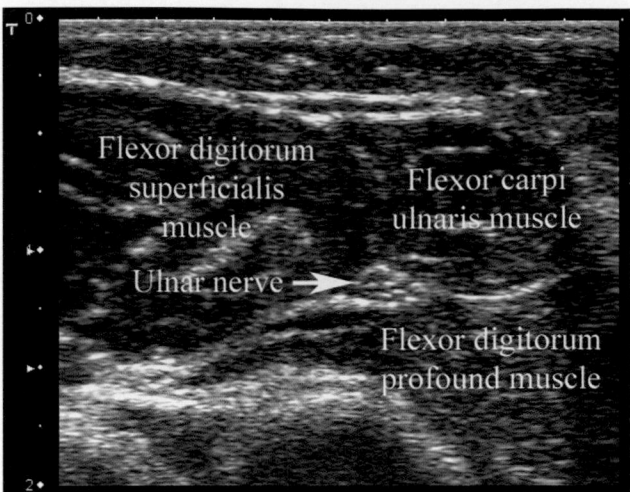

Figure 52–19. Sonographic visualization of the ulnar nerve in the proximal forearm region between the flexor carpi ulnaris, flexor digitorum superficialis, and flexor digitorum profound muscles (right side = ulnar; Toshiba Aplio ultrasound unit with a 14-MHz linear probe).

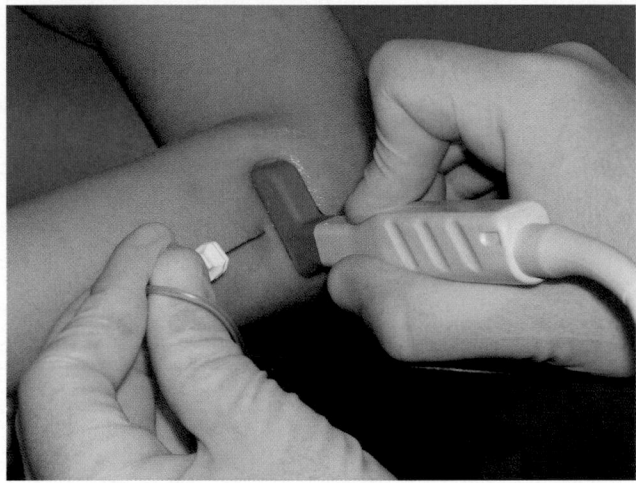

Figure 52–20. Puncture technique for ulnar nerve blockade in the proximal forearm region.

a very superficial level as it proceeds from the axillary region in a distal direction. In the area of the ulnar nerve sulcus, its visualization is impeded by bone artifacts. Farther distally, it comes close to the ulnar artery. Figure 52–19 illustrates the ulnar nerve distal to the ulnar nerve sulcus. Sometimes, it is helpful to use the ulnar artery, which is located more distally, as reference. Subsequently, the nerve can be tracked back in a proximal direction to the selected puncture site. Figure 52–20 shows the position of the ultrasound probe relative to the needle; the puncture site is located distal to the ulnar nerve sulcus.

Median Nerve

The median nerve is formed from both the lateral and medial fascicles and is located between the axillary and cubital areas. There is, invariably, a close anatomic relationship to the ax-

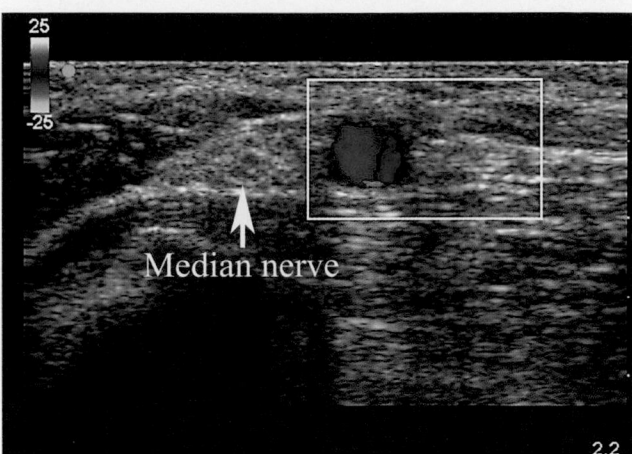

Figure 52–21. Sonographic visualization of the median nerve ulnar to the axillary artery (marked by color Doppler; SonoSite MicroMaxx ultrasound unit with a 13 MHz probe).

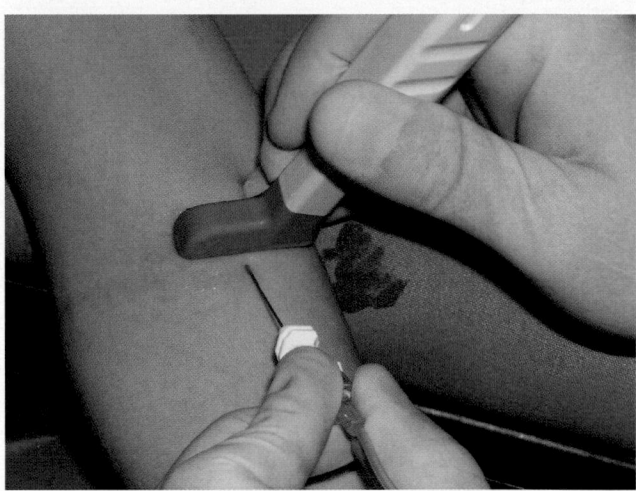

Figure 52–22. Puncture technique for blockade of the median nerve ulnar to the brachial artery in the cubital area.

illobrachial artery. As a general rule, it is located ventral to the artery in the axillary area and medial (hence, ulnar) to the artery in the cubital area. Its level in the cubital area is very superficial, and sometimes it is larger than the artery in diameter (Figure 52–21). The position of the probe relative to the needle is shown in Figure 52–22. For nerve blockade, the needle is first advanced to a point ulnar to the nerve. If the local anesthetic fails to spread in an adequate manner, the needle is repositioned between the artery and the nerve, making sure that these structures are not damaged in the process. With superficial blocks, a skin-nick can facilitate insertion of the short-beveled needle.

LOWER-LIMB BLOCKS

Traditionally, lower limb PNBs have not been popular for use in children; caudal blocks are more frequently used.[1] Nevertheless, selective blockade of children's lower limbs can be very useful in a number of clinical scenarios. Because the available data on lower limb blocks were collected mostly in adults, the volumes of local anesthetic used in children frequently were derived from adult studies. The insertion techniques used in children are typically extrapolated from the data in adults as well. All available techniques that rely on ultrasound guidance for lower limb nerve blockade in children are described in the section that follows.

Psoas Compartment Block

Some 30 years ago, Chayen and coworkers[20] and Winnie and colleagues[21] described a posterior approach to the lumbar plexus in adults. The clinical term *psoas compartment block* was coined by the Chayen group at that time.[20] Although it is normally inappropriate by both physiologic and anatomic criteria to think of children as "small adults," the lumbar plexus is usually characterized by almost identical anatomic and topographic conditions, except that it is naturally less deep in children. Using either the technique described by Winnie or one modified from Chayen, Dalens and coworkers[22] investigated two posterior approaches to the lumbar plexus in children undergoing surgical procedures of the hip and femur and found a considerable age-dependent variability. More recently, Dalens provided data on the depth of the lumbar plexus based on body weight.[23]

Dadure and investigators used CT scanning in an attempt to measure the depth of the lumbar plexus, but their attempts to visualize neural structures failed in most children.[24] Therefore, they had no choice but to take an educated guess as to the depth of the plexus inside the posterior segment of the psoas major muscle. With the help of ultrasonography, we were able to visualize the lumbar plexus and its surrounding structures, and to measure its distance, in an accurate manner.[25] The fact that the neural structures can be visualized in children while they cannot be visualized in adults is due to the ability to use higher resolution probes because of the shallower depth of the plexus. Note that the lumbar plexus is located in the transition zone between the posterior and medal thirds of the psoas major muscle both in adults and in children.

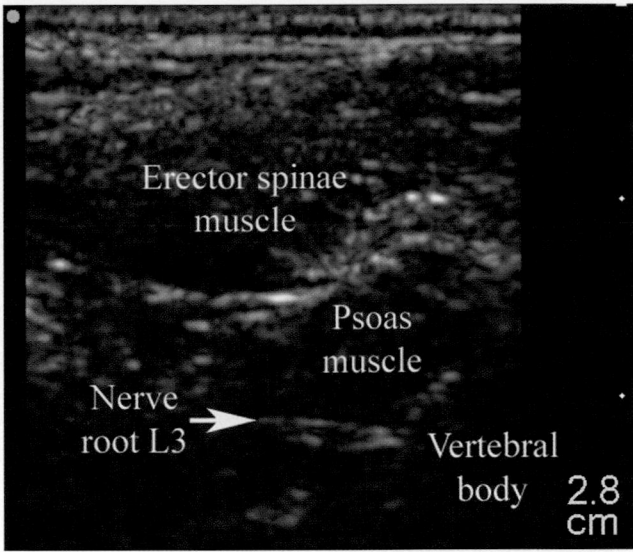

Figure 52–23. Ultrasound image of the lumbar plexus inside the psoas muscle (left side = lateral; SonoSite 180plus ultrasound unit with a 5-10-MHz linear probe).

ducers in the lumbar paravertebral region, since the convex geometry of the ultrasound field allows for better imaging of the paravertebral structures. In newborns and infants, however, linear transducers with a small array surface are preferable.

The first step toward visualizing the lumbar plexus by ultrasonography is to locate the access level (usually L4 or L5). In a paravertebral longitudinal section, the costal processes of the lumbar vertebrae are visualized and counted one by one in a caudocranial direction, beginning at the dorsal ultrasound reflection of the sacrum. The transducer is then gradually shifted parallel to the spinous processes in a cranial direction. Once the L4-5 intervertebral space is reached, the transducer is turned by 90 degrees to a transversal plane (Figure 52–23). Based on this configuration, the lumbar plexus can be targeted inside the posterior segment of the psoas major muscle. In infants and small children, a perpendicular needle orientation transverse to the transducer should be selected because of the limited space and short distance to the plexus (only 2–3 cm; Figure 52–24). By contrast, the in-line technique, as used in adults, is also the method of choice in larger children and adolescents.[26]

Potential indications for posterior blockade of the lumbar plexus in children include surgical treatment of the hip, femur, and knee joint. The use of ultrasonography in psoas compartment blocks is justified by the risk of epidural/intrathecal injection. Damage to the kidney is another potential risk (the kidneys extend down to the L4 to L5 level in small children).[27]

Clinical Pearls

- Peripheral nerves are usually visualized with linear transducers.
- Linear transducers with a small array surface are preferable in newborns and infants.
- Convex transducers are preferable in the lumbar paravertebral region because the convex geometry of the ultrasound field allows for better imaging of the paravertebral structures.

The 3-in-1 Block

The technique of inguinal perivascular blockade of the femoral, obturator, and lateral cutaneous femoral nerves was

Although peripheral nerves are usually visualized with linear transducers, better results were obtained with convex trans-

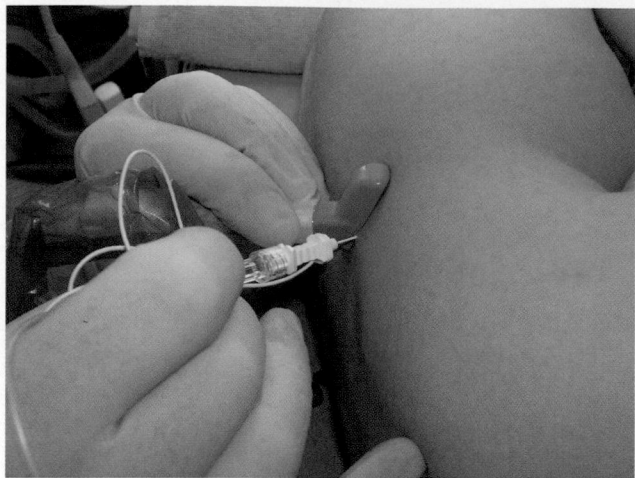

Figure 52–24. Puncture technique for psoas compartment block in a 2-year-old child using a linear ultrasound probe and a cross-sectional technique.

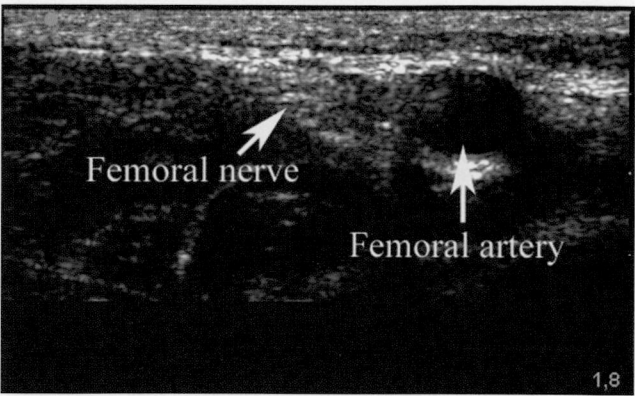

Figure 52–25. Sonographic visualization of the femoral nerve lateral to the femoral artery (SonoSite MicroMaxx ultrasound unit with a 13-MHz probe).

first described by Winnie and colleagues in 1973.[28] Much debate ensued about whether this technique was really capable of blocking all three nerves and on the spread direction of the local anesthetic. Originally, it was assumed that the local anesthetic spread proximally from the inguinal puncture site to the lumbar plexus along a muscle–fascia sheath. This assumption was clearly refuted by our study group in an MRI investigation that demonstrated that the local anesthetic exclusively spread in a lateral and medial direction with this technique.[29] The quality of sensory blockade depends more on the needle insertion technique than on the volume of local anesthetic.[4,30] This finding in particular has important implication in children, in whom the use of large doses of local anesthetic may be prohibitive in this technique.

Unlike other lower limb peripheral blocks, however, the 3-in-1 technique is relatively well documented with conventional methods of nerve identification in children. Most commonly, this technique is used for muscle biopsy in children (eg, in making the diagnosis of malignant hyperthermia or neuromuscular diseases).[31–33] Various investigators used the technique for both single-shot and continuous applications of perioperative pain therapy in femoral fractures.[34–38] They obtained respectable success rates (up to 96%) with this approach.[37] However, an ultrasound-guided 3-in-1 block offers a number of advantages:

1. The volumes of local anesthetic can be further reduced, and combined nerve blocks can be performed more safely. For example, the sensory nerve supply to the femoral shaft is affected by both the femoral and sciatic nerves; hence the sciatic nerve should be additionally blocked for effective pain therapy in femoral shaft fractures.
2. Because the femoral nerve is located very close to the femoral artery, there is also a risk of arterial puncture.
3. Using ultrasound guidance, it should be possible to direct the spread of the local anesthetic in a lateral and (to a smaller extent) medial direction, such that a true 3-in-1

block is achieved. Also, it should be possible to selectively block the femoral nerve only by reducing the amount of local anesthetic (*volume-dependent differential blockade*).

A high-frequency ultrasound probe is advanced to a point in the immediate distal vicinity of the inguinal ligament to visualize the femoral artery and, more laterally, the femoral nerve. The weight of the transducer alone is usually sufficient to compress the femoral vein, which is located medial to the artery. The space between the artery and the nerve harbors the iliopectineal fascia, representing the deep folium of the inguinal ligament. The femoral nerve is usually very close to the skin and it can be visualized in its entirety only from a position immediately distal to the inguinal ligament (Figure 52–25) because it soon divides into its distal branches.

Clinical Pearl

■ With 3-in-1 block, the blockade of the obturator nerve is limited to only the anterior (cutaneous) ramus; consequently, a better name for the obturator block should be the 2.5-in-1 block.

As in most peripheral blocks, the needle is inserted perpendicular to the transducer (Figure 52–26). The needle can be placed either lateral or medial to the femoral nerve. Note that the nerve is often located very close to the artery, so the needle must be advanced with care if a medial position (toward the artery) is selected. It is, therefore, usually better to select a lateral position. The amount of local anesthetic to be injected depends on how many nerves are targeted. For selective blockade of the femoral nerve, it is sufficient if the injectate covers just the surface of the nerve. However, if a 3-in-1 block is required, a larger volume must be injected, so that the local anesthetic visibly spreads in a lateral and medial direction. Note that blockade of the obturator nerve is usually confined to its anterior ramus. Therefore, the 3-in-1 block is

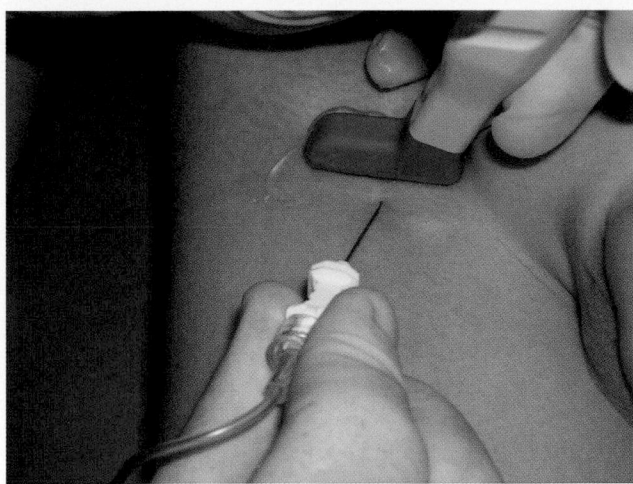

Figure 52–26. Puncture technique for femoral nerve, or 3-in-1, blockade.

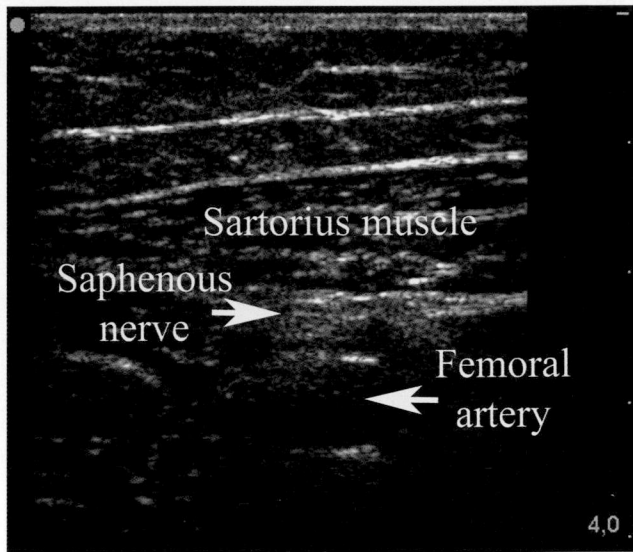

Figure 52–27. Sonographic visualization of the saphenous nerve below the sartorius muscle (SonoSite MicroMaxx ultrasound unit with a 13-MHz probe).

really a "2.5-in-1" block (refer to Chapter 36). Direct visualization of the lateral cutaneous femoral nerve requires the use of a high-resolution transducer and is only possible in larger children. A limitation to this technique is that the ultrasound-assisted technique for 3-in-1 blocks still relies on the lateral and medial distribution pattern of the local anesthetic to reach the obturator nerve because this nerve normally cannot be visualized by ultrasonography due to its position between the adductor muscles and the small diameter of its two branches.

The 3-in-1 technique is particularly well suited for continuous nerve blockade. This approach was described for conventional methods of needle guidance as well.[34,35] The same puncture technique is used as with the single-shot approach. Following injection of the local anesthetic, the catheter is placed underneath the iliopectineal fascia under ultrasound guidance. It is also possible to selectively block the femoral nerve in this way. The catheter is not directly visible in the majority of cases; however, a small amount of local anesthetic injected on a preliminary basis will be enough to foresee the spread direction and whether successful blockade can be expected, once the full volume is used. It is essential to decide beforehand whether a selective femoral nerve block or a complete 3-in-1 block is required. For selective femoral nerve blockade, the local anesthetic can be applied continuously through the catheter (eg, 0.1–0.2 mL/kg of local anesthetic in a low concentration). For 3-in-1 blockade, an initial bolus dose is recommended, although low concentrations of a long-acting substance, such as levobupivacaine (0.125%) or ropivacaine (0.2% twice daily), usually is sufficient. Ultrasound monitoring can be performed while the bolus is being applied through the catheter to identify its position.

Selective Saphenous Nerve Block

The saphenous nerve is best located with a high-resolution ultrasound probe at the distal-medial thigh level in the transition zone between the sartorius and gracilis muscles and

their attachment of their respective tendons (Figure 52–27). The puncture should be transverse to the proximal aspect toward the transducer (Figure 52–28) or performed using the in-line technique. Only small amounts of local anesthetic are required for blockade. In addition, smaller volumes are advisable because a larger volume of local anesthetic may cause excessive pressure in this tissue compartment and, consequently, increase the risk of nerve injury.

Sciatic Nerve Block

Sciatic nerve blocks should form an integral part of every well-trained anesthesiologist's repertoire. It is desirable that several approaches to the sciatic nerve are mastered because the need for various approaches is dictated by the nature of the surgical procedure, as well as by the positioning of the child and the

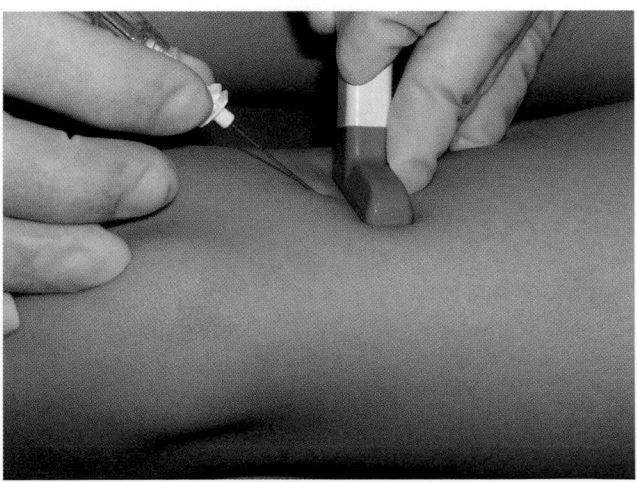

Figure 52–28. Cross-sectional puncture technique for saphenous nerve blockade.

affected limb. In clinical practice, good results were obtained with the subgluteal, the midfemoral, and the popliteal access route. A clear-cut distinction between these three approaches cannot always be made. Perhaps the greatest advantage of ultrasound guidance for sciatic blockade is that it enables the anesthesiologist to block nerves at any location without the need to use surface landmarks as reference. Therefore, selecting a site of optimal sonographic visibility is the only consideration in addition to selecting the level of blockade depending on the type of surgery and patient positioning. The sciatic nerve is not uniformly accessible to ultrasound imaging over its entire course.

The success rates achieved with conventional guidance techniques (mainly identification of the nerve with a nerve stimulator) for sciatic nerve blockade in children are excellent. For instance, Konrad and Jöhr[39] and Tobias and Mencio[40] reported successful blocks in over 90% of cases. However, the large volumes of local anesthetic (0.75–1.0 mL/kg) used in these studies may not allow for the use the additional combined blocks (eg, femoral or 3-in-1 blocks). Furthermore, nerve stimulation or other indirect techniques of nerve identification carry a certain risk of damaging the targeted nerve during puncture due to the shear size of the sciatic nerve. Ultrasound guidance may be superior in this regard because, theoretically, it should allow the needle to be safely inserted, avoiding direct nerve contact.

When it comes to ultrasound-guided sciatic nerve block, the choice of approach is different from those used with the nerve stimulator-guided techniques. For instance, the approach described by Labat, which enjoys widespread popularity in adults, should not be used in children because ultrasound visualization may be limited in this area. This is because the nerve is located underneath several muscle layers, such that the high-frequency ultrasound probes cannot be used. A similar problem is encountered with the anterior approach, in which the sciatic nerve is overlapped by the trochanter minor. In addition, the anterior approach is very uncomfortable due to the deep location of the nerve. For these reasons, we do not use the anterior approach, even though Aizenberg and investigators reported on its use in children.[41] Dalens and coworkers demonstrated, in a comparative study, that the posterior and lateral access routes were both more reliable and more practical than the anterior approach in children.[42] Their findings are generally in agreement with the following discussion of meaningful approaches to ultrasound-guided sciatic nerve blocks.

Subgluteal Approach

The subgluteal approach is the most proximal approach we use for sciatic nerve blockade under ultrasound guidance. Bösenberg employed a nerve stimulator for this access route,[38] thereby achieving good success rates despite injecting relatively small amounts of local anesthetic (0.5 mg/kg for unilateral and 0.3 mg/kg for bilateral blocks). Gray and coworkers mention ultrasonography as an alternative option to guide sciatic blocks through the subgluteal approach.[43]

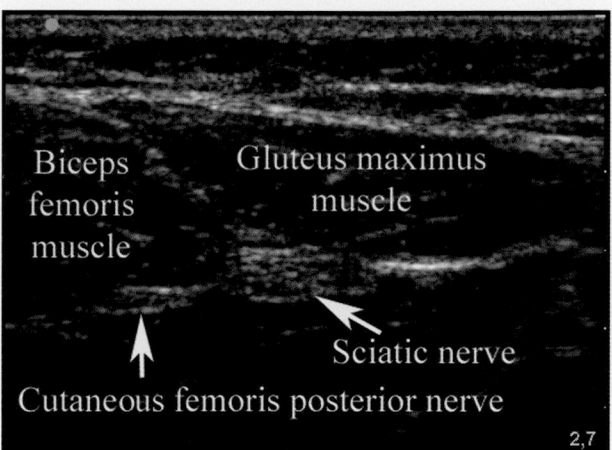

Figure 52–29. Sonographic visualization of the sciatic and cutaneous femoris posterior nerves (left side = medial; SonoSite MicroMaxx ultrasound unit with a 13-MHz probe).

The child may remain in a supine position for this technique, but a prone or side position is also possible. We always try to meet individual requirements, thus selecting the most comfortable position for the child.

The sciatic nerve is located close to the surface in the immediate subgluteal area, requiring the use of a high-frequency linear ultrasound probe. Figure 52–29 illustrates the position of the sciatic nerve between the gluteus maximus and quadratus femoris muscles (lateral) on the one hand and the biceps femoris muscles (medial) on the other. The posterior cutaneous femoral nerve usually can be visualized medial and slightly more superficial to the sciatic nerve. In association with a thigh tourniquet, this nerve should also be blocked. Therefore, indications for this approach include not only situations in which good ultrasound visibility is required but also the use of a tourniquet.

Figure 52–30 illustrates the needle position relative to the ultrasound transducer, the child being in a supine position with the hip and knee flexed. After the needle has been

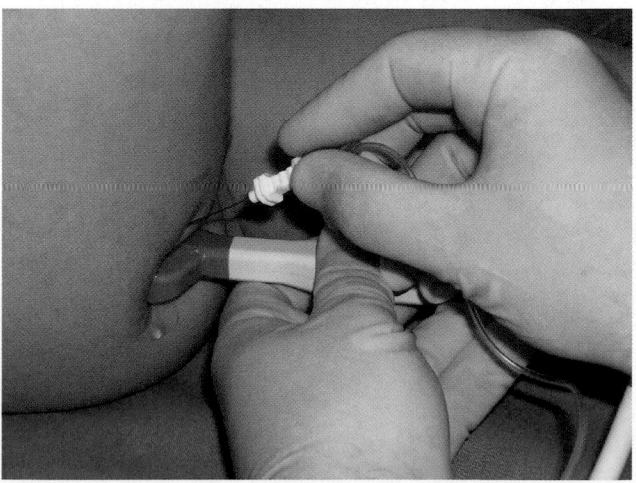

Figure 52–30. Puncture technique for sciatic nerve blockade from a subgluteal route with the hip and knee flexed.

placed medial to the sciatic nerve, the local anesthetic usually spreads to the posterior cutaneous femoral nerve. If the initial injection fails to reach the nerve, the needle is repositioned more medial to the posterior cutaneous femoral nerve to optimize the distribution of local anesthetic. As a rule, however, a single shot will suffice.

Midfemoral Approach

The midfemoral approach to the sciatic nerve is usually selected only if a subgluteal or popliteal approach is not possible, usually because some segments of the sciatic nerve are not accessible to ultrasonography. A clear-cut distinction between the midfemoral and popliteal approach cannot always be made.

The same needle position is selected as with the subgluteal approach (Figure 52–31). The in-line technique is a viable option for this type of puncture. With increasing displacement of the transducer in a distal (popliteal) direction, practical considerations will dictate that the needle insertion be parallel to the long axis of the transducer.

It is essential to track the route of the sciatic nerve in a distal direction, thereby visualizing its separation into the tibial and peroneal nerves. Schwemmer and coworkers reported that the level at which this separation takes place varies widely,[44] which is in accordance with our own observations. This variability is not known to correlate with body weight or body height. Therefore, if complete blockade of the sciatic nerve is required, the needle insertion site should be proximal to this point of separation. Again, this requirement can only be accurately met through direct sonographic visualization.

Figure 52–32 illustrates anatomic conditions in the midfemoral access area proximal to the furcation site of the sciatic nerve as visualized by ultrasound. The puncture itself is carried out in the same way as the subgluteal puncture. It should be placed between the biceps femoris and semimembranous muscles. Puncturing the muscles should be avoided

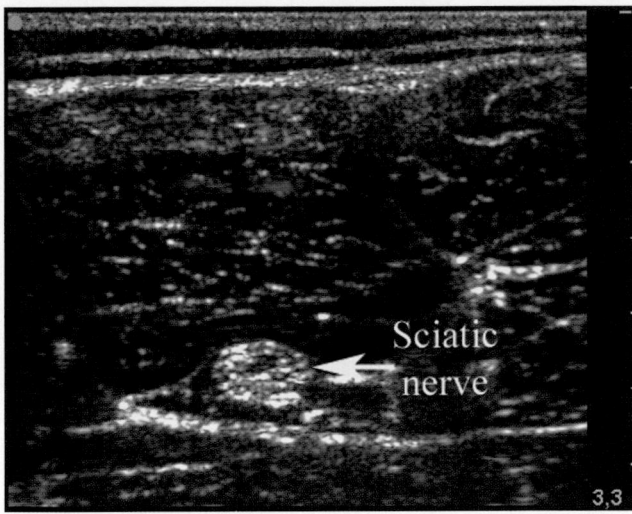

Figure 52–32. Sonographic visualization of the sciatic nerve at the midfemoral level (left side = lateral, SonoSite MicroMaxx ultrasound unit with a 13-MHz probe).

to reduce the risk of hematoma during blockade. Depending on how deep the nerve is located, the use of a longer needle (70 mm) may be indicated. In the overwhelming majority of cases, the needle has to be repositioned several times to optimize the distribution of the local anesthetic.

Popliteal Sciatic Block

The popliteal approach to the sciatic nerve, also referred to as a *fossa popliteal block*, is very useful in pediatric anesthesia. One of its advantages is that blockade from a dorsal route is relatively painless in this rhombus-shaped knee area (whose upper sides are formed laterally by the femoral biceps muscle and medially by the semimembranous and semitendinous muscles), as no muscle bellies are perforated during puncture. One shortcoming of conventional guidance by nerve stimulation is, however, that no reliable information is obtained about at which level the sciatic nerve bifurcates into the tibial and peroneal nerves. The only practical way to identify this level, which varies widely between children, is by ultrasonography.[44]

The conventional technique is described as proximal to the fold of the popliteal fossa, with the puncture in a somewhat lateral position to the midline at a 45-degree angle relative to the skin, using 0.75–1.0 mL/kg of local anesthetic.[45] According to Konrad and Jöhr, body weight shows the best correlation with tibial nerve depth in children.[39]

A high-frequency probe should be used for popliteal access to the sciatic nerve in order to accurately identify the point at which the nerve furcates into its two branches, Figure 52–33 illustrates the sciatic nerve proximal to this furcation site. More distally, the peroneal nerve divides at a very superficial level, and the tibial nerve courses distally and deeper. The lateral approach to popliteal block is particularly suitable (Figure 52–34) because the child may remain in a supine position during the blockade, similarly to the technique in adult patients.[46,47] The exact puncture site is selected based

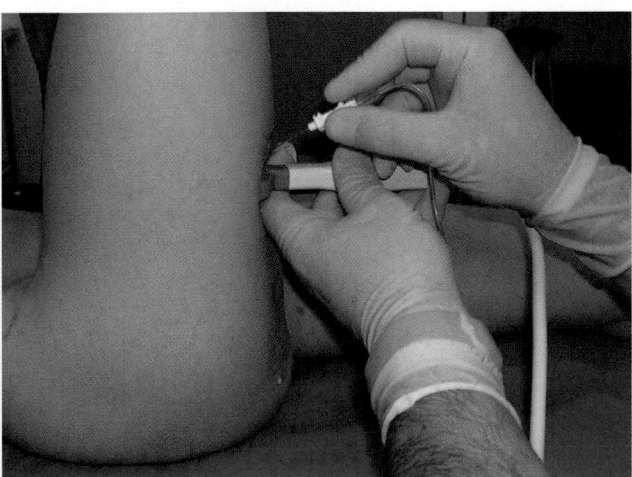

Figure 52–31. Cross-sectional puncture technique for midfemoral sciatic nerve blockade with the hip and knee flexed.

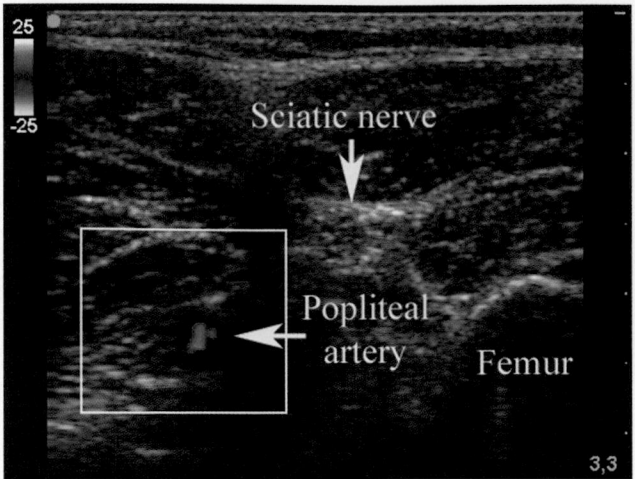

Figure 52–33. Sonographic visualization of the sciatic nerve slightly proximal to the furcation into the peroneal and tibial nerves (left side = medial; SonoSite MicroMaxx ultrasound unit with a 13-MHz probe).

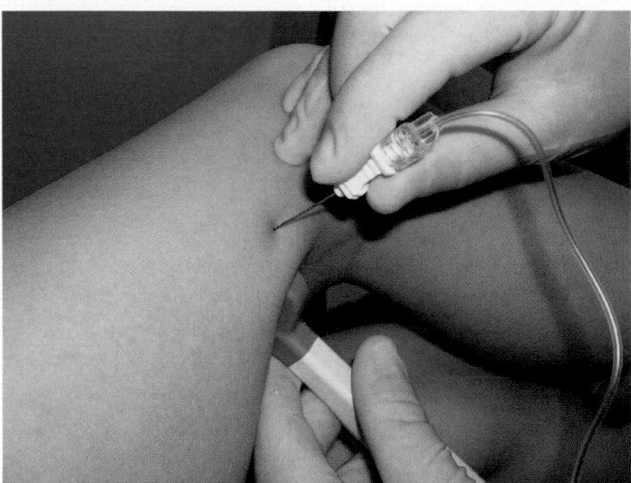

Figure 52–34. Lateral (in-line) puncture technique for sciatic nerve blockade above the popliteal fossa.

on the depth of the nerve visualized in the ultrasound image. The needle tip is first positioned above and then below the sciatic nerve, which will ensure an optimal distribution pattern of the local anesthetic. Naturally, the advantage of not transversing the muscles is lost with this technique. Therefore, a distinction must be made between the lateral (in-line) and dorsal (cross-sectional) techniques.

ABDOMINAL WALL BLOCKS

Blockade of the ilioinguinal/iliohypogastric nerves is the only documented application for ultrasound-guided techniques performed through the abdominal wall. Since this technique is used very frequently in clinical practice, a detailed discus-

sion of its anatomic implications is provided, with the focus on ultrasound-guided puncture techniques.

Ilioinguinal/Iliohypogastric Nerve Block

Blockade of the ilioinguinal/iliohypogastric nerves is a frequently used regional anesthetic technique for surgical procedures carried out in the sensory regions supplied by both nerves. For procedures in the inguinal region (inguinal hernia, orchiopexy), the effectiveness of this technique is similar to that for caudal blocks.[48] The needle insertion site for ilioinguinal/iliohypogastric blockade is usually located 1 cm medial to the anterior superior iliac spine, and the exact needle position is identified by a fascial click.[49] Considering the inaccuracy of this approach, it is not surprising that ilioinguinal/iliohypogastric nerve blocks yielded failure rates of 20% to 30%.[50] Furthermore, severe complications, such as intestinal puncture or pelvic hematoma, were reported.[51–53]

These introductory remarks illustrate that the safety and effectiveness of ilioinguinal/iliohypogastric nerve blockade can be greatly improved by direct visualization.[5]

The following paragraphs illustrate the anatomic and sonographic principles of this technique. The anatomy of the lateral abdominal wall is more complicated than one might assume. Back in 1952, Jamieson and coworkers indicated that the position of these nerves relative to the muscles is subject to great anatomic variability.[54] Therefore, it is not surprising that blind needle insertion yields a relatively low success rate. Schoor and colleagues demonstrated this point in an anatomic study performed with children,[55] in which most of the failed injections in that study were too medial.

The anatomic relationships can be summarized as follows. Both the ilioinguinal and the iliohypogastric nerves pass through the fascia lumborum at the lateral border of the quadratus lumborum muscle and then extend to the area between the internal oblique and the transverse abdominal muscles. The iliohypogastric nerve is located superior and medial to the ilioinguinal nerve and, in the area of the anterior superior iliac spine, furcates into the lateral and medial cutaneous rami at its two terminal branches. The lateral cutaneous ramus passes through the internal and external abdominal obliques and provides sensory supply to the skin in the anterior buttocks region. The medial cutaneous ramus passes both through the internal abdominal oblique muscle and the aponeurosis of the external abdominal oblique and supplies the skin in the abdominal wall region above the symphysis. The ilioinguinal nerve supplies the skin region underneath the area supplied by the iliohypogastric nerve as well as the anterior region of the scrotum.

The ultrasound examination should be performed with a high-frequency linear probe. The ilioinguinal nerve is best visualized immediately medial to the anterior superior iliac spine. (Figure 52–35) From our studies, we found that the anterior superior iliac spine is located at a mean distance of 7 mm to the nerve. The iliohypogastric nerve is located very

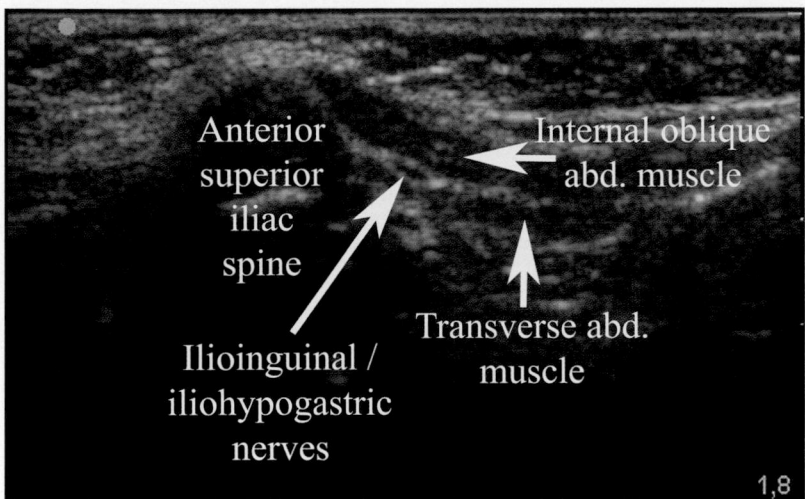

Figure 52–35. Sonographic visualization of the ilioinguinal/iliohypogastric nerves medial to the anterior superior iliac spine and between the internal oblique abdominal and transverse abdominal muscles. In many patients, the external oblique abdominal muscle is only present in the form of an aponeurosis in this area (SonoSite MicroMaxx ultrasound unit with a 13-MHz probe).

close to the ilioinguinal nerve (3 mm on average). It is important to note that in 50% of cases, only two muscle layers are present in the puncture area, representing the internal abdominal oblique and the transverse abdominal muscles. Very often, the external abdominal oblique muscle is only present as an aponeurosis in the puncture area. Note that the nerves are located close to the peritoneum. In our investigations, we observed a mean distance of 3 mm (the shortest distance measured was 1 mm).

As illustrated in Figure 52–36, the needle is inserted perpendicular to the ultrasound probe and it is placed between the internal abdominal oblique and the transverse abdominal muscles. The volume of local anesthetic required to anesthetize both nerves is 0.2 mL/kg. These doses are considerably smaller than those recommended in other reports, which, especially in infants, adds greatly to the safety of the procedure, considering that very high serum levels were reported for this technique.[56] There is rarely a need to reposition the needle for blockade of the iliohypogastric nerve.

Ultrasound-guided blockade of the ilioinguinal/iliohypogastric nerves—using surgical analgesia with a combined approach consisting of inhalation anesthesia with 1 monitored anesthesia care (MAC) unit of anesthetic gas and nerve blockade—yields a 96% success rate, even at low doses of local anesthetic (0.2 mL/kg). In addition, potential complications, such as intestinal puncture, are avoided safely with this approach. Furthermore, the risk of accidental femoral paresis is eliminated at lower doses of local anesthetic.[57] In addition, the work of Willschke and colleagues clearly demonstrated that body weight, body height, or similar parameters correlate neither with the distance between the anterior superior iliac spine and the ilioinguinal nerve nor with the depth of the ilioinguinal/iliohypogastric nerves nor with the distance between the nerves and the peritoneum.[5]

Ultrasound guidance for ilioinguinal/iliohypogastric nerve blocks offers several advantages over traditional, blind techniques because it decreases the risk of complications and increases the success rate.

SUMMARY

In summary, most regional anesthetic techniques used in adult patients can be used in children. Table 52–1 lists various nerve block techniques used in children along with their indications, suggested transducer frequencies, and some techniques details. Numerous published study results are available on the subject; however, many of the various puncture techniques used with conventional guidance techniques are not described very precisely. The widely held view, that local anesthetic spreads extensively and in all directions in very small children, making optimally exact puncture techniques unnecessary, is inaccurate. Ultrasound guidance is an excellent tool to optimize these nerve blocks. Ultrasound-guided nerve blocks require an adequate level of additional training. Workshops to convey the elementary hands-on skills are indispensable; however, competent supervision must also be available in the early phase of the practical application.

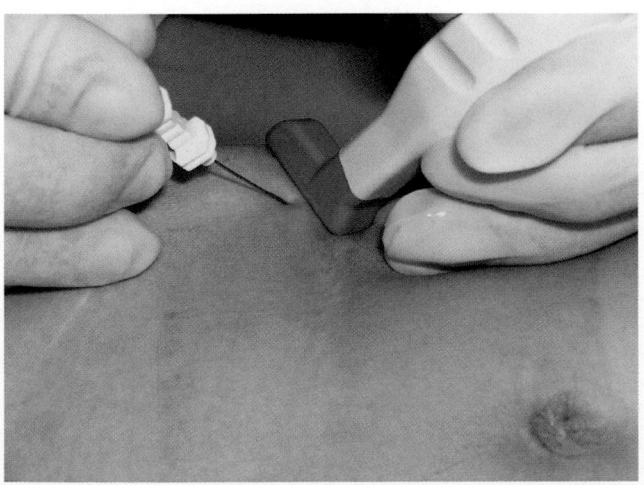

Figure 52–36. Puncture site for ilioinguinal nerve blockade.

Table 52–1.

Summary of Nerve Blocks

Type of Nerve Block	Indications	Transducer (MHz)	Puncture Technique	Comments	Figure References
Scalene block	Shoulder, upper arm	Linear 10–15	Cross sectional, tangential	Rarely indicated	52–6 to 52–8
Supraclavicular brachial plexus block	Entire upper limb, including the proximal upper-arm area	Linear 10–15	In-line	Risk of pleural injury; our preferred position for catheters	52–9, 52–10
Infraclavicular brachial plexus block	Cubital fossa and its distal vicinity	Linear 5–10	Cross sectional	To be performed in an area where the nerve structures can be optimally visualized	52–11, 52–12
Axillary brachial plexus block	Proximal forearm and its distal vicinity	Linear 10–15	Cross sectional; the needle may need to be repositioned several times depending on the distribution pattern	Structures very close to the surface; nerves should be tracked in a distal direction for correct identification	52–13 to 52–16
Radial, ulnar, and median nerves	Surgical procedures in the corresponding sensory regions	Linear 10–15	Cross sectional	—	52–17 to 52–22
Psoas compartment block	Hip joint, thigh, abdominal wall	Linear 5–10 in small children Sector 2–4/4–7 in larger children	Cross sectional or in-line	Relatively deep block; for experienced users only	52–23, 52–24
3-in-1 block	Thigh, knee, sensory region	Linear 10–15	Cross sectional; immediately below the inguinal ligament	Blockade very close to the surface	52–25, 52–26
Saphenous nerve	Sensory area, knee (ramus infrapatellaris)	Linear 10–15	Cross sectional or in-line	Blockade very close to the surface	52–27, 52–28
Subgluteal sciatic nerve block	Entire lower limb combined with 3-in-1 block; high tourniquet (posterior cutaneous femoral nerve)	Linear 10–15	Cross sectional	Sometimes requires needle repositioning	52–29, 52–30
Midfemoral sciatic nerve block	Lower leg	Linear 5–10	Cross sectional or in-line	To be performed in an area where the nerve can be optimally visualized	52–31, 52–32
Popliteal block	Lower leg	Linear 10–15	In-line	Visualization of cleavage into tibial and peroneal nerves	52–33, 52–34
Ilioinguinal/ iliohypogastric nerve blocks	Inguinal hernia, orchidopexy, hydrocele	Linear 10–15	Cross sectional	Nerves very close to the peritoneum; one needle position is usually sufficient for both nerves	52–35, 52–36

References

1. Giaufré E, Dalens B, Gombert A: Epidemiology and morbidity of regional anesthesia in children: A one-year prospective survey of the French-Language Society of Pediatric Anesthesiologists. Anesth Analg 1996;83:904–912.

2. Bosenberg A, Thomas J, Lopez T, et al: Validation of a six-graded faces scale for evaluation of postoperative pain in children. Paediatr Anaesth 2003;13:708–713.

3. Bosenberg AT, Raw R, Boezaart AP: Surface mapping of peripheral nerves in children with a nerve stimulator. Paediatr Anaesth 2002;12:398–403.

4. Marhofer P, Schrogendorfer K, Wallner T, et al: Ultrasonographic guidance reduces the amount of local anesthetic for 3-in-1 blocks. Reg Anesth Pain Med 1998;23:584–588.

5. Willschke H, Marhofer P, Bosenberg A, et al: Ultrasonography for ilioinguinal/iliohypogastric nerve blocks in children. Br J Anaesth 2005;95:226–230.

6. Mazoit JX, Dalens BJ: Pharmacokinetics of local anaesthetics in infants and children. Clin Pharmacokinet 2004;43:17–32.

7. Bricker SR, McLuckie A, Nightingale DA: Gastric aspirates after trauma in children. Anaesthesia 1989;44:721–724.

8. Bartholdy J, Holm-Knudsen RJ: [Brachial plexus blockade via the interscalene port–for regional anesthesia/analgesia of upper extremities; use, application and risks]. Ugeskr Laeger 1994;156:5676–5679.

9. Tobias JD: Brachial plexus anaesthesia in children. Paediatr Anaesth 2001;11:265–275.

10. Büttner J, Meier G: *Kontinuierliche periphere Techniken zur Regionalanästhesie und Schmerztherapie—Obere und untere Extremität.* Uni-Med Verlag, 1999, pp 93–96.

11. Dalens B, Vanneuville G, Tanguy A: A new parascalene approach to the brachial plexus in children: Comparison with the supraclavicular approach. Anesth Analg 1987;66:1264–1271.

12. Pande R, Pande M, Bhadani U, et al: Supraclavicular brachial plexus block as a sole anaesthetic technique in children: An analysis of 200 cases. Anaesthesia 2000;55:798–802.

13. Fleischmann E, Marhofer P, Greher M, et al: Brachial plexus anaesthesia in children: Lateral infraclavicular vs axillary approach. Paediatr Anaesth 2003;13:103–108.

14. de Jose Maria B, Tielens LK: Vertical infraclavicular brachial plexus block in children: A preliminary study. Paediatr Anaesth 2004;14:931–935.

15. Greher M, Retzl G, Niel P, et al: Ultrasonographic assessment of topographic anatomy in volunteers suggests a modification of the infraclavicular vertical brachial plexus block. Br J Anaesth 2002;88:632–636.

16. Marhofer P, Sitzwohl C, Greher M, et al: Ultrasound guidance for infraclavicular brachial plexus anaesthesia in children. Anaesthesia 2004;59:642–646.

17. Fisher WJ, Bingham RM, Hall R: Axillary brachial plexus block for perioperative analgesia in 250 children. Paediatr Anaesth 1999;9:435–438.

18. Jöhr M: *Axilläre Plexusanästhesie Kinderanästhesie.* Urban & Fischer, 2001, pp 200–203.

19. Carre P, Joly A, Cluzel Field B, et al: Axillary block in children: Single or multiple injection? Paediatr Anaesth 2000;10:35–39.

20. Chayen D, Nathan H, Chayen M: The psoas compartment block. Anesthesiology 1976;45:95–99.

21. Winnie AP, Ramamurthy S, Durrany Z, et al: Plexus blocks for lower extremity surgery. Anesth Rev 1974;1:11–16.

22. Dalens B, Tanguy A, Vanneuville G: Lumbar plexus block in children: A comparison of two procedures in 50 patients. Anesth Analg 1988;67:750–758.

23. Dalens B: Regional anesthesia in children. In *Miller's Anesthesia.* Churchill Livingstone, 2000.

24. Dadure C, Raux O, Gaudard P, et al: Continuous psoas compartment blocks after major orthopedic surgery in children: A prospec-

25. Kirchmair L, Enna B, Mitterschiffthaler G, et al: Lumbar plexus in children. A sonographic study and its relevance to pediatric regional anesthesia. Anesthesiology 2004;101:445–450.

26. Kirchmair L, Entner T, Kapral S, et al: Ultrasound guidance for the psoas compartment block: An imaging study. Anesth Analg 2002;94:706–710 (table of contents).

27. Leonhardt H: *Anatomie des Menschen Stuttgart.* Thieme, 1987.

28. Winnie A, Ramamurthy S, Durrani Z: The inguinal perivascular technique of lumbar plexus anesthesia. "The 3-in-1 block." Anesth Analg 1973;52:989–993.

29. Marhofer P, Nasel C, Sitzwohl C, et al: Magnetic resonance imaging of the distribution of local anesthetic during the three-in-one block. Anesth Analg 2000;90:119–124.

30. Marhofer P, Schrögendorfer K, Koinig H, et al: Ultrasonographic guidance improves sensory block and onset time of three-in-one blocks. Anesth Analg 1997;85:854–857.

31. Gielen M, Viering W: Lumbar plexus block for muscle biopsy in malignant hyperthermia patients. Amide local anaesthetics may be used safely. Acta Anaesthesiol Scand 1986;30:581–583.

32. Maccani RM, Wedel DJ, Melton A, et al: Femoral and lateral femoral cutaneous nerve block for muscle biopsies in children. Paediatr Anaesth 1995;5:223–227.

33. Rosen K, Broadman LM: Anaesthesia for diagnostic muscle biopsy in an infant with Pompe's disease. Can Anaesth Soc J 1986;33:790–794.

34. Johnson C: Continuous femoral nerve blockade for analgesia in children with femoral fractures. Anaesth Intensive Care 1994;22:281–283.

35. Tobias JD: Continuous femoral nerve block to provide analgesia following femus fracture in a paediatric ICU population. Anaesth Intensive Care 1994;22:616–618.

36. Rosenblatt R: Continuous femoral anesthesia for lower extremity surgery. Anesth Analg 1980;59:631–632.

37. McNicol L: Lower limb blocks for children: Lateral cutaneous and femoral nerve blocks for postoperative pain relief in paediatric patients. Anaesthesia 1986;41:27–31.

38. Bösenberg A: Lower limb nerve blocks in children using unsheathed needles and a nerve stimulator. Anaesthesia 1995;50:206–210.

39. Konrad C, Johr M: Blockade of the sciatic nerve in the popliteal fossa: A system for standardization in children. Anesth Analg 1998;87:1256–1258.

40. Tobias JD, Mencio GA: Popliteal fossa block for postoperative analgesia after foot surgery in infants and children. J Pediatr Orthop 1999;19:511–514.

41. Aizenberg VL, Tarasov VI, Ovchinnikov VI, et al: [Regional anesthesia of the sciatic nerve with anterior approach in children: New landmarks]. Anesteziol Reanimatol 2004;Jan-Feb:35–38.

42. Dalens B, Tanguy A, Vanneuville G: Sciatic nerve blocks in children: Comparison of the posterior, anterior, and lateral approaches in 180 pediatric patients. Anesth Analg 1990;70:131–137.

43. Gray AT, Collins AB, Schafhalter-Zoppoth I: Sciatic nerve block in a child: A sonographic approach. Anesth Analg 2003;97:1300–1302.

44. Schwemmer U, Markus CK, Greim CA, et al: Sonographic imaging of the sciatic nerve and its division in the popliteal fossa in children. Paediatr Anaesth 2004;14:1005–1008.

45. Jöhr M: *Periphere Blockaden Kinderanästhesie München.* Urban und Fischer Verlag, 2001, p 207.

46. McLeod DH, Wong DH, Vaghadia H, et al: Lateral popliteal sciatic nerve block compared with ankle block for analgesia following foot surgery. Can J Anaesth 1995;42:765–769.

47. McLeod DH, Wong DH, Claridge RJ, et al: Lateral popliteal sciatic nerve block compared with subcutaneous infiltration for analgesia following foot surgery. Can J Anaesth 1994;41:673–676.

48. Markham SJ, Tomlinson J, Hain WR: Ilioinguinal nerve block in children. A comparison with caudal block for intra and postoperative analgesia. Anaesthesia 1986;41:1098–1103.

tive computed tomographic scan and clinical studies. Anesth Analg 2004;98:623–628.

49. Dalens B: Regional Anesthetic Techniques. In Bissonnette B DB, BJ Dalens (eds): *Pediatric Anesthesia—Principles and Practice*. McGraw-Hill, 2002, pp 563–565.

50. Lim SL, Ng Sb A, Tan GM: Ilioinguinal and iliohypogastric nerve block revisited: Single shot versus double shot technique for hernia repair in children. Paediatr Anaesth 2002;12:255–260.

51. Johr M, Sossai R: Colonic puncture during ilioinguinal nerve block in a child. Anesth Analg 1999;88:1051–1052.

52. Amory C, Mariscal A, Guyot E, et al: Is ilioinguinal/iliohypogastric nerve block always totally safe in children? Paediatr Anaesth 2003;13:164–166.

53. Vaisman J: Pelvic hematoma after an ilioinguinal nerve block for orchialgia. Anesth Analg 2001;92:1048–1049.

54. Jamieson RW, Swigart LL, Anson BJ: Points of parietal perforation of the ilioinguinal and iliohypogastric nerves in relation to optimal sites for local anaesthesia. Q Bull Northwest Univ Med Sch 1952;26:22–26.

55. Schoor AN, Boon JM, Bosenberg AT, et al: Anatomical considerations of the pediatric ilioinguinal/iliohypogastric nerve block. Paediatr Anaesth 2005;15:371–377.

56. Smith T, Moratin P, Wulf H: Smaller children have greater bupivacaine plasma concentrations after ilioinguinal block. Br J Anaesth 1996;76:452–455.

57. Notaras MJ: Transient femoral nerve palsy complicating preoperative ilioinguinal nerve blockade inguinal for herniorrhaphy. Br J Surg 1995;82:854.

Regional Anesthesia for Obstetric & Gynecologic Surgery

53

Obstetric Regional Anesthesia

Philippe Gautier, MD • Edward Jew, MD • Bonnie Deschner, MD • Alan C. Santos, MD

INTRODUCTION

Most women experience moderate to severe pain during labor and delivery, often requiring some form of pharmacologic analgesia.[1] The lack of proper psychological preparation combined with fear and anxiety can greatly enhance the patient's sensitivity to pain and further add to the discomfort during labor and delivery. However, skillfully conducted obstetric analgesia, in addition to relieving pain and anxiety, may benefit the mother in many other ways. This chapter focuses on management of an obstetric patient with primary focus on regional anesthesia techniques.

Physiologic Changes of Pregnancy

Pregnancy results in significant changes affecting most maternal organ systems (Table 53–1). These changes are initiated by hormones secreted by the corpus luteum and the placenta. Such changes have important implications for the anesthesiologist caring for the pregnant patient. This chapter reviews the most relevant physiologic changes of pregnancy and discusses the approach to obstetric management using regional anesthesia.

Changes in the Cardiovascular System

Oxygen consumption increases during pregnancy, requiring the maternal cardiovascular system to meet the increasing metabolic demands of a growing fetus. The end result of these changes is an increase in heart rate (15–25%) and cardiac output (up to 50%) compared with values before pregnancy. In addition, lower vascular resistance is found in the uterine, renal, and other vascular beds. These changes result in a lower arterial blood pressure because of a decrease in peripheral resistance, which exceeds the increase in cardiac output. Decreased vascular resistance is mostly due to the secretion of estrogens, progesterone, and prostacyclin.[2] Particularly significant increase in cardiac output occurs during labor and in the immediate postpartum period owing to added blood volume from the contracted uterus.

Clinical Pearls

Cardiovascular changes and pitfalls in advanced pregnancy are:

- Increase in heart rate (15–25%) and cardiac output (up to 50%).
- Decrease in vascular resistance in the uterine, renal, and other vascular beds.
- Compression of the lower aorta in the supine position may further decrease uteroplacental perfusion and result in fetal asphyxia.
- For the above reason, significant hypotension is more likely to occur in the pregnant than in the nonpregnant woman having regional anesthesia, necessitating uterine displacement or lateral pelvic tilt maneuvers, intravascular preloading, and ready availability of vasopressors.

From the second trimester, aortocaval compression by the enlarged uterus becomes progressively more important, reaching its maximum effect at 36–38 weeks, after which it may decrease as the fetal head descends into the pelvis.[3] Cardiac output may decrease when patients are in the supine position but not in the lateral decubitus position. Venous occlusion by the growing fetus causes supine hypotensive syndrome in 10% of pregnant women and manifests as maternal tachycardia, arterial hypotension, faintness, and pallor.[4] Compression of the lower aorta in this position may further decrease uteroplacental perfusion and result in fetal asphyxia. Uterine displacement or lateral pelvic tilt should be applied routinely during anesthetic management of the pregnant patient.

Changes in the electrocardiogram are common in late pregnancy and consist of left axis deviation (caused by the upward displacement of the heart by the gravid uterus). There is also a tendency toward premature atrial contractions, sinus tachycardia, and paroxysmal supraventricular tachycardia.

Changes in the Respiratory System

Minute ventilation increases from the beginning of pregnancy to a maximum of 50% above normal by term.[5] This

Table 53–1.

Summary of Physiologic Changes of Pregnancy at Term

Variable	Change	Amount
Total blood volume	Increase	25–40%
Plasma volume	Increase	40–50%
Fibrinogen	Increase	50%
Serum cholinesterase activity	Decrease	20–30%
Cardiac output	Increase	30–50%
Minute ventilation	Increase	50%
Alveolar ventilation	Increase	70%
Functional residual capacity	Decrease	20%
Oxygen consumption	Increase	20%
Arterial carbon dioxide tension	Decrease	10 mm Hg
Arterial oxygen tension	Increase	10 mm Hg
Minimum alveolar concentration	Decrease	32–40%

is mostly a result of a 40% increase in tidal volume and a small increase in respiratory rate. Dead space does not change significantly during pregnancy; thus, alveolar ventilation is increased by 70% at term. After delivery, as blood progesterone levels decline, ventilation returns to normal within 1–3 weeks.[6]

Elevation of the diaphragm occurs with increase in the size of the uterus. Expiratory reserve volume, residual volume, and functional residual capacity decrease by the third semester of pregnancy.[5] However, because there is also an increase in inspiratory reserve volume, total lung capacity remains unchanged. A decreased functional residual capacity is typically asymptomatic in healthy parturients. Those with preexisting alterations in closing volume as a result of smoking, obesity, scoliosis, or other pulmonary disease may experience early airway closure with advancing pregnancy, leading to hypoxemia. The Trendelenburg and supine positions also exacerbate the abnormal relationship between closing volume and functional residual capacity. The residual volume and functional residual capacity return to normal shortly after delivery.

Pregnant women often have difficulty with nasal breathing. Friability of the mucous membranes during pregnancy can cause severe bleeding, especially on airway instrumentation. These changes are caused by increase in extracellular fluid and vascular engorgement. It may also be difficult to perform a laryngoscopy in obese, short-necked parturients with enlarged breasts. Use of a short-handled laryngoscope has proved helpful.

Clinical Pearls

- Airway edema may be particularly severe in pregnant women and those with preeclampsia, those in the Trendelenburg position for prolonged periods, and those with concurrent use of tocolytic agents.

Metabolic Changes

Oxygen consumption increases during early pregnancy, with an overall increase of 20% by term. Regardless, increased alveolar ventilation occurring during pregnancy actually leads to a reduction in the partial pressure of carbon dioxide in arterial blood ($Paco_2$) to 32 mm Hg and an increase in the partial pressure of oxygen in arterial blood (Pao_2) to 106 mm Hg. The plasma buffer base decreases from 47 to 42 mEq; consequently, the pH remains practically unchanged. The maternal uptake and elimination of inhalational anesthetics are enhanced because of the increased alveolar ventilation and decreased FRC. However, the decreased functional residual capacity and increased metabolic rate predispose the mother to development of hypoxemia during periods of apnea/hypoventilation.[7]

Changes in the Gastrointestinal System

Enhanced progesterone production causes decreased gastrointestinal motility and slower absorption of food. Gastric secretions are more acidic, lower esophageal sphincter one is decreased, and a delay in gastric emptying can be demonstrated by the end of the first trimester.[8] Uterine growth leads to upward displacement and rotation of the stomach, with increased pressure and a further delay in gastric emptying. By the 34th week, evacuation of a watery meal may be prolonged by 60%.[9] Pain, anxiety, and administration of opioids (systemic or neuraxial) and belladonna alkaloids may further exacerbate this delay.

The risk of regurgitation on induction of general anesthesia depends, in part, on the gradient between the lower esophageal sphincter and intragastric pressures. In parturients with "heartburn," the lower esophageal sphincter tone is greatly reduced.[10] The efficacy of prophylactic nonparticulate antacids is diminished by inadequate mixing with gastric contents, improper timing of administration, and the tendency for antacids to increase gastric volume. Administration of histamine (H_2)-receptor antagonists, such as cimetidine and ranitidine, requires careful timing. A good case can be made for the administration of IV metoclopramide before elective cesarean section delivery. This dopamine antagonist hastens gastric emptying and increases resting lower esophageal sphincter tone in both nonpregnant and pregnant women.[11] However, conflicting reports have appeared on its efficacy and on the frequency of side effects, such as extrapyramidal reactions and transient neurologic dysfunction.[12,13] No routine prophylactic regimen can be recommended with certainty.

Endocrine Changes Influencing Plasma Volume, Blood Composition, & Glucose Metabolism

Plasma volume and total blood volume begin to increase in early gestation, resulting in an increase of 40–50% and 25–40% respectively, at term. These changes are due to an increased mineralocorticoid activity during pregnancy, which results in sodium retention and increased body water content.[14] The relatively smaller increase in red blood cell volume (20%) accounts for a relative reduction in hemoglobin (to 11–12 g/L and hematocrit (to 35%); the platelet count, however, remains unchanged. Plasma fibrinogen concentrations increase during normal pregnancy by approximately 50%, whereas clotting factor activity is variable.[15] Serum cholinesterase activity declines to a level of 20% below normal by term and reaches a nadir in the puerperium. The net effects of these changes in the serum cholinesterase is of negligible relevance to the metabolism of clinically used doses of succinylcholine or ester-type local anesthetics (2-choloroprocaine).[16,17] The albumin–globulin ratio declines because of the relatively greater reduction in albumin concentration. A decrease in serum protein concentration may be clinically significant in that the free fractions of protein-bound drugs can be expected to increase.

Human placental lactogen and cortisol increase the tendency to hyperglycemia and ketosis, which may exacerbate preexisting diabetes mellitus. The patient's ability to handle a glucose load is decreased, and the transplacental passage of glucose may stimulate fetal secretion of insulin, leading in turn to neonatal hypoglycemia in the immediate postpartum period.[18]

Altered Drug Responses in Pregnancy

Pregnancy results in a progesterone-mediated increase in neural sensitivity to local anesthetics.[19] Lower doses of local anesthetic are needed per dermatomal segment of epidural or spinal block. This has been attributed to an increased spread of local anesthetic in the epidural and subarachnoid spaces as a result of epidural venous engorgement and enhanced sensitivity to local anesthetic block due to progesterone. The minimum alveolar concentration for inhalational agents is decreased by 8–12 weeks of gestation and may be related to an increase in progesterone levels.[20]

Clinical Pearls

- During pregnancy, there is a progesterone-mediated increase in neural sensitivity to local anesthetics.
- Doses of local anesthetic need to be lowered per dermatomal segment of epidural or spinal block.

PLACENTAL TRANSFER OF LOCAL ANESTHETICS

Local anesthetics readily cross the placenta by simple diffusion. Several factors influence the placental transfer of drugs, including the physicochemical characteristics of the drug itself, maternal drug concentrations in the plasma, properties of the placenta, and hemodynamic events within the fetomaternal unit.

Highly lipid-soluble drugs, such as local anesthetics, cross biologic membranes more readily, and the degree of ionization is important because the nonionized moiety of a drug is more lipophilic than the ionized drug. Local anesthetics are weak bases, with a relatively low degree of ionization and considerable lipid solubility. The relative concentrations of drug existing in the nonionized and ionized forms can be estimated from the Henderson-Hasselbalch equation:

$$pH = pKa + \log (base)/(cation) \qquad (53.1)$$

The ratio of base to cation becomes particularly important with local anesthetics because the nonionized form penetrates tissue barriers, whereas the ionized form is pharmacologically active in blocking nerve conduction. The pKa is the pH at which the concentrations of free base and cation

are equal. For the amide local anesthetics, the pKa values (7.7–8.1) are sufficiently close to physiologic pH so that changes in maternal or fetal biochemical status may significantly alter the proportion of ionized and nonionized drug (Figure 53–1). At steady state, the concentrations of nonionized local anesthetics in the fetal and maternal plasma are equal. With fetal acidosis, there is a greater tendency for drug to exist in the ionized form, which cannot diffuse back across the placenta. This causes a larger total amount of local anesthetic to accumulate in the fetal plasma and tissues. This is called **ion trapping.**[21]

Clinical Pearl

- Prolonged administration of highly protein-bound drugs (eg, bupivacaine) may lead to substantial fetal accumulation of the drugs.

The effects of maternal plasma protein binding on the rate and amount of local anesthetic accumulating in the fetus are inadequately understood. Animal studies have shown that the transfer rate is slower for drugs that are extensively bound to maternal plasma proteins such as bupivacaine.[22,23] However, with prolonged administration of highly protein-bound drugs such as bupivacaine, substantial accumulation of drug can occur in the fetus.[24]

The concentration gradient of free drug between the maternal and fetal blood is a significant factor. On the maternal side, the dose administered, the mode and site of administration, and the use of vasoconstrictors can influence fetal exposure. The rates of distribution, metabolism, and excretion of the drug, which may vary, are equally important. Higher doses result in higher maternal blood concentrations. The absorption rate can vary with the site of injection. For instance, an IV bolus results in the highest blood concentrations. It was believed that intrathecal administration resulted in negligible plasma concentrations of local anesthetics. However, we now know that spinal anesthesia induced with 75 mg lidocaine results in maternal plasma concentrations that are similar to those reported by others after epidural anesthesia.[25] Furthermore, significant levels of the drug can be found in the umbilical vein at birth.

Repeated administration can result in high maternal blood concentrations, depending on the dose and frequency of reinjection, in addition to the kinetic characteristics of the drug. The half-life of amide local anesthetic agents is relatively long, so that repeated injection may lead to accumulation in the maternal plasma[26] (Figure 53–2). In contrast, 2-chloroprocaine, an ester local anesthetic, undergoes rapid enzymatic hydrolysis in the presence of pseudocholinesterase. After epidural injection, the mean half-life in the mother is approximately 3 minutes; after reinjection, 2-chloroprocaine can be detected in the maternal plasma for only 5–10 minutes, and no accumulation of this drug has occurred.[27]

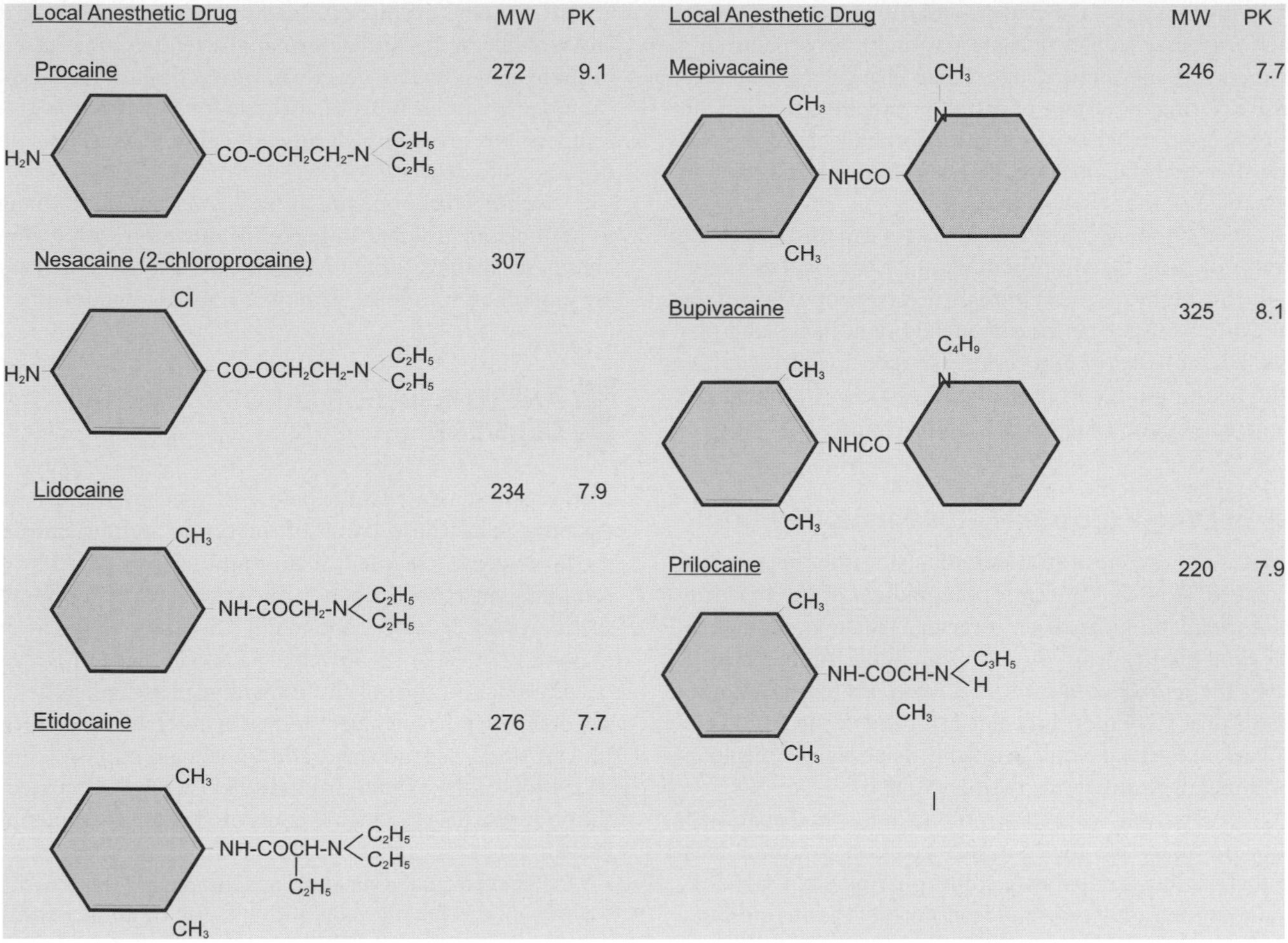

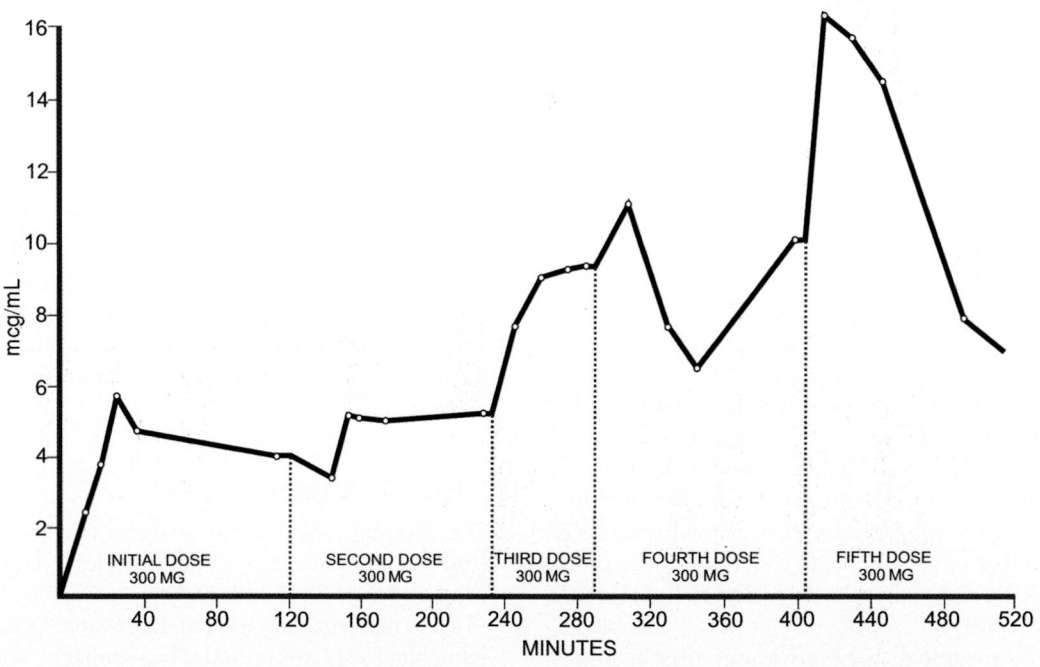

Local Anesthetic Drug	MW	PK
Procaine	272	9.1
Nesacaine (2-chloroprocaine)	307	
Lidocaine	234	7.9
Etidocaine	276	7.7
Mepivacaine	246	7.7
Bupivacaine	325	8.1
Prilocaine	220	7.9

Figure 53–1. Chemical structures of local anesthetics.

Figure 53–2. Increased maternal blood concentration after repeated doses of mepivacaine.

Pregnancy is associated with physiologic changes, which also may influence maternal pharmacokinetics and the action of anesthetic drugs. These changes may be progressive during the course of gestation and are often difficult to predict. Nonetheless, the elimination half-life of bupivacaine after epidural injection has been shown to be similar in pregnant and nonpregnant women.[28]

Fetal regional blood flow changes can also affect the amount of drug taken up by individual organs. For example, during asphyxia and acidosis, a greater proportion of the fetal cardiac output perfuses the fetal brain, heart, and placenta. Infusion of lidocaine resulted in increased drug uptake in the heart, brain, and liver of asphyxiated baboon fetuses compared with nonasphyxiated control fetuses.[29]

Risk of Drug Exposure: Fetus versus Newborn

The fetus can excrete local anesthetics back into the maternal circulation after the concentration gradient of the free drug across the placenta has been reversed. This may occur even if the total plasma drug concentration in the mother exceeds that in the fetus, because there is lower protein binding in fetal plasma.[23] 2-Chloroprocaine is the only drug that is metabolized in the fetal blood so quickly that even with acidosis, substantial exposure in the fetus is avoided.[27]

Term as well as preterm infants have the hepatic enzymes necessary for the biotransformation of amide local anesthetics. In a comparative study, pharmacokinetics of lidocaine among adult ewes and fetal/neonatal lambs indicated that the metabolic clearance in the newborn was similar to, and renal clearance greater than, that in the adult.[30] However, the half-life was longer in the newborn related to a greater volume of distribution and tissue uptake, so that at any given moment the neonate's liver and kidneys are exposed to a smaller fraction of lidocaine accumulated in the body. Similar results have been reported in another study involving lidocaine administration to human infants in a neonatal intensive care unit.[31]

Neonatal depression occurs at blood concentrations of mepivacaine or lidocaine that are approximately 50% less than those producing systemic toxicity in the adult. However, infants accidentally injected in utero with mepivacaine (intended for maternal caudal anesthesia) stopped convulsing when the mepivacaine level decreased below the threshold for convulsions in the adult.[32] The relative central nervous toxicity and cardiorespiratory toxicity of local anesthetics have been studied in sheep.[33] The doses required to produce toxicity in the fetus and newborn lamb were greater than those required in the ewe. In the fetus, this difference was attributed to placental clearance of drug into the mother and better maintenance of blood gas tensions during convulsions, whereas in the newborn lamb, a larger volume of distribution was probably responsible for the higher doses needed to induce toxic effects.

It has been suggested that bupivacaine may be implicated as a possible cause of neonatal jaundice because its high affinity for fetal erythrocyte membranes resulting in a decrease in filterability and deformability renders subjects more prone to hemolysis. However, a more recent study has failed to show demonstrable bilirubin production in newborns whose mothers were given bupivacaine for epidural anesthesia during labor and delivery.[34]

Neurobehavioral studies have revealed subtle changes in newborn neurologic and adaptive function with regional anesthesia. In the case of most anesthetic agents, these changes are minor and transient, lasting for only 24–48 hours.[35]

ANESTHESIA FOR LABOR & VAGINAL DELIVERY

In the first stage of labor, pain is caused by uterine contractions related to dilation of the cervix and distention of the lower uterine segment. Pain impulses are carried in visceral afferent type C fibers, which accompany the sympathetic nerves. In early labor, only the lower thoracic dermatomes (T11-12) are affected. However, with progressive cervical dilation during the transition phase, adjacent dermatomes may be involved and pain referred from T10 to LI. During the second stage, additional pain impulses due to distention of the vaginal vault and perineum are carried in the pudendal nerve, which is composed of lower sacral fibers (S2-4).

Regional analgesia may benefit the mother in other ways beyond relieving pain and anxiety. In animal studies, pain may cause maternal hypertension and reduced uterine blood flow.[36] Epidural analgesia blunts the increases in maternal cardiac output, heart rate, and blood pressure that occur with painful uterine contractions and "bearing-down" efforts.[37] By reducing maternal secretion of catecholamines, epidural analgesia may convert a previously dysfunctional labor pattern to a normal one.[38] Regional analgesia can benefit the fetus by eliminating maternal hyperventilation with pain, which often leads to a reduced fetal arterial oxygen tension owing to a leftward shift of the maternal oxygen–hemoglobin dissociation curve.[39]

The most frequently chosen methods for relieving the pain of parturition are psychoprophylaxis, systemic medication, and regional analgesia. Inhalational analgesia, conventional spinal analgesia, and paracervical blockade are less commonly used. General anesthesia is rarely necessary but may be indicated for uterine relaxation in some complicated deliveries.

Systemic Analgesia

The advantages of systemic analgesics include ease of administration and patient acceptability. However, the drug, dose, time, and method of administration must be chosen carefully to avoid maternal or neonatal depression. Drugs used for systemic analgesia are opioids, tranquilizers, and occasionally ketamine.

Systemic Opioids

In the past, meperidine was the most commonly used systemic analgesic to ameliorate pain during the first stage of labor. It can be administered by IV injection (effective analgesia in 5–10 minutes) or intramuscularly (peak effect in 40–50 minutes). It was also commonly used for postoperative pain in the general population. But with the popularity of its administration, disturbing side effects began to emerge. One of the most serious side effects was the occurrence of seizures both from the primary drug effect and from its metabolite, normeperidine. In the pregnant patient at risk for seizures—that is, with pregnancy-induced hypertension or preeclampsia—confusing the picture by the administration of a drug known to cause seizures complicates patient care.[40,41] Other side effects are nausea and vomiting, dose-related depression of ventilation, orthostatic hypotension, the potential for neonatal depression, and euphoria out of proportion to the analgesic effect, leading to misuse of the drug.[42] Meperidine may also cause transient alterations of the fetal heart rate, such as decreased beat-to-beat variability and tachycardia. Among other factors, the risk of neonatal depression is related to the interval from the last drug injection to delivery.[43] The placental transfer of an active metabolite, normeperidine, which has a long elimination half-life in the neonate (62 hours), has also been implicated in contributing to neonatal depression and subtle neonatal neurobehavioral dysfunction. Consequently, the use of meperidine has fallen out of favor as an analgesic for labor.

Experience with the newer synthetic opioids, such as fentanyl and alfentanil, has been limited. Although they are potent, their use during labor is restricted by their short duration of action. For example, a single IV injection of fentanyl, up to 1 mcg/kg, results in prompt pain relief without severe neonatal depression.[44] These drugs offer an advantage when analgesia of rapid onset but short duration is necessary (eg, with forceps application). For more prolonged analgesia, fentanyl can be administered with patient-controlled delivery devices.[45] More commonly, fentanyl (15–25 mcg) and sufentanil (5–10 mcg) have been used with local anesthetics in an initial spinal dose with a local anesthetic during the placement of a continuous spinal–epidural for labor with excellent relief of pain.[46,47]

Remifentanil is an opioid that is rapidly metabolized by serum and tissue cholinesterases, and consequently, has a short (3-minute), context-sensitive half-time.[48] When used in bolus dosing (0.3–0.8 mcg/kg per bolus), remifentanil has been found to have an acceptable level of maternal side effects and minimal effect on the neonate. Remifentanil crosses the placenta and appears to be either rapidly metabolized or redistributed in the neonate.[49] In one study, Apgar and neurobehavioral scores were good in neonates whose mothers were given an intravenous infusion of remifentanil, 0.1 mcg-kg/min during cesarean section delivery under epidural anesthesia.[50] When administered by patient-controlled analgesia, remifentanil has been found to provide better pain relief, equivalent hemodynamic stability, less sedation, and a

lesser degree of oxygen desaturation when compared with meperidine.[49,51] In countries outside the United States, intermittent nitrous oxide has been used for labor analgesia. When comparing remifentanil with nitrous oxide, remifentanil was found to provide better pain relief with fewer side effects.[52]

Opioid agonists–antagonists, such as butorphanol and nalbuphine, have also been used for obstetric analgesia. These drugs have the proposed benefits of a lower incidence of nausea, vomiting, and dysphoria, as well as a "ceiling effect" on depression of ventilation.[53] Butorphanol is probably the most popular; unlike meperidine, it is biotransformed into inactive metabolites and has a ceiling effect on depression of ventilation in doses exceeding 2 mg. A potential disadvantage is a high incidence of maternal sedation. The recommended dose is 1–2 mg by IV or IM injection. Nalbuphine 10 mg IV or IM is an alternative to butorphanol.

Naloxone, a pure opioid antagonist, should not be administered to the mother shortly before delivery to prevent neonatal ventilatory depression because it reverses maternal analgesia at a time when it is most needed. In some instances, naloxone has been reported to cause maternal pulmonary edema and even cardiac arrest. If necessary, the drug should be given directly to the newborn IM (0.1 mg/kg.

Ketamine

Ketamine is a potent analgesic. However, it may also induce unacceptable amnesia that may interfere with the mother's recollection of the birth. Nonetheless, ketamine is a useful adjuvant to incomplete regional analgesia during vaginal delivery or for obstetric manipulations. In low doses (0.2–0.4 mg/kg), ketamine provides adequate analgesia without causing neonatal depression.

Regional Analgesia Techniques

Regional techniques provide excellent analgesia with minimal depressant effects in mother and fetus. The techniques most commonly used for labor anesthesia include central neuraxial blocks (spinal, epidural, and combined spinal/epidural), paracervical, and pudendal blocks, and, less frequently, lumbar sympathetic blocks. Hypotension resulting from sympathectomy is the most common complication that occurs with central neuraxial blockade. Therefore, maternal blood pressure must be monitored at regular intervals, typically every 2–5 minutes for approximately 15–20 minutes after the initiation of the block and at routine intervals thereafter. Regional analgesia may be contraindicated in the presence of severe coagulopathy, acute hypovolemia, or infection at the site of needle insertion. Chorioamnionitis without sepsis, is not a contraindication to central neuraxial blockade.

Epidural Analgesia

Effective analgesia for the first stage of labor is achieved by blocking the T10-Ll dermatomes with a low concentrations

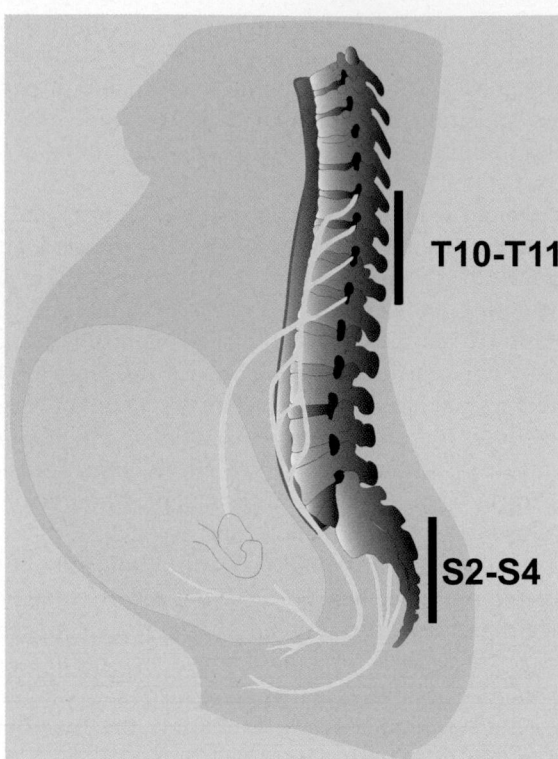

Figure 53–3. Pain pathways in a parturient.

T10-T11

S2-S4

of local anesthetic, often in combination with a lipid-soluble opioid. For the second stage of labor and delivery, because of pain due to vaginal distention and perineal pressure, the block should be extended to include the pudendal segments, S2-4 (Figures 53–3 and 53–4).

There has been concern that early initiation of epidural analgesia during the latent phase of labor (2–4 cm cervical dilation) may result in prolongation of the first stage of labor and a higher incidence of dystocia and cesarean section delivery, particularly in nulliparous women.[54–57] Generally speaking, the first stage of labor is not prolonged by epidural analgesia, provided that aortocaval compression is avoided.[54–56,58,59] Chestnut et al.[58,59] demonstrated that the incidence of cesarean section delivery was no different in nulliparous women having epidural analgesia initiated during the latent phase (at 4 cm dilation) compared with women whose analgesia was initiated during the active phase. Others have shown that epidural analgesia is not associated with an increased incidence of cesarean section delivery compared with IV patient-controlled analgesia in nulliparous women.[55,56] However, a prolongation of the second stage of labor has been reported in nulliparous women, possibly owing to a decrease in expulsive forces or malposition of the vertex.[54,59] Thus, with use of epidural analgesia, the American College of Obstetricians and Gynecologists (ACOG) has defined an abnormally prolonged second stage of labor as longer than 3 hours in nulliparous and 2 hours in multiparous women.[60] A longer second stage of labor may be minimized by the use of an ultra-dilute local anesthetic solution in combination with opioid.[61] Long-acting amides such as bupivacaine, ropiva-

caine, and levobupivacaine are most frequently used because they produce excellent sensory analgesia while sparing motor function, particularly at the low concentrations used for epidural analgesia.

Clinical Pearls

- Analgesia during the **first stage** of labor is achieved by blocking the T10-Ll dermatomes anesthetic (see Figure 53–3).
- Analgesia for the **second stage** of labor and delivery requires the block of the S2-4 segments because of pain due to vaginal distention and perineal pressure.

Analgesia for the first stage of labor may be achieved with 5–10 mL of bupivacaine, ropivacaine, or levobupivacaine (0.125–0.25%) followed by a continuous infusion (8–12 mL/h) of 0.0625% bupivacaine or levobupivacaine, or 0.1% ropivacaine. Fentanyl 1–2 mcg/mL or sufentanil 0.3–0.5 mcg/mL may be added. During the actual delivery, the perineum may be blocked with 10 mL of 0.5% bupivacaine, 1% lidocaine, or, if a rapid effect is required, 2% chloroprocaine in the semirecumbent position.

There is controversy regarding the need for a test dose when using a dilute solution of local anesthetic.[62,63] Catheter aspiration alone is not always diagnostic. For that reason, some authors believe that a test dose should be administered to improve detection of an intrathecally or intravascularly placed epidural catheter. If injected into a blood vessel, 15 mcg epinephrine results in a change in heart rate of 20–30 bpm with a slight increase in blood pressure within 30 seconds of administration. The duration is approximately 30 seconds. The anesthesiologist should observe the tachometer during the first minute after injection to determine whether an accidental intravascular injection has occurred. Other subtle signs of intravascular injection may include a feeling of apprehension, unease, or palpitations. It is important to fractionate the total dose of local anesthetic and observe the patient at 1-minute intervals.

Patient-controlled epidural analgesia is a safe and effective alternative to conventional bolus or infusion techniques.[64] Maternal acceptance is excellent, and demands on anesthesia manpower may be reduced. Initial analgesia is achieved with bolus doses of local anesthetic. Once the mother is comfortable, patient-controlled epidural analgesia may then be started with a maintenance infusion (4–8 mL/h) of local anesthetic (bupivacaine, levobupivacaine, ropivacaine 0.0625–0.125%) with or without opioid (fentanyl 1–2 mcg/mL; sufentanil 0.3–0.5 mcg/mL). The machine may be programmed to administer an epidural demand bolus of 4 mL with a lockout period of 10 minutes between doses.[64] The caudal rather than the lumbar approach may result in a faster onset of perineal analgesia and therefore may be preferable to the lumbar epidural approach when an imminent

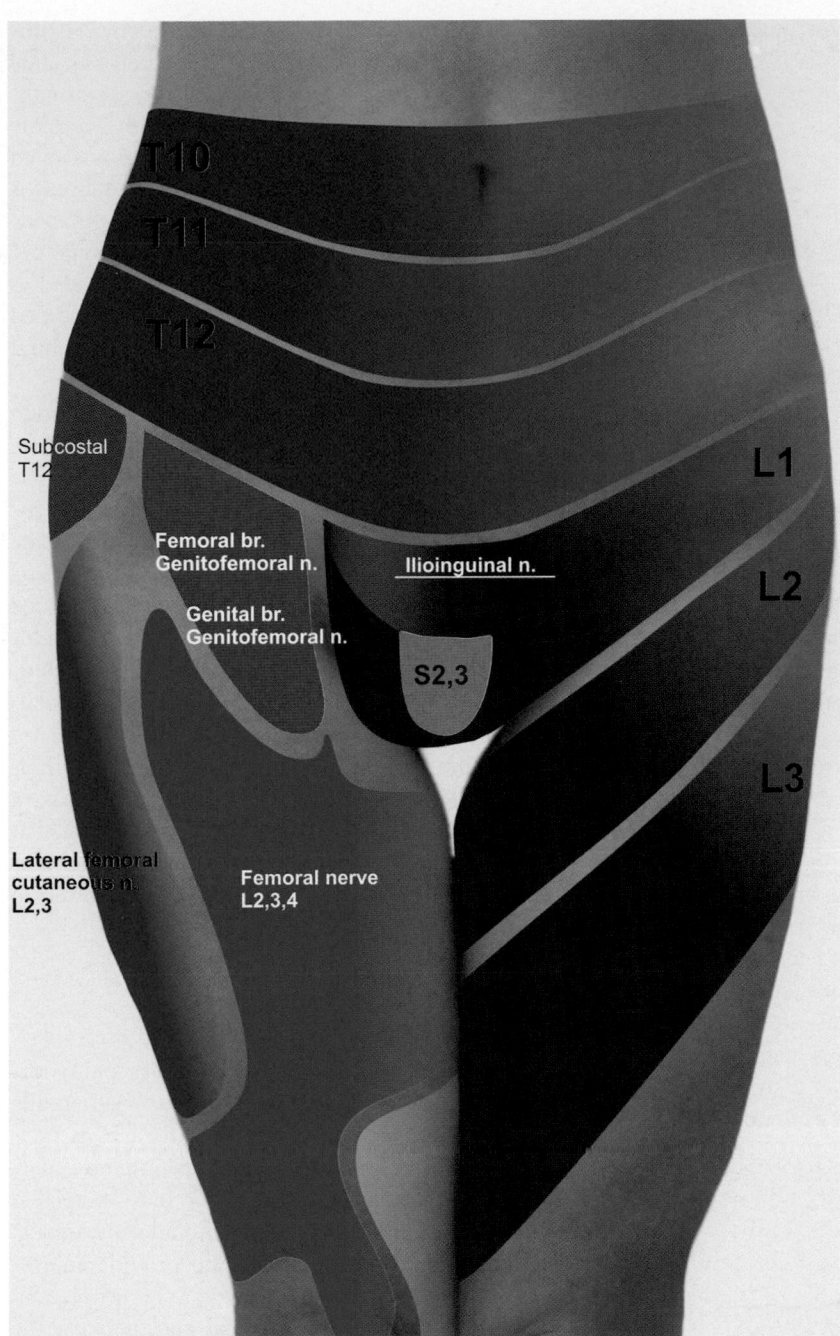

Figure 53–4. Dermatomal level of the lower abdomen, perineal area, hip, and thighs.

vaginal delivery is anticipated. However, caudal analgesia is no longer popular because of occasionally painful needle placement, a high failure rate, potential contamination at the injection site, and risks of accidental fetal injection. Before caudal injection, a digital rectal examination must be performed to exclude needle placement in the fetal presenting part. Low spinal "saddle block" has virtually eliminated the need for caudal anesthesia in modern practice.

Spinal Analgesia

A single intrathecal injection for labor analgesia has the benefits of a reliable and rapid onset of neural blockade.

However, repeated intrathecal injections may be required for a long labor, thus increasing the risk of postdural puncture headache. In addition, motor block may be uncomfortable for some women and may prolong the second stage of labor.

Microcatheters were introduced for continuous spinal anesthesia in the 1980s. They were subsequently withdrawn when found to be associated with neurologic deficits, possibly related to maldistribution of local anesthetic in the cauda equina region.[65] Fortunately, in a recent multi-institutional study, no cases of neurologic symptoms occurred after the use of 28-gauge microcatheters for continuous spinal analgesia in laboring women.[66] Spinal anesthesia is also a safe and effective alternative to general anesthesia for instrumental delivery.

Combined Spinal–Epidural Analgesia

Combined spinal–epidural analgesia is an ideal analgesic technique for use during labor. It combines the rapid, reliable onset of profound analgesia resulting from spinal injection with the flexibility and longer duration of epidural techniques.

Technique

After identification of the epidural space using a conventional (or specialized) epidural needle, a longer (127-mm), pencil-point spinal needle is advanced into the subarachnoid space through the epidural needle (more detail on this technique can be found in Chapter 16). After intrathecal injection, the spinal needle is removed and an epidural catheter inserted. Intrathecal injection of fentanyl 10–25 mcg or sufentanil 2.5–5 mcg, alone or in combination with 1 mL of isobaric bupivacaine 0.25%, produces profound analgesia lasting for 60–120 minutes with minimal motor block.[67] Opioid alone may provide sufficient relief for the early latent phase, but almost always the addition of bupivacaine is necessary for satisfactory analgesia during advanced labor. An epidural infusion of bupivacaine 0.03–0.0625% with opioid may be started within 10 minutes of spinal injection. Alternatively, the epidural component may be activated when necessary. Women with hemodynamic stability and preserved motor function who do not require continuous fetal monitoring may ambulate with assistance.[68,69] Before ambulation, women should be observed for 30 minutes after intrathecal or epidural drug administration to assess maternal and fetal well-being. A recent study indicated that early administration of combined spinal–epidural analgesia to nulliparous women did not increase the cesarean section delivery rate.[70]

Clinical Pearls

- Intrathecal injection of fentanyl 10–25 mcg or sufentanil 5–10 mcg alone or more commonly in combination with 1 mL isobaric bupivacaine 0.25% produces profound analgesia lasting for 90–120 minutes with minimal motor block.

The most common side effects of intrathecal opioids are pruritus, nausea, vomiting, and urinary retention. Rostral spread resulting in delayed respiratory depression is rare with fentanyl and sufentanil and usually occurs within 30 minutes of injection.[71] Transient nonreassuring fetal heart rate patterns may occur because of uterine hyperstimulation, presumably as a result of a rapid decrease in maternal catecholamines or because of hypotension after sympatholysis.[72] A preliminary study by O'Gorman et al.[73] suggests that fetal bradycardia may occur in the absence of uterine hyperstimulation or hypotension and is unrelated to uteroplacental insufficiency. The incidence of fetal heart rate abnormalities may be greater in multiparous woman with a rapidly progressing, painful labor.[74] Most studies have demonstrated that the incidence of emergency cesarean section delivery is no greater with combined spinal–epidural analgesia than after conventional epidural analgesia.[75,76] Postdural puncture headache is always a risk after intrathecal injection. However, the incidence of headache is no greater with combined spinal–epidural analgesia compared with standard epidural analgesia.[77]

Unintentional intrathecal catheter placement through the dural puncture site is also rare after use of a 26-gauge spinal needle for combined spinal–epidural analgesia. The potential exists for epidurally administered drug to leak intrathecally through the dural puncture, particularly if large volumes of drug are rapidly injected. In fact, epidural drug requirements are approximately 30% less with combined spinal–epidural analgesia than with standard lumbar epidural techniques for cesarean section delivery.[78] Some clinicians do not advocate the combined spinal–epidural analgesia technique for labor because of the concern for an "unproven" epidural catheter that may need to be used emergently for cesarean section delivery. The patient may have a partial block insufficient for surgery with an epidural that may or may not work. An algorithm for patient management in the event of an incomplete spinal can be found in Figure 53–5.

Paracervical Block

Although paracervical block effectively relieves pain during the first stage of labor, it is now rarely used in the United States because of its association with a high incidence of fetal asphyxia and poor neonatal outcome, particularly with the use of bupivacaine. This may be related to uterine artery constriction or increased uterine tone.[79] Paracervical block is a useful technique to provide analgesia for uterine curettage. The technique is very simple and involves a submucosal injection of local anesthetic at the vaginal fornix near the neural fibers innervating the uterus (Figure 53–6).

Paravertebral Lumbar Sympathetic Block

Paravertebral lumbar sympathetic block is a reasonable alternative when contraindications exist to central neuraxial techniques. Lumbar sympathetic block interrupts the painful transmission of cervical and uterine impulses during the first stage of labor.[80] Although there is less risk of fetal bradycardia with lumbar sympathetic block compared with paracervical blockade, technical difficulties associated with the performance of the block and risks of intravascular injection have hampered its routine use. Hypotension may also occur with lumbar sympathetic blocks.

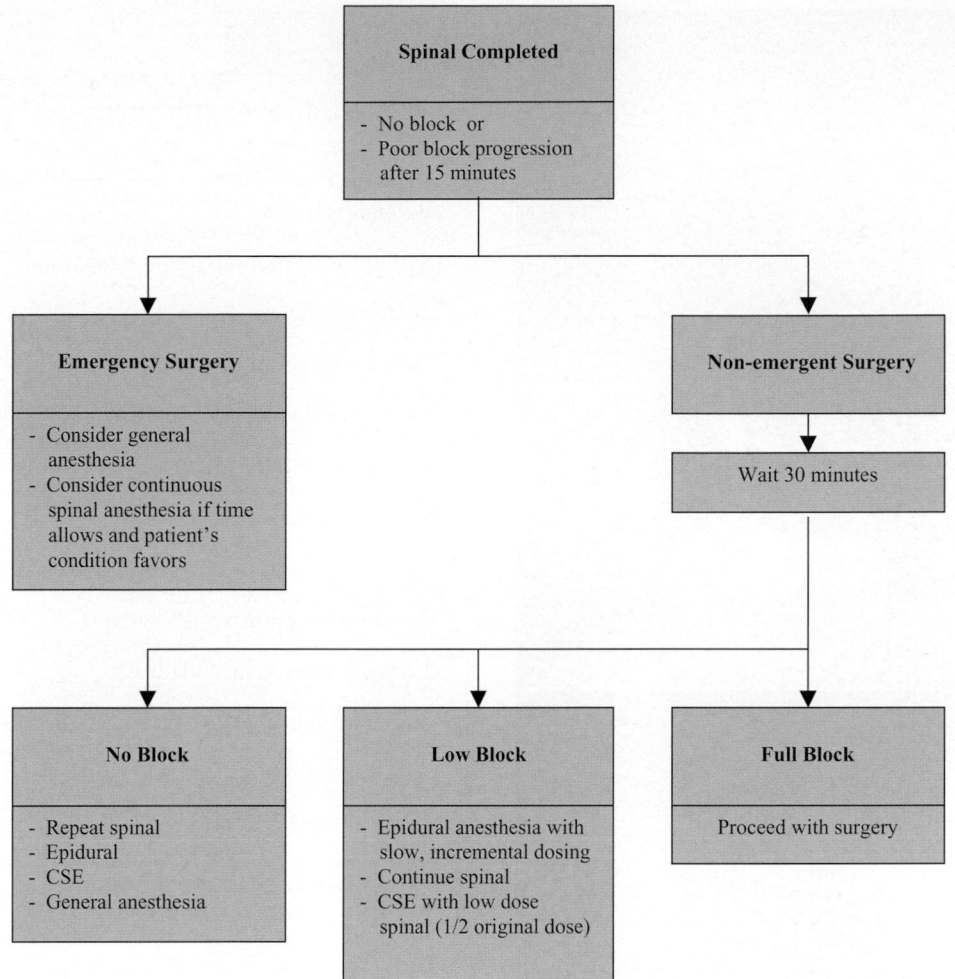

Figure 53–5. Management algorithm for an obstetric patient with inadequate neuraxial anesthesia. CSE, combined spinal–epidural.

Pudendal Nerve Block

The pudendal nerves are derived from the lower sacral nerve roots (S2-4) and supply the vaginal vault, perineum, rectum, and sections of the bladder. The nerves are easily blocked transvaginally where they loop around the ischial spines. Local anesthetic, 10 mL, deposited behind each sacrospinous ligament can provide adequate anesthesia for outlet forceps delivery and episiotomy repair.

ANESTHESIA FOR CESAREAN SECTION DELIVERY

The most common indications for cesarean section delivery include failure to progress, nonreassuring fetal status, cephalopelvic disproportion, malpresentation, prematurity, and prior uterine surgery involving the corpus. The choice of anesthesia should depend on the urgency of the procedure in addition to the condition of the mother and fetus. After a comprehensive discussion of the risks and benefits of all anesthesia options, the mother's desires should be considered.

Before the initiation of any anesthetic technique, resuscitation equipment for mother and neonate should be available (Table 53–2).

Advantages of Regional Anesthesia in the Obstetric Patient

A 1992 survey of obstetric anesthesia practices in the United States demonstrated that most patients undergoing cesarean section delivery do so under spinal or epidural anesthesia.[81] Regional techniques have several advantages: They reduce the risk of gastric aspiration, avoid depressant anesthetic drugs, and allow the mother to remain awake during delivery. Operative blood loss may also be reduced with regional compared with general anesthesia. Generally speaking, with regional techniques the duration of antepartum anesthesia does not affect neonatal outcome, provided that there is no protracted aortocaval compression or hypotension.[82] The risk of hypotension may be greater than during vaginal delivery because the sensory block must extend to at least the T4 dermatome. Proper positioning and prehydration with

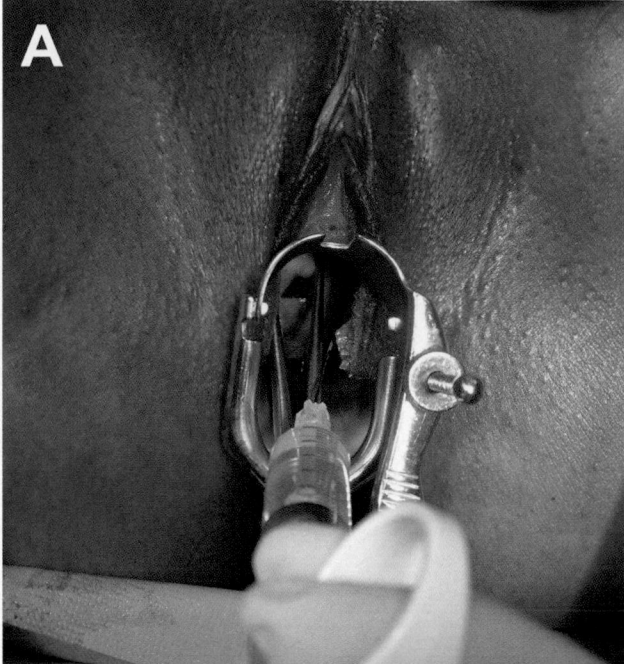

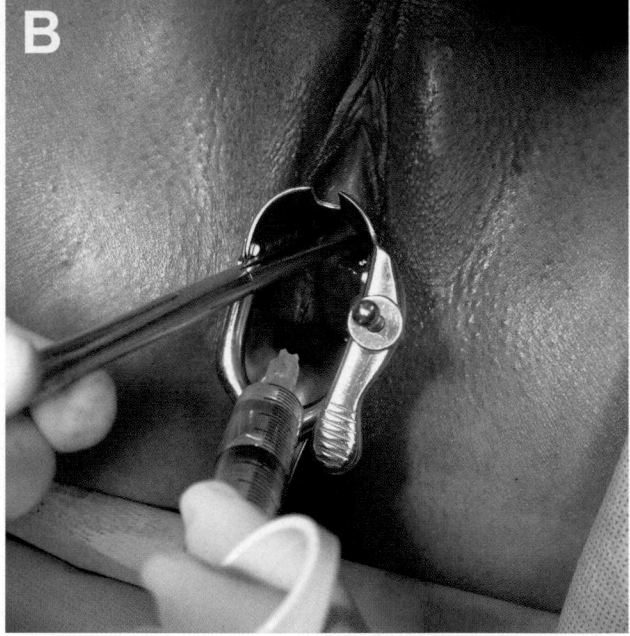

Figure 53–6. A and **B:** Paracervical block is a useful technique to provide analgesia for uterine curettage. The technique is very simple and involves a submucosal injection of local anesthetic at the vaginal fornix, near the neural fibers innervating the uterus.

Table 53–2.
Resuscitation Equipment in the Delivery Room
Radiant warmer
Suction with manometer and suction trap
Suction catheters
Wall oxygen with flow meter
Resuscitation bag ($\leq$750 mL)
Infant face masks
Infant oropharyngeal airways
Endotracheal tubes 2.5, 3.0, 3.5, and 4.0 mm
Endotracheal tube stylets
Laryngoscope(s) and blade(s)
Sterile umbilical artery catheterization tray
Needles, syringes, three-way stopcocks

Medications and solutions
      1:10,000 epinephrine
      Naloxone hydrochloride
      Sodium bicarbonate
      Volume expanders

reports of ineffectiveness and pulmonary edema, especially in patients with preeclampsia.

Spinal Anesthesia

Subarachnoid block is probably the most commonly administered regional anesthetic for cesarean section delivery because of its speed of onset and reliability. It has become an alternative to general anesthesia for emergency cesarean section.[84] Hyperbaric solutions of lidocaine 5%, tetracaine 1.0%, or bupivacaine 0.75% have been used. However, bupivacaine has now become the most widely used drug for spinal anesthesia for cesarean delivery. Using 0.75% hyperbaric bupivacaine, Norris[85] has shown that it is not necessary to adjust the dose of drug based on the patient's height. Hemodynamic monitoring during cesarean section should be similar to that used for other surgical procedures with the exception that blood pressure should be monitored at a minimum of every 3 minutes before the birth of the baby. Before delivery, oxygen should be routinely administered to optimize fetal oxygenation. Reports of transient neurologic syndrome and/or cauda equina syndrome have been associated with lidocaine in doses greater than 60 mg, whether it is in a 5% or a 2% preparation.

at least 10–15 mL/kg of dextrose crystalloid solution is recommended, particularly if a volume deficit exists.[83] If hypotension occurs despite these measures, left uterine displacement should be increased, the rate of IV infusion augmented, and IV ephedrine 5–15 mg (or phenylephrine 25–50 mcg) administered incrementally. Note, however, that routine aggressive prehydration has become controversial because of

Table 53–3.

Local Anesthetics Commonly Used for Cesarean Section Delivery with Subarachnoid Block

Dosage per Height of Patient (cm)	Bupivacaine 0.75% in 8.25% Dextrose (mg)	Bupivacaine 0.5% (Isobaric) (mg)
150–160 cm	8	8
160–180	10	10–12.5
>180 cm	12	12.5–15
Onset of action	2–4 min	5–10 min

This has led some clinicians to avoid the use of lidocaine for intrathecal administration (see Local Anesthetic Toxicity). See Table 53–3 for local anesthetics and their dosages that are commonly used for cesarean section delivery with subarachnoid block.

Clinical Pearls

- Even with an adequate dermatomal level for surgery, women may experience visceral discomfort, particularly during exteriorization of the uterus and traction on abdominal viscera.
- Perioperative analgesia can be provided more favorably by the addition of fentanyl 6.25 mcg or 0.1 mg of preservative-free morphine to the local anesthetic solution.

Despite an adequate dermatomal level, women may experience varying degrees of visceral discomfort, particularly during exteriorization of the uterus and traction on abdominal viscera. Improved perioperative analgesia can be provided by the addition of fentanyl 10 mcg or 0.1 mg of preservative-free morphine to the local anesthetic solution.[86] Nausea and vomiting may be alleviated by the administration of droperidol or metoclopramide. Maternal sedation should be avoided, if possible. If the initial block is not adequate, concern exists regarding a repeat spinal injection and the potential for inadvertent high spinal anesthesia. Figure 53–5 presents a range of options that are available in situations in which spinal anesthesia fails to prove adequate for surgery.

Lumbar Epidural Anesthesia

Epidural anesthesia has a slower onset of action and a larger drug requirement to establish an adequate sensory block com-

pared with spinal anesthesia. The advantages are a perceived reduced risk of postdural puncture headache and the ability to titrate the local anesthetic through the epidural catheter. However, correct placement of the epidural catheter and avoidance of inadvertent intrathecal or intravascular injection are essential.

Clinical Pearls

- Aspiration of the epidural catheter for blood or cerebrospinal fluid is not absolutely reliable for detection of catheter misplacement.
- A "test dose" is often used to rule out inadvertent intravascular or intrathecal catheter placement.
- A small dose of local anesthetic, lidocaine 45 mg or bupivacaine 5 mg, produces a readily identifiable sensory and motor block if injected intrathecally.
- Addition of epinephrine (15 mcg) with careful hemodynamic monitoring may signal intravascular injection when followed by a transient increase in heart rate and blood pressure.
- However, the use of an epinephrine test dose is controversial because false-positive results do occur in the presence of uterine contractions.

Aspiration of the epidural catheter for blood or cerebrospinal fluid is not 100% reliable for detection of catheter misplacement. For this reason, a "test dose" is often used to rule out inadvertent intravascular or intrathecal catheter placement. A small dose of local anesthetic, lidocaine 45 mg or bupivacaine 5 mg, produces a readily identifiable sensory and motor block if injected intrathecally. Addition of epinephrine (15 mcg) with careful heart rate and blood pressure monitoring may signal intravascular injection with transient increase in heart rate and blood pressure. However, an epinephrine test dose is controversial because false-positive results do occur in the presence of uterine contractions. In addition, epinephrine may reduce uteroplacental perfusion. Electrocardiography and application of a peak-to-peak heart rate criterion may improve detection (10 beats over maximum heart rate preceding epinephrine injection). Rapid injection of 1 mL of air with simultaneous precordial Doppler monitoring appears to be a reliable indicator of intravascular catheter placement.[87] A negative test, although reassuring, does not eliminate the need for fractional administration of local anesthetic.

Local Anesthetic Choices

The most commonly used agents are 2-chloroprocaine 3%, bupivacaine 0.5%, and lidocaine 2% with epinephrine 1:200,000.

Adequate anesthesia can be usually achieved with 15–25 mL of local anesthetic given in divided doses. The patient should be monitored as with spinal anesthesia. Because of its extremely high rate of metabolism in maternal and fetal plasma, 2-chloroprocaine provides a rapid-onset, reliable block with minimal risk of systemic toxicity.[27] It is the local anesthetic of choice in the presence of fetal acidosis and when a preexisting epidural block is to be rapidly extended for an urgent cesarean section delivery.[84] Neurologic deficits after massive inadvertent intrathecal administration of the drug have occurred with the formulation containing a relatively high concentration of sodium bisulfite, at a low pH.[88] In a new formulation of 2-chloroprocaine (Nesacaine-MPF), ethylene diaminetetraacetic acid (EDTA) has been substituted for sodium bisulfite. However, severe spasmodic back pain has been described after epidural injection of large volumes of Nesacaine-MPF in surgical patients, but not in parturients.[89] This has been attributed to EDTA-induced leaching of calcium from paravertebral muscles. The most recent formulation of 2-chloroprocaine contains no additives and is packaged in an amber vial to prevent oxidation.

Bupivacaine 0.5% provides profound anesthesia of slower onset for cesarean section delivery but of longer duration of action. Considerable attention has been focused on the drug because it was reported that unintentional intravascular injection could result not only in convulsions but also in almost simultaneous cardiac arrest, with patients often refractory to resuscitation.[90] The greater cardiotoxicity of bupivacaine (and etidocaine) compared with other amide local anesthetics has been well established.

When using potent long-acting amide local anesthetics, fractioning the induction dose is critical. Lidocaine has an onset and duration intermediate to those of 2-chloroprocaine and bupivacaine. The need to include epinephrine in the local anesthetic solution to ensure adequate lumbosacral anesthesia limits the use of lidocaine in women with maternal hypertension and uteroplacental insufficiency.

Prolonged postoperative pain relief can be provided by epidural administration of an opioid, such as morphine 4 mg or using patient-controlled epidural anesthesia. Delayed respiratory depression may occur with the use of morphine; hence the patient must be monitored carefully in the postoperative period. Recently, a lipid-encapsulated preparation of morphine (Depo Dur) has been approved for postcesarean section delivery analgesia. It can only be used epidurally and can last up to 48 hours, and the patient must be monitored for delayed respiratory depression.

ANESTHETIC COMPLICATIONS

Maternal Mortality

A study of anesthesia-related deaths in the United States between 1979 and 1990 showed that the case fatality rate with general anesthesia was 16.7 times greater than that with regional anesthesia. Most anesthesia-related deaths were a result of cardiac arrest due to hypoxemia when difficulties securing the airway were encountered.[81] Pregnancy-induced anatomic and physiologic changes, such as reduced functional residual capacity, increased oxygen consumption, and oropharyngeal edema, may expose the patient to serious risks of desaturation during periods of apnea and hypoventilation.

Pulmonary Aspiration

The risk of inhalation of gastric contents is increased in pregnant women, particularly if difficulty is encountered establishing an airway or if airway reflexes are obtunded. Measures to decrease the risks of aspiration include comprehensive airway evaluation, prophylactic administration of nonparticulate antacids, and preferred use of regional anesthesia.

Hypotension

Regional anesthesia may be associated with hypotension, which is related to the degree and rapidity of local anesthetic-induced sympatholysis. Thus, greater hemodynamic stability may be observed with epidural anesthesia, where gradual titration of local anesthetic allows for better control of the block level as well as for adequate time for administration of vasopressors in anticipation of blood pressure reduction.

The risk of hypotension is lower in women who are in labor compared with nonlaboring women.[91] Maternal prehydration with 15 mL/kg of lactated Ringer's solution before initiation of regional anesthesia and avoidance of aortocaval compression may decrease the incidence of hypotension. It has been demonstrated that for effective prevention of hypotension, the blood volume increase from preloading must be sufficient to result in a significant increase in cardiac output.[92] This was possible only with the administration of hetastarch, 0.5–1 liter.[92] Nonetheless, controversy exists regarding the efficacy of volume loading in the prevention of hypotension.[81,93] If hypotension does occur despite prehydration, therapeutic measures should include increasing displacement of the uterus, rapid infusion of IV fluids, titration of IV ephedrine (5–10 mg), and oxygen administration. In the presence of maternal tachycardia, phenylephrine 25–50 mcg may be substituted for ephedrine in women with *normal uteroplacental function*. Continued vigilance and active management of hypotension can prevent serious sequelae in both mother or neonate.[91,94]

Total Spinal Anesthesia

High or total spinal anesthesia is a rare complication of intrathecal injection in modern day practice. It occurs with excessive cephalad spread of local anesthetic in the subarachnoid space. Unintentional intrathecal administration of epidural medication as a result of dural puncture or catheter migration may also result in this complication. Left uterine displacement and continued fluid and vasopressor administration may be necessary to achieve hemodynamic stability. Reverse Trendelenburg position does not prevent cephalad spread and may cause cardiovascular collapse because of venous pooling related to sympathectomy. Rapid control of the airway is essential, and endotracheal intubation may be necessary to ensure oxygenation without aspiration.

Clinical Pearls

- Obstetric patients often complain of difficulty breathing during cesarean section delivery under neuraxial anesthesia.

- Although most common reasons are inability to feel "breathing" as the abdominal and thoracic segments are anesthetized (including the stretch receptors), practitioners must rule out an impending "high spinal" anesthesia by repetitive examinations.

- The following maneuvers are useful to rule out the possibility of high neuraxial anesthesia:
  1. *Ability of the patient to phonate*
  2. *Ability to squeeze the practitioner's hand (indicates that the block level is below the level of the brachial plexus (C6-T1)*

Systemic Toxicity of Local Anesthetics

Unintended intravascular injection or drug accumulation after repeated epidural injection can result in high serum levels of local anesthetic. Rapid absorption of local anesthetic from highly vascular sites of injection may also occur after paracervical and pudendal blocks.

Resuscitation equipment should always be available when any major nerve block is undertaken. Intravenous access, airway equipment, emergency drugs, and suction equipment should be immediately accessible. To avoid systemic toxicity of local anesthetic agents, strict adherence to recommended dosages and avoidance of unintentional intravascular injection are essential.

Despite these precautions, life-threatening convulsions and, more rarely, cardiovascular collapse may occur. Seizure activity has been treated with IV thiopental 25–50 mg or diazepam 5–10 mg. In current clinical practice, propofol 20–50 mg or midazolam 2–4 mg are more commonly used. The airway should be evaluated and oxygenation maintained. If cardiovascular collapse does occur, the Advanced Cardiac Life Support (ACLS) algorithm should be followed. Cesarean delivery may be required to relieve aortocaval compression and to ensure the efficiency of cardiac massage.[95]

Postdural Puncture Headache

Pregnant women have a higher risk for developing postdural puncture headache. The reduced epidural pressure also increases the risk of cerebrospinal fluid leakage through the dural opening. The pathophysiology and management of postdural puncture headache are discussed in greater detail in Chapter 73.

Neurologic Complications

Neurologic sequelae of central neuraxial blockade, although rare, have been reported. Pressure exerted by a needle or catheter on spinal nerve roots produces immediate pain and necessitates repositioning. Infections such as epidural abscess and meningitis are very rare and may be a manifestation of systemic sepsis. Epidural hematoma can also occur, usually in association with coagulation defects. Nerve root irritation may have a protracted recovery, lasting weeks or months. Peripheral nerve injury as a result of instrumentation, lithotomy position, or compression by the fetal head may occur even in the absence of neuraxial technique.

REGIONAL ANESTHESIA IN COMPLICATED PREGNANCY

Pregnancy and parturition are considered "high risk" when accompanied by conditions unfavorable to the well-being of the mother or fetus, or both. Maternal problems may be related to the pregnancy, that is, preeclampsia-eclampsia, hypertensive disorders of pregnancy, or antepartum hemorrhage resulting from placenta previa or abruptio placentae. Diabetes mellitus; cardiac, chronic renal, and neurologic problems; sickle cell disease; asthma; obesity; and drug abuse are not related to pregnancy but often are affected by it. Prematurity (gestation of less than 37 weeks), postmaturity (42 weeks or longer), intrauterine growth retardation, and multiple gestation are fetal conditions associated with risk. During labor and delivery, fetal malpresentation (eg, breech, transverse lie), placental abruption, compression of the umbilical cord (eg, prolapse, nuchal cord), precipitous labor, or intrauterine infection (eg, prolonged rupture of membranes) may increase the risk to the mother or fetus.

In general, the anesthetic management of the high-risk parturient is based on the same maternal and fetal considerations as for the management of healthy mothers and fetuses. However, there is less room for error because many of these functions may be compromised before the induction of anesthesia. For example, significant acidosis is prone to develop in fetuses of diabetic mothers when delivered by cesarean section with spinal anesthesia complicated by even brief maternal hypotension.

Preeclampsia-Eclampsia

Pathophysiology and Signs and Symptoms

Hypertensive disorders occur in approximately 7% of all pregnancies and are a major cause of maternal mortality. The most recent diagnostic criterion for preeclampsia is referred to as "proteinaceous increase in blood pressure."[96] The presence or absence of edema is no longer considered on of the required criteria. Rather than a specific blood pressure elevation, a blood pressure that is consistently 15% above baseline is now considered diagnostic. The added appearance of convulsions is diagnostic for eclampsia.[96] Preeclampsia-eclampsia is a

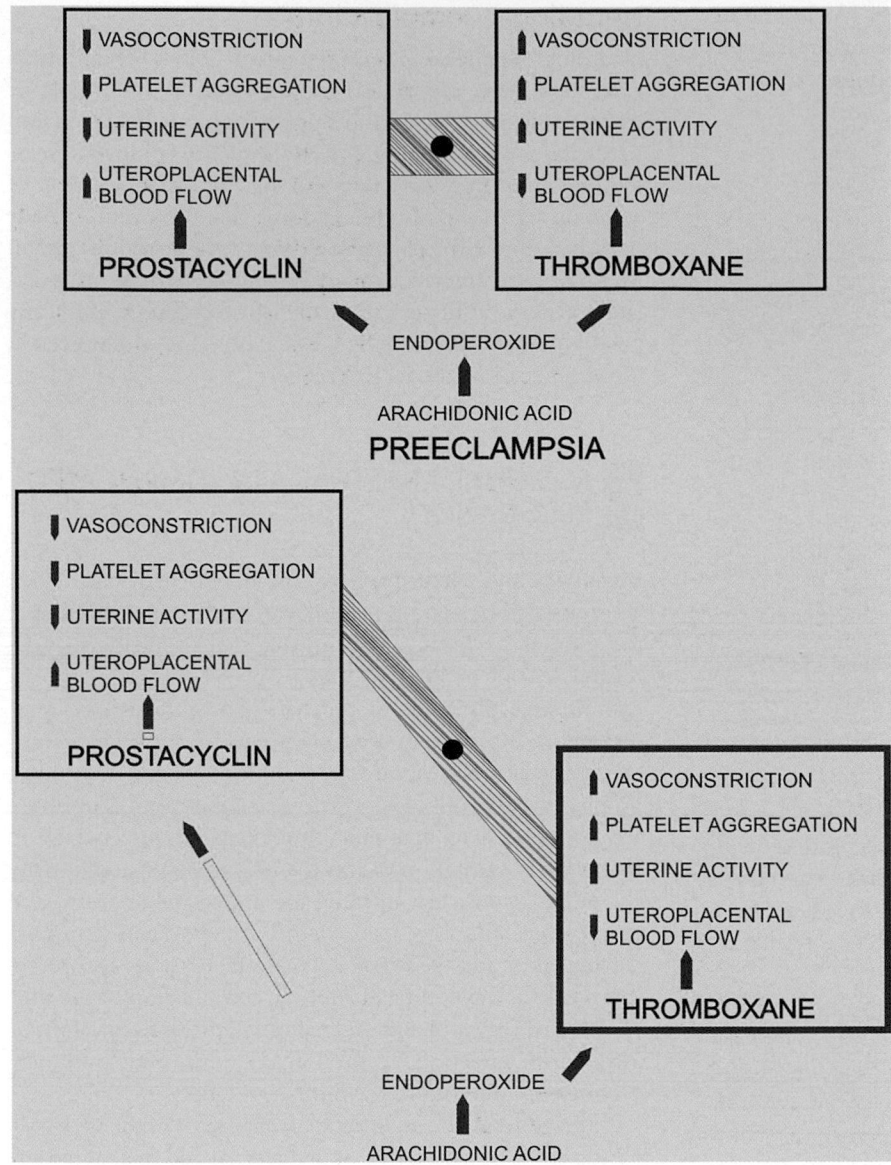

PROSTACYLIN
↓ VASOCONSTRICTION
↓ PLATELET AGGREGATION
↓ UTERINE ACTIVITY
↑ UTEROPLACENTAL BLOOD FLOW

THROMBOXANE
↑ VASOCONSTRICTION
↑ PLATELET AGGREGATION
↑ UTERINE ACTIVITY
↓ UTEROPLACENTAL BLOOD FLOW

ENDOPEROXIDE
ARACHIDONIC ACID
PREECLAMPSIA

PROSTACYLIN
↓ VASOCONSTRICTION
↓ PLATELET AGGREGATION
↓ UTERINE ACTIVITY
↑ UTEROPLACENTAL BLOOD FLOW

THROMBOXANE
↑ VASOCONSTRICTION
↑ PLATELET AGGREGATION
↑ UTERINE ACTIVITY
↓ UTEROPLACENTAL BLOOD FLOW

ENDOPEROXIDE
ARACHIDONIC ACID

Figure 53–7. Pathophysiology of preeclampsia and eclampsia.

disease unique to humans, occurring predominantly in young nulliparous women. Symptoms usually appear after the 20th week of gestation, occasionally earlier with a hydatidiform mole.

The origin of preeclampsia-eclampsia is unknown, but all patients manifest placental ischemia. Placental ischemia results in a release of uterine renin, an increase in a release of uterine renin, an increase in angiotensin activity, and a widespread arteriolar vasoconstriction causing hypertension, tissue hypoxia, and endothelial damage (Figure 53–7). Fixation of platelets at sites of endothelial damage results in coagulopathies, occasionally in disseminated intravascular coagulation. Enhanced angiotensin-mediated aldosterone secretion leads to an increased sodium reabsorption and edema. Proteinuria, a sign of preeclampsia, is also attributed to placental ischemia, which would lead to local tissue degeneration and a release of thromboplastin with subsequent deposition of fibrin in constricted glomerular vessels. As a result,

increased permeability to albumin and other plasma proteins occurs. Furthermore, there is a decreased production of prostaglandin E, a potent vasodilator secreted in the trophoblast, which normally balances the hypertensive effects of the rennin–angiotensin system.

Many of the symptoms associated with preeclampsia, including placental ischemia, systemic vasoconstriction, and increased platelet aggregation, may result from an imbalance between the placental production of prostacyclin and thromboxane. During normal pregnancy, the placental produces equal amounts of these two, but in a preeclamptic pregnancy, there is seven times more thromboxane than prostacyclin.[97] According to the latest theory, endothelial cell injury is central to the development of preeclampsia.[98] This injury occurs as a result of reduced placental perfusion, leading to a production and release of substances (possibly lipid peroxidases) causing endothelial cell injury. Abnormal endothelial cell function contributes to an increase in peripheral resistance and other abnormalities noted in preeclampsia through a release of fibronectin, endothelin, and other substances.

Clinical Pearls

Preeclampsia is classified as severe if it is associated with any of the following:

- Systolic BP *consistently* >15% above baseline
- Diastolic BP *consistently* >15% above baseline
- Proteinuria of 5 g/24 h
- Oliguria (400 mL/24 h)
- Cerebrovisual disturbances
- Pulmonary edema or cyanosis
- Epigastric pain
- Intrauterine growth retardation

In severe preeclampsia-eclampsia, all major organ systems are affected because of widespread vasospasm. Global cerebral blood flow is not diminished, but focal hypoperfusion cannot be ruled out. Postmortem examination has revealed hemorrhagic necrosis in the proximity of thrombosed precapillaries, suggesting intense vasoconstriction. Edema and small foci of degeneration have been attributed to hypoxia. Petechial hemorrhages are common after the onset of convulsions. Symptoms related to the above changes include headache, vertigo, cortical blindness, hyperreflexia, and convulsions. Cerebral hemorrhage and edema are the leading causes of death in preeclampsia-eclampsia, which together account for approximately 50% of deaths. Heart failure may occur in severe cases as a result of peripheral vasoconstriction and increased blood viscosity from hemoconcentration. Decreased blood supply to the liver may lead to periportal necrosis of variable extent and severity. Subcapsular hemorrhages account for the epigastric pain encountered in severe cases.

In the kidneys, there is swelling of glomerular endothelial cells and deposition of fibrin, leading to a constriction of the capillary lumina. Renal blood flow and glomerular filtration rate decrease, resulting in reduced uric acid clearance and, in severe cases, reduced clearance of urea and creatinine. Although preeclampsia is accompanied by exaggerated retention of water and sodium, the shift of fluid and proteins from the intravascular into the extravascular compartment may result in hypovolemia, hypoproteinemia, and hemoconcentration, which may be further aggravated by proteinuria. The risk of uteroplacental hypoperfusion and poor fetal outcome correlates with the degree of maternal plasma and protein depletion. The mean plasma volume in women with preeclampsia was found to be 9% less than normal, and in those with severe disease it was as much as 30–40% below normal.[99]

Adherence of platelets at sites of endothelia damage may result in consumption coagulopathy, which develops in approximately 20% of patients with preeclampsia. Mild thrombocytopenia, with platelet count of 100,000–150,000 per mm, is the most common finding. Prolongation of prothrombin and partial throboplastin times indicates consumption of procoagulants. Bleeding time, prolonged in approximately 25% of patients with normal platelet counts, is no longer considered a reliable test of clotting.[100] The HELLP syndrome is a particular form of severe preeclampsia characterized by **h**emolysis, **e**levated **l**iver enzymes, and **l**ow **p**latelets.

The goals of the management of the patient with preeclampsia-eclampsia are to prevent or control convulsions, improve organ perfusion, normalize blood pressure, and correct clotting abnormalities. The mainstay of anticonvulsant therapy in the United States is magnesium sulfate. Its efficacy in preventing seizures has been well substantiated, but its mechanism of action remains controversial. The patient usually receives a loading dose of 4 g in a 20% solution, administered over 5 minutes followed by a continuous infusion of 1–2 g/h.

Antihypertensive therapy in preeclampsia is used to lessen the risk of cerebral hemorrhage in the mother while maintaining, even improving, tissue perfusion. Plasma volume expansion combined with vasodilation fulfills these goals.[101] Hydralazine is the most commonly used vasodilator because it increases uteroplacental and renal blood flows. Nitroprusside is used during laryngoscopy and intubation to prevent dangerous elevations in blood pressure. Trimethaphan, a ganglion blocking agent, is useful in hypertensive emergencies when cerebral edema and increased intracranial pressure are a concern because it does not cause vasodilation in the brain. Other agents that have been used to control maternal blood pressure include α-methyldopa, nitroglycerine, and now more frequently, labetalol.[102]

Consumption coagulopathy may require infusion of fresh whole blood, platelet concentrates, fresh frozen plasma, and cryoprecipitate. Delivery is indicated in refractory cases or if the pregnancy is close to term. In severe cases, aggressive management should continue for at least 24–48 hours after delivery.

Anesthesia Management

There are very few contraindications for epidural anesthesia in labor and delivery. In the presence of severe clotting abnormalities or severe plasma volume deficit, the risk:benefit ratio favors other forms of anesthesia.[103] In volume-depleted patients positioned with left uterine displacement, epidural anesthesia does not cause an unacceptable reduction in blood pressure and leads to a significant improvement in placental perfusion.[104] With the use of radioactive xenon, it was shown that the intervillous blood flow increased by approximately 75% after the induction of epidural analgesia (10 mL bupivacaine 0.25%).[105] The total maternal body clearance of amide local anesthetics is prolonged in preeclampsia, and repeated administration of these drugs can lead to higher blood concentrations than in normotensive patients.[106]

For cesarean section delivery, the sensory level of regional anesthesia must extend to T3-4, making adequate fluid therapy and left uterine displacement even more vital.

Epidural anesthesia has been preferred to spinal anesthesia in preeclamptic women because of its slower onset of action and controllability. The rapid onset of spinal anesthesia may be associated with hypotension, particularly in a volume-depleted patient. However, in two recent studies, the incidence of hypotension, perioperative fluid and ephedrine administration, and neonatal conditions were found to be similar in preeclamptic women who received either epidural or spinal anesthesia for cesarean delivery.[107,108] There is an increased sensitivity to vasopressors in preeclampsia; therefore, lower doses of ephedrine are usually required to correct hypotension.

Antepartum Hemorrhage

Antepartum hemorrhage occurs most commonly in association with placenta previa (abnormal implantation on the lower uterine segment and partial to total occlusion of the internal cervical os) and abruptio placentae. Placenta previa occurs in 0.11% of all pregnancies, resulting in up to 0.9% incidence of maternal and a 17–26% incidence of perinatal mortality. It may be associated with abnormal fetal presentation, such as transverse lie or breech. Placenta previa should be suspected whenever a patient presents with painless, bright red vaginal bleeding, usually after the seventh month of pregnancy. The diagnosis is confirmed by ultrasonography. If the bleeding is not profuse and the fetus is immature, obstetric management is conservative to prolong the pregnancy. In severe cases or if the fetus is mature at the onset of the symptoms, prompt delivery is indicated, usually by cesarean section. An emergency hysterectomy may be required because of severe hemorrhage, even after the delivery of the placenta, because of uterine atony. In patients who have undergone prior uterine surgery, the risk of severe hemorrhage is even greater owing to a higher incidence of placenta acreta (penetration of myometrium by placental villi).

Abruptio placentae occurs in 0.2–2.4% of pregnant women, usually in the final 10 weeks of gestation and in association with hypertensive diseases. Complications include Couvelaire uterus (ie, when extravasated blood dissects between the myometrial fibers), renal failure, disseminated intravascular coagulation, and anterior pituitary necrosis (ie, Sheehan syndrome). The maternal mortality is high (1.8–11.0%), and the perinatal mortality rate is even higher (excess of 50%). The diagnosis of abruptio placentae is based on the presence of uterine tenderness, hypertonus, and vaginal bleeding of dark, clotted blood. Bleeding may be concealed if the placental margins have remained attached to the uterine wall. Changes in the maternal blood pressure and pulse rate, indicative of hypovolemia, may occur if the blood loss is severe. Fetal movements may increase during acute hypoxia and decrease if hypoxia is gradual. Fetal bradycardia and death may ensue.

Anesthesia Management

Establishment of invasive monitoring (arterial line, central venous catheter) and blood volume replacement via a 14- or 16-gauge stimulating needle is usually required. If clotting abnormalities exist, blood components and fresh frozen plasma, cryoprecipitate, and platelet concentrates may be required. Epidural anesthesia may be considered, but general anesthesia is indicated in the presence of uncontrolled hemorrhage and coagulation abnormalities.[109]

Preterm Delivery

Preterm labor and delivery present a significant challenge to the anesthesiologist because the mother and the infant may be at risk. The definition of prematurity was altered to distinguish between the preterm infant, born before the 37th week of gestation, and the small-for-gestational-age infant, who may be born at term but whose weight is more than 2 standard deviations below the mean. Although preterm deliveries occur in 8–10% of all births, they account for approximately 80% of early neonatal deaths. Severe problems, such as respiratory distress syndrome, intracranial hemorrhage, hypoglycemia, hypocalcemia, and hyperbilirubinemia, are prone to develop in preterm infants.

Obstetricians frequently try to inhibit preterm labor to enhance fetal lung maturity. Delaying delivery be even 24–48 hours may be beneficial if glucocorticoids are administered to the mother to enhance fetal lung maturity. Various agents have been used to suppress uterine activity (tocolysis) such as ethanol, magnesium sulfate, prostaglandin inhibitors, β-sympathomimetics, and calcium channel blockers. β-Adrenergic drugs, such as ritodrine and terbutaline, are the most commonly used tocolytics. Their predominant effect is β_2 receptor stimulation, which results in myometrial inhibition, vasodilation, and bronchodilation. Numerous maternal complications, that is, hypotension, hypokalemia, hyperglycemia, myocardial ischemia, pulmonary edema, and death, have been reported.

Anesthesia Management

Complications may occur because of interactions with anesthetic drugs and techniques. With the use of regional anesthesia, peripheral vasodilation caused by β-adrenergic stimulation increases the risk of hemodynamic instability in the presence of preexisting tachycardia, hypotension, and hypokalemia. The premature infant is known to be more vulnerable than the term newborn to the effects of drugs used in obstetric analgesia and anesthesia. However, there have been few systemic studies to determine the maternal and fetal pharmacokinetics and dynamics of drugs throughout gestation.

There are several postulated causes of enhanced drug sensitivity in the preterm newborn: less protein available for drug binding; higher levels of bilirubin, which may compete with the drug for protein binding; greater drug access to the central nervous system because of a poorly developed blood–brain barrier; greater total body water and lower fat content; and a decreased ability to metabolize and excrete drugs. However, most drugs used in anesthesia exhibit low to moderate degrees of binding in the fetal serum: approximately 50%

for bupivacaine, 25% for lidocaine, 52% for meperidine, and 75% for thiopental.

In selection of the anesthetic drugs and techniques for delivery of a preterm infant, concerns regarding drug effects on the newborn are far less important than prevention of asphyxia and trauma to the fetus. For labor vaginal delivery, well-conducted epidural anesthesia is advantageous in providing good perineal relaxation. Before induction of epidural blockade, the anesthesiologist should ascertain that the fetus is neither hypoxic nor acidotic. Asphyxia results in a redistribution of fetal cardiac output, which increases oxygen delivery to vital organs such as the brain, heart, and adrenals. Regardless, these changes in the preterm fetus may be better preserved with bupivacaine or chloroprocaine than with lidocaine.[110,111] Preterm infants with breech presentation are usually delivered by cesarean section. Regional anesthesia can be successfully used, with nitroglycerin available for uterine relaxation if needed.

Clinical Pearls

- In selecting the anesthetic drugs and techniques for delivering a preterm infant, concerns about drug effects on the newborn are far less important than prevention of asphyxia and trauma to the fetus.
- Before induction of epidural blockade, the anesthesiologist should ascertain that the fetus is neither hypoxic nor acidotic.

Regional analgesia during labor and vaginal delivery has become the preferred technique of pain relief in selected high-risk patients because it prevents obtundation of the mother and depression of the fetus and reduces many of the potential adverse physiologic effects of labor, such as increased oxygen consumption and hemodynamic alterations. For cesarean section delivery, regional anesthesia has emerged as a safe and effective technique in high-risk parturients, partly because of the added ability to provide prolonged postoperative analgesia.

NONOBSTETRIC SURGERY IN THE PREGNANT WOMAN

Approximately 1.6–2.2% of pregnant women undergo surgery for reasons unrelated to parturition. Apart from trauma, the most common emergencies are abdominal, intracranial aneurysms, cardiac valvular disease, and pheochromocytoma. Surgery to correct an incompetent cervix with Shirodkar or McDonald sutures is a procedure directly related to surgery.

When the necessity for surgery arises, anesthetic considerations are related to the alterations in maternal physiologic condition with advancing pregnancy, the teratogenicity of anesthetic drugs, the indirect effects of anesthesia on uterplacental blood flow, and the potential for abortion or premature delivery. The risks must be balanced to provide the most favorable outcome for mother and child. Five major studies have attempted to relate surgery and anesthesia during human pregnancy to fetal outcome as determined by anomalies, premature labor, or intrauterine death.[112–115] Although they failed to correlate surgery and anesthetic exposure with congenital anomalies, all the studies demonstrated an increased incidence of fetal death, particularly after operations performed in the first trimester. A particular anesthetic agent of technique was not implicated. The condition that necessitated surgery was the most relevant factor, with fetal mortality greatest after pelvic surgery or procedures performed for obstetric indications, that is, cervical incompetence.

The cytotoxicity of anesthetic agents is closely associated with biodegradation, which, in turn, is influenced by oxygenation and hepatic blood flow. Thus, the complications associated with anesthesia—maternal hypoxia, hypotension, administration of vasopressors, hypercarbia, hypocarbia, and electrolyte disturbances—may be greater factors in teratogenesis than the use of the agents themselves.[116,117]

Experimental evidence on exposure to specific drugs and agents is discussed briefly, with the understanding that it is difficult to extrapolate laboratory data to the clinical situation in humans. Very large numbers of patients must be exposed to a suspected teratogen before its safety can be ascertained. Complicating factors include the frequency of maternal exposure to a multiplicity of drugs; the difficulty in separating the effects of the underlying disease process and surgical treatment from those of the drug administered; differing degrees of risk with stage of gestation; and the variety, rather than the consistency, of anomalies that appear in association with one agent. With regard to regional anesthetic agents, local anesthetics have not been shown to be teratogenic in animals or humans.

Caution has been exercised with sedatives before block placement because of several reports describing a specific relationship between diazepam and oral clefts; however, other studies have not confirmed this.[118,119] When appropriate, regional techniques are a viable alternative to general anesthesia in the pregnant patient presenting for nonobstetric surgery. As maternal pain and apprehension may result in decreased uterine blood flow and deterioration of the fetus (similar to infusions of epinephrine or norepinephrine), early intervention for pain with regional techniques, ie, peripheral nerve blocks or epidural infusions, can be substantiated especially in the compromised patient.[120]

Clinical Pearl

- Local anesthestics have not been shown to be teratogenic in animals or humans.

SUMMARY

Pregnancy results in a number of significant physiologic changes that require adjustment in anesthesia and analgesia techniques for safe and effective management of the pregnant patient. It is prudent to delay surgeries, when possible, until after the birth of the fetus. Only emergency surgery should be considered during the first trimester.

Regional techniques have become the most accepted for pain relief during labor and vaginal delivery. Likewise, neuraxial techniques are now the most frequently administered anesthetics for cesarean section delivery. Advances in regional anesthesia and its widespread routine use have resulted in significantly enhanced maternal safety compared with general anesthesia.

References

1. Melzack R, Taenzer P, Feldman P, Kinch RA: Labour is still painful after prepared childbirth training. Can Med Assoc J 1981;125: 357.
2. Goodman RP, Killom AP, Brash AR, Branch RA: Prostacyclin production during pregnancy: Comparison of production during normal pregnancy and pregnancy complicated by hypertension. Am J Obstet Gynecol 1982;142:817.
3. Kerr MG, Scott DB, Samuel E: Studies of the inferior vena cava in late pregnancy. BMJ 1964;1:532.
4. Howard BK, Goodson JH, Mengert WE: Supine hypotensive syndrome in late pregnancy. Obstet Gynecol 1953;1:371.
5. Prowse CM, Gaensler EA: Respiratory and acid-base changes during pregnancy. Anesthesiology 1965;26:381.
6. Moya F, Smith BE: Uptake, distribution and placental transport of drugs and anesthetics. Anesthesiology 1965;26:465.
7. Archer GW, Marx GF: Arterial oxygenation during apnoea in parturient women. Br J Anaesth 1974;46:358.
8. Simpson KH, Stakes AF, Miller M: Pregnancy delays paracetamol absorption and gastric emptying in patients undergoing surgery. Br J Anaesth 1988;60:24.
9. Davison JS, Davison MC, Hay DM: Gastric emptying time in late pregnancy and labour. J Obstet Gynaecol Br Commonw 1970;77:37.
10. Brock-Utne JG, Dow TGB, Dimopoulos GE, et al: Gastric and lower oesophageal sphincter (LOS) pressures in early pregnancy. Br J Anaesth 1981;53:381.
11. Wyner J, Cohen SE: Gastric volume in early pregnancy: Effect of metoclopramide. Anesthesiology 1982;57:209.
12. Cohen SE, Woods WA, Wyner J: Antiemetic efficacy of droperidol and metoclopramide. Anesthesiology 1984;60:67.
13. Scheller MS, Sears KL: Post-operative neurologic dysfunction associated with preoperative administration of metoclopramide. Anesth Analg 1987;66:274.
14. Lund CJ, Donovan JC: Blood volume during pregnancy. Am J Obstet Gynecol 1967;98:393.
15. Pritchard J, Macdonald P: Maternal adaptation to pregnancy. In: Pritchard J, Macdonald P (editors): *Williams Obstetrics*. Appleton-Century-Crofts, 1980, pp. 236.
16. Wildsmith JAW: Serum pseudocholinesterase, pregnancy and suxamethonium. Anaesthesia 1972;27:90.
17. Coryell MN, Beach EF, Robinson AR, et al: Metabolism of women during the reproductive cycle: XVII. Changes in electrophoretic patterns of plasma proteins throughout the cycle and following delivery. J Clin Invest 1950;29:1559.
18. Datta S, Kitzmiller JL, Naulty JS, et al: Acid-base status of diabetic mothers and their infants following spinal anesthesia for cesarean section. Anesth Analg 1982;61:662.

19. Datta S, Lambert DH, Gregus J, et al: Differential sensitivities of mammalian nerve fibers during pregnancy. Anesth Analg 1983;62:1070.
20. Gin T, Chan MTV: Decreased minimum alveolar concentration of isoflurane in pregnant humans. Anesthesiology 1994;81:829.
21. Brown WU, Bell GC, Alper MH: Acidosis, local anesthetics and the newborn. Obstet Gynecol 1976;48:27.
22. Hamshaw-Thomas A, Rogerson N, Reynolds F: Transfer of bupivacaine, lignocaine and pethidine across the rabbit placenta: Influence of maternal protein binding and fetal flow. Placenta 1984;5:61.
23. Kennedy RL, Miller RP, Bell JU, et al: Uptake and distribution of bupivacaine in fetal lambs. Anesthesiology 1986;65:247.
24. Kuhnert PM, Kuhnert BR, Stitts JM, Gross TL: The use of a selected ion monitoring technique to study the disposition of bupivacaine in mother, fetus and neonate following epidural anesthesia for cesarean section. Anesthesiology 1981;55:611.
25. Kuhnert BR, Philipson EH, Pimental R, et al: Lidocaine disposition in mother, fetus, and neonate after spinal anesthesia. Anesth Analg 1986;65:139.
26. Morishima HO, Daniel SS, Finster M, et al: Transmission of mepivacaine hydrochloride (Carbocaine) across the human placenta. Anesthesiology 1966;27:147.
27. Kuhnert BR, Kuhnert PM, Prochaska AL, Gross TL: Plasma levels of 2-chloroprocaine in obstetric patients and their neonates after epidural anesthesia. Anesthesiology 1980;53:21.
28. Pihlajamaki K, Kanto J, Lindberg R, et al: Extradural administration of bupivacaine: Pharmacokinetics and metabolism in pregnant and non-pregnant women. Br J Anaesth 1990;64:556.
29. Morishima HO, Covino BG: Toxicity and distribution of lidocaine in nonasphyxiated and asphyxiated baboon fetuses. Anesthesiology 1981;54:182.
30. Morishima HO, Finster M, Pedersen H, et al: Pharmacokinetics of lidocaine in fetal and neonatal lambs and adult sheep. Anesthesiology 1979;50:431.
31. Mihaly GW, Moore RG, Thomas J, et al: The pharmacokinetics and metabolism of the anilide local anaesthetics in neonates. Eur J Clin Pharmacol 1978;13:143.
32. Finster M, Poppers PJ, Sinclair JC, et al: Accidental intoxication of the fetus with local anesthetic drug during caudal anesthesia. Am J Obstet Gynecol 1965;92:922.
33. Morishima HO, Pedersen H, Finster M, et al: Toxicity of lidocaine in adult, newborn and fetal sheep. Anesthesiology 1981;55:57.
34. Gale R, Ferguson JE II, Stevenson D: Effect of epidural analgesia with bupivacaine hydrochloride on neonatal bilirubin production. Obstet Gynecol 1987;70:692.
35. Brockhurst NJ, Littleford JA, Halpern SH: The neurological and adaptive capacity score: A systematic review of its use in obstetric anesthesia research. Anesthesiology 2000;92:237.
36. Morishima HO, Yeh M-N, James LS: Reduced uterine blood flow and fetal hypoxemia with acute maternal stress: Experimental observation in the pregnant baboon. Am J Obstet Gynecol 1979;134:270.
37. Ueland K, Hansen JM: Maternal cardiovascular dynamics: III. Labor and delivery under local and caudal analgesia. Am J Obstet Gynecol 1969;103:8.
38. Moir DD, Willocks J: Management of incoordinate uterine action under continuous epidural analgesia. BMJ 1967;2:396.
39. Miller FC, Petrie RH, Arce JJ, et al: Hyperventilation during labor. Am J Obstet Gynecol 1974;120:489.
40. Beaule PE, Smith MI, Nguyen VN: Meperidine-induced seizure after revision hip arthroplasty. J Arthroplasty 2005;19:516–519.
41. Hagmeyer KO, Mauro LS, Mauro VF: Meperidine-related seizures associated with patient-controlled analgesia pumps. Ann Pharmacother 1993;27:29–32.
42. Kaiko RF, Grabinski PY, Heidrick G, et al: Central nervous system excitatory effects of meperidine in cancer patients. Ann Neurol 1983;13:180–185.
43. Kuhnert BR, Linn PL, Kennard MJ, Kuhnert PM: Effect of low doses of meperidine on neonatal behavior. Anesth Analg 1985;64:335.

44. Eisele JH, Wright R, Rogge P: Newborn and maternal fentanyl levels at cesarean section. Anesth Analg 1982;61:179.

45. Muir HA, Breen T, Campbell DC, et al: Is intravenous PCA fentanyl an effective method for providing labor analgesia? Anesthesiology 1999;(Suppl):A28.

46. Vercauteren M, Bettens K, Van Springel G, et al: Intrathecal labor analgesia: Can we use the same mixture as is used epidurally? Int J Obstet Anesth 1997;6:242–246.

47. Breen TW, Giesinger Cm, Halpern SH: Comparison of epidural lidocaine and fentanyl to intrathecal sufentanil for analgesia in early labor. Int J Obstet Anesth 1999;8:226–230.

48. Kapila A, Glass PS, Jacobs JR, et al: Measured context-sensitive half times of remifentanil and alfentanil. Anesthesiology 1995;83:968.

49. Evron S, Glezerman M, Sadan O, et al: Remifentanil: A novel systemic analgesic for labor pain. Anesth Analg 2005;100:233–238.

50. Kan RE, Hughes SC, Rosen M, et al: Intravenous remifentanil: Placental transfer, maternal and neonatal effects. Anesthesiology 1998;88:1467.

51. Thurlow JA, Laxton CH, Dick A, et al: Remifentanil by patient-controlled analgesia compared with intramuscular meperidine for pain relief in labor. Br J Anaesth 2002;88:374–378.

52. Volmanen P, Akural E, Raudaskoski T, et al: Comparison of remifentanil and nitrous oxide in labour analgesia. Acta Anaesthesiol Scand 2005;49:453–458.

53. Maduska AL, Hajghassemali M: A double blind comparison of butorphanol and meperidine in labor: Maternal pain relief and effect on newborn. Can Anaesth Soc J 1978;25:398.

54. Thorp JA, Hu DH, Albin RM, et al: The effect of intrapartum epidural analgesia on nulliparous labor: A randomized, controlled, prospective trial. Am J Obstet Gynecol 1993;169:851.

55. Sharma SK, Sidawi JE, Ramin SM, et al: Cesarean delivery: A randomized trial of epidural versus patient controlled meperidine analgesia during labor. Anesthesiology 1997;87:487.

56. Halpern SH, Leighton BL, Ohlsson A, et al: Effect of epidural vs parenteral opioid analgesia in the progress of labor: A meta-analysis. JAMA 1998;280:2105.

57. Ramin SM, Gambling DR, Lucas MJ, et al: Randomized trial of epidural versus intravenous analgesia in labor. Obstet Gynecol 1995;86:783.

58. Chestnut DH, Vincent RD, McGrath JM, et al: Does early administration of epidural analgesia affect obstetric outcome in nulliparous women who are receiving intravenous oxytocin? Anesthesiology 1994;80:1193.

59. Chestnut DH, McGrath JM, Vincent RD, et al: Does early administration of epidural analgesia affect obstetric outcome in nulliparous women who are in spontaneous labor? Anesthesiology 1994;80:1201.

60. American College of Obstetrics and Gynecology: Obstetric forceps. AGOG Committee on Obstetrics Maternal and Fetal Medicine, Committee Opinion, 1989.

61. Chestnut DH, Laszewski LJ, Pollack RL, et al: Continuous epidural infusion of 0.0625% bupivacaine-0.0002% fentanyl during the second stage of labor. Anesthesiology 1990;72:613.

62. Birnbach DJ, Chestnut DH: The epidural test dose in obstetric practice: Has it outlived its usefulness? Anesth Analg 1999;88:971.

63. Norris MC, Ferrenbach D, Dalman H, et al: Does epinephrine improve the diagnostic accuracy of aspiration during labor epidural analgesia? Anesth Analg 1999;88:1073.

64. Visconti C, Eisenach JC: Patient-controlled epidural analgesia during labor. Obstet Gynecol 1991;77:348.

65. Rigler ML, Drasner K, Krejcie TC, et al: Cauda equina syndrome after continuous spinal anesthesia. Anesth Analg 1991;72:275.

66. Arkoosh VA, Palmer CM, Van Maren GA, et al: Continuous intrathecal labor analgesia: Safety and efficacy. Anesthesiology 1998;(Suppl):A8.

67. Campbell DC, Camann WR, Datta S: The addition of bupivacaine to intrathecal sufentanil for labor analgesia. Anesth Analg 1995;81:305.

68. Collis RE, Davies DWL, Aveling W: Randomized comparison of combined spinal epidural and standard epidural analgesia in labour. Lancet 1995;345:1413.

69. McLeod A, Fernando R, Page F, et al: An assessment of maternal balance and gait using computerized posturography. Anesthesiology 1999;(Suppl):A8.

70. Wong CA, Scavone BM, Peaceman AM, et al: The risk of cesarean delivery with neuraxial analgesia given early versus late labor. N Engl J Med 2005;352:655.

71. Cohen SE, Cherry CM, Holbrook RH, et al: Intrathecal sufentanil for labor analgesia: Sensory changes, side-effects and fetal heart rate changes. Anesth Analg 1993;77:1155.

72. Clarke VT, Smiley RM, Finster M: Uterine hyperactivity after intrathecal injection of fentanyl for analgesia during labor: A cause of fetal bradycardia? Anesthesiology 1994;81:1083.

73. O'Gorman DA, Birnbach DJ, Kuczkowski KM, et al: Use of umbilical flow velocimetry in the assessment of the pathogenesis of fetal bradycardia following combined spinal epidural analgesia in parturients. Anesthesiology 2000;(Suppl):A2.

74. Riley ET, Vogel TM, EI-Sayed YY, et al: Patient selection bias contributes to an increased incidence of fetal bradycardia after combined spinal epidural analgesia for labor. Anesthesiology 1999;91:A1054.

75. Nielson PE, Erickson R, Abouleish E, et al: Fetal heart rate changes after intrathecal sufentanil or epidural bupivacaine for labor analgesia: Incidence and clinical significance. Anesth Analg 1996;83:742.

76. Albright GA, Forester RM: Does combined epidural analgesia with subarachnoid sufentanil increase the incidence of emergency cesarean section? Reg Anesth 1997;22:400.

77. Norris MC, Grieco WM, Borkowski M, et al: Complications of labor analgesia: Epidural versus combined spinal epidural techniques. Anesth Analg 1995;79:529.

78. Leighton BL, Arkoosh VA, Huffnagle S, et al: The dermatomal spread of epidural bupivacaine with and without prior intrathecal sufentanil. Anesth Analg 1996;83:526.

79. Baxi LV, Petrie RH, James LS: Human fetal oxygenation following paracervical block. Am J Obstet Gynecol 1979;135:1109.

80. Leighton BL, Halpern SH, Wilson DB: Lumbar sympathetic blocks speed early and second stage induced labor in nulliparous women. Anesthesiology 1999;90:1039.

81. Hawkins JL, Gibbs CP, Orleans M, et al: Obstetric anesthesia workforce survey 1992 vs 1981. Anesthesiology 1994;81:A1128.

82. Shnider SM, Levinson G: Anesthesia for cesarean section. In: Shnider SM, Levinson G (editors): *Anesthesia for Obstetrics.* Williams & Wilkins, 1987, pp. 159.

83. Rout CC, Rocke DA, Levin J, et al: A reevaluation of the role of crystalloid preload in the prevention of hypotension associated with spinal anesthesia for elective cesarean section. Anesthesiology 1993;79:262.

84. Marx GF, Luykx WM, Cohen S: Fetal-neonatal status following cesarean section for fetal distress. Br J Anaesth 1984;56:1009.

85. Norris MC: Height, weight and the spread of subarachnoid hyperbaric bupivacaine in the term parturient. Anesth Analg 1988;67:555.

86. Hunt GO, Naulty S, Bader AM, et al: Perioperative analgesia with subarachnoid fentanyl-bupivacaine for cesarean delivery. Anesthesiology 1989;71:535.

87. Leighton BL, Norris MC, Sosis M, et al: Limitations of epinephrine as a marker of intravascular injection in laboring women. Anesthesiology 1987;66:688.

88. Gissen AJ, Datta S, Lambert D: The chloroprocaine controversy: Is chloroprocaine neurotoxic? Reg Anaesth 1984;9:135.

89. Hynson JM, Sessler DI, Glosten B: Back pain in volunteers after epidural anesthesia with chloroprocaine. Anesth Analg 1991;72:253.

90. Albright GA: Cardiac arrest following regional anesthesia with etidocaine or bupivacaine. Anesthesiology 1979;51:285.

91. Brizgys RV, Dailey PA, Shnider SM, et al: The incidence and neonatal effects of maternal hypotension during epidural anesthesia for cesarean section. Anesthesiology 1987;67:782.

92. Ueyama H, He YL, Tanigami H, et al: Effects of crystalloid and colloid preload or blood volume in the parturient undergoing spinal anesthesia for elective cesarean section. Anesthesiology 1999;91:1571.

93. Rout CC, Roche DA: Spinal hypotension associated with cesarean section: Will preload ever work? Anesthesiology 1999;91:1565.

94. Ramanathan S, Grant GJ: Vasopressor therapy for hypotension due to epidural anaesthesia. Acta Anaesthesiol Scand 1988;32:559.

95. Kasten GW, Martin ST: Resuscitation from bupivacaine-induced cardiovascular toxicity during partial inferior vena cava occlusion. Anesth Analg 1986;65:341.

96. Bodurka D: What's new in Gynecology and Obstetrics. J Am Coll Surg 2005;201:265–274.

97. Walsh S: Preeclampsia: An imbalance in placental prostacyclin and thromboxane production. Am J Obstet Gynecol 1985;152:335.

98. Roberts J, Taylor R, Musci T, et al: Preeclampsia: An endothelial cell disorder. Am J Obstet Gynecol 1989;152:1200.

99. Chesley L: Plasma and red cell volumes during pregnancy. Am J Obstet Gynecol 1972:112:440.

100. Rodgers R, Levin J: A critical reappraisal of the bleeding time. Semin Thromb Hemost 1990:16:1–20.

101. Groenendijk R, Trimbos M, Wallenburg H: Hemodynamic measurements in preeclampsia: Preliminary observations. Am J Obstet Gynecol 1984;150:232.

102. Cotton D, Gonik B, Dorman K, Harris R: Cardiovascular alterations in severe pregnancy-induced hypertension: Relationship of central venous pressure to pulmonary capillary wedge pressure. Am J Obstet Gynecol 1985;151:762.

103. Hogg B, Hauth J, Caritis S, et al: Safety of labor epidural anesthesia for women with severe hypertensive disease. Am J Obstet Gynecol 1999;181:1099.

104. Newsome L, Bramwell R, Curling P: Hemodynamic effects of lumbar epidural anesthesia. Anesthesia and Analgesia 1986;65:31.

105. Jouppila P, Jouppila R, Hollmen A, Koivula A: Lumbar epidural analgesia to improve intervillous blood flow during labor in severe preeclampsia. Obstet Gynecol 1982;52:158.

106. Ramanathan J, Botorff M, Jeter J, et al: The pharmacokinetics and maternal and neonatal effects of epidural lidocaine in preeclampsia. Anesth Analg 1986;65:120.

107. Wallace D, Leveno KJ, Cunningham F, et al: Randomized comparison of general and regional anesthesia for cesarean delivery in pregnancies complicated by severe preeclampsia. Obstet Gynecol 1995;86:193.

108. Hood D, Curry R: Spinal versus epidural anesthesia for cesarean section in severely preeclamptic patients: A retrospective survey. Anesthesiology 1999;90:1276.

109. Chestnut DH, Dewan D, Redick L, et al: Anesthetic management for obstetric hysterectomy: A multi-institutional study. Anesthesiology 1989;70:607.

110. Santos A, Tun E, Bobby P, et al: The effects of bupivacaine, L nitro-L-arginine-methyl-ester and phenylephrine on cardiovascular adaptations to asphyxia in the preterm fetal lamb. Anesth Analg1997;84:1299.

111. Morishima HO, Pedersen H, Snatos AS, et al: Adverse effects of maternally administered lidocaine on the asphyxiated preterm fetal lamb. Anesthesiology 1989;71:110.

112. Shnider SM, Webster G: Maternal and fetal hazards of surgery during pregnancy. Am J Obstet Gynecol 1965;92:891.

113. Brodsky J, Cohen E, Brown BJ, et al: Surgery during pregnancy and fetal outcome. Am J Obstet Gynecol 1980;138:1165.

114. Smith B: Fetal prognosis after anesthesia during gestation. Anesth Analg 1963;42:521.

115. Duncan P, Pope W, Cohen M, Greer N: Fetal risk of anesthesia and surgery during pregnancy. Anesthesiology 1986;64:790.

116. Heinonen O, Slone O, Shapiro S: Birth defects and drugs in pregnancy. In: *Birth Defects and Drugs in Pregnancy.* Publishing Sciences Group, 1977, pp. 516.

117. Grabowski C, Paar J: The teratogenic effects of graded doses of hypoxia on the chick embryo. Am J Anat 1958;103:313.

118. Saxen I, Saxen L: Association between maternal intake of diazepam and oral clefts. Lancet 1975;2:498.

119. Safra M, Oakley G: Association between cleft lip with or without cleft palate and prenatal exposure to diazepam. Lancet 1975;2:478.

120. Adamsons K, Mueller-Heubach E, Myers R: Production of fetal asphyxia in the rhesus monkey by administration of catecholamines to the mother. Am J Obstet Gynecol 1971;109:148.

Regional Anesthesia for Pediatric Surgery

54

Regional Anesthesia in Pediatric Patients

A. General Concepts

Santhanam Suresh, MD • Giorgio Ivani, MD

INTRODUCTION

Dating back to ancient Egypt of 2500 BC, regional anesthesia was emphasized for circumcision. Traditional Chinese medicine has touted the use of needles and acupuncture for pain management for centuries. August Bier reported in 1899 the first study on regional anesthesia in children. This was followed by a report by Bainbridge on the use of spinal anesthesia in children.[1] The use of caudal analgesia in children was described in the urology literature in the early 1930s.[2] In the past two decades, numerous studies have demonstrated the need for analgesia in newborn children and infants.[3] This

has resulted in significant changes and advances in clinical anesthesia care for infants, children, and adolescents. In particular, the decrease in stress has resulted in better outcomes in infants and children. Infants exposed to significant pain in the neonatal period may experience biobehavioral changes with advancing age.[4] This and other related research have led the medical community to improve analgesia in infants. Although research in regional anesthesia in adults continues to be performed and is written about prolifically in literature, there seems to be a relative lack of publications in regional anesthesia in children. Most work in regional anesthesia has been carried out by a few researchers with a firm commitment to the use of regional techniques in children. Although the usual dictum that children are just small adults may apply to regional analgesia in the adolescent population, it is much less applicable to infants and toddlers. The goal of this chapter is to provide general principles of practice of regional anesthesia in children.

Anatomic Differences Between Children & Adults

Significant anatomic variations exist between infants and older adolescents and adults. Differences in anatomy between children and adults are described in greater detail elsewhere in this chapter. CT-guided mechanisms and the use of other imaging techniques including ultrasound have led to a better understanding of the anatomy of infants and children.[5] This has facilitated a more accurate placement of needles in children with less risk of complications. The epidural space is superficial compared with that in adults, and this requires greater skill and care while placing a needle.[6] Numerous formulas are available for estimating the distance of the epidural space from the skin.[6] However, this should not alter the judgment of the skilled anesthesiologist placing a needle in the spinal or epidural space.

Assessment & Consent

Parents typically provide consent for a procedure for their child. However, if the child has the cognitive ability to discern right from wrong, it is suggested that the child's consent for performance of a regional technique be obtained as well.[7] There is growing debate as to when or what this age may be. We routinely obtain consent for children over the age of 12 years. If a child refuses to have a regional procedure despite the parents' insistence, it is important for the anesthesiologist to provide an alternative modality of pain relief.

Regional Anesthesia: Awake or Asleep?

Whether the patient should be kept awake or asleep during regional anesthesia has been a controversial area in adults, which has recently permeated into pediatric regional anesthesia practice. The difficulty in placing a regional block in a child is the inability of the child to cooperate as well as the cognitive inability of the child to relate to symptoms such as paresthesia or pain. We feel that the child is best provided with a regional technique under deep sedation or after induction of general anesthesia. Although still controversial in adults, this practice has been the consensus of pediatric anesthesiologists in the United States as well as abroad.[1,8] Prospective data collected from the French group demonstrated a very low incidence of regional anesthesia-related complications in children, with most of them being performed in children who were under general anesthesia.[9] In our practice, we attempt to place thoracic epidural catheters in the older children with response-titrated sedation. All other regional techniques are carried out under heavy sedation or under general anesthesia. As more regional techniques are being performed in children, we will have greater insight into associated complications.

Clinical Pearls

The following are considerations in children for regional anesthesia:

- It is mostly done with the patient asleep.
- The dose is far less than for adults (calculate in mg/kg).
- Look for changes in ECG rather than physiologic parameters to test dose.
- Always get patient consent if the child is older.
- Reported complications with regional anesthesia are far fewer in children than in adults.

Pharmacology of Local Anesthetics in Pediatric Patients

The two main classes of local anesthetics used in infants and children include the amino-amides (amides) and the amino-esters (esters). The amino-amides undergo enzymatic degradation by the liver, whereas the esters are hydrolyzed by plasma cholinesterases. These actions may play a very important role, particularly in neonates and infants.

Amides

These are the most commonly used local anesthetic solution in infants and children. The local anesthetics belonging to this class include lidocaine, bupivacaine, ropivacaine, and levobupivacaine. The choice of local anesthetic solution is based on the desired duration of local anesthetic action and the toxic effects of the local anesthetic solution that is used. Unlike in adult patients, neonates are not able to oxidize and reduce amide local anesthetic agents and hence differ vastly in their ability to reduce toxicity related to local anesthetics.[10,11] The conjugation of local anesthetics in the liver reaches peak adult levels at approximately 3 months of age.[12,13] Some local anesthetics can have higher blood concentrations in adolescents than in adults owing to increased vascular absorption[14]; hence, caution must be exercised in older children. Peak plasma concentrations are obtained in children in about 30 minutes after caudal blockade.[15] Although clearance is similar in older children and adolescents, the steady-state volume of distribution (Vd_{SS} is increased in children compared with that in adults.[16] All amide local anesthetics have been shown to have diminished clearance in neonates and infants younger than 3 months of age, with steady maturation until they reach adult clearance at about 8 months of age.[17] The risk of toxicity associated with repeated doses of local anesthetics is greater in children than in adults.[18] Amino–esters may have a rapid clearance in neonates.[19]

DOSING OF LOCAL ANESTHETICS IN PEDIATRIC PATIENTS

Most pediatric drug doses are based on the weight of the patient[60] (Table 54–1). However, this may not be applicable

Table 54–1.

Maximum Recommended Doses and Approximate Duration of Action of Commonly Used Local Anesthetic Agents

Local Anesthetic	Class	Max Dose (mg/kg)	Duration of Action (min)
Procaine	Ester	10	60–90
2-Chloroprocaine	Ester	20	30–60
Tetracaine	Ester	1.5	180–600
Lidocaine	Amide	7	90–200
Bupivacaine	Amide	2–4	180–600
Ropivacaine	Amide	2–4	180–600
Levobupivacaine	Amide	2–4	180–600

When used in IV regional anesthesia, the dose of lidocaine should be reduced to 3–5 mg/kg.

Table 54–2.

Systemic Toxicity of Local Anesthetic Solution

Central Nervous System

Dizziness and light-headedness
Visual and auditory disturbances
Muscle twitching and tremors
Generalized convulsions

Cardiovascular

Direct cardiac effects
Depressed rapid phase of repolarization of Purkinje fibers
Depressed spontaneous firing of the sinoatrial node
Negative inotropic effect on cardiac muscle
Calcium influx altered leading to decreased myocardial contractility

Effects on vascular tone
Low concentrations-vasoconstriction
High concentrations-vasodilatation
Increased pulmonary vascular resistance

to local anesthetic solution. Studies done on infants undergoing spinal anesthesia demonstrated a larger requirement of local anesthetic solution (weight-scaled) compared with their adult counterparts using bupivacaine or tetracaine.[20] However, studies on rat sciatic nerve models demonstrated similar trends in the neonatal, adolescent, and adult rat.[21]

Tachyphylaxis

Tachyphylaxis is a clinical phenomenon whereby repeated dosing of local anesthetics leads to decreasing effects. There seems to be a correlation between dosing intervals and the presence of pain; dosing intervals that are short enough to avoid breakthrough pain result in a lesser chance of tachyphylaxis.

Toxicity of Local Anesthetic Solutions

Toxicity of local anesthetics solutions includes cardiac, peripheral vascular, neurologic, and allergic reactions[60] (Table 54–2). Dose is always calculated in children on a milligram per kilogram basis rather than predicted volumes as in adult regional anesthesia. Children given local anesthetic solutions, particularly when used as continuous infusions, should be monitored continuously for adverse effects. Toxicity of local anesthetics in children include cardiovascular[22–24] and central nervous system toxicity[25] and allergic reactions to ester local anesthetic solutions. The risk of severe toxicity can be decreased by limiting the local anesthetic dosage in children[26] (see Table 54–2).

SPECIFICS OF LOCAL ANESTHETICS IN PEDIATRIC REGIONAL ANESTHESIA

Bupivacaine

Bupivacaine is the most commonly used local anesthetic solution in infants and children in North America. The pharmacokinetics and pharmacodynamics of bupivacaine have been well documented in the literature.[27,28] It is imperative for the surgeon to consider using a supplemental local anesthetic solution because the infiltration anesthesia adds to the total dosage of local anesthetic solution in the systemic circulation. The preferred concentration for children is 0.25–0.5% for peripheral nerve blocks and 0.1% for continuous infusions. Older children can tolerate a higher dose of local anesthetic solution (0.4 mg/kg/h) compared with neonates and infants (0.2 mg/kg/h).[18]

Metabolism: Bupivacaine is well bound to α-1 glycoprotein. Because of low levels of albumin and α-1 glycoprotein in neonates, the free fraction of bupivacaine may be greater, thereby leading to a greater risk of toxicity.[29] Bupivacaine is an isomer with both L- and D-enantiomer, the D-enantiomer causing most of the adverse effects that are seen in humans. The incidence of cardiac toxicity is greater than neurotoxicity in children. This is due to the concomitant use of general anesthesia, which masks the neurotoxicity; hence, cardiac toxicity is first seen with overdosing of local anesthetic or intravascular placement.

Dosage: The dosage of bupivacaine is limited to 2–4 mg/kg for a single-dose injection and 0.2–0.4 mg/kg for a continuous infusion. It is always judicious to use intermittent and slow bolus injections of bupivacaine to detect intravascular injection. A test dose with epinephrine-containing solution is often used. This facilitates detection of intravascular placement. Besides the use of the usual cardiovascular signs including increase in heart rate and blood pressure, the increasing amplitude of T waves is suggestive of intravascular placement.[30] This is particularly useful in infants whose baseline heart rate may be higher and in whom subtle increases to heart rate may go undetected.

Ropivacaine

Ropivacaine is a newer amide local anesthetic that is being used more frequently in pediatric surgery. It is an L-enantiomer with fewer cardiovascular and central nervous system side effects compared with bupivacaine. The lethal dose of ropivacaine in rats is higher than bupivacaine.[31] Ropivacaine in an equipotent dose may offer less of a motor block compared with that of bupivacaine.[32] Pediatric trials have demonstrated a longer duration of action with ropivacaine than with mepivacaine when used for peripheral nerve blockade.[33] Caution should be exercised while using ropivacaine in children as well, because cases of cardiovascular toxicity have been reported.[34]

Pharmacokinetics: Pharmacokinetic data are available in children on the use of ropivacaine in continuous infusions as well as for single-shot injections.[35–38,39] Although ropivacaine is safer in children owing to its L-enantiomer structure, caution must be exercised because complications from intravascular injections have been reported. α_1-Acid glycoprotein is an acute-phase reactant that increases in the phase of injury such as surgery. In neonates and infants, this response is not surmountable because of the decreased amount of α_1-acid glycoprotein. This facilitates the metabolism of local anesthetic solution. As a result, the free fraction of the local anesthetic is increased in the plasma,[39] which contributes to the greater toxicity of local anesthetics in infants and neonates compared with that in older children and adults.

Levobupivacaine

Levobupivacaine is a newer L-enantiomer with fewer adverse effects than bupivacaine. Pharmacokinetic data are available in children, and the dosage interval is not very different from that of bupivacaine.[40–43] The prevalent use of levobupivacaine is not seen in children owing to nonavailability of the drug in the United States.

Toxicity: Levobupivacaine has been shown to be less toxic in the animal model compared with bupivacaine.[44] Although this drug provides the practitioner with an option to use a drug that is less cardiotoxic, caution should be exercised in use of this drug and adequate care should be taken to avoid intravascular injection. Animal experiments have shown that levobupivacaine has less myocardial depression and a decreased incidence of inducing fatal dysrhythmias compared with bupivacaine.

ESTER-TYPE LOCAL ANESTHETICS

Ester local anesthetics differ from amide local anesthetics in that they are metabolized by plasma cholinesterases.[45–47] As a result, metabolism of ester local anesthetics depends on plasma cholinesterase levels.[48–51] Hence in populations with decreased plasma cholinesterase levels, such as neonates and infants, the plasma level of these drugs may be increased and lead to potentially toxic drug levels. The presence of plasma cholinesterase also limits the duration of activity of these drugs, leading to a shortened activity. The most common ester local anesthetics used in infants and children are chloroprocaine and tetracaine. These drugs, however, are not commonly used in children except as an adjuvant to spinal anesthesia in formerly premature infants undergoing spinal anesthesia or as the sole anesthetic solution for caudal analgesia.[52] Tetracaine is used for spinal anesthesia, especially in premature infants, as the sole anesthetic for inguinal hernia repair.[53] 2-Chloroprocaine has been used extensively in children for analgesia in the central neuraxial space.[54]

TOPICAL ANESTHESIA

It is important to discuss the use of topical anesthesia in children because it is commonly used in clinical practice to provide analgesia for intravenous catheter placements, lumbar punctures, and other invasive procedures in children. The most common preparations include lidocaine, tetracaine, benzocaine, and prilocaine. The topical anesthetic solution permeates through the skin to provide analgesia. The two most common preparations that are available include EMLA (**E**utectic **M**ixture of **L**ocal and **A**nesthetics) and LMX-4, a 4% liposomal lidocaine solution used as a topical anesthetic. Both drugs have undergone extensive trials and have been used in children for repeated painful procedures.[55–58] The introduction of other modalities for pain control including iontophoretic local anesthetic drug delivery can be used for pain control in simple procedures including intravenous catheter placements.[59]

SUMMARY

In summary, regional anesthesia in infants and children has been a well-established entity, although it remains vastly underutilized. Adequate education of the anesthesiology trainees on the use of regional anesthesia, its advantages, and its side effects are of paramount importance for its successful and safe application in the pediatric population.

References

1. Bainbridge W: Analgesia in children by spinal injection with a report of a new method of sterilization of the injection fluid. Med Rec 1900;58:937–940.
2. Campbell MF: Caudal analgesia in children and infants. J Urol 1933;30:245.

3. Anand KJ, Sippell WG, Aynsley-Green A: Randomised trial of fentanyl anaesthesia in preterm babies undergoing surgery: Effects on the stress response. Lancet 1987;1:62–66.

4. Taddio A, Katz J, Ilersich AL, Koren G: Effect of neonatal circumcision on pain response during subsequent routine vaccination [see comments]. Lancet 1997;349:599–503.

5. Marhofer P, Sitzwohl C, Greher M, Kapral S: Ultrasound guidance for infraclavicular brachial plexus anaesthesia in children. Anaesthesia 2004;59:642–646.

6. Suresh S, Wheeler M: Practical pediatric regional anesthesia. Anesthesiol Clin North Am 2002;20:83–113.

7. Tait AR, Voepel-Lewis T, Malviya S: Do they understand? (Part II): Assent of children participating in clinical anesthesia and surgery research. Anesthesiology 2003;98:609–614.

8. Krane EJ, Dalens BJ, Murat I, Murrell D: The safety of epidurals placed during general anesthesia. Reg Anesth Pain Med 1998;23:433–438.

9. Giaufre E, Dalens B, Gombert A: Epidemiology and morbidity of regional anesthesia in children: A one-year prospective survey of the French-Language Society of Pediatric Anesthesiologists. Anesth Analg 1996;83:904–912.

10. Besunder JB, Reed MD, Blumer JL: Principles of drug biodisposition in the neonate. A critical evaluation of the pharmacokinetic-pharmacodynamic interface (Part I). Clin Pharmacokinet 1988;14:189–216.

11. Besunder JB, Reed MD, Blumer JL: Principles of drug biodisposition in the neonate. A critical evaluation of the pharmacokinetic-pharmacodynamic interface (Part II). Clin Pharmacokinet 1988;14:261–286.

12. Rane A, Sjoqvist F: Drug metabolism in the human fetus and newborn infant. Pediatr Clin North Am 1972;19:37–49.

13. Levy G: Pharmacokinetics of fetal and neonatal exposure to drugs. Obstet Gynecol 1981;58:9S–16S.

14. Rothstein P, Arthur GR, Feldman HS, et al: Bupivacaine for intercostal nerve blocks in children: Blood concentrations and pharmacokinetics. Anesth Analg 1986;65:625–632.

15. Ecoffey C, Desparmet J, Maury M, et al: Bupivacaine in children: Pharmacokinetics following caudal anesthesia. Anesthesiology 1985;63:447–448.

16. Murat I, Montay G, Delleur MM, et al: Bupivacaine pharmacokinetics during epidural anaesthesia in children. Eur J Anaesthesiol 1988;5:113–120.

17. Mazoit JX, Denson DD, Samii K: Pharmacokinetics of bupivacaine following caudal anesthesia in infants. Anesthesiology 1988;68:387–391.

18. Berde CB: Toxicity of local anesthetics in infants and children. [Review]. J Pediatr 1993;122(Pt 2):S14–S20.

19. Henderson K, Sethna NF, Berde CB: Continuous caudal anesthesia for inguinal hernia repair in former preterm infants. J Clin Anesth 1993;5:129–133.

20. Frumiento C, Abajian JC, Vane DW: Spinal anesthesia for preterm infants undergoing inguinal hernia repair. Arch Surg 2000;135:445–451.

21. Kohane DS, Sankar WN, Shubina M, et al: Sciatic nerve blockade in infant, adolescent, and adult rats: A comparison of ropivacaine with bupivacaine. Anesthesiology 1998;89:1199–1208.

22. Kasten GW, Martin ST: Bupivacaine cardiovascular toxicity: Comparison of treatment with bretylium and lidocaine. Anesth Analg 1985;64:911–916.

23. Murat I, Esteve C, Montay G, et al: Pharmacokinetics and cardiovascular effects of bupivacaine during epidural anesthesia in children with Duchenne muscular dystrophy. Anesthesiology 1987;67:249–252.

24. Graf BM: The cardiotoxicity of local anesthetics: The place of ropivacaine. Curr Top Med Chem 2001;1:207–214.

25. Bergman BD, Hebl JR, Kent J, Horlocker TT: Neurologic complications of 405 consecutive continuous axillary catheters (table). Anesth Analg 2003;96:247–252.

26. Berde CB: Convulsions associated with pediatric regional anesthesia [editorial comment] [see comments]. Anesth Analg 1992;75:164–166.

27. Ecoffey C, Desparmet J, Maury M, et al: Bupivacaine in children: Pharmacokinetics following caudal anesthesia. Anesthesiology 1985;63:447–448.

28. Murat I, Montay G, Delleur MM, et al: Bupivacaine pharmacokinetics during epidural anaesthesia in children. Eur J Anaesthesiol 1988;5(2):113–120.

29. Ecoffey C, Desparmet J, Maury M, et al: Bupivacaine in children: Pharmacokinetics following caudal anesthesia. Anesthesiology 1985;63:447–448.

30. Freid EB BAVR: Electrocardiographic and hemodynamic changes associated with unintentional intravascular injection of bupivacaine with epinephrine in infants. Anesthesiology 1993;79:394–398.

31. Dony P, Dewinde V, Vanderick B, et al: The comparative toxicity of ropivacaine and bupivacaine at equipotent doses in rats. Anesth Analg 2000;91:1489–1492.

32. Da Conceicao MJ, Coelho L: Caudal anaesthesia with 0.375% ropivacaine or 0.375% bupivacaine in paediatric patients. Br J Anaesth 1998;80:507–508.

33. Fernandez-Guisasola J, Andueza A, Burgos E, et al: A comparison of 0.5% ropivacaine and 1% mepivacaine for sciatic nerve block in the popliteal fossa. Acta Anaesthesiol Scand 2001;45:967–970.

34. Petitjeans F, Mion G, Puidupin M, et al: Tachycardia and convulsions induced by accidental intravascular ropivacaine injection during sciatic block. Acta Anaesthesiol Scand 2002;46:616–617.

35. Ivani G, Mereto N, Lampugnani E, et al: Ropivacaine in paediatric surgery: Preliminary results. Paediatr Anaesth 1998;8:127–129.

36. Ivani G, Mazzarello G, Lampugnani E, et al: Ropivacaine for central blocks in children. Anaesthesia 1998;53:Suppl 6.

37. Ala-Kokko TI, Partanen A, Karinen J, et al: Pharmacokinetics of 0.2% ropivacaine and 0.2% bupivacaine following caudal blocks in children. Acta Anaesthesiol Scand 2000;44:1099–1102.

38. Dalens B, Ecoffey C, Joly A, et al: Pharmacokinetics and analgesic effect of ropivacaine following ilioinguinal/iliohypogastric nerve block in children. Paediatr Anaesth 2001;11:415–420.

39. Mazoit JX, Dalens BJ: Pharmacokinetics of local anaesthetics in infants and children. Clin Pharmacokinet 2004;43:17–32.

40. Ivani G, De Negri P, Lonnqvist PA, et al: A comparison of three different concentrations of levobupivacaine for caudal block in children (table). Anesth Analg 2003;97:368–371.

41. Lerman J, Nolan J, Eyres R, et al: Efficacy, safety, and pharmacokinetics of levobupivacaine with and without fentanyl after continuous epidural infusion in children: A multicenter trial. Anesthesiology 2003;99:1166–1174.

42. Ala-Kokko TI, Raiha E, Karinen J, et al: Pharmacokinetics of 0.5% levobupivacaine following ilioinguinal-iliohypogastric nerve blockade in children. Acta Anaesthesiol Scand 2005;49:397–400.

43. Foster RH, Markham A: Levobupivacaine: A review of its pharmacology and use as a local anaesthetic. Drugs 2000;59:551–579.

44. Mather LE, Huang YF, Veering B, Pryor ME: Systemic and regional pharmacokinetics of levobupivacaine and bupivacaine enantiomers in sheep. Anesth Analg 1998;86:805–811.

45. Tobias JD, O'Dell N: Chloroprocaine for epidural anesthesia in infants and children. AANA J 1995;63:131–135.

46. Raj PP, Ohlweiler D, Hitt BA, Denson DD: Kinetics of local anesthetic esters and the effects of adjuvant drugs on 2-chloroprocaine hydrolysis. Anesthesiology 1980;53:307–314.

47. Tobias JD, Rasmussen GE, Holcomb GW III, et al: Continuous caudal anaesthesia with chloroprocaine as an adjunct to general anaesthesia in neonates. Can J Anaesth 1996;43(1):69–72; 69–72.

48. Crowhust JA: Cholinesterase deficiency. Anaesth Intensive Care 1983;11:7–9.

49. Kuhnert BR, Philipson EH, Pimental R, Kuhnert PM: A prolonged chloroprocaine epidural block in a postpartum patient with abnormal pseudocholinesterase. Anesthesiology 1982;56:477–478.

50. Monedero P, Hess P: High epidural block with chloroprocaine in a parturient with low pseudocholinesterase activity. Can J Anaesth 2001;48:318–319.

51. Kuhnert BR, Kuhnert PM, Prochaska AL, Gross TL: Plasma levels of 2-chloroprocaine in obstetric patients and their neonates after epidural anesthesia. Anesthesiology 1980;53: 21–25.

52. Henderson K, Sethna NF, Berde CB: Continuous caudal anesthesia for inguinal hernia repair in former preterm infants. J Clin Anesth 1993;5:129–133.

53. Krane EJ, Haberkern CM, Jacobson LE: Postoperative apnea, brady-cardia, and oxygen desaturation in formerly premature infants: Prospective comparison of spinal and general anesthesia. Anesth Analg 1995;80:7–13.

54. Henderson K, Sethna NF, Berde CB: Continuous caudal anesthesia for inguinal hernia repair in former preterm infants. J Clin Anesth 1993;5:129–133.

55. Acharya AB, Bustani PC, Phillips JD, et al: Randomised controlled trial of eutectic mixture of local anaesthetics cream for venipunc-ture in healthy preterm infants. Arch Dis Child Fetal Neonatal Ed 1998;78:F138–F142.

56. Benini F, Johnston CC, Faucher D, Aranda JV: Topical anesthesia during circumcision in newborn infants. JAMA 1993;270:850–853.

57. Gourrier E, Karoubi P, el Hanache A, et al: Use of EMLA cream in a department of neonatology. Pain 1996;68:431–434.

58. Eichenfield LF, Funk A, Fallon-Friedlander S, Cunningham BB: A clinical study to evaluate the efficacy of ELA-Max (4% liposomal lidocaine) as compared with eutectic mixture of local anesthetics cream for pain reduction of venipuncture in children. Pediatrics 2002;109:1093–1099.

59. Sethna NF, Verghese ST, Hannallah RS, Solodiuk JC, Zurakowski D, Berde CB: A randomized controlled trial to evaluate S-Caine patch for reducing pain associated with vascular access in children. Anes-thesiology 2005;102:403–408.

60. Suresh S, Cote CJ: Local anesthetics for infants and children. In: Yaffe SJ, Aranda JV (editors): *Neonatal and Pediatric Pharmacology, Therapeutic Principles in Practice,* 3rd ed. Lippincott Williams & Wilkins, 2004, pp. 663–668.

B. Pediatric Epidural & Caudal Analgesia & Anesthesia

Ban C.H. Tsui, MD • Michael Fredrickson, MD • Santhanam Suresh, MD

EPIDURAL BLOCKADE TECHNIQUE FOR PEDIATRIC SURGERY (TECHNICAL)

Introduction

Epidural analgesia has many beneficial effects in the pediatric patient population. In clinical practice, it is commonly used to augment general anesthesia and to manage postoperative pain. Effective postoperative pain relief from epidural analgesia has numerous benefits including earlier ambulation, rapid weaning from ventilators, reduced time spent in a catabolic state and lowered circulating stress hormone levels.[1] Precise placement of epidural needles and catheters for single-shot and continuous epidural anesthesia ensures that the dermatomes involved in the surgical procedure are selectively blocked, allowing for lower doses of local anesthetics and sparing of unnecessary blockade in the regions where blockade is not desired.[2–4]

Anatomic Considerations

Significant anatomic differences in children compared with adults should be considered in using regional anesthesia in children. For instance, in neonates and infants, the conus medullaris is located lower in the spinal column (at approximately the L3 vertebra) compared with that in adults, in whom it is situated at approximately the L1 vertebra. This dissimilarity is a result of different rates of growth between the spinal cord and the bony vertebral column in infants. However, at approximately 1 year of age the conus medullaris reaches an L1 level similar to that in an adult.

The sacrum of children is also more narrow and flat compared with that in the adult population. At birth, the sacral plate, which is formed by five sacral vertebrae, is not completely ossified and continues to fuse until the child is approximately 8 years of age. The incomplete fusion of the sacral vertebral arch forms the sacral hiatus. The caudal epidural space can be accessed easily in infants and children through the sacral hiatus. Because of the continuous development of the sacral canal roof, there is considerable variation in the sacral hiatus. In children, the sacral hiatus is located more cephalad compared with that in adults. Therefore, caution is warranted when placing caudal blocks in infants because the dura may end more caudad and thereby increase the risk of accidental dural puncture.

It has also been suggested that the epidural fat is less densely packed in children than in adults.[5] This loosely packed epidural fat may not only facilitate the spread of local anesthetic, but it may also allow the unimpeded advancement of epidural catheters from the caudal epidural space to the lumbar and thoracic levels.

Clinical Pearls

 In the neonate, the intercristal line bisects L5 (compare L4 or L3-4 interspace in the adult), and the spinal cord ends at L3 in first year of life (compare L1 in the adult).

 As a general rule the epidural space is found at 1 mm/kg of body weight; however, there is considerable individual variation.

Considerations for Choosing Local Anesthetic Solutions for Epidural & Caudal Anesthesia & Analgesia

Newer local anesthetics with favorable potencies, durations of effect, and decreased toxicity profiles have been introduced in the past decade. Local anesthetic concentration and volume are important factors in determining the density and level of blockade. Because most pediatric patients receive epidural analgesia in conjunction with a general anesthetic, the main purpose of the epidural catheter is to deliver sufficient local anesthetic solution for effective intraoperative and postoperative analgesia. Knowledge of total drug dose is important to avoid local anesthetic toxicity, particularly in pediatric patients.

Clinical Pearls

- High concentrations of local anesthetics such as 0.5% bupivacaine or 0.5% ropivacaine are rarely used in the pediatric population.
- Instead, larger volumes of more dilute local anesthetic are more commonly used to cover multiple dermatomes.

A more detailed description of local anesthetic solutions, their characteristics and toxic potential has been described in Chapters 6 and 7. As a general rule, however, high concentrations of local anesthetics such as 0.5% bupivacaine or 0.5% ropivacaine are seldom used in pediatric populations, particularly in the epidural space. Instead, larger volumes of more dilute local anesthetic are more commonly used to cover multiple dermatomes. Opioids prolong the duration of analgesia of local anesthetic, but have also been associated with unacceptable side effects, particularly in pediatric outpatients. Various nonopioid adjuncts such as clonidine and α_2-agonists offer more favorable side-effect profiles; however, relatively little information is available regarding their use pediatric patients.

Selection of Epidural Local Anesthetic Solutions

Clinical Pearls

- In the pediatric population, body weight is a better correlate than patient age in predicting spread of local anesthetic after a caudal block.
- For caudal use, the optimum concentration of bupivacaine is 0.125–0.175%.
- The maximal safe dose of bupivacaine is 2.5–4 mg/kg.
- For continuous epidural infusion, bupivacaine 0.2 mg/kg/h for neonates, and 0.4 mg/kg/h for older children is often used.

- For a single-shot caudal block, a bolus of 1 mL/kg of 0.2% ropivacaine is recommended.
- A continuous infusion of ropivacaine 0.2 mg/kg/h of 0.1% in infants and 0.4 mg/kg/h in older children for 48 hours has been shown to be an effective and safe regimen.

Bupivacaine and ropivacaine are the two most commonly used local anesthetics for neuraxial anesthesia in children. Lidocaine is not often used because of its short duration of action and excessive motor block. Body weight is usually a better correlate than patient age in predicting spread of local anesthetic after a caudal block.[6] The maximal safe dose of bupivacaine is 2.5–4 mg/kg.[7] For caudal use, the optimum concentration of bupivacaine is 0.125–0.175%.[9] Compared with the 0.25% preparation, this concentration provides a similar duration of postoperative analgesia (4–8 hours) but with less motor blockade.[8] Some clinicians prefer administering doses on a volume-per-weight basis. A dose of 1.0 mL/kg of a dilute solution such as 0.125% bupivacaine to a maximum volume of 30 mL can reliably provide T10 sensory block without exceeding maximum levels recommended in the literature.[9] Higher doses such as 1.25 mL/kg, or even 1.5 mL/kg, may be administered to provide a more cephalad block without the risk of local anesthetic toxicity.[9] For continuous epidural infusion, a commonly accepted dosage guideline of bupivacaine is 0.2 mg/kg/h for neonates and 0.4 mg/kg/h for older children.[10] Cumulative toxicity is a concern even at lower rates of local anesthetic solution infusions.[3] The alternate use of 2-chloroprocaine may be well tolerated by neonates.[11]

Newer local anesthetic agents include the L-enantiomers ropivacaine and levobupivacaine. Ropivacaine has a higher therapeutic index than the older local anesthetic bupivacaine.[12–15] At low concentrations, ropivacaine may produce less motor block and comparable analgesia when compared with bupivacaine with a decreased incidence of cardiac and central nervous system toxicity.[9] Because of its possible vasoconstricting properties, ropivacaine may undergo slower systemic absorption than bupivacaine.[16,17] This may have clinical implications when a prolonged local anesthetic infusion is used in children with impaired hepatic function.[18] For a single-shot caudal block, a bolus of 1 mL/kg of 0.2% ropivacaine is recommended.[19,20] An infusion of 0.1% ropivacaine at 0.2 mg/kg/h in infants and 0.4 mg/kg/h in older children lasting no longer than 48 hours has also been shown to be effective and safe.[20]

Levobupivacaine, the $S(-)$-isomer of bupivacaine, is less likely to cause myocardial depression and fatal arrhythmias and is also less toxic to the central nervous system than racemic bupivacaine. A dose of 0.8 mL/kg of 0.25% levobupivacine injected caudally provides analgesia in children having penile or groin surgery.[21] For continuous epidural infusions, the dose for levobupivacaine is similar to that for racemic bupivacaine.[10]

Adjuvants to Local Anesthetic Solutions

Adjuvants may be used to prolong the duration of blockade, particularly for single-shot caudal epidural blocks.[22] Single-shot caudal block is used mainly for ambulatory surgery. The major problem associated with this technique is the limited duration of analgesia and unwanted motor blockade. Recent research has focused on trying to resolve these problems with the addition of various adjuvants.

Epinephrine

The most commonly used adjuvant for single-shot caudal anesthesia is epinephrine in a concentration of 1:200,000. Epinephrine has the added benefit of serving as a marker for an inadvertent intravascular injection.

Opioids

Epidural opioids may enhance and prolong analgesia. However, opioid use in an ambulatory setting may not be advisable because of the potential for respiratory depression and other unfavorable side effects (eg, nausea and vomiting, itching, urinary retention).[7] As a result, the use of caudal epidural opioids in children should be restricted to special clinical situations.[23–25] Fentanyl has been used with desirable effects for epidural analgesia in adults for a number of years. Whether there is benefit for fentanyl as an additive in children undergoing single-shot caudal blockade is still debated amongst clinicians.[26,27] One study found an increased incidence of nausea and vomiting when fentanyl was added to the local anesthetic solution for a single-shot caudal block.[27] A dose of 2 mcg/kg of fentanyl for single-shot caudal anesthesia along with the standard local anesthetic solution has been recommended for more extensive or painful procedures or in patients who have a urinary catheter in the postoperative period. The addition of 1 mcg/mL to 2 mcg/mL of fentanyl to 0.1% bupivacaine for continuous epidural infusions has also been used with success in neonates and children in a well-monitored inpatient setting.[28]

Clonidine

Clonidine, an α_1-agonist, acts by stimulating descending noradrenergic medullospinal pathways; this inhibits the release of nociceptive neurotransmitters in the dorsal horn of the spinal cord. The addition of clonidine (1–5 mcg/kg) can improve the analgesic effect of local anesthetics for single-shot caudal blockade as well as prolong its duration of action without the unwanted side effects of epidural opioids.[29] For continuous epidural infusions, clonidine 0.1 mcg/kg/h has been used with good effect.[30] It should be cautioned that higher doses have been associated with sedation and hemodynamic instability in the form of hypotension and bradycardia, and doses as low as 2 mcg/kg have been associated with postoperative sedation.[31] In addition, epidural clonidine blunts the ventilatory response to increasing levels of end-tidal carbon dioxide (P_{CO_2}). Although respiratory depression does not appear to be a common problem,[32] apnea has been reported in a term neonate who received a caudal block consisting of 1 mL/kg of

0.2% ropivacaine with clonidine 2 mcg/kg.[33] Caution should be exercised while using clonidine in very young infants because of the sedation and hypotension that may ensue.

Ketamine

The addition of ketamine or *S*-ketamine to single-shot caudal block prolongs the analgesic effect of local anesthetics. The main disadvantages of ketamine are its psychomimetic effects. However, at low doses (0.25–0.5 mg/kg), ketamine is effective without noticeable behavioral side effects.[29] Ketamine 1 mg/kg can also be used as an effective caudal analgesic solely without the addition of local anesthetic solution.[34,35] The combination of *S*(+)-ketamine (0.5–1 mg/kg) and clonidine (1 or 2 mcg/kg) has been shown to provide effective analgesia after inguinal herniotomy in children with prolonged duration of effect (>20 hours) without any adverse CNS effects or motor impairment.[35,36] However, the safety of ketamine for central neuraxial block has been questioned, particularly with the racemic formulations that contain preservatives. Results from a small clinical trial and case series indicate that a single-bolus administration of preservative-free *S*-ketamine appears to be safe and effective.[7,10] Regardless, these reports lack statistical power and detailed postoperative evaluations to draw definitive conclusions regarding the safety of ketamine for neuraxial use. An additional concern regarding use of ketamine in neonates relates to a controversial series of animal studies suggesting that ketamine can produce apoptotic neurodegeneration in the developing brain.[37,38] Other infant animal studies have demonstrated that ketamine may have a neuroprotective effect.[39,40] Nevertheless, many anesthesiologists are hesitant to introduce caudal *S*-ketamine into their routine clinical practice, and ketamine is unlikely to be widely adopted in countries where preservative-free formulas are not available.

Midazolam

Epidural midazolam (50 mcg/kg), when used alone, produces postoperative analgesia without motor weakness or behavioral changes.[29] This is due to its ability to inhibit GABA receptors in the spinal cord. When added to local anesthetic solutions, midazolam can prolong the duration of analgesia, but this effect has not been consistently demonstrated.[41] The safety of midazolam for neuraxial use, similar to that of ketamine has not been established, and a preservative-free formulation is not universally available.[7]

Neostigmine

Neostigmine (2 mcg/kg) alone produces postoperative analgesia by inhibiting the breakdown of acetylcholine at muscarinic receptors in the dorsal horn.[1] When combined with bupivacaine, a significant synergistic effect is observed. The addition of neostigmine (2 mcg/kg) to 0.25% bupivacaine prolongs the duration of analgesia from 5 to 20 hours after hypospadias repair.[1,42] However, it is associated with an unacceptably high incidence of vomiting (20–30%).[42] This likely precludes its use particularly in an ambulatory setting.

Preservative–free neostigmine has not been widely available and has limited applications in pediatric regional anesthesia.

Complications Associated with Epidural and Caudal Analgesia

Neurologic Injury

Major complications from either single-shot or continuous epidural blocks are rare if proper technique is used.[43,44] A large prospective study, which summarized data from over 15,000 central blocks in children, reported no incidence of permanent neurologic injuries and concluded that the incidence of complications is rare.[45] However, three infant deaths and two other incidences of paraplegia and quadriplegia were reported in another large retrospective report published in 1995 with over 24,000 epidural blocks in children.[46] This study also reported two cases of transient paresthesia.[46] Although the overall risk seems very low, devastating complications from direct damage to the spinal cord can occur during direct thoracic and high lumbar epidural needle placement. Because the placement of epidural needles/catheters is usually performed with the patient under sedation or general anesthesia, the fact that unconscious patients are unable to report pain or paresthesias (the currently accepted warning sign of needle encroachment on the spinal cord) raises concern.[47–50] Recently, a case report described a spinal cord injury after placing single shot thoracic epidural under general anesthesia for appendectomy.[51] This case report highlights the need for clinicians to routinely assess risk/benefit ratio of placing direct thoracic epidurals for less extensive surgery. Thoracic and high lumbar epidural catheter placement in particular should be limited to extensive thoracic and abdominal procedures and should be performed by anesthesiologists with experience in thoracic epidural placement. Before using a direct thoracic approach in patients younger than 2 years old, some prefer to make an attempt to thread the epidural catheter from the lumbar or caudal space with a proper epidural confirmation technique.

Epidural Hematoma

Epidural hematoma associated with epidural analgesia is extremely rare. This may be because anticoagulation protocols are rarely indicated during the perioperative period in pediatric patients, Nonetheless, epidural analgesia should be avoided in patients with clinically significant coagulopathy or thrombocytopenia. The guidelines for use of epidural anesthesia in anticoagulated adult patients should probably also be applied in pediatric patients.

Infection

Compared with lumbar epidural catheters, there is some concern regarding catheter infection with the prolonged use of caudally placed catheters owing to the proximity of the sacral hiatus to the rectum. Although studies have not found clinical evidence of higher infection rates with the caudal approach, bacterial colonization has been reported as higher. *Staphylococcus epidermidis* is the predominant microorganism colonized on the skin and catheters of lumbar and caudal epidurals.[52] Gram-negative bacteria have also been demonstrated on the tips of the caudal catheter.[52] Although the overall infection rate associated with caudal epidural catheters appears to be low, isolated case reports exist of infection related to epidural catheters in children. Even with widely used single-shot caudal blocks, infection such as sacral osteomyelitis can still occur.[53]

Perforation of the rectum may occur if the caudal needle is angled too steeply.[54] To reduce the risk of contamination by stool and urine, techniques such as catheter tunneling and fixing the catheter with occlusive dressing in a cephalad direction can be used.[28,55] A strict aseptic technique including the use of a sterile closed-infusion system should also be used, and care should be taken to avoid local tissue trauma. Daily inspection of the dressing and entry site are also important.

Dural Puncture and Postdural Headache

Dural puncture during caudal epidural analgesia is uncommon if caution is taken to avoid advancing the needle too far into the sacral canal. Treatment for postdural puncture headache (PDPH) includes bed rest, oral or intravenous hydration, simple analgesia such as regular acetaminophen, nonsteroidal antiinflammatory agents, and antiemetics. Bed rest, although relieving the severity of the headache, has no effect on the incidence or duration of PDPH. Hydration should be maintained to continue cerebrospinal fluid production and to avoid dehydration, which may alleviate symptoms. Simple analgesics may be all that is required until there is spontaneous resolution of symptoms.

In adults, caffeine has been used for both prophylaxis and treatment for PDPH. Caffeine causes cerebral vasoconstriction by blocking adenosine receptors, which dilate vessels when activated. Reducing cerebral blood flow decreases the amount of blood in the brain and may lessen the traction on pain-sensitive intracranial structures, relieving PDPH.[56] Caffeine is not frequently used in children for relief of PDPH, and an optimal dose is not known. Side effects are usually mild and may include nausea, insomnia, restlessness, and lightheadedness.

The use of epidural blood patch to treat PDPH has been used with success in adults since 1960.[57] There are now many reports of its successful use in children as well.[57] An epidural blood patch is thought to be effective through the formation of a gelatinous cover over the dural hole by the injected blood. In the short term, the epidural blood patch seals the hole and relieves cerebrospinal fluid hypotension both by mass effect from cerebrospinal fluid cranial displacement and by increasing the intracranial volume and pressure.[58] Actual healing takes place over the longer term. In children, it is recommended that approximately 0.3 mL/kg is injected in the awake or mildly sedated patient, if possible, to detect the appearance of radicular symptoms.

Hemodynamic Effects and Total Spinal Anesthesia

Significant changes in blood pressure are uncommon in pediatric patients after the proper administration epidural analgesia. A high sympathetic single-shot caudal block to

Table 54–3.

Test-Dosing for Epidural Blockade

Recommendations

1. Use test dosing routinely, even while recognizing that test dosing with all available agents is not 100% sensitive. In addition, because the true incidence of intravascular placement is relatively low, most of the positive tests (heart rate increases) will be false-positives. When there is a borderline response, repeating the test dose may increase the specificity and sensitivity.

2. Continuously monitor the ECG and cycle the blood pressure cuff repeatedly. With epinephrine-containing solutions, if the heart rate does not increase, an increase in blood pressure should also raise suspicion of intravascular placement.

3. Avoid performing test dosing when the child is in a very light plane of anesthesia or when there is stimulation (eg, repositioning the patient on the operating table, instrumentation of the airway, incision). Performing the test dose under these conditions increases the likelihood of false-positive, stimulation-induced increases in heart rate or blood pressure.

4. After the test dose, the remainder of the full dose should be administered incrementally. Incremental dosing and continuous monitoring helps increase the odds that intravascular placement will be detected, and further injection will be halted before full cardiodepressant doses are administered.

5. Selective α_1-antagonists such as tamsulosine.

6. Substitute clonidine for opioids in the epidural infusion.

Adapted with permission from Tsui B, Berde C: Caudal analgesia and anesthesia techniques in children. Curr Opin Anaesthesiol 2005, 18:283–288.

T6 evoked no significant changes in heart rate, cardiac index, or blood pressure in children.[59,60] Even when thoracic epidural block is combined with general anesthesia, cardiovascular stability is usually maintained in otherwise healthy pediatric patients. Hypotension should prompt anesthesiologists to immediately rule out a total spinal and/or intravascular injection leading to local anesthetic toxicity. After these complications are ruled out, other causes such as hydration status, intravascular filling pressure, inotropic state, and the depth of anesthesia should be assessed. If a total spinal occurs, supportive measures must be provided until the effect of the block has dissipated. However, in the event of life-threatening extensions of total spinals and if attempted supportive measures are neither effective nor an option, cerebrospinal lavage can be considered as a last maneuver. A recent case report, suggested that 20–30 mL of cerebrospinal fluid can be withdrawn and replaced with 30 to 40 mL of preservative-free normal saline, Ringer's lactate or Plasma-lyte via the epidural catheter.[61] This intervention may shorten the recovery times, minimize potential neurotoxic insult, and reduce the incidence of postdural puncture. In light of the limited experiences and information on cerebrospinal lavage, the potential risks and benefits should be evaluated on a case-by-case basis before using this technique.

Local Anesthetic Toxicity

Local anesthetic toxicity often stems from accidental intravascular injection into epidural blood vessels. This complication can often be avoided by using careful aspiration and test dosing (Table 54–3).

For single-shot caudal, toxicity is more likely to occur when needles are advanced too far into the caudal canal

or when sharp-tipped needles are used.[62] For continuous epidural infusion, neonates and very young infants are at greater risk for local anesthetic toxicity.[3] Seizures have been reported in children receiving continuous infusions of local anesthetics.[2,63] This can be avoided by using dilute solutions of local anesthetics ($\leq 0.125\%$ bupivacaine) and by following current dosing recommendations (see local anesthetic section).[64] More important, vigilant monitoring during the administration of epidural analgesia should be a priority.

Other Adverse Effects

In a retrospective review based on a prospective collected data from 286 pediatric patients; pruritus (26.1%), nausea and vomiting (16.9%), and urinary retention (20.8%) were the most common side effects encountered during epidural anesthesia using an infusion of bupivacaine and fentanyl infusion.[28] Sedation and excessive block each occurred in less than 2% of patients. The incidence of respiratory depression was 4.2%, but the administration of naloxone for severe respiratory depression was never necessary. Table 54–4 summarizes the recommended treatment for the common adverse effects.

EPIDURAL BLOCKADE FOR PEDIATRIC SURGERY (TECHNICAL)

Epidural analgesia can be delivered via a single-shot or continuous-infusion technique. These needles and catheter can be inserted at the caudal, lumbar, or thoracic level. Aspiration tests and test doses indicate possible inadvertent intravascular or intrathecal needle/catheter placement. Other

Table 54–4.

Side Effects of Epidural Analgesia and Suggested Treatment

Itching

1. Exclude and/or fix other remediable causes
2. Low-dose naloxone infusions or partial agonist-antagonists (nalbuphine) are both more effective and less sedating than antihistamines
3. If itching persists despite naloxone or nalbuphine, consider substituting clonidine for opioid in the epidural infusion

Nausea

1. Exclude and/or fix other remediable causes
2. 5-HT Antagonists, eg, ondansetron, dolasetron
3. Low-dose naloxone infusions or nalbuphine
4. Substitute clonidine for opioids in epidural infusion

Ileus and Bowel Dysfunction

1. Exclude and/or fix other remediable causes
2. Give laxatives, if not otherwise contraindicated
3. Substitute clonidine for opioids in epidural infusion
4. Low-dose naloxone infusions or nalbuphine
5. Peripherally or enterally constrained opioid antagonists, including methylnaltrexone or alvimopan (investigational)

Sedation or Hypoventilation

Exclude and/or fix other remediable causes:

1. Depending on severity, reduce or hold dosing of opioids or clonidine
2. Awaken, stimulate, encourage deep breathing
3. If severe, consider naloxone or assisted ventilation as needed

Urinary Retention

1. Exclude and/or fix other remediable causes
2. Avoid use of anticholinergics or antihistaminics if alternatives are available
3. Low-dose naloxone infusions or nalbuphine
4. Bladder catheterization

Adapted with permission from Tsui B, Berde C: Caudal analgesia and anesthesia techniques in children. Curr Opin Anaesthesiol 2005, 18:283–288.

advances in the field of epidural analgesia have focused on accurately positioning continuous epidural catheters. Epidural stimulation, epidural ECG, and ultrasound techniques have been developed in addition to conventional x-ray imaging to assist with accurate epidural needle/catheter placement.

Confirmation of Proper Epidural Needle/Catheter Placement

Aspiration/Test Dose

An aspiration test performed before local anesthetic injection is used to avoid a total spinal and intravascular injection.

Table 54–5.

Confirmation of the Epidural Catheter Position

Intraoperatively (while the patient is under general anesthesia)

1. Radiography with contrast
2. Electrical stimulation
3. ECG
4. Ultrasonography (infant)

Postoperatively (while the patient is awake, whether or not they can give verbal responses)

1. Electrical stimulation
2. Radiography with contrast
3. Chloroprocaine test: Incremental dosing of chloroprocaine 3% solution to demonstrate analgesia (by self-report or behavioral measures as appropriate) *and* signs of segmental effect
   a. Lumbar catheter tip:
      – At least partial sensory and motor blockade in both legs
      – Warming of the volar surface of the toes
   b. Lower thoracic catheter tip:
      – Reduced strength in hip flexion
      – Reduced abdominal skin reflexes
      – Some reduction in heart rate and blood pressure
   c. Upper thoracic catheter tip:
      – Some reduction in heart rate and blood pressure
      – Warming of the volar surface of the hands
      – Unilateral or bilateral Horner syndrome

Dosing is given in four increments at 60-second intervals according to body weight:

0–10 kg	0.2 mL/kg increments (0.8 mL/kg total)
10–25 kg	0.15 mL/kg increments (0.6 mL/kg total)
25–40 kg	0.1 mL/kg increments (0.4 mL/kg total)
>40 kg	0.075 mL/kg increments (0.3 mL/kg total, to a maximum of 20 mL)

Adapted with permission from Tsui B, Berde C: Caudal analgesia and anesthesia techniques in children. Curr Opin Anaesthesiol 2005, 18:283–288.

However, a negative aspiration of blood or cerebrospinal fluid should not be considered as an absolute indicator of proper needle and catheter placement.[9] The specificity of ECG changes (ie, >25% increase in T wave) after the injection of an epinephrine test dose (0.5 mcg/kg), on the other hand, can help predict intravascular injection.[10,65] When used, the ECG should be continuously monitored while injecting local anesthetic via the caudal space (Table 54–5).

Radiographic Methods

X-ray imaging in conjunction with a contrasting agent precisely identifies the tip of the catheter at a specific spinal level.[66] However, without contrast, a radiograph cannot distinguish inadvertent intrathecal or subdural catheter placement from proper epidural placement. In addition, standard x-ray does not allow the anesthesiologist to adjust the position of the catheter during insertion unless fluoroscopy is used. Although fluoroscopy permits the real-time monitoring and adjustment of advancing catheters, it requires additional set-up, incurs increased expense, and increases a patient's exposure to ionizing radiation. As a result, fluoroscopy is not routinely used and is usually limited to difficult and/or special circumstances such as long-term epidural catheter placement for cancer pain.

Ultrasound-Guided Techniques

Ultrasound allows the real-time visualization of anatomic structures and offers the potential to guide epidural needle and catheter placement. Ultrasound can be beneficial for guiding peripheral nerve block placement in both in adult patients,[67,68] and in children. Although the images produced by ultrasound can be used to guide caudal needle placement, they may be of limited value in older children.[69,70] Calcification of the posterior vertebral bodies in children older than 6 months prevents reliable imaging of the spinal cord.[70] At the present time, ultrasound guidance can be helpful for caudal and epidural blocks only in infants and small children, because the sacrum and vertebrae are not fully ossified.

Epidural Stimulation Test

Recently, low-current electrical stimulation has been suggested to monitor and guide the position of the of the epidural catheter during insertion.[28,71] The epidural stimulation test (Table 54–6) can be used to confirm the epidural catheter placement through stimulation of the spinal nerve roots (not the spinal cord) with low electrical current conducted through normal saline in the epidural space via an electrically conducting catheter.[71]

The stimulating catheter set-up requires the cathode lead (*black* for *block*) of the nerve stimulator to be connected to the epidural catheter via an electrode adapter while the anode lead is connected to an electrode on patient's skin as the

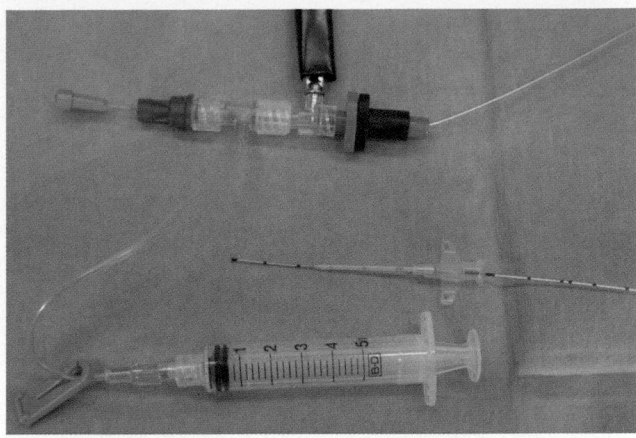

Figure 54–1. Epidural stimulation test. Equipment. The stimulating catheter set-up requires the cathode lead (*black* for *block*) of the nerve stimulator to be connected to the epidural catheter via an electrode adapter while the anode lead is connected to an electrode on patient's skin as the grounding site.

grounding site (Figure 54–1). To avoid misinterpretation of the stimulation response (eg, local muscle contraction may be confused with epidural stimulation), the ground electrode is placed on the lower extremity for thoracic epidurals and on the upper extremity for lumbar epidurals. Correct placement of the epidural catheter tip (1–2 cm from the nerve roots) is indicated by a motor response elicited with a current between 1 and 10 mA.[71–73] A motor response observed with a significantly lower threshold current (<1 mA) suggests that the catheter is in the subarachnoid or subdural space, or is in close proximity to a nerve root.[74,75] In these (rare) cases, a motor response is elicited with a significantly lower threshold current because the stimulating catheter may be very close (<1 cm) to the nerve roots or because it may be in direct contact with highly conductive cerebrospinal fluid.

Although chronic spinal cord stimulation is a safe and effective means of pain management,[76–79] the safety of this epidural stimulation test is not completely known. However,

Table 54–6.

Electrical Stimulation Test

Catheter Location	Motor Response	Current
Subcutaneous	None	>10 mA
Subdural	Bilateral (many segments)	<1 mA
Subarachnoid	Unilateral or bilateral	<1 mA
Epidural space		
Against nerve root	Unilateral	<1 mA
Nonintravascular	Unilateral or bilateral	1–10 mA (threshold current increase after local anesthetic injected)
Intravascular	Unilateral or bilateral	1–10 mA (no change in threshold current after local anesthetic injected)

it is anticipated that the risk of a brief intermittent electrical stimulation used in this test would be even lower than the risk of chronic epidural stimulation used in long-term pain management. In addition, epidural stimulation uses milliamperes (mA) within the range used for patients with chronic pain disorders (4–30 mA)[80] and for intraoperative monitoring during spinal surgery (2–40 mA).[81–83] Although no known complications or patient discomfort have resulted from the epidural stimulation test, it has been recommended to keep the current below 15 mA and the stimulation time as brief as possible.[28,71,73,84] In particular, the current output must be carefully increased from zero and stopped once motor activity is visible to ensure that all motor responses, even those elicited with low current (<1 mA), are detected. The nerve stimulator must be sensitive enough to allow a gradual increase in current output to at least 10 mA. Note that most nerve stimulators currently manufactured for electrolocation of peripheral nerves do not deliver currents greater than 5 mA and therefore are not ideally suited for epidural stimulation.

Pediatric Epidural Stimulation Catheter

A thin metal stylet is essential for effective threading of the epidural catheter from a lower spinal level to the target upper spinal level. A styletted catheter has a soft and flexible tip and is made from a soft polyurethane polymer.[28,85] The stylet of the epidural catheter ends 10 mm proximal to the tip, which allows the tip of the catheter to fold back on itself in a J configuration during insertion (Arrow International). This feature allows retention of the soft and blunted tip of the catheter, while the stylet wire provides stiffness for ease of advancement within the epidural space.

For monitoring advancement, elicited muscle twitches are observed from the lower limbs to the intercostal muscles as the catheter is advanced cranially. This minimizes the concerns of the catheter coiling or kinking by immediately

identifying these events at the time of insertion, allowing for any necessary adjustments.[28,85] The absence of muscle twitches or resistance to the advancing epidural catheter may be indicative of a curled or kinked catheter.

The epidural stimulation test relies on a small electrical current being transmitted through a conducting fluid injected into the epidural space. An ionic solution such as normal saline is used as the priming solution for the catheter. Normal saline dissociates into ions that are sufficient for effective electrical conduction over a short distance. The long length of the epidural catheter or any air lock within its lumen increases the resistance to current flow. Consequently, the lumen of the catheter must contain a metal element to reduce the impedance of the conducting solutions and to ensure proper conduction of electricity through the entire length of the catheter.[71–73,86] Many commercial epidural catheters with metal elements are now available through a number of major manufacturers and can be used for the purpose of epidural stimulation test.[86]

Epidural ECG Technique

One disadvantage of the epidural stimulation technique is that it cannot be performed reliably if any significant clinical neuromuscular blockade is present or local anesthetics have been administered in the epidural space. To overcome this limitation, an alternative monitoring technique using ECG monitoring has been suggested.[87,88] Using the epidural ECG monitoring lead, the anatomic position of the epidural catheter is determined by comparing the ECG signal from the tip of the catheter with a signal from a surface electrode positioned at the "target" segmental level. A standard reference ECG (lead II) is recorded by connecting the right-arm electrode (white) to a skin electrode on the patient's back at the target spinal level, while the left-arm electrode (black) and left-leg electrode (red) are placed at their standard position[88] (Figure 54–2).

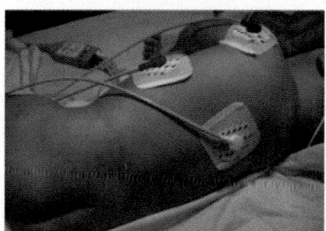

Place right-arm electrode (white) on patient's back to obtain reference surface ECG tracing.

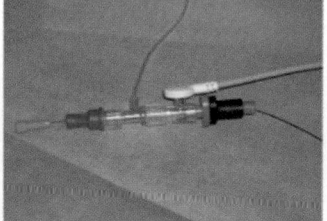

Connect right-arm electrode (white) to the epidural catheter to obtain Epidural ECG tracing.

Match the reference surface ECG tracing to epidural ECG tracing (bottom).

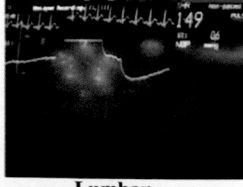

Lumbar

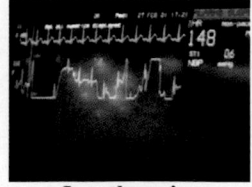

Low thoracic

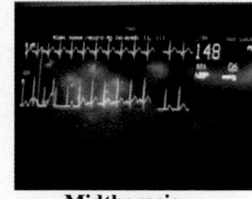

Midthoracic

Figure 54–2. Epidural ECG technique. Using epidural ECG monitoring lead, the anatomic position of the epidural catheter is determined by comparing the ECG signal from the tip of the catheter with a signal from a surface electrode positioned at the target segmental level. As the epidural tip advances toward the thoracic region, the amplitude of the QRS complex increases as the recording electrode comes closer to the heart and the ECG recording becomes more parallel with the cardiac electrical impulse.

Next, the right-arm electrode is connected to the metal hub of the electrode adapter (Johans ECG Adapter, Arrow International, Reading, Pennsylvania) to record a tracing from the epidural catheter. When the epidural catheter tip is positioned in the lumbar and sacral regions, the amplitude of the QRS complex is relatively small, because the recording electrode (epidural tip) is far away from the heart and the vector of the cardiac electrical impulse is at approximately a 90-degree angle. As the epidural tip advances toward the thoracic region, the amplitude of the QRS complex increases as the recording electrode comes closer to the heart and the ECG recording becomes more parallel with the cardiac electrical impulse. The amplitude should match the reference surface electrode amplitude as it passes the target level. Based on these observations, the advancement of an epidural catheter from the lumbar or sacral region into the thoracic region can easily be monitored and placed within two vertebral spaces of the targeted level under ECG guidance.[87] However, unlike the epidural stimulation test, the ECG technique cannot warn of a catheter placed in the subarachnoid or intravascular space. In addition, this technique may not be suitable when threading catheters for a short distance because the reference ECG and epidural ECG may be too similar to compare.

Epidural Approaches

Several epidural approaches currently used in children are described in this chapter. The most common types of epidural analgesia are (1) caudal analgesia, which constitutes the most commonly used regional technique in children; (2) lumbar epidural analgesia; and (3) thoracic epidural analgesia.

Single-Shot Caudal Technique

Single-shot caudal epidural blockade ("kiddy caudals") is widely used to provide perioperative analgesia in pediatric practice. As a single injection, it offers a reliable and effective block for patients undergoing urologic, general, and orthopedic surgery involving the lower abdomen and lower limbs. A single-shot caudal epidural may not be suitable for every case because it has a limited dermatomal distribution and a short duration of action. New local anesthetics and adjuvants, as well as continuous catheter approaches may overcome these limitations.

Choice of Needle for Caudal Analgesia

A variety of needles are available for single-shot caudal blockade. The size or type of needle does not appear to affect the rate of success or the incidence of complications of caudal blockade. Short-bevel 22-gauge needles (<4 cm in length) with stylets are believed to offer a better tactile sensation when the sacrococcygeal ligament is punctured.[43] Theoretically, the use of a styletted needle may reduce the risk of introducing a dermal plug into the caudal space, although an epidermal cell graft tumor in the epidural space has yet to be reported. The use of a 22-gauge Angiocath is also advocated because, with the advancement of these catheters into the caudal space,

it may indicate proper positioning.[44] There are also indications that it is easier to detect intravascular placement and interosseous placement with angiocatheters.[9] To avoid tissue coring with these angiocatheters, the needle must be removed before any injection is made.[89]

Technique for Performing Caudal Epidural Block

Patients are placed either in a lateral decubitus position with the knees drawn up to the chest or in a prone position with a roll under the hips for caudal epidural block placement (Figure 54–3). After proper positioning, the landmarks for caudal epidural block are easily identified in children. After initially identifying the coccyx and continuing to palpate in the midline in a cephalad fashion, the sacral cornua can be felt on either side of the midline approximately one centimeter apart (Figure 54–4). The sacral hiatus is felt as a depression between two bony prominences of the sacral cornua. Under sterile conditions, the needle is inserted and advanced into the

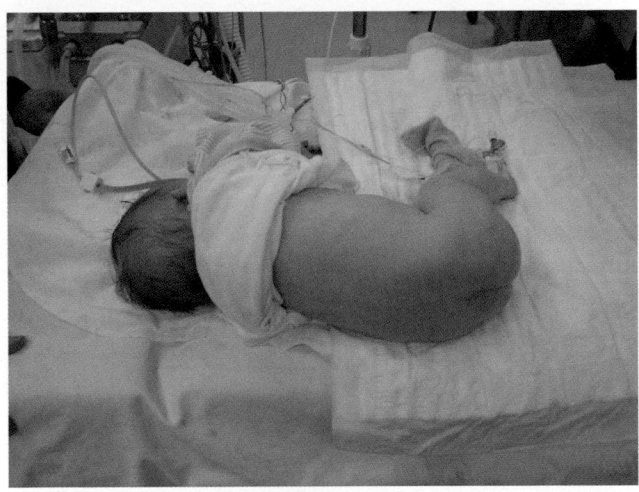

Figure 54–3. Patient positioning. Shown is left lateral position with patient's hips maximally flexed.

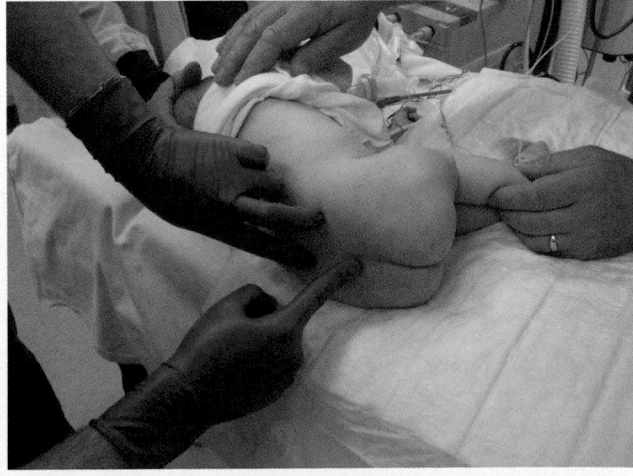

Figure 54–4. Landmarks for caudal anesthesia. Shown are posterior superior iliac spines (two fingers), which form an equilateral triangle with the sacral cornua (single finger).

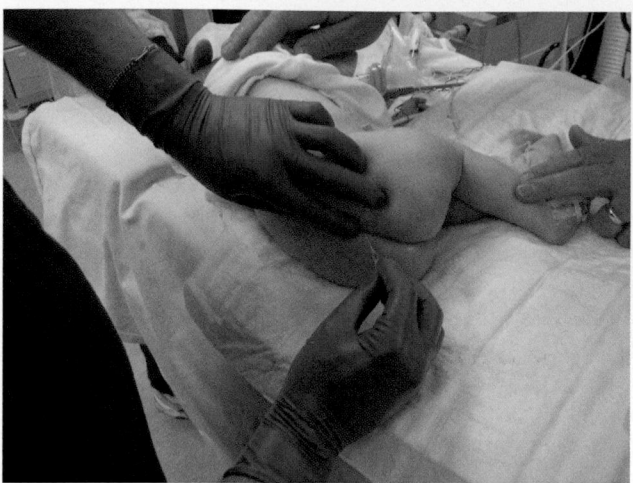

Figure 54–5. Needle advancement in caudal block. The needle is advanced in a cephalad direction. Occasionally, a pop is felt as the sacrococcygeal ligament is penetrated. At this point, the catheter is advanced a centimeter off the needle.

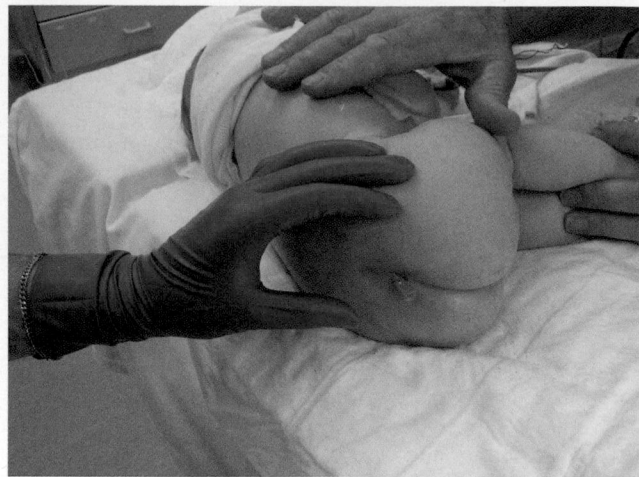

Figure 54–6. Catheter placement. Easy passage of the stimulating needle confirms correct placement.

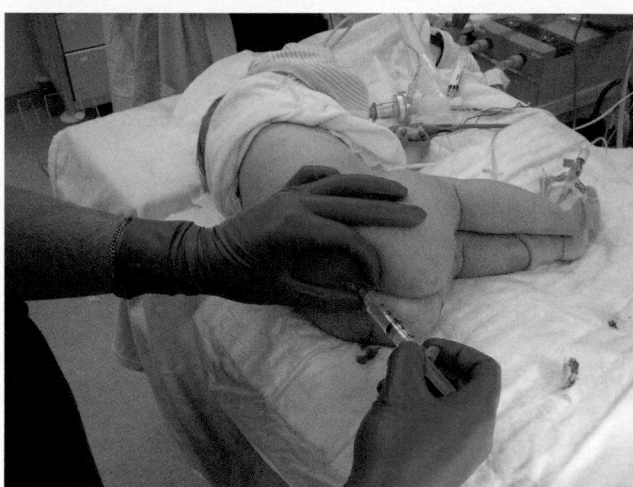

Figure 54–7. The catheter is stabilized with the left hand while the local anesthetic syringe is connected and subsequently injected in divided doses. The ECG is monitored during injection for an increase in heart rate of 10 beats/min or a 20% change in T-wave amplitude. The reliability of these signs without ECG strip monitoring remains untested. The area of skin immediately over the sacrum should be visible to observe for inadvertent subcutaneous injection.

sacral hiatus at approximately a 70-degree angle to the skin until a distinctive "pop" is felt as the sacrococcygeal ligament is punctured (Figure 54–5). After this puncture, the angle of the needle should be reduced to approximately 20 to 30 degrees while the needle is advanced 2 to 4 mm into the caudal canal. If using an angiocatheter (Figure 54–6), the plastic catheter of the needle should easily advance into the caudal epidural space. Any advancement past this point is not recommended because the risk of an inadvertent dural puncture increases significantly.

Clinical Pearls

- Posterior superior iliac spines and sacral hiatus form equilateral triangle.
- Sacral cornua are on either side of hiatus (0.5–1.0 cm apart).
- Dural sac extends to S4 in the infant younger than 1 year (S2 in the adult).

Confirmation of Needle Placement

The classic "pop" felt as sacrococcygeal membrane is pierced is usually sought for proper caudal needle placement. The absence of subcutaneous bulging and the lack of resistance upon injection of local anesthetic are additional signs of proper needle placement (Figure 54–7). Aspiration of the needle should be clear of blood and cerebrospinal fluid and a negative response to a test dose of epinephrine should also be used to rule out intrathecal and intravascular placement (Figure 54–8).

Other tests to confirm proper needle placement include the whoosh test, the swoosh test, and the use of nerve stimulation.[90,91] The whoosh test requires the injection of

2.5 mL of air through the caudal needle, with a "whoosh" being heard with a stethoscope placed over the thoracolumbar spine. However, this can lead to a patchy block. More important, it can cause a venous air embolism if the needle is inserted into an epidural vessel, especially in small infants. The swoosh technique avoids these problems by injecting local anesthetic or saline in place of air, but the benefit of confirming needle placement before local anesthetic injection is lost. Excessive saline injection may dilute subsequent local anesthetic injections and lead to an inadequate block. When using nerve stimulation, proper needle placement is confirmed by motor activity in the anal sphincter with 1–10 mA of current through an insulated needle.[91] The sensitivity and specificity of predicting proper needle placement approach 100%

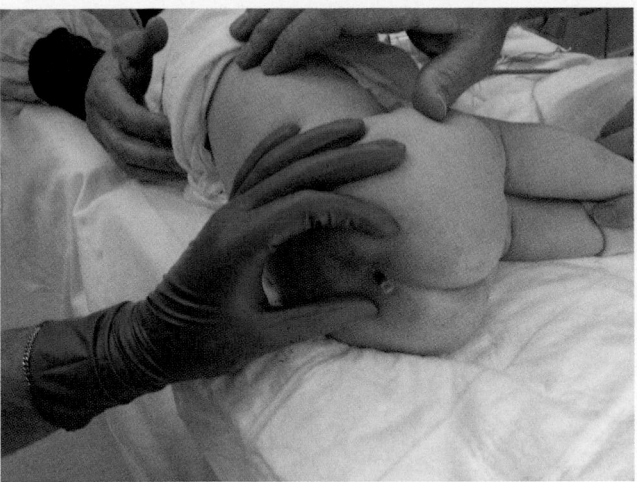

Figure 54–8. Bloody tap. In the infant shown, an epidural vein is inadvertently cannulated as evidenced by the free flow of venous blood. The catheter is consequently removed and the process repeated.

with this approach, although the requirement for an insulated sheathed needle limits its use.[91] Furthermore, most insulated needles lack a stylet and may be more expensive than standard noninsulated needles. Ultrasound has been used to provide real-time images to guide needles into the caudal space.[69] Other predictors of accurate block placement after the injection of local anesthetic have been attempted. Relaxation of the anal sphincter predicts successful caudal blockade,[92] but pupillary reflex dilation and skin temperature changes are not clinically useful.[93]

Clinical Pearls

- Formulas exist for the volume of local anesthetic required to achieve a given dermatomal spread. In practice, a dose of 1 mL/kg of 0.25% bupivacaine with epinephrine gives 4 hours of postoperative analgesia with a low incidence of motor block.
- The only additives that have been shown to prolong analgesia without increasing side effects are:
  1. *Clonidine 1–2 mcg/kg (approximately 8 hours postoperative analgesia)*
  2. *Ketamine (preservative-free) 0.5 mg/kg (up to 12 hours postoperative analgesia)*
- These agents have been shown to prolong the time to first analgesic after minor surgery. In our experience, after the local anaesthetic block has warn off, these agents provide only mild analgesia.

Continuous Caudal Epidural to Lumbar or Thoracic Space

Continuous caudal epidural analgesia overcomes the limited duration and segmental effect of a single-shot technique.

Caudal catheters advanced to a lumbar or thoracic level can be used for surgery involving dermatomes above T10. This technique may carry a smaller risk of dural puncture or spinal cord trauma than a direct thoracic epidural approach.[94]

The technique for needle insertion for continuous caudal analgesia is very similar to the single-shot caudal approach. An intravenous catheter (an 18-gauge angiocatheter for a 20-gauge epidural catheter or a 16-gauge angiocatheter for a 19-gauge epidural catheter) or an 18-gauge Crawford needle is inserted through the sacrococcygeal ligament as described for the single-shot technique. The complete angiocatheter with the needle set should then be advanced no more than 1 cm into the sacral canal. After withdrawing the metal needle, the plastic sheath is gently advanced completely into the caudal space. This allows the epidural catheter to easily pass through the plastic sheath.

The appropriate length of epidural catheter is measured against the back of the child from sacral to the target spinal level or approximate dermatomal coverage required for the surgical procedure. The epidural catheter is then advanced carefully from the caudal space to the target level. Minor resistance to the passage of the catheter can usually be overcome by simple flexion or extension of the patient's vertebral column and/or by simultaneously injecting normal saline through the advancing specialized stimulation epidural catheter (Epidural Positioning System using Tsui test, Arrow International).[28] The location of the catheter tip should be verified using an objective test described as in the previous section (radiography,[66] nerve stimulation,[28] electrocardiography,[87,88] or ultrasound.[69])

Some may criticize these techniques as cumbersome or redundant, but these tests are valuable teaching aids and may prevent extensive follow-up on patients with inadequate analgesia as a result of poorly situated catheters. Studies have suggested that caudal catheter placement should be limited to patients younger than 1 year, owing to the development of a lumbar curve during infancy that prevents easy cephalad advancement of the catheter.[66] However, recent reports have demonstrated that cephalad advancement is possible in older children using epidural stimulation.[28,95,96] The improved success rate in older children has been attributed to the use of a styletted catheter, which allows the simultaneous injecting of saline during advancement, and, more important, to the stimulation test, which monitors the advancement of the catheter tip.[28]

Clinical Pearls

Advantages of a cannula over a needle are:

- Confidence with placement if the cannula slides off the needle easily
- Possible reduced intraosseous injection risk
- Possible reduced intravascular injection risk
- Possible reduced dural puncture risk

Lumbar Epidural Anesthesia

Lumbar epidural analgesia is commonly used for continuous infusions and is rarely used as a single-shot technique. A direct lumbar approach is primarily indicated for providing pain control during and after lower extremity surgery. Lumbar epidural placement, particularly in young children, is performed after the induction of general anesthesia. However, this approach may also be performed awake in a select group of cooperative children and adolescents. The risk/benefit ratio of inserting thoracic epidural catheters in children under general anesthesia is controversial.[47,95] Although this issue is not as controversial for lumbar epidural analgesia as thoracic epidural analgesia,[47] caution should be exercised whenever performing lumbar epidural analgesia above the level of spinal cord to avoid direct needle trauma.

Technique for Placement of Lumbar Epidural Analgesia

A midline approach to lumbar epidural needle placement is preferred. Identification of the epidural space is commonly achieved by loss of resistance to saline. LOR to air should be avoided due to the risk of introducing a venous air embolism particularly in neonates and infants. Children should be positioned in the lateral decubitus position for direct lumbar epidural placement (Figure 54–9). An 18-gauge Tuohy needle with a 20-gauge epidural catheter is often used in children (Figures 54–10 and 54–11). Although identification of the intervertebral space and ligamentum flavum in most pediatric patients is easy, the ligamentum flavum can be less tensile in children; hence a distinctive "pop" may not be easily felt when penetrating this layer. In addition, the distance from the skin to the epidural space can be shallow. Formulas for estimating the distance from skin to epidural space distance have been proposed[97–99] (Table 54–7). Formulas are only a guideline and change according to the angle of placement of the epidural needle.

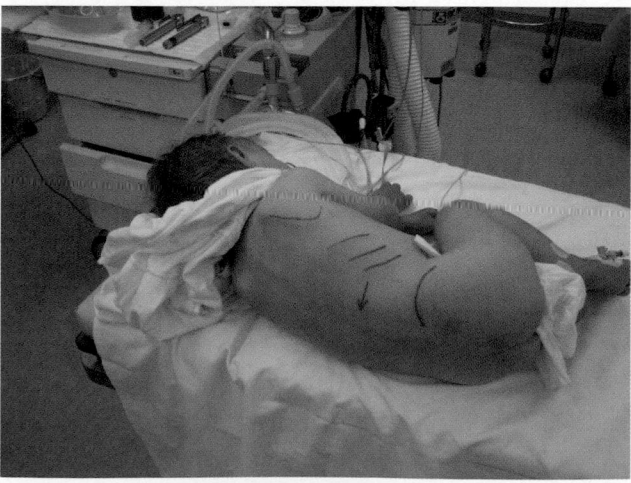

Figure 54–9. Landmarks for epidural anesthesia in small children. The landmarks are similar in adult population except that the intercristal line bisects L5. In this child, the L1 spinous process is marked with an arrow.

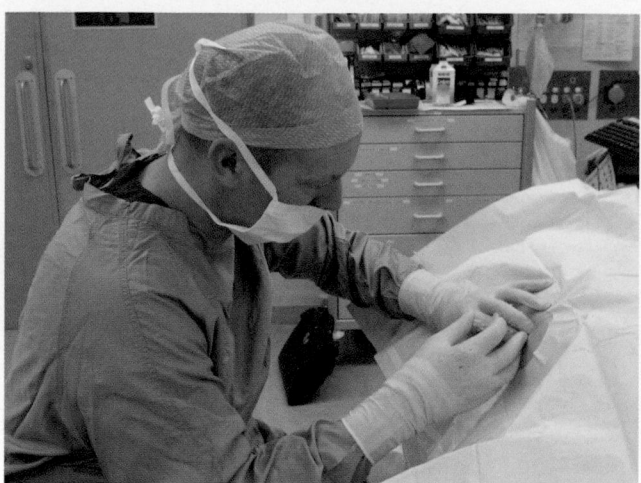

Figure 54–10. Epidural anesthesia in children: Hand position. Patient in the left lateral position. Left-hand index and middle fingers are on either side of chosen interspace. The right hand holds the needle hub.

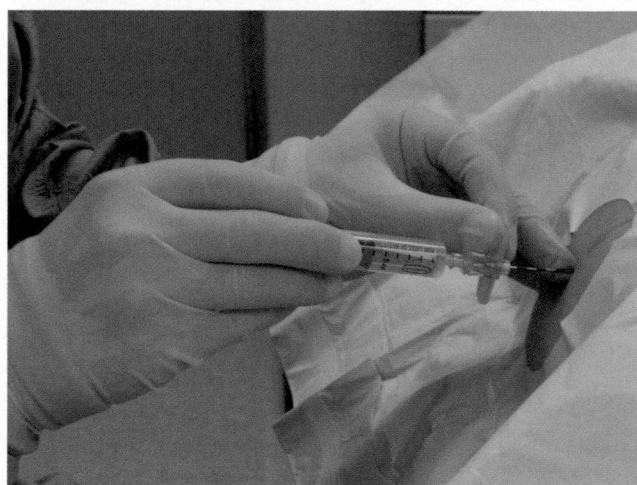

Figure 54–11. Epidural anesthesia in children: Needle advancement. The needle is advanced with stylet in place until interspinous ligament is reached. The stylet is removed and a saline-filled loss-of-resistance syringe is connected to the needle. Both plunger and needle are continuously advanced. Initially an increase in resistance is felt as the ligamentum flavum is entered before a loss of resistance. These sensations are very subtle in the small infant.

Table 54–7.

Formula for Depth of Epidural Space From Skin

1. Rough estimate 1 mm/kg body weight
2. Depth (cm) = $1 + 0.15 \times$ age (years)
3. Depth (cm) = $0.8 + 0.05 \times$ weight (kg)
4. Mean depth in neonates = 1 cm

Lumbar-to-Thoracic Approach

Catheters placed via the lumbar route may be advanced cephalad to thoracic vertebral levels (Figures 54–12 through 54–16. Similar to the problems encountered when advancing catheters in the caudal space in older children, significant resistance also prevents the easy advancement of lumbar epidural catheters to the thoracic levels Despite favorable results using stimulation via a caudal approach, only one recent case report demonstrated the successful placement of a thoracic epidural catheter via the lumbar route with epidural stimulation guidance.[100] Further research and study are warranted for using the stimulating technique for this approach.

Clinical Pearls

- Various formulas exist for calculating the volume of local anesthetic required to block a given number of segments. Because sympathetic blockade is well tolerated in children with very little change in both heart rate and blood pressure, in practice (after an appropriate test dose) a bolus of 0.5–1.0 mL/kg of 0.25% bupivacaine is administered to establish the block.

- For postoperative analgesia, the most common agent used is a combination of bupivicaine 0.125% with fentanyl 2 mcg/mL at the following rates:
  1. *Age >3 months: 0.20–0.35 mL/kg/h (<0.4 mg/kg/h Bupivacaine*
  2. *Age <3 months: 0.1–0.15 mL/kg/h (<0.2 mg/kg/h bupivacaine)*

- In preschool-aged children and especially infants, irritability/agitation may occur despite an apparently well-functioning epidural. This is most likely the result of the IV line, nasogastric tube, urinary catheter, or even the hospital environment. Satisfactory sedation can be achieved with either of the following:
  (a) IV boluses of morphine 25 mcg/kg as required or
  (b) adding clonidine 0.5 mcg/mL to the epidural mixture

- PCEA may result in less motor block than an infusion only prescription without compromising analgesia.
  – Infusion 0.15 mL/kg/h
  – Bolus 0.07 mL/kg lockout 20 minutes

Thoracic Epidural Analgesia

Controversy exists concerning the safety of placing thoracic epidurals under heavy sedation or general anesthesia, because unconscious patients are unable to report symptoms that may warn the anesthesiologist of potential neurologic complications.[47–50] Direct needle trauma to the spinal cord during epidural insertion is rare but can cause devastating complications. Recent reports have detailed cases of direct needle trauma to the spinal cord during epidural placement in both awake and anesthetized patients.[51,101,102] The advancement of catheters from the lumbar and caudal epidural spaces to the thoracic level can be through an alternative approach.

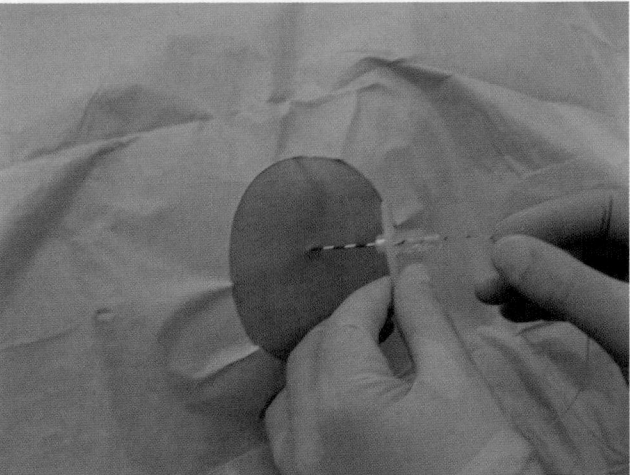

Figure 54–12. Epidural anesthesia in children: Catheter insertion. Catheter advancement is associated with greater resistance than in the adult. The catheter stabilizing attachment may help (not used here).

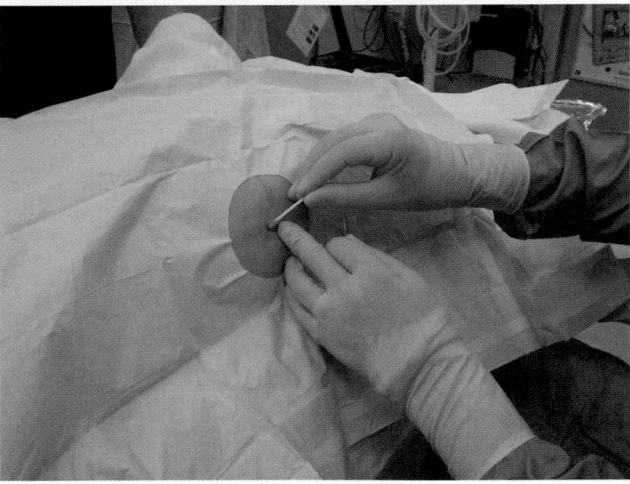

Figure 54–13. Epidural anesthesia in children: Preventing the leakage. Preventing the leakage of local anesthetic in pediatric patients is important because this can consist of a significant percentage of the total drug delivered. The puncture site can be sealed using several methods, one of which is with Liquid Bandage (Johnson & Johnson) using the supplied product applicator.

However, for reasons poorly understood, the advancement of catheters in the epidural space becomes increasingly difficult with advancing age. The reason for this is poorly understood, but it has been suggested that the increase in resistance to catheter advancement parallels the development of the lumbar curvature.[66]

Direct placement of thoracic epidural catheters are still used but more commonly at tertiary care centers, which are limited to extensive procedures involving thoracic and abdominal surgery with well-trained personnel. A recent study in pediatric patients suggested that electrical stimulation applied to an advancing epidural needle may be used

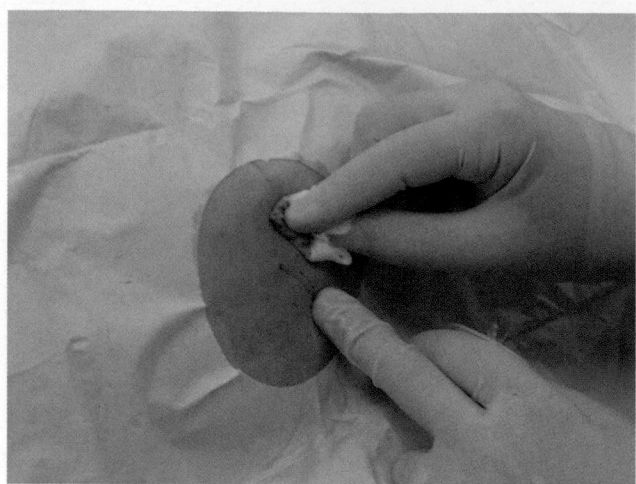

Figure 54–14. Epidural anesthesia in children: Securing the catheter. Tincture of benzoin is applied to improve adhesion of the fixation device.

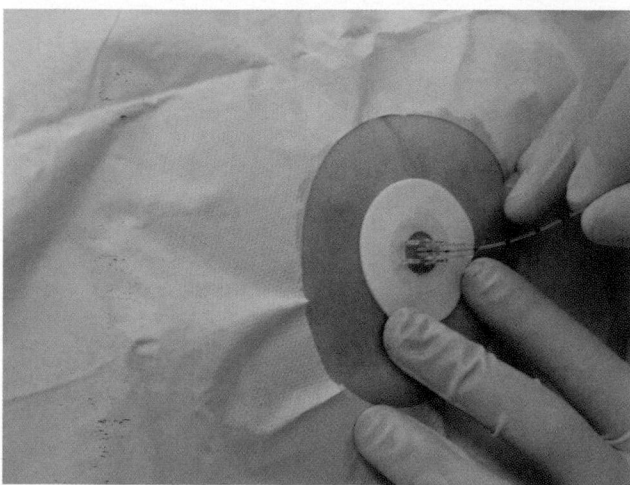

Figure 54–15. Epidural anesthesia in children: Securing the catheter. Epidural catheters that are not secured well in small children dislodge very easily. The device used here is the Simms Portex lockit device. In the small child/infant, allowance should be made for the relatively small distance between adjacent vertebrae. Leaving 3 cm of catheter in the epidural space means the tip of the catheter may be three segments higher (or lower) than the needle insertion point. In this child, the epidural space was located 2 cm deep to the skin. Leaving the catheter at 5 cm (3 cm in space) results in the catheter being situated at approximately T10 (three segments above the T12-L1 interspace).

as an additional safety measure to warn of needle proximity to the intrathecal space, spinal cord, or nerve root.[103] This study demonstrated that the mean current necessary to elicit a motor response with insulated needles in the epidural space is much higher than that in the intrathecal space (5.2 ± 2.4 mA versus 0.6 ± 0.3 mA, respectively).[103] Individually, electrical stimulation and loss of resistance have their limitations, but together both these techniques may compensate for each other's weaknesses to facilitate opti-

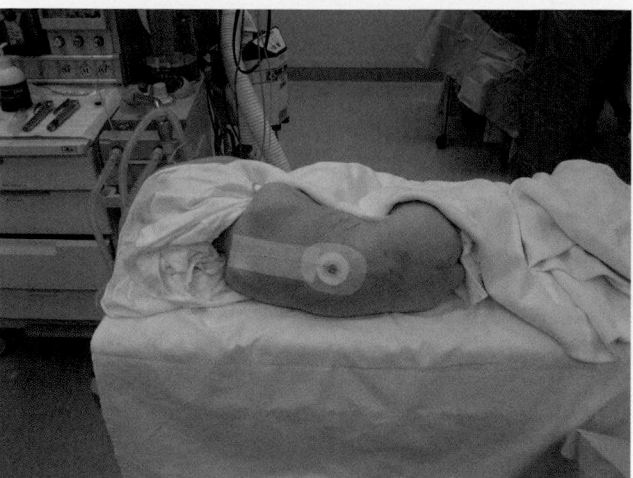

Figure 54–16. Epidural anesthesia in children: Securing the catheter. The epidural fixation device is covered with a clear occlusive dressing.

mal needle placement. A similar concept using electrophysiologic monitoring is common practice in spinal surgery, but currently there is no clear evidence that electrical stimulation would directly benefit thoracic epidural placement.[104] This concept is still in its infancy and further research is warranted.

Clinical Pearls

- Because children require a significantly higher volume/dose of local anesthetic compared with adults to achieve the same dermatome spread, it is important to have the tip of the catheter at the intended surgical site.
- Intended high thoracic catheter advancement from a lumbar insertion site is rarely successful.
- Thoracic epidural insertion should be performed only by practitioners experienced in pediatric lumbar epidural technique.
- Epidural needle insertion in pediatric patients can be performed at any thoracic interspace using either a midline or paramedian approach. The paramedian approach is preferred in adults, whereas a midline approach is often used in children.

Midline Approach

Using midline approach, insertion of the needle is easier at the lower thoracic level (T10 to T12) than at the midthoracic (T4 to T7) level. The lower border of the shoulder blade, which is level with 7th thoracic vertebra, is commonly used as an anatomic landmark. After the patient is placed in the lateral decubitus position, the spinous process of the targeted vertebral level is identified. A 20-gauge Tuohy epidural needle is then inserted at the interspace at a cephalad angle of approximately 70 degrees to the longitudinal axis of the spine (see Figure 54–10). Continuous resistance should be felt as the needle is inserted through the supraspinous and interspinous ligaments. In pediatric patients, the resistance met at the ligamentum flavum may not be noticeably different from that of the other ligaments. The thoracic epidural space is identified with loss of resistance to saline. The advantage of the midline approach is that its technique is very similar to lumbar epidural insertion with the needle angulated only in one plane.

Paramedian Approach

The paramedian approach permits entry to the epidural space at any spinal level. This approach is usually performed with patients in the lateral decubitus position. Right-handed clinicians may prefer to use a right paramedian approach because it increases the working space and it may facilitate needle placement with the patient on the same side as the needle. The needle is initially inserted next to the spinal process and slowly advanced in a direction perpendicular to the skin until lamina is contacted. It is important to take note of lamina depth as it provides an estimated depth of the epidural space from the skin.[105,106] (see Figure 54–5) The needle is redirected medial before being inclined cephalad toward the interspace. Again, loss of resistance to saline identifies the epidural space. Many believe that this approach requires more skill and experience

because the needle must be angled in two planes (ie, medially and cephahad). Thus, anesthesiologists with extensive experience and confidence in epidural analgesia should perform this technique.

Managing Epidural Infusions Postoperatively

For epidural analgesia to be effective and safe, systematic and regulated approaches to patient care must be practiced. A dedicated pediatric acute pain team, consisting of anesthesiologists and nurses, is vital to ensure standardized assessments of pain, vigilant patient monitoring and the proper treatment of any adverse effects. Recommendations for epidural troubleshooting and managing inadequate analgesia are summarized in Table 54–8. Precise placement of epidural needles and catheters is the key to successful epidural analgesia. This requires the use of a reliable method to confirm the location of the catheter tip (eg, x-ray, epidural stimulation). The use of opioids or α_2-agonists in the epidural space may lead to better analgesia. An average length of epidural infusion is about 72 hours, although it may be necessary to continue the infusion for longer periods, especially in children with complicated medical histories and prolonged need for analgesia. A team of dedicated personnel with a focus on pain management should care for these children. When plans to discontinue the epidural infusion are in place, an oral opioid

---

Table 54–8.

Tips for Improving Epidural Analgesia

Inadequate analgesia

1. If there is any doubt about the adequacy of analgesia or the position of the catheter, prove the catheter's position using one of the approaches outlined in Table 54–7. Chloroprocaine can provide catheter tip position and rapidly provide analgesia in most cases.

2. If the epidural infusion does not already include either an opioid or clonidine or $S(+)$ ketamine along with the local anesthetic, consider inclusion of one of these additives, unless there are specific contraindications or unmanageable side-effects.

3. Use bolus dosing to produce analgesia relatively promptly (while staying within maximum allowable local anesthetic dosing parameters). Simply increasing an infusion rate by 10% or 20% requires hours to reach a steady state and subjects the patient to prolonged pain.

4. Titrate the local anesthetic upward into the acceptable range if not done already, unless specifically contraindicated or unless limited by motor or autonomic blockade.

5. For adolescents and young adults with thoracic catheter tips for upper abdominal or thoracic surgery, if there is inadequate analgesia when the local anesthetic infusion is titrated upward to >12 mL/h, consider next increasing the local anesthetic concentration, eg, increasing bupivacaine to 0.15% while maintaining a maximum hourly dosing within the 0.4 mg/kg/h limit.

6. If the catheter tip is in lumbar dermatomes and the surgery is thoracic or upper abdominal, add a hydrophilic opioid, such as hydromorphone or morphine, unless there are specific contraindications.

7. If the catheter is in the epidural space, but the block is preferentially one-sided to the wrong side, consider addition of a hydrophilic opioid—either hydromorphone or morphine—unless there are specific contraindications.

Adapted with permission from Tsui B, Berde C: Caudal analgesia and anesthesia techniques in children. Curr Opin Anaesthesiol 2005, 18:283–288.

Table 54–9.

Sample Order Form: Anesthesia Order—Epidural Analgesia

1.	No additional sedatives/opioids without discussing with anesthesia pain service	
2.	Patient weight = _____ kg	
3.	Allergies:	
4	Solution:_____% (0.125%) bupivacaine with fentanyl_____mcg/mL (0–10 mcg/mL) Other solutions:_____	
5.	Mode:_____ Continuous infusion _____ PCEA and Continuous	
6.	Administer above solution @ _____ mL/hr	
7.	PCEA bolus dose:_____mL (0.5 mL–3 mL)	
8.	Lock-out interval:_____min (15–30 min)	
9.	One-hour limit:_____mL *Dose:* Bupivacaine: ≤0.4 mg/kg/h for children >3 months ≤0.2 mg/kg/h for children <3 months	
10.	PCEA operator: _____Patient_____Parent_____Nurse	
11.	Cardiorespiratory monitor:_____Yes_____No	
12.	Continuous pulse oximetry	
13.	If respiratory rate ≤12, SpO$_2$ ≤92%; patient unarousable, **stop infusion and page anesthesia at pager#_____stat**	
14.	If patient is ambulating, monitors may be disconnected during ambulation	
15.	Assess all dependent skin areas for bed sores (heels)	
16.	For itching, administer diphenhydramine 0.1–0.5 mg/kg _____mg (max 25 mg) IV over 5 min q4h	
17.	For nausea and vomiting, administer ondansetron 0.1 mg/kg_____(max 4 mg) over 5 min q6h prn	
18.	Diazepam 0.02–0.04 mg/kg_____mg IV prn q6h for muscle spasm or anxiety	
19.	If no urine output in 8 hours, page surgical service to evaluate for urinary retention	
20.	Stop infusion and page anesthesia stat at pager#_____ a. If systolic BP < 60 mm Hg b. If patient has increasing weakness or has signs of local anesthetic toxicity including ringing in ears, lip numbness, slurred speech	
21.	Please consult anesthesia pain service for discontinuation of the epidural catheter	
22.	Thank you for consulting the Anesthesia Pain Service	

should always be administered to enable the patient to continue to have excellent analgesia. Finally, the success of the process is based on properly written orders—a crucial part of executing adequate analgesia. A sample order sheet for managing epidural analgesia is shown in Table 54–9.

References

1. Peutrell JM, Lonnqvist PA: Neuraxial blocks for anaesthesia and analgesia in children. Curr Opin Anaesthesiol 2003;461–470.
2. Berde CB: Convulsions associated with pediatric regional anesthesia. Anesth Analg 1992;75:164–166.

3. Larsson BA, Lonnqvist PA, Olsson GL: Plasma concentrations of bupivacaine in neonates after continuous epidural infusion. Anesth Analg 1997;84:501–505.

4. Luz G, Innerhofer P, Bachmann B, et al: Bupivacaine plasma concentrations during continuous epidural anesthesia in infants and children. Anesth Analg 1996;82:231–234.

5. Gunter JB, Eng C: Thoracic epidural anesthesia via the caudal approach in children. Anesthesiology 1992;76:935–938.

6. Takasaki M, Dohi S, Kawabata Y, Takahashi T: Dosage of lidocaine for caudal anesthesia in infants and children. Anesthesiology 1977;47:527–529.

7. De Beer DA, Thomas ML: Caudal additives in children—solutions or problems? Br J Anaesth 2003;90:487–498.

8. Gunter JB, Dunn CM, Bennie JB, et al: Optimum concentration of bupivacaine for combined caudal–general anesthesia in children. Anesthesiology 1991;75:57–61.

9. Tsui BC, Berde CB: Caudal analgesia and anesthesia techniques in children. Curr Opin Anaesthesiol 2005;18:283–288.

10. Bosenberg A: Pediatric regional anesthesia update. Paediatr Anaesth 2004;14:398–402.

11. Henderson K, Sethna NF, Berde CB: Continuous caudal anesthesia for inguinal hernia repair in former preterm infants. J Clin Anesth 1993;5:129–133.

12. Da Conceicao MJ, Coelho L, Khalil M: Ropivacaine 0.25% compared with bupivacaine 0.25% by the caudal route. Paediatr Anaesth 1999;9:229–233.

13. Eledjam JJ, Gros T, Viel E, et al: Ropivacaine overdose and systemic toxicity. Anaesth Intensive Care 2000;28:705–707.

14. Ivani G, Lampugnani E, Torre M, et al: Comparison of ropivacaine with bupivacaine for paediatric caudal block. Br J Anaesth 1998;81:247–248.

15. Reiz S, Haggmark S, Johansson G, Nath S: Cardiotoxicity of ropivacaine—a new amide local anaesthetic agent. Acta Anaesthesiol Scand 1989;33:93–98.

16. Karmakar MK, Aun CS, Wong EL, et al: Ropivacaine undergoes slower systemic absorption from the caudal epidural space in children than bupivacaine (table). Anesth Analg 2002;94:259–265.

17. Ia-Kokko TI, Karinen J, Raiha E, et al: Pharmacokinetics of 0.75% ropivacaine and 0.5% bupivacaine after ilioinguinal-iliohypogastric nerve block in children. Br J Anaesth 2002;89:438–441.

18. Gunter JB: Benefit and risks of local anesthetics in infants and children. Paediatr Drugs 2002;4:649–672.

19. Bosenberg A, Thomas J, Lopez T, et al: The efficacy of caudal ropivacaine 1, 2 and 3 mg × l(-1) for postoperative analgesia in children. Paediatr Anaesth 2002;12:53–58.

20. Ivani G: Ropivacaine: Is it time for children? Paediatr Anaesth 2002;12:383–387.

21. Taylor R, Eyres R, Chalkiadis GA, Austin S: Efficacy and safety of caudal injection of levobupivacaine, 0.25%, in children under 2 years of age undergoing inguinal hernia repair, circumcision or orchidopexy. Paediatr Anaesth 2003;13:114–121.

22. Cook B, Doyle E: The use of additives to local anaesthetic solutions for caudal epidural blockade. Paediatr Anaesth 1996;6:353–359.

23. Attia J, Ecoffey C, Sandouk P, et al: Epidural morphine in children: Pharmacokinetics and CO2 sensitivity. Anesthesiology 1986;65:590–594.

24. Karl HW, Tyler DC, Krane EJ: Respiratory depression after low-dose caudal morphine. Can J Anaesth 1996;43:1065–1067.

25. Lonnqvist PA, Ivani G, Moriarty T: Use of caudal-epidural opioids in children: Still state of the art or the beginning of the end? Paediatr Anaesth 2002;12:747–749.

26. Campbell FA, Yentis SM, Fear DW, Bissonnette B: Analgesic efficacy and safety of a caudal bupivacaine-fentanyl mixture in children. Can J Anaesth 1992;39:661–664.

27. Constant I, Gall O, Gouyet L, et al: Addition of clonidine or fentanyl to local anaesthetics prolongs the duration of surgical analgesia after single shot caudal block in children. Br J Anaesth 1998;80:294–298.

28. Tsui BC, Wagner A, Cave D, Kearney R: Thoracic and lumbar epidural analgesia via the caudal approach using electrical stimulation guidance in pediatric patients: A review of 289 patients. Anesthesiology 2004;100:683–689.

29. Ansermino M, Basu R, Vandebeek C, Montgomery C: Nonopioid additives to local anaesthetics for caudal blockade in children: A systematic review. Paediatr Anaesth 2003;13:561–573.

30. De NP, Ivani G, Visconti C, et al: The dose-response relationship for clonidine added to a postoperative continuous epidural infusion of ropivacaine in children. Anesth Analg 2001;93:71–76.

31. Ivani G, De NP, Conio A, et al: Ropivacaine-clonidine combination for caudal blockade in children. Acta Anaesthesiol Scand 2000;44:446–449.

32. Penon C, Ecoffey C, Cohen SE: Ventilatory response to carbon dioxide after epidural clonidine injection. Anesth Analg 1991;72:761–764.

33. Fellmann C, Gerber AC, Weiss M: Apnoea in a former preterm infant after caudal bupivacaine with clonidine for inguinal herniorrhaphy. Paediatr Anaesth 2002;12:637–640.

34. Almenrader N, Passariello M, D'Amico G, et al: Caudal additives for postoperative pain management in children: S(+)-ketamine and neostigmine. Paediatr Anaesth 2005;15:143–147.

35. Passariello M, Almenrader N, Canneti A, et al: Caudal analgesia in children: S(+)-ketamine vs S(+)-ketamine plus clonidine. Paediatr Anaesth 2004;14:851–855.

36. Hager H, Marhofer P, Sitzwohl C, et al: Caudal clonidine prolongs analgesia from caudal S(+)-ketamine in children. Anesth Analg 2002;94:1169–1172.

37. Hayashi H, Dikkes P, Soriano SG: Repeated administration of ketamine may lead to neuronal degeneration in the developing rat brain. Paediatr Anaesth 2002;12:770–774.

38. Olney JW: New insights and new issues in developmental neurotoxicology. Neurotoxicology 2002;23:659–668.

39. Anand A, Charney DS, Oren DA, et al: Attenuation of the neuropsychiatric effects of ketamine with lamotrigine: Support for hyperglutamatergic effects of N-methyl-D-aspartate receptor antagonists. Arch Gen Psychiatry 2000;57:270–276.

40. Proescholdt M, Heimann A, Kempski O: Neuroprotection of S(+) ketamine isomer in global forebrain ischemia. Brain Res 2001;904:245–251.

41. Baris S, Karakaya D, Kelsaka E, et al: Comparison of fentanyl-bupivacaine or midazolam-bupivacaine mixtures with plain bupivacaine for caudal anaesthesia in children. Paediatr Anaesth 2003;13:126–131.

42. Abdulatif M, El-Sanabary M: Caudal neostigmine, bupivacaine, and their combination for postoperative pain management after hypospadias surgery in children (table). Anesth Analg 2002;95:1215–1218.

43. Giaufre E: Risks and complications of regional anaesthesia in children. Bailliere's Clinical Anaesthesiology 2000;14:659–671.

44. Suresh S, Wheeler M: Practical pediatric regional anesthesia. Anesthesiol Clin North Am 2002;20:83–113.

45. Giaufre E, Dalens B, Gombert A: Epidemiology and morbidity of regional anesthesia in children: A one-year prospective survey of the French-Language Society of Pediatric Anesthesiologists. Anesth Analg 1996;83:904–912.

46. Flandin-Blety C, Barrier G: Accidents following extradural analgesia in children. The results of a retrospective study. Paediatr Anaesth 1995;5:41–46.

47. Krane EJ, Dalens BJ, Murat I, Murrell D: The safety of epidurals placed during general anesthesia. Reg Anesth Pain Med 1998;23:433–438.

48. Broadman LM: Where should advocacy for pediatric patients end and concerns for patient safety begin? Reg Anesth 1997;22:205–208.

49. Fischer HB: Regional anaesthesia—before or after general anaesthesia? Anaesthesia 1998;53:727–729.

50. Fischer HB: Performing epidural insertion under general anaesthesia. Anaesthesia 2000;55:288–289.

51. Kasai T, Yaegashi K, Hirose M, Tanaka Y: Spinal cord injury in a child caused by an accidental dural puncture with a single-shot thoracic epidural needle. Anesth Analg 2003;96:65–67.

52. Kost-Byerly S, Tobin JR, Greenberg RS, et al: Bacterial colonization and infection rate of continuous epidural catheters in children. Anesth Analg 1998;86:712–716.

53. Wittum S, Hofer CK, Rolli U, et al: Sacral osteomyelitis after single-shot epidural anesthesia via the caudal approach in a child. Anesthesiology 2003;99:503–505.

54. Giaufre E: Single-shot caudal block, In: Saint-Maurice C, Steinberg OS (editors): *Regional Anesthesia in Children.* Mediglobe, 1990, pp. 81–87.

55. Bubeck J, Boos K, Krause H, Thies KC: Subcutaneous tunneling of caudal catheters reduces the rate of bacterial colonization to that of lumbar epidural catheters. Anesth Analg 2004;99:689–693.

56. Oliver A: Dural punctures in children: What should we do? Paediatr Anaesth 2002;12:473–477.

57. Janssens E, Aerssens P, Alliet P, et al: Post-dural puncture headaches in children. A literature review. Eur J Pediatr 2003;162:117–121.

58. Liley A, Manoharan M, Upadhyay V: The management of a post-dural puncture headache in a child. Paediatr Anaesth 2003;13:534–537.

59. Dalens B, Hasnaoui A: Caudal anesthesia in pediatric surgery: Success rate and adverse effects in 750 consecutive patients. Anesth Analg 1989;68:83–89.

60. Tsuji MH, Horigome H, Yamashita M: Left ventricular functions are not impaired after lumbar epidural anaesthesia in young children. Paediatr Anaesth 1996;6:405–409.

61. Tsui BC, Malherbe S, Koller J, Aronyk K: Reversal of an unintentional spinal anesthetic by cerebrospinal lavage (table). Anesth Analg 2004;98:434–436.

62. McGown RG: Caudal analgesia in children. Five hundred cases for procedures below the diaphragm. Anaesthesia 1982;37:806–818.

63. Agarwal R, Gutlove DP, Lockhart CH: Seizures occurring in pediatric patients receiving continuous infusion of bupivacaine. Anesth Analg 1992;75:284–286.

64. Berde C: Local anesthetics in infants and children: An update. Paediatr Anaesth 2004;14:387–393.

65. Tobias JD: Caudal epidural block: A review of test dosing and recognition of systemic injection in children. Anesth Analg 2001;93:1156–61.

66. Valairucha S, Seefelder C, Houck CS: Thoracic epidural catheters placed by the caudal route in infants: The importance of radiographic confirmation. Paediatr Anaesth 2002;12:424–428.

67. Chan VW, Perlas A, Rawson R, Odukoya O: Ultrasound-guided supraclavicular brachial plexus block. Anesth Analg 2003;97:1514–1517.

68. Chan VW: Applying ultrasound imaging to interscalene brachial plexus block. Reg Anesth Pain Med 2003;28:340–343.

69. Chen CP, Tang SF, Hsu TC, et al: Ultrasound guidance in caudal epidural needle placement. Anesthesiology 2004;101:181–184.

70. Chawathe MS, Jones RM, Gildersleve CD, et al: Detection of epidural catheters with ultrasound in children. Paediatr Anaesth 2003;13:681–684.

71. Tsui BC, Gupta S, Finucane B: Confirmation of epidural catheter placement using nerve stimulation. Can J Anaesth 1998;45:640–644.

72. Tsui BC, Gupta S, Finucane B: Determination of epidural catheter placement using nerve stimulation in obstetric patients. Reg Anesth Pain Med 1999;24:17–23.

73. Tsui BC, Guenther C, Emery D, Finucane B: Determining epidural catheter location using nerve stimulation with radiological confirmation. Reg Anesth Pain Med 2000;25:306–309.

74. Tsui BC, Gupta S, Finucane B: Detection of subarachnoid and intravascular epidural catheter placement. Can J Anaesth 1999;46:675–678.

75. Tsui BC, Gupta S, Emery D, Finucane B: Detection of subdural placement of epidural catheter using nerve stimulation. Can J Anaesth 2000;47:471–473.

76. North RB, Kidd DH, Zahurak M, et al: Spinal cord stimulation for chronic, intractable pain: Experience over two decades. Neurosurgery 1993;32:384–394.

77. Hoppenstein R: Percutaneous implantation of chronic spinal cord electrodes for control of intractable pain: Preliminary report. Surg Neurol 1975;4:195–198.

78. Krainick JU, Thoden U, Riechert T: Spinal cord stimulation in postamputation pain. Surg Neurol 1975;4:167–170.

79. Richardson RR, Nunez C, Siqueira EB: Histological reaction to percutaneous epidural neurostimulation: Initial and long-term results. Med Prog Technol 1979;6:179–184.

80. Sherwood AM: Biomedical engineering aspects of spinal cord stimulation. Appl Neurophysiol 1981;44:126–132.

81. Komanetsky RM, Padberg AM, Lenke LG, et al: Neurogenic motor evoked potentials: A prospective comparison of stimulation methods in spinal deformity surgery. J Spinal Disord 1998;11:21–28.

82. Nagle KJ, Emerson RG, Adams DC, et al: Intraoperative monitoring of motor evoked potentials: A review of 116 cases. Neurology 1996;47:999–1004.

83. Pereon Y, Bernard JM, Fayet G, et al: Usefulness of neurogenic motor evoked potentials for spinal cord monitoring: Findings in 112 consecutive patients undergoing surgery for spinal deformity. Electroencephalogr Clin Neurophysiol 1998;108:17–23.

84. Tsui BC, Seal R, Koller J, et al: Thoracic epidural analgesia via the caudal approach in pediatric patients undergoing fundoplication using nerve stimulation guidance. Anesth Analg 2001;93:1152–1155.

85. Banwell BR, Morley-Forster P, Krause R: Decreased incidence of complications in parturients with the arrow (FlexTip Plus) epidural catheter. Can J Anaesth 1998;45:370–372.

86. Tsui BC, Sze CK. An in vitro comparison of the electrical conducting properties of multiport versus single-port epidural catheters for the epidural stimulation test. Anesth Analg 2005;101:1528–1530.

87. Tsui BC, Seal R, Koller J: Thoracic epidural catheter placement via the caudal approach in infants by using electrocardiographic guidance. Anesth Analg 2002;95:326–330.

88. Tsui BC: Thoracic epidural catheter placement in infants via the caudal approach under electrocardiographic guidance: Simplification of the original technique. Anesth Analg 2004;98:273.

89. Baris S, Guldogus F, Baris YS, et al: Is tissue coring a real problem after caudal injection in children. Paediatr Anaesth 2004;14:755–758.

90. Orme RM, Berg SJ: The "swoosh" test—an evaluation of a modified "whoosh" test in children. Br J Anaesth 2003;90:62–65.

91. Tsui BC, Tarkkila P, Gupta S, Kearney R: Confirmation of caudal needle placement using nerve stimulation. Anesthesiology 1999;91:374–378.

92. Verghese ST, Mostello LA, Patel RI, et al: Testing anal sphincter tone predicts the effectiveness of caudal analgesia in children (table). Anesth Analg 2002;94:1161–1164.

93. Emery J, Ho D, MacKeen L, et al: Pupillary reflex dilation and skin temperature to assess sensory level during combined general and caudal anesthesia in children. Paediatr Anaesth 2004;14:768–773.

94. Seefelder C: The caudal catheter in neonates: Where are the restrictions? Curr Opin Anaesthesiol 2002;15:343–348.

95. Suresh S: Thoracic epidural catheter placement in children: Are we there yet? Reg Anesth Pain Med 2004;29:83–85.

96. Tamai H, Sawamura S, Kanamori Y, et al: Thoracic epidural catheter insertion using the caudal approach assisted with an electrical nerve stimulator in young children. Reg Anesth Pain Med 2004;29:92–95.

97. Bosenberg AT, Gouws E: Skin-epidural distance in children. Anaesthesia 1995;50:895–897.

98. Hasan MA, Howard RF, Lloyd-Thomas AR: Depth of epidural space in children. Anaesthesia 1994;49:1085–1087.

99. Yamashita M: Mathematical formulae for assessing the depth of the epidural space in children. Anaesthesia 1997;52:94–95.

100. Tsui BC, Entwistle L: Thoracic epidural analgesia via the lumbar approach using nerve stimulation in a pediatric patient with Down syndrome. Acta Anaesthesiol Scand 2005;49:712–714.

101. Bromage PR, Benumof JL: Paraplegia following intracord injection during attempted epidural anesthesia under general anesthesia. Reg Anesth Pain Med 1998;23:104–107.

102. Rose JB: Spinal cord injury in a child after single-shot epidural anesthesia. Anesth Analg 2003;96:3–6.

103. Tsui BC, Wagner AM, Cunningham K, et al: Threshold current of an insulated needle in the intrathecal space in pediatric patients. Anesth Analg 2005;100:662–665.

104. Shi YB, Binette M, Martin WH, et al: Electrical stimulation for intraoperative evaluation of thoracic pedicle screw placement. Spine 2003;28:595–601.

105. Tsui BC, Faccenda KA, Wong V. Prediction of thoracic epidural depth using lamina depth. Abstract Reg Anesth Pain Med 26(2S);74:2005.

106. Murat I: Continuous thoracic epidural block. In: Saint-Maurice C, Steinberg OS (editors): *Regional Anaesthesia in Children.* Mediglobe, 1990, pp. 113–125.

C. Spinal Anesthesia in Children

Santhanam Suresh, MD • Tetsu Uejima, MD

INTRODUCTION

Spinal anesthesia is perhaps one of the oldest and most studied modalities for providing pain relief in patients undergoing surgery. J. Leonard Corning[1] is credited with discovering and administering the first spinal anesthetic in 1885, and his experience was published in a medical journal. Although the use of spinal or intrathecal anesthesia administration in children was described in the early twentieth century,[2–4] this technique was seldom used in the pediatric population until Melman,[4] later followed by Abajian et al.,[5] reported in 1984 a series of high-risk infants who underwent successful surgery under spinal anesthesia. Reports of apnea following general anesthesia in preterm infants appeared in the literature in the early 1980s[6–10] and Abajian's series offered practitioners an impetus to offer an alternative technique with reportedly fewer complications. A number of series have since been reported in all age groups for a variety of surgical procedures attesting to the safety and efficacy of spinal anesthesia.[11–13] The use of spinal anesthesia in children is most commonly used in premature infants who would otherwise require a general anesthetic (Table 54–10).

Anatomy

Understanding the anatomic differences between adults and infants is crucial to safely, and in a technically proficient fashion, administer spinal anesthesia in children (Table 54–11).

The spinal cord terminates at a much more caudad level in neonates and infants than in adults (Figure 54–17). The conus medullaris ends at approximately L1 in adults and at the L2 or L3 level in neonates and infants. To avoid potential injury to the spinal cord, dural puncture should be performed below the level of the spinal cord, that is, below L2/L3 in neonates and infants. In adults, spinal anesthesia is often administered at the interspace that is nearest an imaginary line that stretches across the top of both iliac crests, the intercristal or Truffier's line, corresponding to the L3-4 interspace. However, neonates and infants have a proportionately smaller pelvis than adults, and the sacrum is located more cephalad relative to the iliac crests. Therefore, Truffier's line crosses the midline of the vertebral column at the L4-5 or L5-S1 interspace, well below the termination of the spinal cord, making this landmark applicable in all pediatric patients.[14–16] The dural sac in neonates and infants

Table 54–10.

Indications for Spinal Anesthesia

- Hernia repair
- Circumcision
- Exploratory laparotomy
- Meningomyelocele repair
- Muscle biopsy
- Cardiac surgery

Table 54–11.

Anatomic Differences in Spinal Canal

- Conus medullaris ends at L2-L3 compared with L1 in adults
- Small pelvis with sacrum that starts more cephalad
- Dural sac ends more caudad

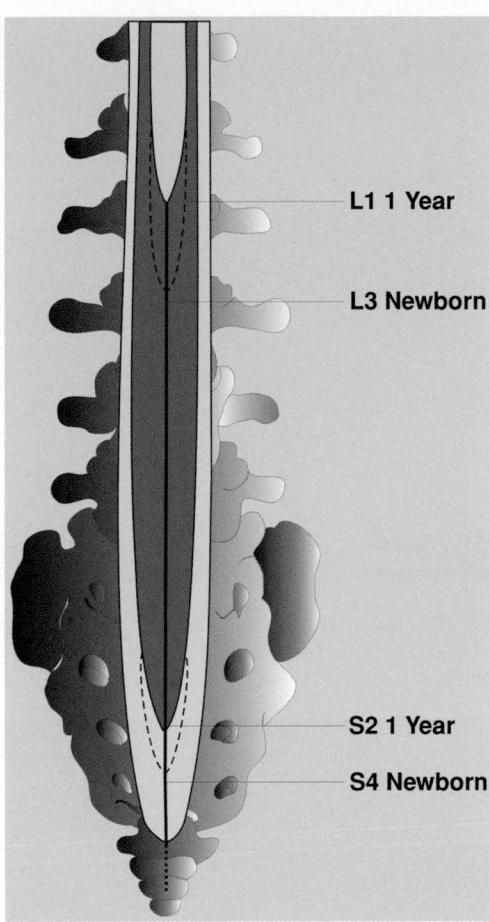

Figure 54–17. The conus medullaris ends at approximately L1 in adults and at the L2 or L3 level in neonates and infants.

also terminates in a more caudad location compared with that in adults, usually at about the level of S3 compared with the adult level of S1. The more caudad termination of the dural sac makes it more likely to have an inadvertent dural puncture during performance of a single-shot caudal block if the caudal needle is advanced too far into the caudal epidural space.[15]

Clinical Pearls

- In infants, Truffier's line crosses the midline of the vertebral column at the L4-5 or L5-S1 interspace.
- The dural sac in neonates and infants terminates at about the level of S3.

Cerebrospinal fluid volume is larger on a milliliter per kilogram basis in infants and neonates (4 mL/kg) compared with their adult counterparts (2 mL/kg). This may, in part, account for the higher local anesthetic dose requirements and shorter duration of action of spinal anesthesia in this population.

TECHNIQUE OF SPINAL ANESTHESIA IN CHILDREN

Preparation

EMLA (eutectic mixture of local anesthetic cream) or LMX (4% lidocaine cream) may be applied to the site of insertion before surgery. The operating room should be warmed before bringing the patient into the room. Warm blankets and radiant heating lamps help to diminish heat loss in infants. With older children, the room should be quiet, and, if possible, surgical instruments should be covered to minimize patient anxiety. Newer operating rooms may be equipped with stereo or video equipment, which may be used to distract older children if the block is performed while the child is awake or sedated. Standard monitoring devices (blood pressure cuff, pulse oximeter, electrocardiogram leads) should be applied before performing the block.

A plan should be made regarding the concomitant use of intravenous sedation or general anesthesia. The approach should be dictated by the medical condition and age of the patient, the comfort level of the anesthesia provider and the nature and anticipated length of the surgical procedure. In former preterm infants undergoing lower abdominal procedures of less than 90 minutes' duration, it is common practice to perform spinal anesthesia without adjuvant sedation and to conduct the anesthetic without supplemental intravenous or general anesthesia. In fact, it has been shown that the use of concomitant sedation may predispose these infants to apnea and bradycardia.[17] Older children may require supplemental sedation or light general anesthesia prior to performing the block. In some cases, spinal anesthesia may be combined with caudal or epidural anesthesia.

Patient Position

Spinal anesthesia is customarily administered in the lateral (Figure 54–18) or sitting position in children (Figure 54–19). Hypobaric solutions are not commonly used in infants. If the

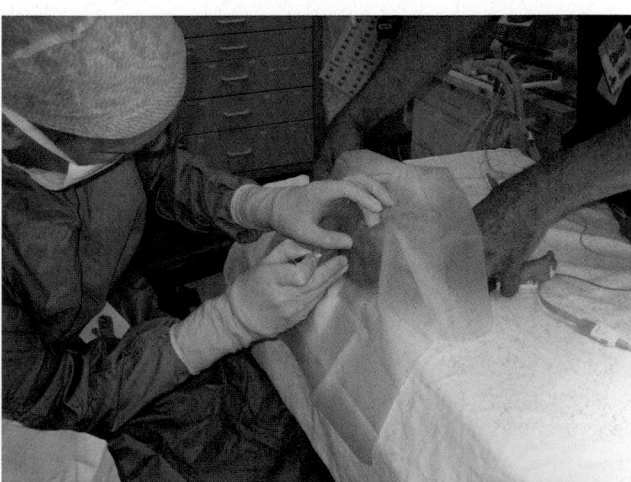

Figure 54–18. Spinal anesthesia in the neonate. Lateral position.

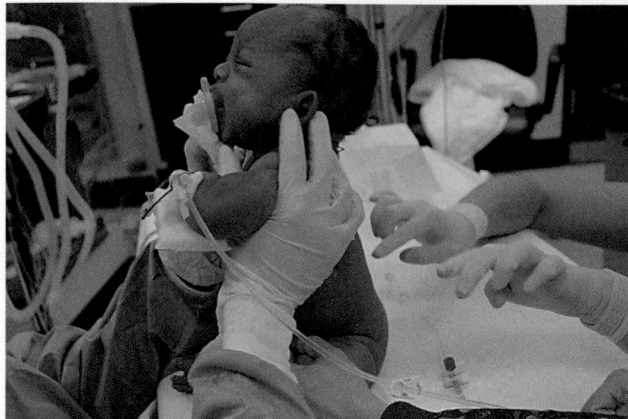

Figure 54–19. Spinal anesthesia in the neonate in the sitting position. Head flexion must be avoided to prevent respiratory obstruction.

sitting position is preferred, special attention must be paid in infants to ensure that the neck is not flexed, which may result in airway obstruction (Figure 54–19). Neck flexion is not necessary because it does not facilitate performance of the block.[18] In older children, an assistant should be present to maintain good positioning and to reassure and distract the child while the block is being performed. It is essential to monitor the oxygen saturation of the infant while performing the spinal to ensure the adequacy and patency of the airway.

Technique

In infants, the L4-5 or L5-S1 interspace should be identified; the L3-4 interspace may be used in older children. The area should be cleared and draped in a sterile fashion. If EMLA or LMX were not applied preoperatively, local anesthesia should be administered before the block in awake or sedated children (Figure 54–20). The desired dose of local anesthetic should be calculated and be prepared in a syringe before dural puncture to ensure that the correct dose is administered. A short 22- or 25-gauge spinal needle is often used. A midline approach is usually recommended over a paramedian approach. The ligamentum flavum is very soft in children and a distinctive "pop" may not be perceived when the dura is penetrated. Once clear CSF is seen exiting the needle, drug(s) should be injected slowly. The barbotage method is not recommended because this may result in unacceptably high levels of motor blockade and a potential for a total spinal blockade. The caudal end of the patient should not be elevated for placement of the electrocautery return electrode because a total spinal can result from spread of local anesthetic solution to a higher spinal level. One of the techniques we have resorted to in our teaching institution to prolong the duration of surgical analgesia is spinal anesthesia using 0.8 mg/kg bupivacaine followed immediately by a caudal block using 0.1% bupivacaine. We turn the patient to the side that has the largest hernia at the time of performance of the block. This prolongs the duration of anesthesia and analgesia. Alternatively, hypobaric solution of local anesthetic can be injected in the lateral position with the operative side up (Figures 54–21 and 54–22).

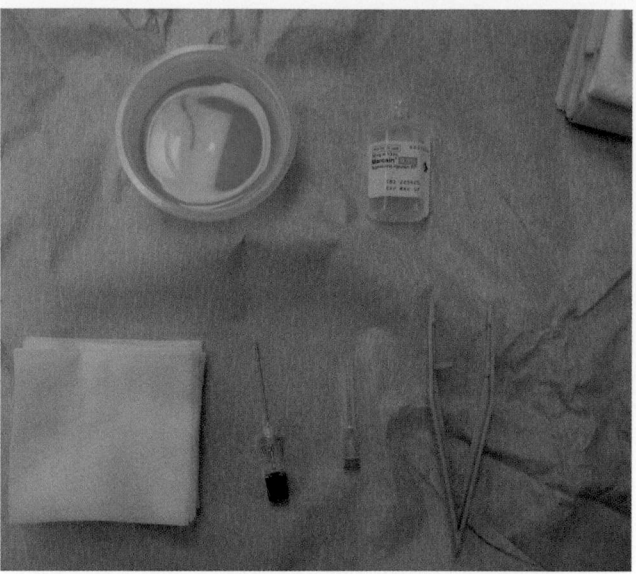

Figure 54–20. Equipment for spinal anesthesia in the neonate: the disinfectant, hypodermic needle for local infiltration, and the spinal needle.

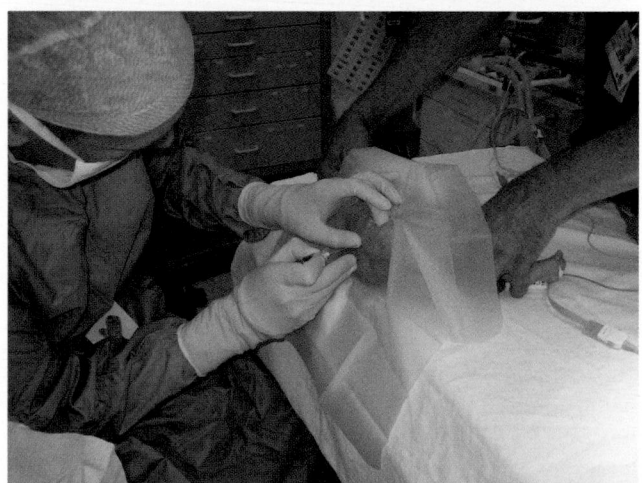

Figure 54–21. Spinal anesthesia in the neonate. Needle insertion.

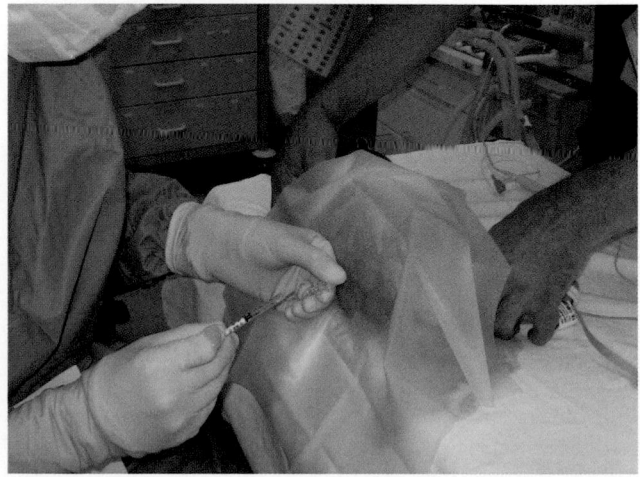

Figure 54–22. Spinal anesthesia in the neonate. Injection of the local anesthetic.

Assessing the Block

Assessing the level of blockade may prove difficult in infants and young children, particularly in patients who have received sedation or those in whom the block is being performed under general anesthesia. In infants, pin prick or their response to cold stimuli (eg, an alcohol swab) may be used as well as observation of their rate and pattern of ventilation. In children older than 2 years, we use the Bromage scale. Care should be taken to avoid placing the patient in the Trendelenburg position after the block because this will result in an extremely high or total spinal, as may occur when placing an electrocautery grounding pad on an infant's back by lifting the lower extremities. In the event of a rapidly rising level of blockade, the patient may be placed in reverse Trendelenburg position.

Clinical Pearls

EVALUATION OF SPINAL ANESTHESIA: BROMAGE SCALE

- No block (0%)—Full flexion of knees and feet possible
- Partial block (33%)—Just able to flex knees, still full flexion of knees possible
- Almost complete block (66%)—Unable to flex knees. Flexion of feet still possible
- Complete block (100%)—Unable to move legs or feet

Adverse Effects

Adverse effects from spinal anesthesia commonly seen in adults are less common in children. These include hypotension, bradycardia, postdural puncture, and transient radicular symptoms.

Hypotension

Hypotension and bradycardia are very rare occurrences when performing spinal anesthesia in children in spite of high levels of blockade and the absence of routine fluid loading prior to blockade (10 mL/kg).[19] However, we do recommend that a venous access be obtained before performing spinal anesthesia in neonates or in infants. Puncuh et al.[25] recently reported their experience with 1132 consecutive spinal anesthetics. Only 27 of 1132 received supplemental analgesia. All spinal blocks were performed with sedation. Hypotension was rarely reported. Mild decrease in blood pressure was reported in 9 of 942 patients who were younger than 10 years of age and in 8 of 190 patients older than 10 years of age. Fluid loading to increase the preload is rarely needed in the child.

Postdural Puncture Headache

The incidence of postdural puncture headache is less in children compared with adults. Large series have been reported after frequent lumbar punctures for spinal tap in children with a lower incidence of postdural puncture headaches.[20] An incidence of 8% was noted in this subgroup of oncology patients with dural puncture. The use of different types of

needles for spinal tap has been studied. This patient group was divided into those for whom either a Quincke needle or a pencil-point Whitacre needle was used. There was no difference in the incidence of headaches between the two needle groups (15% Quincke; 9% Whitacre; $P = .43$)[21] Moreover, the incidence of headaches was not different in different age groups, with 8 of 11 postdural puncture headaches occurring in children under 10 years of age; the youngest was reported in a 23-month-old baby. Transient radicular symptoms have been reported in children after spinal anesthesia with no long-term adverse effects.[22] Postdural puncture headaches have been treated with epidural blood patch (0.3 mL/kg of blood) with very good results.[23] Bed rest and caffeine are initiated followed by blood patch if the headaches do not resolve.[24] In our own practice, we tend to place a prophylactic blood patch if a suspicion of postdural puncture headache is entertained.

LOCAL ANESTHETIC CHOICES & DOSES

A variety of agents and doses have been described in the literature including tetracaine, bupivacaine,[25] lidocaine, amethecaine, levobupivacaine, and ropivacaine[26] (Table 54–12). A dose of 0.5 mg/kg to 1 mg/kg of tetracaine or bupivacaine is generally what we have been using for spinal anesthesia. An epinephrine wash rather than a standard dose of epinephrine for the syringe is preferred in our practice. Hyperbaric solution with glucose or eubaric solution result in the similar quality and duration of the spinal block in children.[27] Although a higher dose is preferred, the risk of a total spinal anesthesia is rare as long as the procedure is carried out diligently. Adjuvants to spinal solution have recently been reported. Clonidine in a dose of 1 mcg/kg added to bupivacaine (1 mg/kg) used in spinal anesthesia in newborn infants has shown to prolong the duration of the block to almost twice the duration of spinal anesthesia without clonidine.[28] We have seen a transient decrease in blood pressures with the use of 2 mcg/kg of clonidine and a propensity to greater sedation in the postoperative period. It may be advisable to use a dose of caffeine (10 mg/kg) intravenously to prevent any potential apnea in the postoperative period, especially if clonidine is used in the spinal anesthetic solution.

Table 54–12.

Dosage for Spinal Anesthesia

Local anesthetic solution
Tetracaine: 0.5–1 mg/kg
Bupivacaine: 0.5–1 mg/kg

Additives
Epinephrine wash
Clonidine: 1–2 mcg/kg
Morphine: 10 mcg/kg (only for cardiac surgical patients who will be ventilated postoperatively)

Table 54–13.

Relative Contraindications to Spinal Anesthesia

- Anatomic abnormalities of the spine
- Degenerative neuromuscular disease
- Patient and family dissent
- Coagulopathy
- Bacterial infection
- Increased intracranial pressure
- Patients with ventriculoperitoneal shunts

Relative Contraindications

Contraindications to the use of spinal anesthesia in children are similar to those in the adult population (Table 54–13). The use of spinal anesthesia in children with neuromuscular diseases, particularly central core disease or congenital neuromuscular disease, is controversial. Other contraindications to spinal anesthesia may include anatomic deformities, infection at the site of insertion, an underlying coagulopathy, hemodynamic instability, presence of a ventriculoperitoneal (or other ventricular) shunt, and poorly controlled seizures. We avoid spinal anesthesia in neonates and children who may have increased intracranial pressures.

Special consideration should be given to the child with a known difficult airway when considering a spinal anesthetic. Although spinal anesthesia may be a reasonable choice in these patients, the first consideration should be the ability of the practitioner to manage the airway. Obviously, the nature of the surgical procedure will dictate the use of regional techniques. Spinal anesthesia has been used for myelomeningocele repair, exploratory laparotomy, and other invasive abdominal procedures in infants. The surgical site, the anticipated length of the procedure, and the surgical position (supine, lateral, prone) are important factors. A third consideration is the age of the child. Spinal anesthesia can be administered in infants who are awake, but preschool and school-age children may require intravenous sedation. This poses its own set of risks in pediatric patients with a difficult airway.

Clinical Uses

Apnea and Former Preterm Infants

The most common indication for spinal anesthesia in pediatric patients is its use in former preterm infants undergoing bilateral inguinal hernia repairs. Apnea can occur in former preterm patients following a general anesthetic.[5,9] A number of small studies have confirmed this finding; however, there is considerable disagreement regarding the incidence of apnea and the conceptual age at which a former preterm infant may safely undergo general anesthesia on an outpatient basis. Lack of uniformity in study design, small patient population

sizes, and variations in methodology probably account for the differences.

Cote et al.[9] performed a meta-analysis of eight studies investigating postoperative apnea in former preterm infants after general anesthesia comprising 255 patients. Overall, the risk of apnea was independently related to both gestational age and conceptual age. Additional risk factors for postoperative apnea were a hematocrit less than 30% and continued apneic episodes at home. The study stratified infants into two risk groups: a 5% risk group and a 1% risk group. The risk of postoperative apnea did not fall below 5% with a 95% statistical confidence interval until patients reached a postconceptual age of 48 weeks with a gestational age of 35 weeks. The risk of apnea did not decrease below 1% with a 95% statistical confidence interval until infants reached 54 weeks conceptual age with a gestational age of 35 weeks or postconceptual age of 56 weeks with a gestational age of 32 weeks.

Regional anesthesia may decrease but not eliminate the incidence of postoperative apnea. The concomitant use of ketamine may increase the incidence of postoperative apnea above that reported in control patients.[17,29] Unfortunately, very little information is available regarding the potential benefits of spinal anesthesia over general anesthesia in this particular population. A small randomized study of former preterm infants who received spinal anesthesia showed a decrease in the incidence of postoperative desaturation and bradycardia compared with those who received general anesthesia for inguinal herniorraphy.[30] They observed no significant difference in the incidence of postoperative apnea between the two groups. An observational study of more than 250 former preterm infants found a 4.9% incidence of postoperative apnea after spinal anesthesia for inguinal herniorraphy.[1] A prospective study from France reported no incidence of postoperative apnea in a subset of 30 former preterm infants who received spinal anesthesia. Craven et al.[31] reviewed several randomized controlled studies and found only borderline statistical advantage of a spinal anesthetic over a general anesthetic.

For Procedures Other Than Herniorrhaphy

Spinal anesthesia has been successfully used for a variety of surgical procedures in children.[12,13] Most of the reported series in the literature involve infants. The early report by Abajian et al.[11] not only included infants undergoing herniorrhaphy but also those undergoing a variety of general, urologic, and orthopedic procedures. It is interesting that the study population included infants with medical conditions the authors felt increased the risk of general anesthesia. These conditions included laryngomalacia, macroglossia, micrognathia, congenital heart disease, Down syndrome, adrenogenital syndrome, failure to thrive, arthrogryposis, and Gordon syndrome.

Blaise et al.[12] reported 30 patients age 7 weeks to 13 years who underwent spinal anesthesia for a variety of surgical procedures. Kokki et al.[26,32] reported satisfactory anesthesia in 92 of 93 children age 1 to 17 years undergoing ropivacaine spinal anesthesia for lower abdominal or lower extremity procedures. Spinal anesthesia has been used in infants for various other procedures including meningomyelocele repair[33] and major abdominal surgery.

Cardiac Surgery

Regional techniques have been used in cardiac surgery to facilitate early extubation.[34] The largest series of use of spinal anesthesia for cardiac surgery comes from a prospective randomized analysis from Stanford University.[35] The group who received spinal anesthesia for postoperative pain relief had less opioid requirement in the postoperative period in children undergoing elective cardiac surgery with early extubation in the operating room.

Clinical Pearls

Special considerations for infants and children undergoing spinal anesthesia:

- Choose patients who are not likely to have a significant decrease in systemic vascular resistance after spinal anesthesia.

- Ability to perform atraumatic spinal anesthesia, especially because these patients will be heparanized in the postoperative period.

- Use of hydrophilic opioid so that a rostral spread can ensure longer duration of analgesia

- Surgeon's motivation

In summary, spinal anesthesia in pediatrics is most commonly used in the preterm infant undergoing anesthesia for hernia repair. Spinal anesthesia can also be used effectively in children for postoperative pain relief, especially if opioids are used. Finally, in some clinical settings, spinal anesthesia may be the only anesthetic option available.

References

1. Corning JL: Spinal anesthesia and local medication of the cord. NY J Med 1885;42:483–485.
2. Gray H: A study of spinal anaesthesia in children and infants: From a series of 200 cases. Lancet 1909;2:913–917.
3. Bainbridge W: Analgesia in children by spinal injection with a report of a new method of sterilization of the injection fluid. Med Rec 1900;58:937–940.
4. Melman E, Penuelas JA, Marrufo J: Regional anesthesia in children. Anesth Analg 1975;54:387–390.
5. Abajian JC, Mellish RW, Browne AF, et al: Spinal anesthesia for surgery in the high-risk infant. Anesth Analg 1984;63:359–362.
6. Gregory GA, Steward DJ: Life-threatening perioperative apnea in the ex-"premie." Anesthesiology 1983;59:495–498.
7. Steward DJ: Postoperative apnea syndrome in premature infants. West J Med 1992;157:567.
8. Steward DJ: Preterm infants are more prone to complications following minor surgery than are term infants. Anesthesiology 1982;56:304–306.
9. Cote CJ, Zaslavsky A, Downes JJ, et al: Postoperative apnea in former preterm infants after inguinal herniorrhaphy. A combined analysis [see comments]. Anesthesiology 1995;82:809–822.
10. Liu LM, Cote CJ, Goudsouzian NG, et al: Life-threatening apnea in infants recovering from anesthesia. Anesthesiology 1983;59:506–510.
11. Frumiento C, Abajian JC, Vane DW: Spinal anesthesia for preterm infants undergoing inguinal hernia repair. Arch Surg 2000;135:445–451.
12. Blaise GA, Roy WL: Spinal anaesthesia for minor paediatric surgery. Can Anaesth Soc J 1986;33(2):227–230.
13. Kokki H, Tuovinen K, Hendolin H: Spinal anaesthesia for paediatric day-case surgery: A double-blind, randomized, parallel group, prospective comparison of isobaric and hyperbaric bupivacaine. Br J Anaesth 1998;81:502–506.
14. Busoni P, Messeri A: Spinal anesthesia in children: Surface anatomy. Anesth Analg 1989;68:418–419.
15. Busoni P, Messeri A: Spinal anesthesia in infants: Could a L5-S1 approach be safer? Anesthesiology 1991;75:168–169.
16. Gray H: *Anatomy of the Human Body: Gray's Anatomy*, 30th ed. Williams & Wilkins, 1985.
17. Welborn LG, Rice LJ, Hannallah RS, et al: Postoperative apnea in former preterm infants: Prospective comparison of spinal and general anesthesia. Anesthesiology 1990;72:838–842.
18. Gleason CA, Martin RJ, Anderson JV, et al: Optimal position for a spinal tap in preterm infants. Pediatrics 1983;71:31–35.
19. Oberlander TF, Berde CB, Lam KH, et al: Infants tolerate spinal anesthesia with minimal overall autonomic changes: Analysis of heart rate variability in former premature infants undergoing hernia repair. Anesth Analg 1995;80:20–27.
20. Ramamoorthy C, Geiduschek JM, Bratton SL, et al: Postdural puncture headache in pediatric oncology patients. Clin Pediatr 1998;37:247–251.
21. Kokki H, Salonvaara M, Herrgard E, Onen P: Postdural puncture headache is not an age-related symptom in children: A prospective, open-randomized, parallel group study comparing a 22-gauge Quincke with a 22-gauge Whitacre needle. Paediatr Anaesth 1999;9:429–434.
22. Salmela L, Aromaa U: Transient radicular irritation after spinal anesthesia induced with hyperbaric solutions of cerebrospinal fluid-diluted lidocaine 50 mg/ml or mepivacaine 40 mg/ml or bupivacaine 5 mg/ml. Acta Anaesthesiol Scand 1998;42:765–769.
23. Ylonen P, Kokki H: Management of postdural puncture headache with epidural blood patch in children. Paediatr Anaesth 2002;12:526–529.
24. Yucel A, Ozyalcin S, Talu GK, et al: Intravenous administration of caffeine sodium benzoate for postdural puncture headache. Reg Anesth Pain Med 1999;24:51–54.
25. Puncuh F, Lampugnani E, Kokki H: Use of spinal anaesthesia in paediatric patients: A single centre experience with 1132 cases. Paediatr Anaesth 2004;14:564–567.
26. Kokki H, Ylonen P, Laisalmi M, et al: Isobaric ropivacaine 5 mg/ml for spinal anesthesia in children. Anesth Analg 2005;100:66–70.
27. Kokki H, Hendolin H: Hyperbaric bupivacaine for spinal anaesthesia in 7-18 yr old children: Comparison of bupivacaine 5 mg ml-1 in 0.9% and 8% glucose solutions. Br J Anaesth 2000;84:59–62.
28. Rochette A, Raux O, Troncin R, et al: Clonidine prolongs spinal anesthesia in newborns: A prospective dose-ranging study. Anesth Analg 2004;98:56–59.
29. Welborn LG, de Soto H, Hannallah RS, et al: The use of caffeine in the control of post-anesthetic apnea in former premature infants. Anesthesiology 1988;68:796–798.
30. Krane EJ, Haberkern CM, Jacobson LE: Postoperative apnea, bradycardia, and oxygen desaturation in formerly premature infants: Prospective comparison of spinal and general anesthesia. Anesth Analg 1995;80:7–13.

31. Craven PD, Badawi M, Henderson-Smart DJ, O'Brien M: Regional (spinal, epidural, caudal) versus general anaesthesia in preterm infants undergoing inguinal herniorrhaphy in early infancy. Cochrane Database Syst Rev 2005.

32. Kokki H, Hendolin H: Comparison of spinal anaesthesia with epidural anaesthesia in paediatric surgery. Acta Anaesthesiol Scand 1995;39:896–900.

33. Viscomi CM, Abajian JC, Wald SL, et al: Spinal anesthesia for repair of meningomyelocele in neonates. Anesth Analg 1995;81:492–495.

34. Zarate E, Latham P, White PF, et al: Fast-track cardiac anesthesia: Use of remifentanil combined with intrathecal morphine as an alternative to sufentanil during desflurane anesthesia. Anesth Analg 2000;91:283–287.

35. Hammer GB, Ramamoorthy C, Cao H, et al: Postoperative analgesia after spinal blockade in infants and children undergoing cardiac surgery (table). Anesth Analg 2005;100:1283–1288.

36. Polaner D, Suresh S, Cote CJ: Pediatric regional anesthesia. In: Cote C, Todres ID, Ryan JF, Goudsouzian NG (editors). *A Practice of Anesthesia for Infants and Children,* 3rd ed. WB Saunders, 2000, pp. 636–675.

D. Peripheral Nerve Blocks for Children

Santhanam Suresh, MD • Michael Frederickson, MD

INTRODUCTION

Peripheral nerve blocks have been regaining significant popularity in the daily practice of most anesthesiologists. Despite the trend toward an increase in the use of regional anesthesia and nerve blocks in adults, peripheral nerve blocks in children remain underused. Common reasons include the concern about neurologic complications and the lack of technical skills required for their successful use. Although performance of peripheral nerve blocks in anesthetized adults is often debated, such practice is well accepted in pediatric patients. A large prospective database collected in France demonstrated no increased incidence of complications when regional anesthesia, particularly when peripheral nerve blocks were performed under general anesthesia.[1] The incidence of regional anesthesia-related complications in one study was less than 0.9 of 1000 anesthetic procedures performed. When peripheral nerve blocks are used with skill, their success and complications of performance in children should not be significantly different from those in adults. In addition, the equipment used in children is similar to that used in adults (see Chapter 17). Although most peripheral nerve blocks are performed in an operating room environment, the use of regional anesthesia in children extends to an emergency department[2] as well as to an intensive care unit setting.[3,4] The key to success of peripheral nerve blockade in children is the proper knowledge of the anatomy, pharmacology, equipment used for regional anesthesia, and effective use of pre-procedure sedation and analgesia.

Equipment

A reliable nerve stimulator is an essential tool to help locate motor nerves for blockade. A nerve stimulator with adequate current output capable of eliciting percutaneous stimulation (eg, 5 mA/1 ms) for surface mapping is suggested.

Clinical Pearls

- Muscle relaxants should be avoided when using a nerve stimulator for motor blockade.

It is crucial to remember that when using a nerve stimulator for motor blockade, muscle relaxants should be avoided and either a deep inhalation induction with placement of an endotracheal tube under general anesthesia or the use of a laryngeal mask airway is preferred. Occasionally, it is feasible to perform a nerve block in an older child with IV sedation without the use of general anesthesia. The negative electrode is attached to the needle (*b*lack to *b*lock), and the positive is attached to the patient (*p*ositive to *p*atient). Once a needle is placed close to a nerve or a plexus and proper stimulation is obtained, the current output is decreased to maintain the motor response at 0.4–0.2 mA to ensure intimate needle–nerve relationship. Objective monitoring of the injection pressures during injection of local anesthetic to decrease the risk of intraneural injection may offset some of the concerns about the use of regional anesthesia in patients under general anesthesia.[5] Similarly, the introduction of ultrasound-guided nerve blocks has significantly increased the accuracy and may decrease the risk of neurologic and systemic complications (see Chapter 52).

Because of the concomitant use of general anesthesia in children, the intraoperative efficacy of nerve blocks is often assessed indirectly using hemodynamic parameters and the required depth of anesthesia. Most regional techniques used in children are primarily used for the purpose of providing postoperative pain control rather than surgical anesthesia. Peripheral nerve blocks are also used in children for chronic painful conditions such as chronic headaches, or CRPS-1.

Local Anesthetics

Section A of this chapter describes the use of local anesthetic solutions in detail. It is imperative, however, to remember that the dosage of local anesthetic solutions should be on a milligram per kilogram basis and not based on total volume used, as is the practice in adult regional anesthesia. Sensory blocks including head and neck blocks require very small volumes of local anesthetic solution. The dosage should be adjusted downward in infants and neonates owing to the decrease in protein binding and α_1-acid glycoprotein, allowing a greater amount of the free fraction of the drug in the systemic circulation. The addition of epinephrine to the local anesthetic solution may offer an additional advantage by (1) revealing intravascular placement, particularly in the child under general anesthesia[6]; and (2) by prolonging local anesthetic action when used for peripheral nerve blockade.

The addition of sodium bicarbonate may offer the advantage of decreasing pain on injection and potentially facilitate a more rapid onset of local anesthetic action.[7] The addition of other additives including clonidine and fentanyl has also been explored in the pediatric population. Clonidine may be effective in prolonging the analgesic effects of local anesthetic solutions.[8–10] However, caution has to be exercised to avoid clonidine in infants and neonates because of the higher incidence of hypotension and excessive sedation in this population. Other local anesthetic solutions including ropivacaine[11,12] and levobupivacaine[13] are effective for providing adequate analgesia when used for peripheral nerve blocks.

Clinical Pearls

Maximum dose of local anesthetics:

- The maximum recommended dose of bupivacaine is 2.5 mg/kg plain and 3.5 mg/kg with epinephrine. The duration of bupivacaine varies from 2–16 hours, depending on the application.
- The maximum recommended dose of 2-chloroprocaine is 8 mg/kg plain and 10 mg/kg with epinephrine. The duration of chloroprocaine is 1–1.5 hours.
- The maximum recommended dose of lidocaine is 5 mg/kg plain and 10 mg/kg with epinephrine. The duration of lidocaine is 2–3 hours.

Volume of local anesthetic for common blocks:

    Axillary block: 0.2–0.6 mL/kg

    Interscalene block: 0.33 mL/kg

    Femoral block: 0.5 mL/kg

    Sciatic block: 0.15–0.2 mL/kg

Nerve Localization Methods

Surface Mapping

The most common method of nerve localization is using a stimulating needle (sheathed needle) with the needle pointed in the direction of the nerve. Because of the need for identifying the location of the nerve before puncture, pediatric patients benefit from surface stimulation or surface mapping.[14] This allows approximation of the site for needle insertion and decreases the need for multiple needle insertions during nerve localization. Surface mapping can be used to facilitate a variety of superficial nerve block procedures such as axillary, radial, median, and ulnar nerve blocks at the axilla and the elbow, as well as for femoral and popliteal fossa blocks. Higher current amperage and/or current duration is required (usually about 5 mA/1 ms) to percutaneously stimulate. A relatively moist surface using either alcohol swabs or lubricating jelly allows for better contact of the negative electrode.

Ultrasonography

Ultrasonography has been introduced into anesthesia practice for over a decade. In recent years, however, interest in this technology to aid in nerve localization has significantly increased coinciding with advances in technology of the ultrasound equipment.[15–17] Although ultrasound may be useful for nerve localization, one of its main benefits is to provide visualization of the dispersion of the local anesthetic within the desired tissue planes. Ultrasound has been shown to provide adequate landmarks for determining the location of nerves in children along with a discriminatory approach to evaluating nerve location and anatomic variations in infants and children.[18] This technology, however, requires significant training and skill for its successful implementation. At the time of publication of this text, there are relatively few practitioners who are adequately skilled and comfortable with the use of ultrasound in children for peripheral nerve blockade. The reader is referred to Chapter 52 for a detailed discussion on this topic.

Sedation

Sedation before performing peripheral nerve blocks in children is imperative for successful use of nerve blocks. Although the performance of regional anesthesia and peripheral nerve blocks in adults is often debated, the use of heavy sedation or general anesthesia before nerve blockade in children is standard practice. The collective opinion of pediatric anesthesiologists has been highlighted in an editorial that encourages the need to continue to perform regional techniques in children under general anesthesia.[19]

Peripheral nerve block in children can be topographically divided to cover all areas of the body (Table 54–14). A short description of the anatomy followed by the technique for performance of nerve blocks is described in this chapter (Table 54–15).

Table 54–14.

Commonly Performed Peripheral Nerve Blocks in Children

Head and neck
Supraorbital and supratrochlear
Occipital
Infraorbital
Superficial cervical plexus

Upper extremity
Brachial plexus
    Parascalene
    Supraclavicular
    Infraclavicular
    Axillary
Elbow
    Median
    Radial
    Ulnar
Wrist
    Median
    Radial
    Ulnar

Lower extremity
Lumbar plexus
Femoral nerve
Lateral femoral cutaneous
Sciatic nerve
    Infragluteal
    Popliteal fossa

Trunk and thorax
Intercostal
Ilioinguinal, iliohypogastric
Rectus sheath block
Penile

Table 54–15.

Suggested Dosing Guidelines for Local Anesthetics for Peripheral Nerve Blocks

Technique	Dose (mL/kg)	Max volume (mL)
Head and neck blocks	0.1 mL/kg	5 mL
Axillary block	0.2–0.3 mL/kg	15 mL
Infraclavicular block	0.2–0.3 mL/kg	15 mL
Intercostal block	0.05–0.1 mL/kg	5 mL
Rectus sheath block	0.2 mL/kg	10 mL
Ilioinguinal nerve block	0.2–0.3 mL/kg	15 mL
Femoral nerve block	0.2–0.4 mL/kg	15 mL
Sciatic nerve block	0.3–0.5 mL	20 mL
Popliteal fossa block	0.3–0.4 mL/kg	15 mL
Lumbar plexus	0.3–0.5 mL/kg	20 mL
Penile block	0.1 mL/kg	10 mL
Digital nerve blocks	0.05–0.1 mL/kg	2–3 mL

for the midportion of the forehead, which is innervated by the supratrochlear nerve. This block can be used for frontal craniotomies[20] as well as for minor surgical procedures including excision of scalp nevus.[21]

Technique: The supraorbital nerve can be easily blocked as it exits the supraorbital foramen. This can be easily correlated in the patient to the midpoint of the pupil (Figure 54–23). When the foramen is located, a subcutaneous injection of local anesthetic solution (1–2 mL 0.25%

ANATOMIC DIVISIONS

Head & Neck Blocks

The use of nerve blocks for various head and neck procedures is gaining popularity, particularly in the pediatric population. Most of these blocks are sensory nerve blocks, which are easy to administer (field blocks) and virtually devoid of complications. They can, however, provide quality analgesia in the postoperative period, facilitating immediate postoperative recovery and pain management. Most of the innervation for the face and scalp are derived from the trigeminal nerve (cranial V) and the cervical plexus (C2-C4).

V1 Division Trigeminal Nerve

The supraorbital and supratrochlear nerves are branches of the first division of the trigeminal nerve that exit from the supraorbital foramen. The supraorbital nerve provides sensory innervation to the anterior portion of the scalp except

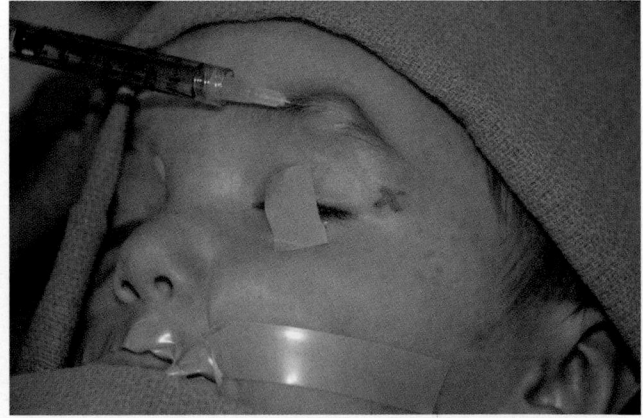

Figure 54–23. Supraorbital nerve block. The supraorbital foramen is located and a local anesthetic (1–2 mL of 0.25% bupivacaine with 1:200,000 epinephrine) is injected subcutaneously.

bupivacaine with 1:200,000 epinephrine) is injected. Once the local anesthetic solution is injected, gentle pressure is maintained to decrease the formation of a hematoma. Complications are rare with this block.

V2 Branch of Trigeminal Nerve

The second division of the trigeminal nerve is also referred to as the maxillary division of the trigeminal nerve. It exits from the maxillary foramen or the infraorbital foramen, which is located about 2 cm from the midline and is usually aligned with the midpoint of the pupils. The nerve provides the sensory supply to the upper lip, the choana, maxillary sinus, part of the nasal septum, and the tip of the nose. This block can be used to provide analgesia for cleft lip surgery,[22] nasal septal repair,[23] and endoscopic sinus surgery.[24–26]

Technique: There are two approaches to the maxillary division of the trigeminal nerve:

Extraoral route: The needle is directed into the infraorbital foramen from an external location of the nerve. The foramen is located externally and a 27-gauge needle is inserted into the foramen. After aspiration to rule out intravascular injection, 1–2 mL of local anesthetic solution is injected.

Intraoral route: The nerve is accessed through the subsulcal area in the buccal mucosa (Figure 54–24). This is our preferred modality for blocking the infraorbital nerve. The upper incisor or the second bicuspid on the side to be blocked is located; a needle is passed through a subsulcal route toward the location of the infraorbital foramen. After careful aspiration, local anesthetic solution is injected. For infants scheduled for cleft lip repairs, we use 0.5 mL of local anesthetic solution for each side; for older children and adolescents, we use 1.5–2 mL of local anesthetic solution. The upper lip is likely to remain numb for several hours after the block and can be disconcerting to patients and older children. Care should also be provided to prevent biting of the upper lip during the emergence period from anesthesia.

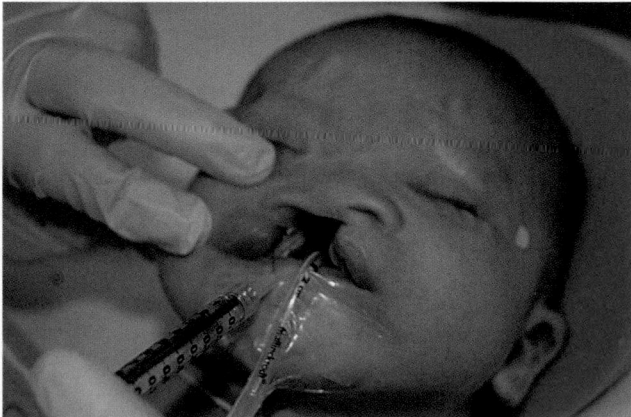

Figure 54–24. Infraorbital nerve block. A needle is passed through a subsulcal route toward the location of the infraorbital foramen. For infants undergoing cleft lip repair, 0.5–1 mL of local anesthetic solution is injected on each side.

V3 Mandibular Division of the Trigeminal Nerve

The mandibular division of the trigeminal nerve provides analgesia for the lower jaw, lower lip, and portions of the temporoparietal portions of the scalp. The most common nerve targeted in children is the mental nerve, which exits from the mental foramen located at the level of the midline in line with the pupil and the supraorbital and infraorbital foramen.

Technique: An intraoral route is again preferred for placement of this nerve block. The needle is directed at the level of the lower incisor toward the infraorbital foramen; 1.5 mL of local anesthetic solution is injected after careful aspiration. Gentle massage of the area is carried out after the injection.

Greater Occipital Nerve

The greater occipital nerve is a branch of cervical root C2. The nerve pierces the aponeurosis and traverses medial to the occipital artery inferiorly and crosses over to the lateral aspect of the artery superiorly by the nuchal line as it innervates the posterior portions of the scalp. This can be used for providing an adequate nerve block of the scalp for posterior fossa craniotomies as well as for patients with chronic occipital neuralgia.[20]

Technique: The occipital protuberance is palpated. The midline is identified and the occipital artery is palpated. A 27-gauge needle is inserted, and a subcutaneous injection of local anesthetic solution is performed (1.5–2 mL of 0.25% bupivacaine with 1:200,000 epinephrine). The area is massaged gently after the injection. Complications are rare with this technique.

Superficial Cervical Plexus Block

The superficial cervical plexus is a pure sensory nerve derived from C2-C4 nerve roots. It wraps around the belly of the sternocleidomastoid at the level of the cricoid and divides into four branches, the lesser occipital supplying the posterior auricular area; the great auricular supplying the mastoid area and the pinna; transverse cervical supplying the anterior portion of the neck; and the superficial cervical supplying the skin over the shoulder in a cape-like distribution over the shoulder joint. Blockade of the superficial cervical plexus can provide good postoperative analgesia for tympanomastoid surgery,[27] otoplasty,[28] thyroid surgery,[29] and for procedures performed on the anterior portion of the neck.[30] The use of this nerve block decreases the use of opioids in the perioperative period, thereby decreasing the incidence of nausea and vomiting.[27]

Technique: The technique is essentially identical with that in the adult patient. The clavicular head of the sternocleidomastoid is identified. A line drawn from the cricoid cartilage to intersect the posterior border of the sternocleidomastoid is identified. A subcutaneous injection of local anesthetic solution (1–2 mL of 0.25% bupivacaine with epinephrine 1:200,000) is performed. Caution must be exercised while injecting because of the close proximity of the nerve to the external jugular vein. Deep injections should be avoided to prevent

```
                          ┌─────────────────┐
                          │ Brachial plexus │
                          └─────────────────┘
         ┌────────────────┬──────────┴───────┬────────────────┐
   ┌───────────┐   ┌──────────────┐   ┌──────────┐   ┌──────────────┐
   │Parascalene│   │Infraclavicular│   │ Axillary │   │ Elbow blocks │
   └───────────┘   └──────────────┘   └──────────┘   └──────────────┘
              ┌──────────┴──────────┐                        │
     ┌─────────────────┐  ┌──────────────────┐      ┌──────────────────┐
     │Anterior approach│  │Para-coracoid approach│  │Median, ulnar, radial│
     └─────────────────┘  └──────────────────┘      └──────────────────┘
```

Figure 54–25. Brachial plexus block in children.

the potential injection into the deep cervical plexus with associated adverse effects including recurrent laryngeal nerve paralysis, paralysis of the hemi-diaphragm, and Horner's syndrome from unilateral sympathetic ganglion blockade. Complications, though rare, are related to deep cervical plexus blockade and intravascular injection. Refer to Chapter 23 for a more detailed description of the technique.

Upper Extremity Blocks

A complete review of the anatomy of the brachial plexus is provided in Chapters 3 and 25. There are multiple approaches to the brachial plexus in children. Although the interscalene block is often used in adults for most surgical procedures of the shoulder, this approach is used infrequently in children. This is due to the increased incidence of complications associated with the use of the interscalene approach, particularly in children who are under general anesthesia.[25] The most common approaches to the brachial plexus in children include the parascalene approach, the infraclavicular approach, and the axillary approach (Figure 54–25).

Local Anesthetic Dose for Upper Extremity Blocks

Local anesthetic dosing for upper extremity peripheral nerve blockade is based on weight. Children younger than 5–8 years should receive 0.3–0.5 mL/kg of bupivacaine 0.25% or ropivacaine 0.2%. Older children may require larger concentrations such as 0.3–0.5 mL/kg of bupivacaine 0.5% or ropivacaine 0.5%. Epinephrine 1:200,000 should be added for detection of inadvertent intravascular injection. For continuous infusion through a peripheral nerve block catheter, the suggested dose of local anesthetic is 0.2 mg/kg/h of ropivacaine 0.1% or levobupivacaine 0.125% in newborns or infants and 0.3–0.4 mg/kg/h of ropivacaine 0.1% or levobupivacaine 0.125% in older children. The maximum dose of ropivacaine for continuous central infusion is 0.4 mg/kg/h, and care should be taken to ensure that the child does not receive more than this amount.

Parascalene approach: This approach has been used extensively in children.[31] It gives the operator the flexibility to approach the plexus with less risk of complications noted with the conventional interscalene approach to the brachial plexus. The roots and trunks of the brachial plexus are blocked in this position, and hence it provides good postoperative analgesia for surgery performed on the shoulder, hand, and arm. Landmarks are the posterior border of the sternocleidomastoid muscle, the midpoint of the clavicle, and the cricoid

cartilage, C6. An imaginary line is drawn between the Chassignac's tubercle and the midpoint of the clavicle. The needle is inserted perpendicularly at the junction of the upper two thirds and lower third of this imaginary line and directed in the anteroposterior plane until twitches are obtained. Then 0.2 mL/kg to a maximum of 10 mL local anesthetic solution is injected after careful aspiration.

Complications: Intravascular injection, intraneural injection, and consequent brachial plexus injury.

Infraclavicular approach: The infraclavicular approach allows an easy approach to the block of the brachial plexus and is suitable for placement of a catheter for continuous plexus anesthesia.

Technique: Following is the classic approach. The midpoint of the clavicle is determined. The axillary artery is palpated in the axilla. Alternatively, ultrasound can be used to localize the plexus (Figure 54–26). A stimulating needle is directed from the midpoint of the clavicle toward the axillary artery at an angle of 45 degrees to the skin. An initial stimulation of the pectoralis muscle is noted, and as the needle approaches the brachial plexus, the flexion or extension of the wrist and elbow is noted. The current is decreased to 0.2–0.3 mA; if a twitch response is still present, after careful aspiration, 0.2 mL/kg of local anesthetic solution to a maximum of 15 mL is injected. This approach is also uniquely suitable for insertion of a catheter and administration of continuous brachial plexus block. The catheter is inserted 3–4 cm beyond the tip of the needle (Figure 54–27) and secured to the anterior chest wall (Figure 54–28).

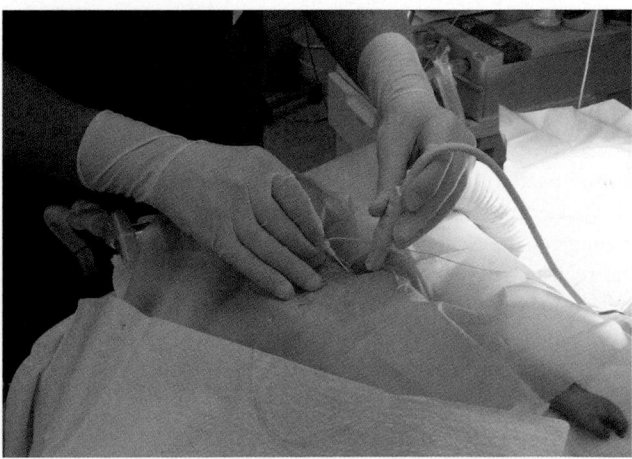

Figure 54–26. Infraclavicular block. Shown is localization of the plexus using ultrasound-guided technique.

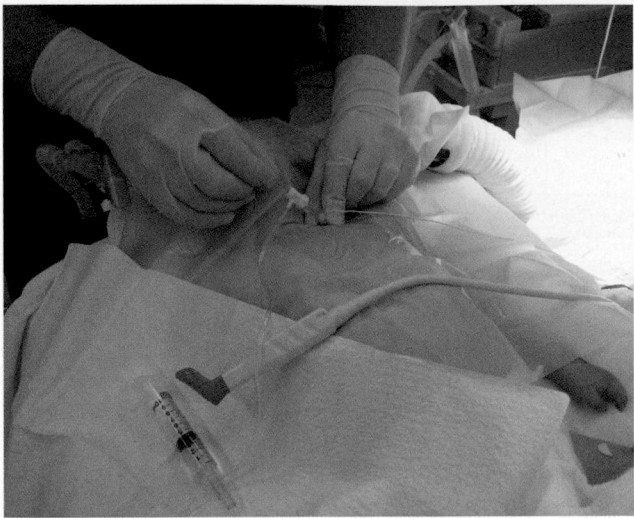

Figure 54–27. Infraclavicular block. Insertion of the catheter.

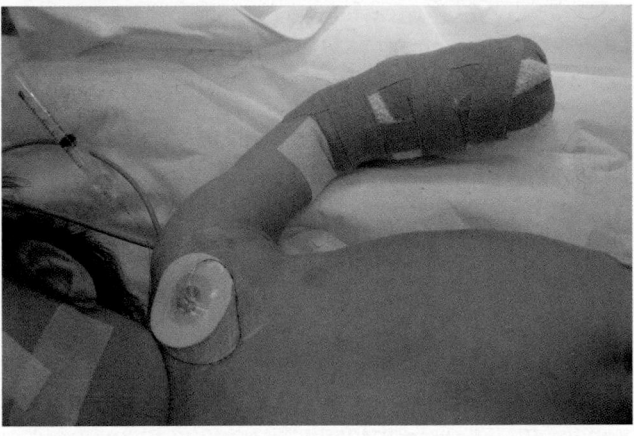

Figure 54–28. Infraclavicular block. The catheter is secured to the anterior chest wall.

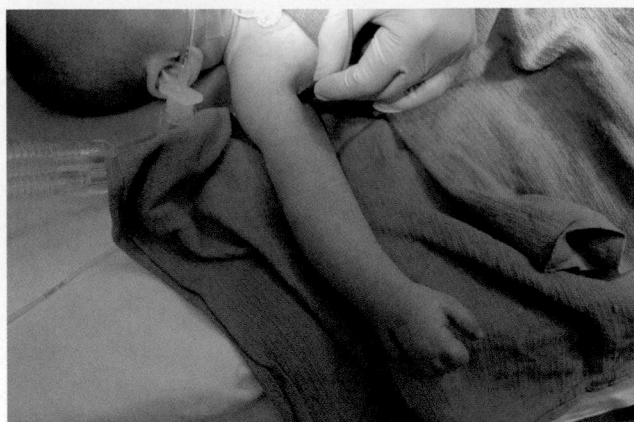

Figure 54–29. Axillary brachial plexus localization using surface stimulation.

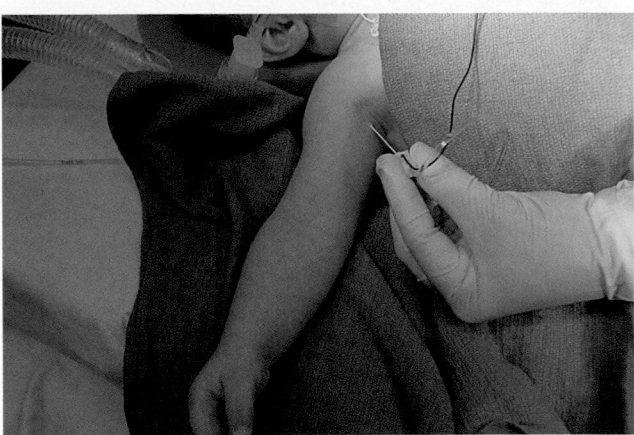

Figure 54–30. Axillary brachial plexus block. Once the brachial plexus is approximated using surface stimulation, nerve stimulator technique is used to accomplish blockade.

Complications: Although rare, the cupola of the lung is in close proximity to the passage of the needle. Hence, caution must be exerted while placing the needle. Intravascular injection is a possible complication because of the close proximity of the subclavian vessels.

Axillary Approach to the Brachial Plexus

The axillary approach to the brachial plexus is the most commonly used approach in children and adolescents. It is used for procedures on the arm and the hand. The primary advantage of the axillary approach is the ease of placement and the relatively lower risk of complications. However, there is a 40–50% potential of missing the musculocutaneous nerve with this approach owing to the proximal exit of this nerve from the axillary sheath. Hence while performing a block using this approach, the musculocutaneous nerve should be blocked separately when analgesia of the biceps and anterior forearm is sought.

Technique: There are several techniques for placing the axillary block. The commonly used approaches include the transarterial approach and the nerve stimulation approach. Although reports of greater success with the transarterial approach are seen in adults,[33] this approach is not often used in children. This is due to the higher incidence of vessel spasm and potential for ischemia in children compared with adults. Surface mapping can be used to approximate the location of the plexus or nerve of interest[14] (Figure 54–29). More recently, ultrasonography has been used for identifying the nerves in the axillary sheath.[34] Although many methods have been reported in adults, the simple common method of using a single injection technique seems to be very effective in children.[35] The patient is positioned with the arm abducted 90 degrees. The elbow is flexed and the arm is placed above the head. After surface mapping to locate the position of the nerve, a stimulating needle is inserted superior to the axillary artery at an angle of 30 degrees with the tip pointed toward the midpoint of the clavicle (Figure 54–30). A "pop" may be felt as the needle enters the axillary sheath. After eliciting the response to nerve stimulation at 0.4 mA, local anesthetic solution is injected. A volume of 0.2–0.4 mL/kg is recommended to a maximum of 20 mL. When anesthesia of the musculocutaneous nerve is required to augment this block, the needle is directed above the pulse of the axillary artery and toward the belly of the coracobrachialis muscle. Contraction of the biceps confirms placement of the needle close to the musculocutaneous nerve.

Complications: Complications from axillary nerve block are uncommon. If the axillary artery is punctured, a hematoma could form. This can be prevented by applying pressure for about 5 minutes after puncture of the vessel.

Nerve Block at the Wrist

Blockade of the radial, ulnar, and median nerves can be accomplished at the level of the wrist. The advantage with these peripheral blocks is the absence of motor blockade. They are primarily used for surgery on the hand, such as syndactyly repair. These are performed in conjunction with general anesthesia since tourniquet pain cannot be eliminated with this block alone. (Refer to Chapter 29 for more information on the technique, which is essentially identical with that in adults.) The following discussion outlines some specifics that relate to application of the wrist blocks in the pediatric patient.

Radial Nerve

The radial nerve is a superficial sensory nerve proximal to the radial head. The radial nerve divides into two branches—a thenar branch and a dorsal branch. This division takes place proximal to the distal end of the radius. This block is performed for children undergoing trigger thumb release or minor surgical procedures involving the thumb and index finger.

Technique: The anatomic "snuff box" is identified. Approximately 2 cm proximal to the anatomic snuff box, local anesthesia is infiltrated subcutaneously. A volume of 2 mL is adequate to provide good analgesia in the postoperative period.

Complications: Rare.

Median Nerve

The median nerve is located between the tendons of the palmaris longus and the flexor carpi radialis. The nerve is usually blocked at the level of the flexor retinaculum. One of the important anatomic advantages of blocking the median nerve at the wrist is the presence of a bursa at the level of the flexor retinaculum. This bursa encompasses the median nerve; hence blockade of this nerve can be carried out without damage to the nerve.

Technique: The tendons of the flexor carpi radialis and the palmaris longus are identified. Flexion of the wrist identifies the tendons. A 27-gauge needle is inserted at the medial border of the palmaris longus tendon. A pop is felt as the bursa is entered. An injection of 2 mL of local anesthetic solution is made. Smaller quantities are required for younger children and infants.

Ulnar Nerve

The palmar cutaneous branch of the ulnar nerve accompanies the ulnar artery to the wrist. It perforates the flexor retinac-

ulum and ends in the palm communicating with the median nerve.

Technique: The nerve is easily blocked at the wrist. The flexor carpi ulnaris tendon is identified. The nerve is blocked under the flexor carpi ulnaris tendon, just proximal to the pisiform bone. A 27-gauge needle is passed under the flexor carpi ulnaris, proximal to the pisiform bone, about 0.5 cm. After aspiration, 2 mL of local anesthetic solution is injected.

Lower Extremity Blocks

The lumbar and sacral plexus supply the lower extremity. The lumbar plexus is contained in the psoas compartment and consists of a small portion of T12 and lumbar nerves L1-L4. The femoral nerve, lateral femoral cutaneous nerve, and obturator nerves are branches of the lumbar plexus that supply most of the thigh and the upper leg. The lower leg is innervated by the sacral plexus, which is derived from the anterior rami of the L4, L5, S1, S2, and S3. This plexus gives rise to the sciatic nerve, which is the largest nerve in the body.

Local Anesthetic Doses for Lower Extremity Blocks

Lower extremity nerve blocks generally require more local anesthetic solution than upper extremity nerve blocks. Children younger than 5–8 years can receive 0.5–1 mL/kg of bupivacaine 0.25% or ropivacaine 0.2%. Older children may require higher concentrations, such as 0.5 mL/kg of bupivacaine 0.5% or ropivacaine 0.5%. Epinephrine 1:200,000 is typically added for detection of inadvertent intravascular injection. If multiple nerve blocks are to be performed, the maximum allowable dose of local anesthetic should not be exceeded when the amount is calculated for both blocks. For continuous infusion through a peripheral nerve block catheter, the suggested dose of local anesthetic is 0.2 mg/kg/h of ropivacaine 0.1% or levobupivacaine 0.125% in newborns or infants and 0.3–0.4 mg/kg/h of ropivacaine 0.1% or levobupivacaine 0.125% in older children.

Femoral Nerve Block

The femoral nerve block is the most commonly performed lower extremity peripheral nerve block in children. It is used for providing pain relief after femoral fractures.[36–38,44] The femoral nerve is located at the level of the crease at the groin, lateral to the pulsation of the femoral artery. Surface mapping must be carried out for locating the position of the nerve before using a sheathed needle.

Technique: The technique is similar to that in the adult (see Chapter 35). The femoral artery pulse is located and the needle is inserted immediately lateral to the pulse to elicit quadriceps muscle contraction. The nerve stimulator is initially set at 1 mA, then reduced to 0.4 mA while observing the quadriceps contraction. Surface mapping electrode can also be used to approximate the location of the nerve. When the location of the needle is stabilized, and after careful aspiration to prevent intravascular injection, local anesthetic solution is injected. A volume of 0.2–0.3 mL/kg is injected.

Complications: Intravascular injection can be prevented by carefully aspirating prior to injection and by injecting graduated doses. The risk of intraneural injection can be reduced by localizing the nerve with a nerve stimulator (>0.2 mA). More recently, the use of injection pressure monitoring has been suggested to add additional information in preventing intraneural injections.[39]

Lateral Femoral Cutaneous Nerve

The lateral femoral cutaneous nerve is derived from L3, L4 segments of the lumbar plexus. It is a pure sensory nerve that passes superficially along the lateral border of the iliac crest as it exits into the fascia iliaca compartment to supply the lateral aspect of the thigh. It is useful for providing analgesia for surgery on the lateral aspect of the thigh including muscle biopsies[40] and graft excisions. This technique is also similar to that in the adult (see Chapter 40). It is a relatively easy block to perform with very few side effects and hence easily applicable in the pediatric population.

Technique: The anterior superior iliac spine is identified. A point 1.5 inches below and medial to the anterior superior iliac spine is identified. After careful aseptic preparation of the area, a blunt needle is introduced into the marked site. An initial pop is felt as the needle enters the skin and the fascia lata; a second pop is felt as the needle enters the fascia iliaca compartment. Once the needle is lodged in this space, loss of resistance can be easily felt as the local anesthetic solution is injected. A total volume of 0.2 mL–0.3 mL of the local anesthetic solution is injected.

Complications: It is very rare to see complications with this block. A hematoma can form at the site of injection, especially if a superficial blood vessel is damaged as the needle enters.

Sciatic Nerve Block

The sacral plexus comprises the sciatic nerve and provides the innervation to the posterior thigh and the leg and most of the foot except the medial portion, which is innervated by the femoral nerve. A number of techniques are used in children for sciatic nerve block (Figure 54–31). We will address two

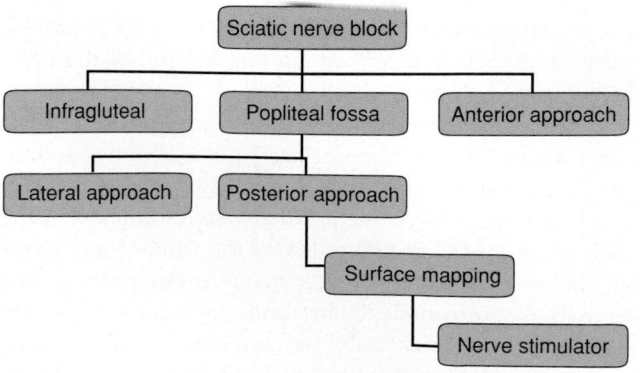

Figure 54–31. Sciatic nerve block in children.

main methods, the infragluteal approach and the popliteal fossa approach.

Infragluteal Sciatic Nerve Block

The infragluteal sciatic nerve block is an easy block to perform in children under general anesthesia because it can be done either in the lateral position or in the supine position with elevation of the limb. The nerve is easily localized for this technique. The infragluteal line where the gluteal crease is present is marked. The biceps femoris tendon is identified and a point inferior to the gluteal crease just medial to the biceps femoris tendon is delineated. A sheathed needle connected to a nerve stimulator is introduced in an anterior plane and cephalad at an angle of 60–70 degrees. Inversion of the foot is indication of blockade of the tibial nerve.[45] The current is reduced to 0.4 mA, and if inversion is still present the local anesthetic solution is injected. If eversion is noted, the needle is withdrawn to the skin and inserted medially. If the biceps femoris tendon is contracting, the needle is drawn back to the skin and the needle is inserted medially away from the muscle belly of the biceps femoris tendon. Plantar flexion is also an indicator of placement of adequate block although this yields a potential for a failed blockade.[45] A volume of 0.5 mL/kg to a maximum of 20 mL is injected into the space. On initial injection of 1 mL of local anesthetic solution, the twitch disappears and confirms the placement of the needle in the right location.

Complications: Absence of complete block, especially if plantar flexion or dorsiflexion are only present without eversion. Intravenous injections are also a complication.

Popliteal Fossa Approach

The popliteal fossa block is our preferred method for blocking the sciatic nerve. There are two approaches to the sciatic nerve in the popliteal fossa—a lateral approach and a posterior approach. The popliteal fossa is a diamond-shaped area with the superior triangle formed by the tendons of the semitendinosus, semimembranosus medially, and the biceps femoris tendon laterally.[46] The sciatic nerve divides into the common peroneal nerve and the tibial nerve. The common peroneal nerve exits the popliteal fossa laterally and the tibial nerve exits medially. The branching of the sciatic nerve takes place about 5–8 cm above the popliteal crease. A common epineural sheath is present that envelops both the tibial and the common peroneal nerve that may lead to complete blockade of both the branches.[47]

LATERAL APPROACH TO THE POPLITEAL FOSSA. Because anesthetized children are typically in the supine position, the lateral approach to popliteal block is particularly advantageous. Although this technique has been well described in children[48] and adults,[6,49] it has not gained wide popularity for use in children.

Technique: After induction of anesthesia and placement of a laryngeal mask airway or mask and strap outfit, the knee is flexed on the side of the block. The biceps femoris tendon is identified, and the needle is placed between the vastus lateralis and the biceps femoris tendon at an angle of about 30 degrees about 5–6 cm above the popliteal crease (Figure 54–32). If the femur is encountered without a twitch response, the needle is pulled back to the skin and inserted at a caudal angle to pass behind the shaft of the femur (Figure 54–33). A response to nerve stimulation at 0.4 mA, usually plantar or dorsiflexion and eversion or inversion, confirms the position of the needle and its proximity to the sciatic nerve. Because at this spot the needle is expected to be above the point at which the sciatic nerve bifurcates into the common peroneal and tibial nerve, response of either tibial or common peroneal nerve is adequate. Cadaveric (adult) studies have shown a wide variation of the position of the sciatic nerve division.[50] This may further vary in children. After aspiration to rule out intravascular placement, local anesthetic solution is injected. A total volume of 0.5 mL/kg is injected with a maximum volume of 20 mL. Alternatively, perineural catheter can be inserted using a similar technique to provide long-lasting analgesia

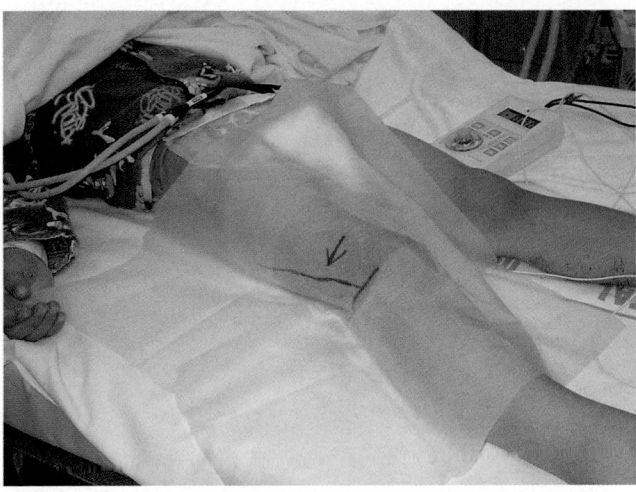

Figure 54–32. Popliteal sciatic block. Landmarks for the lateral approach.

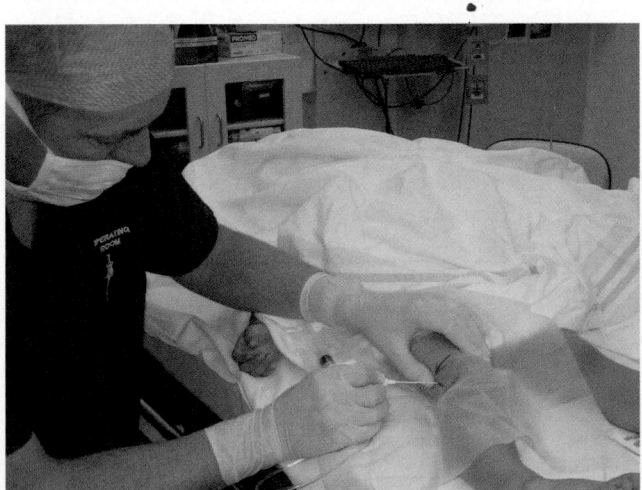

Figure 54–33. Popliteal sciatic block, lateral approach. Needle insertion.

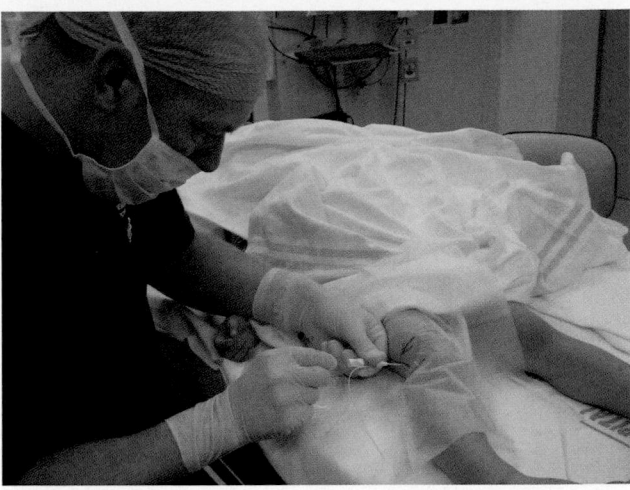

Figure 54–34. Popliteal block, lateral approach. Catheter insertion.

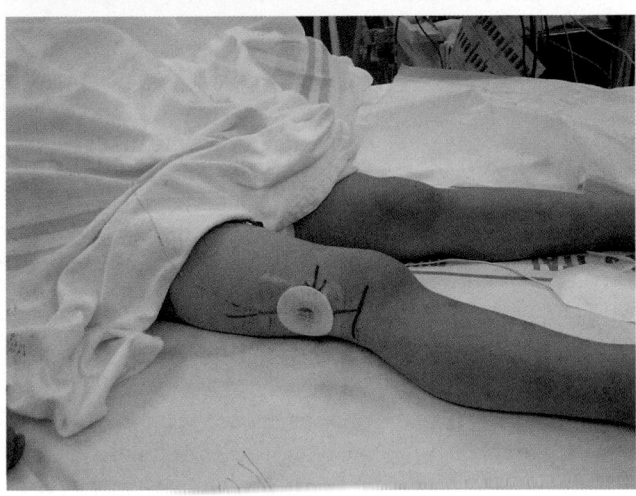

Figure 54–35. Popliteal block, lateral approach. Securing the catheter.

(Figure 54–34). The catheter can be conveniently secured at this position (Figure 54–35).

Complications: Sparing of one of the branches of the sciatic nerve especially if the division takes place proximally.[46] Intravascular injection may be a complication if caution is not exercised before injecting the local anesthetic solution.

POSTERIOR APPROACH TO THE POPLITEAL FOSSA. Although the classic teaching of posterior approach to the popliteal fossa entails placing the patient prone and marking the tendons that make up the "diamond" of the fossa, this may not be needed in the pediatric population because of their weight and the ability to lift the leg easily. We prefer keeping the patient supine and then localizing each individual nerve, tibial nerve, and common peroneal nerve by surface mapping (Figure 54–36). Once each nerve is identified, they are individually blocked using a stimulating needle. The tibial nerve is localized with the presence of inversion and plantar flexion (*i*nternal nerve = *i*nversion); the common peroneal nerve is localized by the presence of

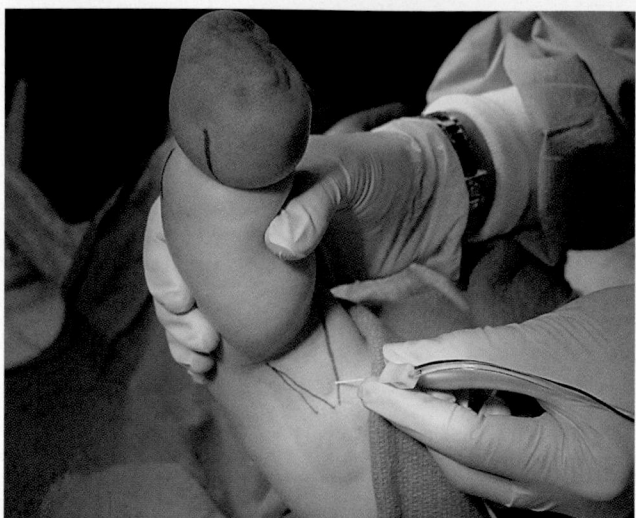

Figure 54–36. Popliteal sciatic block, posterior approach. The needle is inserted between the tendons of the biceps femoris (laterally) and semitendinosus muscles.

eversion and dorsiflexion.(*external nerve = e*version). The total volume can also be reduced to 0.2 mL/kg because individual nerves blocked require less local anesthetic solution. This is particularly valuable in infants, in whom toxicity can be seen at lower doses of local anesthetic solution.

Ankle Block

The ankle block is a very common and easy block to perform for children undergoing foot surgery. The disadvantage is the absence of pain relief during tourniquet application. However, because most procedures are performed under general anesthesia, the presence of adequate pain relief in the postoperative period can be achieved using this block. There are five main nerves to be blocked: the posterior tibial, deep peroneal, superficial peroneal, saphenous, and sural. All of these nerves are distal branches of the sciatic nerve except for the saphenous nerve, which is a branch of the femoral nerve. The nerves are superficial and therefore do not require much volume. Epinephrine should be avoided in the local anesthetic solution because end arteries are present at the site of injection (see Chapter 39 for illustrations and detailed description).

Tibial Nerve

The tibial nerve is the largest nerve that supplies the plantar aspect of the foot and is an important nerve to be blocked for any foot surgery. We routinely use surface mapping with a current of 5 mA to locate the tibial nerve before injection. The nerve is located behind the posterior tibial pulsation below the medial malleolus. A 27-gauge needle is advanced to the bone and slightly withdrawn to avoid injection into the periosteum; 5–8 mL of local anesthetic solution is injected. Alternatively, a sheathed needle can be used and plantar flexion or inversion can be elicited before injection.

Saphenous Nerve

The saphenous nerve is the distal cutaneous branch of the femoral nerve. It is located superficially anterior to the medial malleolus. A superficial ring injected along the medial malleolus and 5 mL of local anesthetic solution is injected. Caution must be exercised to avoid intravascular injection because the saphenous vein courses alongside the nerve. The saphenous nerve supplies the skin over the medial aspect of the leg below the knee and ankle.

Deep Peroneal Nerve

The peroneal nerve innervates the first web space of the foot. It can be blocked by depositing local anesthetic solution lateral to the extensor hallucis longus tendon. The needle is advanced until the periosteum of the tibia is encountered, then drawn back slightly. Local anesthetic solution 2–3 mL is injected.

Superficial Peroneal Nerve

The superficial peroneal nerve supplies the sensory supply to the dorsum of the foot. It is superficial and can be easily blocked by injecting a superficial ring of local anesthesia between the lateral malleolus and the extensor hallucis longus tendon.

Sural Nerve

The sural nerve supplies the sensory innervation to the lateral aspect of the foot. It can be easily blocked by injecting local anesthetic solution between the lateral malleolus and the calcaneus.

The ankle block is a very easy block to perform and has very few side effects. If performed carefully, it can provide excellent analgesia for foot surgery.

Digital Nerve Blocks

Digital nerve blocks are provided for analgesia of the fingers and toes. It is an ideal block for simple procedures such as trigger finger release and ingrown toenail excisions and for foreign body removal and minor lacerations requiring suturing. We have used these blocks successfully for blocking pain after laser therapy for warts in children.[51] This technique is addressed in Chapter 30.

Hand

Anatomy: The common digital nerves of the hand are derived from the median and ulnar nerves and divide in the palm to supply the fingers. All digital nerves are accompanied by digital vessels. The median nerve provides three digital nerves. The first divides into the three palmar digital nerves that supply the side of the thumb; the second common digital nerve supplies the web space between the index and middle finger and the third common palmar digital nerve communicates with the ulnar nerve to supply the web space between the middle and ring finger. These then become the proper digital nerves that supply the skin of the distal phalanx. There are smaller digital nerves derived from the radial and ulnar nerves that supply the dorsum of the fingers. The four dorsal digital nerves are located on the ulnar side of the thumb, the radial side of the index finger, adjacent to the index and middle fingers. All digital nerves terminate in two main branches (1) supplying the skin under the fingertips and (2) supplying the pulp under the nail.

Technique: The digital nerves are blocked using non–epinephrine-containing solution on each side of the finger at the bifurcation between the metacarpal heads. A dorsal or volar injection accomplishes similar results. A needle is inserted into the web space between the thumb and index finger to a distance of about 1 cm. A second needle is inserted into the thenar eminence on the radial aspect of the thumb. For the other fingers, the needle is inserted between the metacarpal heads. A needle is inserted proximal to the thenar web space at the distal palmar crease. After aspiration, 1 mL of local anesthetic solution (without epinephrine) is injected.

Complications: Large volumes of local anesthetic solutions are contraindicated because they can cause vascular compromise.

Feet

Anatomy: The digital nerves to the feet are derived from the plantar cutaneous branch of the tibial nerve. The proper digital nerve of the toe supplies the medial aspect of the great toe. The three common digital nerves split into two proper digital nerves each. The first supplies the adjacent areas of the great and second toes, the second supplies the adjacent sides of the second and third toes, and the third supplies the adjacent sides of the third and fourth toes. Each of these terminates at the tip of the toe. A branch from the superficial peroneal nerve supplies the dorsum of the foot. These are derived from two nerves: (1) The dorsal cutaneous nerve divides into two branches, a medial branch supplying the great toe and a lateral branch supplying the adjacent sides of the second and third toes; and (2) the intermediate dorsal cutaneous nerve that passes along the lateral part of the foot supplying the lateral aspect of the foot and communicating with the sural nerve. The two dorsal digital terminal branches supply the adjacent parts of the third and fourth toes and another branch supplying the adjacent sides of the fourth and fifth toes.

Technique: It is easy to block the digital nerves by accessing the web space on the dorsolateral aspect of the foot. It is best to avoid these blocks in children who may have compromised blood flow to the toes. Vasoconstrictors are to be avoided for all these blocks.

Trunk Blocks

Ilioinguinal Nerve Block

For most hernia surgery in children, a caudal block is the block of choice. However, if there is a relative contraindication to a caudal block owing to the presence of a sacral dimple or if the child is obese and the caudal space is not easily identified, an ilioinguinal nerve block is used.

Anatomy: The ilioinguinal and iliohypogastric nerves originate from the T12 (subcostal nerve) and L1 (ilioinguinal, iliohypogastric) nerve roots of the lumbar plexus. These nerves pierce the internal oblique aponeurosis 2–3 cm medial

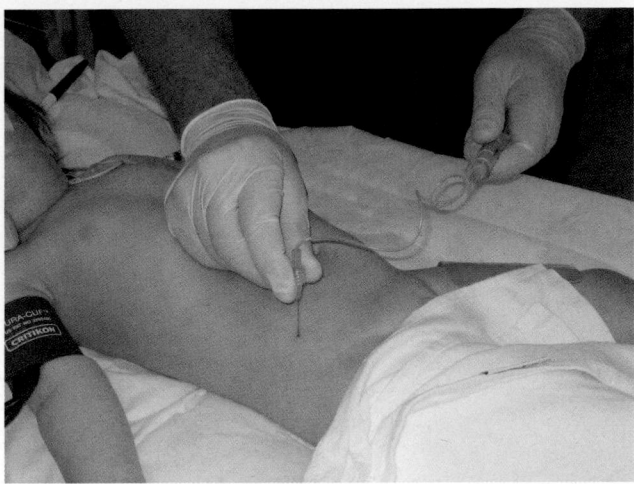

Figure 54–37. Ilioinguinal block. The needle is inserted at the point at which the lateral third meets with the medial two thirds of the line connecting the umbilicus with the anterior superior iliac spine.

to the anterior superior iliac spine. The ilioinguinal nerve travels between the internal oblique and the external oblique aponeurosis. Here, it accompanies the spermatic cord and is part of the neurovascular bundle to the genital area.

Technique: A line is drawn between the umbilicus and anterior superior iliac spine. The line is divided into thirds. The point where the lateral third meets with the medial two thirds is where the needle is inserted. The needle is advanced toward the inguinal canal and passed in until a pop is felt (Figure 54–37). Local anesthetic solution is injected into the area after aspiration. Alternatively, an ilioinguinal nerve block can be performed by having the surgeon flood the site of surgery with 10 mL of local anesthetic solution.

Complications: Ilioinguinal nerve block is relatively safe. Perforation of the bowel wall can occur and has been reported.[52] Occasional femoral nerve blockade can occur while this block is placed.[52]

Rectus Sheath Block

The rectus sheath block was first described in 1899 for surgery performed around the umbilical area. It is particularly useful in children for umbilical area surgery.

Anatomy: The umbilical area is innervated by the 10th thoracoabdominal intercostals nerves from the right and left side. Each nerve then passes behind the costal cartilage and between the transverse abdominis muscle and the internal oblique muscle. The nerve runs between the sheath and the posterior wall of the rectus abdominis muscle and ends at the anterior cutaneous branch supplying the skin of the umbilical area.

Technique: The aim of this block is to deposit local anesthetic solution between the muscle and the posterior aspect of the sheath. The technique has been well described by Ferguson et al.[54] A 23-gauge needle is inserted above or below the umbilicus $^1/_2$ cm medial to the linea semilunaris in a perpendicular plane. The anterior rectus sheath is identified

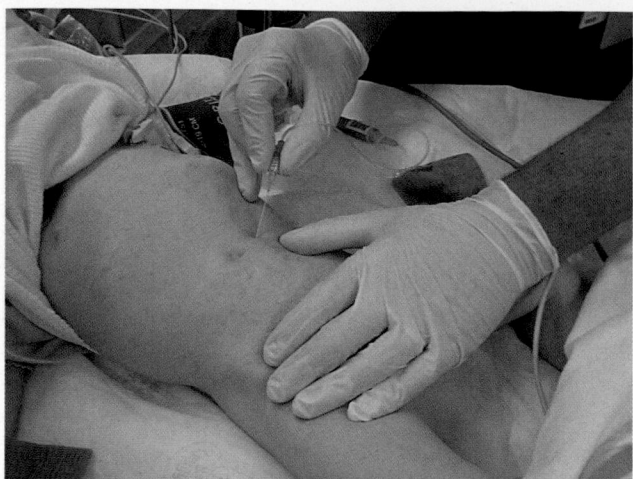

Figure 54–38. Rectus sheath block. A 23-gauge needle is inserted above or below the umbilicus $^1/_2$ cm medial to the linea semilunaris in a perpendicular plane. Once the sheath is entered, local anesthetic solution is deposited posterior to the sheath. The usual depth of needle entry is about 0.5–1.5 cm.

by moving the needle with a back-and-forth motion until a scratching sensation is felt and the rectus sheath is identified and entered (Figure 54–38). After the belly of the muscle is entered, the needle is further advanced until the posterior aspect of the rectus sheath is appreciated with a scratching sensation as the needle is moved again with a back-and-forth motion. Once the sheath is felt, it is entered and local anesthetic solution is deposited posterior to the sheath. The usual depth of needle entry is about 0.5–1.5 cm. After aspiration, 0.2 mL/kg of bupivacaine 0.25–0.5% is injected on each side.

If resistance is felt to injection, the needle is advanced deeper because it may be in the body of the muscle. This block can be performed with a greater degree of precision with the assistance of ultrasound as the muscle is readily visualized (Figures 54–39 and 54–40). A sharp needle is used in a direction perpendicular to the skin.

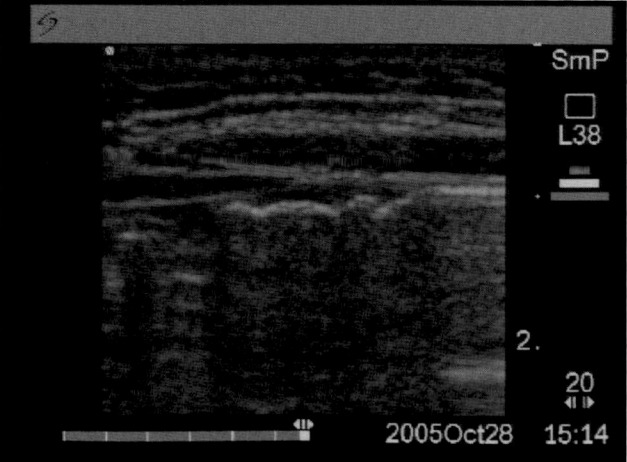

Figure 54–39. Rectus sheath block. The ultrasound image shows the widening space between the muscle and the posterior aspect of the rectus sheath.

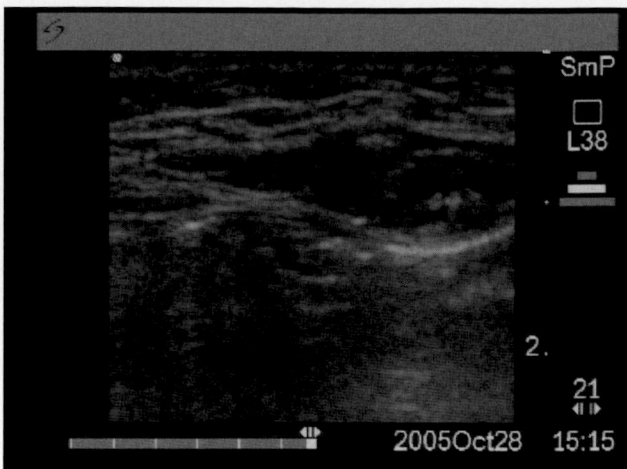

Figure 54–40. Rectus sheath block. As the larger volume of local anesthetic is injected, the space between the muscle and the posterior aspect of the rectus sheath continuous to distend.

Complications: A lateral approach may not allow appreciation of passage of the needle through the various layers, a superficial injection after passage through the anterior rectus sheath may not allow spread of local anesthetic owing to the presence of tendinous bands. The risk of an intravascular injection may be increased when a large volume is injected directly into the rectus muscle.

Penile Nerve Block

The nerve supply to the penis is derived from the pudendal nerve and the pelvic plexus. The dorsal nerves of the penis enter the subpubic space at the level of the symphysis pubis, and supply the sensory innervation to the shaft of the penis.

Technique: Non–epinephrine-containing solution is used for this nerve block. A needle is inserted in the subpubic space 1 cm lateral to the midline and advanced until a pop is felt as the needle enters the fascial compartment bounded superficially by scarpas fascia (Figure 54–41). After careful aspiration, 2 mL + (0.1 mL/kg) to a maximum of 5 mL of plain local anesthetic is injected. The injection is then repeated on the other side of the midline. An alternative approach is to place a subcutaneous ring block around the base of the penile shaft (Figure 54–42). Although this is effective in providing analgesia, complications include the presence of a hematoma and a higher incidence of inadequate postoperative pain relief.[55] Our preferred approach is to use an injection at the base of the penis.

Complications: Hematoma formation.

Thoracic Paravertebral Block

Thoracic paravertebral blocks are used to treat postoperative pain after thoracotomy and unilateral abdominal surgery (open splenectomy, nephrectomy). Contraindications for this technique are rare. A pediatric (5 cm) epidural kit is used.

Anatomy: Approximate distance to the paravertebral space in children (mm) is 20 + (0.5 × weight in kg). The

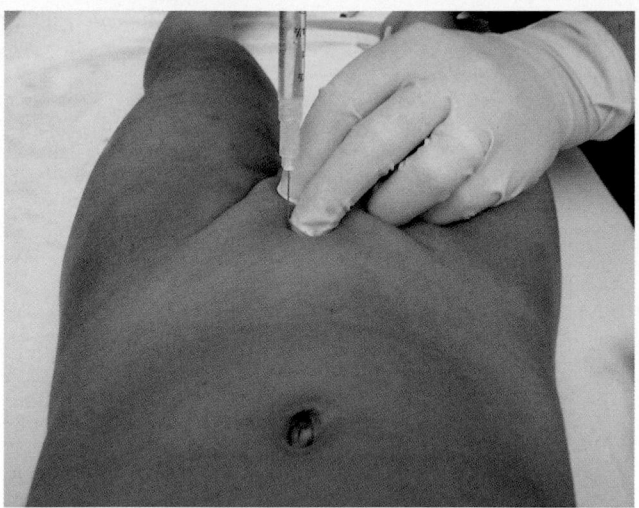

Figure 54–41. Penile nerve block, subpubic approach. A needle is inserted in the subpubic space 1 cm lateral to the midline and advanced until a pop is felt as the needle enters the fascial compartment. After careful aspiration, 2 mL + (0.1 mL/kg) to a maximum of 5 mL of plain local anesthetic is injected. The injection is then repeated on the other side of the midline.

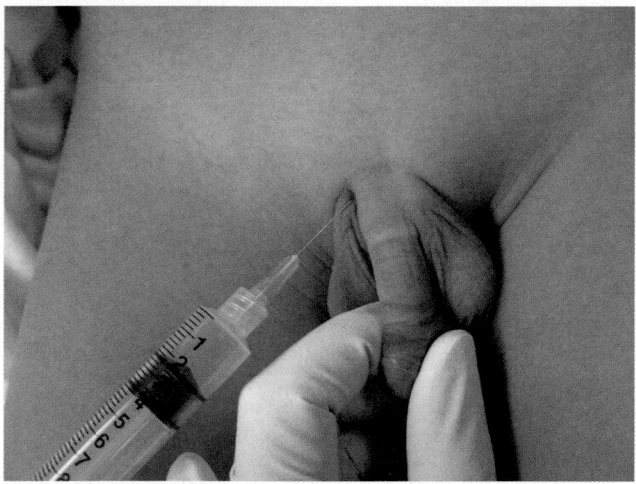

Figure 54–42. Penile block: Subcutaneous ring block. A subcutaneous ring block is accomplished by injecting local anesthetic around the base of the penile shaft.

needle point is typically 1–2 cm lateral to midline; T7-9 level is usually used.

Technique: The patient is positioned in the lateral decubitus position in the neutral position (Figure 54–43). The needle is inserted through the skin; then the stylet is removed. A syringe is attached for assessment of the loss of resistance. The needle is advanced until the transverse process is contacted (Figure 54–44). At this point, the needle is advanced 1 cm past the transverse process. Alternatively, the syringe is advanced until the loss of resistance is appreciated. A bolus of 0.5–1 mL/kg of 0.25% bupivacaine is injected. The same technique can be used to insert a paravertebral catheter for continuous infusion (eg, 0.3 mL/kg/h of 0.125% bupivacaine), similar to other continuous nerve block techniques (Figures 54–45 and 54–46).

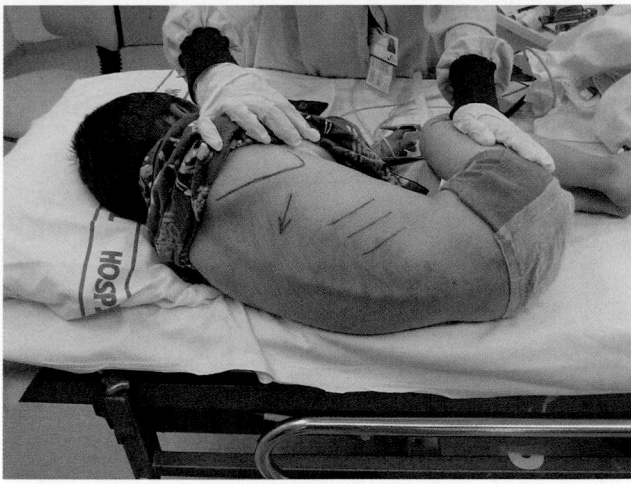

Figure 54–43. Thoracic paravertebral block. The patient is positioned in the lateral decubitus position with slight flexion of the back. The arrow points to T7 (tip of the scapulae).

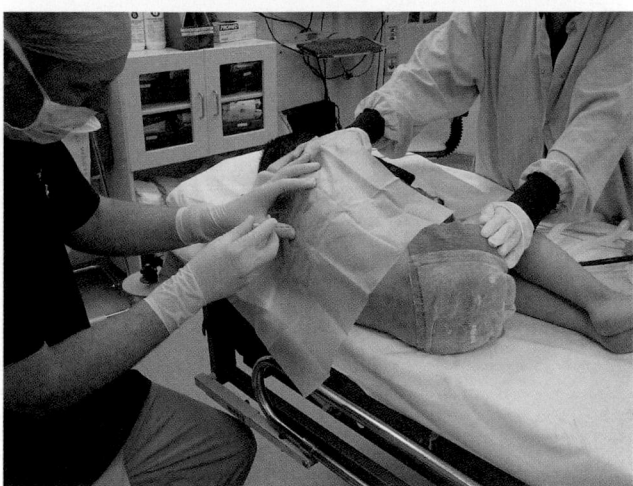

Figure 54–44. Thoracic paravertebral block. The needle is inserted 1–2 cm lateral to the midline and advanced to the transverse process. The needle is then "walked off" superiorly or inferiorly by 1 cm.

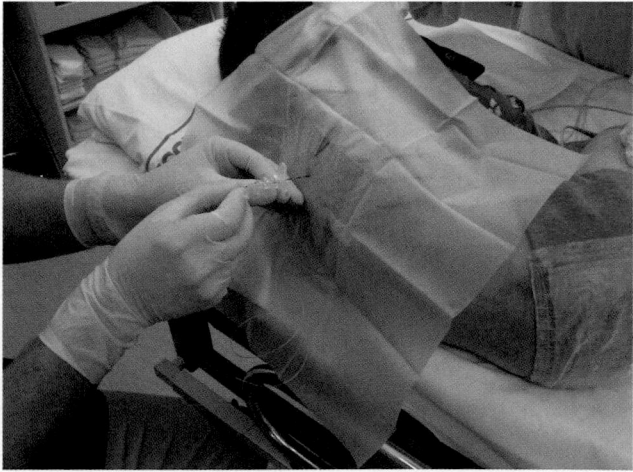

Figure 54–45. Thoracic paravertebral block. After the paravertebral space is identified, the catheter is inserted 2–4 cm beyond the tip of the needle.

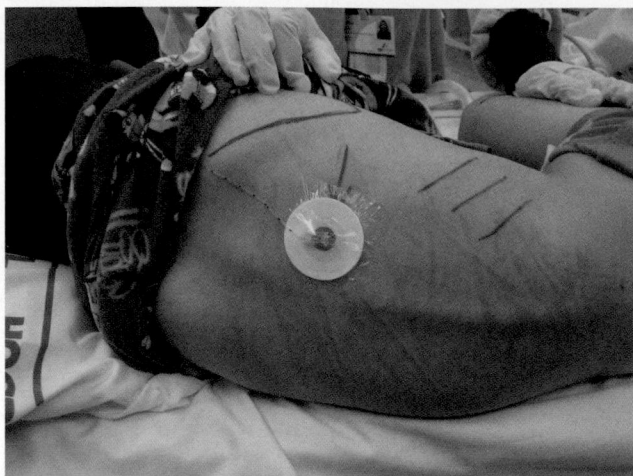

Figure 54–46. Thoracic paravertebral block. The catheter is firmly secured to the patient's back using a locking device.

SUMMARY

Peripheral nerve blocks can be performed with ease in children and adolescents. Adequate knowledge of the anatomy of the area along with appropriate indications and knowledge of complications facilitates the use of peripheral nerve blocks in children. The fear of the use of peripheral nerve blocks in children under general anesthesia is not unfounded, but newer techniques utilizing technology such as ultrasound may make complications even less frequent than reported with current methods.

References

1. Giaufre E, Dalens B, Gombert A: Epidemiology and morbidity of regional anesthesia in children: A one-year prospective survey of the French-Language Society of Pediatric Anesthesiologists. Anesth Analg 1996;83:904–912.
2. Chu RS, Browne GJ, Cheng NG, Lam LT: Femoral nerve block for femoral shaft fractures in a paediatric emergency department: Can it be done better? Eur J Emerg Med 2003;10:258–263.
3. Berde CB, Sethna NF, Levin L, et al: Regional analgesia on pediatric medical and surgical wards. Intensive Care Med 1989;15(Suppl 1):S40–S43.
4. Tobias JD: Continuous femoral nerve block to provide analgesia following femur fracture in a paediatric ICU population. Anaesth Intensive Care 1994;22:616–618.
5. Hadzic A, Dilberovic F, Shah S, et al: Combination of intraneural injection and high injection pressure leads to fascicular injury and neurologic deficits in dogs. Reg Anesth Pain Med 2004;29:417–423.
6. Freid EB, Bailey A, Valley R: Electrocardiographic and hemodynamic changes associated with unintentional intravascular injection of bupivacaine with epinephrine in infants. Anesthesiology 1993;79:394–398.
7. Wong K, Strichartz GR, Raymond SA: On the mechanisms of potentiation of local anesthetics by bicarbonate buffer: Drug structure-activity studies on isolated peripheral nerve. Anesth Analg 1993;76:131–143.
8. Ivani G, Mattioli G, Rega M, et al: Clonidine-mepivacaine mixture vs plain mepivacaine in paediatric surgery. Paediatr Anaesth 1996;6:111–114.

9. Murphy DB, McCartney CJ, Chan VW: Novel analgesic adjuncts for brachial plexus block: A systematic review. Anesth Analg 2000;90:1122–1128.
10. Ivani G, Tonetti F: Postoperative analgesia in infants and children: New developments. Minerva Anestesiol 2004;70:399–403.
11. Dalens B, Ecoffey C, Joly A, et al: Pharmacokinetics and analgesic effect of ropivacaine following ilioinguinal/iliohypogastric nerve block in children. Paediatr Anaesth 2001;11:415–420.
12. Kohane DS, Sankar WN, Shubina M, et al: Sciatic nerve blockade in infant, adolescent, and adult rats: A comparison of ropivacaine with bupivacaine. Anesthesiology 1998;89:1199–1208.
13. Ala-Kokko TI, Raiha E, Karinen J, et al: Pharmacokinetics of 0.5% levobupivacaine following ilioinguinal-iliohypogastric nerve block-ade in children. Acta Anaesthesiol Scand 2005;49:397–400.
14. Bosenberg AT, Raw R, Boezaart AP: Surface mapping of peripheral nerves in children with a nerve stimulator. Paediatr Anaesth 2002;12:398–403.
15. Marhofer P, Sitzwohl C, Greher M, Kapral S: Ultrasound guidance for infraclavicular brachial plexus anaesthesia in children. Anaesthesia 2004;59:642–646.
16. Hadzic A, Vloka JD: A comparison of the posterior versus lateral approaches to the block of the sciatic nerve in the popliteal fossa. Anesthesiology 1998;88:1480–1486.
17. Chan VW: Applying ultrasound imaging to interscalene brachial plexus block. Reg Anesth Pain Med 2003;28:340–343.
18. Kirchmair L, Enna B, Mitterschiffthaler G, et al: Lumbar plexus in children. A sonographic study and its relevance to pediatric regional anesthesia. Anesthesiology 2004;101:445–450.
19. Krane EJ, Dalens BJ, Murat I, Murrell D: The safety of epidurals placed during general anesthesia. Reg Anesth Pain Med 1998;23:433–438.
20. Suresh S, Bellig G: Regional anesthesia in a very low-birth-weight neonate for a neurosurgical procedure. Reg Anesth Pain Med 2004;29:58–59.
21. Suresh S, Wagner AM: Scalp excisions: Getting "ahead" of pain. Pediatr Dermatol 2001;18:74–76.
22. Prabhu KP, Wig J, Grewal S: Bilateral infraorbital nerve block is superior to peri-incisional infiltration for analgesia after repair of cleft lip. Scand J Plastic Reconst Surg Hand Surg 1999;33:83–87.
23. Molliex S Navez M, Baylot, D, et al: Regional anesthesia for outpatient nasal surgery. Br J Anaesth 1996;76:151–153.
24. Suresh S, Patel AS, Dunham, ME, et al. A randomized double-blind controlled trial of infraorbital nerve block versus intravenous morphine sulfate for children undergoing endoscopic sinus surgery: Are postoperative outcomes different? Anesthesiology 2002;97:A-1292.
25. Yasan H, Dogru H: Effect of infraorbital nerve block under general anesthesia on consumption of isoflurane and postoperative pain in endoscopic endonasal maxillary sinus surgery by Higashizawa and Koga. J Anesth 2003;17:68.
26. Higashizawa T, Koga Y: Effect of infraorbital nerve block under general anesthesia on consumption of isoflurane and postoperative pain in endoscopic endonasal maxillary sinus surgery. J Anesth 2001;15:136–138.
27. Suresh S, Barcelona SL, Young NM, et al: Postoperative pain relief in children undergoing tympanomastoid surgery: Is a regional block better than opioids? Anesth Analg 2002;94:859–862.
28. Cregg N, Conway F, Casey W: Analgesia after otoplasty: Regional nerve blockade vs local anaesthetic infiltration of the ear. Can J Anaesth 1996;43(2):141–147.
29. Dieudonne N, Gomola A, Bonnichon P, Ozier YM: Prevention of postoperative pain after thyroid surgery: A double-blind randomized study of bilateral superficial cervical plexus blocks. Anesth Analg 2001;92:1538–1542.
30. Suresh S, Templeton L: Superficial cervical plexus block for vocal cord surgery in an awake pediatric patient. Anesth Analg 2004;98:1656–1657.
31. Dalens B, Vanneuville G, Tanguy A: A new parascalene approach to the brachial plexus in children: Comparison with the supraclavicular approach. Anesth Analg 1987;66:1264–1271.

32. Klaastad O, Smedby O, Kjelstrup T, Smith HJ: The vertical infra-clavicular brachial plexus block: A simulation study using magnetic resonance imaging. Anesth Analg 2005;101:273–278.

33. Aantaa R, Kirvela O, Lahdenpera A, Nieminen S: Transarterial brachial plexus anesthesia for hand surgery: A retrospective analysis of 346 cases. J Clin Anesth 1994;6:189–192.

34. Ting PL, Sivagnanaratnam V: Ultrasonographic study of the spread of local anaesthetic during axillary brachial plexus block. Br J Anaesth 1989;63:326–329.

35. Carre P, Joly A, Cluzel FB, et al: Axillary block in children: Single or multiple injection? Paediatr Anaesth 2000;10:35–39.

36. Grossbard GD, Love BR: Femoral nerve block: A simple and safe method of instant analgesia for femoral shaft fractures in children. Aust N Z J Surg 1979;49:592–594.

37. Johnson CM: Continuous femoral nerve blockade for analgesia in children with femoral fractures. Anaesth Intensive Care 1994;22:281–283.

38. Ronchi L, Rosenbaum D, Athouel A, et al: Femoral nerve blockade in children using bupivacaine. Anesthesiology 1989;70:622–624.

39. Hadzic A, Dilberovic F, Shah S, et al: Combination of intraneural injection and high injection pressure leads to fascicular injury and neurologic deficits in dogs. Reg Anesth Pain Med 2004;29:417–423.

40. Maccani RM, Wedel DJ, Melton A, Gronert GA: Femoral and lateral femoral cutaneous nerve block for muscle biopsies in children. Paediatr Anaesth 1995;5:223–227.

41. Winnie AP, Ramamurthy S, Durrani Z: The inguinal paravascular technic of lumbar plexus anesthesia: The "3-in-1 block." Anesth Analg 1973;52:989–996.

42. Marhofer P, Schrogendorfer K, Koinig H, et al: Ultrasonographic guidance improves sensory block and onset time of three-in-one blocks. Anesth Analg 1997;85:854–857.

43. Chayen D, Nathan H, Chayen M: The psoas compartment block. Anesthesiology 1976;45:95–99.

44. Dalens B, Tanguy A, Vanneuville G: Lumbar plexus block in children: A comparison of two procedures in 50 patients. Anesth Analg 1988;67:750–758.

45. Sukhani R, Candido KD, Doty R Jr, et al: Infragluteal-parabiceps sciatic nerve block: An evaluation of a novel approach using a single-injection technique. Anesth Analg 2003;96:868–873.

46. Vloka JD, Hadzic A, April E, Thys DM: The division of the sciatic nerve in the popliteal fossa: Anatomical implications for popliteal nerve blockade. Anesth Analg 2001;92:215–217.

47. Vloka JD, Hadzic A, Lesser JB, et al: A common epineural sheath for the nerves in the popliteal fossa and its possible implications for sciatic nerve block. Anesth Analg 1997;84:387–390.

48. terRahe CT, Suresh S: Popliteal fossa block: Lateral approach to the sciatic nerve. Reg Anesth Pain Med 2002;6:141–143.

49. Vloka JD, Hadzic A, Kitain E, et al: Anatomic considerations for sciatic nerve block in the popliteal fossa through the lateral approach. Reg Anesth Pain Med 1996;21:414–418.

50. Vloka JD, Hadzic A, April E, Thys DM: The division of the sciatic nerve in the popliteal fossa: Anatomical implications for popliteal nerve blockade. Anesth Analg 2001;92:215–217.

51. Wagner AM, Suresh S: Peripheral nerve blocks for warts: Taking the cry out of cryotherapy and laser. Pediatr Dermatol 1998;15:238–241.

52. Amory C, Mariscal A, Guyot E, et al: Is ilioinguinal/iliohypogastric nerve block always totally safe in children? Paediatr Anaesth 2003;13:164–136.

53. Leng SA: Transient femoral nerve palsy after ilioinguinal nerve block. Anaesth Intensive Care 1997;25:92.

54. Ferguson S, Thomas V, Lewis I: The rectus sheath block in paediatric anaesthesia: New indications for an old technique? Paediatr Anaesth 1996;6:463–466.

55. Holder KJ, Peutrell JM, Weir PM: Regional anaesthesia for circumcision. Subcutaneous ring block of the penis and subpubic penile block compared. Eur J Anaesthesiol 1997;14:495–498.

E. Acute Pain Management in Children

Myron Yaster, MD • Sabine Kost-Byerly, MD

INTRODUCTION

The treatment and alleviation of pain constitute a basic human right that exists regardless of age.[1,2] Although much of this chapter is directed at pediatric pain, which is our area of clinical practice and research, much, if not all, the information is applicable to adult patients as well. Unfortunately, in our quest to treat and cure the underlying disease processes that cause pain, we as physicians have often forgotten about the symptom—pain—that brings patients to us in the first place. What is pain? It is more than simply the physiologic transmission of nociceptive input from a site of injury to the brain. Rather, it is a complex sensation that is integrated and given *value* at higher conscious brain centers. No two people experience pain the same way. Think of symphonic music. The physiology of sound transmission is the same in all of us, but symphonic music to some is simply awful and to others it is glorious. We integrate the neural transmissions and give it personal value based on our age, culture, experience, values, and state of mind. The same is true for pain.

Unfortunately, even when their pain is obvious, children frequently receive no treatment—or inadequate treatment—for pain and for painful procedures. The newborn and critically ill child are especially vulnerable to no treatment or undertreatment.[3,4] No other group would be allowed to undergo surgery without anesthesia; yet even in the year 2006 the newborn male typically undergoes circumcision by being tied down to a papoose. The conventional "wisdom" that children neither respond to, nor remember, painful experiences to the same degree that adults do is simply untrue. Indeed, many of the nerve pathways essential for the transmission and perception of pain are present and functioning by 24–29 weeks of gestation.[5,6] Recent research in newborn animals has revealed that failure to provide analgesia for pain results in "rewiring" the nerve pathways responsible for pain

transmission in the dorsal horn of the spinal cord and also results in increased pain perception for *future* painful insults. This confirms human newborn research in which the failure to provide anesthesia or analgesia for newborn circumcision resulted not only in short-term physiologic perturbations but also in longer-term behavioral changes, particularly during immunization.[7,8]

Nurses are taught to be wary of physicians' orders (and patients' requests) as well. The most common prescription order for potent analgesics, "to give as needed" (*pro re nata*, PRN), in reality means "to give as infrequently as possible." The PRN order also means that either the patient must know or remember to ask for pain medication or the nurse must identify when a patient is in pain. Neither of these requirements may be met by children in pain. Children less than 3 years of age, or critically ill children, may be unable to adequately verbalize when or where they hurt. Alternatively, they may be afraid to report their pain. Many children withdraw or deny their pain in an attempt to avoid yet another terrifying and painful experience—the intramuscular injection or "shot." Finally, several studies have documented the inability of nurses, physicians, and parents to correctly identify and treat pain even in postoperative pediatric patients.

Societal fears of opioid addiction and lack of advocacy are also causal factors in the undertreatment of pediatric pain. Unlike adult patients, pain management in children is often dependent on the ability of parents to recognize and assess pain and on their decision to treat or not treat it. Parental misconceptions concerning pain assessment and pain management, as well as a fear of inducing addiction, may therefore result in inadequate pain treatment. This is particularly true in patients who are too young or too developmentally handicapped to self-report their pain.

Even in hospitalized patients, most of the pain that children experience is managed by the patient's parents. Parents may fail to report pain either because they are unable to assess it or are afraid of the consequences of pain therapy. In one study, false beliefs about addiction and the proper use of acetaminophen and other analgesics resulted in the failure to provide analgesia to children.[9] In another, the belief that pain was useful or that repeated doses of analgesics lead to medication not working well resulted in the failure of the parents to provide or ask for prescribed analgesics to treat their children's pain.[10] Parental education is therefore essential if children are to be adequately treated for pain. Unfortunately, the ability to properly educate parents about this issue is often limited by insufficient resources, time, and personnel.

Fortunately, the past 25 years have seen an explosion in research and interest in pediatric pain management and in the development of pediatric pain services, primarily under the direction of pediatric anesthesiologists. The pain service teams provide the pain management for acute, postoperative, terminal, neuropathic, and chronic pain. Nevertheless, the assessment and treatment of pain in children are important aspects of pediatric care, regardless of who provides it, and failure to provide adequate control of pain amounts to substandard and unethical medical practice.

PAIN ASSESSMENT

The International Association for the Study of Pain defines pain as "an unpleasant and emotional experience associated with actual or potential tissue damage, or described in terms of such damage."[11] As discussed above, the perception of pain is a subjective, conscious experience; operationally, it can be defined as "what the patient says hurts" and exists "when the patient says it does." Infants, preverbal children, and children between the ages of 2 and 7 years may be unable to describe their pain or their subjective experiences. This has led many to conclude incorrectly that children don't experience pain in the same way in which adults do. Clearly, children do not have to know (or to be able to express) the meaning of an experience to have the experience. On the other hand, because pain is essentially a subjective experience, it is becoming increasingly clear that the child's perspective of pain is an indispensable facet of pediatric pain management and an essential element in the specialized study of childhood pain. Indeed, pain assessment and management are interdependent, and one is essentially useless without the other. The goal of pain assessment is to provide accurate data about the location and intensity of pain, as well as the effectiveness of measures used to alleviate or abolish it.

Instruments currently exist to measure and assess pain in children of all ages.[8,12–18] Indeed, the sensitivity and specificity of these instruments have been widely debated and have resulted in a plethora of studies to validate their reliability and validity. The most commonly used instruments measure the quality and intensity of pain and are "self-report measures" that make use of pictures or word descriptors to describe pain. Pain intensity or severity can be measured in children

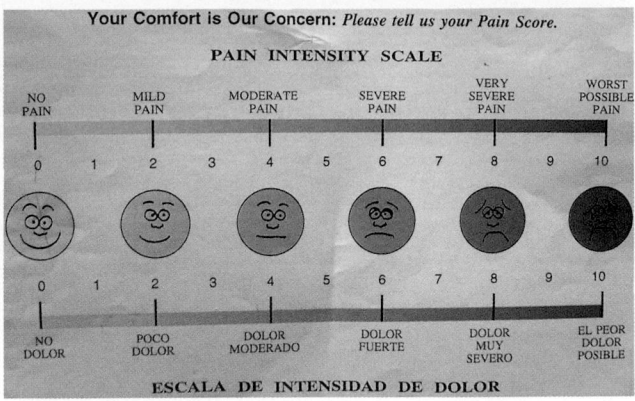

Figure 54–47. Pain intensity scale using faces to rate the intensity of the pain in children. (Reprinted from: Wong DL, Baker CM: Pain in children: Comparison of assessment scales. Pediatr Nurs 1988;14:9–17.)

as young as 3 years of age by using either the Oucher scale (developed by Dr. Judy Beyer)—a two-part scale with a vertical numerical scale (0–100) on one side and six photographs of a young child on the other—or a visual analogue scale, a 10-cm line with a smiling face on one end and a distraught, crying face on the other. In fact, this scale has been validated even by sex and race! In our practice, we use the 6-face pain-scale developed by Dr. Donna Wong primarily because of its simplicity (Figure 54–47).[16] This scale is attached to the vital sign record and nurses are instructed to use it or a more age-appropriate self-report measure whenever vital signs are taken.

PAIN MANAGEMENT

Acute pediatric (and adult) pain management is increasingly characterized by a multimodal or "balanced" approach in which smaller doses of opioid and nonopioid analgesics, such nonsteroidal antiinflammatory drugs (NSAIDs), local anesthetics, NMDA antagonists, and α_2-adrenergic agonists, are combined to maximize pain control and minimize drug-induced adverse side effects. In addition, a multimodal approach utilizes nonpharmacologic, complementary and alternative medicine therapies as well. These techniques include distraction, guided imagery, transcutaneous nerve stimulation, acupuncture, therapeutic massage, and others.[19]

Analgesics with Antipyretic Activity or Nonopioid (or "Weaker") Analgesics

The "weaker" or milder analgesics with antipyretic activity, of which acetaminophen [paracetamol] (Tylenol), salicylate (aspirin), ibuprofen (Motrin), naproxen (Aleve, Naprosyn), diclofenic are the classic examples, make up a heterogeneous group of NSAIDs that are nonopioid analgesics (Table 54–16).[20–22] They provide pain relief primarily by blocking peripheral and central prostaglandin production by inhibiting

Table 54–16.

Oral Dosing Guidelines for Commonly Used Nonopioid Analgesics

Drug (Brand name)	Dose (mg/kg) (<60 kg)	Dose (mg) (>60 kg)	Interval (hours)	Daily Maximum Dose (mg/kg) (<60 kg)	Daily Max Dose (mg) (>60 kg)	Side Effects
Acetaminophen (Tylenol)	10–15[a]	650–1000	4	90[a]	4000	Toxic doses hepatotoxicity lacks anti-inflammatory activity
Ibuprofen (Motrin)	5–10	400–600[c]	6	40[b,c]	2400[c]	GI irritation, bronchospasm; interferes with platelet function, hematuria
Naproxen (Naprosyn)	5–6[c]	250–375[c]	12	24[b,c]	1000[c]	See ibuprofen
Aspirin[d]	10–15[c,d]	650–1000[c]	4	80[b–d]	3600[c]	Reye syndrome,[d] see ibuprofen
Choline Mg Tri-Salicylate[e]	7.5–15[c,d]	500–1000[c]	4–8	80[b–d]	3600[c]	See aspirin

[a] *Maximum daily doses for acetaminophen should be reduced to 80 mg/kg in term neonates and infants and to 60 mg/kg in preterm neonates. Supplied in many liquid formulations ranging from 20 to 100 mg/mL making accidental overdosage easy. Rectal suppositories available, dosing 25–40 mg/kg every 8 hours.*

[b] *Dosing guidelines for neonates and infants have not been established.*

[c] *Higher doses may be used in selected cases for treatment of rheumatologic conditions in children.*

[d] *Aspirin carries a risk of provoking Reye syndrome in infants and children. If other analgesics are available, aspirin use should be restricted to indications in which antiplatelet or antiinflammatory effect is required rather than as a routine analgesic or antipyretic in neonates, infants, or children. Dosing guidelines for aspirin in neonates have not been established.*

[e] *Aspirin-like compound that does not affect platelet adhesiveness or aggregation.*

cyclooxygenase types I and II. These analgesic agents are primarily administered enterally via the oral or, on occasion, the rectal route and are particularly useful for inflammatory, bony, or rheumatic pain. Parenterally administered NSAIDs, such as ketorolac (Toradol), are available for use in children in whom the oral or rectal routes of administration are not possible.[23] Unfortunately, regardless of dose, the nonopioid analgesics reach a "ceiling effect" above which pain cannot be relieved by these drugs alone. Because of this, these weaker analgesics are basic building blocks in a multimodal therapeutic approach and are often administered in oral combination forms with opioids such as codeine, oxycodone, or hydrocodone.

Aspirin, one of the oldest and most effective nonopioid analgesics, has been largely abandoned in pediatric practice because of its possible role in Reye syndrome, its effects on platelet function, and its gastric irritant properties. Despite these problems, a relatively new salicylate product, choline magnesium trisalicylate (Trilisate) is increasingly being used in our pediatric pain management practice, particularly in the management of postoperative pain and in the child with cancer. Choline magnesium trisalicylate is a unique aspirin-like compound that does not bind to platelets and therefore has minimal, if any, effects on platelet function.[21] It is a convenient drug to give to children because it is available in both liquid and tablet form and is administered either twice a day or every 6 hours. The association of salicylates with Reye syndrome limits its use, even though the risk of developing Reye syndrome postoperatively or in cancer is extremely unlikely.

The most commonly used nonopioid analgesic in pediatric practice remains acetaminophen [paracetamol]. Unlike aspirin and the other NSAIDs, acetaminophen works primarily centrally and has minimal, if any, antiinflammatory activity. When administered in normal doses (10–15 mg · kg^{-1}, PO), acetaminophen is extremely safe and has very few serious side effects. It is an antipyretic and, like all enterally administered NSAIDs, takes about 30 minutes to provide effective analgesia. Several investigators have reported that when administered rectally, acetaminophen should be given in significantly higher doses than previous recommendations suggested.[24,25] These authors recommend acetaminophen doses as high as 30–40 mg · kg^{-1} when the drug is administered rectally. Follow-up rectal doses are 30 mg · kg^{-1} every 8 hours. Regardless of route of delivery, to prevent hepatotoxicity, the daily maximum acetaminophen dose in the preterm, term, and older child is 60, 80, 90 mg/kg, respectively (see Table 54–1). The maximum adult dose is 4 g/day.

The discovery of at least 2 cyclooxygenase (COX) isoenzymes, referred to as COX-1 and COX-2, has updated our knowledge of NSAIDs.[26–29] The two COX isoenzymes share structural and enzymatic similarities, but are specifically regulated at the molecular level and may be distinguished by their functions. Protective prostaglandins, which preserve the integrity of the stomach lining and maintain normal renal function in a compromised kidney, are synthesized by COX-1.[26,27,30] COX-2 is an inducible isoform. The inducing stimuli include pro-inflammatory cytokines and growth factors, implying a role for COX-2 in both inflammation and control of cell growth. In addition to the induction of COX-2 in inflammatory lesions, COX-2 is present constitutively in the brain and spinal cord, where it may be involved in nerve transmission, particularly that for pain and fever. Prostaglandins made by COX-2 are also important in ovulation and in the birth process.[26,27,30] The discovery of COX-2 has made possible the design of drugs that reduce inflammation without removing the protective prostaglandins in the stomach and kidney made by COX-1. In fact, developing a more specific COX-2 inhibitor has been the "holy grail" of drug research because this class of drug has all of the antiinflammatory and analgesic properties that one desires in a drug and none of the gastrointestinal and antiplatelet side effects. Unfortunately, the growing controversy regarding the potential adverse cardiovascular risks of prolonged use of the COX-2 inhibitors has dampened much of the enthusiasm for these drugs and has led to the removal of rofecoxib from the market by its manufacturer.[31,32] Finally, many orthopedic surgeons are also concerned about the negative influence of all NSAIDs, both selective and nonselective COX inhibitors, on bone growth and healing.[33–35] Thus, most pediatric orthopedic surgeons have recommended that these drugs not be used in their patients in the postoperative period.

Opioid Drug Selection

Many factors are considered when deciding which is the appropriate opioid analgesic to administer to a patient in pain. These include pain intensity, patient age, coexisting disease, potential drug interactions, treatment history, physician preference, patient preference, and route of administration. The idea that some opioids are "weak" (eg, codeine) and others "strong" (eg, morphine) is outdated. All are capable of treating pain regardless of its intensity if the dose is adjusted appropriately (Table 54–17). And at equipotent doses most opioids have similar effects and side effects. Characteristics of selected μ-agonist opioid drugs are listed for quick reference in Table 54–17. Meperidine is worth a special note of discussion. An entire generation of physicians believe that meperidine causes less respiratory depression and less biliary spasm than morphine. This is simply untrue and was based on a study of postoperative adult patients in whom half received 10 mg morphine and the other half 10 mg of meperidine. The meperidine group had less respiratory depression and biliary spasm than morphine. They also had more pain. The equianalgesic dose of meperidine is 100 mg. When the study was repeated with appropriate dosing, the investigators

found that meperidine had the same side-effect profile as that of morphine.[36] Although meperidine was once among the most commonly prescribed μ-agonist opioids, it no longer is. Meperidine has a neurotoxic metabolite, normeperidine, which possesses no analgesic properties and relies on the kidney for its excretion. Normeperidine accumulation causes central nervous system excitation, resulting in a range of toxic reactions from anxiety and tremors to grand mal seizures.

Commonly Used Oral Opioids: Codeine, Oxycodone, Hydrocodone, and Morphine

Codeine, oxycodone (the opioid in Tylox and Percocet), and hydrocodone (the opioid in Vicodin and Lortab) are opioids that are frequently used to treat pain in children and adults, particularly for less severe pain or when patients are being converted from parenteral opioids to enteral ones (see Table 54–17). Morphine is commonly used in regimens for chronic pain (eg, cancer). Codeine, oxycodone, and hydrocodone are most commonly administered in oral form, usually in combination with acetaminophen or aspirin.[37] Unfortunately, very few, if any, pharmacokinetic or dynamic studies have been performed in children, and most dosing guidelines are anecdotal.

In equipotent doses, codeine, oxycodone, hydrocodone, and morphine are equal both as analgesics and respiratory depressants (see Table 54–17). In addition, these drugs share with other opioids common effects on the central nervous system, including sedation, respiratory depression, and stimulation of the chemoreceptor trigger zone in the brain stem. Indeed, the latter is particularly true for codeine. Codeine is very nauseating; indeed, many patients claim they are "allergic" to it because it so commonly induces vomiting. There are much fewer nausea and vomiting problems with oxycodone and hydrocodone. Indeed, because of this, oxycodone or hydrocodone are now our preferred oral opioids. Codeine, hydrocodone, and oxycodone have a bioavailability of approximately 60% after oral ingestion. The analgesic effects occur as early as 20 minutes after ingestion and reach a maximum at 60–120 minutes. The plasma half-life of elimination is 2.5–4 hours. Codeine undergoes nearly complete metabolism in the liver before its final excretion in urine. Approximately 10% of codeine is metabolized into morphine (CYP 2D6), and it is this 10% that is responsible for codeine's analgesic effect. Interestingly, approximately 10% of the population and most newborn infants cannot metabolize codeine into morphine, and in these patients codeine produces little, if any, analgesia.

Like oxycodone, codeine, and oxycodone, morphine is also very effective when given orally, but only about 20–30% of an oral dose of morphine reaches the systemic circulation. In the past, this led many to conclude that morphine was ineffective when administered orally. This simply isn't true; it was the result of failing to provide sufficient morphine. Therefore, when converting a patient's intravenous morphine requirement to oral maintenance, one must multiply the intravenous dose by a factor of 3 to 4.

Table 54–17.

Opioid Analgesic Initial Dosage Guidelines

Drug	Equianalgesic Dose (mg)		Usual Starting IV (SQ) Doses and Intervals		Parenteral/ Oral Ratio	Usual Starting Oral Doses and Intervals	
	IV, IM, SQ	Oral	<50 kg	>50 kg		<50 kg	>50 kg
Codeine	120	200	NR	NR	1:2	0.5–1 mg/kg q3–4h	30–60 mg q3–4h[a]
Fentanyl	0.1	NA[b]	*Bolus:* 0.5–1 mcg/kg q0.5–2h *Infusion:* 0.5–2 mcg/kg/h	*Bolus:* 25–50 mcg q1–2h *Infusion:* 25–100 mcg/h	NA	NA	NA
Hydrocodone	NA	10–20	NA	NA	NA	0.1 mg/kg q3–4h	5-10 mg q3–4h[a]
Hydromorphone	1.5–2	3–5[c]	*Bolus:* 0.02 mg/kg q0.5–2h *Infusion:* 0.004 mg/kg/h	*Bolus:* 1 mg q0.5–2h *Infusion:* 0.3 mg/h	1:2 1:4[c]	0.03–0.08 mg/kg q3–4h	2–4 mg q3–4h
Meperidine[d]	75–100	150–200	*Bolus:* 1 mg/kg q2–3h	*Bolus:* 50–100 mg q2–3h	1:2	1–2 mg/kg q3–4h	100–150 mg q3–4h
Methadone	10	10–20	0.1 mg/kg q4–8h	5-10 mg q4–8h	1:2	0.2 mg/kg q4–8h	10 mg q4–8h
Morphine	10	30–50	*Bolus:* 0.1 mg/kg q0.5–2h *Infusion:* 0.025 mg/kg/h	*Bolus:* 5–10 mg q0.5–2h *Infusion:* 2 mg/h	1:3 chronic 1:5 single	*Immediate release:* 0.3 mg/kg q3–4h *Sustained release* 20–35 kg: 10–15 mg q8–12h 35–50 kg: 15–30 mg q8–12	*Immediate release:* 15–20 mg q3–4h *Sustained release:* 30–45 mg q8–12h
Oxycodone	NA	10–20	NA	NA	NA	0.1 mg/kg q3–4h	5–10 mg q3–4h[a,e]

[a] *Commercial preparations are often combined with acetaminophen or ibuprofen; must be converted to morphine by CYP 2D6 for analgesic effect.*

[b] *Oral transmucosal form available (Actiq): dose 10–15 mcg/kg.*

[c] *The equianalgesic oral dose and parenteral/oral dose ratio is not well established.*

[d] *Also called pethidine. Meperidine should generally be avoided if other opioids are available, especially with chronic use, because its metabolite, normeperidine can produce seizures.*

[e] *A sustained-release preparation is available.*

Whereas oral morphine is prescribed alone, oral codeine, hydrocodone, and oxycodone are usually prescribed in combination with either acetaminophen or aspirin (Tylenol and codeine elixir, Percocet, Tylox, Vicodin, Lortab). Typically, codeine is prescribed in a dose of 0.5–1 mg/kg. Elixirs, which are available in virtually every pharmacy, contain 120 mg acetaminophen and 12 mg codeine per teaspoon (5 mL).[37] Acetaminophen potentiates the analgesia produced by codeine (and other opioids) and allows the practitioner to use less opioid and yet achieve satisfactory analgesia. Codeine and acetaminophen are also available as "numbered" tablets, eg, Tylenol number 1, 2, 3, or 4. The number refers to how much codeine is in each tablet. Tylenol number 4 has 60 mg codeine, number 3 has 30 mg, number 2 has 15 mg, and number 1 has 7.5 mg. "In all 'combination preparations,' beware of inadvertently administering a hepatotoxic acetaminophen dose when increasing opioid doses

for uncontrolled pain."[38] Acetaminophen toxicity may result from a single toxic dose, from repeated ingestion of large doses of acetaminophen (eg, in adults, 7.5–10 g daily for 1–2 days, children 60–420 mg/kg/day for 1–42 days), or from chronic ingestion. Because of this, we prefer to prescribe the opioid and acetaminophen (or ibuprofen) separately. Although it is an effective analgesic when administered parenterally, intramuscular codeine has no advantage over morphine or any other opioid. Why it is used in neurosurgical and some otorhinolaryngology practices defies logic.

Hydrocodone is prescribed in a dose of 0.05–0.1 mg/kg. The elixir is available as 2.5 mg/5 mL combined with acetaminophen 167 mg/5 mL. As a tablet, it is available in hydrocodone doses between 2.5 mg and 10 mg, combined with 500–650 mg acetaminophen. Oxycodone is prescribed in a dose of 0.05–0.1 mg/kg. Unfortunately, the elixir is not available in most pharmacies. When it is, it comes either as 1 mg/mL *or* 20 mg/mL. This can obviously result in catastrophic dispensing errors. In tablet form, oxycodone is commonly available as a 5-mg tablet or as Tylox (500 mg acetaminophen and 5 mg oxycodone) or Percocet (325 mg acetaminophen and 5 mg oxycodone).

Oxycodone is also available without acetaminophen in a sustained-release tablet for use in chronic pain. Like many other timed-release tablets, it must *not* be crushed and therefore cannot be administered through a gastric tube. Breaking the tablet results in the immediate release of a huge amount of oxycodone. Drug addicts have discovered this and have made this drug a drug of abuse. Like sustained-release morphine (see below), sustained-release oxycodone is only for use in opioid-tolerant patients with chronic pain, and *not* for routine postoperative pain. Also, note that in patients with rapid gastrointestinal transit, sustained-release preparations may not be absorbed at all (liquid methadone may be an alternative.)

Oral morphine is available as a liquid in various concentrations (as much as 20 mg/mL), a tablet (such as MSIR, for **m**orphine **s**ulfate **i**mmediate **r**elease; available in 15- and 30-mg tablets), and as a sustained-release preparation (MS Contin and Oramorph tablets, and Kadian sprinkle capsules, which may be opened and sprinkled on applesauce). Because it is so concentrated, the liquid in particularly easy to administer to children and severely debilitated patients. Indeed, in terminal patients who cannot swallow, liquid morphine provides analgesia when simply dropped into the patient's mouth. [37]

Patient (Parent- and Nurse-)-Controlled Analgesia

Among the many reasons for the undertreatment of pain is the lack of familiarity of physicians (and nurses) with appropriate drugs, drug dosing, and routes of administration. When drugs are given on demand (PRN), there is a lag time between the time the patient's nurse responds, prepares, and administers analgesia. Around-the-clock administration interval administration (eg, q4h) is not the answer either because of the enormous individual variations in pain perception and opioid metabolism. Indeed, fixed doses and time intervals make little sense. Based on the pharmacokinetics of the opioids, it should be clear that intravenous boluses of morphine may need to be given at intervals of 1–2 hours to avoid marked fluctuations in plasma drug levels.

Continuous intravenous infusions may provide steady analgesic levels, are preferable to intramuscular injections, and have been used with great safety and effectiveness in children. However, they are not a panacea because the perception and intensity of pain are not constant. For example, a postoperative patient may be very comfortable resting in bed and may require little adjustment in pain management. This same patient may experience excruciating pain when coughing or voiding or getting out of bed. Thus, rational pain management requires some form of titration to effect whenever any opioid is administered. To give patients, and in some cases parents and nurses, some measure of control over their, or

their children's, pain therapy, demand analgesia or patient-controlled analgesia (PCA) devices have been developed.[39,40] These are microprocessor-driven pumps with a button that the patient presses to self-administer a small dose of opioid.

PCA devices allow patients to administer small amounts of an analgesic whenever they feel a need for more pain relief. The opioid, usually morphine, hydromorphone, or fentanyl is administered either intravenously or subcutaneously. The dosage of opioid, number of boluses per hour, and the time interval between boluses (the "lock-out period") are programmed into the equipment by the pain service physician and nurse to allow maximum patient flexibility and sense of control with minimal risk of overdosage. Generally, because older patients know that if they have severe pain they can obtain relief immediately, many prefer dosing regimens that result in mild to moderate pain in exchange for fewer side effects such as nausea or pruritus. Typically, we initially prescribe morphine, 20 mcg/kg per bolus (or hydromorphone 3–4 mcg/kg/h or fentanyl 0.5 mcg/kg/h), at a rate of 5 boluses/h, with a 6- to 8-minute lock-out interval between each bolus. Variations include larger boluses (30–50 mcg/kg), shorter time intervals (5-minute), and so on.

The PCA pump computer stores within its memory the number of boluses the patient has received as well as the number of attempts the patient has made at receiving boluses. This allows the physician to evaluate how well the patient understands the use of the pump and provides information to program the pump more efficiently. Most PCA units allow low "background" continuous infusions (morphine 20–30 mcg/kg/h, hydromorphone 3–4 mcg/kg/h, fentanyl 0.5 mcg/kg/h) in addition to self-administered boluses. A continuous background infusion is particularly useful at night and often provides more restful sleep by preventing the patient from awakening in pain. It also increases the potential for overdosage.[39–41] Although the adult literature on pain does not support the use of continuous background infusions, our experience has been that continuous infusions are essential both for the patient and for us (fewer phone calls, problems, and so on). Indeed, in our practice, we almost always use continuous background infusions when we prescribe IV (or epidural) PCA.

PCA requires a patient with enough intelligence and manual dexterity and strength to operate the pump. Thus, it was initially limited to adolescents and teenagers, but the lower age limit in whom this treatment modality can be used continues to fall. In fact, it has been our experience that any child able to play Nintendo can operate a PCA pump (age 5–6). Allowing surrogates such as parents or nurses to initiate a PCA bolus is controversial. We recently demonstrated that nurses and parents can be empowered to initiate PCA boluses and to use this technology safely in children even those younger than 1 year of age.[41] In this study, the incidence of common opioid-induced side effects is similar to that observed in older patients. Interestingly, respiratory depression is very rare, but does occur, reinforcing the need for close monitoring and established nursing protocols. Difficulties with PCA include its increased costs, patient age limitations, and the bureaucratic (physician, nursing, and pharmacy) obstacles (protocols, education, storage arrangements) that must be overcome before its implementation.

Contraindications to the use of PCA include inability to push the bolus button (weakness, arm restraints), inability to understand how to use the machine, and a patient's (or parent's) desire not to assume responsibility for his/her own care.

Transmucosal, Intranasal and Transdermal Fentanyl

Because fentanyl is extremely lipophilic, it can be readily absorbed across any biologic membrane including the skin. Thus, it can be given painlessly by new, nonintravenous routes of drug administration including the transmucosal (nose and mouth) and transdermal routes. The transmucosal route of fentanyl administration is extremely effective for acute pain relief. When given intranasally (2 mcg/kg), it produces rapid analgesia that is equivalent to intravenously administered fentanyl.[42]

Alternatively, fentanyl has been manufactured in a candy matrix (Actiq) attached to a plastic applicator (it looks like a lollipop) for transoral/transmucosal absorption. As the child sucks on the candy, fentanyl is absorbed across the buccal mucosa and is rapidly (over 10–20 minutes) absorbed into the systemic circulation.[43–48] If excessive sedation occurs, the fentanyl is removed from the child's mouth by the applicator. It is more efficient than ordinary oral–gastric intestinal administration because transmucosal absorption bypasses the efficient first-pass hepatic metabolism of fentanyl that occurs after enteral absorption into the portal circulation. Actiq has been approved by the FDA for use in children for premedication before surgery and for procedure-related pain (eg, lumbar puncture, bone marrow aspiration).[49] It is also useful in the treatment of cancer pain and as a supplement to transdermal fentanyl.[50] When administered transmucosally, fentanyl is given in doses of 10–15 mcg/kg, is effective within 20 minutes, and lasts approximately 2 hours. Approximately 25–33% of the given dose is absorbed. Thus, when administered in doses of 10–15 mcg/kg, blood levels equivalent to 3–5 mcg/kg IV fentanyl are achieved. The major side effect, nausea and vomiting, occurs in approximately 20–33% of patients who receive it.[51]

The transdermal route is frequently used to administer chronically administered drugs including scopolamine, clonidine, and nitroglycerin. Many factors, such as body site, skin temperature, skin damage, ethnic group, or age affect the absorption of transdermally administered drug. Placed in a selective semipermeable membrane patch, a reservoir of drug provides slow, steady-state absorption of drug across the skin. The patch is attached to the skin by a contact adhesive, which often causes skin irritation.

The use of transdermal fentanyl has revolutionized adult cancer pain management. As fentanyl is painlessly absorbed across the skin, a substantial amount is stored in the upper skin layers, which then act as a secondary reservoir. The presence of a skin depot has several implications: It dampens the fluctuations of fentanyl effect; it needs to be reasonably filled before significant vascular absorption occurs; and it contributes to a prolonged residual fentanyl plasma concentration after patch removal. Indeed, the amount of fentanyl remaining within the system and skin depot after removal of the patch is substantial. At the end of a 24-hour period approximately 30% of the total delivered dose from the patch remains in the skin depot. Thus, removing the patch does not stop the continued absorption of fentanyl into the body.[52]

Because of its long onset time, inability to rapidly adjust drug delivery, and long elimination half-life, transdermal fentanyl is *contraindicated* for *acute* pain management. As stated above, the safety of this drug delivery system is compromised even further, because fentanyl continues to be absorbed from the subcutaneous fat for almost 24 hours after the patch is removed. In fact, the use of this drug delivery system for acute pain has resulted in the death of an otherwise healthy patient. Transdermal fentanyl is applicable only for patients with chronic pain (eg, cancer) or in opioid-tolerant patients. Even when transdermal fentanyl is appropriate, the vehicle imposes its own constraints: The smallest denomination of fentanyl "patch" delivers 25 mcg fentanyl per hour; the others deliver 50, 75, and 100 mcg of fentanyl per hour. Patches *cannot* be physically cut in smaller pieces to deliver less fentanyl. This often limits usefulness in smaller patients, and like other opioids, this drug delivery system has neither been tested nor approved for use in children.

A new noninvasive method of transdermal PCA is on the horizon. Using iontophoresis (electrotransport), small doses of fentanyl (40 mcg) can be self-administered across the skin (E-Trans, ALZA Corp, Mountain View, CA).[53] Transdermal PCA may offer logistic advantages for patients and nursing staff by eliminating the need for venous access, IV tubing, and specialized pumps.

Complications

Regardless of method of administration, all opioids produce common, unwanted side effects, such as pruritus, nausea and vomiting, constipation, urinary retention, cognitive impairment, tolerance, and dependence.[54] Indeed, many patients suffer needlessly from agonizing pain because they would rather suffer than experience these opioid-induced side effects.[55] In addition, physicians are often reluctant to prescribe opioids because of these side effects and because of their fear of other less common, but more serious side effects such as respiratory depression. Several clinical and laboratory studies have demonstrated that low-dose naloxone infusions (0.25–1 mcg/kg/h) can treat or prevent opioid-induced side effects without affecting the quality of analgesia or opioid requirements.[56] We recently confirmed this in a study in children and adolescents and now routinely start a concomitant low-dose naloxone infusion (0.25 mcg/kg/h) whenever we initiate IV PCA therapy.[57]

Transition to Oral Medication

Successful transition from intravenous (or epidural) analgesics to oral medication depends on the clinician's ability to provide alternative therapy that is palatable, acceptable, and above all, equally effective in treating pain. There are many advantages in providing pain medication by the oral route. Enteral therapies are a less invasive route of drug administration and enable children to more rapidly return to their normal lives. Moreover, they are easier and cheaper to deliver than the routes of drug administration they are replacing.

Certain criteria are essential for the successful transition to oral medication. Obviously, normal gastrointestinal function must be present before attempting enteral therapy. Thus, the child must be able to drink and/or eat (or have a functioning gastric tube). A child who is nauseous or vomits after eating will simply not tolerate oral analgesics. Second, severe pain is difficult, if not impossible, to control with oral analgesics alone. Therefore, oral analgesics should be reserved for the treatment of mild to moderate pain during the latter part of the recovery process. Assessment of the degree of pain and existing treatment modalities are steps that aid the transition process. Third, an oral formulation that is palatable and appropriate must be available. Finally, one must convert the current parenteral opioid dosing into a roughly equianalgesic oral dose.

This conversion is fairly straightforward even when patients are receiving multiple forms and doses of parenteral opioids. As a first step, we convert the entire daily dose of administered opioids into IV morphine equivalents (Example 1). We then convert that morphine dose to an equianalgesic dose of oxycodone, our preferred oral opioid, using the formula: 0.1 mg/kg IV morphine = 0.1 mg/kg PO oxycodone. As an astute reader, you should realize that this formula actually underestimates the bioequivalence of the drugs. We do this to minimize the risk of overdosing patients during the transition. Finally, in our practice, we use the IV PCA pump to ease the transition to oral medication. Indeed, the PCA pump provides the child with the option to self-administer a bolus demand dose as a "rescue dose" if the equianalgesic dosing calculations are in error and thereby acts as a "safety net" during the transition.

Example 1: A 5-year-old, 20-kg boy was the victim of a motor vehicle accident and sustained a pelvic fracture. He has been on IV PCA morphine for 2 weeks and will be discharged home for further outpatient therapy and recovery. He receives morphine 2 mg/h and averages 1 bolus of 0.5 mg morphine every hour. He cannot swallow pills.

> Step 1: 2 mg/h for 24 hours = 48 mg morphine/24 hours
>
> Step 2: 0.5 mg/bolus for 24 bolus/day = 12 mg morphine
>
> Step 3: total 24 hour morphine = 48 + 12 mg = 60 mg
>
> Step 4: 60 mg IV morphine = 60 mg PO oxycodone (actually this represents a 25–40% decrease in bioequivalence)
>
> Step 5: Prescribe oxycodone elixir (1 mg/mL) 10 mg every 4 hours and an analgesic with antipyretic activity (such as acetaminophen or ibuprofen).
>
> Step 6: 20–30 minutes after administering the first oral analgesic dose stop the basal opioid infusion.

> Step 7: The IV PCA device is discontinued if no further IV PCA demand doses are used in the next 6–12 hours. Increase the oral analgesic dose by approximately 25% if 1–3 demand doses are recorded in 6 hours.

Local Anesthetics

Over the past 25 years, the use of local anesthetics and regional anesthetic techniques in pediatric practice has undergone a dramatic change. Unlike most drugs used in medical practice, local anesthetics must be physically deposited at their site of action by direct application. This requires patient cooperation and the use of specialized needles and equipment. Because of this, for decades children were considered poor candidates for regional anesthetic techniques because of their overwhelming fear of needles. However, once it was recognized that regional anesthesia could be used as an adjunct, and not a replacement for general anesthesia, its use has increased exponentially. Regional anesthesia offers the anesthesiologist and pain specialist many benefits. It modifies the neuroendocrine stress response, provides profound postoperative pain relief, ensures a more rapid recovery, and may shorten hospital stay. Furthermore, because catheters placed in the epidural, upper or lower extremity or lumbar plexi, and other spaces can be used for days or months, local anesthetics are increasingly being used not only for postoperative pain relief, but also for medical (eg, sickle cell vasoocclusive crisis), neuropathic, and terminal pain.[58-62] Peripheral nerve blocks can also provide significant pain relief after many common pediatric procedures. These techniques range from simple infiltration of local anesthetics to neuraxial blocks, such as spinal and epidural analgesia. To be used safely, a working knowledge of the differences in how local anesthetics are metabolized in infants and children is necessary (Table 54–18).[58,63,64]

Effects of Age on Metabolism of Local Anesthetics

The ester local anesthetics are metabolized by plasma cholinesterase. Neonates and infants up to 6 months of age have less than half of the adult levels of this plasma enzyme. Clearance may thereby be reduced and the effects of ester local anesthetics prolonged. Amides, on the other hand, are metabolized in the liver and bound by plasma proteins. Neonates and young infants (<3 months of age) have reduced liver blood flow and immature metabolic degradation pathways. Thus, larger fractions of local anesthetics are unmetabolized and remain active in the plasma longer than in the adult. More local anesthetic is excreted in the urine unchanged. Furthermore, neonates and infants may be at increased risk for the toxic effects of amide local anesthetics because of lower levels of albumin and α_1-acid glycoproteins, which are proteins essential for drug binding.[65] This leads to increased concentrations of free drug and potential toxicity, particularly with bupivacaine. On the other hand, the larger volume of distribution at steady state seen in the neonate for these (and other) drugs may confer some clinical protection by lowering plasma drug levels.

The metabolism of the amide local anesthetic prilocaine is unique in that it results in the production of oxidants that

Table 54–18.

Maximum Local Anesthetic Dosing Guidelines

Drug	Dose mg/kg without Epinephrine	Dose mg/kg with Epinephrine	Duration in hours	Contraindications	Comments
Bupivacaine[a]	2	3	3–6		Reduce dose by 50% in neonates
Chloroprocaine[b]	8	10	1	Plasma cholinesterase deficiency	Short acting, rapid metabolism, useful in neonates and ? patients with seizures or liver disease
Lidocaine	5	7	1		
Ropivacaine	2	3	3–6		Less cardiotoxicity than bupivacaine

[a] *When given by epidural continuous infusion: 0.2–0.4 mg/kg/h.*
[b] *In neonatal epidural continuous infusion: 10–15 mg/kg/h.*

can lead to the development of methemoglobinemia. This occurs in adults with doses of prilocaine greater than 600 mg. Because premature and full-term infants have decreased levels of methemoglobin reductase, they are more susceptible to developing methemoglobinemia.[66] An additional factor rendering newborns more susceptible to methemoglobinemia is the relative ease by which fetal hemoglobin is oxidized compared with adult hemoglobin. Because of this, prilocaine has not been recommended for *routine* use in neonates.[67–69] Unfortunately, this has limited the use of the topical local anesthetic, EMLA (eutectic mixture of local anesthetics) in the newborn.

Recent evidence suggests that the fear of using EMLA in neonates may be unfounded. Single doses have been shown to be safe and effective in the management of newborn circumcision.[65,70] In 1999, Essink-Tjebbes et al.[71] published an efficacy and safety review of studies involving EMLA in neonates (excluding circumcision) and found that EMLA was safe when used once a day in both full-term and preterm neonates. They subsequently showed that using 0.5 g up to four times a day on the heels of preterm infants did not raise methemoglobin levels.[72] A study in term neonates using 1 g of EMLA on intact skin found that methemoglobin concentrations were significantly higher in the EMLA group in the intervals from 3.5 to 13 hours after application but were well below potentially harmful levels.[73] Fortunately, several alternative topical local anesthetics (lidocaine 4% creams) are now available (and more are coming to the marketplace) that are equally effective and do not contain prilocaine.[74,75]

Local Anesthetic Dosing

It is beyond the scope of this chapter to discuss in detail the many nerve blocks and regional anesthetic that

can be easily and safely performed in pediatrics. However, a brief discussion of local anesthetic dosing is warranted, particularly for the most commonly used local anesthetics for local infiltration, topical application, and neural blockade. These include lidocaine, bupivacaine, ropivacaine, and chloroprocaine.

As in adults, local anesthetic toxicity is primarily related to how rapidly and how much local anesthetic is absorbed (or deposited) in the blood. Toxicity can be limited by careful attention to dose and route of administration and by limiting the rate of rise of local anesthetic into the systemic circulation. Therefore, careful attention to detail is mandatory, particularly when these drugs are used in newborns and younger infants. Usually, no more than 2–2.5 mg/kg of bupivacaine (and ropivacaine) or 5–7 mg/kg lidocaine should be used (see Table 54–18). When given by continuous infusion, the maximum hourly bupivacaine infusion rate should not exceed 0.4 mg/kg/h in the older child and adolescent and 0.2 mg/kg/h in the newborn.[76] Dilute solutions of the local anesthetics can be used to provide adequate spread of the anesthetic solution without exceeding the maximum dose. Epinephrine can also be added to the solution in vascular areas to slow the uptake of the anesthetic and to prolong its action. However, epinephrine must never be used in procedures involving end arteries, such as the penis or distal extremities, to avoid ischemic injury to these areas.

Finally, the pain of local anesthetic administration can be minimized by using small-gauge needles (25–30) and warm, buffered anesthetic solutions and by injecting slowly. Adding bicarbonate to local anesthetic solutions shortens the onset time (faster block) and reduces the pain of injection.[77,78] This is best accomplished by adding 1 mL (1 mEq) of 8.4% sodium bicarbonate to 9 mL lidocaine or by adding 1 mL (1 mEq) of 8.4% sodium bicarbonate to 29 mL bupivacaine.[63,79]

CONCLUSION

The past 25 years have seen an explosion in research and interest in pediatric (and adult) pain management. In this brief review, we have tried to consolidate in a comprehensive manner some of the most commonly used agents and techniques in current practice.

References

1. Schechter NL, Berde CB, Yaster M: *Pain in Infants, Children, and Adolescents,* 2nd ed. Lippincott Williams & Wilkins, 2003, pp. 1–892.
2. Yaster M, Krane EJ, Kaplan RF, et al: *Pediatric Pain Management and Sedation Handbook.* Mosby Year Book, 1997, pp. 1–674.
3. Anand KJ, Hickey PR: Pain and its effects in the human neonate and fetus. N Engl J Med 1987;317:1321–1329.
4. Stevens B, Gibbins S, Franck LS: Treatment of pain in the neonatal intensive care unit. Pediatr Clin North Am 2000;47:633–650.
5. Fitzgerald M: Neurobiology of fetal and neonatal pain. In: Wall PD, Melzack R (editors): *Textbook of Pain,* 3d ed. Churchill Livingstone, 1994, pp. 153–164.
6. Lee SJ, Ralston HJ, Drey EA, et al: Fetal pain: A systematic multidisciplinary review of the evidence. JAMA 2005;294:947–954.
7. Taddio A, Katz J, Ilersich AL, Koren G: Effect of neonatal circumcision on pain response during subsequent routine vaccination. Lancet 1997;349:599–603.
8. Taddio A, Katz J: The effects of early pain experience in neonates on pain responses in infancy and childhood. Paediatr Drugs 2005;7:245–257.
9. Forward SP, Brown TL, McGrath PJ: Mothers' attitudes and behavior toward medicating children's pain. Pain 1996;67:469–474.
10. Finley GA, McGrath PJ, Forward SP, et al: Parents' management of children's pain following 'minor' surgery. Pain 1996;64:83–87.
11. Merskey H, Albe-Fessard DG, Bonica JJ: Pain terms: A list with definitions and notes on usage. Recommended by the IASP Subcommittee on Taxonomy. Pain 1979;6:249–252.
12. Varni JW, Thompson KL, Hanson V: The Varni/Thompson Pediatric Pain Questionnaire. I. Chronic musculoskeletal pain in juvenile rheumatoid arthritis. Pain 1987;28:27–38.
13. Thompson KL, Varni JW: A developmental cognitive-biobehavioral approach to pediatric pain assessment. Pain 1986;25:283–296.
14. Beyer JE, Wells N: The assessment of pain in children. Pediatr Clin North Am 1989;36:837–854.
15. Beyer JE, Denyes MJ, Villarruel AM: The creation, validation, and continuing development of the Oucher: A measure of pain intensity in children. J Pediatr Nurs 1992;7:335–346.
16. Wong DL, Baker CM: Pain in children: Comparison of assessment scales. Pediatr Nurs 1988;14:9–17.
17. Franck LS, Greenberg CS, Stevens B: Pain assessment in infants and children. Pediatr Clin North Am 2000;47:487–512.
18. Anthony KK, Schanberg LE: Pediatric pain syndromes and management of pain in children and adolescents with rheumatic disease. Pediatr Clin North Am 2005;52:611–639, vii.
19. Rusy LM, Weisman SJ: Complementary therapies for acute pediatric pain management. Pediatr Clin North Am 2000;47:589–599.
20. Berde CB, Sethna NF: Analgesics for the treatment of pain in children. N Engl J Med 2002;347:1094–1103.
21. Yaster M: Non-steroidal antiinflammatory drugs. In: Yaster M, Krane EJ, Kaplan RF (editors): *Pediatric Pain Management and Sedation Handbook.* Mosby Year Book, 1997, pp. 19–28.
22. Tobias JD: Weak analgesics and nonsteroidal anti-inflammatory agents in the management of children with acute pain. Pediatr Clin North Am 2000;47:527–543.
23. Maunuksela EL, Kokki H, Bullingham RE: Comparison of intravenous ketorolac with morphine for postoperative pain in children. Clin Pharmacol Ther 1992;52:436–443.
24. Birmingham PK, Tobin MJ, Henthorn TK, et al: Twenty-four-hour pharmacokinetics of rectal acetaminophen in children: An old drug with new recommendations. Anesthesiology 1997;87:244–252.
25. Rusy LM, Houck CS, Sullivan LJ, et al: A double-blind evaluation of ketorolac tromethamine versus acetaminophen in pediatric tonsillectomy: Analgesia and bleeding. Anesth Analg 1995;80:226–229.
26. Vane JR, Botting RM: Mechanism of action of nonsteroidal anti-inflammatory drugs. Am J Med 1998;104:2S–8S;discussion 21S–2.
27. Vane JR, Botting RM: Mechanism of action of aspirin-like drugs. Semin Arthritis Rheum 1997;26:2–10.
28. Jouzeau JY, Terlain B, Abid A, et al: Cyclo-oxygenase isoenzymes. How recent findings affect thinking about nonsteroidal anti-inflammatory drugs. Drugs 1997;53:563–582.
29. Cashman JN: The mechanisms of action of NSAIDs in analgesia. Drugs 1996;52(Suppl 5):13–23.
30. Vane JR, Bakhle YS, Botting RM: Cyclooxygenases 1 and 2. Annu Rev Pharmacol Toxicol 1998;38:97–120.
31. Johnsen SP, Larsson H, Tarone RE, et al: Risk of hospitalization for myocardial infarction among users of rofecoxib, celecoxib, and other NSAIDs: A population-based case-control study. Arch Intern Med 2005;165:978–984.
32. Levesque LE, Brophy JM, Zhang B: The risk for myocardial infarction with cyclooxygenase-2 inhibitors: A population study of elderly adults. Ann Intern Med 2005;142:481–9.
33. Dahners LE, Mullis BH: Effects of nonsteroidal anti-inflammatory drugs on bone formation and soft-tissue healing. J Am Acad Orthop Surg 2004;12:139–143.
34. Simon AM, Manigrasso MB, O'Connor JP: Cyclo-oxygenase 2 function is essential for bone fracture healing. J Bone Miner Res 2002;17:963–976.
35. Einhorn TA: Cox-2: Where are we in 2003? The role of cyclooxygenase-2 in bone repair. Arthritis Res Ther 2003;5:5–7.
36. Radnay PA, Duncalf D, Novakovic M, Lesser ML: Common bile duct pressure changes after fentanyl, morphine, meperidine, butorphanol, and naloxone. Anesth Analg 1984;63:441–444.
37. Krane EJ, Yaster M: Transition to less invasive therapy. In: Yaster M, Krane EJ, Kaplan RF, et al (editors): *Pediatric Pain Management and Sedation Handbook.* Mosby Year Book, 1997, pp. 147–162.
38. Heubi JE, Barbacci MB, Zimmerman HJ: Therapeutic misadventures with acetaminophen: Hepatoxicity after multiple doses in children. J Pediatr 1998;132:22–27.
39. Berde CB, Lehn BM, Yee JD, et al: Patient-controlled analgesia in children and adolescents: A randomized, prospective comparison with intramuscular administration of morphine for postoperative analgesia. J Pediatr 1991;118:460–466.
40. Yaster M, Billett C, Monitto C: Intravenous patient controlled analgesia. In: Yaster M, Krane EJ, Kaplan RF, et al (editors): *Pediatric Pain Management and Sedation Handbook.* Mosby Year Book, 1997, pp. 89–112.
41. Monitto CL, Greenberg RS, Kost-Byerly S, et al: The safety and efficacy of parent-/nurse-controlled analgesia in patients less than six years of age. Anesth Analg 2000;91:573–579.
42. Galinkin JL, Fazi LM, Cuy RM, et al: Use of intranasal fentanyl in children undergoing myringotomy and tube placement during halothane and sevoflurane anesthesia. Anesthesiology 2000;93:1378–1383.
43. Schechter NL, Weisman SJ, Rosenblum M, et al: The use of oral transmucosal fentanyl citrate for painful procedures in children. Pediatrics 1995;95:335–339.
44. Goldstein-Dresner MC, Davis PJ, Kretchman E, et al: Double-blind comparison of oral transmucosal fentanyl citrate with oral meperidine, diazepam, and atropine as preanesthetic medication in children with congenital heart disease. Anesthesiology 1991;74:28–33.
45. Streisand JB, Stanley TH, Hague B, et al: Oral transmucosal fentanyl citrate premedication in children. Anesth Analg 1989;69:28–34.
46. Stanley TH, Hague B, Mock DL, et al: Oral transmucosal fentanyl citrate (lollipop) premedication in human volunteers. Anesth Analg 1989;69:21–27.

47. Ashburn MA, Lind GH, Gillie MH, et al: Oral transmucosal fentanyl citrate (OTFC) for the treatment of postoperative pain. Anesth Analg 1993;76:377–381.

48. Streisand JB, Varvel JR, Stanski DR, et al: Absorption and bioavailability of oral transmucosal fentanyl citrate. Anesthesiology 1991;75:223–229.

49. Dsida RM, Wheeler M, Birmingham PK, et al: Premedication of pediatric tonsillectomy patients with oral transmucosal fentanyl citrate. Anesth Analg 1998;86:66–70.

50. Portenoy RK, Payne R, Coluzzi P, et al: Oral transmucosal fentanyl citrate (OTFC) for the treatment of breakthrough pain in cancer patients: A controlled dose titration study. Pain 1999;79:303–312.

51. Epstein RH, Mendel HG, Witkowski TA, et al: The safety and efficacy of oral transmucosal fentanyl citrate for preoperative sedation in young children. Anesth Analg 1996;83:1200–1205.

52. Grond S, Radbruch L, Lehmann KA: Clinical pharmacokinetics of transdermal opioids: Focus on transdermal fentanyl. Clin Pharmacokinet 2000;38:59–89.

53. Chelly JE, Grass J, Houseman TW, et al: The safety and efficacy of a fentanyl patient-controlled transdermal system for acute postoperative analgesia: A multicenter, placebo-controlled trial (table). Anesth Analg 2004;98:427–433.

54. Yaster M, Kost-Byerly S, Maxwell LG: Opioid agonists and antagonists. In: Schechter NL, Berde CB, Yaster M (editors): *Pain in Infants, Children, and Adolescents,* 2nd ed. Lippincott Williams & Wilkins, 2003, pp. 181–224.

55. Watcha MF, White PF: Postoperative nausea and vomiting. Its etiology, treatment, and prevention. Anesthesiology 1992;77:162–84.

56. Gan TJ, Ginsberg B, Glass PS, et al: Opioid-sparing effects of a low-dose infusion of naloxone in patient-administered morphine sulfate. Anesthesiology 1997;87:1075–1081.

57. Maxwell LG, Kaufmann SC, Bitzer S, et al: The effects of a small-dose naloxone infusion on opioid-induced side effects and analgesia in children and adolescents treated with intravenous patient-controlled analgesia: A double-blind, prospective, randomized, controlled study. Anesth Analg 2005;100:953–958.

58. Dalens B: Regional anesthesia in children. Anesth Analg 1989;68:654–672.

59. Giaufre E, Dalens B, Gombert A: Epidemiology and morbidity of regional anesthesia in children: A one-year prospective survey of the French-Language Society of Pediatric Anesthesiologists. Anesth Analg 1996;83:904–912.

60. Yaster M, Maxwell LG: Pediatric regional anesthesia. Anesthesiology 1989;70:324–338.

61. Ross AK, Eck JB, Tobias JD: Pediatric regional anesthesia: Beyond the caudal. Anesth Analg 2000;91:16–26.

62. Golianu B, Krane EJ, Galloway KS, Yaster M: Pediatric acute pain management. Pediatr Clin North Am 2000;47:559–587.

63. Yaster M, Tobin JR, Maxwell LG: Local anesthetics. In: Schechter NL, Berde CB, Yaster M (editors): *Pain in Infants, Children, and Adolescents.* Williams & Wilkins, 1993, pp. 179–194.

64. Dalens B: *Regional Anesthesia in Infants, Children, and Adolescents.* Williams & Wilkins, 1995.

65. Lerman J, Strong HA, LeDez KM, et al: Effects of age on the serum concentration of alpha 1-acid glycoprotein and the binding of lidocaine in pediatric patients. Clin Pharmacol Ther 1989;46:219–225.

66. Lloyd CJ: Chemically induced methaemoglobinaemia in a neonate. Br J Oral Maxillofac Surg 1992;30:63–65.

67. Brisman M, Ljung BM, Otterbom I, et al: Methaemoglobin formation after the use of EMLA cream in term neonates. Acta Paediatr 1998;87:1191–1194.

68. Engberg G, Danielson K, Henneberg S, Nilsson A: Plasma concentrations of prilocaine and lidocaine and methaemoglobin formation in infants after epicutaneous application of a 5% lidocaine-prilocaine (EMLA). Acta Anaesthesiol Scand 1987;31:624–628.

69. Nilsson A, Engberg G, Henneberg S, et al: Inverse relationship between age-dependent erythrocyte activity of methaemoglobin reductase and prilocaine-induced methaemoglobinaemia during infancy. Br J Anaesth 1990;64:72–76.

70. Taddio A, Stevens B, Craig K, et al: Efficacy and safety of lidocaine-prilocaine cream for pain during circumcision. N Engl J Med 1997;336:1197–1201.

71. Essink-Tjebbes CM, Hekster YA, Liem KD, van Dongen RT: Topical use of local anesthetics in neonates. Pharm World Sci 1999;21:173–176.

72. Essink-Tjebbes CM, Wuis EW, Liem KD, et al: Safety of lidocaine-prilocaine cream application four times a day in premature neonates: A pilot study. Eur J Pediatr 1999;158:421–423.

73. Brisman M, Ljung BM, Otterbom I, et al: Methaemoglobin formation after the use of EMLA cream in term neonates. Acta Paediatr 1998;87:1191–1194.

74. Koh JL, Harrison D, Myers R, et al: A randomized, double-blind comparison study of EMLA and ELA-Max for topical anesthesia in children undergoing intravenous insertion. Paediatr Anaesth 2004;14:977–982.

75. Lehr VT, Cepeda E, Frattarelli DA, et al: Lidocaine 4% cream compared with lidocaine 2.5% and prilocaine 2.5% or dorsal penile block for circumcision. Am J Perinatol 2005;22:231–237.

76. Berde CB: Convulsions associated with pediatric regional anesthesia. Anesth Analg 1992;75:164–166.

77. Christoph RA, Buchanan L, Begalla K, Schwartz S: Pain reduction in local anesthetic administration through pH buffering. Ann Emerg Med 1988;17:117–120.

78. Orlinsky M, Hudson C, Chan L, Deslauriers R: Pain comparison of unbuffered versus buffered lidocaine in local wound infiltration. J Emerg Med 1992;10:411–415.

79. Yaster M, Tobin JR, Fisher QA, Maxwell LG: Local anesthetics in the management of acute pain in children. J Pediatr 1994;124:165–176.

55

Local & Regional Anesthesia in Pediatric General Dentistry

Ilija Škrinjarić, DMD

INTRODUCTION

The practice of modern dentistry is inconceivable without the application of local anesthesia. The dentist has various devices and procedures available for achievement of local anesthesia at his/her disposal. However, it is a paradox that the local anesthesia procedure enables painless work in the mouth also causes patients the most discomfort and fear. Research has shown that the administration of the injection is the primary fear-inducing stimulus in children, and in patients in general.[1-5]

The painful experience of the injection is the most frequent reason for fear of the dentist in children. Local anesthesia in children's dentistry not only enables the therapeutic procedure in the child, but also enables the child to experience the procedure as pleasant and to remain relaxed. Of interest, studies have also shown that not only does the child fear the painful procedure and discomfort during treatment, but that dentists are also more apprehensive.[5]

Successfully administered local anesthesia is of crucial importance allowing the dentist to perform a number of therapeutic procedures on the tooth and in the oral cavity. Unfortunately, the administration of the injection of local anesthesia remains the main problem connected with painful sensation and the occurrence of dental anxiety in the patients, particularly children. Consequently, numerous studies in the field of pain control and fear have concentrated on reducing or completely eliminating pain when administering local anesthesia.[3,6,7]

Indeed, many techniques of local anesthesia administration can be made nontraumatic and without significant discomfort for the patient. This goal is possible also for mandibular blockade and infiltration anesthetic in the palatal mucosa. For administration of painless anesthesia, the dentist must possess certain knowledge, readiness, and skill. In this respect, concentrated efforts of the dentist to learn painless local anesthesia techniques are of exceptional importance.

Injection of local anesthesia is still the most common and effective method of anesthesia in clinical dental pediatric practice, in spite of many attempts to find an alternative less painful and more pleasant procedure for dental treatment. The application of jet injections without needles is only a partial solution of the problem because many areas in the oral cavity cannot be adequately anesthetized without the use of the traditional needle/syringe system.

Dental procedures are associated with pain and discomfort by the patient. This is the main reason for the development of dental fear and anxiety in children, with additional possible serious consequences for future dental treatment. For this reason alone, the painless administration of anesthetic is an important step in avoiding the development of fearful and uncooperative patients.

To control or reduce the patient's pain perception during the administration of intraoral injection, dentists must focus on the factors that influence that perception. The pain of intraoral injection is attributed primarily to the following:

1. Tissue damage by the needle
2. Pressure created by the anesthetic solution
3. Flow rate of the anesthetic
4. Temperature of the drug solution
5. pH of the anesthetic solution

To control the pain sensation during anesthetic administration, all of these factors must be controlled.

This chapter examines the specific aspects of administration of local anesthesia in dental practice and currently available procedures and devices for this application in dental practice with special emphasis to achieving painless local anesthesia in children.

SPECIFICS OF LOCAL & REGIONAL ANESTHESIA IN PEDIATRIC DENTISTRY

When administering local anesthesia the clinician should start with the assumption that nobody likes to receive an injection of any type. This is particularly the case for children. Thus, the method of administering the anesthesia to a child is of extreme importance, not only for performing a specific operation in the mouth, but also for future cooperation from the child. Carefully administered local anesthesia can be almost painless and acceptable for the child. On the other hand, painful local anesthesia can be unpleasant and a frightening experience

for the child, and the treatment is made difficult or even impossible.

Before administering local anesthesia, it is necessary to determine whether the child has had any experience of local anesthesia and what he or she feels about it. If the child has no experience and is cooperative and positive, the procedure of administering anesthesia can usually be performed with less difficulty.

Administration of anesthesia to children of preschool age is a particular problem because they are, in general, less tolerant of pain and discomfort than older children. It should be kept in mind that although it is possible to give an injection almost painlessly, it is impossible to avoid the strange sensation as the local anesthesia takes effect, which causes anxiety in some children.

FACTORS INFLUENCING THE OCCURRENCE OF PAIN DURING INJECTIONS OF ANESTHESIA

The dentist can control the discomfort and fear of local anesthesia. To ensure this outcome, it is necessary to acknowledge many factors that have a significant influence on the degree of pain during the administration of anesthesia. Some of the most important are the patient's fear and anticipation of pain, perception of the needle and syringe, technique and method used, condition of local tissue, and how well the surface anesthesia is applied.

Fear & Anticipation of Pain

Most children consider the injection of anesthesia to be the most undesirable intervention in the mouth.[1,5] The administration of local anesthesia is not only a stressful experience for the patient, but also for the dentist. This is particularly

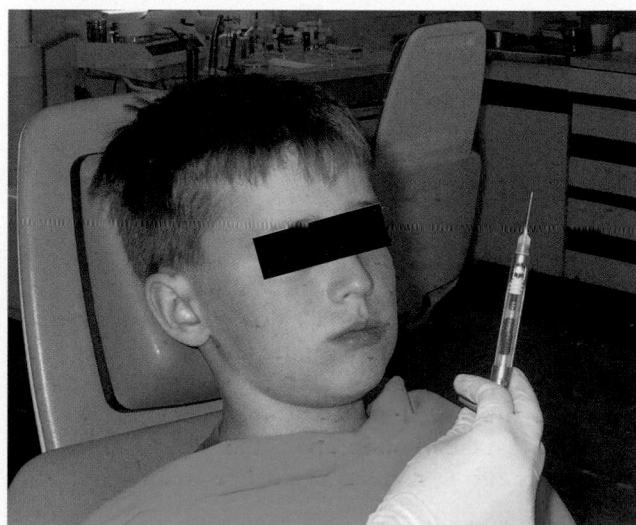

Figure 55–1. Waving the syringe in front of the child before the administration of local anesthesia as a common mistake in dental practice.

the case when the patient anticipates pain and unwillingly accepts the procedure of anesthesia[2,8,9] (Figure 55–1).

There are two important aspects of administering painless anesthesia: (1) communication and (2) technical. The occurrence of fear and a negative experience of local anesthesia are most frequently found in children.[4,5]

A calm and relaxed child is not only important for easier administration of anesthesia but also for its success, that is, the effect of the anesthetic.[5,10,11] Psychological and pharmacologic techniques can both be used to prepare the child for the administration of local anesthesia.

It should be stressed that a tense patient with an increased anticipation of pain usually feels more intense pain during local anesthesia. Acquainting the patient with surface (topical) anesthesia and the subsequent anticipation that there will be no pain, can reduce the anticipation of pain to a great extent. It is also important to stress that **suggestion** can be used, with the aim of reducing anticipation of pain. Suggestion and relaxation before the injection are also important for the effect of the local anesthesia.[5,11]

Verbal communication with the patient is essential, and it should be maintained during the preparation and administration of local anesthesia. It is important to emphasize that surface anesthesia is given initially to ensure that all other procedures are painless and pleasant. The patient should be encouraged while administering the anesthesia. It should be stressed that this is done slowly so that the administration is more pleasant and the anesthesia is maximally effective.

Conversation with the patient achieves better relaxation before and during administration. If this is not possible by psychological means, **sedation** (eg, nitrous oxide or midazolam) can be used. However, sedation cannot replace local anesthesia; it is merely preparation for easier and more successful administration of the local anesthesia.[11]

Injection Needle

The main reason for fear of local anesthesia for most patients is the needle. In the case of patients with strong fears or phobias of the needle, a needleless technique of local anesthesia can be applied (eg, jet injection).

During administration of needle injection anesthesia attention should be paid to ensure that the discomfort of needle insertion is minimal or completely prevented. Factors that influence the discomfort during the penetration of the needle include diameter (gauge) of the needle, type of needle, method of penetration through tissue, and quality of the topical anesthesia of the mucous membrane. For instance, a thinner needle causes less tissue trauma and less pain during penetration of the tissue (Figure 55–2). Needles thicker than 27 gauge (optimal 27 and 30 gauge) are not recommended for use in children.[11] Also, a slow injection of small amounts of anesthetic is less painful to patients. The site of the needle penetration should be prepared with the application some form of surface anesthesia.

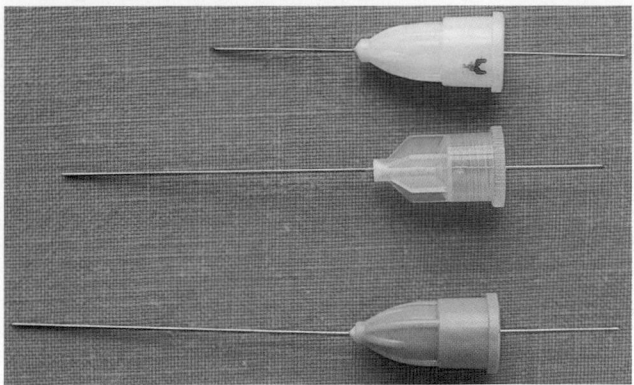

Figure 55–2. Recommended sizes of the local anesthetic needles: **A:** Intraligamentar anesthesia: 30 gauge, 12 mm; **B:** Infiltration anesthesia: 27 gauge or 30 gauge; **C:** Mandibular block: 27 gauge, 25 mm.

Anesthetic

Two features of local anesthetic have an influence on pain during injection: temperature and pH. Prior to administering anesthesia, the local anesthetic should be at room temperature. If the anesthetic is kept in a refrigerator, it should be warmed up to body temperature prior to use by holding it in the hand or better yet, in a warming device[10,11] (Figure 55–3).

Local anesthetic that contains a vasoconstrictor (epinephrine) has an appreciably **lower pH** than plain

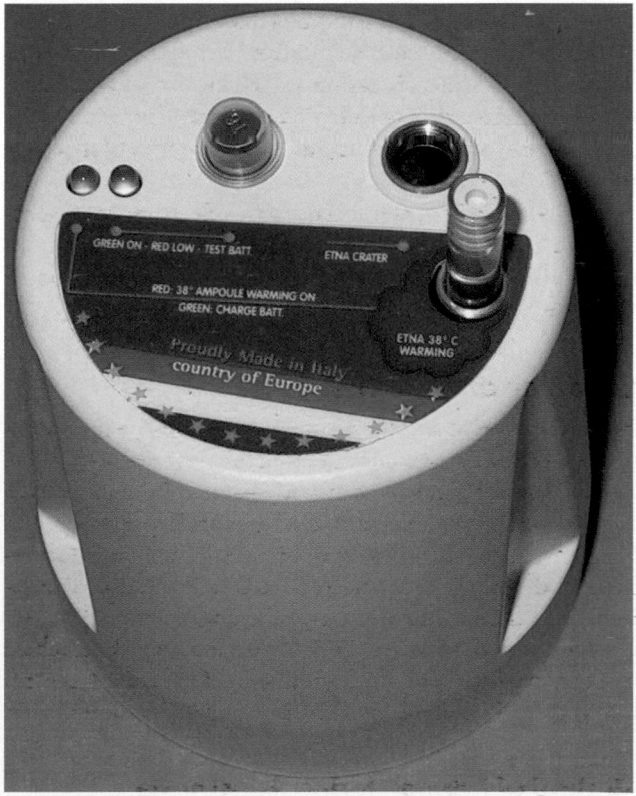

Figure 55–3. A device for warming up a refrigerated cartridge of local anesthetic prior to use.

solutions of local anesthetic. The lower the pH of the anesthetic, the **more painful** is the injection. Consequently, the use of local anesthetic without a vasoconstrictor is appropriate in children (eg, plain solutions of mepivacaine or prilocaine). Indeed, studies have shown that pain associated with the intraoral administration of local anesthesia can be significantly reduced if a plain anesthetic without vasoconstrictor is used.[10,12]

Syringe

The level of anxiety in the patient before administration of local anesthesia also depends to a large extent on the **appearance of the syringe.** The traditional needle-injection assembly automatically induces fear of dental treatment in a child. To avoid fear of the needle or tension in the patient prior to anesthesia, it is possible to successfully use **jet injection** in some areas. This method then can be extended by additional administration of injection anesthesia, if necessary.

Technique

Infiltration anesthesia in loose tissue is less painful than for instance, mandibular block anesthesia, in which the needle penetrates into the denser tissues. In small children, infiltration anesthesia in the mandible, can be used and thus avoid mandibular blockade, which is more painful.

Anesthesia of the palatal mucous membrane can be achieved by the application of palatal nontraumatic injections (a combination with intrapapillary anesthesia), application of jet injections, or computerized anesthesia (eg, Wand method). Slow and steady injection is most important to decrease pain, which is easiest to achieve by an automated method. Alternatively objective assessment of injection pressure can be used to avoid forceful, traumatic injection of local anesthetic.

A combination of transcutaneous electrical nerve stimulation (TENS) and infiltration anesthesia can reduce or completely eliminate pain from injection (either infiltration or blockade).

Condition of Local Tissue

Administration of anesthesia into inflamed tissue may result in less successful local anesthesia because of the high pH of the tissue and because of other mediators of the inflammation. Nerve endings in an inflamed area are hyperalgesic, and conduct painful impulses on minimal stimulation.[11] Consequently, the entrance of a needle and administration of anesthetic into an inflamed area is considerably more painful. Hyperalgesia of the nerves in the inflamed area can be remedied by the administration of an anesthetic of greater concentration (eg, 4% instead of 2% articaine, or 5% lidocaine).[11]

Method of Administering Anesthesia

Slow injection of the anesthetic is extremely important to decrease pain on injection. To decrease pain one 1.8-mL

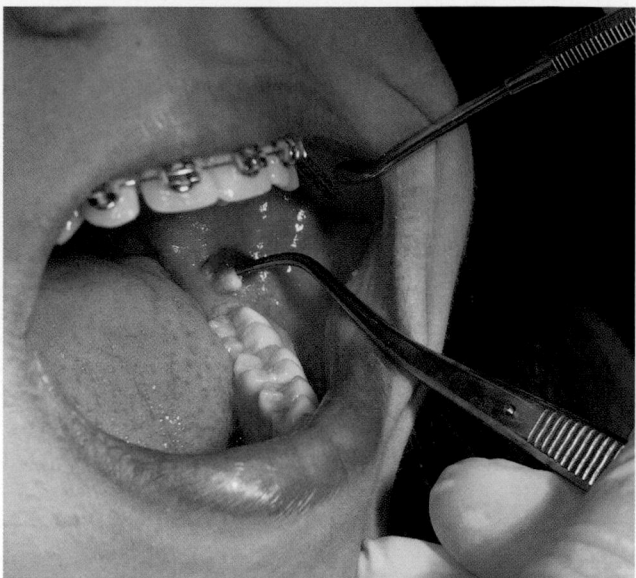

Figure 55–4. Application of topical anesthetic gel before alveolar nerve block injection.

cartridge is injected over 1 to 2 minutes. Faster injection is painful because it results in greater trauma injection pressure, and painful stretching of the local tissue.

Topical Anesthesia

Topical anesthesia is a fundamental part of the administration of infiltration local anesthesia because it has both psychological and pharmacologic importance. Skillfully and patiently applied topical anesthesia can reduce or completely eliminate the pain from the needle penetration (Figure 55–4).

METHODS & DEVICES FOR ADMINISTERING PAINLESS LOCAL ANESTHESIA

Various methods are used with the aim of reducing pain when administering local anesthesia in children. Among the most frequent are surface anesthesia of the site of the needle penetration, anesthesia by jet injection, and sedation of the child prior to administering the injection. More recently, a specific technique of a computerized local anesthesia device (eg, WAND) was developed.[10,13–18]

Jet Injection

The most important aspect of its application is the elimination of fear of the injection needle. For this reason, jet injection is especially suitable for application in children and adults with a phobia of needle injection. Using a jet injection, it is often possible to achieve reliable anesthesia of the working area for an entire range of intraoral procedures. For those patients in whom jet injection is insufficient, it is almost always possible to accomplish adequate local anesthesia to allow

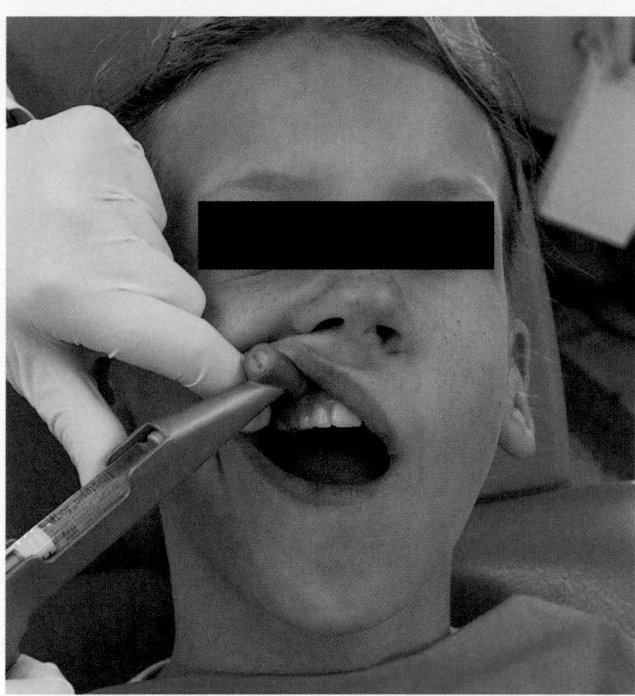

Figure 55–5. Administration of topical anesthesia in a child with a jet injector.

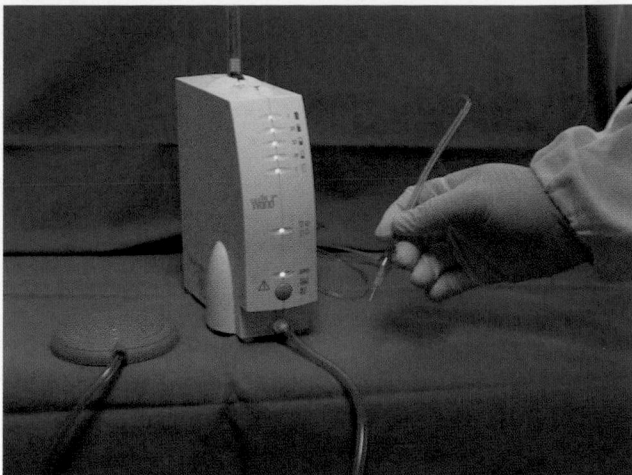

Figure 55–6. Example of computer-controlled anesthesia delivery system: WAND, Milestone Scientific, Livingstone, NJ.

painless administration of additional, traditional needle injection anesthesia (Figure 55–5).

Jet injection offers a great advantage in ensuring local anesthesia in patients with a phobia of classic injection (needle penetration). This is particularly the case in pediatric dentistry, where, because of lower bone density, much better anesthetic effect can be achieved than in adults. Consequently, in children, a small amount of anesthetic can be used to achieve good anesthesia for almost all procedures on the teeth in primary dentition. Used alone or in combination with sedation jet injection allows pleasant and virtually painless dental treatment in children and adults.

Computer-Controlled Anesthesia Delivery System

An example of a computer-controlled anesthesia delivery system is shown in Figure 55–6. The system shown allows practically painless administration of local anesthesia, even in an area with dense connective tissue, such as the mucous membrane of the hard palate.[13,14,16–18]

The device functions by injecting anesthetic at a constant, slow rate and controlled pressure, regardless of the type and resistance of the tissue (loose connective or firm connective palatal mucous membrane). Slow, intermittent injection is maintained by a computer controlled piston. The appliance also enables electronic control of the rate of injection during the entire procedure. Administration of the anesthetic into the tissue is performed very slowly so as to enable the anesthetic to enter the tissue before the needle and to create a passage for it. It is believed that the maintenance of constant pressure and passage of the anesthetic, with an ideal rate of injection of the

anesthetic, are the main reasons for achievement of pleasant and almost painless injections with this system.[13,14,16]

The appearance of the system for administering anesthesia has an important role in the total perception and attitude toward anesthesia. The hand piece with the needle looks like a stick, which is why the system is often called "anesthesia with a stick." It can be presented to the children picturesquely as "anesthesia with a magic stick" and not injection, which children are far more willing to accept (Figure 55–7). Such a device does not induce a feeling of anxiety in children, and children with experience with it report the procedure as pleasant.[15,19,20] Multiple studies have demonstrated that computer-controlled anesthesia for children, particularly those of preschool age, is associated with significantly less discomfort, when compared to the needle-injection method.

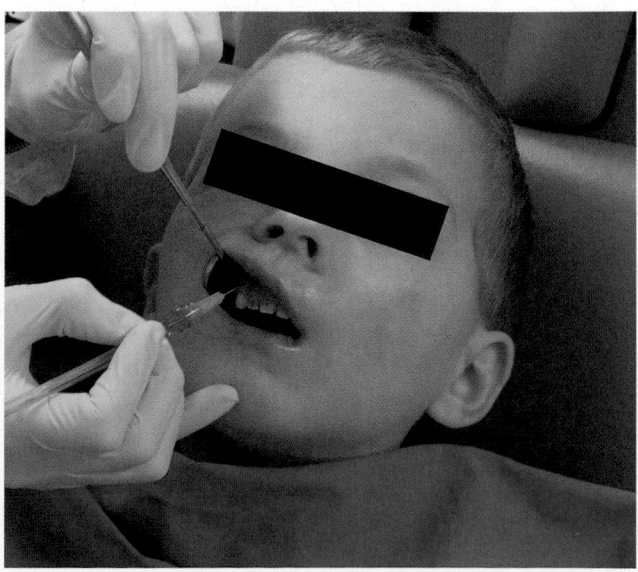

Figure 55–7. Administration of infiltration anesthesia in a child using the Wand delivery system.

SUMMARY

In summary, the use of modern methods and devices makes it possible to ensure an almost painless administration of intraoral local anesthesia in children. It is important to take into account all of the factors that influence pain including the perception of pain with the intraoral injection of anesthetic. The injection of anesthesia in a relaxed child, with prior application of surface anesthesia, plays an important role in making dental procedures more pleasant experiences. In patients with significant fear of the needle, application of jet injection followed by classic infiltration anesthesia, when necessary, is extremely useful.

References

1. Bedi R, Sutcliffe P, Donnan P, et al: The prevalence of dental anxiety in a group of 13- and 14-year-old Scottish children. Int J Paediatr Dent 1992;2:17–24.
2. Dower JS Jr, Simon JF, Peltier B, et al: Patients who make a dentist most anxious about giving injections. J Californ Dent Assoc 1995;23:35–40.
3. Jones CM, Heidmann J, Gerrish AC: Children's ratings of dental injection and treatment pain, and the influence of the time taken to administer the injection. Int J Paediatr Dent 1995;5:81–85.
4. Milgrom P, Coldwell SE, Getz T, et al: Four dimensions of fear of dental infections. J Am Dent Assoc 1997;128:756–766.
5. Ram D, Peretz B: Administering local anaesthesia to paediatric dental patients—Current status and prospects for the future. Int J Paediatr Dent 2002;12:80–89.
6. Houpt M, Heins P, Lamster I, et al: Evaluation of intraoral lidocaine patches in reducing needle-insertion pain. Compendium 1997;18:309–317.
7. Maragakis G, Musselman R: The time used to administer local anesthesia to 5- and 6-year-olds. J Pediatr Dent 1996;20:321–323.
8. Borea G, Montebugnoli G, Braiato A: The effects of patient anxiety on the cardiovascular stress of dentists. Quintessence Int 1989;20:853–857.
9. Poiset M, Johnson R, Nakamura R: Pulse rate and oxygen saturation in children during routine dental procedures. J Dent Child 1990;57:279–293.
10. Malamed SF: *Handbook of Local Anesthesia*. Mosby, 1997.
11. Meechan JG: *Practical Dental Local Anaesthesia*. Quintessence Publishing, 2002.
12. Kramp LF, Eleazer PD, Scheetz JP: Evaluation of prilocaine for the reduction of pain associated with transmucosal anesthetic administration. Anesth Prog 1999;46:52–55.
13. Friedman MJ, Hochman MN: A twenty-first century computerized injection system for local pain control. Compendium 1997;18:995–1003.
14. Hochman M, Chiarello D, Hochman C, et al: Computerized local anesthetic delivery vs. traditional syringe technique. NY State Dent J 1997;8/9:24–29.
15. Lieberman WH: The Wand. Pediatr Dent 1999;21:2.
16. Friedman MJ, Hochman MN: The AMSA injection: A new concept for local anesthesia of maxillary teeth using a computer-controlled injection system. Quintessence Int 1998;29:297–303.
17. Friedman MJ, Hochman MN: P-ASA block injection: A new palatal technique to anesthetize maxillary anterior teeth. J Esthet Dent 1999;11:63–71.
18. Milestone Scientific: The Wand: Computer controlled anaesthetic delivery system. *Operating Manual*. 1999, pp 1–14.
19. Asarch T, Allen K, Petersen B, et al: Efficacy of a computerized local anesthesia device in pediatric dentistry. Pediatr Dent 1999;21:421–424.
20. Allen KD, Kotil D, Larzelere RE, et al: Comparison of a computerized anesthesia device with a traditional syringe in preschool children. Pediatr Dent 2002;24:315–320.

Regional Anesthesia in Patients with Special Considerations

56

Regional Anesthesia in the Elderly

Bernadette Veering, MD, PhD

INTRODUCTION

In many developed countries, the proportion of the population that is older is growing. The oldest old (80 years or older) are the fastest growing segment of the older population. Currently, this group accounts for 11% of those 60 years of age and older. By the year 2030, 17% of the population in the United States will be older than 65 years.[1] Improvements in surgical techniques, anesthesia, and intensive care units make surgical interventions in older and sicker patients possible. It is estimated that over half of the population older than 65 years will require surgical intervention at least once during the remainder of their lives[2] (Figure 56–1). Consequently, elderly patients are becoming an even larger part of anesthetic practice. Regional anesthesia is frequently used in elderly patients, especially during orthopedic surgery, genitourologic and gynecologic procedures, and hernia repair. Although age can no longer be considered as a contraindication to anesthesia

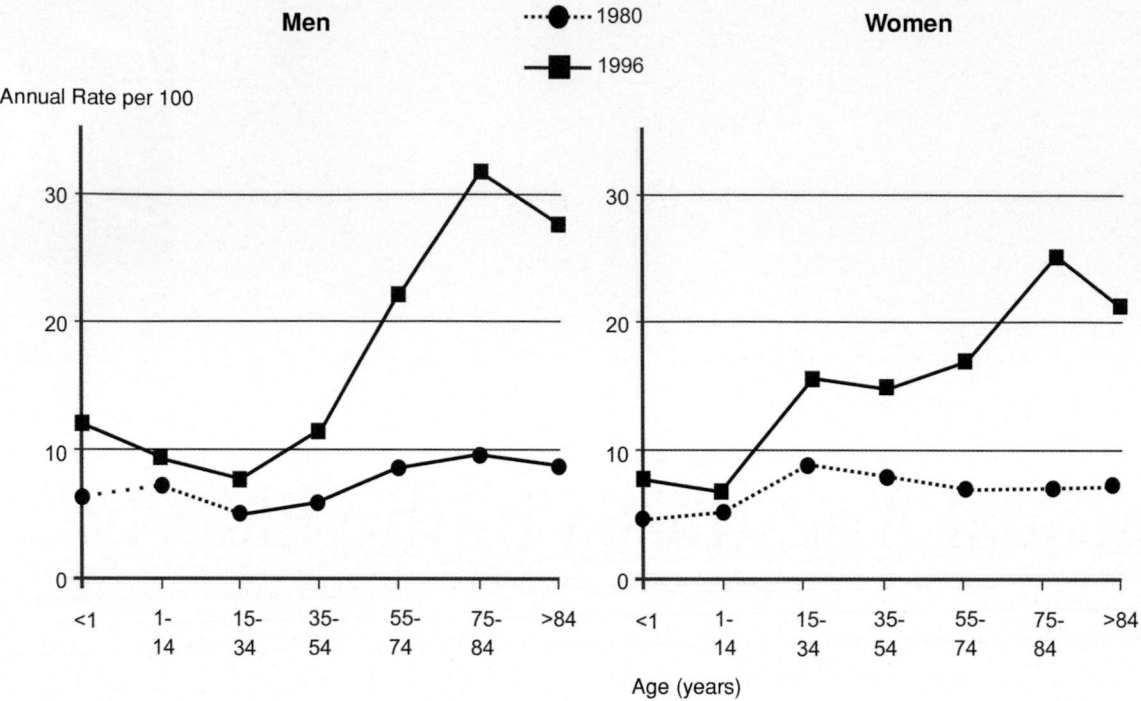

Figure 56–1. Annual rate of anesthesia per 100 population within the different age groups from 1980 to 1996 in France (Reprinted, with permission, from Clerque F, Auroy Y, Pequinot F, et al: French survey of anesthesia in 1996. Anesthesiology 1999;91:1509).

and surgery, anesthesia-related morbidity and mortality remain higher among elderly than among young adult surgical patients.

DEFINITION OF AGING

To effectively treat elderly patients, clinicians must have an understanding of aging, how it occurs, how it affects specific organ systems, and how it influences clinical care when a patient is subjected to surgery. Aging is a normal phenomenon, although the basic mechanisms that cause aging are still poorly understood. Aging per se is represented by those manifestations of irreversibly altered organ function that are common in all elderly persons and are usually progressive. The physiologic process of aging varies considerably from person to person; hence variation in organ capabilities

increases with age. Different organs in the same individual may age at different rates; each system has its own temporal pattern of age change. The organ reserves, which are so essential to ensure homeostasis, gradually decrease, resulting in an increased sensitivity to internal and external environmental stressful stimuli[3] (Figure 56–2).

INCREASING AGE & RISK OF ANESTHESIA-RELATED PERIOPERATIVE COMPLICATIONS

Age alone is not a major factor in predicting the risks to a patient undergoing anesthesia and operation. The overall physical status or disease state or both are better predictors of outcome. Risk is directly related to the number and extent of coexisting preoperative diseases. Ischemic heart disease,

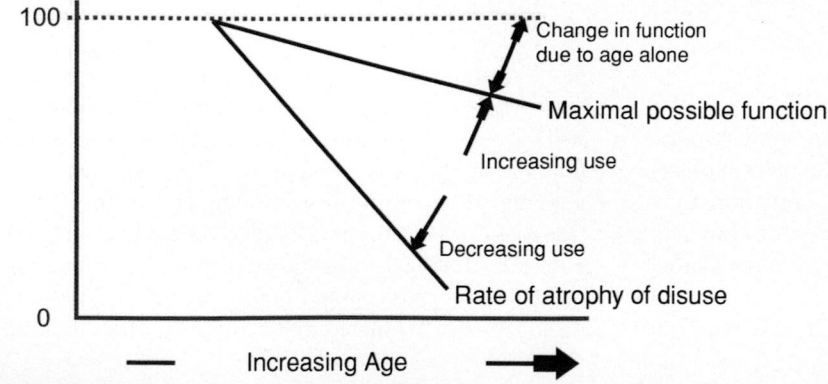

Figure 56–2. Effects of aging on organ function (Reprinted, with permission, from Williams ME: Clinical implications of aging physiology. Am J Med 1984;76:1049).

diabetes mellitus, and hypertension are the preoperative conditions most indicative of a higher risk of peri- and postoperative morbidity and mortality.[4] The type of operation appears to be important; upper abdominal surgery procedures are associated with the highest morbidity and mortality, followed by open-heart surgery procedures. The importance of the site as a major determinant of perioperative risk in the elderly applies equally to both emergency and elective surgery. The anesthetic complication rate increases very little with advancing age in the absence of coexisting disease. As a group, elderly surgical patients are at increased risk of perioperative morbidity and mortality because of the high incidence of coexisting diseases. One third of older patients have three or more preexisting diseases or complicating conditions, and four fifths have at least one complicating condition. Underlying medical diseases and the type, duration, and urgency are more important predictors of outcome than chronologic age.

Clinical Pearls

- The overall physical status or disease state or both are better predictors of perioperative outcome than age.
- The risk of adverse outcome is directly related to the number and extent of coexisting preoperative diseases.
- Preoperative conditions most indicative of a higher risk of peri- and postoperative morbidity and mortality include ischemic heart disease, diabetes mellitus, and uncontrolled arterial hypertension.
- The type of surgical intervention appears to be important, with upper abdominal surgery procedures associated with the highest morbidity and mortality, followed by open-heart surgery procedures.

AGE-RELATED ANATOMIC & PHYSIOLOGIC CHANGES OF SIGNIFICANCE TO THE ADMINISTRATION OF REGIONAL ANESTHESIA

Central & Peripheral Nervous Systems

The central and peripheral nervous systems degenerate with advancing age. The diameter of the myelinated fibers in the dorsal and ventral roots becomes smaller, and the number of these fibers decreases. By the age of 90 years, more than one third of the myelinated nerve population has disappeared. The connective tissue sheaths that cover the nerve tissues become weakened by the general deterioration in the mucopolysaccharides of the ground substance, allowing local anesthetic solution to penetrate the sheaths more readily.[5] These changes may affect the neural block characteristics and the pharmacology of local anesthetic agents. However, currently, it is well understood how these changes may affect pharmacodynamics of neuraxially or perineurally administered local anesthetics.

Clinical Pearls

- By the age of 90 years, more than one third of the myelinated nerve population has disappeared.
- The connective tissue sheaths that cover the nerve tissues become weakened by the general deterioration in the mucopolysaccharides of the ground substance, allowing local anesthetic solution to penetrate the sheaths more readily.
- These changes may affect the neural block characteristics and the pharmacology of local anesthetic agents; however, no clinical studies have as yet elucidated the significance of these changes.

The abovementioned factors are accelerated by arteriosclerosis and diabetes, both of which cause premature aging. After the third decade, there is a steady slowing of the conduction velocity in peripheral nerves, especially in motor nerves.[6] The dura becomes more permeable to local anesthetic agents because of a significant increase in the size of the arachnoid villi.[7] This change is accompanied by a decrease in the thickness of the root dura. Aging is possibly associated with a reduction in the volume of cerebrospinal fluid (CSF) and with an increase of the specific gravity of the CSF, both of which may influence the distribution of intrathecally injected local anesthetics.[8]

Autonomic Nervous System

Changes in the autonomic nervous system with age may alter the course of a regional anesthetic block. Normal aging is associated with a progressive impairment of autonomic homeostasis, that is, there is a delayed restabilization during hemodynamic stress.[9] Aging is accompanied by a variety of neurohormonal changes. One example is that tonic parasympathetic outflow declines, while the basal sympathetic nervous system activity increases. Elderly people respond to stresses of different degrees with a larger increase in norepinephrine levels. The beta-receptor affinity for adrenergic agonists and antagonists appears to be blunted, probably because of a reduced affinity of the beta-receptor for agonists.[10] The changes in autonomic function are referred to as physiologic beta-blockade.

Clinical Pearls

- Baroreceptors are autonomic reflex responses that maintain cardiovascular homeostasis.
- Sensitivity of the baroreceptors declines progressively with age; this decline results in reduced compensatory blood pressure and heart rate responses when the carotid blood pressure alters.
- These factors are of clinical importance when the sympathetic blockade of central neural blockade is associated with a decrease in systemic blood pressure (see section on Hypotension).

Baroreceptors are autonomic reflex responses that maintain cardiovascular homeostasis. Their sensitivity declines progressively with age,[11] resulting in reduced compensatory blood pressure and heart rate responses when the carotid blood pressure alters. These factors are of clinical importance when the sympathetic blockade or central neural blockade is associated with a decrease in systemic blood pressure.

Cardiovascular System

Aging is associated with a variety of morphologic and functional changes of the cardiovascular system.[9] With aging, the large arteries progressively lose elasticity. This loss of elasticity leads to increased systolic pressure, which results in increased afterload for the left ventricle and finally, to mild generalized hypertrophy of the left ventricular wall, which is characterized by increased end-diastolic left ventricular volume.[12] The diminished elasticity and fibrotic changes of the heart muscle make the aged heart noncompliant and thus both volume-sensitive and volume-intolerant. All of these observations have important clinical implications for the treatment of patients undergoing regional anesthesia.

Clinical Pearls

- Elderly patients are unable to respond to stress by significantly increasing the left ventricular ejection fraction.
- In elderly patients, cardiac output is maintained by increasing end-diastolic volume, resulting in an increased stroke volume.
- Elderly patients may, therefore, not maintain blood pressure as effectively as younger patients when challenged by relatively minor hypovolemia and additional cardiovascular stress.
- These factors have considerable importance when administering neuraxial anesthesia; sympathetic blockade can result in severe hypotension in the setting of hypovolemia.

The elderly are unable to respond to stress by significantly increasing the left ventricular ejection fraction. In elderly patients, cardiac output is maintained by increasing end-diastolic volume, which results in increased stroke volume.[12] Elderly patients may, therefore, not maintain blood pressure as effectively as younger patients when challenged by relatively minor hypovolemia and additional cardiovascular stress. These factors have considerable importance when administering neuraxial anesthesia. Sympathetic

blockade can result in severe hypotension in the setting of hypovolemia.

CENTRAL NEURAL BLOCKADE

Epidural Anesthesia

Older age is associated with a higher upper level of analgesia after thoracic and lumbar epidural administration of a fixed dose of a local anesthetic solution[13–15] (Figure 56–3, Table 56–1). The influence of age on the upper level of analgesia varies with different volumes and also depends on variability between individuals.

Higher levels of analgesia with advancing age are attributed to reduced leakage of local anesthetic solution because of progressive sclerotic closure of intervertebral foramina.[16] In the younger individual, the areolar tissue around the intervertebral foramina is soft and loose. In the elderly, the areolar tissue becomes dense and firm, partially sealing the intervertebral foramina. As the fatty tissue degenerates and the content reduces with advancing age, the epidural space becomes more compliant and less resistant; this may also contribute to the greater longitudinal spread of injected solutions in elderly patients.[17] The clinical course of epidural anesthesia may be influenced by a shift in the site of action,

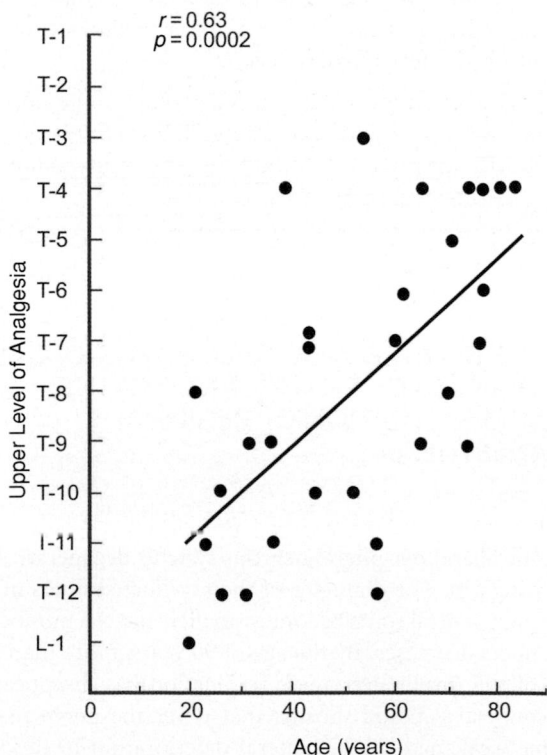

Figure 56–3. Relationship between the upper level of analgesia and age after epidural administration of 0.5% bupivacaine (Reprinted, with permission, from Veering BT, Burm AGL, Van Kleef JW, et al: Epidural anesthesia with bupivacaine: Effects of age on neural blockade and pharmacokinetics. Anesth Analg 1987;66:589).

Table 56–1.			

Effects of Age on the Neural Blockade After Epidural Administration of Bupivacaine,[13,31] Ropivacaine,[14] and Levobupivacaine[15]

	Bupivacaine 0.5%	Ropivacaine 1%	Levobupivacaine 0.75%
Analgesia			
Initial onset time (min)	≈	≈	≈
Time to maximal cephalad spread (min)	≈	≈	≈
Time to maximal caudad spread (min)	↓	≈	≈
Maximal number of segments blocked	↑	↑	↑
Highest level ($T_{dermatome}$)	↑	↑	↑
Two-segment regression (min)	≈	↑	≈
Time to recovery at T12 (min)	≈↑	≈	≈
Time to total recovery (min)	≈	≈	≈
Motor Blockade			
Initial onset time (min)	≈↓	≈	≈
Maximal degree of block	≈↑	↑	≈
Time to total recovery (min)	≈	≈	≈

↑ *increased*; ↓ *decreased*; ≈ *unchanged*.

from a predominantly paravertebral site in the young, to a subdural or transdural site in the elderly. The shift may be caused partly by an increased permeability for local anesthetics of the dura because of an increased size of the arachnoid villi.[7] With increasing age, changes in the connective tissue ground substances may result in changes in local distribution, that is, in the distribution rate of the local anesthetic from the site of injection (the epidural space) to the sites of action.[16]

In older patients the onset time to maximal caudad spread and motor blockade decreases together with an enhanced intensity of motor blockade following epidural administration of bupivacaine.[13] With the relatively new, long-acting local anesthetic agents ropivacaine and levobupivacaine, the spread of analgesia and the intensity of motor block increases with advancing age as well.[14,15]

Often, epinephrine is used in the epidural test dose as a marker of intravascular injection. A given dose of epinephrine may be less reliable in older patients, owing to decreased β-adrenergic responsiveness.[18] Lumbar epidural anesthesia with lidocaine does not affect the resting ventilation parameters, such as minute ventilation and tidal volume, in older patients or stimulate the ventilatory response to hypercapnia to the same degree as in younger patients.[19] Therefore, lumbar epidural anesthesia appears to be a suitable alternative technique in elderly patients. To limit the extent of analgesic and sympathetic blockade after epidural administration, the dose should be reduced. The relationship between the epidural segmental dose requirement and the analgesic spread is not linear and still unclear in older patients. Further studies are required to determine the optimum dose to provide epidural anesthesia in the elderly patient.

Clinical Pearls

- Older age is associated with a higher upper level of analgesia after thoracic and lumbar epidural administration of a fixed dose of a local anesthetic solution.

- Higher levels of analgesia with advancing age were attributed to reduced leakage of local anesthetic solution because of progressive sclerotic closure of the intervertebral foramina.

- The clinical course of epidural anesthesia may be influenced by a shift of the site of action from a predominantly paravertebral site in the young, to a subdural or transdural site in the elderly.

- Epinephrine as a marker of intravascular injection may be less reliable in older patients, owing to decreased β-adrenergic responsiveness.

- Lumbar epidural anesthesia with lidocaine does not affect the resting ventilation parameters, such as minute ventilation and tidal volume, in older patients, making lumbar epidural anesthesia a suitable alternative technique in elderly patients.

- To limit the extent of analgesic and sympathetic blockade after epidural administration, the dose should be reduced; the relationship between the epidural segmental dose requirement and the analgesic spread is not linear and not well delineated.

- Geriatric patients show an increased responsiveness to opioids; the dose of epidural neuraxial opioids should be decreased in the elderly.

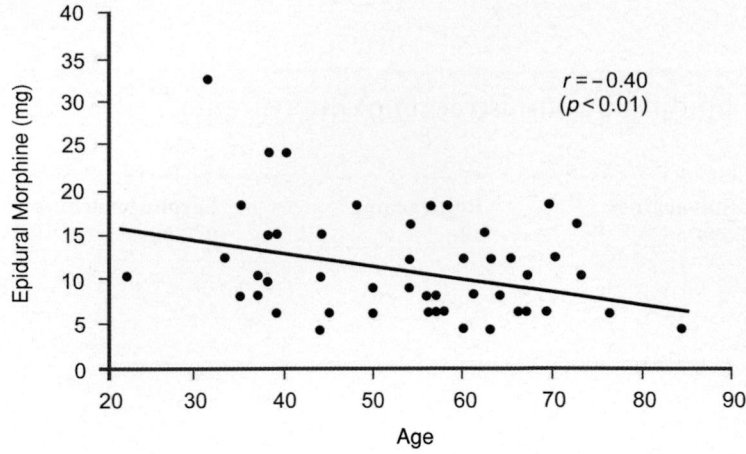

Figure 56–4. The 24-h dose of epidural morphine required for effective analgesia after abdominal hysterectomy decreases with age (Reprinted, with permission, from Ready LB, Chadwick HS, Ross B, et al: Age predicts effective morphine dose after abdominal hysterectomy. Anesth Analg 1987;66:1215).

Geriatric patients show an increased responsiveness to opioids. Epidural opioids are administered to surgical patients to provide prolonged postoperative analgesia. A reduction in the requirements of epidural morphine in older patients was reported. The cause is thought to be related to higher CSF concentrations[20] (Figure 56–4). Patient-controlled epidural analgesia (PCEA) provides effective management of postoperative pain via the epidural route. It was suggested that the bolus dose and infusion rate of opioids be reduced up to 50% when administered to the elderly.

Spinal Anesthesia

The effect of age on the maximal height of spinal analgesia with isobaric solutions is marginal.[21,22] The complete, profound, long-lasting motor blockade and the increased duration of analgesia with glucose-free bupivacaine spinal anesthesia in elderly patients provide satisfactory conditions for orthopedic and vascular surgical procedures in the lower limbs. On the other hand, use of a hyperbaric solution increased the level of analgesia with age, extending some three to four segments higher in elderly patients than occurred in young adult patients[22,23] (Table 56–2). Both with glucose-free and hyperbaric bupivacaine solutions, the prolongation of action at the T12 dermatome allows more time for operations in the lower abdominal or inguinal region in older patients. In addition, a more rapid development of motor blockade was reported in older patients. Spinal anesthesia with hyperbaric bupivacaine is very suitable for lower abdominal and urologic procedures of intermediate duration in elderly patients. The reduction of the volume of CSF and the changes in the anatomic configuration of the lumbar and thoracic spine with advancing age may all contribute to the more extensive block using hyperbaric solutions in elderly patients.

Intrathecal opioids are administered to surgical patients to provide prolonged postoperative analgesia. Respiratory depression is a concern in elderly patients receiving spinal opioids. A reduction in the requirements of epidural morphine in older patients was reported and thought to be related to higher CSF concentrations.[24] Spinal anesthesia with

bupivacaine and fentanyl is well tolerated in nonpremedicated elderly patients.[25] Caution should be used when benzodiazepines are given as premedication and concomitantly in geriatric patients.

Table 56–2.

Effects of Age on the Characteristics of Neural Blockade After Subarachnoid Administration of Bupivacaine[22,23]

	Bupivacaine 0.5% Glucose-Free	Hyperbaric
Analgesia		
Initial onset time (min)	≈	≈
Time to maximal cephalad spread (min)	≈	↑
Time to maximal caudad spread (min)	↓	≈
Maximal number of segments blocked	≈	↑
Highest level ($T_{dermatome}$)	≈	↑
Two-segment regression (min)	≈	≈
Time to recovery at T12 (min)	↑	↑
Time to total recovery (min)	↑	≈
Motor blockade		
Initial onset time (min)	≈	↓
Maximal degree of block	≈	≈
Time to total recovery (min)	≈	≈

↑ *increased;* ↓ *decreased;* ≈ *unchanged.*

Clinical Pearls

- Both epidural and spinal techniques are applicable and allow satisfactory conditions for lower abdominal, pelvic, or lower limb surgery.
- Spinal anesthesia with glucose-free bupivacaine provides the most satisfactory conditions for lower limb surgery in elderly patients.
- Epidural administration of the longer-acting local anesthetic solutions, for example, bupivacaine, ropivacaine, and levobupivacaine, at the L3-4 interspace allows the longest time for the performance of lower abdominal surgery, whereas spinal anesthesia with hyperbaric bupivacaine is very suitable for lower abdominal and urologic procedures of intermediate duration in elderly patients.

In conclusion, when establishing a central neural blockade in elderly patients who are cooperative, both epidural and spinal techniques are applicable and allow satisfactory conditions for lower abdominal, pelvic, or lower limb surgery. Comparing both techniques, spinal anesthesia with glucose-free bupivacaine provides the most satisfactory conditions for lower limb surgery in elderly patients. Epidural administration of the longer-acting local anesthetic solutions, bupivacaine, ropivacaine, and levobupivacaine, at the L3-4 interspace allows the longest time for the performance of lower abdominal surgery, whereas spinal anesthesia with hyperbaric bupivacaine is very suitable for lower abdominal and urologic procedures of intermediate duration in elderly patients.

PERIPHERAL NERVE BLOCKS

Peripheral nerve blocks are used frequently in elderly patients, especially as a satisfactory supplementary analgesic technique for upper limb trauma and hip and knee surgery. For instance, a femoral 3-in-1 nerve block appeared to be a successful block for prolonged pain relief without local anesthetic toxicity in elderly patients.[26]

However, few studies have investigated peripheral nerve block characteristics in elderly patients. After a midhumeral block performed with a small volume of ropivacaine, complete sensory and motor blocks lasted longer in elderly than in younger patients (approximately 2.5 times longer). A positive relationship was found between age and duration of complete sensory and motor blockade.[27] These alterations in the clinical profile may partly be attributed to a decrease in the conduction velocity of the peripheral nerves, especially the motor nerves, and to a gradual degeneration of the peripheral nervous system.[6] By the age of 90 years, one third of the myelinated fibers have disappeared from peripheral nerves.

PHARMACOLOGY

Effects of regional anesthesia comprise a complex combination of pharmacokinetics, pharmacodynamics, the physiologic consequences of neural blockade, and the physiologic status of the patient. Serum concentrations of local anesthetics are of clinical importance with respect to the risk for systemic side effects and toxicity. The concentrations depend on vascular uptake (absorption) of these agents from the extravascular injection site into the bloodstream and systemic disposition (distribution into the bloodstream and elimination from the body). Changes in the pharmacokinetics may be responsible, in part, for the observed changes in the clinical profile.

Pharmacokinetics of Central Neural Blockade & Age

Systemic Absorption

The process of drug removal from the site of administration influences the duration of anesthesia.[28] Peak plasma concentrations of lidocaine and bupivacaine after epidural or caudal administration change little, if at all, with increasing age.[29] Peak plasma concentrations are indirectly related to the rate of absorption. Details on the absorption cannot be derived from the plasma concentration profiles because these depend on the systemic disposition also. The use of a stable isotope method allows the simultaneous study of absorption and disposition.[30]

The absorption of local anesthetic agents following epidural and subarachnoid administration is biphasic: a rapid initial phase followed by a much slower one. With epidural anesthesia the initial fast absorption rate is a reflection of the high initial concentration gradient and the large vascularity of the epidural space. The slower, second absorption phase is attributed to the slow uptake of local anesthetics from the epidural fat depending on the blood partitioning. The initial absorption is much slower after subarachnoid administration, as a result of poor perfusion of the subarachnoid space and a lower drug gradient. The systemic absorption of bupivacaine was unchanged with advancing age as was the total duration of epidural anesthesia.[31] The early absorption of epidural levobupivacaine was less in the elderly.[15] This fact may decrease the risk of systemic toxicity in the elderly.

Clinical Pearls

- The absorption of local anesthetic agents following epidural and subarachnoid administration follows a biphasic pattern.
- With epidural anesthesia the initial fast absorption rate is a reflection of the high initial concentration gradient and the large vascularity of the epidural space.
- The slower, second absorption phase is attributed to the slow uptake of local anesthetics from the epidural fat depending on the blood partitioning.

After subarachnoid administration, the mean absorption time was shorter in elderly patients because of a faster late absorption rate.[32] This characteristic does not translate clinically into a shorter duration of spinal anesthesia. The underlying mechanism of this observation is unknown, but the reduced sensitivity of older patients to the intrinsic vasoactive properties of bupivacaine may modulate local perfusion and, hence, uptake into the systemic circulation.

The changes in clinical effects do not appear to be related to impairment of vascular absorption, leaving more drug available to block nerves, but are more likely related to changes in intrinsic neuronal sensitivity or local distribution or both.

Systemic Disposition

Age-related changes in drug distribution may result from changes in body composition or changes in drug binding and tissue perfusion. The influence of age on the distribution of local anesthetic agents is almost negligible. Local anesthetic agents are primarily eliminated by metabolism. The effect of age on the metabolism and excretion of local anesthetics is related to changes in hepatic function. Hepatic blood flow declines with age.[33] As a consequence, the clearance of local anesthetics with a high hepatic extraction ratio depending on hepatic blood flow may decrease. Accordingly, the clearance of lidocaine decreases with increasing age.[29] There is also a gradual decline in hepatic mass. As a result, the clearance of local anesthetics with relatively low hepatic extraction ratios, which mostly depend on metabolizing hepatic enzyme activity, may decrease with age. Such a decrease has been demonstrated for bupivacaine[13] (Figure 56–5). The consequences of

the reduced clearance will be most relevant during administration of repeated doses and continuous blockade. Probably, plasma concentrations will rise to higher levels in older patients, with consequent reduction in the safety margin. Infusion rates or top-up doses may need to be adjusted in older patients. This need should not necessarily affect the quality of blockade because of the increased sensitivity to local anesthetic agents in older patients.

TECHNICAL DIFFICULTIES IN PERFORMING REGIONAL ANESTHETICS

It can be difficult to perform neuraxial anesthesia in the geriatric age group. Positioning patients for regional anesthetic techniques becomes increasingly difficult with age. The anatomic configuration of the lumbar and thoracic spine is changed. Elderly individuals often have dorsal kyphosis and a tendency to flex the hips and knees because of osteoarthritic changes and cartilage calcification. In advanced age with degenerative disk and joint changes, distortion and compression of the epidural space are common. The ligamentum flavum probably changes into a form that is easily ossified. Attempts to accomplish dural puncture for spinal anesthesia are often unsuccessful because needle placement and advancement may not be easy, especially through calcified ligaments. Similarly, the presence of osteophytes decreases the size of the intervertebral foramina, limiting the access to the subarachnoid space. There are no easy solutions to the technical difficulties that these anatomic changes present. The largest intervertebral foramina are in the L5-S1 interspace; this anatomic characteristic can be used clinically to gain access to the epidural or subarachnoid space (Taylor's approach) in patients with severe osteoarthritis and ossified ligaments. A lateral approach of the needle to the epidural and subarachnoid space may avoid both the increased calcification in the midline and the tendency of the dorsal vertebrae to impact on one another.

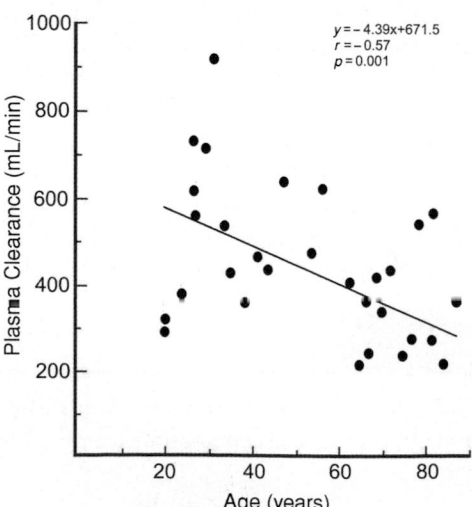

Figure 56–5. Relationship between total plasma clearance and age (Reprinted, with permission, from Veering BT, Burm AGL, Van Kleef JW, et al: Epidural anesthesia with bupivacaine: Effects of age on neural blockade and pharmacokinetics. Anesth Analg 1987;66:589).

Clinical Pearls

- Placement of the needle epidurally or intrathecally may not be easy in elderly patients; calcified interspinous ligaments, osteophytes in the intervertebral foramina, other anatomic changes, and deformities limit the access to the neuraxis.

- The largest intervertebral foramina are in the L5-S1 interspace; this anatomic characteristic can be used clinically to gain access to the epidural or subarachnoid space using a lateral approach (Taylor's approach) in patients with severe osteoarthritis and ossified ligaments.

POTENTIAL DISADVANTAGES OF REGIONAL ANESTHESIA IN THE ELDERLY

Hypotension

Hypotension is perhaps the most adverse effect of central neural blockade in the elderly. Hypotension occurs as the result of a decrease in systemic vascular resistance and central venous pressure from blockade of the preganglionic sympathetic nerve fibers with vasodilatation and redistribution of central blood volume to lower extremities and splanchnic beds.[34] Hypotension is deleterious because elderly patients have decreased physiologic reserve and an increased incidence of systemic disease. The incidence of hypotension following spinal anesthesia is 10–40%. High levels of sensory anesthesia and increasing age appear to be the two main risk factors for the development of hypotension with spinal anesthesia.[35] Decreased cardiac reserves, structural changes in the arterioles, and changes in the autonomic nervous system with increasing age may contribute to substantial hypotension in elderly patients. Marked hypotension is especially harmful to elderly patients with limited cardiac reserve. Normal aging is associated with a reduction in the baroreceptor-reflex–mediated, heart rate response to hypotensive stimuli; consequently, elderly patients may not respond with the same degree of sympathetic activity as younger patients. A given dose of epidural ropivacaine produces a higher level of analgesia in elderly than in younger patients. It is associated with a greater incidence and degree of hypotension and bradycardia[14] (Figure 56–6).

Treatment of Hypotension During Regional Anesthesia

Optimal treatment for central neural blockade—induced hypotension continues to be a matter of debate. Ideally, the treatment of hypotension should correct any alterations in systemic vascular resistance and venous pooling. Whether fluid administration or drug treatment is more physiologic remains debatable. The efficacy of intravenous fluid preloading to support arterial pressure during regional anesthesia in an aging population is questioned because volume loading does not prevent the decrease in systemic vascular resistance caused by spinal anesthesia, but, in fact, may cause a further decrease.[36] Irrespective of whether crystalloid, colloid, or no prehydration is used, hypotension is common following the administration of spinal anesthesia in normovolemic elderly patients undergoing elective procedures.[37] The combination of modest administration of a colloid during the induction phase of the block plus an α-agonist (eg, phenylephrine) appears to restore both blood pressure and cardiac output to baseline levels.[38] It should be emphasized, however, that rapid volume preloading constitutes a potential risk in older patients with limited cardiopulmonary reserve.

Continuous spinal anesthesia allows the titration of small amounts of local anesthetics to achieve the desired level of anesthesia and greater control over hemodynamic changes. The approach may be preferable in elderly patients in whom the development of hypotension is of particular concern (see Chapter 57, Regional Anesthesia in Patients with Cardiovascular Disease). The synergism between intrathecal opioids and local anesthetics may allow a reduction in the dose of local anesthetic and reduce hypotension, while still maintaining

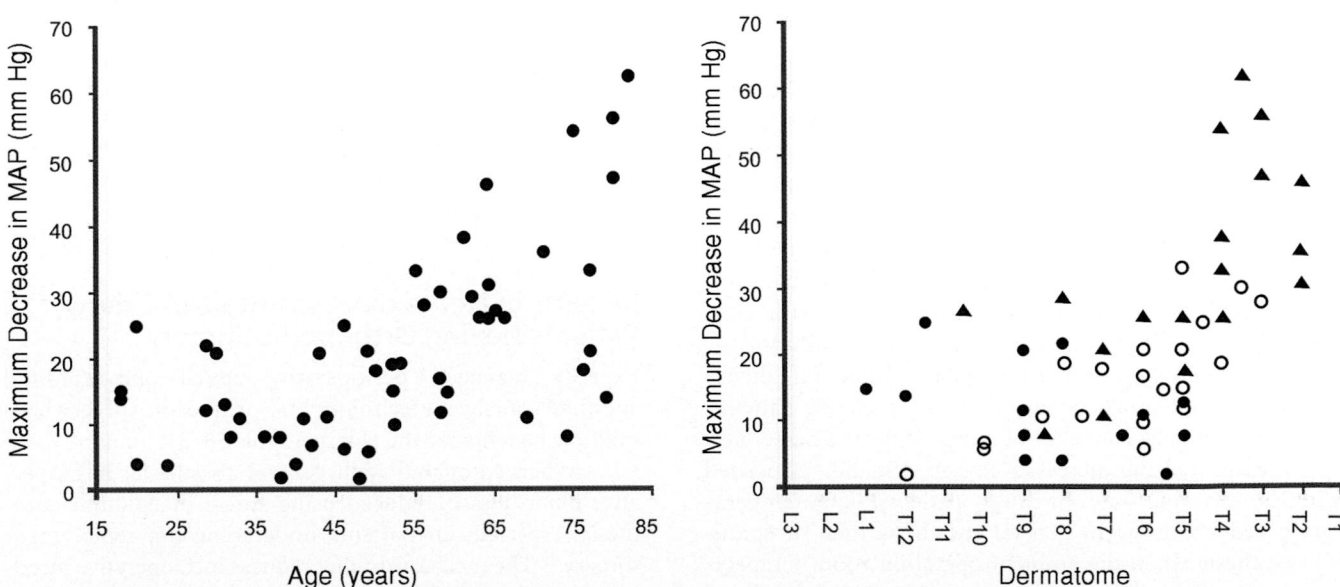

Figure 56–6. *Left:* Effects of age on the decrease of the mean arterial blood pressure (MAP; mm Hg) after the induction of epidural anesthesia. *Right:* Maximum decrease of the mean arterial blood pressure (MAP; mm Hg) during the first hour after the induction of epidural anesthesia and the highest level of analgesia (by dermatome) for the three age groups. Group 1: 19–40 years. Group 2: 41–60 years. Group 3: >61 years.

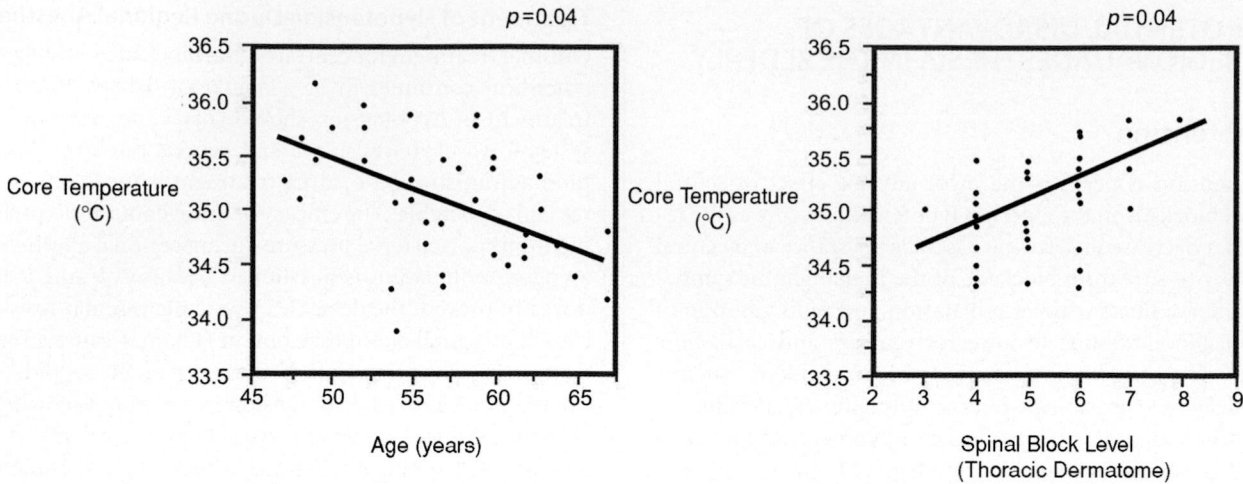

Figure 56–7. Advanced age (*left*) and high level of spinal block (*right*) pose risk of hypothermia (Reprinted, with permission, from Frank SM, El-Rahmany HK, Cattaneo CG, et al: Predictors of hypothermia during spinal anesthesia. Anesthesiology 2000;92:1330).

adequate anesthesia. Therefore, a reduced dose of hyperbaric bupivacaine (7.5 mg) in combination with sufentanil[39] or a minidose of plain bupivacaine (4 mg) in combination with fentanyl (20 mcg) can provide reliable spinal anesthesia for the repair of hip fracture in aged patients with few events of hypotension and little need for vasopressor support of blood pressure.[40]

Hypothermia

Both accidental and perioperative hypothermia (a decrease in core temperature) are common in the elderly during general, epidural, and spinal anesthesia. Because of age-related changes in temperature regulation, the elderly are prone to hypothermia during surgery. Thus, low core temperature may not trigger protective autonomic responses. Elderly patients have a lower shivering and vasoconstriction threshold than younger patients during spinal anesthesia that is proportionate to the level of spinal anesthesia[41] (Figure 56–7). In addition, higher levels of analgesia result in higher levels of peripheral sympathetic and motor nerve blockade, which prevents thermoregulatory vasoconstriction and shivering. The higher the level of blockade, the more significant the expected impairment of thermoregulatory function. Shivering is also a potentially greater problem in elderly patients, who, with a higher incidence of ischemic heart disease, may not tolerate well the increased oxygen demands associated with the shivering state. In elderly patients, body temperature is reduced more by general anesthesia than by epidural anesthesia when the ambient operation room temperature is cold. This difference between general anesthesia and epidural anesthesia is not significant when ambient operating room temperature is relatively warm.[42] The time required for postoperative rewarming to recover normal body temperature also appears to increase directly with advancing age.

Spinal Headache

The decreased incidence of headache in the elderly population is due to physiologic factors (aging, dehydration, arthritis, etc), which contribute to increased tissue density and needle resistance. These factors result in more needle bending, a more tangential puncture, and thus, a lower incidence of postspinal headache in the elderly.

ORTHOPEDIC SURGERY

Hip fractures occur often in the frail elderly who may have multiple medical conditions. The majority of these fractures occur in patients with an average age of around 80 years. Most hip fracture patients are treated surgically and require anesthesia. Anesthesia for hip fracture usually involves either a general or regional anesthetic. Spinal anesthesia is the most commonly used method for hip fracture surgery.

Benefits of Neuraxial Anesthesia in Elderly Patients Having Orthopedic Surgery

Expertly managed perioperative spinal and epidural anesthesia–analgesia techniques for orthopedic surgery have multiple benefits for the elderly (Table 56–3).

When compared with general anesthesia, intraoperative blood loss is reduced using spinal or epidural anesthesia, especially in patients undergoing hip replacement surgery.[43] The mechanism that reduces intraoperative bleeding, amounting to about 50%, is probably a reduction in the central venous pressure. Postoperative blood loss, however, does not seem to depend on the anesthetic technique used. The neuroendocrine stress response to major orthopedic surgery, illustrated by the rise in blood cortisol and glucose concentrations, can be suppressed partially or completely by

Table 56–3.

Advantages of Epidural and Spinal Anesthesia and Postoperative Analgesia in Elderly Orthopedic Patients

Fewer thromboembolic complications

Reduced intraoperative blood loss

Decreased stress responses to surgery

Preservation of pulmonary gas exchange

Improved immediate postoperative pain relief

Reduced immediate postoperative morbidity

Reduced 1-month mortality rates

spinal or epidural anesthesia.[44] The clinical benefits of these findings, however, remain uncertain.

Other benefits of central neural blockade include a lower incidence of pulmonary embolism, respiratory complications, and deep vein thrombosis. Direct favorable changes in the coagulation cascade, increased blood flow in lower extremities due to sympathectomy, and possible direct effect of local anesthetics on endothelial elements may be responsible for the reduced incidence of venous thromboembolism following regional anesthesia.[45] Continuous epidural catheter techniques provide safe and excellent postoperative analgesia in elderly patients, facilitating early postoperative mobilization for a faster convalescence.[44] Early postoperative cognitive dysfunction is particularly common in elderly orthopedic patients; there appears to be no difference in the effects of general, epidural, or spinal anesthesia in the incidence of postoperative cognitive dysfunction following total knee arthroplasty. The dysfunction may result from the cumulative stress of hospitalization, trauma, and pain.[46] A systemic review of randomized trials showed that regional anesthesia for hip fracture surgery was associated with a reduced mortality rate at 1-month as well as a reduced incidence of deep vein thrombosis in comparison with the occurrence under general anesthesia.[47] No conclusions can be drawn for longer term morbidity and mortality (2 months to 1 year).[43]

▮ SUMMARY

As the percentage of the elderly in the population increases, the number of elderly patients requiring surgery climbs. Elderly patients have an increased risk for perioperative morbidity and mortality due to the higher incidence of coexisting, age-related diseases. Age per se is not a major factor in predicting the risk of anesthesia and operation; age-related disease, rather then aging, is primarily responsible for the progressive increase in morbidity and mortality with elderly

surgical patients. Factors other than the choice of anesthesia may be crucial for long-term survival. Older patients experience slightly higher levels of sensory and motor blockade following epidural and spinal anesthesia. Elderly patients also have a somewhat greater risk for arterial hypotension due to the sympatholytic consequences of acute peripheral autonomic blockade impairment in the autonomic reflexes maintaining cardiovascular homeostasis. Safe regional anesthesia in elderly patients requires expert care and reduced doses of agents for the same effect. Regional anesthesia offers several advantages to elderly patients because it provides postoperative analgesia with minimal sedative side effects; however, intrathecal opioids can produce significant respiratory depression in elderly surgical patients. Also, epidural and spinal anesthesia may reduce the incidence of thromboembolic complications in geriatric patients, especially following orthopedic and lower extremity vascular surgery.

References

1. Kinsella K, Velkoff VA: US Census Bureau, Series P95/01-1, *An Aging World*, 2001.
2. Clerque F, Auroy Y, Pequinot F, et al: French survey of anesthesia in 1996. Anesthesiology 1999;91:1509.
3. Williams ME: Clinical implications of aging physiology. Am J Med 1984;76:1049.
4. Leung JM, Dzankic S: Relative importance of preoperative health status versus intraoperative factors in predicting postoperative adverse outcomes in geriatric surgical patients. J Am Ger Soc 2001;49:1080.
5. Bromage PR: Mechanism of action of extradural analgesia. Br J Anaesth 1975;47:199.
6. Dorfman LJ, Bosley TM: Age related changes in peripheral and central nerve conduction in man. Neurology 1979;29:38.
7. Shanta TR, Evans JA: The relationship of epidural anesthesia to neural membranes and arachnoid villi. Anesthesiology 1972;37:543.
8. May C, Kaye JA, Atack JR, et al: Cerebrospinal fluid production is reduced in healthy aging. Neurology 1990;40:500.
9. Rooke GA, Robinson BJ: Cardiovascular and autonomic nervous system aging. Probl Anesth 1997;9:482.
10. Vestal RE, Wood AJJ, Shand DG: Reduced beta-adrenoceptor sensitivity in the elderly. Clin Pharmacol Ther 1979;26:181.
11. James MA, Potter JF: Orthostatic blood pressure changes and arterial baroreflex sensitivity in elderly subjects. Age Ageing 1999;28:522.
12. Lakatta EG: Cardiovascular regulatory mechanisms in advanced age. Physiol Rev 1993;73:413.
13. Veering BT, Burm AGL, Van Kleef JW, et al: Epidural anesthesia with bupivacaine: Effects of age on neural blockade and pharmacokinetics. Anesth Analg 1987;66:589.
14. Simon MJ, Veering BT, Stienstra R, et al: The effects of age on neural blockade and hemodynamic changes after epidural anesthesia with ropivacaine. Anesth Analg 2002;94:1325.
15. Simon MJ, Veering BT, Stienstra R, et al: Effect of age on the clinical profile and systemic absorption and disposition of levobupivacaine after epidural administration. Br J Anaesth 2004;93:512.
16. Bromage PR: *Epidural Analgesia*. WB Saunders, 1978, pp 40–42.
17. Hirabayashi Y, Shimizu R, Matsuda J, et al: Effect of extradural compliance and resistance on spread of extradural analgesia. Br J Anaesth 1990;65:508.
18. Guinard JP, Mulroy MF, Carpenter RL: Aging reduces the reliability of epidural epinephrine test doses. Reg Anesth 1995;20:193.
19. Sakura S, Saito Y, Kosaka Y: The effects of epidural anesthesia on ventilatory response to hypercapnia and hypoxia in elderly patients. Anesth Analg 1996;82:306.

20. Ready LB, Chadwick HS, Ross B, et al: Age predicts effective morphine dose after abdominal hysterectomy. Anesth Analg 1987;66:1215.

21. Pitkänen M, Haapaniemi L, Tuominen M, et al: Influence of age on spinal anaesthesia with isobaric 0.5% bupivacaine. Br J Anaesth 1984;56:279.

22. Veering BT, Burm AGL, Van Kleef JW, et al: Spinal anesthesia with glucose-free bupivacaine: Effects of age on neural blockade and pharmacokinetics. Anesth Analg 1987;66:965.

23. Veering BT, Burm AGL, Spierdijk J: Spinal anaesthesia with hyperbaric bupivacaine: Effects of age on neural blockade and pharmacokinetics. Br J Anaesth 1988;60:187.

24. Racle JP, Benkhadra A, Poy JY, et al: Spinal analgesia with hyperbaric bupivacaine: Influence of age. Br J Anaesth 1986;60:508.

25. Fernandez-Galinski D, Rué M, Moral V, et al: Spinal anaesthesia with bupivacaine and fentanyl in geriatric patients. Anesth Analg 1996;83:537.

26. Snoeck MM, Vree TB, Gielen MJ, et al: Steady state bupivacaine plasma concentrations and safety of a femoral '3-in-1' nerve block with bupivacaine in patients over 80 years of age. Int J Clin Pharmacol Ther 2003;41:107.

27. Paqueron X, Boccara G, Bendahou M, et al: Brachial plexus nerve block exhibits prolonged duration in the elderly. Anesthesiology 2002;97:1245.

28. Tucker GT: Pharmacokinetics of local anaesthetics. Br J Anaesth 1986;58:717.

29. Veering BT: Pharmacological aspects of local anesthics in the elderly. Acta Anaesth Belg 1998;49:117.

30. Burm AGL, Van Kleef JW, Vermeulen NPE, et al: Pharmacokinetics of lidocaine and bupivacaine following subarachnoid administration in surgical patients: Simultaneous investigation of absorption and disposition kinetics using stable isotopes. Anesthesiology 1988;69:584.

31. Veering BT, Burm AGL, Vletter AA, et al: The effect of age on the systemic absorption and systemic disposition of bupivacaine after epidural administration. Clin Pharmacokinet 1992;22:75.

32. Veering BT, Burm AGL, Vletter AA, et al: The effect of age on systemic absorption and systemic disposition of bupivacaine after subarachnoid administration. Anesthesiology 1991;74:250.

33. Wynne HA, Cope LH, Mutch E, et al: The effect of age upon liver volume and apparent liver blood flow in healthy man. Hepatology 1989;9:297.

34. Veering BT, Cousins MJ: Cardiovascular and pulmonary effects of epidural anesthesia. Anaesth Intensive Care 2000;28:620.

35. Carpenter RL, Caplan RA, Brown DL, et al: Incidence and risk factors for side effects of spinal anesthesia. Anesthesiology 1992;76:906.

36. Rooke GA: Cardiovascular aging and anesthetic implications. J Cardiothorac Vasc Anesth 2003;17:512.

37. Buggy D, Higgins P, Moran C, et al: Prevention of spinal anesthesia-induced hypotension in the elderly: Comparison between preanesthetic administration of crystalloids, colloids and no prehydration. Anesth Analg 1997;84:106.

38. Critchley LAH: Hypotension, subarachnoid block and the elderly patient. Anaesthesia 1996;51:1139.

39. Olofsen C, Nygards EB, Bjersten AB, et al: Low-dose bupivacaine with sufentanil prevents hypotension after spinal anaesthesia for hip repair in elderly patients. Acta Anaesthsiol Scand 2004;48:1240.

40. Ben-David B, Frankel R, Arzumonov T, et al: Minidose bupivacaine-fentanyl spinal anesthesia for surgical repair of hip fracture in the aged. Anesthesiology 2000;92:6.

41. Frank SM, El-Rahmany HK, Cattaneo CG, et al: Predictors of hypothermia during spinal anesthesia. Anesthesiology 2000;92:1330.

42. Frank SM, Beattie C, Christopherson R, et al: Epidural versus general anesthesia, ambient operating room temperature, and patient age as predictors of inadvertent hypothermia. Anesthesiology 1992;77:252.

43. Parker MJ, Handoll HHG, Griffiths R: Anaesthesia for hip fracture surgery in adults. Cochrane Database Syst Rev 2004;18:CD000521.

44. Kehlet H, Holte K: Effect of postoperative analgesia on surgical outcome. Br J Anaesth 2001;87:62.

45. Donadoni R, Baele G, Devulder J, et al: Coagulation and fibrinolytic parameters in patients undergoing total hip replacement: Influence of anaesthesia technique. Acta Anaesthesiol Scand 1989;33:588.

46. Williams-Russo P, Urquhart RN, Sharrock NE, et al: Postoperative delirium: Predictors and prognosis in elderly orthopedic patients. J Am Geriatr Soc 1992;40:759.

47. Urwin SC, Parker MJ, Griffiths R: General versus regional anaesthesia for hip fracture surgery: a meta-analysis of randomized trials. Br J Anaesth 2000;84:450.

57

Regional Anesthesia & Cardiovascular Disease

Navin A. Mallavaram, MD • Daniel M. Thys, MD

INTRODUCTION

The decision to use regional anesthesia can be a complex medical choice. Preexisting medical conditions, type of surgery, anesthetic risks, and patient characteristics all may have a profound impact on anesthetic choice and perioperative management. In patients with cardiovascular disease, regional anesthesia techniques (either alone or in conjunction with general anesthesia) can offer the potential perioperative benefits of stress response attenuation, cardiac sympathectomy, earlier extubation, shorter hospital stay, and intense postoperative analgesia.

Neuraxial anesthesia has been shown to be useful in treating patients with coronary artery disease. This includes treatment of anginal symptoms, primary (or part of a combined) anesthetic for the surgical procedure, and acute postoperative pain management. Its use in the high-risk patient during noncardiac surgery can offer reduced blood loss and need for transfusion and a decreased incidence of thromboembolic events.

Regional anesthetic options are not limited to neuraxial techniques when dealing with patients with cardiovascular disease. Paravertebral block has also been used as an adjunct to general anesthesia in the management of patients undergoing cardiac surgery. In addition, intercostal nerve blockade and parasternal block can be used for postoperative pain relief in patients after cardiac surgery. Cervical plexus block can be used in the anesthetic management of patients undergoing carotid endarterectomy. Lower extremity blocks, such as combined sciatic–femoral nerve block can also be used in high-risk patients in whom even modest alterations in hemodynamics would not be tolerated.

Local anesthetics alone or in combination with narcotics are used for regional anesthesia in patients with cardiovascular disease. Ropivacaine is a commonly used local anesthetic during neuraxial anesthesia for cardiac surgery. Although its pharmacologic properties, including onset of action and duration of action, are essentially the same as those of bupivacaine, ropivacaine possesses less cardiotoxic properties, produces less central nervous system depression, and is associated with less motor blockade. Ropivacaine is often combined with sufentanil when used during epidural administration for cardiac surgery. Intrathecal narcotics in combination with general anesthesia can provide intraoperative and postoperative analgesia. The most common undesirable effects of intrathecal opioids are respiratory depression, nausea and vomiting, pruritus, and urinary retention. However, advances in narcotic formulations may allow for sustained-release delivery and target-specific affinity, which may reduce the potential of common narcotic side effects. Standard local anesthetic preparations are used in performing upper and lower extremity blocks in patients with cardiovascular disease.

The most severe complication from neuraxial anesthesia is epidural hematoma formation. The incidence of hematoma formation ranges from 1:150,000 after epidural instrumentation to 1:220,000 for intrathecal instrumentation. Risk of hematoma formation after either technique is increased if performed before systemic heparinization. Currently, only a minority of practicing anesthesiologists use neuraxial blockade in the management of patients undergoing cardiac surgery. Patients presenting for major noncardiac surgery often receive anticoagulation to prevent venous thrombosis and pulmonary embolism. It appears that anesthesiologists more frequently perform neuraxial blockade on these patients after weighing the risk of hematoma formation against the benefits.

THORACIC EPIDURAL ANESTHESIA

Physiologic Effects on the Cardiovascular System

Thoracic epidural anesthesia (TEA) blocks the cardiac afferent and efferent sympathetic fibers with loss of chronotropic and inotropic drive to the myocardium.[1] The level of sympathetic blockade that follows a TEA depends in part on the degree of sympathetic tone before the block. This may explain why different studies report different effects of TEA on the cardiovascular system. Goertz et al.[2] used transesophageal echocardiography to assess the effects of TEA on cardiac function in healthy volunteers. TEA was not shown to produce significant changes in systolic or diastolic arterial pressures, heart rate, left ventricular end-systolic and end-diastolic cross-sectional areas and left ventricular wall stress as measured under general anesthesia. However, left ventricular maximum elastance, as a measure of left ventricular contractility, was significantly reduced. This observation led the investigators to conclude that TEA severely alters left ventricular contractility even in healthy subjects without preexisting cardiac disease. In another study of healthy subjects, left ventricular ejection and diastolic filling performance were unchanged, but a decrease in cardiac output and fractional area shortening were observed[3] (Table 57–1).

Ottesen[4] reported that TEA does not affect oxygen consumption (Vo_2) during exercise. However, even at moderate workloads, systemic arterial blood pressures were significantly lower with TEA than during control exercise in healthy subjects. No other changes in systemic or pulmonary circulatory parameters were observed. In another exercise study, Wattwil et al.[5] reported that after administration of TEA, heart rate, systolic blood pressure, stroke volume, and cardiac output decreased. They also injected local anesthetic (0.5% bupivacaine) intramuscularly and observed similar cardiovascular effects, leading them to the conclusion that the changes may be due in part to systemic effects.

Several studies have documented the effects of TEA on cardiovascular function in patients with heart disease. In a small study of 10 patients scheduled for thoracotomy, a TEA with a mean analgesic level of C7 to T5 had only minor effects on the cardiovascular system.[6] In patients with severe coronary artery disease and unstable angina pectoris, Blomberg et al.[7] observed that TEA relieved chest pain. It also significantly decreased heart rate, systolic arterial, and pulmonary arterial and pulmonary capillary wedge pressures without any significant changes in coronary perfusion pressure, cardiac output, stroke volume, and systemic or pulmonary vascular resistances.

Intraoperatively, Reinhart et al.[8] observed lower cardiac index and oxygen delivery (Qo_2) in patients receiving TEA and general anesthesia than in those receiving general anesthesia alone; Vo_2 were similar. They also reported that the oxygen supply-demand ratio (Qo_2/Vo_2) was less in the TEA group throughout the perioperative period and about 30% below baseline values during early recovery. The authors attributed the reduced adaptation of cardiac output to tissue oxygen needs during TEA to negative inotropic and chronotropic effects of sympathetic blockade. In patients on chronic β-adrenergic blocking medication, TEA has been reported to induce a moderate decrease in mean arterial pressure and coronary perfusion pressure, but without producing clinically significant cardiovascular effects.[9]

Table 57–1.				

Acoustic Quantification-Derived Echocardiographic Variables During Thoracic Epidural Anesthesia

	High Thoracic Epidural		Low Thoracic Epidural	
	Before Block	**After Block**	**Before Block**	**After Block**
EDA(cm^2)	9.4 ± 1.4	10.3 ± 1.1^a	8.8 ± 1.1	8.8 ± 0.9
ESA (cm^2)	4.8 ± 1.3	6.0 ± 1.1^b	4.8 ± 1.2	4.8 ± 0.9
FAC (%)	50 ± 11	37 ± 11^a	51 ± 9	51 ± 9
PFR (EDA/sec)	3.7 ± 09	3.3 ± 1.2	3.7 ± 1.2	3.9 ± 1.1
PER (EDA/sec)	3.4 ± 1.3	2.9 ± 0.8	3.8 ± 1.5	4.0 ± 1.2
D1/D2	2.3 ± 1.0	2.0 ± 0.8	1.8 ± 0.5	1.6 ± 0.5

^{a} $p < 0.01$ *vs before block.*
^{b} $P < 0.05.$
EDA, end-diastolic area; ESA, end-systolic area; FAC, fractional area change; PFR, peak filling rate; PER, peak ejection rate; D1/D2, ratio of peak dA/dt (change in area of left ventrical versus time) in the rapid filling phase (D1) to the peak dA/dt in the atrial contraction phase (D2).
Reproduced, with permission, from Niimi Y, Ichinose F, Saegusa H, et al: Echocardiographic evaluation of global left ventricular function during high thoracic epidural anesthesia. J Clin Anesth 1997;9(2):118–124.

Berendes et al.[10] reported that in patients undergoing coronary artery bypass grafting (CABG) with combined TEA and general anesthesia, regional left ventricular function was significantly improved, and cardiac troponin I concentrations were reduced when compared with patients receiving general anesthesia alone (Figure 57–1). In addition, TEA reduced the concentrations of atrial and brain natriuretic peptides. The authors concluded that cardiac sympathectomy by TEA improves regional left ventricular function and reduces postoperative ischemia after CABG. In another study of CABG patients, TEA was associated with better hemodynamic stability before and after cardiopulmonary bypass when compared with general anesthesia.[11] In addition, TEA may provide improvement in pulmonary function, possibly because of more profound postoperative analgesia after cardiac surgery.[12]

Cardiac function was also evaluated in patients with two- or three-vessel coronary artery disease who were treated with β-adrenergic blocking agents. Systolic and diastolic arterial pressures, heart rate, and global and regional ejection fractions using equilibrium radionuclide angiography were measured at rest and during maximal exercise before and after TEA. During TEA exercise, systolic arterial pressure, diastolic arterial pressure, and the rate–pressure product, but not heart rate, were significantly lower when compared with control exercise. The global and anterolateral ejection fractions were significantly higher, and the regional wall motion score was significantly lower during TEA exercise than during control exercise. ST-segment depression was significantly lower during TEA exercise.[13] Schmidt et al.[14] noted that in patients with coronary artery disease, TEA induced a significant improve-

ment in left ventricular diastolic function, whereas indices of systolic function did not change (Figures 57–2 through 57–4).

Patients with cardiac disease are prone to hemodynamic changes during laryngoscopy and intubation, thus placing them at risk for ischemic events. TEA has been associated with stable hemodynamics and preservation of baroreflex sensitivity, suggesting withdrawal of vagal activity. Licker et al.[15] reported that patients who received TEA in addition to general anesthesia had smaller increases in mean arterial pressure and heart rate during laryngoscopy and tracheal intubation than those who received general anesthesia only; this would suggest that TEA affords hemodynamic protection during these maneuvers.

Clinical Pearls

- TEA can significantly decrease heart rate and systolic arterial, pulmonary arterial, and pulmonary capillary wedge pressures without any significant changes in coronary perfusion pressure, cardiac output, stroke volume, and systemic or pulmonary vascular resistances in patients with coronary artery disease.

- In patients with unstable angina, TEA can decrease the frequency of anginal attacks and nitroglycerin intake, and increase self-rated quality of life.

- As an anesthetic for CABG, TEA offers thoracic and cardiac sympathectomy, attenuation of the stress response, analgesia for surgery, and postoperative analgesia, which may improve outcome after CABG surgery.

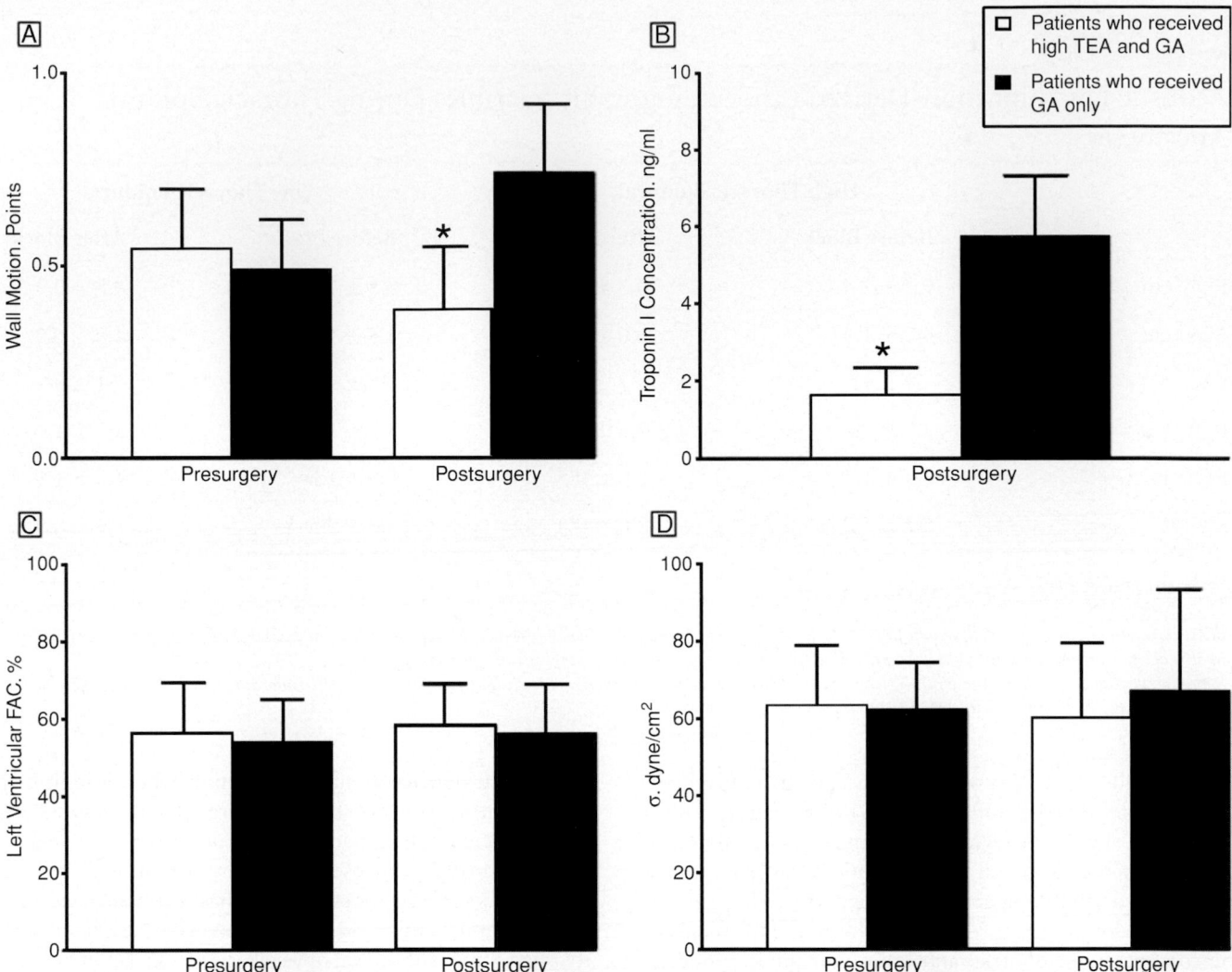

Figure 57–1. Patients' global and regional left ventricular function and afterload. **A:** Preoperative and postoperative values of global left ventricular wall motion index. **C:** Left ventricular fractional area change (FAC). **D:** Left ventricular end-systolic meridional wall stress(es) as well as postoperative concentrations of cardiac troponin I in patients who received general anesthesia (GA) only or GA and high thoracic epidural anesthesia (TEA) (**B**). Values are given as mean (SD). Asterisks indicate *P* <.05. (Reproduced, with permission, from Berendes E, Schmidt C, Van Aken H, et al: Arch Surg 2003;138[12]:1283–1290.)

■ More rapid tracheal extubation, decreased pulmonary complications and cardiac arrhythmias, and reduced pain scores are other benefits of TEA.

■ The use of a set of standard safety measures, such as preoperative testing of activated partial thromboplastin time (aPTT), platelet count, and prothrombin time, and the cessation of antiplatelet drugs before surgery may avert the occurrence of symptomatic epidural hematomas.

■ For major vascular surgery, TEA can provide more hemodynamic stability and better pain control than general anesthesia or monitored anesthesia care with local anesthesia.

Management of Cardiac Disease

TEA has been used in the management of cardiac disease (Figure 57–5). Cardiac sympathetic blockade by TEA dilates stenotic coronary arteries and has been used to control pain in patients with unstable angina.[16] The mechanism by which TEA reduces angina during long-term treatment is unclear. It has been reported that the improvement in symptoms probably results partly from an anesthetic effect and does not appear to be related to a change in myocardial blood flow or a reduction in stress-induced ischemia. In addition, new myocardial infarctions are not masked or missed in patients receiving TEA for symptomatic treatment of angina.[17] The effects of long-term, home self-treatment with TEA on angina, quality of life, and safety were studied by Richter et al.[18] Thirty-seven

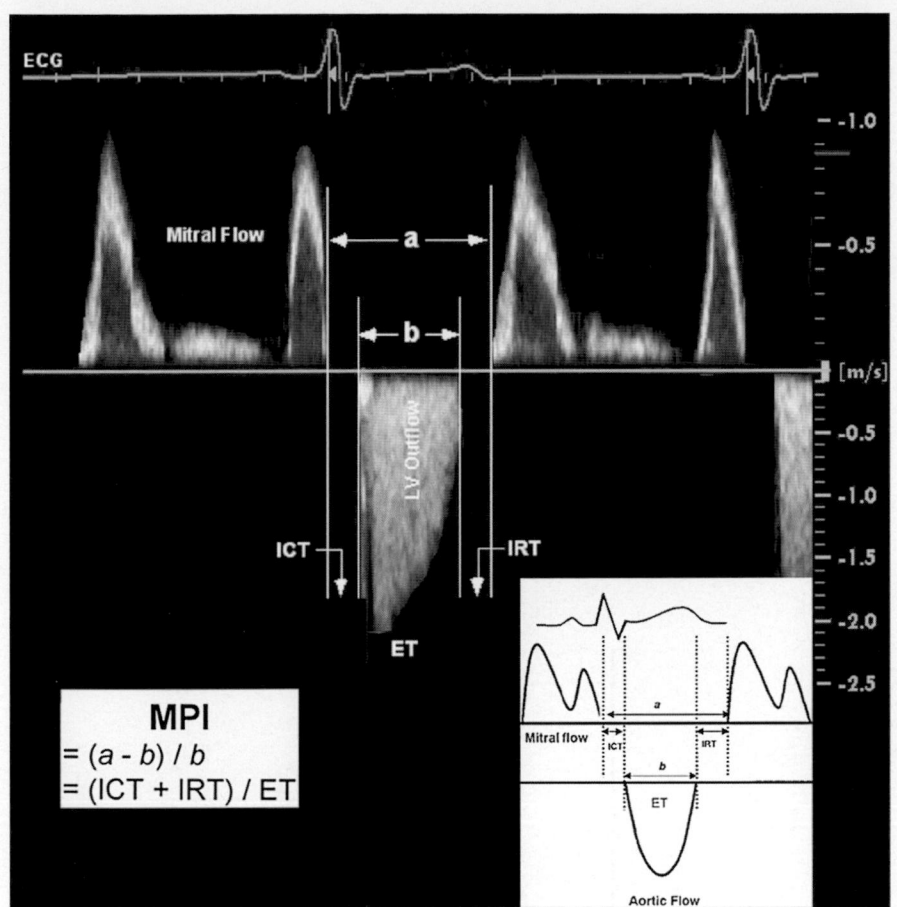

Figure 57–2. Estimation of the myocardial performance index (MPI; Tei index). MPI is calculated from two time intervals as a–b/b. Interval a: from cessation to next onset of mitral flow. Interval b: from onset to cessation of aortic flow. Time intervals a and b are indicated in milliseconds. A typical example of measuring the MPI using Doppler ECG registration of mitral and aortic flow velocity profiles is demonstrated. For illustrative purposes, the original Doppler tracings of mitral inflow and left ventricular (LV) outflow are plotted together. ET, ejection time of LV outflow; ICT, isovolumic contraction time; IRT, isovolumic relaxation time. (Reproduced, with permission, from Schmidt C, Hinder F, Van Aken H, et al: The effect of high thoracic epidural anesthesia on systolic and diastolic left ventricular function in patients with coronary artery disease. Anesth Analg 2005;100[6]:1561–1569.)

patients with refractory angina began treatment with TEA, using a subcutaneously tunneled epidural catheter and a bupivacaine solution. All but one of the patients improved symptomatically. The improvement was maintained throughout the treatment period (4 days to 3 years). The authors reported that the frequency of anginal attacks and nitroglycerin intake decreased, whereas the overall self-rated quality of life assessed by visual analog scale (VAS) increased.

Studies have looked at the number of anginal attacks and the severity of myocardial ischemia assessed by 48-hour ambulatory Holter monitoring in patients with severe, refractory unstable angina receiving TEA or standard antianginal therapy. Olausson et al.[19] reported that the incidence of myocardial ischemia was lower in the TEA group (22% versus 61%; $P < .05$). The number of ischemic episodes per patient was 1.0 ± 0.6 in the TEA group and 3.6 ± 0.9 in the control group ($P < .05$), and the episode duration per patient was 4.1 ± 2.5 minutes and 19.7 ± 6.2 minutes in the TEA and the control groups, respectively ($P < .05$).

Cardiac Surgery

Coronary Artery Bypass Grafting

As an anesthetic for CABG, TEA offers thoracic and cardiac sympathectomy, attenuation of the stress response, analgesia for surgery, and postoperative analgesia, which may improve outcome after CABG. One review suggests that for patients undergoing CABG surgery, the risk:benefit ratio is in favor of epidural and spinal anesthesia, provided no specific contraindications exist and the guidelines for the use of regional techniques in cardiac surgery are followed.[20] Patients managed with regional anesthetic techniques seem to benefit from superior postoperative analgesia, shorter postoperative ventilation, reduced incidence of supraventricular arrhythmias, and lower rates of perioperative myocardial infarction. The results of this particular analysis suggest that for each episode of neurologic complication that might occur, 20 myocardial infarctions and 76 episodes of atrial fibrillation would be prevented. Thus, regional anesthesia and analgesia would be considered an effective strategy that improves perioperative morbidity.

As an adjunct to general anesthesia, TEA can be useful in off-pump CABG. Salvi et al.[21] reported on 106 patients receiving TEA combined with sevoflurane general anesthesia. The mean time to extubation was 4.6 ± 2.9 hours. VAS scores for pain during the first 24-hour period were less than 2 in all patients. The average intensive care unit (ICU) stay was 1.5 ± 0.8 days. Incidences of perioperative myocardial infarction, myocardial ischemia, and atrial fibrillation were 2.8%, 7.5%, and 10.6%, respectively. Two patients died—one from multiorgan failure and the other from myocardial infarction. Heart rate, mean arterial pressure, cardiac index, and systemic vascular resistance were not affected by TEA alone. Mean arterial pressure and cardiac index decreased ($P < .05$)

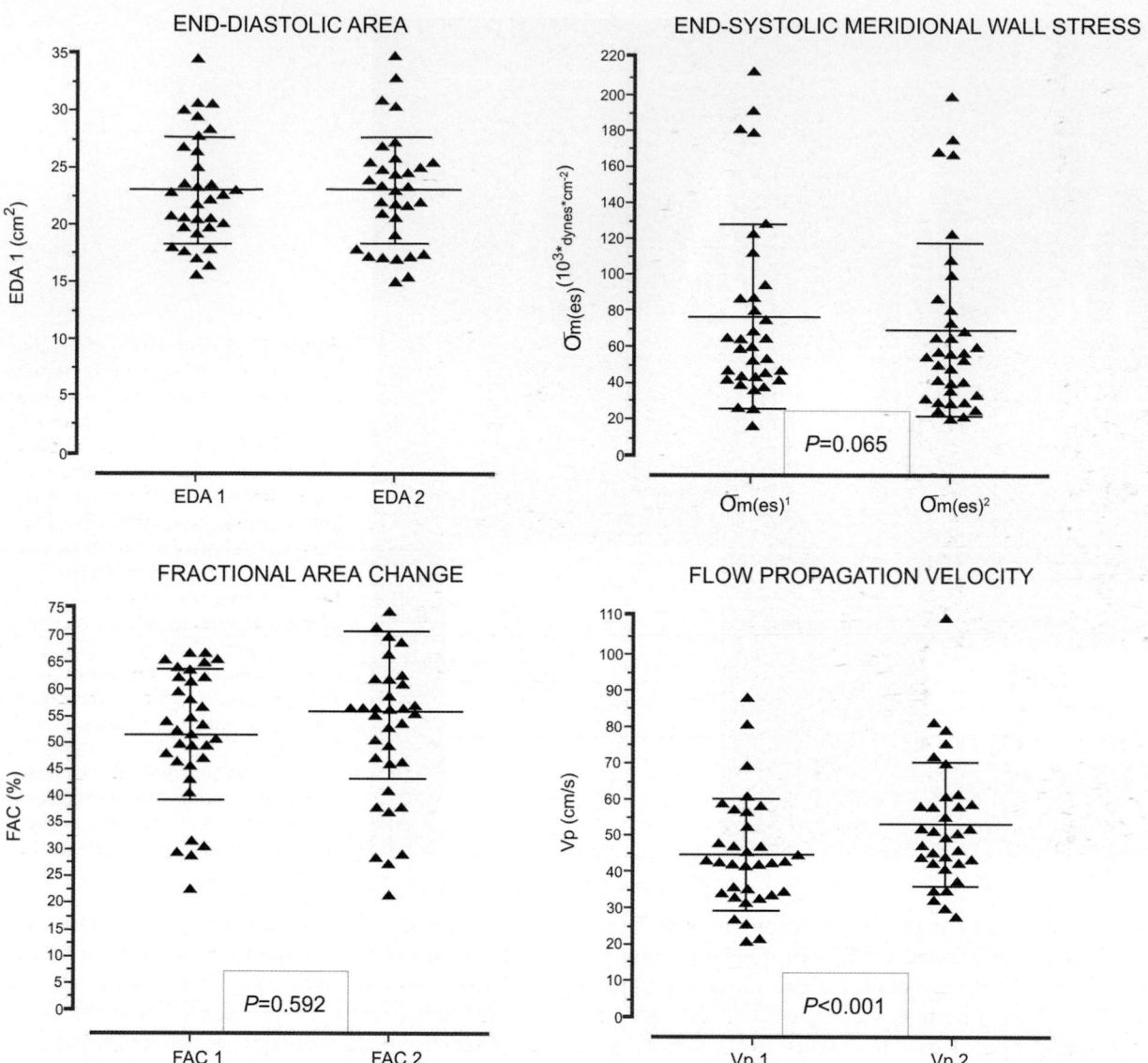

Figure 57–3. Estimates of left ventricular preload (EDA; end-diastolic cross-sectional area [cm^2]), afterload ($\sigma_{m(es)}$; end-systolic meridional wall stress [10^3/dynes/cm^2)] global systolic function (fractional area change [FAC] [%]), and global diastolic function (flow propagation velocity [V$_p$] [cm/s]). Data are represented as scatterplots. Mean values are superimposed as horizontal lines and SD as vertical lines. The *P* values denote comparisons before (1) and after (2) high thoracic epidural anesthesia (paired *t* test). (Reproduced, with permission, from Schmidt C, Hinder F, Van Aken H, et al: The effect of high thoracic epidural anesthesia on systolic and diastolic left ventricular function in patients with coronary artery disease. Anesth Analg 2005;100[6]:1561–1569.)

when general anesthesia was induced and remained stable thereafter. Neither heart rate nor systemic vascular resistance changed from baseline during the operation. The authors concluded that thoracic epidural block as an adjunct to general anesthesia is a feasible technique in off-pump CABG. It induces intense postoperative analgesia and does not compromise central hemodynamics.

Kessler et al.[22] compared TEA alone (ropivacaine plus sufentanil, n = 30), TEA combined with general anesthesia (n = 30), and general anesthesia alone in patients scheduled for off-pump CABG surgery. The general anesthetic consisted of propofol, remifentanil, and cisatracurium. Intraoperative

heart rate decreased significantly with TEA alone or in combination with general anesthesia. None of the patients with TEA alone was admitted to the ICU; all were monitored in the intermediate care unit for an average of 6 hours postoperatively and were allowed to eat and drink as desired on admission. Postoperative pain scores were lower in both groups with TEA. There were no differences among groups in overall patient satisfaction. The authors concluded that general anesthesia + TEA appeared to be the most comprehensive anesthetic, allowing for revascularization of any coronary artery and providing good hemodynamic stability and reliable postoperative pain relief.

$$MPI = \frac{ICT + IRT}{ET}$$

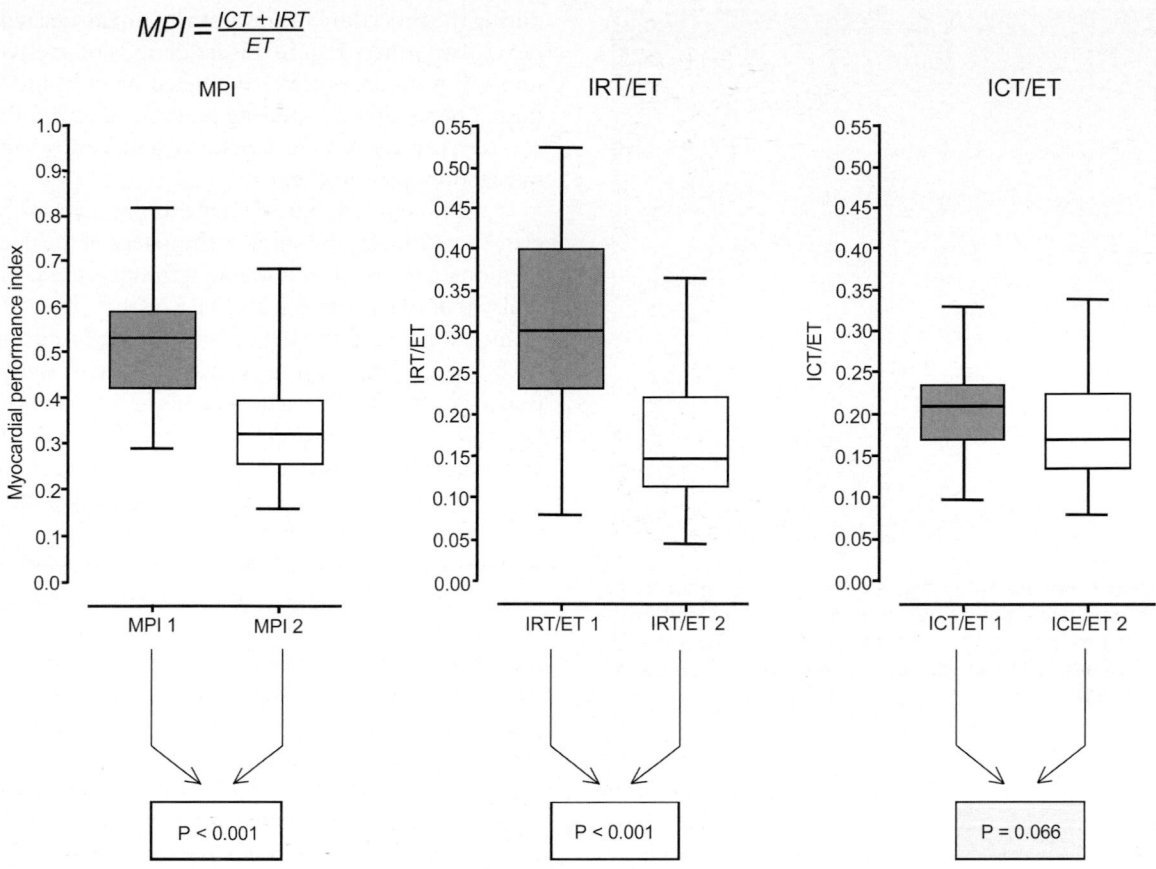

Figure 57–4. Comparison of the myocardial performance index (MPI), the ratio of isovolumic relaxation time versus ejection time (IRT/ET), and the ratio of isovolumic contraction time versus ejection time (ICT/ET) before (1) and after (2) high thoracic epidural anesthesia (HTEA). The boxes extend from the 25th to the 75th percentile. The error bars extend down to the smallest value and up to the largest. The lines at the middle of the boxes are the medians. MPI and IRT/ET, but not ICT/ET, changed significantly after HTEA (paired *t* test). (Reproduced, with permission, from Schmidt C, Hinder F, Van Aken H, et al: The effect of high thoracic epidural anesthesia on systolic and diastolic left ventricular function in patients with coronary artery disease. Anesth Analg 2005;100[6]:1561–1569.)

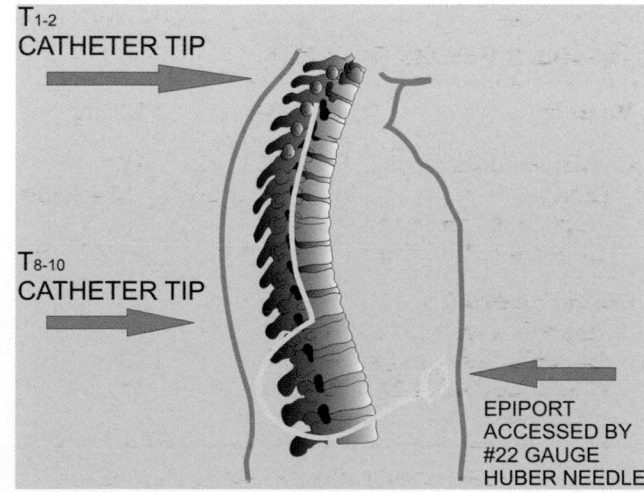

Figure 57–5. The Epiport epidural catheter with subcutaneous access port at T1. (Reproduced, with permission, from Gramling-Babb PM, Zile MR, Reeves ST: Preliminary report on high thoracic epidural analgesia: Relationship between its therapeutic effects and myocardial blood flow as assessed by stress thallium distribution. J Cardiothorac Vasc Anesth 2000;14[6]:657–661.)

Stritesky et al.[23] reported on 129 patients undergoing cardiac surgery awake with spontaneous ventilation using TEA for anesthesia. Ninety patients underwent on-pump surgery and 39 underwent off-pump surgery. A thoracic epidural block was placed 1 hour before skin incision at the T2-T4 level. Forty-two cases had aortic valve replacement, 32 patients underwent on-pump CABG, 12 had off-pump CABG, 12 had mitral valve replacement, 27 underwent sternal wound reexploration, and 4 had combined procedures. There were 10 conversions to general anesthesia and no deaths. Mean duration of stay in the ICU was 7.2 hours; in-hospital stay 5.1 days. Low cardiac output syndrome, stroke, renal insufficiency, and pulmonary dysfunction were not observed in patients who underwent TEA. Less postoperative pain was also demonstrated.

The authors felt that TEA provided rapid recovery and early outpatient care of patients after cardiac surgery and that TEA would be beneficial for patients with preoperative pulmonary dysfunction.

Several other studies have shown TEA to be effective for CABG surgery in the awake patient[24–26] (Figure 57–6).

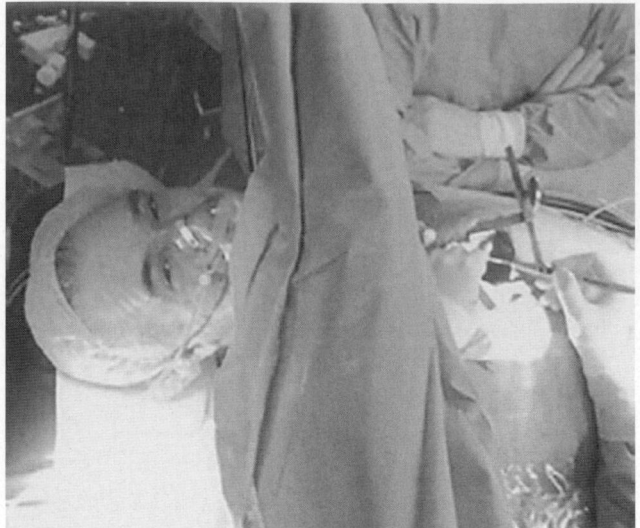

Figure 57–6. Coronary artery bypass grafting through a lower ministernotomy while the patient is awake. (Reproduced, with permission, from Aybek T, Kessler P, Dogan S, et al: Awake coronary artery bypass grafting: Utopia or reality? Ann Thorac Surg 2003;75[4]:1165–1170.)

Kessler et al.[27] reported on the feasibility and complications of TEA as the sole anesthetic in 20 patients undergoing beating-heart arterial revascularization. Minimally invasive direct coronary CABG (MIDCAB) via partial lower sternotomy was used in 10 patients with single-vessel disease, whereas complete median sternotomy with off-pump coronary artery bypass grafting (OPCAB) was chosen for 10 patients with multivessel disease. An epidural catheter was inserted at the T1-2 or T2-3 level. An epidural infusion of ropivacaine 0.5% and sufentanil 1.66 mcg/mL was started to establish anesthetic levels at C5-6 for OPCAB and at T1-2 for MIDCAB. Nine OPCAB and eight MIDCAB procedures were completed while the patients were awake and spontaneously breathing during the entire procedure. Three patients required intraoperative conversion to GA because of surgical pneumothorax (OPCAB), insufficient anesthesia, or phrenic nerve palsy (both MIDCAB).

In both groups, the heart rate decreased significantly ($P < .05$) by 10–15% during the procedure. Compared with baseline, mean arterial blood pressure was decreased significantly only during coronary anastomosis. $Paco_2$ increased from 42 ± 2 mm Hg to 46 ± 7 mm Hg ($P < .05$) throughout the perioperative course during OPCAB, whereas it remained almost unaltered during MIDCAB procedures. All patients rated TEA as "good" or "excellent" and reported a high degree of satisfaction with the procedure.

Anderson et al.[28] found similar results when studying the use of TEA for awake cardiac surgery. He reported on a total of 10 operations including 7 MIDCAB, 2 transmyocardial revascularizations (TMR) and 1 MIDCAB/TMR hybrid. The mean preoperative forced expiratory volume for 1 second (FEV_1) was 1.9 liters. Significant intraoperative hypoxia or hypercarbia was not seen. One patient required intubation during the procedure for restlessness not associated with hypoxia. Two others required brief periods of assisted ventilation. All procedures were completed without incident. The mean operating time and length of stay were 70 minutes and 4.7 days, respectively. Postoperative pain control and patient satisfaction were excellent.

Although ischemic damage to the myocardium is inevitable during CABG surgery, the extent of the damage may be influenced by the anesthetic technique used. Barrington et al.[29] reported on the effect of TEA on the release of troponin I, time to tracheal extubation, and analgesia during elective CABG surgery. One hundred twenty patients were randomized to general anesthesia or general anesthesia plus TEA. The general anesthesia group received fentanyl (7–15 mcg/kg) and a morphine infusion. The TEA group received fentanyl (5–7 mcg/kg) and an epidural infusion of ropivacaine 0.2% and fentanyl 2 mcg/mL until postoperative day 3. Researchers found no differences in troponin I levels between the study groups. The time to tracheal extubation in the TEA group was 15 minutes (range 10–20) compared with 430 minutes (range 284–590) in the general anesthesia group ($P < .0001$). Analgesia was improved in the TEA group compared with the general anesthesia group. Mean arterial blood pressure and systemic vascular resistance in the ICU were lower in the TEA group. They concluded that TEA for CABG had no effect on troponin release but improved postoperative analgesia and was associated with a reduced time to extubation (Table 57–2; Figure 57–7). Kendall et al.[30] conducted a prospective, randomized study to determine the baseline values of troponin T release after off-pump CABG in 30 patients randomly allocated to receive propofol, isoflurane, or isoflurane plus TEA. All other treatments were standardized. They found

Table 57–2.

Troponin Results (n = 60)

Variable	GA	HTEA
Continuous data, median (IQR)	17.2 (10.7–26.4)	17.0 (10.4–27.9)
Troponin I 12 h (mcg/L)	9.1	9.1
Troponin I 24 h (mcg/L)	(4.9–25.9)	(6.0–21.0)
Categorical data (n)		
Troponin I 12 > 15 (mcg/L)	32	35
Troponin I 12 > 15 (mcg/L)	19	20
Q wave/troponin I 24 > 15 (mcg/L)	2	1

GA, general anesthesia; HTEA, high thoracic epidural anesthesia; IQR, interquartile range; troponin I 12 h and 24 h, samples are taken 12 and 24 hours after release of aortic cross-clamp; Q wave, new persistent Q wave on day 5.

Reproduced, with permission, from Barrington MJ, Kluger R, Watson R, et al: Epidural anesthesia for coronary artery bypass surgery compared with general anesthesia alone does not reduce biochemical markers of myocardial damage. Anesth Analg 2005;100(4):921–928.

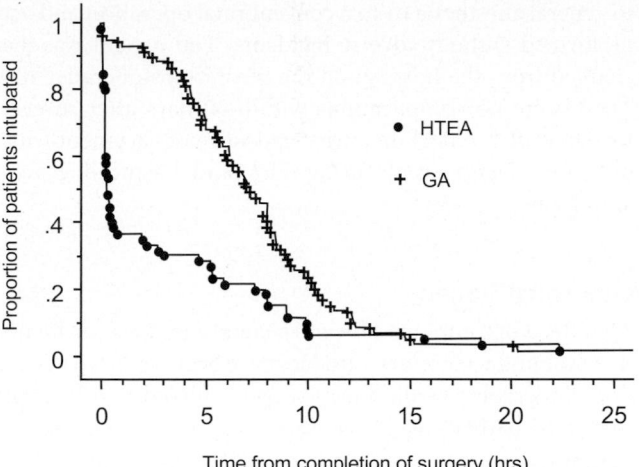

Figure 57–7. Kaplan-Meier survival plot for time to extubation. ● = high thoracic epidural anesthesia (HTEA) group; + = general anesthesia (GA) group ($P < .0001$). (Reproduced, with permission, from Barrington MJ, Kluger R, Watson R, et al: Epidural anesthesia for coronary artery bypass surgery compared with general anesthesia alone does not reduce biochemical markers of myocardial damage. Anesth Analg 2005;100[4]:921–928.)

that mean troponin T levels at 24 hours were not significantly different between the groups ($P = .41$).

Loick et al.[31] investigated the effects of general anesthesia with TEA or with intravenous clonidine on the stress response and incidence of myocardial ischemia in patients undergoing CABG surgery. Seventy patients scheduled for elective CABG surgery received general anesthesia with sufentanil and propofol. In 25 patients, TEA was induced before general anesthesia and continued during the entire study period. Another 24 patients received intravenous clonidine as a bolus of 4 mcg/kg before the induction of general anesthesia. Clonidine was then infused at a rate of 1 mcg/kg/h during surgery and at 0.2–0.5 mcg/kg/h postoperatively. The control group consisted of 21 patients who underwent general anesthesia as performed routinely. Hemodynamics, plasma epinephrine and norepinephrine, cortisol, troponin T, and other cardiac enzymes were measured pre- and postoperatively. Both TEA and clonidine reduced the postoperative heart rate compared with the control group without jeopardizing cardiac output or perfusion pressure. Plasma epinephrine increased perioperatively in all groups but was significantly lower in the TEA group. Neither TEA nor clonidine affected the increase in plasma cortisol. The release of troponin T was attenuated by TEA. New ST-segment elevation or depression occurred in more than 70% of the control patients but only in 40% of the clonidine group and in 50% of the TEA group. The investigators concluded that TEA, but not intravenous clonidine, combined with general anesthesia for CABG demonstrated a beneficial effect on the perioperative stress response and decreased postoperative myocardial ischemia.

Liu et al.[32] recently conducted a meta-analysis of 15 trials that studied the effects of perioperative central neu-

raxial analgesia on outcome after CABG. The total number of patients was 1178. According to the analysis, TEA does not affect the incidences of mortality (0.7% TEA vs 0.3% general anesthesia) or myocardial infarction (2.3% TEA vs 3.4% general anesthesia). However, TEA does significantly reduce the risk of arrhythmias (odds ratio 0.52), pulmonary complications (odds ratio 0.41), and time to tracheal extubation (by 4.5 hours). TEA reduces analog pain scores at rest by 7.8 mm and with activity by 11.6 mm. The authors concluded that there were no differences in the rates of mortality or myocardial infarction after CABG surgery with central neuraxial analgesia. More rapid tracheal extubation, decreased pulmonary complications and cardiac arrhythmias, and reduced pain scores were, however, benefits of TEA.

Fillinger et al.[33] conducted a prospective, randomized, nonblinded clinical trial assessing the effects of anesthetic on recovery from cardiac surgery. Sixty patients scheduled for elective cardiac surgery with cardiopulmonary bypass were randomly assigned to 1 of 2 study groups. One group was to receive general anesthesia during surgery and intravenous opioid analgesia after surgery, whereas the second group received TEA combined with general anesthesia during surgery and epidural analgesia for the first 24 postoperative hours. They found no statistically significant differences in time to tracheal extubation, duration of postoperative ICU stay, duration of postoperative hospitalization, pain control, urinary free cortisol, cardiopulmonary complication rate, or total hospital charges.

The most feared complication of TEA is epidural hematoma. Studies have found that, in the setting of cardiac surgery, following a set of standard safety measures averts the occurrence of symptomatic epidural hematomas. These measures consist of preoperative coagulation tests including aPTT, platelet count, and prothrombin time and the cessation of antiplatelet drugs before surgery.[34,35] Scott et al.[36] conducted a prospective, randomized, controlled study of the incidence of major organ complications in 420 patients undergoing routine CABG with or without TEA. All patients received a standardized general anesthetic. Patients in the TEA group received TEA for 96 hours. Patients in the general anesthesia group received narcotic analgesia for 72 hours. Both groups received supplementary oral analgesia. New supraventricular arrhythmias occurred in 21 of 206 patients (10.2%) in the TEA group compared with 45 of 202 patients (22.3%) in the general anesthesia group ($P = .0012$). Pulmonary function (maximal inspiratory lung volume) was better in the TEA group ($P < .0001$). Extubation was achieved earlier ($P < .0001$) and with significantly fewer lower respiratory tract infections in the TEA group (TEA = 31 of 206, general anesthesia = 59 of 202; $P = .0007$). Significantly fewer patients had acute confusion (general anesthesia = 11 of 202, TEA = 3 of 206; $P = .031$) and acute renal failure (general anesthesia = 14 of 202, TEA = 4 of 206; $P = .016$) in the TEA group. The incidence of stroke was insignificantly less in the TEA group (general anesthesia = 6 of 202, TEA = 2 of 206; $P = .17$). No neurologic complications were associated with TEA. The researchers concluded that continuous TEA significantly improved the quality of recovery after CABG surgery compared with general anesthesia and conventional narcotic analgesia.

Turfrey et al.[37] reported similar results after performing a retrospective analysis of the perioperative course of 218 patients who underwent routine CABG. All patients received a standardized general anesthesia, using target-controlled infusions of alfentanil and propofol. One hundred patients also received TEA with bupivacaine and clonidine, started before surgery and continued for 5 days after surgery. The remaining 118 patients received a target-controlled infusion of alfentanil for analgesia for the first 24 hours after surgery, followed by intravenous patient-controlled morphine analgesia for a further 48 hours. New arrhythmias requiring treatment occurred in 18% of the TEA group of patients compared with 32% of the general anesthesia group ($P = .02$). There was also a trend toward a reduced incidence of respiratory complications in the TEA group. The time to tracheal extubation was decreased in the TEA group, with 21% of the patients being extubated immediately after surgery compared with 2% in the general anesthesia group ($P < .001$). No serious neurologic problems resulted from the use of TEA.

Valvular Surgery

Although most studies on the use of TEA in cardiac surgery have focused on CABG, a few investigations and case reports describe its use in valvular surgery. Hemmerling et al.[38] have reported on the feasibility and hemodynamic stability of immediate extubation after simple or combined aortic valve surgery using TEA and general anesthesia. Thirty patients with an ejection fraction of more than 30% undergoing aortic valve surgery were studied prospectively. After initiation of TEA, general anesthesia was induced with fentanyl 2–4 mcg/kg, propofol 1–2 mg/kg, and endotracheal intubation was facilitated by rocuronium. Anesthesia was maintained with sevoflurane titrated according to bispectral index (target = 50). Perioperative analgesia was provided by TEA (bupivacaine 0.125% at 6–14 mL/h). Patients underwent simple aortic valve surgery (n = 17) or combined aortic valve surgery (n = 13) with additional CABG (n = 8), replacement of the ascending aorta (Bentall procedure; n = 4), and repair of open foramen ovale (n = 1). All 30 patients were extubated within 15 minutes after surgery at 36.5°C. There was no need for reintubation. Pain scores were low immediately after surgery and at 6, 24, and 48 hours after surgery. During and up to 6 hours after surgery, there was no significant hemodynamic change due to TEA. Fifteen of the 30 patients needed temporary pacemaker activation. There were no complications related to TEA. The authors concluded that immediate extubation is feasible after aortic valve surgery with TEA and maintenance of hemodynamic stability throughout surgery.

Klokocovnik et al.[39] describe a patient who underwent aortic valve replacement through a ministernotomy while awake under TEA. The procedure was not converted to general anesthesia or to a conventional operation and was performed without adverse incidents. The patient was discharged from the hospital on the second postoperative day. There were no complications within 30 days after surgery. Kozian et al.[40] report on a tricuspid valve replacement without any adverse events using TEA and balanced general anesthesia.

Congenital Surgery

The effects of combined TEA and general anesthesia on hemodynamic and respiratory variables have been reported in children undergoing cardiac heart surgery. Slin'ko et al.[41] report that in 55 patients age 1–14 years, TEA was used in combination with oxygen-air-halothane anesthesia. In one group, lidocaine and fentanyl were used for TEA, and in another clonidine and lidocaine. In a control group, standard intravenous fentanyl-diazepam anesthesia was combined with oxygen-air-halothane anesthesia. In the clonidine-lidocaine group, the endocrine stress response was decreased in comparison with other groups, even without narcotics. Hemodynamics remained stable even in patients with NYHA (New York Heart Association) class III–IV heart disease. These same investigators also report that TEA has been found to be safe and effective for postoperative pain in children after heart surgery.[42] In one study, 40 children received epidural analgesia after open-heart surgery. Lidocaine was injected in a dose of 1.5–2 mg/kg every 1.5–2 hours. Controls (n = 16) received intravenous fentanyl + diazepam analgesia. Respiratory response and awakening were significantly earlier ($P < .001$) in the epidural group. Cooperation with nurses was much better in this group, too. No side effects were observed in the epidural group.

Peterson et al.[43] report on a retrospective study describing the results of the use of regional anesthesia in 220 pediatric cardiac operations. They indicate that tracheal extubation in the operating room could be achieved for 89% of the patients. Ninety-five percent of the patients had pain scores less than or equal to 4.0 at all intervals postoperatively. Adverse effects of regional anesthesia included emesis, pruritus, urinary retention, postoperative transient paresthesia, and respiratory depression (Table 57–3). The incidence of peridural hematoma was zero. The rate of adverse effects was lower using the TEA approach compared with various caudal, lumbar epidural, and spinal approaches. Hospital stay was not prolonged because of regional anesthetic complications. In this study, regional anesthesia was found to be safe and effective in the management of pediatric patients undergoing cardiac surgery.

Hammer et al.[44] evaluated whether spinal anesthesia or TEA in combination with general anesthesia was associated with circulatory stability, satisfactory postoperative sedation/analgesia, and a low incidence of adverse effects. They found no significant differences in the incidence of clinically significant changes in vital signs, oxygen desaturation, hypercarbia, or vomiting when comparing TEA with spinal anesthesia for children undergoing cardiac surgery.

Absolute Incidence of Complications Attributable to Regional Anesthesia

Complication	L/C SSE	L/C Cath	Intrath	Thorac Cath	Total
Emesis	45	24	9	8	86
Pruritus	1	14	1	5	21
Urinary retention	6	8	1	1	16
Paresthesias	0	7	0	0	7
Respiratory depression	4	0	0	0	4
Site/CNS infection	0	0	0	0	0
Peridural hematoma	0	0	0	0	0

L/C SSE, lumbar/caudal single-shot epidural; L/C Cath, lumbar/caudal catheter epidural; Intrath, intrathecal single-shot; Thorac Cath, thoracic catheter epidural; CNS, central nervous system.
Reproduced, with permission, from Peterson KL, DeCampli WM, Pike NA, et al: A report of two hundred twenty cases of regional anesthesia in pediatric cardiac surgery. Anesth Analg 2000;90(5):1014–1019.

Noncardiac Surgery in Patients with Cardiovascular Disease

When TEA is used for major vascular surgery, it is reported to provide more hemodynamic stability and better pain control than general anesthesia or monitored anesthesia care with local anesthesia.[45] TEA has been found safe and effective for endovascular aortic aneurysm repair, especially in patients with severe coexisting diseases. In addition, TEA minimizes sedation and postoperative analgesic requirements, decreases cardiopulmonary complications, and decreases overall hospital stay, thereby reducing cost.

Bonnet et al.[46] investigated the hemodynamic consequences of abdominal aortic surgery with infrarenal cross-clamping in 21 patients randomized to one of two groups. In group I (n = 11), neuroleptanesthesia was used, whereas group II (n = 10) received TEA at the T8-T9 level. In all patients, hemodynamic measurements were performed using pulmonary artery catheters. The use of TEA was characterized by greater hemodynamic stability during surgery. Patients in the neuroleptanesthesia group experienced significant lability of blood pressure, heart rate, and cardiac index.

Her et al.[47] compared intraoperative hemodynamic variables and postoperative morbidity between a group of patients undergoing abdominal aortic surgery—one with combined TEA and general anesthesia (n = 30) and one with general anesthesia alone (n = 19). Patients in the combined group were given epidural bupivacaine intraoperatively and epidural morphine postoperatively. After cross-clamping of the aorta, cardiac index and pulmonary capillary wedge pressure did not change in the combined group, whereas cardiac index decreased (mean change, 0.30 L/min/m^2; $P = .006$) and pulmonary capillary wedge pressure increased (mean change 1 mm Hg; $P = .007$) in the group with general anesthesia alone. After unclamping of the aorta, cardiac index increased in both groups (mean change, 0.26 L/min/m^2, $P = .002$ and 0.30 L/min/m^2 $P = .001$, respectively). Postoperatively, the necessity for ventilatory support and the incidence of respiratory failure were lower in the combined group than in the general anesthesia alone group ($P = .0002$ and $P = .018$, respectively). In addition, vasodilator therapy was required less frequently in the combined group ($P = .002$). Duration of ICU stay was shorter in the combined group (2.7 days vs 3.8 days; $P = .003$). The authors concluded that for infrarenal abdominal aortic surgery, combined TEA and general anesthesia is associated with more stable intraoperative hemodynamics and significantly less postoperative morbidity than general anesthesia alone.

Different results, however, were obtained by Garnett et al.,[48] who studied the incidence of perioperative myocardial ischemia in patients undergoing elective aortic surgery. Patients were randomly assigned to one of two groups. One group (n = 48) received combined general anesthesia and epidural anesthesia and postoperative epidural analgesia for 48 hours; the other group (n = 51) received general anesthesia followed by postoperative intravenous analgesia. The authors reported that myocardial ischemia was common because it occurred in 55% of patients. In the hospital, preoperative ischemia was uncommon (combined = 8; general anesthesia = 3). Ischemic events were common intraoperatively (combined = 25; general anesthesia = 18), with mesenteric traction producing the largest number of events (combined = 11; general anesthesia = 11). Postoperative ischemia was most common on the day of surgery. Termination of epidural analgesia produced rebound ischemia (60 events in 9 patients). The authors concluded that combined general anesthesia and epidural anesthesia and postoperative epidural analgesia do not reduce the incidence of myocardial ischemia or morbidity compared with general anesthesia and postoperative intravenous analgesia.

Norris et al.[49] studied patient outcomes in 168 patients undergoing surgery of the abdominal aorta using different types of anesthesia. Patients were randomly assigned to receive either TEA combined with general anesthesia or general anesthesia alone intraoperatively and either intravenous or epidural patient-controlled analgesia (PCA) postoperatively (four treatment groups). PCA was continued for at least 72 hours. Length of stay and direct medical costs for patients surviving to discharge were similar among the four treatment groups. Postoperative outcomes were also similar among the groups with respect to death, myocardial infarction, myocardial ischemia, reoperation, pneumonia, and renal failure. Postoperative pain scores were the same for the four groups, but epidural PCA was associated with a significantly shorter time to extubation ($P = .002$). Times to ICU discharge, ward admission, first bowel sounds, first flatus, tolerating clear liquids, tolerating regular diet, and independent ambulation were also equivalent for the four groups. The authors concluded that in patients undergoing surgery of the abdominal aorta, TEA combined with general anesthesia and followed by either intravenous or epidural PCA, offers no major advantage or disadvantage when compared with general anesthesia alone followed by either intravenous or epidural PCA.

Davies et al.[50] prospectively studied intraoperative hemodynamics and outcomes in 50 patients undergoing elective abdominal aortic surgery who were randomized to receive either combined epidural (T9-T10 level) and general anesthesia and postoperative epidural analgesia or general anesthesia and postoperative intravenous morphine infusion. The use of intraoperative vasopressors was significantly higher in the combined group ($P < .01$), but the use of intravenous glyceryl trinitrate was significantly lower ($P < .01$). No significant difference was found between groups in regard to blood loss, volume replacement, and the number of patients requiring postoperative ventilation. Two patients in the combined group died postoperatively compared with one in the general anesthesia group (nonsignificant). There was no significant difference between groups in the total number or type of postoperative complications. The authors concluded that combined epidural anesthesia with general anesthesia altered intraoperative cardiovascular management but did not affect postoperative outcome.

Gelman et al.[51] studied the effect of TEA on the cardiovascular function of morbidly obese patients undergoing gastric bypass surgery. Patients were given general anesthesia alone or a combination of TEA and general anesthesia. Circulatory function was measured and calculated using radial artery cannulation and pulmonary artery catheterization with pulmonary artery thermodilution catheters. During surgery, the TEA group demonstrated greater decreases in cardiac index, left and right ventricular stroke work, systolic blood pressure–heart rate product, arteriovenous oxygen content difference, oxygen consumption, and intrapulmonary shunt compared with the general anesthesia group. Postoperatively, epidural analgesia was associated with decreases in left ventricular stroke work, systolic pressure–heart rate product, arteriovenous oxygen content differences, and oxygen consumption compared with values observed when patients experienced pain. Morphine given for relief of postoperative pain was not associated with significant changes in cardiovascular function. The authors concluded that continuous TEA used for upper abdominal surgery in morbidly obese patients benefits intraoperative cardiovascular function, as reflected by a decrease in left ventricular stroke work, and postoperatively by relief of pain.

Acute Pain Management

In patients with cardiac disease undergoing cardiac surgery, good pain management is an important goal to improve out-

comes and reduce postoperative complications. The value of TEA in this setting has been studied extensively. Royse et al.[52] studied 80 patients who were randomized to TEA or intravenous morphine analgesia for postoperative pain control after CABG with cardiopulmonary bypass. A thoracic epidural catheter was inserted the night before surgery at either the T1-T2 or T2-T3 level. Eight milliliters of 0.5% ropivacaine with 20 mcg fentanyl was administered before induction of anesthesia. Ropivacaine 0.2% with 2 mcg/mL fentanyl was then infused at a rate of 5–14 mL/h to attain a sensory block of T1 to T10. Pain was measured using a VAS scale from 0 to 10. Psychological morbidity, intraoperative hemodynamics, ventricular function, lung function, and physiotherapy cooperation were also assessed. On the third postoperative day, TEA and morphine were stopped, and only oral medications were used. Acetaminophen, indomethacin, and tramadol were allowed as supplemental analgesics in both groups. Pain scores were significantly less with TEA on postoperative days 1 and 2 at rest and with coughing. When TEA and morphine were stopped on day 3, there were no significant differences. Secondary endpoints of postoperative depression and posttraumatic stress subscales of the Minnesota Multiphasic Personality Inventory were lower with TEA. In addition, extubation occurred earlier with TEA (2.6 vs 5.4 hours; $P < .001$). TEA showed improved physiotherapy cooperation ($P < .001$), arterial oxygen tension ($P = .041$), and peak expiratory flow rate ($P = .001$). Mean arterial pressure was lower with TEA ($P = .036$); otherwise, no differences were found in intraoperative hemodynamics or ventricular function.

Liem et al.[53] studied the effects of intraoperative and postoperative epidural pain management during and after CABG on the recovery time, postoperative pulmonary and cardiac parameters, VAS scores, and sedation scores. They compared the findings with those of patients anesthetized with general anesthesia whose postoperative pain was relieved with intermittent intravenous administration of nicomorphine. Fifty-four patients were studied postoperatively after uncomplicated CABG surgery. In the TEA group (n = 27), intraoperative analgesia was based on TEA in combination with general anesthesia. In the general anesthesia group (n = 27), intravenous anesthesia with high-dose sufentanil and midazolam was used. Postoperative pain management in the general anesthesia group consisted of intermittent intravenous administration of nicomorphine 0.1 mg/kg every 6 hours, whereas in the TEA group patients received a continuous high TEA with 0.125% bupivacaine plus sufentanil. Patients in the TEA group awakened earlier (148 minutes vs 335 minutes), resumed spontaneous respiration earlier (326 minutes vs 982 minutes), and were extubated earlier (463 minutes vs 1140 minutes). VAS scores, sedation scores, and postoperative Pao$_2$ were significantly ($P \leq .01$) better in the TEA group. The incidence of tachycardia (15 vs 2 patients) and postoperative myocardial ischemia (12 vs 4 patients) was higher in the general anesthesia group. The authors concluded that intraoperative and postoperative pain treatment with epidurally administered bupivacaine plus sufentanil improved the recovery time, as well as pulmonary and cardiac outcomes after

CABG, when compared with intravenous postoperative pain treatment after intraoperative general anesthesia with sufentanil and midazolam.

Hemmerling et al.[54] studied 100 consecutive patients undergoing OPCAB surgery to examine the feasibility of immediate extubation after using opioid-based analgesia or TEA and compare postoperative analgesia between continuous TEA versus PCA. Perioperative analgesia was provided by TEA (n = 63) using bupivacaine 0.125% at a continuous rate of 8–14 mL/h and repetitive boluses of bupivacaine 0.25% during surgery. In the other group (n = 37), perioperative analgesia was achieved by intravenous fentanyl boluses (up to 15 mcg/kg) and remifentanil 0.1–0.2 mcg/kg/min, followed by morphine PCA after surgery. Ninety-five patients were extubated within 25 minutes after surgery (TEA n = 62; PCA n = 33). Five patients were not extubated immediately because their core temperature was lower than 35°C. One patient was reintubated because of agitation (TEA group); one was reintubated because of severe pain and morphine-induced respiratory depression (PCA group). Pain scores were generally low after surgery, with pain scores in the TEA group being significantly lower immediately, at 6 hours, 24 hours, and 48 hours after surgery ($P < .05$) (Figure 57–8). The authors concluded that immediate extubation is possible after OPCAB surgery using either opioid-based analgesia or TEA, but TEA provides significantly lower pain scores after surgery compared with morphine PCA.

However, when Bois et al.[55] studied 124 patients to assess the role of postoperative analgesia on myocardial ischemia after aortic surgery using intravenous PCA or TEA, different results were obtained. In the PCA group, a bolus of morphine, 0.05 mg/kg, was given, followed by 0.02 mg/kg of

morphine on demand every 10 minutes. Bupivacaine 0.125% and fentanyl 10 mcg/mL were used in the TEA group. Analgesics were titrated to maintain a VAS score ≤ 3. The overall incidence of myocardial ischemia was 18.4–18.2% for TEA and 18.6% for PCA (P = not significant). There were no differences between the groups in the total duration of ischemia per patient (22.2 ± 119.8 minutes for TEA and 20.5 ± 99 minutes for PCA) and the number of episodes per patient (0.69 ± 2.1 for TEA and 1.2 ± 4.9 for PCA). Twenty-three patients had an adverse cardiac outcome, but there were no differences between the groups. Although the postoperative pain control was superior with TEA, its use did not result in a lower incidence of early myocardial ischemia when compared with intravenous PCA with morphine.

In patients who underwent CABG, a comparative audit of the use of TEA versus intravenous opioids for postoperative pain control showed no significant differences in the frequency or intensity of persistent pain (defined as pain still present 2 or more months after surgery).[56] Similarly in patients undergoing cardiac valve replacement, TEA was shown to provide excellent analgesia in the peri- and postoperative period, but did not offer a protective effect on chronic post-sternotomy pain.[57]

LUMBAR EPIDURAL ANESTHESIA

Physiologic Effects on the Cardiovascular System

The influence of lumbar epidural anesthesia (LEA) without cardiac sympathectomy on global and regional left ventricular function was investigated before surgery in healthy subjects and in patients suffering from stable mild effort-related angina.[58] In both groups, epidural blockade was performed with 10 mL of 0.5% bupivacaine. Radionuclide angiography was used to determine cardiac output, left ventricular ejection fraction, and end-systolic and end-diastolic volumes and to analyze left ventricular wall motion. Throughout the procedure, patients with a history of angina exhibited neither chest pain nor ECG evidence of myocardial ischemia. At control, left ventricular ejection fraction and systolic pressure-volume ratio were lower in the patients with angina. These patients also had evidence of regional left ventricular dysfunction. Epidural blockade without volume loading resulted in slight improvements in left ventricular ejection fraction and regional function. Such changes were not observed in normal patients. After volume loading, the improvements in ventricular function subsided. These observations led the authors to conclude that LEA may improve global and regional ventricular function in patients with angina provided that volume loading is limited.

Another study reported that LEA enhances cardiac vagal tone mainly through a decrease in venous return.[59] In hypertensive patients, LEA has been shown to cause decreases in mean arterial pressure, with associated decreases in systemic vascular resistance and cardiac output.[60]

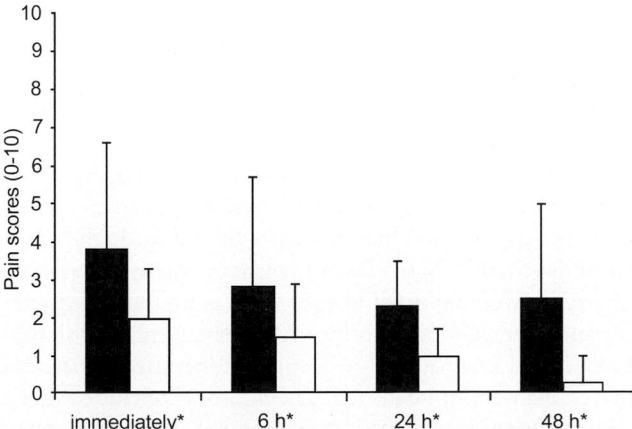

Figure 57–8. Mean postoperative pain scores at rest by group (PCA, black; TEA, white) and time (the highest pain score immediately after surgery and within 6, 24, and 48 hours after surgery). Data are presented as means ± standard deviation. PCA, patient-controlled analgesia with morphine; TEA, high thoracic epidural analgesia; *P* < .05. (Reproduced, with permission, from Hemmerling TM, Prieto I, Choiniere JL, et al: Ultra-fast-track anesthesia in off-pump coronary artery bypass grafting: A prospective audit comparing opioid-based anesthesia vs thoracic epidural-based anesthesia. Can J Anaesth 2004;51[2]:163–168.)

Clinical Pearls

- LEA in the high-risk patient during noncardiac surgery can offer reduced blood loss and need for transfusion and a decreased incidence of thromboembolic events.
- LEA has been shown to provide excellent postoperative analgesia in patients after vascular and orthopedic surgery.
- LEA may reduce the incidence of myocardial ischemia in elderly patients with coronary artery disease undergoing vascular or orthopedic procedures compared with that associated with general anesthesia.

Noncardiac Surgery

Perioperative myocardial ischemia occurs frequently in elderly patients undergoing hip fracture surgery. Matot et al.[61] prospectively studied 68 patients with known coronary artery disease or those at high risk for coronary artery disease undergoing hip fracture surgery. On admission to the emergency room, patients were assigned to receive a usual care analgesic regimen (intramuscular meperidine control group, n = 34) or continuous epidural infusion of local anesthetic and opioid (epidural group, n = 34). Preoperative adverse cardiac events were significantly more prevalent in the control group compared with the epidural group (7 of 34 vs 0 of 34; $P = .01$). Adverse cardiac events included fatal myocardial infarction in three patients, fatal congestive heart failure in one, nonfatal congestive heart failure in one, and new-onset atrial fibrillation in two (Table 57–4). The incidence of intraoperative and postoperative adverse cardiac events was similar for the two groups. The significant difference between groups in the incidence of preoperative cardiac events prompted interruption of the study after the planned interim analysis. The authors concluded that compared with conventional analgesia, early administration of continuous epidural analgesia is associated with a lower incidence of preoperative adverse cardiac events in elderly patients with hip fracture who have or are at risk for coronary artery disease.

Scheinin et al.[62] also looked at the impact of analgesic management on the incidence and severity of cardiac ischemia in at-risk patients. Seventy-seven elderly patients undergoing surgical treatment of traumatic hip fractures were randomized to conventional analgesic regimen (intramuscular oxycodone, OPI group) or continuous epidural infusion of bupivacaine/fentanyl (LEA group). The analgesic regimens were started preoperatively. Patients were operated under spinal anesthesia, and the treatments were continued 3 days postoperatively. The ECG was continuously recorded by Holter monitor. Any ST-segment depression of ≥ 0.1 mV or elevation of ≥ 0.2 mV lasting 1 minute or more was considered an ischemic episode. Nocturnal arterial oxygen saturation (Sao_2) was recorded perioperatively, and subjective pain was assessed every morning using a VAS scale. Fifty-nine (OPI

Table 57–4.

Outcomes by Type of Analgesia Received

Outcome	Control (%)	Epidural
Primary outcome, total patients (n)	34	34
		0
Preoperative cardiac events	7[a] (20)	0
Congestive heart failure	1 (2.9)	0
New-onset atrial fibrillation	2 (5.9)	0
Death	4 (11.7)	
Secondary outcome, total patients (n)	30	34
Postoperative cardiac events	4 (13.3)	2 (5.9)
Myocardial infarction	1 (3.3)	1 (2.9)
Congestive heart failure	0	1 (2.9)
New-onset atrial fibrillation	3 (10)	0
Postoperative noncardiac events		
Bronchopneumonia	2 (6.6)	2 (5.9)
Pulmonary embolism	1 (3.3)	1 (2.9)

[a] $P = .011$.
Reproduced, with permission, from Matot I, Oppenheim-Eden A, Ratrot R, et al: Preoperative cardiac events in elderly patients with hip fractures randomized to epidural or conventional analgesia. Anesthesiology 2003; 98(1):156–163.

30; LEA 29) patients were evaluated for efficacy. Thirteen patients (43%) in the OPI and 12 patients (41%) in the LEA group had ischemic episodes; the difference was not significant. However, significantly more patients in the OPI group had ischemic episodes during the surgery (8 vs 0 in the LEA group; $P = .005$). The median total ischemic burden (ie, the integral of ST change over time) in patients with ischemic episodes was 10 times larger in the OPI group (340 mm $\times$ minutes) compared with the LEA group (30 mm $\times$ minutes) ($P = .002$) (Table 57–5). There were no significant differences between the groups in average heart rates or in heart rates at the start of ischemic episodes or in maximal heart rates during the attacks. Average nocturnal Sao_2 was similar in the two groups, and there were no differences in the number of hypoxemic ($Sao_2 < 90\%$) episodes. Preoperatively, no differences were reported of subjective pain, but postoperative and average perioperative VAS scores were almost 40% lower in the LEA group ($P = .006$). Perioperative myocardial infarctions were not detected. The authors concluded that a continuous epidural bupivacaine/fentanyl analgesic regimen that is started preoperatively reduces perioperative pain and the amount of myocardial ischemia in elderly patients with hip fracture.

Perler et al.[63] evaluated the records of 78 consecutive patients undergoing elective femoropopliteal or femorotibial bypass grafts to assess the impact of the anesthetic management on graft patency. They were randomized to receive general anesthesia and postoperative PCA (general anesthesia, n = 41), or epidural anesthesia and postoperative continuous

Table 57–5.

Characteristics of Perioperative Myocardial Ischemia

	OPI (n = 30)	EPI (n = 29)	P value
Patients with Ischemia (%)			
Preoperative period	8 (27)	3 (10)	0.18
Intraoperative period	8 (27)	0 (0)	0.005
Postoperative period	13 (43)	10 (34)	0.60
Total perioperative period	13 (43)	12 (41)	1.0
Area Under the Curve for Ischemia (mm/min) (Patients with ischemia only)			
Preoperative period	65 (51)	18 (53)	0.41
Intraoperative period	31 (34)	0 (0)	NA
Postoperative period	252 (317)	30 (26)	0.011
Total perioperative period	340 (342)	30 (36)	0.002
Heart Rate (beats/min)			
Mean perioperative	83 (9)	82 (9)	0.48
At start of ischemia	94 (11)	98 (11)	0.38
Max during attack	98 (1)	102 (14)	0.36

Data are presented as number (%).
EPI, epidural group; NA, not applicable; OPI, intramuscular oxycodone group.
Reproduced, with permission, from Scheinin H, Virtanen T, Kentala E, et al: Epidural infusion of bupivacaine and fentanyl reduces perioperative myocardial ischaemia in elderly patients with hip fracture—a randomized controlled trial. Acta Anaesthesiol Scand 2000;44(9):1061–1070.

epidural analgesia (LEA, n = 37). Graft occlusion occurred in 11 cases within the first 7 postoperative days, including 9 general anesthesia and 2 LEA patients ($P < .05$). There were two femoropopliteal occlusions—both in patients who had received general anesthesia. Nine femorotibial occlusions were observed; 7 were in patients receiving general anesthesia and 2 in LEA patients. Graft occlusion occurred in 11 of the 64 limb salvage cases, including 9 general anesthesia and 2 LEA cases ($P < .05$). Seven of 55 greater saphenous vein grafts occluded; 6 were in patients who had general anesthesia versus 1 LEA patient ($P < .05$).

Another study compared the effects of general anesthesia with postoperative PCA and LEA with epidural PCA on hemostatic function and postoperative arterial thrombotic complications in patients undergoing elective lower extremity vascular reconstruction.[64] The findings indicate that LEA may decrease the risk of arterial thrombotic complications in patients undergoing lower extremity revascularization.

Bode et al.[65] studied the effects of general anesthesia versus LEA on cardiac outcome in patients undergoing peripheral vascular surgery who had a high likelihood of associated coronary artery disease. Four hundred twenty-three patients were randomly assigned to receive general anesthesia

(n = 138), LEA (n = 149), or spinal anesthesia (n = 136) for femoral-to-distal artery bypass surgery. All patients were monitored with radial and pulmonary arterial catheters. Postoperatively, patients were in a monitored setting for 48–72 hours and had daily ECGs for 4–5 days and creatine phosphokinase/isoenzymes every 8 hours for 3 days, then daily for 4 days. The recorded cardiac outcomes were myocardial infarction, angina, and congestive heart failure. The authors found that cardiovascular morbidity and overall mortality were not significantly different among groups when analyzed by either intention to treat or type of anesthesia received. In the intention-to-treat analysis, the incidences of cardiac events or death for the general anesthesia, spinal, and LEA groups were 16.7%, 21.3%, and 15.4%, respectively. The absolute risk difference observed between general anesthesia and all regional anesthesia groups for cardiac event or death was −1.6% (95% confidence interval −9.2%, 6.1%). The authors concluded that the choice of anesthesia does not significantly influence cardiac morbidity and overall mortality in patients undergoing peripheral vascular surgery.

Cohen et al.[66] investigated postoperative cardiac outcomes in patients with congestive heart failure undergoing femoral-to-distal artery bypass surgery, comparing LEA with general anesthesia. One hundred and six patients with prior or persistent congestive heart failure undergoing femoral-to-distal artery bypass surgery were randomized to general anesthesia (n = 29) or regional anesthesia (LEA n = 42; or spinal anesthesia, n = 3). The primary endpoint was death or adverse cardiac events (myocardial infarction, unstable angina, or congestive heart failure). The authors found no statistically significant difference among groups in the incidence of combined cardiac events, death, myocardial infarction, death or myocardial infarction combined, unstable angina, or congestive heart failure.

To determine whether tight hemodynamic control would decrease intraoperative myocardial ischemia and major postoperative cardiac morbidity, Christopherson et al.[67] maintained blood pressure and heart rate within predetermined limits in patients randomized to LEA or general anesthesia for peripheral vascular surgery. One hundred patients undergoing elective lower extremity revascularization for atherosclerotic peripheral vascular disease were randomized to receive either LEA or general anesthesia. Blood pressure and heart rate limits were determined before randomization. Hemodynamic monitoring and management of anesthesia were standardized. Myocardial ischemia and major cardiac morbidity were diagnosed by a "blinded" cardiologist, based on continuous ambulatory ECG monitoring, cardiac enzymes, and 12-lead ECGs. Intraoperative blood pressure and heart rate were analyzed by investigators masked to the type of anesthesia given. The authors found that in a greater percentage of the patients randomized to general anesthesia the intraoperative blood pressures were above the predefined limits when compared with the LEA patients. They also noted that the patients had more rapid changes in heart rate and blood pressure. Intraoperative ischemia and major cardiac morbidity were similar in the two groups. Patients experiencing intraoperative ischemia, regardless of anesthetic type, more frequently had blood pressures more than 10% above their upper limit and/or more rapid heart rate changes compared with patients without ischemia. The investigators concluded that prevention of elevated intraoperative blood pressure and/or rapid changes in blood pressure or heart rate may be more successful with LEA than with general anesthesia. Vital sign abnormalities may occur more frequently in patients who have had intraoperative ischemia or are at risk for having it later in the procedure.

Another study compared outcomes between LEA and general anesthesia in a group of patients with a high risk for cardiac and other morbidity who were undergoing elective vascular reconstruction of the lower extremities.[68] The results showed comparable rates of cardiac and most other morbidity between the two groups, but LEA was associated with a lower incidence of reoperation for inadequate tissue perfusion.

Acute Pain Management

The data that support the use of LEA for postoperative pain management in patients with cardiac disease are limited. Mehta et al.[69] compared the effect of buprenorphine through the lumbar and thoracic epidural routes for postoperative analgesia after CABG. Forty patients with normal left ventricular ejection fraction scheduled for CABG were randomly divided into two groups: a TEA group (n = 19) and a LEA group (n = 20). For postoperative pain relief, they received epidural 0.15 mg of buprenorphine at the first demand for pain relief after extubation. A top-up dose of 0.15 mg of buprenorphine was administered in patients whose VAS score was higher than 3 at 1 hour after the first dose. Subsequent breakthrough pain was treated with ketorolac 30 mg intramuscularly. Pain, assessed by VAS scores on a 0–10 scale, respiratory rate, FEV_1, forced vital capacity, mean arterial blood pressure, cardiac index, Pao_2, and $Paco_2$ were measured at frequent intervals. Side effects of epidural opioids were noted. Both groups were comparable in demographic characteristics, had similar VAS scores from 1 to 24 hours postoperatively, required similar amounts of intramuscular ketorolac for break-through pain, and had comparable pulmonary functions and side effects. The authors concluded that buprenorphine given by the lumbar epidural route after CABG compares favorably in terms of quality of analgesia and incidence of side effects with the same drug given via the thoracic epidural route.

Shayevitz et al.[70] compared the effects of LEA compared with intravenous opioids for postoperative pain control in children who had undergone cardiac surgery for palliation or repair of congenital heart disease. In the LEA patients (n = 27), epidural catheters were placed after anesthetic induction, but before anticoagulation. A bolus of 50 mcg/kg of preservative-free morphine sulfate was administered through the catheter, followed by a continuous infusion at 3–4 mcg/kg/h for 22–102 (median, 46) hours postoperatively. The intravenous opioid patients received 50 mcg/kg of intravenous fentanyl before incision, followed by a continuous infusion at 0.3 mcg/kg/min. The fentanyl infusion rate was decreased to 0.1 mcg/kg/min postoperatively and maintained for 24 hours. Times to tracheal extubation, transfer from the ICU, and resumption of regular diet were significantly shorter in LEA patients. LEA and intravenous opioid patients received similar amounts of fentanyl during surgery. However, during the postoperative recovery, LEA patients who were extubated late received significantly less supplemental opioid medication than intravenous opioid patients extubated late during the first 5 postoperative days. No complications related to dural puncture, bleeding into the epidural space, or respiratory depression were encountered. Pruritus and nausea/vomiting were the most commonly reported morbidities in both groups. Fifty-six percent of LEA patients and 41% of intravenous opioid patients reported pruritus ($P = .4$). There was no significant difference in the incidence of nausea and vomiting between the groups (34% vs 30%, respectively). The authors found improved outcomes only in LEA patients extubated late compared with intravenous opioid patients.

INTRATHECAL ANESTHESIA

Adult Cardiac Surgery

Although some anesthesiologists perform spinal anesthesia in adult patients undergoing cardiac surgery, its use is probably limited by the concern for postheparinization lumbar hematoma. In one survey of 892 cardiac anesthesiologists, only 68 (7.6%) reported using of spinal techniques.[71]

The hemodynamic response to lumbar spinal anesthesia using hyperbaric bupivacaine or lidocaine with morphine has been evaluated in cardiac surgical patients by Kowalewski et al.[72] These investigators observed that induction of general anesthesia produced a decrease in mean arterial pressure. The addition of spinal anesthesia produced a decrease in heart rate. Heart rate and mean arterial pressure did not change with sternotomy. In almost all patients, the arterial blood pressure needed to be supported with phenylephrine at some time during the operation. High-dose intrathecal bupivacaine, when combined with general anesthesia has been shown to result in less β-receptor dysfunction and a lower stress response (serum epinephrine, norepinephrine, and cortisol concentrations) during the CABG procedure than with general anesthesia alone[73] (Figure 57–9). However, other studies have reported that although large-dose intrathecal morphine initiates reliable postoperative analgesia, it does not reliably attenuate the stress response during and after cardiac surgery.[74,75]

Vanstrum et al.[76] assessed the use of intrathecal morphine compared with placebo during cardiac surgery on hemodynamics and postoperative pain to determine whether intrathecal morphine is effective in decreasing analgesic and antihypertensive drug requirements after CABG in a prospective, randomized, double-blind study. Approximately

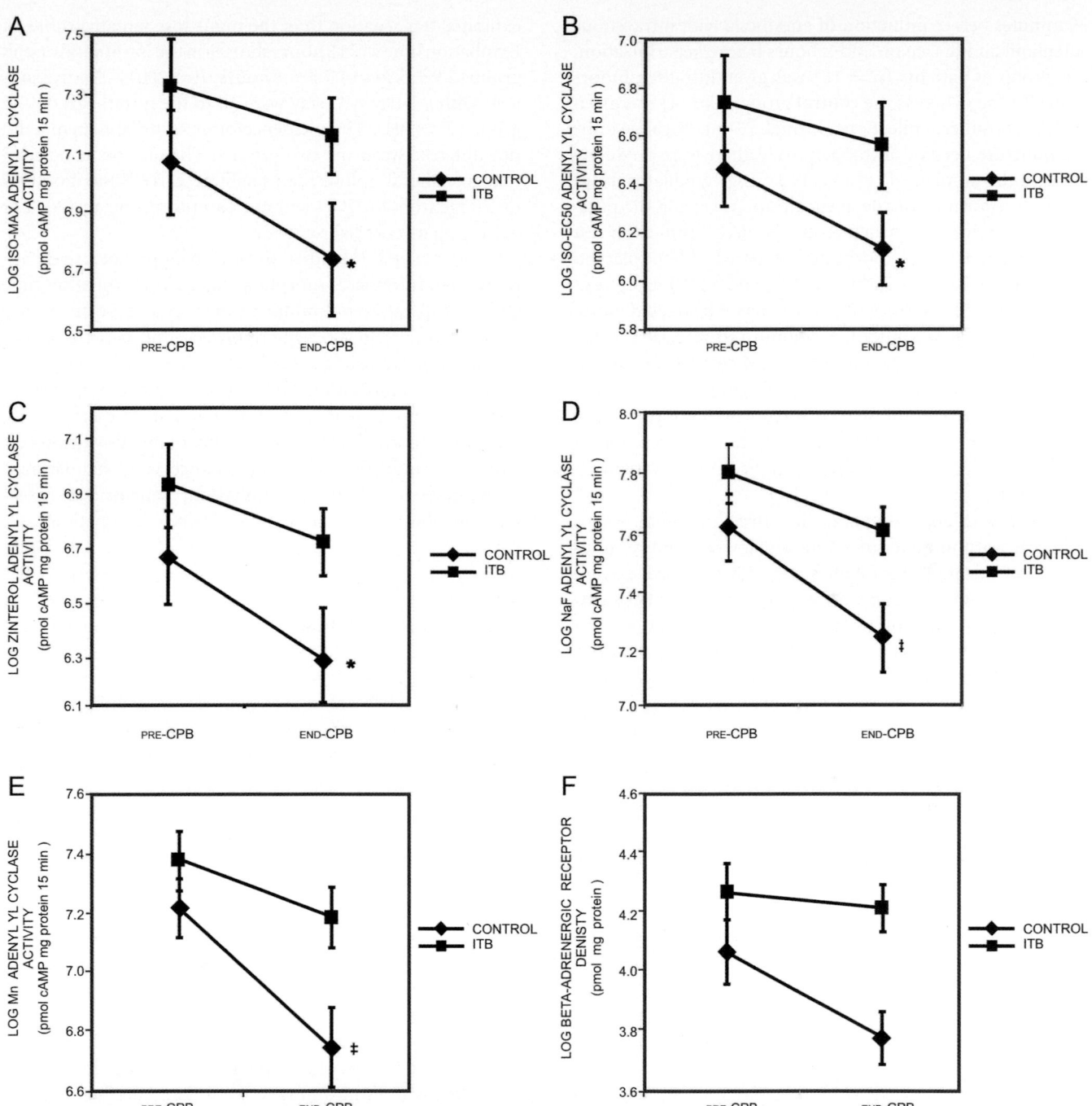

Figure 57–9. **A:** Maximal isproteronol (ISO MAX). **B:** 50% maximal isoproterenol (ISO EC$_{50}$. **C:** Zinterol. **D:** Sodium fluoride (NaF)-stimulated. **E:** Manganese (Mn)-stimulated β-adrenergic receptor (βAR) responsiveness, as measured by adenylyl cyclase activity in control and intrathecal bupivacaine (ITB) groups with cardiopulmonary bypass (CPB) times from 61–120 minutes. The control group shows a significant decline in adenylyl cyclase activity in each of these measures, whereas the ITB group does not. **F:** βAR density in control and ITB groups with CPB times from 61–120 minutes. The control group shows a significant decline in βAR density at $P = .02$. Adenylyl cyclase activity and βAR density (βAR Bmax) are reported as picomoles of cyclic adenosine monophosphate per milligram of protein per 15 minutes and femtomoles per milligram of protein, respectively. The data were log-transformed. Results are expressed as mean $\pm$ SEM (*$P < .05$, ‡$P < .005$). (Reproduced, with permission, from Lee TW, Grocott HP, Schwinn D, Jacobsohn E: High spinal anesthesia for cardiac surgery: Effects on beta-adrenergic receptor function, stress response, and hemodynamics. Anesthesiology 2003;98[2]:499–510.)

30 minutes before induction of anesthesia with intravenous sufentanil and diazepam and 2 hours before heparinization, one group of patients (n = 16) was given intrathecal morphine 0.5 mg, whereas the control group (n = 14) was given placebo intrathecal injections through 22- or 25-gauge lumbar puncture needles. Intraoperatively, there were no differences in the number of patients requiring vasodilator drugs or those requiring volatile agent titration. During the postoperative period, the treated group required significantly less (P < .05) intravenous morphine compared with the placebo group during the first 24 hours (1.8 ± 0.7 vs 5.4 ± 1.5 mg) and 30 hours (2.4 + 0.8 vs 8.3 ± 1.9 mg). The treated group also required significantly less sodium nitroprusside in the first 24 hours (58.1 ± 29.0 vs 89.1 ± 18.4 mg). There were no differences in pain scores, and the only complications (itching, nausea, and vomiting) were infrequent. It was concluded that an intrathecal dose of 0.5 mg morphine is efficacious in reducing analgesic and antihypertensive drug requirements after CABG.

Bettex et al.[77] compared the effects of combined intrathecal morphine and sufentanil with low-dose intravenous sufentanil during propofol anesthesia for fast-track cardiac surgery. Twenty-four consecutive patients with normal cardiopulmonary function who were scheduled for elective cardiac surgery were randomized to receive either a continuous intravenous infusion of sufentanil 0.9–1.8 mcg/kg/min (n = 13) or a single lumbar intrathecal dose of sufentanil 50 mcg and morphine 500 mcg (n = 11). Intrathecal sufentanil and morphine allowed a shorter duration of intubation (104 ± 56.5 vs 213 ± 104 min; P = .01), reduced the need for postoperative analgesia with nicomorphine (equipotent to morphine) (0.7 ± 0.4 vs 1.2 ± 0.4 mg/h; P = .008), and improved postoperative maximal inspiratory capacity (53.4 ± 16.1 vs 38.4 ± 12.5% of the norm; P = .05). The authors concluded that in low-risk patients undergoing CABG or valvular surgery, combined intrathecal sufentanil and morphine with a target-controlled infusion of propofol satisfies the goals of fast-track cardiac surgery. Shorter intubation times and superior postoperative analgesia have also been reported with the intrathecal use of remifentanil, morphine, and clonidine after cardiac surgery.[78–80]

Shroff et al.[81] studied 21 ASA physical status III and IV men scheduled for elective CABG. Patients were randomized to receive intrathecal 10 mcg/kg morphine and 25 mcg fentanyl preoperatively (n = 12) or no intrathecal opioid (n = 9). The latter group received 25–50 mcg/kg fentanyl and 0.05 to 0.1 mg/kg midazolam intraoperatively, whereas the intrathecal opioid group received intravenous fentanyl and midazolam only as needed. Both groups were administered intravenous morphine and midazolam postoperatively as needed. For the first 24 hours postoperatively, pain levels (0 = none to 10 = most severe) and sedation levels (1 = none to 5 = unconscious) were measured hourly. The time to extubation and discharge from the ICU was recorded. ECG evidence of myocardial ischemia was noted. Pain scores were low for both groups (1.5), but the intrathecal opioid subjects

exhibited less sedation than the high-dose fentanyl subjects. Extubation time was 12 hours shorter in the intrathecal opioid group (2.9 ± 5.3 vs 14.7 ± 6.8 hours, P = .001). The five subjects with a 1-day ICU stay were all in the intrathecal opioid group (P = .04). The incidence of myocardial ischemia did not differ between the two groups. The authors concluded that intrathecal opioids can facilitate early extubation and discharge from the ICU without compromising analgesia or increasing myocardial ischemia.

Mehta et al.[82] studied the effects of preoperatively administered intrathecal morphine sulfate on extubation time and postoperative pulmonary function and postoperative analgesia after OPCAB. One hundred adult patients scheduled for elective primary OPCAB were randomized to preoperative administration of 8 mcg/kg intrathecal morphine sulfate (group 1) with a 25-gauge spinal needle or to receive sterile normal saline placebo subcutaneously (group 2). Anesthetic induction and maintenance were standardized to facilitate early tracheal extubation; patients were extubated in the ICU. Postoperative times to extubation were 9.47 ± 3.83 hours in group 1 versus 11.25 ± 3.94 hours in group 2 (P = .025). Postextubation bedside spirometric lung volumes, expressed as percentage of preoperative lung volume, showed significant differences in group 1 compared with group 2 in forced vital capacity (39.66% ± 15.42% vs 31.85% ± 11.65%; P = .016), FEV$_1$ (44.8% ± 16.18% vs 35.97% ± 13.32%; P = .013), maximum voluntary ventilation (39.40% ± 13.57% vs 33.11% ± 14.80%; P = .056), and expiratory flow rate (47.76% ± 24.61% vs 37.37% ± 4.33%; P = .031). There was no mortality or neurologic complication in either group. They concluded that intrathecal morphine provided superior quality of analgesia, which translated into better maintenance of postoperative lung volume as determined by spirometry.

Another study suggests that intrathecal morphine provides better analgesia after cardiac surgery than conventional intravenous analgesia and that a lower dose (1 mg) is associated with less postoperative depression as assessed by Paco$_2$ measurements.[83] In a different study, the use of intrathecal opioids did not, however, facilitate earlier tracheal extubation or improve intraoperative hemodynamic stability compared with intravenous sufentanil and desflurane alone for fast-track cardiac anesthesia.[84] Latham et al.[84] prospectively studied 40 patients undergoing elective primary CABG, aortic valve replacement, or mitral valve replacement. After a standardized anesthetic induction, anesthesia was maintained with a remifentanil infusion, 0.1 mcg/kg/min and desflurane 3–10%, inspired (group I, n = 20) or a sufentanil infusion 0.3 mcg/kg/h and desflurane 3–10%, inspired (group II, n = 20). Patients receiving remifentanil were administered 8 mcg/kg of intrathecal morphine for postoperative analgesia. Both anesthetic regimens provided comparable intraoperative hemodynamic stability and similar recovery profiles, with extubation times of 5.1 ± 4.3 hours (group I) and 5.8 ± 6.7 hours (group II). The authors concluded that the use of remifentanil in combination with intrathecal morphine did not facilitate earlier tracheal extubation or improve intraoperative hemodynamic stability compared with sufentanil alone for fast-track cardiac anesthesia.

Alhashemi et al.[85] studied the effects of low doses of intrathecal morphine on extubation time and on postoperative analgesic requirements after CABG. Fifty patients scheduled for elective primary CABG were randomized to receive placebo, 250 mcg, or 500 mcg of intrathecal morphine preoperatively. Intraoperative fentanyl and midazolam were limited to 15 mcg/kg and 20 mcg/kg intravenously. Patients were extubated in the ICU. There were no significant differences in extubation times for the three groups. Postoperative morphine requirements in the 250 mcg and 500 mcg groups were 13.6 ± 7.8 mg and 11.7 ± 7.4 mg, compared with 21.3 ± 6.2 mg in the placebo group ($P = .001$). The requirements for postoperative midazolam, nitroglycerin, and sodium nitroprusside were also similar among the three groups. The authors concluded that despite decreased postoperative morphine requirements, intrathecal morphine administration did not have a clinically relevant effect on extubation time after CABG surgery.

Chaney et al.[86] found that the mean time from ICU arrival to extubation was significantly prolonged in patients who received intrathecal morphine when compared with patients who received intrathecal placebo. Extubation was substantially delayed because of prolonged ventilatory depression in some patients who had received intrathecal morphine. Although postoperative intravenous morphine use was less in patients who received intrathecal morphine than in those receiving placebo, the difference between the groups was not significant.

The hemodynamic effects of spinal anesthesia in combination with general anesthesia were studied prospectively in infants and children undergoing open-heart surgery by Finkel et al.[87] After premedication with midazolam and an inhalation induction with sevoflurane, 30 patients, 7 months to 13 years of age, who were undergoing open-heart surgery, received intrathecal injections with 0.5% tetracaine D10 mixed with morphine. The spinal blocks were placed at the L2-3 or L3-4 interspace, and cephalad spread was promoted by positioning the patients in 30 degrees of Trendelenburg position for a minimum of 10 minutes. Maintenance of anesthesia was with isoflurane 0.2–0.5% in 70% nitrous oxide to maintain heart rate and blood pressure within 20% of postinduction baseline values. Hemodynamic values were recorded at predetermined timed intervals and intraoperative events up to and including aortic cannulation. Patients were divided into four age groups (<1 years, 1–3 years, 4–6 years, and >7 years).

The authors reported that hemodynamic stability was demonstrated in all four age groups. Statistically significant slowing of the heart rate did occur in the groups older than 1 year at 25 minutes, although clinically significant bradycardia requiring treatment never occurred. Hypotension did occur during specific surgical manipulations but recovered spontaneously. Atropine, fluid boluses, and vasopressors were never used. At the conclusion of surgery, all patients met extubation criteria and could move all four extremities.

Pirat et al.[88] prospectively studied the cardiovascular and neurohumoral responses during intrathecal or intravenous fentanyl anesthesia for pediatric cardiac surgery. Thirty children 6 months to 6 years old were anesthetized with an intravenous fentanyl bolus of 10 mcg/kg. This was followed by a fentanyl infusion of 10 mcg/kg/h in the intravenous group (n = 10), 2 mcg/kg of intrathecal fentanyl in the intrathecal group (n = 10), or a combination of intravenous and intrathecal fentanyl in the combined group (n = 10). The findings in all three groups were statistically similar except for higher blood glucose levels during cardiopulmonary bypass in the intrathecal group compared with the intravenous group ($P < .004$). The combined intravenous–intrathecal group was the only group in whom the increases in heart rate and mean arterial blood pressure from presurgery to poststernotomy were not significant. The 24-hour urinary cortisol excretion rates were lowest in the combined group. A single intrathecal injection of fentanyl 2 mcg/kg offered no advantage over systemic fentanyl with regard to hemodynamic stability or suppression of the stress response. The combination of these two regimens may provide better hemodynamic stability during the pre-bypass period and may be associated with a decreased 24-hour urinary cortisol excretion rate.

To analyze the feasibility of immediate extubation, Figueira Moure et al.[89] studied 29 ASA I-II pediatric patients undergoing surgery to correct simple heart defects. These patients were compared with a control group of 23 patients who had not received caudal morphine or had been selected for early extubation. Anesthesia was provided with sevoflurane, midazolam, rocuronium, fentanyl (maximum dose 10 mcg/kg), and a bolus of caudal morphine (50–60 mcg/kg) after anesthetic induction. All patients were extubated satisfactorily in the operating room. None required reintubation or reoperation. Postoperative pain was controlled with metamizol alone for 79.3% of patients. No episodes of respiratory depression or neurologic complications were observed. Pediatric ICU and hospital stays were significantly shorter in the study group than in the control group.

Williams and Abajian[90] reported on the use of spinal anesthesia in high-risk neonates for the repair of patent ductus arteriosus. Spinal anesthesia with tetracaine was used as an alternative to general anesthesia in a series of 15 consecutive patients. The average dose of tetracaine was 2.4 mg/kg. Two patients early in the series had an inadequate level and received supplemental isoflurane. The remainder of the patients received either no or minimal supplementation to the basic technique. The cardiovascular status of the group was very stable with minimal changes in blood pressure, and recovery was rapid. The three patients who had not been intubated before surgery were extubated soon after surgical repair was completed. No complications of the technique were noted.

Clinical Pearls

- Intrathecal morphine is efficacious in reducing analgesic and antihypertensive drug requirements after CABG.
- Earlier extubation and maintenance of postoperative lung volume as determined by spirometry are benefits of intrathecal anesthesia after cardiac surgery.
- When used for noncardiac surgery in the high-risk patient, intrathecal anesthesia is associated with fewer episodes of hypotension and less need for vasopressor support compared with general anesthesia.

Noncardiac Surgery

Juelsgaard et al.[91] studied 43 patients with coronary artery disease divided into three groups. Group A was allocated to receive either incremental spinal anesthesia (bupivacaine 0.5% plain); group B was allocated to receive single-dose spinal anesthesia (2.5 mL of bupivacaine 0.5% plain); and group C received general anesthesia (fentanyl, thiopentone, atracurium, enflurane, N_2O/O_2) for hip surgery. The number of patients who developed ST-segment depression was not significantly different among the three groups, but the number of ST-segment depression episodes differed. In group A, a total of 7 ST-segment depressions occurred in the observation period compared with 125 in group B and 16 in group C ($P < .05$). Intraoperative ST-segment depression occurred only in group B. Hypotensive events also varied among the groups: There were three events in group A, 33 in group B, and 40 in group C ($P < .002$). Altogether, 56% of hypotensive patients developed ST-segment depression compared with 10% of normotensive patients ($P < .003$). In group A, 1.6 mL of 0.5% bupivacaine were used as opposed to the fixed dose of 2.5 mL in group B ($P < .001$). In the first postoperative week, mortality rate was higher in group B ($P < .05$), but after 1 month there was no significant difference in mortality rates among the three groups. The incidence of hypotension and myocardial ischemia was lowest in the group receiving incremental spinal anesthesia.

Olofsson et al.[92] reported that for the repair of hip fractures in aged patients, a reduced dose of hyperbaric bupivacaine (7.5 mg) in combination with sufentanil (5 mcg) provides reliable spinal anesthesia with few episodes of hypotension and little need for vasopressor support of the blood pressure. Ben-David et al.[93] studied 20 patients 70 years or older undergoing surgical repair of hip fracture who were randomized into two groups of 10 patients each. Group A received a spinal anesthetic of bupivacaine 4 mg plus fentanyl 20 mcg, and group B received 10 mg bupivacaine. Hypotension was defined as a systolic pressure of less than 90 mm Hg or a 25% decrease in mean arterial pressure from baseline. Hypotension was treated with intravenous ephedrine boluses of 5–10 mg to a maximum of 50 mg and thereafter with phenylephrine boluses of 100–200 mcg. All patients had satisfactory anesthesia. One of 10 patients in group A required ephedrine as a single dose of 5 mg. Nine of 10 patients in group B required vasopressor support of blood pressure. Group B patients required an average of 35 mg ephedrine, and 2 patients required phenylephrine. The lowest recorded systolic, diastolic, and mean blood pressures as fractions of the baseline pressures were, respectively, 81%, 84%, and 85% for group A compared with 64%, 69%, and 64% for group B. The authors concluded that a "minidose" of 4 mg bupivacaine in combination with 20 mcg fentanyl provides adequate spinal anesthesia for surgical repair of hip fractures in the elderly.

In a retrospective study to determine whether spinal anesthesia can be safely used for patients undergoing endoluminal abdominal aortic aneurysm repair, Huang[94] concluded that spinal anesthesia was safe. However, the major disadvantage of spinal anesthesia was its limited duration of anesthesia because 25% of patients had to be converted to general anesthesia owing to the extended length of surgery and 8% owing to anxiety. Continuous spinal anesthesia is a better choice for such procedures because it allows continuous intrathecal analgesia in the postoperative period and provides effective pain relief that is reflected by the favorable surgical outcome.[95,96]

Fleron et al.[97] studied 217 patients scheduled to undergo abdominal aortic surgery who were randomly allocated to receive either general anesthesia alone (control) or general anesthesia combined with intrathecal narcotics (1 mcg/kg sufentanil with 8 mcg/kg preservative-free morphine injected at the L4-5 interspace). The administration of intrathecal opioid provided more intense analgesia than PCA during the first 24 hours postoperatively ($P < .05$). There was no difference between the groups for the incidence of combined major cardiovascular, respiratory, and renal complications or mortality rate. The incidence of myocardial damage or infarction, as evidenced by abnormal plasma concentrations of troponin I, did not differ between the two groups. The authors concluded that intense postoperative analgesia via intrathecal opioids does not alter the combined incidence of major cardiovascular, respiratory, and renal complications compared with general anesthesia alone.

Backlund et al.[98] randomized 40 elderly patients (>65 years) to either spinal or general anesthesia, who were scheduled to undergo hip arthroplasty or peripheral vascular surgery and were at high risk for postoperative myocardial ischemia. Ambulatory ECG recordings until the third postoperative morning, a daily 12-lead ECG, and serum creatine kinase and troponin concentrations were obtained. The number of ischemic episodes, total duration of ischemia, and ischemic minutes per hour were noted for each patient perioperatively. Sixteen of the patients (40%) had postoperative myocardial ischemia. An intraoperative increase in the plasma concentration of norepinephrine but not epinephrine was detected in the patients who later developed postoperative myocardial ischemia. There were no differences between the groups, and the authors concluded that the type of anesthesia had no effect on the incidence of myocardial ischemia during or after surgery.

Similarly, Windsor et al.[99] studied the incidence of myocardial ischemia in patients undergoing transurethral resection of the prostate who had either spinal or general anesthesia. Ninety-four patients undergoing transurethral resection of the prostate underwent Holter ECG monitoring pre- and postoperatively. There was no difference in the incidence of silent myocardial ischemia between the spinal (n = 60) and the general anesthesia (n = 34) groups. Others have reported similar findings.[100] A number of case reports have been published on the usefulness of spinal anesthesia in patients with a variety of cardiac diseases. Velickovic et al.[101,102] successfully used continuous spinal anesthesia for two patients with recurrent peripartum cardiomyopathy presenting in congestive heart failure for emergent cesarean section delivery. The spinal anesthesia not only provided adequate anesthesia but also markedly reduced the patients' symptoms. Others have reported similar success with spinal anesthesia in obstetric patients with hypertrophic obstructive cardiomyopathy,[103] severe pulmonary stenosis,[104] and coronary artery disease.[105]

Acute Pain Management

Zarate et al.[106] compared remifentanil combined with intrathecal morphine with sufentanil for postoperative pain control in patients receiving desflurane anesthesia for elective CABG or valve replacement. Before entering the operating room, patients in the remifentanil group (n = 20) received morphine 8 mcg/kg intrathecally. Anesthesia was induced using a standardized anesthetic technique in all patients. In the remifentanil group, anesthesia was maintained with remifentanil, 0.1 mcg/kg/min in combination with desflurane 3–10%. In the sufentanil group (n = 20), patients received sufentanil 0.3 mcg/kg/h and desflurane 3–10%. There were no differences between the two groups with respect to time from arrival in the ICU to tracheal extubation (5.1 ± 4.3 hours vs 5.8 ± 6.7 hours for remifentanil and sufentanil groups, respectively). After extubation, patients in the remifentanil group had significantly lower VAS scores, reduced PCA requirements, and greater satisfaction with their perioperative pain management compared with patients in the sufentanil group. The researchers concluded that remifentanil combined with intrathecal morphine provided superior pain control after cardiac surgery compared with a sufentanil-based general anesthesia technique.

Boulanger et al.[107] assessed whether intrathecal analgesia facilitates early extubation and provides superior pain control after cardiac surgery compared with PCA or nurse-administered subcutaneous injections. Sixty-two patients undergoing elective cardiac surgery participated in this prospective, randomized, partly blinded study. Perioperative care was standardized, and patients were assigned to receive intrathecal morphine (ITM group) followed by PCA, intrathecal placebo (ITP group) followed by PCA, or subcutaneous injections of morphine every 4 hours as needed (SC group). Rating scales and questionnaires were used to assess clinical outcomes. The authors found that the use of intrathecal morphine did not favor earlier extubation, and there was even a tendency for

longer extubation times in the intrathecal morphine group compared with the intrathecal placebo and subcutaneous groups. Pain scores, adverse effects, postoperative recovery, and patient satisfaction were comparable in the three groups. The report concluded that intrathecal morphine is not indicated in patients undergoing cardiac surgery if early extubation is planned.

Suominen et al.[108] assessed the analgesic effect and safety of intrathecal morphine in postoperative pain control in children after heart surgery with a sternotomy incision. Eighty children, 3–55 kg, who were undergoing elective cardiac surgery with opioid-based anesthesia were randomly divided into a treatment group who received 20 mcg/kg intrathecal morphine at induction of anesthesia and a control group. Thirty-five patients were enrolled in the intrathecal morphine group and 36 in the control group. The mean time for the first intravenous morphine dose from intrathecal morphine administration or equivalent time zero in the control group was significantly longer ($P = .003$) in the intrathecal morphine group compared with the control group (12.3 vs 8.7 hours). Time from pediatric ICU admission to the start of intravenous morphine was also significantly longer ($P = .01$) in the intrathecal morphine group (6.0 vs 3.4 hours). The total intravenous morphine consumption over the mean 19 postoperative hours was significantly lower ($P = .03$) in the intrathecal morphine group. However, the use of intrathecal morphine did not result in earlier extubation or earlier discharge from the pediatric ICU. Of the 35 patients who received intrathecal morphine at induction of anesthesia, 20% (n = 7) did not require any additional morphine in the pediatric ICU compared with 3 of 36 control group patients. This did not reach statistical significance. The incidence of adverse events was low in both groups.

THORACIC BLOCKS (PARAVERTEBRAL & INTERCOSTAL)

Physiologic Effects

Saito et al.[109] studied the effects of paravertebral blocks in healthy volunteers. Twenty-two milliliters of 1% lidocaine were injected at the T11 level into the ventral area of the right-sided paravertebral space in 16 volunteers. A week later, the procedure was repeated with a saline injection. Unilateral analgesia (with no contralateral element) was induced in every subject injected with lidocaine; there was no block after saline injection. Loss of pinprick sensation was observed within 10 minutes after injection and involved a mean of 12 (range 8–13) dermatomes. A sympathetic block was indicated by cutaneous temperature increase within at least six dermatomes (Figure 57–10). Increase of arterial blood pressure was obtained in all volunteers with no change in pulse rate. No side effects or complications occurred. Epidural spread of the local anesthetic was unlikely because of the absence of contralateral cutaneous analgesia and temperature increase.

Cheema et al.[110] studied six patients undergoing paravertebral block for chronically painful conditions of the chest

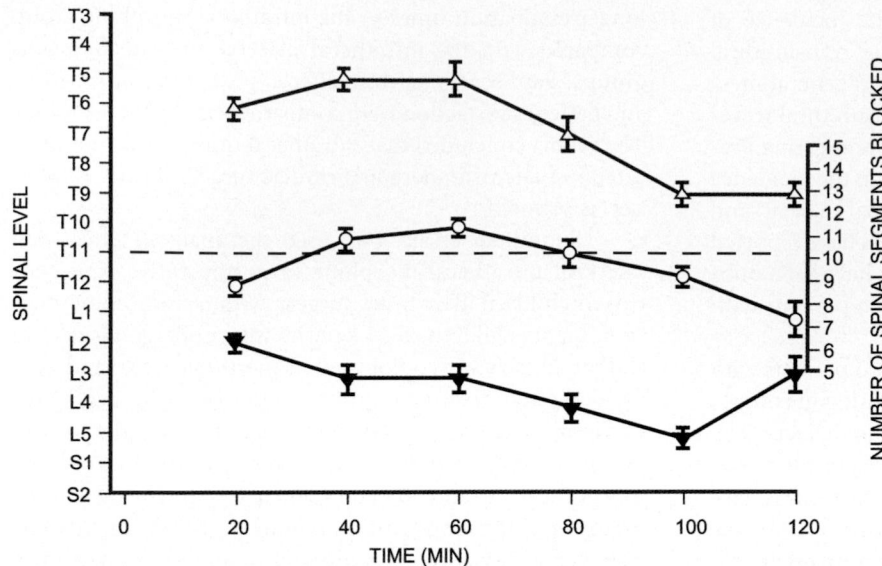

Figure 57–10. Somatic distribution of paravertebral block. The upward-pointing open triangles indicate the mean upper level of the block with 95% confidence intervals. The downward-pointing solid triangles show the mean lower level of the block with 95% confidence intervals. The dashed line passing through T11 is the level of the injections. The open circles indicate the mean of the total number of blocked segments with 95% confidence intervals. (Reproduced, with permission, from Saito T, Den S, Cheema SP, et al: A single-injection, multi-segmental paravertebral block-extension of somatosensory and sympathetic block in volunteers. Acta Anaesthesiol Scand 2001;45[1]:30–33.)

wall, who were thermographically imaged so that the extent of cutaneous vasodilatation—hence sympathetic blockade—could be correlated with the distribution of the somatic block. All blocks were performed by a single experienced operator with a single percutaneous entry, using 15 mL of 0.5% bupivacaine at a mean level of T9-10 (range T7-8, T10-11). Correct needle placement was confirmed radiologically. There was a mean distribution of the somatic block over five dermatomes (range 1–8), as evidenced by the loss of pinprick sensation; the upper and lower limits of blockade were T6 and L3, respectively. The mean distribution of the sympathetic blockade was eight dermatomes (range 6–10), as evidenced by ipsilateral skin warming with upper and lower limits of T5 and L3, respectively. No bilateral spread was observed. No significant postural changes in blood pressures were seen, although there was a small but significant decrease in supine heart rate ($P = .05$).

There is anecdotal evidence that paravertebral blocks can be beneficial in patients with ischemic heart disease and can relieve angina. Ho et al.[111] reported on the intraoperative resolution of ST-segment depression after a right thoracic paravertebral block (Figure 57–11).

Clinical Pearls

- Paravertebral block with indwelling catheters can provide good hemodynamic stability, good postoperative analgesia, and short times to extubation, with few significant complications after cardiac surgery.

- Intercostal nerve blockade can provide early extubation and a decreased need for postoperative narcotic analgesia after cardiac surgery.

- Parasternal block is associated with less postoperative narcotic analgesia requirements and better oxygenation after cardiac surgery.

Cardiac Surgery

Canto et al.[112] prospectively studied the feasibility and efficacy of bilateral continuous paravertebral block combined with general anesthesia in cardiac surgery. One hundred and-eleven elective patients had two paravertebral catheters inserted: one on either side of the midline within 2.5 cm of the spinous process of the third or fourth thoracic vertebrae. A mixture of ropivacaine and fentanyl was infused through the catheters during and after surgery. The technique was associated with good hemodynamic stability, good postoperative analgesia, and short times to tracheal extubation with few significant complications.

Exadaktylos et al.[113] evaluated the preoperative application of intercostal nerve blockade (ICB), combined with general anesthesia for peri- and postoperative pain control. They also assessed its efficacy for early extubation. Nine consecutive patients undergoing MIDCAB surgery were evaluated. Preoperative ipsilateral ICB intercostal nerve block was used in all patients. After induction, isoflurane (0.4–0.8%) and nitrous oxide in combination with the preoperative nerve blockade provided sufficient anesthesia throughout the procedure. Only 2 of 9 patients required additional small doses of narcotics. All patients could be safely extubated within 15 minutes of skin suture. Postoperative discomfort and pain were minimal.

McDonald et al.[114] investigated the effects of a parasternal block on postoperative analgesia, respiratory function, and extubation times in 20 patients having cardiac surgery via median sternotomy. Seventeen patients completed the study. A desflurane-based, small-dose opioid anesthetic was used. Before sternal wire placement, the surgeons performed the parasternal block as well as local anesthetic infiltration of the sternotomy and mediastinal tube sites with either 54 mL of saline placebo or 54 mL of 0.25% levobupivacaine with 1:400,000 epinephrine. Effects on pain and respiratory function were studied over 24 hours. Patients in the levobupivacaine group used significantly less morphine in the first

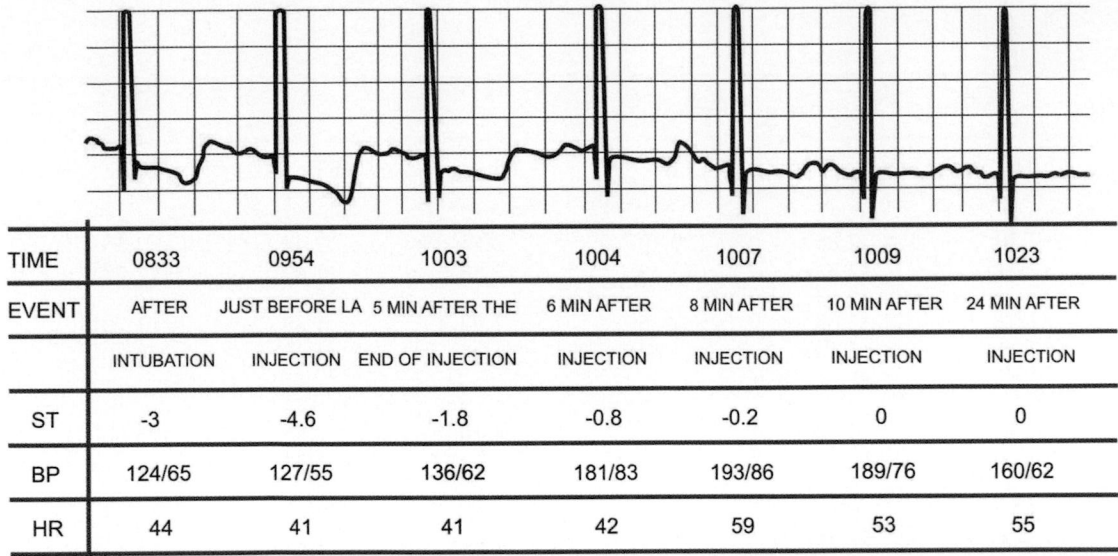

TIME	0833	0954	1003	1004	1007	1009	1023
EVENT	AFTER	JUST BEFORE LA	5 MIN AFTER THE	6 MIN AFTER	8 MIN AFTER	10 MIN AFTER	24 MIN AFTER
	INTUBATION	INJECTION	END OF INJECTION	INJECTION	INJECTION	INJECTION	INJECTION
ST	-3	-4.6	-1.8	-0.8	-0.2	0	0
BP	124/65	127/55	136/62	181/83	193/86	189/76	160/62
HR	44	41	41	42	59	53	55

Figure 57–11. Intraoperative ECG changes before and after right thoracic paravertebral block at T3-4 using 6 mL of bupivacaine 0.5%. All ECG tracings were recorded with the patient in the supine position. Events were at 3 minutes after tracheal intubation (8:33 AM) and just before the bupivacaine injection (9:54 AM). The injection of 6 mL of bupivacaine local anesthetic (LA) completed at 9:58 AM. BP, blood pressure [mm Hg]; HR, heart rate [bpm]; ST, = ST-segment change [mm], as displayed numerically on the ECG monitor. The ECG at 8:33 AM shown here is lead II; the rest are lead III. (Reproduced, with permission, from Ho AM, Lim HS, Yim AP, et al: The resolution of ST segment depressions after high right thoracic paravertebral block during general anesthesia. Anesth Analg 2002;95[1]:227–228.)

4 hours after surgery (20.8 ± 6.2 mg vs 33.2 ± 10.9 mg in the placebo group; $P = .013$). They also had better oxygenation at the time of extubation. Four of 9 in the placebo group needed rescue pain medication, versus none of 8 in the levobupivacaine group ($P = .08$). Peak serum levobupivacaine concentrations were below potentially toxic levels in all patients (0.64 ± 0.43 mcg/mL; range 0.24–1.64 mcg/mL). They concluded that parasternal block and local anesthetic infiltration of the sternotomy wound and mediastinal tube sites with levobupivacaine can be a useful analgesic adjunct for patients who are expected to undergo early tracheal extubation after cardiac surgery.

Noncardiac Surgery

Ohkado et al.[115] describe the case of a 74-year-old woman with aortitis syndrome who was scheduled for mastectomy. She also had severe peripheral vascular disease. Anesthesia consisted of a combination of TEA and intercostal blocks, which were performed with bupivacaine 15 mg (0.5%, 3 mL) at the T3 and T4 levels. During the surgery, the patient remained hemodynamically stable, and no neurologic symptoms were observed.

Another report describes the case of a 72-year-old woman with a significant medical history of hypertrophic obstructive cardiomyopathy requiring breast cancer surgery.[116] Paravertebral blocks were performed at T1-T6 with 5 mL of 0.5% ropivacaine and epinephrine 1:400,000 injected at each level. Intraoperatively, the patient required no other medication for analgesia and was comfortable and conversant

during the 2-hour procedure. She remained pain-free after the operation and did not require any opioid medication until the following day.

Pain Management

Behnke et al.[117] evaluated PCA and intercostal block for postoperative pain relief in patients undergoing MIDCAB procedures. Forty-three patients were included in the study. Anesthesia was induced and maintained in a standardized total intravenous manner with propofol, remifentanil, cisatracurium; glyceroltrinitrate, clonidine, and esmolol were given as needed. After revascularization, patients were randomly assigned to one of two groups receiving either 7.5 mg piritramid intravenously before extubation and continuing a PCA with a 2-mg bolus and a 10-minute lockout, or an intercostal block with 20-mL ropivacaine 1% (4 × 5 mL). In addition, all patients received 1 g of paracetamol rectally before induction of anesthesia and 1 g of metamizol intravenously at the end of surgery. A rescue medication of 3.75 mg piritramid intravenously was allowed. Pain scores, Aldrete scores (AS 0–12), and oxygen saturation were obtained at 1, 4, and 8 hours after extubation. The intercostal block group showed a significantly greater pain reduction in the first (5.8 ± 1.8 vs 7.3 ± 1.9; $P < .02$) and fourth hours (3.6 ± 1.3 vs 4.6 ± 1.4; $P < .02$), respectively. Transfer to an intermediate care ward 1 hour after extubation was achieved more often in the intercostal block group (ICB 9.6 ± 1.5 vs PCA 8.9 ± 1.2; $P < .05$). There was no difference between the groups with respect to oxygen saturation. The additional

Table 57–6.

Pain at Rest and While Coughing (VAS Scores)

	0 h	2 h	4 h	6 h	8 h	10 h	12 h
At Rest							
TEA	2.20 (2.21)	2.85 (2.38)	3.10 (2.88)	2.75 (2.88)	2.48 (1.82)	2.55 (2.28)	2.35 (1.98)
PVB	2.63 (2.41)	2.68 (2.10)	2.25 (1.62)	1.95 (1.43)	1.85 (1.35)	1.70 (0.80)	1.63 (0.74)
When Coughing							
TEA	4.70 (2.86)	4.50 (2.24)	4.20 (2.18)	4.10 (2.12)	3.75 (1.97)	3.80 (2.17)	3.90 (1.83)
PVB	5.22 (2.29)	5.10 (2.25)	4.50 (2.19)	4.50 (1.61)	4.15 (1.81)	4.35 (1.81)	3.83 (1.62)

Values are mean (SD).
PVB, paravertebral block; TEA, thoracic epidural.
Reproduced, with permission, from Dhole S, Mehta Y, Saxena H, et al: Comparison of continuous thoracic epidural and paravertebral blocks for postoperative analgesia after minimally invasive direct coronary artery bypass surgery. J Cardiothorac Vasc Anesth 2001;15(3):288–292.

piritramid demand was 9.3 mg in the intercostal block group and 5 mg in the PCA group in the first 8 hours postoperatively. The authors concluded that compared with PCA, intercostal block gives better pain relief in the early postoperative phase after MIDCAB procedures.

Dowling et al.[118] evaluated whether a continuous regional infusion of a local anesthetic delivered to the operative site would result in decreased levels of postoperative pain and narcotic requirements for patients who undergo a standard median sternotomy for cardiac surgery. Patients undergoing elective CABG alone or in combination with laser transmyocardial revascularization received bilateral intercostal block with either ropivacaine or saline. At wound closure, two catheters with multiple side openings were inserted percutaneously and placed directly over the sternum. The same agent was then administered as a continuous regional infusion for 48 hours. The total amount of narcotic analgesia required by the ropivacaine group was significantly less than for the control group (47.3 vs 78.7 mg, respectively; $P = .038$). The ropivacaine group required less narcotics on postoperative day 2 as well (15.5 vs 29.4 mg; $P = .025$). The mean overall pain scores for the ropivacaine group were significantly less than the mean overall scores for the normal saline group (1.6 vs 2.6, respectively; $P = .005$). Patients receiving ropivacaine had a mean length of stay of 5.2 days compared with 8.2 days for patients in the normal saline group ($P = .001$). Even after excluding outliers (length of stay = 39 days), the normal saline group mean length of stay was still longer at 6.3 days ($P < .01$). No difference in pulmonary function was seen. The authors concluded that continuous delivery of local anesthetics significantly improved postoperative pain control while decreasing the amount of narcotic analgesia

required. There was also a significant decrease in hospital length of stay, which is likely to result in significant cost reductions.

Dhole et al.[119] compared continuous TEA and paravertebral block for postoperative analgesia in patients undergoing MIDCAB surgery. They evaluated the quality of analgesia, complications, compliance to chest physiotherapy, hemodynamics, and respiratory effects. Patients in the TEA group had an epidural catheter inserted at the T4-5 interspace, whereas patients in the paravertebral block group had a catheter inserted in the paravertebral space on the left side at the T4-5 level. There was no statistically significant difference in VAS scores and requirement of supplemental analgesia between the two groups (Table 57–6). Cardiac index at 4 hours and 6 hours was significantly higher in the TEA group. Patients in the paravertebral block group had significantly lower respiratory rates at 8, 10, and 12 hours. All other parameters were comparable. The authors concluded that paravertebral block is as effective as TEA for postoperative analgesia after MIDCAB.

UPPER EXTREMITY REGIONAL ANESTHESIA & CARDIAC DISEASE

Fiorani et al.[120] compared the influence of anesthetic technique on perioperative complications in patients undergoing carotid endarterectomy in a retrospective study of 1020 consecutive patients; 337 patients (33%) were treated under general anesthesia and 683 (67%) under cervical block. The overall perioperative stroke rate was 1.9%, the death–stroke rate was 0.7%, and the cardiac complication rate was 0.8%.

The perioperative stroke rate was higher in the general anesthesia group than in the cervical block group (3.2% vs 1.3%, $P = .01$). Cardiac complication rates were similar in the two groups. A carotid artery shunt was used in 75 patients (22%) receiving general anesthesia and in 92 patients (13%) receiving a cervical block ($P = .0004$). The causes of stroke in the cervical block group were intraoperative embolism (4 cases, 26%), perioperative thromboembolism (7 cases, 58%) and clamping ischemia (1 case, 16%). Mechanisms causing stroke in the general anesthesia group remained unidentified or uncertain. The authors concluded that cervical block anesthesia yields better perioperative results than general anesthesia, probably because it allows more reliable cerebral monitoring. It thereby reduces or even eliminates perioperative strokes related to clamping ischemia. It also facilitates detection of the mechanism underlying intraoperative strokes, allowing surgical techniques and intraoperative management to be modified accordingly. Finally, cervical block anesthesia significantly reduces the need for internal carotid artery shunting.

Sternbach et al.[121] studied the differences in perioperative hemodynamics and associated outcomes in patients who underwent carotid endarterectomy with regional and general anesthesia. Carotid endarterectomy was performed in 527 patients (226 with cervical block and 324 with general anesthesia). The patients who underwent the operation under general anesthesia had significantly greater intraoperative and postoperative hemodynamic variability and received more vasoactive medications during surgery (87% vs 51%; $P < .001$) and in the recovery room (36% vs 21%; $P = .0009$). Major postoperative blood pressure derangements were more common in the general anesthesia group (18% vs 10%; $P < .05$). Patients who underwent the operation under general anesthesia more frequently needed ICU admission (16% vs 7%; $P = .01$) and had more frequent delays in discharge (20% vs 11%; $P = .008$) with a postoperative length of stay of 2.1 days vs 1.6 days for the regional group ($P = .01$). Although no difference was seen in neurologic morbidity rates between groups (combined major stroke/death rate, 1.8%), the major cardiac morbidity rate was noted to be lower in the cervical block group (1% vs 4%; $P = .05$). The total in-room time was shorter in the cervical block group (108 vs 122 minutes; $P < .001$). The authors concluded that carotid endarterectomy performed under cervical block is associated with significantly less perioperative hemodynamic instability than when performed under general anesthesia. This results in fewer major adverse cardiac events. Ultimately, the use of critical care resources is decreased, as is the hospital length of stay.

Bowyer et al.[122] studied the outcomes of 489 patients undergoing 500 carotid endarterectomy, comparing general anesthesia with cervical block anesthesia. Overall, the perioperative mortality was 0.8%. Compared with the regional anesthesia group, the general anesthesia group had greater overall morbidity (23.3 vs 13.6%; $P < .008$) and more frequent use of postoperative vasoactive drugs to control blood pressure (40.4 vs 26.1%; $P < .001$). Furthermore, anesthesia time, operative time, and frequency of shunt use were significantly greater in the general anesthesia group ($P < .03$).

Prough et al.[123] report on 185 carotid endarterectomies that were performed on 153 patients under regional anesthesia. Of these patients, 38 (25 %) had suffered a previous myocardial infarction, 63 (41 %) had documented coronary artery disease, and 115 (75 %) had hypertension. Anesthesia was provided by a superficial cervical plexus block. Monitoring consisted of measurement of direct arterial pressure and continuous display of the ECG. Oxygen was administered by nasal cannula throughout the procedure. Mean arterial pressure was elevated, when necessary, by infusion of phenylephrine. No patient in this study suffered an acute myocardial infarction. The only cardiac complications consisted of eight episodes of non–life-threatening arrhythmias. The authors concluded that regional anesthesia for carotid endarterectomy is associated with a low risk of perioperative myocardial infarction.

Davies et al.[124] studied 128 patients having carotid endarterectomy under superficial and deep cervical plexus blocks to determine the incidence of intraoperative and postoperative neurologic and cardiovascular complications. Twenty-seven patients who had intraoperative neurologic changes after carotid artery clamping responded to shunt insertion. Six patients had transient neurologic changes after the operation but no permanent neurologic complications. Tachycardia (55%) and hypertension (67%) were the most common intraoperative cardiovascular changes, and one patient had clinical postoperative myocardial infarction. Ninety-two percent of patients who could be adequately assessed preferred to have the same method of anesthesia for a future carotid endarterectomy. The authors concluded that carotid endarterectomy under superficial and deep cervical plexus blocks was associated with a high patient acceptance, low neurologic complication rate, and an acceptable rate of cardiac complications.

Ombrellaro et al.[125] investigated the effects of anesthetic technique on cardiac morbidity after carotid artery surgery. Two-hundred-sixty-six consecutive carotid endarterectomies were performed under local/regional (n = 140) or general anesthesia (n = 126). The effects of anesthetic technique on postoperative adverse cardiac events were assessed retrospectively. Forty-seven adverse cardiac events (4 myocardial infarction, 9 congestive heart failure, 7 angina, and 27 new ventricular arrhythmias) occurred postoperatively in 38 patients (14.3%). There were no deaths. The relative risks of general anesthesia for arrhythmias, myocardial infarction, angina, congestive heart failure, and total adverse cardiac events were 2.22, 0.37, 0.83, 1.38, and 1.5, respectively. The only statistically significant difference between the two groups was an increased risk of postoperative arrhythmias after general anesthesia ($P < .03$). The authors concluded that major cardiac morbidity after carotid endarterectomy is independent of anesthetic technique.

Clinical Pearls

- Cervical block can provide significantly less perioperative hemodynamic instability, resulting in fewer major adverse cardiac events compared with general anesthesia during carotid endarterectomy.
- Cervical block can also allow reliable cerebral monitoring, thereby reducing the chance of perioperative strokes.
- Cervical block can decrease the frequency of shunt use during carotid endarterectomy.

LOWER EXTREMITY REGIONAL ANESTHESIA & CARDIAC DISEASE

Fanelli et al.[126] assessed cardiovascular function in 20 ASA I–II patients scheduled for elective orthopedic surgery with tourniquet. The principal objective of the study was to compare the hemodynamic changes induced by unilateral spinal anesthesia and combined sciatic–femoral nerve block. Spinal anesthesia was obtained by 8 mg of hyperbaric bupivacaine 0.5% (group S, n = 10). Combined sciatic–femoral nerve block was obtained by 7 mg/kg of mepivacaine 2% (group NB, n = 10). The duration of surgery and acceptability of anesthetic techniques were similar in the two groups. In eight patients of group S, spinal block was restricted to the operated side (pinprick test and Bromage scale), whereas the other two patients developed bilateral spinal block after being turned supine. The NB group showed no hemodynamic changes during the study, whereas patients in group S showed a small but significant decrease of mean arterial blood pressure ($P < .002$ vs baseline and $P < .04$ vs NB), cardiac index ($P < .01$ vs baseline and $P < .01$ vs NB), and stroke volume index ($P < .01$ vs baseline and $P \leq .01$ vs NB). They concluded that both sciatic–femoral and unilateral spinal blockade provide adequate anesthesia for unilateral leg surgery with tourniquet. The sciatic–femoral technique affects cardiovascular performance less than unilateral spinal.

Peripheral nerve blocks are associated with minimal hemodynamic disturbances. They are perhaps ideal for high-risk surgical patients who cannot tolerate the adverse consequences of even the slightest alteration of hemodynamics. Several case reports illustrate these benefits. Chia et al.[127] presented the practical benefits of a combined sciatic–femoral nerve block on a 56-year-old man with severe sepsis and recent myocardial infarction requiring an urgent above-knee amputation. Ho and Karmakar[128] report the use of a combined paravertebral lumbar plexus and parasacral sciatic nerve block for reduction of a hip fracture in an elderly patient with severe aortic stenosis. Tanaka and Negoro[129] describe the use of a psoas compartment block in a 72-year-old woman with severe heart failure due to rheumatoid myocarditis who required an open reduction of a left femoral neck (trochanteric) fracture. With the patient in the lateral position with the fractured

side up, they performed the block at L3-4 using a 22-gauge Tuohy needle to inject 10 mL of normal saline and 20 mL of 2% mepivacaine. No complications were reported. Rizzo et al.[130] used regional anesthesia to anesthetize a 32-year-old man suffering from Eisenmenger's syndrome with left-type-only ventricle, who needed an extirpation of meniscus by arthroscopic surgery. They used sciatic, femoral, and lateral cutaneous of thigh nerve blocks with ropivacaine without complications.

Clinical Pearls

- In high-risk patients undergoing lower extremity surgery, combined sciatic–femoral nerve block can provide excellent hemodynamic stability and prevent the perils of endotracheal intubation and mechanical ventilation.

CONCLUSIONS

Numerous studies have been undertaken to determine the effects of regional anesthesia on the cardiovascular system during cardiac and noncardiac surgery in the high-risk patient. Epidural and intrathecal anesthesia have been shown to provide stress response attenuation, cardiac sympathectomy, improved cardiac performance, and intense postoperative analgesia for cardiac and noncardiac surgery. Conflicting data remain regarding whether neuraxial anesthesia techniques are associated with earlier extubation times and shorter ICU and hospital stays. In addition, few studies have used clinical outcomes as primary endpoints, although the benefits reported may translate into improved patient outcome. Other regional anesthesia techniques such as paravertebral block, intercostal nerve block, parasternal block, cervical plexus block, and combined sciatic–femoral nerve block all have been successfully used in the anesthetic management of patients with cardiovascular disease. In addition, the application of regional anesthesia, especially neuraxial techniques, in anticoagulated patients remains an area of controversy. However, the use of a set of standard safety measures has been shown to avert the occurrence of symptomatic hematomas. Well-designed randomized controlled studies with large patient numbers may help resolve some of the controversies surrounding regional anesthesia's impact on outcome after cardiac and noncardiac surgery in the high-risk patient. Despite the controversies, regional anesthetic techniques have gained popularity in both the anesthesiology and surgical communities and are increasingly considered valuable resources in managing patients with cardiovascular disease.

References

1. Veering BT, Cousins MJ: Cardiovascular and pulmonary effects of epidural anaesthesia. Anaesth Intensive Care 2000;28(6):620–635.
2. Goertz AW, Seeling W, Heinrich H, et al: Influence of high thoracic epidural anesthesia on left ventricular contractility assessed

using the end-systolic pressure-length relationship. Acta Anaesthesiol Scand 1993;37(1):38–44.

3. Niimi Y, Ichinose F, Saegusa H, et al: Echocardiographic evaluation of global left ventricular function during high thoracic epidural anesthesia. J Clin Anesth 1997;9(2):118–124.

4. Ottesen S: The influence of thoracic epidural analgesia on the circulation at rest and during physical exercise in man. Acta Anaesthesiol Scand 1978;22(5):537–547.

5. Wattwil M, Sundberg A, Arvill A, Lennquist C: Circulatory changes during high thoracic epidural anaesthesia—influence of sympathetic block and of systemic effect of the local anaesthetic. Acta Anaesthesiol Scand 1985;29(8):849–855.

6. Hasenbos M, Liem TH, Kerkkamp H, Gielen M: The influence of high thoracic epidural analgesia on the cardiovascular system. Acta Anaesthesiol Belg 1988;39(1):49–54.

7. Blomberg S, Emanuelsson H, Ricksten SE: Thoracic epidural anesthesia and central hemodynamics in patients with unstable angina pectoris. Anesth Analg 1989:69(5):558–562.

8. Reinhart K, Foehring U, Kersting T, et al: Effects of thoracic epidural anesthesia on systemic hemodynamic function and systemic oxygen supply-demand relationship. Anesth Analg 1989;69(3):360–369.

9. Stenseth R, Berg EM, Bjella L, et al: The influence of thoracic epidural analgesia alone and in combination with general anesthesia on cardiovascular function and myocardial metabolism in patients receiving beta-adrenergic blockers. Anesth Analg 1993;77(3):463–468.

10. Berendes E, Schmidt C, Van Aken H, et al: Reversible cardiac sympathectomy by high thoracic epidural anesthesia improves regional left ventricular function in patients undergoing coronary artery bypass grafting: A randomized trial. Arch Surg 2003;138(12):1283–1290.

11. Liem TH, Booij LH, Hasenbos MA, Gielen MJ: Coronary artery bypass grafting using two different anesthetic techniques. Part I: Hemodynamic results. J Cardiothorac Vasc Anesth 1992;6(2):148–155.

12. Stenseth R, Bjella L, Berg EM, et al: Effects of thoracic epidural analgesia on pulmonary function after coronary artery bypass surgery. Eur J Cardiothorac Surg 1996;10(10):859–865.

13. Kock M, Blomberg S, Emanuelsson H, et al: Thoracic epidural anesthesia improves global and regional left ventricular function during stress-induced myocardial ischemia in patients with coronary artery disease. Anesth Analg 1990;71(6):625–630.

14. Schmidt C, Hinder F, Van Aken H, et al: The effect of high thoracic epidural anesthesia on systolic and diastolic left ventricular function in patients with coronary artery disease. Anesth Analg 2005;100(6):1561–1569.

15. Licker M, Farinelli C, Klopfenstein CE: Cardiovascular reflexes during anesthesia induction and tracheal intubation in elderly patients: The influence of thoracic epidural anesthesia. J Clin Anesth 1995;7(4):281–287.

16. Gramling-Babb P, Miller MJ, Reeves ST, et al: Treatment of medically and surgically refractory angina pectoris with high thoracic epidural analgesia: Initial clinical experience. Am Heart J 1997;133:648–655.

17. Gramling-Babb PM, Zile MR, Reeves ST: Preliminary report on high thoracic epidural analgesia: Relationship between its therapeutic effects and myocardial blood flow as assessed by stress thallium distribution. J Cardiothorac Vasc Anesth 2000;14(6):657–661.

18. Richter A, Cederholm I, Jonasson L, et al: Effect of thoracic epidural analgesia on refractory angina pectoris: Long-term home self-treatment. J Cardiothorac Vasc Anesth 2002;16(6):679–684.

19. Olausson K, Magnusdottir H, Lurje L, et al: Anti-ischemic and anti-anginal effects of thoracic epidural anesthesia versus those of conventional medical therapy in the treatment of severe refractory unstable angina pectoris. Circulation 1997;96(7):2178–2182.

20. Djaiani G, Fedorko L, Beattie WS: Regional anesthesia in cardiac surgery: A friend or a foe? Semin Cardiothorac Vasc Anesth 2005;9(1):87–104.

21. Salvi L, Sisillo E, Brambillasca C, et al: High thoracic epidural anesthesia for off-pump coronary artery bypass surgery. J Cardiothorac Vasc Anesth 2004;18(3):256–262.

22. Kessler P, Aybek T, Neidhart G, et al: Comparison of three anesthetic techniques for off-pump coronary artery bypass grafting: General anesthesia, combined general and high thoracic epidural anesthesia, or high thoracic epidural anesthesia alone. J Cardiothorac Vasc Anesth 2005;19(1):32–39.

23. Stritesky M, Semrad M, Kunstyr J, et al: On-pump cardiac surgery in a conscious patient using a thoracic epidural anesthesia—an ultra fast track method. Bratisl Lek Listy 2004;105(2):51–55.

24. Karagoz HY, Kurtoglu M, Bakkaloglu B, et al: Coronary artery bypass grafting in the awake patient: Three years' experience in 137 patients. J Thorac Cardiovasc Surg 2003;125(6):1401–1404.

25. Aybek T, Kessler P, Khan MF, et al: Operative techniques in awake coronary artery bypass grafting. J Thorac Cardiovasc Surg 2003;125(6):1394–1400.

26. Aybek T, Kessler P, Dogan S, et al: Awake coronary artery bypass grafting: Utopia or reality? Ann Thorac Surg 2003;75(4):1165–1170.

27. Kessler P, Neidhart G, Bremerich DH, et al: High thoracic epidural anesthesia for coronary artery bypass grafting using two different surgical approaches in conscious patients. Anesth Analg 2002;95(4):791–797.

28. Anderson MB, Kwong KF, Furst AJ, Salerno TA: Thoracic epidural anesthesia for cardiac surgery via left anterior thoracotomy in the conscious patient. Heart Surg Forum 2002;5(2):105–108.

29. Barrington MJ, Kluger R, Watson R, et al: Epidural anesthesia for coronary artery bypass surgery compared with general anesthesia alone does not reduce biochemical markers of myocardial damage. Anesth Analg 2005;100(4):921–928.

30. Kendall JB, Russell GN, Scawn ND, et al: A prospective, randomised, single-blind pilot study to determine the effect of anaesthetic technique on troponin T release after off-pump coronary artery surgery. Anaesthesia 2004;59(6):545–549.

31. Loick HM, Schmidt C, Van Aken H, et al: High thoracic epidural anesthesia, but not clonidine, attenuates the perioperative stress response via sympatholysis and reduces the release of troponin T in patients undergoing coronary artery bypass grafting. Anesth Analg 1999;88(4):701–709.

32. Liu SS, Block BM, Wu CL: Effects of perioperative central neuraxial analgesia on outcome after coronary artery bypass surgery: A meta-analysis. Anesthesiology 2004;101(1):153–161.

33. Fillinger MP, Yeager MP, Dodds TM, et al: Epidural anesthesia and analgesia: Effects on recovery from cardiac surgery. J Cardiothorac Vasc Anesth 2002;16(1):15–20.

34. Pastor MC, Sanchez MJ, Casas MA, et al: Thoracic epidural analgesia in coronary artery bypass graft surgery: Seven years' experience. J Cardiothorac Vasc Anesth 2003;17(2):154–159.

35. Sanchez R, Nygard E: Epidural anesthesia in cardiac surgery: Is there an increased risk? J Cardiothorac Vasc Anesth 1998;12(2):170–173.

36. Scott NB, Turfrey DJ, Ray DA, et al: A prospective randomized study of the potential benefits of thoracic epidural anesthesia and analgesia in patients undergoing coronary artery bypass grafting. Anesth Analg 2001;93(3):528–535.

37. Turfrey DJ, Ray DA, Sutcliffe NP, et al: Thoracic epidural anaesthesia for coronary artery bypass graft surgery. Effects on postoperative complications. Anaesthesia 1997;52(11):1090–1095.

38. Hemmerling TM, Choiniere JL, Basile F, et al: Immediate extubation after aortic valve surgery using high thoracic epidural anesthesia. Heart Surg Forum 2004;7(1):16–20.

39. Klokocovnik T, Hollan J, Sostaric M, et al: Minimally invasive aortic valve replacement under thoracic epidural anesthesia in a conscious patient: Case report. Heart Surg Forum 2004;7(3):E196—E197.

40. Kozian A, Schilling T, Tiede T, et al: Open heart tricuspid valve replacement in a heroin addict. Anaesthetist 2005;54(6):578–581.

41. Slin'ko SK: State of the sympathoadrenal system and hemodynamics in children during congenital heart defect surgery with high thoracic

epidural anesthesia using lidocaine-clofelin. Anesteziol Reanimatol 2000;(1):10–13.

42. Slin'ko SK: High thoracic epidural analgesia in the postoperative period after correction of congenital heart defects in children. Anesteziol Reanimatol 1999;(4):44–46.

43. Peterson KL, DeCampli WM, Pike NA, et al: A report of two hundred twenty cases of regional anesthesia in pediatric cardiac surgery. Anesth Analg 2000;90(5):1014–1019.

44. Hammer GB, Ngo K, Macario A: A retrospective examination of regional plus general anesthesia in children undergoing open heart surgery. Anesth Analg 2000;90(5):1020–1024.

45. Lippmann M, Lingam K, Rubin S, et al: Anesthesia for endovascular repair of abdominal and thoracic aortic aneurysms: A review article. J Cardiovasc Surg (Torino) 2003;44(3):443–451.

46. Bonnet F, Touboul C, Picard AM, et al: Neuroleptanesthesia versus thoracic epidural anesthesia for abdominal aortic surgery. Ann Vasc Surg 1989;3(3):214–219.

47. Her C, Kizelshteyn G, Walker V, et al: Combined epidural and general anesthesia for abdominal aortic surgery. J Cardiothorac Anesth 1990;4(5):552–557.

48. Garnett RL, MacIntyre A, Lindsay P, et al: Perioperative ischaemia in aortic surgery: Combined epidural/general anaesthesia and epidural analgesia vs general anaesthesia and i.v. analgesia. Can J Anaesth 1996;43(8):769–777.

49. Norris EJ, Beattie C, Perler BA, et al: Double-masked randomized trial comparing alternate combinations of intraoperative anesthesia and postoperative analgesia in abdominal aortic surgery. Anesthesiology 2001;95(5):1054–1067.

50. Davies MJ, Silbert BS, Mooney PJ, et al: Combined epidural and general anaesthesia versus general anaesthesia for abdominal aortic surgery: A prospective randomised trial. Anaesth Intensive Care 1993;21(6):790–794.

51. Gelman S, Laws HL, Potzick J, et al: Thoracic epidural vs balanced anesthesia in morbid obesity: An intraoperative and postoperative hemodynamic study. Anesth Analg 1980;59(12):902–908.

52. Royse C, Royse A, Soeding P, et al: Prospective randomized trial of high thoracic epidural analgesia for coronary artery bypass surgery. Ann Thorac Surg 2003;75(1):93–100.

53. Liem TH, Hasenbos MA, Booij LH, Gielen MJ: Coronary artery bypass grafting using two different anesthetic techniques: Part 2: Postoperative outcome. J Cardiothorac Vasc Anesth 1992;6(2):156–161.

54. Hemmerling TM, Prieto I, Choiniere JL, et al: Ultra-fast-track anesthesia in off-pump coronary artery bypass grafting: A prospective audit comparing opioid-based anesthesia vs thoracic epidural-based anesthesia. Can J Anaesth 2004;51(2):163–168.

55. Bois S, Couture P, Boudreault D, et al: Epidural analgesia and intravenous patient-controlled analgesia result in similar rates of postoperative myocardial ischemia after aortic surgery. Anesth Analg 1997;85(6):1233–1239.

56. Ho SC, Royse CF, Royse AG, et al: Persistent pain after cardiac surgery: An audit of high thoracic epidural and primary opioid analgesia therapies. Anesth Analg 2002;95(4):820–823.

57. Jensen MK, Andersen C: Can chronic poststernotomy pain after cardiac valve replacement be reduced using thoracic epidural analgesia? Acta Anaesthesiol Scand 2004;48(7):871–874.

58. Baron JF, Coriat P, Mundler O, et al: Left ventricular global and regional function during lumbar epidural anesthesia in patients with and without angina pectoris. Influence of volume loading. Anesthesiology 1987;66(5):621–627.

59. Baron JF, Decaux-Jacolot A, Edouard A, et al: Influence of venous return on baroreflex control of heart rate during lumbar epidural anesthesia in humans. Anesthesiology 1986;64(2):188–193.

60. Dagnino J, Prys-Roberts C: Studies of anaesthesia in relation to hypertension. VI: Cardiovascular responses to extradural blockade of treated and untreated hypertensive patients. Br J Anaesth 1984;56(10):1065–1073.

61. Matot I, Oppenheim-Eden A, Ratrot R, et al: Preoperative cardiac events in elderly patients with hip fracture randomized to epidural or conventional analgesia. Anesthesiology 2003;98(1):156–163.

62. Scheinin H, Virtanen T, Kentala E, et al: Epidural infusion of bupivacaine and fentanyl reduces perioperative myocardial ischaemia in elderly patients with hip fracture—a randomized controlled trial. Acta Anaesthesiol Scand 2000;44(9):1061–1070.

63. Perler BA, Christopherson R, Rosenfeld BA, et al: The influence of anesthetic method on infrainguinal bypass graft patency: A closer look. Am Surg 1995;61(9):784–789.

64. Rosenfeld BA, Beattie C, Christopherson R, et al: The effects of different anesthetic regimens on fibrinolysis and the development of postoperative arterial thrombosis. Perioperative Ischemia Randomized Anesthesia Trial Study Group. Anesthesiology 1993;79(3):435–443.

65. Bode RH Jr, Lewis KP, Zarich SW, et al: Cardiac outcome after peripheral vascular surgery. Comparison of general and regional anesthesia. Anesthesiology 1996;84(1):3–13.

66. Cohen MC, Pierce ET, Bode RH, et al: Types of anesthesia and cardiovascular outcomes in patients with congestive heart failure undergoing vascular surgery. Congest Heart Fail 1999;5(6):248–253.

67. Christopherson R, Glavan NJ, Norris EJ, et al: Control of blood pressure and heart rate in patients randomized to epidural or general anesthesia for lower extremity vascular surgery. Perioperative Ischemia Randomized Anesthesia Trial (PIRAT) Study Group. J Clin Anesth 1996;8(7):578–584.

68. Christopherson R, Beattie C, Frank SM, et al: Perioperative morbidity in patients randomized to epidural or general anesthesia for lower extremity vascular surgery. Perioperative Ischemia Randomized Anesthesia Trial Study Group. Anesthesiology 1993;79(3):422–434.

69. Mehta Y, Juneja R, Madhok H, Trehan N: Lumbar versus thoracic epidural buprenorphine for postoperative analgesia following coronary artery bypass graft surgery. Acta Anaesthesiol Scand 1999;43(4):388–393.

70. Shayevitz JR, Merkel S, O'Kelly SW, et al: Lumbar epidural morphine infusions for children undergoing cardiac surgery. J Cardiothorac Vasc Anesth 1996;10(2):217–224.

71. Goldstein S, Dean D, Kim SJ, et al: A survey of spinal and epidural techniques in adult cardiac surgery. J Cardiothorac Vasc Anesth 2001;15(2):158–168.

72. Kowalewski RJ, MacAdams CL, Eagle CJ, et al: Anaesthesia for coronary artery bypass surgery supplemented with subarachnoid bupivacaine and morphine: A report of 18 cases. Can J Anaesth 1994;41(12):1189–1195.

73. Lee TW, Grocott HP, Schwinn D, Jacobsohn E: High spinal anesthesia for cardiac surgery: Effects on beta-adrenergic receptor function, stress response, and hemodynamics. Anesthesiology 2003;98(2):499–510.

74. Chaney MA, Smith KR, Barclay JC, Slogoff S: Large-dose intrathecal morphine for coronary artery bypass grafting. Anesth Analg 1996;83(2):215–222.

75. Hall R, Adderley N, MacLaren C, et al: Does intrathecal morphine alter the stress response following coronary artery bypass grafting surgery? Can J Anaesth 2000;47(5):463–46

76. Vanstrum GS, Bjornson KM, Ilko R:Postoperative effects of intrathecal morphine in coronary artery bypass surgery. Anesth Analg 1988;67(3):261–26

77. Bettex DA, Schmidlin D, Chassot PG, Schmid ER: Intrathecal sufentanil-morphine shortens the duration of intubation and improves analgesia in fast-track cardiac surgery. Can J Anaesth 2002;49(7):711–717.

78. Lena P, Balarac N, Arnulf JJ, et al: Fast-track coronary artery bypass grafting surgery under general anesthesia with remifentanil and spinal analgesia with morphine and clonidine. J Cardiothorac Vasc Anesth 2005;19(1):49–53.

79. Lena P, Balarac N, Arnulf JJ, et al: Intrathecal morphine and clonidine for coronary artery bypass grafting. Br J Anaesth 2003;90(3):300–303.

80. Bowler I, Djaiani G, Abel R, et al: A combination of intrathecal morphine and remifentanil anesthesia for fast-track cardiac anesthesia and surgery. J Cardiothorac Vasc Anesth 2002;16(6):709–714.

81. Shroff A, Rooke GA, Bishop MJ: Effects of intrathecal opioid on extubation time, analgesia, and intensive care unit stay following coronary artery bypass grafting. J Clin Anesth 1997;9(5):415–419.

82. Mehta Y, Kulkarni V, Juneja R, et al: Spinal (subarachnoid) morphine for off-pump coronary artery bypass surgery. Heart Surg Forum. 2004;7(3):E205–E210.

83. Fitzpatrick GJ, Moriarty DC: Intrathecal morphine in the management of pain following cardiac surgery. A comparison with morphine i.v. Br J Anaesth 1988;60(6):639–644.

84. Latham P, Zarate E, White PF, et al: Fast-track cardiac anesthesia: A comparison of remifentanil plus intrathecal morphine with sufentanil in a desflurane-based anesthetic. J Cardiothorac Vasc Anesth 2000;14(6):645–651.

85. Alhashemi JA, Sharpe MD, Harris CL, et al: Effect of subarachnoid morphine administration on extubation time after coronary artery bypass graft surgery. J Cardiothorac Vasc Anesth 2000;14(6):639–644.

86. Chaney MA, Furry PA, Fluder EM, Slogoff S: Intrathecal morphine for coronary artery bypass grafting and early extubation. Anesth Analg 1997;84(2):241–248.

87. Finkel JC, Boltz MG, Conran AM: Haemodynamic changes during high spinal anaesthesia in children having open heart surgery. Paediatr Anaesth 2003;13(1):48–52.

88. Pirat A, Akpek E, Arslan G: Intrathecal versus IV fentanyl in pediatric cardiac anesthesia. Anesth Analg 2002;95(5):1207–1214.

89. Figueira Moure A, Pensado Castineiras A, Vazquez Fidalgo A, et al: Early extubation with caudal morphine after pediatric heart surgery. Rev Esp Anestesiol Reanim 2003;50(2):64–69.

90. Williams RK, Abajian JC: High spinal anaesthesia for repair of patent ductus arteriosus in neonates. Paediatr Anaesth 1997;7(3):205–209.

91. Juelsgaard P, Sand NP, Felsby S, et al: Perioperative myocardial ischaemia in patients undergoing surgery for fractured hip randomized to incremental spinal, single-dose spinal or general anaesthesia. Eur J Anaesthesiol 1998;15(6):656–663.

92. Olofsson C, Nygards EB, Bjersten AB, Hessling A: Low-dose bupivacaine with sufentanil prevents hypotension after spinal anesthesia for hip repair in elderly patients. Acta Anaesthesiol Scand 2004;48(10):1240–1244.

93. Ben-David B, Frankel R, Arzumonov T, et al: Minidose bupivacaine-fentanyl spinal anesthesia for surgical repair of hip fracture in the aged. Anesthesiology 2000;92(1):6–10.

94. Huang JJ: Spinal anesthesia for endoluminal abdominal aortic aneurysm repair. J Clin Anesth 2002;14(3):176–178.

95. Mathes DD, Kern JA: Continuous spinal anesthetic technique for endovascular aortic stent graft surgery. J Clin Anesth 2000;12(6):487–490.

96. Michaloudis D, Petrou A, Fraidakis O, et al: Continuous spinal anaesthesia/analgesia for abdominal aortic aneurysm repair and post-operative pain management. Eur J Anaesthesiol 1999;16(11):810–815.

97. Fleron MH, Weiskopf RB, Bertrand M, et al: A comparison of intrathecal opioid and intravenous analgesia for the incidence of cardiovascular, respiratory, and renal complications after abdominal aortic surgery. Anesth Analg 2003;97(1):2–12.

98. Backlund M, Lepantalo M, Toivonen L, et al: Factors associated with post-operative myocardial ischaemia in elderly patients undergoing major non-cardiac surgery. Eur J Anaesthesiol 1999;16(12):826–833.

99. Windsor A, French GW, Sear JW, et al: Silent myocardial ischaemia in patients undergoing transurethral prostatectomy. A study to evaluate risk scoring and anaesthetic technique with outcome. Anaesthesia 1996;51(8):728–732.

100. Edwards ND, Callaghan LC, White T, Reilly CS: Perioperative myocardial ischaemia in patients undergoing transurethral surgery: A pilot study comparing general with spinal anaesthesia. Br J Anaesth 1995;74(4):368–372.

101. Velickovic IA, Leicht CH: Continuous spinal anesthesia for cesarean section in a parturient with severe recurrent peripartum cardiomyopathy. Int J Obstet Anesth 2004;13(1):40–43.

102. Velickovic IA, Leicht CH: Peripartum cardiomyopathy and cesarean section: Report of two cases and literature review. Arch Gynecol Obstet 2004;270(4):307–310.

103. Okutomi T, Kikuchi S, Amano K, et al: Continuous spinal analgesia for labor and delivery in a parturient with hypertrophic obstructive cardiomyopathy. Acta Anaesthesiol Scand 2002;46(3):329–331.

104. Ransom DM, Leicht CH: Continuous spinal analgesia with sufentanil for labor and delivery in a parturient with severe pulmonary stenosis. Anesth Analg 1995;80(2):418–421.

105. Honig O, Winter H, Baum KR, et al: Cesarean section with continuous spinal anesthesia in a cardiopulmonary high-risk patient. Anaesthesist 1998;47(8):685–689.

106. Zarate E, Latham P, White PF, et al: Fast-track cardiac anesthesia: Use of remifentanil combined with intrathecal morphine as an alternative to sufentanil during desflurane anesthesia. Anesth Analg 2000;91(2):283–287.

107. Boulanger A, Perreault S, Choiniere M, et al: Intrathecal morphine after cardiac surgery. Ann Pharmacother 2002;36(9):1337–1343.

108. Suominen PK, Ragg PG, McKinley DF, et al: Intrathecal morphine provides effective and safe analgesia in children after cardiac surgery. Acta Anaesthesiol Scand 2004;48(7):875–882.

109. Saito T, Den S, Cheema SP, et al: A single-injection, multi-segmental paravertebral block-extension of somatosensory and sympathetic block in volunteers. Acta Anaesthesiol Scand 2001;45(1):30–33.

110. Cheema SP, Ilsley D, Richardson J, Sabanathan S: A thermographic study of paravertebral analgesia. Anaesthesia 1995;50(2):118–121.

111. Ho AM, Lim HS, Yim AP, et al: The resolution of ST segment depressions after high right thoracic paravertebral block during general anesthesia. Anesth Analg 2002;95(1):227–228.

112. Canto M, Sanchez MJ, Casas MA, Bataller ML: Bilateral paravertebral blockade for conventional cardiac surgery. Anaesthesia 2003;58(4):365–370.

113. Exadaktylos AK, Trampitsch E, Mares P, et al: Pre-operative intercostal nerve blockade for minimally invasive coronary bypass surgery: A standardised anaesthetic regimen for rapid emergence and early extubation. Cardiovasc J S Afr 2004;15(4):178–181.

114. McDonald SB, Jacobsohn E, Kopacz DJ, et al: Parasternal block and local anesthetic infiltration with levobupivacaine after cardiac surgery with desflurane: The effect on postoperative pain, pulmonary function, and tracheal extubation times. Anesth Analg 2005;100(1):25–32.

115. Ohkado S, Nishiyama T, Tamai H, et al: Combined intercostal nerve block and epidural anesthesia in a patient with severe aortitis syndrome. Masui 2000;49(7):782–784.

116. Buckenmaier CC III, Steele SM, Nielsen KC, Klein SM: Paravertebral somatic nerve blocks for breast surgery in a patient with hypertrophic obstructive cardiomyopathy. Can J Anaesth 2002;49(6):571–574.

117. Behnke H, Geldner G, Cornelissen J, et al: Postoperative pain therapy in minimally invasive direct coronary arterial bypass surgery. I.V. opioid patient-controlled analgesia versus intercostals block. Anaesthetist 2002;51(3):175–179.

118. Dowling R, Thielmeier K, Ghaly A, et al: Improved pain control after cardiac surgery: Results of a randomized, double-blind, clinical trial. J Thorac Cardiovasc Surg 2003;126(5):1271–1278.

119. Dhole S, Mehta Y, Saxena H, et al: Comparison of continuous thoracic epidural and paravertebral blocks for postoperative analgesia after minimally invasive direct coronary artery bypass surgery. J Cardiothorac Vasc Anesth 2001;15(3):288–292.

120. Fiorani P, Sbarigia E, Speziale F, et al: General anaesthesia versus cervical block and perioperative complications in carotid artery surgery. Eur J Vasc Endovasc Surg 1997;13(1):37–42.

121. Sternbach Y, Illig KA, Zhang R, et al: Hemodynamic benefits of regional anesthesia for carotid endarterectomy. J Vasc Surg 2002;35(2):333–339.

122. Bowyer MW, Zierold D, Loftus JP, et al: Carotid endarterectomy: A comparison of regional versus general anesthesia in 500 operations. Ann Vasc Surg 2000;14(2):145–151.

123. Prough DS, Scuderi PE, Stullken E, Davis CH Jr: Myocardial infarction following regional anaesthesia for carotid endarterectomy. Can Anaesth Soc J 1984;31(2):192–196.

124. Davies MJ, Murrell GC, Cronin KD, et al: Carotid endarterectomy under cervical plexus block—a prospective clinical audit. Anaesth Intensive Care 1990;18(2):219–223.

125. Ombrellaro MP, Freeman MB, Stevens SL, Goldman MH: Effect of anesthetic technique on cardiac morbidity following carotid artery surgery. Am J Surg 1996;171(4):387–390.

126. Fanelli G, Casati A, Aldegheri G, et al: Cardiovascular effects of two different regional anaesthetic techniques for unilateral leg surgery. Acta Anaesthesiol Scand 1998;42(1):80–84.

127. Chia N, Low TC, Poon KH: Peripheral nerve blocks for lower limb surgery—a choice anaesthetic technique for patients with a recent myocardial infarction? Singapore Med J 2002;43(11):583–586.

128. Ho AM, Karmakar MK: Combined paravertebral lumbar plexus and parasacral sciatic nerve block for reduction of hip fracture in a patient with severe aortic stenosis. Can J Anaesth 2002;49(9):946–950.

129. Tanaka Y, Negoro T: Psoas compartment block for surgery of the femoral neck (trochanteric) fracture in a patient with severe heart failure due to rheumatoid myocarditis. Masui 2000;49(10):1133–1135.

130. Rizzo D, Giustiniano E, Pellicori D, et al: Sciatic, femoral and cutaneous nerve block for arthroscopic meniscectomy in a patient with Eisenmenger's syndrome. Case report. Minerva Anestesiol 1999;65(10):733–736.

58

Regional Anesthesia & Systemic Disease

Jeffrey Gadsden, MD • Admir Hadzic, MD

INTRODUCTION

Patients with coexisting severe systemic disease may be at a higher risk for perioperative complications related to surgery and administration of anesthesia. Regional anesthesia is often touted as beneficial in many patients who have pulmonary, cardiac, renal, and other disease. However, the physiologic changes that occur with various regional anesthesia techniques must be understood and viewed within the context of an individual patient's pathophysiology so that the technique benefits the patient fully and reduces the risk of complications from the patient' disease. This chapter focuses on the pathophysiology of several common systemic diseases frequently encountered by the regional anesthesiologist and discusses the interplay between common regional anesthesia techniques and patient disease.

PULMONARY DISEASE

Surgical patients with coexisting pulmonary impairment are at risk for intraoperative or postoperative pulmonary complications, regardless of anesthetic technique.[1] However, increasing evidence suggests that regional anesthesia may be associated with improved pulmonary outcomes compared with those associated with general anesthesia.[2–4] A thorough understanding of respiratory physiology and the implications of regional anesthetic techniques is crucial to the safe and effective use of regional anesthesia in these patients.

Epidural & Spinal Anesthesia

Most of the pulmonary effects of neuraxial anesthesia are due to motor block of the intercostal and abdominal musculature. If a significant systemic uptake of local anesthetic occurs, some central and direct myoneural respiratory depression can also be seen, although this plays a minor role overall.[5] Since neuraxial anesthesia produces a "differential" blockade of motor, sensory, and autonomic fibers, the degree to which respiratory function is impaired depends on the relative extent of segmental motor blockade. Using dilute concentrations of epidural local anesthetic may provide adequate sensory block as high as the cervical levels, while sparing the motor function of the respiratory muscles in the lower somatic segments.[6] Achieving diaphragmatic paralysis via a phrenic nerve (C3 through C5) block in the absence of a total spinal anesthesia is difficult in practice, since even a sensory block as high as C3 will only produce a motor block at approximately T1 through T3.[5] However, high neuraxial blocks may precipitate hypotension sufficient to decrease blood flow to the respiratory center in the medulla, leading to respiratory arrest.

With **higher levels of epidural** or **spinal anesthesia**, chest wall musculature, and in particular the intercostal muscles, become segmentally weakened and contribute less to the respiratory effort. This in turn, may eventually lead to altered chest wall motion during spontaneous respiration. For instance, some studies have suggested that during high neuraxial anesthesia, the more compliant chest wall is retracted during inspiration and may actually display paradoxical rib cage motion.[7,8] Others, however, have found that epidural blockade to sensory levels of T6 or even T1 do not lead to rib cage constriction with inspiration and may in fact increase the contribution that chest wall expansion makes to tidal volume.[9,10] This may be explained by an incomplete motor block of high, intercostal muscles or the compensatory role played by the "accessory" muscles of respiration such as the anterior and middle scalene muscles.[11]

Lumbar epidural anesthesia does not impair resting minute ventilation, tidal volume, or respiratory rate.[12–14] Furthermore, functional residual capacity (FRC) and closing capacity appear to be relatively unchanged during lumbar epidural anesthesia.[15–17] Effort-dependent tests of respiratory function, such as forced expiratory volume in one second (FEV$_1$), forced vital capacity, and peak expiratory flow rate, do exhibit modest decreases in the setting of lumbar epidural blockade, reflecting the reliance of these indices on intercostal and abdominal musculature.[18] In contrast, the effect of thoracic epidural anesthesia on pulmonary mechanics is less clear, with studies showing both a decrease[14,19] and increase[20] in minute ventilation and tidal volumes. One volunteer study found that high thoracic epidural anesthesia (T1 sensory level) led to an increase in FRC of approximately 15% with no change in tidal volume or respiratory rate.[10] This somewhat surprising finding may be explained by two mechanisms offered by the investigators. First, most volunteers exhibited a decrease in their intrathoracic blood volume, a physiologic occurrence confirmed by Arndt and colleagues.[21] Second, the study also found that the end-expiratory position of the diaphragm was shifted caudally, which is possibly related to a relative increase in diaphragmatic tonic activity or a reduction in intraabdominal pressure. Thoracic epidural anesthesia results in a modest decrease in vital capacity (VC), FEV$_1$, total lung capacity, and maximal midexpiratory flow rate.[15]

The ventilatory response to hypercarbia and hypoxia is preserved with neuraxial anesthesia.[9,14] Partial pressures of both oxygen (Po$_2$) and carbon dioxide (Pco) are essentially unchanged during epidural or spinal anesthesia.[9,10] In addition, bronchomotor tone is not altered to any significant degree, despite theoretical concerns of bronchoconstriction secondary to sympatholysis.[21] Indeed, epidural anesthesia has been used successfully for high-risk patients with chronic obstructive pulmonary disease and asthma undergoing abdominal operations.[22,23]

Neuraxial anesthesia has been shown in a number of settings to lead to reduced postoperative pulmonary complications compared with general anesthesia. The reasons behind this are probably multifactorial, owing in part to superior analgesia, reduced diaphragmatic impairment, altered stress response, and a decreased incidence of postoperative hypoxemia.[24,25] Epidural anesthesia provides better pain control than general anesthesia for abdominal and thoracic surgery, which leads to reduced splinting, a more effective cough mechanism, and preserved postoperative lung volumes, including FRC and VC.[26] One study directly comparing epidural and general anesthesia in high-risk patients concluded that overall outcomes, including the need for prolonged postoperative ventilation, were improved with the regional technique.[27] Another trial in patients undergoing lower limb vascular surgery reported a greater than 50% reduction in the incidence of respiratory failure in the group randomized to epidural anesthesia.[28] A more recent meta-analysis of 141 randomized trials (including over 9000 patients) comparing regional and general anesthesia for hip surgery showed a risk reduction for pulmonary embolism, pneumonia, and respiratory depression of 55%, 39%, and 59%, respectively, with the regional anesthesia.[29] Interestingly, these outcomes were unchanged regardless of whether neuraxial anesthesia was continued into the postoperative period, illustrating that the beneficial effect of epidural and spinal anesthesia on pulmonary physiology occurs, at least in part, at the time of surgical insult.

Brachial Plexus Block

In the absence of inadvertent complications such as pneumothorax, alterations in respiratory mechanics seen with brachial plexus block are due primarily to phrenic nerve blockade and hemidiaphragmatic paralysis. This has been shown to occur in 100% of patients receiving interscalene blockade,[29] and leads to a reduction by 27% in both FVC and FEV_1.[30] While the clinical significance of this reduction in healthy patients is not entirely clear, it may be useful to risk-stratify patients about to undergo interscalene blocks as one would a patient undergoing lung resection. In other words, ask the question: "Will this patient tolerate a perioperative FEV_1 reduction of 27%?" Some investigators have attempted to reduce the incidence of phrenic nerve palsy by decreasing the volume of local anesthetic; however, volumes as little as 10–20 mL still result in diaphragmatic paralysis.[31,32] In fact, one case report illustrated clinically significant respiratory compromise requiring tracheal intubation following an interscalene block using a volume of 3 mL of 2% mepivacaine.[33]

Clinical Pearls

- Interscalene brachial plexus block causes phrenic nerve paralysis in 100% of cases and reduces FVC and FEV_1 by 27%.
- The clinical significance of this finding in healthy patients is probably negligible.

The risk of phrenic nerve blockade decreases as one moves more distally along the plexus. Axillary nerve block has no effect on diaphragm function and presents a good choice for those patients with marginal pulmonary reserve (ie, cannot tolerate a 27% reduction in lung function). On the other hand, the supraclavicular block is associated with a 50–67% incidence of hemidiaphragm paralysis.[34–36] The infraclavicular approach is probably sufficiently distant from the course of the phrenic nerve so as to spare the diaphragm,[37,38] although there are case reports of phrenic nerve involvement.[39] These discrepancies probably relate to the different approaches to the infraclavicular block—for instance the "coracoid block" is performed with a relatively lateral or distal puncture site, whereas the vertical infraclavicular block begins at a more medial location. Although the infraclavicular or axillary blocks may be desirable for their relative pulmonary-sparing profiles, they carry the disadvantage of providing incomplete anesthesia for the upper arm and shoulder. However, creative solutions have been employed to get around this issue. Martinez and coworkers combined an infraclavicular block with a suprascapular nerve block for emergent humeral head surgery in a patient who was acutely asthmatic and had a baseline FEV_1 of 1.13 L (32% predicted). Therefore, a knowledgeable combination of peripheral nerve blocks can provide complete anesthesia of the upper limb while avoiding respiratory complications in patient with a pulmonary disease.[40]

Continuous brachial plexus blocks with perineural catheters are an attractive method of maintaining the advantages of plexus blockade into the postoperative period and have been shown to reduce postoperative pain, oral opioid requirements and their side effects, and sleep disturbances after shoulder surgery.[41] However, there have been reports of complications attributed to the prolonged phrenic nerve paresis that invariably occurs with this technique. These have included chest pain, atelectasis, pleural effusion, and dyspnea.[42,43] This is of particular concern because many patients are being discharged home with catheters and may not have access to timely intervention should these complications arise. On the other hand, the degree of clinically significant respiratory impairment with continuous interscalene blockade varies among patients and, in fact, may be well tolerated, especially if using relatively dilute concentrations of local anesthetic that only provide a partial phrenic paresis.[44]

Clinical Pearls

- Phrenic paresis in patients with good respiratory function is questionable.
- Regardless, the use of continuous brachial plexus techniques should be carefully considered in patients with preexisting significant pulmonary disease.

Maurer and associates reported a case of a patient with no preexisting pulmonary disease who underwent bilateral shoulder arthroplasty under combined bilateral continuous interscalene blockade and general anesthesia.[45] Postoperative analgesia was maintained in the hospital for 72 h via the catheters using infusions of 7 mL/h of 0.2% ropivacaine for each side (total 14 mL/h). Despite a marked postoperative reduction in FVC (60%) from baseline as well as sonographic evidence of diaphragmatic impairment, the patient had an uneventful postoperative course (with excellent analgesia) and good recovery. This anecdotal example illustrates that the clinical significance of phrenic paresis in patients with good respiratory function is questionable. Regardless the use of continuous brachial plexus techniques should be carefully considered in patients with preexisting pulmonary disease, especially if they are to be discharged home with the catheters in situ.

Paravertebral & Intercostal Nerve Blocks

Several studies investigated the effects of paravertebral and intercostal blocks on pulmonary function in patients with rib fractures or those undergoing thoracotomy. Intercostal blockade has been shown to improve arterial oxygen saturation (Sao_2) and peak expiratory flow rate (PEFR) in patients with traumatic rib fractures associated with severe pain.[46] Likewise, Karmakar and investigators found that continuous paravertebral blockade over a period of 4 days in patients with multiple fractured ribs led to significant improvement in respiratory rate, FVC, PEFR, Sao_2, and the Pao_2 fraction of inspired oxygen ratio.[47] These findings are probably related to the favorable effect of analgesia on respiratory efforts by the patient and improved respiratory mechanics.

Paravertebral blocks are very effective for management of pain following thoracotomy and can significantly improve postoperative spirometry. One review of 55 randomized, controlled trials of analgesic techniques following posterolateral thoracotomy revealed that paravertebral blockade was the method that best preserved pulmonary function compared with either intercostal or epidural analgesia.[48] The combined results showed an average preservation of approximately 75% of preoperative pulmonary function when paravertebral analgesia was used versus 55% for both intercostal and epidural analgesia. It is unclear why paravertebral blockade might result in improved PEFR and Sao$_2$ compared with epidural analgesia in this and other studies, but it may be related to increased utilization of opioids, higher incidence of nausea and vomiting, and the presence of **bilateral** intercostal muscle blockade (and therefore diminished chest wall mobility) in the epidural cohorts.[49]

Clinical Pearls

- Paravertebral or intercostal blockade provides excellent analgesia following both rib fractures and thoracotomy.
- These blocks also result in improved spirometry and pulmonary outcomes.

Pulmonary Complications Not Related to Conduction Blockade

Pulmonary complications related to the use of regional anesthetic techniques fall into two categories. The first is those related directly or indirectly to the physiologic changes that occur with the blockade itself. Examples include atelectasis and pneumonia resulting from an inability to mobilize secretions. The second category comprises those that are independent of the effect of blockade, and although there are sporadic reports of rare complications such as pulmonary hemorrhage[50] and chylothorax,[51] the most common of these is pneumothorax. Not surprisingly, pneumothoraces occur most frequently when the puncture site overlies the pleura, and especially when performing supraclavicular and intercostal blocks. The overall incidence is low, however,[52–55] and refinements of previously published techniques based on MRI studies and ultrasound guidance can decrease the incidence further.[56,57] Nevertheless, techniques with a risk of pneumothorax should be carefully considered or avoided in patients with borderline pulmonary function.

RENAL DISEASE

Renal dysfunction is commonly present in the surgical population. Perioperative renal failure accounts for approximately 50% of all patients requiring acute hemodialysis in the United States. Patients with chronic renal insufficiency frequently present for procedures, such as creation of vascular shunts and revascularization of the lower limbs. Regional anesthetic techniques are frequently ideal options to provide anesthesia for these patients and procedures.

Effect of Regional Anesthesia on Renal Function

The treatment of patients at risk for perioperative renal dysfunction should focus on two principles: avoiding nephrotoxic agents and maintaining kidney perfusion. Local anesthetics do not possess any nephrotoxic properties per se, and in fact the coadministration of procaine has been shown to mitigate some of the nephrotoxic effects of cisplatin in rats.[58] Of greater relevance is the effect of anesthetic-induced hypotension on renal blood flow. The kidneys are capable of autoregulation over a wide variety of mean arterial pressures (approximately 80–180 mm Hg) and maintain glomerular filtration rate (GFR) by autonomous changes in renal vascular resistance.[59] Below the so-called lower limit of autoregulation, the kidney begins to shut down its energy-dependent physiologic processes, and the GFR and urinary output fall as a result. Ultimately, if left unchecked, renal ischemia develops, especially in the sensitive renal medulla. Although neuraxial anesthesia and the concurrent sympathectomy can reduce mean arterial pressure (MAP), renal blood flow is often preserved.[60] This is believed to reflect an increase in left ventricular stroke volume in response to the drop in systemic vascular resistance (SVR). Rooke and investigators studied hemodynamic responses and abdominal organ perfusion (as measured by scintigraphy) in 15 patients undergoing lidocaine spinal anesthesia with a sensory block ranging from T1 to T10.[61] Whereas the MAP and SVR fell on average by 33% and 26%, respectively, blood volume in the kidneys increased by approximately 10%. There may be limits to the degree of compensation afforded by cardiac output, however. One study using a primate model showed that although renal blood flow was minimally affected by T10 spinal anesthesia, it was significantly reduced by a T1 sensory block.[62] This illustrates again that lumbar and low thoracic levels of neuraxial anesthesia in patients with renal disease are well tolerated physiologically and significant changes do not begin to manifest until higher levels are achieved.

Clinical Pearl

- Lumbar and low-thoracic levels of neuraxial anesthesia do not exhibit a significant effect on renal hemodynamics.

The renin–angiotensin system, which is initiated in the kidney in response to a reduction in renal perfusion, plays an important role in blood pressure homeostasis. It serves as a complementary humoral mechanism to the sympathetic nervous systems. Hopf and colleagues conducted a study to determine if thoracic epidural anesthesia suppressed the renin response to induced hypotension.[63] Plasma renin and vasopressin concentrations were measured before, during, and after a hypotensive challenge with nitroprusside in patients with and without thoracic epidural anesthesia (sensory level T1 through T11). With an intact sympathetic nervous system (ie, no epidural), plasma renin levels doubled in response to the hypotensive challenge lasting 15 min. In contrast, there was no change in the renin concentration when hypotension was induced to the same MAP in the epidural cohort. This suggests that sympathetic fibers play a key role in the renin–angiotensin system and that thoracic epidural anesthesia interferes with the functional integrity of that system.

For obvious reasons, postoperative renal function is of foremost concern when administering anesthesia for recipients of renal transplantation. Several studies have looked at the effect of general versus regional (or combined epidural/general) anesthesia on postoperative renal function in this setting. The choice of anesthetic technique was not shown to have an effect on graft outcome in either adult or pediatric populations.[64,65] Also, the choice of anesthetic technique for living donors was shown to be independent of recipient graft outcome.[66] Other nontransplant outcomes data, including those from the large meta-analysis by Rodgers and coworkers, indicate that regional anesthesia is associated with a lower risk for postoperative renal failure than general anesthesia. However, the authors cautioned that the confidence intervals were wide and were compatible with both no effect and a two-thirds risk reduction.[25] Overall, it appears that a well-conducted regional anesthetic does not negatively affect perioperative kidney function and renal outcome compared with general anesthesia.

Considerations for Regional Anesthesia in Chronic Renal Failure

Patients with chronic renal failure often manifest a large number of pathophysiologic changes that may influence regional anesthetic care. These may include the presence of an anion-gap metabolic acidosis, electrolyte disturbances such as hyperkalemia, and coagulopathies due to uremia-induced platelet dysfunction. Plasma concentrations of local anesthetic following peripheral nerve blocks are often high enough to cause central nervous system or cardiac toxicity in any patient, even when no obvious intravascular injection has occurred. This is probably related to the large dose used when performing "high-volume blocks" such as brachial plexus blocks. Some authors have recommended that dosages be adjusted in patients with chronic renal insufficiency based on observations of toxicity presumed to be related to concurrent acidosis or hyperkalemia.[67,68] Indeed, experimental evidence suggests that acidemia decreases the protein binding of bupivacaine, thereby increasing the free fraction and risk of toxicity.[69] In addition, hyperkalemia (5.4 vs 2.7 mEq/L) has been shown in dogs to *halve* the dose of bupivacaine required to induce cardiotoxicity.[70] Interestingly, the potassium level had no effect on seizure dose in the same animals. This is an ominous finding, as it suggests that the so-called safety margin of plasma levels between CNS and cardiac toxicity, which is already relatively narrow with bupivacaine, is even less re-

liable in the presence of hyperkalemia. Even in the absence of acid–base or electrolyte disturbances, plasma levels of local anesthetics following peripheral nerve block are often higher in patients with chronic renal failure.[71,72] The reason for this is not entirely clear, but may relate to increased blood flow (and hence uptake at the injection site) due to the hyperdynamic circulation often seen in uremic patients.[73] On the other hand, α_1-acid glycoprotein (AAG) levels are increased in uremia[74] and may lend a protective effect by binding more local anesthetic in the bloodstream.[75] The increased levels of AAG also result in both a reduced free fraction available for hepatic metabolism and in a reduced volume of distribution. These two pharmacokinetic consequences appear to balance each other so that the serum half-life is not significantly changed.[71] Hemodialysis is ineffective in removing lidocaine from plasma, and therefore cannot be relied on to treat toxicity.[76]

Clinical Pearls

- Acidemia decreases the protein binding of bupivacaine, thereby increasing the free fraction and the risk of toxicity.
- Patients with uremia often exhibit higher plasma levels of local anesthetic following peripheral nerve block.

No significant difference exists between patients with chronic renal failure and healthy patients with respect to peripheral nerve block latency, duration, or quality.[71,77,78] In one study of spinal anesthesia properties in patients with chronic renal failure versus healthy patients, Orko and associates found that block quality was similar, but that both onset time and duration of the block were reduced in the patients with uremia.[79] The authors postulated a volume-contracted intrathecal space in uremic patients as a mechanism for the quicker onset, but the actual cause remains speculative. The shorter duration of sensory block may again be related to enhanced uptake in the setting of a hyperdynamic circulation.

Uremic coagulopathy is characterized by a defect of platelet aggregation that is probably due to a toxic effect by uremic substances on the binding of fibrinogen to the platelet glycoprotein IIb/IIIa receptor.[80] This often manifests in clinically appreciable bleeding, and at least one case of subarachnoid hematoma leading to paraplegia after a spinal anesthetic in a chronic renal failure patient has been published.[81] Patients undergoing hemodialysis require intermittent anticoagulation and may present to the operating room with an unclear coagulation status. Care must be taken to delineate heparin or other anticoagulant regimens. Despite this platelet dysfunction, uremic patients are at higher risk for thrombotic events.[82] One case of hypoxia following a brachial plexus block in a uremic patient was later found to be secondary to pulmonary embolism.[83] The authors of the report suggested that a likely mechanism was dislodgement of a preexisting thrombus from the proximal arm, facilitated by block-related manipulation and vasodilation of the upper extremity.

Several studies have compared anesthetic techniques for the creation of arteriovenous fistulae, a procedure that is common in patients with end-stage renal disease and is well suited to brachial plexus block.[84] Although some investigators have concluded that little difference exists in outcome between general, local, and brachial plexus anesthesia for this operation,[85] Mouquet and colleagues specifically studied the effects of these three techniques on brachial artery blood flow and concluded that both general anesthesia and brachial plexus block improved blood flow through the fistula during surgery, whereas local infiltration did not.[86]

HEPATIC DISEASE

Liver injury or dysfunction can range from a mild, asymptomatic "transaminitis" to frank hepatic failure. There are many causes of liver disease, both acquired and congenital, but all manifest as either failure of parenchymal cell function (ie, acute and chronic hepatitis, cirrhosis) or cholestasis.[87] Considerations for regional anesthesia in patients with liver disease include the potential for altered disposition and metabolism of local anesthetics, the effect of regional anesthesia on hepatic perfusion, and concerns regarding coagulopathy related to liver dysfunction.

Pharmacokinetics of Local Anesthetics in Liver Disease

Amide local anesthetics are metabolized in liver microsomes by the cytochrome P-450 system.[88] A decrease in microsomal function, as may be seen in acute or chronic liver disease, can lead to a reduction in biotransformation and clearance of these drugs, putting the patient at risk for local anesthetic toxicity. As with other drugs that are metabolized in the liver, the hepatic extraction ratio determines the relative importance of hepatic perfusion versus intrinsic enzyme activity in the overall clearance of the drug. For example, bupivacaine has a low extraction ratio (ie, its clearance is more sensitive to alterations in hepatic enzyme activity), whereas etidocaine exhibits a relatively high extraction ratio and depends on adequate liver perfusion for clearance.[89] Lidocaine has an intermediate hepatic extraction ratio and therefore relies on both perfusion and enzymatic activity. Severe hepatic disease such as cirrhosis can affect both liver perfusion and intrinsic enzyme function. In this scenario, the clearance of all amide local anesthetics, regardless of their extraction ratio, is likely to be reduced. Because the volume of distribution of local anesthetics (and many other drugs) is increased in hepatic disease, the actual plasma levels may not differ significantly from healthy patients with a single dose, despite the diminished clearance.[90–92] The altered distribution may be related to decreased levels of plasma AAG, which are reduced in proportion to the severity of liver disease.[93] Clinically, it appears that single-dose peripheral nerve blocks with amide local anesthetics probably do not require a dosage adjustment in this population, whereas continuous infusions have the potential to accumulate to toxic levels.[94]

The cytochrome P-450 enzyme system is subject to induction or inhibition by a variety of drugs and dietary nutrients. This may play a role in the subsequent metabolism of amide local anesthetics. For example, substances that inhibit microsomal enzymes, such as cimetidine or grapefruit juice, may lead to an accumulation of local anesthetic, augmenting the risk of toxicity, especially in the setting of preexisting hepatic dysfunction.[95]

Ester local anesthetics are cleared by plasma cholinesterases in the blood and liver. Severe hepatic disease may result in decreased levels of cholinesterase and result in prolonged plasma half-lives of esters such as procaine.[96] On the other hand, red cell esterases remain intact during liver disease and are able to provide some hydrolytic function.[97] Because plasma cholinesterase is extremely efficient, it is unlikely that an enzyme deficiency secondary to hepatic disease could impair the hydrolysis of ester-type local anesthetics to a degree sufficient to cause toxicity.[89]

Effect of Regional Anesthesia on Hepatic Blood Flow

The hepatic blood supply is unique in that it relies on both portal venous return and hepatic artery blood flow, which make up approximately 75% and 25% of the total flow, respectively. The regulation of hepatic blood flow is complex. The portal system is passive and not subject to autoregulation, whereas the hepatic artery can increase or decrease its contribution to flow in response to alterations in portal venous flow.[98] The hepatic artery also autoregulates in response to MAP, in much the same way as cerebral or renal vessels do, but may rely on an intact sympathetic response for effect.[99]

General anesthesia has been shown to cause a decrease in hepatic blood flow, which may lead to ischemia and postoperative liver dysfunction.[100] Less is known about the effects of regional anesthesia on hepatic perfusion. Grietz and coworkers performed a high epidural (block level T1 through T4) in 16 dogs and examined the effect on systemic and hepatic hemodynamics.[101] MAP and portal venous flow were both reduced compared with control values, by 52% and 26%, respectively. In contrast, hepatic artery flow was unchanged, probably relating to a reduction in hepatic artery resistance of 51%. In addition, hepatic oxygen uptake was preserved through an increased oxygen extraction. Another study by Vagts and colleagues found that thoracic epidural anesthesia

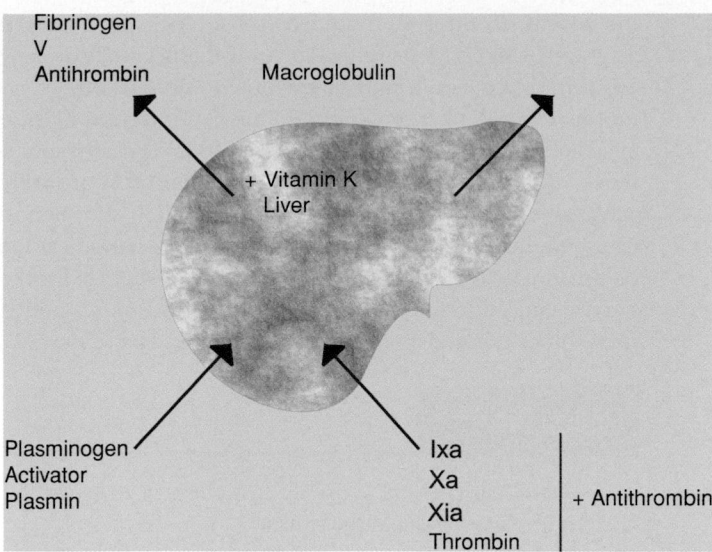

Figure 58–1. The central role of the liver in coagulation.

in anesthetized pigs was associated with decreased mean arterial blood pressure and hepatic artery blood flow, but no change in hepatic oxygen delivery or uptake, or tissue oxygen partial pressure compared with pigs receiving general anesthesia alone.[102] Taken together, these findings should reassure the clinician that high neuraxial anesthesia may be well tolerated with respect to hepatic oxygenation, despite a modest reduction in MAP. Care should be taken to maintain cardiac output and perfusion pressure during anesthesia to ensure the adequate perfusion of *all* the vital organs.

Hepatic Coagulopathy

Severe hepatic disease is associated with abnormalities of the coagulation system. The cause is multifactorial and may include the decreased synthesis of procoagulant proteins, impaired clearance of activated coagulation factors, nutritional deficiency (eg, vitamin K, folate), the synthesis of functionally abnormal fibrinogen, splenomegaly secondary to portal hypertension (sequestrational thrombocytopenia), qualitative platelet defects, and bone marrow suppression of thrombopoiesis (eg, by alcohol, hepatitis virus infection) (Figure 58–1).[103] Because of the potential complexity of the coagulopathy, it may be necessary to perform additional laboratory tests such as clotting factor and fibrinogen assays to completely delineate the nature of the problem. Clotting factor deficiencies can be treated with vitamin K supplementation or fresh frozen plasma transfusion or both. Platelet transfusion may be necessary in the case of thrombocytopenia. Newer therapies such as recombinant factor VIIa have also been used to correct bleeding associated with liver failure.[104] Because the vitamin K–dependent clotting factors are more susceptible to hepatocellular disease, the prothrombin time (PT) and international normalized ratio (INR) are often used as markers of coagulation system integrity. However, the predictive value of PT/INR on hemorrhage during bedside procedures such as lumbar puncture or central line placement has been shown to be poor.[105] As such, it is important to carefully weigh

the risks and benefits of a neuraxial anesthetic technique in a patient with suspected hepatic-induced coagulopathy. Although an INR of less than 1.5 "should be associated with normal hemostasis" according to the ASRA consensus guidelines on anticoagulation,[106] this statement applies primarily to warfarin-induced anticoagulation and may not be a reliable indicator of the likelihood of problematic bleeding in liver failure. The risks associated with performing peripheral nerve blocks in patients with abnormal coagulation parameters is less clear. Obviously the risk of bleeding is increased with techniques in which the needle is laced in the vicinity to a major blood vessel. Deep blocks, such as the sciatic nerve block, should probably be avoided in a coagulopathic patient due to the risk of deep muscular hemorrhage. Likewise, care should be taken when performing blocks in the vicinity of noncompressible blood vessels (ie, the subclavian artery in the case of supraclavicular block) in patients who have coagulation abnormality. The risks of regional anesthesia in the setting of a coagulable disorder are elaborated in Chapter 7.

Clinical Pearl

- Deep blocks, such as anterior sciatic or lumbar plexus blocks, should be practiced with special care in patients who are coagulopathic. Similarly, blocks in the vicinity of noncompressible blood vessels such as the subclavian artery should be carefully considered.

DIABETES MELLITUS

Diabetes is a multisystem disease characterized by carbohydrate intolerance and insulin dysregulation that has many implications for the regional anesthesiologist.[107] Besides the usual anesthetic concerns such as the presence of coronary artery, cerebrovascular, and renal disease, diabetics have a high incidence of preexisting peripheral neuropathy, which has implications for block performance, success, and risk for neurologic complications. Other considerations are the effect of regional anesthesia on glucose homeostasis and the increased risk of infection in diabetic patients.

Peripheral Neuropathy in Diabetics

Diabetic neuropathy is one of the most common neurologic diseases, affecting up to 100% of patients with long-standing disease.[108] Patients can be asymptomatic, but in affected patients symptoms are typically described as paresthesias, sensory loss, or neuropathic pain. The mechanism of diabetic neuropathy is thought to be related to either a direct metabolic and osmotic effect of chronic hyperglycemia on neurons or a microvascular insult leading to nerve ischemia.[109]

Performing nerve blocks on diseased nerves has been a source of concern. Kalichman and Calcutt studied sciatic nerve histology in rats following blockade with lidocaine and found significantly more nerve edema in diabetic versus control cohorts.[110] The reason for the edema is probably multifactorial and may include the presence of an altered blood–nerve barrier or decreased uptake of local anesthetic, leading to a longer duration of nerve bathing. An increase in endoneural fluid pressure due to edema may constrict small transperineural vessels, precipitating ischemia in an already compromised nerve. This may translate to an increased incidence of postoperative paresthesias following nerve blocks, including neuraxial blocks, in diabetics. Al-Nasser reported a case of a prolonged (>8 weeks) bilateral lower limb paresthesias and pain following lumbar epidural analgesia with 0.2% ropivacaine in a diabetic patient undergoing radical prostatectomy.[111] Postoperative electromyographic studies showed widespread sensory neuropathy of both upper and lower limbs, indicating that the patient, although asymptomatic, had preexisting neuropathy that may have predisposed to this rare complication. The actual prevalence of neurologic complications in diabetics receiving nerve blocks is unknown, but is probably quite low. Diabetes is a common disease, and reports of this complication in the literature are sparse, suggesting that in the vast majority of cases, recovery from peripheral nerve blocks is uneventful.

A perhaps more practical issue for regional anesthesiologists is the effect of diabetic neuropathy on electrolocation of nerves while using a nerve stimulator. Diabetic patients may have altered response to nerve localization. In one case report, authors were unable to elicit motor response in a patient with diabetes even with current intensity as high as 2.5–5 mA.[112] Indeed, nerve conduction studies in diabetics with neuropathy consistently show a reduction in conduction velocity and amplitude, for both motor and sensory nerves, which may help explain this phenomenon.[113] However, in our tertiary center where we perform nearly all foot and amputation surgery exclusively under lower extremity nerve blocks, the overwhelming majority of patients still have a normal response to nerve stimulation, and low current stimulation (0.5 mA) is almost always obtained even in patients with overt diabetic neuropathy. Nevertheless, with

the advent of ultrasound-guided nerve blocks, it has been shown that in certain circumstances if the needle is directly adjacent to a nerve, it may be possible to obtain little or no motor response to stimulation, even when injection of local anesthetic through that needle results in a clinically sound block.[114] For these reasons, in this population it is probably acceptable to inject local anesthetic even when stimulation cannot be obtained with currents <0.5–0.7 mA as long as the obtained motor response is well defined and specific for the nerve being blocked. Where applicable, ultrasound-guided nerve blocks should also be beneficial in these patients.

Clinical Pearls

- Diabetic patients are prone to a metabolic neuropathy that impairs nerve conduction.
- Stimulating current of greater intensity is occasionally needed to obtain visible muscle twitches when using a nerve stimulator to electrolocate nerves.

Effect of Regional Anesthesia on Glucose Homeostasis

It is well known that surgery performed in combination with general anesthesia provokes a counterregulatory response that significantly increases plasma levels of glucose, as well as levels of cortisol and catecholamines. This so-called stress response has long been considered a homeostatic defense mechanism that is important in an organism's adaptation to harmful stimuli. However, recent evidence has suggested that the avoidance or even treatment of hyperglycemic states in the perioperative and critical care settings can lead to improved morbidity and mortality rates. For example, Van Den Berghe and coworkers randomized over 1500 critically ill surgical patients to receive either aggressive (goal blood glucose 80–110 mg/dL) or standard (goal blood glucose 180–200 mg/dL) insulin therapy while in the intensive care unit.[115] At 12 months, the mortality rate with aggressive therapy was markedly reduced from 8.0% to 4.6%. These outcomes data were supported in a similar study by Krinsley involving a heterogeneous group of critically ill patients, both surgical and medical.[116] Cardiac surgical patients have been shown to have a 30% higher risk of an adverse outcome (including cardiac, neurologic, pulmonary, infectious, or death) when intraoperative mean glucose levels are 20 mg/dL higher than those in controls.[117] The exact mechanism by which tight glycemic control improves outcomes in these populations is unclear, but may involve decreased hepatic glucose production, positive influences on immune function with alteration in inflammatory cytokines, or enhanced glucose transport to intracellular sites.[118]

Regional anesthesia has been shown to ameliorate the hyperglycemic response to surgery and therefore may play a role in this protective phenomenon. An intraoperative glucose tolerance test resulted in markedly elevated plasma glucose levels in patients receiving general versus epidural anesthesia for such procedures as inguinal herniorrhaphy and hysterectomy.[119-120] Likewise, abdominal hysterectomy performed under spinal anesthesia is associated with lower intra- and postoperative glucose levels compared with those for neurolept anesthesia.[121] Retrobulbar block reduces the hyperglycemic stress response to both cataract[122] and scleral buckle[123] surgery.

Glucose homeostasis is rather complex and several factors likely contribute to the salutary action of regional anesthesia on glycemic control. These may include the inhibition of hepatic gluconeogenesis, as well as the inhibition of catecholamine and cortisol responses to surgery.[124] In addition, the "absence of general anesthesia" may be a causative factor in glycemic control, as volatile agents such as halothane and enflurane have been shown to impair glucose tolerance in dogs.[125] It seems clear from the available data that to improve outcomes from major surgery anesthesiologists must prevent as much nociceptive input from reaching the central nervous and neuroendocrine system as possible.[126] The use of regional anesthesia can easily facilitate this and may be especially pertinent for "brittle" diabetics in whom tight glycemic control is difficult at the best of times.

Clinical Pearls

- "Tight" perioperative glycemic control is associated with better outcomes.
- Regional anesthesia blocks nociceptive input from reaching the central nervous system and helps prevent the usual hyperglycemic response to surgery.

THYROID NEUROPATHY

Diabetes and uremia are the most common metabolic neuropathies; however, several other less common causes have implications for the regional anesthesiologist. These include those neuropathies that result from the use of certain medications; exposure to toxins; and those related to connective tissue, autoimmune, and vascular diseases.[127] One of the most prevalent causes of metabolic neuropathy is that associated with overt hypothyroidism. Thyroid neuropathy is a largely sensory phenomenon that is poorly understood, but is present in approximately 40% of patients diagnosed with hypothyroidism.[128] It is most obvious in frank myxedema, but nerve conduction studies have shown evidence of velocity impairment in subclinical hypothyroidism.[129] Thyroid neuropathy is most likely to present as peripheral nerve entrapment, particularly the median nerve, and these patients are frequently referred for carpal tunnel decompression.[130] Entrapment of the eighth cranial nerve leading to deafness is also not uncommon. Patients may complain of dysesthesias in a glove-and-stocking pattern, as well as lancinating pains suggestive of nerve root compression. "Hung" deep tendon reflexes (brisk reflex response with a delayed return to normal

tone) are a hallmark of hypothyroidism and probably relate to both neuropathy and myopathy. Pathologically, affected nerves exhibit mucinous deposition and, in advanced cases, segmental demyelination with loss of large myelinated nerve fibers.[131]

Little data exist on the effect preexisting thyroid neuropathy may have on the management of regional anesthesia in this population. It may be reasonable to predict that electrolocation responses may be diminished, as is seen in diabetes, resulting in an inability to elicit twitches at desired levels (eg, 0.3–0.4 mA) of current, although no direct data support this. Another potential consequence of performing regional anesthesia in patients with nerve entrapment is what has been termed the "double-crush syndrome."[132] This refers to the enhanced susceptibility of nerves to injury or impairment at one anatomic location, when already compressed or otherwise injured at another, separate location. A classic example is the patient with symptoms of carpal tunnel syndrome after seemingly minor trauma or injury to the median nerve, who is later found to have compression of the C6 nerve root. Although originally described in terms of mechanical injury, it has been recognized that metabolic and pharmacologic factors can contribute to the double-crush syndrome,[133] including hypothyroidism. Thus, it may be that patients with thyroid neuropathy are at increased risk for neurologic injury when receiving regional anesthesia blocks, as minor needle trauma to a susceptible nerve may produce functional neurologic deficits. Although this remains speculative at present, it reinforces the need for a detailed history and documentation of preexisting neurologic deficit in patients with hypothyroidism and the careful consideration of techniques in these patients. Finally, if suspected, thyroid neuropathy has been shown to be correctable in many cases by prompt treatment with thyroid replacement therapy, which may allow for some degree of risk reduction from this complication.[134,135]

OBESITY

Obesity is an increasingly prevalent problem worldwide. Between 1980 and 2000 in the United States, obesity rates doubled for adults and children and tripled for adolescents.[136] In addition to the usual anesthetic considerations for morbidly obese patients, such as the presence of various cardiopulmonary, gastrointestinal, and endocrine comorbidities, the abundance of extra tissue can present a challenge to regional anesthesiologists. Obesity has been shown to impair the ability of anesthesiologists to correctly identify lumbar spinal interspaces.[137] Outcomes are similarly affected in overweight patients. In a study of over 9000 blocks at a single institution, patients with a body mass index (BMI) >30 kg/m^2 were 1.62 times more likely to experience a failed regional block than were those with a BMI >25 kg/m^2.[138] Not surprisingly, the investigators cited difficulty in landmark identification, patient positioning, and insufficient length of needle used as the main impediments to successful block placement. Despite this, regional anesthesia often remains an attractive option for obese patients, because it may reduce the incidence of cardiopulmonary and airway complications compared with those experienced during general anesthesia.

Clinical Pearls

- Obese patients are significantly more likely to experience a failed regional block than are slim patients.
- Reasons for this include loss of surface landmarks, difficulty in patient positioning, and the use of insufficiently long needles.

Several groups have sought to overcome the challenge of increased tissue mass with the use of novel radiologic techniques while performing regional blocks. Although fluoroscopy has been used extensively by interventional pain management physicians to increase the reliability and precision of various nerve blocks, its application in facilitating blocks for surgical anesthesia has been less practical. Nevertheless, fluoroscopy has been used in the placement of axillary brachial plexus catheters,[139] the performance of sciatic nerve blocks,[140] and as an aid in facilitating spinal anesthesia in morbidly obese patients.[141] However, its use is limited by the need to relate neural anatomy to structures that appear radiodense, such as bones, needles, or contrast-injected vessels.

Ultrasound is another promising technology that is being utilized with increasing frequency in regional anesthesia and that may aid the placement of peripheral and neuraxial blocks in the morbidly obese. Proponents of ultrasound-guided regional anesthesia cite the potential advantage of direct visualization of both the needle and the nerve structures,[142] which may be especially useful in obese patients with obscured surface landmarks. Studies conducted in obese parturients have verified the utility of ultrasound in identifying the epidural space and other spinal structures prior to introduction of an epidural needle.[143,144] One potential limitation of ultrasound-guided blocks in the obese is the penetration depth of the transducer, which becomes smaller as the frequency (and thus the resolution) increases. To date, little evidence has been published that directly addresses the use of ultrasound for regional anesthesia in the obese population.

Obesity may have an effect on the dosing of spinal medications, although the issue is somewhat controversial. A common notion is that increased abdominal mass leads to compression of intrathecal volume by engorgement of epidural plexuses, leading to an increased, and potentially dangerous, block height during spinal anesthesia. This is supported by data correlating block height with patient weight during standardized spinal anesthesia for cystoscopy.[145] Indeed, some authors have advocated the consideration of "low-dose" spinal anesthesia in the morbidly obese, due to wide variations in their dosing requirements. In one extremely overweight parturient (BMI = 66 kg/m^2), cesarean section was completed successfully with a 5-mg spinal dose of bupivacaine as the sole anesthetic agent.[146] However, patient weight does not necessarily correlate with degree of compression of the intrathecal sac, and many investigators have argued that weight alone is not a reliable predictor of block height during spinal anesthesia.[147–149] It is probably reasonable to approach the spinal dosing of obese patients with a degree of caution, and when practical, incrementally adjust the anesthetic dose.

References

1. Mitchell CK, Smoger SH, Pfiefer MP, et al: Multivariate analysis of factors associated with postoperative pulmonary complications following general elective surgery. Arch Surg 1998;133:194–198.
2. Cuschieri R, Morran C, Howie J, et al: Postoperative pain and pulmonary complications: Comparison of three analgesia regimens. Br J Surg 1985;72:495–498.
3. Ballantyne JC, Carr DB, deFerranti S, et al: The comparative effects of postoperative analgesic therapies on pulmonary outcome: Cumulative meta-analyses of randomized, controlled trials. Anesth Analg 1998;86:598–612.
4. Slinger P, Shennib H, Wilson S: Post-thoracotomy pulmonary function: A comparison of epidural versus intravenous meperidine infusions. J Cardiothorac Vasc Anesth 1995;9:128–134.
5. Cousins MJ, Veering BT: Epidural neural blockade. In Cousins MJ, Bridenbaugh PO (eds): *Neural Blockade in Clinical Anesthesia and Management of Pain*, 3 ed. Lippincott-Raven, 1998, pp 243–321.
6. Michalek P, David I, Adamec M, et al: Cervical epidural anesthesia for combined neck and upper extremity procedure: A pilot study. Anesth Analg 2004;99:1833–1836.
7. Eisele J, Trenchard D, Burki N, et al: The effect of chest wall block on respiratory sensation and control in man. Clin Sci 1968;35:23–33.
8. Kochi T, Sako S, Nishino T, et al: Effect of high thoracic extradural anaesthesia on ventilatory response to hypercapnia in normal volunteers. Br J Anaesth 1989;62:362–367.
9. Yamakage M, Namiki A, Tsuchida H, et al: Changes in ventilatory pattern and arterial oxygen saturation during spinal anaesthesia in man. Acta Anaesthesiol Scand 1992;36:569–571.
10. Warner DO, Warner MA, Ritman EL: Human chest wall function during epidural anesthesia. Anesthesiology 1996;85:761–773.
11. De Troyer A, Kelly S: Action of neck accessory muscles on rib cage in dogs. J Appl Physiol 1984;56:326–332.
12. Labaille T, Clergue F, Samii K, et al: Ventilatory responses to CO_2 following intravenous and epidural lidocaine. Anesthesiology 1985;63:179–183.
13. Sakura S, Saito Y, Kosaka Y: Effect of lumbar epidural anesthesia on ventilatory response to hypercapnia in young and elderly patients. J Clin Anesth 1993;5:109–113.
14. Sakura S, Saito Y, Kosaka Y: The effects of epidural anesthesia on ventilatory response to hypercapnia and hypoxia in elderly patients. Anesth Analg 1996;82:306–311.
15. McCarthy GS: The effect of thoracic extradural analgesia on pulmonary gas distribution, functional residual capacity and airway closure. Br J Anaesth 1976;48:243–247.
16. Lundh R, Hedenstierna G, Johansson H: Ventilation–perfusion relationships during epidural analgesia. Acta Anaesthesiol Scand 1983;27:410–416.
17. Reber A, Bein T, Högman M, et al: Lung aeration and pulmonary gas exchange during lumbar epidural anaesthesia and in the lithotomy position in elderly patients. Anaesthesia 1998;53:854–861.
18. Moir D. Ventilatory function during epidural analgesia. Br J Anaesth 1963;35:3–7.
19. Takasaki M, Takahashi T: Respiratory function during cervical and thoracic extradural analgesia in patients with normal lungs. Br J Anaesth 1980;52:1271–1276.
20. Gruber EM, Tschernko EM, Kritzinger M, et al: The effects of thoracic epidural analgesia with bupivacaine 0.25% on ventilatory mechanics in patients with severe chronic obstructive pulmonary disease. Anesth Analg 2001;92:1015–1019.

21. Arndt JO, Hock A, Stanton-Hicks M, et al: Peridural anesthesia and the distribution of blood in supine humans. Anesthesiology 1985;63:616–623.

22. Groeben H, Schafer B, Pavlakovic G, et al: Lung function under high thoracic segmental epidural anesthesia with ropivacaine or bupivacaine in patients with severe obstructive pulmonary disease undergoing breast surgery. Anesthesiology 2002;96:536–541.

23. Kolker AR, Hirsch CJ, Gingold BS, et al: Use of epidural anesthesia and spontaneous ventilation during transabdominal colon and rectal procedures in selected high-risk patient groups. Dis Colon Rectum 1997;40:339–343.

24. Liu S, Carpenter R, Neal J: Epidural anesthesia and analgesia: Their role in postoperative outcome. Anesthesiology 1995;82:1474–1506.

25. Rodgers A, Walker N, Schug S, et al: Reduction of postoperative mortality and morbidity with epidural or spinal anesthesia: Results from overview of randomized trials. BMJ 2000;321:1–12.

26. Wahba WM, Don HF, Craig DB: Post-operative epidural analgesia: Effects on lung volumes. Can Anaesth Soc J 1975;22:519–527.

27. Yeager MP, Glass DD, Neff RK, et al: Epidural anesthesia and analgesia in high-risk surgical patients. Anesthesiology 1987;66:729–736.

28. Christopherson R, Beattie C, Frank SM, et al: Perioperative morbidity in patients randomized to epidural or general anesthesia for lower extremity vascular surgery. Anesthesiology 1993;79:422–434.

29. Urmey WF, Talts KH, Sharrock NE: One hundred percent incidence of hemidiaphragmatic paresis associated with interscalene brachial plexus anesthesia as diagnosed by ultrasonography. Anesth Analg 1991;72:498–503.

30. Urmey WF, McDonald M: Hemidiaphragmatic paresis during interscalene brachial plexus block: Effects on pulmonary function and chest wall mechanics. Anesth Analg 1992;74:352–357.

31. Al-Kaisy AA, Chan VW, Perlas A: Respiratory effects of low-dose bupivacaine interscalene block. Br J Anaesth 1999;82:217–220.

32. Sala-Blanch X, Lazaro JE, Correa J, et al: Phrenic block caused by interscalene brachial plexus block: Effects of digital pressure and a low volume of local anesthetic. Reg Anesth Pain Med 1999;24:231–235.

33. Koscielniak-Nielsen ZJ: Hemidiaphragmatic paresis after interscalene supplementation of insufficient axillary block with 3 mL of 2% mepivacaine. Acta Anaesth Scand 2000;44:1160–1162.

34. Knoblanche GE: The incidence and aetiology of phrenic nerve blockade associated with supraclavicular brachial plexus block. Anaesth Intensive Care 1979;7:346–349.

35. Mak PH, Irwin MG, Ooi CG, et al: Incidence of diaphragmatic paralysis following supraclavicular brachial plexus block and its effect on pulmonary function. Anaesthesia 2001;56:352–356.

36. Neal JM, Moore JM, Kopacz DJ, et al: Quantitative analysis of respiratory, motor, and sensory function after supraclavicular block. Anesth Analg 1998;86:1239–44.

37. Rodriguez J, Barcena M, Rodriguez V, et al: Infraclavicular brachial plexus block effects on respiratory function and extent of the block. Reg Anesth Pain Med 1998;23:564–568.

38. Dullenkopf A, Blumenthal S, Theodorou P, et al: Diaphragmatic excursion and respiratory function after the modified Raj technique of the infraclavicular plexus block. Reg Anesth Pain Med 2004;29:110–114.

39. Gentili ME, Deleuze A, Estèbe JP, et al: Severe respiratory failure after infraclavicular block with 0.75% ropivacaine: A case report. J Clin Anesth 2002;14:459–461.

40. Martinez J, Sala-Blanch X, Ramos I, et al: Combined infraclavicular plexus block with suprascapular nerve block for humeral head surgery in a patient with respiratory failure: An alternative approach. Anesthesiology 2003;98:784–785.

41. Ilfeld BM, Morey TE, Wright TW, et al: Continuous interscalene brachial plexus block for postoperative pain control at home: A randomized, double-blinded, placebo-controlled study. Anesth Analg 2003;96:1089–1095.

42. Souron V, Reiland Y, Delaunay L: Pleural effusion and chest pain after continuous interscalene brachial plexus block. Reg Anesth Pain Med 2003;28:535–538.

43. Sardesai AM, Chakrabarti AJ, Denny NM. Lower lobe collapse during continuous interscalene brachial plexus local anesthesia at home. Reg Anesth Pain Med 2004;29:65–68.

44. Borgeat A, Perschak H, Bird P, et al: Patient-controlled interscalene analgesia with ropivacaine 0.2% *versus* patient-controlled intravenous analgesia after major shoulder surgery: Effects on diaphragmatic and respiratory function. Anesthesiology 2000;92:102–108.

45. Maurer K, Ekatodramis G, Hodler J, et al: Bilateral continuous interscalene block of brachial plexus for analgesia after bilateral shoulder arthroplasty. Anesthesiology 2002;96:762–764.

46. Osinowo O, Zahrani M, Softah A: Effect of intercostal nerve block with 0.5% bupivacaine on peak expiratory flow rate and arterial oxygen saturation in rib fractures. J Trauma 2004;56:345–347.

47. Karmakar MK, Critchley LA, Ho AM: Continuous thoracic paravertebral infusion of bupivacaine for pain management in patients with multiple fractured ribs. Chest 2003;123:424–431.

48. Richardson J, Sabanathan S, Shah R: Post-thoracotomy spirometric lung function: The effect of analgesia. A review. J Cardiovasc Surg (Torino) 1999;40:445–456.

49. Richardson J, Sabanathan S, Jones J, et al: A prospective, randomized comparison of preoperative and continuous balanced epidural or paravertebral bupivacaine on post-thoracotomy pain, pulmonary function and stress responses. Br J Anaesth 1999;83:387–392.

50. Thomas PW, Sanders DJ, Berrisford RG: Pulmonary haemorrhage after percutaneous paravertebral block. Br J Anaesth 1999;83:668–669.

51. Fine PG, Bubela C: Chylothorax following celiac plexus block. Anesthesiology 1985;63:454–456.

52. Shanti CM, Carlin AM, Tyburski JG: Incidence of pneumothorax from intercostal nerve block for analgesia in rib fractures. J Trauma 2001;51:536–539.

53. Naja Z, Lonnqvist PA: Somatic paravertebral nerve blockade. Incidence of failed block and complications. Anaesthesia 2001;56:1184–1188.

54. Borgeat A, Ekatodramis G, Kalberer F, et al: Acute and nonacute complications associated with interscalene block and shoulder surgery: A prospective study. Anesthesiology 2001;95:875–880.

55. Brown DL, Bridenbaugh LD: The upper extremity. Somatic block. In Cousins MJ, Bridenbaugh PO (eds): *Neural Blockade in Clinical Anesthesia and Management of Pain*, 3 ed. Lippincott-Raven Publishers, 1998, pp 345–371.

56. Klaastad O, Smith HJ, Smedby O: A novel infraclavicular brachial plexus block: The lateral and sagittal technique, developed by magnetic resonance imaging studies. Anesth Analg 2004;98:252–256.

57. Chan VW, Perlas A, Rawson R, et al: Ultrasound-guided supraclavicular brachial plexus block. Anesth Analg 2003;97:1514–1517.

58. Fenoglio C, Boicelli CA, Ottone M, et al: Protective effect of procaine hydrochloride on cisplatin-induced alterations in rat kidney. Anticancer Drugs 2002;13:1043–1054.

59. Navar LG: Renal autoregulation: Perspectives from whole kidney and single nephron studies. Am J Physiol Renal Physiol 1978;234:F357–F370.

60. Suleiman MY, Passannante AN, Onder RL, et al: Alteration of renal blood flow during epidural anesthesia in normal subjects. Anesth Analg 1997;84:1076–1080.

61. Rooke GA, Freund PR, Jacobson AF: Hemodynamic response and change in organ blood volume during spinal anesthesia in elderly men with cardiac disease. Anesth Analg 1997;85:99–105.

62. Sivarajan M, Amonry DW, Lindbloom LE, et al: Systemic and regional blood-flow changes during spinal anesthesia in the rhesus monkey. Anesthesiology 1975;43:78–88.

63. Hopf HB, Schlaghecke R, Peters J: Sympathetic neural blockade by thoracic epidural anesthesia suppresses renin release in response to arterial hypotension. Anesthesiology 1994;80:992–999.

64. Akpek EA, Kayhan Z, Donmez A, et al: Early postoperative renal function following renal transplantation surgery: Effect of anesthetic technique. J Anesth 2002;16:114–118.

65. Coupe N, O'Brien M, Gibson P, et al: Anesthesia for pediatric renal transplantation with and without epidural analgesia—A review of 7 years experience. Paediatr Anaesth 2005;15:220–228.

66. Sener M, Torgay A, Akpek E, et al: Regional versus general anesthesia for donor nephrectomy: Effects on graft function. Transplant Proc 2004;3:2954–2958.

67. Gould DB, Aldrete JA: Bupivacaine cardiotoxicity in a patient with renal failure. Acta Anaesthesiol Scand 1983;27:18–21.

68. Lucas LF, Tsueda TF: Cardiovascular depression after brachial plexus block in two diabetic patients with endstage renal failure. Anesthesiology 1990;73:1032–1035.

69. Coyle DE, Denson DD, Thompson GA, et al: The influence of lactic acid on the serum potassium binding of bupivacaine: Species differences. Anesthesiology 1984;61:127–133.

70. Avery P, Redon D, Schaenzer G, et al: The influence of serum potassium on the cerebral and cardiac toxicity of bupivacaine and lidocaine. Anesthesiology 1984;61:134–138.

71. Pere P, Salonen M, Jokinen M, et al: Pharmacokinetics of ropivacaine in uremic and nonuremic patients after axillary brachial plexus block. Anesth Analg 2003;96:563–569.

72. Rodriguez J, Quintela O, Lopez-Rivadulla M, et al: High doses of mepivacaine for brachial plexus block in patients with end-stage chronic renal failure. A pilot study. Eur J Anaesth 2001;18: 171–176.

73. Mostert JW, Evers JL, Hobika GH, et al: The haemodynamic response to chronic renal failure as studied in the azotaemic state. Br J Anaesth 1970;42:397–411.

74. Vasson MP, Baguet JC, Arveiller MR, et al: Serum and urinary alpha-1 acid glycoprotein in chronic renal failure. Nephron 1993;65:299–303.

75. Mather LE, Thomas J: Bupivacaine binding to plasma protein fractions. J Pharm Pharmacol 1978;30:653–654.

76. Vaziri ND, Saiki JK, Hughes W: Clearance of lidocaine by hemodialysis. South Med J 1979;72:1567–1568.

77. Rice AS, Pither CE, Tucker GT: Plasma concentrations of bupivacaine after supraclavicular brachial plexus blockade in patients with chronic renal failure. Anaesthesia 1991;46:354–357.

78. McEllistrem RF, Schell J, O'Malley K, et al: Interscalene brachial plexus blockade with lidocaine in chronic renal failure—A pharmacokinetic study. Can J Anaesth 1989;36:59–63.

79. Orko R, Pitkanen M, Rosenberg PH: Subarachnoid anaesthesia with 0.75% bupivacaine in patients with chronic renal failure. Br J Anaesth 1986;58:605–609.

80. Gawaz MP, Dobos G, Spath M, et al: Impaired function of platelet membrane glycoprotein IIb-IIIa in end-stage renal disease. J Am Soc Nephrol 1994;5:36–46.

81. Grejda S, Ellis K, Arino P: Paraplegia following spinal anesthesia in a patient with chronic renal failure. Reg Anesth 1989;14:155–157.

82. Boccardo P, Remuzzi G, Galbusera M: Platelet dysfunction in renal failure. Semin Thromb Hemost 2004;30:579–589.

83. Rose M, Ness TJ. Hypoxia following interscalene block. Reg Anesth Pain Med 2002;27:94–6.

84. Alsalti RA, el-Dawlatly AA, al-Salman M, et al: Arteriovenous fistula in chronic renal failure patients: Comparison between three different anesthetic techniques. Middle East J Anesthesiol 1999;15:305–314.

85. Solomonson MD, Johnson ME, Ilstrup D: Risk factors in patients having surgery to create an arteriovenous fistula. Anesth Analg 1994;79:694–700.

86. Mouqet C, Bitker MO, Bailliart O, et al: Anesthesia for creation of a forearm fistula in patients with end-stage renal failure. Anesthesiology 1989;70:909–14.

87. Stoelting RK: Diseases of the liver and biliary tract. In Stoelting RK, Dierdorf SF (eds): *Anesthesia and Co-existing Disease,* 4 ed. Churchill-Livingstone, 2002, pp 218–296.

88. Tucker GT, Mather LE: Clinical pharmacokinetics of local anesthetics. Clin Pharmacokinet 1979;4:241–278.

89. Tucker GT, Mather LE: Properties, absorption, and disposition of local anesthetic agents. In Cousins MJ, Bridenbaugh PO (eds): *Neural Blockade in Clinical Anesthesia and Management of Pain,* 3 ed. Lippincott-Raven, 1998, pp 55–95.

90. Rosenberg PH, Veering BT, Urmey WF: Maximum recommended doses of local anesthetics: A multifactorial concept. Reg Anesth Pain Med 2004;29:564–575.

91. Magorian T, Wood P, Caldwell J, et al: The pharmacokinetics and neuromuscular effects of rocuronium bromide in patients with liver disease. Anesth Analg 1995;80:754–759.

92. Servin FS, Cockshott JD, Farinotti R, et al: Pharmacokinetics of propofol infusions in patients with cirrhosis. Br J Anaesth 1990;65:177–183.

93. Barry M, Keeling PWN, Weir D, et al: Severity of cirrhosis and the relationship of alpha-1 acid glycoprotein concentration to plasma binding of lidocaine. Clin Pharmacol Ther 1990;47:366–370.

94. Thomson PD, Melmon KL, Richardson JA, et al: Lidocaine pharmacokinetics in advanced heart failure, liver disease, and renal failure in humans. Ann Intern Med 1973;78:499–508.

95. Naguib M, Magboul MM, Samarkandi AH, et al: Adverse effects and drug interactions associated with local and regional anaesthesia. Drug Saf 1998;18:221–250.

96. Reidenberg MM, James M, Dring LG. The rate of procaine hydrolysis in serum of normal subjects and diseased patients. Clin Pharmacol Ther 1972;13:279–284.

97. Calvo R, Carlos R, Erill S: Effects of disease and acetazolamine on procaine hydrolysis by red cell enzymes. Clin Pharmacol Ther 1980;27:179–183.

98. Lautt WW, Greenway CV: Conceptual review of the hepatic vascular bed. Hepatology 1987;7:952–963.

99. Lautt WW, Macedo MP: Hepatic circulation and toxicology. Drug Metab Rev 1997; 29:369–395.

100. Gelman S. General anesthesia and hepatic circulation. Can J Physiol Pharmacol 1987;65:1762–179.

101. Greitz T, Andreen M, Irestedt L: Haemodynamics and oxygen consumption in the dog during high epidural block with special reference to the splanchnic region. Acta Anaesthesiol Scand 1983;27:211–217.

102. Vagts DA, Iber T, Puccini M, et al: The effects of thoracic epidural anesthesia on hepatic perfusion and oxygenation in healthy pigs during general anesthesia and surgical stress. Anesth Analg 2003;97:1824–1832.

103. Kelly DA, Tuddenham EG: Haemostatic problems in liver disease. Gut 1986;27:339–349.

104. Shami VM, Caldwell SH, Hespenheide EE, et al: Recombinant activated factor VII for coagulopathy in fulminant hepatic failure compared with conventional therapy. Liver Transpl 20039:138–143.

105. Dzik WH: Predicting hemorrhage using preoperative coagulation screening assays. Curr Hematol Rev 2004;3:324–330.

106. Horlocker TT, Wedel DJ, Benzon H, et al: Regional anesthesia in the anticoagulated patient: Defining the risks (The second ASRA consensus conference on neuraxial anesthesia and anticoagulation). Reg Anesth Pain Med 2003;28:172–197.

107. Coursin DB, Connery LE, Ketzler JT: Perioperative diabetic and hyperglycemic management issues. Crit Care Med 2004;32:S116–S125.

108. Greene DA, Stevens MJ, Feldman EL: Diabetic neuropathy: Scope of the syndrome. Am J Med 1999;107(2B):2S–8S.

109. Feldman EL, Stevens MJ, Greene DA: Pathogenesis of diabetic neuropathy. Clin Neurosci 1997;4:365–370.

110. Kalichman MW, Calcutt NA: Local anesthetic-induced conduction block and nerve fiber injury in streptozotocin-diabetic rats. Anesthesiology 1992;77:941–947.

111. Al-Nasser B: Toxic effects of epidural analgesia with ropivacaine 0.2% in a diabetic patient. J Clin Anesth 2004;16:220–223.

112. Sites BD, Gallagher J, Sparks M: Ultrasound guided popliteal block demonstrates an atypical motor response to nerve stimulation in two patients with diabetes mellitus. Reg Anesth Pain Med 2003;28:479–482.

113. Partanen J, Niskanen L, Lehtinen J, et al: Natural history of peripheral neuropathy in patients with non-insulin dependent diabetes mellitus. N Engl J Med 1995;333:89–94.

114. Minville V, Zetlaoui PJ, Fessenmeyer C, et al: Ultrasound guidance for difficult lateral popliteal catheter insertion in a patient with peripheral vascular disease. Reg Anesth Pain Med 2004;29:368–370.

115. Van Den Berghe G, Wouters P, Weekers F, et al: Intensive insulin therapy in critically ill patients. N Engl J Med 2001;345:1359–1367.

116. Krinsley JS: Effect of an intensive glucose management protocol on the mortality of critically ill adult patients. Mayo Clin Proc 2004;79:992–1000.

117. Ghandi GY, Nuttall GA, Abel MD, et al: Intraoperative hyperglycemia and perioperative outcomes in cardiac surgery patients. Mayo Clin Proc 2005;80:862–866.

118. Annane D, Melchior JC: Hormone replacement therapy for the critically ill. Crit Care Med 2003;31:634–635.

119. Jensen CH, Berthelsen P, Kuhl C, Kehlet H: Effect of epidural analgesia on glucose tolerance during surgery. Acta Anaesthesiol Scand 1980;24:472–474.

120. Houghton A, Hickey JB, Ross SA, et al: Glucose tolerance during anaesthesia and surgery. Comparison of general and extradural anaesthesia. Br J Anaesth 1978;50:495–499.

121. Moller IW, Hjortso E, Krantz T, et al: The modifying effect of spinal anaesthesia on intra- and postoperative adrenocortical and hyperglycaemic response to surgery. Acta Anaesthesiol Scand 1984;28:266–269.

122. Barker JP, Robinson PN, Vafidis GC, et al: Local analgesia prevents the cortisol and glycaemic responses to cataract surgery. Br J Anaesth 1990;64:442–445.

123. Vogt G, Heiden M, Losche CC, et al: A preoperative retrobulbar block in patients undergoing scleral buckling reduces pain, endogenous stress response, and improves vigilance. Reg Anesth Pain Med 2003;28:521–527.

124. Kehlet H: Modification of responses to surgery by neural blockade: Clinical implications. In Cousins MJ, Bridenbaugh PO (eds): *Neural Blockade in Clinical Anesthesia and Management of Pain*, 3 ed. Lippincott-Raven, 1998, pp 129–175.

125. Camu F: Carbohydrate intolerance during halothane anesthesia in dogs. Acta Anaesthesiol Belg 1973:24:177–188.

126. Richardson J, Jones J, Atkinson R: The effect of thoracic paravertebral blockade on intercostal somatosensory evoked potentials. Anesth Analg 1998;87:373–376.

127. Mendell JR, Sahenk Z: Painful sensory neuropathy. N Engl J Med 2003;348:1243–1255.

128. Duyff RF, Van den Bosch J, Laman DM, et al: Neuromuscular findings in thyroid dysfunction: A prospective clinical and electrodiagnostic study. J Neurol Neurosurg Psychiatry 2000;68:750–755.

129. Misiunas A, Niepomniszcze H, Ravera B: Peripheral neuropathy in subacute hypothyroidism. Thyroid 1995;5:283–286.

130. Khedr EM, El Toony LF, Tarkhan MN, et al: Peripheral and central nervous system alterations in hypothyroidism: Electrophysiological findings. Neuropsychobiology 2000;41:88–94.

131. Shirabe T, Tawara S, Terao A, et al: Myxoedematous polyneuropathy: A light and electron microscopic study of the peripheral nerve and muscle. J Neurol Neurosurg Psychiatry 1975;38:241–247.

132. Upton AR, McComas AJ: The double crush in nerve entrapment syndromes. Lancet 1973;2:359–362.

133. Hebl JR, Horlocker TT, Pritchard DJ: Diffuse brachial plexopathy after interscalene blockade in a patient receiving cisplatin chemotherapy: The pharmacologic double crush syndrome. Anesth Analg 2001;92:249–251.

134. Schenker M, Kraftsik R, Glauser L, et al: Thyroid hormone reduces the loss of axotomized sensory neurons in dorsal root ganglia after sciatic nerve transection in adult rat. Exp Neurol 2003;184:225–236.

135. Norcross-Nechay K, Richards GE, Cavallo A: Evoked potentials show early and delayed abnormalities in children with congenital hypothyroidism. Neuropediatrics 1989;20:158–163.

136. Centers for Disease Control and Prevention: CDC's National Leadership Role in Addressing Obesity. http://www.cdc.gov/doc.do/id/0900f3ec803207fd

137. Broadbent CR, Maxwell WB, Ferrie R, et al: Ability of anaesthetists to identify a marked lumbar interspace. Anaesthesia 2000;55:1122–1126.

138. Nielsen KC, Guller U, Steele SM, et al: Influence of obesity on surgical regional anesthesia in the ambulatory setting: An analysis of 9038 blocks. Anesthesiology 2005;102:181–187.

139. Pham-Dang C, Meunier JF, Poirier P, et al: A new axillary approach for continuous brachial plexus block. A clinical and anatomic study. Anesth Analg 1995;81:686–693.

140. Tan WS, Spigos DG: Sciatic nerve block under fluoroscopic guidance. Cardiovasc Intervent Radiol 1986;9:59–60.

141. Eidelman A, Shulman MS, Novak GM: Fluoroscopic imaging for technically difficult spinal anesthesia. J Clin Anesth 2005;17:69–71.

142. Marhofer P, Greher M, Kapral S: Ultrasound guidance in regional anesthesia. Br J Anaesth 2005;94:7–17.

143. Wallace DH, Currie JM, Gilstrap LC, et al: Indirect sonographic guidance for epidural anesthesia in obese pregnant patients. Reg Anesth 1992;17:233–236.

144. Grau T, Leipold RW, Horter J, et al: The lumbar epidural space in pregnancy: Visualization by ultrasonography. Br J Anaesth 2001;86:798–804.

145. McCulloch WJ, Littlewood DG: Influence of obesity on spinal analgesia with isobaric 0.5% bupivacaine. Br J Anaesth 1986;58:610–614.

146. Reyes M, Pan PH: Very low-dose spinal anesthesia for cesarean section in a morbidly obese preeclamptic patient and its potential implications. Int J Obstet Anesth 2004;13:99–102.

147. Norris MC: Patient variables and the subarachnoid spread of hyperbaric bupivacaine in the term parturient. Anesthesiology 1990;72:478–482.

148. Greene NM: Distribution of local anesthetic solutions within the subarachnoid space. Anesth Analg 1985;64:715–730.

149. Stienstra R, Greene NM: Factors affecting the subarachnoid spread of local anesthetic solutions. Reg Anesth 1991;16:1–6.

59

Regional Anesthesia in the Patient with Preexisting Neurologic Disease

Steven Deschner, MD

INTRODUCTION

Patients with preexisting neurologic disease present a unique challenge to the anesthesiologist. Knowledge of the pathophysiology of the disease and the effect of anesthetic drug therapy on the disease process is essential for the safe management of anesthesia for these patients. Both active and dormant neurologic diseases may worsen in the perioperative period, independent of the chosen anesthetic method. However when regional techniques are used, the cause of postoperative neurologic deficits may be difficult to evaluate as neural injury can be related to a wide variety of reasons, ie, surgical trauma, tourniquet pressure, improper positioning, or anesthetic technique.[1] The possibility of needle-induced trauma, local anesthetic toxicity, or neural tissue ischemia or damage during regional anesthesia has led many anesthesiologists to avoid regional techniques in patients with underlying neurologic diseases.

Many of these patients can benefit from regional techniques. Greater autonomic stability, the ability to provide selective anesthesia and analgesia, greater hemodynamic stability (especially with peripheral nerve block anesthesia in patients with concurrent cardiomyopathy), and the avoidance of side effects related to general anesthetics and opioids are a few of the advantages.[2,3] Careful preoperative neurologic evaluation, evaluation of the risk/benefit ratio, and a comprehensive discussion with the patient about the anesthetic plan and the possibility of worsening neurologic signs and symptoms unrelated to the anesthetic technique is important for successful implementation of regional techniques in this patient population.

INCIDENCE OF NEUROLOGIC COMPLICATIONS RELATED TO REGIONAL ANESTHESIA

Although perioperative nerve injuries have been well recognized as a complication of spinal and epidural anesthesia, severe or disabling neurologic complications occur relatively rarely. In 1999, Cheney and colleagues examined the American Society of Anesthesiologists Closed Claims database to determine what percentage of the claims were related to nerve damage in malpractice cases.[4] Of the 4183 claims reviewed, 670 (16%) were anesthesia-related nerve injuries. Ulnar neuropathies were the most frequently reported, followed by other injuries to the brachial plexus, lumbosacral nerve roots, and spinal cord. The injuries were bilateral in 14% of the ulnar injuries and in 12% of the brachial plexus injuries. The important factor in this analysis is that the incidence of ulnar and brachial plexus injuries was greater with general anesthesia than with regional anesthesia.[5,6] Horlocker and coworkers examined the cause of perioperative nerve injury in a review of 607 patients undergoing 1614 axillary blocks for upper extremity surgery. Various surgical variables (direct trauma, stretch, hematoma, vascular compromise, case or tourniquet ischemia) were thought to be the cause of neurologic complications in the majority of the cases (89%).[7]

In the Closed Claims Analysis 189 (4%) involved either the lumbosacral root or the spinal cord. Injuries to these areas were more frequently associated with regional anesthesia. The lumbosacral root injuries were thought to be related to paresthesias during needle or catheter placement or pain on injection of local anesthetic. The spinal cord injuries were related to blocks for chronic pain or neuraxial blocks on patients receiving systemic anticoagulation. These injuries were not related to the presence of preexisting neurologic disease. In another review of over 50,000 spinal and epidural anesthetics, the incidence of persistent peripheral neuropathy, including paresthesia and sensory or motor dysfunction ranged from 0% to 0.16% for spinal anesthetics and 0% to 0.06% for epidural anesthetics, still appreciably lower than the incidence of nerve injuries reported with general anesthetic cases.[8-11]

Although the reported incidence of nerve injuries with regional anesthesia is very low, the use of regional techniques in patients with preexisting neuropathies is often considered controversial. The possibility of needle- or catheter-induced nerve trauma, neural ischemia, or local anesthetic toxicity placing the patient with an underlying neurologic deficit at greater risk has limited the use of regional techniques in this patient population. In a retrospective study of over 300 patients with preexisting ulnar neuropathy undergoing ulnar nerve transposition, it was demonstrated that anesthetic technique did not affect neurologic outcome in the immediate postoperative period or up to 6 weeks after surgery.[6] The authors did not find any evidence that the use of a peripheral nerve block increased the risk of new or worsening neurologic symptoms in patients with preexisting ulnar nerve

neuropathy. They concluded that regional anesthesia is as safe as general anesthesia in these patients with mononeuropathy.

In patients with other serious neurologic diseases, regional anesthesia is often avoided for a variety of reasons, including lack of understanding of the disease process, the risk of unknown or unpredicted effects of local anesthetics in abnormal nervous tissue, concerns regarding possibly worsening preexisting symptoms, limited experience using regional techniques, and limited data to support its utilization.

The following paragraphs discuss many of the neurologic conditions the anesthesiologist may encounter. The approach to the management of anesthesia is included with a discussion of various regional techniques that can be safely used in these patients. When information in the literature is sparse, suggestions for anesthetic techniques are included based on available neurologic research, case reports, and experience of clinicians in institutions performing large volume regional anesthesia techniques.

CENTRAL NERVOUS SYSTEM DISEASE

Degenerative Diseases

Parkinson's Disease

Parkinson's disease is a disabling neurologic disease affecting 3% of the population older than age 65 years. The peak onset is in the sixth decade, but the disease can begin to manifest from age 20 to age 80 with the male to female ratio of 3:2. Parkinson's disease is caused by loss of dopamine-containing nerve cells in the substantia nigra.[13] The presence of Lewy bodies, eosinophilic cytoplasmic inclusions in pigmented neurons, are a characteristic feature. The cause of the disease is unknown although multiple theories have been proposed, including a defect in the gene for α-synuclein, mitochondrial dysfunction, excitotoxicity secondary to persistent activation of N-methyl-D-aspartate (NMDA) receptors, and oxidative stress secondary to catabolism of dopamine.[12,13]

Four clinical features are characteristic of Parkinson's disease: rigidity "cogwheel," bradykinesia, resting tremor, and postural instability.

These patients may have depression and dysautonomia. Patients with Parkinson's disease may suffer from orthostatic hypotension and urinary dysfunction. Clinical assessment should include an evaluation of these systems to identify potential problems. Measurements of blood pressure in the lying and standing position should be obtained to assess the degree of autonomic dysfunction as evidenced by orthostatic hypotension.

Treatment is directed at increasing dopamine levels in the brain.[12] The mainstay of treatment is levodopa or dopamine receptor agonists. Monoamine oxide inhibitors are used to prolong the action of dopamine in the striatum. Catechol-O-methyl transferase (COMT) inhibitors are used to inhibit the breakdown of dopamine in the periphery and increase its bioavailability. Anticholinergics are effective in treating tremor, but because of many side effects (worsening dementia, psychosis, dry mouth, constipation), they are reserved for younger patients in the early phase of disease.

Anesthetic Considerations

Patients with Parkinson disease most commonly present for urologic, ophthalmologic, or orthopedic procedures. In addition to the routine history, physical examination, and preoperative testing, assessment of systems specifically affected by Parkinson disease should be evaluated. See Table 59–1 for specific systems affected.

Regional Anesthesia in Parkinson's Disease

Autonomic dysfunction is exacerbated by inhalational anesthetics, resulting in more hemodynamic instability.[14] Halothane, although less commonly used today, sensitizes the heart to catecholamines and should be avoided in patients on levodopa.[14] Isoflurane and sevoflurane are less arrhythmogenic; however, hypotension from catecholamine depletion, autonomic dysfunction, and the coadministration of other medications remains a concern.[14] Muscle relaxants and positive pressure ventilation can lead to prolonged postoperative ventilatory support in a patient with respiratory impairment, common in the Parkinson patient.[15] There are numerous reports of opioid-induced muscle rigidity in patients with an established diagnosis of Parkinson's disease.[15] Postoperative nausea and vomiting related to opioids, reversal agents, and

Table 59–1.

Specific System Assessment for Parkinson's Disease

System	Assessment
Head and neck	Pharyngeal muscle dysfunction Dysphagia Sialorrhea Blepharospasm
Respiratory	Respiratory dysfunction from rigidity, or uncoordinated movement of the respiratory muscles
Cardiovascular	Orthostatic hypotension Cardiac dysrhythmias Hypertension
Gastrointestinal	Susceptibility to reflux
Urologic	Difficulty in micturation
Musculoskeletal	Muscle rigidity
Central nervous system	Akinesia Tremor Confusion/hallucinations Depression

inhalation anesthetics may be more common.[17] Patients with Parkinson's disease are more prone to postoperative confusion and hallucinations.[17]

Regional anesthesia may have advantages over general anesthesia as the effects of inhalation anesthetics, muscle relaxants, high-dose opioids, and anesthetic medications that may exacerbate the symptoms of Parkinson's disease are eliminated. By utilizing peripheral nerve block anesthesia or appropriate segmental epidural anesthesia with limited sedation, the autonomic instability can be controlled, the incidence of nausea and vomiting limited, and muscle rigidity resulting from doses of narcotics used for general anesthesia can be avoided. Careful titration of sedation with limited use of opioids is suggested in this patient population.

Alzheimer's Disease

Alzheimer's disease is the major cause of dementia in the United States.[16] If affects 10% of people older than age 65 with the female to male ratio of 2:1. Risk factors include female sex, advanced age, family history, Down syndrome, and African American or Hispanic descent. Patients with a history of brain trauma may have an increased risk of developing the disease.[16]

The cause is unknown. Pathologic changes in the brain include the accumulation of tau protein with formation of neurofibrillary tangles, deposition of β-amyloid with formation of neuritic plaques, and selective loss of cholinergic neurons, leading to cortical atrophy. It is theorized that these changes may arise as a result of excitotoxicity involving the NMDA receptor. Current drug therapy is directed at increasing the levels of acetylcholine, cholinesterase inhibition, cholinergic receptor stimulation, and blocking NMDA receptors with the intent of reducing excitotoxicity.[16]

The clinical features of the patient with Alzheimer's disease are a gradual decline of intellectual function, progressive loss of short-term memory, disorientation, language and speech problems, and seizures in 10% of the patients. Paranoid delusions with hallucinations and personality changes are common.[16]

Anesthetic Considerations

The choice of anesthetic technique for patients with Alzheimer's disease should be guided by the patient's general physiologic condition, the degree of neurologic deterioration, and the potential for drug interactions between the anesthetics and the patient's treatment. Detection of early symptoms may be difficult. Administration of sedatives or anticholinergics could precipitate delirium. Inhalation agents must be administered with care as the elderly patient is more sensitive to the depressant cerebral and cardiovascular effects of these agents.[17] Anesthetics with short durations of action and rapid recovery are advantageous.

Regional Anesthesia in Alzheimer Disease

Regional anesthesia can be a challenge because these patients are often uncooperative preoperatively. The advantage of regional techniques is the ability to selectively anesthetize the area of interest without subjecting the patient to systemic effects of general anesthetic agents. For block placement, a short-acting sedative/hypnotic, such as propofol or midazolam, at a low dose is effective. Depending on the type of block, a short-acting narcotic (eg, alfentanil) may be administered just before the block placement. Avoiding postoperative confusion and delirium caused by inhalation agents, narcotics, muscle relaxants, and reversal agents may be beneficial to this patient population.[17] Postoperative pain control without narcotics may be an even greater benefit of peripheral nerve blocks. Educating the staff and the caregivers about protection of the insensate extremity, requiring assistance with mobilization, and the duration of the block is a necessary part of the anesthetic management. Although these patients can be challenging to treat without general anesthesia, they can benefit from regional techniques.

Amyotrophic Lateral Sclerosis (Lou Gehrig Disease)

Amyotrophic lateral sclerosis (ALS) is a progressive degenerative disease of motor cells throughout the central nervous system (CNS). It involves destruction of cortical, brainstem, and spinal motor neurons. Progression of the disease is relentless. Death occurs within 3 to 5 years of the diagnosis, most commonly precipitated by aspiration. The onset is usually after the age of 50 with a male to female ration of 2:1. The cause is unknown, but theories include glutamate excitotoxicity, oxidative stress, mitochondrial dysfunction, paraneoplastic tumors, autoimmune disease, and viral infection.[18] The prevalence of the disease is 6:100,000, making it a rare but profound disease.

Initially, the disease presents as atrophy, weakness, and fasciculations in the intrinsic hand muscles. As the disease progresses, atrophy and weakness develop in all skeletal muscles including those of the tongue, pharynx, larynx, and respiratory muscles of the chest. Patients lose the ability to cough, increasing the risk of aspiration. Eventually, respiratory failure ensues, requiring mechanical ventilation. Autonomic dysfunction may be evident and is manifested by orthostatic hypotension and an increased resting heart rate. The cause of death is usually related to respiratory failure.[18]

Anesthetic Considerations

Patients with ALS present a challenge to the anesthesiologist. Neuromuscular transmission is markedly abnormal leading to the up-regulation of nicotinic acetylcholine receptors (nAChRs).[19] The up-regulation makes these patients vulnerable to hyperkalemia in response to succinylcholine.[20] They have presynaptic impairment of neuromuscular transmission, making them hypersensitive to nondepolarizing muscle relaxants.[21] If general anesthesia is used, intubation with a deep inhalation agent without the administration of muscle relaxants is recommended.[22] As the disease progresses, respiratory muscles weaken, placing these patients at high risk for respiratory depression and aspiration. They can be exquisitely sensitive to sedatives and anesthetic drugs. Postoperative ventilatory support after general anesthesia is usually necessary.[23]

Regional Anesthesia in ALS

Regional anesthesia has been used on patients with ALS. There have been several case reports of successful epidural anesthesia for abdominal surgeries, ie, hysterectomy, bowel obstruction, and orthopedic procedures.[24–26] Case studies and reports of the use of peripheral nerve blocks in patients with ALS are not available, probably because the condition is so rare. Given the importance of preserving the laryngeal reflexes and respiratory failure due to the weakness of the respiratory muscles, the judicious use of selective peripheral nerve blocks may be beneficial for these patients. In patients with advanced weakness of the respiratory muscles, interscalene nerve block should be used with caution due to the resultant diaphragmatic paralysis.

Spinal Cord Injury

Spinal cord injury after trauma affects over 10,000 Americans each year. Of these, approximately one half occur at the cervical level. Complete neurologic deficit occurs in about 3500 patients per year, and partial deficits in another 4500 patients per year.[27] The majority of the injuries are secondary to blunt trauma, with a smaller percentage the result of penetrating injuries. Advances in the care of patients with acute spinal cord injury have reduced the mortality rate to less than 7% per year.[28]

The clinical presentation varies depending on the chronicity, the magnitude, and the level of the injury. Acutely, the patient appears flaccid with spinal shock. Hypotension, bradycardia, dysrhythmias, hypoxemia, and alveolar hypoventilation are common presenting symptoms. There is high risk of aspiration. When the injury becomes chronic, as manifested by the return of spinal reflexes, multiple complications arise including involuntary skeletal muscle spasms, overactivity of the sympathetic nervous system, chronic respiratory and genitourinary infections, altered thermoregulation, and pain.[29]

A major problem that appears after the resolution of spinal shock is autonomic dysreflexia. It is a life-threatening syndrome resulting from cutaneous or visceral stimulation below the level of the spinal cord injury and leading to extreme vascular instability. The syndrome has been shown to develop if the level of injury is at T7 or above, although some cases have been reported in patients with lesions below T7.[30] The trigger for the syndrome is a cutaneous, proprioceptive, or visceral stimulus below the level of the spinal cord injury lesion, ie, a full bladder or bowel. Activation of sympathetic nerves cause vasoconstriction and subsequent hypertension. The increase in the blood pressure is sensed in the aortic bodies and carotid sinus, resulting in vagal hyperactivity. Exaggerated vagal stimulation causes bradycardia, heart block, and ventricular dysrhythmias. Reflex vasodilation can be observed above the level of the lesion causing flushing in the head and neck. Hypertension can be so severe that subarachnoid hemorrhage, seizures, and acute left ventricular failure can occur.[29] In the obstetric patient, it can result in significant maternal–fetal morbidity including hypertensive encephalopathy, stroke, intraventricular hemorrhage, and death. It may occur in up to 85% of pregnant women with spinal cord lesions at or above T6 to T7.[31]

Other abnormalities occur with spinal cord injury. Retention of urine and feces are common. Abdominal distension can be severe enough to impair respiration. Acute spinal cord injury is associated with the highest risk of venous thromboembolism among all hospital admissions. If there is no DVT prophylaxis or the patient is noncompliant with prophylactic therapy, DVTs will occur in more than half (40–100%) of the patients within the first 3 months after injury.[32]

Anesthetic Considerations

The care of the patient with spinal cord injury depends on the timing, the location, and any associated injuries the patient may have. In the acute phase, the spinal cord is vulnerable to secondary injury from hypotension and hypoxia. Thermoregulation is impaired. Prompt recognition and treatment with early intubation and oxygenation, vasopressor therapy, and warming measures is indicated. During the acute phase, well-controlled general anesthesia is usually the best option as an anesthetic plan if there is any indication of respiratory compromise. Because of the high risk of deep venous thrombosis in the acute injury phase, most patients will be on prophylactic medication, either low-molecular-weight heparin or unfractionated heparin subcutaneously, which serves as a potential contraindication to neuraxial anesthesia. Most urgent orthopedic trauma cases are often performed under general anesthesia because the majority of these patients are already intubated, the mental status is altered by the trauma, or multiple procedures are going to be performed at one time involving multiple areas of the body. The use of succinylcholine should be avoided after the first 24 h of injury to avoid the massive hyperkalemic response that has been well documented.[33]

Patients with either quadriplegia or paraplegia may be hemodynamically unstable acutely as a result of initial spinal shock or occult injury. Computed tomographic scans, radiographs, and laboratory studies should be reviewed prior to surgery and blood samples drawn for either type and screen or type and cross match. Invasive monitoring, such as arterial lines, may be necessary to manage blood pressure changes. Vasopressors may be necessary to stabilize the blood pressure. Complicating the hemodynamic picture at this time with neuraxial anesthesia may not be the best option.

Regional Anesthesia in Patients with Spinal Cord Injuries

Regional anesthesia techniques can be a valuable tool in the treatment of patients with chronic spinal cord injury. Central neuraxial anesthesia has been used successfully for extracorporeal shockwave lithotripsy, for gynecologic procedures to prevent autonomic hyperreflexia, and in obstetrics for labor and delivery.[34–36] Peripheral nerve blocks have been used successfully to facilitate lithotomy positioning required for gynecologic or urologic examinations in spastic paraplegics.[37]

LESIONS BELOW T7. For patients with lesions below T7, the risk of hemodynamic instability from autonomic dysreflexia is reduced, but not eliminated. The incidence has been reported for lesions as low as T10.[38] In obstetrics, spinal or epidural anesthesia for labor, delivery, and cesarean section is preferred after the period of spinal shock has passed to attempt to avoid the complications associated with autonomic dysreflexia, as the occurrence is reduced with regional techniques.[35,36]

Pulmonary dysfunction, although more prevalent in lesions above T7, is still a concern with the paraplegic patient.[39]

Peripheral nerve blocks on the lower extremities may be an excellent anesthetic choice in these patients, providing adequate anesthesia while avoiding the known effects of general anesthesia, ie, respiratory compromise, overall muscle relaxation, nausea, and sedation from narcotics. Because of the uncertain risk of autonomic hyperreflexia in lesions below T7, peripheral nerve block or central neuraxial blocks reduce the risk of its occurrence by blocking the sensory limb of the reflex. An added advantage to peripheral nerve blocks is prevention of chronic pain, common in patients with spinal cord injuries.[40] Patients with spinal cord injury are prone to the development of spasticity. In the dysreflexive spinal cord of a paraplegic patient, pain has been shown to increase the level of spasticity.[40] Pain from surgical procedures may, therefore, precipitate spasticity. Utilizing peripheral nerve block anesthesia may prevent this from occurring. Nerve blocks must be performed with a nerve stimulator or ultrasound rather than paresthesia techniques as the patient with paraplegia may not have sensory (paresthesia) perception.

Upper extremity blocks can be performed safely in the paraplegic patient, as spinal cord functions above the lesion is intact and normal. Careful evaluation of the patient for coexisting medical problems or to ascertain the absolute level of the lesion is recommended. The development of syringomyelia has been reported in these patients, creating deficits above the established lesion which can cause unforeseen problems for the anesthesiologist.

LESIONS ABOVE T7. The risk of autonomic hyperreflexia has been reported to be 85% or higher in this patient population.[41] Light general anesthesia does not offer protection against its occurrence. Deep general anesthesia is effective, but the associated hemodynamic instability associated may not be tolerated in many of these patients. Pulmonary dysfunction is common and accounts for the largest percentage of morbidity in this population. General anesthesia with intubation may result in prolonged mechanical ventilation with increased risk of pulmonary infection. These patients are prone to the development of neurogenic pulmonary edema. It has been reported that certain anesthetic agents, ie, barbiturates, can provoke its occurrence.[42] General anesthesia-induced bowel and bladder dysfunction can compound the preexisting dysfunction associated with the disease.

Regional anesthesia, eg, spinal and epidural blockade, are effective in preventing autonomic hyperreflexia and have been used successfully in obstetrics for spinal cord-injured patients, even with high cord lesions.[36,43] However, concerns about the ability to determine the anesthetic level, exaggerated hypotension, and difficulties with placing the block secondary to spinal deformities from injury or prior surgery make many clinicians reluctant to use neuraxial anesthesia in this setting.

Peripheral nerve blocks, especially on the lower extremities, are a theoretically acceptable form of anesthesia for the properly evaluated patient with a high-level spinal cord injury. Selective nerve blocks on the lower extremities, ie, femoral-sciatic or ankle blocks, are an effective alternative to exposing the patient to general anesthesia. Providing adequate anesthesia is even more important with a high spinal cord lesion to avoid the stimulus for autonomic hyperreflexia. Avoiding systemic hypotension with general anesthesia or an exaggerated hypotensive response with neuraxial anesthesia is possible with selective nerve blocks. Again, paresthesia techniques cannot be used; nerve stimulation or ultrasound-guided technique are required for proper localization of the nerve(s) to be blocked.

Upper extremity peripheral nerve blocks should be approached on an individual basis. For a patient with a low cervical injury, who is not ventilator-dependent, performing an interscalene block with subsequent unilateral phrenic nerve paresis and up to 30% reduction in pulmonary function volumes, may create the need for respiratory support. However, an infraclavicular or axillary block may be beneficial both for surgical anesthesia and for reducing spasticity without creating further respiratory compromise in the appropriate patient.

Demyelinating Central Nervous System Diseases

Multiple Sclerosis

Multiple sclerosis (MS) is the most common demyelinating disease of the CNS, affecting over a million people worldwide.[44] Of the people affected, 75% are women in young adulthood (ages 20–40). It is characterized by random, multiple sites of demyelination in the brain and spinal cord. The peripheral nervous system is not involved. The cause of the disease is unknown, but is thought to involve a complex series of immunologic events in a genetically susceptible person. Infectious agents (especially viral), may predispose the disease.[44,45] The autoimmune mechanism is supported by laboratory findings in many patients. Often, cerebrospinal fluid (CSF) in patients with MS have elevated IgG with oligoclonal bands. Sodium channels are also redistributed along the demyelinated axon, leading to an increase in the influx of sodium and sodium-calcium exchange and ultimately destruction of axons.[46,47]

The presentation of the disease can vary. The symptoms of MS depend on the sites of demyelination. The most common clinical signs and symptoms are visual disturbances, ataxia, limb paresthesias and weakness, and autonomic disturbances including bowel and bladder dysfunction. The course of the disease is characterized by recurrent exacerbations of the symptoms (**relapsing remitting MS**). After

a period of approximately 20 years, patients do not fully recover from the symptoms. Deficits persist and disability progresses (**secondarily progressive MS**). In severe cases, some patients may be wheelchair-bound or develop respiratory failure.[48–50] Pregnancy is associated with an improvement in symptoms, but relapses generally occur in the first 6 months postpartum.[51]

Treatment consists of corticosteroids, interferon, glatiramer, and mitoxantrone used to modulate the immunologic and inflammatory responses.[44] Side effects of the treatment therapy include adrenal suppression, liver function test abnormalities, anemia, leukopenia, and dose-related cardiotoxicity.[44]

Anesthetic Considerations in Patients with MS

Autonomic dysfunction can be seen in patients with MS.[49] They exhibit an increased sensitivity to sympathomimetics used to manage hypotension.[52] Preload should be adequately maintained for hemodynamic stability. Increases in temperature as well as metabolic and hormonal changes associated with surgery are thought to be responsible for exacerbation of symptoms that may occur postoperatively.[48] A temperature change of as little as 0.5°C may block impulse conduction in demyelinated fibers.[48] Stress dose steroids may be necessary, depending on the dose and length of time steroids have been used preoperatively. Although the effect of surgery and anesthesia on the course of MS is controversial, (ie, reports support and refute the exacerbation of symptoms from anesthesia), the patient should be advised that regardless of the anesthetic technique, there is a possibility that a relapse of symptoms may occur after surgery.[54]

Regional Anesthesia in Patients with MS

The use of regional anesthesia, ie, central neuraxial blocks, in patients with MS is controversial. Both spinal and epidural anesthesia have been used safely, but unpredictable progression of the neurologic symptoms has been observed.[54] The mechanism by which spinal anesthesia may exacerbate MS is unknown, but it is speculated that demyelinated areas of the spinal cord might be more sensitive to the effects of local anesthetics.[55] In fact, it has been suggested that lidocaine can be used to unmask silent demyelinating lesions in MS, making it a diagnostic tool.[56] Epidural anesthesia has been found to be innocuous in obstetric analgesia and anesthesia. However, in one study, patients who received concentrations of bupivacaine greater than 0.25% experienced postpartum relapses.[55,57]

Because MS is a disorder of the central nervous system, peripheral nerve block anesthesia should be a more appropriate choice then spinal anesthesia. Peripheral nerve block anesthesia may be considered the technique of choice for patients with MS when the surgical procedure allows it.[58]

Although not contraindicated, lumbar plexus blocks and paravertebral blocks may have a prolonged duration of action in patients with MS. In one report, a patient who received a paravertebral block for an inguinal hernia repair developed a flaccid paralysis of both lower extremities. The block regressed slowly, with full recovery, in 12.5 h. It was postulated that in peripheral blocks near the central neuraxis, uptake of local anesthetics into the spinal cord may cause a prolonged duration or unpredictable response in patients with MS, similar to spinal anesthetics.[59]

PERIPHERAL NERVOUS SYSTEM DISEASES: PERIPHERAL NEUROPATHIES

Peripheral neuropathies involve motor, sensory, and autonomic fibers outside of the CNS. They produce variable motor, sensory, and autonomic symptoms. They can be divided into disorders producing focal (ie, mononeuropathy) or widespread (ie, polyneuropathy) nerve dysfunction. The polyneuropathies may be symmetrical [ie, the distribution of deficits is symmetrical and usually distal (Guillain–Barré)] or asymmetrical (ie, diabetic, uremic, or vasculitic).

The causes of peripheral neuropathies are multiple, ie, metabolic, vasculitic, hereditary, infectious, neoplastic, paraneoplastic, trauma, toxins, or medication-induced. The most common cause is diabetic neuropathy, affecting nearly 100% of patients with long-standing disease.[60] Diabetic neuropathy is discussed in Chapter 58.

Treatment for peripheral neuropathies involves identification of the cause and attempting to mitigate or remove it. Painful neuropathies have been treated with many agents, including antiepileptic drugs, antidepressants, sodium channel-blocking agents, tramadol, and capsaicin ointment.[61] It is important for the anesthesiologist to understand the disease process, the potential interaction of anesthetic agents with chronic treatment medications, and the differences in response to local anesthetics or nerve stimulation if regional anesthetics are to be employed.

Inherited Peripheral Neuropathies

Charcot–Marie–Tooth Disease

Charcot–Marie–Tooth (CMT) disease is the most common inherited peripheral neuropathy. The incidence is 1:2500. It is both a motor and sensory peripheral neuropathy, classically presenting as distal skeletal muscle weakness and wasting (quadriceps muscle wasting, peroneal muscle atrophy). Peroneal nerve atrophy causing weakness in the anterior and lateral compartments of the leg is the most common presentation, but considerable variations in the presentation are common. The sensory deficit is usually milder than the motor deficits. Exacerbations of the disease during pregnancy is thought to be related to hormonal changes.[62] A variety of respiratory problems, including respiratory insufficiency and vocal cord paresis, have been associated with CMT disease.[62] Cardiac conduction defects can occur, although they are not common.[62]

Anesthetic Considerations

Primary concerns with anesthesia include responses to muscle relaxants, increased incidence of malignant hyperthermia, and postoperative respiratory failure. There is no evidence of a prolonged response to muscle relaxants, and these patients seem to tolerate anesthesia without incident. However, because episodes of malignant hyperthermia have been reported, agents that trigger this life-threatening problem should be avoided.[63,64] Respiratory function, including a review of pulmonary function studies, blood gases, or evaluations by consultants should be evaluated prior to the initiation of anesthesia. A history of hospital admissions requiring mechanical ventilation or frequent exacerbations of pneumonia will alert the anesthesiologist to the risk of postoperative respiratory complications.

Regional Anesthesia for Patients with CMT Disease

The main advantage of regional anesthesia over general anesthesia in the patient with CMT disease is in eliminating the triggers for malignant hyperthermia. Subjecting the patient with a tendency toward respiratory failure to general anesthesia is avoided. Further vocal cord damage is also avoided by eliminating the need for airway manipulation. Even though pregnancy may cause exacerbations, epidural anesthesia for labor and delivery have been performed successfully without adverse effects.[65]

There is very little data in the literature about peripheral nerve block anesthesia or analgesia in patients with this disease. Upper extremity blocks avoid exposing the patient to potentially harmful anesthetic agents, intubation, and mechanical ventilation. It is prudent to remember that in patients with respiratory dysfunction, interscalene blocks will result in a 30% reduction in pulmonary volumes. Probably this block should be avoided in the presence of severe pulmonary dysfunction. Lower extremity blocks are more controversial. In the presence of peroneal and quadriceps muscle wasting, lower extremity blocks are probably best avoided, although they can be used with for selective cases.

Inflammatory-Immune Peripheral Neuropathies

Guillain–Barré Syndrome

Guillain-Barré syndrome (GBS) is an acute inflammatory demyelinating polyradiculoneuropathy. The incidence is 4 in 10,000, with men affected slightly more often than women. The disease is rare in pregnancy with only 29 reported cases in the literature from 1986 to 2002, but the risk of GBS increases for the mother during the postpartum period.[67,68] Death from Guillain-Barré syndrome is usually secondary to respiratory failure or autonomic nervous system dysfunction (ie, labile systemic blood pressure, cardiac conduction disturbances, sudden death).

The cause of GBS is unknown. It has been associated with a variety of bacterial and viral infections in two thirds of the cases. Other possible precipitants include vaccinations (polio, rabies), malignancies (most commonly Hodgkin lymphoma), hyperthyroidism, and drugs (heroin).[66,69,70] It is theorized that an infection triggers an immune response that targets myelin components of the nerve cells, resulting in macrophage-induced demyelination. In addition to the demyelination seen in GBS, channelopathies have been identified.[70] A sodium channel-blocking factor, similar to that seen in MS, has been found in the cerebrospinal fluid of patients with GBS, possibly contributing to the paralysis seen in this syndrome.[71]

The most common clinical presentation is an acute onset of progressive, symmetrical motor weakness, paralysis, and areflexia.[70] It usually begins in the legs, then ascends cephalad. Intercostal and pharyngeal muscle weakness may require intubation and mechanical ventilation. The incidence of dull, aching, burning low back or lower extremity pain occurs in approximately 90% of these patients. The condition worsens for several days to a peak at approximately 4 weeks. A period of stability follows for 1 to 2 weeks, then gradual improvement to normal or nearly normal function. Complications include aspiration pneumonia, respiratory and cardiac arrest, deep vein thrombosis, pulmonary embolism, and persistent motor weakness. The mortality rate ranges from 3% to 12%. Treatment is primarily supportive. Plasmapheresis or intravenous immunoglobulin (IVIG) therapy has been used successfully to reduce the duration of symptoms, but there is no cure.[70]

Anesthetic Considerations

It is highly recommended that patients with Guillain–Barré syndrome have a complete neurologic evaluation both before and after anesthesia is administered. A knowledge of the course of the disease, associated medical conditions, and expected time and quality of recovery will aid the anesthesiologist in choosing the anesthetic technique that best meets the needs of the patient. A thorough preoperative discussion with the patient, when possible, should include the risk/benefit ratio of general anesthesia vs regional anesthesia.

Up-regulation of the acetylcholine postsynaptic receptor occurs as a result of demyelination or axonal degeneration of nerve fibers.[72] Succinylcholine should be avoided due to the increased risk of a hyperkalemic response leading to cardiac arrest.[72] The response to nondepolarizing muscle relaxants varies from extreme sensitivity to resistance, depending on the phase of the disease.

Autonomic dysfunction, occurring in approximately 60% of the patients with GBS, indicates that the compensatory mechanisms for cardiovascular stability are defective.[72] Postural changes, blood loss, or positive pressure ventilation may result in an exaggerated hypotensive response. Asystole has been reported with eyeball pressure and tracheal suctioning in patients with GBS.[73] Systemic hypertension with noxious stimulation (ie, laryngoscopy), and an exaggerated response to indirect-acting vasopressors can occur.[52]

Respiratory and pharyngeal muscle involvement may predispose a loss of airway patency, decrease cough response, and increase risk of aspiration following general anesthesia.[73,74] The need for postoperative mechanical support should be anticipated when general anesthesia is provided.

Regional Anesthesia in Patients with GBS

Regional anesthetics may be beneficial for the patient with GBS.

In the pregnant patient, regional analgesia has been utilized to limit the exaggerated hemodynamic response to labor pain.[73] Sensitivity to local anesthetics may occur, possibly secondary to the sodium channel-blocking factor found in the CSF of these patients.[46,74,75] Because of the increased autonomic instability, epidural anesthesia may be preferable over spinal anesthesia because of its slower onset and more stable hemodynamic profile.[74,75] Theoretically, smaller doses of local anesthetics may be required and higher levels may be achieved secondarily to the effects of denervation.[53] Complications associated with neuraxial anesthesia in GBS patients, such as worsening neurologic symptoms, prolonged duration of action of local anesthetics, triggering underlying disease, and cardiac arrest after low subarachnoid block have been reported in the literature.[74–76]

The use of peripheral nerve block anesthesia in the patient with Guillain-Barré syndrome has not been reported. Theoretical advantages of regional anesthetic include the ability to provide excellent selective anesthesia, minimize sedation, eliminate the need for general anesthetic medications, and avoid intubation and ventilation. The hemodynamic instability associated with central neuraxial blocks is also avoided. The block should be performed utilizing a nerve stimulator or ultrasound technique. Objective monitoring of injection pressures may also be useful to prevent injection into a tight compartment space (eg nerve fascicle) and for objective procedure documentation.

Entrapment Neuropathies

Carpal Tunnel Syndrome

Carpal tunnel syndrome is the most common entrapment neuropathy.[77] Causes include wrist trauma, diabetes, hypothyroidism, rheumatoid arthritis, oral contraceptives, repetitive motion of the wrist, and pregnancy.[77] It results from compression of the median nerve between the transverse carpal ligament (flexor retinaculum) and the carpal bones of the wrist. Either a reduction in the size of the space in the carpal tunnel or an increase in the volume of its contents leading to an increased carpal tunnel pressure engenders the symptoms commonly associated with the disease.[77] The common clinical presentation is tingling; numbness; and pain in the thumb, index finger, long finger, and radial side of the ring finger.[69,77] Patients may complain of pain and paresthesias spreading to the affected arm and shoulder. Thenar weakness and loss of two-point discrimination may be observed.[77]

Treatment is directed at immobilization of the wrist when the cause is transient or related to a medically treatable disease, such as pregnancy or hypothyroidism. Splinting keeps the wrist in a neutral position, decreasing pressure on the carpal tunnel. Other treatments (ie, physical therapy, diuretics, steroid injection) have been tried with varying levels of success. *Definitive* treatment is surgical decompression of the median nerve by dividing the flexor retinaculum.[77]

Anesthetic Considerations in CTR

Anesthetic options for carpal tunnel release (CTR) surgery are numerous.[78] General anesthesia, local anesthetic infiltration, intravenous regional anesthesia, and peripheral nerve blocks of the brachial plexus or more distally at the peripheral nerves are some of the options. The choice of anesthetic technique is the same as with any type of surgical procedure. The goal is to provide the safest, most efficient anesthesia that affords the greatest benefit to the patient while offering coverage for the operative procedure. Because a bloodless operative field is required to enable clear identification of the anatomy to avoid damage to surrounding nerve fibers, an arm tourniquet is usually required. If the tourniquet is inflated longer than 30 min, however, intolerable tourniquet pain may occur and must be addressed.[78]

Local anesthetic infiltration is the simplest method of anesthesia, but it does not limit tourniquet pain, and may cause anatomic distortion of the surgical site from the infiltrating solution.[79] Intravenous regional anesthesia is another simple technique, but if the tourniquets are not applied properly, venous engorgement after tourniquet inflation can distort surgical exposure.[80] General anesthesia fulfills all of the surgical requirements for carpal tunnel release, but with the risk/benefit ratio for a relatively minor surgical procedure it may not be warranted, especially for ambulatory surgery.[81]

Regional Anesthesia for CTR

Peripheral nerve block anesthesia is an excellent means of anesthesia for CTR. Several peripheral block options are available to meet the anesthetic requirements for CTR surgery. At the brachial plexus, infraclavicular and axillary blocks provide excellent anesthesia as well as tourniquet tolerance beyond 30 min. Surgical site distortion does not occur. The disadvantage of a brachial plexus block is that both motor and sensory block occurs. If the surgeon is not concerned about an intraoperative sensory block, then a short-acting local anesthetic can be used that would allow return of motor–sensory function prior to the patient's discharge home.[80]

Peripheral blocks can be performed at or distal to the elbow for CTR surgery. The advantage of this technique is that selective sensory blocks can be performed while limiting the motor block (most motor fibers have already divided at this level). The disadvantages to selective lower peripheral nerve blocks is that multiple nerves must be located and blocked. Although the median nerve provides the predominant innervation of this area, there is overlap from the ulnar and radial nerves. To provide complete anesthesia, all three terminal branches of the brachial plexus should be blocked.

If the incision is extended to the forearm, cutaneous branches of the musculocutaneous nerve are involved. Tourniquet pain is still an issue with distal peripheral nerve blocks, but most of these procedures do not extend beyond 30 min. The administration of additional light sedation is usually adequate for patient comfort.[82]

Ulnar Nerve Entrapment

Ulnar nerve entrapment can occur either at the elbow or at the wrist. Ulnar-sided wrist pain is often vague and chronic in nature, has an insidious onset, and its symptoms are often intermittent. Diagnosis can be frustrating both for the patient and for the physician. Ulnar wrist pain is usually related to acute traumatic injuries, chronic overuse injuries, or chronic degenerative problems.[83] Depending on the nature and timing of the injury, treatment includes rest, immobilization, nonsteroidal antiinflammatory drugs (NSAIDs), steroids, or surgical decompression.[84]

Ulnar nerve entrapment at the elbow, "cubital entrapment syndrome," is the second most frequent upper extremity compression neuropathy.[85] The ulnar nerve is at increased risk because of its superficial location in the regional of the medial elbow. Injury to the nerve may occur as a result of acute trauma, compression, repetitive traction, subluxation of the nerve, osteoarthritis, gout, or following surgical treatment of an upper extremity injury. The initial symptoms include intermittent hypersthesia in the ulnar nerve distribution, elbow pain, and paresthesias in the ring and small fingers. These symptoms are often intermittent and may occur for months or years. In the later stages of the disease, weakness of the intrinsic muscles of the hand with or without visible atrophy may be observed.[85] Initial treatment of closed injuries to the ulnar nerve include physical therapy and NSAIDs. Open injuries with evidence of ulnar nerve disruption associated with fractures or lacerations are commonly treated with early surgical repair or grafting. Surgical decompression has a high success rate if performed prior to the occurrence of chronic signs and symptoms.[86]

Anesthetic Considerations for Ulnar Nerve Entrapment Surgery

General, regional, or local anesthesia can be used for surgical decompression of an entrapped ulnar nerve. The choice of anesthetic depends on the surgical procedure, whether nerve function will be tested intraoperatively, and the extent of injury accompanying the nerve injury. The most conservative approach is local anesthesia with sedation (in selective cases). General anesthesia is often used for more involved procedures.[6]

Regional Anesthesia for Ulnar Nerve Entrapment

The use of regional anesthetic techniques in patients with preexisting neuropathies is controversial, but is gaining acceptance as a safe method of anesthesia in centers that perform large numbers of regional blocks. The primary concern in these patients is that needles or catheters used for regional blocks may place the patient at a greater risk of nerve injury from trauma, local anesthetic toxicity, or neural ischemia, especially in the face of preexisting neurologic derangements.[6] In a 2001 study of 360 patients with pre-existing ulnar neuropathy undergoing ulnar nerve transposition, Hebl and colleagues found that anesthetic technique did not affect the neurologic outcome immediately after surgery or 2–6 weeks postoperatively in patients undergoing ulnar nerve transposition surgery.[6] Depending on the surgical site, a supraclavicular, infraclavicular, or axillary block will provide effective anesthesia for the procedure. The block may be performed using a nerve stimulator, with the understanding that the ulnar distribution may be impaired. If the inner aspect of the upper extremity is part of the operative site (T1, T2 distribution), local infiltration by the surgeon or additional sedation is usually all that is required for patient comfort. A preoperative discussion with the surgeon to determine the intraoperative plan, specific concerns related to the patient's disease process, and the extent of the operative field (to determine the coverage required with a peripheral nerve block) will assist the anesthesiologist in making the most appropriate choice of anesthetic.

NEUROMUSCULAR JUNCTION DISEASE

The neuromuscular junction is an area of primary interest for the anesthesiologist because it holds the key to skeletal muscle function. The large number of nAChRs (1–10 million) in the postsynaptic muscle membrane (the motor end-plate) is critical for maintaining normal neuromuscular function. Under normal circumstances, only a small portion of the available receptors must bind to acetylcholine to trigger a muscle contraction. Therefore, there is an excess of receptors available providing a "wide margin of safety" for muscle contraction in the event that the postsynaptic receptors are blocked, damaged, or destroyed.

Neuromuscular blocking agents that interact with the nicotinic cholinergic receptor to prevent muscle contraction are commonly used during many surgical procedures. A large number of receptors must be occupied by neuromuscular blocking agents before muscle paralysis occurs. In the patient with a neuromuscular junction defect the effects of these anesthetic agents are markedly altered

Skeletal muscle relaxation can also be produced by deep inhalational anesthesia or by local anesthetics. The mechanism of action is different. Inhaled anesthetics produce muscle relaxation by altering physiology of the brain and spinal cord, as well as the nAChRs.[87] Local anesthetics produce muscle relaxation by their effect on voltage-dependent sodium channels on nerve and muscle membranes.[88] When a neuromuscular junction defect is present, as is the case in the myasthenic syndromes, the anesthesiologist must carefully choose the anesthetic agent that will provide the greatest benefit without potentiating the skeletal muscle weakness or causing a myasthenic crisis.

Myasthenia Gravis

Myasthenia gravis (MG) is a chronic, acquired autoimmune disease caused by antibodies that destroy or inactivate the nAChRs at the neuromuscular junction. The antibodies specifically target the α-subunit of the receptor in 80% of the cases of the disease. In the other 20% of the patients (seronegative patients), autoantibodies target a muscle-specific tyrosine kinase (MuSK).[89] Weakness and easy fatigability are the hallmark symptoms, with either discrete muscle groups affected (ie, ocular MG), or generalized weakness with life-threatening respiratory muscle dysfunction (ie, myasthenia crisis).[90] The antibodies do not affect the nAChRs in the autonomic nervous system or the CNS because of differences in protein structure, therefore limiting autonomic and CNS symptoms in the disease process.[91]

MG has a prevalence of 14 per 100,000, without an ethnic predominance. The most common age at onset is the second and third decade in women (childbearing age) and the sixth to seventh decade in men. Family members of patients with MG are 1000 times more likely to have the disease than the general population. The effects of pregnancy on MG are variable; symptoms can remain unchanged, worsen, or improve. Of the 30–40% of patients whose symptoms worsen with pregnancy, primigravidas usually experience exacerbations in the first trimester. In subsequent pregnancies, exacerbations in the third trimester and in the postpartum period are more common.[92]

Skeletal muscles innervated by cranial nerves are especially vulnerable. In 70% of the cases, the initial complaint is diplopia, with over 90% of the patients demonstrating extraocular muscle weakness during the course of the disease. The vast majority will have bulbar muscle involvement (laryngeal, pharyngeal muscles), leading to airway compromise, dysphagia, and the increased risk of aspiration. Other signs and symptoms of the disease include asymmetrical skeletal muscle weakness with exercise, myocarditis (leading to cardiomyopathy, atrial fibrillation and heart block), hypothyroidism, and isolated respiratory failure from diaphragmatic and thoracic intercostal muscle weakness.[90]

The clinical course of the disease is marked by periods of exacerbations and remissions. Most patients whose initial symptoms are limited to ptosis or diplopia will develop generalized muscle weakness within the first 3 years.[93] Muscle strength characteristically improves with rest but deteriorates rapidly with exertion. The life-threatening result of the disease is called a myasthenic crisis. It is a severe exacerbation of weakness often associated with respiratory compromise precipitated by menses, infection, noncompliance with treatment, or the introduction of new medications (ie, aminoglycosides to treat infection, beta-blockers).[93]

Treatment for MG can be medical or surgical, depending on the patient's age, the presence of a thymoma, and the extent of the disease. Medical treatment is aimed at (1) enhancing neuromuscular transmission by anticholinesterases, (2) suppressing the immune system with corticosteroids, immunosuppressants (cyclosporine/azathioprine), and (3) modulating the circulating antibody level with plasmapheresis or IVIG. Elective thymectomy is the preferred treatment for patients with generalized MG, those younger than 60 years of age, and in all patients with a thymoma (33% risk of malignancy). MG patients undergoing thymectomy are twice as likely to attain a medication-free remission and 1.7 times as likely to have an improvement in symptoms.[94] Beneficial effects of thymectomy may be delayed for months or years, and most patients will continue to have symptoms to a varying degree. Prior to surgery, effective immunosuppressant therapy must be used to make the patient asymptomatic to reduce postoperative morbidity and mortality.[70]

Anesthetic Considerations for patients with MG

Anesthetic management of the patient with MG is complicated because the response to commonly used drugs is variable.[95,96] Cautious use of sedatives, muscle relaxants, and general anesthetics must be considered for all patients with a diagnosis of MG.

A thorough preoperative evaluation is necessary for the safe delivery of anesthesia for these patients. Preoperative evaluation should include (1) consultation with the patient's neurologist to review the course of the patient's disease, treatment, and any recent changes in status, (2) review of the patient's preoperative drug therapy, changes in dose or type of medication, and response to medications as well as potential interactions with anesthetic agents, (3) counseling the patient and the family about the potential for postoperative mechanical ventilation.

Optimizing the patient's condition preoperatively can improve outcome. Anticholinesterase agents are usually discontinued preoperatively unless the patient is physically dependent on them. Preoperative plasmapheresis has been used successfully to optimize the patient's condition and reduce perioperative morbidity and mortality.[96]

The most important preoperative factor predicting the need for postoperative mechanical ventilation is the degree and severity of bulbar involvement, especially when associated with a prior history of respiratory failure.[97] Other factors that have been identified as predictors for postoperative respiratory support include disease duration of >6 years, concomitant pulmonary disease, peak inspiratory pressure of −25 cm H_2O, and vital capacity of <4 mL/kg.[97]

Anesthetic medications need to be used with caution. Because of the reduced number of nAChRs, myasthenic patients are resistant to succinylcholine.[98] However, they are exquisitely sensitive to nondepolarizing muscle relaxants.[99] Short- and intermediate-duration nondepolarizing muscle relaxants can be used with careful titration and monitoring with a nerve stimulator. Long-acting muscle relaxants should be avoided. If the patient has been on pyridostigmine therapy, the response to muscle relaxants changes. The patient will be less sensitive to nondepolarizing muscle relaxants, the response to succinylcholine or mivacurium will be prolonged

(plasma cholinesterase effect), and reversal of the block at the end of the case is unpredictable.[98,99]

General anesthesia has been provided with total intravenous anesthesia (remifentanil) and high thoracic epidural, or inhaled anesthetic without neuromuscular blockers.[100] It is important to remember that these patients are more sensitive to inhaled anesthetics (leading to a slower recovery from anesthesia), and to the neuromuscular depressant effects of isoflurane and halothane.[100] Drugs that interfere with neuromuscular transmission (ie, aminoglycoside antibiotics, antiarrhythmics, beta-blockers, phenytoin) should be limited or avoided when possible. Usually, opioids are avoided or limited. During the postoperative period, abrupt reduction in skeletal muscle strength may occur, necessitating the need for mechanical ventilation. Diligent postoperative monitoring in the surgical intensive care unit is therefore necessary for the myasthenic patient.

Regional Anesthesia in Patients with MG

Because of the numerous problems associated with perioperative sedation, general anesthetic agents, and muscle relaxants, regional anesthesia may be a better choice for anesthesia in the myasthenic patient. Because local anesthetics do not directly affect the nAChRs, regional anesthesia offers greater predictability with fewer complications.

Epidural anesthesia has been used in myasthenic patients. High thoracic epidural with either total intravenous anesthesia or a balanced general anesthesia provides excellent anesthesia for the MG patient undergoing thymectomy.[101,102] In the pregnant patient with MG, epidural anesthesia has been used successfully to reduce the physical and emotional stress that may potentiate a crisis.[103] Many of the drugs used to treat the disease are continued during pregnancy to avoid a crisis, but these may have an effect on platelet function and number. Prior to placing a central neuraxial block, it is important to obtain a coagulation profile as well as a platelet count.[103] Amide local anesthetics may be a better choice than ester local anesthetics because the metabolism of amides is not dependent on cholinesterase activity.[103]

Very little data are available on the use of peripheral nerve blocks in the patient with MG. The successful use of a paravertebral block for inguinal hernia surgery, infraclavicular block for a dislocated elbow, and various central neuraxial blocks for surgery on the lower extremities have been reported.[104,105]

Interscalene blocks should be avoided in patients with bulbar or respiratory compromise because the phrenic nerve can be blocked during the procedure. Infraclavicular or axillary blocks in selected cases will provide anesthesia for the upper extremity without compromising respiratory function. Isolated digital nerve blocks for injuries to the fingers, hand, wrist, or ankle are excellent methods for providing anesthesia without involving other muscle groups. Lumbar plexus blocks should probably be avoided in patients with dysfunctional platelet function. The anesthesiologist should be prepared for the possibility of epidural spread causing a more profound motor block. Femoral, popliteal sciatic, and ankle blocks are effective blocks for surgery on the lower extremities. Reduced doses of sedatives and opioids during block placement are necessary due to the sensitivity of the myasthenic patient to these medications.

Lambert–Eaton Myasthenic Syndrome

Lambert–Eaton myasthenic syndrome (LEMS) is a rare autoimmune disease in which autoantibodies target voltage-gated calcium channels.[106] Sixty-six percent of the cases are associated with carcinomas (usually small cell carcinomas of the lung), but the symptoms of LEMS may precede the discovery of the cancer by as much as 5 years. The autoantibodies are directed at calcium channels in the tumor, but because of antigenic similarity, they cross-react with calcium channels at the presynaptic neuromuscular junction responsible for the release of acetylcholine. Consequently, acetylcholine release is reduced.[106]

The typical patient is a male, smoker, 50–70 years of age, who presents with slowly progressive proximal muscle weakness and fatigue that affects gait and the ability to stand and climb stairs.[106] Muscle pain and paresthesias can occur, although the sensory examination is usually normal. Over 75% of the patients with LEMS have symptoms of autonomic dysfunction, including dry mouth, constipation, blurred vision, orthostatic hypotension, and impotence.[106] Ocular and bulbar symptoms (ptosis, dysphagia, diplopia) are less prominent than in MG, but may occur in up to 30% of the patients. Unlike in MG, exercise improves strength.[106]

Treatment of LEMS is geared toward identification and treatment of the underlying neoplasm, medications that enhance neuromuscular transmission, and alteration of the autoantibodies. Early and successful treatment of the lung cancer usually results in clinical improvement.[70,107] Treatment includes 3,4-diaminopyridine (enhances acetylcholine release by blocking potassium channels), pyridostigmine (inhibits acetylcholinesterase, resulting in more available acetylcholine), immunosuppressants, plasmapheresis or IVIG.[107]

Medications that interfere with neuromuscular transmission can worsen the symptoms of LEMS should be avoided. These include aminoglycoside antibiotics, beta-blockers, neuromuscular blocking agents, quinidine, and iodinated contrast agents.[107]

Anesthetic Considerations

Patients with LEMS are sensitive to the effects of both depolarizing and nondepolarizing muscle relaxants. Therefore, doses of these drugs should be reduced.[108] Neuromuscular function should be carefully assessed with a nerve stimulator. Because the syndrome is difficult to diagnose, it may be unmasked perioperatively when the patient demonstrates prolonged paralysis after receiving the usual dose of neuromuscular blockers.[108] In patients with LEMS, antagonism with anticholinesterases may be inadequate.[108] The possibility of postoperative mechanical ventilation must be considered. Because of the autonomic dysfunction related to the syndrome, hemodynamic instability may occur with inhaled anesthetics.[108] Anticipating and preparing for orthostatic changes is prudent.

Regional Anesthesia for Patients with LEMS

LEMS is a rare disease, much less common than MG. Literature regarding the use of regional anesthesia in these patients is absent. Given the complications associated with general anesthesia, selective nerve blocks may be advantageous in specific cases.

SUMMARY

The current literature regarding regional anesthesia in patients with preexisting neurologic disease is limited. Many neurologic conditions pose a risk to patients undergoing general anesthesia. Problems could arise with autonomic dysfunction, airway and respiratory complications, abnormal responsiveness to anesthetic drugs, and delirium. For these reasons, the use of regional techniques should be considered after careful evaluation of the patient's disease processes, neurologic evaluation, consideration of the risk/benefit ratio, and the surgical procedure. Peripheral nerve blocks may be the safest and most appropriate method of anesthesia. However, the risk of nerve block-related neurologic complications has prevented many from employing regional anesthesia in these patients. Practitioners of regional anesthesia have been particularly vulnerable to the blame for postoperative neurologic impairment. However, recent developments in nerve localization with ultrasound-assisted nerve blocks, and injection pressure monitoring have decreased the risk of causing nerve damage. With these developments, regional anesthesia will have an increasingly important role in management of patients with preexisting neurologic conditions.

References

1. Horlocker TT, Wedel D: Neurologic complications of spinal and epidural anesthesia. Reg Anesth Pain Med 2000;25:83–98.
2. Backman E, Nylander E: The heart in Duchenne muscular dystrophy: A progressive longitudinal study. Eur Heart J 1992;13:1239–1244.
3. Baur CP, Schlecht R, Jurkay-Rott K, et al: Anesthesia in neuromuscular disorders. Anasthesiol Intensivmed Notfallmed Schmerzther 2002;37:77–83.
4. Cheney FW, Domino KB, Caplan RA, et al: Nerve injury associated with anesthesia. A closed claims analysis. Anesthesiology 1999;90:1062–1069.
5. Borgeat A: Neurologic deficit after peripheral nerve block: What to do? Minerva Anestesiol 2005;71:353–355.
6. Hebl JR, Horlocker TT, Sorenso EJ, et al: Regional anesthesia does not increase the risk of postoperative neuropathy in patients undergoing ulnar nerve transposition. Anesth Analg 2001;93:1606–1611.

7. Horlocker TT, Kufner RP, Bishop AT, et al: The risk of persistent paresthesia is not increased with repeated axillary block. Anesth Analg 1999;88:382–387.

8. Sadove MS, Levin MJ, Rant-Sejdinaj I: Neurological complications of spinal anesthesia. Can Anaesth Soc J 1961;8:405–416.

9. Moore DC, Bridenbaugh LD: Spinal block: A review of 11,574 cases. JAMA 1966;195:123–128.

10. Dripps Rd, Vandam LD: Long-term follow-up of patients who received 10,098 spinal anesthetics: Failure to discover major neurological sequelae. JAMA 1954;156:1486–1491.

11. Kane RE: Neurologic deficits following epidural or spinal anesthesia. Anesth Analg 1981;60:150–161.

12. Olanow CW: A rationale for using dopamine agonists as a primary symptomatic therapy in Parkinson's disease. In Obeso JA (ed): *Dopamine Agonists in Early Parkinson's Disease.* Wells Medical, 1997, pp 37–48.

13. Lang AE, Lozano AM: Parkinson's disease: First of two parts. New Engl J Med 1998; 339: 1044.

14. Mantz J, Varlet C, Lecharny JB, et al: Effects of volatile anaesthetics, thiopental, and ketamine on spontaneous and depolarization-evoked dopamine release from striatum. Anesthesiology 1994;80:352–363.

15. Klausner JM, Caspi J, Lelcuk S, et al: Delayed muscle rigidity and respiratory depression following fentanyl anesthesia. Arch Surg 1988;123:66–67.

16. Mayeux R, Sano M: Treatment of Alzheimer's disease. N Engl J Med 1999;341:1670.

17. Burton DA, Nicholson G, Hall GM: Anaesthesia in elderly patients with neurodegenerative disorders: Special considerations. Drugs Aging 2004;21:229–242.

18. Jackson CE, Bryan WW: Amyotrophic sclerosis. Semin Neurol 1998;18:27.

19. Maselli RA, Wollman RL, Leung C, et al: Neuromuscular transmission in amyotrophic lateral sclerosis. Muscle Nerve 1993;16:1193–1203.

20. Beach TP, Stone WA, Hamelberg W: Circulatory collapse following succinylcholine. Report of a patient with diffuse lower motor neuron disease. Anesth Analg 1971;50:431–437.

21. Rosenbaum KJ, Neigh JL, Strobel GE: Sensitivity to nondepolarizing muscle relaxants in amyotrophic lateral sclerosis. Anesthesiology 1971;35:638–641.

22. Mishima Y, Katsuki s, Sawada M, et al: Anesthetic management of a patient with amyotrophic lateral sclerosis. Masui 2002;51:762–764.

23. Moser B, Lirk P, Lechner M, et al: General anaesthesia in a patient with motor neuron disease. Eur J Anaesthesiol 2004;21:921–923.

24. Otsuka N, Igarashi M, Shimodate Y, et al: Anesthetic management of two patients with amyotrophic lateral sclerosis. Masui 2004;53:1279–1281.

25. Chen LK, Chang Y, Liu CC, et al: Epidural anesthesia combined with propofol sedation for abdominal hysterectomy in a patient with ALS. Acta Anaesthesiol Sin 1998;36:103–106.

26. Kochi T, Oka T, et al: Epidural anesthesia for patients with amyotrophic lateral sclerosis. Anesth Analg 1989; 68: 410–412.

27. Albin MS, White RJ: Epidemiology, physiopathology and experimental therapeutics of acute spinal injury. Crit Care Clin 1987;3:441–452.

28. Burney RE, Maio RF, Maynard F, et al: Incidence, characteristics and outcome of spinal cord injury at trauma centers in North America. Arch Surg 1993;128:596–599.

29. Stowe DF, Bernstein JS, Madsen KE, et al: Autonomic hyperreflexia in spinal cord patients during extracorporeal shock wave lithotripsy. Anesth Analg 1989;68:788.

30. Kendrick WW, Scott JW, Jousse AT, et al: Reflex sweating and hypertension in traumatic transverse myelitis. Treat Serv Bull 1953;8:437.

31. Pope CS, Markenson GR, Bayer-Zwirello LA, et al: Pregnancy complicated by chronic spinal cord injury and history of autonomic hyperreflexia. Obstet Gynecol 2001;97:802–805.

32. Geerts WH, Heit JA, Clagett GP, et al: Prevention of venous thromboembolism. Chest 2001;119:132–175.

33. Gronert GA, Theye RA: Pathophysiology of hyperkalemia induced by succinylcholine. Anesthesiology 1975;1975:89.

34. Silbert BS, Kluger R, Dixon GC, et al: Anaesthesia for extracorporeal shockwave lithotripsy at the Victorian Lithotripsy Service—the first 300 patients. Anaesth Intensive Care 1988;16:310–317.

35. Gilson GJ, Miller AC, Clevenger FW, et al: Acute spinal cord injury and neurogenic shock in pregnancy. Obstet Gynecol Sur 1995;50:556–560.

36. Kang AH: Traumatic spinal cord injury: Neurologic disorders in pregnancy. Clin Obstet Gynecol 2005;48:67–72.

37. Muralidhar V: Blocks to facilitate lithotomy positioning in spastic paraplegics. Anesth Analg 1996;82:219.

38. Samuels SI, Jaffe RA, Schendel SA: Functional restoration. In Jaffe RA, Samuels SI (eds): *Anesthesiologist's Manual of Surgical Procedures,* 2nd ed. Lippincott Williams & Wilkins, 1999, pp 836–838.

39. Fishburn MJ, Marino RJ, Ditunno JF Jr: Atelectasis and pneumonia in acute spinal cord injury. Arch Phys Med Rehabil 1990;71:197–200.

40. Stanton-Hicks M, Baron R, Boas R, et al: Complex regional pain syndromes: Guidelines for therapy. Clin J Pain 1998;14:155–166.

41. Baker ER, Cardenas DD, Benedettik TJ: Risks associated with pregnancy in spinal cord-injured women. Obstet Gynecol 1992;80:425–528.

42. Filho L, Morandin RC, de Almeida AR, et al: Importance of anesthesia for the genesis of neurogenic pulmonary edema in spinal cord injury. Neurosci Lett 2005;373:165–170.

43. Burns R, Clark VA: Epidural anesthesia for caesarean section in a patient with quadriplegia and autonomic hyperreflexia. Int J Obstet Anesth 2004;13:120–123.

44. Noseworthy JH: Progress in determining the causes and treatment of multiple sclerosis. Nature 1999;399:A40–A47.

45. Meinl E: Concepts of viral pathogenesis of multiple sclerosis. Curr Opin Neurol 1999;12:303–307.

46. Brinkmeier H, Aulkemeyer P, Wollinsky KH, et al: An endogenous pentapeptide acting as a sodium channel blocker in inflammatory autoimmune disorders of the central nervous system. Nat Med 2000;6:808–811.

47. Craner MJU, Newcombe JA, Black JA, et al: Molecular changes in neurons in multiple sclerosis: Altered axonal expression of Na 1.2 and N 1.6 sodium channels and Na+/Ca++ exchanger. Proc Nat Acad Sci USA 2004;101:8167–8173.

48. Kuwaira I, Kondo T, Ohto Y, et al: Acute respiratory failure in multiple sclerosis. Chest 1990;97:246.

49. Vita G, Fazio MC, Milone S, et al: Cardiovascular autonomic dysfunction in multiple sclerosis is likely related to brainstem lesions. J Neurol Sci 1993;120:1993.

50. Buyse B, Demedts M, Meekers J, et al: Respiratory dysfunction in multiple sclerosis: A prospective analysis of 60 patients. Eur Respir J 1997;10:139.

51. Cook SD, Troiano RE, Bansil S, et al: Multiple sclerosis and pregnancy. Adv Neurol 1994;64:83.

52. Bannister R, Davies B, Holly E, et al: Defective cardiovascular reflexes and supersensitivity to sympathomimetic drugs in autonomic failure. Brain 1979;102:163–176.

53. Naguib M, Flood P, McArdle JJ, et al: Advances in neurobiology of the neuromuscular junction: Implications for the anesthesiologist. Anesthesiology 2002;96:202–231.

54. Jones RM, Heal TEJ: Anaesthesia and demyelinating disease. Anaesthesia 1980;35:879.

55. Bader AM, Hunt CO, Datta S, et al: Anesthesia for the obstetric patient with multiple sclerosis. J Clin Anesth 1988;1:21–24.

56. Sakurai M, Mannen T, Kanazawa I, et al: Lidocaine unmasks silent demyelinative lesions in multiple sclerosis. Neurology 1992;42:2088–2093.

57. Damas AF, Texier C, Ducloy-Bouthors AS, et al: Obstetrical analgesia and anaesthesia in multiple sclerosis. Ann Fr Anesth Reanim 2003;22:861–864.

58. Ingrosso M, Cirillo V, Papasso A, et al: Femoral and sciatic nerve block in orthopedic traumatologic lower limbs surgery in patients with multiple sclerosis. Minerva Anestesiol 2004;71:223–226.

59. Finucane BAT, Terblanche OC: Prolonged duration of anesthesia in a patient with multiple sclerosis following paravertebral block. Can J Anaesth 2005;52:454–458.

60. Greene DA, Stevens MJ, Feldman EL: Diabetic neuropathy: Scope of the syndrome. Am J Med 1999;107:2S–8S.

61. Hughes R: Treatment of peripheral nerve disorders. Curr Opin Neurol 2005;18:554–556.

62. Rudnick-Schoneborn S, Rohrig D, Nicholson G, et al: Pregnancy and delivery in Charcot–Marie–Tooth disease Type I. Neurology 1993;43:2011–2016.

63. Ducart A, Adnet P, Renaud B, et al: Malignant hyperthermia during sevoflurane administration. Anesth Analg 1995;80:609–611.

64. Roelofse JA, Shipton EA: Anaesthesia for abdominal hysterectomy in Charcot–Marie–Tooth disease: A case report. S Afr Med J 1985;67:605–606.

65. Sugai L, Sugai Y: Epidural anesthesia in a patient with Charcot–Marie–Tooth disease, bronchial asthma and hypothyroidism. Masai 1989;38:688–691.

66. Rudnicki SA, Dalmau J: Paraneoplastic syndromes of the peripheral nerves. Curr Opin Neurol 2005;18:598–603.

67. Cheng Q, Jiang GX, Fredrickson S, et al: Increased incidence of Guillain–Barre syndrome postpartum. Epidemiology 1998;1998:601–604.

68. Chan LY, Tsui MH, Leung TN: Guillain–Barre syndrome in pregnancy. Acta Obstet Gynecol Scand 2004;83:319–325.

69. Mabie WC: Peripheral neuropathies during pregnancy. Clin Obstet Gynecol 2005;48:57–66.

70. Lynn DJ, Newton HB, Rae-Grant MD: Neurologic diseases and disorders. In Newton L, Newton HB, Rae-Grant MD(eds): *Five Minute Neurology Consult,* 1st ed. Lippincott Williams & Wilkins, 2004, pp 206–207.

71. Brinkmeier H, Seewald MJ, Wollinsky KH, et al: On the nature of endogenous antiexcitatory factors in the CSF of patients with demyelinating neurological disease. Muscle Nerve 1996;19: 54–62.

72. Dalman JE, Verhagen WI: Cardiac arrest in Guillain-Barre syndrome and the use of suxamethonium. Acta Neurol Belg 1994;94:259–261.

73. Martz DG, Schreibman DL, Matjasko MJU: Neurologic diseases. In Benumof JL (ed): *Anesthesia and Uncommon Diseases.* WB Saunders, 1998, pp 3–37.

74. Perel A, Reches A, Davidson JT: Anaesthesia in the Guillain-Barre syndrome. A case report and recommendations. Anaesthesia 1977;32:257–609.

75. Vassiliev DV, Nystrom, EU, Leicht CH: Combined spinal and epidural anesthesia for labor and cesarean delivery in a patient with Guillain–Barre syndrome. Reg Anesth Pain Med 2001;26:174–176.

76. Steiner I, Argov Z, Cahan C, et al: Guillain–Barre syndrome after epidural anesthesia: Direct nerve root damage may trigger disease. Neurology 1985;35:1473–1475.

77. Turgut F, Cetinsahin M, Turgut M, et al: The management of carpal tunnel syndrome in pregnancy. J Clin Neurosci 2001;8:332–334.

78. Sinba A, Chan V, Anastakis DJ: Anesthesia for carpal tunnel release. Can J Anaesth 2003;50:323–327.

79. Hutchinson DT, McClinton, MA: Upper extremity tourniquet tolerance. J Hand Surg 1993;18A:206–210.

80. Chan VWS, Peng PWH, Kaszas Z: A comparative study of general anesthesia, intravenous regional anesthesia, and axillary block for outpatient hand surgery: Clinical outcome and cost analysis. Anesth Analg 2001;93:1181–1184.

81. Chung F, Mezei G: Factors contributing to a prolonged stay after ambulatory surgery. Anesth Analg 1999;89:1352–1359.

82. Delaunay L, Chelly JE: Blocks at the wrist provide effective anesthesia for carpal tunnel release. Can J Anaesth 2001;48:656–660.

83. Shin AY, Deitch MA, Sachar K, Boyer, MI: Ulnar-sided wrist pain: Diagnosis and treatment. J Bone Joint Surg 2004;86:1560–1574.

84. Bottke CA, Louis DS, Braunstein EM: Diagnosis and treatment of obscure ulnar-sided wrist pain. Orthopedics 1989;12:1075–1079.

85. Antoniadis G, Richter HP: Pain after surgery for ulnar neuropathy at the elbow: A continuing challenge. Neurosurgery 1997;41:585–591.

86. Dellon AL: Review of treatment results for ulnar nerve entrapment at the elbow. J Hand Surg1989;14–A:688–700.

87. Franks NP, Lieb WR: Molecular and cellular mechanisms of general anesthesia. Nature 1994;367:607–614.

88. Usubiaga JE, Standaert F: The effects of local anesthetics on motor nerve terminals. J Pharmacol Exper Ther 1968;159:353–361.

89. Hoch W, McConville J, Helms S: Auto-antibodies to the receptor tyrosine kinase MuSK in patients with myasthenia gravis without acetylcholine receptor antibodies. Nat Med 2001;7:365–368.

90. Stevens RD: Neuromuscular disorders and anesthesia. Curr Opin Anesthesiol 2001;14:693–698.

91. Vernino S, Adamski J, Kryzer TJ: Neuronal nicotinic ACh receptor antibody in subacute autonomic neuropathy and cancer-related syndromes. Neurology 1998;50:1806–1813.

92. Karnad DR, Guntupalli KK: Neurologic disorders in pregnancy. Crit Care Med 2005;33:s362–s371.

93. Baraka AS, Jalbout MI: Anesthesia and myopathy. Curr Opin Anesthesiol 2002;15:371–376.

94. Gronseth S, Barohn RJ: Practice parameter: Thymectomy for autoimmune myasthenia gravis (an evidence-based review). Report of the Quality Standards Subcommittee of the American Academy of Neurology. Neurology 2000;55:7–15.

95. Baraka AS, Jalbout MI: Anesthesia and myopathy. Curr Opin Anesthesiol 2002; 15: 371–376.

96. Baraka A: Anaesthesia and myasthenia gravis. Can J Anaesth 1992;39:476–486.

97. Eisenkraft JB, Papatestas AE, Pozner JN: Predictors of respiratory failure following transcervical thymectomy. Ann NY Acad Sci 1987;505:888–890.

98. Eisenkraft JB, Book WJ, Mann SM: Resistance to succinylcholine in myasthenia gravis: A dose-response study. Anesthesiology 1988;69:760–763.

99. Eisenkraft JB, Book WJ, Papatestas AE: Sensitivity to vecuronium in myasthenia gravis: A dose-response study. Can J Anaesth 1990;37:301–306.

100. Nilsson E, Muller K: Neuromuscular effects of isoflurane in patients with myasthenia gravis. Acta Anaesthesiol Scand 1990;33:126–131.

101. Mekis D, Kamenik M: Remifentanil and high thoracic epidural anesthesia: A successful combination for patients with myasthenia gravis undergoing transsternal thymectomy. Eur J Anaesthsiol 2005;22:397–399.

102. Stevens RD: Neuromuscular disorders and anesthesia. Curr Opin Anesthesiol 2001;14:693–6989.

103. Ferrero S, Pretta S, Nicoletti A: Myasthenia gravis: Management issues during pregnancy. Eur J Obstet Gynecol Reprod Biol 2005;104:21–25.

104. Sinha A, Ahmad K, Harrop-Griffiths W: The use of a vertical infraclavicular brachial plexus block in a patient with myasthenia gravis: Effects on lung function. Anaesthesia 2001;56:165–168.

105. Baur CP, Schlecht R, Jurkat-Rott K, et al: Anesthesia is neuromuscular disorders. Part I. Anaesthesiol Intensive Med 2002;37:77–83.
106. Takamori M, Maruta Komai K: Lambert–Eaton myasthenic syndrome as an autoimmune calcium-channelopathy. Neurosci Res 2000;36:183–191.
107. Kokontis L, Gutmann L: Current treatment of neuromuscular disease. Arch Neurol 2000;57:939–943.
108. Small S, Ali HH, Lennon VA: Anesthesia for an unsuspected Lambert–Eaton myasthenic syndrome with autoantibodies and occult small cell lung carcinoma. Anesthesiology 1992;76:142–145.

60

Acute Compartment Syndrome of the Limb: Implications for Regional Anesthesia

Xavier Sala-Blanch, MD • José De Andrés, MD • Alton Barron, MD • Paul Hobeika, MD • Adam Cohen, MD • Lakshmanasamy Somasundaram, MD

INTRODUCTION

Compartment syndrome is an orthopedic emergency. It is an acute condition of the limbs in which the pressure of isolated or groups of compartments increases dramatically and limits local soft tissue perfusion to the point of ischemic necrosis. Regional anesthesia may mask the signs and symptoms of compartment syndrome, so practitioners should be alert to patient risk factors, clinical presentation, and management of this potentially limb-threatening condition. The musculoskeletal structures of the limbs are enclosed within compartments created by investing, inelastic sheets of fascia that have a limited ability to expand. These compartments contain skeletal muscles that form the bulk of their contents, along with the neurovascular structures that pass through the compartment. If missed, compartment syndrome[1] can be a life- and limb-threatening condition.

Compartment syndrome is most common in the lower leg and forearm, although it can also occur in the hand, foot, thigh, and upper arm. In theory, the upper leg muscles are at a lower risk for injury than are the smaller muscles of the lower leg, because the muscles of the thigh can dissipate the large forces of direct trauma, causing less muscle injury and resultant edema.[2] Acute compartment syndrome occurs more commonly in one of the four smaller compartments of the lower leg.

Historically, the consequences of persistently elevated intracompartmental pressures was first described by Richard von Volkmann,[3] who documented nerve injury and late muscle contracture from compartment syndrome after supracondylar fracture of the distal humerus. Jepson[4] described ischemic contractures in dog hind legs, resulting from limb hypertension after experimentally induced venous obstruction. Only after almost 30 years (1970s) has the importance of measuring compartmental pressures become apparent.

Etiology

Any condition that can reduce the volume of the compartment or increase the size of the contents of the compartment can lead to an acute compartment syndrome. Examples of factors leading to these changes are presented in Table 60–1.

Pathophysiology

Compartment syndrome is essentially soft tissue ischemia; however, the exact mechanism of compartment syndrome is unclear. Because various osseofascial compartments have a relatively fixed volume, introduction of excess fluid or external constriction increases pressure within the compartment and decreases tissue perfusion (Figure 60–1). As the

Table 60–1.

Factors Leading to Compartment Syndrome

Conditions That Increase the Content of the Compartment

- Direct soft tissue trauma with or without long bone fracture (10–20% incidence after closed fracture)
- Closed tibial shaft fractures (40%) and closed forearm fractures (12%)
- Soft tissue crush injuries without fractures in 23% of cases of compartment syndrome[5,6]
- Open fractures, which should theoretically decompress the adjacent compartments, may lead to compartment syndrome[7]
- Hemorrhage: Vascular injury, coagulopathy
- Anticoagulation therapy[8]
- Revascularization of limb after ischemia
- High-energy trauma, as from high-speed motor vehicle accident or crush injury
- Increased capillary permeability after burns (especially circumferential)
- Infusions or high-pressure injections (eg, regional blocks, paint guns)
- Extravasations of arthroscopic fluid (eg, after routine knee arthroscopy[9])
- Reperfusion after prolonged periods of ischemia
- Anabolic steroid use, resulting in muscle hypertrophy[10]
- Decreased serum osmolarity (eg, nephritic syndrome[11])
- Strenuous exercise, especially in previously sedentary people

Conditions That Lead to Reduction in Volume of Tissue Compartments

- Tight circumferential dressings (eg, can occur with cotton cast padding alone)
- Closure of fascial defects[12]
- Cast or splint, especially if placed before removal of surgical tourniquet
- Prolonged limb compression, as in Trendelenburg and lateral decubitus positions[6,13] or in patients obtunded from alcohol or drug abuse
- Excessive traction to fractured limbs[14]

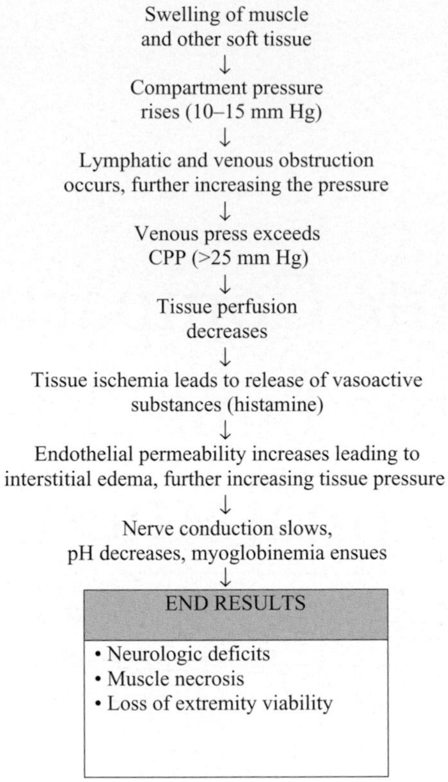

Swelling of muscle
and other soft tissue
↓
Compartment pressure
rises (10–15 mm Hg)
↓
Lymphatic and venous obstruction
occurs, further increasing the pressure
↓
Venous press exceeds
CPP (>25 mm Hg)
↓
Tissue perfusion
decreases
↓
Tissue ischemia leads to release of vasoactive
substances (histamine)
↓
Endothelial permeability increases leading to
interstitial edema, further increasing tissue pressure
↓
Nerve conduction slows,
pH decreases, myoglobinemia ensues
↓

END RESULTS
• Neurologic deficits • Muscle necrosis • Loss of extremity viability

Figure 60–1. Pathophysiology of acute compartment syndrome. CPP, capillary perfusion pressure.

compartmental pressure increases, the tissue hypoperfusion results in tissue hypoxia impeding cellular metabolism. If prolonged, permanent myoneural tissue damage occurs.[14–16] Under physiologic circumstances, the venous pressure exceeds that of the interstitial tissue pressure, sustaining venous outflow.[14] However, as tissue pressure increases, extrinsic venous luminal pressure is exceeded, resulting in collapse of the vein. The pressure at which this occurs is not known; however, it is generally agreed that compartmental pressures greater than 30 mm Hg require emergent intervention because ischemia is imminent.

Hypoxic injury causes cells to release free radicals, which increases endothelial permeability. This, in turn, leads to a vicious cycle of continued fluid loss, further increasing tissue pressure and injury. Diminished blood flow to local nerves first manifests as sensory changes. Paresthesias develop within 30 minutes of onset of ischemia. Irreversible nerve damage begins after 12–24 hours of total ischemia.[14] Irreversible changes in the muscles begin after only 4–8 hours, leading to muscle fiber death and late myocontracture.[17]

DIAGNOSIS OF COMPARTMENT SYNDROME

Compartment syndrome is a clinical diagnosis that must be based primarily on the patient's clinical signs and symptoms. Pain out of proportion to the injury, especially with passive

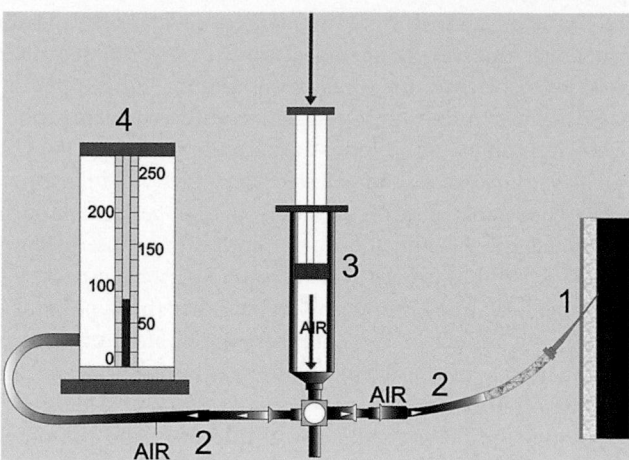

Figure 60–2. Intramuscular pressure measurement by the Whiteside technique. (1) Intramuscular needle, 18 gauge. (2) Perfusion line. (3) 20-mL Syringe. (4) Mercury manometer.

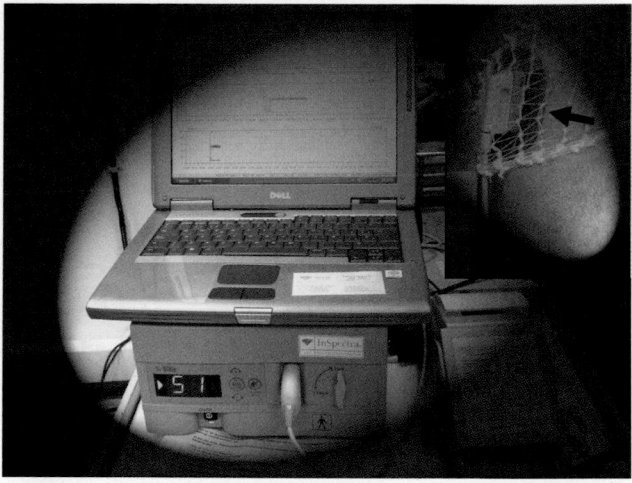

Figure 60–4. Near infrared spectroscopy is a noninvasive method for monitoring the oxygen saturation of hemoglobin and myoglobulin.

stretch of the muscles in the suspicious compartment or limb, is one of the most reliable indicators. A palpably tense extremity compared with the uninjured limb is also an important finding. The classic other P's of **p**allor, **p**ulselessness, and **p**aresis are not useful. Pallor and pulselessness are rarely present in compartment syndrome and by the time paresis manifests, the damage is largely irreversible.

Clinical Pearls

- Diagnosis of compartment syndrome must be based primarily on the patient's clinical signs and symptoms.
- Pain out of proportion to the injury is one of the most reliable indicators.

In the unresponsive, obtunded, or anesthetized patient, measurement of compartmental pressures with a needle and arterial line transducer or other pressure-measuring device is useful (Figures 60–2 and 60–3). An absolute value above 30 mm Hg in the normotensive patient is consistent with compartment syndrome. This value is diminished in the hypotensive patient as the lower arterial pressure renders the

limbs even more susceptible to ischemic injury. Near infrared spectroscopy is another noninvasive method suggested for monitoring the oxygen saturation of hemoglobin and myoglobulin in the tissue at risk (Figure 60–4).

The Upper Limb

There are several compartments of the upper extremity that, when injured, may result in compartment syndrome requiring fasciotomy in the arm, forearm, or hand.

The *arm* has two compartments: anterior and posterior (Figure 60–5).

The *forearm* has three compartments: the volar and dorsal compartments and the compartment containing the muscles of the mobile wad. Mubarak et al.[18] have demonstrated that these compartments are interconnected, unlike the compartments of the leg (Figures 60–6 and 60–7). Consequently, decompression of the volar compartment alone may decrease the pressure in the other two compartments. Regardless, dorsal compartment fasciotomy should still be performed if it remains tight after volar decompression.[19] The muscles of the volar compartment of the forearm include the digital and wrist flexors and the forearm pronators. These muscles are tested by passive extension of the digits and wrist and by supination of the forearm.

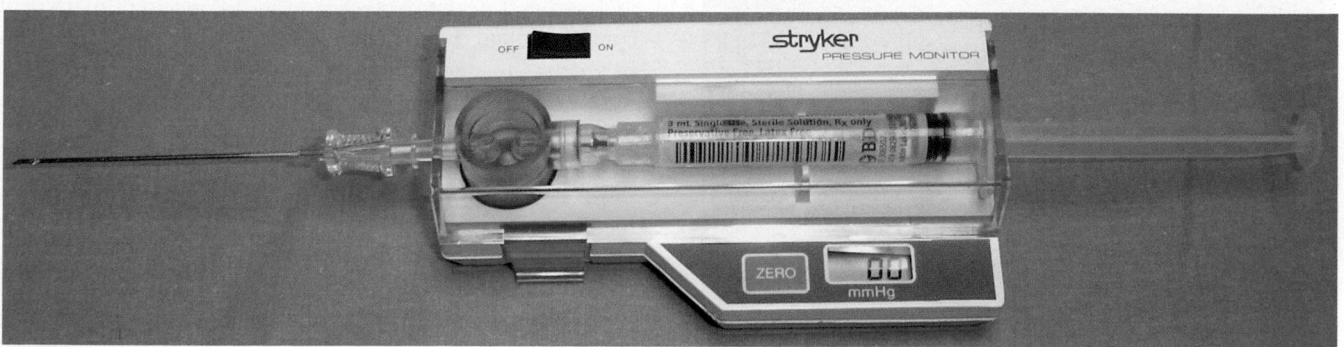

Figure 60–3. Intracompartmental pressure-monitoring device with digital display.

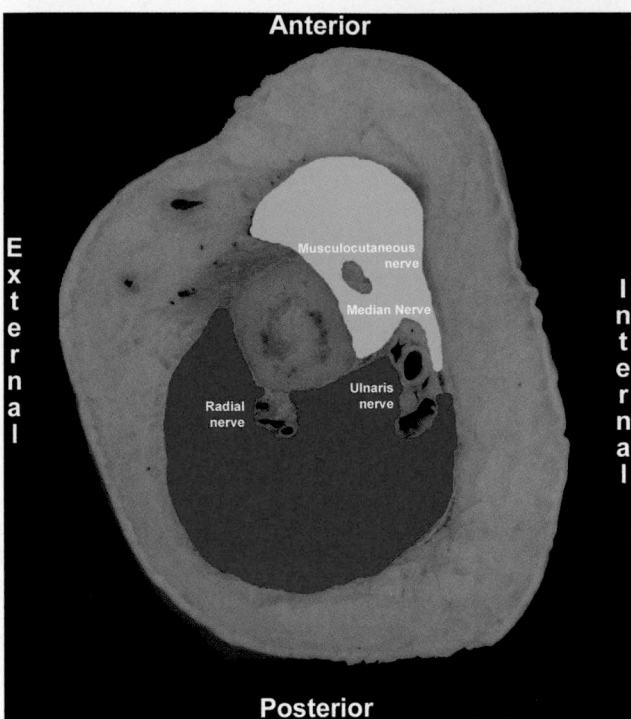

Figure 60–5. Tissue compartments of the arm.

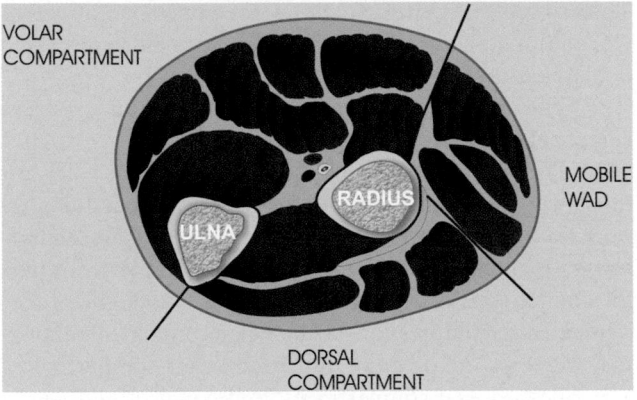

Figure 60–6. Tissue compartments of the forearm.

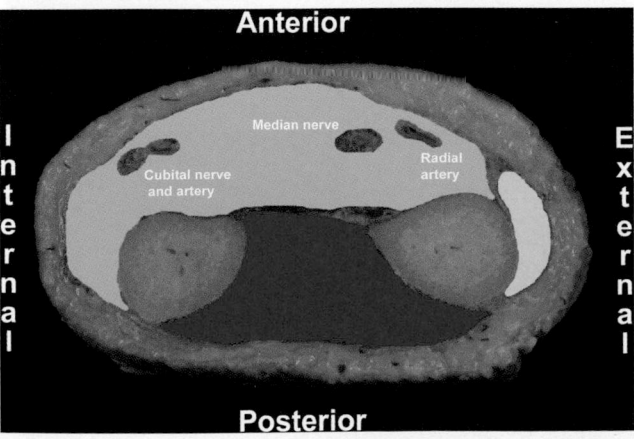

Figure 60–7. Forearm compartments.

The dorsal forearm compartment contains the thumb and finger metacarpophalangeal joint extensors, the ulnar wrist extensors, and the forearm supinators and is tested by passive finger, thumb, and wrist flexion and by forearm pronation. The mobile wad includes the brachioradialis and the two radial wrist extensors and is tested by passive wrist flexion.

There are 10 compartments in the *hand*, the most prominent ones being the dorsal and palmar interosseous compartments, of which there are four and three, respectively (Figure 60–8). The other compartments are the hypothenar, thenar, and adductor. The compartment containing the adductor muscle of the thumb is often overlooked when doing fasciotomies. Studies using renograffin dye had shown no connection between the dorsal interossei and the other compartments, showing that each compartment has to be decompressed separately.

The finger is enclosed in a tight investing fascia and is compartmentalized by the fascia and the volar skin at the flexor crease. Although no muscle bellies are distal from the metacarpophalangeal joints, ischemia and engorgement can lead to tissue loss (Figure 60–9).

The Lower Limb

Thigh

The thigh muscles are divided into three compartments invested by thick fascia: the anterior, medial, and posterior (Figures 60–10 and 60–11). Because thigh compartment syndrome is uncommon, it may go unrecognized. A history of anticoagulant use is common in patients with thigh compartment syndrome. Signs and symptoms include a history of thigh swelling and/or hematoma and pain after a minor injury in a patient who is anticoagulated.[20,21] Although rare, the thigh syndrome can also occur in patients after joint replacement surgery. The combination of minor trauma and anticoagulation produces bleeding into muscle and tissue spaces, leading to increased compartment pressure. Pain ranges from mild to severe and may be elicited only when the hip and knee are flexed and extended. Other findings of vascular occlusion—loss of pulse, pallor, paresthesias, and paralysis—are frequently absent.

Lower Leg

The lower leg contains four compartments, each invested by inelastic fascia (Figures 60–12 and 60–13). Each compartment contains a major nerve: the deep peroneal in the anterior compartment, the superficial peroneal in the lateral compartment, the saphenous in the superficial posterior compartment, and the tibial in the deep posterior compartment. Swelling in the lateral or the anterior compartment can compress both the deep and superficial peroneal nerves against the neck of the fibula. The superficial peroneal nerve usually lies in the interval between the two peroneal muscles for a short distance and then emerges anterior to the peroneus brevis. It pierces the lateral compartment fascia at the junction of the middle and distal third of the leg. The anatomy of the superficial

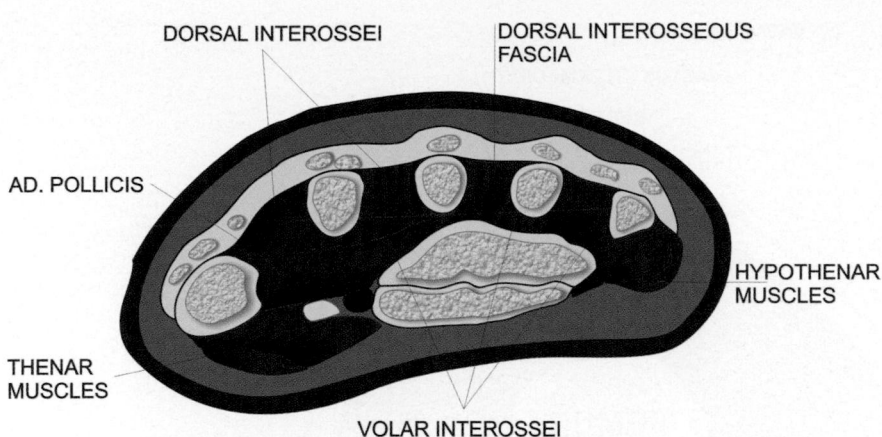

DORSAL INTEROSSEI DORSAL INTEROSSEOUS FASCIA

AD. POLLICIS

HYPOTHENAR MUSCLES

THENAR MUSCLES

VOLAR INTEROSSEI

Figure 60–8. Cross-section through the palm to show the compartments of the hand.

and deep posterior compartments is somewhat variable, but both compartments, and especially the deep compartment, are frequently involved in compartment syndrome.

The Foot

The foot has numerous rigidly bound compartments, and even mild bleeding into these spaces can elevate the pressures dramatically (Figure 60–14). According to Manoli and Weber,[22] there are nine compartments in the foot. Three compartments run the entire length of the foot (medial, lateral, and superficial). Five compartments are contained within the forefoot (adductor and four interossei). The calcaneal compartment is confined to the hind foot, but communicates with the posterior compartment of the leg. This compartment contains the quadratus muscle and the lateral plantar neurovascular bundle. The clinically most relevant compartments are the medial, central, lateral, and interossei.[23,24]

A wide spectrum of injuries can result in compartment syndrome of the foot; the most likely ones are crush injuries, especially those associated with multiple metatarsal fractures. Often, the only reliable method of diagnosis is by clinical suspicion and measurement of the intracompartmental pressures. Loss of posterior tibial or dorsalis pedis pulse is notoriously unreliable in the early diagnosis of the compartment

syndrome. The earliest clinical findings are muscle and nerve ischemia and pain. Although this pain might be confused with that of pain from the injury itself, it may be exacerbated by gentle, passive dorsiflexion of the toes, which stretches the intrinsic muscles of the foot. Lack of sensation is generally accepted as an important sign of nerve ischemia, but it is less reliable when compared with a two-point discrimination and light touch over the plantar aspect of the foot and toes.

Compartment pressure measurements are the only objective and accurate tests to diagnose and record compartment syndrome, particularly because the changes in the compartment pressures can precede the clinical signs of the compartment syndrome.

The **central compartment** can be measured by passing the needle between the metatarsal and abductor hallucis muscle at the base of the first metatarsal. The **interossei**

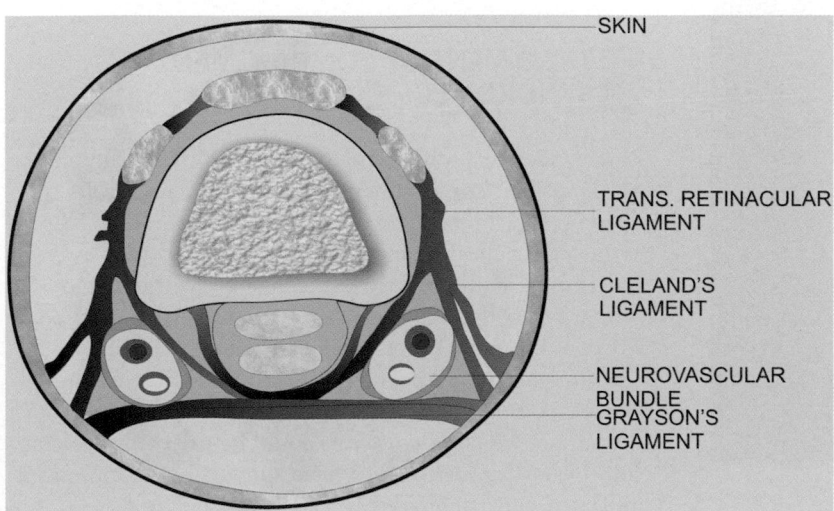

SKIN

TRANS. RETINACULAR LIGAMENT

CLELAND'S LIGAMENT

NEUROVASCULAR BUNDLE GRAYSON'S LIGAMENT

Figure 60–9. Cross-section through the finger.

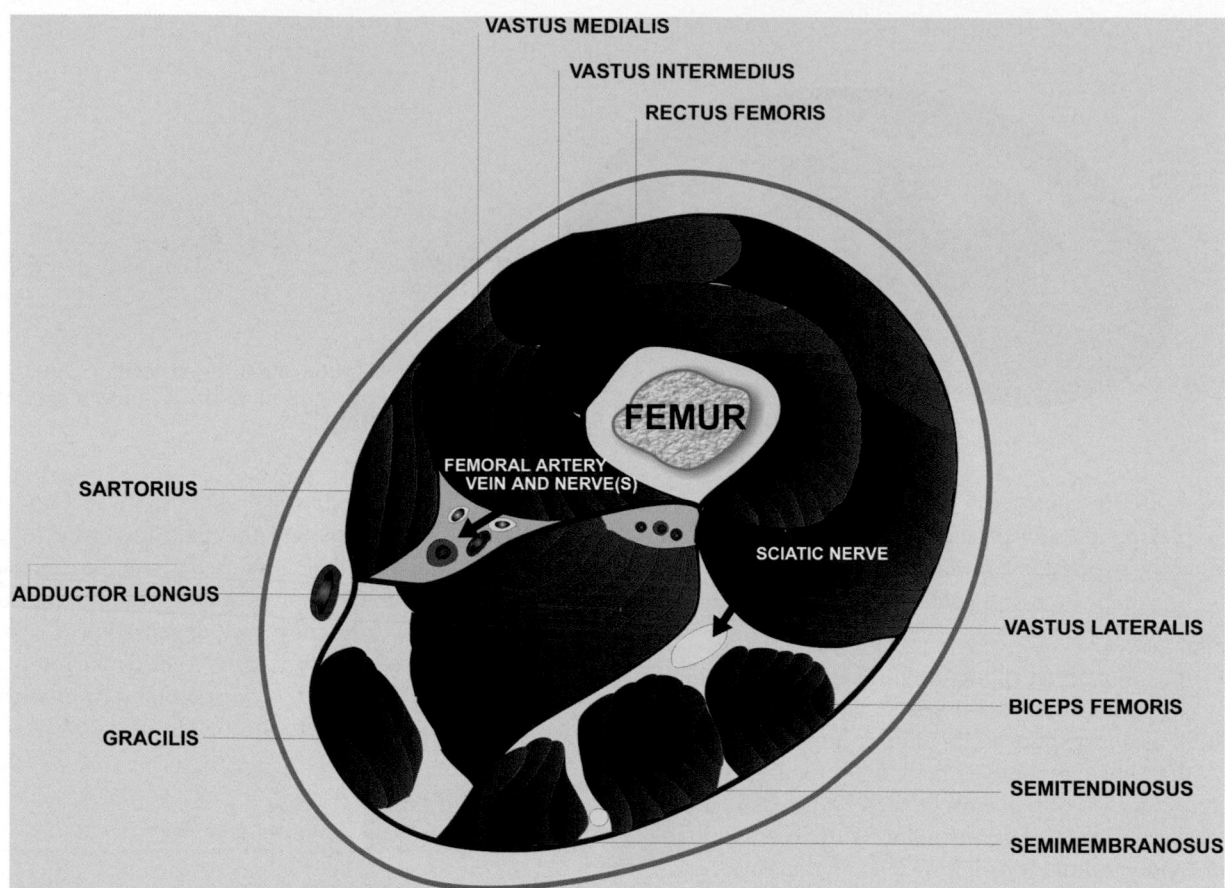

Figure 60–10. Compartments of the upper thigh.

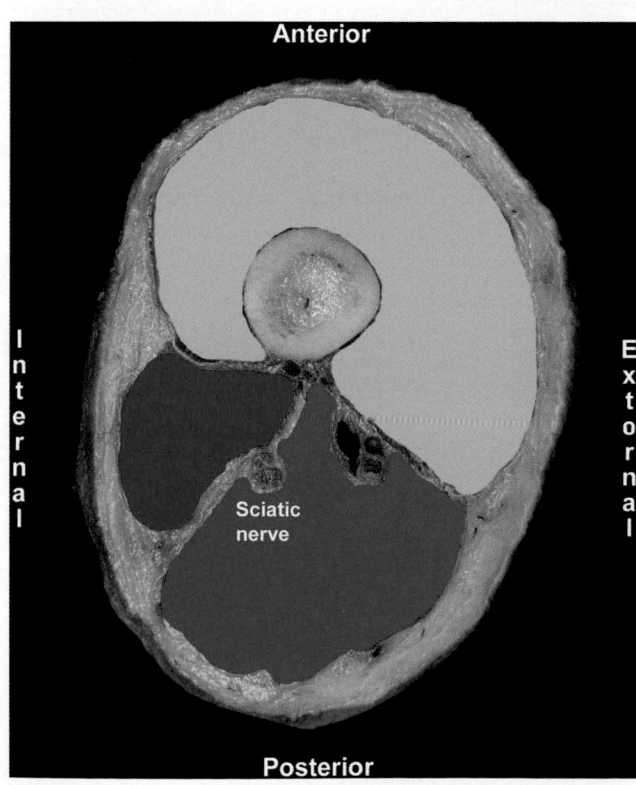

Figure 60–11. Thigh compartments.

compartment is measured in two positions by introducing the needle through the intermetatarsal spaces, preferably between the second and forth web spaces to avoid punctures to the dorsalis pedis within the first intermetatarsal region.

The **calcaneal** or **quadratus compartment** is measured by inserting the needle 5 cm distal and 2 cm inferior to the medial malleolus and advancing through the abductor muscle.

TREATMENT OF COMPARTMENT SYNDROME

Emergency fasciotomy remains the definitive treatment for a diagnosis of compartment syndrome because of its well-documented, limb-saving results. It is universally accepted as being the best chance for complete recovery and for prevention of further tissue necrosis. Treatment is based primarily on the clinical picture together with corroborative compartmental pressure measurements (Figure 60–15). The surgeon should proceed emergently with a decompression fasciotomy when clinically indicated because the exact pressure at which fasciotomy should be performed remains controversial. Most studies have shown that fasciotomy is indicated when the compartment pressure reaches 30 mm

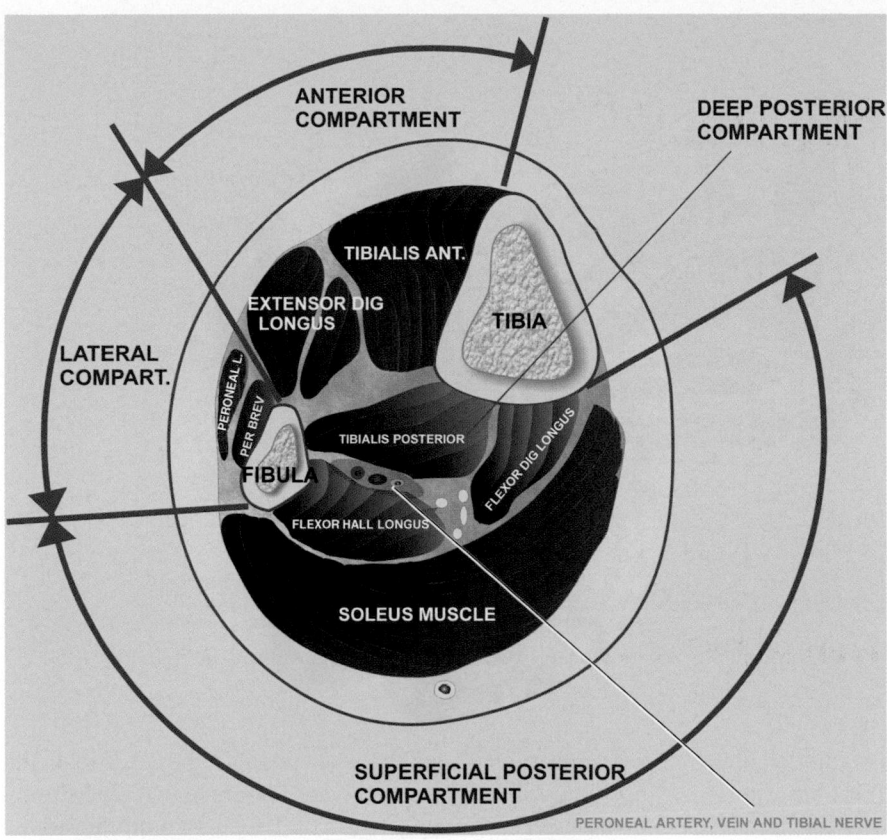

Figure 60–12. Contents of the four compartments of the lower leg.

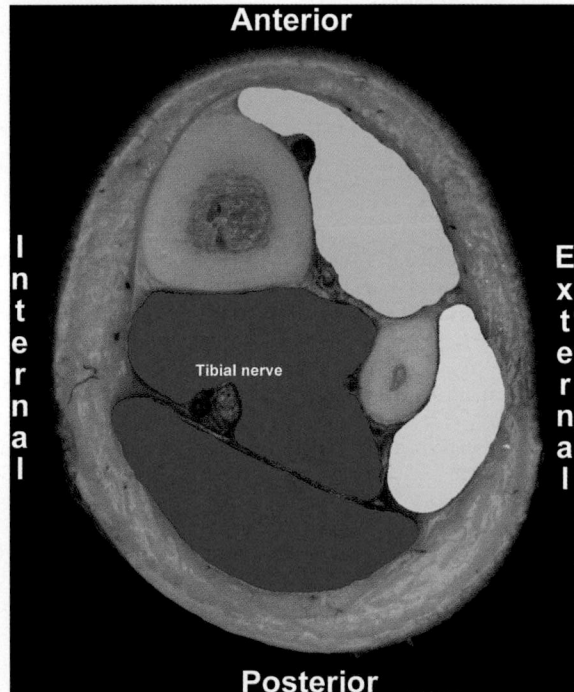

Figure 60–13. Lower leg compartments: Spatial distribution.

Hg.[24–26] Fasciotomy is also recommended when the compartmental pressure is within 30 mm Hg of the patient's diastolic pressure.[26]

Clinical Pearls

- Emergency fasciotomy remains the definitive treatment for compartment syndrome.
- Its limb-saving results make it universally accepted as being the best chance for complete recovery and for prevention of further tissue necrosis.
- Fasciotomy is indicated when the compartment pressure reaches 30 mm Hg.
- After a complete fasciotomy is performed, additional release is rarely needed.

After a complete fasciotomy, there is rarely a need for additional releases. The fasciotomy incisions are always left open with wound closure delayed for a minimum of 5 days. The patient is followed up clinically unless anesthetized or obtunded, in which case regular compartment pressure measurements should be made.

SUMMARY

Because regional anesthesia may mask pain in compartment syndrome, regional blocks should be performed in consultation with the surgical team, and shorter-acting local anesthetics should be used in uncertain circumstances.

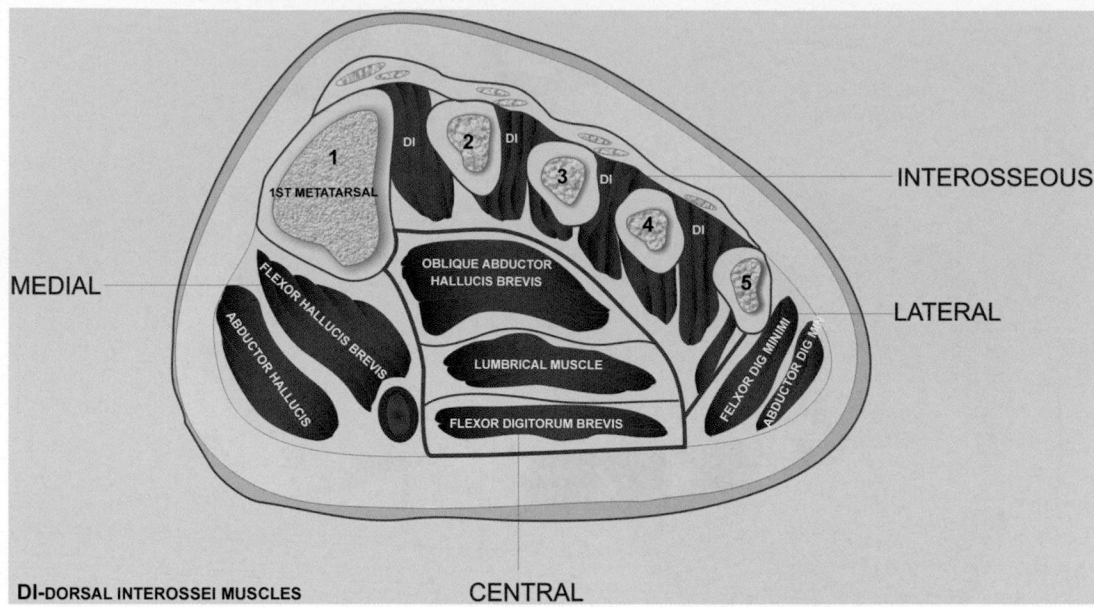

Figure 60–14. Coronal section of the foot through base of metatarsals depicting the medial, central, lateral, and interosseous compartments.

Prolonged surgery, especially in patients undergoing procedures in the Trendelenburg or lateral decubitus positions, poses a risk of compartment syndrome. The Trendelenburg position requires that the legs are strapped at a higher level than the heart. This can be avoided by repositioning and redraping the legs, or if this is not possible, the head-down tilt position should be reversed every 2 hours so that reperfusion of the lower limbs can occur. In the lateral decubitus position, the down arm and the down leg must be well padded to avoid excessive compression.

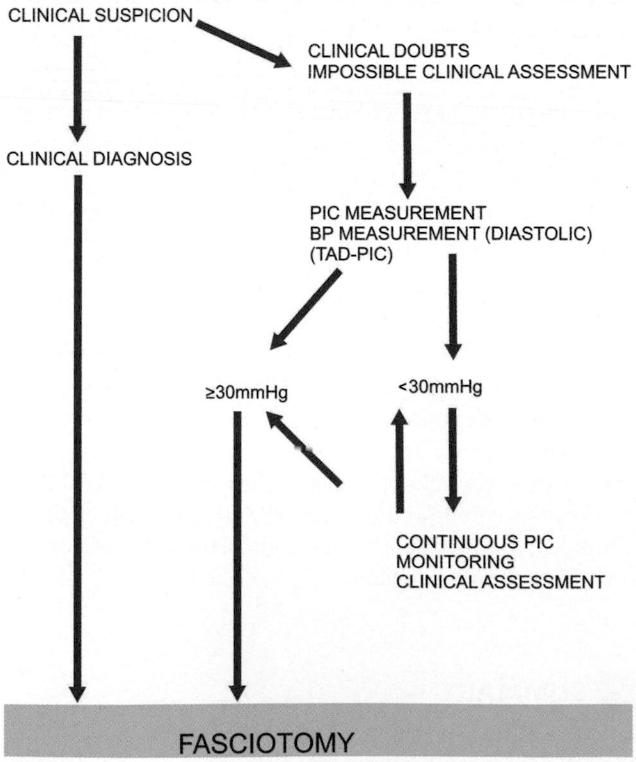

Patients on anticoagulation medication tend to have a higher risk of thigh compartment syndrome, even with relatively minor trauma or surgical interventions. This clinical scenario must be approached with a high index of suspicion.

CLINICAL SUSPICION

CLINICAL DOUBTS
IMPOSSIBLE CLINICAL ASSESSMENT

CLINICAL DIAGNOSIS

PIC MEASUREMENT
BP MEASUREMENT (DIASTOLIC)
(TAD-PIC)

≥30mmHg   <30mmHg

CONTINUOUS PIC
MONITORING
CLINICAL ASSESSMENT

FASCIOTOMY

Figure 60–15. Diagnosis and management of compartment syndrome. PIC, pressure within the compartment; TAD-PIC, diastolic blood pressure.

References

1. Matsen F, Winquist R, Krugmire R: Diagnosis and management of compartment syndromes. J Bone Joint Surg 1980;62A:286.
2. Schwartz J, Brumback R, Lakatos R: Acute compartment syndrome of the thigh: A spectrum of injury. J Bone Joint Surg 1989;71(3):392–400.
3. von Volkmann R: Die ischamischen Kontakturen. Zentralbl Chir 1881;8:801.
4. Jepson P: Ischemic contracture, experimental study. Ann Surg 1926;68A:820.
5. McQueen M, Gaston P, Court-Brown C: Acute compartment syndrome: Who is at risk? J Bone Joint Surg 2000;82B:200–203.
6. Rorabeck C: The treatment of the compartment syndromes of the leg. J Bone Joint Surg 1984;66B:93–97.
7. De Lee J, Stichi J: Open tibia fracture with compartment syndrome. Clin Orthop 1981;160:175–183.
8. Macon W, Futrell J: Median nerve neuropathy after percutaneous puncture of brachial artery in patients receiving anticoagulation. N Engl J Med 1973;288:1396.
9. Peek R, Haynes D: Compartment syndrome as a complication of arthroscopy: A case report and a study of interstitial pressures. Am J Sports Med 1984;12(6):464–468.
10. Halpern A, Nagel D: Bilateral compartment syndrome associated with androgen therapy: A case report. Clin Orthop 1977;128:54–61.
11. Sweeney H, O'Brien G: Bilateral anterior tibial syndrome in association with nephrotic syndrome: Report of a case. Arch Intern Med 1965;116:487–490.

12. Wolfort F, Mogelvang L, Filtzer H: Anterior tibial compartment syndrome following muscle hernia repair. Arch Surg 1973;106:97–99.

13. Chase J, Harford F, Pinzur M, Zussman M: Intraoperative lower extremity compartment pressures. Dis Colon Rectum 2000;43:678–680.

14. Matsen F: Compartmental syndrome. A unified concept. Clin Orthop 1975;113:8–14.

15. Botte M, Santi M, Prestianni C, Abrams R: Ischemic contracture of the foot and ankle: Principles of management and prevention. Orthopedics 1996;19(3):235–244.

16. Ziv I, Mosheiff R, Zeligowski A, et al: Crush injuries of the foot with compartment syndrome: Immediate one-stage management. Foot Ankle 1989;9(4):185–189.

17. Whitesides T, Harada H, Morimoto K: The response of skeletal muscle to temporary ischemia: An experimental study. J Bone Joint Surg 1971;53A:1027–1028.

18. Gelberman R, Zakaib G, Mubarak S, et al: Decompression of the forearm compartments. Clin Orthop 1978;134:225–229.

19. Allen M, Steingold R, Kotecha M: The importance of volar compartment in crush injuries in the forearm. Injury 1985;16:173–175.

20. Choyce A, Chan V, Middleton W, et al: What is the relationship between paresthesia and nerve stimulation for axillary brachial plexus block? Reg Anesth Pain Med 2001;26:100–104.

21. An H, Simpson M, Gale S, Jackson W: Acute anterior compartment syndrome in the thigh: A case report and review of the literature. J Orthop Trauma 1987;1:180–183.

22. Manoli A II, Weber T: Fasciotomy of the foot: An anatomical study with special reference to release of the calcaneal compartment. Foot Ankle 1990;10(6):267–275.

23. Sarraffian S: *Anatomy of the Foot and Ankle.* JB Lippincott, 1983.

24. Myerson M: Experimental decompression of the fascial compartment of the foot: The basis for fasciotomy in an acute compartment syndromes. Foot Ankle 1988;8:308–314.

25. Mubarak S, Owen C: Compartment syndrome and its relationship to the crush syndrome: A spectrum of disease—a review of 11 cases of prolonged limb compression. Clin Orthop 1975;113:81–89.

26. Whitesides T, Haney T, Morimoto K: Tissue pressure measurements as a determinant for the need of fasciotomy. Clin Orthop 1975;113:43–51.

Perioperative Management of Patients Having Regional Anesthesia

61

Perioperative Management with Peripheral Nerve Block Anesthesia

Bonnie Deschner, MD • Admir Hadzic, MD

INTRODUCTION

Regional anesthesia offers multiple clinical advantages that contribute to both an improved patient outcome and lower overall health care costs.[1-4] Peripheral nerve blocks provide excellent anesthesia, postoperative pain relief, reduced complications of wound healing compared with infiltration anesthesia, fewer side effects than general anesthesia, and facilitate early physical activity.[5-8] Peripheral nerve blocks are frequently used in elderly patients to limit excessive sedation while providing excellent pain control.[9] Nerve blocks are associated with reduced use of opioids for postoperative pain, fewer postoperative complications, and earlier discharges.[6,10-12] Single-injection regional blocks and continuous peripheral catheters play a valuable role in a multimodal approach to pain management in the critically ill patient, providing excellent patient comfort while reducing the physiologic stress response.[13]

However, compared with neuraxial and general anesthesia, success with peripheral nerve blocks is undoubtedly more anesthesiologist-dependent.[14-16] Technical skills and determination are required for the successful implementation of peripheral nerve blocks. Factors such as accurate identification of surface landmarks and an adequate number of supervised, successful attempts at each block are necessary for safe, effective peripheral nerve block implementation.[14,16-18] A dedicated team of well-trained anesthesiologists is a prerequisite to ensure consistent peripheral nerve block service in any institution.[19,20] Intraoperative management, once the block has been placed, requires diligent observation and judicious

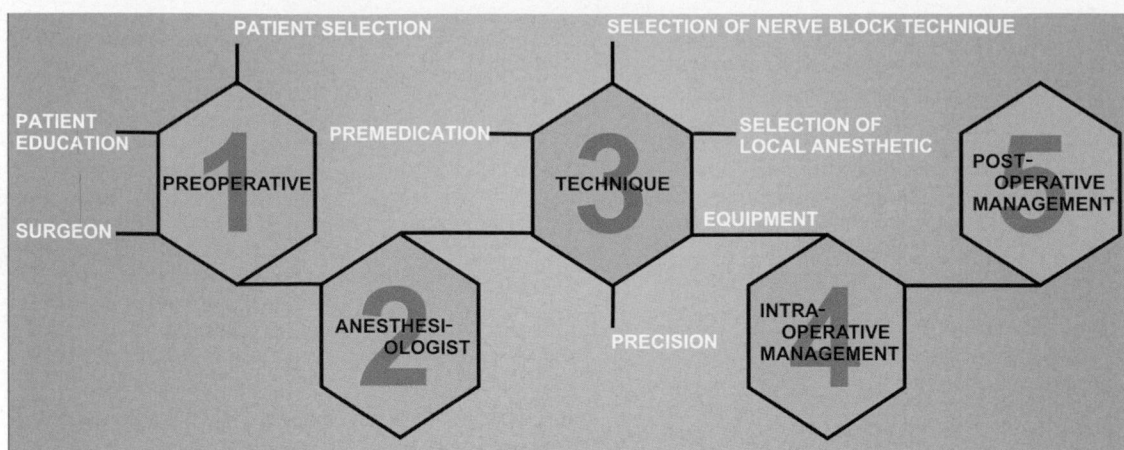

Figure 61–1. Five elements for success with nerve blocks.

use of supplemental drugs for anxiolysis and sedation. Postoperative management, including patient and nursing education, discussion of the block duration, expected sensory and motor deficits, and a plan for pain management as the block diminishes, is the final element required for success with nerve blocks (Figure 61–1).

PREANESTHETIC MANAGEMENT

Even before the anesthesiologist meets the patient, planning for anesthetic management begins with a review of the operative schedule. Attention to the procedure, what portion of the patient's body is involved, the patient's name and age, and the surgeon's preference direct the anesthesiologist toward the choice of general, regional, or combined techniques. Knowing the surgeon's abilities plays a role in selecting both the block technique and the local anesthetic to be used if regional techniques are to be implemented. Advance planning includes placing equipment and supplies necessary for the chosen technique in the block area or the operating room (OR) prior to the patient's arrival, increasing the efficiency of the anesthetic experience.

Medical Record Review

The patient's chart should be reviewed for relevant history, physical examination findings, and laboratory studies that may influence the anesthetic plan. The chart review should be conducted with as much care as is taken with surgery involving general anesthesia. Laboratory tests, the electrocardiogram (ECG), tests of cardiovascular risk, radiographic reports, and any additional consultations should be reviewed.

Routine laboratory studies are not indicated for the low-risk patient undergoing low-risk procedures. Selective laboratory tests, such as hematocrit, coagulation profile, and blood urea nitrogen (BUN)/creatinine, should be checked in select, high-risk patients, when significant blood loss is ex-

pected, or in patients known to have been on anticoagulant therapy.[21,22] Prolongation of the elements of the coagulation profile (prothrombin time, partial thromboplastin time, international normalized ration [INR]) can be a contraindication to neuraxial blocks, but specific peripheral nerve blocks may still be performed safely. Guidelines for the application of regional anesthetic techniques in the anticoagulated patient can be found in Chapter 70 (Regional Anesthesia in Patients on Anticoagulants). In general, blocks associated with a higher risk of bleeding because of proximity to major vessels or those that traverse major muscle layers may be performed 4 h after the last dose of subcutaneous heparin, 12 h after the last dose of low-molecular-weight heparin (LMWH), 7 days after clopidogrel (Plavix), and 4 weeks after the discontinuation of GIIa/IIIb inhibitors.[23] Nonsteroidal antiinflammatory drugs (NSAIDs) and aspirin are not contraindications to block placement.

Clinical Pearls

- Deep nerve blocks, or those close to large vessels can be performed 4 h after subcutaneous heparin, and 12 h after LMWH.
- Although caution should be used with Plavix and GIIa/IIIb inhibitors, NSAIDs and aspirin are *not* contraindications to nerve block placement.

An ECG may be obtained and evaluated for high-risk patients or for those known to have cardiovascular disease.[24,25] The ECG should be reviewed for changes suggestive of myocardial ischemia, infarction, new dysrhythmias, or conduction defects that may require additional evaluation prior to surgery.

Chest radiographs are usually not warranted for an asymptomatic patient without risk factors who is younger than 75 years of age.[26] If a chest radiograph has been completed in a high-risk patient, it should be reviewed in the same manner as would be done prior to general anesthesia. The anesthesiologist must be cognizant of the fact that the co-administration of general anesthesia may be necessary.

The medication profile is important for alerting the anesthesiologist to the presence of drug allergies, the presence and treatment of disease, anticoagulation therapy, pain therapy, and chronic treatment states. Herbal and vitamin therapy should be reviewed, as some of these over-the-counter medications can affect the patient's response to medication as well as platelet function.[27] Tobacco, illicit drug, and alcohol use should be included in the evaluation. For instance, the history of cocaine abuse may preclude the use of epinephrine in the solution of local anesthetics or dictate the use of direct-acting vasoconstrictors (eg, phenylephrine) in case of neuraxial anesthesia–induced hypotension.

Patient Selection

Any patient scheduled for surgery on an extremity should be considered a candidate for peripheral nerve block anesthesia.[28–30] Regional anesthesia, alone or in combination with general anesthesia, is feasible and desirable in most surgical patients for almost any operative site. Factors such as the primary indication for surgery, the presence of coexisting diseases, potential contraindications, and the patient's psychological state should all be considered.[31]

Regional anesthesia can be particularly challenging in high-risk surgical patients undergoing orthopedic, thoracic, abdominal, or vascular surgery. Diabetics and the elderly benefit from the selective anesthesia provided by peripheral nerve blocks. The isolated vasodilation provided by sympathetic blockade in the operative extremity in the patient with severe peripheral vascular disease is of benefit to both the surgeon and the patient.[32,33] Patients with asthma in whom airway instrumentation is best avoided are also excellent candidates for peripheral nerve block anesthesia.[34]

Obese patients, those with sleep apnea, confusion or delirium, and the elderly need special consideration. Regional anesthesia can be used with success in most of these patients; however, the risk/benefit ratio must be evaluated. Obesity provides a challenge to all forms of anesthesia, including intravenous access, identification of surface landmarks, airway obstruction with sedation, more rapid oxygen desaturation secondary to a reduced functional residual capacity, and difficult intubations.[35,36] In an analysis of more than 9000 blocks, Nielsen and colleagues found that patients with a body mass index (BMI) of greater than or equal to 30 kg/m^2 were 1.62 times more likely to have a failed block. Because other variables such as increased risk with general anesthesia, difficulty in alleviating postoperative pain, and unanticipated admissions, obese patients should not be automatically excluded from regional anesthesia procedures.[37] Overall satisfaction with regional techniques has been similar to that for patients with a normal BMI.

Careful evaluation of the patient's overall health, the ability to handle surgery with minimal sedation (to avoid airway obstruction from heavy sedation), and benefits of regional techniques over general techniques can help the anesthesiologist to determine the best form of anesthesia.

Clinical Pearls

- Obesity provides a challenge for any anesthetic technique; however, carefully chosen and expertly performed peripheral nerve blocks often prove to be the best and safest anesthetic option for this patient population.
- Patients with obstructive sleep apnea are at a higher risk for perioperative morbidity and mortality. If regional anesthesia with sedation is performed in these patients, diligence by the anesthesiologist is required to recognize and promptly treat obstruction.
- Reducing the dose and using shorter-acting sedatives are of benefit in these patients.[38] The use of dexmedetomidine may prove an excellent alternative in this patient population (see Chapter 11, Sedation–Analgesia During Local and Regional Anesthesia, for more information on pharmacologic choice for sedation).

Confused, demented, and disoriented or uncooperative patients present a particular challenge when regional anesthesia is considered. Although regional anesthesia can be performed in a comfortably sedated patient, these patients may require continued deep sedation throughout the operative period. Factors such as the patient's size, airway function, emergent vs nonemergent case (ie, full stomach), combativeness vs confusion should be considered when choosing the anesthetic technique. General and regional techniques have been compared in two large randomized trials in patients with preoperative mental status changes. In both groups, regional techniques were performed safely without significant differences in morbidity or cognitive function intraoperatively and postoperatively.[39–41]

Clinical Pearl

- Regional anesthesia may be the safest choice of anesthesia for the patient with limited mental capacity. After initial sedation for the block, additional medications can be limited so as not to confuse the postoperative neurologic examination.

As the population ages, the number of elderly patients presenting for anesthesia and surgery has increased exponentially. Regional anesthesia is frequently used in these patients because minimal sedation can be used for the procedure, and the patients receive excellent postoperative pain control. Factors specific to the elderly patient, such as coexisting disease, mental status changes, and type and duration of surgery, should be evaluated prior to instituting peripheral nerve blocks.[9] Aging affects the pharmacokinetics and pharmacodynamics of local anesthetics. Changes in

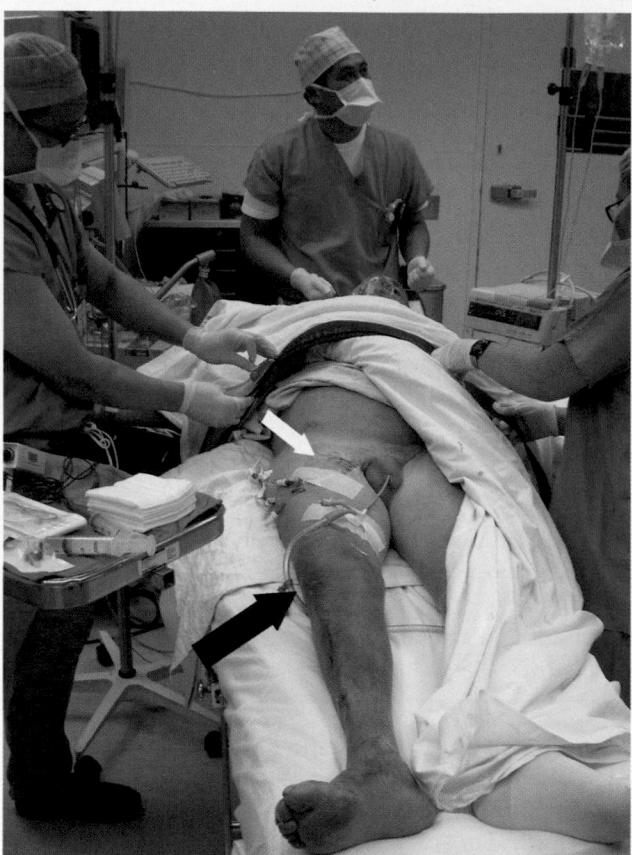

Figure 61–2. An example of how a nerve block may be the most suitable anesthetic option even in the presence of severe coagulation abnormality. Shown is an elderly patient who was emergently brought from the intensive care unit for washout of the septic knee (*black arrow*). He sustained a massive myocardial infarction several days prior and was extubated after a difficult weaning just 24 h prior this surgery. His INR was 2.4 and his left femoral vein was cannulated with a triple-lumen catheter (*white arrow*). He was profoundly hypotensive in the ICU and treated with multiple vasopressors.

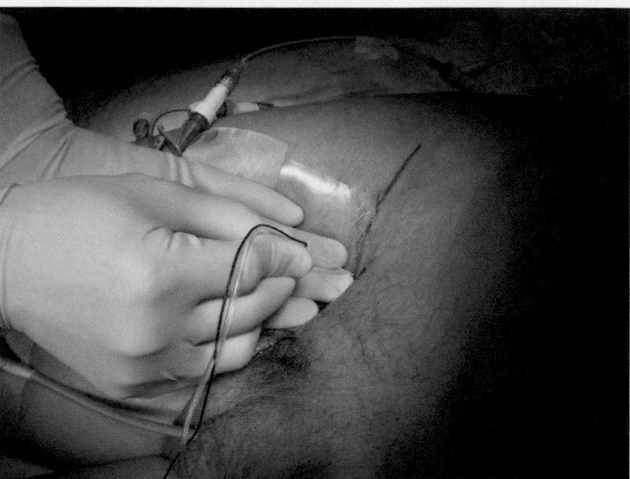

Figure 61–3. Femoral nerve block was stimulated immediately lateral to the pulse of the femoral artery and 15 mL of mepivacaine 1.5% was injected, which was all that was required for the planned surgery. This avoided the need for reintubation as the spinal or epidural anesthesia was contraindicated in the setting of anticoagulation.

systemic absorption, distribution, and clearance of local anesthetics cause an increased sensitivity, decreased dose requirements, and a change in the onset and duration of action.[42,43] Epinephrine can prolong the duration of the block, but it creates a greater risk of ischemic neurotoxicity in peripheral nerves of the elderly.[44]

Perhaps the only absolute contraindications to regional anesthesia are patient refusal, an active infection at the site of puncture, severe systemic coagulopathy, and a true allergy to local anesthetics (Figures 61–2 and 61–3).

Patient education by an informed anesthesiologist will nearly always assure a reluctant patient to consent to a block procedure. However, a patient adamantly opposed to regional blocks for whatever reason should never be coerced.[45,46] True allergies to local anesthetics are extremely rare and have been found to be toxic responses or non–drug-related responses in the majority of the cases.[47]

Postoperative neuropathy may be difficult to assess in the presence of a peripheral nerve block performed with a

long-acting local anesthetic. If the neurologic examination must be done immediately postoperatively, then a shorter-acting local anesthetic can be administered, thereby allowing the patient the choice of anesthetic techniques.[42] Because of their lower potential for cardiovascular toxicity, shorter-acting, less toxic local anesthetics are also preferred in hemodynamically frail patients. In some patients or clinical scenarios when the level of anxiety is high concerning the neurologic outcome, general anesthesia may indeed be the most practical option instead of labor-intensive perioperative management and interaction with the rest of the medical team. Ultimately, the use of regional anesthesia in patients with preexisting neurologic disease is a matter of judgment and experience. For more in-depth discussion on this topic, the reader is referred to Chapter 59 (Regional Anesthesia in Patients with Neurologic Disease).

Clinical Pearl

- The only absolute contraindication to peripheral nerve blockade is patient refusal!

Patient Interview/Education

Patient education is vital to successful regional anesthesia. Among the general public and particularly the elderly, there is a common lack of awareness regarding the potential uses and benefits of regional anesthesia. Patients are commonly offered the choice between two overly simplistic descriptions of anesthesia options: "a needle in the neck" or "go to sleep." Neither of these descriptions accurately describes the nature of the anesthetic care. Many patients, therefore, have a tendency to choose general anesthesia due to the lack of understanding of what regional anesthesia comprises and the anxiety over needle insertion during block performance. Another common misconception is that nerve blocks are associated with an increased risk of nerve injury. In fact, the data from the closed-claims studies suggest that the majority of reported neurologic complications are actually associated with general anesthesia due to problems with patient positioning.[48]

During the preoperative visit, the anesthesiologist should help the patient to understand the basics of the anesthetic management and to establish realistic expectations. The anesthesiologist must be personally convinced that the proposed technique is the best choice, or it will be difficult to provide assurance to the patient. Patients should be educated about the principal benefits of regional anesthesia—avoidance of general anesthesia and airway management, improved pain control, and reduced incidence of nausea and vomiting—all of which are evident immediately in the postoperative period.[7,49]

Clinical Pearls

- The anesthesiologist must be *personally* convinced that peripheral nerve blockade is the best anesthetic technique for the patient to be successful with this type of anesthesia.
- A choice between a "needle in the neck" or "going to sleep" is overly simplistic and inaccurate and predisposes patients to choose general anesthesia.
- Patients can be instructed that they will be sedated or lightly asleep while the blocks are being placed and that they are not likely to remember the block procedure. This promise then should be fulfilled by using a combination of midazolam and a short-acting narcotic to accomplish the promised amnesia and analgesia during the block procedure.

The patient should be informed about the duration of the blockade, the need for analgesic therapy as the block is wearing off, and the care of the insensate extremity. Informing patients about what to expect and helping them understand that incremental sedation or analgesia ("light sleep") will be given before and during the procedure encourages most patients to consent to regional blockade. The amount of information given varies with each patient. It should be tailored to the patient's desire and the type of the nerve block procedure planned followed by obtaining the informed consent.[50] A review of the patient's prior record of pain management, including chronic states and treatment, may alert the anesthesiologist to unrealistic expectations that the patient may have that should be addressed before premedication is administered. This will also alert the anesthesiologist that larger doses of sedatives or narcotics may be required for the patient's comfort.

Clinical Pearls

- Patients need to know what the block will and will not cover.
- Chronic pain patients need to be reassured that their pain needs, unrelated to the surgical site, will be met.

Anesthesia Consent

A consent for anesthesia should be obtained before sedation is administered. This should include the proposed method of anesthesia, the benefits, risks, and complications of regional anesthesia specifically related to the patient. The consent should include the possibility of general anesthesia in the event that the regional technique is incomplete or ineffective, changes in the surgical plan surgical exposure, and patient comfort considerations. Many institutions have adopted specific anesthesia consent forms separate from those for surgery, although this practice varies depending on the institution. Regardless of the individual institution's consent practices, once the consent is signed, it is advisable to write a brief, specific note in the patient's chart that describes the discussion the anesthesiologist had with the patient. The note simply states whether any specific patient concerns were discussed. Here is an example of such note:

"An interscalene block for anesthesia was discussed with the patient. The risks, benefits, alternatives, and complications were discussed. Questions were answered. The patient expressed understanding of the proposed anesthetic plan, and the consent was signed."

Such note is far more valuable as a medicolegal document that a proper consulting procedure took place than any preformated, institutional consent signed by the patient.

Clinical Pearl

- Following the discussion about risks, benefits, and complications of peripheral nerve blockade, it is advisable that the anesthesiologist write a short note in the patient's chart documenting the discussion and any additional concerns the patient may have.

Surgical Considerations

An insightful and educated surgeon is often the greatest advocate of regional anesthesia. Patients undergoing various orthopedic, vascular, hand, and podiatric surgical procedures can be anesthetized using regional anesthesia techniques. Surgeons will quickly adopt and demand regional anesthesia to facilitate patient care when it is implemented in an efficient, consistent manner. Some surgeons, however, may have reservations about utilizing regional techniques until they are shown that OR efficiency can be increased, patient satisfaction enhanced, postoperative pain issues reduced or alleviated, and that favorable outcomes are associated with expertly performed regional anesthesia procedures.[51,52] Surgeons who have accepted the value of regional techniques often introduce the techniques to their patients during the preoperative visit. However, an adequate number of the faculty in the anesthesia department must be trained in regional techniques in order to provide a continuous service and maintain the confidence of the surgical team and the patients.[14,53]

Preoperatively, a discussion with the surgeon about the proposed procedure is essential. The discussion must include considerations regarding the site, nature, extent, and duration of the planned surgical procedure. Issues such as patient positioning, field avoidance, and the use of a tourniquet should be discussed to make sure that the intended technique will be adequate and appropriate for the planned surgery and for the particular patient.

In general, procedures involving the upper body, head, and neck create more anxiety in many patients secondary to the claustrophobic effect of drapes and proximity of the surgical site to the patient's head. Adequate sedation without compromising airway protection will usually alleviate the problem if the anesthesiologist is prepared. When the surgical team has to surround the head, effectively blocking access by the anesthesiologist, in some instances it may be safer to secure the airway prior to proceeding with surgery.[54,55]

Clinical Pearl

- The greatest advocate an anesthesiologist can have for successful peripheral nerve block anesthesia is an informed, supportive surgeon.
- Understanding the surgical procedure and the individual surgeon's approach allows the anesthesiologist to wisely choose the best anesthetic technique.

Anesthesiologist

The anesthesiologist's confidence and ability to establish a rapport with the patient are the most important factors for convincing a patient to accept the proposed anesthetic technique. Presenting the patient with a wide range of anesthetic options for the particular procedure is confusing for the patient. Instead, a better approach is to present the patient with the regional anesthetic plan that best meets his needs based on his physical and emotional status, coincides with the surgeon's plan, and is within the realm of the anesthesiologists expertise. As the number and complexity of regional anesthesia techniques keep increasing, it is becoming clear that regional anesthesia is a training-intensive and a distinct subspecialty of anesthesiology. Thorough training during residency is necessary to obtain consistent results and avoid complications.[53,56] A well-structured regional anesthesia fellowship is by far the best path toward success in academic endeavor in this area.[57,58]

Physical Examination

Physical examination with assessment of the block site is essential to determining whether the block can be performed safely. For example, performing an interscalene block in a patient with severe chronic obstructive pulmonary disease could result in the need for mechanical ventilation due to hemidiaphragmatic paresis on the ipsilateral side.[59] On the other hand, unhealthy patients requiring urgent or emergent surgery for lower extremity fractures clearly benefit from peripheral nerve blocks because general anesthesia in these circumstances would be poorly tolerated.[60] Once the decision has been made to proceed with the regional technique, certain anatomic landmarks can be used to enhance the success of the block despite the physical habitus of the patient. The following paragraphs briefly describe physical examination clues to improve the success rate of some of the peripheral nerve blocks.

Interscalene Brachial Plexus Block

Evaluation of the neck is the key examination for the interscalene block. The proportions of the shoulder girdle, size of the neck, and prominence of the muscles vary greatly among patients. The three bony landmarks that should be observed are the sternal notch, the clavicle, and the mastoid process. Even in the obese or stocky patient with a short neck, these landmarks can be evaluated. In addition, locating the clavicular head of the sternocleidomastoid muscle and the external jugular vein are important in estimating the site for needle insertion. Even though the external jugular vein has a highly variable course, the interscalene groove is almost always immediately in front of or behind the external jugular vein.[61] In patients with difficult anatomy, the clavicle and external jugular vein often prove to be the most reliable landmarks.[62] In the patient with difficult anatomy (ie, short, thick neck), a single-shot interscalene block may be a better choice than attempting a continuous catheter technique. If it is difficult to locate the interscalene groove, transcutaneous stimulation can be used by employing a higher stimulus intensity and scanning the skin surface of the neck (Figure 61–4). Once the twitches are obtained, the current is decreased to the minimum at which the twitch is still observed. For this purpose, a nerve stimulator with higher current output is used (models made for monitoring the neuromuscular junction blockade). Commercial models made specifically for surface localization have also become available in recent years. This technique provides a better idea of where the stimulating needle should be inserted. Where equipment and expertise is available, ultrasound-guided interscalene block may be a better choice.

Clinical Pearl

- The clavicle and the external jugular vein often prove to be the most reliable landmarks for location of the brachial plexus in the neck.

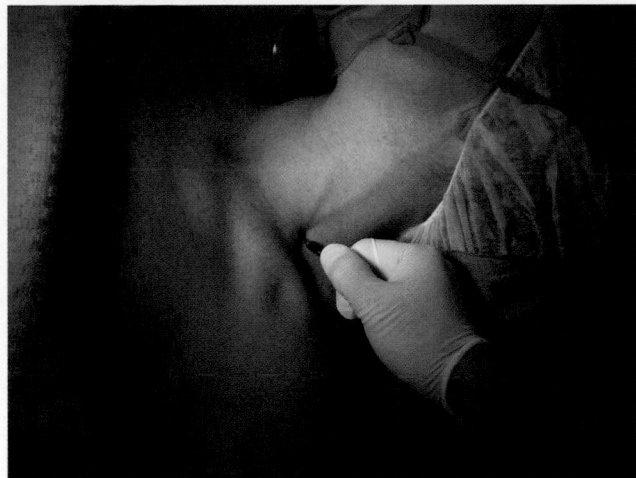

Figure 61–4. Transcutaneous localization of the brachial plexus in the interscalene groove. The negative lead (–) of the nerve stimulator (a model used for monitoring neuromuscular blockade) can be used to approximate the site of needle insertion by applying 10–20 mA over the area of interest. Once a twitch of the brachial plexus is obtained, the current is progressively decreased while the negative lead is moved medially or laterally to identify the location where the brachial plexus can be stimulated with the lowest current intensity (typically 5–10 mA). That place is then labeled as an approximate site for needle insertion.

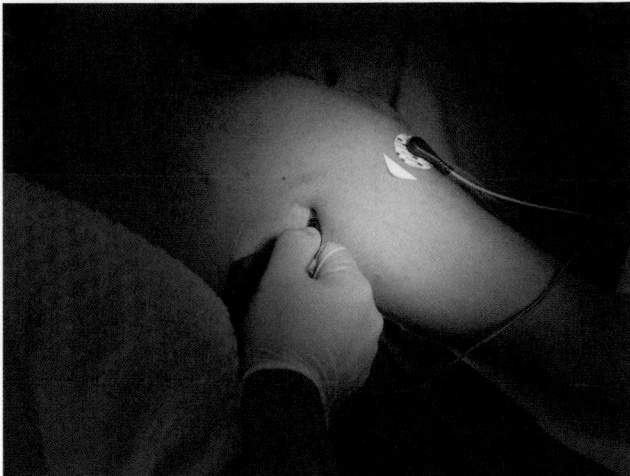

Figure 61–5. Transcutaneous localization of the axillary brachial plexus. The negative lead (–) of the nerve stimulator (a model used for monitoring neuromuscular blockade) can be used to approximate the site of needle insertion by applying 10–20 mA over the area of interest. Once a twitch of the hand is obtained, the current is progressively decreased while the negative lead is moved medially or laterally to identify the location where the brachial plexus can be stimulated with the lowest current intensity (typically 5–10 mA). This is then labeled as an approximate site for needle insertion.

Infraclavicular Brachial Plexus Block

Evaluation of the upper chest, clavicle, and shoulder area is important in performing the infraclavicular block. The primary landmarks are the coracoid process and the medial clavicular head. The most difficult process to identify, especially in an obese patient or a patient with a muscular chest, is the coracoid process.[63,64] To find the coracoid process, follow the clavicle from the medial to the distal end. Toward the distal end, a groove or depression is felt just below the clavicle, the deltopectoral triangle or groove. Drop the fingers of the palpating hand into the groove, then abduct the shoulder (raise the arm in a forward position). As the arm is lowered, the coracoid process will be felt by the fingers of the palpating hand. Once the coracoid process is located, many of the techniques described to stimulate the brachial plexus using the infraclavicular approach can be initiated.[65,66] If the patient has too much tissue in the upper chest area, another approach to the brachial plexus (eg, low interscalene approach) might be a better option.

In obese patients or those who have large chest muscles or breasts, it may be easier to perform this block in the semisitting position to "unload" the soft tissues using gravity and provide better access to the infraclavicular area. Of note, percutaneous stimulation as electroprelocation is often not useful in infraclavicular block due to the deep location of the brachial plexus at this point.

Axillary Brachial Plexus Block

The key physical examination finding is the location of the axillary artery. To find the axillary artery, the patient should be placed supine with the head facing away from the side to be blocked. On the side to be blocked, the shoulder should be abducted with the elbow flexed at a 90-degree angle. If the shoulder is excessively abducted, palpation of the axillary artery may be more difficult. Even in an obese patient, the axillary artery can be palpated if the shoulder and forearm are properly adjusted.[14,67] When palpation of the axillary artery proves difficult, the use of a Doppler probe or ultrasound is useful. Similar to the interscalene block, transcutaneous stimulation can be used to approximate the position of the individual elements of the brachial plexus (Figure 61–5).

Blocks Involving the Spine: Spinal, Epidural, Plexus Blocks

It is not uncommon to see trainees who are evaluating patients before planned regional anesthesia perform extensive airway and other systemic examinations but pay no attention to the characteristics of the anatomy where the entire anesthetic will be administered (eg, spine). Evaluation of the spine preoperatively will allow the anesthesiologist to decide whether neuraxial anesthesia or a lumbar plexus block will prove easier to perform. In addition, such an examination will help the clinician to decide whether the patient should be placed in a supine or lateral position for a neuraxial block, or whether a different method of anesthesia is more appropriate. In the elderly patient, the evidence of severe kyphoscoliosis or arthritic changes in joints may direct the clinician to using the lateral paramedian approach for the block. In the obese patient, the midline approach may be the best for a successful block. Other examination findings of importance for regional anesthesia involving the spine include evidence of localized

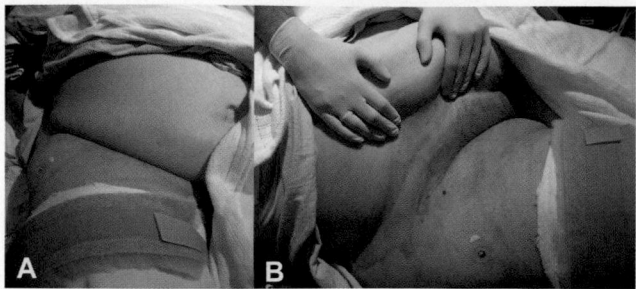

Figure 61–6. A pendant abdomen (***A***) obscures the femoral triangle. Retraction of the lower abdomen by a helper (***B***) is useful in exposing the femoral triangle during femoral nerve blockade.

infection, scoliosis, and congenital defects or scars that may affect either the placement or the choice of technique.[68,69]

Blocks Involving the Lower Extremities

Physical examination of the groin and lower extremity should occur prior to implementation of nerve blocks of the femoral or sciatic nerves or their branches. It is pointless to obtain a patient's consent for a block procedure and discuss the anesthetic plan with the surgical team without examining the site of needle insertion because a local pathology can prevent the performance of the planned technique. The presence of infection, neuropathy, severe peripheral vascular disease, or trauma will guide the anesthesiologist to the best procedure for the patient. In a patient with vascular disease, the anesthesiologist should evaluate the lower extremity for scars that may indicate vascular grafts involving the femoral artery, a relative contraindication to femoral blockade. The area around the ankle should be evaluated for presence of disease, infection, excessive lipidema, or edema that may present a contraindication or make an ankle block impossible. Obesity can make palpating landmarks such as the femoral artery for a femoral nerve block or the quadriceps muscles for a lateral popliteal sciatic nerve block more challenging. Physical examination of the areas to be blocked allow alteration in the anesthetic plan (ie, a change from a lateral or subgluteus posterior approach to sciatic) or a change in equipment (ie, longer stimulating needle) to be made prior to instituting the block.[70,71] Similar to the procedure for an axillary block, a Doppler probe can be used to facilitate localization of the femoral artery when palpation proves difficult. Retraction of the lower abdomen in morbidly obese patients can substantially facilitate the performance of the femoral block (Figure 61–6).

■ ANESTHETIC CONSIDERATIONS

The goals of the anesthetic plan are to ensure that the patient is properly evaluated, (ie, the choice of the anesthetic technique is the best for the patient based on the surgical procedure), the patient's physical and mental status has been assessed, and that the patient will remain hemodynamically stable when her inherent protective reflexes are blunted or abolished. Additional considerations with regional anesthesia include providing adequate premedication, placing the block efficiently so as not to compromise valuable OR time, providing complete anesthesia for the surgical site, planning for an inadequate or incomplete block, and patient comfort during long procedures.[72]

Laterality Issues

Wrong-side anesthetic procedures have been reported in patients receiving peripheral nerve blocks, especially when the patient changes position for the block.[73] Wrong-sided blocks probably occur more frequently than reported. Despite multiple checks, laterality errors can occur, particularly in institutions where large numbers of nerve blocks are performed. Risk factors that may contribute to these errors include delay between obtaining the patient's consent and the block performance, different anesthesiologists performing the block and managing the patient intraoperatively (resident "block rotations"), time pressure to administer the block without delaying surgery, and covering the patient's involved extremity with blankets to maintain warmth, effectively obscuring the marked site of surgery.

A rigid laterality protocol prior to the block placement should substantially reduce the risk of wrong-sided blocks. In our institution the following procedure is followed:

1. The surgical staff is required to mark the surgical site immediately prior to taking the patient to the OR using a wide marker and marking the site as "YES."
2. Once the patient is in the OR, the surgical and anesthesia staff confirm the laterality with the OR nurse immediately on arrival in the OR.
3. Both of the patient's extremities are uncovered and examined for laterality prior to the block procedure.
4. A "time-out" for confirmation between two caregivers is required before block performance as well as before the surgical incision.

Fortunately, long-term sequalae after laterality errors typically do not occur, but there is an increased risk of performing surgery on the wrong side when the wrong limb is anesthetized. Careful attention to the surgical consent, the marked extremity, and following procedures to double-check the surgical site are important in preventing laterality errors in patients receiving peripheral nerve block anesthesia.

Premedication of Patients for Neural Blockade

Premedication is one of the essential elements for successful neural blockade, whether it is for neuraxial blocks or peripheral nerve blocks. Anxiety causes feelings of uneasiness, tension, and nervousness and has been associated with a higher degree of intraoperative movement and sedation requirements. Utilizing anxiolytic premedication does not delay hospital discharge and is associated with a greater degree of patient satisfaction.[74,75] A patient's previous experience with regional anesthesia is a significant factor in acceptance of a regional technique for future surgery. Fear of needle puncture has been cited as a major cause for patient dissatisfaction or refusal of regional anesthesia.[76,77] If a paresthesia technique is utilized for placement of a peripheral nerve block, less sedation is used as patient cooperation is necessary, but it should not be eliminated. When a nerve stimulator is employed for placement, a greater amount of sedation can be used for patient comfort.

Premedication with an anxiolytic should be administered preoperatively just as it is given prior to general anesthetics.[78–80] In addition to the benefits mentioned, premedication prevents patients from having an unpleasant recollection of the anesthetic experience. Inadequately premedicated patients move during the block placement, making it difficult to interpret responses to nerve stimulation and possibly dislodge the needle from its intended position.

All peripheral nerve blocks can be divided into two major groups: blocks associated with minor patient discomfort (superficial blocks) and blocks associated with more patient discomfort (deep blocks). A sedation protocol should be chosen according to the regional anesthesia technique planned and according to individual patient characteristics. For instance, an interscalene brachial plexus block can be administered to a minimally sedated, fully alert patient. On the other hand, an infraclavicular, sciatic, or lumbar plexus block necessitates, for most patients, a greater degree of sedation and analgesia to ensure the patient's comfort and acceptance. Regardless of the sedation technique chosen, the goal of sedation is to provide maximum patient comfort while maintaining meaningful patient contact throughout the procedure.

Clinical Pearl

- Adequate premedication is one of the key ingredients to successful peripheral nerve practice. Fear of needles is a major reason for patient refusal of regional anesthesia. Blocks associated with more patient discomfort (eg, infraclavicular, sciatic) require more sedation.

The pharmacology of drugs commonly used for premedication in regional anesthesia is discussed in greater detail in Chapter 11 (Sedation–Analgesia During Local and Regional Anesthesia). The discussion here will be limited only to salient features of immediate relevance to the practice of regional anesthesia.

Midazolam is one of the most common anxiolytics used for premedication. Midazolam is effective given orally, intranasaly, sublingually, intramuscularly, intravenously, and as a continuous infusion.[81] It has been used in combination with a variety of medications, such as narcotics, propofol, and dexmedetomidine, for intraoperative and postoperative pain management. Benzodiazepines bind specific receptors in the central nervous system, enhancing the inhibitory effect of various neurotransmitters. For example, benzodiazepines facilitate GABA-receptor binding, leading to an increase in the membrane conductance of chloride ions. The subsequent change in membrane polarization inhibits normal neuronal function. The advantages of midazolam compared with other drugs in this class include flexibility in administration methods, lack of pain on administration either intravenously or intramuscularly, and its favorable onset and duration of action. It has been suggested that midazolam may also have a favorable effect on postoperative nausea and vomiting.[80]

A narcotic analgesic is introduced only at the time of needle placement. For example, alfentanil provides intense analgesia of short duration, making it an excellent choice for administration just prior to block placement. Alfentanil is a less potent (1/5 to 1/10) analog of fentanyl. It penetrates the brain rapidly with an onset time to peak effect of 1 to 2 min. Recovery from alfentanil is more rapid than from fentanyl or sufentanil.[82] Prolongation of drug effect after large or repeated doses is less likely because of its increased protein binding, lower lipid solubility, and smaller volume of distribution. Unlike fentanyl, there are no secondary increases in alfentanil plasma concentrations after large or repeated doses.[83] When alfentanil is used for block placement, evaluation of the block can be conducted with return of full patient cooperation within minutes.[84] Fentanyl and sufentanil have also been used effectively as part of the block sedation regimen. Fentanyl, in titrated doses of 25 to 100 mcg, provides satisfactory analgesia for block placement with minimal untoward side effects (eg, hemodynamic instability or severe respiratory depression), but plasma levels can increase with large or repeated doses.[85]

When multiple nerve blocks are necessary, low-dose sufentanil has been suggested to be an effective alternative to alfentanil, providing satisfactory pain relief without alterations in consciousness.[79] Regardless of the narcotic chosen, timing of the administration of the narcotic depends on its onset and peak effect, which should coincide with needle insertion through deeper tissues. The dose and type of premedication used depend on the procedure, the patient, and the anesthesiologist's knowledge of the pharmacodynamics of the drugs chosen. Commonly used regimens for sedation during various regional anesthesia procedures are listed in Table 61–1.

Clinical Pearls

- Midazolam is an excellent anxiolytic for sedation prior to nerve block placement because of its multiple modes of administration, quick onset, and duration.
- Narcotics (eg, alfentanil) are usually given only at the time of block placement.
- The choice of medication, its dosage, and mode of administration should take into consideration the individual patient's characteristics, response to drugs, and overall medical status.

Table 61–1.

Suggested Sedation Before Nerve Blocks Placement

Block Placement	Sedation
Blocks resulting in mild patient discomfort	
Cervical blocks	
Interscalene block	
Supraclavicular block	Midazolam 2–4 mg ±
Axillary block	alfentanyl 250–500 mcg
Posterior popliteal block	
Blocks resulting in more patient discomfort	
Infraclavicular block	
Wrist blocks	
Paravertebral blocks	Midazolam 4–6 mg ±
Lumbar plexus block	alfentanyl 500–1000 mcg
Lateral popliteal block	
Saphenous block	

Performance of Neural Blockade: Block Area vs Blocks in the OR

Peripheral nerve blocks are often thought to result in decreased OR efficiency. In contrast to this popular belief, when actual OR times are compared in that manner, several studies have demonstrated that OR times are actually reduced with the utilization of regional anesthesia.[86] In a study by Williams and coworkers comparing general anesthesia with peripheral nerve blockade or to a combination of both, regional anesthesia was associated with the lowest anesthesia-controlled time, the lowest turnover time, and the lowest incidence of unplanned hospital admission.[87]

Whether a designated block room is needed depends on the skill and experience of the anesthesiologist as well as the local anesthesiology practice and layout of the holding area and ORs. Studies evaluating OR efficiency with peripheral nerve block anesthesia performed in an induction room vs in the OR have demonstrated conflicting results.[86,88] Advantages of an induction room include reduction in OR time (arrival to beginning of surgery), less stressful environment for resident education and training, and the ability to change the anesthetic plan or redo an inadequate block without delaying surgery. Disadvantages of a designated block or induction room include the need for qualified personnel to monitor the patient once the block is placed, additional expenses related to the physical space and equipment, and lack of utilization of the space (first case of the day, outside regular OR hours, next patient not ready for a variety of reasons)[89,90] Patient anxiety levels are unchanged whether the block is placed in the OR or in a dedicated induction area.[91] In teaching institutions where peripheral nerve blocks are routinely administered in the OR,

anesthesia induction time improves with the skill level of the anesthesiologist.[92]

Regardless of where the actual procedure is performed, adequate space, equipment, and monitoring are imperative to ensure time-efficient care of the patient. If a block room is used, the physical size should allow enough space for proper monitoring, emergency access, and resuscitation of the patient. All supplies, drugs, and other equipment for the block procedure should be readily available in the room and prepared at the bedside. Proper lighting, administration of oxygen, and emergency airway management equipment with suction must be available whenever a nerve block is performed.

Intraoperative Management

Almost any anesthesiologist with skill and determination can become proficient in neuraxial and peripheral nerve blocks, but the intraoperative treatment of the patient can be the most challenging aspect of the practice of regional anesthesia. Sedation appropriately adjusted for patient comfort is always beneficial and improves the quality of the anesthesia achieved with peripheral nerve blocks. Most surgeons prefer patients to be lightly asleep during surgery so that they can better concentrate on the technical aspects of the operation. Similarly, the majority of patients also prefer not to be aware of activities in the OR. The choice and amount of sedation depends on the patients' desire for sedation, their tolerance, and any medical problems that may affect the ability to tolerate deeper levels of sedation.

Intraoperative Sedation

Many choices are available for intraoperative sedation once the block has been placed. For an in-depth discussion on these medications see Chapter 11 (Sedation–Analgesia During Local and Regional Anesthesia). Here we will briefly discuss advantages and disadvantages to many of the medications often used in conjunction with regional anesthesia. The anesthesiologist should be comfortable with the mechanism of action, onset and duration, side effects, and hemodynamic effects of the medications used. It is prudent to remember that not all patients require significant additional sedation beyond that used for initial block placement.

Propofol, a diisoprophenol, is commonly used for induction, sedation, and maintenance of anesthesia. Because of its water insolubility, it is prepared in an emulsion that can cause pain on injection especially through small veins. Advantages of propofol include rapid onset, elimination, and low incidence of side effects. It has an antiemetic quality, making it a desirable medication for ambulatory surgery. Disadvantages in addition to the incidence of pain on injection include significant cardiovascular depression, especially in the elderly or debilitated patient. Propofol can either be given as repeated bolus doses every 5–15 min or, more commonly, as a continuous infusion. The usual dose for sedation during regional anesthesia is between 10 and 50 mcg/kg/min.

Dexmedetomidine, an α_2-receptor agonist, has been used in critical care settings to effectively provide sedation with less hemodynamic instability than with propofol. It is gaining popularity as an effective agent for intraoperative sedation. Dexmedetomidine is approximately eight times more selective toward the α_2-adrenoreceptors than clonidine. It decreases anesthetic requirements by up to 90% as well as inducing analgesia.[93] At therapeutic doses, dexmedetomidine is not associated with respiratory depression, despite the profound levels of sedation that occur. It has the advantage of reducing postoperative narcotic requirements because of its analgesic properties. Compared with propofol, it has a slower onset and offset of sedation. Intraoperative mean arterial pressure is not reduced to the degree seen with propofol. Heart rate is decreased because of its sympatholytic and vagal-mimetic effects.[94] The average infusion rate for intraoperative sedation is 0.5–0.8 mcg/kg/h. It is important for the clinician to note that errors with dexmedetomidine infusion have occurred because the drug was infused in micrograms per kilogram per *minute* instead of micrograms per kilogram per *hour*.[95]

Clonidine, an α_2-adrenoreceptor agonist, has been advocated as another effective agent for intraoperative sedation. In a study on patients undergoing prolonged dental surgery, it was infused at a rate of 2 mcg/kg. It did not induce significant bradycardia, hypotension, or other severe side effects in healthy volunteers and provided an analgesic effect similar to that for dexmedetomidine.[96]

Low-dose midazolam infusions (0.03–1 mg/kg/h), combinations of ketamine and midazolam, and propofol and ketamine have been used effectively for intraoperative sedation after block placement. Ketamine has potent analgesic effects, provides hemodynamic stability (sympathomimetic action), and has minimal effect on the ventilatory drive, making it an excellent choice for debilitated patients or as a supplement for incomplete regional anesthesia. Analgesia can persist up to 40 min after ketamine administration has been terminated. Its association with postanesthetic confusion, disorientation, bad dreams, or hallucinations has limited its use in ambulatory surgery. Premedicating the patient with midazolam, limiting the dose, and allowing the patient to recover quietly will circumvent some of the untoward effects of ketamine.[97,98]

The use of narcotics during the intraoperative treatment of patients receiving regional anesthesia should be limited unless the patient has a chronic condition causing discomfort unrelated to the blocked surgical site. Narcotics should be used for analgesia and patient confort, not for anesthesia. They should not used to "rescue" an incomplete or failed block. Patient complaints should be investigated to determine if the discomfort is from positioning, prior chronic conditions, or in the surgical area not completely covered by the block. Because anesthesia of the skin is often the last to occur, local infiltration by the surgeon, when possible, and deeper levels of sedation at the beginning of the procedure are often all that is required for the procedure to proceed while the block is "setting up." Providing adequate padding for extremities; support for the upper back, shoulders, and head; prewarming the OR table; and providing continued warmth with forced air heating, heated blankets, and warmed intravenous infusions will decrease the discomfort caused by the cold OR and firm OR table. Deeper levels of sedation or opioids may be required for patients with chronic pain conditions. Using a short-acting sedative (eg, propofol) is a better choice than continued narcotic boluses that will compromise the patient's ability to protect the airway. If the block is inadequate or these measures are ineffective, it is safer to induce a light general anesthesia and control the airway rather than resorting to oversedation and intravenous narcotics. However, patients who chronically use oral opioids to treat their osteoarthritic or other pain needs may require and benefit from the judicious intraoperative use of opioids for their comfort.

Finally, some patients can be well sedated by the administration of low concentrations of nitrous oxide, similarly to the practice widely used in dental offices. Others, however, may be very intolerant of the effects of nitrous oxide. Nitrous oxide has analgesic and sedative properties and can be easily discontinued if the patient is not tolerating it.

Clinical Pearls

- A variety of drugs can be used successfully for intraoperative sedation. The anesthesiologist should develop a protocol he or she is comfortable with, then adjust the medications according to the physical and medical condition of the patient.

- Managing the appropriate amount of sedation is the art of a successful regional anesthesia practice.

- Successful regional anesthesia still provides the key elements of general anesthesia: analgesia, amnesia, muscle relaxation, and hypnosis. The major difference lies in the different ratios and different means of providing those elements.

Intraoperative Monitoring

Intraoperative monitoring is essential to the safety of regional anesthesia. Before any local or regional anesthetic is administered, equipment and medications should be available to support full resuscitation. The same equipment used for general anesthesia should be checked and be immediately available in the event that the anesthetic is converted to general. If the block is placed in the OR, blood pressure, electrocardiography, pulse oximetry, and end-tidal carbon dioxide monitoring should be instituted before the block is placed. A face mask (6 L of oxygen) or nasal cannula (up to 5 L of oxygen) should be applied once sedation is begun and continued throughout the case. It is of utmost importance that a properly functioning bag–mask device capable of delivering positive–pressure ventilation be immediately available in the area where regional anesthesia is practiced. The CO_2-sampling line can be connected to the face mask or to the nasal prongs to provide continuous end-tidal CO_2 measurement. Temperature monitoring should follow ASA standards.[99] For longer cases in which large areas of the patient's body are exposed, the patient's temperature should be monitored continuously.

Monitoring the patient under light or deep sedation requires vigilance on the part of the anesthesiologist. The potential problem of hypoventilation induced by sedatives is ever present. End-tidal CO_2 monitoring and pulse oximetry help guide the depth of sedation that is safe for the patient. In one study of plastic surgery patients, 39% of the patients developed oxygen saturations below 89%, despite appropriately administered sedation.[100]

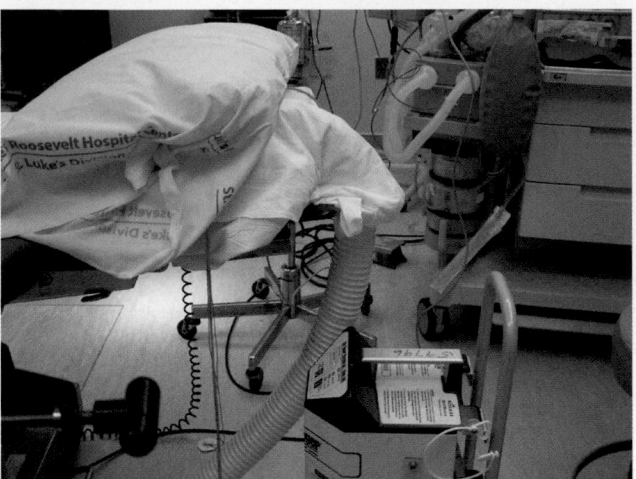

Figure 61–7. Warming the operating room table and blankets with force air prior to positioning the patient can provide significant patient comfort.

vent uncomfortable postoperative shivering and delays in discharge from the recovery room. Making the OR table as comfortable as possible with additional padding and positioning will make longer procedures more tolerable, especially for the arthritic patient or the patient with chronic axial pain.

Clinical Pearl

- Intraoperative monitoring of the patient with peripheral nerve block anesthesia is no different from that for general anesthesia. Back-up medications and supplies for general anesthesia should always be available.

Clinical Pearl

- Keeping the patient comfortable and warm takes vigilance on the part of the anesthesiologist. Remember that only the blocked extremity is protected from discomfort from the hard OR table or uncomfortable positions.

Intraoperative Patient Care

In addition to hemodynamic monitoring, other needs of the patient need to be addressed whether the patient is under light or deep sedation. Noxious stimuli and uncomfortable positioning may make a pleasant experience potentially intolerable.

Significant noise levels are often present in the OR due to discussion among the staff, handling of instruments, or the use of various pneumatic instruments. In a study on noise levels during various orthopedic surgical procedures, noise levels up to 118 decibels (dB)—a level that is potentially damaging to the hearing—were recorded when pneumatic drills and saws were used. Suction tips were found to yield levels up to 96 dB.[101] In another study on the effect of noise on the bispectral index, noise levels over 100 dB resulted in an appreciable increase in the bispectral index, despite propofol sedation.[102] Shielding the patient's ears from the unwanted noise should be done routinely to help reduce the patient's anxiety.

Warming the OR table with forced air prior to positioning the patient on the table, then covering the patient with a warm blanket helps to relax the patient and provide comfort prior to sedation for the block injection (Figure 61–7). Preventing hypothermia during the operation will help pre-

Transition of Patients from the OR to Postoperative Care

After surgery, most patients are fully alert and able to meaningfully discuss the findings with the surgeon in the OR while a wound dressing is being applied. On arrival in the recovery room, most ambulatory surgery patients are fast-tracked to the postanesthesia care unit and prepared for discharge. Inpatients are often more comfortable, especially in the early recovery period, due to the lasting effects of the local anesthetics chosen for the regional technique.

Transfer of Care to the Nursing Staff

To prevent unnecessary concerns by anyone involved in treating the patient, it is important, on completion of the surgical procedure, to discuss with the surgeons, patient, and nursing staff the expected duration of the motor and sensory blockade. A proper multimodal pain management protocol should be developed and thoroughly discussed with the nursing staff and the patients and their families. An understanding of the need to provide pain relief for surgical areas not covered by the nerve block and to avoid severe pain when the block wears off is important for a satisfactory postoperative recovery. To avoid unnecessary consultations, it is important for the staff and patient to understand that the block may last longer in some patients than in others because of the variability in the duration of action of local anesthetics.

Clinical Pearl

- Patients will need either intravenous patient-controlled analgesia (PCA) or oral analgesics for pain relief of areas not covered by the block, even if a continuous nerve block is used postoperatively. Most nerve blocks will yield excellent analgesia but may not eliminate the need for multimodal approach to pain management resulting from residual neural blockade.

Outpatient Acute Pain Management

Standard verbal and written instructions regarding pain management at home and protection of the anesthetized extremity are commonly provided for outpatients to ensure continued safe and satisfactory recovery.[52] Additional instructions are necessary for patients with continuous peripheral nerve block analgesia. Both verbal and written instructions about the infusion pump, its safety mechanisms, signs and symptoms of local anesthetic toxicity, and contact information should any questions arise should be given to the patient before discharge. Most centers utilizing continuous peripheral nerve block infusions at home have developed protocols for patient follow-up and evaluation, patient and nursing education, and emergency contact information. When home health nurses can be involved, extensive patient education and home evaluation can be conducted. The home health nurses can be trained to evaluate the patient for adjustments in drug delivery and assess catheter sites, dressings, and infusion devices. They can be trained to remove the peripheral nerve catheters, saving the need for the patient to return to the hospital for care. Telephone follow-up within the first 24 h is a necessary part of patient care when continuous catheters are utilized. Depending on the length of time the catheter is left in place, continued regular follow-up by telephone or a postoperative visit should be instituted until the catheter is removed.[103]

It is beyond the scope of this chapter to discuss various local anesthetic protocols for continuous outpatient nerve blocks (the reader is directed to Chapter 10 [Local Anesthetic Solutions for Continuous Nerve Blocks] for more information on this subject). In general, a continuous infusion of dilute ropivacaine (0.2%) at a continuous rate of 5–10 mL/h has been suggested by some authors as it provides excellent sensorimotor dissociation with better preservation of motor function than bupivacaine.[104] Other administration protocols include PCA (bolus technique) or a low background continuous infusion combined with a smaller boluses of PCA. It has been suggested that PCA techniques reduce the local anesthetic consumption by 64 to 73%.[105]

Inpatient Acute Pain Management

The same education is important for the patient who is to be admitted after a surgical procedure with regional anesthesia. Because longer-acting local anesthetics can be used for the patient who is to be admitted, it is important for the nursing and surgical staff to understand that the duration of the sensory and motor block will be prolonged. Again, educating the staff and the patient will prevent unnecessary consultations for neurologic defects. Even surgical staff comfortable with regional techniques need to be educated about the duration and effect of the peripheral nerve blocks. For example, when a patient has a total knee replacement, often a continuous femoral nerve catheter is placed for postoperative pain control. The femoral nerve block will cover a large portion of the area causing pain, but the sciatic distribution is not blocked. Pain control for the sciatic distribution is usually best accomplished by prescribing intravenous PCA or oral analgesia. This multimodal approach to pain management is especially important for the inpatient as the surgical procedures are usually more involved. Educating the staff about the benefits and limitations of the block as well as the need for additional pain medication will prevent misconceptions about patient pain complaints.[106,107]

Other factors related to the block also require staff education for the safety of the patient. If the block is going to affect lower extremity motor function, the patient will not be able to get out of bed by himself or bear weight on the blocked lower extremity. This should be explained to the patient and the caregivers. If an upper extremity block has been performed, then measures to protect the blocked upper extremity (eg, sling for interscalene blocked extremity) need to be instituted. The patient and family need to be reminded that the full function of the extremity will return when the block wears off.

SUMMARY

Regional anesthesia is an exciting, expanding subspecialty of anesthesiology. For the safe and efficient practice of regional anesthesia, dedication, experience, and perseverance are all necessary. It is a subspecialty as diverse as any other in anesthesia, requiring the same degree of advanced training from the resident to the fellowship level and beyond. Placing the block is only one aspect of the regional anesthesia practice. Appropriate patient selection and education, staff education, intraoperative management, and postoperative patient care are all important factors that must be included in the development of a successful regional anesthesia program.

References

1. Wu C, Naqibuddin M, Rowlingson A, et al: The effect of pain on heath-related quality of life in the immediate postoperative period. Anesth Analg 2003;97:1078–1085.
2. Klein S, Nielsen K, Greengrass R, et al: Ambulatory discharge after long-acting peripheral nerve blockade: 2382 blocks with ropivacaine. Anesth Analg 2002;94:65–70.

3. Chung F, Mezei G: Factors contributing to a prolonged stay after ambulatory surgery. Anesth Analg 1000;89:1352–1361.

4. Schuster M, Gottschalk A, Berger J, et al: A retrospective comparison of costs for regional and general anesthesia techniques. Anesth Analg 2005;100:786–794.

5. Hadzic A, Kraca P, Hobeika P, et al: Peripheral nerve blocks result in superior recovery profile compared with general anesthesia in outpatient knee arthroscopy. Anesth Analg 2005;100:976–981.

6. Luber M, Greengrass R, Vail TP: Patient satisfaction and effectiveness of lumbar plexus and sciatic nerve block for total knee arthroplasty. J Arthroplasty 2001;16:17–21.

7. Hadzic A, Williams B, Karaca P, et al: For outpatient rotator cuff surgery, nerve block anesthesia provides superior same-day recovery over general anesthesia. Anesthesiology 2005;102:1001–1007.

8. Pilny J, Kubes J: Forefoot surgery under regional anesthesia. Acta Chir Orthop Traumatol Cech 2005;72:122–124.

9. Tsui B, Wagner A, Finucane B: Regional anesthesia in the elderly: A clinical guide. Drugs Aging 2004;21:895–910.

10. Evans H, Steele S, Nielsen K, et al: Peripheral nerve blocks and continuous catheter techniques. Anesthesiol Clin North Am 2005;23:141–162.

11. Chakravarthy V, Arya V, Dhillon M, et al: Comparison of regional nerve block to epidural anaesthesia in day care arthroscopic surgery of the knee. Acta Orthop Belg 2004;70:551–559.

12. Navas A, Gutierrez T, Moreno M: Continuous peripheral nerve blockade in lower extremity surgery. Acta Anaesthesiol Scand 2005;49:1048–1055.

13. Schulz-Stübner S, Boezaart A, Hata J: Regional analgesia in the critically ill. Crit Care Med 2005;33:1400–1407.

14. Perris T, Watt J: The road to success: A review of 1000 axillary brachial plexus blocks. Anaesthesia 2003;58:1220–1224.

15. Reilley T, Gerhardt M: Anesthesia for foot and ankle surgery. Clin Podiatr Med Surg 2002;19:125–147.

16. Rosenblatt M, Fishkind D: Proficiency in interscalene anesthesia—How many blocks are necessary. J Clin Anesth 2003;15:285–288.

17. de Andres J, Bolinches R, Nalda M: Importance of the needle in regional anesthesia. Rev Esp Anestesiol Reanim 1990;37:71–74.

18. Grant S, Breslin D, MacLeod D, et al: Variability in determination of point of needle insertion in peripheral nerve blocks: A comparison of experienced and inexperienced anaesthetists. Anaesthesia 2003;58:688–692.

19. Martin G, Lineberger C, MacLeod D, et al: A new teaching model for resident training in regional anesthesia. Anesth Analg 2002;95:1837–1838.

20. Sites B, Gallagher J, Cravero J, et al: The learning curve associated with a simulated ultrasound-guided interventional task by inexperienced anesthesia residents. Reg Anesth Pain Med 2004;29:544–548.

21. Narr B, Hansen T, Warner M: Preoperative laboratory screening in healthy Mayo patients: Cost-effective elimination of tests and unchanged outcomes. Mayo Clin Proc 1991;66:155.

22. Alsumait B, Alhumood S, Ivanova T, et al: A prospective evaluation of preoperative screening laboratory tests in general surgical patients. Med Princ Pract 2002;11:42.

23. Horlocker T, Wedel D, Benzon H, et al: Regional anesthesia in the anticoagulated patient: Defining the risks. Reg Anesth Pain Med 2003;28:172–197.

24. Blery C, Charpak Y, Szatan M: Evaluation of a protocol for selective ordering of preoperative tests. Lancet 1986;1:139–141.

25. Rabkin S, Horne J: Properative electrocardiography: Effect of new abnormalities on clinical decisions. Can Med Assoc J 1983;128:146.

26. Gupta S, Gibbons F, Sen I: Routine chest radiography in the elderly. Age Ageing 1985;14:11.

27. Ang-Lee M, Moss J, Yuan C: Herbal medicines and perioperative care. JAMA 2001;286:208.

28. Provenzano D, Viscusi E, Adams S, et al: Safety and efficacy of the popliteal fossa nerve block when utilized for foot and ankle surgery. Foot Ankle Int 2002;23:394–399.

29. Casati A, Grispigni C, Aldegheri G, et al: Peripheral or central nerve blocks for foot surgery: A prospective, randomized clinical comparison. Foot Ankle Surg 2002;8:95–100.

30. Brown D: Brachial plexus anesthesia: An analysis of options. Yale J Biol Med 1993;66:415–431.

31. Regel H, Rose W, Hahnel S, et al: Evaluation of psychological stress before general anesthesia. Psychiatr Neurol Med Psychol 1985;37:151–155.

32. Davies M, McGlade D: One hundred sciatic nerve blocks: A comparison of localization techniques. Anesth Intensive Care 1993;21:76–78.

33. Misiolek H, Dobosz J, Grzanka A: Anesthesia for axillofemoral bypass surgery in the patient with multivessel coronary artery disease. Wiad Lek 2004;57:516–519.

34. Mulroy M, McDonald S: Regional anesthesia for outpatient surgery. Anesthesiol Clin North Am 2003;21:289–303.

35. Adams J, Murphy P: Obesity in anaesthesia and intensive care. Br J Anesth 2000;85:91–108.

36. Davies K, Houghton K, Montgomery J: Obesity and day-case surgery. Anaesthesia 2001;56:1112–1115.

37. Nielsen K, Guller U, Steele S, et al: Influence of obesity on surgical regional anesthesia in the ambulatory setting: An analysis of 9,038 blocks. Anesthesiology 2005;102:181–187.

38. Jain S, Dhand R: Perioperative treatment of patients with obstructive sleep apnea. Curr Opin Pulm Med 2004;10:482–488.

39. Williams-Russo P, Sharrock N, Mattis S, et al: Cognitive effects after epidural vs general anesthesia in older adults. A randomized trial. JAMA 1995;274:44–50.

40. Somprakit P, Lertakyamanee J, Satraratanamai C, et al: Mental state change after general and regional anesthesia in adults and elderly patients, a randomized clinical trial. J Med Assoc Thai 2002;85:S875–S883.

41. Kamitani K, Higuchi A, Asahi T, et al: Postoperative delirium after general anesthesia vs. spinal anesthesia in geriatric patients. Masui 2003;52:972–975.

42. Selander D, Brattsand R, Lundborg G, et al: Local anesthetics: Importance of mode of application, concentration, and adrenaline for the appearance of nerve lesions. Acta Anaesthesiol Scand 1979;23:127.

43. Covino B, Wildsmith J: Clinical pharmacology of local anesthetic agents. In Cousins B (ed): Neural Blockade in Clinical Anesthesia and Management of Pain, 3rd ed. Lippincott-Raven, 1998, p 97.

44. Hall J, Ferro A: Myocardial ischaemia and ventricular arrhythmias precipitated by physiologic concentrations of adrenaline in patients with coronary artery disease. Br Heart J 1992;67:419.

45. Paci E, Barneschi M, Miccinesi G, et al: Informed consent and patient participation in the medical encounter: A list of questions for an informed choice about the type of anesthesia. Eur J Anesth 1999;16:160–165.

46. Papanikolaou M, Voulgari A, Lykouras L: Psychological factors influencing the surgical patients' consent to regional anaesthesia. Acta Anaesthesiol Scand 1994;38:607–611.

47. Whalen J, Dufresne R: Delayed-type hypersensitivity after subcutaneous administration of amide anesthetic. Arch Dermatol 1996;132:1256–1257.

48. Lee L, Posner K, Domino K, et al: Injuries associated with regional anesthesia in the 1980s and 1990s: A closed claim analysis. Anesthesiology 2004;101:143–152.

49. Evans H, Steele S, Nielsen KC: Peripheral nerve blocks and continuous catheter techniques. Anesthesiol Clin North Am 2005;23:141–162.

50. Del Carmen M, Joffe S: Informed consent for medical treatment and research: A review. Oncologist 2005;10:636–641.

51. Hadzic A, Vloka JD: Keys to success with peripheral nerve blocks. In Hadzic A (ed): Peripheral Nerve Blocks: Principles and Practice. McGraw-Hill, 2004, pp 79–89.

52. Nielsen K, Steele S: Management of outpatient orthopedic surgery. Anaesthesiology 2001;14:611–616.

53. Rosenblatt M, Fishkind D: Proficiency in interscalene anesthesia—How many blocks are necessary. J Clin Anesth 2003;15:285–288.

54. Munte S, Adams H: Stand-by and conscious sedation—Possibilities and limits of anesthesiological management. Anaesthesiol Reanim 2001;26:44–49.

55. Mitchell J: Recommendations for standards of monitoring during anaesthesia and recovery. Anaesthesia 2001;56:488.

56. Hadzic A, Vloka JD, Santos A, et al: Training requirements for peripheral nerve blocks. Anesthesiology 2000;93:1541–1544.

57. Neal J, Kopac D, Liguori G, et al: The training and careers of regional anesthesia fellows: 1983–2002. Reg Anesth Pain Med 2005;30:215–217.

58. Brown D: Fellowship training in regional anesthesia. Reg Anesth Pain Med 2005;30:215–217.

59. Urmey W, Talts K, Sharrock N: 100% incidence of hemidiaphragmatic paresis associated with interscalene brachial plexus anesthesia as diagnosed by ultrasonography. Anesth Analg 1991;72:498–503.

60. Shah S, Tsai T, Iwata T, et al: Outpatient regional anesthesia for foot and ankle surgery. Int Anesthesiol Clin 2005;43:143–151.

61. Bishop J, Sprague M, Gelber J, et al: Interscalene regional anesthesia for shoulder surgery. J Bone Joint Surg [Am] 2005;87:874–879.

62. Wong G, Brown D, Miller G, et al: Defining the cross-sectional anatomy important to interscalene brachial plexus block with magnetic resonance imaging. Reg Anesth Pain Med 1998;23:77–80.

63. Minville V, N'Guyen L, Chassery C, et al: A modified coracoid approach to infraclavicular brachial plexus blocks using a double-stimulation technique in 300 patients. Anesth Analg 2005;100:263–265.

64. MacLeod D, Grant S, Martin G, et al: Identification of coracoid process for infraclavicular blocks. Reg Anesth Pain Med 2003;5:485.

65. Neuburger M, Kaiser H, Ass B, et al: Vertical infraclavicular blockade of the brachial plexus. A modified method to verify the puncture point under consideration of the risk of pneumothorax. Anaesthesia 2003;52:619–624.

66. Desroches J: The infraclavicular brachial plexus block by the coracoid approach is clinically effective: An observational study of 150 patients. Can J Anaesth 2003;50:253–257.

67. Porter J, McCartney C, Chan V: Needle placement and injection posterior to the axillary artery may predict successful infraclavicular brachial plexus block: A report of three cases. Can J Anaesth 2005;52:69–73.

68. McLeod A, Roche A, Fennelly M: Case series: Ultrasonography may assist epidural insertion in scoliosis patients. Can J Anaesth 2005;52:717–720.

69. Cook T: Combined spinal-epidural techniques. Anaesthesia 2000;55:42–64.

70. Donohue C, Goss L, Metz S, et al: Combined popliteal and saphenous nerve blocks at the knee: An underused alternative to general or spinal anesthesia for foot and ankle surgery. J Am Podiatr Med Assoc 2004;94:368–374.

71. Taboada M, Alvarez J, Cortes J, et al: The effects of three different approaches on the onset time of sciatic nerve blocks with 0.75% ropivacaine. Anesth Analg 2004;98:242–247.

72. Osborn T, Sandler N: The effect of preoperative anxiety on intravenous sedation. Anesth Prog 2004;51:46–51.

73. Edmonds C, Liguori G, M Stanton, et al: Two cases of a wrong-site peripheral nerve block and a process to prevent this complication. Reg Anesth Pain Med 2005;30:99–103.

74. Smith A, Pittaway A: Premedication for anxiety in adult day surgery. Cochrane Database Systems Review 2000;3:CD002192.

75. Hasen K, Samartzis D, Casas L, et al: An outcome study comparing intravenous sedation with midazolam/fentanyl (conscious sedation) versus propofol infusion (deep sedation) for aesthetic surgery. Plast Reconstr Surg 2003;112:1690–1691.

76. Gajaraj M, Sharma S, Souter A, et al: A survey of obstetrical patients who refuse regional anaesthesia. Anaesthesiology 1995;50:740–741.

77. Kinirons BP, H Bouaziz, Paqueron X, et al: Sedation with sufentanil and midazolam decreases pain in patients undergoing upper limb surgery under multiple nerve block. Anesth Analg 2000;90:1118–1121.

78. Smith A, Pittaway A: Premedication for anxiety in adult day surgery. Cochrane Database Systems Review 2000;1:2192.

79. Kinirons B, Bouaziz H, Paqueron X, et al: Sedation with sufentanil and midazolam decreases pain in patients undergoing upper limb surgery under multiple nerve block. Anesth Analg 2000;90:1118–1121.

80. Bauer K, Dom P, Ramirez A: Preoperative intravenous midazolam: Benefits beyond anxiolysis. J Clin Anesth 2004;16:177–183.

81. Feldman S, Paton W, Scurr C: Mechanisms of drugs in anaesthesia. In Feldmna S (ed): Mechanisms of Drugs in Anaesthesias. Oxford University Press, 1993.

82. From R, Warner D, Todd M, et al: Anesthesia for craniotomy: A double-blind comparison of alfentanil, fentanyl, and sufentanil. Anesthesiology 1990;73:896–904.

83. Hudson R, Stanski D: Metabolism versus redistribution of fentanyl and alfentanil. Anesthesiology 1983;59:A243.

84. McHardy F, Fortier J, Chung F, et al: A comparison of midazolam, alfentanil and propofol for sedation in outpatient intraocular surgery. Can J Anaesth 2000;47:211–214.

85. Adams A, Pybus D: Delayed respiratory depression after use of fentanyl during anesthesia. Br J Med 1978;1:278.

86. Chelly J, Greger J, Samsam T, et al: Reduction of operating and recovery room times and overnight hospital stays with interscalene blocks as sole anesthetic technique for rotator cuff surgery. Minerva Anesthesiol 2001;67:613–619.

87. Williams B, Kentor M, Williams J, et al: Process analysis in outpatient knee surgery: Effects of regional and general anesthesia on anesthesia-controlled time. Anesthesiology 2000;93:529–538.

88. Armstrong K, Cherry R: Brachial plexus anesthesia compared to general anesthesia when a block room is available. Can J Anaesth 2004;51:41–44.

89. Dalens B: More on regional anesthesia induction rooms. Can J Anaesth 2004;51:741.

90. Drolet P, Girard M: Regional anesthesia, block room and efficiency: Putting things in perspective. Can J Anaesth 2004;51:1–5.

91. Soni JC, Thomas D: Comparison of anxiety before induction of anesthesia in the anaesthetic room or operating theatre. Anaesthesia 1989;44:651–655.

92. Overdyk F, Harvey S, Fishman R, et al: Successful strategies for improving OR efficiency at academic institutions. Anesth Analg 1998;86:896–906.

93. Memis D, Turan A, Karamanlioghlu B, et al: Adding dexmedetomidine to lidocaine for intravenous regional anesthesia. Anesth Analg 2004;98:835–840.

94. Arain SR, Ebert TJ: The efficacy, side effects, and recovery characteristics of dexmedetomidine versus propofol when used for intraoperative sedation. Anesth Analg 2002;95:461–466.

95. Jorden V, Pousman R, Sanford M, et al: Dexmedetomidine overdose in the perioperative setting. Ann Pharmacother 2004;38:803–807.

96. Ise T, Yamashiro M, Furuya H: Clonidine as a drug for intravenous conscious sedation. Odontology 2002;90:57–63.

97. Wresch K: Analgesia and sedation to supplement incomplete regional anesthesia. Anesthetist 1995;44:S580–S587.

98. Deng X, Xiao W, Luo M, et al: The use of midazolam and small-dose ketamine for sedation and analgesia during local anesthesia. Anesth Analg 2001;93:1174–1177.

99. Brodsky J: What intraoperative monitoring makes sense. Chest 1999;115:101S–105S.

100. Singer R, Thomas P: Pulse oximeter in the ambulatory aesthetic surgical facility. Plast Reconstr Surg 1988;82:111.

101. Ray C, Levinson R: Noise pollution in the operating room: A hazard to surgeons, personnel, and patients. J Spinal Disord 1992;5:485–488.

102. Kim D, Kil H, White P: The effect of noise on the bispectral index during propofol sedation. Anesth Analg 2001;93:1170–1173.

103. Grant S, Nielsen K, Greengrass R, et al: Continuous peripheral nerve block for ambulatory surgery. Reg Anesth Pain Med 2000;26:209–214.

104. Borgeat A, Kalberer F, Jacob H: Continuous peripheral nerve block for ambulatory surgery. Reg Anesth Pain Med 2001;26:209–214.

105. Singelyn F, Vanderelst P, Gouverneur J: Extended femoral nerve sheath block after total hip arthroplasty: Continuous vs. patient-controlled techniques. Anesth Analg 2001;92:455–459.

106. Karflsten R, Strom K, Gunningberg L: Improving assessment of postoperative pain in surgical wards by education and training. Qual Saf Health Care 2005;14:332–335.

107. Larijani G, Sharaf I, Warshal D, et al: Pain evaluation in patients receiving intravenous patient controlled analgesia after surgery. Pharmacotherapy 2005;25:1168–1173.

Regional Anesthesia in Specific Patient Populations

62

Peripheral Nerve Blocks for Outpatient Surgery

Robert J. Schlosser, MD • Karen C. Nielsen, MD • Holly Evans, MD • Stephen M. Klein, MD •
Marcy S. Tucker, MD • Susan M. Steele, MD

GENERAL CONSIDERATIONS AND BRIEF HISTORY: ADVANTAGES OF NERVE BLOCKS IN AMBULATORY SURGERY

The development of ambulatory surgery and that of peripheral nerve blocks (PNBs) occurred over two separate historic timelines. The performance of outpatient or ambulatory surgeries commenced in the mid-1800s, and its utilization rapidly escalated throughout the next century.

By 1980, 16.3% of all surgeries were performed on an outpatient basis. By 1984 this number rose to 30% and the Society for Ambulatory Anesthesia (SAMBA) was born. The total outpatient rate approached 50% by 1990, 60% in 1997, and may have hit 70% in 2003.[1,2] During the same span of time, techniques for PNBs were also being discovered. The decades from 1884, (when Koller and Brettauer first instilled ocular cocaine in Heidelberg, Germany[3]) to 1912 and 1914, (when Kappis and Heidenhein described the interscalene block,[4]) marked the birth of PNBs. Despite the coexistence of both ambulatory anesthesia and PNB techniques for over a century, they were not typically used concurrently.

As ambulatory surgery acquired today's popularity and widespread use, the scope of surgical procedures similarly expanded to become more invasive and pain-inducing. Suddenly, physicians were faced with a dual challenge: provide short-acting anesthesia thus achieving home-readiness within hours of surgery, concurrent with long-acting postoperative analgesia permitting the patient to remain discharged to the home environment. The differences between these dual desires have proven irreconcilable with modern opiate analgesia. This has been recently documented by Apfelbaum and colleagues, who quantified the shortcomings of ambulatory analgesic regimens. They found that 78% of those queried had felt pain of moderate (52%), severe (22%) or extreme (7%) intensity.[5]

In response to ambulatory anesthesia's dilemma, PNB techniques offer solutions ideal for an outpatient anesthetic: site-specific surgical anesthesia and a decreased dependency on general anesthesia (GA). In so doing, PNBs buffer the response to surgical stress, better maintain functional residual capacity, defend against loss of immunologic function, and avoid or shorten the period of postoperative ileus.[6] By providing effective analgesia, PNBs can reduce patient exposure to opioids and their side effects. This allows for a more rapid discharge of satisfied patients to their home environment, resulting in cost savings for the ambulatory surgery center. As a cornerstone of multimodal analgesia, PNBs with long-acting local anesthetic (LA) help reduce patient readmission for pain or other side effects. Extending the effect of LA through continuous peripheral nerve blocks (CPNBs) further lengthens the period of low side-effect postoperative analgesia in the home environment.

Despite the advances in PNBs and CPNBs, these techniques remain underutilized skills in ambulatory anesthesia. As recently as the year 2000, Dexter and Macario[7] revealed that ambulatory surgeries utilized regional anesthesia in only 8% of cases. A 1997 survey by Hadzic and coworkers found that although 98% of anesthesiologists used some regional techniques, less than half of respondents placed at least five PNBs per month.[8] A 2001 survey by Klein and colleagues concurred that although interscalene, axillary, and ankle blocks were performed more often, major conduction PNBs of the lower extremity were not commonly employed. Further analysis indicated that 85% of anesthesiologists discharged patients with long-acting PNBs of the three aforementioned types, but only 36% were willing to place a long-acting femoral nerve block. Many factors contribute to avoidance of long-lasting PNBs including fear of patient injury or self-care deficits at home, logistical issues related to the time needed for performance and onset of the PNB, as well as unfamiliarity with techniques.[9] Concerns regarding unfamiliarity with techniques will persist as long as inadequacies exist in resident education.[10–12] But the issues of perceived outcome benefits versus risks, time required for PNB performance, and PNB reliability will

likely remain the deciding factors in its use for outpatients. Regardless of the reason, the result remains the same: outpatient PNB remains a vastly underutilized technique. The real history of PNB and ambulatory surgery remains to be written.

Clinical Pearls

- Ambulatory surgery procedures have grown in scope and complexity, requiring more specialized regional anesthesia procedure for faster patient recovery and better postoperative pain control.
- PNBs provide a robust alternative to general ambulatory anesthesia.
- PNB still remains a vastly underutilized technique.

PATIENT SELECTION

Several factors, both negative and positive, aid the anesthesiologist in excluding or selecting an ambulatory patient for a nerve block. The primary absolute negative factor is patient refusal of PNB. Assuming acceptance of the technique however, patient selection depends on benefits outweighing the risks to patient safety during placement of the block and, secondarily, on patient safety after discharge with an insensate extremity. Primary patient exclusion begins with a stated allergy to LA. Another reason to reconsider PNBs involves deep or noncompressible nerve block sites in a sufficiently anticoagulated patient. Although central neuraxial blockade can certainly be used in patients receiving a variety of anticoagulants,[13] the rules governing its use are likely too stringent to be applied to all PNB techniques. If a patient can accept the traumatic risk of an elective direct laryngoscopy, they can likely also weather the risk of a femoral nerve block from an experienced operator.

Immunologic concerns warrant exclusion if an infection is present at the nerve block site. Patients with sever pulmonary disease are not often scheduled to have procedures in an ambulatory facility, however, moderate to severe chronic obstructive pulmonary disease (COPD) in a patient warrants cautious consideration prior to selection of paravertebral block (PVB) or brachial plexus blockade. Although PNB techniques offer potential benefits over GA and narcotic analgesia, the consequences of pneumothorax and phrenic nerve paralysis must be weighed cautiously. Another screening consideration surrounds the patient with nerve injury. This is especially true in patients with either a worsening or improving nerve deficit that is under consideration for blockade. Although the literature provides no evidence that administration of PNBs in patients with preexisting neuropathy carries a risk of worsening the neurologic deficit, the complexity of the management and neurologic follow-up of these patients may outweigh the benefits of nerve blocks. Central nervous lesions can also cause anxiety in the consideration of peripheral block. Some advocate steering clear of patients with fluctuating central lesions like multiple sclerosis to avoid perceived liability surrounding the patient's natural disease progression; these opinions are not substantiated in the literature, however. The final consideration of acute risks versus benefits applies not to patient physiology, but to the environment in which the PNB is placed. If it is to occur outside of the operating room, standard American Society of Anesthesiology monitors, suction, oxygen and resuscitative gear and medicines are required. More information on application of regional anesthesia in patients with coexisting disease can be found in Part VIII of this textbook (Regional Anesthesia in Patients with Special Considerations).

After excluding patients in whom the immediate risks outweigh potential benefits of PNBs, concerns still remain regarding patient safety after discharge home with an insensate extremity. However, concerns of rendering the patients immobile in their home environment can be abated by the well-developed social support network that usually surrounds this subset of patients. In sharp contrast to these patients would be the patient with a weak nonoperative leg who has received a lower extremity block. Lower extremity block must also be carefully weighed in the morbidly obese, the frail elderly, and the patient with Parkinson disease because they are at a higher risk of falling. Postoperative surgical issues occasionally intrude on selection of long-duration PNB with the need for functional nerve assessment.

Conversely, PNBs should be actively encouraged for patients about to undergo an invasive or extensive surgery on an extremity, such as open joint reconstruction or replacement, osteotomies, tendon transfers, fracture repair, or manipulation of arthrofibrosis. PNBs should also be sought for patients with chronic pain conditions and opioid tolerance to aid them in management of postoperative pain. Patients with complex regional pain syndrome (CRPS) have demonstrated a pattern of abnormal nerve healing and are prone to redevelopment of CRPS in the operative extremity. Regional anesthesia has been shown to be beneficial in preventing a recurrence when clonidine is used with intravenous regional anesthesia (IVRA) or when the most proximal and sympatholytic PNB is employed.[14,15] PNBs can also be of great benefit for patients undergoing surgeries that are particularly emetogenic, such as mastectomy, or for those with histories of postoperative nausea and vomiting (PONV) or opioid intolerance. Long-acting or continuous PNBs can also help patients avoid other side effects of opioids. Respiratory depression can be avoided in the COPD patient, and ileus or constipation can be limited after herniorrhaphy. Regional anesthesia (RA) can help prevent the need for airway manipulation in patients with asthma. PNBs can reduce surgical blood loss,[16] assuaging concerns of the anemic or Jehovah's Witness patient. A final (and controversial) benefit also exists in using PNB to help the anesthesiologist sidestep the issue of an anticipated difficult airway.

Clinical Pearls

- PNB should be avoided in patients who refuse it, in those with LA allergy or unstable neuropathies, and when the safety infrastructure is lacking.
- Caution is warranted with anticoagulation, upper extremity block with COPD, lower extremity block with morbid obesity, frailty, Parkinson disease, or a weak nonoperative leg.
- PNB should be advocated in patients who undergo painful procedures; are prone to PONV, ileus, or respiratory depression; or are tolerant of opioids.

TECHNIQUE SELECTION

Interscalene Brachial Plexus Block

Interscalene PNB anesthetizes the brachial plexus, typically at the C6 nerve root. The popularity of this block relates to its utility in providing long-lasting analgesia after painful ambulatory orthopedic shoulder surgery. When Hadzic[17] compared interscalene block to GA in 50 patients for outpatient rotator cuff surgery, he found that patients with PNB had more frequent postanesthesia care unit (PACU) bypass (76% vs 16%), suffered less pain, ambulated earlier, met discharge criteria sooner (123 min vs 286 min), had fewer unplanned readmissions (0 vs 16%), and were more satisfied with their care. Brown coworkers[18] found similar results and fewer postoperative side effects after interscalene block versus GA (pain 14% vs 45%, PONV 8% vs 43%, urinary retention 0% vs 25%, hospital admissions 17% vs 48%). In a large retrospective review comparing interscalene block with GA, D'Alessio and colleagues[19] further demonstrated reductions in nonsurgical intraoperative time (29 ± 9 min vs 49 ± 12 min) and PACU time (72 ± 24 min vs 102 ± 40 min), as well as decreased anesthetic side effects in PACU.

Al-Kaisy's group[20] prospectively compared interscalene block with 10 mL 0.125% bupivacaine against placebo for outpatient shoulder arthroscopy done under GA. They found decreased pain and morphine use (2.7 ± 2.6 mg vs 9.5 ± 5.2 mg) during the PACU stay and a faster achievement of discharge criteria (139 ± 34 min vs 193 ± 59 min) with the nerve block. They also noted no difference between patient groups in their 24-h opioid use following PNB resolution at 2 h. In a similar study, Laurila and associates[21] compared a low-volume interscalene block with a subacromial bursa block and placebo. They also found the interscalene block to be the most effective for early postoperative pain control.

Singelyn and coworkers[22] compared patients undergoing arthroscopic acromioplasty with interscalene PNB, isolated suprascapular nerve block, intraarticular LA, or systemic opioids. They concluded that interscalene PNB was most proficient, that suprascapular block was an alternative option, but that intraarticular LA injection offered no benefit to intravenous (IV) opioids.

Failure to achieve surgical anesthesia with interscalene PNB ranges from 0 to 9.5%,[18−20,23] requiring conversion of 16% of cases to GA.[18] Although side effects often include shortness of breath, dysphonia, and Horner's syndrome[18,24] they rarely thwart discharge planning. More importantly, studies on inpatients have demonstrated a low risk of neurologic injury. In a series of 520 patients having single-injection or continuous interscalene block, Borgeat and colleagues[25] found that 14% had paresthesia, dysesthesia, or nonsurgical pain 10 days after surgery. The majority of these symptoms gradually resolved, leaving only one patient symptomatic with a plexus injury 9 months after surgery. The combination of an efficacious PNB, its relatively benign clinical application, and demonstrated benefits compared with GA ensure ongoing use of the interscalene block.

Clinical Pearls

Interscalene brachial plexus block

- This block is useful for shoulder and upper arm surgery.
- It has an excellent clinical efficacy.
- The risk of block inadequacy and similar risk of transient neuropathy is ≤10%.
- Horner's syndrome and transient dyspnea are common.

Supraclavicular Brachial Plexus Block

The supraclavicular PNB approaches the brachial plexus trunks between the clavicle and the first rib. Due to the close proximity of the trunks at this level and the close apposition of the surrounding fascia, the supraclavicular block can provide more reliable anesthesia with faster onset distal to the shoulder than the axillary approach. Bedder and associates[26] showed that supraclavicular block using 0.5% bupivacaine provided onset of sensory anesthesia in 4.0 ± 1.2 min and peak effect in 17.7 ± 1.8 min. Consequently, supraclavicular block is ideal for rapid-turnover outpatient procedures of the elbow, wrist, and hand. Because the axillary nerve may be spared with this PNB, supraclavicular block is not always reliable for shoulder surgeries.[27] With the supraclavicular block, the needle insertion site is near the dome of the lung. Anecdotal reports have associated the "plumb-bob" technique with an unacceptably high risk of pneumothorax, leading many practitioners to avoid this block. Nevertheless, no study supports this concern or warrants prolonged observation of a patient after an uneventful anesthetic and recovery. To the contrary, Franco and Vieira[28] demonstrated the safety of supraclavicular PNB in a series of 1001 patients anesthetized by both consultants and residents. Touting a clinical efficacy of 97.2%, no major complications were reported. These data highlight the potential usefulness and safety profile of this as yet underutilized technique.

Clinical Pearls

Supraclavicular block

- Supraclavicular block has the fastest onset of any brachial plexus block.
- The success rate is high.
- Supraclavicular block is suitable for upper extremity procedures, excepting those for the shoulder.
- The risk of pneumothorax is low with adequate training.

Infraclavicular Brachial Plexus Block

Infraclavicular PNB is approached at the division and cord level of the brachial plexus. PNB at this level provides anesthesia appropriate for procedures done on the mid to distal upper extremity. As with supraclavicular PNB, this block has a high success rate and a low risk of pneumothorax.[29−31]

Hadzic and coworkers[32] contrasted patients who underwent ambulatory wrist surgery with GA with those who received infraclavicular PNB. As a group, those patients with GA had lower PACU bypass rates (24% vs 76%), higher rates of PONV (32% vs 8%), and more numerous requests for analgesia (48% vs 0%). Fewer patients in the infraclavicular group reported inability to concentrate in the PACU (8% vs 56%), though statistical significance was lost by the time that discharge criteria were met. Although the infraclavicular block performed in the operating room prolonged induction by 5 min, total operative time was similar to GA. Discharge criteria were met more quickly in the PNB group (100 ± 44 min vs 203 ± 91 min), and opioid use was similar in both groups over the first 48 h.

Desroches[33] used infraclavicular PNB to achieve surgical anesthesia in 91% of outpatients and required 7 min or less for block execution. The risk of pneumothorax remained low at 0.7%, although published rates of vascular puncture can be as high as 17%.[34] The newer techniques with needle redirection laterally should reduce the risk of pneumothorax to practically negligible.

Clinical Pearls

Infraclavicular Block

- This techniques is time-efficient.
- It is suitable for upper extremity procedures distal to the shoulder.
- The success rate is high.
- The risk of noncompressible vascular puncture is low.

Axillary Brachial Plexus Block

The brachial pulse allows for facile location of the axillary artery and the common sheath that invests the branches of the brachial plexus. This reliable landmark, the low risk of pneumothorax, and the usefulness of this PNB for surgical anesthesia of the mid to distal upper extremity has helped to make the axillary block the most popular PNB in the United States.[8,9] Axillary PNB can be successfully executed with a nerve stimulator, paresthesia, or the transarterial technique.

Septa within the fascial sheath[35,36] may limit the rate of diffusion of LA to terminal nerves and result in individual nerve sparing. This can in turn lead to nerve sparing as well as delayed anesthetic set-up. In an attempt to overcome this problem, the stimulation and injection of individual nerves has been studied.[37] Bouaziz and associates[38] attempted to make an additional improvement in outcome by utilizing 0.5% bupivacaine to anesthetize the ulnar and median nerves and 2% lidocaine for the others. This strategy resulted in long-lasting anesthesia of a palmar incision with faster recovery of the remaining arm. Koscielniak-Nielsen and coworkers[39] investigated success and patient perceptions using multiple-stimulation in unmedicated outpatients. They found that electrolocation was uncomfortable for 80%, but that 98% would have the same technique in the future. Thirteen percent would request sedation in the future, and 95% were comfortable being discharged with an insensate extremity. Despite this success, although block performance only took an average of 9.8 min, block onset took an additional 23 min using a 1:1 mixture of 0.75% ropivacaine and 2% mepivacaine. Utilization of a preoperative "block room" can eliminate the delay of LA set-up, decrease nonsurgical operating room time, and improve overall efficiency.[40,41]

Outpatient axillary PNB is not without the risk of block failure or complication. Davis and colleagues[42] reviewed 530 such blocks and found a 7% incidence of block failure requiring GA and a 2 % incidence of inadequate postoperative analgesia requiring admission. Complications were rare, with a less than 1% incidence of LA toxicity and no persistent neurologic deficits. Cooper's group[43] reviewed the anesthetics of 1149 outpatients and found that 93% of those who responded would have an axillary block in the future. Those who were reluctant to have another block were more likely to have experienced any side effect (ie, bruising or pain in the axilla).

Chan and coworkers[44] prospectively compared axillary block with IVRA and GA in 126 individuals having outpatient hand surgery. The RA groups required less opioids and had a decreased incidence of PONV ($p < 0.05$). But the induction time, overall discharge time, and cost were least in the IVRA group ($p < 0.05$).

Clinical Pearls

Axillary Block
- Axillary block is efficacious for elbow, forearm, and hand procedures.
- It is easy to perform with minimal risk of complications.
- The possibility of nerve sparing exists, with up to 7% risk of block failure.
- Axillary block has the slowest onset time of all brachial plexus techniques.

Iliohypogastric–Ilioinguinal Nerve Block

The iliohypogastric (T12, L1) and ilioinguinal (L1) nerves provide sensory innervation to the inferior abdomen and buttocks, the superomedial thigh, and part of the external genitalia. Block of these nerves is easily and efficiently performed 2 cm medial and 2 cm superior to the anterior superior iliac spine. Alternatively, the surgeon can apply LA to the nerves directly during an inguinal hernia repair. In the literature, the iliohypogastric–ilioinguinal nerve block has been used successfully as an adjunct to GA in surgeries such as inguinal herniorrhaphy and varicocelectomy.[45] When compared with placebo,[46] local wound infiltration,[47] subarachnoid block (SAB),[48] or GA alone,[48] ilioinguinal–iliohypogastric nerve block has been associated with decreases in postoperative pain scores,[46-48] postoperative opioid requirements,[46,47] PONV,[48] cost,[48] and discharge times.[48] Complications with this nerve block are usually related to the proximity of these nerves to the femoral nerve. Inadvertent femoral nerve block[49,50] can result in difficulty with ambulation and may be difficult to differentiate from direct surgical trauma to the nerve. Overall, although data demonstrate its usefulness as an adjunct for hernia surgery, the magnitude of benefit seen may not support its routine use when compared with the simple alternative of surgical wound infiltration and multimodal analgesia.

Clinical Pearls

ILIOINGUINAL–ILIOHYPOGASTRIC NERVE BLOCKS
- These blocks are and easy to perform adjunct for inguinal herniorrhaphy or varicocelectomy.
- There is a risk of inadvertent femoral nerve block.

Lumbar Plexus Block

The lumbar plexus block anesthetizes the femoral, obturator, and lateral femoral cutaneous nerves more reliably than more distal approaches to the femoral nerve.[51] Although lumbar plexus block is useful for procedures that range from hip[52] to knee[53-55] arthroplasty, the expansiveness of this block may be disadvantageous to outpatients unless a short-acting local anesthetic is used (eg, chloroprocaine). Loss of iliopsoas muscle function prevents flexion at the hip and increases the difficulty of ambulating with crutches or even a walker. Furthermore, there exists a risk of epidural spread of LA, ranging between 1.8% to 8.9%.[56,57] This may be caused by injecting LA too medially after eliciting the muscular response of a single nerve root. Such a mishap may prevent a patient from walking and delay discharge when long-acting local anesthetics are used.

Knee arthroscopy remains a commonly performed ambulatory surgical procedure for which lumbar plexus PNB may be useful. Two randomized prospective trials compared lumbar plexus PNB with SAB or GA for this procedure. Jankowski and associates[58] found that more than twice the number of GA patients (45%) required analgesics in PACU versus those who received lumbar plexus PNB (21%) or SAB

(14%). Although pain scores were higher at all points in the GA group, because mean scores were low even in this group they questioned whether lumbar plexus block was really necessary for this procedure. Hadzic and coworkers[59] presented compelling support for a lumbar plexus block and sciatic nerve block over GA for knee arthroscopy. By utilizing lumbar plexus and sciatic PNBs they were able to decrease severe PONV from 62% to 12%, odynophagia from 60% to 28% and time to achieve discharge criteria from 205 ± 94 min to 131 ± 62 min. The percent achieving PACU bypass increased with PNBs from 24% to 72%. Although PNBs (placed in the operating room) lengthened the time required for induction by 7 min, there was no overall increase in length of time spent in the operating room.

Clinical Pearls

Lumbar Plexus Blocks

- Lumbar plexus blocks can provide anesthesia for hip arthroscopy and, in combination with sciatic nerve blockade, for extensive knee surgery.
- This is the only consistent technique for coverage of "3-in-1" distribution.
- The risk of epidural spread is ≤10%.
- Weakness of hip flexors can impede patient discharge.

Femoral Nerve Block & Fascia Iliaca Block

Anesthesia of the proximal lower extremity including the anterior knee and medial calf can be achieved with a femoral nerve block or a fascia iliaca block. Both of these PNBs can be performed on a supine patient with easily identified landmarks. Because anesthesia of the lateral femoral cutaneous and obturator nerves are often desired in addition to femoral block, individual anesthesiologists have attempted to increase LA volumes and to apply distal pressure to achieve these ends.[60] The "3-in-1" technique, however, fails to consistently block the lateral femoral cutaneous and especially the obturator nerve.[51,61–63]

Femoral PNB has been employed for knee arthroscopy with varying success.[64,65] More impressive results have been obtained for painful procedures, such as anterior cruciate ligament (ACL) reconstruction. Mulroy and coworkers[66] compared femoral PNB to sham block in 55 patients who had already received either epidural or intraarticular analgesia after ACL repair. Overall, the best analgesia was seen in patients with femoral PNB, whereas half of patients in the sham group reported pain VAS ≥5/10. Furthermore, a trend of lower opioid use over 36 h was identified. This was substantiated in a retrospective study by Williams and colleagues,[67] who found that outpatients garnered some benefit from femoral PNB for minor knee surgery but large benefit from more invasive procedures. Not only did femoral PNB provide improved analgesia in these individuals, it also reduced unanticipated hospital admissions. Further analysis found that the addition of sciatic PNB for invasive knee surgery augmented those advantages. Of note, without PNBs, invasive knee surgery held a four to six times greater risk of the patient being admitted to the hospital. In a more recent study,[68] this group estimated the cost savings afforded by PNBs for ACL repairs. Assuming a PACU bypass rate of 82% and an unplanned admission rate of 4%, their institution would save $98,600 after 250 procedures.

When femoral PNB is used for minor knee surgery, such as knee arthroscopy, it has been shown that providing broader coverage of the lumbar plexus is beneficial. Bonicalzi and Gallino[69] increased femoral PNB volume from 10 to 20 mL in an attempt to broaden "3-in-1" coverage, which resulted in better operative conditions and decreased postoperative discomfort. Patel and coworkers[65] divided knee arthroscopy patients into those receiving GA, combined femoral and lateral femoral cutaneous PNB, and femoral PNB with sham lateral femoral cutaneous block. Again, operative conditions were improved, and postoperative complaints of pain decreased (from 27% to 3%) with broader nerve block coverage.

Although PNB of the femoral nerve group remains an effective mode of anesthesia for knee surgeries ranging from knee arthroscopy to ACL reconstruction, arguing its use for less invasive surgeries of the knee on grounds of postoperative analgesia alone is difficult. For more invasive lower extremity surgeries, however, the studies do warrant as broad an application of LA to this nerve group as can be reasonably afforded.

Clinical Pearls

Femoral Nerve Block and Fascia Iliaca Block

- These blocks are easy to perform for anteromedial thigh and medial calf.
- They afford improved postoperative analgesia for invasive knee procedures.
- Variable blockade of lateral femoral cutaneous and obturator nerves limits anesthetic applicability and analgesic efficacy for extensive lower extremity surgery.

Proximal Sciatic Nerve Block

Proximal blockade of the sciatic nerve proves a useful adjunct to PNB of the thigh. Several studies have evaluated the utility of combined PNBs for knee arthroscopy. In one such investigation, Sansone and colleagues[70] utilized combined femoral–sciatic nerve block in 601 patients and were required to provide further intraoperative pain relief only 12% of the time and sedation 20% of the time. Out of this group, only 0.7% required conversion to GA. No neurologic deficits were revealed at 1 month's follow-up.

Other studies have demonstrated effective use of a femoral–sciatic nerve block for knee arthroscopy but failed to show a prolonged analgesic benefit from mepivacaine compared with "fast track" GA[71] and unilateral[72] or bilateral[73] SAB. When compared with propofol–remifentanil GA, the femoral–sciatic nerve block group had less intraoperative bradycardia (0% vs 21%) and hypotension (0% vs 36%) as well as lower postoperative pain VAS scores in PACU (0 vs 7 out of 10). However, 12% of patients receiving femoral–sciatic block complained of mild pain during surgery, one patient required fentanyl and one a GA. Addition of a sciatic nerve block to a femoral or lumbar plexus nerve block likely provides better tourniquet anesthesia than femoral or lumbar plexus nerve block alone. This may be useful for the patient who requests little or no intraoperative sedation.

Similar to the data discussed with femoral nerve blocks, the analgesic benefit from combined femoral–sciatic nerve block is more apparent when more invasive procedures are performed with long-acting LA.[67] Nakamura and colleagues[74] compared recipients of GA ($n = 36$) to patients who underwent femoral–sciatic nerve block ($n = 31$) for ACL reconstruction. The combined PNB allowed 90% of patients to avoid hospitalization postoperatively, and as a result saved $2,907 per patient.

Clinical Pearls

Proximal Sciatic Nerve Block

■ Proximal sciatic nerve block is an anesthetic and analgesic adjunct to lumbar plexus nerve block for complex knee surgery and an adjunct to saphenous nerve block for surgery below the knee.

■ It blocks the posterior cutaneous nerve of the thigh needed for thigh tourniquet.

■ The risk of neuropathic complications is low.

■ It blocks hamstring musculature, augmenting operative extremity weakness.

■ It can inhibit parasympathetic control of bladder emptying.

Distal Sciatic Nerve Block

Both proximal and distal sciatic nerve blocks have broad application for foot and ankle surgery. Utilization of a more distal PNB preserves the function of the hamstring muscle group. A more distal approach, however, typically necessitates the use of either a calf tourniquet or potent sedation in the presence of a thigh tourniquet. With either sciatic nerve block approach, a femoral or saphenous nerve PNB can provide anesthesia to the spared distal extremity territory of the medial calf or ankle.

Posterior[75] or lateral[76,77] popliteal fossa PNB interrupts sciatic conduction prior to the division of the tibial and peroneal branches of the nerve. Since this PNB is relatively safe and easy to perform with a high degree of patient satisfaction,

it proves a model block for ambulatory surgery of the distal lower extremity.[78]

Reliability was demonstrated by Singelyn and co-workers,[79] who investigated the posterior popliteal fossa sciatic nerve block with 1% mepivacaine or 0.5% bupivacaine in 507 patients having 625 blocks. Femoral nerve anesthesia was provided separately when needed. Surgical anesthesia occurred in 92%, supplemental analgesia was necessary in 5%, and GA in only 3% of cases. Discomfort associated with the block procedure was minimal in 89%, moderate in 9%, and severe in 2%. Of the 466 patients who rated their satisfaction with perioperative analgesia, 95% were completely satisfied, 4% expressed moderate reservations, and 1% expressed major reservations.

Although some in busy ambulatory practices find it challenging to achieve adequate popliteal fossa sciatic nerve block in a timely fashion, Fernandez-Guisasola associates[80] have provided promising data comparing two LA solutions for outpatient foot and ankle surgery. They found rapid onset of anesthesia using either 40 mL of 0.5% ropivacaine (6.5 ± 5.1 min) or 1% mepivacaine (6.2 ± 3.7 min). As expected, sensory block following ropivacaine significantly outlasted that from mepivacaine (20.7 ± 6.2 h vs 6.5 ± 1.7 h).

The analgesic duration of a popliteal fossa sciatic nerve block can exceed that for an ankle block or wound infiltration, two alternative anesthetics for foot surgery. McLeod and colleagues[81] compared popliteal fossa PNB with ankle block in 40 patients undergoing GA for foot surgery. Bupivacaine (20 mL of 0.5%) was utilized to provide postoperative analgesia. Both techniques proved to be efficacious, though popliteal fossa PNB yielded 1080 min of analgesia versus 690 min with ankle block. The same group[77] further studied lateral popliteal fossa PNB versus subcutaneous infiltration of the wound with similar results lateral popliteal fossa provided 1082 min of analgesia versus 373 min with wound infiltration.

A novel use of popliteal fossa sciatic nerve block was described by Vloka and associates[82] when they combined this block with a posterior cutaneous nerve block of the thigh for short saphenous vein stripping. This technique provided an acceptable alternative to SAB and was associated with fewer requests for analgesia in PACU (21% vs 64%), faster recovery (67 ± 10 min vs 122 ± 50 min in PACU), and earlier discharge (total time in hospital 222 ± 53 min vs 294 ± 68 min). Thus it appears, in principle as well as in practice, that preserved hamstring muscle function combined with dense postoperative analgesia allow for early mobilization of ambulatory patients and support the use of distal sciatic PNB in this setting.

Clinical Pearls

Distal Sciatic Nerve Block

■ This block is easy to perform for foot or ankle surgery.

■ It provides longer lasting analgesia than an ankle block.

■ It preserves hamstring function.

Paravertebral Block

Dermatomal anesthesia of the thoracolumbar trunk can be achieved by injecting LA into the paravertebral space deep to the transverse processes to bathe the nerve roots after their exit from the intervertebral foramina. Performance of PVBs has provided anesthesia as well as postoperative analgesia for outpatient breast,[41,83–87] inguinal hernia,[88–91] and ileostomy revision surgery.[92]

Decreased opioid requirements and subsequent PONV are important benefits of PVBs when used for potentially emetogenic surgery. Klein and coworkers utilized PVB with 0.5% bupivacaine for hernia[89] surgery and for mastectomy.[41] After mastectomy, the PVBs served to reduce the number of patients requiring postoperative analgesia from 97.8% to 25% compared with those who received GA.[87] Because the technique is typically performed as a "blind" technique, without the use of nerve stimulation, a clear endpoint is not always achieved prior to injection of LA. This may be the source of the published variability in rates of successful blocks.[41,85,87] This variability, combined with the proximity of the needle tip to the lung, with consequent risk of pneumothorax (0–6.7%),[41,83–87] warrants at a minimum operator experience with PVBs prior to routine use of this block in the ambulatory setting.

Clinical Pearls

Paravertebral Block

- Paravertebral block is useful for anesthesia of the thoracolumbar dermatomes.
- It provides the longest lasting analgesia after breast or hernia surgery.
- Variable success rates have been reported.
- Some risk of pneumothorax exists.

AMBULATORY CONTINUOUS PERIPHERAL NERVE BLOCKS

Although single-injection PNBs have numerous advantages, one limitation is the rapid resolution of the nerve block after an invasive surgery in a patient who may not have sufficient blood levels of opioids present for adequate ongoing analgesia. Wilson and coworkers[23] followed patient's home course after interscalene block for shoulder surgery and found that one third experienced extreme VAS pain scores of 4 or 5 out of 5 and that 5.3% of patients contacted their surgical team because of unbearable pain.

In response to these concerns, there have been several case reports and a limited number of trials that reported using CPNB with outpatients. Rawal and associates[93] first described an elastomeric balloon pump that allowed self-administration of LA at home. Subsequently, patients having upper[94–100] and lower extremity[101–103] surgery of varying

invasiveness have been discharged home with CPNB. There has been an overall low incidence of reported neurologic side effects with this therapy in the inpatient setting,[25] offering limited support to the progressive use of CPNB in the home environment. Despite the lack of extensive patient safety data, initial reports demonstrate that patients are indeed comfortable with home CPNB infusions.[97]

Rotator cuff repair is a common outpatient procedure often felt to justify placement of an interscalene brachial plexus catheter. Compared with interscalene brachial plexus infusion of saline, opioid requirements have been diminished by 50%[97] and analgesia sustained for as long as 4 days.[104] Concurrently, other measures of comfort (pain scores, satisfaction, and fragmented sleep) have been consistently favorable.[95–97]

Similar success has also been reported with axillary[100] and infraclavicular[99] CPNB after hand surgery. Rawal and coworkers[100] noted few technical problems and high outpatient satisfaction with the use of continuous axillary PNB after hand surgery. Similar analgesic success and limited motor block followed resolution of initial surgical anesthesia when both dilute bupivacaine (0.125%) and ropivacaine (0.125–0.2%) were infused through axillary and infraclavicular CPNB catheters.[99,100]

Perhaps the greatest effect of home CPNB has been for major lower extremity surgery such as ankle fusions, multiligament knee reconstructions, and forefoot procedures that historically have required a hospital stay for IV analgesia. A continuous popliteal fossa PNB has been shown to decrease the rate of hospital admission after foot and ankle surgery and to hasten discharge time while reducing pain and opioid consumption by up to 70%.[102,103] Lumbar plexus and sciatic CPNB have also been utilized to enable multiligament knee reconstructions[104] as well as to provide analgesia to reduce the length of stay for total knee arthroplasty (at our institution).

Establishment of an efficacious CPNB infusion necessitates an individualized regimen based on patient physiology and surgical procedure. Competing interests that affect this decision include the desire to provide quality analgesia, to avoid undesired motor blockade, to avoid LA toxicity, and to maximize the pump's LA reservoir to prolong the infusion duration. Differing strategies have involved intermittent boluses without basal infusion,[93] basal infusion only,[94,95,97] or basal infusion with intermittent patient-controlled bolus.[96,99] While citing the need for ongoing research, a review by Ilfeld and Enneking[105] concluded that a basal infusion (5–10 mL/h) decreased breakthrough pain and increased satisfaction, whereas a patient-controlled bolus (2–5 mL/20–60 min) allowed for a lower infusion rate and longer infusion time of the LA pump.

An area that requires further investigation is the proper treatment of the patient after discharge. Strategies to avoid patient injury, LA toxicity, and insertion site infection are essential. Several studies have advocated.

1. Careful catheter testing for intravascular placement prior to discharge

2. Patient and caretaker education (focusing on safety, pump function and complications)
3. Written instructions on extremity care and warning signs and symptoms of LA toxicity as well as appropriate analgesic expectations
4. Health care provider contact information to answer questions or problems
5. Daily health care provider contact by telephone to monitor side effects, determine efficacy, and follow the integrity of the insertion site, and
6. An individualized decision regarding at-home or in-hospital catheter removal.

Rigorous patient selection, education, and close follow-up have led to few adverse events with CPNB. A recent report from the US Food and Drug Administration,[106] however, has drawn attention to problems with continuous wound infusions using disposable pumps in the home. They reported details on 40 adverse event reports, in which 15 patients developed surgical wound infections and 17 patients exhibited tissue necrosis, an extremely rare surgical complication. Although parallels from wound catheters cannot be extrapolated to CPNB, vigilance in this area seems warranted.

A variety of home infusion pumps are available that have improved accuracy, infusion pressure, and bolus capabilities, as well as larger reservoir volumes than previous models. Ilfeld and Enneking[105] highlighted the major differences between commercially available models, including greatest infusion accuracy (electronic), patient bolus capability (some elastomeric and electronic), ease of depressing patient bolus button (electronic), programmability (electronic), disposability (elastomeric and some electronic), and price (variable). Audible alarms (electronic—previously noted to be detrimental due to a high false-alarm rate—may, with redesigned electronic pumps prove advantageous since elastomeric pumps cannot indicate an inability to deliver a set infusion rate.

Clinical Pearls

Continuous Nerve Blocks
- Continuous nerve blocks are useful for managing pain, especially after open-joint repair or replacement.
- A basal infusion plus bolus regimen is most beneficial.
- Multiple delivery systems are available to tailor care.
- Careful patient selection, education and daily follow-up are required.

PREMEDICATION & SEDATION

Sedation is an intrinsic part of RA that helps ensure its success and popularity with patients. Patients often approach the operative theater with significant anxiety, which can influence their choice of anesthetic technique. Gajraj and colleagues[107]

found that fear of the needle (28%) and fear seeing or hearing operative events (10%) were cited by obstetric patients refusing RA. De Andres and associates[108] also found anxiety in the awake patient significant in both the patient's preoperative attitude toward RA and as a predictor of use of regional anesthesia in the future. Fanelli and coworkers[109] similarly found that a quarter of patients undergoing PNB would refuse PNB in the future due to discomfort during the procedure. Clearly, reassurance about the use of sedation and appropriate premedication is necessary to minimize pain and ensure patients' acceptance of PVBs.

A variety of pharmacologic agents can be used for sedation during block placement. Although any combination of agents can be employed successfully, it is important that the medications and their side effects are concordant with the following goals:

1. Patients should be competent to sign missing consent forms and participate in the marking of their operative extremity prior to block placement and surgery.
2. Pharmaceuticals should provide rapid onset of sedation and analgesia, the persistence of which should not preclude patient discharge.
3. Pharmaceuticals should be appropriately titratable such that the apneic threshold is not too easily breached.
4. They should minimize the risk of PONV.
5. They should be appropriately amnestic to satisfy patient desires.
6. They should not be too costly in comparison with their alternatives.

Pharmacokinetics and cost issues offer some bias for selecting midazolam, fentanyl, or alfentanyl as agents for block placement, although fentanyl is certainly emetogenic, particularly if repeated doses are given throughout the surgery. Keeping the fentanyl dose to a minimum (no more than 100 mcg) or substituting low-dose propofol is a viable strategy that can meet all of the previously mentioned goals. For intraoperative sedation, the ability to titrate, the antiemetic effect, and amnesia (with loss of consciousness) of propofol argue for its use.

Clinical Pearls

- Appropriate sedation titrated to patients wishes increases the patient's acceptance of PNB since most patients approach the topic with significant anxiety. Adequate premedication, including sedatives and analgesics, should be a part of every successful modern PVB anesthetic plan.
- Midazolam, fentanyl, alfentanyl, and propofol are most suitable for a satisfactory regional anesthesia experience.

Local Anesthetic Drugs

Choice of which of the commonly employed LA drugs to utilize is determined by safety profile, duration of action,

Table 62–1.

Local Anesthetic Characteristics

Local Anesthetic (with Epinephrine 1:400,000)	Duration of PNB Anesthesia (h)	Duration of PNB Analgesia (h)	Speed of Onset for PNB (minutes)
Lidocaine 2%	1.5–2	2–5	5–15[a]
Mepivacaine 1%	2–3	4–6	12–20[a]
Mepivacaine 1.5%	2–3	4–6	8–15[a]
Ropivacaine 0.5%	6–8	11–13	15–40

[a] *Hastened by addition of bicarbonate (1:10 v/v).*
Reprinted, with permission, from Brown DL: Atlas of Regional Anesthesia. W. B. Saunders, 1992.

and speed of onset. Since PNB for outpatients often occurs outside the auspices of a hospital setting, safety (avoiding toxicity, resuscitability after toxicity) is a primary concern. Choosing commercially available anesthetics based on safety profile provides a rank order of: lidocaine > mepivacaine > ropivacaine > bupivacaine. Because of the decreased margin of cardiac safety and increased difficulty of successful resuscitation, bupivacaine is no longer recommended as the first agent for ambulatory care.[110,111]

Of the remaining drugs, anticipated duration of action for anesthesia and analgesia when injected around a nerve or plexus and speed of onset is shown in Table 62–1.

The motor-sparing analgesia of ropivacaine makes it an ideal candidate for long-lasting ambulatory PNB as well as for home perineural infusions.

Clinical Pearls

- Based on safety profile, the best substitute for bupivacaine is l-bupivacaine or ropivacaine for ambulatory PNB.
- The choice of LA is then based on desired duration of action.

Postoperative Recovery

Depending on the depth and duration of intraoperative sedation, PACU bypass may or may not be feasible for patients who received PNB. Several scoring systems have been proposed to judge a patient's bypass eligibility. Of the reported systems, the White–Song criteria was not designed to accommodate PNB and allows bypass for transient vomiting or retching or IV control of moderate to severe pain if other scores are perfect.[112] Accepting a modified Aldrete score of 9[32] (patients with PNB cannot move a blocked extremity) or a Mayo Modified Discharge Scoring System score of 8 or higher[58] can successfully allow for PACU bypass, although neither of these

systems address patient pain scores or PONV. Williams[113] offers an alternative, similar to the modified Aldrete score, which demands at the outset no need for IV intervention (for pain, nausea, vomiting, pruritus, shivering, or hypotension/orthostasis) and no pain greater than 3 on a 10-point scale.

Clinical Pearl

- Patients not needing IV intervention and scoring high on PACU discharge scoring systems are ideal candidates for PACU bypass.

Multimodal Pain Management

The more methodologies employed to treat postoperative pain, the higher the chances of success and the lower the chances of significant side effects. The concept behind this approach to postoperative analgesia is known as multimodal pain management. With long-acting LA from PNB or CPNB as a basis for analgesia, acetaminophen and nonsteroidal antiinflammatory drugs (NSAIDs) can prove useful and inexpensive adjuncts. Even if surgical concerns about bone healing predominate,[114,115] there is no evidence that a single dose of a potent NSAID alters bone healing outcomes. Although a minimal opioid dose may be needed for postoperative pain management after surgeries ranging from cyst removals to mastectomies performed under PNB, they are typically required for more invasive procedures. Avoiding formulations containing acetaminophen will avoid the ceiling restrictions it otherwise places on home opioid use and can maximize the benefits of a simple every 6-h dosing of acetaminophen and ibuprofen. Other strategies such as limb elevation and cryotherapy should be employed routinely. Deep-tissue electrical stimulation via electrodes placed under the dressings by the surgeons have also shown recent promise, though these devices should not be utilized until after PNB resolution.[116] Written discharge instructions should be given to the patient, highlighting all of these points.

Clinical Pearl

- Multimodal analgesia should involve the use of LA, NSAIDs, acetaminophen, and opioids, as well as cryotherapy when possible.

Discharge Criteria and Patient Instructions

Determining home readiness after ambulatory PNB involves meeting some extra criteria in addition to the standard checklist required of day surgery patients (normal vital signs, absence of moderate to severe pain, PONV, or bleeding). This is especially the case when the patient is to go home with a long-acting PNB. It remains controversial to shift responsibility for care of the insensate extremity to patients in their home environment. Extremity numbness theoretically increases the risk of injury from either a fall at home or from direct injury to the limb lacking protective reflexes. To date, large prospective studies of this issue have been few in number. Davis and colleagues[42] succeeded in discharging 526 patients after axillary PNB with no subsequent injury. Our group[117] prospectively followed 2382 ambulatory patients who had received ropivacaine PNB to either an upper or lower extremity. One patient in this group did fall while exiting his car, but he did not sustain an injury. Seven patients from this group (0.29%) developed a new paresthesia in the operative limb that could have been anesthesia-related. These studies suggest that proper education of patients prior to discharge with an insensate extremity can help avoid most if not all problems.

It is postulated that the reason for such a safe track record relates to careful screening by anesthesiologists and explicit instructions reinforced by PACU staff. Patients must be educated not to use their insensate extremity, to pad and protect it, to visually inspect it, and to avoid direct skin contact with heat or ice. Patients with a lower extremity PNB must be instructed not to weight bear on an insensate limb, must demonstrate proficiency with the use of crutches or a walker, and must be able to iterate a plan for dealing with obstacles such as stairs. Those who are discharged home with a CPNB pump must live within a certain distance of the medical center (ie, ~2 h), must have a caregiver present with them for the entire duration of LA infusion, and must be available for daily postoperative follow-up while the catheter is in use. They must be instructed to call immediately if the catheter site displays signs of infection, if the extremity exhibits signs and symptoms of compartment syndrome, or if the patient demonstrates any signs or symptoms of LA toxicity. Patients and their caregivers must be taught about catheter hygiene and care and catheter removal and be given detailed instructions about pump use, including how to stop the infusion.

Clinical Pearls

- Discharging patients with long-acting PNB has a short but positive track record.
- Patients and their caregivers must be educated to safely care for a numb extremity.
- Home care instructions for CPNB must be extensive.

SUMMARY

The rapid expansion of surgical case variety and complexity has resulted in the inability of GA to provide quality care for all ambulatory patients. This has been evidenced by frequent readmissions for pain and PONV. In contrast, the successes of ambulatory PNBs referenced in this chapter support their emerging role. For upper extremity procedures, the use of PNB has demonstrated improved analgesia, faster patient discharge readiness, and decreased opioid-related side effects compared with that for GA. For surgery involving lower extremity procedures of greater complexity the benefits of dense analgesia from PNB become more apparent. The use of lower extremity PNB appears to be critical to same-day discharge and lower rates of readmission in patients undergoing more invasive same-day surgery on the lower extremity.

The use of multimodal analgesia with long-acting LA provides extended analgesic benefit. The addition of CPNB can significantly expand this benefit at home. However, the slow onset time associated with long-acting LA and the time needed to place continuous catheters can adversely affect ambulatory efficiency. Although effective strategies do exist to diminish this impact, timely administration of RA may still be challenging and represent an impediment to use in some institutions. Developing additional solutions to this obstacle will be important in broadening the use of PNB in the ambulatory population. Another potential impediment results from patient anxiety and apprehension regarding RA. Reassurance about the use of sedation for PNB placement and intraoperative course should alleviate this problem.

Selection of appropriate patients for PNBs and CPNBs and detailed discharge instructions are important for continuing the track record of safety with these techniques. Ongoing positive patient experiences with RA will beget future successes. Whether ambulatory anesthesiologists will be prepared for this success remains to be determined. Improvements in residency training and intensive workshops for current practitioners will likely be necessary to keep up with future demand for outpatient PNBs.

References

1. Hammons T, Piland NF, Small SD, et al: Ambulatory patient safety. What we know and need to know. J Ambul Care Manage 2003;Jan-Mar 26(1):63–82.
2. Hospital Cost Trends. BCBShealthissues.com; June 19, 2003.
3. Fink BR: Leaves and needles: The introduction of surgical local anesthesia. Anesthesiology 1985;63(1):77–83.
4. Winnie AP, Ramamurthy S, Durrani Z, et al: Interscalene cervical plexus block: A single-injection technic. Anesth Analg 1975;54(3):370–375.
5. Apfelbaum JL, Chen C, Mehta SS, et al: Postoperative pain experience: Results from a national survey suggest postoperative pain continues to be undermanaged. Anesth Analg 2003;97(2):534–540.
6. Greengrass RA. Regional anesthesia for ambulatory surgery. Anesthesiol Clin North Am 2000;18(2):341–353, vii.
7. Dexter F, Macario A: What is the relative frequency of uncommon ambulatory surgery procedures performed in the United States with an anesthesia provider? Anesth Analg 2000;90(6):1343–1347.
8. Hadzic A, Vloka JD, Kuroda MM, et al: The practice of peripheral nerve blocks in the United States: A national survey. Reg Anesth Pain Med 1998;23(3):241–246.
9. Klein SM, Pietrobon R, Nielsen KC, et al: Peripheral nerve blockade with long-acting local anesthetics: A survey of the Society for Ambulatory Anesthesia. Anesth Analg 2002;94(1):71–76.
10. Smith MP, Sprung J, Zura A, et al: A survey of exposure to regional anesthesia techniques in American anesthesia residency training programs. Reg Anesth Pain Med 1999;24(1):11–16.
11. Kopacz DJ, Neal JM: Regional anesthesia and pain medicine: Residency training–the year 2000. Reg Anesth Pain Med 2002;27(1):9–14.

12. Martin G, Lineberger CK, MacLeod DB, et al: A new teaching model for resident training in regional anesthesia. Anesth Analg 2002;95(5):1423–1427.

13. Horlocker TT, Bajwa ZH, Ashraf Z, et al: Risk assessment of hemorrhagic complications associated with nonsteroidal antiinflammatory medications in ambulatory pain clinic patients undergoing epidural steroid injection. Anesth Analg 2002;95(6):1691–1697.

14. Reuben SS, Rosenthal EA, Steinberg RB, et al: Surgery on the affected upper extremity of patients with a history of complex regional pain syndrome: The use of intravenous regional anesthesia with clonidine. J Clin Anesth 2004;16(7):517–522.

15. Reuben SS: Preventing the development of complex regional pain syndrome after surgery. Anesthesiology 2004;101(5):1215–1224.

16. Tetzlaff JE, Yoon HJ, Brems J: Interscalene brachial plexus block for shoulder surgery. Reg Anesth 1994;19(5):339–343.

17. Hadzic A, Karaca PE, Hobeika P et al: Peripheral nerve blocks result in superior recovery profile compared with general anesthesia in outpatient knee arthroscopy. Anesth Analg 2005;100:976–81.

18. Brown AR, Weiss R, Greenberg C, et al: Interscalene block for shoulder arthroscopy: Comparison with general anesthesia. Arthroscopy 1993;9(3):295–300.

19. D'Alessio JG, Rosenblum M, Shea KP, et al: A retrospective comparison of interscalene block and general anesthesia for ambulatory surgery shoulder arthroscopy. Reg Anesth 1995;20(1):62–68.

20. Al-Kaisy A, McGuire G, Chan VW, et al: Analgesic effect of interscalene block using low-dose bupivacaine for outpatient arthroscopic shoulder surgery. Reg Anesth Pain Med 1998;23(5):469–473.

21. Laurila PA, Lopponen A, Kanga-Saarela T, et al: Interscalene brachial plexus block is superior to subacromial bursa block after arthroscopic shoulder surgery. Acta Anaesthesiol Scand 2002;46(8):1031–1036.

22. Singelyn FJ, Lhotel L, Fabre B: Pain relief after arthroscopic shoulder surgery: A comparison of intraarticular analgesia, suprascapular nerve block, and interscalene brachial plexus block. Anesth Analg 2004;99(2):589–592.

23. Wilson AT, Nicholson E, Burton L, et al: Analgesia for day-case shoulder surgery. Br J Anaesth 2004;92(3):414–415.

24. Krone SC, Chan VW, Regan J, et al: Analgesic effects of low-dose ropivacaine for interscalene brachial plexus block for outpatient shoulder surgery—A dose-finding study. Reg Anesth Pain Med 2001;26(5):439–443.

25. Borgeat A, Ekatodramis G, Kalberer F, et al: Acute and nonacute complications associated with interscalene block and shoulder surgery: A prospective study. Anesthesiology 2001;95(4):875–880.

26. Bedder MD, Kozody R, Craig DB: Comparison of bupivacaine and alkalinized bupivacaine in brachial plexus anesthesia. Anesth Analg 1988;67(1):48–52.

27. Lanz E, Theiss D, Jankovic D: The extent of blockade following various techniques of brachial plexus block. Anesth Analg 1983;62(1):55–58.

28. Franco CD, Vieira ZE. 1,001 subclavian perivascular brachial plexus blocks: Success with a nerve stimulator. Reg Anesth Pain Med 2000;25(1):41–46.

29. Borgeat A, Ekatodramis G, Dumont C: An evaluation of the infraclavicular block via a modified approach of the Raj technique. Anesth Analg 2001;93(2):436–441.

30. Jandard C, Gentili ME, Girard F, et al: Infraclavicular block with lateral approach and nerve stimulation: Extent of anesthesia and adverse effects. Reg Anesth Pain Med 2002;27(1):37–42.

31. Kilka HG, Geiger P, Mehrkens HH: Infraclavicular vertical brachial plexus blockade. A new method for anesthesia of the upper extremity. An anatomical and clinical study. Anaesthesist 1995;44(5):339–344.

32. Hadzic A, Arliss J, Kerimoglu B, et al: A comparison of infraclavicular nerve block versus general anesthesia for hand and wrist day-case surgeries. Anesthesiology 2004;101(1):127–132.

33. Desroches J: The infraclavicular brachial plexus block by the coracoid approach is clinically effective: An observational study of 150 patients. Can J Anaesth 2003;50(3):253–257.

34. Koscielniak-Nielsen ZJ, Rotboll Nielsen P, Risby Mortensen C: A comparison of coracoid and axillary approaches to the brachial plexus. Acta Anaesthesiol Scand 2000;44(3):274–279.

35. Partridge BL, Katz J, Benirschke K: Functional anatomy of the brachial plexus sheath: Implications for anesthesia. Anesthesiology 1987;66(6):743–747.

36. Thompson GE, Rorie DK: Functional anatomy of the brachial plexus sheaths. Anesthesiology 1983;59(2):117–122.

37. Gaertner E, Kern O, Mahoudeau G, Freys G, et al: Block of the brachial plexus branches by the humeral route. A prospective study in 503 ambulatory patients. Proposal of a nerve-blocking sequence. Acta Anaesthesiol Scand 1999;43(6):609–613.

38. Bouaziz H, Narchi P, Mercier FJ, et al: The use of a selective axillary nerve block for outpatient hand surgery. Anesth Analg 1998;86(4):746–748.

39. Koscielniak-Nielsen ZJ, Rotboll-Nielsen P, Rassmussen H: Patients' experiences with multiple stimulation axillary block for fast-track ambulatory hand surgery. Acta Anaesthesiol Scand 2002;46(7):789–793.

40. Armstrong KP, Cherry RA: Brachial plexus anesthesia compared to general anesthesia when a block room is available. Can J Anaesth 2004;51(1):41–44.

41. Greengrass R, O'Brien F, Lyerly K, et al: Paravertebral block for breast cancer surgery. Can J Anaesth 1996;43(8):858–861.

42. Davis WJ, Lennon RL, Wedel DJ: Brachial plexus anesthesia for outpatient surgical procedures on an upper extremity. Mayo Clin Proc 1991;66(5):470–473.

43. Cooper K, Kelley H, Carrithers J: Perceptions of side effects following axillary block used for outpatient surgery. Reg Anesth 1995;20(3):212–216.

44. Chan VW, Peng PW, Kaszas Z, et al: A comparative study of general anesthesia, intravenous regional anesthesia, and axillary block for outpatient hand surgery: Clinical outcome and cost analysis. Anesth Analg 2001;93(5):1181–1184.

45. Yazigi A, Jabbour K, Jebara SM, et al: Bilateral ilioinguinal nerve block for ambulatory varicocele surgery. Ann Fr Anesth Reanim 2002;21(9):710–712.

46. Toivonen J, Permi J, Rosenberg PH: Effect of preincisional ilioinguinal and iliohypogastric nerve block on postoperative analgesic requirement in day-surgery patients undergoing herniorrhaphy under spinal anaesthesia. Acta Anaesthesiol Scand 2001;45(5):603–607.

47. Ding Y, White PF: Post-herniorrhaphy pain in outpatients after preincision ilioinguinal-hypogastric nerve block during monitored anaesthesia care. Can J Anaesth 1995;42(1):12–15.

48. Song D, Greilich NB, White PF, et al: Recovery profiles and costs of anesthesia for outpatient unilateral inguinal herniorrhaphy. Anesth Analg 2000;91(4):876–881.

49. Ghani KR, McMillan R, Paterson-Brown S: Transient femoral nerve palsy following ilio-inguinal nerve blockade for day case inguinal hernia repair. J R Coll Surg Edinb 2002;47(4):626–629.

50. Rosario DJ, Jacob S, Luntley J, et al: Mechanism of femoral nerve palsy complicating percutaneous ilioinguinal field block. Br J Anaesth 1997;78(3):314–316.

51. Parkinson SK, Mueller JB, Little WL, et al: Extent of blockade with various approaches to the lumbar plexus. Anesth Analg 1989;68(3):243–248.

52. Stevens RD, Van Gessel E, Flory N, et al: Lumbar plexus block reduces pain and blood loss associated with total hip arthroplasty. Anesthesiology 2000;93(1):115–121.

53. Luber MJ, Greengrass R, Vail TP: Patient satisfaction and effectiveness of lumbar plexus and sciatic nerve block for total knee arthroplasty. J Arthroplasty 2001;16(1):17–21.

54. Horlocker TT, Hebl JR, Kinney MA, et al: Opioid-free analgesia following total knee arthroplasty—A multimodal approach

using continuous lumbar plexus (psoas compartment) block, acetaminophen, and ketorolac. Reg Anesth Pain Med 2002;27(1):105–108.

55. Greengrass RA, Klein SM, D'Ercole FJ, et al: Lumbar plexus and sciatic nerve block for knee arthroplasty: Comparison of ropivacaine and bupivacaine. Can J Anaesth 1998;45(11):1094–1096.

56. Farny J, Girard M, Drolet P: Posterior approach to the lumbar plexus combined with a sciatic nerve block using lidocaine. Can J Anaesth 1994;41(6):486–491.

57. De Biasi P, Lupescu R, Burgun G, et al: Continuous lumbar plexus block: Use of radiography to determine catheter tip location. Reg Anesth Pain Med 2003;28(2):135–139.

58. Jankowski CJ, Hebl JR, Stuart MJ, et al: A comparison of psoas compartment block and spinal and general anesthesia for outpatient knee arthroscopy. Anesth Analg 2003;97(4):1003–1009, table of contents.

59. Hadzic A, Karaca PE, Hobeika P, et al: Peripheral nerve blocks result in superior recovery profile compared with general anesthesia in outpatient knee arthroscopy. Anesth Analg 2005;100(4):976–981.

60. Winnie AP, Ramamurthy S, Durrani Z: The inguinal paravascular technic of lumbar plexus anesthesia: The "3-in-1 block". Anesth Analg 1973;52(6):989–996.

61. Lang SA, Yip RW, Chang PC, et al: The femoral 3-in-1 block revisited. J Clin Anesth 1993;5(4):292–296.

62. Seeberger MD, Urwyler A: Paravascular lumbar plexus block: Block extension after femoral nerve stimulation and injection of 20 vs. 40 ml mepivacaine 10 mg/ml. Acta Anaesthesiol Scand 1995;39(6):769–773.

63. Marhofer P, Nasel C, Sitzwohl C, et al: Magnetic resonance imaging of the distribution of local anesthetic during the three-in-one block. Anesth Analg 2000;90(1):119–124.

64. Goranson BD, Lang S, Cassidy JD, et al: A comparison of three regional anaesthesia techniques for outpatient knee arthroscopy. Can J Anaesth 1997;44(4):371–376.

65. Patel NJ, Flashburg MH, Paskin S, et al: A regional anesthetic technique compared to general anesthesia for outpatient knee arthroscopy. Anesth Analg 1986;65(2):185–187.

66. Mulroy MF, Larkin KL, Batra MS, et al: Femoral nerve block with 0.25% or 0.5% bupivacaine improves postoperative analgesia following outpatient arthroscopic anterior cruciate ligament repair. Reg Anesth Pain Med 2001;26(1):24–29.

67. Williams BA, Kentor ML, Vogt MT, et al: Femoral–sciatic nerve blocks for complex outpatient knee surgery are associated with less postoperative pain before same-day discharge: A review of 1,200 consecutive cases from the period 1996–1999. Anesthesiology 2003;98(5):1206–1213.

68. Williams BA, Kentor ML, Vogt MT, et al: Economics of nerve block pain management after anterior cruciate ligament reconstruction: Potential hospital cost savings via associated postanesthesia care unit bypass and same-day discharge. Anesthesiology 2004;100(3):697–706.

69. Bonicalzi V, Gallino M: Comparison of two regional anesthetic techniques for knee arthroscopy. Arthroscopy 1995;11(2):207–212.

70. Sansone V, De Ponti A, Fanelli G, et al: Combined sciatic and femoral nerve block for knee arthroscopy: 4 years' experience. Arch Orthop Trauma Surg 1999;119(3-4):163–167.

71. Casati A, Cappelleri G, Berti M, et al: Randomized comparison of remifentanil–propofol with a sciatic–femoral nerve block for out-patient knee arthroscopy. Eur J Anaesthesiol 2002;19(2):109–114.

72. Cappelleri G, Casati A, Fanelli G, et al: Unilateral spinal anesthesia or combined sciatic–femoral nerve block for day-case knee arthroscopy. A prospective, randomized comparison. Minerva Anestesiol 2000;66(3):131–136; discussion 137.

73. Casati A, Cappelleri G, Fanelli G, et al: Regional anaesthesia for outpatient knee arthroscopy: A randomized clinical comparison of two different anaesthetic techniques. Acta Anaesthesiol Scand 2000;44(5):543–547.

74. Nakamura SJ, Conte-Hernandez A, Galloway MT: The efficacy of regional anesthesia for outpatient anterior cruciate ligament reconstruction. Arthroscopy 1997;13(6):699–703.

75. Rorie DK, Byer DE, Nelson DO, et al: Assessment of block of the sciatic nerve in the popliteal fossa. Anesth Analg 1980;59(5):371–376.

76. Vloka JD, Hadzic A, Kitain E, et al: Anatomic considerations for sciatic nerve block in the popliteal fossa through the lateral approach. Reg Anesth 1996;21(5):414–418.

77. McLeod DH, Wong DH, Claridge RJ, et al: Lateral popliteal sciatic nerve block compared with subcutaneous infiltration for analgesia following foot surgery. Can J Anaesth 1994;41(8):673–676.

78. Hansen E, Eshelman MR, Cracchiolo A 3rd: Popliteal fossa neural blockade as the sole anesthetic technique for outpatient foot and ankle surgery. Foot Ankle Int 2000;21(1):38–44.

79. Singelyn FJ, Gouverneur JM, Gribomont BF: Popliteal sciatic nerve block aided by a nerve stimulator: A reliable technique for foot and ankle surgery. Reg Anesth 1991;16(5):278–281.

80. Fernandez-Guisasola J, Andueza A, Burgos E, et al: A comparison of 0.5% ropivacaine and 1% mepivacaine for sciatic nerve block in the popliteal fossa. Acta Anaesthesiol Scand 2001;45(8):967–970.

81. McLeod DH, Wong DH, Vaghadia H, et al: Lateral popliteal sciatic nerve block compared with ankle block for analgesia following foot surgery. Can J Anaesth 1995;42(9):765–769.

82. Vloka JD, Hadzic A, Mulcare R, et al: Combined popliteal and posterior cutaneous nerve of the thigh blocks for short saphenous vein stripping in outpatients: an alternative to spinal anesthesia. J Clin Anesth 1997;9(8):618–622.

83. Weltz CR, Greengrass RA, Lyerly HK: Ambulatory surgical management of breast carcinoma using paravertebral block. Ann Surg 1995;222(1):19–26.

84. Terheggen MA, Wille F, Borel Rinkes IH, et al: Paravertebral blockade for minor breast surgery. Anesth Analg 2002;94(2):355–359, table of contents.

85. Klein SM, Bergh A, Steele SM, et al: Thoracic paravertebral block for breast surgery. Anesth Analg 2000;90(6):1402–1405.

86. Pusch F, Freitag H, Weinstabl C, et al: Single-injection paravertebral block compared to general anaesthesia in breast surgery. Acta Anaesthesiol Scand 1999;43(7):770–774.

87. Coveney E, Weltz CR, Greengrass R, et al: Use of paravertebral block anesthesia in the surgical management of breast cancer: Experience in 156 cases. Ann Surg 1998;227(4):496–501.

88. Weltz CR, Klein SM, Arbo JE, et al: Paravertebral block anesthesia for inguinal hernia repair. World J Surg 2003;27(4):425–429.

89. Klein SM, Greengrass RA, Weltz C, et al: Paravertebral somatic nerve block for outpatient inguinal herniorrhaphy: An expanded case report of 22 patients. Reg Anesth Pain Med 1998;23(3):306–310.

90. Klein SM, Pietrobon R, Nielsen KC, et al: Paravertebral somatic nerve block compared with peripheral nerve blocks for outpatient inguinal herniorrhaphy. Reg Anesth Pain Med 2002;27(5):476–480.

91. Wassef MR, Randazzo T, Ward W: The paravertebral nerve root block for inguinal herniorrhaphy—A comparison with the field block approach. Reg Anesth Pain Med 1998;23(5):451–456.

92. Kalady MF, Fields RC, Klein S, et al: Loop ileostomy closure at an ambulatory surgery facility: A safe and cost-effective alternative to routine hospitalization. Dis Colon Rectum 2003;46(4):486–490.

93. Rawal N, Axelsson K, Hylander J, et al: Postoperative patient-controlled local anesthetic administration at home. Anesth Analg 1998;86(1):86–89.

94. Klein SM, Steele SM, Nielsen KC, et al: The difficulties of ambulatory interscalene and intra-articular infusions for rotator cuff surgery: A preliminary report. Can J Anaesth 2003;50(3):265–269.

95. Nielsen KC, Greengrass RA, Pietrobon R, et al: Continuous interscalene brachial plexus blockade provides good analgesia at home after major shoulder surgery-report of four cases. Can J Anaesth 2003;50(1):57–61.

96. Ilfeld BM, Morey TE, Wright TW, et al: Continuous interscalene brachial plexus block for postoperative pain control at home: A randomized, double-blinded, placebo-controlled study. Anesth Analg 2003;96(4):1089–1095.

97. Klein SM, Grant SA, Greengrass RA, et al: Interscalene brachial plexus block with a continuous catheter insertion system and a disposable infusion pump. Anesth Analg 2000;91(6):1473–1478.

98. Corda DM, Enneking FK: A unique approach to postoperative analgesia for ambulatory surgery. J Clin Anesth 2000;12(8):595–599.

99. Ilfeld BM, Morey TE, Enneking FK: Continuous infraclavicular brachial plexus block for postoperative pain control at home: A randomized, double-blinded, placebo-controlled study. Anesthesiology 2002;96(6):1297–1304.

100. Rawal N, Allvin R, Axelsson K, et al: Patient-controlled regional analgesia (PCRA) at home: Controlled comparison between bupivacaine and ropivacaine brachial plexus analgesia. Anesthesiology 2002;96(6):1290–1296.

101. Klein SM, Greengrass RA, Grant SA, et al: Ambulatory surgery for multi-ligament knee reconstruction with continuous dual catheter peripheral nerve blockade. Can J Anaesth 2001;48(4):375–378.

102. White PF, Issioui T, Skrivanek GD, et al: The use of a continuous popliteal sciatic nerve block after surgery involving the foot and ankle: Does it improve the quality of recovery? Anesth Analg 2003;97(5):1303–1309.

103. Ilfeld BM, Morey TE, Wang RD, et al: Continuous popliteal sciatic nerve block for postoperative pain control at home: A randomized, double-blinded, placebo-controlled study. Anesthesiology 2002;97(4):959–965.

104. Ilfeld BM, Enneking FK: A portable mechanical pump providing over four days of patient-controlled analgesia by perineural infusion at home. Reg Anesth Pain Med 2002;27(1):100–104.

105. Ilfeld BM, Enneking FK: Continuous peripheral nerve blocks at home: A review. Anesth Analg 2005;100(6):1822–1833.

106. Brown SL, Morrison AE: Local anesthetic infusion pump systems adverse events reported to the Food and Drug Administration. Anesthesiology 2004;100(5):1305–1307.

107. Gajraj NM, Sharma SK, Souter AJ, et al: A survey of obstetric patients who refuse regional anaesthesia. Anaesthesia 1995;50(8):740–741.

108. De Andres J, Valia JC, Gil A, et al: Predictors of patient satisfaction with regional anesthesia. Reg Anesth 1995;20(6):498–505.

109. Fanelli G, Casati A, Garancini P, et al: Nerve stimulator and multiple injection technique for upper and lower limb blockade: Failure rate, patient acceptance, and neurologic complications. Study Group on Regional Anesthesia. Anesth Analg 1999;88(4):847–852.

110. Ohmura S, Kawada M, Ohta T, et al: Systemic toxicity and resuscitation in bupivacaine-, levobupivacaine-, or ropivacaine-infused rats. Anesth Analg 2001;93(3):743–748.

111. Groban L, Deal DD, Vernon JC, et al: Cardiac resuscitation after incremental overdosage with lidocaine, bupivacaine, levobupivacaine, and ropivacaine in anesthetized dogs. Anesth Analg 2001;92(1):37–43.

112. White PF, Song D: New criteria for fast-tracking after outpatient anesthesia: A comparison with the modified Aldrete's scoring system. Anesth Analg 1999;88(5):1069–1072.

113. Williams BA: For outpatients, does regional anesthesia truly shorten the hospital stay, and how should we define postanesthesia care unit bypass eligibility? Anesthesiology 2004;101(1):3–6.

114. Goodman S, Ma T, Trindade M, et al: COX-2 selective NSAID decreases bone ingrowth in vivo. J Orthop Res 2002;20(6):1164–1169.

115. Aspenberg P: Don't administer NSAID after bone surgery! Lakartidningen 2002;99(22):2554.

116. Jarit GJ, Mohr KJ, Waller R, et al: The effects of home interferential therapy on post-operative pain, edema, and range of motion of the knee. Clin J Sport Med 2003;13(1):16–20.

117. Klein SM, Nielsen KC, Greengrass RA, et al: Ambulatory discharge after long-acting peripheral nerve blockade: 2382 blocks with ropivacaine. Anesth Analg 2002;94(1):65–70.

63

Neuraxial Anesthesia in Outpatients

Michael F. Mulroy, MD • Francis V. Salinas, MD

INTRODUCTION

Since the first description of subarachnoid anesthesia by Bier, it has remained the simplest and most effective technique of regional anesthesia. The use of neuraxial techniques in outpatients has been a more recent development, awaiting ready availability of newer needles that reduced the side effect of postdural puncture headache to an acceptable level in the ambulatory setting. The last 10 years have seen a dramatic increase in the use of these techniques in outpatients, for several reasons.

Simplicity and effectiveness should make central neuraxial techniques (either spinal or epidural) ideal in the outpatient setting. Both spinal and epidural anesthesia are more familiar to practitioners than peripheral nerve blocks and are easier to perform because they do not require nerve localization techniques. They can be performed rapidly and without assistance. Neuraxial techniques are effective for lower abdominal, perineal, and lower extremity surgery, and are among the best choices for practitioners who are just starting to incorporate regional anesthetic techniques in an outpatient practice. They also provide optimal outcomes in most of the important aspects of outpatient anesthesia. Patients with neuraxial blocks have lower pain scores on admission to PACU than patients receiving general anesthesia (GA).[1-5] Their frequency of postoperative nausea and vomiting (PONV) appears to be at most one-third of that after GA.[6] Most importantly, the frequency of phase 1 PACU bypass is high,[1,6,7] and discharge times are comparable to even the fastest for GA techniques if appropriate local anesthetic agents and dosages are chosen.[8] Modern small-gauge rounded point needles and short-acting drugs have reduced the side effects that were of concern in the past. With propofol infusions available to provide light but transient sedation, the objection to "being awake" during regional techniques has also disappeared, leaving neuraxial techniques as an excellent choice.

This chapter will focus on the advantages, disadvantages, and practical points associated with spinal and epidural anesthesia in the outpatient setting.

GENERAL CONSIDERATIONS

Advantages

Spinal Anesthesia

Spinal anesthesia (SA) is one of the simplest and most reliable of regional anesthesia techniques. The external anatomic landmarks are easily identified. The block can be performed with minimal discomfort, the end-point of cerebrospinal fluid flow is unmistakable, and the onset of anesthesia is more rapid than with any other regional technique. Because of the rapidity of onset, the block can be performed in the operating room without the requirement for additional personnel or a block room. The efficient performance of the block does not add substantially to operating room time any more than for the induction of GA. The onset of the sensory blockade is sufficiently rapid to attain surgical anesthesia by the time the positioning and preparation of the patient are completed. A variety of local anesthetic agents are available that can provide a wide range of duration of surgical anesthesia. The risk of nausea can be reduced if systemic opioids are avoided. Likewise, nausea and vomiting[2,9,10] and residual somnolence associated with general anesthetics or heavy premedication can be avoided, allowing a rapid return to full alertness in the PACU. SA is also a technique with a high degree of patient familiarity because of its use in obstetrics and thus is more likely to be accepted by many patient populations. In addition, it employs the lowest dose of local anesthetic of any major regional anesthetic technique and has minimal potential for systemic toxicity.

Epidural Anesthesia

Epidural anesthesia (EA) shares many of the advantages of SA, particularly clinician familiarity, simplicity of superficial landmarks, and ease of performance of the block. It has the additional advantage of allowing a continuous catheter to be placed in the epidural space, which creates the potential for tailoring both the segmental spread and duration of the block. Although it is a more flexible technique, this advantage is attained at the price of a slower onset of surgical anesthesia.

Combined Spinal--Epidural Anesthesia

Combined spinal–epidural anesthesia (CSEA) is also a useful technique in the outpatient setting. The procedure is technically more challenging: once the epidural space is identified, the spinal needle must be introduced through the epidural needle and advanced further into the subarachnoid space. After the local anesthetic is injected, the spinal needle is withdrawn and the epidural catheter is inserted into the epidural space and taped in place. This technique requires more time and technical skill, but CSEA provides the advantages of the rapid onset and dense block of SA along with the flexibility of an indwelling catheter to allow incremental and repeated injections to achieve the desired segmental spread and duration of surgical anesthesia. This technique has been used effectively for extracorporeal shock wave lithotripsy procedures, where the duration of treatment may be unpredictable. Another advantage of the combined technique is the rapid onset of dense perineal anesthesia, which may not be provided by lumbar EA alone. It has also been used for knee arthroscopies when low doses of subarachnoid local anesthesia are used to provide a predictable short duration, but may be supplemented by epidural injection of local anesthetic if further spread or duration of blockade are needed.[11] Although the technique combines some of the disadvantages of both neuraxial procedures, it also maximizes the advantages and positive aspects of both SA and EA.

Drawbacks

Neuraxial anesthesia does have potential disadvantages. SA is typically a single-injection blockade, and thus careful attention must be paid to selection of the appropriate local anesthetic agent and dose. If the surgical duration was underestimated or becomes prolonged for unexpected reasons, supplemental GA may be needed. The "single-injection" aspect of SA frequently induces clinicians to give "just a little bit more" drug to ensure adequate distribution and duration; however, this tendency must be resisted, as the downside of this increased dosing pattern is a prolonged recovery and discharge time.[6]

Postdural puncture headache (PDPH) remains a risk with SA. Newer pencil-point, smaller gauge needles have significantly reduced this frequency to less than 3%.[12] It is even less frequent in patients older than age 40. Although PDPH does not result in long-term neurologic damage and usually is not a prolonged inconvenience for the patient, it must be acknowledged in the discussion of SA with the outpatient. If it is inconvenient for a patient to return for an epidural blood patch or essential that the patient not have this debility, alternative anesthetic techniques should be considered.

The most recent concerns about SA for outpatients have revolved around potential toxicity of local anesthetic drugs. A major concern was the reporting of permanent neurologic damage associated with very high doses of concentrated lidocaine injected through spinal microcatheters. This has not been a problem with standard doses of the local anesthetics used for single-injection spinal anesthetics, although all anesthetics injected in the subarachnoid space are potentially neurotoxic.[13] A more common, relevant concern has been the symptoms of neurologic irritation associated primarily with lidocaine. This syndrome of "transient neurologic symptoms" (TNS) consists of a burning type of back pain radiating into the buttocks or legs that appears 6–24 h after the resolution of SA and can persist for 1 to 6 days.[14] TNS occurs approximately 15–30% of the time, with the highest frequency following lidocaine SA.[15] Obese outpatients are more susceptible, especially those having procedures performed in the lithotomy or knee arthroscopy positions.[16] Although no sensory or motor deficits are associated with this syndrome,[17] and to date no persistent neurologic deficits, it is nevertheless a significant source of morbidity in some patients. Many practitioners have sought alternatives to lidocaine to reduce the incidence of TNS (see section on Lidocaine).

EA also has some potential drawbacks in the outpatient setting. Its slower onset of blockade compared with SA may cause a slight delay. However, if induction of EA is performed in a block room outside the operating room, the onset of anesthesia with drugs such as chloroprocaine (2-CP) or lidocaine is so rapid that there is little delay in the onset of surgery, and the use of EA may even promote operating room efficiency.[18] Other drawbacks associated with EA include the greater risk for postdural headache if an unintentional dural puncture occurs. Since the potential for headache is directly related to the size of the needle, the use of the larger gauge epidural needles may represent a greater risk, although the incidence of PDPH from an unintentional dural puncture in experienced hands should be less than 0.5%. EA involves the use of larger doses of local anesthetic drugs, and thus represents a greater potential for systemic toxicity than occurs with SA. The careful use of safety steps is just as appropriate for the outpatient as for the inpatient.[19]

Another limitation of both neuraxial techniques is the absence of residual analgesia. Multiple randomized comparisons of neuraxial techniques to GA show that early pain is significantly less with the regional techniques,[1–3,20,21] but once the block has resolved, some alternative mode of analgesia must be provided for the patient. This may be accomplished by the use of local anesthetic infiltrated into the wound, intraarticular injection of local anesthetic, or even a supplemental peripheral nerve block (eg, a femoral nerve or ankle block). The need for additional analgesia may not be an issue after relatively less painful procedures, such as diagnostic knee arthroscopy. Nevertheless, the possibility for breakthrough pain must be considered in the planning of the central neuraxial anesthesia for the outpatient.

A common concern is the potential for difficulty with urination following neuraxial blockade. With higher doses of longer acting local anesthetics, the bladder is distended beyond its normal cystometric capacity during the prolonged duration of neural blockade and may be unable to return to normal function once the sensory blockade dissipates.[22] Fortunately, with the short-duration central neuraxial blockades that are usually employed in the outpatient setting, bladder function returns promptly following complete resolution of the blockade. Patients can be successfully discharged home after short-duration spinal anesthetics with procaine, 2-CP, lidocaine, and even low doses of bupivacaine.[23] The use of certain additives, such as epinephrine, may impede this recovery.[24,25] The requirement for postoperative voiding is not essential with short-acting local anesthetics or low dose (<6 mg) bupivacaine spinal anesthetic techniques.

SPECIFIC OUTPATIENT SURGICAL PROCEDURES SUITABLE FOR NEURAXIAL ANESTHESIA

Hernia Repair

Inguinal herniorrhaphy is one of the most common procedures performed on an outpatient basis. Neuraxial anesthesia provides excellent anesthesia and motor relaxation for this operation.[26] SA with procaine or lidocaine in a *hyperbaric solution* (to give cephalad spread to the T4 through T6 level) is usually sufficient to provide high enough block with appropriate discharge times. The heavier solution (created by the addition of glucose to the local anesthetic) promotes spread to the "lowest" portion of the spinal canal, which is actually the midthoracic region when the patient is in the supine position. Using this technique creates higher spread of the dose, may allow a slightly lower dose to achieve anesthesia,[27] and can provide a more rapid resolution of blockade compared with the same dose of local anesthetic injected as an isobaric solution. This more rapid resolution can be negated if higher doses of local anesthetic are used because of insecurity regarding adequate spread of anesthesia. Inappropriately high doses increase the risk of prolonged blockade and delayed discharge.

Although postoperative voiding is not usually a problem after short-acting or low-dose bupivacaine, patients with hernia repairs frequently have urinary retention simply because of the postoperative pain that produces reflex inhibition of the voiding pathway. Generous use of local anesthetic infiltration during and after the procedure may help prevent this, but many centers still require hernia patients to void before discharge regardless of the anesthetic technique. EA offers an alternative for this surgical procedure because of the segmental band of anesthesia and the opportunity to use shorter acting drugs such as 2-CP or lidocaine, but with the ability to administer these agents via the indwelling epidural catheter to ensure an adequate distribution, depth, and duration of surgical anesthesia as dictated by the nature of the surgical procedure.

Anorectal Procedures

Whereas EA may have a delayed onset in the sacral fibers, intrathecal anesthesia limited to specific dermatomal fibers is an ideal application of SA. For lithotomy procedures, a traditional "saddle block" technique with hyperbaric 2-CP or procaine in small doses (20–30 mg) is appropriate. This may add some time to the procedure because of the need to keep the patient in the sitting position for at least 5 min to concentrate the local anesthetic in the sacral area. Because of the risk of TNS, lidocaine may not be an ideal choice. An excellent alternative is the use of the prone jackknife position, where procaine or 2-CP, as well as lidocaine can be made *hypobaric*.[28] This is easily accomplished by adding an equal volume of sterile water to the local anesthetic solution, usually 2 mL of each. This technique is efficient in the operating room because the block can be performed with the patient in the operating position, and onset is fast enough to allow surgery to begin as soon as the surgical preparation is complete. One hazard is that the level of anesthesia may rise if the patient is turned supine with the head elevated after a short procedure. Patients should be recovered form this technique in the full supine position for the first hour. Again, provision for adequate postoperative analgesia should be made by generous injection of local anesthetics during the procedure by the surgeon. The choice of an appropriate short-duration local anesthetic is important to provide competitive discharge times.[20]

Laparoscopy

Although laparoscopic procedures of the upper abdomen are not tolerated well with regional techniques, pelvic laparoscopy appears to be suitable with neuraxial blockade in some hands. Vaghadia and colleagues have shown the successful use of low-dose SA for outpatient gynecologic laparoscopy. For this situation, lidocaine 25 mg combined with fentanyl 20 mcg injected in the sitting position produces adequate sensory anesthesia with minimal motor blockade, which was well tolerated by their patients.[29] This is another example of the use of a hypobaric solution, this time providing upward spread of the solution by the dilution to a total volume of 3 mL with sterile water. In this case, the dilution also creates a lower dose of local anesthetic at each dermatome, and thus allows a less dense block and a more rapid resolution of the dilute anesthetic. The combination of low total dose and dilution provides rapid discharge and a high degree of patient satisfaction. This SA dosing strategy requires a gentle and skilled surgeon capable of performing the operation with less extensive distention of the peritoneum. If such a partnership can be arranged, patients appear to benefit from this technique.

Knee Surgeries

Knee surgeries are excellent situations for using neuraxial techniques, because they provide good surgical conditions and rapid recovery. Epidural blockade with a continuous technique is especially useful for providing a variable length of anesthesia for unpredictable or longer procedures, such as cruciate ligament repairs. With short- or intermediate-duration local anesthetics, timing of dosage can be managed to allow rapid and competitive discharge times.[3,4,8,30] The drawback is that larger initial doses are required to provide the lower lumbar spread to anesthetize the knee, especially the posterior portion. With the short-duration drugs, the onset time is usually rapid enough that surgical anesthesia is present by the time the surgical preparation and draping is completed.

SA provides even more rapid onset, and has been used successfully, especially for the short predictable procedures such as diagnostic arthroscopy or partial meniscectomy. The challenge here is choosing the correct drug and dose to provide adequate anesthesia but competitive recovery. Lidocaine had been the drug of choice before the TNS controversy and is still used in many institutions and provides competitive early discharge.[5] Hodgson has used procaine as an alternative, with lower TNS but other side effects.[31] Others have reported success with low-dose bupivacaine spinal block, with a low incidence of TNS.[32] This technique requires addition of 20 to 25 mcg of fentanyl to 5 mg bupivacaine to provide sufficient density of anesthesia with a low enough dose to permit rapid resolution. The high variability of spread and duration of bupivacaine, however, makes this a challenging technique.[33] Another approach to reduce TNS has been the use of very low dose lidocaine. Ben-David reported a 10-fold decrease in TNS (incidence comparable to bupivacaine) when he used 20 mg of lidocaine with 25 mcg of fentanyl,[34] but others have not been able to confirm his results.[35] Most recently, the investigation of 2-CP as a spinal anesthetic has provided both rapid discharge and a suggestion of a low incidence of TNS;[36] it may therefore be a useful alternative in the future.

Another variation of spinal technique is **unilateral spinal blockade.** This approach uses a hyperbaric solution, keeping the patient in the lateral decubitus position for 10 to 15 min after injection to allow concentration of the local anesthetic in the dependent nerve roots. This reduces the usual spread of the drug to the midthoracic level and allows smaller doses and less sympathetic blockade, and thus a shorter duration with fewer side effects. This technique has been employed with low-dose bupivacaine, ropivacaine, and levobupivacaine[37,38] and has been shown to have advantages compared with conventional hyperbaric techniques and to GA.[2,39–42] The main disadvantage of this technique is the longer time for induction of anesthesia, but this may be overcome if the block can be performed in a holding area while the operating room is being prepared.

Most diagnostic and minor knee procedures do not include significant postoperative pain, and thus the patient is usually free to leave when the neuraxial anesthetic resolves. With the more painful procedures, such as patellar tendon cruciate ligament repair, the use of supplemental peripheral nerve blocks can provide significant analgesia and speedy discharge.[43,44]

Foot Surgery

Foot surgery requires more sacral anesthesia, and thus EA may not be as useful. Spinal blockade has been used successfully, including the unilateral techniques described previously.[45] The major problem with foot surgery is that it can be extremely painful, and SA provides no residual analgesia when the block resolves. This is an excellent opportunity for the combination of a dense spinal blockade for the surgery, followed by a long-acting peripheral nerve blockade, or even the insertion of a continuous peripheral nerve catheter on the sciatic nerve to provide postoperative analgesia.[46]

SELECTION OF LOCAL ANESTHETICS & ADJUVANTS

Chloroprocaine

For epidural injection, 2-CP has been the standard drug for the outpatient setting because of its short duration (complete resolution within 2 h, with a narrow variation [Figure 63–1]). 2-CP provides discharge times that are competitive with short-acting GA techniques.[47,48] The onset of blockade is sufficiently rapid that if the block is performed in a preoperative holding area, the patient usually has obtained surgical anesthesia during the time of transition to the operating room and patient positioning, preparation, and draping. The major drawback with 2-CP as the epidural agent has been the issue of back pain associated with this drug. Back pain appears to be dose-related.[49] The use of single-injection techniques, limited to less than 25 mL, decreases the incidence of back pain. The introduction of preservative-free preparations also appears to have eliminated the risk of neurotoxicity that was previously associated with this drug when unintentional high-dose subarachnoid injection was performed.

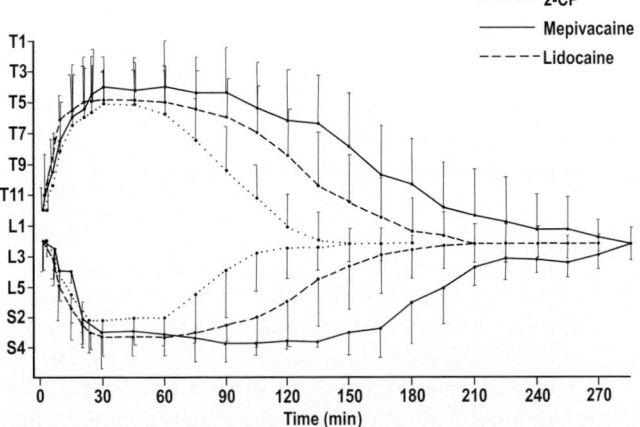

Figure 63–1. Duration of epidural anesthesia. Dermatomal spread and resolution after injection of three different local anesthetics for outpatient extracorporeal lithotripsy. (Adapted, with permission, from Kopacz DJ, Mulroy MF: Chloroprocaine and lidocaine decrease hospital stay and admission rate after outpatient epidural anesthesia. Reg Anesth 1990;15:19.)

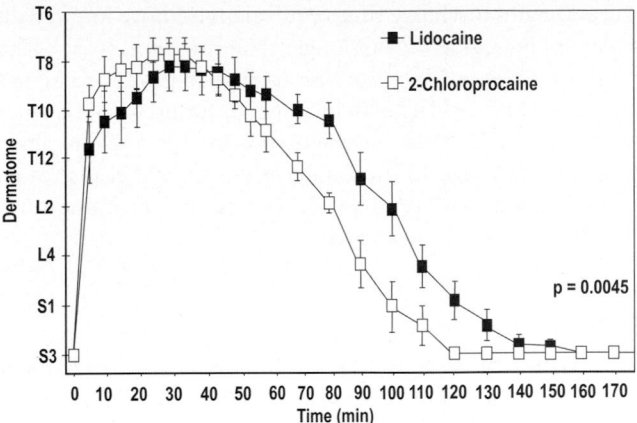

Figure 63–2. Chloroprocaine spinal anesthesia. Comparison of onset and resolution of 40 mg of lidocaine or 2-chloroprocaine in healthy volunteers. (Reprinted, with permission, from Kouri ME, Kopacz DJ: Spinal 2-chloroprocaine: A comparison with lidocaine in volunteers. Anesth Analg 2004;98:75.)

2-CP had originally been introduced for SA in the 1950s,[50] and the advent of the new preservative-free solutions has allowed its reexamination for subarachnoid use. The current 2% and 3% preservative-free preparations are slightly hyperbaric at 37°C and reliably produce sensory block (to pinprick) to the T8 through T4 level when used in a dose range of 40 to 60 mg.[51,52] Kouri and Kopacz demonstrated in a volunteer model that 40 mg of 2-CP provides tolerance to simulated surgical stimulus for up to 60 min at the T12 dermatome, which was equivalent to anesthesia provided by 40 mg of 2% lidocaine (Figure 63–2).[53] More importantly, 40 mg 2-CP resulted in complete resolution of sensory block and the ability to spontaneously void (103 min) sooner than with equipotent doses of lidocaine (126 min), procaine (151 min),[54] or low-dose bupivacaine (191 min).[55] The duration of surgical anesthesia can be reliably prolonged by 20 min by the addition of 20 mcg of fentanyl.

Concern has been raised about potential neurotoxicity of 2-CP in an animal model in extremely high doses (equivalent to 1000 mg in a 70-kg man),[56] but this level of toxicity does not appear to be any greater than that seen in the same model with lidocaine or prilocaine.[57] Although further investigation will be required to confirm that this drug is safe and effective for clinical use, initial experience has not identified a problem of TNS[36] and 2-CP may prove to be a suitable alternative to lidocaine.

Procaine

An older alternative for short-duration SA has been the aminoester drug procaine. This drug is available in a commercial 10% solution, which should be diluted by at least 50% before injection. Procaine can be made hyperbaric, isobaric, or hypobaric by the addition of appropriate additives. It has been used in doses of 75 to 100 mg for procedures such as knee arthroscopy and hernia repair with good results, with surgical duration and discharge times equivalent to those found with 50 mg of lidocaine,[8,31] but longer than those for 2-CP.[54] The addition of fentanyl to procaine appears to produce a higher frequency and severity of itching than is found with the other local anesthetics.[58] Nevertheless, procaine is a useful alternative to lidocaine in the United States today because of its lower incidence of TNS than with lidocaine.[15] Procaine is not reliable as an epidural anesthetic.

Lidocaine

The traditional short-acting local anesthetic for outpatient SA has been lidocaine. In dosages in the 50-mg range, this local anesthetic provides 60–90 min of surgical anesthesia, with a predictable resolution within 2.5 h, which allows for an acceptable discharge home after most outpatient procedures on the lower abdomen and lower extremity. For patients having procedures not in the lithotomy or arthroscopy positions, the incidence of TNS is <15% and is relatively mild, making lidocaine still an acceptable choice of procedures in the supine position.[14] It can also be diluted with sterile water and injected as a hypobaric solution in the prone jackknife position in a 40-mg dose, to provide excellent surgical anesthesia for most anorectal procedures.[28]

Although diluting the concentration of lidocaine does not reduce the frequency of TNS,[59] there has been enthusiasm for the use of small doses of lidocaine potentiated by small doses of fentanyl to provide anesthesia for lithotomy or knee procedures. Vaghadia and colleagues have used 20 mg of lidocaine with fentanyl for SA for gynecologic laparoscopic surgery and have reported no instances of TNS in several of their case series.[10,60,61] Ben-David studied a group at high-risk group for TNS (knee arthroscopy patients) and reported an incidence of only 3% TNS with a 20-mg dose of lidocaine potentiated by 25 mcg of fentanyl.[62] Other studies have found an incidence of 12% of TNS with 25 mg of lidocaine plus fentanyl in this high-risk population.[35] Although many practitioners have changed to using a low dose of lidocaine, many have looked for other alternatives such as procaine and 2-CP.

Lidocaine has also been used for EA in the outpatient setting. Its duration of action is approximately 30 min longer than that of 2-CP,[47] and thus epidural lidocaine may be more suitable for surgical procedures in the 60- to 90-min range.

Mepivacaine

Mepivacaine is an aminoamide local anesthetic similar in structure to lidocaine, with a slightly longer duration of action. Mepivacaine has been used successfully for SA for knee arthroscopies in 40-mg doses, with discharge time slightly longer than for lidocaine. There are conflicting reports about the frequency of TNS associated with this drug, with some authors claiming a reduced incidence, and others finding an equivalent frequency of TNS following mepivacaine (vs lidocaine).[15]

Prilocaine

Although prilocaine is not available in the United States as a local anesthetic for spinal use, it has produced effective SA in clinical trials and a lower incidence of TNS than seen with lidocaine.

Bupivacaine

Bupivacaine is a more potent and longer acting aminoamide local anesthetic and has received interest as a potential alternative to lidocaine for outpatient SA because of the lower incidence of TNS. Unfortunately, in addition to a longer duration, bupivacaine also has a wider variability in the duration of anesthetic action. Liu and coworkers showed in a series of volunteers that each additional milligram of bupivacaine added to SA provides approximately an average 10-min prolongation of surgical anesthesia, but a 20-min prolongation of discharge time.[33] More importantly, the standard deviation of the readiness for discharge time was almost an hour, which can translate into unacceptably long discharge times for some outpatients when doses greater than 6 mg are used. This wide standard deviation has also been confirmed at low doses.[32] The variability in the height of the block as well as the duration make bupivacaine not easily predictable for outpatient surgical procedures. Nevertheless, many practitioners are willing to accept this variability and potentially prolonged block in exchange for the very low rate of TNS associated with this drug, which is at 3% or less in clinical trials.

Ropivacaine and Levobupivacaine

The aminoamide ropivacaine has been studied for outpatient anesthesia. Although it is effective as a subarachnoid local anesthetic, it appears to be less potent than bupivacaine by approximately 50%.[63–65] Although this drug has enjoyed popularity because of its reduced risk of cardiac toxicity in large doses and less motor blockade when used on peripheral nerve blockade, these two advantages are not clinically relevant in its use in a subarachnoid space. Levobupivacaine is another less cardiotoxic enantiomer equivalent to bupivacaine studied for outpatient use,[66] but its additional cardiac safety is not a relevant factor in SA. None of the longer acting aminoamides are useful for EA in the outpatient.

Adjuvants

Additives have been used with SA over the years to prolong the duration or to intensify blockade, and thus allow a lower dose of the local anesthetic drug itself.

Changing the *baricity* of a subarachnoid local anesthetic solution by the addition of either sterile water or dextrose can allow greater control of the spread of local anesthetic to specific areas within the intrathecal space, as described in previous sections. Such manipulations can produce "unilateral" SA, allowing lower doses of local anesthetic and faster same-day discharge. The block frequently crosses over to the opposite side when the patient is finally turned supine, although it is less dense and of shorter duration on the opposite side. The use of such a lower dose allows for more rapid recovery and less chance of urinary retention, but the additional time required to perform this unilateral technique presents a challenge in a rapid-turnover ambulatory surgical setting. In this context, the RA induction room is of tremendous benefit for the safe and efficient placement of unilateral hyperbaric SA for patients undergoing lower extremity surgery.

Epinephrine

Epinephrine was, but is no longer, the classic drug additive for SA. Epinephrine provides prolongation and potentiation for all local anesthetics. It has been shown to be safe in standard doses of 100 to 200 mcg, but it is associated with a significant increase in the time to voiding in patients receiving both bupivacaine and lidocaine.[22,24] Epinephrine also produces an unusual flu-like syndrome when added to 2-CP.[67] In general, epinephrine does not appear to be a useful additive for outpatient SA unless used in extremely low doses[68] and is probably best avoided altogether.

Fentanyl

Fentanyl has been used extensively as an additive in outpatient SA. Fentanyl prolongs and intensifies the block produced by lidocaine and 2-CP without a delay in urination. Thus, intrathecal fentanyl in doses of 20 to 25 mcg may be a useful adjunct for ambulatory SA.[25,32,68,69] Unfortunately, fentanyl is associated with pruritus: 100% of volunteers receiving lidocaine or 2-CP SA with fentanyl experienced itching. In the clinical setting, where other factors such as surgical pain and systemic sedatives and analgesics are added, the itching is reported less frequently by patients. Patients receiving lidocaine SA with fentanyl appear to have an incidence of about 25% of mild pruritus. When fentanyl is added to bupivacaine, the incidence appears to double, but again the symptoms remain mild. When fentanyl is added to procaine, itching becomes more noticeable and unpleasant and may even require systemic treatment.[58] The itching usually responds to small doses of nalbuphine or diphenhydramine. Nevertheless, the use of fentanyl is effective in reducing the total dose of local anesthetic and allowing a shorter discharge time.[32] The longer acting intrathecal hydrophilic opioids such as morphine provide extended postoperative analgesia for monitored inpatients. However, morphine's slow onset of action and low risk of respiratory depression make it an undesirable intrathecal drug in the outpatient setting.

Clonidine

Clonidine is an α_2-agonist that potentiates local anesthetics in the subarachnoid space and on peripheral nerves. Doses of 15 to 45 mcg are effective without side effects, but larger doses may produce bradycardia and sedation.[70,71] The addition of 15 mcg to 2-CP SA, for example, prolongs motor and sensory block without systemic side effects.[71] Unfortunately, in the United States the drug is marketed in relatively expensive large-dose vials, in contrast to the European market where

it is available in more practical smaller incremental dosages. For that reason, it has not attained great popularity in the United States, but is worth considering for potentiation of SA. Another additive that has been tested is **neostigmine,** but it is associated with severe intractable nausea, which makes it unacceptable as an additive at the present time.[72]

POSTOPERATIVE RECOVERY

Although peripheral nerve blocks can provide excellent postoperative analgesia if patients are allowed to be discharged before resolution of the block, neuraxial techniques generally require that the patient's block be completely resolved before discharge in order to allow successful ambulation. Spinal and EA regress in slightly different patterns. With lumbar EA, the regression is generally both upward and downward from the points of maximum caudad and cephalad spread, and thus results in the final resolution of sensory anesthesia usually occurring somewhere in the lumbar dermatomes near the level of the original injection. Because of this, patients with epidurals are generally able to ambulate and void as soon as the sensory block is resolved on the thigh. On the other hand, SA tends to resolve in a cephalad-to-caudad fashion, with disappearance of sensory and motor block in the sacral dermatomes occurring last. There has been concern in the past about residual sympathetic blockade with subarachnoid anesthesia even after the sensory block is resolved. It has been shown that if perianal sensation has returned, along with proprioception in the big toe, sympathetic activity is generally back to normal and orthostatic hypotension is not a risk when these patients are ambulated.[73] Thus, the resolution of neuraxial blockade can be fairly easily determined with either technique.

Two major issues with recovery are the timing of discharge and postoperative analgesia. As mentioned earlier, careful attention must be paid to the selection of the drug and dose in order to allow a rapid resolution of the block at the appropriate time following the surgery. This requires a familiarity with the procedure and the surgeon. More importantly, when the blockade is resolved, some alternative form of analgesia must be provided. The best choice is the use of local infiltration with long-acting local anesthetics by the surgeon at the time of the operation. Other alternatives include injection of peripheral nerve blocks in the PACU as the spinal or epidural is resolving. Examples of this are the use of bupivacaine for ankle blocks after foot surgery or for femoral nerve blocks following anterior cruciate ligament repair. The next best alternative is to rely on nonopioid analgesia for patients who will have mild postoperative pain, such as the use of ketorolac or other nonsteroidal antiinflammatory drugs for patients having mild pain associated with diagnostic knee arthroscopy. If patients are having more severe pain, the use of more potent oral opioids may be required, but this may negate the advantages of regional anesthesia because of the potential for nausea, pruritus, or sedation when these drugs are administered in the PACU.

Discharge Criteria

In general, the discharge criteria, including alertness, hemodynamic stability, and freedom from nausea and vomiting, are the same for patients receiving neuraxial blockade on an outpatient basis as for all other outpatients. The need for an accompanying adult and overnight supervision is also the same. The two central special features of neuraxial blockade patients are the issue of postoperative analgesia and of voiding.

As mentioned previously, postoperative analgesia, in the form of supplemental local anesthesia or systemic analgesic techniques, is necessary. These analgesics need to be tailored to the individual patient. If local anesthesia or a peripheral nerve block is used, they need to be placed early enough to allow adequate analgesia as the spinal or epidural anesthetic wears off. Occasionally, the resolution of neuraxial block reveals that the previous management plan was not adequate, and a subsequent reinjection of local anesthetic or peripheral nerve block (or adjustment of medications) is needed. This may delay discharge, but generally most outpatient anesthesiologists have developed a good sense of the appropriate regimen for patients in these situations.

The issue of voiding is a controversial topic. For outpatients, the use of short-acting neuraxial techniques (SA with 2-CP, procaine, lidocaine, or low-dose bupivacaine or EA with 2-CP or lidocaine) is not associated with overdistention of the bladder. For patients without known risk factors for postoperative urinary retention (PUR), it does not appear necessary to require them to demonstrate an ability to void after resolution of a short-acting neuraxial block. There are several exceptions to this in high-risk groups. This may include patients with previous history of urinary retention, elderly men with prostate symptoms or likelihood of prostate symptoms, or specific surgical procedures that place them at risk for PUR. Those procedures are generally associated with pelvic or groin surgeries such as hernia repair or perirectal procedures after which voiding may be impaired by the pain produced by lower abdominal straining. In general, these patients are regarded as high risk and are usually required to void before discharge in most ambulatory surgery settings. Patients having urologic surgery are also frequently required to void by their surgeon in order to demonstrate absence of bleeding and return of normal bladder function. Other than these exceptions, most patients with neuraxial blockade can be discharged with the same criteria as patients receiving GA. If there is any concern about bladder distension, the use of a bladder ultrasound can easily identify distended bladders and lead to a prophylactic drainage before discharge. Such ultrasound units are frequently available in ambulatory surgery centers.

Patient Instructions

Postoperative instructions for patients receiving neuraxial blockade are the same as for other outpatients. If a supplemental peripheral nerve block has been given, the patients need to be instructed to protect the insensate extremity until the numbness wears off. Nausea and vomiting should be far less common at discharge than with GA techniques. Patients who have not voided before discharge need to be carefully instructed to report back to an emergency room if they are unsuccessful in voiding within 8 h after discharge. They may be one of the rare patients with voiding difficulties who will need subsequent catheterization to relieve an overdistended bladder. But as mentioned earlier, this is no indication for delaying discharge in the low-risk group.

Problems that are specific to neuraxial blockade include the potential for PDPH and neurologic symptoms following resolution of the block. The first of these is the most common, yet should still occur at less than 1% frequency with the appropriate equipment and patient selection. Nevertheless, all patients receiving spinals (or unintentional dural puncture during EA) need to be given a specific telephone number to call for follow-up and a detailed description of the potential symptoms of a PDPH. They need to be advised about the potential need to return to the hospital for an epidural blood patch if severe symptoms do develop. Questioning for symptoms of such a headache needs to be part of the routine phone call follow-up that is performed in outpatient units. If a headache does develop, conservative therapy at home is usually the most appropriate. If it persists for several days or is severe enough to interfere with daily function of the patient, the performance of an epidural blood patch on an outpatient basis is usually sufficient to cure the symptoms.

Neurologic symptoms are also possible and need to be evaluated in the follow-up phone call. The most common is the description of TNS following SA. Although it occurs more frequently with lidocaine, it also has been reported after every local anesthetic, so it should be searched for in every postspinal anesthetic patient. The symptoms may occur 6–24 h following discharge and traditionally are back pain radiating to the buttocks or legs. Fortunately, most of the symptoms are mild and transient. Although NSAIDs have been recommended for the therapy, there is really no effective treatment at the current time. The patient should be reassured that these symptoms usually regress spontaneously within 48 h, and that they do not represent any permanent neurologic deficit, nor is there any expectation that they will recur again if the patient has another spinal in the future.

A much less frequent complication, but still a possibility in the outpatient, is the development of nerve compression symptoms related to epidural hematoma formation. Although this symptom is primarily a phenomenon of inpatients receiving anticoagulants, it has been reported in the outpatient setting.[74] The unique feature of this syndrome is the development of back pain *associated with motor weakness.* This is distinctly different from the TNS syndrome, which does not include any motor symptoms. This syndrome may also develop immediately after discharge. Presentation of any motor weakness mandates an immediate return to the hospital and evaluation of the patient with a CAT scan or (preferably) an MRI to eliminate the possibility of epidural clot formation.

SUMMARY

Overall, neuraxial techniques have an important role in the outpatient setting. They are simple to perform and highly reliable and are generally associated with a faster onset of action than peripheral nerve blockade discussed elsewhere. They carry the disadvantage that the block must be resolved before patient discharge, and thus other methods of postoperative analgesia must be planned to provide for pain relief on discharge. It is critical to select the dose and drug that is most appropriate for the specific surgical procedure in order to provide an appropriate duration of blockade to allow a timely discharge from the outpatient unit. Nevertheless, with these cautions and appropriate choices, neuraxial blockade has a strong role to play in the outpatient surgical setting.

References

1. Jankowski CJ, Hebl JR, Stuart MJ, et al: A comparison of psoas compartment block and spinal and general anesthesia for outpatient knee arthroscopy. Anesth Analg 2003;97:1003–1009.
2. Korhonen AM, Valanne JV, Jokela RM, et al: A comparison of selective spinal anesthesia with hyperbaric bupivacaine and general anesthesia with desflurane for outpatient knee arthroscopy. Anesth Analg 2004;99:1668–1673.
3. Dahl V, Gierloff C, Omland E, et al: Spinal, epidural or propofol anaesthesia for out-patient knee arthroscopy? Acta Anaesthesiol Scand 1997;41:1341–1345.
4. Parnass SM, McCarthy RJ, Bach BR Jr, et al: Beneficial impact of epidural anesthesia on recovery after outpatient arthroscopy. Arthroscopy 1993;9:91–95.
5. Wong J, Marshall S, Chung F, et al: Spinal anesthesia improves the early recovery profile of patients undergoing ambulatory knee arthroscopy. Can J Anaesth 2001;48:369–374.
6. Liu SS, Strodbeck WM, Richman JM, et al: Comparison of regional versus general anesthesia for ambulatory anesthesia: A meta-analysis of randomized controlled trials. Anesth Analg 2005;101:1634–1642.
7. Casati A, Cappelleri G, Aldegheri G, et al: Total intravenous anesthesia, spinal anesthesia or combined sciatic-femoral nerve block for outpatient knee arthroscopy. Minerva Anestesiol 2004;70:493–502.
8. Mulroy MF, Larkin KL, Hodgson PS, et al: A comparison of spinal, epidural, and general anesthesia for outpatient knee arthroscopy. Anesth Analg 2000;91:860–864.
9. Lennox PH, Chilvers C, Vaghadia H: Selective spinal anesthesia versus desflurane anesthesia in short duration outpatient gynecological laparoscopy: A pharmacoeconomic comparison. Anesth Analg 2002;94:565–568.
10. Lennox PH, Vaghadia H, Henderson C, et al: Small-dose selective spinal anesthesia for short-duration outpatient laparoscopy: Recovery characteristics compared with desflurane anesthesia. Anesth Analg 2002;94:346–350.
11. Urmey WF, Stanton J, Peterson M, et al: Combined spinal-epidural anesthesia for outpatient surgery. Dose-response characteristics of intrathecal isobaric lidocaine using a 27-gauge Whitacre spinal needle. Anesthesiology 1995;83:528–534.
12. Mulroy MF, Wills RP: Spinal anesthesia for outpatients: Appropriate agents and techniques. J Clin Anesth 1995;7:622–627.
13. Hodgson PS, Neal JM, Pollock JE, et al: The neurotoxicity of drugs given intrathecally (spinal). Anesth Analg 1999;88:797–809.
14. Pollock JE: Transient neurologic symptoms: Etiology, risk factors, and management. Reg Anesth Pain Med 2002;27:581–586.
15. Zaric D, Christiansen C, Pace NL, et al: Transient neurologic symptoms after spinal anesthesia with lidocaine versus other local anesthetics: A systematic review of randomized, controlled trials. Anesth Analg 2005;100:1811–1816.
16. Freedman JM, Li DK, Drasner K, et al: Transient neurologic symptoms after spinal anesthesia: An epidemiologic study of 1,863 patients. Anesthesiology 1998;89:633–641.
17. Pollock JE, Burkhead D, Neal JM, et al: Spinal nerve function in five volunteers experiencing transient neurologic symptoms after lidocaine subarachnoid anesthesia. Anesth Analg 2000;90:658–665.
18. Williams BA, DeRiso BM, Figallo CM, et al: Benchmarking the perioperative process: III. Effects of regional anesthesia clinical pathway techniques on process efficiency and recovery profiles in ambulatory orthopedic surgery. J Clin Anesth 1998;10:570–578.
19. Mulroy MF, Norris MC, Liu SS: Safety steps for epidural injection of local anesthetics: review of the literature and recommendations. Anesth Analg 1997;85:1346–1356.
20. Li S, Coloma M, White PF, et al: Comparison of the costs and recovery profiles of three anesthetic techniques for ambulatory anorectal surgery. Anesthesiology 2000;93:1225–1230.
21. Toivonen J, Permi J, Rosenberg PH: Analgesia and discharge following preincisional ilioinguinal and iliohypogastric nerve block combined with general or spinal anaesthesia for inguinal herniorrhaphy. Acta Anaesthesiol Scand 2004;48:480–485.
22. Axelsson K, Mollefors K, Olsson JO, et al: Bladder function in spinal anaesthesia. Acta Anaesthesiol Scand 1985;29:315–321.
23. Mulroy MF, Salinas FV, Larkin KL, et al: Ambulatory surgery patients may be discharged before voiding after short-acting spinal and epidural anesthesia. Anesthesiology 2002;97:315–319.
24. Chiu AA, Liu S, Carpenter RL, et al: The effects of epinephrine on lidocaine spinal anesthesia: a cross-over study. Anesth Analg 1995;80:735–739.
25. Liu S, Chiu AA, Carpenter RL, et al: Fentanyl prolongs lidocaine spinal anesthesia without prolonging recovery. Anesth Analg 1995;80:730–734.
26. Ryan JA Jr, Adye BA, Jolly PC, et al: Outpatient inguinal herniorrhaphy with both regional and local anesthesia. Am J Surg 1984;148:313–316.
27. Van Gessel EF, Forster A, Schweizer A, et al: Comparison of hypobaric, hyperbaric, and isobaric solutions of bupivacaine during continuous spinal anesthesia. Anesth Analg 1991;72:779.
28. Bodily MN, Carpenter RL, Owens BD: Lidocaine 0.5% spinal anaesthesia: a hypobaric solution for short-stay perirectal surgery. Can J Anaesth 1992;39:770–784.
29. Vaghadia H, McLeod DH, Mitchell GW, et al: Small-dose hypobaric lidocaine-fentanyl spinal anesthesia for short duration outpatient laparoscopy. I. A randomized comparison with conventional dose hyperbaric lidocaine. Anesth Analg 1997;84:59–64.
30. Horlocker TT, Hebl JR: Anesthesia for outpatient knee arthroscopy: Is there an optimal technique? Reg Anesth Pain Med 2003;28:58–63.
31. Hodgson PS, Liu SS, Batra MS, et al: Procaine compared with lidocaine for incidence of transient neurologic symptoms. Reg Anesth Pain Med 2000;25:218–222.
32. Ben-David B, Solomon E, Levin H, et al: Intrathecal fentanyl with small-dose dilute bupivacaine: better anesthesia without prolonging recovery. Anesth Analg 1997;85:560–565.
33. Liu SS, Ware PD, Allen HW, et al: Dose-response characteristics of spinal bupivacaine in volunteers. Clinical implications for ambulatory anesthesia. Anesthesiology 1996;85:729–736.
34. Ben-David B, DeMeo PJ, Lucyk C, et al: A comparison of minidose lidocaine-fentanyl spinal anesthesia and local anesthesia/propofol infusion for outpatient knee arthroscopy. Anesth Analg 2001;93:319–325.
35. Pollock JE, Mulroy MF, Bent E, et al: A comparison of two regional anesthetic techniques for outpatient knee arthroscopy. Anesth Analg 2003;97:397–401.
36. Yoos JR, Kopacz DJ: Spinal 2-chloroprocaine for surgery: An initial 10-month experience. Anesth Analg 2005;100:553–558.

37. Cappelleri G, Aldegheri G, Danelli G, et al: Spinal anesthesia with hyperbaric levobupivacaine and ropivacaine for outpatient knee arthroscopy: A prospective, randomized, double-blind study. Anesth Analg 2005;101:77–82.

38. Kiran S, Upma B: Use of small-dose bupivacaine (3 mg vs 4 mg) for unilateral spinal anesthesia in the outpatient setting. Anesth Analg 2004;99:302–303.

39. Borghi B, Stagni F, Bugamelli S, et al: Unilateral spinal block for outpatient knee arthroscopy: A dose-finding study. J Clin Anesth 2003;15:351–356.

40. Esmaoglu A, Karaoglu S, Mizrak A, et al: Bilateral vs unilateral spinal anesthesia for outpatient knee arthroscopies. Knee Surg Sports Traumatol Arthrosc 2004;12:155–158.

41. Fanelli G, Borghi B, Casati A, et al: Unilateral bupivacaine spinal anesthesia for outpatient knee arthroscopy. Italian Study Group on Unilateral Spinal Anesthesia. Can J Anaesth 2000;47:746–751.

42. Valanne JV, Korhonen AM, Jokela RM, et al: Selective spinal anesthesia: a comparison of hyperbaric bupivacaine 4 mg versus 6 mg for outpatient knee arthroscopy. Anesth Analg 2001;93:1377–1379.

43. Mulroy MF, Larkin KL, Batra MS, et al: Femoral nerve block with 0.25% or 0.5% bupivacaine improves postoperative analgesia following outpatient arthroscopic anterior cruciate ligament repair. Reg Anesth Pain Med 2001;26:24–29.

44. Williams BA, Kentor ML, Williams JP, et al: Process analysis in outpatient knee surgery: Effects of regional and general anesthesia on anesthesia-controlled time. Anesthesiology 2000;93:529–538.

45. Casati A, Fanelli G, Cappelleri G, et al: Effects of speed of intrathecal injection on unilateral spinal block by 1% hyperbaric bupivacaine. A randomized, double-blind study. Minerva Anestesiol 1999;65:5–10.

46. Zaric D, Boysen K, Christiansen J, et al: Continuous popliteal sciatic nerve block for outpatient foot surgery—A randomized, controlled trial. Acta Anaesthesiol Scand 2004;48:337–341.

47. Kopacz DJ, Mulroy MF: Chloroprocaine and lidocaine decrease hospital stay and admission rate after outpatient epidural anesthesia. Reg Anesth 1990;15:19–25.

48. Neal JM, Deck JJ, Kopacz DJ, et al: Hospital discharge after ambulatory knee arthroscopy: A comparison of epidural 2-chloroprocaine versus lidocaine. Reg Anesth Pain Med 2001;26:35–40.

49. Stevens RA, Urmey WF, Urquhart BL, et al: Back pain after epidural anesthesia with chloroprocaine. Anesthesiology 1993;78:492–498.

50. Foldes FF, Mc NP: 2-Chloroprocaine: A new local anesthetic agent. Anesthesiology 1952;13:287–296.

51. Kopacz DJ: Spinal 2-chloroprocaine: Minimum effective dose. Reg Anesth Pain Med 2005;30:36–42.

52. Na KB, Kopacz DJ: Spinal chloroprocaine solutions: Density at 37 degrees C and pH titration. Anesth Analg 2004;98:70–74.

53. Kouri ME, Kopacz DJ: Spinal 2-chloroprocaine: A comparison with lidocaine in volunteers. Anesth Analg 2004;98:75–80.

54. Gonter AF, Kopacz DJ: Spinal 2-chloroprocaine: A comparison with procaine in volunteers. Anesth Analg 2005;100:573–579.

55. Yoos JR, Kopacz DJ: Spinal 2-chloroprocaine: A comparison with small-dose bupivacaine in volunteers. Anesth Analg 2005;100:566–572.

56. Taniguchi M, Bollen AW, Drasner K: Sodium bisulfite: Scapegoat for chloroprocaine neurotoxicity? Anesthesiology 2004;100:85–91.

57. Kishimoto T, Bollen AW, Drasner K: Comparative spinal neurotoxicity of prilocaine and lidocaine. Anesthesiology 2002;97:1250–1253.

58. Mulroy MF, Larkin KL, Siddiqui A: Intrathecal fentanyl-induced pruritus is more severe in combination with procaine than with lidocaine or bupivacaine. Reg Anesth Pain Med 2001;26:252.

59. Pollock JE, Liu SS, Neal JM, et al: Dilution of spinal lidocaine does not alter the incidence of transient neurologic symptoms. Anesthesiology 1999;90:445.

60. Chilvers CR, Vaghadia H, Mitchell GW, et al: Small-dose hypobaric lidocaine-fentanyl spinal anesthesia for short duration outpatient laparoscopy. II. Optimal fentanyl dose. Anesth Analg 1997;84:65–70.

61. Vaghadia H, Collins L, Sun H, et al: Selective spinal anesthesia for outpatient laparoscopy. IV: Population pharmacodynamic modelling. Can J Anaesth 2001;48:273–278.

62. Ben-David B, Maryanovsky M, Gurevitch A, et al: A comparison of minidose lidocaine-fentanyl and conventional-dose lidocaine spinal anesthesia. Anesth Analg 2000;91:865–870.

63. Gautier PE, De Kock M, Van Steenberge A, et al: Intrathecal ropivacaine for ambulatory surgery. Anesthesiology 1999;91:1239–1245.

64. Kallio H, Snall EV, Tuomas CA, et al: Comparison of hyperbaric and plain ropivacaine 15 mg in spinal anaesthesia for lower limb surgery. Br J Anaesth 2004;93:664–669.

65. McDonald SB, Liu SS, Kopacz DJ, et al: Hyperbaric spinal ropivacaine: a comparison to bupivacaine in volunteers. Anesthesiology 1999;90:971–977.

66. Alley EA, Kopacz DJ, McDonald SB, et al: Hyperbaric spinal levobupivacaine: A comparison to racemic bupivacaine in volunteers. Anesth Analg 2002;94:188–193.

67. Smith KN, Kopacz DJ, McDonald SB: Spinal 2-chloroprocaine: A dose-ranging study and the effect of added epinephrine. Anesth Analg 2004;98:81–88.

68. Turker G, N UC, Yilmazlar A, et al: Effects of adding epinephrine plus fentanyl to low-dose lidocaine for spinal anesthesia in outpatient knee arthroscopy. Acta Anaesthesiol Scand 2003;47:986–992.

69. Vath JS, Kopacz DJ: Spinal 2-chloroprocaine: the effect of added fentanyl. Anesth Analg 2004;98:89–94.

70. De Kock M, Gautier P, Fanard L, et al: Intrathecal ropivacaine and clonidine for ambulatory knee arthroscopy: A dose-response study. Anesthesiology 2001;94:574–578.

71. Davis BR, Kopacz DJ: Spinal 2-chloroprocaine: The effect of added clonidine. Anesth Analg 2005;100:559–565.

72. Liu SS, Hodgson PS, Moore JM, et al: Dose-response effects of spinal neostigmine added to bupivacaine spinal anesthesia in volunteers. Anesthesiology 1999;90:710–717.

73. Pflug AE, Aasheim GM, Foster C: Sequence of return of neurological function and criteria for safe ambulation following subarachnoid block (spinal anaesthetic). Can Anaesth Soc J 1978;25:133–1339.

74. Gilbert A, Owens BD, Mulroy MF: Epidural hematoma after outpatient epidural anesthesia. Anesth Analg 2002;94:77–78.

64

Continuous Peripheral Nerve Blocks in Outpatients

Brian M. Ilfeld, MD, MS • Elizabeth M. Renehan, MD • F. Kayser Enneking, MD

INTRODUCTION

Over 40% of ambulatory patients experience moderate-to-severe postoperative pain at home following orthopedic procedures.[1] Single-injection peripheral nerve blocks with long-acting local anesthetics can provide excellent postoperative analgesia. However, the analgesic benefit of single-injection blocks is typically limited to the duration of the blockade and, subsequently, patients must usually rely on oral opioids to control pain. Unfortunately, opioids are associated with undesirable side effects, such as pruritus, nausea and vomiting, sedation, and constipation. To improve postoperative analgesia following ambulatory surgery, increasing interest has focused on providing perineural local anesthetic infusions, also called, continuous peripheral nerve blocks, to outpatients. This technique involves a percutaneous insertion of a catheter directly adjacent to the peripheral nerve(s) supplying the surgical site. Local anesthetic is then infused via the catheter, providing prolonged, site-specific analgesia.

HISTORY

In 1946, Ansbro first described continuous regional blockade using a cork to stabilize a needle placed adjacent to the brachial plexus divisions to provide a continuous supraclavicular block.[2] However, for decades, patients were required to remain hospitalized because the available pumps used to infuse local anesthetic were large, heavy, and technically sophisticated. It was not until 52 years later that outpatient perineural infusion using a percutaneous catheter and a small, lightweight, portable infusion pump was described.[3]

ADVANTAGES & EVIDENCE

The first report of continuous infusion of local anesthetics at home was reported by Rawal and colleagues.[3] Shortly thereafter, numerous reports or series of ambulatory perineural infusions were published, which described the use of catheters in various anatomic locations, including paravertebral,[4] interscalene,[5–7] intersternocleidomastoid,[8] infraclavicular,[6] axillary,[9] psoas compartment,[9,10] femoral,[9,11] fascia iliaca,[5] sciatic,[9,10] popliteal,[6,12] and tibial nerve.[6] Ambulatory continuous peripheral nerve blocks in pediatric patients also were reported.[13]

Klein and colleagues were first to study and *quantify* the benefits of perineural infusion of local anesthetic.[14] In their randomized, double-blind, placebo-controlled investigation, patients undergoing open rotator cuff repair who received an interscalene block and perineural catheter preoperatively, were randomized to receive either perineural ropivacaine 0.2% or normal saline postoperatively (10 mL/h). Patients receiving perineural placebo averaged a 3 on a 0–10 visual analog pain scale (VAS), compared with a 1 for subjects receiving ropivacaine. Although a portable pump was used, patients remained hospitalized during local anesthetic infusion of less than 24 h, and catheters were removed by the investigators prior to home discharge.[14] Consequently, while these data suggested that perineural infusion may improve postoperative analgesia following hospital discharge, the actual advantages of continuous nerve blocks for patients *at home* remained unknown.

Data from perineural infusion in outpatients subsequently were provided in four randomized, double-blind, placebo-controlled studies.[15–18] Patients receiving perineural local anesthetic achieved significantly lower resting and breakthrough pain scores than did those using exclusively oral opioids for analgesia (Figure 64–1). In addition, they required significantly fewer oral analgesics to achieve their improved level of analgesia (see Figure 64–1). Preoperatively, patients scheduled for moderately painful procedures had a perineural catheter placed: an infraclavicular catheter for hand/forearm procedures,[15] a popliteal catheter for foot/ankle surgeries,[16,18] or an interscalene catheter for shoulder procedures.[17] Postoperatively, patients received either perineural local anesthetic or normal saline and were followed at home for up to 60 h. All patients were instructed to use a bolus from their infusion pump for breakthrough pain, and oral analgesics if this maneuver failed. In patients with an interscalene catheter following shoulder surgery, the local anesthetic infusion provided analgesia so effective that 80% of patients receiving ropivacaine required one or fewer opioid tablets per day during their infusion and reported average resting pain as less than 1.5 on a scale of 0 to 10.[17] This compares with all patients

receiving placebo, who required four or more opioid tablets per day, beginning the evening of surgery. These patients reported average resting pain scores between 3 and 4. For breakthrough pain, the differences between treatment groups were even more pronounced in all of these four placebo-controlled studies (see Figure 64–1).

Improved analgesia provided several additional benefits in patients who received perineural local anesthetic. Of patients receiving perineural ropivacaine, 0 to 30% reported insomnia due to pain, compared with 60% to 70% of patients receiving placebo.[15–17] Additionally, awakenings from sleep because of pain averaged 0.0 to 0.2 times on the first postoperative night, compared with 2.0 to 2.3 times for patients using only oral opioids.[15–17] Lower doses of oral opioid intake translated into a lower rate of nausea, vomiting, pruritus, and sedation.[15–18] Satisfaction with postoperative analgesia was both clinically and statistically higher for patients receiving local anesthetic.[15–18] Finally, patients with popliteal local anesthetic infusion rated their quality of recovery significantly higher than patients receiving placebo.[18] Whether these demonstrated benefits resulted in a tangible improvement in patients' health-related quality of life remains unanswered.[19] Additionally, more work is required to determine the optimal location of catheter placement for common surgical procedures (eg, axillary vs infraclavicular for hand surgery).

Additional possible advantages of using outpatient perineural infusion to allow earlier discharge of patients who require potent analgesia may include other benefits of a shorter hospitalization, such as decreases in nosocomial infection,[20,21] harmful medical error,[22,23] and increases in health-related quality of life.[19] Societal benefits include tangible cost savings[24–26] arising from the ability to discharge patients home directly from the recovery room after surgeries such as total elbow and shoulder replacement[27] and on the first postoperative day following total hip and knee replacement.[28] Additional data are required to define the appropriate subset of patients and assess the benefits and incidence of complications associated with this practice.

PATIENT SELECTION

Clinical Pearls

- Outpatient infusion should be reserved for patients expected to have moderate-to-severe postoperative pain (low pain tolerance or surgical procedure resulting in significant postoperative pain).
- Appropriate patient selection is the key for successful and safe use of continuous peripheral nerve blocks in outpatients.

Most investigators limit the use of ambulatory infusion to patients who are expected to have *moderate* or *severe* postoperative pain of a duration greater than 24 h that is not

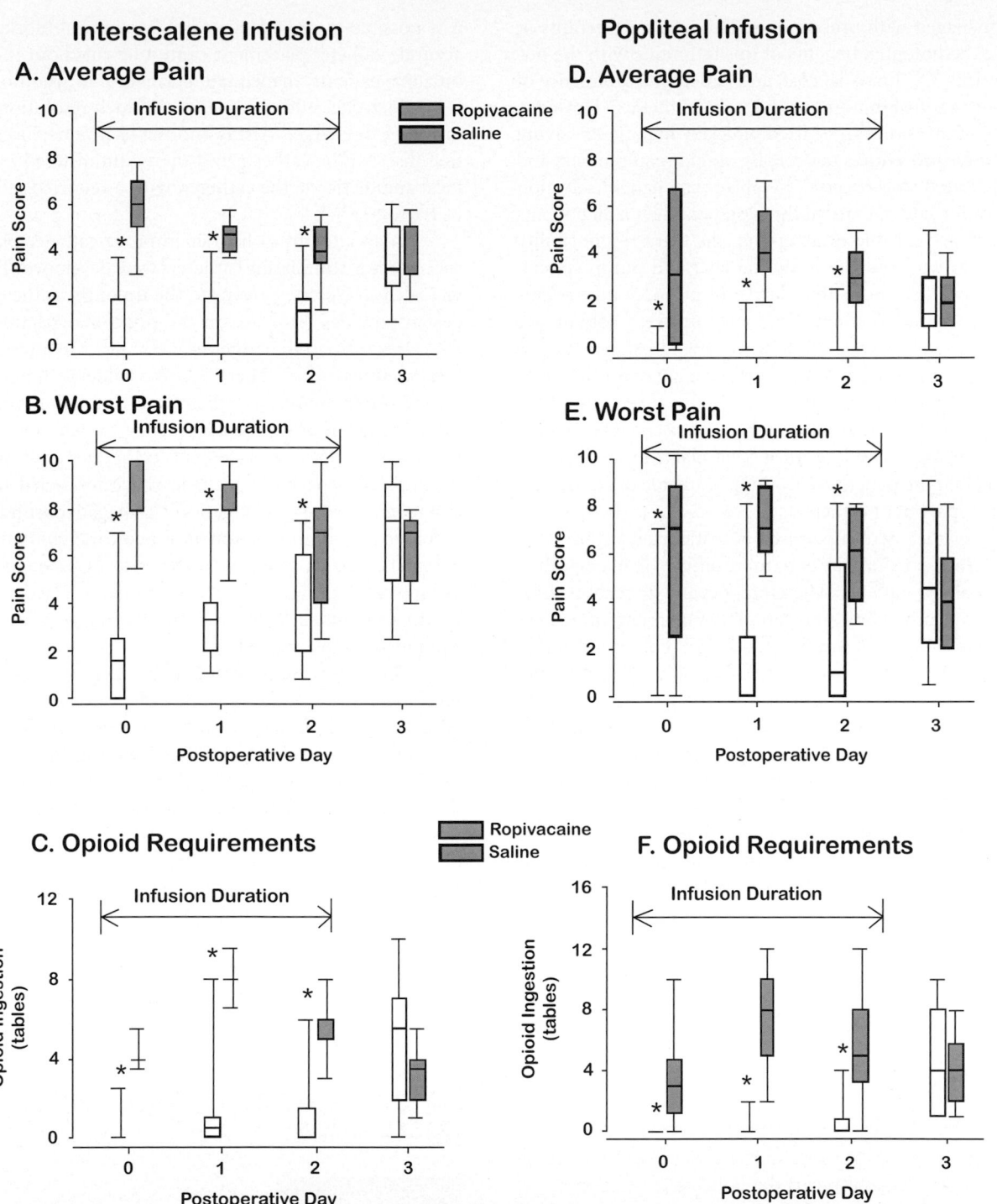

Figure 64–1. Effects of interscalene and sciatic/popliteal perineural infusion of either ropivacaine or placebo on average pain at rest (**A** and **D**), worst pain overall (**B** and **E**), and opiate use (**C** and **F**) following moderately painful shoulder or lower extremity surgery (scale: 0–10). Each opiate tablet consisted of oxycodone, 5 mg. *Note:* The infusion was discontinued after postoperative day 2, as indicated by the horizontal lines. Data are expressed as median (horizontal bar) with twenty-fifth to seventy-fifth (box) and tenth to ninetieth (whiskers) percentiles for patients randomly assigned to receive either 0.2% ropivacaine or 0.9% saline placebo. For tightly clustered data (eg, panel A, postoperative days 0 and 1, ropivacaine group), the median approximated the tenth and twenty-fifth percentile values. In this case, the median is 0 and only the seventy-fifth and ninetieth percentiles are clearly noted ($p < 0.05$: *, compared to saline for a given postoperative day. (Adapted, with permission, from Ilfeld BM, Morey TE, Wang RD, et al: Continuous popliteal sciatic nerve block for postoperative pain control at home: A randomized, double-blinded, placebo-controlled study. Anesthesiology 2002;97:959–965; Ilfeld BM, Morey TE, Wright TW, et al: Continuous interscalene brachial plexus block for postoperative pain control at home: A randomized, double-blinded, placebo-controlled study. Anesth Analg 2003;96:1089–1095.)

easily managed with oral opioids. This practice attempts to balance the potential benefits of this technique with the potential risks,[29,30] financial cost, and patient inconvenience of carrying an infusion pump with local anesthetic.[27] However, outpatient infusion can be used judicially in patients having *less invasive* procedures to decrease opioid requirements and opioid-related side effects.[3,31] Appropriate patient selection is crucial for safe outpatient infusion because not all patients desire, or are capable of accepting, the extra responsibility that comes with the use of the catheter and pump system. For instance, because some degree of postoperative cognitive dysfunction is common following surgery,[32] patients are often required to have a caretaker during infusion.[15–17,33–36] Whether a caretaker is necessary for one night or for the entire duration of infusion remains unresolved.[37] If removal of the catheter is expected to occur at home, then a caretaker willing to perform this procedure must be available at the infusion conclusion if the patient is unwilling or unable to do this (eg, psoas compartment catheter).

In medically unsupervised outpatients, complications may take longer to identify or be more difficult to manage than in hospitalized patients. Therefore, hepatic or renal insufficiency is a relative contraindication to outpatient infusion in an effort to avoid local anesthetic toxicity.[38] For infusions that may affect the phrenic nerve and ipsilateral diaphragm function (eg, interscalene or cervical paravertebral catheters), patients with lung disease (eg, reactive airway disease, chronic obstructive pulmonary disease) are often excluded because *continuous* interscalene local anesthetic infusions can result in ipsilateral diaphragm paralysis.[39] Consequently, conservative application of continuous interscalene block is suggested until additional investigation of hospitalized, medically supervised patients documents its safety,[40,41] although the effect on overall pulmonary function may be minimal for relatively healthy patients.[42]

SELECTION OF INSERTION TECHNIQUE

Clinical Pearls

- A negative aspiration test and "test dose" of local anesthetic and epinephrine via the catheter are suggested.
- Securing the catheter adequately is of crucial importance to avoid dislodgment.

In a substantial number of cases—as high as 40% in some reports[43]—inaccurate catheter placement may occur.[17,44,45] This issue is of critical importance for outpatients because catheter replacement is not an option after leaving the medical facility. Many techniques and types of equipment have been described for catheter insertion. Using one common technique, the initial local anesthetic bolus is given via the needle, followed by catheter placement. Using this method,

it is possible to provide a successful surgical block, but inaccurate catheter placement cannot be ruled out.[17] For ambulatory patients, inadequate perineural infusion often will not be detected until after surgical block resolution following home discharge.[17] Using another technique, investigators first inserted the catheter and then administered a bolus of local anesthetic via the catheter, with a reported failure rate of 1% to 8%.[46,47]

In an attempt to further improve catheter placement success rates, stimulating catheters were developed. These devices deliver electric current to the tip of the catheter.[48] The design provides feedback on the positional relationship of the catheter tip to the target nerve(s) prior to administering local anesthetics.[33,34] There is some evidence that confirming the placement of the catheter via stimulation *through* the catheter may improve the accuracy of catheter placement.[49] However, the optimal placement techniques and equipment for ambulatory perineural infusion have not been determined and require further investigation.[50] A negative aspiration test for blood and administration of epinephrine-containing local anesthetic (*test dose*) via the catheter is suggested to rule out intrathecal,[51] epidural,[52] or intravascular[53] placement prior to initiating infusion of local anesthetics, regardless of the equipment or technique used.

For patients at home, daily inspection of the catheter insertion site and reinforcement, when needed, may not be possible without home nursing care. Therefore, in an effort to minimize the risk of accidental dislodgement, every effort to optimally secure the catheter must be made prior to discharge. Such maneuvers include the use of sterile liquid adhesive (eg, benzoin), sterile tape (eg, Steri-Strips), securing of the catheter–hub connection with either tape or specifically designed devices (eg, StatLock), subcutaneous tunneling of the catheter,[48,54] and the use of 2-octyl cyanoacrylate glue.[55] Using a combination of these techniques, investigators have reported a catheter retention rate of 95% to 100% for over 60 h[33,34,36] and 85% for up to 7 days[27] in ambulatory patients.

LOCAL ANESTHETIC & ADJUVANT SELECTION

Clinical Pearls

- Most reports on outpatient perineural infusions involved the use of dilute concentrations of ropivacaine or bupivacaine.
- No adjuvant to local anesthetic infusion has demonstrated conclusive benefits.

Although perineural infusions of levobupivacaine[56] and shorter acting agents have been reported,[57–59] the majority of publications involve techniques using ropivacaine

0.2% or bupivacaine 0.125% to 0.25%. Currently, there is insufficient information to determine if there is an optimal local anesthetic (or concentration) for ambulatory infusions.[31,56,60] Although higher concentrations of local anesthetic provide additional analgesia, they also increase the risk of local anesthetic toxicity, undesirable motor blockade, and the incidence of a completely insensate extremity, and they may mask possible subsequent nerve compression injury.[16,18,36,59] In ambulatory patients, the degree of motor block provided by the infusion is an important consideration. The optimal concentration and infusion rate for a particular catheter site in relationship to the degree of motor block are not established. The only studies investigating local anesthetics and motor block involved patients with an interscalene catheter, and results suggested that 0.2% ropivacaine and 0.15% bupivacaine are associated with a low incidence of motor block and complete sensory block.[60,61] However, practitioners should note that even when using a low concentration of local anesthetic, complete motor and sensory block can occur.

Clonidine has been added to long-acting local anesthetic (1–2 mcg/mL) for *continuous* perineural femoral,[62] anterior lumbar plexus,[63–65] interscalene,[66] and popliteal[67] inpatient infusions. Although clonidine added to intermediate-acting local anesthetics increases the duration of *single-injection* nerve blocks,[68] the only available controlled investigations of adding clonidine to a *continuous* ropivacaine infusion (1 or 2 mcg/mL) do not reveal any clinically relevant benefits in outpatients.[35,69] Currently, there is little data to suggest any benefits from the addition of opioids and epinephrine to local anesthetic infusions.

Patient-Controlled Regional Analgesia

Clinical Pearls

- Providing patients with the ability to self-administer bolus doses maximizes the benefits of continuous perineural infusions.
- The optimal basal rate, bolus volume, and lockout time have not been determined.
- Commonly suggested infusion regimen: Basal 5–10 mL/h, bolus 2–5 mL, and lockout time 20–60 min.

Available inpatient and outpatient data suggest that following procedures producing moderate-to-severe pain, providing patients with the ability to self-administer local anesthetic doses (patient-controlled regional analgesia [PCRA]) increases perioperative benefits or decreases local anesthetic consumption (or both).[33–36,63,65,66] However, no information is available to base recommendations on the optimal basal rate, bolus volume, or lockout period, other than for interscalene catheters.[33] In all probability, these factors will also be influenced by the variables noted previously, such as surgical

pain intensity and choice of local anesthetic infusion. Until recommendations based on prospectively collected data are published, practitioners should be aware that investigators have reported successful analgesia using the following with long-acting local anesthetics: basal rate of 5 to 10 mL/h, bolus volume of 2 to 5 mL, and lockout duration of 20 to 60 min. The maximum safe doses for the long-acting local anesthetics remain unknown. However, multiple investigations involving patients free of renal or hepatic disease reported blood concentrations within acceptable limits following up to 5 days of perineural infusion with similar dosing schedules.[38,70–72] Extrapolating from data from patients receiving epidural bupivacaine infusion, a maximum infusion rate of 0.5 mg/kg/h of bupivacaine may be considered.[38]

Following ambulatory shoulder surgery with an interscalene catheter, infusion duration may be increased and similar baseline analgesia can be provided by decreasing the basal rate from 8 to 4 mL/h when patients supplement their block with large bolus doses (6 mL).[33] However, patients experience an increase in breakthrough pain incidence and intensity and sleep disturbances and a decrease in satisfaction with their analgesia. Therefore, if ambulatory patients do not return for additional local anesthetic, practitioners are left with the dilemma of superior analgesia for a shorter duration versus a lesser degree of analgesia for a longer period of time. Of note, the infusion duration can be increased by progressively decreasing the basal infusion rate with a reprogrammable infusion pump, thus theoretically maximizing postoperative analgesia.[7]

Studies that investigated the optimal dosing regimen for outpatients involved surgical procedures producing moderate postoperative pain. For procedures resulting in relatively *mild* postoperative pain, it is possible—even probable—that adequate analgesia would be adequately achieved with a bolus-only dosing regimen.[51] It is possible that the optimal dosing regimens, basal rates, and bolus doses may vary among different catheter types.[49] More data are necessary, however, before any such recommendations can be made.

Clinical Pearls

- Continuous peripheral nerve blocks often require supplemental analgesics.
- Oral opioids, NSAIDs, acetaminophen are suggested pharmacologic adjuncts for use with continuous peripheral nerve blocks in outpatients.
- Cryotherapy and elevation are common nonpharmacologic adjuncts.

Multimodal analgesia is an approach to pain control that combines a variety of pharmacologic and physical modalities. By combining modalities that have different mechanisms, clinicians can target multiple levels of the pathways that mediate postoperative pain. The goal of this approach is to optimize pain control by taking advantage of additive or synergistic analgesic effects between modalities while minimizing the unwanted side effects of individual agents.[73] Although continuous peripheral nerve blocks provide potent analgesia, they do not eliminate the need for other modalities. Randomized, placebo-controlled investigations demonstrated a decreased requirement for supplemental analgesia in outpatients with a perineural local anesthetic infusion; however, no protocol has eliminated the necessity for supplemental analgesia for all patients.[15–18] Systemic analgesics as well as nonpharmacologic modalities are important for optimizing analgesia and minimizing adverse effects.

Oral medications from several pharmacologic classes often are used in multimodal outpatient analgesic regimens. Common opioids used with continuous nerve blocks are oxycodone, hydrocodone, and codeine.[15–18] Nonsteroidal antiinflammtory drugs (NSAIDs) are an attractive addition to ambulatory multimodal analgesic regimens because of their unique mechanism, opioid-sparing effects, and lack of opioid-related side effects. Both traditional NSAIDs, such as ibuprofen and ketorolac, as well as COX2 inhibitors, such as celecoxib, have been used for outpatients.[15–17,27] However, with the recent controversy surrounding the safety of COX2 inhibitors, their future role as an adjunctive analgesic is now unclear.[74] Combining an NSAID with acetaminophen provides better analgesia than acetaminophen alone.[75,76] In contrast, study results are conflicting on whether the addition of acetaminophen to an analgesic regimen already including a traditional NSAID offers improved analgesia.[75–77] Although a formulation of opioid combined with acetaminophen or traditional NSAID adds to patient convenience, it also limits the amount of opioid available because of the maximum recommended doses of the nonopioid medications.

Nonpharmacologic techniques for pain control are simple and effective means of improving postoperative analgesia. Elevation, cryotherapy, ultrasound, transcutaneous electrical nerve stimulation (TENS), acupuncture, massage, biofeedback, and hypnosis have all been evaluated as postoperative analgesic adjuncts.[78–84] However, the concurrent use of these modalities with regional anesthesia remains unanswered. With respect to cooling, patients with decreased sensation or insensate extremities should be cautioned about the risk of cold injury to their skin when ice or cooling pads are applied to the blocked area, although there have been no case reports of complications due to cryotherapy. More discussion on the selection of local anesthetic solutions and multimodal analgesia may be found in Chapters 10 (Local Anesthetic Solutions for Continuous Nerve Blocks), 11 (Pharmacologic Considerations for Conscious Sedation and Nonopioid Analgesics in the Perioperative Period), 59 (Regional Anesthesia in the Patient with Preexisting Neurologic Disease), and 61 (Perioperative Management with Peripheral Nerve Block Anesthesia).

MEANS OF DELIVERY OF LOCAL ANESTHETICS: TECHNICAL CONSIDERATIONS

Clinical Pearls

- Commercially available infusion pumps vary in their infusion characteristics.
- When selecting an infusion pump, the technical characteristics should be taken into account.

A number of small, portable infusion pumps are currently available (Table 64–1, Figures 64–2 and 64–3), each with its benefits and limitations (Table 64–2). Many factors must be taken into account when determining the optimal device for a given clinical situation. The provided list of infusion devices includes those for which performance data are available from independent sources. The list is not inclusive of all available units.

Bolus Dose Capability

Various pumps allow for both patient-controlled local anesthetic boluses and a basal infusion (see Table 64–2), whereas others allow for only one of these.[85–89] Bolus dose capability (also termed PCRA) offers two significant benefits over a continuous infusion alone. First, higher doses of oral opiates are often required to control breakthrough pain without patient-controlled bolus doses.[34,88] Second, for outpatients using a limited local anesthetic reservoir, PCRA allows a provider to minimize the basal rate and, in turn, provide maximum infusion duration and minimal motor block,[7] yet also permits bolus dosing to control breakthrough pain[34] and use during physical therapy.[27,27,28,33,36] Compared with continuous infusions alone, equivalent or superior analgesia with a lower rate of local anesthetic consumption can be provided by using patient-controlled boluses of local anesthetic.[34,63,65,66]

The means by which the bolus dose is provided may also be an important factor in patient safety and convenience. A number of elastomeric pumps provide bolus-only dosing by having the patient release an occluding clamp on the tubing connecting the pump and catheter. Investigators provided these units to patients with the instructions to initiate the bolus by releasing the clamp, watch a clock and reclamp the tubing after a preset number of minutes.[3,31] However, it is possible for the entire contents of the local anesthetic reservoir to be administered in under an hour if the patient forgets to reclamp the tubing. This potentially dangerous scenario has been reported, although no apparent adverse results have occurred.[5] In contrast, electronic pumps offer easily depressed buttons that deliver a controlled volume and are easily used by patients who have difficulty applying force to a clamp or bolus button (eg, patients with arthritis). Practitioners should consider the

Table 64–1.

Distributors and Manufacturers of Infusion Pumps

Pump (Reference)	Distributor	City	State
6060 MT[89]	Baxter Healthcare	Deerfield	IL
Accufuser[85] and Accufuser Plus XL[86,87,89]	McKinley Medical	Wheat Ridge	CO
ambIT LPM[89] and ambIT PCA[89]	Sorenson Medical	West Jordan	UT
AutoMed 3200[89] and AutoMed 3400[87]	Algos, LC	Salt Lake City	UT
BlockIt (WalkMed)[86]	McKinley Medical	Wheat Ridge	CO
CADD-Legacy PCA[86] and CADD-Prism PCS[86]	Smiths Medical	St. Paul	MN
C-Bloc[85]	I-Flow Corporation	Lake Forest	CA
Infusor LV5[87]	Baxter Healthcare	Deerfield	IL
Ipump[89]	Baxter Healthcare	Deerfield	IL
Microject PCA[85,86] and Microject PCEA[87]	Sorenson Medical	West Jordan	UT
On-Q C-Bloc with OnDemand[89]	I-Flow Corporation	Lake Forest	CA
Pain Care 3200[87]	Breg, Inc.	Vista	CA
Pain Pump I[85]	Stryker Instruments	Kalamazoo	MI
Pain Pump II[87]	Stryker Instruments	Kalamazoo	MI
Sgarlato[85]	Sgarlato Labs	Los Gatos	CA

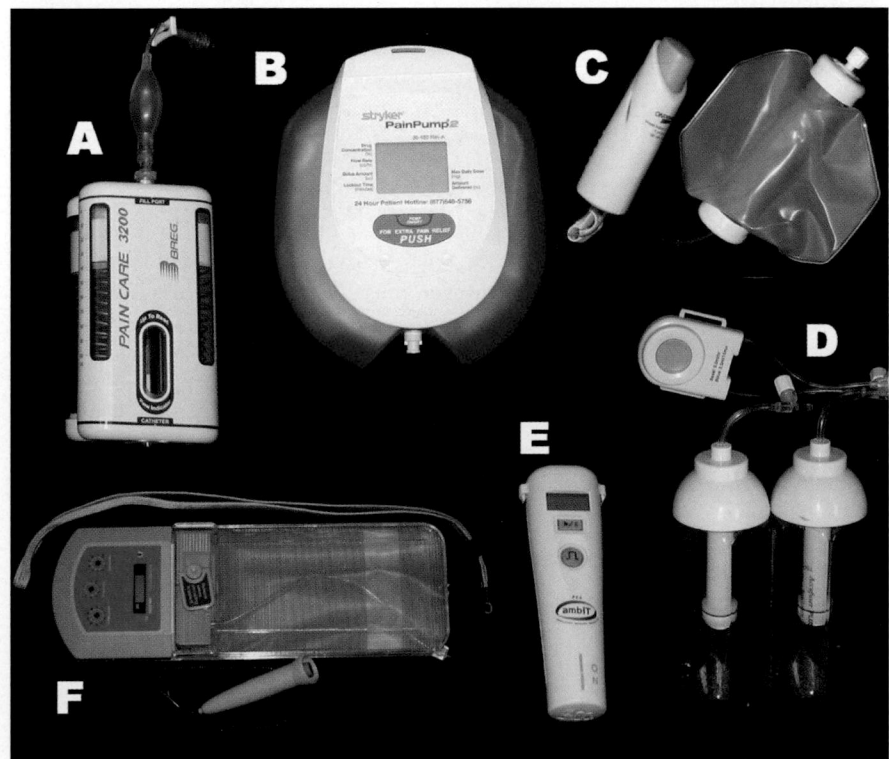

Figure 64–2. Examples of portable *disposable* basal- and bolus-capable infusion pumps. Pain Care 3200 (**A**), Pain Pump II (**B**), On-Q C-Bloc with OnDemand (**C**), Accufuser Plus XL (**D**), ambIT PCA (**E**), and AutoMed 3200 (**F**). Distributor information and pump attributes are included in the Appendix and Table 64–2. Note that the ambIT PCA is produced as a disposable model as well as a more expensive reusable unit. It appears in both Figures 64–2 and 64–3.

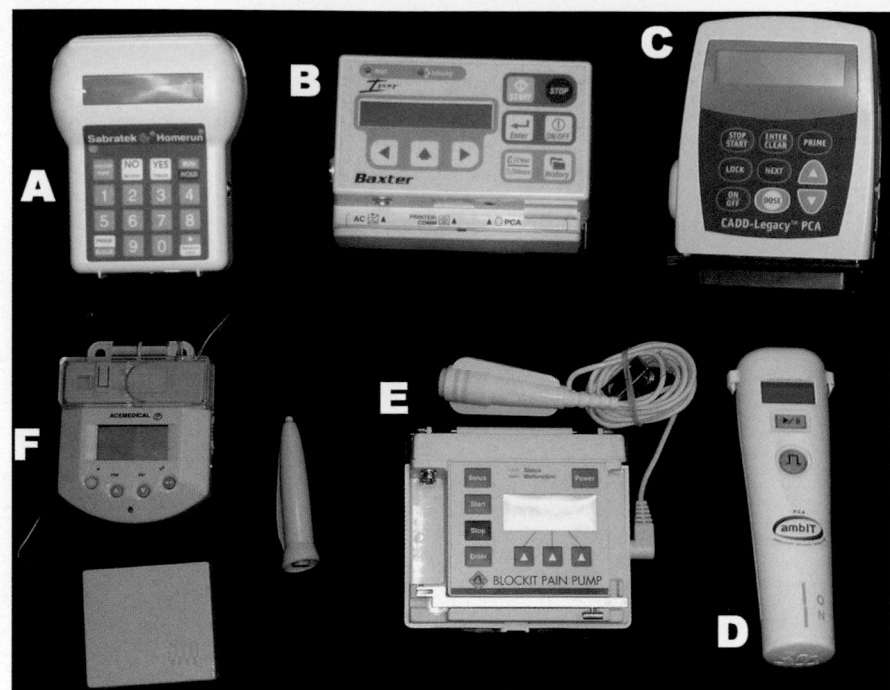

Figure 64–3. Examples of portable *reusable* basal- *and* bolus-capable infusion pumps. 6060 MT (**A**), Ipump PMS (**B**), CADD-Legacy PCA (**C**), ambIT PCA (**D**), BlockIt (**E**), and AutoMed 3400 (**F**). Distributor information and pump attributes are included in Table 64–2. Note that the ambIT PCA is produced as a disposable model as well as a more expensive reusable unit. It appears in both Figures 64–2 and 64–3.

relative risks and benefits now that multiple pumps are available for the provision of *controlled* bolus dosing (see Table 64–2).

Programmability

If various rates of infusion, bolus volumes, and lockout times are desired, an electronic pump is preferred. Most of the non-electronic pumps can be ordered at various infusion rates, however, the infusion rate and bolus volume are usually fixed by the manufacturer and cannot be adjusted (Baxter Healthcare International manufactures an elastomeric pump with an adjustable basal rate; however, this pump is unavailable in the United States). Just as found with epidural infusions, the optimal basal infusion rate for perineural catheters varies greatly among patients.[15,35] Analgesia can be optimized by allowing patients to vary their basal rate with instructions from a health care provider via the telephone.[7,35]

Accuracy, Consistency, Reliability

For the purposes of this chapter, *accuracy* is defined as infusing at the set/expected rate, while *consistency* is infusing at the same rate for the majority of the time of infusion. For these attributes, there are currently no government-defined minimum standards. In general, elastomeric devices provide a higher-than-expected basal rate initially (110%–150% expected), returning to their expected rate within 2 to 12 h, and again increasing to a higher rate prior to reservoir exhaustion.[85–87,89,90] Electronic infusion pumps provide highly accurate (90%–100% expected) and consistent (±5% baseline) basal rates over the entire infusion duration.[85–87,89] Spring-powered pumps initially provide a higher-than-expected basal rate (115%–135% expected),

which steadily decreases to a lower-than-expected rate (70%–75% expected) by reservoir exhaustion.[85,87,90] There are insufficient data to determine the clinical situations in which the typical basal rate variation of nonelectronic pumps would be clinically relevant. In studies using elastomeric pumps, it remained unknown if providing a more uniform basal rate would have affected outcomes.[6,14,17]

There are little available data regarding infusion pump *reliability* (eg, failure rates).[91] While irritating alarms cannot be triggered by nonelectronic pumps,[92] there is also no warning of a pump malfunction or catheter occlusion.[16] Some electronic pumps were noted to infuse without an erroneous alarm for over 10,000 cumulative hours of clinical use.[33,34,36]

Disposability & Cost

Reusable electronic infusion pumps are generally more expensive than the available single-use/disposable models (see Table 64–2). However, reusable pumps that use relatively inexpensive disposable "cassettes" for each new patient (cost usually ~US $10) may be more cost-effective for practitioners who use these devices repeatedly (see Table 64–2). But, a reusable unit requires the patient to return the infusion pump by either the mail service or revisiting the surgical center.[33,34,36]

Miscellaneous Factors

A temperature-dependent device regulates the infusion rate of most elastomeric pumps.[85–87,89] Current units are more resistant to temperature variations than older pump models, which responded to a 4°C increase in ambient temperature with an increase up to 35% in their basal rate.[85–87,89] Therefore, if patients are instructed to avoid temperature

Table 64–2.

Technical Characteristics of Available Infusion Pumps

Pump Model (References)	Wt.[a] (g)	Reservoir Volume (max mL)	Basal Infusion (mL/h)	Bolus Dose (mL)	Bolus Lockout (min–h)	Retail Price (U.S. $)	Power Source
6060 MT[89]	525	IV bag[b]	0.1–50.0	0–50	0–60	3995	Electronic
ambIT PCA[89]	133	IV bag[b]	0–20	0–20	5–24	500–800[c]	Electronic
AutoMed 3400[87]	325	IV bag[b]	0–50	0–50	0–60	675	Electronic
BlockIt (WalkMed)[86]	323	IV bag[b]	0–30	0–30	0–24	1750–2300	Electronic
CADD-Legacy PCA[86]	372	IV bag[b]	0–50	0–9.9	5–24	3595	Electronic
CADD-Prism PCS[86]	547	IV bag[b]	0–30	0–9.9	5–24	4125	Electronic
Ipump PMS[89]	415	IV bag[b]	0–19.9[d]	0–9.9	1–6	4295	Electronic
Microject PCA[e85,86]	198	IV bag[b]	0–9.9	0–2	6–1	N/A[e]	Electronic
Microject PCEA[e87]	198	IV bag[b]	0–29	0–10	10–120	N/A[e]	Electronic
ambIT LPM[89]	133	IV bag[b]	0–20	0–20	5–24	250–350[c]	Electronic
AutoMed 3200[89]	350	250	0–10	0–5	2–60	255	Electronic
Pain Pump II[87]	408	400	0.5–15	0–15	10–2	250[c]	Electronic
Accufuser Plus XL[86,87,89]	109	550	5, 8, or 10[f]	2	15, 60 min[f]	260	Elastomeric
Pain Care 3200[87]	290	200	5.7–2.9[f,g]	4–6[f,g]	40–1.3[f,g]	175	Spring
On-Q C-Bloc with OnDemand[89]	135	400[h]	5	5	60 min[f]	250–500	Elastomeric
Accufuser[85]	95	275	2, 4, 5, 8, 10[f]	N/A	N/A	150–225	Elastomeric
C-Bloc[85]	65	400	5 or 10[f]	N/A	N/A	395[c]	Elastomeric
Infusor LV5[87]	65	275	2, 5, 7, 10[f]	N/A	N/A	55	Elastomeric
Pain Pump I[85]	104	120	0.8, 2.1, 4.2[f]	N/A	N/A	150[c]	Vacuum
Sgarlato[85]	225	200	0.5, 1, 2, 4[f]	N/A	N/A	225[c]	Spring

N/A: Not applicable.

[a] *Including batteries and disposable cassette in electronic pumps; and excluding infusate for all pumps.*

[b] *Local anesthetic reservoir is an external syringe or IV-style bag of any size.*

[c] *Approximate price for Florida (US): other regions may vary.*

[d] *If a bolus dose is not provided, the maximum basal rate is 90 mL/h.*

[e] *The Microject pumps are reusable because disposable cassettes are used with the mechanical pump, but the pumps themselves are less expensive than some "disposable" pumps, and may thus be considered disposable, if desired. Not available in the United States.*

[f] *Fixed during manufacture.*

[g] *Basal infusion rate described as "4 mL/h continuous flow" on product packaging and marketing materials. However, product information contained within the instruction manual specifies that the rate is 5.7 mL/h at the beginning of the infusion, and steadily declines to 2.9 mL/h by reservoir exhaustion. Bolus dose is variable, and lock-out increases as infusion progresses.[87]*

[h] *On-Q C-Block with OnDemand may be "overfilled" to 500 mL, decreasing the basal rate for a portion of the infusion, but allowing for a longer infusion duration.[89]*

extremes, infusion rate variability is easily minimized. Elastomeric pump infusion rates are reduced at high altitude (hypobaric conditions).[93] It should also be noted that the basal infusion rate, patient-administered bolus dose volume and frequency, and infusion duration determine the required local anesthetic reservoir volume (see Table 64–2). Most spring-powered and electronic pumps are refillable; however, elastomeric pumps may not function properly if simply refilled. For more discussion on equipment for continuous peripheral nerve blocks the reader is referred to Chapter 49 (Stimulating Catheters).

DISCHARGE CRITERIA & PATIENT INSTRUCTIONS

Discharge criteria and patient instructions include the following considerations.

Clinical Pearls

- Discharge of the patient with an insensate extremity is associated with a low degree of risk.
- A prescription for oral opioids should be filled by patients following discharge.
- Oral and written instructions, including health care provider contact numbers, should be provided.

Obviously, mobilization is a requirement for home discharge. For this reason, discharge with a peripheral nerve block of the lower extremity remains controversial.[94] Following a single-injection nerve block for ambulatory surgery, discharge with an insensate extremity results in minimal complications.[95] However, whether patients should weight-bear with a continuous peripheral nerve block remains unexamined. Therefore, conservative management may be optimal, and some investigators recommended that patients avoid using their surgical limb for weight bearing.[8,16,36] This is usually accomplished with the use of crutches, and the patient's ability to use these aids without syncope or difficulty must be demonstrated prior to discharge. Protecting the surgical extremity must be emphasized, and except during physical therapy sessions, any removable brace or splint should remain in place.

Postoperative analgesic requirements cannot be assessed if the initial surgical block remains unresolved prior to discharge. Most patients require oral analgesics to supplement their perineural local anesthetic infusion.[33,34,36] Supplemental oral opioid use depends on many factors, such as the type of surgery, other analgesic adjuvants such as cryotherapy, the local anesthetic infused, and the dosing regimen provided, as well as patient's pain tolerance and preoperative analgesic therapy. Furthermore, the possibility of catheter misplacement during the initial insertion or subsequent dislodgement or equipment failure mandates that oral analgesics be immediately available. Unfortunately, there are no means to accurately *predict* which patients will require oral opioids. Therefore, a prescription for oral analgesics should be provided to all patients, and the importance of filling the prescription immediately after leaving the surgical center should be emphasized. If patients wait to fill the prescription until after they have determined that oral analgesics are required, a period of inadequate analgesia may result.

Most investigators educate both the patient and his or her caretaker at the same time prior to discharge because most patients have some degree of postoperative cognitive dysfunction. Both verbal and written instructions should be provided, along with contact numbers for health care providers who are available throughout the infusion duration.[6,15,31,96] In addition to standard outpatient instructions, topics reviewed often include expectations regarding surgical block resolution, infusion pump instructions, breakthrough pain treatment, catheter site care, limb protection, and the plan for catheter removal. Forewarning the patient that pain in the operative limb is anticipated following surgical block resolution and fluid leakage at the catheter site is common (and what to do if these are experienced) often proves helpful. Signs and symptoms of possible catheter- and local anesthetic-related complications include, but are not limited to, pulmonary compromise,[40,41] nerve injury,[97] site infection,[98] and local anesthetic toxicity.[53] Although there are case reports of *initially* misplaced catheters, *migration* following a documented correct placement has not been described, but remains a theoretical risk.[51–53,99,100] Possible complications of an unidentified initially misplaced catheter or of a catheter migration include intravascular or interpleural catheterization resulting in local anesthetic toxicity, intramuscular catheterization resulting in myonecrosis, and epidural/intrathecal catheterization when using interscalene, paravertebral, or psoas compartment catheters. As is the standard of care for inpatients, health care providers may want to consider documenting each patient contact (Figure 64–4).

Catheter removal is achieved with various techniques: patients may be discharged with written instructions,[12] a health care provider may perform this procedure,[101] or patients' caretakers (or occasionally the patients themselves) may remove the catheters with instructions given by a provider over the telephone.[15–17,33,34,36] One survey suggested that with instructions given by phone, 98% of patients felt comfortable removing their catheter at home, only 4% would have preferred to return for a health care provider to remove the catheter, and 43% responded that they would have felt comfortable even with written instructions only.[102] Nonsterile gloves can be given to patients for catheter removal at home.[15–17]

SUMMARY

Data from prospective, randomized studies suggest that perineural local anesthetic infusion is a technique that can provide excellent postoperative analgesia, letter sleep quality, and patient satisfaction while decreasing supplemental opioid

Florida Surgical Center
AT SHANDS HOSPITAL AT THE UNIVERSITY OF FLORIDA

Progress Note for Ambulatory Perineural Local Anesthetic Infusion

Surgery Date_____/_____/200__   Surgeon:_____   Home phone: (_____) _____ - _____

Procedure: _____   Other phone: (_____) _____ - _____

Post-op in PACU
- ☐ Catheter w/ neg. aspiration & _____ mL of _____ w/ _____ µg epinephrine/mL to catheter w/ neg. aspiration q2 mL
- ☐ No heart rate or sensory changes within 3 minutes
- ☐ Verbal and written instructions given to patient/care-taker & all questions answered, MD phone #s provided
- ☐ Pump tubing secured to catheter, pump programmed & infusion begun

Notes: _____
                                                                          Physician Signature

POD #0 _____:_____
- ☐ Patient or patient's caretaker contacted by phone
- ☐ Symptoms of local anesthetic toxicity, catheter migration and infection denied
- ☐ Appropriate sensory/motor function of affected extremity acknowledged
- ☐ Surgical pain under control
- ☐ Patient would like to have catheter remain in situ at this time
- ☐ All questions answered

Notes: _____
                                                                          Physician Signature

POD #1 _____:_____
- ☐ Patient or patient's caretaker contacted by phone
- ☐ Symptoms of local anesthetic toxicity, catheter migration and infection denied
- ☐ Appropriate sensory/motor function of affected extremity acknowledged
- ☐ Surgical pain under control
- ☐ Patient would like to have catheter remain in situ at this time
- ☐ All questions answered

Notes: _____
                                                                          Physician Signature

POD #2 _____:_____
- ☐ Patient or patient's caretaker contacted by phone
- ☐ Symptoms of local anesthetic toxicity, catheter migration and infection denied
- ☐ Appropriate sensory/motor function of affected extremity acknowledged
- ☐ Surgical pain under control
- ☐ Patient would like to have catheter remain in situ at this time
- ☐ Catheter removed by patient's caretaker with MD on phone, tip reported to be blue/silver
- ☐ All questions answered

Notes: _____
                                                                          Physician Signature

POD #3 _____:_____
- ☐ Patient or patient's caretaker contacted by phone
- ☐ Symptoms of local anesthetic toxicity, catheter migration and infection denied
- ☐ Appropriate sensory/motor function of affected extremity acknowledged
- ☐ Surgical pain under control
- ☐ Patient would like to have catheter remain in situ at this time
- ☐ Catheter removed by patient's caretaker with MD on phone, tip reported to be blue/silver
- ☐ All questions answered

Notes: _____
                                                                          Physician Signature

POD #4 _____:_____
- ☐ Patient or patient's caretaker contacted by phone
- ☐ Symptoms of local anesthetic toxicity, catheter migration and infection denied
- ☐ Appropriate sensory/motor function of affected extremity acknowledged
- ☐ Surgical pain under control
- ☐ Patient would like to have catheter remain in situ at this time
- ☐ Catheter removed by patient's caretaker with MD on phone, tip reported to be blue/silver
- ☐ All questions answered

Notes: _____
                                                                          Physician Signature

Figure 64–4. An example of a progress note that can be used to record telephone contacts with ambulatory patients. (Reproduced, with permission, from Ilfeld BM, Enneking FK: Continuous peripheral nerve blocks at home: A review. Anesth Analg 2005;100:1822–1823.)

requirements and opioid-related side effects. A basal infusion maximizes infusion benefits, while providing patient-controlled bolus doses allows for a decreased basal rate and increased duration of infusion (less local anesthetic consumption). Perineural infusion in outpatients is a relatively new concept, and many aspects of this analgesic technique are awaiting more clarification. In keeping with evidence-based medical practice, optimal techniques, equipment, and patient selection should be determined by prospective, controlled trials, and not merely by institutional preference.

References

1. Rawal N, Hylander J, Nydahl PA, et al: Survey of postoperative analgesia following ambulatory surgery. Acta Anaesthesiol Scand 1997;41:1017–1022.
2. Ansbro FP: A method of continuous brachial plexus block. Am J Surg 1946;71:716–722.
3. Rawal N, Axelsson K, Hylander J, et al: Postoperative patient-controlled local anesthetic administration at home. Anesth Analg 1998;86:86–89.
4. Buckenmaier CC III, Klein SM, Nielsen KC, et al: Continuous paravertebral catheter and outpatient infusion for breast surgery. Anesth Analg 2003;97:715–717.
5. Ganapathy S, Amendola A, Lichfield R, et al: Elastomeric pumps for ambulatory patient controlled regional analgesia. Can J Anaesth 2000;47:897–902.
6. Macaire P, Gaertner E, Capdevila X: Continuous post-operative regional analgesia at home. Minerva Anestesiol 2001;67:109–116.
7. Ilfeld BM, Enneking FK: A portable mechanical pump providing over four days of patient-controlled analgesia by perineural infusion at home. Reg Anesth Pain Med 2002;27:100–104.
8. Corda DM, Enneking FK: A unique approach to postoperative analgesia for ambulatory surgery. J Clin Anesth 2000;12:595–599.
9. Grant SA, Nielsen KC, Greengrass RA, et al: Continuous peripheral nerve block for ambulatory surgery. Reg Anesth Pain Med 2001;26:209–214.
10. Klein SM, Greengrass RA, Grant SA, et al: Ambulatory surgery for multi-ligament knee reconstruction with continuous dual catheter peripheral nerve blockade. Can J Anaesth 2001;48:375–378.
11. Chelly JE, Gebhard R, Coupe K, et al: Local anesthetic delivered via a femoral catheter by patient-controlled analgesia pump for pain relief after an anterior cruciate ligament outpatient procedure. Am J Anesthesiol 2001;28(4):192–194.
12. Klein SM, Greengrass RA, Gleason DH, et al: Major ambulatory surgery with continuous regional anesthesia and a disposable infusion pump. Anesthesiology 1999;91:563–513.
13. Ilfeld BM, Smith DW, Enneking FK: Continuous regional analgesia following ambulatory pediatric orthopedic surgery. Am J Orthop 2004;33:405–408.
14. Klein SM, Grant SA, Greengrass RA, et al: Interscalene brachial plexus block with a continuous catheter insertion system and a disposable infusion pump. Anesth Analg 2000;91:1473–1478.
15. Ilfeld BM, Morey TE, Enneking FK: Continuous infraclavicular brachial plexus block for postoperative pain control at home: A randomized, double-blinded, placebo-controlled study. Anesthesiology 2002;96:1297–1304.
16. Ilfeld BM, Morey TE, Wang RD, et al: Continuous popliteal sciatic nerve block for postoperative pain control at home: A randomized, double-blinded, placebo-controlled study. Anesthesiology 2002;97:959–965.
17. Ilfeld BM, Morey TE, Wright TW, et al: Continuous interscalene brachial plexus block for postoperative pain control at home: A randomized, double-blinded, placebo-controlled study. Anesth Analg 2003;96:1089–1095.
18. White PF, Issioui T, Skrivanek GD, et al: The use of a continuous popliteal sciatic nerve block after surgery involving the foot and ankle: Does it improve the quality of recovery? Anesth Analg 2003;97:1303–1309.
19. Wu CL, Naqibuddin M, Rowlingson AJ, et al: The effect of pain on health-related quality of life in the immediate postoperative period. Anesth Analg 2003;97:1078–1085.
20. Public health focus: Surveillance, prevention, and control of nosocomial infections. MMWR CDC Surveill Summ 1992;41:783–787.
21. Wenzel RP, Edmond MB: The impact of hospital-acquired bloodstream infections. Emerg Infect Dis 2001;7:174–177.
22. Relman AS: The institute of medicine report on the quality of health care. N Engl J Med 2001;345:702–703.
23. Leape LL: Institute of Medicine medical error figures are not exaggerated. JAMA 2000;284:95–97.
24. Mushinski M: Average charges for hip replacement surgeries: United States, 1997. Stat Bull Metrop Insur Co 1999;80:32–40.
25. Mushinski M: Average charges for a total knee replacement: United States, 1994. Stat Bull Metrop Insur Co 1996;77:24–30.
26. Weinstein J: *The Dartmouth Atlas of Musculoskeletal Health Care*. AHA Press, 2000.
27. Ilfeld BM, Wright TW, Enneking FK, et al: Effect of interscalene perineural local anesthetic infusion on postoperative physical therapy following total shoulder replacement. Reg Anesth Pain Med 2004;29:A18.
28. Ilfeld BM, Gearen PF, Enneking FK, et al: Effect of femoral perineural local anesthetic infusion on postoperative functional ability following total knee arthroplasty. Anesthesiology 2004;101:A945.
29. Ekatodramis G, Macaire P, Borgeat A: Prolonged Horner syndrome due to neck hematoma after continuous interscalene block. Anesthesiology 2001;95:801–803.
30. Ribeiro FC, Georgousis H, Bertram R, et al: Plexus irritation caused by interscalene brachial plexus catheter for shoulder surgery. Anesth Analg 1996;82:870–872.
31. Rawal N, Allvin R, Axelsson K, et al: Patient-controlled regional analgesia (PCRA) at home: Controlled comparison between bupivacaine and ropivacaine brachial plexus analgesia. Anesthesiology 2002;96:1290–1296.
32. Johnson T, Monk T, Rasmussen LS, et al: Postoperative cognitive dysfunction in middle-aged patients. Anesthesiology 2002;96:1351–1357.
33. Ilfeld BM, Morey TE, Wright TW, et al: Interscalene perineural ropivacaine infusion: A comparison of two dosing regimens for postoperative analgesia. Reg Anesth Pain Med 2004;29:9–16.
34. Ilfeld BM, Morey TE, Enneking FK: Infraclavicular perineural local anesthetic infusion: A comparison of three dosing regimens for postoperative analgesia. Anesthesiology 2004;100:395–402.
35. Ilfeld BM, Morey TE, Enneking FK: Continuous infraclavicular perineural infusion with clonidine and ropivacaine compared with ropivacaine alone: A randomized, double-blinded, controlled study. Anesth Analg 2003;97:706–712.
36. Ilfeld BM, Thannikary LJ, Morey TE, et al: Popliteal sciatic perineural local anesthetic infusion: A comparison of three dosing regimens for postoperative analgesia. Anesthesiology 2004;101:970–907.
37. Klein SM, Steele SM, Nielsen KC, et al: The difficulties of ambulatory interscalene and intra-articular infusions for rotator cuff surgery: A preliminary report: [Difficultes des perfusions interscalenes et intra-articulaires ambulatoires pour la reparation de la coiffe des rotateurs: Un rapport preliminaire]. Can J Anaesth 2003;50:265–269.
38. Denson DD, Raj PP, Saldahna F, et al: Continuous perineural infusion of bupivacaine for prolonged analgesia: Pharmacokinetic considerations. Int J Clin Pharmacol Ther Toxicol 1983;21:591–597.
39. Pere P: The effect of continuous interscalene brachial plexus block with 0.125% bupivacaine plus fentanyl on diaphragmatic motility and ventilatory function. Reg Anesth 1993;18:93–97.

40. Smith MP, Tetzlaff JE, Brems JJ: Asymptomatic profound oxyhemoglobin desaturation following interscalene block in a geriatric patient. Reg Anesth Pain Med 1998;23:210–213.

41. Sardesai AM, Chakrabarti AJ, Denny NM: Lower lobe collapse during continuous interscalene brachial plexus local anesthesia at home. Reg Anesth Pain Med 2004;29:65–68.

42. Borgeat A, Perschak H, Bird P, et al: Patient-controlled interscalene analgesia with ropivacaine 0.2% versus patient-controlled intravenous analgesia after major shoulder surgery: Effects on diaphragmatic and respiratory function. Anesthesiology 2000;92:102–108.

43. Salinas FV: Location, location, location: Continuous peripheral nerve blocks and stimulating catheters. Reg Anesth Pain Med 2003;28:79–82.

44. Coleman MM, Chan VW: Continuous interscalene brachial plexus block. Can J Anaesth 1999;46:209–214.

45. Ganapathy S, Wasserman RA, Watson JT, et al: Modified continuous femoral three-in-one block for postoperative pain after total knee arthroplasty. Anesth Analg 1999;89:1197–1202.

46. Borgeat A, Dullenkopf A, Ekatodramis G, et al: Evaluation of the lateral modified approach for continuous interscalene block after shoulder surgery. Anesthesiology 2003;99:436–442.

47. Borgeat A, Blumenthal S, Karovic D, et al: Clinical evaluation of a modified posterior anatomical approach to performing the popliteal block. Reg Anesth Pain Med 2004;29:290–296.

48. Boezaart AP, de Beer JF, du TC, et al: A new technique of continuous interscalene nerve block. Can J Anaesth 1999;46:275–281.

49. Salinas FV, Neal JM, Sueda LA, et al: Prospective comparison of continuous femoral nerve block with nonstimulating catheter placement versus stimulating catheter-guided perineural placement in volunteers. Reg Anesth Pain Med 2004;29:212–220.

50. Chelly JE, Williams BA: Continuous perineural infusions at home: Narrowing the focus. Reg Anesth Pain Med 2004;29:1–3.

51. Litz RJ, Vicent O, Wiessner D, et al: Misplacement of a psoas compartment catheter in the subarachnoid space. Reg Anesth Pain Med 2004;29:60–64.

52. Cook LB: Unsuspected extradural catheterization in an interscalene block. Br J Anaesth 1991;67:473–475.

53. Tuominen MK, Pere P, Rosenberg PH: Unintentional arterial catheterization and bupivacaine toxicity associated with continuous interscalene brachial plexus block. Anesthesiology 1991;75:356–358.

54. Ekatodramis G, Borgeat A: Subcutaneous tunneling of the interscalene catheter. Can J Anaesth 2000;47:716–717.

55. Klein SM, Nielsen KC, Buckenmaier CC, III, et al: 2-Octyl cyanoacrylate glue for the fixation of continuous peripheral nerve catheters. Anesthesiology 2003;98:590–591.

56. Casati A, Borghi B, Fanelli G, et al: Interscalene brachial plexus anesthesia and analgesia for open shoulder surgery: A randomized, double-blinded comparison between levobupivacaine and ropivacaine. Anesth Analg 2003;96:253–259.

57. Buettner J, Klose R, Hoppe U, et al: Serum levels of mepivacaine-HCl during continuous axillary brachial plexus block. Reg Anesth 1989;14:124–127.

58. Wajima Z, Shitara T, Nakajima Y, et al: Comparison of continuous brachial plexus infusion of butorphanol, mepivacaine and mepivacaine–butorphanol mixtures for postoperative analgesia. Br J Anaesth 1995;75:548–551.

59. Bergman BD, Hebl JR, Kent J, et al: Neurologic complications of 405 consecutive continuous axillary catheters. Anesth Analg 2003;96:247–252.

60. Borgeat A, Kalberer F, Jacob H, et al: Patient-controlled interscalene analgesia with ropivacaine 0.2% versus bupivacaine 0.15% after major open shoulder surgery: The effects on hand motor function. Anesth Analg 2001;92:218–223.

61. Casati A, Vinciguerra F, Scarioni M, et al: Lidocaine versus ropivacaine for continuous interscalene brachial plexus block after open shoulder surgery. Acta Anaesthesiol Scand 2003;47:355–360.

62. Capdevila X, Barthelet Y, Biboulet P, et al: Effects of perioperative analgesic technique on the surgical outcome and duration of rehabilitation after major knee surgery. Anesthesiology 1999;91:8–15.

63. Singelyn FJ, Gouverneur JM: Extended "three-in-one" block after total knee arthroplasty: Continuous versus patient-controlled techniques. Anesth Analg 2000;91:176–180.

64. Singelyn FJ, Deyaert M, Joris D, et al: Effects of intravenous patient-controlled analgesia with morphine, continuous epidural analgesia, and continuous three-in-one block on postoperative pain and knee rehabilitation after unilateral total knee arthroplasty. Anesth Analg 1998;87:88–92.

65. Singelyn FJ, Vanderelst PE, Gouverneur JM: Extended femoral nerve sheath block after total hip arthroplasty: Continuous versus patient-controlled techniques. Anesth Analg 2001;92:455–459.

66. Singelyn FJ, Seguy S, Gouverneur JM: Interscalene brachial plexus analgesia after open shoulder surgery: Continuous versus patient-controlled infusion. Anesth Analg 1999;89:1216–12120.

67. Singelyn FJ, Aye F, Gouverneur JM: Continuous popliteal sciatic nerve block: An original technique to provide postoperative analgesia after foot surgery. Anesth Analg 1997;84:383–386.

68. Iskandar H, Guillaume E, Dixmerias F, et al: The enhancement of sensory blockade by clonidine selectively added to mepivacaine after midhumeral block. Anesth Analg 2001;93:771–775.

69. Ilfeld BM, Morey TE, Thannikary LJ, et al: Clonidine added to a continuous interscalene ropivacaine perineural infusion to improve postoperative analgesia: A randomized, double-blind, controlled study. Anesth Analg 2005;100:1172–1178.

70. Ekatodramis G, Borgeat A, Huledal G, et al: Continuous interscalene analgesia with ropivacaine 2 mg/mL after major shoulder surgery. Anesthesiology 2003;98:143–150.

71. Kaloul I, Guay J, Cote C, et al: Ropivacaine plasma concentrations are similar during continuous lumbar plexus blockade using the anterior three-in-one and the posterior psoas compartment techniques: [Les concentrations plasmatiques de ropivacaine sont similaires pendant le bloc continu du plexus lombaire realise par voie anterieure trois-en-un et par voie posterieure de la loge du psoas]. Can J Anaesth 2004;51:52–56.

72. Anker-Moller E, Spangsberg N, Dahl JB, et al: Continuous blockade of the lumbar plexus after knee surgery: A comparison of the plasma concentrations and analgesic effect of bupivacaine 0.250% and 0.125%. Acta Anaesthesiol Scand 1990;34:468–472.

73. Kehlet H, Dahl JB: The value of "multimodal" or "balanced analgesia" in postoperative pain treatment. Anesth Analg 1993;77:1048–1056.

74. FitzGerald GA: Coxibs and cardiovascular disease. N Engl J Med 2004;351:1709–1711.

75. Hyllested M, Jones S, Pedersen JL, et al: Comparative effect of paracetamol, NSAIDs or their combination in postoperative pain management: A qualitative review. Br J Anaesth 2002;88:199–214.

76. Montgomery JE, Sutherland CJ, Kestin IG, et al: Morphine consumption in patients receiving rectal paracetamol and diclofenac alone and in combination. Br J Anaesth 1996;77:445–447.

77. Dahl V, Dybvik T, Steen T, et al: Ibuprofen vs. acetaminophen vs. ibuprofen and acetaminophen after arthroscopically assisted anterior cruciate ligament reconstruction. Eur J Anaesthesiol 2004;21:471–475.

78. Tyler E, Caldwell C, Ghia JN: Transcutaneous electrical nerve stimulation: An alternative approach to the management of postoperative pain. Anesth Analg 1982;61:449–456.

79. Hashish I, Hai HK, Harvey W, et al: Reduction of postoperative pain and swelling by ultrasound treatment: A placebo effect. Pain 1988;33:303–311.

80. Carroll D, Tramer M, McQuay H, et al: Randomization is important in studies with pain outcomes: Systematic review of transcutaneous electrical nerve stimulation in acute postoperative pain. Br J Anaesth 1996;77:798–803.

81. Montgomery GH, David D, Winkel G, et al: The effectiveness of adjunctive hypnosis with surgical patients: A meta-analysis. Anesth Analg 2002;94:1639–1645.

82. Webb JM, Williams D, Ivory JP, et al: The use of cold compression dressings after total knee replacement: A randomized controlled trial. Orthopedics 1998;21:59–61.

83. Singh H, Osbahr DC, Holovacs TF, et al: The efficacy of continuous cryotherapy on the postoperative shoulder: A prospective, randomized investigation. J Shoulder Elbow Surg 2001;10:522–525.

84. Saito N, Horiuchi H, Kobayashi S, et al: Continuous local cooling for pain relief following total hip arthroplasty. J Arthroplasty 2004;19:334–337.

85. Ilfeld BM, Morey TE, Enneking FK: The delivery rate accuracy of portable infusion pumps used for continuous regional analgesia. Anesth Analg 2002;95:1331–1336.

86. Ilfeld BM, Morey TE, Enneking FK: Delivery rate accuracy of portable, bolus-capable infusion pumps used for patient-controlled continuous regional analgesia. Reg Anesth Pain Med 2003;28:17–23.

87. Ilfeld BM, Morey TE, Enneking FK: Portable infusion pumps used for continuous regional analgesia: Delivery rate accuracy and consistency. Reg Anesth Pain Med 2003;28:424–432.

88. Ilfeld BM, Morey TE: Use of term "patient-controlled" may be confusing in study of elastometric pump. Anesth Analg 2003;97:916–917.

89. Ilfeld BM, Morey TE, Enneking FK: New portable infusion pumps: Real advantages or just more of the same in a different package? Reg Anesth Pain Med 2004;29:371–376.

90. Valente M, Aldrete JA: Comparison of accuracy and cost of disposable, nonmechanical pumps used for epidural infusions. Reg Anesth 1997;22:260–266.

91. Sawaki Y, Parker RK, White PF: Patient and nurse evaluation of patient-controlled analgesia delivery systems for postoperative pain management. J Pain Symptom Manage 1992;7:443–453.

92. Capdevila X, Macaire P, Aknin P, et al: Patient-controlled perineural analgesia after ambulatory orthopedic surgery: A comparison of electronic versus elastomeric pumps. Anesth Analg 2003;96:414–417.

93. Mizuuchi M, Yamakage M, Iwasaki S, et al: The infusion rate of most disposable, non-electric infusion pumps decreases under hypobaric conditions. Can J Anaesth 2003;50:657–662.

94. Klein SM, Pietrobon R, Nielsen KC, et al: Peripheral nerve blockade with long-acting local anesthetics: A survey of the Society for Ambulatory Anesthesia. Anesth Analg 2002;94:71–76.

95. Klein SM, Nielsen KC, Greengrass RA, et al: Ambulatory discharge after long-acting peripheral nerve blockade: 2382 blocks with ropivacaine. Anesth Analg 2002;94:65–70.

96. Grant SA, Neilsen KC: Continuous peripheral nerve catheters for ambulatory anesthesia. Curr Anesthesiol Rep 2000;99:304–307.

97. Borgeat A, Ekatodramis G, Kalberer F, et al: Acute and nonacute complications associated with interscalene block and shoulder surgery: A prospective study. Anesthesiology 2001;95:875–880.

98. Cuvillon P, Ripart J, Lalourcey L, et al: The continuous femoral nerve block catheter for postoperative analgesia: Bacterial colonization, infectious rate and adverse effects. Anesth Analg 2001;93:1045–1049.

99. Souron V, Reiland Y, De Traverse A, et al: Interpleural migration of an interscalene catheter. Anesth Analg 2003;97:1200–1201.

100. Hogan Q, Dotson R, Erickson S, et al: Local anesthetic myotoxicity: A case and review. Anesthesiology 1994;80:942–947.

101. Chelly JE, Greger J, Gebhard R: Ambulatory continuous perineural infusion: Are we ready? [letter; comment]. Anesthesiology 2000;93:581–582.

102. Ilfeld BM, Esener DE, Morey TE, et al: Ambulatory perineural infusion: The patients' perspective. Reg Anesth Pain Med 2003;28:418–423.

65

Regional Anesthesia in Community Practice

Joseph Marino, MD

INTRODUCTION

A renewed interest in the treatment of postoperative pain, together with the need for expedient operating room management, creates a professional mandate for the development of safe anesthetic alternatives to the ubiquitous general anesthesia. It is well documented that regional anesthesia helps to decrease opioid-related side effects, facilitates the bypass of the postanesthesia care unit, shortens the turnover times, facilitates early patient discharge, and decreases the risk of unanticipated hospital admissions.[1-5] However, a variety of factors germane to the private practice of anesthesiology hinders the wider application of a regional anesthesia-driven service to the community setting. These factors include increased production pressure due to an accelerated surgical pace and volume and a demand for efficiency. In addition, the lack of resources, a shortfall in assistance, and the capricious state of third-party reimbursement often force the specialty to question whether these services can be implemented and offered in a community setting.

Establishment of an effective service involves changing the existing medical practice culture. This change can be accomplished only by effectively communicating the measurable advantages of newer techniques to patients, surgeons, and other medical and anesthesia colleagues. With the assistance of written orders and flow sheets, nurses are empowered to assume an important role in assessing and caring for the inpatient with a regional anesthetic. Collaboration with other disciplines (internal medicine, surgery, and physical therapy) ensures that lapses in care are avoided. Extending the unparalleled analgesic benefits of regional anesthesia to the outpatient setting further expands the range of surgical procedures performed and facilitates home readiness.

Spreading the Word to Patients

In their survey results, Matthey and coworkers[1] found reasons why patients avoid regional anesthetics and confirmed that patients' perceptions of regional anesthesia were greatly distorted. Fears of being awake during surgery, experiencing pain during the procedure, needle placement, back injury, and paralysis constituted the main unfounded reasons why patients opted for general anesthesia.[1] The efforts of anesthesiologists have been inadequate in correcting these misconceptions and addressing patient's concerns. Converting such misconceptions into a greater acceptance of regional anesthesia involves an organized approach to educating patients. The preoperative anesthesia visit is an ideal opportunity for the anesthesia care team to discuss expectations and assuage these fears.

Delineating the advantages of regional anesthesia combined with assurances that patients can be made comfortable during administration of the regional anesthetic or asleep throughout the surgical procedure effectively addresses a patient's primary preoccupation with hearing, feeling, or seeing the anesthesia procedure or surgery. Preprinted pamphlets and a patient instruction sheet help to reinforce the information disseminated during the preoperative anesthesia interview.

An example of a particularly effective tool for educating patients is a class given by the orthopedic nursing staff for patients considering joint replacement surgery. As part of a patient education seminar, monthly hour-long classes are given in our institution. Topics can include all major aspects of a typical hospital stay for a patient undergoing joint replacement surgery. Patients find this informal setting an ideal place to review various aspects of their care. Discussion includes the benefits of aggressive thromboprophylaxis, the opioid-sparing advantages of continuous perineural blockade, and block-related side effects, such as postoperative numbness. Instruction on the use of ambulatory assistive devices (eg, knee immobilizers) combined with the assistance of physical therapists further allay fears that motor blockade will impede ambulation. Patients learn that regional anesthesia and analgesia techniques permit more aggressive physiotherapy, thus enhancing outcome and comfort during recovery.

Educated patients become valuable and formidable assistants in the interventional aspects of their care. For example, patients informed of the possibility of posterior knee pain after a continuous femoral block for a total knee replacement are empowered with the knowledge to request a supplemental block (popliteal or sciatic block) rather than worrying about the prospect that "this block in my groin" is ineffective. Patients become proactive participants, rather than passive, stoic individuals hopeful that their experience will be uncomplicated by inadequate pain management.

Reeling in the Gatekeepers

Before going to a surgeon for an orthopedic consultation, seeing an internist is usually the first step in the patient's procession toward joint reconstruction. The primary care physician is an integral part of targeted efforts to educate the medical community. Misconceptions not only exist among patients and their families but may be propagated by inadequately informed medical professionals. Medical community support cannot be expected if time is not taken to build interest in the part that modern regional anesthesia plays in patient care.

A medical grand rounds format highlighting the advantages of regional techniques can be an efficacious tool for educating medical practitioners. These educational efforts arm primary care physicians with the necessary information to debunk occasional negative regional anesthesia myths. In other words, educating the gatekeeper is a valuable step in efforts to change the public's perception and to increase acceptance of regional analgesic techniques.

Surgeon Perception

Surgeon preference is an important factor influencing patient choice.[2] Imagine the scenario of a patient entering an orthopedist's office and requesting a regional block as the primary anesthetic. Visions of significant operating room delay together with concerns of failed block outcome and the potential for adverse block-related sequelae (eg, seizure and nerve injury) may lead an uniformed surgeon to dissuade the patient from this anesthetic alternative. Increased turnover times, unpredictable success, and fear of complications are traditional barriers that decreased the popularity of regional block techniques among surgeons.[2] Advocating for regional techniques in a grand rounds format can increase surgical awareness; however, evidence-based presentations and improved dialogue will do little to gain surgeon support if an infrastructure capable of promoting operating room efficiency is not created.

Clinical Pearls

GETTING THE SURGEONS ON BOARD IN THE OUTPATIENT SETTING

The following are suggestions to avoid delays:

- Preoperative block placement is ideal and does not require a designated block room (Figure 65–1); the monitoring capabilities and availability of staff make the postanesthesia care unit (PACU) a reasonable alternative.

- Using a regional block as the primary anesthetic need not result in delays in scheduled start times. If the PACU is unavailable, consider block placement during room "set-up" because the time used to drape the operative field is adequate to achieve the level of block progression essential for surgical trespass.

- Interventions performed to supplement a general anesthetic (analgesic versus anesthetic blocks such as interscalene block for shoulder surgery or femoral block for anterior cruciate ligament reconstruction) can be easily executed in the PACU after adequate emergence from general anesthesia. Patient satisfaction is enhanced and

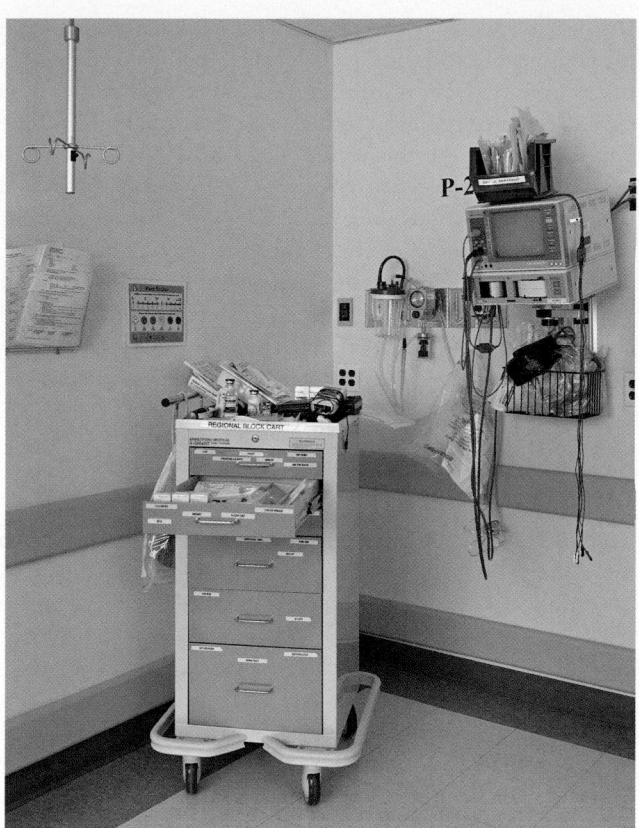

Figure 65–1. A preoperative block placement area with monitoring and regional anesthesia cart.

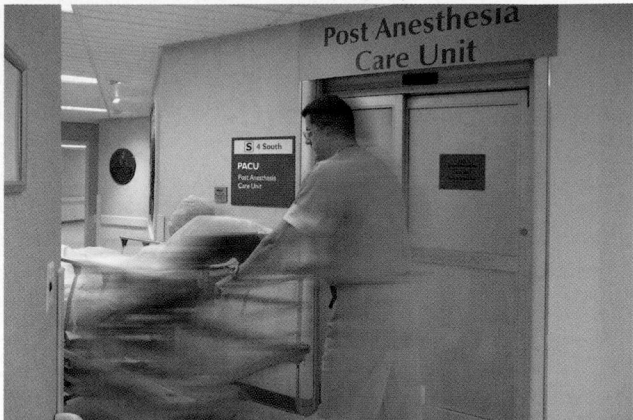

Figure 65–2. Regional anesthesia techniques can substantially help "fast-tracking" by allowing the awake and comfortable patients to bypass the postanesthesia care unit (Phase 1).

of newer, more labor-intensive techniques require specific technical skill and a time investment that may not be adequately reimbursed (Table 65–1) and, thus, may be met with resistance or a lack of enthusiam by practitioners in a community practice setting.

One of the barriers to the use of regional techniques among anesthesiologists in community practice is the perception that these techniques (beyond neuraxial techniques) require lengthy, specialized training. Indeed, inadequate exposure to these techniques during residency training leads to a low comfort level with these procedures. Rather than

PACU discharge times are improved because concurrent doses of side effect–prone opioids are avoided.

■ Regional techniques result in a superior recovery profile by improving home readiness in the ambulatory setting compared with "fast-track" general anesthesia techniques (Figure 65–2).

The following are suggestions on how to make an impact on quality of analgesia:

■ The superior analgesia provided by perineural infusion techniques allows for an increase in the scope and complexity of surgical cases performed on an outpatient basis. Before the analgesic advances of peripheral nerve blockade, postoperative pain constituted a major limitation to the expansion of ambulatory surgery.[6]

■ Severe postoperative pain no longer needs to result in unanticipated hospital admissions.

■ Witnessing these improvements in analgesia, anesthetic efficiency, recovery profile, and home readiness, surgeons are rapidly embracing perineural techniques as a very potent analgesic strategy.

Training Requirements

Fear of litigation and compensation issues have forced private practitioners to reevaluate their practices. Introduction

Table 65–1.

Regional Anesthesia—Acute Pain Management Procedure Billing Codes

Procedure	CPT Code
Brachial plexus, single shot	64415
Brachial plexus, continuous	64416
Sciatic, single shot	64445
Sciatic, continuous	64446
Femoral, single shot	64447
Femoral, continuous	64448
Psoas, continuous	64449
Thoracic epidural	62318
Lumbar epidural	62319
Epidural blood patch	62273
Intravenous PCA	01997

PCA, patient-controlled analgesia.

risk failure, many practitioners avoid these procedures and abandon any opportunity for achieving block proficiency.

However, an anesthesiologist should be able to perform a regional anesthetic with the same degree of skill as a general anesthetic. Contrary to the common belief, fellowship training in regional anesthesia is not mandatory to develop proficiency in peripheral block technique. This is analogous to the training in other anesthesia subspecialties. The expertise acquired through formal, fellowship training is useful in the practice of pediatric, ambulatory, obstetric, neurologic, cardiac, and regional anesthesia and is instrumental in advancing the subspeciality but not a prerequisite for successful practice. In contrast, confidence and comfort with regional techniques can be achieved through motivated self-study workshops, and regular practice. Although the prospect of "practicing" peripheral blockade in the private setting may be unattractive to some anesthesiologists, it is no different from acquiring experience with a new general anesthetic drug machine or technique.[7]

Practitioners should develop proficiency with easy techniques (single-injection) before moving on to more advanced blocks (continuous catheter techniques). Because of its readily identifiable landmarks, ease of insertion, and low risk-profile,[8] a femoral block is considered the ideal technique to develop familiarity with perineural procedures.

A variety of educational tools and on-line teaching sites exist to help the regional enthusiast perfect their craft. For instance, the New York School of Regional Anesthesia (htpp://www.NYSORA.com) website has been a state-of-the-art on-line educational source for more than a decade. It is easy to follow, downloadable, and comprehensive. The American Society of Regional Anesthesia (htpp://www.asra.com), Regional Anesthesia Study Center of Iowa (RASCI, http://www.uianesthesia.com/rasci/), and ARL francophone (htpp://www.alrf.asso.fr) are only a few among several other excellent sites that offer on-line information on practice of regional anesthesia. Consistent review followed by practical application leads to the optimizing consistent success in clinical practice. Although texts and CD-ROMs provide valuable information, the practical application of these skills in a hands-on cadaver workshop may prove to be the training technique with the greatest clinical yield.

SETTING UP A REGIONAL ANESTHESIA PRACTICE

Getting the Word Out

The term "marketing" is defined as the prospect of selling goods or services to actualize a sales transaction.[9] The term may be viewed as offensive to some practitioners because physicians are often reluctant to *sell* their services. However, because the public's perception of regional anesthetic techniques is distorted by a lack of understanding, efforts made to increase the acceptance of these techniques must communicate the message proficiently.

A hospital newsletter is a marketing tool circulated throughout the community to provide patients with information on available resources. Hospital newsletters can be used to explain regional anesthesia services and highlight the physicians skilled in this technique. A hospital newsletter is not a tool to sell goods or services but rather a way to inform the community about the availability of an advanced modern service and a vehicle to change the public's perception. Without concrete information, patients rely on conjecture. If a hospital newsletter does not exist in an institution, hospital administrators should be lobbied to create one by reminding them that an educated consumer makes the best customer.

Role of the Nursing Staff Members and Around-the-clock Acute Pain Coverage

Nursing staff member support is an implicit prerequisite to the viability of a regional analgesia-based service. The focus of educational in-services should not only effectively prepare the nurse for the nuances of peripheral nerve blockade but should also delineate nursing responsibilities in the entire process

The success of a regional anesthesia service is predicated on a coordinated effort among all nursing disciplines (Figure 65–3). As the healthcare provider with the greatest level of in-house patient contact, an orthopedic floor nurse spearheads the effectiveness of the service by proficiently evaluating analgesic efficacy as well as monitoring for block-related side effects. Working documents, such as acute pain flow sheets and specific block-related order forms, provide clear guidelines to assist nursing staff members making the assessments. (Refer to Chapter 79 for information on regional analgesia forms and flow charts.) Daily correspondence with and immediate access to the anesthesia staff for any catheter-related issues are required to allay any nursing-related concerns associated with the implementation of a new service.[10] An acute pain service pager serves as a valuable nursing resource by permitting access to the anesthesia care provider assigned acute pain duties. If in-house anesthesia coverage is available, then the on-call physician manages overnight block–related issues. If in-house overnight coverage is not available, then a mechanism that provides for timely patient evaluation is needed. The implementation of standardized flow sheets and order forms facilitates documentation, actualizes reimbursement, and applies a structured and organized flow to the service. This organizational structure and team approach translate into optimal patient care.

The results of a regional analgesia-based service include decreased nursing interventions and enhanced patient care. Instead of tending to patients with nausea, administering opioid injections and rescue antiemetics, nurses are able to concentrate on pain assessment, diagnosis, and documentation of patient response to therapy. A nurse that is given the responsibility of removing femoral and interscalene catheters is instructed to document catheter tip visualization and call the anesthesiologist if catheter removal is met with any resistance. This structure has been proved to be a safe and effective

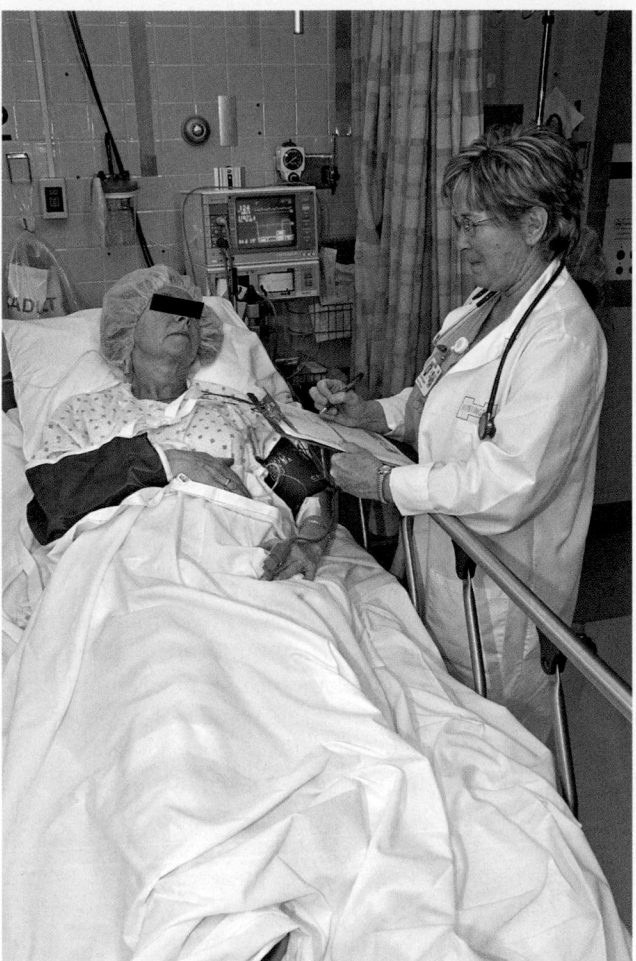

Figure 65–3. A perioperative nurse interviews the patient before administration of regional anesthesia.

Table 65–2.

Description of Nursing Roles

Preadmission
- Communicate instructions to patients and escorts
- Distribute patient instruction sheet
- Discuss informed consent

Admission
- Verify informed consent
- Confirm operative side

Operating Room
- Confirm operative side
- Coordinate block placement during room set-up if needed
- Assist with block placement

Postanesthesia Care Unit
- Assist with block placement if needed
- Evaluate efficacy of analgesia
- Adjust pain therapy and treatment of side effects
- Monitor for block-related side effects

Medical-Surgical Unit
- Reevaluate efficacy of analgesia
- Monitor for block-related side effects
- Inspect catheter dressing
- Troubleshoot technical issues with infusion devices
- Communicate with anesthesiologist on catheter-related issues
- Remove catheters according to guidelines
- Interface with physical therapy
- Coordinate expeditious patient discharge

practice that empowers the nursing staff to coordinate efficient and timely discharges (Table 65–2; Figure 65–4).

A physical therapy program is an essential step in the transition from convalescence to anticipated postoperative outcome. Physical therapists need to be in-serviced regarding the potential for motor blockade with lower extremity perineural techniques and its impact on ambulation. Initially, surgeons may be concerned that a partially blocked extremity would lead to an increase in patient falls during ambulation; however, the vigilance of a well-informed physical therapy team combined with the use of ambulatory-assist devices (eg, knee immobilizers) helps substantially reduce the risk of iatrogenic injuries. As a result of coordinated efforts by the members of the departments of nursing and physical therapy, a more aggressive physiotherapy regimen, together with earlier ambulation, results in a decrease in the length of hospital stay.[11]

Collectively, fulfillment of these roles enhances the department's ability to provide a state-of-the-art effective pain management service to all patients. However, without a proactive nursing staff, this goal would be reached with great difficulty.

Management of Complications

Complications after regional anesthesia are relatively rare; however, they can occur with all medical interventions, including regional anesthesia and analgesia. Because the fear of complications is often present among patients and surgeons alike, a well-developed system for detection and follow-up of such complications should be in place in spite of their low risk. Meticulous technique combined with a thorough knowledge

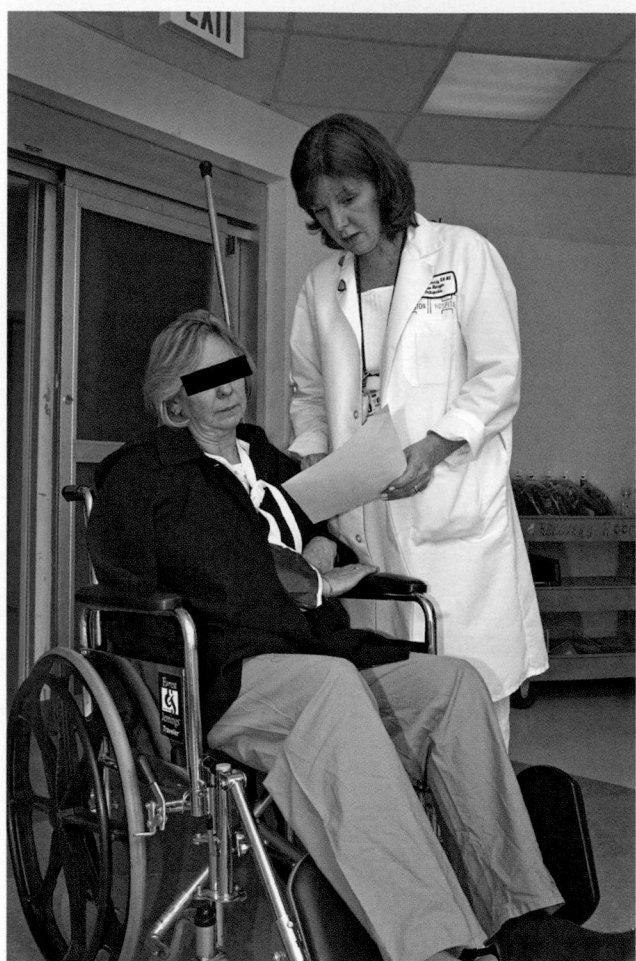

Figure 65–4. A perioperative nurse discusses the discharge instructions with the patients.

of anatomy should significantly decrease their occurrence. A review of the risks with an appropriately executed informed consent and patient follow-up, should be an integral element of every intervention.

Surgeons and other involved medical staff cannot be expected to advocate the use of regional anesthesia and analgesia techniques if a mechanism for prevention, assessment, diagnosis, and treatment of potential nerve injury is not in place. Developing a system in which each patient who received an intervention is contacted at 24 hours and 1 week after discharge will avoid the perception of "dumping" the responsibility for follow-up of postblock complications into the surgeon's lap, which inevitably creates resentment. Maintaining a patient log that documents each intervention, the time of correspondence, and neurologic status is an easy and effective way to track the block outcome. A postprocedure follow-up record that is mailed to the surgeon's office on a monthly basis can be combined with these efforts. The orthopedic surgeon can use this document during the patient's postoperative visit to assist in the assessment and diagnosis of any block-related sequelae.

Identification of potential injury followed by appropriate neurologic referral can allay any feelings of abandonment or disregard by patients and surgeons alike. Interfacing with

the neurology and chronic pain department members establishes a valuable alliance necessary for the subsequent care of patients with block-related sequelae. Patients appreciate this comprehensive system of follow-up care. As a result of these efforts, surgeons now view the anesthesiology practice as an implicit part of their postoperative clinical algorithm and act as vociferous advocates.

FORMS, DOCUMENTATION, & REIMBURSEMENT

Before instituting regional anesthesia service, appropriate policies, procedures, and guidelines must be written and reviewed by the respective hospital committees. A working document, such as the nursing pain flow sheet, promotes a high quality of care and optimizes efficiency by maintaining structure and organization. Dedicated continuous perineural block order forms should be distinct from epidural order forms (see Chapter 7). Perineural block forms outline guidelines of care specific to perineural infusions and emphasize a multimodal treatment of pain. Breakthrough pain therapy and orders for sedation are included on the order form.

Each time an intervention is performed, documentation in the patient's medical record is required. A combined peel-and-stick carbon copy progress note that serves as both progress note and billing sheet can be used. The peel-off sticker can be placed in the patient's medical record, and the rear carbon copy can be distributed to the respective third-party payer for reimbursement. This method obviates the need for any after-the-fact chart copying and provides the payer with all the necessary patient information, including diagnosis and procedure (ICD-9 and CPT) codes. Documentation of informed consent, block placement characteristics, and daily stick-and-peel progress notes in a **SOAP** (**s**ubjective, **o**bjective, **a**ssessment, **p**lan) format are features that make it a highly effective and user-friendly reimbursement procurement tool.

A documentation form can be standardized (see Chapter 80, Documentation of Regional Procedures) to satisfy the medical, legal, billing, and compliance goals.[12] The key elements of such a form include methods of sedation, monitoring, nerve localization, and various aspects of injection administration, such as pressure and pain on injection, and others. This form can be customized to better meet individual institutional practices and include documentation. Application of these elements into the community setting can only enhance a clinical practice that will ultimately benefit patient care.

TYING IT ALL TOGETHER

Acceptance of regional techniques as either the primary anesthetic or as a central component of a multimodal postoperative pain service is predicated on effectively communicating their benefits to those involved. After extolling the virtues of regional techniques to an audience through a formalized educational process, a detailed infrastructure capable of providing a safe and efficient practice of these techniques is necessary for success. Once the advantages of these techniques are instituted and realized, a culture fixated on general anesthesia followed by opiates-based pain management can begin to change to a better alternative.

Technical perfection in perineural blockade for the regional anesthesiologist is characterized by a high success rate of block with diminutive risk. Recent developments of a variety of clinical aids, such as percutaneous nerve electrolocation, injection pressure monitors, stimulating catheters, electrolocation needles with built-in disconnect and current indicators, and ultrasound-assisted nerve blocks are just some of the technical refinements that will imminently improve the block success rate and decrease the risk of complications.[13–18]

References

1. Matthey PW, Finegan BA, Finucaine BT: The public's fears about and perceptions of regional anesthesia. Reg Anesth Pain Med 2003;29:96–101.
2. Oldman M, McCartney CJL, Leung A, et al: A survey of orthopedic surgeons' attitudes and knowledge regarding regional anesthesia. Anesth Analg 2004;98:1486–1490.
3. Hadzic A, Karaca PE, Hobeika P, et al: Peripheral nerve blocks result in superior recovery profile compared with general anesthesia in outpatient knee arthroscopy. Anesth Analg 2005;100:976–981.
4. Pavlin DJ, Rapp SE, Polissar NL, et al: Factors affecting discharge time in adult outpatients. Anesth Analg 1998;87:816–826.
5. D'Alessio JG, Rosenblum M, Shea KP, Freitas DG: A retrospective comparison of interscalene block and general anesthesia for ambulatory surgery shoulder arthroscopy. Reg Anesth 1995;20:62–68.
6. Nielsen KC, Steele SM: Ambulatory continuous regional anesthesia: Ambulatory evaluation and safety considerations. Tech Reg Anesth Pain Manage 2004;8:99–103.
7. Bonica JJ: Regional anesthesia in private practice. Anesthesiology 1960;Sept-Oct:554–556.
8. Cuivillion P, Ripart J, Lalourcey L, et al: The continuous femoral nerve block catheter for postoperative analgesia: Bacterial colonization, infectious rate and adverse effects. Anesth Analg 2001;93:1045–1049.
9. *Webster's New Universal Dictionary of the English Language,* Business Encyclopedic Edition. Library Guild, 1971, p. 583.
10. Sevarino FB, Preble LM: *A Manual for Acute Postoperative Pain Management.* Raven Press, 1992, pp. 7–39.
11. Chelly JE, Greger J, Gebhard R, et al: Continuous femoral blocks improve recovery and outcome of patients undergoing total knee arthroplasty. J Arthroplasty 2001;16:436–445.
12. Gerancher JC, Viscusi ER, Liguori G, et al: Development of a standardized peripheral nerve block procedure note form. Reg Anesth Pain Med 2005;30:67–71.
13. Williams SR, Chouinard P, Arcand G, et al: Ultrasound guidance speeds execution and improves the quality of supraclavicular block. Anesth Analg 2003;97:1518–1523.
14. Yang WT, Chui PT, Metreweli C: Anatomy of the normal brachial plexus revealed by sonography and the role of sonographic guidance in anesthesia of the brachial plexus. AJR 1998;171(6):1631–1636.
15. Sinha A, Chan V: Ultrasound imaging for popliteal sciatic nerve block. Reg Anesth Pain Med.2004;29:130–134.
16. Hogan Q. Finding nerves is not simple. Reg Anesth Pain Med 2003;28:367–371.
17. Choyce A, Chan V, Middleton W, et al: What is the relationship between paresthesia and nerve stimulation for axillary brachial plexus block. Reg Anesth Pain Med 2001;26:100–104.
18. Sites BD, Gallagher J, Sparks M: Ultrasound-guided popliteal block demonstrates an atypical motor response to nerve stimulation in 2 patients with diabetes mellitus. Reg Anesth Pain Med 2003;28:479–482.

66

Regional Anesthesia in Austere Environment Medicine

Chester C. Buckenmaier, III, MD

I. INTRODUCTION

II. AUSTERE ENVIRONMENT ANESTHESIOLOGY

III. ADVANTAGES OF REGIONAL ANESTHESIA IN AUSTERE ENVIRONMENTS

IV. ACCEPTANCE OF ADVANCED REGIONAL ANESTHESIA IN AEA

V. PERIOPERATIVE MEDICINE & ACUTE PAIN CONTROL

VI. PEARLS & PITFALLS OF REGIONAL ANESTHESIA IN AN AUSTERE ENVIRONMENT

VII. SUMMARY

INTRODUCTION

Regional anesthesia has played a pivotal role in the development of anesthesiology as a medical specialty since the discovery of the local anesthetic properties of cocaine by Carl Köller in 1884. In the decades since this landmark discovery, surgeons and anesthesia providers have appreciated the advantages of regional anesthesia in their patients, particularly in surgical situations complicated by limited resources and austere environmental conditions. War, more than any other human endeavor, has driven the need to provide effective anesthesia for surgery in austere environments. Indeed, the development of anesthesiology as a distinct specialty has been attributed to the medical experience obtained in World War II.[1] The physician–anesthetists of that era quickly recognized that regional anesthesia imparted the least physiologic insult to the wounded soldier and allowed a more awake patient

to be returned to the recovery ward, thus reducing the burden on limited wartime medical resources.[1] As anesthesiology matured as a medical specialty and departments of anesthesiology began to break away from departments of surgery in academic centers, regional anesthesia continued to evolve. During the Vietnam War, the value of regional anesthesia in harsh medical conditions was reestablished. In one series of 1000 battle casualties, nerve block, spinal, or local anesthesia was used in 49% of cases. "This allowed increased anesthesia coverage of more surgical procedures at any one time as well as decreasing the demands on postoperative ward personnel in a multiple casualty situation."[2] The role of regional anesthesia in combat casualty care continues to expand in modern conflicts. Consequently, military medical planners are understandably interested in austere environment anesthesia due to the realities of military wartime missions. Civilian anesthesiologists are also interested in the advantages of regional anesthesia in austere environments for disasters, civil defense, or missions to medically underserved regions of the world.

In the last 15 years regional anesthesia has undergone a renaissance. New equipment, such as peripheral nerve stimulators and ultrasound technology have facilitated block placement and enhanced resident training in regional anesthesia. Continuous peripheral nerve block catheters and peripheral nerve infusion pumps have extended the benefits of regional block techniques beyond the immediate perioperative period to days after an operation and even into the home.[3] In this chapter the advantages and application of advanced regional anesthesia in austere environment medicine will be examined. The role of recent advances in regional anesthesia equipment and techniques in facilitating anesthesia in less than ideal conditions will also be discussed.

AUSTERE ENVIRONMENT ANESTHESIOLOGY

The practice of medicine in an austere environment requires a significantly different approach than that used for medicine practiced in the major medical centers or in developed countries in general. This is especially true for the practice of anesthesiology. In developed countries, the anesthesiologist has a tremendous resource base that is readily available and largely transparent to the production of an anesthetic plan. The utilities, roads, computers and other wonders of modern infrastructure common to developed nations are rarely noticed by anesthesiologists, but they impart a tremendous advantage in ensuring a successful anesthetic outcome. In contrast, the anesthesiologist practicing austere environment anesthesiology (AEA) becomes very aware of the effect limited resources can have on anesthetic decisions. In AEA, the anesthesiologist must factor local infrastructure realities into anesthetic plans. Anesthetic choices and plans that work well in state-of-the-art operating rooms can have disastrous consequences if applied to austere environments without due consideration of local resources and conditions. The available roads; electrical, sanitation, medical gas services; climactic conditions; and operating room facilities, among other issues, will greatly affect the anesthetic plan in AEA.

The influence of local environmental and weather conditions on AEA is a particularly important consideration, especially during medical missions following natural disasters. Temperature and terrain extremes, along with dangerous faunae and disease must be included in any successful anesthetic plan in these environments. Temperature extremes can affect patient health directly and degrade equipment, medication, and anesthesiologist function. Rough terrain can affect practitioner and patient travel, impede communication, and limit resupply of consumable medical supplies. Finally, local geopolitics, in its most extreme form, war, can have a tremendous influence on AEA.

One approach to overcoming the realities of AEA is to surmount local resource limitations by transporting the modern anesthesia infrastructure to the AEA location, thus freeing

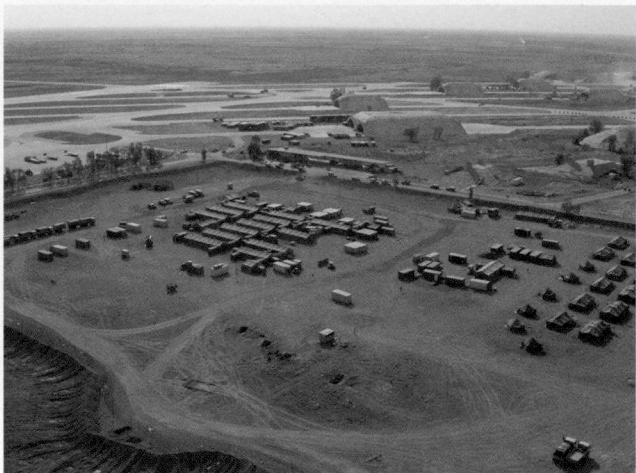

Figure 66–1. Twenty-first Combat Support Hospital, Balad, Iraq, 2003. The hospital is on the left with living quarters on the right of the photograph.

the anesthesiologist from many if not all of these considerations. This approach is best illustrated by the U.S. military in caring for wounded soldiers on the battlefields of Iraq and Afghanistan through the fielding of combat support hospitals (CSH) that have capabilities similar to civilian hospitals in developed countries (Figure 66–1). While the CSH is a successful approach to caring for injured patients anywhere in the world, the logistics required to place and support such a facility are well beyond the capability of most humanitarian medical mission planners or disaster medicine planners.

ADVANTAGES OF REGIONAL ANESTHESIA IN AUSTERE ENVIRONMENTS

Because of the logistical constraints and the environmental realities inherent to AEA, anesthesiologists involved in these types of missions must find anesthetic and analgesic techniques that require minimal logistical support, provide adequate surgical conditions, afford postoperative pain control, and result in a patient that is alert in the postoperative recovery room. Modern advanced regional anesthesia has many characteristics that make it an attractive choice for AEA missions (Table 66–1).

Clinical Pearls

- Compared with general anesthesia using a volatile anesthetic, regional anesthesia is particularly suited for anesthesia in austere environments because of its smaller logistical needs.

- The equipment for regional anesthesia (peripheral nerve stimulator, single-injection or continuous peripheral nerve block needle and tubing, local anesthetic, and infusion pump) is compact, lightweight, and easily transported.

Table 66–1.

Advantages of Regional Anesthesia in Austere Environmental Conditions

Excellent operating conditions

Profound perioperative analgesia

Stable hemodynamics

Limb specific anesthesia

Reduced need for other anesthetics

Improved postoperative alertness

Minimal side effects

Rapid recovery from anesthesia

Simple, easily transported equipment needed

Reprinted, with permission, from Buckenmaier CC III, Lee EH, Shields CH, et al: Regional anesthesia in austere environments. Reg Anesth Pain Med 2003;28:321–327.)

Compared with general anesthesia using a volatile anesthetic, regional anesthesia is particularly suited for AEA because of its small logistics footprint. The equipment for regional anesthesia (peripheral nerve stimulator, single-injection or continuous peripheral nerve block needle and tubing, local anesthetic, and infusion pump) is compact, lightweight, and easily transported. In contrast, the equipment used to deliver volatile anesthetics does not posses these attributes (Figure 66–2). Though general anesthesia remains the gold standard for AEA, this capability must be planned for and surgical cases that demand general anesthesia carefully triaged. The availability of compressed oxygen can often dictate the number and types of cases that can be managed in austere environments. Many anesthetic ventilators are pneumatically driven and can consume significant quantities of compressed oxygen during a typical general anesthetic. Oxygen cylinders or oxygen generation equipment (eg, the portable oxygen generation system [POGS] shown in Figure 66–2B which required six men to lift into place) can represent a significant logistics challenge to any AEA mission. Possible alternatives to pneumatically driven volatile anesthetics include draw-over anesthesia or total intravenous anesthesia (TIVA) using target-controlled infusion (TCI) pumps. These alternatives remain in development and may not be available to many anesthesiologists. Whenever possible, regional anesthesia is the preferred technique for most cases during an AEA mission because it allows conservation of resources that may be required for more complicated surgeries or emergencies.[4]

Regional anesthesia provides excellent operating conditions for the surgeon. With the establishment of a surgical block, motor, sensory, and sympathetic nerves to a

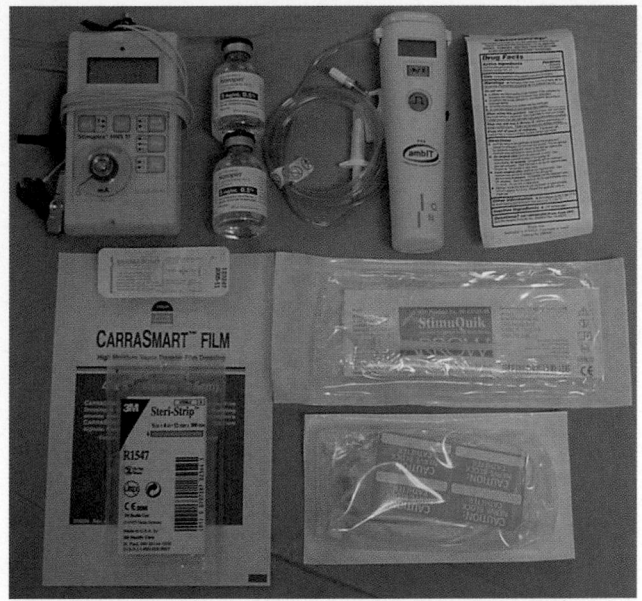

A

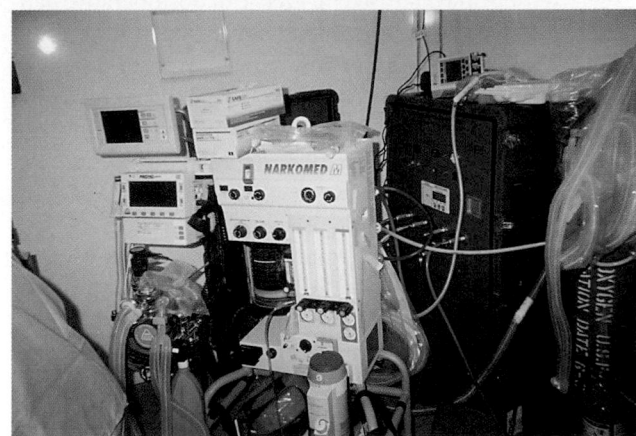

B

Figure 66–2. Equipment scale comparison between typical equipment used for regional anesthesia and equipment used for a general anesthetic using volatile gas. **A:** Equipment for single-injection or continuous peripheral nerve block displayed on top. Items include Stimuplex HNS-11 nerve stimulator (B. Braun Medical Inc., Bethlehem, PA), Naropin 0.5% (ropivacaine HCL, AstraZeneca, Wilmington, DE), Ambit infusion pump (Sorenson Medical, Inc, West Jordan, UT), Chloraprep (Medi-Flex Hospital Products, Inc, Overland Park, KS), Dermabond (Ethicon Inc, Cornelia, GA), Steri-Strip (3M Health Care, St. Paul, MN), CarraSmart (Carrington Laboratories, Inc, Irving, TX), StimuQuick insulated peripheral block needle (Arrow International Inc., Reading, PA), and Contiplex Tuohy continuous nerve block set (B. Braun Medical Inc, Bethlehem, PA). **B:** Photograph displays equipment for a general anesthetic (with volatile anesthetics) used at the Twenty-eighth Combat Support Hospital, Iraq. Items include Narcomed M (Dräger Medical Inc, Lübeck, Germany) connected to a Portable Oxygen Generation System (POGS—On Site Gas Systems, Inc., Newington, CT).

body region are blocked. This provides muscle relaxation,[5] preemptive analgesia,[6] reduced overall stress response to surgery,[7] a reduction in thromboembolic complications,[8] and reduced blood loss.[9,10] Because afferent nociceptive stimulation from the surgical site is greatly attenuated or eliminated during the operative procedure, stable hemodynamics are characteristic of regional anesthesia. In AEA, when monitoring capability is often constrained, intraoperative hemodynamic stability is important. Regional anesthetic techniques allow the procedure to be performed on an awake or lightly sedated patient who can communicate with the anesthesiologist, providing the best monitor of patient well-being.

Postoperatively, the advantages of regional anesthesia in AEA become even more apparent. Unlike general anesthesia, which provides for little to no postoperative analgesia, regional techniques with long-acting local anesthetics maintain analgesia for hours following the operation. If continuous peripheral nerve block (CPNB) techniques are employed, analgesia can be extended for days postoperatively. Another important benefit of regional anesthesia in the postsurgical recovery area is the improved alertness and reduced nausea and vomiting associated with these techniques compared with the affects from general anesthesia. In the modern ambulatory surgery setting, the increased incidence of postoperative nausea and vomiting, drowsiness, and pain are the most frequent causes of prolonged postoperative stay.[11,12] Although these issues have economic significance in developed countries, in the resource-limited practice of AEA, difficult recovery can have a profoundly negative effect on mission success. Recovery area personnel and monitoring capability are usually limited in AEA. Anesthesiologists working in this environment favor techniques, like regional anesthesia, that facilitate sending alert patients, free of pain and nausea, who can be active proponents in their recovery despite limited resources. Rapid recovery of the patient's own airway protective reflexes is a significant advantage of regional compared with general anesthesia in AEA.

ACCEPTANCE OF ADVANCED REGIONAL ANESTHESIA IN AEA

Effective perioperative pain management is an important consideration following any operative procedure regardless of the location and conditions under which it is performed. Since Serturner, a German pharmacist, first identified and isolated morphine from opium in 1803, morphine and other opioid drugs have played a major role in pain management in austere environments, especially in the military. Although the preeminence and success of opioid medications in pain management is well established, their use is not without significant side effects that are undesirable in the best medical environments but can be potentially devastating in AEA. International regulations concerning the transportation of opioids and limited monitoring capability can further complicate the use of these drugs in AEA. Studies have demonstrated a reduced requirement for opioid pain medication following surgery when regional anesthesia techniques are used.[3,13] Using CPNB techniques, pain relief can

be extended for days, further reducing the need for opioid pain medications. The efficacy of CPNB infusions have been demonstrated in the ambulatory surgery setting, allowing anesthesiologists to extend the benefits of peripheral nerve block following surgery well into the patient's recovery at home.[14–16]

Despite the benefits of regional anesthesia techniques, information regarding the use of CPNB in AEA is limited. Recently, the use of CPNB for surgical anesthesia and analgesia on the modern battlefield and throughout the evacuation chain back to the United States has been demonstrated successfully.[17] Since this first success, CPNB catheters have been increasingly used to treat a number of patients within the Iraq combat theater. The application of regional anesthesia, CPNB in particular, has been one of the medical success stories to emerge from the military's experience in the Iraq war. Although the technology remains new to the modern battlefield and is far from being universally accepted, many soldiers have enjoyed the benefits of advanced regional anesthesia and CPNB in the management of their combat wounds in the austere battlefield environment of Iraq. Advances in soldier body armor and the Iraq insurgent's preference for using improvised explosive devices has resulted in a preponderance of extremity wounds and traumatic amputations. The application of CPNB catheters in many of these patients has facilitated the multiple operative procedures they often undergo since reestablishment of a surgical block can be easily accomplished via the existing catheter(s). Additionally, the analgesic block provided by CPNB allows for far superior pain control on the long, jarring evacuation flights to Germany and the United States compared with morphine alone, which until recently was the only option for pain control on an evacuation aircraft.

Despite this initial success, the military has been slow to embrace advanced regional anesthesia as a viable battlefield medicine standard of care. The reasons for this reluctance are numerous and not easily defined, but worth exploring since the military medical community's concerns over advanced regional anesthesia will also provide insight into why, despite its many advantages, advance regional anesthesia is not the predominate anesthetic for AEA. First, general anesthesia with volatile anesthetics is the "gold standard" anesthetic in developed countries. The safety and efficacy of general anesthesia has been established over the decades with countless successful applications. Anesthesiology training programs focus on general anesthesia techniques, and most practitioners are very comfortable with its use for all surgical indications. Unfortunately, the technology and personnel support needed to employ general anesthesia successfully can quickly exhaust the resources available during AEA as previously noted. In the U.S. military, a tremendous investment has been made in technology to safely provide general anesthesia to war casualties, regardless of the environment. Additional requirements on the military medical supply system, such as advanced regional anesthesia, are less attractive to medical logistical planners when so much effort has been directed toward volatile-anesthetic-based general anesthesia. Although the capability to perform general anesthesia in AEA is vital, general anesthesia is not necessarily the best choice for every clinical situation encountered on the mission. The availability of other options is a key to AEA mission success.

Lack of training in advanced regional anesthesia has also hampered the development of this anesthetic in the AEA environment.[18,19] Advanced regional anesthesia training, at least in U.S. anesthesiology residency programs, is far from what it needs to be for these techniques to become ubiquitous within the anesthesia community and not just the domain of a select few regional anesthesia specialists. A considerable investment is required by the anesthesiologist to learn block techniques and detailed human anatomy before advanced regional anesthesia can become part of routine anesthesia practice. The increased availability of regional anesthesia courses, the development of regional anesthesia fellowship training programs, and the explosion of interest in the medical literature suggests that this issue may become moot in the not too distant future. In the military, the Army Regional Anesthesia and Pain Management Initiative, a Congressionally sponsored program established in 2000, has done much to establish advanced regional anesthesia and other modern pain management techniques on the modern battlefield.

During the last decade, along with and complimentary to the resurgence of interest in regional anesthesia, there has been an upsurge in available technology to support and enhance the practice of advanced regional anesthesia. Although these technologies, such as peripheral nerve stimulators, stimulating catheters, portable infusion pumps, and ultrasound, to name just a few, have revolutionized the practice of regional anesthesia, the plethora of equipment to choose from can be confusing. This situation is made worse by the lack of consensus among regional anesthesiologists as to what technologies and practices are best for physician and patient alike. Stimulating versus nonstimulating catheters, ultrasound-directed versus stimulating needle placement, needle sharpness and design, CPNB catheter infusion rates, and bolus parameters are just a few of the topics that often pervade regional anesthesia conference floor discussions. Unlike general anesthesia, modern regional anesthesia (particularly CPNB) does not enjoy decades of safe application and experience in use. This relatively new frontier in anesthesiology and perioperative analgesia attracts many anesthesiologists to the study of advanced regional anesthesia techniques, but it is the discomfort of challenging new technologies and ideas that deters many. Considerable effort is needed to take the "art" out of regional anesthesia and establish its "science" before these techniques can become generally accepted.

Finally, perhaps the most unusual reason for the slow acceptance of regional anesthesia in AEA and in the military is our professional and social attitudes toward pain. The science of understanding pain and its management is a relatively new phenomenon. Before the advent of modern anesthesia practice, surgeons were instructed to not display excessive concern over a patient's discomfort during surgery and to operate fast, since a speedy surgery limited suffering.[20] Even after the development of anesthesiology as a medical specialty, pain has been, and still is, considered an unfortunate and unavoidable consequence of surgical intervention. In the AEA environment, expending limited medical resources on the management of pain can seem a luxury. As evidence mounts on the destructive aspects of pain, particularly as it contributes to the overall surgical stress response and postoperative morbidity, effective pain control is fast becoming less a luxury and more a necessary component of successful surgical care.[21,22] Though compassion and the relief of suffering is reason enough to provide good pain control, in the twenty-first century it is just good medicine.

PERIOPERATIVE MEDICINE & ACUTE PAIN CONTROL

The successful application of regional anesthesia in austere environments requires anesthesiologists to embrace their role as physicians of perioperative medicine. Simply put, the anesthesiologist must accept responsibility for the patient's operative care before, during, and long after his or her surgical procedure. Although this extended role for the anesthesiologist beyond the operating room and recovery area is nontraditional, the anesthesiologist is uniquely trained to manage perioperative pain and enhance recovery using a multimodal approach that includes advanced regional anesthesia techniques and technologies. The anesthesiologist's perioperative role is enhanced through the establishment of a regional anesthesia/acute pain section. The anesthesiologist working outside of the operating room in the regional anesthesia/acute pain section facilitates the introduction of advanced regional anesthesia both in modern hospitals and in AEA. This location is equipped with regional anesthesia supplies and should have basic monitors, oxygen, suction, airway and resuscitation equipment and medications in the event of an emergency. This investment in resources has profound advantages in the AEA environment. The regional anesthesia section facilitates patient preparation for surgery, and, if appropriate, blocks with long-acting local anesthetics or CPNB can be established before previous surgery patients are out of the operating room, thus improving efficiency. The block area anesthesiologist is also available to serve as a perioperative medical consultant, critical care provider, and acute pain specialist for recovering patients.

The need for this expanded role of anesthesiologists in perioperative analgesia is exemplified by the austere military medical environment that currently exists in Iraq. In previous conflicts, wounded American soldiers often spent days recovering from combat wounds before they were deemed fit to be evacuated to higher levels of medical care outside of the war theater. In the current War on Terror a soldier's evacuation from point of injury to a major medical facility outside of the combat theater is often measured in hours. This aggressive evacuation policy has contributed significantly to the salvage of many soldiers who likely would have died in previous conflicts. Unfortunately, traditional opioid-based pain management techniques alone are not well suited to the difficult air evacuation environment that makes rapid removal of casualties to distant major medical facilities possible. Medical personnel on evacuation flights are often faced with many wounded patients in significant pain. In the low light, high noise, high vibration, and difficult monitoring environment of evacuation aircraft, the significant side effects associated with opioid-only pain control become magnified. The advantage of CPNB and modern peripheral nerve infusion pumps that allow patients to manage their own pain control is obvious. These catheters also facilitate repeated operations and dressing changes by allowing reestablishment of surgical blocks through bolus administration of local anesthetic via established CPNB catheters. Military anesthesiologists are actively pursuing this technology.

PEARLS & PITFALLS OF REGIONAL ANESTHESIA IN AN AUSTERE ENVIRONMENT

Patients receiving regional anesthesia, as part of their care, should be warned to avoid weight bearing on blocked extremities. They should also be advised to take special precautions to avoid further injury to the blocked region of the body since normal protective sensations and proprioception will be diminished or absent. Patients should also be cautioned about possible side effects that may be associated with specific block procedures. For example, patients receiving an interscalene block should be warned of the possibility of developing Horner's syndrome and a hoarse voice. They should be reassured that these conditions are temporary and will resolve completely with resolution of the block. These warnings are especially important in AEA where cultural differences can heighten patient fears and negatively affect the patient's perception of their anesthetic care. Planning for adequate translator resources is vital for any medical mission in which language differences exist between caregivers and patients.

Using CPNB, the benefits of regional anesthesia can be extended for days into a patient's recovery from surgery. This advantage can have a profoundly positive influence on the care of patients who require evacuation over long distances or have injuries that necessitate frequent surgical interventions or dressing changes. Although this technique has important advantages in AEA, it also presents the medical team with unique management challenges that are best addressed by the regional anesthesia/acute pain anesthesiologist working outside of the operating room. The decision to use CPNB on AEA patients must be individualized to each patient's clinical situation. During the clinical evaluation of the patient for anesthesia, the anesthesiologist will be able to ascertain if the patient is a suitable candidate for CPNB. Not all patients are willing or able to tolerate CPNB infusions despite the relative simplicity of the technology. If a patient remains resistant to CPNB therapy after thoughtful discussion with a physician, then the technique should be abandoned in favor of more traditional anesthetic and pain management techniques. Additionally, personnel resources must be available to monitor and appropriately manage any development of local anesthetic toxicity following a block. The anesthesiologist must also weigh the benefits of applying CPNB for each surgical situation against the risks of the technique. In the author's practice, all patients are warned, "The use of a block needle can result in injury or infection and because we are working near nerves the possibility of nerve damage does exist, though these complications are rare." The least invasive intervention that can adequately control a patient's pain should always be sought for each clinical situation. Finally, the anesthesiologist must have an established plan for a follow-up of CPNB patients. Follow-up can be as simple as a telephone call, but CPNB patients and their catheters should be evaluated daily. Patients treated with CPNB catheters should also be educated on signs and symptoms of local anesthetic toxicity. The patient must have 24-h access to an anesthesia provider should problems occur during the infusion. Fortunately, the answer for any CPNB infusion problem is the same, stop the infusion, resort to back-up pain medications, seek medical help. The U.S. Air Force has developed a series of infusion pump labels to provide CPNB patients and their caregivers basic instructions during air evacuation to manage infusion problems when an anesthesiologist may not be immediately available (Figure 66–3). Internet e-mail is also a valuable communication tool when physicians and nurses are required to treat CPNB patients that are being transferred to medical facilities separated by great distance. E-mail can often be accessed in the most remote areas where other forms of long-distance communication are unavailable. Although these CPNB management principles may seem burdensome to apply in the AEA environment, the advantages in pain relief for patients are clear and consistent with compassionate anesthetic care. With proper planning, CPNB works well in austere environments.

One of the frequent complaints concerning CPNB infusions is catheter dislodgement. Poorly secured catheters can migrate or fall out, reducing the effectiveness of the technique, especially when patients require evacuation to other medical facilities. Although many devices and procedures are available to secure catheters, in the military evacuation environment and in military hospitals the following CPNB catheter-securing procedures seem to work best. After placement, all catheters are gently aspirated for blood and 5 mL of local anesthetic containing epinephrine 1:400,000 is injected

• **Will be placed on the pump at initial catheter insertion**

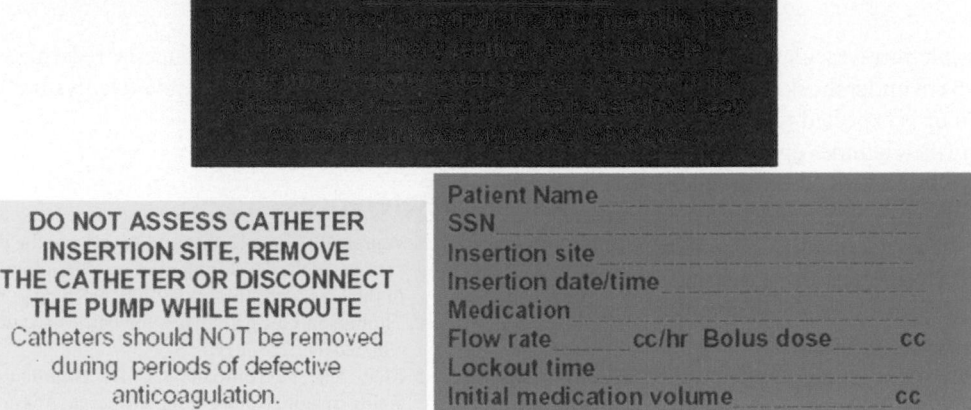

DO NOT ASSESS CATHETER
INSERTION SITE, REMOVE
THE CATHETER OR DISCONNECT
THE PUMP WHILE ENROUTE
Catheters should NOT be removed
during periods of defective
anticoagulation.

Patient Name_____
SSN_____
Insertion site_____
Insertion date/time_____
Medication_____
Flow rate_____ cc/hr Bolus dose_____ cc
Lockout time_____
Initial medication volume_____ cc

Figure 66–3. Military and US Air Force AeroEvacuation-specific labels for continuous peripheral nerve block infusions.

Table 66–2.

Standard Adult Ropivacaine Dosages for Single-Injection and Continuous Regional Anesthesia at Walter Reed Army Medical Center.[a]

Regional Anesthesia Technique	Adult Single-Injection Dose of Ropivacaine (mL 0.5% ropivacaine, except as noted)	Continuous Infusion of 0.2% Ropivacaine (mL)	Patient-Controlled Bolus Rate of 0.2% Ropivacaine[b] (mL bolus/20 min lockout)	Notes
Interscalene	35–40	8–10	2	Often supplemented with an intercostal brachial nerve block
Supraclavicular	35–40	8–10	2	Shortest latency block of the brachial plexus
Infraclavicular	35–40	10–12	2	Catheter techniques less effective than supraclavicular catheters
Axillary	40	10–12	2	Catheter techniques less common
Paravertebral	3–5 per level blocked	8–10	2	Catheters effective in thoracic region only
Lumbar plexus (posterior approach)	35–40	8–10	2	Epidural spread is a concern
Femoral	20–30	8–10	2	Catheter techniques less effective than lumbar plexus catheters
Sciatic (anterior or posterior approach)	20–30	8–10	2	Proximal approaches to the sciatic nerve preferable for catheters
Sciatic (lateral or popliteal approach)	35–40	10–12	2	Catheter techniques less common
Lumbar plexus or femoral + sciatic	50–60 mL between both sites	5–10 for both catheters	2 mL on one catheter	Infusion rates divided between catheters based on distribution of patient's pain
Epidural	20–25	6–10	2	Opioids often added to infusions
Spinal	5–15 mg of 1.0% ropivacaine	NA	NA	Opioids often added to injections

[a] *Information is based on the authors' experience with ropivacaine in a successful and busy regional anesthesia practice. Mepivacaine 1.5% can be used in place of ropivacaine at the volumes noted when a shorter duration block is desirable.*

[b] *Occasionally, 5 mL bolus/30-min lockout is used in selected patients. Generally, total infusion (continuous plus bolus) > 20 mL/h are avoided.*

NA = not applicable.

to diagnose possible intravascular placement. Catheters are tunneled for 3 to 5 cm under the skin in any CPNB patient who will be evacuated or is expected to maintain the catheter for longer then 72 h (this includes epidural catheters). Whether tunneled or not, all catheters are secured with cyanoacrylate glue at the skin puncture site,[23] followed by a medical spray adhesive. The catheter is looped at the puncture site and further secured with Steri-Strips and a transparent dressing. All catheters are labeled with the site of the block and the date and time of catheter placement.

A variety of excellent peripheral nerve infusion pumps are available. A discussion of infusion pump technology is beyond the scope of this chapter, more information on comparison and contrasting the devices can be found in Chapter 48 (Equipment for Continuous Nerve Blocks).[24,25] Currently in the military two different infusion pumps are in use. The Stryker PainPump II (Stryker Instruments, Kalamazoo, MI) is a single-use, disposable electronic infusion pump and is currently the only peripheral nerve infusion pump approved for flight on military aircraft. The amBit (Sorenson Medical, Inc, West Jordan, Utah) is a multiuse, adjustable electronic infusion pump that is currently being used in fixed military medical facilities in Iraq. These devices were selected because of their consistent infusion performance in temperature extremes and at altitude.

A variety of local anesthetics are available for use in AEA regional anesthesia. Ropivacaine is the long-acting local anesthetic preferred by the author for single-injection blocks and CPNB catheter infusions. Compared with other long-acting local anesthetics such as bupivacaine and levobupivacaine, ropivacaine is the safest long-acting local anesthetic available.[26,27] Mepivacaine is the intermediate-acting local anesthetic often selected when a shorter duration block is desirable or when catheters are bolused to reestablish a surgical level block for dressing changes or surgery. Table 66–2 provides some examples of effective single-injection and CPNB infusion rates for a variety of regional anesthetic blocks.

SUMMARY

In summary, regional anesthesia has characteristics that make its application in the AEA desirable. Although the rewards for the patient in improved postoperative alertness, pain control, and possibly enhanced recovery are apparent, these benefits are only realized through a significant investment by anesthesiologists in the education and the increased effort advanced regional anesthesia requires for successful application. Anesthesiologists who embrace the challenge of advanced regional anesthesia become more versatile anesthesia providers whether their practice is in a modern, high-technology hospital or an isolated, austere tent. As recent events involving terrorism and natural disaster have demonstrated, the ability to provide safe anesthesia and effective analgesia regardless of environmental circumstances is a valuable twenty-first century skill for all anesthesiologists.

References

1. Waisel DB: The role of World War II and the European theater of operations in the development of anesthesiology as a physician specialty in the USA. Anesthesiology 2001;94(5):907–914.
2. Thompson GE: Anesthesia for battle casualties in Vietnam. JAMA 1967;201(7):215–219.
3. Klein SM, Buckenmaier CC III: Ambulatory surgery with long acting regional anesthesia. Minerva Anestesiol 2002;68(11):833–841.
4. Buckenmaier CC III, Lee EH, Shields CH, et al: Regional anesthesia in austere environments. Reg Anesth Pain Med 2003;28(4):321–327.
5. Brown AR, Weiss R, Greenberg C, et al: Interscalene block for shoulder arthroscopy: Comparison with general anesthesia. Arthroscopy 1993;9(3):295–300.
6. Kelly DJ, Ahmad M, Brull SJ: Preemptive analgesia I: Physiological pathways and pharmacological modalities. Can J Anaesth 2001;48(10):1000–1010.
7. Greengrass RA: Regional anesthesia for ambulatory surgery. Anesthesiol Clin North Am 2000;18(2):341–353, vii.
8. Tuman KJ, McCarthy RJ, March RJ, et al: Effects of epidural anesthesia and analgesia on coagulation and outcome after major vascular surgery. Anesth Analg 1991;73(6):696–704.
9. Buckenmaier CC III, Xenos JS, Nilsen SM: Lumbar plexus block with perineural catheter and sciatic nerve block for total hip arthroplasty. J Arthroplasty 2002;17(4):499–502.
10. Twyman R, Kirwan T, Fennelly M: Blood loss reduced during hip arthroplasty by lumbar plexus block. J Bone Joint Surg Br 1990;72(5):770–771.
11. Chung F, Mezei G: Factors contributing to a prolonged stay after ambulatory surgery. Anesth Analg 1999;89(6):1352–1359.
12. Pavlin DJ, Rapp SE, Polissar NL, et al: Factors affecting discharge time in adult outpatients. Anesth Analg 1998;87(4):816–826.
13. Wang H, Boctor B, Verner J: The effect of single-injection femoral nerve block on rehabilitation and length of hospital stay after total knee replacement. Reg Anesth Pain Med 2002;27(2):139–144.
14. Buckenmaier CC III, Klein SM, Nielsen KC, et al: Continuous paravertebral catheter and outpatient infusion for breast surgery. Anesth Analg 2003;97(3):715–717.
15. Klein SM, Buckenmaier CC III: Ambulatory continuous interscalene brachial plexus blockade. Tech Reg Anesth Pain Manage 2004;8(2):58–62.
16. Nielsen KC, Greengrass RA, Pietrobon R, et al: Continuous interscalene brachial plexus blockade provides good analgesia at home after major shoulder surgery-report of four cases. Can J Anaesth 2003;50(1):57–61.
17. Buckenmaier CC, McKnight GM, Winkley JV, et al. Continuous peripheral nerve block for battlefield anesthesia and evacuation. Reg Anesth Pain Med 2005;30:202–205.
18. Brown DL, Boezaart A: Regional training circa 2000: What's really new. Reg Anesth Pain Med 2002;27(1):1–2.
19. Kopacz DJ, Neal JM: Regional anesthesia and pain medicine: Residency training–the year 2000. Reg Anesth Pain Med 2002;27(1):9–14.
20. Condon-Rall ME: A brief history of military anesthesia. In Zajtchuk R, Grande CM (eds): Part IV: *Anesthesia and Perioperative Care of the Combat Casualty.* Washington DC: Office of the Surgeon General, 1995, pp 855–896.
21. Kehlet H: Multimodal approach to control postoperative pathophysiology and rehabilitation. Br J Anaesth 1997;78(5):606–617.

22. Kelly DJ, Ahmad M, Brull SJ: Preemptive analgesia II: Recent advances and current trends. Can J Anaesth 2001;48(11):1091–1101.

23. Klein SM, Nielsen KC, Buckenmaier CC III, et al: 2-Octyl cyanoacrylate glue for the fixation of continuous peripheral nerve catheters. Anesthesiology 2003;98(2):590–591.

24. Ilfeld BM, Morey TE, Enneking FK: The delivery rate accuracy of portable infusion pumps used for continuous regional analgesia. Anesth Analg 2002;95(5):1331–1336, table.

25. Ilfeld BM, Morey TE, Enneking FK: Portable infusion pumps used for continuous regional analgesia: Delivery rate accuracy and consistency. Reg Anesth Pain Med 2003;28(5):424–432.

26. Graf BM: The cardiotoxicity of local anesthetics: The place of ropivacaine. Curr Top Med Chem 2001;1(3):207–214.

27. Wang RD, Dangler LA, Greengrass RA: Update on ropivacaine. Expert Opin Pharmacother 2001;2(12):2051–2063.

67

Regional Analgesia in the Critically Ill

Sebastian Schulz-Stübner, MD

INTRODUCTION

Intensive care specialists have become increasingly more interested in the prevention and treatment of physiologic and psychological stress in critically ill patients[1,2] in order to prevent detrimental consequences ranging from systemic inflammatory response syndrome,[4] to cardiac complications,[5,6] to posttraumatic stress disorder.[7-9] Studies have addressed the questions of an optimal sedation regimen and several evidence-based guidelines and strategies have been published.[10-14] The analgesic component for sufficient stress relief, however, has not been addressed extensively, and few recommendations, primarily based on individual clinical practices, are currently available.[15]

In view of the side effects of opioids, especially respiratory depression, altered mental status, and reduced bowel function, regional analgesia utilizing neuraxial and peripheral nerve blocks offer significant advantages. The lack of a universally reliable pain assessment tool ("analgesiometer") in the critically ill contributes to the dilemma of adequate analgesia. Many patients in the critical care unit are not able to communicate or use a conventional visual or numeric analog scale to quantify pain. Alternative assessment tools derived from pediatric[16-18] or geriatric[19] practice that rely on grimacing and other physiologic responses to painful stimuli might be useful, but have been inadequately studied in the intensive care unit (ICU). Changes in heart rate and blood pressure in response to nursing activities, dressing changes, or wound care can also serve as indirect measurements of pain,[20] and sedation scores like the Ramsey or Riker and colleagues[21,22] scale might be helpful, although not specifically designed for pain assessment.

The objective of this chapter is to describe the indications, limitations, and practical aspects of continuous regional analgesic techniques in the critically ill based on the available evidence, which at the moment is limited to case reports, cohort studies, expert opinion, and extrapolation from studies looking primarily at intraoperative use of regional anesthesia extending into the postoperative ICU stay. The evidence level of our recommendation is therefore mostly grade C and D according to the "Grades of Recommendation" published by the Oxford University Centre for Evidence Based Medicine (http://www.cebm.net/index.asp).

EPIDURAL ANALGESIA

Epidural analgesia is probably the most commonly used regional analgesic technique in the ICU setting.[23] Some indications, in which epidural analgesia may not improve mortality rates but facilitates management and improves patient comfort in the ICU, include chest trauma,[24–27] thoracic[28,29] and abdominal surgery,[5,30,31] major vascular surgery,[32,33] major orthopedic surgery,[34] acute pancreatits,[35] paralytic ileus,[36–39] cardiac surgery,[40,41] and intractable angina pain.[42,43] Although high-risk patients seem to profit most from epidural analgesia,[44,45] the current literature does not address the specific circumstances of the critically ill patient with multiple comorbidity and organ failure. For that reason, an individual approach is necessary when considering application of epidural analgesia in this population.[46]

In a survey of 216 general ICUs in England, Low[47] found that 89% of the responding units used epidural analgesia, but only 32% had a written policy governing its use. Although 68% of the responding units would not place an epidural catheter in a patient with positive blood cultures, only 52% considered culture-negative sepsis, or systemic inflammatory response syndrome (SIRS), to be a contraindication. The majority of respondents did not list lack of consent or the need for anticoagulation after the catheter was placed as contraindications to the insertion an epidural catheter. Although the issues of consent, possible coagulopathy, and infection can be addressed rather easily in elective procedures, they become major problems in newly admitted patients, for example, those with multiple trauma or painful intraabdominal processes, especially acute pancreatitis. There is also controversy about the safety of placing epidural catheters in sedated patients,[48,49] and confirmation of a good catheter position can be difficult in the critically ill patient if sensory level testing is not reliable.

Positioning the patient for the procedure can be a problem, depending on the underlying injury, the number and position of tubes and catheters, or external fixation devices. Table 67–1 summarizes indications, contraindications, and practical problems with the placement of epidural catheters.

The help of trained nursing staff is essential for good positioning and safe handling of tubes and catheters during the procedure. Maximum barrier precautions similar to the placement of central lines should be considered for placing epidural catheters in the critically ill as well. Tunneling the catheter should be considered to prevent dislocation and reduce possible catheter site infections.[50] To confirm the correct position of the epidural catheter, electrical stimulation during placement or a postplacement radiograph with a small amount of nonneurotoxic contrast medium may be beneficial.[51,52]

Table 67–1.

Epidural Analgesia in the Critically Ill

Indications	Contraindications	Practical Problems	Dose Suggestions
Thoracic epidurals:			
Chest trauma	Coagulopathy or current use	Positioning of patient	*Bolus regimen:*
Thoracic surgery	of anticoagulants during	Monitoring of neurologic	5–10 mL 0.125–0.25%
Abdominal surgery	catheter placement and	function (consider	bupivacaine or 0.1–0.2%
Paralytic ileus	removal[59,60]	MEP/SSEP[a])	ropivacaine q 8–12 h
Pancreatitis	Sepsis/bacteremia		Consider addition of 1–2 meg
Intractable angina	Local infection at puncture		clonidine in hemodynamically
Lumbar epidurals:	site		stable patients
Orthopedic surgery	Severe hypovolemia		*Continuous infusion:*
or trauma of lower	Acute hemodynamic		0.0625% bupivacaine or 0.1%
extremities	instability		ropivacaine at 5 mL/h
Peripheral vascular	Obstructive ileus		Consider addition of opioids (eg,
disease of lower			hydromorphone, sufentanil) or
extremities			clonidine if high systemic opioid
			demands persist

[a] *MEP = motor-evoked potentials, SSEP = somatosensory-evoked potentials.*
Source: Reprinted with permission from Schulz-Stübner S et al: Crit Care Med 2005;33:1400–1407.

Clinical Pearls

- The most common side effects of epidural blocks are bradycardia and hypotension related to sympathetic block.

- Hemodynamic changes can be more pronounced with intermittent bolus dosing, in patients with hypovolemia, or those with reduced venous return secondary to high positive end-expiratory pressure ventilation.

- Discontinuation of continuous infusion every morning will allow neurologic assessment when necessary.

- There is no compelling evidence of increased risks of epidural bleeding with developing coagulopathy or therapeutic anticoagulation while an epidural catheter is in place. Nevertheless, the benefits of epidural analgesia should be weighed against the risk of this serious complication.

Bolus injections of long-acting local anesthetics such as bupivacaine, ropivacaine, or levobupivacaine or the discontinuation of continuous infusion every morning will allow neurologic assessment when necessary. Monitoring of motor-evoked potentials (MEP) to the lower extremities and somatosensory-evoked potentials (SSEP) of the tibial nerve may serve as indicators when the neurologic examination is doubtful due to the patient's altered mental status. Although routinely used in the operating room for monitoring spinal cord integrity and for diagnosis and prognosis of spinal cord injury, the use of this technology in the ICU in the context of epidural analgesia has not been adequately assessed.

The most common side effects of epidural blocks are bradycardia and hypotension related to sympathetic block. Hemodynamic changes can be more pronounced with intermittent bolus dosing, in patients with hypovolemia, or those with reduced venous return secondary to high positive end-expiratory pressure (PEEP) ventilation. Based on data from lumbar punctures and meningitis from the beginning of the twentieth century,[53] current sepsis and bacteremia are considered contraindications for intrathecal opioid applications and, by analogy, for placement of epidural catheters. However, many ICU patients, especially after trauma and major surgery, present with a clinical picture of SIRS. Fever and increased white blood cell counts alone, that is, in the absence of positive blood cultures, do not provide a reliable diagnosis of bacteremia. The combination of the serum markers C-reactive protein (CRP), procalcitonin, and interleukin-6, on the other hand, have been shown to indicate bacterial sepsis with a high degree of sensitivity and specificity[54−57] and can guide the decision to place an epidural catheter. Regarding the patient's coagulation status, the current recommendations of the American Society of Regional Anesthesia (ASRA)[58,59] should be followed. Adequate safety intervals during the administration of anticoagulative

drugs are equally important for the placement and removal of epidural catheters.[60,61] Although there is no compelling evidence of increased risks of epidural bleeding with developing coagulopathy or therapeutic anticoagulation while an epidural catheter is in place, the benefits of epidural analgesia should be weighed against this potential, highly detrimental complication.

PERIPHERAL NERVE BLOCKS FOR THE UPPER EXTREMITIES

At the time of this writing, there are no randomized, controlled trials or large prospective trials evaluating the use of peripheral nerve blocks for the upper extremity in critically ill patients. Nevertheless, severe trauma to the shoulder or arm is often part of the multiple injuries due to traffic or workplace accidents, often in combination with blunt chest trauma requiring mechanical ventilation. These injuries can contribute to severe pain, especially during positioning of the patient. If the orthopedic injury is part of complex trauma including brain injury in which the mental status of the patient is altered and opioid-based analgesic regimens might mask the neurologic situation, sufficient analgesia can be achieved for the shoulder or upper limb with either continuous interscalene,[62−64] continuous cervical paravertebral,[64−67] or infraclavicular[68] approaches to the brachial plexus.

Particular concerns arise concerning the placement of regional blocks in ICU patients with impaired mental status due to neurologic injury or therapeutic sedation. Benumof reported a small series of serious complications, including spinal cord injury related to the interscalene approach, which might have been associated with sedation or general anesthesia.[69] His case descriptions relate to the spinal cord injury in heavily sedated or anesthetized patients and not to injury of the peripheral nerves. Despite this, performance of blocks anatomically close to the centroneuraxis can indeed carry a higher risk of spinal cord needle or injection injury. In sedated critically ill patients a combination of ultrasound and nerve stimulation for the placement of interscalene catheters and a technique with a less medial needle direction[70,71] should help to minimize the risk of complications. Perhaps most importantly, such blocks should be performed only by clinicians with adequate experience. The unavoidable blocking of the phrenic nerve and the loss of hemidiaphragmatic function[72] should be considered while planning the intervention. Although phrenic nerve blockade has negligible effects in mechanically ventilated patients, it may impair weaning from mechanical ventilation in high-risk patients. Furthermore, the proximity of the insertion site of the interscalene catheter to a tracheostomy tube might increase the risk of infection, and careful, standardized monitoring of the puncture site is therefore needed. Positioning problems might limit the use of the cervical paravertebral approach, which provides good analgesia for shoulder, arm, and hand.

Clinical Pearls

- In patients with altered mental status in whom opioid-based analgesic regimens might make neurologic evaluation difficult, excellent analgesia can be achieved for the shoulder or upper limb with continuous interscalene, cervical paravertebral, or infraclavicular approaches to the brachial plexus.

- Performance of blocks anatomically close to the centroneuraxis can carry a higher risk of spinal cord needle or injection injury. In heavily sedated critically ill patients such blocks should be performed only by clinicians with adequate experience.

- An interscalene brachial plexus block results in the loss of hemidiaphragmatic function. Although phrenic nerve blockade has negligible effects in mechanically ventilated patients, it may impair weaning from mechanical ventilation in high-risk patients.

The continuous infraclavicular[64,68,73–75] and axillary[64,76–78] approaches provide good analgesia for most of the arm, elbow, and hand. Bolus injection of local anesthetic through the catheter should especially be considered in patients who need surgical anesthesia, for example, for painful dressing changes or debridements for burns or large soft tissue wounds in the affected area. The small risk of pneumothorax must be considered against the slightly higher success rate and easier catheter maintenance of the infraclavicular versus the axillary approach, but can be ignored if a chest tube is already in place. A more lateral infraclavicular approach[79–81] might help to reduce the pneumothorax risk further.

PERIPHERAL NERVE BLOCKS FOR THE LOWER EXTREMITIES

Femoral nerve catheters are helpful in the management of acute pain from femoral neck fractures, in the period between the injury to shortly after surgical stabilization of the fracture.[82,83] Skilled use of ultrasound[84] might limit the unavoidable pain with nerve stimulation in this situation, which otherwise can be treated with small doses of intravenous remifentanil (0.3–0.5 mcg/kg) or ketamine (0.2–0.4 mg/kg). A fascia iliaca compartment block[85,86] might be a technical alternative.

Continuous femoral catheters in combination with a sciatic block provide excellent pain relief for the whole leg and even surgical anesthesia for procedures like external fixation.[87] Whether an anterior[88] or posterior approach (midgluteal,[89] subgluteal[90] classical Labat approach with one or two injections[91]) to the sciatic nerve is chosen depends largely on the skills of the operator and the ability to adequately position the patient for the procedure. If a combination of catheter techniques is used, as is often needed for the lower extremity, the total daily dose of local anesthetic should be adjusted based on catheter location, admixtures like epinephrine, drug interactions, and disease states as summarized in a recent review by Rosenberg and coworkers.[92]

Bolus injection of long-lasting local anesthetics in combination with clonidine[93] or buprenorphine[94] may help to reduce the overall amount of local anesthetics needed and minimize the effects of local anesthetic toxicity, although research results about these adjuvants are equivocal at present.[95,96]

OTHER REGIONAL ANALGESIC TECHNIQUES

Celiac plexus blocks may provide excellent analgesia for pancreatitis and cancer-related upper abdominal pain, but technical difficulties in the critically ill (CT guidance, fluoroscopy, or transgastric ultrasound) and the need for repeated injections limit its value for acutely critically ill patients.

Intrapleural catheters for pain control after chest trauma are of limited value secondary to concurrent drainage from chest tubes. The risk of pneumothorax limits their benefits for the management of pain after conventional cholecystectomy compared with the epidural or paravertebral technique in ventilated patients.

Thoracic paravertebral catheters can be a valuable alternative to epidural catheters for the management of unilateral pain restricted to a few dermatomes (eg, rib fractures[97] or zoster neuralgia).

Table 67–2 provides a summary of the most often utilized continuous peripheral catheters.

Single-injection nerve blocks, for example, intercostal blocks for the placement of chest tubes, scalp blocks[98] for the placement of halo fixation, and sufficient local infiltration anesthesia for typical ICU procedures like placement of arterial and central venous catheters, lumbar punctures, or ventriculostomies are often forgotten, although they are easy and safe to perform. If EMLA cream is used for topical anesthesia it needs to be applied 30–45 min before the procedure to achieve an optimal effect.

Intrathecal morphine[99–102] injections as a single shot and via spinal catheters (microcatheters are currently not approved in the United States but are available in Europe) can be an alternative to epidural catheters, especially if only short-term use after surgery is anticipated.

SYSTEMIC EFFECTS & COMPLICATIONS OF LOCAL ANESTHETICS IN THE CRITICALLY ILL PATIENT

Local anesthetics have been shown to have several positive systemic effects (including analgesic, bronchodilatory, neuroprotective, anti-inflammatory, antiarrhythmic, and antithrombotic properties)[103] when given or absorbed in adequate quantities (the exact dose–response relationships are widely unknown). They also have negative effects, such as, neurotoxicity (dose-dependent),

Table 67–2.

Continuous Peripheral Nerve Blocks in the Critically Ill

Block	Indications	Contraindications	Practical Problems	Dose Suggestions
Interscalene	Shoulder/arm pain	Untreated contralateral pneumothorax Dependence on diaphragmatic breathing Contralateral vocal cord palsy Local infection at puncture site	Horner syndrome may obscure neurologic assessment Block of ipsilateral phrenic nerve Close proximity to tracheostomy and jugular vein line sites	*Bolus regimen:*[a] 10 mL 0.25% bupivacaine or 0.2% ropivacaine q 8–12 h and on demand *Continuous infusion:* 0.125% bupivacaine or 0.1–0.2% ropivacaine at 5 mL/h
Cervical paravertebral	Shoulder/elbow/wrist pain	Severe coagulopathy Dependence on diaphragmatic breathing Contralateral vocal cord palsy Local infection at puncture site	Horner syndrome may obscure neurologic assessment Block of ipsilateral phrenic nerve Patient positioning	*Bolus regimen:*[a] 10 mL 0.25% bupivacaine or 0.2% ropivacaine q 8–12 h and on demand *Continuous infusion:* 0.125% bupivacaine or 0.1–0.2% ropivacaine at 5 mL/h
Infraclavicular	Arm/hand pain	Severe coagulopathy Untreated contralateral pneumothorax Local infection at puncture site	Pneumothorax risk Steep angle for catheter placement Interference with subclavian lines	*Bolus regimen:*[a] 10–20 mL 0.25% bupivacaine or 0.2% ropivacaine q 8–12 h and on demand *Continuous infusion:* 0.125% bupivacaine or 0.1–0.2% ropivacaine at 5–10 mL/h
Axillary	Arm/hand pain	Local infection at puncture site	Arm positioning Catheter maintenance	*Bolus regimen:*[a] 10–20 mL 0.25% bupivacaine or 0.2% ropivacaine q 8–12 h and on demand *Continuous infusion:* 0.125% bupivacaine or 0.1–0.2% ropivacaine at 5–10 mL/h
Paravertebral Thoracic Lumbar	Unilateral chest or abdominal pain restricted to few dermatomes	Severe coagulopathy Untreated contralateral pneumothorax Local infection at puncture site	Patient positioning Stimulation success sometimes hard to visualize	*Bolus regimen:*[a] 10–20 mL 0.25% bupivacaine or 0.2% ropivacaine q 8–12 h and on demand *Continuous infusion:* 0.125% bupivacaine or 0.1–0.2% ropivacaine at 5–10 mL/h
Femoral or sciatic	Unilateral leg pain	Severe coagulopathy Local infection at puncture site	Patient positioning Interference of femoral nerve catheters with femoral lines	*Bolus regimen:*[a] 10 mL 0.25% bupivacaine or 0.2% ropivacaine q 8–12 h and on demand *Continuous infusion:* 0.125% bupivacaine or 0.1–0.2% ropivacaine at 5 mL/h

[a]*Consider addition of 50–100 mcg clonidine in hemodynamically stable patient or 150–300 mcg buprenorphine*[94,114] *to each bolus dose q 12–24 h to prolong duration of action.*
Source: Reprinted with permission from Schulz-Stübner S et al: Crit Care Med 2005;33:1400–1407.

myotoxicity,[104,105] inhibition of wound healing, cardiotoxicity (dose-dependent), and central nervous excitation or depression (dose-dependent).[106]

To prevent local anesthetic systemic toxicity from accidental intravascular injection, a test dose of local anesthetic or saline with 1:200,000 epinephrine can be used with catheter placement, but the sensitivity of heart rate, blood pressure increase, and T wave changes[103] might be altered in ICU patients, especially those treated with beta-blockade and α_2-agonists or catecholamines. Careful aspiration to check for blood return should be performed before each bolus injection.

Most studies examining plasma levels of local anesthetics were not performed in critically ill patients. Scott and colleagues described the safe use of epidural ropivacaine 0.2% for 72 h with plasma levels far below the toxic threshold,[107] and Gottschalk and associates observed safe plasma levels after 96 h in patients treated with thoracic epidural ropivacaine 0.375%, indicating no significant accumulation over time.[108]

GENERAL MANAGEMENT ASPECTS OF CONTINUOUS REGIONAL ANALGESIA CATHETERS IN CRITICALLY ILL PATIENTS

In general, given the lack of cooperation and communication in many ICU patients, regional analgesia techniques using continuous catheters in the ICU require a higher level of vigilance than needed for regular ward patients. A close cooperation between the ICU team and the acute pain or anesthesia service of the hospital is required.

Critical care nursing personnel should be specifically trained in handling regional analgesia catheters and must be aware of the potential complications and their early warning signs. Because of the frequently large and confusing numbers of various infusion catheters in critically ill patients, the risk of drug errors and wrong administration of drugs through continuous regional analgesia catheters may be higher in these patients. Well-trained and highly qualified personnel are the best safeguard against these complications besides eye-catching labels, standardized care protocols, and perhaps specially designed connectors for those catheters.

Comprehensive diagnostic approaches, including magnetic resonance imaging or computed tomography, should be undertaken when there are clinical signs of possible bleeding complications (eg, suspected epidural or retroperitoneal hematoma). Structured observations of catheters for infectious complications and careful adherence to aseptic technique during placement and tunneling of the catheters, as well as the possible use of antibiotic-coated catheters in the future may reduce possible infectious complications. Catheters should not be removed routinely after certain time intervals, but only when clinical signs of infection appear.

If catheters get disconnected a study by Langevin[109] suggests that when the fluid in the catheter is static the proximal 25 cm of the catheter can be immersed in a disinfectant, cut, and reconnected to a sterile connector. This technique is only feasible for catheters in which the fluid column can be observed. Stimulating catheters should never be cut because of the danger of unwinding the internal metal spiral wire, which conducts electrical current. No study has looked at the risk of reconnecting these catheters after thorough disinfection of the outer surface, which is likely a common practice in many institutions. Cuvillon and colleagues[110] reported a high overall incidence of colonization (57%) of femoral catheters without septic complications. Therefore the decision to reconnect or remove the catheter must be based on a case-by-case basis and specific clinical circumstances. The overall risk of permanent neurologic damage (from direct trauma, bleeding, or serious infections) or death from regional anesthesia and analgesia seems to be low in the perioperative setting as shown by large surveys by Auroy and coworkers[111,112] and Moen and associates.[113] Although both studies certainly include critically ill patients, there are no specific subgroup data available.

SUMMARY

In summary, regional analgesia, whether utilizing single-injection regional blocks or continuous neuraxial and peripheral catheters, can play a valuable role in a multimodal approach to pain management in the critically ill patient to achieve optimum patient comfort and to reduce physiologic and psychological stress. By avoiding high systemic doses of opioids, several complications like withdrawal syndrome, delirium, mental status changes, and gastrointestinal dysfunction can be reduced or minimized. Because of limited patient cooperation during placement and monitoring of continuous regional analgesia, indications for their use must be carefully chosen based on anatomy, clinical features of pain, coagulation status, and logistic circumstances. High-quality, trained nursing care and well-trained physicians are essential prerequisites when using these techniques safely in the critical care environment. These recommendations are based on small series, uncontrolled trials, or extrapolated from controlled trials in the perioperative setting (grade C and D recommendations); further research on the use of regional analgesia techniques in the critically ill is needed before definitive guidelines can be recommended.

References

1. Brodner G, Pogatzki E, Van Aken H, et al: A multimodal approach to control postoperative pathophysiology and rehabilitation in patients undergoing abdominothoracic esophagectomy. Anesth Analg 1998;86:228–234.
2. Brodner G, Mertes N, Buerkle H, et al: Acute pain management: Analysis, implications and consequences after prospective experience with 6349 surgical patients. Eur J Anaesthesiol 2000;17:566–575.
3. Herridge MS: Long-term outcomes after critical illness. Curr Opin Crit Care 2002;8:331–336.
4. Afessa B, Green B, Delke I, et al: Systemic inflammatory response syndrome, organ failure, and outcome in critically ill obstetric patients treated in an ICU. Chest 2001;120:1271–1277.

5. Peyton PJ, Myles PS, Silbert BS, et al: Perioperative epidural analgesia and outcome after major abdominal surgery in high-risk patients. Anesth Analg 2003;96:548.

6. De Leon-Casasola OA, Lema MJ, Karabella D, et al: Postoperative myocardial ischemia: Epidural versus intravenous patient-controlled analgesia. A pilot project. Reg Anesth 1995;20:105–112.

7. Jones C, Skirrow P, Griffiths RD, et al: Rehabilitation after critical illness: A randomized, controlled trial. Crit Care Med 2003;31:2456–2461.

8. Cuthbertson BH, Hull A, Strachan M, et al: Post-traumatic stress disorder after critical illness requiring general intensive care. Intensive Care Med 2004;30:450–455.

9. Campbell AS: Recognising post-traumatic stress in intensive care patients. Intensive Crit Care Nurs 1995;11:60–65.

10. Dellinger RP, Carlet JM, Masur H, et al: Surviving sepsis campaign guidelines for management of severe sepsis and septic shock. Crit Care Med 2004;32:858–873.

11. Brattebo G, Hofoss D, Flaatten H, et al: Effect of a scoring system and protocol for sedation on duration of patients' need for ventilator support in a surgical intensive care unit. Qual Saf Health Care 2004;13:203–205.

12. Nasraway SA Jr, Jacobi J, Murray MJ, et al: Sedation, analgesia, and neuromuscular blockade of the critically ill adult: Revised clinical practice guidelines for 2002. Crit Care Med 2002;30:117–118

13. Jacobi J, Fraser GL, Coursin DB, et al: Clinical practice guidelines for the sustained use of sedatives and analgesics in the critically ill adult. Crit Care Med 2002;30:119–141.

14. Gehlbach BK, Kress JP: Sedation in the intensive care unit. Curr Opin Crit Care 2002;8:290–298.

15. Pasero C, McCaffery M: Multimodal balanced analgesia in the critically ill. Crit Care Nurs Clin North Am 2001;13:195–206.

16. Dilworth NM, MacKellar A: Pain relief for the pediatric surgical patient. J Pediatr Surg 1987;22:264–266.

17. Manworren RC, Hynan LS: Clinical validation of FLACC: Preverbal patient pain scale. Pediatr Nurs 2003;29:140–146.

18. Breau LM, Finley GA, McGrath PJ, et al: Validation of the Non-communicating Children's Pain Checklist-Postoperative Version. Anesthesiology 2002;96:528–535.

19. Feldt KS: The checklist of nonverbal pain indicators (CNPI). Pain Manag Nurs 2000;1:13–21.

20. Blenkharn A, Faughnan S, Morgan A: Developing a pain assessment tool for use by nurses in an adult intensive care unit. Intensive Crit Care Nurs 2002;18:332–341.

21. Riker RR, Picard JT, Fraser GL: Prospective evaluation of the Sedation-Agitation Scale for adult critically ill patients. Crit Care Med 1999;27:1325–1329.

22. Riker RR, Fraser GL: Sedation in the intensive care unit: Refining the models and defining the questions. Crit Care Med 2002;30:1661–1663

23. Naber L, Jones G, Halm M: Epidural analgesia for effective pain control. Crit Care Nurse 1994;14:69–72, 77–83; quiz 84–85.

24. Holcomb JB, McMullin NR, Kozar RA, et al: Morbidity from rib fractures increases after age 45. J Am Coll Surg 2003;196:549–555.

25. Karmakar MK, Ho AM: Acute pain management of patients with multiple fractured ribs. J Trauma 2003;54:615–625.

26. Luchette FA, Radafshar SM, Kaiser R, et al: Prospective evaluation of epidural versus intrapleural catheters for analgesia in chest wall trauma. J Trauma 1994;36:865-9;discussion 869–870.

27. Catoire P, Bonnet F: [Locoregional analgesia in thoracic injuries]. Can Anesthesiol 1994;42:809–814.

28. Asantila R, Rosenberg PH, Scheinin B: Comparison of different methods of postoperative analgesia after thoracotomy. Acta Anaesthesiol Scand 1986;30:421–425.

29. Licker M, Spiliopoulos A, Frey JG, et al: Risk factors for early mortality and major complications following pneumonectomy for non-small cell carcinoma of the lung. Chest 2002;121:1890–1897.

30. Carli F, Trudel JL, Belliveau P: The effect of intraoperative thoracic epidural anesthesia and postoperative analgesia on bowel function

after colorectal surgery: A prospective, randomized trial. Dis Colon Rectum 2001;44:1083–1089.

31. Jorgensen H, Wetterslev J, Moiniche S, et al: Epidural local anaesthetics versus opioid-based analgesic regimens on postoperative gastrointestinal paralysis, PONV and pain after abdominal surgery. Cochrane Database Syst Rev 2000:CD001893.

32. Albani A, Renghi A, Gramaglia L, et al: Regional anaesthesia in vascular surgery: A multidisciplinary approach to accelerate recovery and postoperative discharge. Minerva Anestesiol 2001;67:151–154.

33. Bush RL, Lin PH, Reddy PP, et al: Epidural analgesia in patients with chronic obstructive pulmonary disease undergoing transperitoneal abdominal aortic aneurysmorraphy—A multi-institutional analysis. Cardiovasc Surg 2003;11:179–184.

34. Wu CL, Anderson GF, Herbert R, et al: Effect of postoperative epidural analgesia on morbidity and mortality after total hip replacement surgery in Medicare patients. Reg Anesth Pain Med 2003;28:271–278.

35. Niesel HC, Klimpel L, Kaiser H, et al: [Epidural blockade for analgesia and treatment of acute pancreatitis]. Reg Anaesth 1991;14:97–100.

36. Baig MK, Wexner SD: Postoperative ileus: A review. Dis Colon Rectum 2004;47:516–526.

37. Kreis ME, Kasparek MS, Becker HD, et al: [Postoperative ileus: Part II (Clinical therapy)]. Zentralbl Chir 2003;128:320-8.

38. Holte K, Kehlet H: Postoperative ileus: progress towards effective management. Drugs 2002;62:2603–2615.

39. Kehlet H, Holte K: Review of postoperative ileus. Am J Surg 2001;182:3S–10S.

40. Peterson KL, DeCampli WM, Pike NA, et al: A report of two hundred twenty cases of regional anesthesia in pediatric cardiac surgery. Anesth Analg 2000;90:1014–1019.

41. Aybek T, Kessler P, Dogan S, et al: Awake coronary artery bypass grafting: Utopia or reality? Ann Thorac Surg 2003;75:1165–1170.

42. Svorkdal N: Pro: anesthesiologists' role in treating refractory angina: Spinal cord stimulators, thoracic epidurals, therapeutic angiogenesis, and other emerging options. J Cardiothorac Vasc Anesth 2003;17:536–545.

43. Marchertiene I: [Regional anesthesia for patients with cardiac diseases]. Medicina (Kaunas) 2003;39:721–729.

44. Thompson JS: The role of epidural analgesia and anesthesia in surgical outcomes. Adv Surg 2002;36:297–307.

45. Rodgers A, Walker N, Schug S, et al: Reduction of postoperative mortality and morbidity with epidural or spinal anaesthesia: Results from overview of randomised trials. BMJ 2000;321:1493.

46. Burton AW, Eappen S: Regional anesthesia techniques for pain control in the intensive care unit. Crit Care Clin 1999;15:77–88, vi.

47. Low JH: Survey of epidural analgesia management in general intensive care units in England. Acta Anaesthesiol Scand 2002;46:799–805.

48. Bromage PR, Benumof JL: Paraplegia following intracord injection during attempted epidural anesthesia under general anesthesia. Reg Anesth Pain Med 1998;23:104–107.

49. Krane EJ, Dalens BJ, Murat I, et al: The safety of epidurals placed during general anesthesia. Reg Anesth Pain Med 1998;23:433–438.

50. Herwaldt LA PJ, Coffin SA, Schulz-Stübner S: Nosocomial infections associated with anesthesia. In Mayhall CG (ed): Hospital Epidemiology and Infection Control, 3rd ed. Lippincott Williams & Wilkins, 2004, pp 1073–1117.

51. Tsui BC, Gupta S, Finucane B: Confirmation of epidural catheter placement using nerve stimulation. Can J Anaesth 1998;45:640–644.

52. Tsui BC, Guenther C, Emery D, et al: Determining epidural catheter location using nerve stimulation with radiological confirmation. Reg Anesth Pain Med 2000;25:306–309.

53. Wegeforth P LJ: Lumbar puncture as a factor in the pathogenesis of meningitis. Am J Med Sci 1919;158:183–202.

54. Bell K, Wattie M, Byth K, et al: Procalcitonin: A marker of bacteraemia in SIRS. Anaesth Intensive Care 2003;31:629–636.

55. Du B, Pan J, Chen D, et al: Serum procalcitonin and interleukin-6 levels may help to differentiate systemic inflammatory response of infectious and non-infectious origin. Chin Med J (Engl) 2003;116:538–542.

56. Luzzani A, Polati E, Dorizzi R, et al: Comparison of procalcitonin and C-reactive protein as markers of sepsis. Crit Care Med 2003;31:1737–1741.

57. Delevaux I, Andre M, Colombier M, et al: Can procalcitonin measurement help in differentiating between bacterial infection and other kinds of inflammatory processes? Ann Rheum Dis 2003;62:337–340.

58. Kaplan R: ASRA consensus statements for anticoagulated patients. American Society of Regional Anesthesia. Reg Anesth Pain Med 1999;24:477–478.

59. Horlocker TT, Wedel DJ, Benzon H, et al: Regional anesthesia in the anticoagulated patient: Defining the risks (the second ASRA Consensus Conference on Neuraxial Anesthesia and Anticoagulation). Reg Anesth Pain Med 2003;28:172–197.

60. Gogarten W, Van Aken H, Büttner J, et al: Regional anesthesia and thromboembolism prophylaxis/anticoagulation. Revised guidelines of the German Society of Anesthesiology and Intensive Care Medicine. Anaesth Intesivmed 2003;44:218–230.

61. Vandermeulen E, Gogarten W, Van Aken H: [Risks and complications following peridural anesthesia]. Anaesthesist 1997;46 Suppl 3:S179–186.

62. Boezaart AP, de Beer JF, du Toit C, et al: A new technique of continuous interscalene nerve block. Can J Anaesth 1999;46:275–281.

63. Brown DL: Brachial plexus anesthesia: An analysis of options. Yale J Biol Med 1993;66:415–431.

64. Schulz-Stubner S: [Brachial plexus. Anesthesia and analgesia]. Anaesthesist 2003;52:643–657.

65. Boezaart AP, De Beer JF, Nell ML: Early experience with continuous cervical paravertebral block using a stimulating catheter. Reg Anesth Pain Med 2003;28:406–413.

66. Boezaart AP, Koorn R, Borene S, et al: Continuous brachial plexus block using the posterior approach. Reg Anesth Pain Med 2003;28:70–71.

67. Boezaart AP, Koorn R, Rosenquist RW: Paravertebral approach to the brachial plexus: An anatomic improvement in technique. Reg Anesth Pain Med 2003;28:241–244.

68. Ilfeld BM, Enneking FK: Brachial plexus infraclavicular block success rate and appropriate endpoints. Anesth Analg 2002;95:784.

69. Benumof JL: Permanent loss of cervical spinal cord function associated with interscalene block performed under general anesthesia. Anesthesiology 2000;93:1541–1544.

70. Meier G, Bauereis C, Maurer H, et al: [Interscalene plexus block. Anatomic requirements—Anesthesiologic and operative aspects]. Anaesthesist 2001;50:333–341.

71. Meier G, Bauereis C, Heinrich C: [Interscalene brachial plexus catheter for anesthesia and postoperative pain therapy. Experience with a modified technique]. Anaesthesist 1997;46:715–719.

72. Sala-Blanch X, Lazaro JR, Correa J, et al: Phrenic nerve block caused by interscalene brachial plexus block: Effects of digital pressure and a low volume of local anesthetic. Reg Anesth Pain Med 1999;24:231–235.

73. Neuburger M, Kaiser H, Rembold-Schuster I, et al: [Vertical infraclavicular brachial-plexus blockade. A clinical study of reliability of a new method for plexus anesthesia of the upper extremity]. Anaesthesist 1998;47:595–599.

74. Borene SC, Edwards JN, Boezaart AP: At the cords, the pinkie towards: Interpreting infraclavicular motor responses to neurostimulation. Reg Anesth Pain Med 2004;29:125–129.

75. Sandhu NS, Capan LM: Ultrasound-guided infraclavicular brachial plexus block. Br J Anaesth 2002;89:254–259.

76. Ang ET, Lassale B, Goldfarb G: Continuous axillary brachial plexus block—A clinical and anatomical study. Anesth Analg 1984;63:680–684.

77. Sia S, Lepri A, Campolo MC, et al: Four-injection brachial plexus block using peripheral nerve stimulator: A comparison between axillary and humeral approaches. Anesth Analg 2002;95:1075–1079, table of contents.

78. Retzl G, Kapral S, Greher M, et al: Ultrasonographic findings of the axillary part of the brachial plexus. Anesth Analg 2001;92:1271–1275.

79. Kapral S, Jandrasits O, Schabernig C, et al: Lateral infraclavicular plexus block vs. axillary block for hand and forearm surgery. Acta Anaesthesiol Scand 1999;43:1047–1052.

80. Greher M, Retzl G, Niel P, et al: Ultrasonographic assessment of topographic anatomy in volunteers suggests a modification of the infraclavicular vertical brachial plexus block. Br J Anaesth 2002;88:632–636.

81. Jandard C, Gentili ME, Girard F, et al: Infraclavicular block with lateral approach and nerve stimulation: Extent of anesthesia and adverse effects. Reg Anesth Pain Med 2002;27:37–42.

82. Finlayson BJ, Underhill TJ: Femoral nerve block for analgesia in fractures of the femoral neck. Arch Emerg Med 1988;5:173–176.

83. Tan TT, Coleman MM: Femoral blockade for fractured neck of femur in the emergency department. Ann Emerg Med 2003;42:596–597;author reply 597.

84. Marhofer P, Schrogendorfer K, Koinig H, et al: Ultrasonographic guidance improves sensory block and onset time of three-in-one blocks. Anesth Analg 1997;85:854–857.

85. Lopez S, Gros T, Bernard N, et al: Fascia iliaca compartment block for femoral bone fractures in prehospital care. Reg Anesth Pain Med 2003;28:203–207.

86. Cuignet O, Pirson J, Boughrouph J, et al: The efficacy of continuous fascia iliaca compartment block for pain management in burn patients undergoing skin grafting procedures. Anesth Analg 2004;98:1077–1081, table of contents.

87. Kaden V, Wolfel H, Kirsch W: [Experiences with a combined sciatic and femoral block in surgery of injuries of the lower leg]. Anaesthesiol Reanim 1989;14:299–303.

88. Barbero C, Fuzier R, Samii K: Anterior approach to the sciatic nerve block: Adaptation to the patient's height. Anesth Analg 2004;98:1785–1788, table of contents.

89. Franco CD: Posterior approach to the sciatic nerve in adults: Is euclidean geometry still necessary? Anesthesiology 2003;98:723–728.

90. Di Benedetto P, Casati A, Bertini L, et al: Posterior subgluteal approach to block the sciatic nerve: Description of the technique and initial clinical experiences. Eur J Anaesthesiol 2002;19:682–686.

91. Bailey SL, Parkinson SK, Little WL, et al: Sciatic nerve block. A comparison of single versus double injection technique. Reg Anesth 1994;19:9–13.

92. Rosenberg PH, Veering BT, Urmey WF: Maximum recommended doses of local anesthetics: A multifactorial concept. Reg Anesth Pain Med 2004;29:564–575.

93. Casati A, Magistris L, Fanelli G, et al: Small-dose clonidine prolongs postoperative analgesia after sciatic-femoral nerve block with 0.75% ropivacaine for foot surgery. Anesth Analg 2000;91:388–392.

94. Gao F, Waters B, Seager J, et al: Comparison of bupivacaine plus buprenorphine with bupivacaine alone by caudal blockade for postoperative pain relief after hip and knee arthroplasty. Eur J Anaesthesiol 1995;12:471–476.

95. Culebras X, Van Gessel E, Hoffmeyer P, et al: Clonidine combined with a long acting local anesthetic does not prolong postoperative analgesia after brachial plexus block but does induce hemodynamic changes. Anesth Analg 2001;92:199–204.

96. Picard PR, Tramer MR, McQuay HJ, et al: Analgesic efficacy of peripheral opioids (all except intra-articular): A qualitative systematic review of randomised controlled trials. Pain 1997;72:309–318.

97. Wehling MJ, Koorn R, Leddell C, et al: Electrical nerve stimulation using a stimulating catheter: What is the lower limit? Reg Anesth Pain Med 2004;29:230–233.

98. Costello TG, Cormack JR, Hoy C, et al: Plasma ropivacaine levels following scalp block for awake craniotomy. J Neurosurg Anesthesiol 2004;16:147–150.

99. Rawal N, Tandon B: Epidural and intrathecal morphine in intensive care units. Intensive Care Med 1985;11:129–133.

100. Shroff A, Rooke GA, Bishop MJ: Effects of intrathecal opioid on extubation time, analgesia, and intensive care unit stay following coronary artery bypass grafting. J Clin Anesth 1997;9:415–419.

101. Hall R, Adderley N, MacLaren C, et al: Does intrathecal morphine alter the stress response following coronary artery bypass grafting surgery? Can J Anaesth 2000;47:463–466.

102. Bowler I, Djaiani G, Abel R, et al: A combination of intrathecal morphine and remifentanil anesthesia for fast-track cardiac anesthesia and surgery. J Cardiothorac Vasc Anesth 2002;16:709–714.

103. Schulz-Stubner S: *Regionalanästhesie und -Analgesie.* Schattauer, 2003.

104. Zink W, Seif C, Bohl JR, et al: The acute myotoxic effects of bupivacaine and ropivacaine after continuous peripheral nerve blockades. Anesth Analg 2003;97:1173–1179, table of contents.

105. Zink W, Graf BM: Local anesthetic myotoxicity. Reg Anesth Pain Med 2004;29:333–340.

106. Zink W, Graf BM: [Toxicology of local anesthetics. Clinical, therapeutic and pathological mechanisms]. Anaesthesist 2003;52:1102–1123.

107. Scott DA, Emanuelsson BM, Mooney PH, et al: Pharmacokinetics and efficacy of long-term epidural ropivacaine infusion for postoperative analgesia. Anesth Analg 1997;85:1322–1330.

108. Gottschalk A, Burmeister MA, Freitag M, et al: [Plasma levels of ropivacaine and bupivacaine during postoperative patient controlled thoracic epidural analgesia]. Anasthesiol Intensivmed Notfallmed Schmerzther 2003;38:705–709.

109. Langevin PB, Gravenstein N, Langevin SO, et al: Epidural catheter reconnection. Safe and unsafe practice. Anesthesiology 1996;85:883–888.

110. Cuvillon P, Ripart J, Lalourcey L, et al: The continuous femoral nerve block catheter for postoperative analgesia: Bacterial colonization, infectious rate and adverse effects. Anesth Analg 2001;93:1045–1049.

111. Auroy Y, Benhamou D, Bargues L, et al: Major complications of regional anesthesia in France: The SOS Regional Anesthesia Hotline Service. Anesthesiology 2002;97:1274–1280.

112. Auroy Y, Narchi P, Messiah A, et al: Serious complications related to regional anesthesia: Results of a prospective survey in France. Anesthesiology 1997;87:479–486.

113. Moen V, Dahlgren N, Irestedt L: Severe neurological complications after central neuraxial blockades in Sweden 1990–1999. Anesthesiology 2004;101:950–959.

68

Regional Anesthesia & Acute Pain Management in the Emergency Department

Jeffrey Gadsden, MD • Knox H. Todd, MD

INTRODUCTION

Emergency physicians are called on to provide care for a variety of emergent, urgent, and often complex conditions. Many patients present with pain as a component of their illness or require diagnostic and/or therapeutic interventions that are inherently painful to perform. As a result, the management of analgesia in the emergency department (ED) is a critical skill and an important element in the overall care of patients in this setting. This chapter is an overview of acute pain in the context of the ED as well as potential therapies, including regional anesthetic techniques for the emergency physician.

OLIGOANALGESIA: PAIN AS A PROBLEM IN THE ED

Pain is the single most common reason patients seek care in the ED, and it accounts for up to 79% of visits.[1] Given the prevalence of pain as a presenting complaint, one might expect emergency physicians to assign its treatment a high priority. However, pain is seemingly invisible to providers of emergency medical care. *Oligoanalgesia*, a term coined by Wilson and Pendleton[2] in 1989, is the inadequate use of methods to relieve pain. Multiple studies in the emergency medicine literature have observed that oligoanalgesia is a common occurrence.[3] Notwithstanding the issue of providing compassionate care, pain that is not acknowledged and managed appropriately causes anxiety, depression, sleep disturbances, increased oxygen demands with the potential for end-organ ischemia, and decreased movement with an increased risk of venous thrombosis.[4,5] Failure to recognize and treat pain may also result in dissatisfaction with medical care, hostility toward the physician, unscheduled returns to the ED, delayed full return to full function, and a potential increased risk of litigation.[6]

Several studies have attempted to define the prevalence of pain and oligoanalgesia in ED settings. Johnston and coworkers[7] investigated the incidence and severity of pain among patients presenting to noncritical treatment areas within the EDs of two urban hospitals in Canada. Fifty-eight percent of adults and 47% of children reported pain on ED arrival. Approximately 50% of these patients described the pain as moderate to severe. At the time of discharge, one third of both groups continued to report pain of moderate to severe intensity. In fact, 11% of children and adults in this study actually reported clinically important increases in pain intensity during their stay in the ED.

Another prospective study found that among adults treated at one Chicago ED, 78% presented with pain as a chief complaint.[8] Fifty-eight percent of all patients received analgesics or nonpharmacologic intervention, but only 15% received opioids, despite high levels of pain intensity. Guru and Dubinsky[9] found that 50% of patients who were treated for acutely painful conditions did not receive prescriptions for pain management at discharge. Another review of urban, university-based EDs reported that 69% of patients with painful conditions, including thermal burns, long-bone fractures, and vaso-occlusive crises, received no pain medication at all and that 55% were discharged with no analgesic prescription.[10]

A study by Brown et al.[11] revealed that pain medications were frequently not part of ED treatment for fractures, even for visits with documented moderate or severe pain.

Despite a tendency for undertreatment of pain in the ED, patients continue to expect analgesia. Fosnocht and coworkers[12] used a 100-mm visual analog-type scale (VAS) to gauge patient expectation of pain relief in the ED (0 mm = no relief; 100 mm = complete relief). Patients with pain reported a mean expectation for pain relief of 72%, with 18% of patients expecting complete relief of their pain. It is interesting that this value was seemingly independent of the initial pain severity, so that those with mild pain expected the same degree of relief as those with severe pain. Other studies have suggested that patient expectations are very influential on both the patient's experience of pain and satisfaction with their care.[13,14]

Why is pain being undertreated in the ED? Several factors may play a role. Difficulty in accurately assessing pain is a well-known problem to providers of emergency medical care. Caregivers have been shown in several studies to underestimate pain scores when compared with those reported by the patients themselves.[9,15] The assessment may also be hindered by the limitations of commonly used verbal scales. For example, Rupp and Delaney[3] point out that asking a patient to describe his or her pain in relation to the "worst pain imaginable" obviously results in different answers, depending on the patient's particular frame of reference. Other factors leading to oligoanalgesia may include apprehension about dependency when prescribing opioids (both on the part of the patient and the physician),[16] concern regarding side effects such as respiratory depression,[17] and the desire to withhold pain medication until informed consent for a procedure has been obtained, and concern about not obscuring a diagnosis (eg, an acute abdomen). Attitudes toward this last practice are changing, although slowly, because of mounting evidence that adequate analgesia in these situations allows patients to relax. This removes voluntary guarding as a confounding factor and allows for a more precise evaluation of localized sensitivity.[3,18–20]

Some patient groups are known to carry a higher risk for oligoanalgesia (Figure 68–1). For example, multiple studies

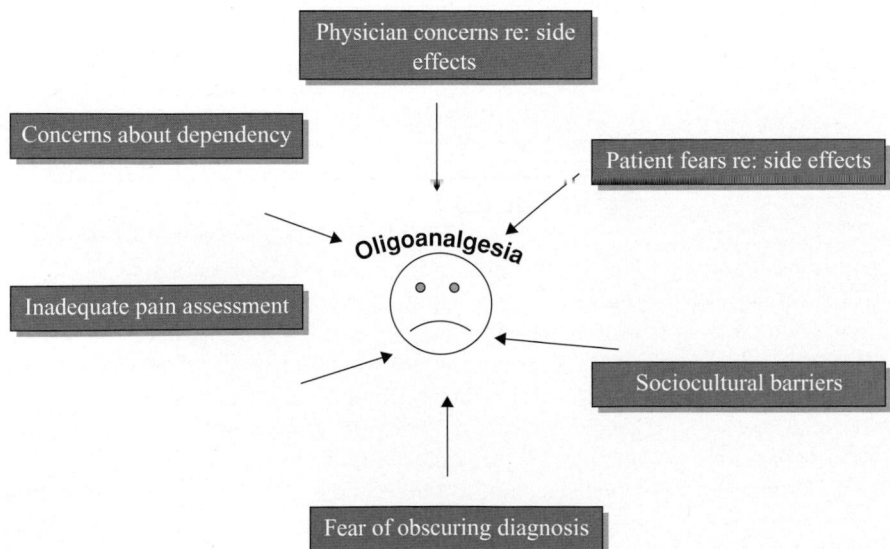

Figure 68–1. Factors contributing to oligoanalgesia in the emergency department.

Table 68–1.

JCAHO Standards for Pain Management

- Recognize the right of patients to appropriate assessment and management of pain
- Assess the existence and, if so, the nature and intensity of pain in all patients
- Record the results of the assessment in a way that facilitates regular reassessment and follow-up
- Determine and ensure staff competency in pain assessment and management, and address pain assessment and management in the orientation of all new staff
- Establish policies and procedures that support the appropriate prescription or ordering of effective pain medications
- Educate patients and their families about effective pain management
- Address patient needs for symptom management in the discharge planning process

have documented lower rates of analgesic administration for both young children and the elderly when compared with other patients in pain.[10,21,22] Kozlowski and colleagues[23] reported that in patients with isolated lower extremity injuries, those with fractures were twice as likely to receive pain medication as those without fractures, even when controlling for the severity of pain. Patient gender appears to be unimportant with respect to analgesia in the ED according to one prospective study.[24]

Patient ethnicity is perhaps the best-studied risk factor for oligoanalgesia in the ED. In 1993, Todd and colleagues[25] examined the medical records of all patients with acute, isolated, long-bone fractures seen at the UCLA Emergency Medicine Center in 1991 and 1992. Hispanic patients in this study were twice as likely as non-Hispanic white patients to receive no pain medications during their ED stay (RR 2.1; 95% CI 1.4–3.3). This relative risk for ethnicity remained significant after controlling for covariates related to patient (gender, language, and insurance coverage), injury (open versus closed fracture, admittance versus discharge, need for reduction), and physician characteristics (ethnicity, gender, specialty). After multiple logistic regression analyses, patient ethnicity remained the strongest predictor of ED analgesic administration. In a follow-up study performed at a large, community, university-affiliated ED in urban Atlanta, Todd and colleagues[26] found similar disparities in analgesic treatment between white and African-American patients with isolated long-bone fractures despite similar documentation of pain complaints.

The solution to these disparities may involve more than simply addressing cultural biases, however. Research into the genomic basis of pain sensation is beginning to show that different individuals, as well as groups of individuals, process

pain signals differently.[27] This may help guide providers of analgesia as to which individuals may be experiencing more intense pain for the same injury or illness. In addition, response to analgesics may also be attributable in part to gene expression, just as cytochrome P450 receptor differences determine a patient's ability to utilize codeine.[28]

PAIN ASSESSMENT IN THE ED

Recognizing that pain is a major public health problem, the Joint Commission on Accreditation of Healthcare Organizations (JCAHO) has placed a great deal of emphasis on the importance of pain management, in part by implementing standards that create new expectations for the assessment and management of pain[29] (Table 68–1). These standards have been endorsed by the American Pain Society.

One of the key take-home points of the JCAHO recommendations focuses on the usefulness of standardized scales so that frequent reassessment of a patient's pain can be progressively documented and treated. Indeed, many hospital EDs have begun to include pain as the "fifth vital sign," to encourage frequent and standardized reassessment.

Several pain assessment tools are available for use in the ED. One of the most common is the visual analog scale (VAS)—easy to use and convenient for statistical analysis. Patients are asked to make a mark on a horizontal line corresponding to the intensity of their pain (Figure 68–2). This scale is attractive for acute care settings in which short-term changes in VAS can be used to guide titration of analgesic therapy. Todd and coworkers[30] conducted serial interviews with patients reporting acute pain and concluded that a change of less than 13 mm in the VAS is clinically insignificant. Another

Least Possible Pain	Worst Pain Imaginable

Indicate the severity of your pain by placing a **single mark** through the line above at the appropriate point.

Figure 68–2. Visual Analog Scale.

similar tool is the numeric rating scale (NRS), which asks the patient to verbally rate the pain on a numerical scale—usually 1–10. Both the VAS and NRS have been shown to be reliable and valid tools for assessing acute pain.[31,32]

Mandated reporting of pain scores has been shown to result in improved frequency of analgesic administration for ED patients presenting with acute pain.[33]

MONITORING DURING SEDATION & ANALGESIA

Opioids are the most frequently used analgesic for moderate-to-severe pain in the ED, but they carry a risk of dose-dependent respiratory depression as well as sedation and hypotension. In addition to treating pain as a presenting complaint, emergency physicians are often called on to perform diagnostic or therapeutic procedures that are associated with a brief but intense amount of pain. In these cases, sedatives such as benzodiazepines, opioids, and other anesthetic drugs are sometimes used to facilitate an expeditious and painless procedure. As such, emergency physicians must be skilled at monitoring patients who are sedated and must be able to manage potential complications resulting from sedation such as the need for advanced airway management.[34] In 2005, the American College of Emergency Physicians (ACEP) updated their guidelines for procedural sedation and analgesia in the ED, replacing guidelines set out in 1998. The recommendations appear as a series of "critical questions." Key elements are as follows:

1. **What are the personnel requirements needed to provide procedural sedation and analgesia in the ED?**

    -   During moderate and deep sedation, a qualified support person should be present for continuous monitoring of the patient.
    -   Patient must be supervised by an emergency physician or other appropriately trained and credentialed specialist.

    The literature is unclear about the number of personnel required during light sedation in addition to the physician performing the procedure.

2. **Is preprocedural fasting necessary before initiating procedural sedation?**

    -   Recent food intake is not a contraindication for administering procedural sedation and analgesia, but should be considered in choosing the timing and target level of sedation.

    This guideline is based on the assertion that the combination of vomiting and loss of airway protective reflexes is an extremely rare occurrence with procedural sedation and analgesia. The American Society of Anesthesiologists recommends a minimum fast of 2 hours for clear liquids and 6 hours for solids, but it should be noted that both groups base their recommendations on consensus opinion rather than firm evidence.

It is prudent to weigh the risks of sedation versus delaying the procedure when considering this issue for nonfasted ED patients.

3. **What equipment and supplies are required to provide sedation and analgesia?**

    -   Oxygen, suction, reversal agents, and advanced life support medications and equipment should be available.

    These items should include immediate access to a bag-valve-mask device, oral and nasal airways, laryngoscopes, and endotracheal tubes.

4. **How should respiratory status be assessed?**

    -   Pulse oximetry should be used in patients at increased risk of developing hypoxemia, such as patients on high doses or multiple drugs are used and when patients with significant comorbidity.
    -   Consider capnography to provide additional information regarding early identification of hypoventilation.

    Pulse oximetry is a low-risk, high-yield intervention that is unobtrusive, is easy to apply, and does not cause patient discomfort. The guidelines recommend obtaining and documenting vital signs (heart rate, respiratory rate, blood pressure and pulse oximetry) before, during, and after procedural sedation, but do not specify a recommended time interval. Response to verbal stimuli is a valuable monitor that is useful during sedation to monitor depth and guide further drug administration.

    It is convenient to classify depth of sedation into three categories: sedation/analgesia (formerly conscious sedation), in which patients can respond purposefully to verbal and tactile stimuli; deep sedation, in which patients with depressed consciousness are not easily arousable and do not respond to stimuli in a purposeful manner; and general anesthesia, which is a medically controlled state of unconsciousness accompanied by a loss of protective airway reflexes.[35] In reality, sedation and anesthesia are part of the same continuum, and using escalating doses of any sedative drug can push a patient into the next "level." The ACEP guidelines state that a key to minimizing complications is the titration of drugs to the desired effect. Because of familiarity with the pharmacokinetic properties of commonly used drugs such as midazolam and fentanyl, this is usually achieved without incident. There is some controversy regarding the use of more potent anesthetic drugs such as etomidate[36] and, in particular, propofol,[37] in the ED setting. The extremely rapid onset of action and potent cardiorespiratory depressant effects of propofol have led some emergency physicians to caution against its widespread use in the ED,[38] citing studies showing an inability of physicians in the ED to avoid overshooting their sedation target when using the drug.[39] On the other hand, there is a growing body of evidence that propofol can be used safely by ED physicians for procedural sedation; it is likely that it will continue to gain popularity for this role.[40,41]

PHARMACOLOGIC STRATEGIES FOR ACUTE PAIN

Although many analgesic drugs are available to the emergency physician, it is important to tailor a pharmacologic regimen to each patient. For mild pain, simple analgesics often are all that is required. In contrast, moderate or severe pain may demand a more multifaceted approach to analgesia. We now know that pain is an extremely complex process involving many different classes of mediators and receptors. For this reason, the concept of multimodal analgesia is a crucial one in pain medicine. Multimodal analgesia is the combining of different classes of drugs to improve pain relief while minimizing the potential for side effects due to reduced reliance on one agent.[42]

Acetaminophen

Acetaminophen has analgesic and antipyretic, but no antiinflammatory, properties. Its mechanism is unclear, but acetaminophen probably works via inhibiting prostaglandin synthesis. It is a good analgesic for mild to moderate pain, especially pain due to osteoarthritis, musculoskeletal pain, headache, earache, and dysmenorrhea. It is frequently used in combination with nonsteroidal antiinflammatories (NSAIDs) or opioids. The most serious adverse effect is hepatotoxicity, which is rarely seen except in the case of an overdose far exceeding the daily recommended limits. Because of its long safety record and low incidence of adverse effects, acetaminophen is the most frequently used analgesic in North America and is often the base on which to build multimodal analgesia.

NSAIDs

"Nonsteroidals" are also very common in the management of acute pain. In addition to analgesic and antipyretic properties, these drugs are antiinflammatories and function by inhibiting cyclooxygenase (COX), an enzyme responsible for prostaglandin synthesis. This property renders NSAIDs useful for treating inflammatory and prostaglandin-related pain such as rheumatoid arthritis and dysmenorrhea, as well as renal and biliary colic, headache, and musculoskeletal injuries. The inhibition of COX is also responsible for its side-effect profile, which includes nephrotoxicity via decreased renal perfusion and an increased risk of gastroduodenal ulcer formation. These side effects are dose-dependent and are more likely to occur in the elderly and those with preexisting renal or peptic ulcer disease.[43] Other adverse effects include hypersensitivity, platelet dysfunction, and asthmatic exacerbation in sensitive individuals.[44]

There are many NSAIDs to choose from, and they appear to be relatively interchangeable as a class. In other words, with the correct dosing, ibuprofen is as effective as indomethacin or diclofenac. Ketorolac is unique in that it may be used parenterally, thereby ensuring a rapid onset, which is an attractive attribute in the ED. Ketorolac has been used favorably in emergency medicine for various types of acute pain.[45] The COX-2 inhibitor class of NSAIDs have not been adequately studied in the ED setting.[42] This class of drugs has recently been associated with adverse cardiovascular outcomes in major clinical trials, and two of the major COX-2 inhibitors have been voluntarily withdrawn from the market pending further investigation.

Opioids

Intravenous opioids, titrated to effect, are the treatment of choice for patients with moderate-to-severe, acute pain in the ED.[46] Morphine is the standard against which most analgesic interventions are compared, although emergency physicians are using an increasingly wide spectrum of opioids, such as fentanyl and sufentanil, for their rapid onset and limited duration of action during procedural sedation and analgesia.[47] Other commonly used parenteral opioids are meperidine and hydromorphone, although use of the former is declining owing to its neurotoxic and anticholinergic side effects. Oral opioids such as codeine and oxycodone are a popular choice when prescribing discharge medications for moderate pain, especially in combination with acetaminophen or NSAIDs. Major side effects common to all opioids include dose-dependent respiratory depression, nausea, constipation, pruritus, and urinary retention. Owing to concerns about serious adverse effects as well as fear of punitive action by regulatory agencies, many physicians suffer from "opiophobia," and underprescribe this potent and effective class of analgesics.[3]

Other Adjuvants

Many other nontraditional strategies have been used in the perioperative period to reduce the duration and severity of postoperative pain. Few of these have been applied to the acute pain setting in the ED. One example of a drug that has been used is ketamine, an NMDA (*N*-methyl-D-aspartate)-receptor **antagonist** that has a unique dissociative–anesthetic effect and is known for having potent analgesic properties. Ketamine is occasionally used for procedural sedation in children.[48] Inhaled nitrous oxide has both sedative and analgesic properties, but its popularity for use in the ED has waxed and waned over the years.[49] Other pharmacologic adjuvants that have promise in other areas of pain management but are infrequently used in the ED are clonidine, dexmedetomidine, gabapentin, neostigmine, and magnesium.

Combination or Multimodal Analgesia

Combining two or more drugs of different classes has been shown to reduce the side-effect profile of each and particularly for opioids, an effect termed "opioid-sparing."

For example, ketorolac plus morphine allows for less morphine use and a reduction in opioid-related side effects for postoperative pain.[50] Acetaminophen plus oxycodone provides more superior analgesia than controlled-release oxycodone after oral surgery.[51] After adenoidectomy, children who received ibuprofen plus acetaminophen required less analgesia at home than those who received either drug alone.[52] Techniques that aim at opioid sparing have been shown to reduce time to discharge from the ED and improve patient satisfaction.

Although most of this research has been carried out in the perioperative setting, much of it is applicable to acute pain in the ED, despite barriers to adequate pain management, such as crowding and lack of continuity of care. Other techniques used by anesthesiologists that have potential applications for acute pain in the ED are aggressive titration protocols, continuous infusion pumps, and patient-controlled analgesia.[53]

LOCAL & REGIONAL ANESTHETIC TECHNIQUES IN THE ED

Whereas many pain relievers work by altering the transmission, perception or modulation of pain impulses at the spinal or brain level, local anesthetics primarily exert their effect by blocking axonal transmission in peripheral nerves, thereby preventing nociceptive signals from reaching the central nervous system. By stopping the pain impulses before they arrive at the dorsal horn of the spinal cord, regional anesthetic techniques reduce the degree of central sensitization, or "wind-up," and allow for high-quality pain relief with minimal side effects.

Regional and local anesthesia is particularly well suited to the ED, where many patients present with acute, localized painful injuries that are amenable to a short-term, selective peripheral blockade.

Topical Anesthetics

Topical anesthesia involves the application of local anesthetic directly to a mucosal or skin surface. It has the advantage of a needle-less technique, and many small lacerations and injuries can be effectively anesthetized by the application of these agents. Several studies have shown that the application of a topical local anesthetic mixture significantly reduced the severity of pain on injection and the time to discharge in patients with simple lacerations required suturing.[54,55]

For mucous membranes, lidocaine 1–4% provides adequate anesthesia after topical application and can be administered several different ways. Viscous jelly can be swished around the mouth; lidocaine can be nebulized for anesthesia of the oropharynx and airway; pledgets can be soaked and then applied directly to a mucosal area. Care must be taken when using local anesthetics on mucosal surfaces because uptake is rapid, especially when higher concentrations are used (eg, 4% lidocaine). Safe dosages should be calculated in advance and adhered to.

For intact skin, the most common form of topical anesthesia is eutectic mixture of local anesthesia (EMLA). EMLA cream is a 1:1 mixture of 2.5% lidocaine and 2.5% prilocaine and has been well established as a means to decrease pain from venipuncture and intravenous cannulation in children.[56] It is usually applied to skin, then covered with a barrier dressing while waiting for its anesthetic effect. Adverse effects are minimal, although cases of methemoglobinemia have been reported secondary to prilocaine toxicity.[57] One disadvantage with EMLA is the duration of application required for effective local anesthesia, usually between 45 and 60 minutes. EMLA has also been used for minor procedures such as infant penile circumcision.[58]

ELA-Max is a relatively new product that contains 4% lidocaine cream in a liposomal matrix. It is applied to the skin in a manner similar to that of EMLA and has been shown to be as effective as EMLA but with a faster onset of action (30 minutes versus 60 minutes).[59] Other methods of topical anesthesia for intact skin include the delivery of lidocaine by iontophoresis[60] and the use of jet injectors.[61] Both have been used in the ED with success.

Nonintact skin can be effectively anesthetized by the application of a liquid mixture of local anesthetic and vasoconstrictor. Examples include TAC (tetracaine 0.5%, adrenaline 0.05%, and cocaine 11.8%), LET (lidocaine 4%, epinephrine 0.1%, and tetracaine 0.5%), and MAC (marcaine, adrenaline, and cocaine).[62,63] The mixture is applied to the wound and covered with moist gauze. Adequate anesthesia usually results after 25–30 minutes.

Local Infiltration

Injecting local anesthetics subcutaneously can result in sufficient anesthesia to allow for minor superficial procedures, such as suturing of wounds. Because anticipation of a needle stick is often emotionally traumatic for patients, especially children, the use of techniques to lessen the pain on injection is always appreciated. These include the use of small needles (ie, 27- to 30-gauge), slow administration of the anesthetic (1 mL over 30 seconds), and the buffering of local anesthetic by sodium bicarbonate.[64,65] Bartfield and colleagues[66] studied pain on injection at wound sites and found that local anesthesia is less painful when injected from within a laceration than through intact skin. Vasoconstrictors such as epinephrine added to local anesthetic increase the duration of the anesthesia (by decreasing local uptake) and provide better hemostasis at the wound site. Vasoconstrictors should not be used on the ear, nose, penis, fingers, or toes because ischemia and tissue necrosis may result.

Intravenous Regional Anesthesia or Bier's Block

Intravenous regional anesthesia (IVRA) was first performed in 1908 by Karl August Bier, and the procedure has changed little since that time.[67] It has been shown to have an excellent safety record, to provide effective anesthesia of the isolated limb, and to be easy to perform.[68] The method for establishing the block is described elsewhere but essentially involves exsanguinating a limb using a compressive device, inflating a double tourniquet on the proximal end of the limb, then injecting local anesthetic intravenously into the isolated limb. The local anesthetic spreads throughout the venous channels of the arm or leg, diffusing out to act on both the free nerve endings in the tissues and the larger peripheral nerve branches. It is a popular form of anesthesia for reducing fractures in the ED, especially in children.[69] Complications are rare with IVRA but are usually caused by inappropriate management of the double cuff, leading to "washout" of local anesthetic into the central circulation and subsequent toxicity. Most authors recommend a minimum tourniquet time of 20–30 minutes before deflating, regardless of the duration of the procedure. Some also advocate a staged tourniquet deflation to allow for partial washout in an attempt to lower peak blood local anesthetic concentrations.

The most common agent for IVRA is lidocaine, but other local anesthetics such as prilocaine have been used. Bupivacaine has fallen out of favor owing to the unnecessary risk of systemic toxicity. Some practitioners add narcotics or other adjuvants to the mixture such as ketorolac, tramadol, or clonidine. The traditional preparation is a high-volume, dilute concentration of lidocaine (eg, 40 mL of 0.5% for an upper arm tourniquet), but good results can be achieved with a low-volume, high-concentration technique (eg, 12–15 mL of 2% lidocaine). Onset of either is usually less than 5 minutes for full anesthesia.

Peripheral Nerve Blocks

In general, blocks of peripheral nerves have several advantages over local infiltration.[70] They are often less painful to perform and may cause less anxiety for the patient, especially when the procedure involves sensitive areas such as the palm or sole. Tissue distortion of the wound is usually avoided. Also, depending on the area, less local anesthetic may be required, reducing the risk of systemic toxicity. Compared with parenteral or oral analgesics, nerve blocks have been shown to provide superior analgesia and greater patient satisfaction for treatment of pain associated with femoral neck or shaft fractures.[71]

Peripheral nerve blocks require some degree of specialized training but, with practice, can be implemented in the ED setting to great effect. Nerve blockade is often performed in the ED as a blind technique or one in which paresthesias are sought as confirmation of correct needle placement.[70] Nerve stimulation as a means of locating peripheral nerves has been slow to catch on in the ED setting, despite its almost universal use among anesthesiologists. This may be due in part to lack of experience with the nerve stimulators, and unfamiliarity with the technique. However, it has been shown to be both easy to learn and effective when performed by emergency physicians.[72]

Ultrasound-guided nerve blockade is a relatively new trend that is showing promise as a way to improve accuracy and block success.[73] This technique may be particularly attractive to emergency physicians, because most have experience in both performing ultrasound exams and using ultrasound for placement of intravenous lines.

Regardless of the technique used, there is evidence that peripheral nerve blocks in the ED are underused as a means of acute pain management.[74] Emergency physicians should have an armamentarium of nerve blocks that can be used for the relief of acute pain in the ED. Finally, nerve blocks require proper patient education before the block is performed.

Some blocks can be associated with some degree of discomfort (eg, ankle block). Adequate pre-block analgesia improves patient cooperation and ultimately satisfaction. The following is a brief overview of peripheral nerve blocks that are commonly performed in the ED setting. For a complete description of individual techniques, please refer to the respective chapter.

Digital Blocks

Digital blocks of the fingers and toes are more comfortable and easier to perform than local infiltration. Four nerves enter each digit—two on the volar aspect and two on the dorsal aspect—approximately at the 2, 4, 8, and 10 o'clock positions. The most consistent method for anesthetizing the finger or toe is to insert a fine-gauge (ie, 27-gauge) needle into the dorsal web space, just lateral to the bone. After raising a subcutaneous wheal with 0.5–1 mL of local anesthetic, the needle is advanced toward the palm or sole until it is just past the bone on the volar side. After negative aspiration, a further 1–1.5 mL is injected. Then the procedure is repeated on the other side of the digit. In this manner, all four nerves are blocked. Epinephrine-containing solutions should never be used in digital blocks as ischemia and necrosis may result.

Wrist Blocks

These blocks are appropriate for minor procedures on the palm or dorsum of the hand, or on the fingers when more than one digit is involved. The technique involves blocking the terminal branches of the median, ulnar, and radial nerves or any appropriate combination of these nerves, depending on the anatomic location of the injury. Most practitioners use a blind technique based on the relatively consistent location of these nerves at the wrist,[75] but they can also be performed using a nerve stimulator technique.[76] Wrist blocks are safe and easy to perform, but they require a good working knowledge of the anatomy of the hand and wrist.

Ankle Blocks

Ankle blocks are similar to wrist blocks to the extent that it is a blockade of the terminal branches of several peripheral nerves just before entering the foot. This block is suitable for relieving pain and/or performing procedures anywhere on the foot. Like the wrist block, selective blockade of individual peripheral nerves can be performed (eg, posterior tibial nerve block for suturing a sole laceration). On the other hand, blocking all five nerves (posterior tibial, sural, saphenous, and superficial and deep peroneal) provides complete anesthesia of the foot below the ankle. Some practitioners advocate five separate injections, whereas others recommend a three-puncture technique. The latter approach is carried out by first performing separate posterior tibial and sural blocks behind the medial and lateral malleoli, respectively, then using a single puncture site just lateral to the extensor hallucis longus tendon. With this maneuver, the deep peroneal nerve is blocked, followed by withdrawing the needle to just below the skin and redirecting both laterally and medially while depositing local anesthetic in a subcutaneous wheal to block the saphenous and superficial peroneal nerves. Ankle blocks are extremely useful but are somewhat uncomfortable and therefore require a moderate degree of sedation and analgesia.

Femoral Nerve Blocks

The femoral nerve block has been used for many years in the ED for treatment of pain associated with fractures of the femoral shaft or neck. It is also useful for pain associated with patellar and patellar tendon injuries as well as superficial injuries to the anterior thigh. This block confers anesthesia to the entire anterior thigh and most of the femur and knee joint. Because the saphenous nerve is a superficial sensory branch of the femoral nerve that extends along the medial aspect of the lower leg, anesthesia of this area is also achieved. The popularity of the femoral nerve block in the ED is probably due to its reliability and ease of performance. The femoral nerve is a superficial nerve at the level of the inguinal crease, and its reliable position next to the femoral vessels makes it easy to locate.[77] The block is often performed using a "double pop" technique, which corresponds to the penetration of both the fascia lata and the fascia iliaca layers, under which the femoral nerve resides. The clinician should feel two clicks or pops as the needle, preferably with a noncutting tip, passes through these fascial sheets.

Alternatively, paresthesia may be sought in the femoral nerve distribution. Proximity to the femoral nerve with a nerve stimulator and stimulating needle results in quadriceps twitches and a jerking of the patella. Usually, 15–20 mL of local anesthetic are enough to provide quality anesthesia. Winnie and coworkers[78] described the 3-in-1 block in 1973, which was designed to augment femoral nerve anesthesia with simultaneous blockade of the lateral femoral cutaneous nerve and the obturator nerve. The technique is performed by applying pressure to the femoral sheath just distal to the injection point and using a relatively high volume of local anesthetic, thereby forcing a proximal migration of the solution. The usefulness of the 3-in-1 block has been questioned, because the blockade of the other two components is unreliable, probably owing to fascial septa in the femoral sheath.[79] Another approach, called a **fascia iliaca block**, involves a needle insertion site several centimeters lateral to the femoral nerve, thereby reducing concerns about vascular or nerve injury.[80] The distribution of anesthesia is similar to that of femoral nerve block. Overall, the complication rate is low for femoral nerve block. Some anecdotal reports of femoral nerve blockade masking the symptoms of a compartment syndrome of the thigh have been investigated and found to be lacking in evidence.[81]

Intercostal Nerve Blocks

The intercostal nerve block is most commonly used in the ED to provide analgesia for patients with broken or contused ribs. In this population, it has been shown to provide excellent analgesia for most rib fractures, but also to improve respiratory mechanics (as measured by peak expiratory flow rate) and arterial oxygen saturation.[82] It should not be performed in patients with flail chest. Pneumothorax is the primary concern when performing this block, and it occurs in approximately 1.4% of nerves blocked.[83] This incidence increases in patients with obstructive lung disease. The block anesthetizes only the anterior and lateral chest wall because it is usually performed distal to where the posterior cutaneous diverges from the main intercostal nerve.

The safest location to perform the intercostal nerve block is at the posterior axillary line, because it is here that the internal intercostal muscle lies between the nerve and the pleura. The ribs are used as landmarks, and a mobile needle is carefully walked off the inferior edge where the neurovascular bundle lies in the costal groove. Proper stabilization of the hands on the posterior chest wall is important to prevent inadvertent slipping of the needle into the intrapleural. After advancing 1–2 mm past the edge of the rib, the clinician aspirates to check for blood or air, and then injects 3–5 mL of local anesthetic slowly. Care must be taken with local anesthetic dosing because systemic uptake is high, owing to the close presence of the intercostal vessels. After 30 minutes, if no clinical signs of pneumothorax are present, the patient may be discharged with advice to return if dyspnea or chest pain appears.[70]

Axillary Brachial Plexus Blocks

The brachial plexus is formed by the union of spinal roots C5 to T1. These pass under the clavicle and through the axilla to form the peripheral branches of the nerves supplying the upper limb, namely, the musculocutaneous, radial, ulnar, and median nerves (as well as several smaller nerves). Although there are many approaches to the brachial plexus used in clinical anesthesia, such as the interscalene, supraclavicular, and infraclavicular, few emergency physicians have the level of comfort performing these without supplemental training.

In contrast, the axillary approach is a favorable one for regional anesthesia novices owing to the presence of good landmarks, the close bundling of the nerves in a neurovascular sheath, and the low incidence of serious complications. The axillary arterial pulse is used as the primary landmark for all approaches, whether for seeking paresthesia, using a nerve stimulator, or performing a transarterial technique. The latter approach may in fact be the easiest because it requires no extra equipment apart form a 23-gauge needle and a small length of IV tubing attached to the local anesthetic syringe. With the nondominant hand palpating the axillary pulse, the needle is passed through the skin and into the axillary artery, which is evidenced by the return of bright red blood through the IV tubing. The needle is slowly advanced until the aspiration of blood ceases, which corresponds to the passage of the

Table 68–2.

Miscellaneous Nerve Blocks and their Indications

Peripheral Nerve Block	Indication
Interscalene brachial plexus block	• Pain at the shoulder or upper arm • Manipulation of frozen shoulder or painful elbow
Lumbar plexus block	• Fractured neck/shaft of femur • Wounds of the thigh that include obturator and/or lateral femoral cutaneous distribution
Sciatic nerve block	• Pain of the posterior thigh and/or leg below the knee • Tibia/fibula fracture, ankle/foot fracture
Popliteal nerve block	• Pain below the knee • Tibia/fibula fracture, ankle/foot fracture

needle through the back wall of the artery. At this point, the needle tip should be within the fascial sheath that contains the radial, ulnar, and median nerves. After negative aspiration, the local anesthetic is injected. Some clinicians deposit local anesthetic in front of the artery as well after withdrawing back through the vessel. This block provides dense anesthesia of the forearm and hand and is useful for treating pain associated with fractures and deeper wounds of those areas. Note that the musculocutaneous nerve has already left the sheath at this point and, if desired, requires a separate blockade by injecting 5–10 mL of local anesthetic into the belly of the coracobrachialis muscle.

Other Peripheral Nerve Blocks

Often, a case arises in which a patient is a candidate for a peripheral nerve block that falls outside the scope of the emergency physician. In these instances, it may be appropriate to consult an anesthesiologist to provide advice and perhaps perform the block, given the expertise in this area. Table 68–2 outlines some blocks typically not performed by ED personnel but may be of value in specific circumstances.

EPIDURAL & SPINAL ANESTHESIA

Spinal anesthesia is rarely used in the ED. Epidural techniques, however, may be used occasionally. Epidural blocks are usually associated with conditions requiring longer durations of action (up to several days for postoperative patients) and may not immediately be considered for the acute pain seen in the ED. However, given the frequent shortage of in-patient hospital beds, patients may remain in the ED for hours or days awaiting intensive care or intermediate care beds. In these cases, it may be appropriate to begin epidural analgesia in the ED.

Epidural analgesia may be used for conditions that are expected to be extremely painful for periods of 48–96 hours. During this time window, other methods of analgesia are implemented and the epidural analgesia can be discontinued. Indications for epidural analgesia include the presence of relatively discrete pain with contiguous dermatomes that can be alleviated with segmental neural blockade. Patients must be able to tolerate seated or lateral decubitus positioning while the epidural is being placed. Hemodynamic instability, coagulopathy, and sepsis are contraindications to epidural analgesia, given the hemodynamic consequences of sympathetic blockade and the potential for precipitating an epidural hematoma or abscess, respectively.

Multiple rib fractures resulting from blunt trauma are the most common indication for epidural techniques in the ED.[84,85] As with intercostal blocks, thoracic epidurals have a favorable effect on pulmonary mechanics, and patients are more likely to avoid endotracheal intubation and positive-pressure ventilation and the concomitant sedation, which precludes the monitoring of mental status. Rarely, patients suffering from pain in the anorectal region benefit from a low lumbar or caudal epidural block. Lower limb crush injuries and intractable renal colic have also been considered indications for epidural analgesia during the ED stay.

SUMMARY

Acute pain is a problem in the emergency department that is well recognized. Emergency physicians must develop an approach to the management of acutely ill patients that includes the assessment and treatment of pain as well as the treatment of the underlying illness. Multimodal analgesia, with a combination of oral, parenteral, and nerve block techniques, is the most effective way to provide quality pain relief in the emergency department while minimizing dangerous and otherwise adverse effects. Regional anesthesia is a powerful adjunct to acute pain management that has been traditionally underused in the emergency department, and more attention should be given to providing pain relief through the thoughtful use of peripheral nerve blocks.

References

1. Cordell WH, Keene KK, Giles BK, et al: The high prevalence of pain in emergency medical care. Am J Emerg Med 2002;20:165–169.
2. Wilson JE, Pendleton JM: Oligoanalgesia in the emergency department. Am J Emerg Med 1989;7:620–623.
3. Rupp T, Delaney KA: Inadequate analgesia in emergency medicine. Ann Emerg Med 2004;43:494–503.
4. Gureje O, Von Korff M, Simon Ge, et al: Persistent pain and well-being: A World Health Organization Study in Primary Care. JAMA 1998;280:147–151.
5. Anderson FA Jr, Spencer FA: Risk factors for venous thromboembolism. Circulation 2003;107(23 Suppl 1):I9–I16.
6. Furrow BR: Pain management and provider liability: No more excuses. J Law Med Ethics 2001;29:28–51.
7. Johnston CC, Gagnon AJ, Fullerton L, et al: One-week survey of pain intensity on admission to and discharge from the emergency department; a pilot study. J Emerg Med 1998;16:377–382.
8. Tanabe P, Buschmann M: A prospective study of ED pain management practices and the patient's perspective. J Emerg Nurs 1999;25:171–177.
9. Guru V, Dubinsky I: The patient versus caregiver perception of acute pain in the emergency department. J Emerg Med 2000;18:7–12.
10. Selbst SM, Clark M: Analgesic use in the emergency department. Ann Emerg Med 1990;19:1010–1013.
11. Brown JC, Klein EJ, Lewis CW, et al: Emergency department analgesia for fracture pain. Ann Emerg Med 2003;42:197–205.
12. Fosnocht DE, Heaps ND, Swanson ER: Patient expectations for pain relief in the ED. Am J Emerg Med 2004;22:286–288.
13. Afilalo M, Tselios C: Pain relief versus patient satisfaction. Ann Emerg Med 1996;27:436–438.
14. Carragee EJ, Vittom D, Truong TP, et al: Pain control and cultural norms and expectations after closed femoral shaft fractures. Am J Orthop 1999;28:97–102.
15. Choiniere M, Melzack R, Girard N, et al: Comparisons between patients' and nurses' assessment of pain and medication efficacy in severe burn injuries. Pain 1990;40:143–152.
16. Potter M, Schafer S, Gonzalez-Mendez E, et al: Opioids for chronic nonmalignant pain: attitudes and practices of primary care. J Fam Pract 2001;50:145–151.
17. Bailey PL, Pace NL, Ashburn MA: Frequent hypoxemia and apnea after sedation with midazolam and fentanyl. Anesthesiology 1990;73:826–830.
18. Attard AR, Corlett MJ, Kidner NJ, et al: Safety of early pain relief for acute abdominal pain. BMJ 1992;305:554–556.
19. LoVecchio F, Oster N, Sturmann K, et al: The use of analgesics in patients with acute abdominal pain. J Emerg Med 1997;15:775–779.
20. Silen W. *Cope's Early Diagnosis of the Acute Abdomen,* 20th ed. Oxford University Press, 2000.
21. Friedland LR, Kulick RM: Emergency department analgesic use in pediatric trauma victims with fractures. Ann Emerg Med 1994;23:203–207.
22. Jones JS, Johnson K, McNinch M: Age as a risk factor for inadequate emergency department analgesia. Am J Emerg Med 1996;14:157–160.
23. Kozlowski MJ, Wiater JG, Pasaqual RG, et al: Painful discrimination: The differential use of analgesia in isolated lower limb injuries. Am J Emerg Med 2002;20:502–505.
24. Raftery KA, Smith-Coggins R, Chen AH: Gender-associated differences in emergency department pain management. Ann Emerg Med 1995;26:313–321.
25. Todd KH, Samaroo N, Hoffman JR: Ethnicity as a risk factor for inadequate emergency department analgesia. JAMA 1993;269:1537–1539.
26. Todd KH, Deaton C, D'Adamo AP, Goe L: Ethnicity and analgesic practice. Ann Emerg Med 2000;35:11–16.
27. Carpenter KJ, Dickenson AH: Molecular aspects of pain research. Pharacogenomics J 2002;2:87–95.
28. Dresser GK, Bailey DG: A basic conceptual and practical overview of interactions with highly prescribed drugs. Can J Clin Pharmacol 2002;9:191–198.
29. JCAHO: Pain Management Standards for 2001: Joint Commission on Accreditation of Healthcare Organizations, 2001;1.2.7–1.2.8.
30. Todd KH, Funk KG, Funk JP, Bonacci R: Clinical significance of reported changes in pain severity. Ann Emerg Med 1996;27:485–489.
31. Bijur PE, Silver W, Gallagher EJ: Reliability of the visual analog scale for measurement of acute pain. Acad Emerg Med 2001;8:1153–1157.
32. Bijur PE, Latimer CT, Gallagher EJ: Validation of a verbally administered numerical rating scale of acute pain for use in the emergency department. Acad Emerg Med 2003;10:390–392.
33. Nelson BP, Cohen D, Lander O, et al: Mandated pain scales improve frequency of ED analgesic administration. Am J Emerg Med 2004;22:582–585.
34. Miller MA, Levy P, Patel MM: Procedural sedation and analgesia in the emergency department: What are the risks? Emerg Med Clin North Am 2005;23:551–572.
35. American Society of Anesthesiologists: Practice guidelines for sedation and analgesia by non-anesthesiologists. Anesthesiology 1996;84:459–471.
36. Dursteler BB, Wightman JM: Etomidate-facilitated hip reduction in the emergency department. Am J Emerg Med 200;18:204–208.
37. Frazee BW, Park RS, Lowery D, Baire M: Propofol for deep procedural sedation in the ED. Am J Emerg Med 2005;23:190–195.
38. Green SM: Propofol for emergency department procedural sedation—not yet ready for prime time. Acad Emerg Med 1999;6:975–978.
39. Havel CJ Jr, Strait RT, Hennes H: A clinical trial of propofol vs midazolam for procedural sedation in a pediatric emergency department. Acad Emerg Med 1999;6:989–997.
40. Bassett KE, Anderson JL, Pribble CG, et al: Propofol for procedural sedation in children in the emergency department. Ann Emerg Med 2003;42:773–782.
41. Miner JR, Biros M, Krieg S, et al: Randomized clinical trial of propofol versus methohexital for procedural sedation during fracture and dislocation reduction in the emergency department. Acad Emerg Med 2003;10:931–937.
42. Innes GD, Zed PJ: Basic pharmacology and advances in emergency medicine. Emerg Med Clin North Am 2005;23:433–465.
43. Gutthann SP: Nonsteroidal anti-inflammatory drugs and the risk of hospitalization for acute renal failure. Arch Intern Med 1996;156:2433–2439.
44. Berges-Gimeno MP, Stevenson DD: Nonsteroidal anti-inflammatory drug-induced reactions and desensitization. J Asthma 2004;41:375–384.
45. Yealy DM: Ketorolac in the treatment of acute pain. Ann Emerg Med 1992;21:985–986.
46. McQuay H, Moore A, Justins D: Treating acute pain in hospital. BMJ 1997;314:1531–1535.
47. Walsh M, Smith GA, Yount RA: Continuous intravenous infusion fentanyl for sedation and analgesia of the multiple trauma patient. Ann Emerg Med 1991;20:913–915.
48. Muniz AE, Woleben C, Foster RL, Bartle S: Ketamine versus opioids plus midazolam for conscious sedation in children in the emergency department. Ann Emerg Med 2004;44(Suppl 1):S57–S58.
49. Gerhardt RT, King KM, Wiegert RS: Inhaled nitrous oxide versus placebo as an analgesic and anxiolytic adjunct to peripheral venous cannulation. Am J Emerg Med 2001;19:492–494.
50. Cepeda MS, Carr DB, Miranda N, et al: Comparison of morphine, ketorolac, and their combination for postoperative pain. Anesthesiology 2005;103:1225–1232.
51. Gammaitoni AR, Galer BS, Bulloch S, et al: Randomized, double-blind, placebo-controlled comparison of the analgesic efficacy of oxycodone 10 mg/acetaminophen 325 mg versus controlled-release oxycodone 20 mg in postsurgical pain. J Clin Pharmacol 2003;43:296–304.

52. Viitanen H, Tuominen N, Vaaraniemi H, et al: Analgesic efficacy of rectal acetaminophen and ibuprofen alone or in combination for paediatric day-case adenoidectomy. Br J Anaesth 2003;91:363–367.

53. Bijur PE, Kenny MK, Gallagher EJ: Intravenous morphine at 0.1 mg/kg is not effective for controlling severe acute pain in the majority of patients. Ann Emerg Med 2005;46:362–367.

54. Singer AJ, Stark MJ: Pretreatment of lacerations with lidocaine, epinephrine, and tetracaine at triage: A randomized double-blind trial. Acad Emerg Med 2002;7:751—756.

55. Priestly S, Kelly AM, Chow L: Application of topical local anesthetic at triage reduces treatment time for children with lacerations: A randomized controlled trial. Ann Emerg Med 2003;42:34–40.

56. Rogers TL, Ostrow CL: The use of EMLA cream to decrease venipuncture pain in children. J Pediatr Nurs 2004;19:33–39.

57. Couper RT: Methaemoglobinaemia secondary to topical lignocaine/prilocaine in a circumcised neonate. J Paediatr Child Health 2000;36:406–407.

58. Taddio A: Pain management for neonatal circumcision. Paediatr Drugs 2001;3:101–111.

59. Eichenfield LF, Funk A, Fallon-Friedlander S, et al: A clinical study to evaluate the efficacy of ELA-Max (4% liposomal lidocaine) as compared with eutectic mixture of local anesthetics cream for pain reduction of venipuncture in children. Pediatrics 2002;109:1093–1099.

60. Wallace MS, Ridgeway B, Jun E, et al: Topical delivery of lidocaine in healthy volunteers by electroporation, electroincorporation, or iontophoresis: An evaluation of skin anesthesia. Reg Anesth Pain Med 2001;26:229–238.

61. Peter DJ, Scott JP, Watkins HC, Frasure HE: Subcutaneous lidocaine delivered by jet-injector for pain control before IV catheterization in the ED: The patients' perception and preference. Am J Emerg Med 2002;20:562–566.

62. Ernst AA, Marvez-Valls E, Nick TG, et al: LAT (lidocaine-adrenaline-tetracaine) versus TAC (tetracaine-adrenaline-cocaine) for topical anesthesia in face and scalp lacerations. Am J Emerg Med 1995;13:151–154.

63. Kuhn M, Rossi SO, Plummer JL, Raftos J: Topical anaesthesia for minor lacerations: MAC versus TAC. Med J Aust 1996;164:277–280.

64. Scarfone RJ, Jasani M, Gracely EJ: Pain of local anesthetics: Rate of administration and buffering. Ann Emerg Med 1998;31:36–40.

65. Christophe RA, Buchanan L, Begalla K, et al: Pain reduction in local anesthetic administration through pH buffering. Ann Emerg Med 1988;17:117–120.

66. Bartfield JM, Sokaris SJ, Raccio-Robak N: Local anesthesia for lacerations: Pain of infiltration inside vs outside the wound. Acad Emerg Med 1998;5:100–105.

67. Brill S, Middleton W, Brill G, Fisher A: Bier's block: 100 years old and still going strong! Acta Anaesthesiol Scand 2004;48:117–122.

68. Farrell RG, Swanson SL, Walter JR: Safe and effective IV regional anesthesia for use in the emergency department. Ann Emerg Med 1985;14:288–292.

69. Blasier RD, White R: Intravenous regional anesthesia for management of children's extremity fractures in the emergency department. Pediatr Emerg Care 1996;12:404–406.

70. Crystal CS, Blankenship RB: Local anesthetics and peripheral nerve blocks in the emergency department. Emerg Med Clin North Am 2005;23:477–502.

71. McGlone R, Sadhra K, Hamer DW, et al: Femoral nerve block in the initial management of femoral shaft fractures. Arch Emerg Med 1987;4:163–168.

72. Stella J, Ellis R, Sprivulis P: Nerve stimulator-assisted femoral nerve block in the emergency department. Emerg Med 2000;12:322–325.

73. Marhofer P, Greher M, Kapral S: Ultrasound guidance in regional anaesthesia. Br J Anaesth 2005;94:7–17.

74. Chu RSL, Browne GJ, Cheng NG, Lam LT: Femoral nerve block for femoral shaft fractures in a paediatric emergency department: Can it be done better? Eur J Emerg Med 2003;10:258–263.

75. Thompson WL, Malchow RJ: Peripheral nerve blocks and anesthesia of the hand. Mil Med 2002;167:478–482.

76. Macaire P, Choquet O, Jochum D, et al: Nerve blocks at the wrist for carpal tunnel release revisited: The use of sensory-nerve and motor-nerve stimulation techniques. Reg Anesth Pain Med 2005;30:536–540.

77. Vloka JD, Hadzic A, Drobnik L, et al: Anatomical landmarks for femoral nerve block: A comparison of four needle insertion sites. Anesth Analg 1999;89:1467–1470.

78. Winnie AP, Ramamurthy S, Durrani Z: The inguinal paravascular technique of lumbar plexus anesthesia: The "3-in-1 block." Anesth Analg 1973; 52:989–996.

79. Lang SA, Yip RW, Chang P, Gerard M: The femoral 3-in-1 block revisited. J Clin Anesth 1993;5:292–296.

80. Morau D, Lopez S, Biboulet P, et al: Comparison of continuous 3-in-1 and fascia iliaca compartment blocks for postoperative analgesia: Feasibility, catheter migration, distribution of sensory block, and analgesic efficacy. Reg Anesth Pain Med 2003;28:309–314.

81. Karagiannis G, Hardern R: Best evidence topic report. No evidence found that a femoral nerve block in cases of femoral shaft fractures can delay the diagnosis of compartment syndrome of the thigh. Emerg Med J 2005;22:814.

82. Osinowo OA, Zahrani M, Softah A: Effect of intercostal nerve block with 0.5% bupivacaine on peak expiratory flow rate and arterial oxygen saturation in rib fractures. J Trauma 2004;56:345–347.

83. Shanti CM, Carlin AM, Tyburski JG: Incidence of pneumothorax from intercostal nerve block for analgesia in rib fractures. J Trauma 2001;41:536–539.

84. Bulger EM, Edwards T, Klotz P, et al: Epidural analgesia improves outcome after multiple rib fractures. Surgery 2004;13:426–430.

85. Karmakar MK, Ho AM: Acute pain management of patients with multiple fractured ribs. J Trauma 2003;54:615–625.

Neurologic Complications of Regional Anesthesia

69

Neurologic Complications of Peripheral Nerve Blocks: Mechanisms & Management

Steven Deschner, MD • Alain Borgeat, MD • Admir Hadzic, MD

A. Basic Considerations

INTRODUCTION

Although there are relatively few published reports of anesthesia-related nerve injury associated with peripheral nerve blocks (PNBs), it is likely that the commonly cited incidence (0.4%) of neurologic injury is underestimated owing to underreporting.[1-3] Most complications of PNBs were reported with upper extremity blocks. The less frequent clinical application of lower extremity nerve blocks may be the main reason why there are even fewer reports of anesthesia-related nerve injury associated with lower extremity PNBs compared with upper extremity PNBs.[4] Although neurologic complications after PNBs can be related to factors associated with the block technique (eg, needle trauma, intraneuronal injection, neuronal ischemia, and toxicity of local anesthetics), a search for other common causes should include positional and surgical factors (eg, positioning, stretching, retractor injury, ischemia, and hematoma formation). In some instances, the neurologic injury may be a result of a combination of these factors.

In all four sections of this chapter, mechanisms and consequences of acute neurologic injury related to the nerve block procedure are discussed and, where appropriate, methods and techniques to reduce the risk of complications are suggested. Specific nerve injuries with upper and lower nerve block techniques, neuraxial anesthesia, and local anesthetic toxicity are discussed elsewhere in this volume.

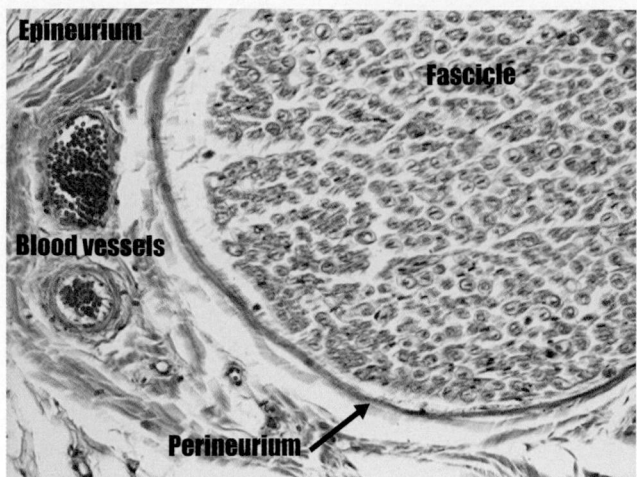

Figure 69–1. Histology of the peripheral nerve. Shown is a large fascicle of the peripheral nerve with its axons, surrounded by perineurium, epineurium, and nourishing blood vessels.

FUNCTIONAL HISTOLOGY OF THE PERIPHERAL NERVES

Knowledge of the functional histology of the peripheral nerve is important to understand the mechanisms of peripheral nerve injury; the reader is referred to Chapters 3 and 4 for more in-depth discussion on this subject. Here we briefly review salient features of the organization of the peripheral nerves. A peripheral nerve is a complex structure consisting of fascicles held together by the **epineurium,** an enveloping, external connective sheath (Figure 69–1). Each fascicle contains many nerve fibers and capillary blood vessels embedded in a loose connective tissue, the **endoneurium.**[5] The **perineurium** is a multilayered epithelial sheath that surrounds individual fascicles and consists of several layers of perineural cells. Therefore, in essence, a fascicle is a group of nerve fibers or a bundle of nerves surrounded by perineurium. Of note, fascicles can be organized in one of three common arrangements: monofascicular (single, large fascicle); oligofascicular (few fascicles of various sizes); and polyfascicular (many fascicles of various sizes).[6]

Nerve fibers can be myelinated or unmyelinated; sensory and motor nerves contain both in a ratio of 4:1, respectively. Unmyelinated fibers are composed of several axons, wrapped by a single Schwann cell. The axons of myelinated nerve fibers are enveloped individually by a single Schwann cell. A thin layer of collagen fibers, the endoneurium, surrounds the individually myelinated or groups of unmyelinated fibers.

Nerve fibers depend on a specific endoneurial environment for their function. Peripheral nerves are richly supplied by an extensive vascular network in which the endoneurial capillaries have endothelial "tight junctions," a peripheral analogy to the blood–brain barrier. The neurovascular bed is regulated by the sympathetic nervous system, and its blood flow can be as high as 30–40 mL/100 g per minute.[7] In addition to conducting nerve impulses, nerve fibers also main-

tain axonal transport of various functionally important substances such as proteins and precursors for receptors and transmitters. This process is highly dependent on oxidative metabolism. Any of these structures and functions can be deranged during a traumatic nerve injury, with the possible result of temporary or permanent impairment or loss of neural function.

The size and number of the fascicles in a peripheral nerve substantially vary from one peripheral nerve to another. In general, the larger the nerve, the greater the number and size of the fascicles. In addition, the larger the fascicle, the greater is the risk of intraneural injection because large fascicles can accommodate the tip of the needle.[8] Of note, the fascicular bundles are not continuous throughout the peripheral nerve. They divide and anastomose with one another as frequently as every few millimeters.[8] However, the axons within a small set of adjacent bundles redistribute themselves so that they remain in approximately the same quadrant of the nerve for several centimeters. This arrangement is of practical concern to the surgeons trying to repair a severed nerve. If the cut is clean, it may be possible to suture individual fascicular bundles together. In such a scenario, there is a good probability that the distal segment of nerves will be sutured to the central stump of motor axons and sensory axons. In such cases, good functional recovery is possible. If a short segment of the nerve is missing, however, the fascicles in the various quadrants of the stump may no longer correspond with one another, good axial alignment may not be possible, and functional recovery is greatly compromised or improbable.[8] This arrangement of the peripheral nerve helps explain why intraneural injections result in more serious consequences as opposed to clean needle nerve cuts, which tend to heal much more readily.

Clinical Pearls

- The larger the nerve, the greater the number and size of the fascicles. The larger the fascicle, the greater is the risk of true intraneural injection because large fascicles can accommodate the tip of the needle.

- The delicate arrangement of the peripheral nerve offers an explanation as to why intraneural injections can result in permanent neurologic injury.

- The connective tissue of a nerve is tough compared with the nerve fibers themselves. The connective tissue of a nerve permits a certain amount of stretch without damage to the nerve fibers. The nerve fibers are somewhat "wavy," and when stretched, the connective tissue around them is also stretched, giving it some protection.[9] This feature perhaps plays a safety role in nerve blockade by allowing the nerves to be "pushed" rather than penetrated by the advancing needle during nerve localization. For this reason, it is prudent to avoid stretching the nerves and nerve plexuses during nerve blockade.

- Nerves receive blood from the adjacent blood vessels running along their course. These feeding branches to larger nerves are of macroscopic size and irregularly arranged, forming anastomoses to become longitudinally running vessel(s) that supply the nerve and give off subsidiary branches.
- Although the connective tissue sheath enveloping nerves serves to protect the nerves from stretching, the neuronal injury after nerve blockade may be due at least partly to the pressure or stretch within poorly compliant connective sheaths and the consequent interference with the vascular supply to the nerve.

MECHANISMS OF PERIPHERAL NERVE INJURY

The cause of peripheral nerve injury related to the use of PNBs falls into one of four categories (Table 69–1). **Laceration** results when the nerve is cut partially or completely, such as by a scalpel or a large-gauge cutting needle. **Stretch injuries** to the nerves may result when nerves or plexuses are stretched in a nonphysiologic or exaggerated physiologic position, such as during shoulder manipulation under an interscalene block. **Pressure,** as a mechanism of nerve injury, is relatively common. A typical example of this mechanism is chronic compression of the nerves by neighboring structures, such as fibrous bands, scar tissue, or abnormal muscles that pass through fibro-osseous spaces if the space is too small, such as the carpal tunnel. Such chronic compression syndromes are called **entrapment neuropathies.** Examples of pressure injuries applicable to PNBs include external pressure over a period of hours (eg, a Saturday night palsy, resulting from pressure of a chair back on the radial nerve of

the insensate arm). The pressure may be repeated and have a cumulative effect (eg, an ulnar neuropathy resulting from habitually leaning on the elbow). Such a scenario is conceivable, for instance, in a patient who positions the anesthetized arm (eg, long-acting or continuous brachial plexus block) in a nonphysiologic position for a few hours. Another example of pressure-related nerve injury is prolonged use of a high-pressure tourniquet. An intraneural injection may lead to sustained high intraneural pressure, which exceeds capillary occlusion pressure, and leads to nerve ischemia.[10] Finally, a forceful injection into a low-compliant connective tissue plane (space) containing a peripheral nerve may lead to nerve ischemia and neurologic dysfunction. **Vascular nerve damage** after nerve blocks can occur when there is acute occlusion of the arteries from which the vasa nervorum are derived or from a hemorrhage within a nerve sheath. With injection injuries, the nerve may be directly impaled and the drug injected directly into the nerve, or the drug may be injected into adjacent tissues, causing an acute inflammatory reaction or chronic fibrosis—both indirectly involving the nerve. **Chemical nerve injury** is the result of tissue toxicity of injected solutions (eg, local anesthetic toxicity, neurolysis with alcohol or phenol).

CLINICAL CLASSIFICATION OF ACUTE NERVE INJURIES

Classification of acute nerve injuries is useful when considering the physical and functional state of damaged nerves. In his

Table 69–1.

Mechanisms of Peripheral Nerve Injury Related to Peripheral Nerve Blocks

Mechanical—acute
  Laceration
  Stretch
  Intraneural injection

Vascular
  Acute ischemia
  Hemorrhage

Pressure
  Extraneural
  Intraneural
  Compartment syndrome

Chemical
  Injection of neurotoxic solutions

Table 69–2.

Classification of Nerve Injuries

Seddon	Sunderland	Structural and Functional Processes
Neuropraxia	1	Myelin damage, conduction slowing, and blocking
Axonotmesis	2	Loss of axonal continuity, endoneurium intact, no conduction
Neurotmesis	3	Loss of axonal and endoneurial continuity, perineurium intact, no conduction
	4	Loss of axonal, endoneurial, and perineurial continuity; epineurium intact; no conduction
	5	Entire nerve trunk separated; no conduction

Based on data from Seddon H: Three types of nerve injury. Brain 1943;66: 236–288; Sunderland S: A classification of peripheral nerve injuries producing loss of function. Brain 1951;74:491–516; and Lundborg G: Nerve Injury and Repair. Churchill Livingstone, 1988.

classification, Seddon[11] introduced the terms neurapraxia, axonotmesis, and neurotmesis (Table 69–2); Sunderland[12] subsequently proposed a five-grade classification system.

Neuropraxia refers to nerve dysfunction lasting several hours to 6 months after a blunt injury to the nerve. In neuropraxia, the nerve axons and connective tissue structures remain intact. The nerve dysfunction probably results from several factors, of which *focal demyelination* is the most important abnormality. Intraneural hemorrhage, pressure ischemia changes in the vasa nervorum, disruption of the blood–nerve barrier and axon membranes, and electrolyte disturbances all may add to the impairment of nerve function. Because the nerve dysfunction is rarely complete, clinical deficits are partial and recovery usually occurs within a few weeks, although some neurapraxic lesions (with minimal or no axonal degeneration) may take several months to recover.

Axonotmesis consists of *physical interruption of the axons* but within intact Schwann cell tubes and intact connective tissue structures of the nerve (ie, the endoneurium, perineurium, and epineurium). Sunderland[12] subdivided this group, depending on which of the three structures were involved (see Table 69–2). With axonotmesis, the nerve sheath remains intact, enabling regenerating nerve fibers to find their way into the distal segment. Consequently, efficient axonal regeneration can eventually take place.

Neurotmesis refers to a *complete interruption of the entire nerve* including the axons and all connective tissue structures (epineurium included). Clinically, there is total nerve dysfunction. With both axonotmesis and neurotmesis, axonal disruption leads to wallerian degeneration, from which recovery occurs through the slow process of axonal regeneration. However, with neurotmesis, the two nerve ends may be completely separated, and the regenerating axons may not be able to find the distal stump. For these reasons, effective recovery does not occur unless the severed ends are sutured or joined by a nerve graft. With closed injuries, the only way to distinguish clearly between axonotmesis and neurotmesis is by surgical exploration and intraoperative inspection of the nerve.

Note that most acute nerve injuries are mixed lesions.[11] Different fascicles and nerve fibers typically sustain different degrees of injury, which may make it difficult to assess the type of injury and predict outcome even by electrophysiologic means. Recovery from a mixed lesion is characteristically biphasic; it is relatively rapid for fibers with neurapraxic damage, but much slower for axons that have been physically interrupted and have undergone wallerian degeneration.

Mechanical Nerve Injury

Intraneural Injection and Its Prevention

Rather than a relatively clear injury caused by sharp needle cuts, intraneural injection has the potential to create structural damage to the fascicle(s) that is more extensive and less likely to heal (Figure 69–2). Indeed, the devastating sequelae of sensory and motor loss after injection of various agents into peripheral nerves has been well documented.[13] Nearly all experimental studies on this subject have demonstrated

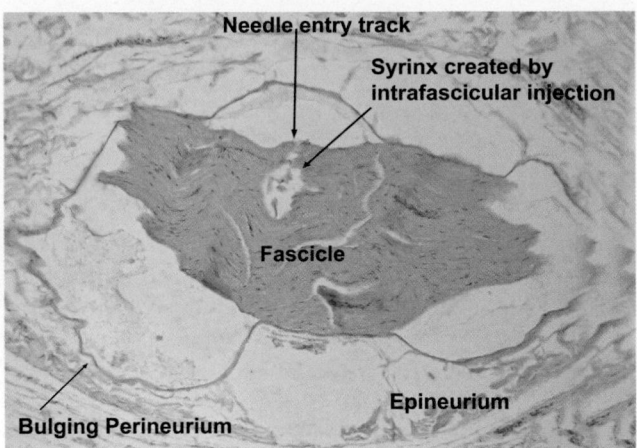

Figure 69–2. Mechanical injection injury to the peripheral nerve. Shown is a large fascicle with a needle track, syrinx created by hydrostatic pressure of the injectate, as well as the needle track into the fascicle. Perineurium is seen bulging off the surface of the fascicle.

that the site of injection is critical in determining the degree and nature of injury. More specifically, to induce neurologic injury, the injectate must be injected intrafascicularly; extrafascicular injections of the same substance typically do not cause nerve injury.[14] Thus, the main factor leading to a substantial peripheral nerve damage associated with injection techniques is injection of local anesthetic into a fascicle. This causes mechanical destruction of the fascicular architecture and sets into motion a cascade of pathophysiologic changes, including inflammation, cellular infiltration, axonal degeneration, and others—all possibly leading to nerve scarring and permanent neurologic impairment.

Histologic features of injury after intraneural injection are rather nonspecific and range from simple mechanical disruption and delamination to fragmentation of the myelin sheath and marked cellular infiltration (Figure 69–3). Using a variety of animal models of nerve injury, a vast array

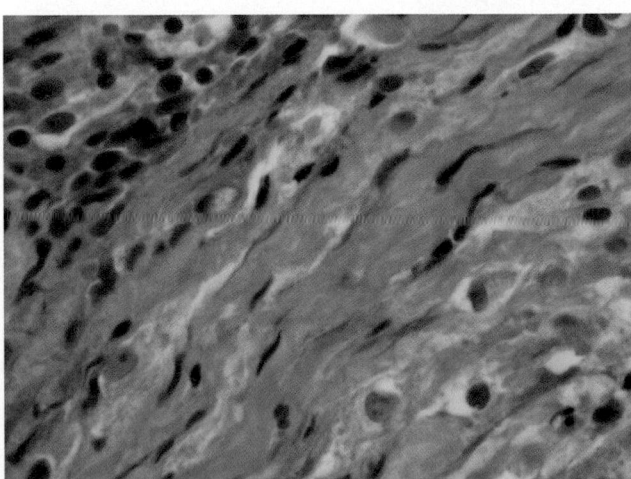

Figure 69–3. Fascicular injury after an intraneural injection. Shown is loss axonal degeneration, extravasation of erythrocytes, and inflammatory cell infiltration.

of cellular changes following peripheral nerve trauma have been documented.[14] The extent of actual neurologic damage after an intrafascicular injection can range from neuropraxia with minimal structural damage to neurotmesis with severe axonal and myelin degeneration, depending on the needle–nerve relationship, the agent injected, and the dose of the drug used.[15–19] In general, subperineural changes tend to be more prominent compared with the central area of the fascicle.[20] In addition, injury to primary sensory neurons that is not detectable histologically causes a shift in membrane channel expression, sensitivity to algogenic substances, neuropeptide production, and intracellular signal transduction both at the injury site and in the cell body in the dorsal root ganglion. This leads to increased excitability and acute or chronic pain often experienced by patients with neurologic injury. It should be noted that intraneural injection and its resultant mechanical injury are merely the inciting mechanisms; a host of additional changes occur involving inflammatory reactions, chemical neuritis, and intraneural hemorrhage, all of which eventually may combine and lead to nerve scarring and chronic neuropathic pain.

Pain on Injection

Little is known about how to avoid an intraneural injection. Pain with injection has long been thought of as the cardinal sign of intraneural injection; consequently, it is commonly suggested that blocks be avoided in heavily premedicated or anesthetized patients. However, numerous case reports have suggested that pain may not be reliable as a sole warning sign of impending nerve injury, and it may present in only a minority of cases.[21–25] Fanelli and colleagues[3] have reported unintended paresthesia in 14% of patients in their study; however, univariate analysis of potential risk factors for postoperative neurologic dysfunction failed to demonstrate paresthesia as a risk factor. In addition, the sensory nature of the pain-paresthesia can be difficult to interpret in clinical practice.[26] For instance, a certain degree of discomfort on injection ("pressure paresthesia") is considered normal and affirmative of impending successful blockade because this symptom is thought to indicate that injection of local anesthetic has been made in the vicinity of the targeted nerve.[26] In clinical practice, however, it can be difficult to discern when pain-paresthesia on injection is normal and when it is the ominous sign of an intraneural injection.[27] Moreover, it is unclear how pain or paresthesia on injection, even when present, can be used clinically to prevent development of neurologic injury. For instance, in a prospective study on neurologic complications of regional anesthesia by Auroy and colleagues,[2] neurologic injuries after paresthesia ensued, although the participating anesthesiologists stopped the injection when pain on injection was reported by the patients.

Intensity of the Stimulating Current

The optimal current intensity resulting in accurate localization of a nerve has been a topic of controversy.[28–31] For instance, stimulation at currents higher than 0.5 mA may result in block failure because the needle tip is positioned outside the fascial sheath that envelopes a nerve, whereas stimulation at currents lower than 0.2 mA theoretically pose a risk of intraneural injection.[32] Other authors suggest that a motor response with a current intensity between 1.0 and 0.5 mA is sufficient for accurate placement of the block needle[28]; still others advise using a current of much lower intensity (0.5– 0.1 mA).[29,31] Others simply suggest stimulating with currents less than 0.75 mA,[33,34] or progressively reducing the current to as low a level as possible while still maintaining a motor response.[30]

Clinical Pearls

- Most authors suggest that nerve stimulation with current intensity of 0.2–0.5 mA (0.1 msec) indicates intimate needle–nerve placement.

- Stimulation with current intensity of ≤0.2 mA may be associated with intraneural needle placement.

- Motor response to nerve stimulation may be absent even when the needle is inserted intraneurally.

Many recently published reports on nerve blocks have suggested obtaining nerve stimulation with currents of 0.2– 0.5 mA (100 msec) before injecting local anesthetics, believing that motor response with current intensities lower than 0.2 mA may be associated with intraneural needle placement. However logical these beliefs may sound, no published clinical reports substantiate these concerns.

In current clinical practice, development of nerve localization and injection monitoring techniques to reliably prevent intraneural injection remains elusive.[22] Nerve stimulators are very useful for nerve localization; however, the needle–nerve relationship cannot be precisely and reliably ascertained adequately, as early literature suggests.[28] Response to nerve stimulation with a commonly used current intensity (1 mA) may be absent even when the needle makes physical contact with or is inserted into a nerve[35–37] (Figure 69–4). Occurrence of nerve injuries despite using nerve stimulation to localize nerves further suggests that nerve stimulators can at best provide only a rough approximation of the needle–nerve relationship.[1] A fundamental problem with the nerve stimulation is that the current flows in all directions, following the path of least resistance and not necessarily only toward the nerve. Miniscule changes at the needle tip–tissue interface can make a substantial difference in the preferential flow of current away from the nerve. This may result in cessation of the motor response even when the needle is in intimate relation with the nerve or when it is placed intraneurally. The current interest for ultrasound-assisted nerve localization holds promise for facilitating nerve localization and administration of nerve blocks. However, the image resolution of this technology is insufficient to visualize nerve fascicles and prevent intrafascicular injection.

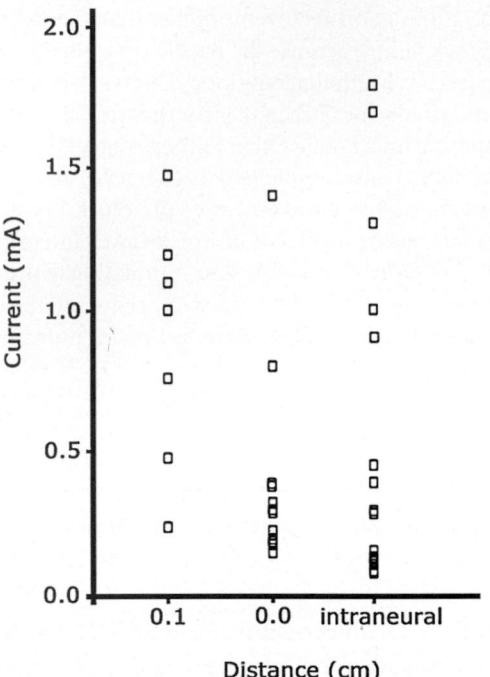

Figure 69–4. Intensity of the electrical current required to obtain a motor response in a sciatic nerve block model in pigs. As the distance of the needle to the nerve decreases from 0.1 mm to the intraneural location of the needle, stimulation can be obtained with a current of progressively lesser intensity (minimum 0.08 mA/0.1 msec with needle intraneurally). However, when the needle was inserted intraneurally, motor response could not be obtained in 25% of the attempts even with currents of 0.5–1.7 mA. (From Hadzic A, et al. 2006. Unpublished data).

Resistance to Injection

Assessing resistance to injection is a common practice, similar to loss of resistance to injection of air or saline using a "syringe feel" during administration of epidural, paravertebral, or lumbar plexus blocks. Similarly, assessing tissue resistance and injection compliance constitute another means of estimating the anatomic location of the needle tip during the practice of PNBs. For this, clinicians use a syringe feel to estimate what may be an abnormal resistance to nerve block injection and thus reduce the risk of intraneural injection.[10,31,38] However, this practice has significant inherent limitations.[39] For instance, the resistance to injection is greater with smaller needles, introducing additional confusion as to what constitutes normal or abnormal resistance. Second, rather than loss of resistance in an epidural injection, there is no baseline pressure information or change in tissue compliance during nerve block injection. In other words, with nerve block injection there is no change in pressure that can be relied on. For instance, in a study by Claudio and colleagues,[39] all anesthesiologists detected a change in pressure of as little as 0.5 psi during a simulated nerve block injection. However, when gauging the absolute pressure, clinicians substantially varied (by as much as 40 psi) in their perception of what constituted an abnormal resistance to injection. Finally, no information has been available on what constitutes normal or abnormal injection

pressure during nerve block injection. For these reasons, subjective estimation of resistance to injection is at least as inaccurate as perhaps estimating blood pressure by palpating radial artery pulse; objective means of assessing resistance to injection should be far superior in standardizing injection force and pressure.

Clinical Pearls

- Injections into epineurium or periepineural tissue do not result in significant resistance to injection.
- When injection proves to be difficult (injection pressures >20 psi), the injection should be stopped.
- Manual assessment of the resistance to injection using a hand-feel method is highly subjective and depends on the speed of injection, needle size, and ability of the person injecting to consistently discern normal from abnormal resistance.

To explain the mechanisms responsible for development of neuraxial anesthesia after an interscalene block,[40,41] Selander and Sjostrand[42] injected solutions of local anesthetic into rabbit sciatic nerves and traced the spread of the anesthetic along the nerve sheet. They postulated that an intraneural injection results in significant intraneural spread of local anesthetic. In their model, these investigators incidentally noticed that intraneural injections often resulted in higher pressures (up to 9 psi) than those required for perineural injections (<4 psi). Injection into a nerve fascicle resulted in rupture of the perineurium and histologic evidence of disruption of the fascicular anatomy. This study, however, used a small animal model, microinjections (10–200 μL), miniature needles, and clinically irrelevant injection rates (100–300 μL/min) and did not study neurologic consequences after intraneural injections. Perhaps for these reasons their results foretelling the possible association of injection pressure with intrafascicular injection did not change the clinical practice.

More recent studies, however, have used clinically more applicable injection speeds and volumes of local anesthetic in a canine model of nerve injury.[4] The results of these studies suggest that intrafascicular injection is associated with high injection pressures (>20 psi) and carry a risk of neurologic injury[20] (Figures 69–5 and 69–6). Only intraneural injections resulting in pressures greater than 20 psi have been associated with clinically detectable neurologic deficits (Figure 69–7) as well as histologic evidence of injury to nerve fascicles.

The current evidence suggests that neurologic injury does not always develop after an intraneural injection.[37] In fact, injection after an intraneural needle placement is more likely to result in deposition of the local anesthetic between and not into the fascicles.[20] Intraneural, but *extrafascicular* (interfascicular) injection probably occurs more commonly than is thought in clinical practice.[37] Such an injection results

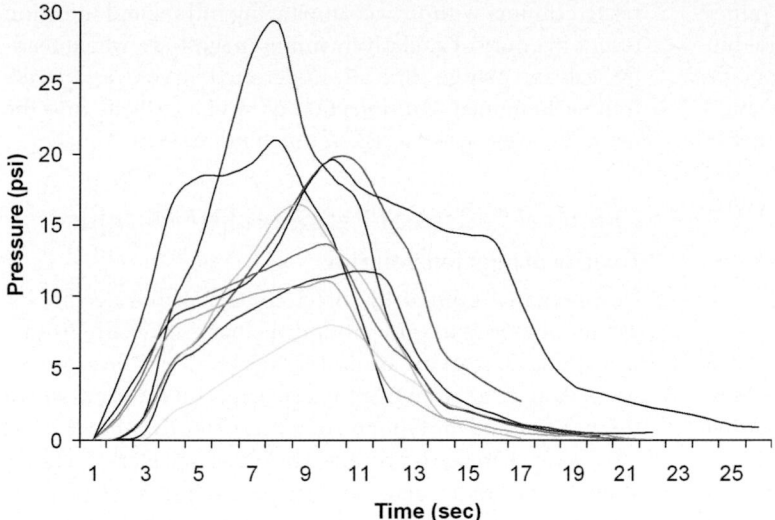

Figure 69–5. Injection pressures recorded during *perineural* injection of 2% lidocaine in a sciatic nerve block model in pigs. Using an injection speed of 15 mL/min and 25-gauge insulated nerve block needle, pressures were at or below 20 psi in all but one injection.

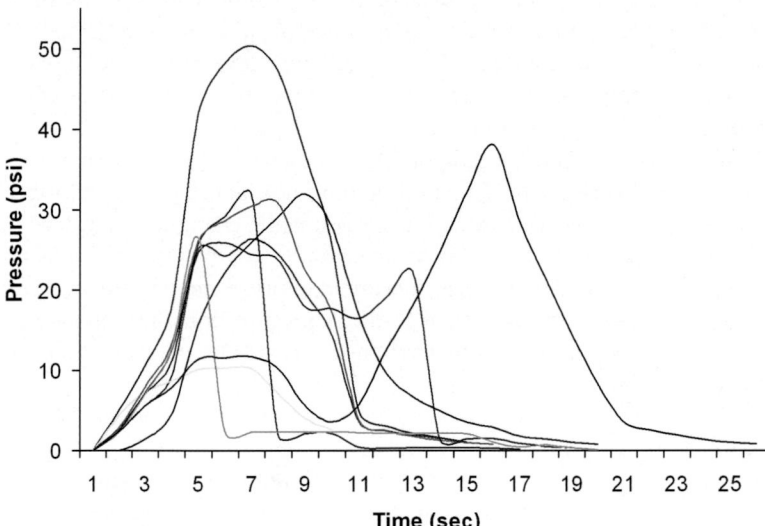

Figure 69–6. Injection pressures recorded during *intraneural* injection of 2% lidocaine in a sciatic nerve block model in pigs. Using an injection speed of 15 mL/min and 25-gauge insulated nerve block needle, pressures were significantly above 20 psi in all but two injections.

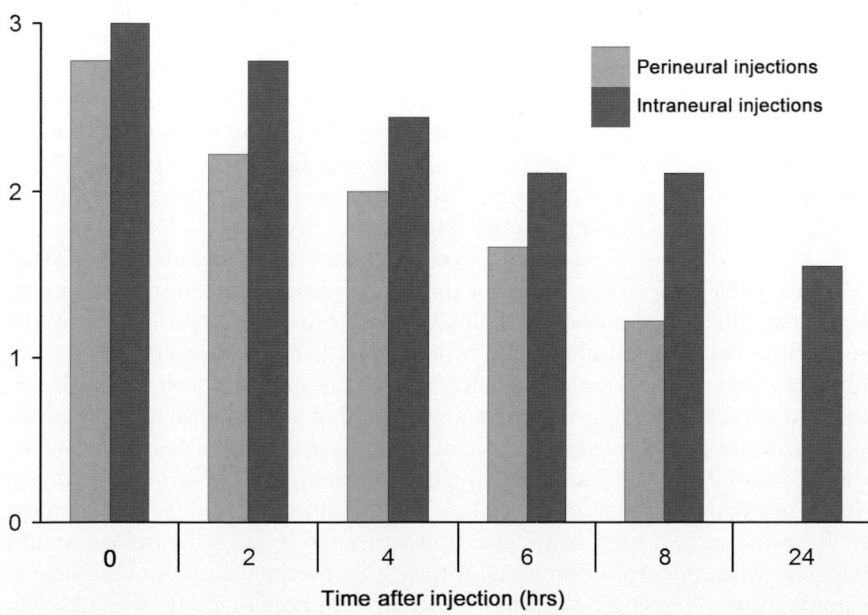

Degree of paresis: 0 - no paresis; 1 - mild paresis; 2 - pronounced paresis; 3 - flaccid extremity

Figure 69–7. Twenty-four hours after perineural or intraneural application of 2% lidocaine in a sciatic nerve block model in pigs, the intraneural group continues to exhibit signs of paresis in the sciatic nerve distribution.

in a block of unusually fast onset and long duration rather than in neurologic injury. This is because an intraneural but extrafascicular injection leads to intimate exposure of nerve fascicles to high concentration and doses of local anesthetics. However, permanent neurologic injury does not develop because the local anesthetic is deposited *outside* the fascicles and the blocks slowly resolve after the injection without evidence of histologic derangement.

Needle Design and Direct Needle Trauma

Needle tip design and risk of neurologic injury have been matters of considerable debate for more than three decades. Nearly 30 years ago, Selander and colleagues[43] suggested that the risk of perforating a nerve fascicle was significantly lower when a short-bevel (eg, angle of 45 degrees) needle was used as opposed to a long-bevel (angle of 12–15 degrees) needle. The results of their work are largely responsible for the currently prevalent trend of using short-bevel needles (ie, angles 30–45 degrees) for most major peripheral nerve conduction blocks. However, the more recent work of Rice and McMahon[44] suggested that when placed intraneurally, short-bevel needles cause more mechanical damage than the long-bevel needles.[44] In their experiment in a rat model, deliberate penetration of the largest fascicle of the sciatic nerve with short-bevel needles resulted in the greatest degree of neural trauma. Their work suggests that sharp needles produce clean, more-likely-to-heal cuts, whereas blunt needles produce irregular and more extensive damage on the microscopic images. In addition, the cuts produced by the sharper needles were more likely to recover faster and more completely than were the irregular, more traumatic injuries caused by the blunter, short-bevel needles.[44]

Although the data on needle design and nerve injury have not been clinically substantiated, the theoretical advantage of short-bevel needles in reducing the risk of nerve penetration has influenced both practitioners and needle manufacturers. Consequently, whenever practical, most clinicians today prefer to use short-bevel needles for major conduction blocks of the peripheral nerves and plexuses. Sharp-beveled, small-gauge needles, however, continue to be used routinely for many nerve block procedures, such as axillary transarterial brachial plexus block, wrist and ankle blocks, cutaneous nerve block, and others.

Regardless of the considerations related to the needle design and risk of nerve injury, the actual clinical significance of isolated, direct needle trauma remains unclear. For instance, it is possible that both paresthesia and nerve stimulation techniques of nerve localization often result in unrecognized intraneural needle placement; yet the risk of neurologic injury remains relatively low. Similarly, during femoral arterial cannulation (arterial line insertion), it is likely that the needle is often inadvertently inserted into the femoral nerve; yet injuries to the femoral nerve are rare, and when they occur, they are usually attributed to hematoma formation rather than needle injury.[45] It is possible that a needle-related trauma without accompanying intraneural injection results in injury of a relatively minor magnitude, which readily heals and may go clinically undetected. In contrast, needle trauma combined with injection of local anesthetic into the nerve fascicles carries a risk of much more severe injury.[20]

Chemical Causes of Peripheral Nerve Injury

Toxicity of Injected Solution

Nerves can be injured by direct contact with a needle, injection of a drug into or around the nerve, pressure from a hematoma, or scarring around the nerve.[9,46–48] The degree of nerve damage after an injection depends on the exact site of the injection and the type and quantity of the drug used.[15] The most severe damage is produced by intrafascicular injections, although extrafascicular (subepineurial) injections of some particularly toxic drugs can also produce nerve damage.[16,17] Benzylpenicillin, diazepam, and paraldehyde are the most damaging; however, a number of other medications, such as antibiotics, analgesics, sedatives, and antiemetic medications, are also capable of damaging peripheral nerves when injected experimentally or accidentally.[15]

Local anesthetics produce a variety of cytotoxic effects in cell cultures, including inhibition of cell growth, motility, and survival, as well as morphologic changes. The extent of these effects is proportionate to the length of time the cells are exposed to the local anesthetic solution and occur using local anesthetic at normal clinical concentrations. Within normal ranges, the cytotoxic changes are greater as concentrations increase.

In the clinical setting, the exact site of local anesthetic deposition plays a critical role in determining the pathogenic potential.[49] After applying local anesthetics outside a fascicle, the regulatory function of the perineural and endothelial blood–nerve barrier is only minimally compromised. High concentrations of extrafascicular anesthetics may produce axonal injury independent of edema formation and elevated endoneurial fluid pressure.[50] As with the effects of local anesthetics in cell cultures, the duration of exposure and the concentration of local anesthetic determine the degree and incidence of local anesthetic—induced residual paralysis. Neurotoxicity of local anesthetics are dealt with in greater detail elsewhere in this chapter.

Neurologic complications after regional anesthesia may also be caused by the direct effects of local anesthetics on the nervous tissue. Toxicity has been reported primarily with the intrathecal use of local anesthetics. However, with the increasing popularity of PNB anesthesia, reports are surfacing about the direct toxic effects of local anesthetics on peripheral nerves.[2] Several theories regarding the mechanism of injury have been suggested. Prolonged exposure, high doses, high concentrations, body positioning, and the specific agent used may cause transient or permanent neurologic injury by a number of intracellular mechanisms. Once the neurologic injury has occurred, it has been suggested that additives such as epinephrine or a preexisting neurologic condition may predispose the patient to the neurotoxic effects of local anesthetics (the "double-crush" concept).

Experimental models of neurotoxicity of local anesthetics have included application of local anesthetic to the sciatic nerve in animals, desheathed nerve preparations, and dorsal root ganglion cells in culture using concentration of local anesthetic comparable to those used clinically.[51] These studies have revealed considerable information about the mechanism of injury. Sakura and colleagues[52] discovered that the mechanism did not involve voltage-dependent sodium channels. They substituted tetrodotoxin for lidocaine and found that tetrodotoxin blocked these channels as effectively as lidocaine without producing the toxicity associated with lidocaine. Johnson and colleagues[53] discovered that cell toxicity may be related to mitochondrial degradation. Local anesthetics caused the mitochondria to depolarize and stop producing adenosine triphosphate (ATP). With the loss of ATP, energy-dependent mechanisms are compromised, leading to the accumulation of calcium intracellularly and activation of enzymes that cause cell degradation. This was unrelated to hypoxia, because lidocaine actually reduced oxygen demand.[51] Cell death or apoptosis was related to the concentration and/or the length of exposure. Exposure to 1% lidocaine for more than 90 minutes was required to kill 50% of the cells. Exposures of less than 1 hour were reversible, but exposure to lidocaine at 5% concentration caused rapid cell death or necrosis.[51]

In addition to electrolyte imbalance (leading to cell death), loss of ATP has been found to cause failure of axonal transport, compromising the ability of the neuron to transport materials synthesized in the perikaryon to the axon terminal.[54] Fast axonal transport moves neurotransmitters from the cell body to the nerve terminal. Lidocaine has been shown to produce a reversible blockade of rapid axonal transport. Recovery is dependent on the concentration and the exposure time of the local anesthetic on the nerve tissue. High concentrations and/or prolonged exposure has been postulated to cause prolonged or permanent nerve injury.[55] Furthermore, the loss of ATP leads to the failure of the sequestration of neurotransmitters within the cells, leading to an increase in the extracellular concentration of glutamate. Excessive glutamate in the extracellular space through NMDA (*N*-methyl-D-aspartate) receptors can exacerbate the elevation of calcium within the cells, ultimately leading to further cell degradation.[56] This effect is noted only in the central neuraxis, where glutamate is found.

Local anesthetics have been shown to cause membrane solubilization at high concentrations. At clinical concentrations, they can form micelles that may act as detergents to disrupt the cell membrane.[57–60] Oda and colleagues[61] demonstrated that 5% lidocaine and 0.5% dibucaine were minimum concentrations causing irreversible neurologic damage. No neurologic damage was seen with 2% lidocaine or 0.2% dibucaine.

Neurotoxicity varies with the local anesthetic solution. In histopathologic, electrophysiologic, and neuronal cell models, lidocaine and tetracaine have been shown to have a greater potential for neurotoxicity than bupivacaine.[62] Additives, that is, epinephrine, can increase the toxicity of both lidocaine and bupivacaine.[63] A preexisting neurologic condition, such as peripheral neuropathy, injury, or surgery, may predispose the patient to nerve injury from toxicity at clinical doses (ie, the double-crush concept).[64]

In summary, local anesthetics have potentially cytotoxic effects. The mechanisms appear to involve disruption of mitochondrial function, electrolyte imbalance leading to detrimental intracellular calcium accumulation, loss of axonal transport, and release of glutamate. The toxicity and ultimate damage to nerve tissue are related to concentration of the agent, site of action, time of exposure, and the specific local anesthetic agent used. Most studies have demonstrated a greater effect on intrathecal use compared with epidural or peripheral nerve exposure. This may reflect the typically higher baricity, more concentrated dose of local anesthetic bathing the spinal cord for a prolonged period of time compared with a large volume, less concentrated solution typically used in epidural, and peripheral nerve blocks.

Vascular Mechanisms Causing Nerve Injury

Neural Ischemia

Lack of blood flow to the primary afferent neuron results in metabolic stress. The earliest response of the peripheral sensory neuron to ischemia is depolarization and generation of spontaneous activity, symptomatically perceived as paresthesias. This is followed by blockade of slow-conducting myelinated fibers and eventually all neurons, possibly through accumulation of excess intracellular calcium, which accounts for the loss of sensation with initiation of limb ischemia. Nerve function returns within 6 hours if ischemic times are less than 2 hours. Ischemic periods of up to 6 hours may not produce permanent structural changes in nerves. However, detailed pathologic examination after ischemia initially shows minimal changes, but with 3 hours or more of reperfusion, edema and fiber degeneration develop and last 1–2 weeks, followed by a phase of regeneration that will last 6 weeks. In addition to neuronal damage, oxidative injury associated with ischemia and reperfusion also affects the Schwann cells, initiating apoptosis.

The perineurium is a tough and resistant tissue layer. An injection into this compartment or a fascicle can cause a prolonged increase in endoneurial pressure exceeding the capillary perfusion pressure. This pressure, in turn, can result in endoneurial ischemia.[10,42] The addition of vasoconstricting agents theoretically can enhance ischemia because of the resultant vasoconstriction and reduction in blood flow. The addition of epinephrine has been shown in vitro to decrease the blood supply to intact nerves in the rabbit.[65] However, in patients undergoing lower extremity surgery, addition of epinephrine to the local anesthetic solution used in combined femoral and sciatic nerve blocks has not been shown to be a risk factor for developing post-block nerve dysfunction.[3]

Pressure Mechanisms Causing Nerve Injury

Tourniquet Neuropathy

Tourniquet-induced neuropathy is well documented in the orthopedic literature and ranges from mild neuropraxia to permanent neurologic injury.[66–69] The incidence of tourniquet paralysis has been reported as 1 in 8000 operations.[70] A prospective study of lower extremity nerve blockade suggests that higher tourniquet inflation pressure (>400 mm Hg) was associated with an increased risk of transient nerve injury.[3] Current recommendations for appropriate use of the tourniquet include the maintenance of a pressure of no more than 150 mm Hg greater than the systolic blood pressure and deflation of the tourniquet every 90–120 minutes.[69] Even with these recommendations, post-tourniquet-application neuropraxia may occur, particularly in the setting of preexisting neuropathy.[71,72]

Compressive Hematoma

Little data exist regarding the safety of PNB in patients treated with anticoagulants. Compressive hematoma formation leading to neuropathy has been associated with needle misadventures when performing lower extremity PNB, particularly with concomitant treatment with anticoagulants.[73,74] However, in contrast to spinal or epidural hematoma, peripheral neuropathy from compressive hematoma typically resolves completely.[75–78] Regardless, these reports emphasize the important differences in the risk-benefit ratio of PNBs compared with neuraxial blocks in patients receiving anticoagulant therapy.

B. Peripheral Nerve Blocks in Anesthetized Patients

INTRODUCTION

Regional anesthesia-associated nerve injury is a significant source of concern for patients, surgeons, and anesthesiologists alike. In addition, nerve injury is a potential medicolegal liability for anesthesiologists.[79] PNBs, in particular, are of significant concern because the typical technique involves placing the needle tip in the immediate vicinity of the nerve or plexus. Consequently, any postoperative neurologic impairment is automatically, and often unjustly, attributed to the PNB procedure.

Few issues in regional anesthesia have been the subject of such intense controversy as whether PNBs carry a higher risk of neurologic complications when performed in anesthetized patients compared with awake patients. Opinions vary from heavy premedication being essential to the success of regional anesthesia to its being equated with negligence. Unfortunately, no large-scale controlled studies of the safety of PNBs in awake versus anesthetized patients exists, nor are such studies likely to be available in the future. Without randomized, controlled studies, experts are left to draw conclusions and make logical recommendations solely on their interpretation of the few available case reports and anecdotal experiences. However, any such recommendations regarding the use of sedation or general anesthesia in patients receiving PNBs could have significant medicolegal repercussions. Therefore, the multifaceted purpose of this text is to review the available literature that supports or refutes the practice of administering nerve blocks in anesthetized patients, to discuss the current controversies, and to provide insight into the future of the subspecialty with regard to this issue. Specific concerns regarding performance of PNBs in anesthetized patients are presented and addressed. Although the scientific value of case reports is often discounted, such reports may actually be more informative than large epidemiologic studies because they include a detailed account of periblock events, which is often lacking in epidemiologic studies.

SYMPTOMS OF INTRANEURAL INJECTION

The premise behind the common recommendation that a PNB should be performed only in awake patients is that an awake patient can provide information that can prevent intraneural injection and therefore avoid neurologic injury. This is because it is believed that intraneural injections are excruciatingly painful and an awake protesting patient is the best available monitor. However, there are three significant problems with this logic.

First, the literature does not support the widespread notion that relying on a fully awake patient's report of pain on injection is a reliable method to prevent nerve injury. In fact, most neurologic complications reported in the literature have not been associated with pain on injection.[1–3,23–25,27,79–85] For instance, of 49 cases of nerve injury found in the literature search (Table 69–3), 48 patients (98%) were awake. Of these, 42 cases included specific information about the patient's response to the injection; only 4 (10%) patients reported pain on injection. Some reports specifically state that the patient did not have pain, whereas in most others the authors

Table 69–3.

Reports of Peripheral Nerve Injury with Major Conduction Blocks

Webber S et al. (2002)	Two patients developed brachial plexus injury after interscalene blocks. Both blocks were performed in awake patients using nerve stimulator technique. One patient had paresthesia on injection; this information, however, was not useful in preventing the neurologic complication.
Tsao BE et al. (2004)	A retrospective study of 13 patients with injury to the infraclavicular brachial plexus after axillary brachial plexus block; only 1 patient reported pain during the block (not clear as to whether the pain was during needle insertion or local anesthetic injection).
Ediale KR et al. (2004)	Report of prolonged hemidiaphragmatic paralysis after a nerve stimulator-assisted interscalene brachial plexus in an awake patient; paresthesia or pain on injection not reported.
Al-Nasser B et al. (2004)	Report of femoral nerve injury complicating continuous psoas compartment block. Procedure was performed in an awake patient with a nerve stimulator; there was no pain or paresthesia on needle insertion or injection of local anesthetic.
Stark RH et al. (1996)	Report of 3 cases of severe permanent neurologic injury after axillary block for hand surgery; 2 patients suffered ulnar persistent nerve injury, and the third suffered median nerve injury. Nerve stimulator technique was used in all 3 cases. The report indicates that "no unusual problems were reported in administering the block by the anesthesiologist."
Cheney F et al. (1997)	Report of a closed-claims analysis of anesthesia-related complications. In 13 injuries to the axillary blocks, pain on injection was present in only 2 patients; 1 patient received block under general anesthesia. The remaining patients were awake and asymptomatic.
Auroy Y et al. (2002)	A prospective study on complications of regional anesthesia in 12 nerve injuries associated with PNBs. Of these, all patients were awake, and paresthesia was present in only 2 patients (15%). A nerve stimulator was used to localize nerves in 9 patients with injury.
Lim EK, Pereira R (1984)	Report of a brachial plexus injury after supraclavicular brachial plexus block using a paresthesia technique. The patient was awake, the block performance uneventful, and there was no pain on injection.
Gillespie et al. (1987)	Report of a case of reflex sympathetic dystrophy complicating interscalene block. Their patient was awake, a paresthesia technique was used, and the patient had no pain or discomfort on injection of local anesthetic.
Shah S et al. (2005)	Report of neurologic complication after anterior sciatic block that resulted in common peroneal nerve neuropathy. A nerve stimulator technique had been used in a conversant patient; high resistance on injection was noted, there was no pain on injection.
Bonner SM, Pridie K (1997)	Report of sciatic nerve palsy after uneventful sciatic nerve block in a fully awake patient who had no pain on injection.
Bashein G. (1985)	Report of a case of persistent phrenic nerve injury after an interscalene block in an awake patient. No information on pain on injection was provided; however, it was likely absent since the anesthesiologist was able to complete the injection of 50 mL of local anesthetic.
Kaufman BR et al. (2000)	Report of 7 cases of neurologic injury in which all patients had significant discomfort at some point during block placement and went on to develop neurologic injury and disabling chronic pain. Unfortunately, all information in the report was gathered by retrospective chart review. Consequently, it is not known whether the patients had pain during nerve localization or during actual injection of local anesthetic.
Auroy Y et al. (1997)	Report of results of a prospective study on regional anesthesia complications. In this series, 4 patients had neurologic injury due to PNBs. They reported that 19 epidural anesthetics and 4 PNBs were associated with discomfort. It is not clear whether patients with PNBs had paresthesia or pain on injection.
Walton et al. (2000)	A seemingly uneventful nerve stimulator-guided interscalene brachial plexus block in an awake patient resulted in severe brachial plexus injury. There was no pain on needle placement or injection of local anesthetic.
Candido K et al. (2005)	A prospective study in 693 patients having brachial plexus block standardized to technique, local anesthetic and additives. 31 patients had neurologic symptoms likely related to interscalene block; all patients were awake and no patient had pain on injection.
htpp://www.nysora.com; July 2005	Six cases of nerve injuries are discussed on the on-line forum of the New York School of Regional Anesthesia website (htpp://www.nysora.com; July 2004). All injuries occurred in awake patients; none of the patients had pain on injection of local anesthetic.
Borgeat A et al. (2002)	One patient had a permanent brachial plexus injury. The block was performed with the patient awake; there was no paresthesia or pain on injection; the surgery was complex.

PNBs, peripheral nerve blocks.

commented that the block performance was uneventful. Note that the pain on administration of local anesthetic into nerve tissue may be absent even in the central neuraxial area. For instance, Kao et al.[86] reported a case of neural injury that was clearly related to spinal cord trauma from a thoracic catheter that had been inserted while the patient was anesthetized; the patient did not have pain during administration of local anesthetic postoperatively. More recently, Tripathi et al.[87] reported a case report of paraplegia after an intracordal injection during attempted steroid injection, whereas Tsui and Armstrong[88] reported a case of direct spinal cord injury after epidural injection. Both complications occurred in awake patients, who did not report pain on needle placement and consequent injection. These reports clearly indicate that reliance on pain as a symptom of injection into neurologic tissue is unreliable.

The second problem refers to the value of the pain (if present) as a monitor in preventing nerve injury. For instance, in patients in whom the pain does accompany an intraneural injection, it may already be too late to prevent neurologic injury. For example, in the ASA closed-claims study, Cheney and coworkers[79] indicate that on those occasions when pain did occur during injection, the anesthesiologist stopped the injection. However, the patients still went on to develop nerve injury. Similarly, studies using animal models of intraneural injection suggest that nerve fascicles become injured at the very onset of the injection and with injection of a very small volume of local anesthetic (as little as 0.5–1 mL).[20,42] Thereafter, as injection continues, the fascicle ruptures and the injectate escapes through the ruptured perineurium into the epineurial sheath. At this stage, however, the damage to the fascicle(s) may already have been done.

Third, pain is notoriously difficult to assess in terms of quality and intensity. Therefore, distinguishing between the discomfort that is commonly seen during local anesthetic injection (which is considered normal) and that of intraneural injection can be difficult. As an example, in the study by Borgeat et al.,[81] 21% of patients undergoing interscalene block reported transient, burning pain, but none of these patients went on to develop neurologic complication.

NORMAL VERSUS ABNORMAL DISCOMFORT/PAIN ON INJECTION

Injection of local anesthetic in close proximity to the nerves is often associated with discomfort.[26,81] This is thought to result from mechanical irritation of the nerves or plexi as local anesthetic is injected in the immediate vicinity. Based on his studies of brachial plexus anesthesia, Winnie[26] coined the term "pressure paresthesia" to describe the discomfort patients feel during local anesthetic injection and implied that this was a desirable sign of impending successful blockade. In actual clinical practice, however, the variability of patients' pain thresholds, their ability to verbalize a sensation pain during a procedure, and an anesthesiologist's subjective interpretation of any such response make it very difficult to recommend where a "line" could be drawn between nor-

mal and abnormal pain or paresthesia on injection. In fact, a number of published case reports demonstrate that patients' complaints of pain during PNB may not be helpful in preventing the development of the neurologic complication. For instance, Barutell et al.[27] published a report in which a patient communicated discomfort on injection that was perceived as "normal pressure paresthesia" by the anesthesia team. When the injection was carried out, the patient went on to develop permanent neurologic damage. Similarly, in the report by Kaufman et al.,[89] seven patients had discomfort at some point during block injection; however, this information could not be used to prevent the development of permanent neurologic injury, which occurred in all patients. This, however, may be an example of case-report bias. In other words, it is possible that patients' reports of pain may have prevented injuries but such events are unlikely to get reported.

DOGMAS ON COMPLICATIONS OF REGIONAL ANESTHESIA

Blanket statements and dogmas are common in the field of medicine and in regional anesthesia in particular. Much too often, a wide range of recommendations based on a single observation are inappropriately extrapolated. As an example, Walton et al. reported the occurrence of brachial plexus palsy after total shoulder arthroplasty under an otherwise uneventful interscalene block.[90] However, the authors went on to suggest that, "to minimize the risk of brachial plexus injury with interscalene block," PNBs should not be performed in anesthetized patients, and if paresthesia of "unusual severity" occurs, the injection should be immediately stopped. Ironically, their patient was neither anesthetized before the block injection, nor had paresthesia or pain on injection!

Benumof[91] reported four cases of severe neurologic injury that resulted in cervical paraplegia in patients receiving interscalene brachial plexus blocks under general anesthesia. The discussions that followed, however, often recommended that sedation and general anesthesia be abandoned to reduce the risk of nerve injury. Such recommendations are based on this case report are inappropriate because none of the patients in this report suffered a peripheral nerve injury. Rather, these patients received an intracordal injection, a complication entirely avoidable with restriction of the needle insertion depth and/or use of more lateral approach to interscalene block.[4]

Those who base their criticism of "heavy" premedication or general anesthesia before performing PNBs on the cases reported by Benumof[91] forget that interscalene block is a superficial procedure, devoid of significant discomfort and in which excessive sedation and analgesia are usually unnecessary except in children who otherwise would not hold still during the procedure. In contrast, many other PNB procedures involve deeper placement of the needle and several attempts at nerve localization that result in significant patient discomfort.[20,92] Therefore, generalized recommendations to avoid premedication during PNBs carry the risk of limiting the use of PNBs because of an inevitable decrease in patient acceptance. In our practice at St. Luke's–Roosevelt Hospital Center in New York, patients are sent an anesthesia satisfaction survey after their discharge home. Analyses of more than 5000 patient responses clearly indicate that the most satisfied patients are those with no recollection of any anesthetic procedure being performed on them. Therefore, if PNBs are to be accepted by patients, adequate premedication is necessary to avoid patient discomfort during needle placement.

LITERATURE REVIEW

No study has compared the risk of neurologic complications in awake versus anesthetized patients, and it is unlikely that such studies will ever be done. A review of published reports of injury after PNBs indicates that significant neurologic injury after PNBs in *awake* patients occurs at a rate of 0.06–0.4%.[81] Most of these reports included brachial plexus blocks only, probably because these techniques are used more frequently than lower extremity nerve blocks.[4] In a recent similar prospective evaluation by Bogdanov and Loveland,[93] none of 548 patients who received an interscalene brachial plexus block *after induction of general anesthesia* developed permanent or long-term neurologic complications. Similarly, in a report presented at the 2005 Annual ASRA Spring Meeting, Gadsen et al. (ASRA, 2005) presented the data on 226 PNBs of both upper and lower extremities, all performed in heavily sedated or anesthetized patients, none of whom developed neurologic complications. Bogdanov and Loveland used a modified classic approach to interscalene block that was proposed to reduce complications, whereas Tsai et al. used objective assessment of injection pressures to reduce the risk of intraneural injection during PNBs of both upper and lower extremity[94] (Figure 69–8).

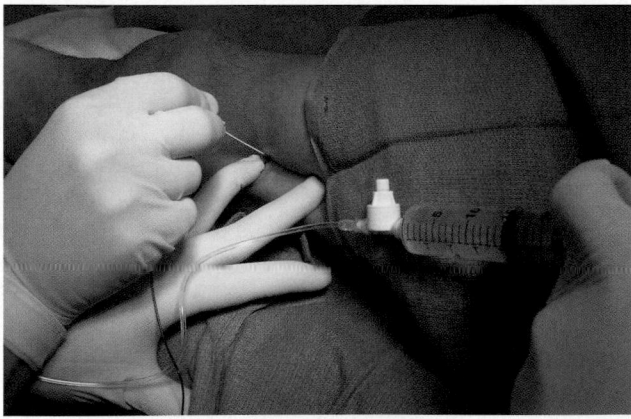

Figure 69–8. Injection of local anesthetic in lateral approach to popliteal block with in-line monitoring of the injection pressure. The goal of the monitoring is to avoid pressures >20 psi, which may be associated with intraneural injection. While the practitioner is performing the block procedure, a helper is injecting the local anesthetic and monitoring the pressure indicated on the piston on the injection monitor (B-Smart, Concert Medical, Needham, MA).

Although the relatively small number of patients in these reports does not allow accurate comparison, these studies at least indicate that the risk of complications of PNBs after general anesthesia may not be substantially more common than complications reported in other similarly powered studies in awake patients.[81] In fact, performance of PNBs in heavily premedicated patients or after induction of general anesthesia is undoubtedly a common practice and a routine in the pediatric anesthesia practice. A recent informal poll conducted during the ASRA 2005 session on complications of PNBs indicated that approximately half of the present attendees performed blocks in heavily sedated or anesthetized patients.

RESCUE BLOCKS, MULTIPLE INJECTION TECHNIQUES, & REVERSE AXIS BLOCKS

Several PNB techniques that are equivalent to a PNB in anesthetized patients are accepted as sound practice. These include "rescue" blocks, multiple injection techniques, and "reverse" axis blocks. They are all similar to the practice of PNBs in anesthetized patients because the PNB is performed in a partially or fully anesthetized limb.

Rescue Blocks

Missed nerve blocks may occur 3–30% of the time and usually involve only one or two of the terminal nerves.[95] Several well-established and universally accepted techniques of PNBs, such as repetition of the block, peripheral injection of the nerve, and others are often used to rescue failed blocks despite the risk that the needle may be inserted or injection made into an anesthetized nerve.[96] Common examples of rescue blocks after failed axillary or interscalene brachial plexus blocks include elbow and wrist blocks.[97,98]

Multiple Injection Techniques

Multiple injection techniques for both upper and lower limb blockade have been introduced relatively recently in clinical practice with the suggestion that they decrease onset time, increase the success rate, and decrease the required dose of local anesthetic.[99–106] The withdrawal and redirection of the needle to elicit multiple motor responses, however, carry a greater risk of direct needle trauma and intraneural injection into already anesthetized nerves. Regardless, this technique has been uniformly accepted by most experts in the field.

Double Blocks and Repeat Blocks

Regional anesthesia for elbow surgery has traditionally been a challenge. The most commonly used brachial plexus blocks—the classic approach to interscalene block and the axillary block—are not ideal because they either do not result in reliable block of the ulnar nerve or do not result in adequate analgesia for the tourniquet. For this reason, in patients undergoing elbow surgery, successful regional anesthesia requires the concomitant use of two separate approaches: an interscalene and an axillary approach.[110] Obviously, performance of brachial plexus block at either level precludes the sensory or motor feedback information during performance of the block at the second level.

CENTRAL NERVOUS SYSTEM TOXICITY IN AWAKE VERSUS ASLEEP PATIENTS

Practice of PNBs involves administering large volumes and doses of local anesthetics. A typical clinical presentation of local anesthetic toxicity is an awake or sedated patient during or immediately after injection of local anesthetic, followed by sudden onset of confusion, seizure, arrhythmias, or cardiac arrest.[23,89] It has been suggested that heavy sedation or general anesthesia increases the risk of severe systemic toxicity of local anesthetics because it diminishes the patient's ability to report early signs and symptoms of rising local anesthetic serum levels. However, there are no reports of local anesthetic toxicity in adult patients under general anesthesia; essentially all reports of toxicity were in awake patients.[108–111] For example, Edde and Deutsch[23,112] reported a cardiac arrest after interscalene brachial plexus block in an awake patient who had no symptoms of toxicity until the entire dose (20 mL of 0.5% bupivacaine) was administered. Conversely, others may argue that premedication offers protection because of its anticonvulsive effects. Moreover, because the critical steps in treating patients with severe toxicity are the establishment of a patent airway, hyperventilation, administration of oxygen, and hemodynamic support, one can argue that anesthetized and ventilated patients who develop systemic toxicity may actually be better off because they already have a secured airway, they are receiving a high concentration of oxygen, and they are typically in an environment that is ideally suited for aggressive resuscitation.

Bernards et al.[113] reported that pigs given an intravenous infusion of bupivacaine failed to demonstrate signs of central nervous system toxicity before cardiovascular collapse if they had been premedicated with benzodiazepines. Indeed, in clinical studies of local anesthetic toxicity, volunteers clearly report an escalating series of symptoms as plasma concentration of local anesthetic rises during continuous, slow intravenous infusion. However, the occurrence of symptoms of local anesthetic toxicity depends on the rate at which the drug is injected. The difficulty in extrapolating this into clinical practice is that local anesthetic for the purpose of neuronal blockade is given as a relatively rapid bolus rather than a slow, escalating continuous infusion, as is the case in animal models.

For these reasons, any suggestion that general anesthesia predisposes to a greater risk of severe systemic toxicity of local anesthetic is purely theoretical, because no data firmly support this belief. Finally, local anesthetic toxicity is of potentially greater concern in the pediatric patient owing to lower

dose requirements and need for stringent adherence to mg/kg dosage rather than a volume dosage, as is the common practice in adult anesthesia. Regardless, the practice of regional anesthesia in anesthetized patients is universally accepted in this patient population.

NERVE BLOCKS IN ANESTHETIZED CHILDREN VERSUS ADULTS

In contrast to PNBs in adults, performing blocks in anesthetized pediatric patients is a universally accepted practice. This is by necessity because pediatric patients are unlikely to be cooperative during needle insertion, nerve stimulation, and manipulation necessary to accomplish PNB. In addition, most pediatric patients require concomitant administration of general anesthesia to allow for immobility during the surgical procedure. However, from the standpoint of risk of complications, this divergence in consensus on PNBs after general anesthesia between adults and pediatric patients does not make much sense. In other words, with the possible exception of infants, no sufficient anatomic or neurophysiologic differences justify this divergence in recommendations.

Although one can argue that complications of PNBs in children are rare, PNBs are not routinely used in the pediatric population, and there are simply no series comparable to those in adults to allow one to draw a clear conclusion regarding the risk of nerve injury in children. However, a large prospective study performed in France in children demonstrated a small risk of complications with PNBs.[114]

MONITORING POSSIBILITIES DURING PNBS

Since this discussion focuses on the impact of heavy sedation or general anesthesia on the risk of neurologic complications, it is important to discuss the monitoring that is available to reduce the risk of nerve injury during PNBs. In general, two phases are amenable to monitoring during PNB placement. These include needle placement guidance (percutaneous stimulation, ultrasound) and avoidance of intraneural injection (report of pain on injection by the patient (when present), nerve stimulation, and assessment of resistance to injection).[115] With regard to intraneural injection, neither percutaneous stimulation nor ultrasound guidance is helpful. Percutaneous stimulation may be helpful for approximating the needle insertion site, but it is useless for estimating the needle–nerve relationship. Ultrasound, on the other hand, offers real-time needle guidance below the skin level. However, in addition to the required skill, expense, and inconvenience of the equipment, the image resolution is simply insufficient to rule out intraneural needle placement.[37] Most practitioners inject a small volume of injectate to determine the location of the tip of the needle. However, injectate as small as 0.2–0.5 mL is adequate to cause nerve injury if injected into a fascicle.

Nerve stimulator-assisted PNBs entered the practice of regional anesthesia with the promise of decreasing the risk of neurologic complications associated with the paresthesia technique.[116] However, it soon became apparent that nerve stimulators could not prevent neurologic injury.[1] More recently, it has been suggested that in many circumstances, the motor response to nerve stimulation may be absent at the point at which the needle makes contact with the nerve[121] and that intraneural needle placement is possible despite the use of nerve stimulators[37] (see Figure 69–4). One possible explanation for this phenomenon is hyperpolarization of the nerve that may occur when the needle is positioned in the vicinity of the nerve and excessively high current intensity is used.

SUMMARY

Few issues in the practice of regional anesthesia have evoked such strong and divergent opinion among clinicians as have the performance of PNBs in anesthetized or deeply sedated patients. This is because administration of PNBs has traditionally been based on individual preferences, clinical impressions, and other subjective criteria rather than on established practice standards. Avoidance of deep sedation and general anesthesia is often suggested to decrease the risk of peripheral nerve injury with PNBs; however, there is no evidence in the literature to suggest that either practice is safer with regard to the risk of nerve injury. Nevertheless, the serious nature of complications resulting from inadvertent injections

into the spinal cord suggests that regional anesthesia techniques close to the centroneuraxis should be practiced with extreme caution and insight into the appropriate depth of the needle insertion, whether the patient is awake, sedated, or anesthetized. It is also important to realize that neurologic injury is not always necessarily related to regional anesthesia technique. With PNBs, nerve injury that occurs postoperatively without pain, paresthesia, or high injection pressure is more likely related to surgery (surgical technique, stretching, positioning), rather than the PNB technique. Adequate proper training and the use of proper techniques and nerve block/monitoring equipment are more likely to decrease the risk of complications than are unfounded blanket statements about the advisability of performing PNBs in anesthetized patients. This is because such statements are unfounded by the relevant literature and can have a potentially negative impact on the practice of regional anesthesia.

Many patients and PNB techniques require appropriate sedation for block performance and patient acceptance. However, clinicians may be reluctant to use them because of the medicolegal concerns engendered by admonitions against performing blocks in sedated or anesthetized patients. Future efforts must be directed toward developing more objective and exacting nerve localization and injection monitoring techniques to more reliably detect and prevent intraneural injection. The results of these efforts will be of far greater importance to the future of PNBs and their role in practice of modern anesthesiology than overreaching, unsubstantiated opinions and statements.

C. Methods and Means of Decreasing the Risk of Neurologic Complications Associated with Nerve Blocks

INTRODUCTION

The published data suggest that neurologic complications of PNBs are relatively rare. However, the severity of consequences and lack of prevention strategies continue to present a source of significant concern for both clinicians and patients. The main inciting mechanism of neurologic injury with PNBs appears to be an intrafascicular or intraneural injection. It is fortunate that peripheral nerves possess an inherent natural protection; intraneural injections often do not result in intrafascicular needle placement and therefore do not necessarily lead to nerve injury. It is commonly suggested that the use of short-bevel needles and avoidance of excessive sedation and general anesthesia should be carried out to decrease the risk of nerve injury. However, these commonly voiced recommendations have been recently challenged. In addition, avoidance of adequate premedication may have a significant negative impact by decreasing the patient's acceptance and satisfaction with PNBs. The relatively low incidence of complications with PNBs, together with the lack of objective documentation and means to more precisely monitor administration of nerve blocks make retrospective analyses of cases of nerve injury largely speculative with regard to the actual mechanism of nerve injury in clinical practice.

RECOMMENDATIONS FOR DECREASING PNB COMPLICATIONS

Aseptic Technique

Most nerve block techniques are merely percutaneous injections. However, infections are known to occur and can result in significant disability. Because this complication is almost entirely preventable, every effort should be made to adhere to strictly aseptic technique.

Short-Bevel Insulated Needles

Insulated needles are now widely available and result in much more precise needle placement. The short-bevel design helps to prevent nerve penetration.

Needles of Appropriate Length for Each Block Technique

Excessively long needles should not be used for nerve blockade. For instance, it is important to never use needles longer than 50 mm for an interscalene block. In addition to the safety reasons, needles of appropriate length are also advanced with far greater precision than excessively long needles.

Surface Localization

In patients with difficult anatomy, surface localization of superficially seated nerves or plexuses can help reduce the number of needle passes.

Needle Advancement

During needle localization, advance and withdraw the needle slowly. Keep in mind that nerve stimulators deliver current of very short duration once (1 Hz) or twice (2 Hz) per second and that no current is delivered between the pulses. Thus, fast insertions and withdrawal of the needle passages may result in failure to stimulate the nerve because the needle may pass nearby or even through the nerve between the stimuli without eliciting nerve stimulation.

Fractionated Injections

Inject smaller doses and volumes of local anesthetics (3–5 mL) with intermittent aspiration to avoid inadvertent intravascular injection. Always observe the patient during the injection of local anesthetic because negative aspiration of blood is not always present with an intravenous injection. This approach may allow detection of the signs of local anesthetic toxicity before the entire dose is injected. Regardless of the monitoring method, slow injection is of paramount importance to avoid massive intravascular injection.

Accuracy of the Nerve Stimulator

Always ensure that the nerve stimulator is operational and delivering the specified current and that the leads are properly connected to the patient and the needle.

Avoidance of Forceful, Fast Injections

Forceful, fast injections are more likely to result in channeling of local anesthetic to the unwanted tissue layers, lymphatic vessels, or small veins that may have been cut during needle advancement. Such injections may result in channeling of the local anesthetic in the systemic circulation with consequent risk of central nervous system and cardiac toxicity. Finally, forceful, fast injections under excessive pressure are more likely to result in an unrecognized intraneuronal injection. Limit the injection speed to 15–20 mL/minute.

Avoidance of High Injection Pressures

Intraneuronal needle placement may result in high resistance (pressure) to injection owing to the compact nature of the neuronal tissue and its connective tissue sheaths. Always use the same syringe and needle size to develop a "feel" during the injection. As a rule, when injection of the first milliliter of local anesthetic proves difficult, the needle should be slightly withdrawn and the injection attempted again. If resistance persists, the needle should be completely withdrawn and flushed before repeating the insertion. Ultimately, objective injection pressure monitoring will likely become a standard monitor to standardize nerve block injections, reduce the risk of intraneural injection, and to be a basis for medicolegal documentation (see Figure 69–8).

Aborting Injection When Pain Is Reported

Severe pain or discomfort on injection may signify intraneuronal placement of the needle and should be avoided. When this occurs, the injection should be abandoned, although chances are that damage may have already been caused at the time when the pain occurs. Lancinating, "shooting" pain on injection should not be confused with a mild "paresthesia-like" feeling reported by the patient when the needle is placed in the immediate vicinity of the nerve or plexus. In this case, local anesthetic can be injected slowly, provided that the resistance to injection is normal (< 20 psi). Resuming the injection after waiting to see whether the pain will go away should not be done under any circumstances.

Choosing the Local Anesthetic Solution Wisely

Always choose a shorter-acting (and less toxic) local anesthetic for short procedures in which long-lasting postoperative analgesia is not required. Local anesthetic toxicity is the most common complication with neuronal blockade. The risk of severe toxicity is substantially lower with chloroprocaine or lidocaine than with bupivacaine.

Blocks in Anesthetized Patients

Without reliable monitoring, blocks in anesthetized patients still should not be common practice. When it is necessary to place blocks in anesthetized patients, this should be done by practitioners with experience. The introduction of ultrasound-guided nerve blocks and injection pressure monitoring is likely to change the practice and allow more routine performance of nerve blocks in anesthetized patients.

Repeating a Block After a Failed Block

Repeating a block after a failed block should be avoided whenever possible. When indicated, it should be done only by those with substantial experience in the planned technique. Avoidance of abnormal resistance to injection or objective injection pressure monitoring is of utmost importance here as the clinician can no longer count on pain on injection as a sign of intraneural injection. Similarly, neurostimulation may no longer be possible once the local anesthetic is injected. Real-time ultrasound imaging is also useful when repeating the failed block, as it allows more accurate placement of the needle.

— D. Management of Patients with Neurologic Injury —

PERIPHERAL NERVE INJURY AFTER PERIPHERAL NERVE BLOCKS

Nerve injury is recognized as a potential complication of peripheral nerve block (PNB) anesthesia, but fortunately, severe or disabling injuries are rare. When they do occur, they can be a frightening complication for patient, surgeon, and anesthesiologist. Fortunately, most symptoms of nerve injury resolve in 4–6 weeks in over 95% of patients and in 99% of the patients by 1 year.[81] Early intervention may help prevent the long-term sequelae that can occur with unrecognized, and therefore improperly treated nerve injuries. With the resurgence of interest and utilization of PNB anesthesia, it is important to develop a coinciding plan for management of postoperative nerve injuries. The plan should include recognition, diagnosis, and treatment of the nerve injury. A working knowledge of the long-term prognosis, understanding the importance of appropriate neurology consultations, and familiarity with available diagnostic tests and treatment options is essential for the proper management of patients with neurologic injury.

With any PNB, inclusive documentation of the block is of utmost importance for diagnostic, therapeutic, and medicolegal purposes. Documentation that includes the nerve(s) stimulated, the minimum current used, the number of attempts, the appearance of pain or paresthesia during the procedure and measures taken, resistance to injection and injection pressure if pressure monitoring is used, type/dose of local anesthetic agent, and patient condition during the block is essential in understanding the mechanism of the injury. This documentation can help the anesthesiologist and/or consulting specialist to determine the possible cause of the injury and any associated conditions and to guide treatment modalities.

Mechanisms of Injury & Symptoms

After peripheral nerve anesthesia, if sensory and/or motor function remains depressed beyond the expected duration of action of the local anesthetic, potential causes for the neurologic deficits should be investigated. Neurologic deficits may be related to vascular injuries, compression injuries, local anesthetic action, or traumatic nerve injury with fascicular disruption. When faced with a neurologic deficit, especially in a patient in whom a PNB has been placed, it is important to remember that many causes of nerve injury are unrelated to the performance of the regional anesthetic.

Other factors, such as, tourniquet use, improper positioning, postoperative swelling, surgical trauma, and pre-existing neurologic deficits may be contributing or causative influences. Proper and objective documentation of the nerve block procedures can go a long way toward deciphering whether the injury was caused by a nerve block, surgery, or other factors.

Vascular Injuries

When symptoms occur early in the postoperative period (within minutes to hours), the anesthesiologist should suspect a vascular or compression-type injury due to disruption of the blood supply from an insult to the vascular structures, from hematoma at the surgical or block site, or from deep venous thrombosis. This is particularly true if a neurologic deficit appears after apparent resolution of the block.

Compression Injuries

Compression neuropathies usually present as a focal mononeuropathy at sites where nerves pass through tissue tunnels, that is, median through carpal tunnel, spinal nerve through vertebral foramina. Acute compression injuries can develop secondary to limb tourniquet paralysis, from retractors used for surgical procedures, from expanding hematomas, or from improper intraoperative positioning, that is, stretching of the cords of the brachial plexus during sternal retraction, or from extending/pronating the forearm causing ulnar nerve compression.[75,117] A compression injury can also occur with PNB anesthesia from increased endoneurial fluid pressure. This can occur with injection into a tight tissue compartment or when high injection pressures are used during nerve block administration.[77] Metabolic diseases such as diabetes mellitus may make nerves more susceptible to compression injuries.[119]

Local Anesthetic Action

It is important to remember that neurologic deficits may be related to the residual neurologic blockade. Long-acting local anesthetics such as ropivacaine or bupivacaine have been reported to last up to 24 hours. It is well recognized that intraneural injections can and do occur without obligatory neurologic injury.[37] Most such injections result in intraneural, but *perifascicular* injection of local anesthetic, and their hallmark is a block of much longer duration than expected.[20] When additives are included in the local anesthetic mixture, particularly in the setting of an intraneural injection, the block can be prolonged up to 48 hours.[120] In the elderly and in those with preexisting neurologic diseases, local anesthetic action can be prolonged secondary to abnormal uptake or reduced perfusion to the nervous tissue.[121] The site of the block may have an effect on the duration of action of the local anesthetic.[122] Therefore, in patients with known or occult preexisting neurologic disease, the elderly, and those treated with long-acting local anesthetics, sufficient time should be allowed for the local anesthetic to be thoroughly metabolized. Physical examination of these patients usually reveals a slowly receding block. Once the return of motor function occurs, the block usually recedes in an accelerated fashion. If motor function returns with persistent sensory deficits, or motor dysfunction persists, further evaluation is necessary.

Traumatic/Toxic Nerve Injury

Nerve injury after PNBs may be caused by direct needle trauma, intraneural injection, or local anesthetic neurotoxicity. Several animal studies have demonstrated that the nerve injury occurs more frequently with long-bevel needles, but the duration and severity of the injury are greater with short-bevel needles. When the bevel orientation is perpendicular rather than parallel with nerve fibers, studies have shown that nerve injury can be more severe.[43] Intraneural intrafascicular injection is characterized by high injection pressures at the onset of injection.[20] Such injections are characterized by a prolong blockade followed by incomplete resolution and residual neurologic deficit. Because a miniscule amount of local anesthetic (as little as 0.5 mL) is required to rupture the fascicle, intraneural injection should be suspected whenever there is resistance to injection or when the patient experiences severe pain on injection.

All local anesthetics are potentially neurotoxic. Neurotoxicity depends on the dose, concentration, and length of exposure to the nerve tissue. Vasoconstrictive additives such as epinephrine, which can affect neural blood flow, may potentiate nerve injuries. Local anesthetic neurotoxicity is more prevalent in patients with preexisting neurologic deficits, especially those with demyelinating diseases. In several studies of patients with occult or diagnosed multiple sclerosis, local anesthetic action was prolonged. The prolonged duration was thought to be related to an abnormal uptake of local anesthetic in demyelinated nerves.[121]

Magnitude of Neural Injury

The degree of neural insult can be defined by the terms neurapraxia, axonotmesis, and neurotmesis. The mildest form, **neurapraxia** denotes a mild degree of neural insult with failure of impulse conduction across the affected segment. The electromyogram (EMG) is normal, but conduction velocity as demonstrated by a nerve conduction study is decreased. Usually when the offending cause has been removed, recovery occurs over a variable amount of time, which may be as long as several weeks. Complete recovery can usually be anticipated. **Axonotmesis**, an intermediate injury, occurs when there is axonal disruption with preservation of the endoneurium. Recovery is dependent on the rate of axonal regeneration (1–3 mm/day). If recovery occurs, it is most likely prolonged and incomplete. The prognosis is better for young, healthy patients with distal lesions. The most severe form of neural injury is **neurotmesis,** a complete transection or crushing of the nerve with disruption of the endoneurium. Surgical repair is usually indicated, but even then, recovery is usually incomplete. Prognosis for full recovery is poor.

PATIENT EVALUATION/PHYSICAL EXAMINATION

Symptoms of Nerve Injury

The symptoms of a nerve lesion after PNB manifest after the block has receded—usually within 48 hours. The perception of symptoms is influenced by the origin of the nerve lesion and other confounding factors, such as postoperative pain, immobility, effects of surgery, position, application of casts, dressing, bandaging, and so forth. The intensity and duration of symptoms may also vary with the severity of the injury—from a light, intermittent tingling and numbness lasting a few weeks to a persistent, painful paresthesia, neuropathic pain, sensory loss, and/or motor weakness lasting for several months or years. Some nerve injuries may even evolve into a severe causalgia or reflex sympathetic dystrophy. Keep in mind that although dermatomes can provide clues to the location of injuries, the loss of sensation at the skin does

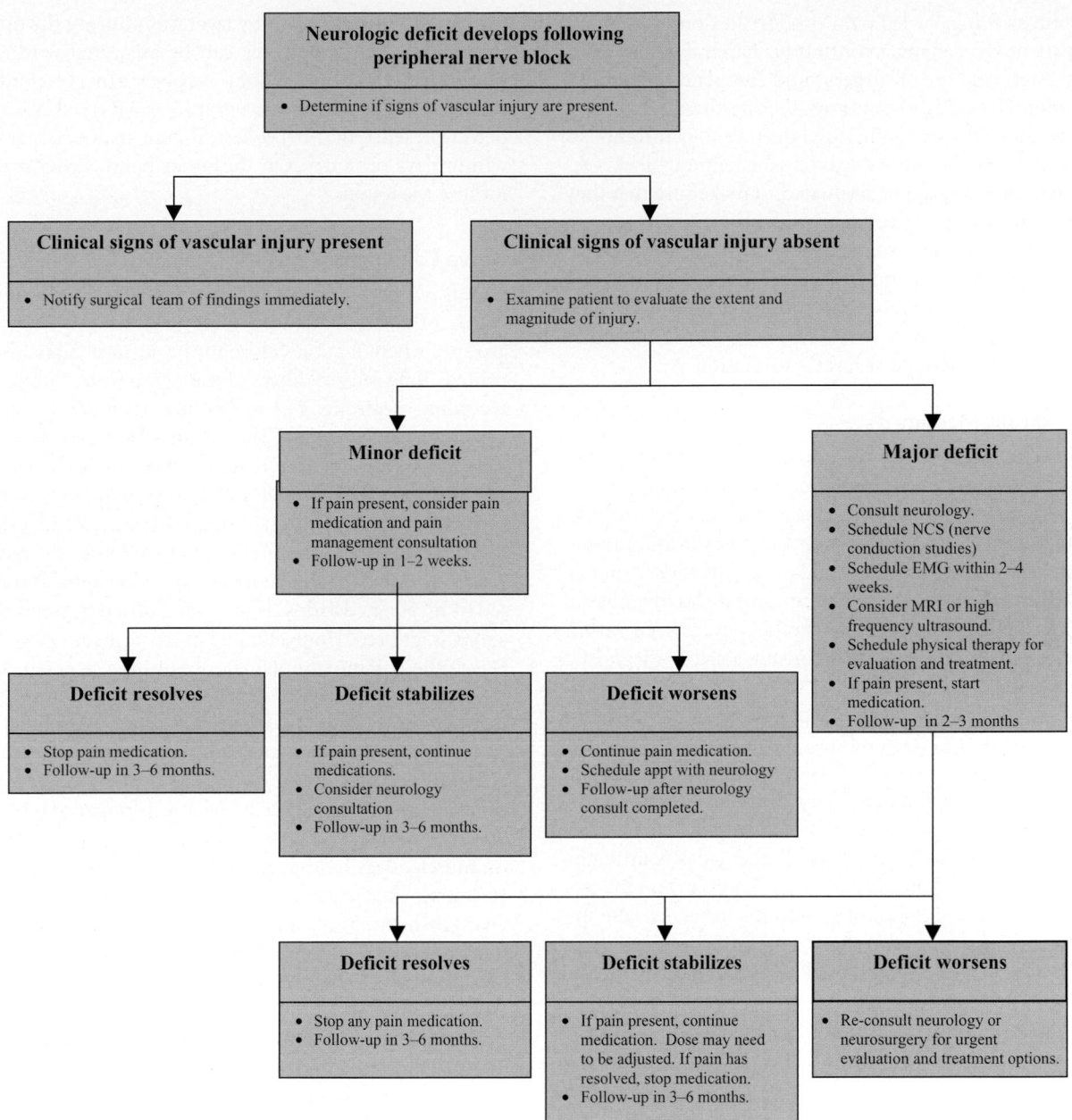

Figure 69–9. Management of neurologic deficit following peripheral nerve block. EMG, electromyography.

not provide precise information concerning the site of injury because the boundaries of dermatomes are not precise, clearly defined lines. More useful information can be obtained from the loss of motor function on the basis of the origin and assessment of motor performance.

Symptoms of neurologic injury range from mild to severe. Typical symptoms are dysesthesia, paresthesia, numbness, weakness, and pain. Symptoms of nerve injury may be acute or may not become clinically apparent for several days to several weeks. The approach to patient evaluation should be indistinguishable, regardless of the timing of the suspected injury (Figure 69–9). Physical examination should include an assessment of vascular integrity, sensory/motor function, and reflexes.

Vascular Mediated

Vascular-mediated injuries include injury to arteries or veins, the formation of deep venous thrombosis, or a combination of any of these, creating vascular compromise.

Vascular injury with associated ischemia should be immediately excluded. The examination should include an assessment of both venous and arterial circulation, skin color changes, the presence of engorgement or edema, hematoma, or pain at the surgical or block site. If a vascular injury is suspected, the surgical team should be consulted immediately to manage and treat the problem. For example, patients with lower extremity joint replacement surgeries are prone to the development of deep venous thrombosis. Patients may be completely asymptomatic, or they may complain of limb

pain, limb swelling, or leg pain on dorsiflexion of the foot. If the patient is receiving a continuous femoral nerve block, (typical after this type of surgery) and complains of pain *behind* the knee (sciatic distribution), the anesthesiologist must be cognizant of the possibility of a deep venous thrombosis versus incisional pain not covered by the femoral block. Occlusive dressings should be evaluated to make sure that they are not contributing to the vascular insult.

With arterial compromise, the patient complains of intense pain, paresthesia, and cold. The onset is usually rapid. A Doppler/vascular study is the most common diagnostic test to aid in the diagnosis. Arterial occlusion or compromise usually requires emergent surgical exploration.

Neurologically Mediated

If the physical examination demonstrates intact circulation, then a more thorough neurologic examination should be initiated. This includes a comprehensive motor and sensory examination as well as assessment of the reflexes. In multiple studies evaluating the incidence and prognosis of nerve injury after PNB anesthesia, most mild symptoms such as dyesthesia, mild paresthesia or numbness, or mild pain resolved within the first few days or weeks of the insult. Further diagnostic testing was not indicated.[2,3,81,123–125]

If the neurologic deficit is persistent or more severe (ie, moderate to severe numbness, weakness and/or pain), then an evaluation by a neurologist may be indicated. For the hospitalized patient, the neurology consultation and subsequent examination should take place during the hospitalization. If the patient has already been discharged, a neurologist can be contacted for an outpatient evaluation. The magnitude or rate of progression of symptoms influences the urgency of the neurology consultation. Temporizing measures for pain control may be initiated until the patient can be evaluated. The neurology assessment involves a more meticulous clinical examination to try to evaluate the degree of deficit and to determine what further diagnostic tests are indicated.

DIAGNOSTIC TESTS

A variety of diagnostic tests are available for the detection of nerve injury. Each test has specific indications, advantages, and disadvantages, depending on the injury, patient characteristics, availability of the diagnostic equipment, and expertise of the operator. The diagnostic tests currently available include electrophysiology, high-resolution ultrasound, and magnetic resonance imaging.

Electrophysiology Testing

When a patient presents with complaints of weakness, numbness, and/or paresthesia, several questions arise. Are these complaints the result of a nerve lesion? Did a lesion exist prior to surgery? Did the lesion result from placement of a nerve block, by nerve compression or traction during or after the surgical procedure, or by laceration during the operative procedure? These questions can be answered with electrophysiology. Electrophysiology involves a nerve conduction study (NCS) and electromyography (EMG). NCS is used to detect presence of a nerve lesion, and it can be performed within days of injury. On the other hand, EMG is used to localize the lesion.

Nerve Conduction Studies

NCS is performed by placing cutaneous electrodes along the course of a nerve. The only places a nerve can be evaluated are sites where it comes close to the surface. Signal is transmitted along sensory fibers of the nerve from stimulating to recording electrode. The amplitude of signal, the time for signal transmission, and the distance between electrodes is measured. From measurements of time and distance, a conduction velocity is calculated. Nerves are composite structures formed by axons of different diameter that conduct signal at different velocities. The first signal to arrive at the recording electrode is the only signal measured. This signal is transmitted by myelinated axons. Signal transmitted by unmyelinated axons is ignored. Unmyelinated axons transmit pain. Therefore if the patient complains only of pain, a nerve conduction study is unlikely to detect any changes in amplitude or conduction velocity. A patient can have a normal NCS and still suffer from legitimate pain. A reduction in conduction velocity indicates myelin damage. A reduction in amplitude indicates axonal damage. Conduction along motor fibers can also be evaluated; however, the recording electrode is placed on muscle. Because the signal involves the entire motor unit (ie, motor axon, neuromuscular junction, and muscle fibers), changes in amplitude and conduction velocity are more difficult to evaluate. A lesion can be detected by NCS within 1–2 days of injury. Therefore, the initial NCS should be scheduled 1–2 days after injury. If the initial study is normal, the patient probably has a neurapraxia that should resolve with time. The patient should be followed clinically for improvement of symptoms. If symptoms persist or worsen, the study should be repeated in 4–6 weeks. If the initial NCS shows abnormality, then the lesion needs to be localized. NCS has a limited ability to do this. However, to localize a lesion within a nerve or plexus, EMG needs to be performed.

Electromyography

EMG records muscle depolarization. Depolarization is detected by a needle electrode placed in the muscle and appears as a deflection on an oscilloscope. The shape and frequency of the deflections provide information about the nerve and muscle. In normal muscle at rest, there should be no spontaneous depolarization or deflections on EMG. Following nerve injury, muscle fibers are released from the control by the nerve and begin to discharge spontaneously. On EMG, this appears as deflections called positive waves and fibrillations. It takes between 2 and 4 weeks for these changes to appear. Therefore, the EMG is scheduled 2–4 weeks following injury. Given the delay in appearance of pathology on EMG, some laboratories may perform EMG at the time the initial NCS is obtained. EMG obtained within the first week of injury is used to determine if there are signs of nerve damage that existed prior to surgery and may be responsible for the patient's complaints. While this may have some merit, it must be tempered with the fact that EMG is an uncomfortable procedure performed without sedation, anesthesia, or analgesia. Some patients may be unable to complete the test. Consequently, many patients will not agree to repeat an EMG. The purpose for EMG is localization of the lesion. The best signal to perform this function appear 2–4 weeks following injury; therefore, to evaluate a lesion that may have occurred during an anesthetic or surgical procedure, the only EMG that must be obtained should be scheduled 2–4 weeks following the injury. If EMG is delayed beyond 4 weeks, signs of reinnervation (long duration, high amplitude, polyphasic motor unit potentials) may appear and complicate the evaluation. To determine the site of lesion on a nerve, a series of muscles are tested. There is no standard set of muscles evaluated. The muscles are selected based on their relationship to the region of the suspected nerve lesion. For example if a lesion is suspected in the posterior cord of the brachial plexus, deltoid and triceps brachii muscles need to be tested. For the injury to be in the posterior cord, positive waves or fibrillations need to be present in both muscles. If they are present only in the deltoid, then the lesion may be in the axillary nerve or in the upper roots of the brachial plexus. The axillary nerve can be further evaluated by testing teres minor. Roots in the upper regions of the brachial plexus can be evaluated by testing supraspinatus. The neurologist performing the EMG selects the muscles to be tested. It is very important to educate the neurologist about the procedures of nerve block and surgery. Sites where nerves may have been placed at risk need to be discussed. Failure to have this discussion could mean an EMG with considerable error.

Once a lesion is localized, inferences can be made about its etiology. For example, a lesion located over a bony prominence may be the result of compression caused by inappropriate or prolonged positioning of a limb during surgery. A lesion located in the region where a nerve block procedure may have been caused by the anesthesiologist. A lesion located in the region of the operative site may have been caused by the surgeon. Therefore, in this context, EMG can be considered as a tool for evaluating the *etiology* of a nerve lesion.

Doppler Ultrasound/High-Frequency Ultrasound

Doppler ultrasound provides structural information about the image being scanned. Most commonly, it is used to study the carotid arteries and major arteries and veins of the lower extremities. It can also be used to examine the arteries at the wrist, in the palms, and in the digits. It is the most common diagnostic test for deep venous thrombosis. A newer type of ultrasound, high-frequency ultrasound, is an effective imaging modality for identifying morphologic changes in the peripheral nerves. It is being used to evaluate nerve rupture, inflammatory processes, and compressive syndromes in peripheral

nerves. It can localize the lesion. It may be a useful tool for initial imaging of a suspected peripheral nerve injury or for follow-up imaging. It is faster and more cost-effective than magnetic resonance imaging. But it has limitations in that the test is operator-dependent, requires an extended learning curve to obtain and interpret images, and is limited to nerves within 2 cm of the skin surface.[126] At greater depths, coarser-quality ultrasound nerve images can be obtained, but they are difficult to distinguish from other tissues such as tendons.[127]

Magnetic Resonance Imaging/Magnetic Resonance Neurography

Magnetic resonance imaging, specifically magnetic resonance neurography, is a relatively new imaging technique that can reliably and selectively image peripheral nerves.[128] By manipulating magnetic resonance imaging parameters, nerves can be made to show up as three-dimensional "neurographic" images, comparable to angiograms. When it is properly implemented, magnetic resonance neurography is capable of providing high-quality information about nerve compression, nerve inflammation, nerve trauma, systemic neuropathies, and recovery of nerves from pathologic states.[129] Direct nerve imaging has been shown to demonstrate nerve continuity, distinguish intraneural from perineural masses, and localize nerve compressions before surgical exploration.[130] Like ultrasound, its indication for acute peripheral nerve injury is in localizing the lesion. In some studies, magnetic resonance signal alterations were shown to occur as early as 24 hours after an axonal nerve lesion, possibly making it the earliest form of detection of nerve injury.[131] Magnetic resonance studies are limited by access to the patient, cost, longer scanning times, and equipment availability.

TREATMENT OPTIONS FOR PERIPHERAL NERVE INJURY

When a nerve injury has occurred, treatment of the patient depends on the severity of the injury. It is prudent to remember that most of these injuries resolve with time. The care of the patient with a nerve injury can be divided into two groups: those with minor deficits and those with major deficits. Regardless of the type of injury, the patient should be evaluated clinically to ascertain whether a more serious or occult injury or correctable contributing condition is not overlooked.

Minor Deficits

If the examination reveals minor deficits, reassurance is key to relieving the patient's anxiety. Further diagnostic testing or therapy is usually not indicated. Weekly to biweekly telephone follow-up to assess resolution of the injury by the pain management team provides reassurance, allows early detection of more serious problems, and instills confidence in the patient. It is important to remember that one bad experience with regional anesthesia often creates a negative attitude toward future application for the patient, his family, and possibly the surgical team. Providing the patient with consistent, caring follow-up despite the injury, helps to rebuild patient confidence in future anesthetic experiences.

Major Deficits

If the clinical examination of the patient reveals a *major* neurologic deficit, early neurologic and/or neurosurgery consultation is advisable. In addition to a complete neurologic examination, the neurologist determines the most appropriate diagnostic test for the patient. For example, if a compression injury is suspected, ultrasonography or magnetic resonance imaging of the involved plexus may be performed. In patients with pain, medication for pain should be started early to prevent nerve sensitization. Physical and occupational therapy consultations are obtained by the neurology department with arrangements made for treatment after the patient is discharged. A consultation for social services may be necessary if the injury will make an impact on the patient's ability to perform activities of daily living. Similarly, early consultation with physical therapy is a must to reduce the risk of contractures, muscle atrophy, and prolonged disability. Close follow-up by neurology clinician should be arranged as well as continued follow-up by an anesthesiology clinician until the injury is completely resolved or is stable.

Drug Therapy

Multiple drugs are effective to treat neurally mediated pain. The more commonly prescribed medications include tricyclic antidepressants, serotonin reuptake inhibitors, anticonvulsants, opioids, and capsaicin cream. These drugs should be administered under the direction of a chronic pain specialist or a neurologist who has evaluated the patient and has the capacity to do follow-up evaluations.

Tricylic Antidepressants

Amitriptyline is among the more efficacious drugs. It has multiple effects including blocking the reuptake of serotonin and norepinephrine, blocking the NMDA receptor, and blocking voltage-dependent sodium channels. A more recent study demonstrated that amitriptyline has an ability to maintain spinal cord GABA(B) receptor activity.[132] The drug can be started at 10–25 mg daily and escalated by 25 mg every week to an effective level. Doses should be limited to 100 mg daily. Side effects include decreased salivation, constipation, urinary hesitancy, blurred vision, orthostatic hypotension, sedation, and cognitive impairment. One very serious side effect in cardiac patients is torsade de pointes from prolongation of the Q-T interval, but this has been shown to occur only in higher doses.

Selective Serotonin Reuptake Inhibitors

Paroxetine is the only selective serotonin reuptake inhibitor that may be effective in the treatment of neurally derived pain. In a study comparing paroxetine with imipramine (another tricyclic antidepressant), paroxetine was as effective in 60–70% of the patients receiving the drug.[133] Because of its marginal effectiveness, it is reserved for patients who are unable to tolerate other classes of medications.

Anticonvulsants

Commonly prescribed anticonvulsants in the treatment of minor neural changes (pain and paresthesia) are gabapentin and carbamazepine. Gabapentin is an amino acid derivative of GABA (gamma-amino butyric acid). The proposed mechanism of analgesic action is related to its effect on sensitized neurons. It is thought to directly or indirectly inhibit excitatory neurotransmitters, block neuronal calcium channels, and augment central nervous system inhibitory pathways by increasing GABA transmission.[134] Gabapentin is usually started at 300 mg daily with increasing doses to 1300–1800 mg per day in divided doses. Side effects of gabapentin include drowsiness, anxiety, visual disturbances, hypertension, and ataxia. Other anticonvulsants that have been used in the treatment of neurally mediated pain are carbamazepine, topiramate, levetiracetam, and oxcarbazepine.

Opioids

Opioid therapy is controversial, but may be effective in alleviating pain of peripheral nerve injury origin. In five randomized, controlled trials of opioid therapy used for neuropathic pain, all demonstrated benefits from opioids in controlling pain.[135,136] Commonly prescribed opioids for short-term therapy include oxycodone, oxycontin, or fentanyl patches. To prevent opioid dependence or tolerance, other therapeutic agents, such as amitriptyline and gabapentin, should be titrated up while titrating off the opioids.

Tramadol

Tramadol is approved for use in the United States for moderate to severe pain. It binds to mu opioid receptors, contributing to its analgesic properties. It inhibits the reuptake of serotonin and norepinephrine into the central nervous system. In recent literature, tramadol has been shown to be effective in the treatment of arthritic and neuropathic pain and in mixed nociceptive-neuropathic pain.[137] It is tolerated by elderly patients, has a low incidence of constipation, is devoid of immunosuppressive activity, and has a low tendency toward tolerance. It has a minimum risk of addiction and abuse.

Capsaicin Ointment

Capsaicin is a vanniloid compound most commonly found in hot peppers. Many of the neuropathies with pain as the predominant symptom involve small afferent fibers resistant to the analgesic action of the more commonly prescribed medications. Capsaicin can deplete the transmitter contents of these small afferent fibers leading to their degeneration and subsequent pain-generating ability. Its application is primarily for cutaneous hyperalgesia states such as postherpetic neuralgia. It is probably not effective for most painful neuropathies of deeper origin. After starting medication therapy, consultant follow-up should be scheduled for 2 weeks after the injury to determine whether the deficit has resolved, persisted, or worsened. If the deficit has resolved, any medication given for pain should be discontinued. The patient should be instructed to notify the consultant if any neurologic changes develop within the next month. If the deficit persists, the dose of pain medication is adjusted as described. During follow-up visits, the patient should be asked about any side effects associated with the prescribed medication. Subsequent follow-up depends on the nature of the deficit. If it is stable but persistent, consultant follow-up should be arranged for 3–6 months. If the deficit has worsened, adjustments are made in the drug therapy to try to alleviate symptoms. Follow-up is determined by the consultant based on the patient's condition and symptoms.

SUMMARY

Despite meticulous care, patient selection, and experience, neurologic deficits after regional anesthesia may occur. The debate over performing blocks in awake or sedated/asleep patients is inconsequential because nerve injuries have occurred in both groups. Understanding the mechanism of injury, the typical clinical course following injury, and the prognosis and obtaining appropriate consults are essential knowledge for the regional anesthesiologist. A basic understanding of diagnostic tests and treatment modalities provide the clinician with information necessary to participate in meaningful discussions with the patient and other specialists involved in the patient's care. Regardless of the consultations obtained, the importance of follow-up by an anesthesiologist cannot be overemphasized. Complete documentation of the initial consult, the block procedure, the postoperative care, and follow-up are extremely important in the event of any legal action as well as in the professional care of the patient.

Few publications have had a greater impact on the clinical practice of anesthesiology than the American Society of Anesthesiologists (ASA) practice guidelines.[138] These practice guidelines have been designed to enhance and promote the safety of anesthetic practice and have made the practice of general anesthesia much safer. Such guidelines are much needed but currently do not exist with regard to the practice of PNBs. This is most likely because administration of PNBs has been traditionally based on individual preferences, clinical impressions, and other subjective methods. Future efforts should be directed toward developing more objective and exacting nerve localization and injection-monitoring techniques to more reliably detect and prevent intraneural intrafascicular injection. The results of these efforts will inevitably be of crucial importance to the future of PNBs and their role in practice of modern anesthesiology.

References

1. Auroy Y, Benhamou D, Bargues L: Major complications of regional anesthesia in France: The SOS regional anesthesia hotline service. Anesthesiology 2002;97:1274–1280.

2. Auroy Y, Narchi P, Messiah A, et al: Serious complications related to regional anesthesia: Results of a prospective survey in France. Anesthesiology 1997;87:479–486.

3. Fanelli G, Casati A, Garancini P, Torri G: Nerve stimulator and multiple injection technique for upper and lower limb blockade: Failure rate, patient acceptance, and neurologic complications. Anesth Analg 1999;88:847–852.

4. Hadzic A, Vloka J, Kuroda M, et al: The practice of peripheral nerve blocks in the United States: A national survey. Reg Anesth Pain Med 1988;23:241–246.

5. Sunderland S: The sciatic nerve and its tibial and common peroneal divisions: Anatomical and physiological features. In: Sunderland S (editor): Nerves and Nerve Injuries, 2nd ed. Churchill Livingstone, 1978, pp. 925—991.

6. Millesi H, Terzis JK: Nomenclature in peripheral nerve surgery. Clin Plast Surg 1984;11:3–8.

7. Selander D: Nerve toxicity of local anesthetics. In: Lofstrom J, Sjostrand U (editors): Local Anesthesia and Regional Blockade. Elsevier Science, 1988, pp. 77.

8. Kingsley R: The gross structure of the nervous system. In: Kingsley R (editor): *Concise Text of Neuroscience.* Lippincott Williams & Wilkins, 2000, pp. 1–15.

9. Sunderland S: Nerve and Nerve Injury. Churchill Livingstone, 1978, pp. 31—2.

10. Selander D: Peripheral nerve injury after regional anesthesia. In: Finucane B (editor): *Complications of Regional Anesthesia.* Churchill Livingstone, 1999, pp. 105–115.

11. Seddon H: Three types of nerve injury. Brain 1943;66:236–288.

12. Sunderland S: A classification of peripheral nerve injuries producing loss of function. Brain 1951;74:491–516.

13. Hudson A, Kline D, Gentili F: Management of peripheral nerve problems. In: Peripheral Nerve Injection Injury. In: Omer G, Spinner M (editors): WB Saunders, 1980, pp. 639—653.

14. Mackinnon S, Dellon A: Classification of nerve injuries as the basis of treatment. In: Mackinnon SE (editor): Surgery of the Peripheral Nerve. Thieme Medical Publishers, 1988, pp. 35–63.

15. Gentili F, Hudson A, Hunter D: Clinical and experimental aspects of injury injuries of peripheral nerves. Can J Neurol Sci 1980;7:143–151.

16. Mackinnon SE, Hudson AR, Gentili F, et al: Peripheral nerve injury with steroid agents. Plast Reconstr Surg 1982;69:482–489.

17. Mackinnon S, Hudson A, Llamas F, et al: Peripheral nerve injury by chymopapain injection. J Neurosurg 1984;61:1–8.

18. Strasberg J, Atchabahian A, Strasberg S, et al: Peripheral nerve injection injury with antiemetic agents. J Neurotrauma 1999;16:99–107.

19. Gentili F, Hudson A, Kline D, Hunter D: Early changes following injection injury of peripheral nerves. Can J Surg 1980;23:177–182.

20. Hadzic A, Dilberovic F, Shah S, et al: Combination of intraneural injection and high injection pressure leads to severe fascicular injury and neurologic deficits in dogs. Reg Anesth Pain Med 2004;29:417–423.

21. Bhananker S, Domino K: What actions can be used to prevent peripheral nerve injury. In: *Evidence-Based Practice of Anesthesiology.* Elsevier, 2004, pp. 228–235.

22. Fremling M, Mackinnon S: Injection injury to the median nerve. Ann Plast Surg 1996;37:561–567.

23. Bashein G, Robertson H, Kenndey W: Persistent phrenic nerve paresis following interscalene brachial plexus block. Anesthesiology 1985;63:102–104.

24. Lim E, Pereira R: Brachial plexus injury following brachial plexus block. Anesth Analg 1984;39:691–694.

25. Gillespie J, Menk E, Middaugh R: Reflex sympathetic dystrophy. A complication of interscalene block. Anesth Analg 1987;66:1316–1317.

26. Winnie A: Interscalene brachial plexus block. Anesth Analg 1970;49:455–466.

27. Barutell C, Vidal F, Raich M, Montero A: A neurological complication following interscalene brachial plexus block. Anaesthesia 1980;35:365–367.

28. Raj P, De Andrés J, Grossi P, et al: Aids to localization of peripheral nerves. In: Raj P (editor): *Textbook of Regional Anesthesia*. Churchill Livingstone, 2002, pp. 251–284.

29. Brown D: Local anesthetics and regional anesthesia equipment In: Brown DL(editor): *Atlas of Regional Anesthesia*. WB Saunders, 1992, pp. 3–11.

30. Chelly J: Nerve stimulator. In Chelly J (editor): *Peripheral Nerve Blocks. A Color Atlas*. Lippincott Williams & Wilkins, 1999, pp. 7–10.

31. Jankovic D, Wells C: Brachial plexus. In: Jankovic D, Wells C (editors): *Regional Nerve Blocks*, 2nd ed. Blackwell Science Berlin, 2001, pp. 58–86.

32. Voelckel W, Klima G, Krismer C, et al: Signs of inflammation after sciatic nerve block in pigs. Anesth Analg 2005;101:1844–1846.

33. Jankowski CJ, Hebl JR, Stuart MJ, et al: A comparison of psoas compartment block and spinal and general anesthesia for outpatient knee arthroscopy. Anesth Analg 2003;97:1003–1009.

34. Tonidandel WT, Mayfield JB: Successful interscalene block with a nerve stimulator may also result after a pectoralis major motor response. Reg Anesth Pain Med 2002;27:491–493.

35. Urmey W, Stanton J: Inability to consistently elicit a motor response following sensory paresthesia during interscalene block administration. Anesthesiology 2002;96:552–554.

36. Choyce A, Chan V, Middleton W, et al: What is the relationship between paresthesia and nerve stimulation for axillary brachial plexus block? Reg Anesth Pain Med 2001;26:100–104.

37. Sala-Blanch X, Pomes J, Matute P, et al: Intraneural injection during anterior approach for sciatic nerve block. Anesthesiology 2004;101:1027–1030.

38. Weaver M, Tandatnick C, Hahn M: Peripheral Nerve Blockade. In: Raj P (editor) *Regional Anesthesia*. Churchill Livingstone, 2002, pp. 857–870.

39. Claudio RE, Hadzic A, Shih H, et al: Injection pressures by anesthesiologists during simulated peripheral nerve block. Reg Anesth Pain Med 2004;29:201–205.

40. Passannante AN: Spinal anesthesia and permanent neurologic deficit after interscalene block. Anesth Analg 1996;82:873–874.

41. Dutton RP, Eckhardt WF III, Sunder N: Total spinal anesthesia after interscalene blockade of the brachial plexus. Anesthesiology 1994;80:939–941.

42. Selander D, Sjostrand J: Longitudinal spread of intraneurally injected local anesthetics. An experimental study of the initial neural distribution following intraneural injections. Acta Anesth Scand 1978;22:622–634.

43. Selander D, Dhuner K, Lundborg G: Peripheral nerve injury due to injection needles used for regional anesthesia. Acta Anaesthesiol Scand 1977;21:182–189.

44. Rice A, McMahon S: Peripheral nerve injury caused by injection needles used in regional anaesthesia: Influence of bevel configuration, studied in a rat model. Br J Anaesth 1992;9.433–438.

45. Kent K, Moscucci M, Mansour K, et al: Retroperitoneal hematoma after cardiac catheterization: Prevalence, risk factors, and optimal management. J Vasc Surg 1994;20:905–910.

46. Rousseau J, Reznik M, LeJeune G, Franck G: Sciatic nerve entrapment by pentazocine-induced muscle fibrosis: A case report. Arch Neurol Psychiatry 1979;36:723–724.

47. Obach J, Aragones J, Ruano D: The infrapiriformis foramen syndrome resulting from intragluteal injection. J Neurol Sci 1983;58:135–142.

48. Napiontek M, Ruszkowski K: Paralytic drop foot and gluteal fibrosis after intramuscular injections. J Bone Joint Surg Br 1993;75:83–85.

49. Selander D: Neurotoxicity of local anesthetics: Animal data. Reg Anesth 1993;18:461–468.

50. Kaneko S, Matsumoto M, Tsuruta S, et al: The nerve root entry zone is highly vulnerable to intrathecal tetracaine in rabbits. Anesth Analg 2005;101:107–114.

51. Johnson M, Uhl C, Spittler K, et al: Mitochondrial injury and caspase activation by the local anesthetic lidocaine. Anesthesiology 2004;101:1184–1194.

52. Sakura S, Bollen A, Ciriales R, Drasner K: Local anesthetic neurotoxicity does not result from blockade of voltage gated sodium channels. Anesth Analg 1995;81:338–346.

53. Johnson M, Saenz J, DaSilva A, et al: Effect of local anesthetic on neuronal cytoplasmic calcium and plasma membrane lysis (necrosis) in a cell culture model. Anesthesiology 2002;96:1466–1476.

54. Kanai A, Hiruma H, Katakura T, et al: Low-concentration lidocaine rapidly inhibits axonal transport in cultured mouse dorsal root ganglion neurons. Anesthesiology 2001;95:675–680.

55. Fagiolini M, Caleo M, Strettoi E, Maffei L: Axonal gtransport blockade in the neonatal rat optic nerve induces limited retinal ganglion cell death. J Neurosci 1997;17:7045–7052.

56. Ohtake K: Glutamate release and neuronal injury after intrathecal injection of local anesthetics. Neuroreport 2000;11:1105–1109.

57. Kitagawa N, Oda M, Totoki T: Possible mechanism of irreversible nerve injury caused by local anesthetics: Detergent properties of local anesthetics and membrane disruption. Anesthesiology 2004;100:962–967.

58. Chazotte B, Vanderkooi G: Multiple sites of inhibition of mitochondrial electron transport by local anesthetics. Biochem Biophys Acta 1981;636:153–161.

59. Kanai Y, Katsuki H, Takasaki M: Graded irreversible changes in crayfish giant axon as manifestations of lidocaine neurotoxicity in vitro. Anesth Analg 1998;86:569–573.

60. Ready L, Plummer M, Haschke R, et al: Neurotoxicity of intrathecal local anesthetics in rabbits. Anesthesiology 1985;63:364–370.

61. Oda M, Kitagawa N, Sakurada T, et al: Is the neurotoxic concentration predicted from solution property of local anesthetics agreement with that obtained from animal study. Anesthesiology 1998;89:A1417.

62. Hodgson P, Neal J, Pollock J, Liu S: The neurotoxicity of drugs given intrathecally (spinal). Anesth Analg 1999;797–809.

63. Myers R, Heckman H: Effects of local anesthesia on nerve blood flow: Studies using lidocaine with and without epinephrine. Anesthesiology 1989;71:757–762.

64. Lynch N, Cofield R, Silbert P, Hermann R: Neurologic complications after total shoulder arthroplasty. J Shoulder Elbow Surg 1996;5:53–61.

65. Selander D, Mansson G, Karlsson L, Svanvik J: Adrenergic vasoconstriction in peripheral nerves of the rabbit. Anesthesiology 1985;62:6–10.

66. Middleton R, Varian J: Tourniquet paralysis. Aust N Z J Surg 1974;44:124–127.

67. Dawson D, Hallet M, Wilbourn A: *Entrapment Neuropathies*, 3rd ed. Lippincott-Raven, 1999.

68. Saunders K, Louis D, Weingarden S, Watkibus G. Effect of tourniquet time on postoperative quadriceps function. Clin Orthop 1979;143:194–199.

69. Sharrock N, Savarese J: Anesthesia for orthopedic surgery. In: Miller R, Cucchiara R, Miller E, et al (editors): *Anesthesia*, 5th ed. Churchill Livingstone, 2000, pp. 2118–2139.

70. Jankowski C, Keegan M, Bolton C, Harrison B: Neuropathy following axillary brachial plexus blocks: Is it the tourniquet? Anesthesiology 2003;99:1230–1232.

71. Schurman DA: Ankle-block anesthesia for foot surgery. 1976;44:348–352.

72. Lichtenfeld N: The pneumatic ankle tourniquet with ankle block anesthesia for foot surgery. Foot Ankle 1992;13:344–349.

73. Adam F, Jaziri S, Chauvin M: Psoas abscess complicating femoral nerve block catheter. Anesthesiology 2003;99:230–231.

74. Capdevila X, Macaire P, Dadure C, et al: Continuous psoas compartment block for postoperative analgesia after total hip arthroplasty: New landmarks, technical guidelines and clinical evaluation. Anesth Analg 2002;94:1606–1613.

75. Klein S, D'Ercole F, Greengrass R, Warner D: Enoxaparin associated with psoas hematoma and lumbar plexopathy after lumbar plexus block. Anesthesiology 1997;87:1576–1579.

76. Weller R, Gerancher J, Crews J, Wade K: Extensive retroperitoneal hematoma without neurologic deficit in two patients who underwent lumbar plexus block and were later anticoagulated. Anesthesiology 2003;98:581–585.

77. Ho KJ, Gawley SD, Young MR: Psoas haematoma and femoral neuropathy associated with enoxaparin therapy. Int J Clin Pract 2003;57:553–554.

78. Crosby ET, Reid DR, DiPrimio G, et al: Lumbosacral plexopathy from iliopsoas haematoma after combined general-epidural anaesthesia for abdominal aneurysmectomy. Can J Anaesth 1998;45:46–51.

79. Cheney F, Domino K, Caplan R, Posner K: Nerve injury associated with anesthesia: A closed claims analysis. Anesthesiology 1999:1062–1069.

80. Bonner S, Pridie A: Sciatic nerve palsy following uneventful sciatic nerve block. Anaesthesia 1997;52:1205–1211.

81. Borgeat A, Ekatodramis G, Kalberer F, Benz C: Acute and nonacute complications associated with interscalene block and shoulder surgery: A prospective study. Anesthesiology 2001;95:875–880.

82. Shah S, Hadzic A, Vloka J, et al: Neurologic complication after anterior sciatic nerve block. Anesth Analg 2005;100:1515–1517.

83. Stark R, Wauwatosa W: Neurologic injury from axillary block anesthesia. J Hand Surg 1996;21A:391–396.

84. Tsao B, Wilbourn A: Infraclavicular brachial plexus injury following axillary regional block. Muscle Nerve 2004;30:44–48.

85. Webber S, Jain R: Scalene regional anesthesia for shoulder surgery in a community setting: An assessment of risk. J Bone Joint Surg 2002;84:775–779.

86. Kao MC, Tsai SK, Tsou MY, et al: Paraplegia after delayed detection of inadvertent spinal cord injury during thoracic epidural catheterization in an anesthetized elderly patient. Anesth Analg 2004;99:580–583.

87. Tripathi M, Nath S, Gupta RK: Paraplegia after intracord injection during attempted epidural steroid injection in an awake patient. Anesthe Analg 2005;101:1209–1211.

88. Tsui B, Armstrong K: Can direct spinal cord injury occur without paresthesia? A report of delayed spinal cord injury after epidural placement in an awake patient. Anesth Analg 2005;101:1212–1214.

89. Kaufman B, Nystrom E, Nath S, et al: Debilitating chronic pain syndromes after presumed intraneural injections. Pain 2000;85:283–286.

90. Walton J, Fol J, Friedman R, Dorman B: Complete brachial plexus palsy after total shoulder arthroplasty done with interscalene block anesthesia. Reg Anesth Pain Med 2000;25:318–821.

91. Benumof J: Permanent loss of cervical spinal cord function associated with interscalene block performed under general anesthesia. Anesthesiology 2000;93:1541–1544.

92. Koscielniak-Nielsen Z, Rasmussen H, Nielsen P: Patients' perception of pain during axillary and humeral blocks using multiple nerve stimulations. Reg Anesth Pain Med 2004;29:328–332.

93. Bogdanov A, Loveland R: Is there a place for interscalane block performed after induction of general anesthesia? Eur J Anesthesiol 2005;22:107–110.

94. Gadsden J, Singh AT, Iwata T, et al: Peripheral Nerve Blocks in Heavily Sedated Patients. Reg Anesth Pain Med 2004;29:A26.

95. Goldberg M, Gregg C, Larijani G, et al: A comparison of three methods of axillary approach to brachial plexus blockade for upper extremity. Anesthesiology 1987;66:814–816.

96. Mulroy F: Brachial plexus blocks. In: Mulory F (editor): *Regional Anesthesia: An Illustrated Procedural Guide*, 3rd ed. Lippincott Williams & Wilkins, 2002, pp. 157–182.

97. Katz J: Ulnar nerve: Block at the elbow. In: Katz J (editor): *Atlas of Regional Anesthesia*. Appleton & Lange, 1994, pp. 84–85.

98. Katz J: Median nerve: Block at the elbow. In: Katz J (editor): *Atlas of Regional Anesthesia*, 2nd ed. Appleton & Lange, 1994, pp. 82–83.

99. Lavoie J, Martin R, Tetrault J, et al: Axillary plexus block using peripheral nerve stimulator: Single or multiple injections. Can J Anaesth 1992;39:583–586.

100. Koscielniak-Nielsen Z, Rotboll Nielsen P, Sorensen T, Stenor M: Low dose axillary block by targeted injections of the terminal nerves. Can J Anaesth 1999;46:658–664.

101. Koscielniak-Nielsen Z, Stens-Pedersen H, Lippert F: Readiness for surgery after axillary block: Single or multiple injection techniques. Eur J Anaesth 1997;14:164–171.

102. Fanelli G, Casati A, Beccaria P, et al: Interscalene brachial plexus anaesthesia with small volumes of ropivacaine 0.75%: Effects of the injection technique on the onset time of nerve blockade. Eur J Anaesthesiol 2001;18:54–58.

103. Paqueron X, Bouaziz H, Macalou D, et al: The lateral approach to the sciatic nerve at the popliteal fossa: One or two injections? Anesth Analg 1999;89:1221–1225.

104. Casati A, Fanelli G, Beccaria P, et al: The effects of the single or multiple injection technique on the onset time of femoral nerve blocks with 0.75% ropivacaine. Anesth Analg 2000;91:181–184.

105. Casati A, Fanelli G, Beccaria P, et al: The effects of single or multiple injections on the volume of 0.5% ropivacaine required for femoral nerve blockade. Anesth Analg 2001;93:183–186.

106. Gaertner E, Estebe J, Zamfir A, et al: Infraclavicular plexus block: Multiple injection versus single injection. Reg Anesth Pain Med 2002;27:590–594.

107. Brown A, Parker G: The use of a "reverse" axis (axillary-interscalene) block in a patient presenting with fractures of the left shoulder and elbow. Anesth Analg 2001;93:1618–1620.

108. Breslin D, Martin G, Macleod D, et al: Central nervous system toxicity following the administration of levobupivacaine for lumbar plexus block: A report of two cases. Reg Anesth Pain Med 2003;28:144–147.

109. Mahli A, Coskun D, Akcali D: Aetiology of convulsions due to stellate ganglion block: A review and report of two cases. Eur J Anaesthesiol 2002;19:376–380.

110. Wedel D, Krohn J, Hall J: Brachial plexus anesthesia in pediatric patients. Mayo Clin Proc 1991;66:583–588.

111. Ould-Ahmed M, Drouillard I, Fouirel D, et al: Convulsions induced by ropivacaine after midhumeral block. Ann Fr Anesth Reanim 2002;21:681–684.

112. Edde R, Deutsch S: Cardiac arrest after interscalene brachial plexus block. Anesth Analg 1977;56:446–447.

113. Bernards C, Carpenter R, Rupp S, et al: Effect of midazolam and diazepam premedication on central nervous system and cardiovascular toxicity of bupivacaine in pigs. Anesthesiology 1989;70:318–323.

114. Giaufre E, Dalens B, Gombert A: Epidemiology and morbidity of regional anesthesia in children: A one-year prospective survey of the French-Language Society of Pediatric Anesthesiologists. Anesth Analg 1996;83:904–912.

115. Gerancher J, Viscusi E, Liguori G, et al: Development of a standardized peripheral nerve block procedure note form. Reg Anesth Pain Med 2005;30:67–71.

116. Selander D, Edshage S, Wolf T: Paresthesiae or no paresthesiae? Acta Anaesth Scand 1979;23:27–33.

117. Ben-David B, Stahl S: Axillary block complicatged by hematoma and radial nerve injury. Reg Anesth Pain Med 1999;24:264–266.

118. Bentley F, Schlapp W: The effects of pressure on the conduction in peripheral nerves. J Physiol 1943;102:72.

119. Burns T: Mechanisms of acute and chronic compression neuropathy. In: Dyck P, Thomas P (editors): *Peripheral Neuropathy*, 4th ed. Elsevier-Saunders, 2005, pp. 1391–1402.

120. Hutschala D, Mascher H, Schmetterer L, et al: Clonidine added to bupivacaine enhances and prolongs analgesia after brachial plexus

block via a local mechanism in healthy volunteers. Eur J Anesth 2004;21:198–204.

121. Finucane B, Terblanche O: Prolonged duration of anesthesia in a patient with multiple sclerosis following paravertebral block. Can J Anesth 2005;52:454–458.

122. Fournier R, Weber A, Gamulin Z: Posterior labat vs. lateral popliteal sciatic block: Posterior sciatic block has quicker onset and shorter duration of anaesthesia. Acta Anaesthesiol Scand 2005;49:683–686.

123. Schroeder L, Horlocker T, Schroeder D: The efficacy of axillary block for surgical procedures about the elbow. Anesth Analg 1996;83:747–751.

124. Horlocker T, Kufner R, Bishop A: The risk of persistent paresthesia is not increased with repeated axillary block. Anesth Analg 1999;88:382–387.

125. Stan T, Krantz M, Solomon D: The incidence of neurovascular complications following axillary brachial plexus block using a transarterial approach. Reg Anesth Pain Med 1995;20:486–492.

126. Fornage B: Peripheral nerves of the extremities: Imaging with US. Radiology 1988;167:179–182.

127. Silvestri E, Martinoli C, Derchi L, et al: Echotexture of peripheral nerves: Correlation between US and histologic findings to differentiate tendons. Radiology 1995;197:291–296.

128. Filler A, Hayes C, Kliot M, et al: Magnetic resonance neurography. Lancet 1993;341:659–661.

129. Filler A, Maravilla K, Tsuruda J: MR neurography and muscle MR imaging for image diagnosis of disorders affecting the peripheral nerves and musculature. Neurol Clin 2004;22:643–682.

130. Filler A, Kliot M, Howe F, et al: Application of magnetic resonance neurography in the evaluation of patients with peripheral nerve pathology. J Neurosurg 1996;85:299–309.

131. Bendszus M, Wessig C, Solymosi L, et al: MRI of peripheral nerve degeneration and regeneration: Correlation with electrophysiology and histology. Exp Neurol 2004;188:171–177.

132. McCarson KE, Ralya A, Reisman SA, Enna SJ: Amitriptyline prevents thermal hyperalgesia and modifications in rat spinal cord GABA(B) receptor expression and function in an animal model of neuropathic pain. Biochem Pharmacol 2005;71:196–202.

133. Sindrup S, Brosen K, Gram L: The mechanism of action of antidepressants in pain treatment: Controlled cross-over studies in diabetic neuropathy. Clin Neuropharmacol 1992;15:380.

134. Rogawski M, Loscher W: The neurobiology of antiepileptic drugs. Nat Rev Neurosci 2004;10:685–692.

135. Watson C, Babul N: Efficacy of oxycodone in neuropathic pain: A randomized trial in postherpatic neuralgia. Neurology 1998;59:1837.

136. Rowbotham M: Mechanisms and Pharmacologic Management of Neuropathic Pain. In: Dyck P, Thomas P (editors): Peripheral Neuropathy, 4th ed. Elsevier, 2005, pp. 2637–2652.

137. Mattia C, Coluzzi F: Tramadol. Focus on musculoskeletal and neuropathic pain. Minerva Anestesiol 2005;71:565–584.

138. Anesthesiologists ASA: Policy statement on practice parameters. In: ASA Standards, Guidelines and Statements. American Society of Anesthesiologists Publication 1999:3.

70

Neuraxial Anesthesia & Peripheral Nerve Blocks in Patients on Anticoagulants

Honorio T. Benzon, MD • Rasha S. Jabri, MD

INTRODUCTION

Intraspinal hematoma is a relatively rare condition resulting from a variety of causes. Its incidence is approximately 0.1 per 100,000 patients per year.[1,2] Traumatic causes include lumbar puncture and neuraxial anesthesia as well as a complication of spinal surgery. It is more likely to occur in anticoagulated or thrombocytopenic patients, patients with neoplastic disease, or in those with liver disease or alcoholism.[3,4] Spontaneous bleeding is rare but may be seen from a spinal arteriovenous malformation or vertebral hemangioma. Approximately one quarter to one third of all cases are associated with anticoagulation therapy.[5,6]

Hemorrhage into the spinal canal commonly occurs in the epidural space because of the presence of a prominent epidural plexus of veins. Puncture of epidural vessels during placement of epidural catheters occurs in approximately 3–12% of cases. The incidence of symptomatic epidural hematoma associated with epidural analgesia is difficult to estimate, but combined case series of more than 100,000 epidural anesthetics have been reported without a single epidural hematoma. Spinal hematoma is a rare but devastating event. The actual incidence of neurologic dysfunction resulting from hemorrhagic complications associated with neuraxial blockade is unknown; the incidence cited in the literature is estimated to be 1 in 150,000 epidural and 1 in 220,000 spinal anesthetics. However, the incidence increased significantly after the introduction of low-molecular-weight heparin (LMWH), before the Food and Drug Administration issued a warning, and before the American Society of Regional Anesthesia (ASRA) issued its initial consensus statement in 1998.[7]

The risk of formation of intraspinal hematoma after administration of neuraxial anesthesia and analgesia is increased in patients who received anticoagulant therapy or have a coagulation disorder.[8] For that reason neuraxial anesthesia is often contraindicated in the presence of a coagulopathy. Other risk factors for development of epidural or spinal hematoma include technical difficulty (multiple attempts) in the performance of the neuraxial procedures due to anatomic abnormalities of the spine and multiple or bloody punctures. Intraspinal hematoma is more often associated with epidural catheter use than with the other neuraxial block techniques.

ASRA has recommended guidelines for the safer performance of neuraxial blocks in patients who are on anticoagulants.[7,9] These guidelines were based on extensive review of the literature and of the pharmacology of the different anticoagulants. Recommendations were made on the timing of the neuraxial block and removal of the epidural catheter and the administration of the anticoagulants. In particular, the use of low concentrations of local anesthetics for epidural infusion (preservation of motor strength for easier monitoring) and subsequent neurologic monitoring were recommended by ASRA. The initial consensus guidelines, published in 1998 and updated in 2003,[7,9] greatly assisted clinicians in

decision making with regard to the use of neuraxial procedures in the setting of anticoagulation therapy and possibly decreased the incidence of epidural and spinal hematoma. In this chapter, we discuss the significance of common antiplatelet, anticoagulation, and fibrinolytic therapy and hope to offer the reader a guide in decision making about the use of neuraxial anesthesia and PNBs in clinical practice.

ANTIPLATELET THERAPY

Antiplatelet medications, including aspirin, nonsteroidal antiinflammatory drugs (NSAIDs), and dipyridamole, have been in the past considered relative contraindications to central neural blockade by some authors due to prolongation of the bleeding time and a theoretically greater risk of formation of spinal hematoma. Antiplatelet medications inhibit the platelet cyclooxygenase enzyme and prevent the synthesis of thromboxane A_2. Thromboxane A_2 is a potent vasoconstrictor and facilitates secondary platelet aggregation and release reactions. Platelets from patients on these medications have normal platelet adherence to subendothelium and normal primary hemostatic plug formation. An adequate, although potentially fragile, clot may form.[10] However, although such plugs may be satisfactory hemostatic barriers for smaller vascular lesions, they may not ensure adequate perioperative hemostatic clot formation. The role of platelets in coagulation and hemostasis is shown in Figures 70–1 and 70–2.

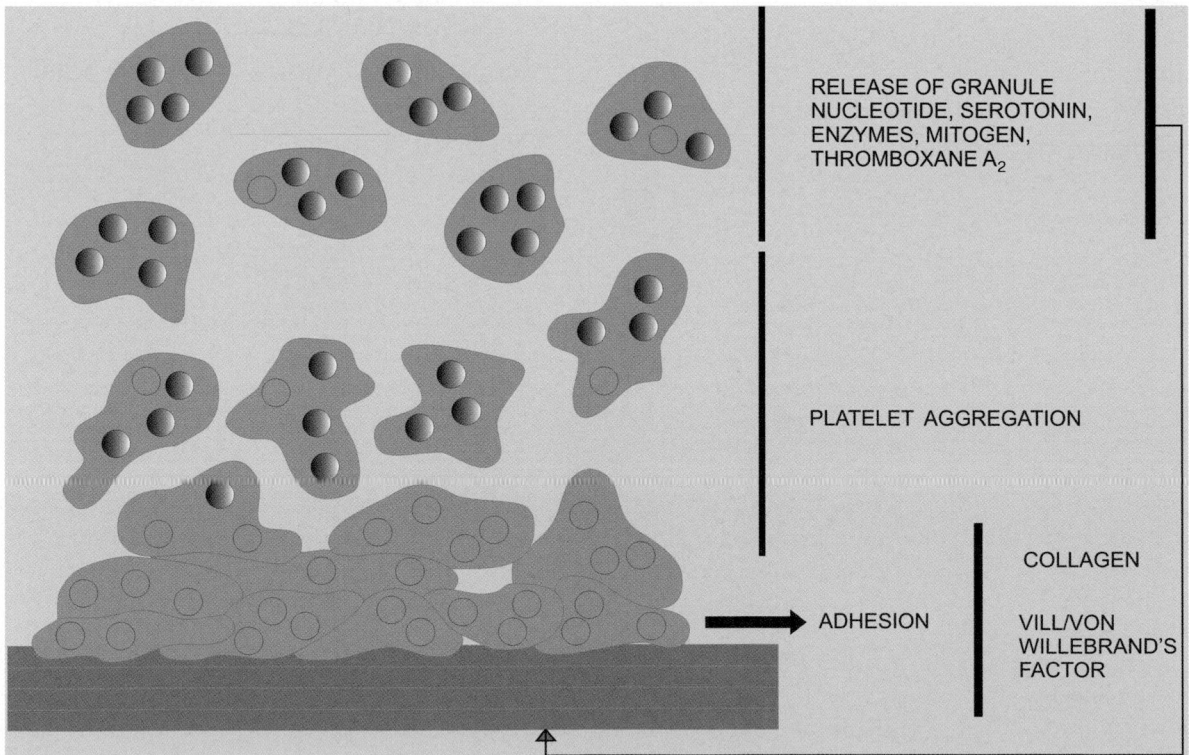

Figure 70–1. Role of platelets in coagulation. Platelets carry out their role in hemostasis through three basic reactions: adhesion, activation (and secretion), and aggregation. When the blood vessels are stripped of endothelium, platelets rapidly bind to the subendothelium by a process termed *adhesion*.

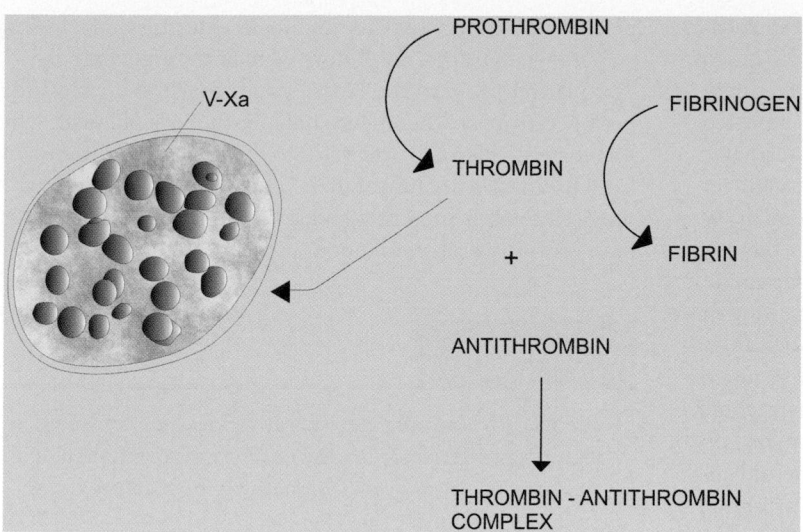

Figure 70–2. Role of platelets in coagulation. Another important task of the platelet is to support plasma coagulation reactions. When activated, platelets bind several important plasma protein complexes. They secrete an activated form of factor V (factor Va), which binds to the platelet surface and binds factor Xa. Platelet-bound factor Xa then markedly accelerates the conversion of prothrombin to thrombin.

The Ivy bleeding time was considered to be a reliable predictor of abnormal bleeding in patients receiving antiplatelet drugs.[11] However, the postaspirin bleeding time is not a reliable indicator of platelet function.[12,13] There is large intra- and interpatient variability in the results of the test. Although the bleeding time may normalize within 3 days after aspirin ingestion, platelet function as measured by platelet response to adenosine diphosphate (ADP), epinephrine, and collagen may take up to a week to return to normal. There is no evidence to suggest that bleeding time can predict hemostatic function, and studies failed to show a correlation between aspirin-induced prolongation of the bleeding time and surgical blood loss.[1,14] Therefore, measurement of an Ivy bleeding time before induction of spinal or epidural anesthesia may not identify those patients at increased risk for hemorrhagic complications. Other NSAIDs (naproxen, piroxicam, ibuprofen) produce only a short-term, mild defect that normalizes within 3 days.[15] Platelet function in patients receiving antiplatelet medications should be assumed to be decreased for 1 week with aspirin and 1–3 days with NSAIDs. This assumption does not take into consideration the continuous formation of new, functional platelets. This continuous production of fresh, normally functioning platelets, combined with the residual function of already circulating platelets may explain the relative safety of performing neuraxial procedures in these patients.

Special platelet function assays are now available to monitor platelet aggregation and degranulation. The platelet function analyzer (PFA) is a test of in vitro platelet function. It is a good screening test for von Willebrand disease and monitors the effect of desmopressin administration. The PFA is prolonged after antiplatelet therapy.[16,17] The test simulates the process of platelet adhesion and aggregation by measuring the ability of platelets to occlude a microscopic aperture in a membrane coated with collagen and epinephrine (C-EPI) or collagen and ADP (C-ADP) under controlled high shear rates. The time required to obtain a complete platelet plug is the closure time in seconds. The normal closure times are 60–160 sec for C-EPI and 50–124 sec for C-ADP. The intake of aspirin and NSAIDs prolongs the closure time of C-EPI, but von Willebrand disease, low platelet count (<100,000/UL), low hematocrit (<30%), and renal failure prolong the closure time for C-ADP.

Possible clinical significance of antiplatelet therapy and the risk of epidural and spinal hematoma in patients on antiplatelet therapy has been raised by a case report of spontaneous epidural hematoma formation in the absence of spinal or epidural anesthesia in a patient with a history of aspirin ingestion.[18] The patient developed severe lower extremity weakness after ingestion of 1500 mg of aspirin in the form of an aspirin-containing antacid. A myelogram revealed intraspinal hematoma and neurologic defect at the T5 to T6 level. The cerebrospinal fluid was clear, although prolonged bleeding from the lumbar puncture site was noted after myelography. A laminectomy was performed, and the intraspinal hematoma was removed. The patient's neurologic function gradually improved. Nevertheless, the risk associated with the administration of spinal or epidural anesthesia to a patient receiving antiplatelet medications remains very controversial. Although Vandermeulen and colleagues implicated antiplatelet therapy in 3 of the 61 cases of spinal hematoma occurring after spinal or epidural anesthesia.[19] Several large studies have demonstrated the relative safety of central neural blockade in combination with antiplatelet therapy. The Collaborative Low-dose Aspirin Study in Pregnancy (CLASP) Group[20] included 1422 high-risk obstetric patients who were administered 60 mg of aspirin daily and underwent epidural anesthesia without any neurologic sequelae. However, no data regarding difficulty of the procedure or bleeding during the placement or removal of the epidural needle or catheter were noted.[20] In a retrospective study of 1013 spinal and epidural anesthetics in which antiplatelet drugs were taken by 39% of the patients including 11% of patients who were on multiple antiplatelet medications, no patient developed signs of spinal hematoma; however, patients on antiplatelet medications showed a higher incidence of blood aspiration through the spinal or epidural needle or the catheter.[21] In a subsequent prospective study in 1000 patients, 39% of whom reported preoperative antiplatelet therapy, there were no hemorrhagic complications.[22] Blood was noted during needle or catheter placement in 22% of patients, and there was frank blood in 7% of the patients. Therefore, preoperative antiplatelet therapy was not a risk factor for bloody needle or catheter placement. Female gender, increased age, history of excessive bruising or bleeding, continuous catheter technique, large needle gauge, multiple attempts, and difficult needle placement were noted to be significant risk factors. Clinical studies in pain clinic patients are similar to those undergoing surgery. Patients on aspirin[10] or NSAIDs[23] who underwent epidural steroid injections did not develop signs and symptoms of intraspinal hematoma.

The lack of correlation between antiplatelet medications and bloody needle or catheter placement provides strong evidence that preoperative antiplatelet therapy does not represent a significant risk factor for the development of neurologic dysfunction from spinal hematoma in patients on antiplatelet therapy. Although there have been case reports of intraspinal hematoma in patients on aspirin and NSAIDs, there were complicating factors in these case reports.[24] These included concomitant heparin administration,[25] coexisting epidural venous angioma,[25] and technical difficulty in performing the procedure.[26–28] Technical difficulties in performing the injection have been identified as major risk factors in the development of intraspinal hematoma after neuraxial injections.

Based on the available evidence, ASRA made several recommendations concerning antiplatelet medications.[9,29] Preoperative antiplatelet therapy does not represent a significant risk factor for the development of neurologic dysfunction from spinal hematoma in patients on antiplatelet therapy. There is no wholly accepted test, including the bleeding time, to guide antiplatelet therapy. Careful preoperative assessment of the patient is important in identifying conditions that might lead to increased risk of bleeding. The timing of intake of the NSAIDs does not represent a specific concern in relation to the placement of single-shot spinal or catheter techniques, postoperative monitoring, or the timing of neuraxial catheter removal. The risk of bleeding complications, however, may be increased in patients on several antiplatelet medications and concurrent use of other medications affecting clotting mechanisms, such as oral anticoagulants, standard heparin, and LMWH.[9,29]

Cyclooxygenase-2 (COX-2) inhibitors gained popularity because of their analgesic properties and lack of platelet and gastrointestinal effects. Studies showed their perioperative analgesic property in a variety of perioperative settings.[30–33] The drugs have minimal gastrointestinal (GI) toxicity and are ideal for patients who are at increased risk for serious upper GI adverse events. Compared with aspirin or NSAIDs, the effects of the COX-2 inhibitors on platelet aggregation and bleeding times were not different from a placebo.[34–36] Blood loss did not increase during spinal fusion surgery when COX-2 inhibitors were given preoperatively.[37] The platelet properties of these drugs make them ideal for perioperative use when neuraxial anesthetic is planned. Unfortunately, rofecoxib and valdecoxib have been withdrawn from the market because of their cardiovascular side effects[38]; only celecoxib is presently being used, but at dosages lower than previously recommended.

Clinical Pearls

- Preoperative antiplatelet therapy does not represent a significant risk factor for the development of neurologic dysfunction from spinal hematoma in patients on antiplatelet therapy.
- There is no wholly accepted test, including the bleeding time, to guide antiplatelet therapy.
- Careful preoperative assessment of the patient is important in identifying conditions that might lead to increased risk of bleeding.
- The timing of intake of the NSAIDs does not represent a specific concern in relation to the placement of single-shot spinal or catheter techniques, postoperative monitoring, or the timing of neuraxial catheter removal.
- The risk of bleeding complications may be increased in patients on several antiplatelet medications and concurrent use of other medications affecting clotting mechanisms, such as oral anticoagulants, standard heparin, and low-molecular-weight heparin.
- COX-2 inhibitors have minimal gastrointestinal toxicity and are ideal for patients who are at increased risk for serious upper GI adverse events. Compared with aspirin or NSAIDS, the effects of the COX-2 inhibitors on platelet aggregation and bleeding times were not different from a placebo.
- It is recommended that clopidogrel (Plavix) be discontinued for 7 days before a neuraxial injection.

The thienopyridine drugs ticlopidine and clopidogrel have no direct effect on arachidonic acid metabolism. These drugs prevent platelet aggregation by inhibiting ADP receptor–mediated platelet activation.[39,40] They also modulate vascular smooth muscle-reducing vascular contraction. Clopidogrel was noted to be 40–100 times more potent than ticlopidine.[41] Clinical doses are usually 75 mg daily for clopidogrel and 250 mg twice a day for ticlopidine. Ticlopidine is rarely used at the present time because it causes neutropenia, thrombocytopenic purpura, and hypercholesterolemia. Clopidogrel is preferred because of its improved safety profile and proven efficacy. It was found to be better than aspirin in patients with peripheral vascular disease.[42] The maximal inhibition of ADP-induced platelet aggregation with clopidogrel occurs 3–5 days after initiation of a standard dose (75 mg), but within 4 to 6 h after the administration of a large loading dose of 300 to 600 mg.[43] The large loading dose is usually given to patients before they undergo percutaneous coronary intervention.[40,44] There has been a case report of spinal hematoma in a patient on ticlopidine.[45] Although there has been no case of intraspinal hematoma in a patient on clopidogrel alone, a case of quadriplegia in a patient on clopidogrel, diclofenac, and aspirin has been reported.[46]

As stated, ASRA concluded that neuraxial blocks may be performed in patients on aspirin, NSAIDs, or COX-2 inhibitors.[9,29] For the thienopyridine drugs, it is recommended that clopidogrel be discontinued for 7 days and ticlopidine for 10 to 14 days before administration of a neuraxial injection. The longer interval for ticlopidine is due to the increase in its half-life with chronic administration; its half-life increases from 12 h after a single dose to 4 to 5 days after a steady state is reached.

ORAL ANTICOAGULANTS

Warfarin exerts its anticoagulant effect by interfering with the synthesis of the vitamin K–dependent clotting factors (VII, IX, X, and thrombin)[47-49] (Figure 70–3).

It also inhibits the anticoagulants protein C and S. Factor VII has a relatively short half-life (6–8 h) and the prothrombin time (PT) may be prolonged into the therapeutic range (1.5–2 times normal) within 24 to 36 h. The anticoag-

ulant protein C also has a short half-life (6–7 h). The initial prolongation of the international normalized ratio (INR) is therefore the result of competing effects of reduced factor VII and protein C and the washout of existing clotting factors. Because of this, the INR is unpredictable during the initial stage of treatment with warfarin.[50,51] Factor VII participates only in the extrinsic pathway, and adequate anticoagulation is not achieved until the levels of biologically active factors II (half-life of 50 h) and X are sufficiently depressed. This requires 4–6 days. High loading doses of warfarin (15 mg) are occasionally employed for the first 2–3 days of therapy, and the desired anticoagulant effect is achieved within 48 to 72 h.[52] The anticoagulant effect of warfarin persists for 4 to 6 days after termination of therapy while new biologically active vitamin K factors are synthesized. The effect of warfarin can be reversed by the transfusion of fresh frozen plasma and vitamin K injections. The risks of warfarin usage are bleeding and the rare occurrence of skin necrosis. Its drawbacks also include the necessity of monitoring its effect with serial monitoring of INR, its interaction with other drugs, and the fact that it has to be discontinued a few days before surgery.[47,48]

Few data exist regarding the risk of spinal hematoma in patients with indwelling spinal or epidural catheters who are subsequently anticoagulated with warfarin. Odoom and Sih[53] performed 1000 continuous lumbar epidural anesthetics in 950 patients who underwent vascular procedures and received preoperative oral anticoagulant. The thrombotest (a test measuring factor IX activity) was decreased and the

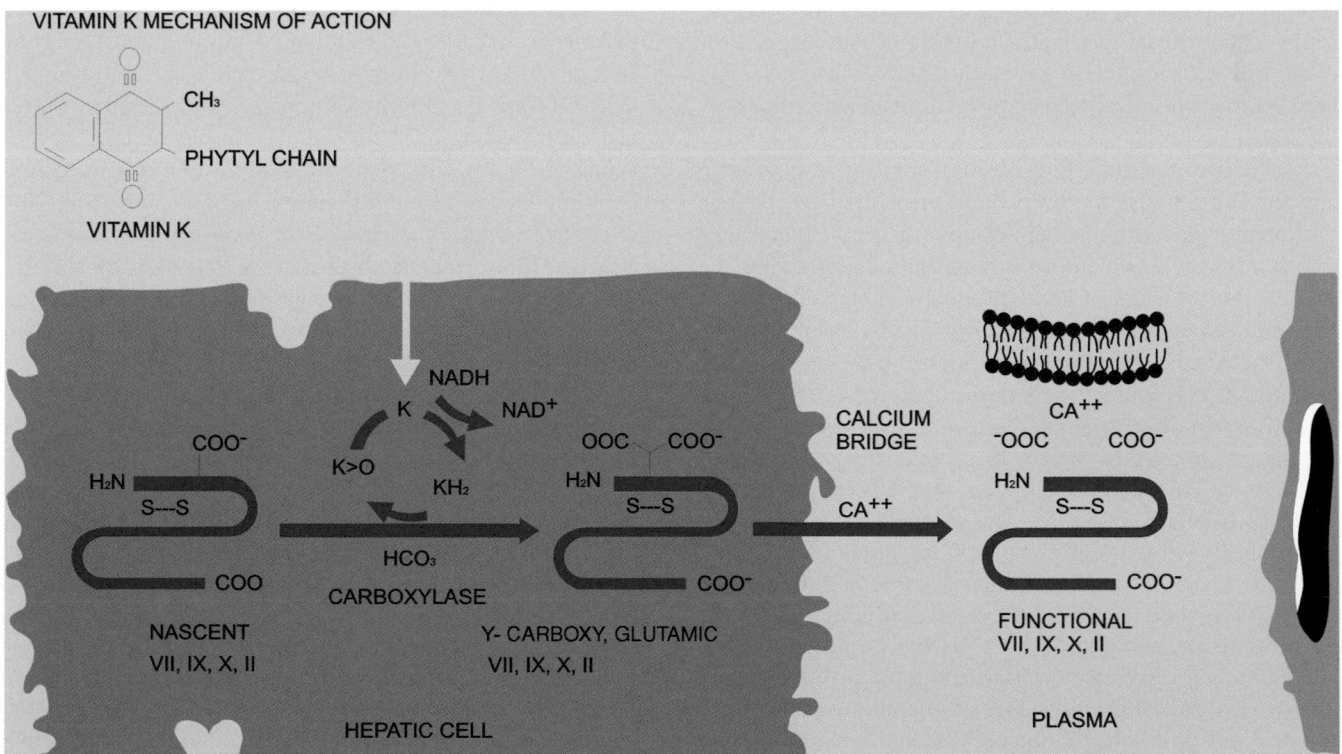

Figure 70–3. Vitamin K–dependent coagulation factor synthesis. Vitamin K is necessary for posttranslational modification of prothrombin, proteins C and S, and factors VII, IX, and X. Vitamin K is stored in hepatocytes.

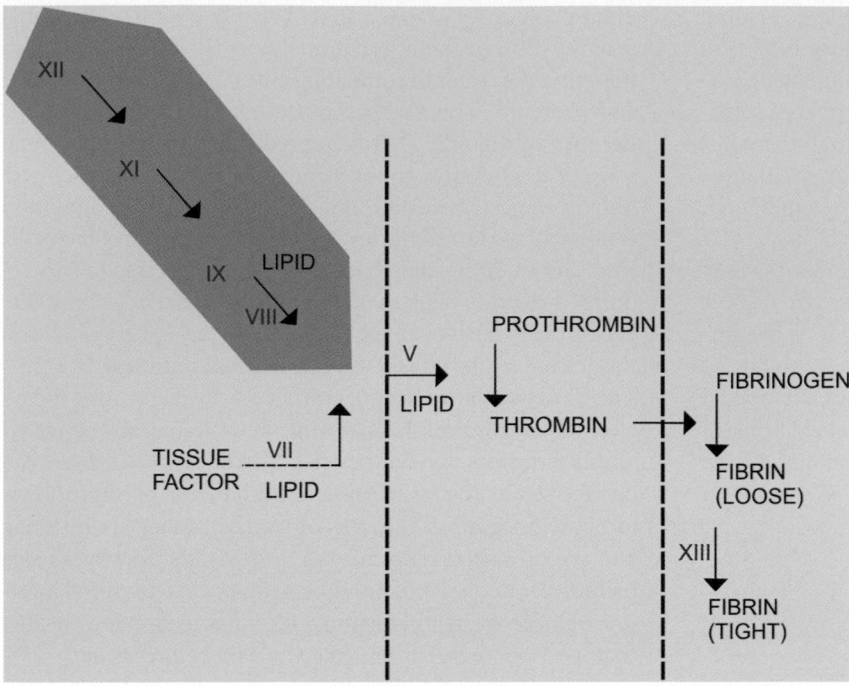

Figure 70–4. Coagulation reaction: Factors responsible for a prolonged PTT are in the shaded area. Patients who have an abnormal PTT but whose PT and other tests are normal can be divided in two groups: those who are prone to bleeding and those that are not. The patients who do not bleed may have an extremely prolonged PTT (90 seconds or more) but do not have a history of bleeding. They will have deficiency in factor XII, prekalikrein, or high-molecular-weight kininogen. These patients should not be denied surgery or epidural anesthesia. The other group, patients who bleed, have both prolonged PTT and a history of bleeding. They will have a deficiency of factor VII (hemophilia A), factor IX (hemophilia B or Christmas disease), or factor XI.

activated partial thromboplastin time (aPTT) was prolonged in all the patients prior to the epidural placement. Heparin was also administered intraoperatively. The epidural catheters remained in place for 48 h postoperatively; the coagulation status of the patients at the time of catheter removal was not described. There were no neurologic complications. Although the results of this study are reassuring, the obsolescence of the thrombotest as a measure of anticoagulation combined with the unknown coagulation status of the patients at the time of catheter removal limits the usefulness of the study.

The use of an indwelling epidural or intrathecal catheter and the timing of its removal in an anticoagulated patient is controversial. Although the trauma of needle placement occurs with both single-dose and continuous catheter techniques, the presence of an indwelling catheter could provoke additional injury to tissues and vascular structures. No spinal hematomas were reported in 192 patients receiving postoperative epidural analgesia in conjunction with low-dose warfarin after total knee arthroplasty.[54] In this study, the patients received warfarin to prolong their PTs to 15.0 to 17.3 sec. The epidural catheters were left indwelling for 37 ± 15 h (range 13–96 h). The mean PT at the time of epidural catheter removal was 13.4 ± 2 s (range 10.6–25.8 s). This and several subsequent studies documented the relative safety of low-dose warfarin anticoagulation in patients with an indwelling epidural catheter.[51,55] However, patients varied greatly in their response to warfarin, and the authors recommended close monitoring of coagulation status to avoid excessive prolongation of the PT. Since intraspinal hematomas have occurred after removal of the catheter,[19] it is recommended that the same laboratory values apply to placement and removal of the epidural catheter.[56] Factors responsible for a pro-

longed PT and PTT are illustrated in Figures 70–4 through 70–6.

The ASRA recommended an INR value of 1.4 or less as acceptable for the performance of neuraxial blocks.[9,48] The value was based on studies that showed excellent perioperative hemostasis when the INR value was ≤ 1.5.[49] Studies on the levels of clotting factors at different INR values showed that the decline of these factors may not be significant at an INR of 1.5. At INR values of 1.5 to 2.0, the concentrations of factor II were noted to be 74% to 82% of baseline, whereas factor VII levels were 27% to 54% of baseline values.[50] At INR values of 2.1 ± 1 during the initial phase of warfarin administration, factors II and VII were $65 \pm 28\%$ and $25 \pm 20\%$ of control values.[57] Levels of 20% of normal are considered adequate for normal hemostasis at the time of major surgery. Another study[58] found that at INRs of 1.3 to 2, under stable anticoagulation with warfarin, the concentrations of the clotting factors VII, IX, and X were within normal limits.

The clinician should be aware of the interactions of warfarin on the coagulation cascade and the role of the INR in monitoring its effect. To minimize the risk of complications, ASRA recommended several precautions.[9,48] Chronic oral therapy should be stopped and the INR measured before a neuraxial block is performed. The concurrent use of other medications, such as aspirin, NSAIDs, and heparins, that affect the clotting mechanism increases the risk of bleeding complications without affecting the INR. If an initial dose of warfarin is given prior to surgery, the INR should be checked if the dose was given more than 24 h earlier. If patients are on low-dose warfarin treatment (mean daily dose approximately 5 mg) during epidural analgesia, the INR should be checked daily and before catheter removal if the initial dose was given more than 36 h previously. Higher daily doses may

PT- THE TEST OF THE EXTRINSIC PATHWAY

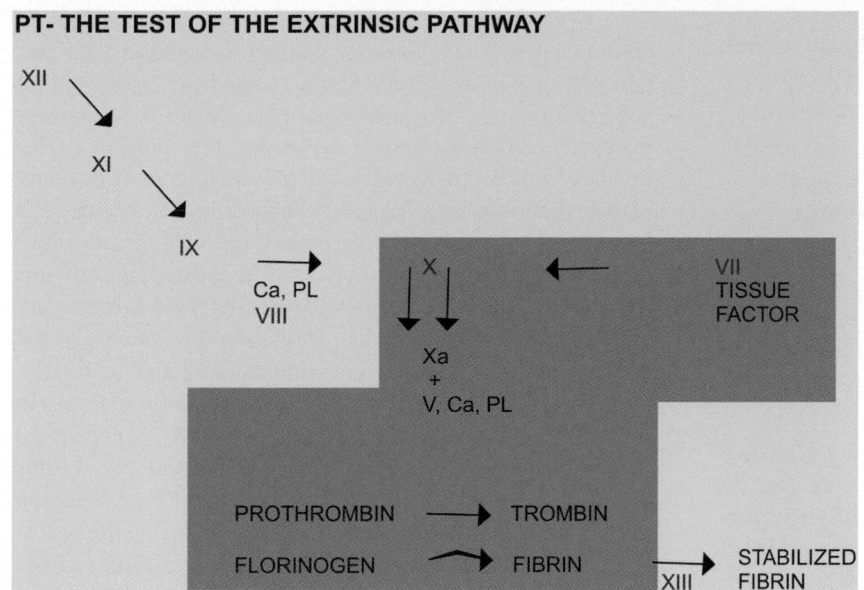

Figure 70–5. Coagulation reaction: Factors involved in prothrombin time (PT) are in the shaded area. The PT is carried out by adding a source of tissue factor to the patient's plasma along with calcium or phospholipid. Tissue factor forms a complex with and activates factor VII. (Ca = calcium; PL = phospholipid.)

PTT- THE TEST OF THE INTRINSIC PATHWAY

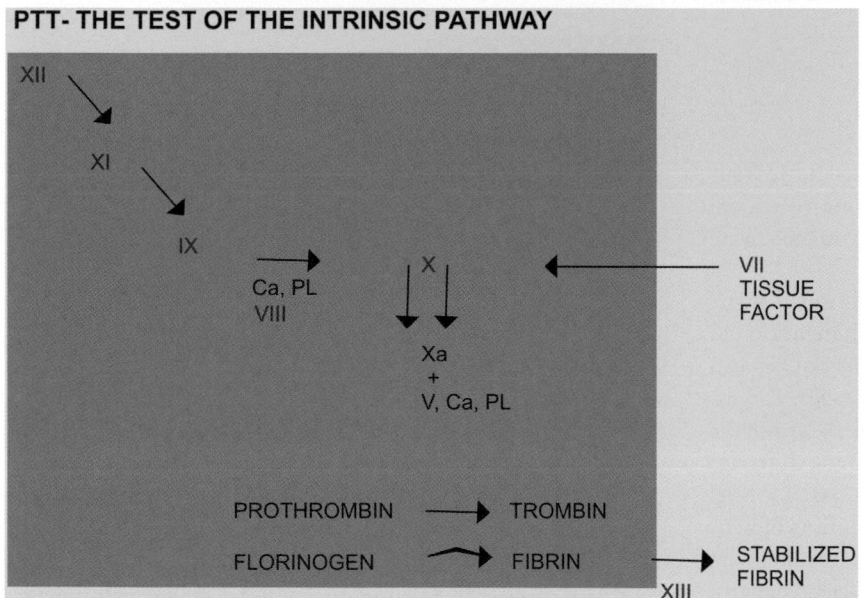

Figure 70–6. Coagulation reaction: Factors involved in partial thromboplastin time (PTT) are in shaded area. In assessing the PTT, coagulation is initiated by an agent that activates the Hageman factor–kininogen–prekalikrein complex. Most coagulation factors are screened by PTT, except factors VII and XIII, the protein that stabilizes fibrin clots by cross-linking them, as well as components of the fibrinolytic system. (Ca = calcium; PL = phospholipid.)

need more intensive monitoring. The warfarin dose should be held or reduced when the INR is >3 in patients with indwelling neuraxial catheters to prevent epidural hematoma and hemarthroma. While on warfarin therapy, the patient's neurologic status should be checked routinely during epidural analgesic infusion, as well as 24 h after the catheter has been removed. Dilute concentrations of local anesthetic should be utilized to minimize the degree of sensory and motor blockade. Clinical judgment must be exercised in making decisions about removing or maintaining neuraxial catheters in patients with therapeutic levels of anticoagulation during neuraxial catheter infusion. The warfarin dose should be reduced for patients who are likely to have an enhanced response to the drug, especially the elderly. For patients on chronic oral anticoagulation, the warfarin must be stopped and the INR measured.

Clinical Pearls

- Chronic oral therapy with warfarin should be stopped and the INR measured before a neuraxial block is performed.
- The concurrent use of other medications, such as aspirin, NSAIDs, and heparins, that affect the clotting mechanism increases the risk of bleeding complications without affecting the INR.
- If an initial dose of warfarin is given prior to surgery, the INR should be checked if the dose was given more than 24 h earlier.
- In patients on low-dose warfarin treatment (mean daily dose approximately 5 mg) during epidural analgesia, the

INR should be checked daily and before catheter removal if the initial dose was given more than 36 h previously. Higher daily doses may need more intensive monitoring.

- The warfarin dose should be held or reduced when the INR is >3 in patients with indwelling neuraxial catheters to prevent epidural hematoma and hemarthroma.

- While on warfarin therapy, the patient's neurologic status should be checked routinely during epidural analgesic infusion, as well as 24 h after the catheter has been removed. Dilute concentrations of local anesthetic should be utilized to minimize the degree of sensory and motor blockade.

- Clinical judgment must be exercised in making decisions about removing or maintaining neuraxial catheters in patients with therapeutic levels of anticoagulation during neuraxial catheter infusion. The warfarin dose should be reduced for patients who are likely to have an enhanced response to the drug, especially the elderly.

HEPARIN

Intravenous Heparin

Heparin is a complex polysaccharide that exerts its anticoagulant effect by binding to antithrombin III. The conformational change in antithrombin accelerates its ability to inactivate thrombin, factor Xa, and factor IXa.[59]

In addition, unfractionated heparin releases a tissue factor pathway inhibitor from endothelium, enhancing its activity against factor Xa.[60] The anticoagulant effect of heparin increases disproportionately with increasing dosages. The anticoagulant effect of subcutaneous heparin takes 1–2 h, but the effect of intravenous heparin is immediate. In fact, the coagulation time is prolonged two to four times the baseline level 5 min after the intravenous injection of 10,000 units of heparin. Heparin has a half-life is 1.5–2 h. It should be noted that patients with acute thromboembolic disease clear heparin more rapidly. Within 4 to 6 h of its administration, the therapeutic dose of heparin ceases. The aPTT is used to monitor the effect of heparin; therapeutic anticoagulation is achieved with a prolongation of the aPTT to greater than 1.5 times the baseline value or a heparin level of 0.2 to 0.4 U/mL.[61] The aPTT is usually not prolonged by the subcutaneous administration of low doses of heparin and is not monitored. Protamine neutralizes the effect of intravenously administered heparin.

Heparin is not the ideal anticoagulant since it is a mixture of molecules only a fraction of which has anticoagulant activity. It binds to platelet factor 4 and to the von Willebrand factor.[62,63] The heparin–antithrombin complex is also not very effective in neutralizing clot-bound thrombin. Finally, heparin is associated with immunologic thrombocytopenia and immune-mediated thrombosis.[62] For patients receiving standard heparin therapy, the risk of bleeding complications is increased in the presence of other medications that affect other clotting mechanisms, including aspirin, NSAIDs, LMWH, and oral anticoagulants.

Several studies demonstrated the safety of spinal or epidural anesthesia followed by systemic heparinization if certain precautions are observed. Rao and El-Etr[64] reported no spinal hematomas in over 4000 patients who underwent lower extremity vascular surgery under continuous spinal or epidural anesthesia. In their study, patients with preexisting coagulation disorders were excluded, heparinization occurred at least 60 min after catheter placement, the level of anticoagulation was carefully monitored, and the indwelling catheters were removed at a time when heparin activity was low. Surgery was canceled in patients when frank blood was noted in the needle and performed the following day under general anesthesia. The same findings were noted in a subsequent report in the neurologic literature. Ruff and Dougherty[65] noted spinal hematomas in 7 of 342 (2%) patients who underwent lumbar puncture and subsequent heparinization for evaluation of cerebral ischemia. The presence of blood during the procedure, concomitant aspirin therapy, and heparinization within 1 h were identified as risk factors in the development of spinal hematoma.

Clinical Pearls

PATIENTS ON HEPARIN THERAPY

- There should be at least a 1-h delay between neuraxial needle placement and heparin administration.

- The epidural catheter should be removed 2–4 h after the last heparin dose and 1 h before subsequent heparin administration.

- Partial thromboplastin time (PTT) or activated coagulation time (ACT) should be monitored to avoid excessive heparin effect.

- Dilute concentrations of local anesthetics are recommended to minimize motor blockade; the patient should be followed postoperatively for early detection of reoccurrence of motor blockade.

- In the event of a traumatic (bloody) or difficult needle placement, there are no data to support mandatory cancellation of surgery.

NEURAXIAL ANALGESIA IN PATIENTS UNDERGOING CARDIOPULMONARY BYPASS

- Neuraxial procedures should be avoided in patients with known coagulopathy.

- Surgery should be delayed 24 h in the patient with a traumatic (bloody) tap.

- The time from the neuraxial procedure to the systemic heparinization should exceed 1 h.

- Heparinization and reversal should be monitored and closely controlled.

- The epidural catheter should be removed when normal coagulation is restored.

- Patients should be monitored closely for signs of spinal hematoma.

ASRA made several recommendations when a neuraxial technique is used in the presence of intraoperative anticoagulation.[9,66] The technique should be avoided in patients with other coagulopathies. There should be at least a 1-h delay between needle placement and heparin administration. The catheter should be removed 2–4 h after the last heparin dose and 1 h before subsequent heparin administration. The PTT or ACT should be monitored to avoid excessive heparin effect. The patient is followed postoperatively for early detection of reoccurrence of motor blockade. Dilute concentrations of local anesthetics are recommended to minimize motor blockade. Although there may be an increased risk in the event of a traumatic (bloody) or difficult needle placement, there are no data to support mandatory cancellation of surgery. The decision to proceed should be based on appropriate clinical judgment and full discussion with the surgeon and the patient.

Neuraxial procedures are occasionally performed in patients who undergo cardiopulmonary bypass. The following precautions have been recommended to prevent the development of intraspinal hematoma[67]:

1. Neuraxial procedures should be avoided in patients with known coagulopathy.
2. Surgery should be delayed 24 h in the patient with a traumatic tap.
3. The time from the neuraxial procedure to the systemic heparinization should exceed 1 h.
4. Heparinization and reversal should be monitored and controlled tightly.
5. The epidural catheter should be removed when normal coagulation is restored, and the patient should be monitored closely for signs of spinal hematoma.

Subcutaneous Heparin

The therapeutic basis of low-dose subcutaneous heparin (5000 units every 8–12 h) is heparin-mediated inhibition of activated factor X. Smaller doses of heparin are required when administered as prophylaxis rather than as treatment for thromboembolic disease. Following intramuscular or subcutaneous injection of 5000 units of heparin, maximum anticoagulation effect is observed in 40 to 50 min and returns to baseline within 4 to 6 h. The aPTT may remain in the normal range and often is not monitored. However, wide variations in individual patient responses to subcutaneous heparin have been reported. Neuraxial techniques are not contraindicated during subcutaneous (minidose) prophylaxis, but the risk of bleeding may be reduced by delaying the heparin administration until after the block. Bleeding may be increased in debilitated patients or after prolonged therapy. The safety of major neuraxial anesthesia in the presence of anticoagulation with subcutaneous doses of unfractionated heparin was documented by several publications.[66] Although the anticoagulant effect of subcutaneous heparin is less significant than that of intravenous heparin, ideally subcutaneous low-dose heparin should also not be administered within 4 to 6 h of neu-

raxial anesthesia to allow for normalization of the heparin effect.

> ## Clinical Pearls
>
> - Neuraxial techniques are not contraindicated in patients receiving subcutaneous (minidose) prophylaxis.
> - Ideally and when practical, the administration of the heparin should be delayed until after spinal or epidural block placement.

Low-Molecular-Weight Heparin

Unfractionated heparin is a heterogeneous mixture of polysaccharide chains that can be separated into fragments of various molecular weights.[68,69] Each low-molecular-weight heparin (LMWH) fractionation contains heparins of different molecular weights, and each is evaluated as a specific pharmacologic substance. The anticoagulant effect of LMWH is similar to that for unfractionated heparin; it activates antithrombin, accelerating antithrombin's interaction with thrombin and factor Xa. LMWH also releases tissue factor pathway from the endothelium. LMWH has a greater activity against factor Xa, whereas unfractionated heparin has equivalent activity against thrombin and factor Xa. The plasma half-life of the LMWHs ranges from 2 to 4 h after an intravenous injection and 3–6 after a subcutaneous injection; its half-life is two to four times that of standard heparin. The longer half-life of LMWH and its dose-independent clearance results in a more predictable anticoagulant response than occurs with heparin,. It has a low affinity for plasma protein, resulting in a greater bioavailability. The advantages of LMWH over unfractionated heparin include a higher and more predictable bioavailability after subcutaneous administration and a longer biological half-life. Also, laboratory monitoring of the anticoagulant response of LMWH is not measured and dose adjustment for weight is not necessary (although an overdose may occur in smaller patients). LMWH exhibits a dose-dependent antithrombotic effect that is accurately assessed by measuring the anti-Xa activity level. The recovery of anti-factor Xa activity after a subcutaneous injection of LMWH approaches 100%,[70] making laboratory monitoring unnecessary except in patients with renal insufficiency or those with body weight less than 50 kg or more than 80 kg.[68] The r time from the thrombelastogram appears to correlate with the serum anti-Xa concentration.[71]

The three commercially available LMWH in the United States are enoxaparin (Lovenox), dalteparin (Fragmin), and tinzaparin (Innohep). Enoxaparin is either given once daily or every 12 h when used as a prophylaxis, and the two other drugs are given once a day. The three drugs appear to have comparable efficacy in the treatment and prevention of venous thromboembolism.[72] Enoxaparin and dalteparin have comparable efficacy in the prevention of death or myocardial infarction among patients with unstable angina.[72]

Clinical Pearls

- The anticoagulant effect of LMWH is similar to that for unfractionated heparin; it activates antithrombin, accelerating antithrombin's interaction with thrombin and factor Xa.

- The plasma half-life of the LMWHs ranges from 2 to 4 h after an intravenous injection and 3–6 h after a subcutaneous injection; its half-life is two to four times that of standard heparin.

- LMWHs do not need laboratory monitoring of their anticoagulant response and do need dose adjustment for weight, although an overdose may occur in smaller patients.

- Numerous cases of neuraxial hematoma occurred in the United States, prompting the FDA to issue a health advisory in December 1997.

The current recommended thromboprophylactic dose in the United States is 30 mg enoxaparin twice daily. The FDA has recently approved enoxaparin 40 mg once daily, which is similar to the European dosing schedule. It should be noted that patients in Europe get their starting dose 12 h before surgery. Since most patients in the United States are admitted on the day of their surgery, it is not practical for them to get their first dose of LMWH 12 h before surgery. Many elderly patients forget to take their medications, and it is not guaranteed that they will take their LMWH at home before their surgery.

Numerous cases of neuraxial hematoma occurred in the United States, prompting the FDA to issue a health advisory in December 1997 and the convening of the first ASRA consensus conference on anticoagulation and neuraxial anesthesia.[73] The smallest effective dose of LMWH should be administered. The postoperative administration of LMWH therapy should be delayed as long as possible, with a minimum of 12 h and ideally 24 h postoperatively. A single-dose spinal anesthetic may be the safest neuraxial technique in patients receiving preoperative LMWH. Waiting for at least 12 h after the LMWH prophylactic dose is recommended before performing a spinal technique. Patients who receive higher doses of LMWH (eg, enoxaparin 1 mg/kg twice daily) require longer delays (24 h). The catheter should be removed when anticoagulation activity is low, at least 12 h after prophylactic LMWH administration and 2–4 h before the next dose. Extreme vigilance of the patient's neurologic status must be observed if LMWH thromboprophylaxis is implemented while an indwelling catheter is infusing. Dilute local anesthetic solution is recommended so that neurologic function can be better monitored. The use of other medications affecting hemostasis, such as antiplatelet drugs, standard heparin, dextran, or oral anticoagulants, in combination with LMWH, creates an additional risk of bleeding complications.

Clinical Pearls

PATIENTS RECEIVING LMWH AND NEURAXIAL ANESTHESIA

- Monitoring of anti-Xa level is not recommended.

- The administration of other anticoagulant medications with LMWHs may increase the risk of spinal hematoma.

- The presence of blood during needle placement and catheter placement does not necessitate postponement of surgery. However, the initiation of LMWH therapy should be delayed for 24 h postoperatively.

- The first dose of LMWH prophylaxis should be given no earlier than 24 h postoperatively and only in the presence of adequate hemostasis.

- In patients who are on LMWH, needle/catheter placement should be performed at least 12 h after the last prophylactic dose of enoxaparin or 24 h after higher doses of enoxaparin (1 mg/kg every 12 h), 24 h after dalteparin (120 U/kg every 12 h or 200 U/kg every 12 h), and 24 h after tinzaparin (175 U/kg daily).

- There should be a 12-h interval between the last prophylactic dose of enoxaparin and removal of the epidural catheter. For higher doses of enoxaparin, a 24-h delay is recommended.

- The LMWH may be administered 2 h after the epidural catheter is removed.

THROMBOLYTIC THERAPY

Thrombolytic agents actively dissolve fibrin clots that have already formed. Exogenous plasminogen activators such as streptokinase and urokinase not only dissolve thrombus but also affect circulating plasminogen, leading to decreased levels of both plasminogen and fibrin. Recombinant tissue-type plasminogen activator (rt-PA), an endogenous agent, is more fibrin-selective and has less effect on circulating plasminogen levels. Clot lysis leads to elevation of fibrin degradation products, which themselves have an anticoagulant effect by inhibiting platelet aggregation. In addition to the fibrinolytic agent, patients frequently receive intravenous heparin to maintain an aPTT of 1.5 to 2 times normal. Patients with acute myocardial infarction who are treated with thrombolytic therapy (streptokinase or rt-PA) and subsequently heparinized have their fibrinogen and plasminogen levels maximally depressed at 5 h after thrombolytic therapy and remain significantly depressed at 27 h.

Although epidural or spinal needle and catheter placement with subsequent heparinization appears relatively safe, the risk of spinal hematoma in patients who receive thrombolytic therapy is not well defined. Two cases of spinal hematoma in patients with indwelling epidural catheters who received thrombolytic agents have been reported in the literature.[74,75] A case of epidural hematoma occurred in a patient with femoral artery occlusion who received an epidural anesthetic for surgical placement of an intraarterial catheter for infusion of urokinase.[74] Three hours postoperatively, the patient complained of back pain that progressed to paraplegia despite discontinuation of the urokinase infusion. An emergency decompressive laminectomy was performed, and a large hematoma compressing the thecal sac was evacuated. The patient recovered full neurologic function within 3 days. Another patient with superficial femoral artery occlusion underwent epidural catheter placement for femoral-popliteal artery bypass.[75] Blood was noted in the epidural catheter during placement. The patient was given 6300 units of heparin 90 min later, and urokinase was also injected intraarterially during the surgical procedure. A heparin infusion of 1000 U/h was initiated and continued postoperatively for 24 h. The epidural catheter was removed in the recovery room. The patient developed paraplegia on the fourth postoperative day. An MRI revealed an epidural hematoma that extended from T10 through L2. An emergency decompressive laminectomy was performed without improvement in the patient's neurologic status.

Clinical Pearls

- Concurrent use of heparin with fibrinolytic and thrombolytic drugs carries a high risk of adverse neuraxial bleeding during spinal or epidural anesthesia.

- Except in highly unusual circumstances, spinal or epidural anesthesia should be avoided in patients receiving fibrinolytic and thrombolytic therapy.

- There are no available data to clearly determine the length of time after discontinuation of these drugs and the safe performance of a neuraxial technique.

Fibrinolytic and thrombolytic agents create a coagulation state that poses a unique problem in performing neuraxial anesthesia. There may also be an increased use of these drugs in the perioperative period due to advances in fibrinolytic or thrombolytic therapy, thus requiring increased vigilance. The ASRA guidelines made recommendations with respect to neuraxial procedures after thrombolytic or fibrinolytic therapy.[9,76] The concurrent use of heparin with fibrinolytic and thrombolytic drugs places patients at high risk of adverse neuraxial bleeding during spinal or epidural anesthesia. Except in highly unusual circumstances, patients receiving fibrinolytic and thrombolytic therapy should be cautioned against receiving spinal or epidural anesthesia. The time frame for avoidance of these drugs and puncture of noncompressible vessels is 10 days. There are no available data to clearly determine the length of time after discontinuation of these drugs and the safe performance of a neuraxial technique. Frequent neurologic monitoring is recommended for an appropriate length of time in patients who have had neuraxial blocks after fibrinolytic or thrombolytic therapy. If a patient has a continuous epidural infusion and received fibri-

nolytic or thrombolytic therapy, drugs that minimize sensory and motor blockade should be used. There has been no definitive recommendation on the timing of removal of neuraxial catheters in patients who unexpectedly receive fibrinolytic or thrombolytic therapy. Measurement of fibrinogen levels may be helpful in guiding a decision about catheter removal or maintenance

Thrombin Inhibitors

Recombinant hirudin derivatives, including desirudin, lepirudin, and bivalirudin, inhibit both free and clot-bound thrombin.[9] Argatroban, an L-arginine derivative, has a similar mechanism of action. These drugs are primarily used in the treatment of heparin-induced thrombocytopenia. There is no pharmacologic reversal to the effect of these drugs. There have been no case reports of spinal hematoma related to neuraxial anesthesia in patients who have received a thrombin inhibitor. However, spontaneous intracranial bleeding has been reported.[9] According to ASRA guidelines, no statement regarding risk assessment and patient management can be made.

Fondaparinux

Fondaparinux is a synthetic anticoagulant that produces its antithrombotic effect through selective inhibition of factor Xa.[77] The drug exhibits consistency in its anticoagulant effect since it is chemically synthesized. It is 100% bioavailable. Rapidly absorbed, it reaches maximum concentration within 1.7 h of administration. Its half-life is 17 h.[77] Fondaparinux is recommended as an antithrombotic agent following major orthopedic surgery[78] and in the initial treatment of pulmonary embolism.[79] The extended half-life (approximately 20 h) allows once-daily dosing. The FDA released fondaparinux with a black box warning similar to that of the LMWHs and heparin.

Clinical Pearls

- The actual risk of spinal hematoma with fondaparinux is unknown. The daily dosing makes safe catheter removal harder to predict.

- The use of fondaparinux in the presence of an indwelling epidural catheter is not recommended.

The actual risk of spinal hematoma with fondaparinux is unknown. The daily dosing makes safe catheter removal harder to predict. Both ASRA[9] and the American College of Chest Physicians recommend against the use of fondaparinux in the presence of an indwelling epidural catheter. Their recommendations were based on the sustained and irreversible antithrombotic effect of fondaparinux, early postoperative dosing, and the spinal hematoma reported during the initial clinical trials of the drug. Close monitoring of the literature for risk factors associated with surgical bleeding may be helpful in risk assessment and patient treatment. Performance of neuraxial techniques should occur under conditions used in clinical trials (single needle pass, atraumatic needle placement, avoidance of indwelling neuraxial catheters).[9] If this is not feasible, an alternative method of prophylaxis should be considered.

HERBAL THERAPY

The most commonly used herbal medications are garlic, ginkgo, and ginseng. Garlic inhibits platelet aggregation, and its effect on hemostasis appears to last 7 days. Ginkgo inhibits platelet-activating factor, and its effect lasts 36 h. Ginseng has a variety of effects: it inhibits platelet aggregation in vitro and prolongs both thrombin time and aPPT in laboratory animals; its effect lasts 24 h.[9] In spite of their effect on platelet function, herbal drugs by themselves appear to present no added significant risk in the development of spinal hematoma in patients having epidural or spinal anesthesia. Mandatory discontinuation of these medications, or cancellation of surgery in patients in whom these medications have been continued, is not supported by available clinical data. However, the concurrent use of other medications that affect clotting mechanisms, such as oral anticoagulants or heparin, may increase the risk of bleeding complications in these patients. There is no accepted test to assess adequacy of hemostasis in the patient who took herbal medication(s). At this time, there appears to be no specific concerns as to the timing of neuraxial block in relationship to the dosing of herbal therapy, postoperative monitoring, or the timing of neuraxial catheter removal.[9]

CLINICAL FEATURES, DIAGNOSIS, & MANAGEMENT OF EPIDURAL HEMATOMA

Patients who develop spinal hematoma usually present with sudden, severe, constant back pain with or without a radicular component. Percussion over the spine aggravates the pain as well as maneuvers that increase intraspinal pressure, including coughing, sneezing, or straining. In addition, the return of the motor weakness and/or sensory deficit after the apparent resolution of the epidural or spinal blockade is highly suggestive of epidural or spinal hematoma formation. Motor and sensory findings depend entirely on the level and size of the hematoma, but may include weakness, paresis, loss of bowel or bladder function, and virtually any sensory deficit. MRI is the diagnostic study of choice. The differential diagnosis includes spinal abscess, epidural neoplasm, acute disk herniation, and spinal subarachnoid hemorrhage. Recovery without surgery is rare, and surgical consultation for consideration of emergent decompressive laminectomy must be obtained. Functional recovery is related primarily to the length of time the symptoms are present, and recovery after 72 h of symptoms is rare. The clinical features, diagnosis and differential

diagnosis, and treatment of a patient with a spinal hematoma are discussed in more detail in Chapter 71 (Diagnosis and Management of Intraspinal, Epidural, and Peripheral Nerve Hematoma).

SUMMARY COMMENTS ON ANTICOAGULANTS & NEURAXIAL BLOCKS

Anesthesiologists are urged to be up to date on their knowledge of new anticoagulant medications, anticoagulation protocols, and updated guideline recommendations (Table 70–1). Since spinal hematoma may occur even in the absence of identifiable risk factors, vigilance in monitoring is critical for early evaluation of neurologic dysfunction and prompt intervention. The decision to perform neuraxial blockade and the timing of catheter removal in a patient receiving anticoagulant therapy should be made on an individual basis, weighing the benefits of regional anesthesia against the small though definite risk of spinal hematoma.

ANTICOAGULATION & PERIPHERAL NERVE BLOCKS

In contrast to neuraxial procedures in the presence of anticoagulants, there have been no studies on peripheral nerve blocks in the presence of anticoagulants. Nevertheless, there have been case reports of hematomas when peripheral blocks are performed in patients who were on these drugs.

One should realize that spontaneous hematomas in various locations have been reported in patients who took anticoagulants. These include hematomas of the abdominal wall, intracranial hemorrhage, and psoas hematoma with enoxaparin[80–82] and intrahepatic hemorrhage with LMWH.[83] In fact, major hemorrhagic complications occur in 1.9% to 6.5% of patients on enoxaparin.[84]

A case of psoas hematoma and lumbar plexopathy was reported in a patient who was on enoxaparin and had a lumbar plexus block.[85] The patient suffered a calcaneal fracture and was placed on enoxaparin 30 mg twice a day for deep vein thrombosis prophylaxis. In addition, she was on aspirin 325 mg a day. She had two surgeries for her calcaneal fracture; the first one was done under sciatic nerve block and the second under lumbar plexus block. She finally had a right below-the-knee amputation. Several attempts were made at lumbar plexus block, but the authors were unsuccessful, so a sciatic nerve block was ultimately performed. The enoxaparin was given 19.5 h before the block and 4.5 h after the block. The patient had hip pain and subsequently was unable to move her right leg. Computed tomography (CT) showed a right retroperitoneal hematoma involving the right psoas muscle. The enoxaparin was stopped and the hematoma was allowed to resorb. The patient regained motor function over the next 5 days and had no sensory or motor deficit at the 4-month follow-up visit.[85] It should be noted that the timing of enoxaparin administrations was within the current

Table 70–1.

Summary of Guidelines on Anticoagulants and Neuraxial Blocks

I. Antiplatelet medications
  1. Aspirin, NSAIDs, COX-2 inhibitors
    May continue
    Pain clinic patients: Aspirin preferably stopped 2–3 days in thoracic and cervical epidurals (author's preference—see text)
  2. Thienopyridine derivatives
    a. Clopidogrel (Plavix)—discontinue for 7 days
    b. Ticlopidine (Ticlid)—discontinue for 14 days
    Do not perform a neuraxial block in patients on more than one antiplatelet drug
  3. GPIIB/IIIA inhibitors: Time to normal platelet aggregation
    a. Abciximab (Reopro) = 24–48 h
    b. Eptifibatide (Integrilin) = 4–8 h
    c. Tirofiban (Aggrastat) = 4–8 h
    Antiplatelet medications (ASA, Plavix) are usually given after GPIIb/IIIa inhibitors. The above guidelines on aspirin and Plavix should be adhered to

II. Warfarin
  Check INR
  INR ≤ 1.5 before neuraxial block or epidural catheter removal

III. Heparin
  1. Subcutaneous heparin (5000 units SQ q 12 h)
    Subcutaneous heparin is not a contraindication against a neuraxial block
    Neuraxial block should preferably be performed before SQ heparin is given
    Risk of decreased platelet count with SQ heparin therapy > 5 days
  2. Intravenous heparin
    Neuraxial block: 2–4 h after the last intravenous heparin dose
    Wait ≥ 1 h after neuraxial block before giving intravenous heparin

IV. Low-molecular-weight heparin (LMWH)
  No concomitant antiplatelet medication, heparin, or dextran
  1. LMWH Preop
    a. Wait 12 h before a neuraxial block:
    b. Enoxaparin (Lovenox) 0.5 mg/kg bid (prophylactic dose)
    c. Wait 24 h before a neuraxial block:
    d. Enoxaparin (Lovenox), 1 mg/kg bid (therapeutic dose)
    e. Enoxaparin (Lovenox), 1.5 mg/kg qd
    f. Dalteparin (Fragmin), 120 units/kg bid
    g. Dalteparin (Fragmin), 200 units/kg qd
    h. Tinzaparin (Innohep), 175 units/kg qd

  2. LMWH Postop:
    a. LMWH should not be started until after 24 h after surgery
    b. LMWH should not be given until ≥ 2 h after epidural catheter removal
  3. Patients with epidural catheter who are given LMWH
    The catheter should be removed at the earliest opportunity.
    Enoxaparin (0.5 mg/kg): Remove the epidural catheter ≥ 12 h after last dose.
    Enoxaparin (1-1.5 mg/kg), dalteparin, tinzaparin: Remove the epidural catheter ≥ 24 h after last dose
    Restart the LMWH ≥ 2 h after the catheter removal
  Summary recommendations for LMWH (preop & postop):
    Wait 24 h except for patients on low-dose enoxaparin (0.5 mg/kg) in which case a 12 h interval is adequate
    Wait 2 h after the catheter is removed before starting LMWH

V. Specific Xa inhibitor: Fondaparinux (Arixtra)
  Short onset, long duration (plasma half-life: 21 h)
  ASRA: No definite recommendation
  If neuraxial procedure *must be performed*, recommend single-needle atraumatic placement, avoid indwelling catheter

VI. Fibrinolytic/Thrombolytic drugs
  No data on safety interval for performance of neuraxial procedure
  Follow fibrinogen levels
  ASRA: No definite recommendation

VII. Thrombin Inhibitors
  Desirudin (Revasc)
  Lepirudin (Refludan)
  Bivalirudin (Angiomax)
  Argatroban (Acova)
    Anticoagulant effect lasts 3 h
    Monitored by aPTT
    ASRA: No recommendation at this time because of paucity of data

VIII. Herbal therapy
  Mechanism of anticoagulant effect and time to normal hemostasis:
  Garlic: Inhibits platelet aggregation, increased fibrinolysis; 7 days
  Ginko: Inhibits platelet-activating factor; 36 h
  Ginseng: Increased PT and PTT; 24 h
    ASRA: Neuraxial block not contraindicated for single herbal medication use
  No data on combined herbal therapy

Note: *The guidelines are the same for the placement and removal of epidural catheters.*
NSAIDs = nonsteroidal antiinflammatory drugs; COX-2 = cyclooxygenese-2; ASA = acetyl salicylic acid (aspirin); GPIIb = glycoprotein IIb receptor; INR = internationalized ratio, SQ = subcutaneous; LMWH = low-molecular-weight heparin; aPTT = activated partial thrompoplastin time; ASRA = American Society for Regional Anesthesiology; PT = prothrombin time; PTT = partial thromboplastin time.
Reprinted, with permission, from Benzon HT: Anticoagulants and neuraxial injections. In Benzon HT, Raja S, Molloy RE, Liu SS, et al: Essentials of Pain Medicine and Regional Anesthesia. Elsevier–Churchill Livingstone, 2005, pp 708–720.

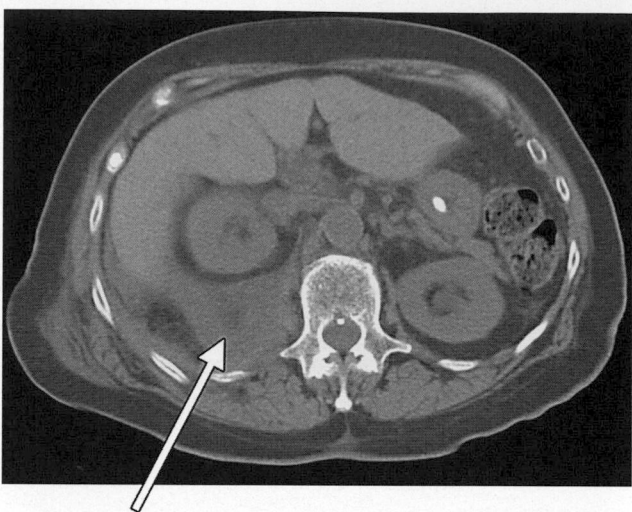

Figure 70–7. Right retroperitoneal hematoma displacing the kidney anteriorly. (Reprinted with permission from: Weller RS, Gerancher JC, Crews JC, Wade K. Extensive retroperitoneal hematoma without neurologic deficit in two patients who underwent lumbar plexus block and were later anticoagulated. Anesthesiology 2003;98:581–585.)

ASRA guidelines.[9] Although aspiration during the procedure showed no blood, bleeding probably occurred during the attempts at lumbar plexus block. The intake of aspirin, in addition to the enoxaparin, probably contributed to the bleeding during the procedure. Other cases of retroperitoneal hematoma were reported after psoas compartment block.[86] One was a patient who was given enoxaparin 30 mg the day after the block (postoperative day 2). The psoas catheter was removed 1 h, 40 min after the enoxaparin, at the peak effect of the drug. Another was a patient who was given heparin infusion 8 h after the block and warfarin (Coumadin) the evening of surgery (postoperative day 1). Both patients complained of paravertebral pain and CT scan showed a large psoas hematomas[86] (Figure 70–7).

Bleeding after sympathetic block in patients on ticlopidine and clopidogrel has been reported.[87] One patient had the block while on ticlopidine; the other patient had the block 3 days after clopidogrel was discontinued. Both patients complained of groin pain; one patient also had medial thigh numbness.[87] Eventually, both patients were found to have retroperitoneal hematoma. Bleeding after intercostal block in a patient on heparin has also been reported.[88]

The symptoms of hematoma formation after peripheral nerve block may include pain (flank or paravertebral pain or groin pain in psoas bleeding), tenderness in the area, steady decline in hemoglobin/hematocrit, hypotension due to hypovolemia, and sensory–motor deficit. Definite diagnosis is made by CT; ultrasound can also be used to detect the presence of renal subcapsular hematoma after psoas compartment block.[89] Treatment may include surgical consultation, reversal of anticoagulation, blood transfusion as necessary, and watchful waiting versus surgical drainage.

It is probably too restrictive to adapt the same ASRA guidelines on neuraxial blocks to patients undergoing peripheral nerve blocks.[9] The ASRA guidelines may be applicable to blocks in vascular and noncompressible areas such as celiac plexus blocks, superior hypogastric plexus blocks, and lumbar plexus blocks. Clinicians should individualize their decision and should discuss the risks and benefits of the block with the patient and the surgeon. Most important, the clinician should follow the patient closely after the block placement. Prospective studies are obviously needed to help guide clinicians in their decision.

References

1. Tekkok IH, Cataltelpe O, Tahta K, et al: Extradural hematoma after continuous extradural anaesthesia. Br J Anaesth 1991;67:112–115.
2. Hejazi N, Thaper PY, Hassler W: Nine cases of nontraumatic spinal epidural hematoma. Neurol Med Chir 1998;38:718–723.
3. Dickman CA, Shedd SA, Spetzler RF, et al: Spinal epidural hematoma associated with epidural anaesthesia: Complications of systemic heparinization in patients receiving peripheral vascular thrombolytic therapy. Anesthesiology 1990;72:947–950.
4. Mattle H, Sieb JP, Rohner M, et al: Nontraumatic spinal epidural and subdural hematomas. Neurology 1987;37:1351–1356.
5. Johnston RA: The management of acute spinal cord compression. J Neurol Neurosurg Psychiatry 1993;56:1046–1054.
6. Wysowski DK, Talarico L, Balsanyi J, et al: Spinal and epidural hematoma and low-molecular-weight heparin. N Engl J Med 1998;338:1774–1775.
7. Heit JA, Horlocker TT (eds). Neuraxial anesthesia and anticoagulation. Reg Anesth Pain Med 1998;23:S129–193.
8. Horlocker TT, Wedel DJ: Anticoagulation and neuraxial block: Historical perspective, anesthetic implications, and risk management. Reg Anesth Pain Med 1998;23:129–134.
9. Horlocker TT, Wedel DJ, Benzon HT: Regional anesthesia in the anticoagulated patient: Defining the risks (The second ASRA consensus conference on neuraxial anesthesia and anticoagulation). Reg Anesth Pain Med 2003;28:171–197.
10. Benzon HT, Brunner EA, Vaisrub N: Bleeding time and nerve blocks after aspirin. Reg Anesth 1984;9:86–90.
11. Rapaport SI: Preoperative hemostatic evaluation: Which tests, if any? Blood 1983;61: 229–231.
12. Hindman BJ: Usefulness of the post-aspirin bleeding time. Anesthesiology 1986;64:368–370.

Clinical Pearls

- The symptoms of hematoma formation after peripheral nerve block may include pain (flank or paravertebral pain or groin pain in psoas bleeding), tenderness in the area, steady decline in hemoglobin/hematocrit, hypotension due to hypovolemia, and sensory–motor deficit.

- Definite diagnosis is made by CT.

- Treatment may include surgical consultation, reversal of anticoagulation, blood transfusion as necessary, and watchful waiting versus surgical drainage.

- It is probably too restrictive to adapt the same ASRA guidelines on neuraxial blocks to patients undergoing peripheral nerve blocks.

13. Rodgers RPC, Levin J: A critical reappraisal of the bleeding time. Semin Thromb Hemost 1990;16:1–20.

14. Ferraris VA, Swanson E: Aspirin usage and perioperative blood loss in patients undergoing unexpected operations. Surg Gynecol Obstet 1983;156:439–442.

15. Cronberg S, Wallmark E, Söderberg I: Effect on platelet aggregation of oral administration of 10 non-steroidal analgesics to humans. Scand J Haematol 1984;33:155–159.

16. Fressinaud E, Veyradier A, Truchaud F, et al: Screening for von Willebrand disease with a new analyzer using high shear stress: A study of 60 cases. Blood 1998;91:1325–1331.

17. Mammen EF, Comp PC, Gossselin R, et al: PFA-100 system. A new method for assessment of platelet dysfunction. Semin Thromb Hemost 1998;24:195–202.

18. Locke GE, Giorgio AJ, Biggers SL Jr, et al: Acute spinal epidural hematoma secondary to aspirin-induced prolonged bleeding. Surg Neurol 1976;5:293–296.

19. Vandermeulen EP, Van Aken H, Vermylen J: Anticoagulants and spinal–epidural anesthesia. Anesth Analg 1994;79:1165–1177.

20. CLASP (Collaborative Low-Dose Aspirin Study in Pregnancy) Collaborative Group. CLASP: A randomized trial of low-dose aspirin for the prevention and treatment of pre-eclampsia among 9364 pregnant women. Lancet 1994;343:619–629.

21. Horlocker TT, Wedel DJ, Offord KP: Does preoperative antiplatelet therapy increase the risk of hemorrhagic complications associated with regional anesthesia? Anesth Analg 1990;70:631–634.

22. Horlocker TT, Wedel DJ, Schroeder DR, et al: Preoperative antiplatelet therapy does not increase the risk of spinal hematoma associated with regional anesthesia. Anesth Analg 1995;80:303–309.

23. Horlocker TT, Bajwa ZH, Ashraft Z, et al: Risk assessment of hemorrhagic complications associated with nonsteroidal antiinflammatory medications in ambulatory pain clinic patients undergoing epidural steroid injection. Anesth Analg 2002;95:1691–1697.

24. Benzon HT: Anticoagulants and neuraxial injections. In: Benzon HT, Raja S, Molloy RE, Liu SS, Fishman FM. *Essentials of pain medicine and regional anesthesia.* Elsevier-Churchill Livingstone, 2005, pp 708–720.

25. Eastwood DW: Hematoma after epidural anesthesia: Relation of skin and spinal angiomas. Anesth Analg 1991;73:352–354.

26. Greensite F, Katz J: Spinal subdural hematoma associated with attempted epidural anesthesia and subsequent spinal anesthesia. Anesth Analg 1980;59:72–73.

27. Mayumi T, Dohi S: Spinal subarachnoid hematoma after lumbar puncture in a patient receiving antiplatelet therapy. Anesth Analg 1983;62:777–779.

28. Gerancher JC, Waterer R, Middleton J: Transient paraparesis after postdural puncture spinal hematoma in a patient receiving ketorolac. Anesthesiology 1997;86:490–494.

29. Urmey WF, Rowlingson JC: Do antiplatelet agents contribute to the development of perioperative spinal hematoma? Reg Anesth Pain Med 1998;23:146–151.

30. Fitzgerald GA, Patrono C: The coxibs, selective inhibitors of cyclooxygenase-2. N Engl J Med 2001;345:433–442.

31. McCrory CR, Lindahl SGE: Cyclooxygenase inhibition for postoperative analgesia. Anesth Analg 2002;95:169–176.

32. Gajraj NM. Cyclooxygenase-2 inhibitors. Anesth Analg 2003;96:1720–1738.

33. Buvanendran A, Kroin JS, Tuman KJ, et al: Effects of perioperative administration of a selective cyclooxygenase 2 inhibitor on pain management and recovery of function after knee replacement: A randomized controlled trial. JAMA 2003;290:2411–2418.

34. Greenberg H, Gottesdiener K, Huntington M, et al: A new cyclooxygenase-2-inhibitor, rofecoxib (VIOXX) did not alter the antiplatelet effects of low-does aspirin in healthy volunteers. J Clin Pharmacol 2000;40:1509–1515.

35. Lessee PT, Hubbard RC, Karim A, et al: Effects of celecoxib, a novel, cyclooxygenase-2-inhibitor, on platelet function in healthy adults: A randomized, clinical trial. J Clin Pharmacol 2000;40:124–132.

36. van Heeken H, Schwartz JI, Depre M, et al: Comparative inhibitory activity of rofecoxib, meloxicam, diclofenac, ibuprofen and naproxen on COX-2 versus COX-1 in healthy volunteers. J Clin Pharmacol 2000;40:1109–1120.

37. Reuben SS, Connelly NR: Postoperative analgesic effects of celecoxib or rofecoxib after spinal fusion surgery. Anesth Analg 2000;91:1221–1225.

38. Psaty BM, Furberg CD: Cox-2 inhibitors—Lessons in drug safety. N Engl J Med 2005;352:1133–1135.

39. Schor K: Antiplatelet drugs: A comparative review. Drugs 1995;50:7–28.

40. Lange RA, Hillis LD: Antiplatelet therapy for ischemic heart disease. N Engl J Med 2004;350:277–280.

41. Boneu B, Destelle G, on behalf of the study group: Platelet antiaggregating activity and tolerance of clopidogrel in atherosclerotic patients. Thromb Haemost 1996;76:939–943.

42. CAPRIE Steering Committee: A randomized blind trial of clopidogrel versus aspirin in patients at risk of ischaemic stroke (CAPRIE). Lancet 1996;348:1329–1339.

43. Helft G, Osende JI, Worthley SG, et al: Acute antithrombotic effect of a front-loaded regimen of clopidogrel in patients with atherosclerosis on aspirin. Arterioscler Thromb Vasc Biol 2000;29:2316–2321.

44. Steinhubl SR, Berger PB, Mann JT, et al: Early and sustained dual oral antiplatelet therapy following percutaneous coronary intervention: A randomized controlled trial. JAMA 2002;288:2411–2420.

45. Mayumi T, Dohi S: Spinal subarachnoid hematoma after lumbar puncture in a patient receiving antiplatelet therapy. Anesth Analg 1983;62:777–779.

46. Benzon HT, Wong HY, Siddiqui T, et al: Caution in performing epidural injections in patients on several antiplatelet drugs. Anesthesiology 1999;91:1558–1559.

47. Shapiro SS: Treating thrombosis in the 21st century. New Engl J Med 2003;349:1762–1764.

48. Enneking FK, Benzon HT: Oral anticoagulants and regional anesthesia: A perspective. Reg Anesth Pain Med 1998;23:140–145.

49. Kearon C, Hirsh J: Management of anticoagulation before and after elective surgery. N Engl J Med 1997;336:1506–1511.

50. Harrison L, Johnston M, Massicote MP, et al: Comparison of 5-mg and 10-mg doses in initiation of warfarin therapy. Ann Intern Med 1997;126:133–136.

51. Benzon HT, Esposito P. Timing of removal of epidural catheters in anticoagulated patients. ASA annual meeting, San Diego, California, October 21, 1997. Anesthesiology 1997;87(3A):A798.

52. Schulman S, Lockner D, Bergstrom K, Blomback M: Intensive initial oral anticoagulation and shorter heparin treatment in deep vein thrombosis. Thromb Haemost 10984;52:276–280.

53. Odoom JA, Sih IL: Epidural analgesia and anticoagulant therapy. Anesthesia 1983;38:254–259.

54. Horlocker TT, Wedel DJ, Schlichting JL: Postoperative epidural analgesia and oral anticoagulant therapy. Anesth Analg 1994;79:89–93.

55. Wu CL, Perkins FM: Oral anticoagulant prophylaxis and epidural catheter removal. Reg Anesth 1996;21:517–524.

56. Horlocker TT: When to remove a spinal or epidural catheter in an anticoagulated patient. Reg Anesth 1993;18:264–265.

57. Weinstock DM, Chang P, Aronson DL, et al: Comparison of plasma prothrombin and factor VII and urine prothrombin F1 concentrations in patients on long-term warfarin therapy and those in initial phase. Am J Hematol 1998;57:193–199.

58. Jerkeman A, Astermark J, Hedner U, et al: Correlation between different intensities of anti-Vitamin K treatment and coagulation parameters. Thromb Res 2000;98:467–471.

59. Rosenberg RD, Bauer KA: The heparin-antithrombin system: A natural anticoagulant mechanism. In Colma RW, Hirsch J, Marder VJ, et al (eds): *Hemostasis and Thrombosis: Basic Principles and Clinical Practice,* 3rd ed. JB Lippincott, 1994, pp 837–860.

60. Abildgaard U, Lindahl AK, Sandset PM: Heparin requires both antithrombin and extrinsic pathway inhibitor for its anticoagulant effect in human blood. Haemostasis 1991;21:254–257.

61. Murray DJ, Brodsnahan WJ, Pennell B, et al: Heparin detection by the activated coagulation time: A comparison of the sensitivity of coagulation tests and heparin assays. J Cardiothorac Vasc Anesth 1997;11:24–28.

62. Shapiro SS. Treating thrombosis in the 21st century. N Engl J Med 2003;349:1762–1764.

63. Weitz JI. Drug therapy: Low-molecular-weight heparins. N Engl J Med 1997;337:688–698.

64. Rao TL, El-Etr AA: Anticoagulation following placement of epidural and subarachnoid catheters: An evaluation of neurologic sequelae. Anesthesisology 1981;55:618–620.

65. Ruff DL, Dougherty JH: Complications of anticoagulation followed by anticoagulation. Stroke 1981;12:879–881.

66. Liu SS, Mulroy MF: Neuraxial anesthesia and analgesia in the presence of standard heparin. Reg Anesth Pain Med 1998;23:157–163.

67. Chaney MA: Intrathecal and epidural anesthesia and analgesia for cardiac surgery. Anesth Analg 1997;84:1211–1221.

68. Weitz JI. Drug therapy: Low-molecular-weight heparins. N Engl J Med 1997;337:688–698.

69. Horlocker TT, Heit JA: Low molecular weight heparin: Biochemistry, pharmacology, perioperative prophylaxis regimens, and guidelines for regional anesthetic management. Anesth Analg 1997;85:874–885.

70. Bara L, Billaud E, Gramond G, et al: Comparative pharmacokinetics of a low molecular weight heparin (PK 10 169) and unfractionated heparin after intravenous and subcutaneous administration. Thromb Res 1985;39:631–636.

71. Klein S, Slaughter T, Vail PT, et al: Thrombelastography as a perioperative measure of anticoagulation resulting from low molecular weight heparin: A comparison with anti-Xa concentrations. Anesth Analg 2000;91:1091–1095.

72. White RH. Low-molecular-weight heparins: Are they all the same? Br J Haematol 2003;121:12–20.

73. Horlocker TT, Wedel DJ: Neuraxial block and low molecular weight heparin: Balancing perioperative analgesia and thromboprophylaxis. Reg Anesth Pain Med 1998;23:164–177.

74. Dickman CA, Shedd SA, Spetzler RF, et al: Spinal epidural hematoma associated with epidural anesthesia: Complications of systemic heparinization in patients receiving peripheral vascular thrombolytic therapy. Anesthesiology 1990;72:947–950.

75. Onishchuk JL, Carlsson C: Epidural hematoma associated with epidural anesthesia: Complications of anticoagulant therapy. Anesthesiology 1992;77:1221–1223.

76. Rosenquist RW, Brown DL. Neuraxial bleeding: Fibrinolytics/thrombolytics. Reg Anesth Pain Med 1998;23S:152–156.

77. Bauer KA: Fondaparinux: Basic properties and efficacy and safety in venous thromboembolism prophylaxis. Am J Orthop 2002;31:4–10.

78. Turpie AG, Bauer KA, Eriksson BL, et al: Fondaparinux vs enoxaparin for the prevention of venous thromboembolism in major orthopedic surgery: A meta-analysis of 4 randomized double-blind studies. Arch Intern Med 2002;162:1833–1840.

79. The Matisse Investigators: Subcutaneous fondaparinux versus intravenous unfractionated heparin in the initial treatment of pulmonary embolism. N Engl J Med 2003;349:1695–1702.

80. Antonelli D, Fares L, Anene C: Enoxaparin associated with huge abdominal wall hematomas: A report of two cases. Am Surgeon 2000;66:797–800.

81. Dickinson LD, Miller L, Patel CP, et al: Enoxaparin increases the incidence of postoperative intracranial hemorrhage when initiated preoperatively for deep vein thrombosis prophylaxis with brain tumors. Neurosurgery 1998;43:1074–1081.

82. Ho KJ, Gawley SD, Young MR: Psoas hematoma and femoral neuropathy associated with enoxaparin therapy. Int J Clin Pract 2003;57:553–554.

83. Houde JP, Steinberg G: Intrahepatic hemorrhage after use of low-molecular-weight heparin for total hip arthroplasty. J Arthroplasty 1999;14:372–374.

84. Noble S, Spencer CM: Enoxaparin: A review of its clinical potential in the management of coronary artery disease. Drugs 1998;56:259–272.

85. Klein SM, D'Ercole F, Greengrass RA, et al: Enoxaparin associated with psoas hematoma and lumbar plexopathy after lumbar plexus block. Anesthesiology 1997;87:1576–1579.

86. Weller RS, Gerancher JC, Crews JC, et al: Extensive retroperitoneal hematoma without neurologic deficit in two patients who underwent lumbar plexus block and were later anticoagulated. Anesthesiology 2003;98:581–583.

87. Maier C, Gleim M, Weiss T, et al: Severe bleeding following lumbar sympathetic blockade in two patients under medication with irreversible platelet aggregation inhibitors. Anesthesiology 2002;97:740–743.

88. Nielsen CH: Bleeding after intercostal nerve block in a patient anticoagulated with heparin. Anesthesiology 1989;71:162–164.

89. Aida S, Takahashi H, Shimoji K: Renal subcapsular hematoma after lumbar plexus block. Anesthesiology 1996;84:452–455.

71

Diagnosis & Management of Intraspinal, Epidural, & Peripheral Nerve Hematoma

Rasha S. Jabri, MD • Steven Deschner, MD • Honorio T. Benzon, MD

INTRODUCTION

Spinal epidural hematoma (SEH) is an accumulation of blood in the potential space between the dura and the bone. Hemorrhage into the spinal canal most commonly occurs in the epidural space because of the prominent epidural venous plexus. SEH may be spontaneous or may follow minor trauma, such as lumbar puncture or neuraxial anesthesia. It is more likely to occur in anticoagulated or thrombocytopenic patients, or in those with liver disease or alcoholism. Approximately one quarter to one third of all cases are associated with anticoagulation therapy.[1,2] Spontaneous bleeding is rare but may be seen with anticoagulation, thrombolysis, blood dyscrasias, coagulopathies, thrombocytopenia, neoplasms, vascular malformations, or vertebral hemagioma.[3,4] The peridural venous plexus is usually involved, though arterial sources of hemorrhage also occur.[5] SEHs are mostly venous in nature because the venous plexus lacks valves, and the plexus has been shown to permit a reversal in blood flow during pressure increase from physical activity.[6] Hematoma sites are usually found in the cervical and thoracic spine.[7]

Most SEHs are located dorsal to the dural sac because of the firm adherence of the dural sac to the posterior longitudinal ligament in the ventral aspect of the spinal canal. The dorsal aspect of the thoracic or lumbar region is involved commonly, and expansion is limited to a few vertebral levels.

Clinical Pearls

- Hemorrhage into the spinal canal most commonly occurs in the epidural space because of the prominent epidural venous plexus.

- SEH may be spontaneous or may follow minor trauma, such as lumbar puncture or neuraxial anesthesia.

- SEH occurs primarily in anticoagulated or thrombocytopenic patients.

- The risk of spinal hematoma in patients without overt risk factors is less than 1 in 150,000 epidural and less than 1 in 220,000 spinal anesthesias.

Incidence

SEH represents a rare spinal emergency, with a frequency of less than 1% of spinal space-occupying lesions.[8] SEH affects 1 per 1,000,000 people annually.[9,10] The actual incidence of neurologic dysfunction resulting from hemorrhagic complications associated with central neural blockade is unknown. In an extensive review of the literature, the calculated incidence was approximated to be less than 1 in 150,000 epidural and less than 1 in 220,000 spinal anesthesias.[11] No racial predilection has been reported, but SEH is more frequent in females. Increased age has been associated with more frequent SEH.

Anticoagulant therapy in association with neuraxial analgesia, as well as the length and intensity of anticoagulation, has been identified as one of the most important risk factors for epidural hematoma.[12] Decreased weight and concomitant hepatic or renal disease, which may exaggerate the anticoagulant response, represent theoretical concerns for bleeding tendency. Thrombolytic therapy represents the greatest risk factor for bleeding complications.[13]

History & Physical Examination

The patient is usually in significant distress and usually presents with a severe, localized constant back pain with or without a radicular component that may mimic disc herniation. Associated symptoms may include weakness, numbness, and urinary or fecal incontinence.[14,15] The onset of pain is occasionally related to minor straining such as with defecation, lifting, coughing, or sneezing, but in the majority of cases the onset of pain is spontaneous.[16,17] Signs of spinal cord and nerve root dysfunction appear rapidly and may progress to paraparesis or paraplegia depending on the level of the lesion. In the lumbar spine, the epidural hematoma may mimic an acute disc herniation. In the cases of epidural hematomas that are related to neuraxial anesthesia or lumbar puncture, the presence of new or progressive postoperative neurologic symptoms should alert the physician to a possible epidural hematoma.

Clinical Pearls

- The patient usually presents with a severe, localized constant back pain with or without a radicular component that may mimic disc herniation.
- Associated symptoms may include weakness, numbness, and urinary or fecal incontinence.
- Return of sensory or motor deficit several hours after spinal or epidural block has worn off (with or without back pain) is highly pathognomonic and should be considered and treated as spinal or epidural hematoma until proven otherwise.

Back pain is enhanced by percussion over the spine, as well as maneuvers that increase intraspinal pressure such as coughing, sneezing, or straining. Depending on the level and the size of the hematoma, physical findings may include unilateral or bilateral weakness, sensory deficits with unilateral or bilateral radicular paresthesias, various alterations in deep tendon reflexes, and alterations of bladder or anal sphincter tone.[18]

Etiology & Location of Hematoma

The proposed factors that can cause spinal epidural hematoma include trauma, anticoagulation, thrombolysis, lumbar puncture, epidural or spinal anesthesia, interventional spine procedures or surgeries, coagulopathy or bleeding diathesis, hepatic disease with portal hypertension, vascular malformation, disk herniation, Paget disease of the vertebral bones, Valsalva maneuver, and hypertension.[19] The most important causes of spontaneous spinal epidural hematoma are clotting disorders, which may be acquired (anticoagulant therapy, malignancies) or congenital (hemophilia).[20,21] Vascular malformations are rarely responsible for spontaneous epidural hematomas; only 4% in a series of 158 cases and 6.5% in a series of 199 cases were reported to be due to vascular malformation.[22,23] Other less common predisposing factors include systemic lupus erythematosus, ankylosing spondylitis, rheumatoid arthritis, Paget disease, disc herniation, and hypertension.[17,24,25] No underlying cause can be identified in about 40% to 50% of cases. The most widely accepted hypothesis is that of venous bleeding. Epidural veins are valveless and are located in the low-pressure epidural space. These veins are unprotected from sudden increases in intraabdominal or intrathoracic pressure (as in the Valsalva maneuver), leading to rupture and hemorrhage.[26,27] It has been proposed that an increase in venous pressure in the epidural space, in association with the hemodynamic changes of pregnancy, may predispose to rupture of a preexisting pathologic venous wall.[28,29] The epidural venous plexus is most prominent in the thoracic spine.[23] Spontaneous SEH most often is located in the thoracic and cervicothoracic region followed by the thoracolumbar location and extends over a few vertebral body levels.[8,15,16,23] Spinal epidural hematoma is usually posterior or posterolateral to the thecal sac (Figure 71–1).[23]

Diagnosis of SEH

Clinical findings of SEH usually include neurologic deficit during the acute stage; the motor and sensory deficits may rapidly develop into paraplegia, quadriplegia, or autonomic dysfunction. Patients usually present with acute axial spine pain that radiates to corresponding dermatomes and evolving focal neurologic deficit with signs of nerve root or spinal cord compression.[30] The epidural hematoma usually presents itself within the first 24–48 h after surgery. Early clinical signs are increased pain or focal neurologic deficit, often in areas not present preoperatively or in areas affected by the surgery. Any new or progressive neurologic symptoms warrant immediate clinical evaluation and diagnostic work-up to rule out any space-occupying lesion including epidural hematoma. A new

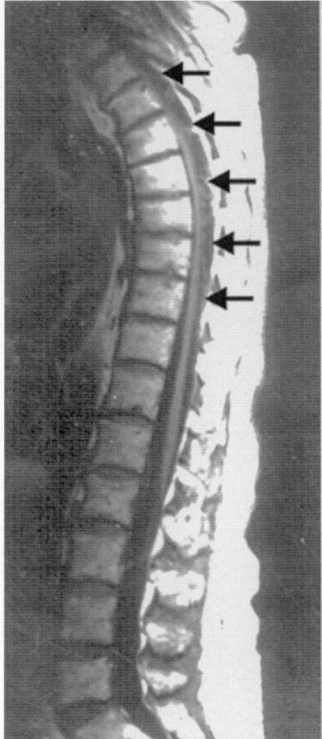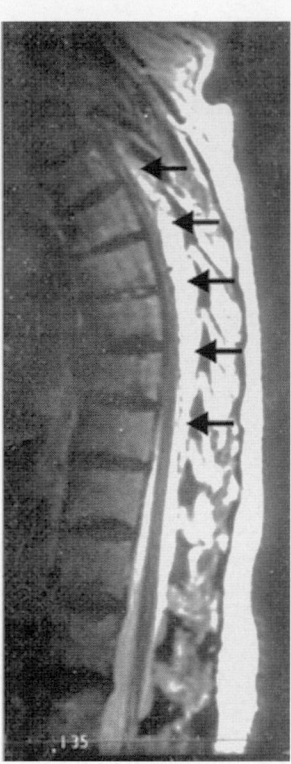

Figure 71–1. Sagittal magnetic resonance images of the thoracolumbar spine. A large complex epidural hematoma extending from T3 to T10 through T11 is seen with hypo- and isodense signal characteristics on a T1-weighted image (*left; arrows*) and hyperintense signal characteristics on a T2-weighted image (*right; arrows*). At the center of the hematoma, the spinal cord abuts the posterior aspect of the thoracic vertebral bodies (*left*). No signal abnormalities of the cord itself are seen. (Reprinted, with permission, from Schwarz SKW, Wong CL, McDonald WN: Spontaneous recovery from a spinal epidural hematoma with atypical presentation in a nonagenarian. Can J Anesth 2004;51:557–561.)

or progressive neurologic deficit occurring in the presence of epidural analgesia mandates immediate discontinuation of the infusion, with the catheter left in place, to rule out any contribution from the local anesthetic. If the epidural infusion is the cause of the neurologic manifestation, a return of sensory and motor function should be noted. Otherwise, an immediate work-up and radiographic imaging studies should be obtained and a consultation with a neurosurgeon sought.

In view of acute axial back pain with deterioration of neurologic deficits, pathologic entities associated with nerve root and spinal cord compression need to be evaluated immediately, to differentiate miscellaneous lesions simulating SEH. The clinical presentation of a patient with suspected epidural hematoma may resemble epidural abscess, spinal cord disease, neoplasms, and acute disc herniation. The differential diagnoses of new or progressive postoperative neurologic symptoms include surgical neuropraxia, prolonged or exaggerated neuraxial block, anterior spinal artery syndrome, exacerbation of a preexisting neurologic disorder, and presentation of a previously undiagnosed neurologic condition.

Complete blood count with platelets should be ordered to assess the extent of bleeding and to determine the presence

of infection. Prothrombin time and activated partial thromboplastin time determine the presence of bleeding diathesis.

Rapid diagnostic radiographic evaluation is essential to minimize delay in treatment of spinal epidural hematoma. Currently, magnetic resonance imaging (MRI) is the diagnostic imaging of choice for spinal emergencies because it allows rapid, noninvasive evaluation of the vertebral column and the spinal cord in all planes. Spinal MRI may delineate the location of an epidural hematoma and identify an associated vascular malformation; it will provide information about the extent of the hematoma as well as the degree of cord compression. MRI is also helpful in determining the age of the hematoma (see Figure 71–1).[17,31,32] The chronologic characteristics of an MRI of a spinal epidural hematoma are similar to those seen with intracranial hemorrhage. In the hyperacute stage (first 6 h), the spinal epidural hematoma appears as isointense as the spinal cord on T1-weighted images and mildly hyperintense and heterogeneous on T2-weighted images, as a result of the presence of intracellular oxyhemoglobin. In an acute stage (7–72 h) the hematoma is still isointense on T1-weighted images and becomes hypointense on T2-weighted images. This is due to the presence of intracellular deoxyhemoglobin, which causes T2 shortening. As the concentration of methemoglobin increases, the hematoma becomes hyperintense and homogeneous on T1- and T2-weighted images. Gadolinium-enhanced magnetic resonance arteriography (MRA) may further define the extent of an arteriovenous malformation.

Conventional CT may diagnose an epidural hematoma, but may give false-negative results if the hematoma is isodense to the thecal sac or the spinal cord and if the image quality is affected by artifacts often seen in upper thoracic region.[32] Spinal computed tomography (CT) scanning may be nondiagnostic in the thoracic spine, where resolution is poorer than in the lumbar and cervical spine because of the high contrast between the lung parenchyma and vertebral bone.

Conventional angiography may be required to definitely demonstrate the presence of a vascular malformation.[17,27] Myelography, and later CT, used to be the main diagnostic modalities for diagnosing epidural hematomas.[33] Myelography and CT-myelography may show an epidural lesion with partial or complete spinal block, but is not specific; it is invasive and may worsen the clinical status. Although myelography can demonstrate signs of compression with visualization of nonspecific contrast blockade or extradural convex compression, it cannot be used to determine the nature and the real extent of the lesion.[34] Combined with spinal CT scanning, SEH can be viewed as an intraspinal biconvex and hyperdense lesion with the density equivalent to blood.[35]

Prevention, Treatment, & Prognosis

Lumbar puncture or epidural anesthesia should be avoided in individuals who are on anticoagulant therapy, following thrombolysis, or when a bleeding diathesis is suspected. Anesthesiologists are urged to be up to date on their knowledge of anticoagulation protocols, new anticoagulant medications,

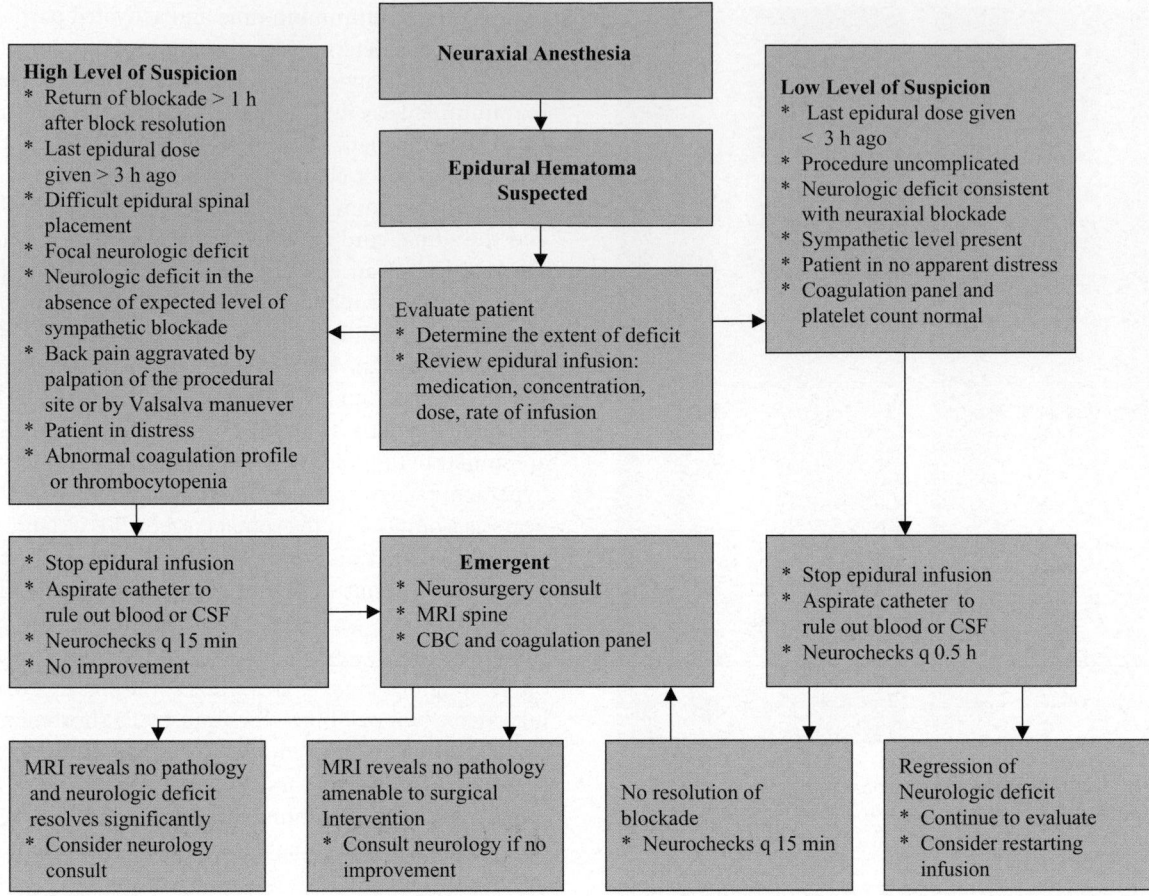

Figure 71–2. Practical approach to decision making in work-up and treatment of a patient with suspected epidural hematoma. CSF = cerebrospinal fluid, MRI = magnetic resonance imaging, CBC = complete blood count.

and new guideline recommendations. The decision to perform neuraxial blockade and the timing of catheter removal in a patient receiving antithrombotic therapy should be made on an individual basis, weighing the risks of spinal hematoma with the benefits of regional anesthesia for a specific patient. The American Society of Regional Anesthesia has published consensus statements on neuraxial anesthesia and anticoagulation with current updates, which provides an up-to-date source for guidelines in the decision-making process in performing neuraxial anesthesia in a patient with risk factors (see Chapter 70, Neuraxial Anesthesia and Peripheral Nerve Blocks in Patients on Anticoagulants).[36]

Although some case reports have described successful conservative management of epidural hematoma, urgent surgical decompression is the treatment of choice for SEH causing acute compromise of cord function.[37] A practical approach to management of suspected epidural hematoma is displayed in Figure 71–2. Nonoperative treatment with good outcome was mainly reported in hematomas localized at the cauda equina level and those with mild neurologic deficit.[20] Although not all spinal hematomas are treated with emergency laminectomy and spontaneous resolution of deficits has been reported in the literature,[38] the decision to observe or surgically intervene is a neurosurgical one. The critical factors for recovery after SEH are the level of preoperative

neurologic deficit and the operative interval.[20,39] In complete preoperative sensorimotor loss, surgery within 36 h of onset of symptoms correlates with favorable outcome.[31] Laminectomy is followed by evacuation of the hematoma, coagulation of bleeding sites, and inspection of the dura. The dura is then tented to the bone and, occasionally, epidural drains are employed for as long as 24 h. The prognosis is worse when there is a delay between the injury and surgical intervention.[31] It was noted that complete neurologic recovery was unlikely if more than 8 h has elapsed between the development of paralysis and surgical intervention.[40] Recovery without surgery is rare, and surgical consultation for consideration of emergent decompressive laminectomy must be obtained as soon as possible. The overall mortality rate is 8%.[41] Functional recovery is related primarily to the length of time the symptoms are present, and recovery after 72 h of symptoms, although rare,[42] has been reported.[43] Prognosis for neurologic recovery primarily depends on the patient's preoperative neurologic status and duration of neurologic dysfunction.[26,44] Since neurologic outcome is linked to early diagnosis and intervention, consultation with a neurosurgeon about the potential emergent evacuation of the hematoma should be obtained as soon as possible.[26] Complications of SEH include neurologic deficits, paraplegia, spasticity, neuropathic pain, and urinary or fecal sphincter dysfunction.

Spinal Epidural Hematoma: Summary

Spinal epidural hematoma comprises a heterogeneous group of disorders with the final common result of hemorrhage in the spinal epidural space. SEH may be acute or chronic, spontaneous, posttraumatic, or iatrogenic. Its occurrence appears to be particularly associated with acquired coagulopathy from medications and disease states. MRI plays an especially important diagnostic role. Surgery needs to be performed as rapidly as possible because the interval between the onset of symptoms and surgery, together with the preoperative clinical status, determine the clinical outcome.

Since spinal epidural hematoma is a rare and potentially reversible cause of spinal cord compression, it is essential that the diagnosis be made as early as possible to enable full recovery. Since spinal hematoma may occur even in the absence of identifiable risk factors, vigilance in monitoring any new neurologic symptoms is critical in allowing early evaluation of neurologic dysfunction and prompt intervention. It is a potentially reversible cause of spinal cord and root compression, and the prompt diagnosis and treatment of this relatively rare condition are important. When accomplished rapidly, surgical decompression can result in full functional recovery.

PERIPHERAL HEMATOMA AFTER NERVE BLOCKS

There have been a few case reports of hematoma after peripheral nerve blocks (Figure 71–3). There were two case reports of psoas hematoma after lumbar plexus block.[45,46]

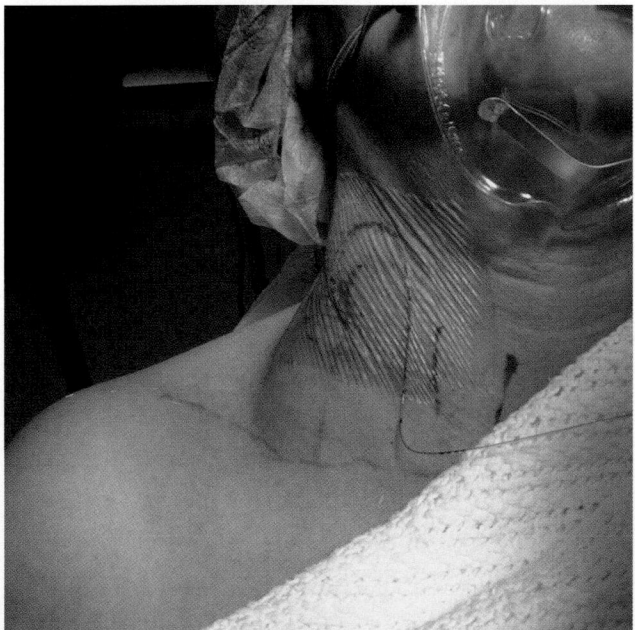

Figure 71–3. Neck hematoma. Sizeable neck hematoma in a patient in whom the external jugular vein was punctured with an 18-gauge Tuohy-style needle during insertion of a catheter in the interscalene groove. The hematoma shown was self-contained and was treated conservatively with local compression.

In one patient, enoxaparin was give 19.5 h before the block and 4.5 h after the block.[45] Note that the intervals between the block and the administration of enoxaparin were within the guidelines recommended by the American Society of Regional Anesthesia,[36] although the patient also took aspirin. The enoxaparin was discontinued, and resorption of the hematoma was observed. In the other reported cases, warfarin and heparin infusion were administered 8 h after the block and, in another patient, enoxaparin was given 40 h after the block.[46] Another case of psoas hematoma was reported after lumbar sympathetic block. One patient was on ticlopidine during the block, and the other patient took clopidogrel 3 days before the block.[47] In these case reports, the blocks were performed near blood vessels in an expandable and noncompressible area. These case reports must also be viewed in the context of spontaneous hematomas in patients who were on anticoagulants.[48–51]

As stated in Chapter 70, the symptoms of hematoma after peripheral nerve block include pain (flank or paravertebral pain or groin pain in psoas bleeding), tenderness in the area, fall in hemoglobin/hematocrit, fall in blood pressure, and sensory and motor deficit. CT scan is used in the diagnosis. In one case report,[52] ultrasound demonstrated the presence of renal subcapsular hematoma. The increased use of ultrasound in peripheral nerve blocks will make it easier for clinicians to follow suspected cases of bleeding after peripheral nerve blocks.

Treatments of hematoma after peripheral nerve blocks usually include surgical consult, blood transfusion as necessary, and watchful waiting versus surgical drainage. In the case reports of psoas hematoma,[45,52] no surgical evacuation of the hematoma was performed. The patients regained their sensory and motor status in a few days to 4 months after the diagnosis. The expandable nature of the site probably helped decreased the possibility of irreversible nerve ischemia. Since there are no published guidelines on anticoagulants and peripheral nerve blocks, anesthesiologists should individualize their decision on the advisability of performing peripheral nerve blocks in patients on anticoagulants. Anesthesiologists should discuss the risks and benefits of the block with the patient and the surgeon. If a block is performed, the patient should be followed very closely after the block and observed for signs and symptoms of peripheral hematoma.

References

1. Johnston RA: The management of acute spinal cord compression. J Neurol Neurosurg Psychiatr 1993;56:1046–1054.
2. Wysowski DK, Talarico L, Bacsanyi J, et al: Spinal and epidural hematoma and low-molecular-weight heparin. N Engl J Med 1998;338:1774–1775.
3. Dickman CA, Shedd SA, Spetzler RF: Spinal epidural hematoma associated with epidural anaesthesia: Complications of systemic heparinization in patients receiving peripheral vascular thrombolytic therapy. Anesthesiology 1990;72:947–950.
4. Mattle H, Sieb JP, Rohner M, et al: Nontraumatic spinal epidural and subdural hematomas. Neurology 1987;37:1351–1356.
5. Beatty RM, Winston KR: Spontaneous cervical epidural hematoma. A consideration of etiology. J Neurosurg 1984;61:143–148.

6. Pan G, Kulkarni M, MacDougall DJ, et al: Traumatic epidural hematoma of the cervical spine: Diagnosis with magnetic resonance imaging. J Neurosurg 1988;68:798–801.

7. Holtas S, Heiling M, Lonntoft M: Spontaneous spinal epidural hematoma: Findings at MR imaging and clinical correlation. Radiology 1996;199:409–413.

8. Alexiadou-Rudolf C, Ernestus R, Nanassis K, et al: Acute nontraumatic spinal epidural hematomas. Spine 1998;23:1810–1813.

9. Tekkok IH, Cataltepe O, Tata K, et al: Extradural hematoma after continuous extradural anaesthesia, Br J Anaesth 1991;67:112–115.

10. Hejazi N, Thaper PY, Hassler W: Nine cases of nontraumatic spinal epidural hematoma. Neurol Med Chir 1998;38:718–723.

11. Tryba M: Epidural regional anesthesia and low molecular heparine: Pro (German). Anasthesiol Intensivmed Notfallmed Schmerzther 1993;28:179–181.

12. Horlocker TT, Wedel DJ: Neuraxial blockade and low molecular weight heparin: Balancing perioperative analgesia and thromboprophylaxis. Reg Anesth 1998;23:164–177.

13. Levine MN, Goldhaber SZ, Gore JM, et al: Hemorrhagic complications of thrombolytic therapy in the treatment of myocardial infarction and venous thromboembolism. Chest 1995;108(Suppl 4):291S–301S.

14. Matsume M, Shimoda M, Shibuya N: Spontaneous cervical epidural hematoma. Surg Neurol 1987;28:381–384.

15. Fukui M, Swarnkar A, Williams R: Acute spontaneous spinal epidural hematomas. Am J Neuroradiol 1999;20:1365–1372.

16. Joseph A, Vinen J: Acute spinal epidural hematoma. J Emerg Med 1993;11:437–441.

17. Packer N, Cummins B: Spontaneous epidural hemorrhage: A surgical emergency. Lancet 1978;1:356–358.

18. Lonjon M, Paquis P, Chanalet S, et al: Nontraumatic spinal epidural hematoma: Report of four cases and review of the literature. Neurosurgery 1997;41:483–487.

19. Graziani N, Bouillot P, Figarella-Bragner D, et al: Cavernous angiomas and arteriovenous malformations of the spinal epidural space: Report of 11 cases. Neurosurgery 1994;35:856–864.

20. Harik S, Raichle M, Reis D: Spontaneously remitting spinal epidural hematoma in a patient on anticoagulants. N Engl J Med 1971;284:1355–1357.

21. Zuccarello M, Scanarini M, D'Avella, et al: Spontaneous spinal extradural hematoma during anticoagulant therapy. Surg Neurol 1980;14:411–413.

22. Chen C, Fang W, Chen C, et al: Spontaneous spinal epidural hematomas with repeated remission and relapse. Neuroradiology 1997;39:737–740.

23. Groen R, Ponssen H: The spontaneous spinal epidural hematoma: A study of the etiology. J Neurolog Sci 1990;98:121–138.

24. Fukui M, Swarnkar A, Williams R: Acute spontaneous spinal epidural hematomas. Am J Neuroradiol 1999;20:1365–1372.

25. Joseph A, Vinen J: Acute spinal epidural hematoma. J Emerg Med 1993;11:437–441.

26. Foo D, Rossier A: Preoperative neurological status in predicting surgical outcome of spinal epidural hematomas. Surg Neurol 1981,15:389–340.

27. David S, Salluzzo RF, Bartfield JM, et al: Spontaneous cervicothoracic epidural hamatoma following prolonged Valsalva secondary to trumpet playing. Am J Emerg Med 1997;15:73–75.

28. Bidzinski J: Spontaneous spinal epidural hematoma during pregnancy. J Neurosurg 1966;24:1017–1018.

29. Carroll S, Malhotra R, Eustace D, et al: Spontaneous spinal extradural hematoma during pregnancy. J Matern Fetal Med 1997;6:218–219.

30. Bruyn GW, Bosma NJ: Spinal extradural hematoma. In Vinken PJ, Bruyn GW (eds): *Handbook of Clinical Neurology.* North-Holland Publishing, 1976, pp 1–30.

31. Lawton M, Porter R, Heiserman J, et al: Surgical management of spinal epidural hematoma: Relationship between surgical timing and neurological outcome. J Neurosurg 1995;83:1–7.

32. Avrahami E, Tadmor R, Ram Z, et al: MR demonstration of spontaneous acute epidural hematoma of thoracic spine. Neuroradiology 1989;31:89–92.

33. Mattle H, Sieb J, Rohner M, et al: Nontraumatic spinal epidural and subdural hematomas. Neurology 1987;37:1351–1356.

34. Cooper DW: Spontaneous spinal epidural hematoma. Case report. J Neurosurg 1967;26:343–345.

35. Beatty RM, Winston KR: Spontaneous cervical epidural hematoma. A consideration of etiology. J Neurosurg 1984;61:143–148.

36. Horlocker TT, Wedel DJ, Benzon HT, et al: Regional anesthesia in the anticoagulated patient: Defining the risks (The second ASRA consensus conference on neuraxial anesthesia and anticoagulation). Reg Anesth Pain Med 2003;28:172–197.

37. Pahapill PA, Lownie SP: Conservative treatment of acute spontaneous spinal epidural hematoma. Can J Anaesth 1998;25:159–163.

38. Schwarz SK, Wong CL, McDonald WN: Spontaneous recovery from a spinal epidural hematoma with atypical presentation in a nonagenarian. Can J Anesth 2004;51:557–561.

39. Wolfgang P, Klaus M: Spinal hematoma unrelated to previous surgery: Analysis of 15 consecutive cases treated in a single institution within a 10-year period. Spine 2004;24:555–561.

40. Vandermeulen EP, Van Aken H, Vermylen J: Anticoagulants and spinal-epidural anesthesia. Anesth Analg 1994;79:1165–1177.

41. Hejazi N, Thaper PY, Hassler W: Nine cases of nontraumatic spinal epidural hematoma. Neurol Med Chir 1998;38:718–723.

42. Groen RT, Van Alphen HA: Operative treatment of spontaneous spinal epidural hematomas: A study of the factors determining postoperative outcome. Neurosurgery 1996;39:494–502.

43. Enomato T, Maki Y, Nakagawa K, et al: Spontaneous spinal epidural hematoma: Report of a case. Neurol Surg 1980;8:875–880.

44. Rohde V, Küker W, Reinges MHT, et al: Microsurgical treatment of spontaneous and non-spontaneous spinal epidural hematomas: Neurological outcome in relation to aetiology. Acta Neurochir 2000;142:787–793.

45. Klein SM, D'Ercole F, Greengrass RA, et al: Enoxaparin associated with psoas hematoma and lumbar plexopathy after lumbar plexus block. Anesthesiology 1997;87:1576–1579.

46. Weller RS, Gerancher JC, Crews JC, et al: Extensive retroperitoneal hematoma without neurologic deficit in two patients who underwent lumbar plexus block and were later anticoagulated. Anesthesiology 2003;98:581–583.

47. Maier C, Gleim M, Weiss T, et al: Severe bleeding following lumbar sympathetic blockade in two patients under medication with irreversible platelet aggregation inhibitors. Anesthesiology 2002;97:740–743.

48. Antonelli D, Fares L, Anene C: Enoxaparin associated with huge abdominal wall hematomas: A report of two cases. Am Surgeon 2000;66:797–800.

49. Dickinson LD, Miller L, Patel CP, et al: Enoxaparin increases the incidence of postoperative intracranial hemorrhage when initiated preoperatively for deep vein thrombosis prophylaxis with brain tumors. Neurosurgery 1998;43:1074–1081.

50. Ho KJ, Gawley SD, Young MR: Psoas hematoma and femoral neuropathy associated with enoxaparin therapy. Int J Clin Pract 2003;57:553–554.

51. Houde JP, Steinberg G: Intrahepatic hemorrhage after use of low-molecular-weight heparin for total hip arthroplasty. J Arthroplasty 1999;14:372–374.

52. Aida S, Takahashi H, Shimoji K: Renal subcapsular hematoma after lumbar plexus block. Anesthesiology 1996;84:452–455.

72

Infection Control in Regional Anesthesia

Sebastian Schulz-Stübner, MD • Jean M. Pottinger, RN, MA • Stacy A. Coffin, MD • Loreen A. Herwaldt, MD

I. INTRODUCTION

II. PATHOGENESIS OF INFECTIONS ASSOCIATED WITH CENTRAL NEURAXIAL BLOCKADE

III. INFECTIONS ASSOCIATED WITH EPIDURAL BLOCKADE

IV. INFECTIONS ASSOCIATED WITH SUBARACHNOID BLOCKADE

V. INFECTIONS ASSOCIATED WITH COMBINED EPIDURAL & SUBARACHNOID BLOCKADE

VI. INFECTIONS ASSOCIATED WITH PERIPHERAL NERVE BLOCKS

VII. PREVENTION OF INFECTIONS ASSOCIATED WITH REGIONAL ANESTHESIA

VIII. SUMMARY

 INTRODUCTION

Infectious complications related to regional anesthesia are rare. Since the only information is available in case reports and retrospective surveys, it is likely that these complications are underreported. The objective of this chapter is to summarize information from the literature on infections associated with regional anesthesia, as well as to discuss the mechanism and to suggest strategies to prevent these complications.

PATHOGENESIS OF INFECTIONS ASSOCIATED WITH CENTRAL NEURAXIAL BLOCKADE

Microorganisms from exogenous or endogenous sources may gain access to the subarachnoid, epidural, or tissue space surrounding peripheral nerves in several ways. Microorganisms from the patient's or anesthesia practitioner's flora can be inoculated directly when a catheter or needle is inserted into those spaces. Several reports in the literature suggest that infections are on occasion caused by the anesthesia practitioner's flora.[1–3] For example, Trautmann and colleagues reported a case of meningitis caused by a *Staphylococcus aureus* strain that was identical by pulsed-field gel electrophoresis to the *S. aureus* isolate from the anesthesiologist's nose.[2] Microorganisms can also enter the epidural space by hematogenous spread from other body sites, such as infected skin,[2,4] or by migrating along the catheter tract.[5,6] Several case reports suggested that infection was caused by spread of bacteria from infected sites through the bloodstream to the epidural space.[7–9] Others maintain that infections at distal sites are *not* contraindications to epidural anesthesia. For example, Newman concluded that distal infections did not increase the risk of epidural infection because traumatic injuries are often infected and no epidural catheter-related infections were identified among over 3000 patients who had epidural neural blockades for postoperative or posttraumatic analgesia.[10] The anesthetic agents injected into the patient's subarachnoid or epidural space are another possible source of infection. Infections from contaminated multidose vials are likely to be rare because most anesthetic drugs are weak bases dissolved in acidic solutions that inhibit growth of bacteria and fungi[11–13]; besides most multidose local anesthetic solutions contain a bacteriostatic agent. Nevertheless, the case report by North and Brophy suggests that contaminated multidose vials still can be a source of infection. These authors reported an infection in which *S. aureus* isolates with matching phage types were recovered from an abscess and a multidose lidocaine vial.[1]

Clinical Pearls

- Streptococcal species, *S. aureus,* and *Pseudomonas aeruginosa* are the most common causative agents.

- Microorganisms from the patient's or anesthesia practitioner's flora can be inoculated directly when a catheter or needle is inserted into the epidural or subarachnoid space.

- Because it is easy to contaminate the needle or the catheters, anesthesiologists must strictly adhere to hygienic measures.

To assess whether contamination of the anesthetic agent or the equipment (needles, syringes, tubing) is related to subsequent infections, investigators have cultured these items after they have been used with patients or during simulations. In four studies, 0–29% of used catheters were contaminated,[14–17] and James and coworkers found that 5 of 101 syringes used to inject anesthetic agents were contaminated.[14] Ross and coworkers drew up 0.25% bupivacaine into control syringes and into syringes used to induce continuous lumbar epidural neural blockade (test syringe) in 18 obstetric patients.[18] After each dose from the test syringe, the investigators cultured the contents of both the test and control syringes. Six of 18 test syringes were contaminated with bacteria, compared with only 1 of 18 control syringes. Raedler and associates cultured 114 spinal and 20 epidural needles after use for single lumbar injections.[19] Twenty-four cultures (17.9%) grew microorganisms: 15.7% coagulase-negative staphylococci, 1.5% yeasts, 0.8% each enterococci, pneumococci, and micrococci. These authors concluded that it is easy to contaminate the needle and that anesthesiologists need to improve their hygienic measures. Despite finding contaminated equipment or anesthetic solutions, these investigators did not identify any infected patients,[14–18] and thus, none of the authors were able to correlate contamination with infection.

INFECTIONS ASSOCIATED WITH EPIDURAL BLOCKADE

There are numerous case reports in the literature of infections occurring after epidural neuraxial blockade, attesting to the fact that such complications can be severe (Table 72–1).[1,7,9,19–55] Thirty-five of 48 patients in these case reports acquired epidural or intraspinal abscesses. Three patients had injections only, 1 patient had injections and several catheters, and 47 patients had catheters. Among the 38 patients who had catheters and for whom the duration of catheterization was specified, the median duration of catheterization was 3 days (range 50 min to 6 weeks). The median time to onset of the first signs or symptoms of infection was 4 days (range 1–4.8 months) after catheter placement. *S. aureus* caused 27 of 42 infections from which bacterial pathogens were isolated. *P. aeruginosa* caused five infections and *Streptococcus* spp. caused five. Three patients died and 27 nearly or fully recovered.

It should be kept in mind that the number of reported cases does not allow us to assess the true frequency of infections after epidural neural blockade. However, several investigators have done studies to assess this risk. When reviewing 350 reports in the literature, Dawkins found no reports of infection after thoracic or lumbar epidural block, but he identified 8 (0.2%) reports of infection after 3767 sacral epidural blocks used for operative procedures and for obstetrics 1969.[56] More recently, Dawson reviewed the literature and found rates of deep infection ranging from 0 to 0.7% and rates of superficial infection ranging from 1.8 to 12%.[57]

Scott and Hibbard surveyed all obstetrics units in the United Kingdom and identified 1 epidural abscess in approximately 506,000 epidural neural blocks.[58] In contrast, Palot and colleagues identified 3 cases of meningitis in 300,000 patients who had undergone epidural blocks.[59] Three smaller series of obstetric epidural neural blockades (some 12,000 patients) did not identify any infections.[60–62] Similarly, in a recent study by the French SOS group on complications of regional anesthesia Auroy and coworkers did not identify any infections in 29,732 epidural neural blocks given for obstetrical procedures.[63] Together, the results of these five studies suggest that 4–5 serious infectious complications (ie, epidural abscesses or meningitis) occur per 1 million obstetric epidural neural blocks.

A number of studies have assessed infections associated with epidural neural blockades done for operative procedures or for short-term pain relief. However, these studies report fewer patients than the studies of epidural neural blockade for obstetric procedures. We summarized findings from nine studies in Table 72–2.[47,51,63–69] Brooks and associates found 4 infections among 4832 (0.08%) patients undergoing epidural neuraxial blockade for surgical procedures or for labor and delivery.[70] All four infections occurred in healthy young women who underwent cesarean sections; two infections were superficial (0.04%), and two involved the epidural space (0.04%). In contrast, Holt and colleagues reported 53 (1.8%)

Table 72–1.

Infections Associated with Epidural Neural Blockade

Author (Reference)	Year	Indication	Epidural Site	Filter used	Catheter Duration	Type of Infection	Time from Insertion to Symptoms	Signs and Symptoms	Micro-organism	Outcome
Edwards[20]	1943	Vaginal delivery	Caudal	NS	NS	Epidural abscess, bacteremia	NS	NS	*Staphylococcus aureus*	Died 31 days after delivery
Ferguson[21][a]	1974	Postoperative analgesia	Thoracic	NS	2 days	Epidural empyema	4 days / 10 days / 14 days	Fever, headache, meningism / Urinary retention / Paraparesis	*S. epidermidis*	Sensory impairment, spastic weakness, walks with crutches
Saady[22][a]	1976	Postoperative analgesia	Thoracic	Yes	1.7 days	Epidural abscess	4 days / 8 days / 9 days / 10 days / 14 days	Fever / Chills, abdominal pain right upper quadrant / Headache, stiff neck / Urinary retention / Lower extremity paraparesis, no anal tone	*S. aureus*	Sensory impairment, walks with minimal assistance
North[1]	1979	1. Priapism	Lumbar	No	3 days	Epidural abscess	1 day / 10 days	Fever / Stiff neck, dysphagia, back pain, absent ankle jerks	*S. aureus*	Full recovery
		2. Fractured ribs, chest injury	Thoracic	Yes	4 days	Epidural abscess	2 days / 4 days	Fever / Stiff neck, sensory loss T2 to T6	*S. aureus*	Sensory impairment
Wenningsted-Torgard[23][b]	1982	Lower back pain	Lumbar	NS	6 days	Skin abscess, spondylitis, bacteremia	10 days	Fever	*S. aureus*	Wedge formation of two vertebral bodies
McDonogh[24]	1984	Fractured ribs	Thoracic	Yes	3.3 days	Epidural abscess	2.5 days / 19 days	Fever Paralysis left leg, weakness, right leg, urinary retention, sensory deficit T7 to 8	*S. aureus*	Residual left-side weakness, uses walking frame, urinary retention
Konig[25]	1985	Knee surgery	Lumbar	NS	4 days	Paravertebral and epidural abscesses, osteomyelitis, phlegmonous duritis, myelitis	2 weeks	Pain, lower extremity paraparesis	*S. epidermidis*	Nearly complete recovery
Sollmann[26]	1987	Phantom limb pain	NS	NS	6 weeks	Large encapsulated "spinal" abscess compressing dura at L4–5	6 weeks / 5 months	Severe back pain Severe sciatica	*Pseudomonas aeruginosa*	Persistent pain

(cont.)

Table 72–1.

Continued

Author (Reference)	Year	Indication	Epidural Site	Filter used	Catheter Duration	Type of Infection	Time from Insertion to Symptoms	Signs and Symptoms	Micro-organism	Outcome
Fine[27]	1988	Neuralgic pain syndrome	Thoracic	Yes	3 days	Site infection, epidural abscess	9 days	Fever, chills, urinary retention	No culture obtained	Sensory impairment
Ready[28]	1989	1. Vaginal delivery	Lumbar	NS	50 min	Meningitis	1 day	Headache, stiff neck, fever, back pain, nuchal rigidity	*Streptococcus uberis*	Full recovery
		2. Cesarean section	NS	NS	3 days	Cellulitis Meningitis	3.5 days 5.5 days	Fever Headache, nuchal rigidity, photo-phobia, hyperacusis	*Enterococcus faecalis*	Full recovery
Berga[29]	1989	Vaginal delivery	Lumbar	NS	NS	Meningitis	1 day	Headache	*Streptococcus sanguis*	Full recovery
Goucke[30]	1990	Back pain	Lumbar	NS	3 epidural injections	Bacteremia, epidural abscess	3.3 weeks after last injection	Back pain, fever, urinary retention	*Staphylococcus aureus*	Died 7 weeks after laminectomy
Lynch[31]	1990	Intra- and postoperative analgesia	Lumbar	Yes	3 days	Spondylitis	3 days	Fever, chills, headache, back pain	*Pseudomonas aeruginosa*	9-month recovery, wears lumbar brace, some lumbar pain
Strong[32]	1991	1. Herpes zoster[b]	Thoracic	Yes	2.5 days 3 days[c]	Epidural abscess	4.4 weeks	Pain, headache, stiff neck, fever, right flank pain	*S. aureus*	Full recovery
		2. Reflex sympathetic dystrophy	Cervical	Yes	5 days 5 days[c]	Cellulitis Epidural abscess	16 days 7 weeks	Cellulitis Neck pain radiating to left arm	Culture negative	Full recovery
Klygis[33]	1991	Vaginal delivery	NS	NS	NS	Epidural abscess	1.5 days	Back pain, paresthesias medial thigh and plantar surface of feet, fever	Group G streptococci	Full recovery
Dawson[34]	1991	Postoperative analgesia	Thoracic	Yes	4 days	Epidural abscess	12 days 18 days	Numbness and weakness in leg, urinary incontinence Paraplegia	*S. aureus*	Loss of motor function, requires indwelling urinary catheter, able to take few steps with help
Waldmann[142]	1991	Cervical radiculopathy	C6	NS	NS	Epidural abscess	72 h	Stiff neck and chills	*S. aureus*	Quadraparetic with partial function of upper extremities and able to walk

Table 72–1.

Continued

Author (Reference)	Year	Indication	Epidural Site	Filter used	Catheter Duration	Type of Infection	Time from Insertion to Symptoms	Signs and Symptoms	Micro-organism	Outcome
Ferguson[35]	1992	Intra- and postoperative analgesia	Lumbar	Yes	4 days	Cellulitis, epidural infection	7 days	Fever, back pain	*S. aureus*	Not specified
NganKee[36]	1992	Cesarean section	Lumbar	Yes	50 h	Epidural abscess	5 days	Fever, back pain, rigors, bacteremia, paresthesias, weakness of both legs	*S. aureus*	Full recovery after 8 weeks
Sowter[37]	1992	Intra- and postoperative analgesia	Thoracic	Yes	5 days	Epidural abscess	3.6 weeks	Back pain, urinary retention, paresthesias and weakness both legs	*S. aureus*	Paraplegic with indwelling urethral catheter
Shintani[38]	1992	Herpes zoster	Lumbar	NS	3 days	Meningitis, epidural abscess	3 days	Headache, nausea, vomiting, fever, somnolence, back pain	Methicillin-resistant *S. aureus*	Full recovery
Nordstrom[39]	1993	Fractured ribs	Thoracic	Yes	6 days	Epidural abscess	19 days	Back pain, numbness both legs, fever, paresis urethral sphincter	*S. aureus*	Incomplete recovery of motor function 4 months after laminectomy
Mamourian[143]	1993	PVD	L3–4	NS	48 h	Epidural abscess	72 h	Lower extremity radicular pain and weakness, urinary retention	*S. aureus*	Full recovery
		Low back pain	NS	NS	Single shot	Epidural abscess	2 weeks	Worsening pain, leg weakness, urinary retention	*S. aureus*	Died from ventricular tachycardia
		PVD	NS	NS	Single shot	Epidural abscess	24 h 4 days	Fever Leg spasm	*S. aureus*	No neurologic deficit
Davis[40]	1993	Vaginal delivery	Lumbar	NS	Less than 1 day	Meningitis	1.7 days	Headache, vomiting, confusion, delirium, fever	Group B β-hemolytic streptococci	Full recovery
Ania[41b]	1994	Lumbar pain	NS	NS	8 days	Meningitis	1 day 3 days	Headache Chills, vomiting	*S. aureus*	Full recovery
Tabo[143]	1994	Herpes zoster	L3–4	NS	3 days	Epidural abscess	4 days	Fever, fatigue, pain	*S. aureus*	Full recovery
Borum[42]	1995	Vaginal delivery	Lumbar	Yes	1 day	Epidural abscess	4 days	Low back pain, tingling both lower extremities	*S. aureus*	Full recovery
							6 days	Weakness both lower extremities		

(cont.)

| Table 72–1. |
| Continued |

Author (Reference)	Year	Indication	Epidural Site	Filter used	Catheter Duration	Type of Infection	Time from Insertion to Symptoms	Signs and Symptoms	Micro-organism	Outcome
Liu[43]	1996	Extracorporeal shockwave lithotripsy	NS	NS	NS	Meningitis	2 days	Headache, photophobia	*Streptococcus pneumoniae*	Full recovery
Dunn[44]	1996	Intra- and postoperative analgesia	NS	NS	1 day	Epidural abscess, osteomyelitis	1 day 14 days	Neck and back pain Back pain, nausea, vomiting, fever	*S. aureus*	Mild hip and loin pain 5 months after the operation
Cooper[45b]	1996	Chronic back pain	Not specified	NS	Injection	Meningitis, cauda equina syndrome	3 days 13 days	Increased back pain, chills, profuse sweating Leg weakness, incontinent of stool	*S. aureus*	Incontinent of stool
Barontini[46]	1996	Transurethral resection of prostate	Lumbar	NS	NS	Epidural abscess	2 days 4 days	Fever, leg weakness Chills, pain, flaccid paraparesis of leg	No culture obtained	Paraplegia
Pinczower[7]	1996	Postoperative analgesia	Lumbar	NS	4 days	L1 vertebral osteomyelitis	3 weeks	Low back pain	*P. aeruginosa*	Full recovery
Wang[144]	1996	RSD	L2–3 and L3–4 (total of 4 catheters during 4 weeks)	NS	4 weeks	Small epidural abscess with meningeal irritation	?	Nuchal rigidity, back pain, nausea, photophobia, severe headache	Not identified	Full recovery
Bengtsson[9]	1997	1. Analgesia after a traumatic amputation	L3–4 T12–L1	Yes	1 day[c] 4 days	Meningitis	4 days	Fever, pain and erythema at 2nd insertion site, stiff neck	*P. aeruginosa*	Full recovery
		2. Analgesia for phantom pains after an amputation	Lumbar	Yes	3 days	Soft tissue and interspinal abscess	3 days	Fever, severe headache, erythema *S. aureus* and swelling at insertions site, back pain radiating to right thigh	No culture obtained	Radicular pain in lower back
		3. Analgesia for painful foot ulcers	Lumbar tunneled catheter	Yes	16 days	Psoas abscess at L2 to L5 tracking to L3–4 intraspinal level	11 days 14 days	Fever Pain radiating from back	*S. aureus*	Full recovery
Sarubbi[47]	1997	1. Analgesia for reflex sympathetic dystrophy	L1–2	NS	3 days	Epidural abscess	3 days	High fever, cloudy drainage at catheter exit site	*S. aureus*	Recovered to her baseline

Table 72–1.

Continued

Author (Reference)	Year	Indication	Epidural Site	Filter used	Catheter Duration	Type of Infection	Time from Insertion to Symptoms	Signs and Symptoms	Micro-organism	Outcome
		2. Surgical anesthesia & postoperative analgesia	NS	NS	2 days	Epidural abscess & meningitis	2 days / 5 days	Bilateral leg weakness and double vision / Flaccid paralysis, double vision from 3rd nerve palsy, meningism, sensory level L1	*S. aureus*	Ambulated with a walker at 3 months
Iseki[48]	1998	Analgesia for herpes zoster	11 epidural injections then catheters at T6–7 T8–9 T7–8	NS	4 days[c] 1 day 6 days	Epidural abscess at T6–7 and inflammation of the perivertebral muscles at T5 to 7	6 days after the final catheterization	Fever, elevated white blood count and C-reactive protein	Methicillin-resistant *S. aureus*	Full recovery
O'Brien[49]	1999	Analgesia for low back pain	1 epidural injection	NS	Not applicable	Epidural abscess	3 months	Back pain, bilateral lower extremity pain	*Mycobacterium fortuitum*	Full recovery
Halkic[50]	2001	Postoperative analgesia	T11–12	NS	4 days	Spondylodiscitis at L5–S1	4 days	Lumbar pain radiating to the groin	*Propionibacterium acnes*	Full recovery
Phillips[51]	2002	1. Postoperative analgesia	Thoracic	NS	3 days	Epidural abscess	4 days 5 days	Fever Low backache, headache, tenderness at insertion site	*S. aureus*	Full recovery
		2. Postoperative analgesia	Thoracic	NS	3 days	Epidural abscess	3 weeks	Pain at insertion site, weakness in lower extremities, urinary retention	Methicillin-resistant *S. aureus*	Died of a pulmonary embolus and cardiac arrest
Royakkers[52]	2002	1. Postoperative analgesia	L2–3	Yes	4 days	Epidural abscess	3 days 4 days 5 days 7 days	Fever Elevated ESR, WBC, C-reactive protein Erythema at exit site Pus at insertion site	*S. aureus*	Full recovery
		2. Postoperative analgesia	T7–8	NS	5 days	Epidural abscess	6 days	Erythema and pus at insertion site	*S. aureus*	Full recovery
		3. Postoperative analgesia	T10–11	NS	3 days	Epidural abscess	7 days	Signs of local infection, back pain, fever to 39°C	*S. aureus*	Full recovery
Hagiwara[53]	2003	Postoperative analgesia	Low thoracic	NS	NS	Epidural abscess	4.8 months	Fever, back pain, neck stiffness, coma, and quadriplegia	Methicillin-resistant *S. aureus*	Nearly full recovery

(cont.)

Table 72–1.

Continued

Author (Reference)	Year	Indication	Epidural Site	Filter used	Catheter Duration	Type of Infection	Time from Insertion to Symptoms	Signs and Symptoms	Micro-organism	Outcome
Evans[54]	2003	Labor analgesia	Lumbar	Yes	NS	Epidural abscess	7 days	Back and leg pain	NS	Incomplete recovery
							9 days	Hot and cold flushes, flu-like illness, pain from back down both legs		
							11 days	Fever, dehydration, tachycardia		
							12 days	Unable to bear weight or pass urine, sensation decreased below knees		
Yue[55]	2003	Low back pain	Caudal	NS in abstract	NS in abstract	Discitis	4 weeks	Low back pain, elevated serum acute-phase reactants, radiographic evidence of L4–L5 discitis	*P. aeruginosa*	Full recovery

[a] *Although discrepancies exist in the two reports, these articles may report the same patient.*
[b] *Patient was given epidural anesthetic agents and epidural steroids.*
[c] *Patient had more than one epidural catheter.*
NS = not specified, PVD = peripheral vascular disease, ESR = erythrocyte sedimentation rate, WBC = white blood cell count.
Adapted, with permission, from Hospital Epidemiology and Infection Control, *3rd ed. C. G. Mayhall (ed): Lippincott Williams & Wilkins, 2004.*

local infections and 11 (0.4%) central nervous system infections related to approximately 3000 epidural catheters.[71,72] The median duration of catheterization was 8 days for patients with local infections and 15 days for those with generalized symptoms ($p = 0.01$). Catheters removed from patients with clinical symptoms were more heavily colonized than those removed from asymptomatic patients. However, 59 of 78 catheters with positive cultures were removed because patients were symptomatic, suggesting that this observation may have been affected by ascertainment bias.

Clinical Pearls

- Studies suggest that 4–5 serious infectious complications (ie, epidural abscesses or meningitis) occur per 1 million epidural blocks.
- Epidural catheters inserted for long-term pain control become infected more frequently than those used for short periods of time.

- Malignancy and reduced immunocompetence might be additional risk factors in the long-term catheter population.
- Case reports of infections occurring after epidural neuraxial blockade point out that complications from infection can be severe and often lead to epidural or intraspinal abscesses.

Given that the number of infections identified in any study has been low, the results reported by investigators who calculated the upper boundaries of the infection risk associated with epidural neural blockade are particularly important because they provide a better estimate of the true risk than do studies that report only the number of infections and the number of procedures. For example, Strafford and coworkers did not identify skin infections or epidural abscesses among 1458 pediatric patients who had epidural analgesia to control perioperative pain.[73] These investigators calculated the incidence of clinical infection to be 0 with a 95%

Table 72–2.

Infections after Epidural Neural Blockades Done for Surgical Procedures or Short-Term Pain Relief

Author (Reference)	Year Published	Number of Patients	Number of Infections
Hunt[17]	1977	102	1 cellulitis
Sethna[64]	1992	1200 children	0
Darchy[65]	1996	75	9 local infections, 4 of which were associated with catheter infections
McNeeley[66]	1997	91	0
Abel[67]	1998	4392	0
Grass[68]	1998	5193	1 exit site infection
Kost-Byerly[69]	1998	210 children	21/170 (12.3%) of caudal catheters, 1/40 (2.5%) lumbar catheters were associated with cellulitis
Phillips[51]	2002	2401	3 epidural infections
Auroy[63]	2002	5561	1 meningitis

Data from Hospital Epidemiology and Infection Control, *3rd ed. C. G. Mayhall (ed): Lippincott Williams & Wilkins, 2004.*

confidence interval from 0% to 0.03%, or 3 infections per 10,000 procedures. Auroy and colleagues, as noted previously, did not identify any infections among 29,732 procedures done for deliveries.[63] They calculated 95% confidence intervals of 0/10,000 to 1/10,000 procedures. Darchy and associates evaluated 75 patients, 9 (12%; incidence density rate of 2.7/100 catheter days) of whom acquired local infections. None of the patients acquired deep infections.[65] Based on these data, Darchy and associates estimated the upper risk of spinal space infections to be 4.8% for catheters that remained in place for 4 days. Of note, these estimates are considerably higher than those of Strafford and coworkers[73] and higher even than the rates found by Du Pen and associates among patients with epidural catheters for long-term pain control[74] (see next paragraph).

In general, epidural catheters inserted for long-term pain control become infected more frequently than those used for short periods of time. Du Pen and associates identified 30 superficial (9.3/10,000 catheter-days), 8 deep catheter track (2.5/10,000 catheter-days), and 15 epidural space (4.6/10,000 catheter-days) infections among 350 patients who had long-term epidural catheters.[74] Similarly, Zenz and colleagues identified two cases of meningitis among 139 patients (1.4%, or 2.1/10,000 catheter-days) treated for pain due to malignancy.[75] Coombs reported that 10 of 92 (10.9%) cancer patients acquired local infections, and 2 (2.2%) acquired meningitis.[76] Malignancy and reduced immunocompetence might be additional risk factors in the long-term catheter population.

INFECTIONS ASSOCIATED WITH SUBARACHNOID BLOCKADE

Case reports in the literature indicate that serious infections can occur as complications of subarachnoid neural blockade (Table 72–3).[2,3,5,6,77–91] Of the 26 infections reported in these case reports, 8 were meningitis, 4 were epidural abscesses, 2 were soft tissue abscesses, and 2 were infections of a disk or of a disk space. The median time to onset of signs or symptoms of infection was 1 day (range 1 h to 2 months) for all infections and 18 h (range 1 h to 10 days for meningitis). Streptococcal species caused 11 of the 23 infections from which bacterial pathogens were identified, and *S. aureus* caused 2 infections and *Pseudomonas* spp. caused 4. Twenty-one patients recovered fully. Compared with infections after epidural neural blockade, infections associated with subarachnoid neural blockade were more likely to be caused by streptococci, and patients were more likely to recover fully. Table 72–4 reviews data from nine studies or reviews, which, if taken together, suggest that the rate of infection is approximately 3.7 per 100,000 subarachnoid neural blockades.[63,91–98]

INFECTIONS ASSOCIATED WITH COMBINED EPIDURAL & SUBARACHNOID BLOCKADE

At present there are few reports in the literature about infectious complications of using combined epidural and subarachnoid neural blockade (CSE). We identified eight case reports of infections (nine infections) after combined procedures[51,99–105] (Table 72–5). The median time to onset of signs or symptoms or infection was 21 h (range 8 h to 9 days) for all infections and 18 h (range 8 h to 3 days) for meningitis. Signs or symptoms of epidural abscesses were first noted 1–9 days after the procedures. Streptococcal species caused three of six cases of meningitis and *S. aureus* caused all three epidural abscesses. Eight of nine patients recovered fully. We identified only one study that assessed rates of infection associated with combined procedures. Cascio and Heath identified 1 case

Table 72–3.

Infections Associated with Subarachnoid Neural Blockade

Author (Reference)	Year	Indication	Type of Infection	Incubation Period	Signs and Symptoms	Micro-organism	Outcome	Comments
Corbett[78]	1971	1. Vaginal delivery	Meningitis	36 h	Fever, headache, stiff neck	*Pseudomonas aeruginosa*	Full recovey	Three patients infected when a physician rinsed the spinal needle stylet in saline used for consecutive deliveries
		2. Vaginal delivery	Meningitis	3 days	Fever, headache, stiff neck, neck pain, nuchal rigidity	*P. aeruginosa*	Full recovery	
		3. Vaginal delivery	Meningitis	4 days	Fever, headache, nausea	*P. aeruginosa*	Full recovery	
Siegel[79]	1974	Vaginal delivery	Left subgluteal abscess	4 h / 14 days	Buttock pain radiating to thigh / Severe pain sacroiliac joint	Mimeae	Full recovery	
Loarie[5]	1978	Debride necrotic heel ulcers	Epidural abscess	2 days / 15 days	Fever, back pain, urinary retention / Bilateral lower extremity weakness, absent anal sphincter tone	*Staphylococcus epidermidis, Bacteroides*	Full recovery	Insulin-dependent diabetic
Berman[6]	1978	Transurethral evacuation of clot from bladder	Meningitis	1 h	Shaking chill, fever, back pain, headache, confusion	*Enterococcus*	Not specified	
Beaudoin[80]	1984	Debride and drain infected foot	Epidural abscess	4 days after last subarachnoid neural blockade	Back pain, pain radiating to upper thighs	*Pseudomonas* spp.	Full recovery	35-year-old insulin-dependent diabetic, received 5 subarachnoid neural blockades in 10 days
Abdel-Magid[81]	1990	Hemorrhoidectomy	Epidural abscess	15 days	Back pain, leg weakness, urinary retention, fever, bilateral absent ankle reflexes	*Proteus* spp.	Full recovery	
Roberts[82]	1990	Remove retained placenta	Meningitis	18 h	Headache, photophobia, fever, chills, positive Kernig's sign, quadriceps weakness	Culture negative	Full recovery	Antibiotics started before the lumbar puncture
Lee[83]	1991	Cesarean section	Meningitis	16 h / 22 h	Severe headache / Nausea, photophobia, decreasing mental status, fever, nuchal rigidity, positive Kernig's sign	Culture negative	Full recovery	
Blackmore[84]	1993	Herniorrhaphy	Meningitis and bacteremia	16 h	Fever, vomiting, obtundation	*Streptococcus mitis*	Full recovery	
Ezri[85]	1994	Hemorrhoidectomy	Meningitis	10 days / 25 days	Fever / Malaise, headache, photophobia, dizziness, fever	*Escherichia coli*	Full recovery	
Mahendru[86]	1994	Foot amputation	Epidural abscess	3 weeks	Back pain, bilateral lower extremity paresis and weakness	No culture obtained	Died from esophageal carcinoma	Insulin-dependent diabetic

Table 72–3.

(*Continued*)

Author (Reference)	Year	Indication	Type of Infection	Incubation Period	Signs and Symptoms	Micro-organism	Outcome	Comments
Gebhard[87]	1994	Knee arthroscopy	Diskitis	2 months	Back and thigh pain, elevated sedimentation rate	*Propioni-bacterium acnes*	Full recovery	
Newton[88]	1994	Vaginal delivery	Meningitis	12 h	Headache, photophobia, declining mental status, fever	*Streptococcus salivarius*	Full recovery	
Schneeberger[3]	1996	1. Knee arthroscopy	Meningitis	12 h	Fever, meningeal signs	*Streptococcus sanguis*	Full recovery	
		2. Knee arthroscopy	Meningitis	12 h 2 days	Headache Fever, meningeal signs	*S. mitis*	Full recovery	
		3. Varicose vein stripping	Meningitis	24 h	Headache, fever, impaired consciousness, meningeal signs	*S. salivarius*	Full recovery	
		4. Varicose vein stripping	Meningitis	12 h	Headache, fever	*Streptococcus cremoris*	Communicating hydro-cephalus	Hydrocephalus may have been preexisting
Horlocker[91]	1997	1. Urologic procedure	Disk space infection	1 day 4 months	Low back pain Incapacitating low back pain	*Staphylococcus aureus*	Full recovery	
		2. Examination under anesthesia	Paraspinal abscess	1 day 11 days	Low back pain Fever	*S. aureus*	Full recovery	
Kaiser[89]	1997	Hysterectomy	Meningitis	12 h	High fever, severe headache, lumbar pain, lethargy, Glasgow score of 12, nuchal rigidity, positive Kernig's and Brudzinski's signs	*S. salivarius*	Full recovery	
Laurila[146]	1998	Arthroscopy	Meningitis	16 h	Headache, nausea, vomiting	*S. salivarius*	Full recovery	Anesthesiologist wore mask, gloves and used chlorhexidine–alcohol solution for skin preparation
Fernandez[90]	1999	Arthroscopic meniscectomy	Meningitis	18 h	Severe headache, nausea, vomiting, high fever, nuchal rigidity	*S. mitis*	Full recovery	
Yaniv[77]	2000	Extracorporeal shock wave lithotripsy for ureterolithiasis	Meningitis	12 h	Fever, severe headache, meningeal signs, elevated white blood cell count	*S. salivarius*	Minor sequelae, mild paresthesia of right thigh	Anesthesiologist wore gown, sterile gloves, face mask
Trautmann[2]	2002	Arthroscopic knee repair	Meningitis	1 day	Fever, nausea, stiff neck	*S. salivarius*	Full recovery	Both patients underwent their operations the same day
		Arthroscopic knee repair	Meningitis	1 day	Headache, nausea, stiff neck	*S. salivarius*	Full recovery	

Adapted, with permission, from Hospital Epidemiology and Infection Control, *3rd ed. C. G. Mayhall (ed): Lippincott Williams & Wilkins, 2004.*

Table 72–4.				
Frequency of Meningitis after Subarachnoid Neural Blockade				
Author (Reference)	**Year**	**Number of patients**	**Number of Infections**	**Rate of Meningitis**
Evans[92]	1945	2,500	0	0
Scarborough[93]	1958	5,000	0	0
Dripps[94]	1954	8,460	0	0
Moore[95]	1966	11,574	0	0
Lund[96]	1968	>21,000	0	0
Sadove[97]	1961	>20,000	3	≈15/100,000
Arner[98]	1952	21,230	1	4.7/100,000
Horlocker[91]	1997	4,217	0	0
Auroy[63]	2002	5,640 Obstetrical	0	0
Auroy[63]	2002	35,439 Nonobstetrical	1	2.8/100,000
TOTAL		>135,060	5	≈3.7/100,000

Adapted, with permission, from Hospital Epidemiology and Infection Control, *3rd ed. C. G. Mayhall (ed): Lippincott Williams & Wilkins, 2004.*

of meningitis after about 700 (≈0.1%) combined epidural and subarachnoid neural blockades.[99]

INFECTIONS ASSOCIATED WITH PERIPHERAL NERVE BLOCKS

Continuous regional anesthetic techniques utilizing peripheral nerve blocks have become more popular in recent years for postoperative pain management especially for orthopedic procedures.[106,107] Only a few studies have addressed infectious complications related to these procedures. The study by Auroy and coworkers of French anesthesiologists did not identify any infections after 43,946 peripheral blocks.[63] Bergman and colleagues identified 1 patient among 368 patients (405 axillary catheters) who had a local *S. aureus* skin infection in the axilla after 48 h of axillary analgesia.[108] The patient recovered fully with antibiotic treatment. Meier and colleagues reported 8 superficial skin infections among 91 patients who had continuous interscalene catheters for an average of 5 days.[109] Nseir describes a case of fatal streptococcal necrotizing fasciitis following axillary brachial plexus block.[110] Adam reported a psoas abscess complicating femoral nerve block catheter.[111]

Cuvillion and coworkers obtained cultures of 208 femoral catheters when they were removed after 48 h.[112] Fifty-four percent of the catheters were colonized with potentially pathogenic bacteria (71% *Staphylococcus epidermidis*, 10% *Enterococcus* spp., and 4% *Klebsiella* spp.). These investigators

also reported three episodes of transient bacteremia, but they did not identify any abscesses or episodes of clinical sepsis.[110] None of the groups provided information about the aseptic techniques used for catheter insertion.

Other reports include cases of osteomyelitis following digital blocks[113] and hematoma block for fracture repair,[114] as well as orbital cellulites from sub-Tenon's anesthesia.[115,116]

All these reports emphasize the importance of maintaining strict asepsis when performing continuing peripheral nerve blocks.

PREVENTION OF INFECTIONS ASSOCIATED WITH REGIONAL ANESTHESIA

To date there is no consensus regarding infection control measures that are necessary when administering central neuraxial blockades. Most anesthesiologists agree that they should prepare the patient's skin with an antimicrobial agent, wash their hands with an antimicrobial soap, and wear sterile gloves. However, anesthesiologists disagree about the necessity of other precautions.[117–123] For example, several surveys indicate that only 50–66% of anesthesia staff wear masks when performing epidural and subarachnoid neural blockades.[124–126]

The review of studies on infections associated with epidural anesthesia indicates that there is no consensus regarding patient risk factors for infectious complications of epidural neural blockade.[107] Few studies have been designed

Table 72–5.

Infections Associated with Combined Subarachnoid and Epidural Neural Blockade

Author (Reference)	Year	Indication	Type of Infection	Time of Symptom Onset	Signs and Symptoms	Micro-organism	Outcome	Comments
Cascio[99]	1995	Vaginal delivery	Meningitis	16 h after delivery, ≈20 h after insertion	Fever, headache, chills, photophobia, mild nuchal rigidity	*Streptococcus salivarius*	Full recovery	Anesthesiologist wore mask, cap, and sterile gloves, and used povidone–iodine spray for skin antisepsis
Harding[100]	1994	1. Vaginal delivery	Aseptic meningitis	21 h after the injection	Severe headache, faint feeling, shortness of breath, urinary retention, aphasia, tingling right side of face, neck stiffness, positive Kernig's sign, low-grade temperature	No growth	Full recovery	Anesthesiologist scrubbed, wore sterile gown and gloves, and used alcoholic chlorhexidine for skin antisepsis
		2. Vaginal delivery converted to emergency cesarean section	Meningitis	3 days after the operation	Headache, fever, vomiting, severe stiff neck, elevated white blood cell count, hypotension, bradycardia	*Staphylococcus epidermidis*	Full recovery	Alcoholic chlorhexidine used for skin antisepsis
Stallard[101]	1994	Analgesia during labor, subsequent cesarean section	Meningitis	18 h after the operation	Acute confusion, fever, aphasia, ignored left side, elevated white blood cell count	No growth	Full recovery	Did three procedures to achieve adequate analgesia; anesthesiologist used alcoholic chlorhexidine for skin antisepsis and wore mask, gown, and gloves
Aldebert[103]	1996	Vaginal delivery	Meningitis	8 h after puncture	Headache, nausea, fever, agitation, nuchal rigidity, positive Babinski sign	Nonhemolytic streptococcus	Full recovery	Anesthesiologist wore mask, gown, cap, and sterile gloves
Dysart[103]	1997	Cesarean section	Epidural abscess	9 days after the operation	Backache, fever, foot drop, weakness of ankle eversion and inversion, absent ankle jerk reflex, decrease pinprick sensation from L5 to perianal region, elevated erythrocyte sedimentation rate	*Staphylococcus aureus*	Nearly full recovery; patient had residual numbness in L5 distribution	Anesthesiologist wore a mask, gown, and gloves and used chlorhexidine for skin antisepsis
Schroter[104]	1997	Anesthesia for vascular surgery	Epidural abscess	1 day after procedure	Back pain, fever, slight nuchal rigidity, erythema and induration at puncture site and purulent drainage from puncture site, elevated white blood cell count	*S. aureus*	Full recovery	Anesthesiologist wore a mask, surgical hood, sterile gloves, and gown and used povidone–iodine for skin antisepsis
Bouhemad[105]	1998	Cesarean section	Meningitis	14 h after delivery	Fever, severe headache, photophobia, drowsiness, stiff neck, positive Kernig's sign	*S. salivarius*	Full recovery	Anesthesiologist wore gown, gloves, face mask, and cap and used tincture of iodine for skin antisepsis
Rathmell[147]	2000	Labor analgesia in pat. with multiple trauma	Epidural abscess	7 days after catheter placement	Back pain, purulent discharge from insertion site	*S. aureus*	Full recovery	
Phillips[51]	2002	Surgical anesthesia and postoperative analgesia	Epidural abscess L1-2	day 6	Discomfort at the epidural site and severe radicular pain in L2 dermatome, erythema and swelling at site, decreased strength, light touch, and pin prick, and loss of ankle jerk reflex	*S. aureus*	Discharged from hospital 3 months after first operation	Anesthesiologist wore a cap, gown, and sterile gloves and used 10% povidone–iodine for skin antisepsis

Adapted, with permission, from Hospital Epidemiology and Infection Control, *3rd ed. C. G. Mayhall (ed): Lippincott Williams & Wilkins, 2004.*

Table 72–6.

Authors' Recommendations for Infection Control Practice

	Single-Shot PNB	Continuous Catheter PNB	Single-Shot Neuraxial Block	Continuous Neuraxial Catheter	Long-Term Implanted Device/Catheter (eg, Intrathecal Pump)
2% Chlorhexidine in 80% alcohol skin prep[a]	+	+	+	+	+
Small sterile drape	(+)		+		
Large sterile drape		+		+	+
Sterile gloves	+	+	+	+	+
Sterile gown		+ (esp. for stimulating catheters)		(+)	+
Mask		(+)	(+)	(+)	+
Hair cover		(+)	(+)	(+)	+
Prophylactic antibiotics	−	−	−	−	(+) single perioperative dose
Filter on injection/infusion system	−	(+)	−	(+)	NA
OR or special procedure room					+
Tunneling of catheter		+ (to prevent dislocation)		+ if used for more than 3 days	
Preparation of injection/infusion solution under sterile conditions (pharmacy)		(+) for continuous infusion		(+) for continuous infusion	

+ *strongly recommended,* (+) *consider,* − *not recommended.*

PNB = peripheral nerve block, NA: Not applicable.

[a]*Alternatively 10% povidone–iodine or 80% alcohol or a mixture of 70–80% alcohol with povidone–iodine for at least 3 min. Choice of agent also depends on type of block (eg, eye blocks etc).*

to assess risk factors for infection associated with epidural or subarachnoid neural blockades, possibly in part because these infections are rare. In fact, we identified only one case-control study that was done to evaluate risk factors for infections associated with epidural neural blockade.[127] Dawson and colleagues evaluated epidural neural blockades done for postoperative pain relief and found that procedures done between April and August had a sixfold higher risk than those done during other months (95% CI 1.28–28.12, $p = 0.009$). The risk of infection was lower if a bag rather than a syringe was used to administer the anesthetic agent (odds ratio 0.17, 95% CI 0.02–1.34, $p = 0.05$). Of the two risk factors identified by this study, only the latter, use of syringes, could be addressed by practice changes.

Assuming that the respiratory tract of anesthesia personnel could be a source of infection, Philips and associates conducted a simulation to assess the efficacy of masks.[128] They seated anesthesia staff in a room with controlled ventilation and asked them to speak directly at blood agar plates placed 30 cm away. The number of bacteria on the plates was significantly lower when masks were worn. However, the clinical significance of this finding is unknown.

Chlorhexidine has been shown to reduce the risk of catheter-associated bloodstream infections significantly compared with povidone–iodine.[129] Several investigators have tried to determine whether a particular disinfectant provides more effective skin antisepsis before epidural neural blocks than do other agents.[130–133] However, none of the studies were large enough to assess rates of infection; instead the outcomes evaluated were catheter or skin colonization. Kasuda and colleagues randomly assigned 70 patients to have their skin prepared with either 0.5% alcoholic solution of chlorhexidine or 10% povidone iodine.[131] After a median of 49 ± 7 h, the investigators removed the catheters and obtained cultures of the insertion sites and catheter tips. There was no difference in rates of positive cultures. Kinirons and associates (the only investigators who reported a power calculation) obtained cultures from catheters removed from 96 children who had epidural catheters longer than 24 h.[132] The colonization rate was lower for catheters removed from children whose skin was prepared with 0.5% alcoholic solution of chlorhexidine (1/52 catheters, 0.9/100 catheter days) than for those removed from children whose skin was prepared with povidone–iodine (5/44 catheters, 5.6/100 catheter days) (relative risk 0.2, 95% CI 0.1–1.0). Sato and coworkers enrolled 60 patients who were undergoing back operations under general anesthesia.[133] After preparing the site with either 0.5% alcoholic chlorhexidine or 10% povidone–iodine, the investigators obtained skin biopsies. Cultures from skin prepared with the alcoholic chlorhexidine were less likely to be positive (5.7%) than were cultures from skin prepared with povidone–iodine (32.4%; $p < 0.01$). However, microscopy was as likely to identify bacteria in the hair follicles of skin prepared with the alcoholic solution of chlorhexidine (14.3%) as skin prepared with povidone–iodine (11.8%).

Clinical Pearls

- Because infections associated with epidural and subarachnoid neural blockade are very infrequent, it is difficult to prove that extreme infection control practices such as wearing masks and using full barrier precautions (ie, the anesthesiologist wears a cap, mask, sterile gloves, and sterile gown and uses a large drape to cover the patient) will reduce the risk of infection.

- Wearing a mask during insertion of indwelling neuraxial or peripheral nerve catheters is suggested because it should allow the anesthesiologist to talk to the patient during the procedure while decreasing the risk of contaminating the insertion site with oral or respiratory flora.

- Surveillance for catheter site infections is one of the most effective methods for reducing the incidence and consequence of indwelling catheter–related infections.

The fact that infections rarely complicate neuraxial blockades suggests that the infection control practices used for these procedures are usually adequate. Given the very low rates of infection associated with epidural and subarachnoid neural blockade, it will be very difficult to prove that additional infection control practices such as wearing masks and using full barrier precautions (ie, the anesthesiologist wears a cap, mask, sterile gloves, and sterile gown and uses a large

drape to cover the patient) reduce the risk of infection. However, bacteria that colonize the skin, respiratory tract, or water caused most reported infections after epidural and subarachnoid neural blockades. Masks have been shown to decrease spread of organisms when anesthesiologists are talking.[128] Thus, a mask would allow the anesthesiologist to talk to the patient while doing the procedure and could decrease the risk of contaminating the insertion site with oral or respiratory flora. Moreover, in the United States, anesthesiologists usually wear masks during operative procedures, even though they are at distance from the operative site. Therefore, it probably makes sense that anesthesia personnel wear masks while performing those procedures.[117] Furthermore, epidural and subarachnoid neural blockades are at least as invasive as placing central venous catheters and the consequences of subsequent infections are at least as bad as those for catheter-associated bloodstream infections. Because the use of full barrier precautions reduces the incidence of catheter-related bloodstream infections,[134] it is possible that hygienic measures similar to those used for placing central venous catheters should be used during the placement of catheters that will remain in place for several days or longer.[57,135]

In addition, we believe that the infusion system should be opened as infrequently as possible and that chlorhexidine should be considered as the agent for preparing the skin before the procedure. Anesthesia personnel should observe their patients closely for signs and symptoms of infection so that infections can be diagnosed and treated immediately. Pegues and coworkers reviewed medical records from 1980 to 1992 of patients who had short-term epidural catheters to identify those who acquired infections. They followed patients prospectively from January 1993 until June 1993.[136] In 1990, they introduced a standardized procedure for inspecting temporary epidural catheters. During the entire 12.5-year period, the investigators identified seven infections, all of which occurred after catheters were inspected routinely. The increased incidence of infection could have resulted from ascertainment or misclassification bias associated with the retrospective review or from increased use of epidural catheters for pain management during the later time period. On the other hand, it could indicate that infections were not diagnosed when catheters were not inspected routinely for signs of infection.

Because it may be difficult to draw up opioids sterilely from ampules, some have suggested that these drugs be drawn through a filter into a syringe that is then double-wrapped and sterilized in ethylene oxide.[137,138] However, the benefit of such extreme precautions is highly hypothetical. Brooks and colleagues implemented the following precautions for continuous central neuraxial blocks done in their hospital:

1. The anesthesiologist should evaluate whether the infusion can be continued if the system becomes disconnected.
2. The exit site should be dressed with a transparent dressing and should be viewed every 8 h or as necessary.
3. A 0.22-μm, 96-h filter should be included in the infusion system.

4. The tubing, filter, and solution should be changed or the system should be discontinued every 96 h.

5. The primary anesthesia and adjuvant bolus dose should be given with a larger syringe that remains attached to the catheter until a continuous analgesia infusion is begun.[70]

To date, there are no published guidelines for placing catheters for peripheral nerve blocks. Recently, new catheter systems have been introduced that require anesthesiologists to perform several manipulations while inserting the catheter.[139] Given the complexity of these manipulations, it is reasonable to assume that aseptic technique similar to that recommended for placement of central venous catheters is warranted.[135]

Other investigators have demonstrated that surveillance for surgical site infections and reporting rates to surgeons is one of the most effective methods for reducing the incidence of and consequence of such infections.[140,141]

SUMMARY

Although rare, infectious complications from regional anesthesia and analgesia do occur and can be serious. Additional studies are necessary to define the rate of infection after different types of regional anesthesia and to identify risk factors for infections. Studies of these are necessary for development of appropriate guidelines for placement and care of catheters used for regional anesthesia. Table 72–6 contains our recommendations for means of decreasing the risk of infections related to regional anesthesia procedures. Future studies and a multicenter surveillance system should be beneficial in addressing some of the unanswered questions about infections after regional anesthesia procedures.

References

1. North JB, Brophy BP: Epidural abscess: A hazard of spinal epidural anaesthesia. Aust N Z J Surg 1979;49:484–485.

2. Trautmann M, Lepper PM, Schmitz FJ: Three cases of bacterial meningitis after spinal and epidural anesthesia. Eur J Clin Microbiol Infect Dis 2002;21:43–45.

3. Schneeberger PM, Janssen M, Voss A: Alpha-hemolytic streptococci: A major pathogen of iatrogenic meningitis following lumbar puncture. Case reports and a review of the literature. Infection 1996;24:29–33.

4. Baker AS, Ojemann RG, Swartz MN, et al: Spinal epidural abscess. N Engl J Med 1975;293:463–468.

5. Loarie DJ, Fairley HB: Epidural abscess following spinal anesthesia. Anesth Analg 1978;57:351–353.

6. Berman RS, Eisele JH: Bacteremia, spinal anesthesia, and development of meningitis. Anesthesiology 1978;48:376–377.

7. Pinczower GR, Gyorke A: Vertebral osteomyelitis as a cause of back pain after epidural anesthesia. Anesthesiology 1996;84:215–217.

8. Wulf H, Striepling E: Postmortem findings after epidural anaesthesia. Anaesthesia 1990;45:357–361.

9. Bengtsson M, Netteblad H, Sjoberg F: Extradural catheter-related infections in patients with infected cutaneous wounds. Br J Anaesth 1997;79:668–670.

10. Newman B: Extradural catheter-related infections in patients with infected cutaneous wounds. Br J Anaesth 1998;80:566.

11. Schmidt RM, Rosenkranz HS: Antimicrobial activity of local anesthetics: Lidocaine and procaine. J Infect Dis 1970;121:597–607.

12. Berry CB, Gillespie T, Hood J, et al: Growth of microorganisms in solutions of intravenous anaesthetic agents. Anaesthesia 1993;48:30–32.

13. Sosis M, Braverman B: Growth of *Staphylococcus aureus* in four intravenous anesthetics. Anesth Analg 1993;77:766–768.

14. James FM, George RH, Naiem H, et al: Bacteriologic aspects of epidural analgesia. Anesth Analg 1976;55:187–190.

15. Shapiro JM, Bond EL, Garman JK: Use of a chlorhexidine dressing to reduce microbial colonization of epidural catheters. Anesthesiology 1990;73:625–631.

16. Barreto RS: Bacteriological culture of indwelling epidural catheters. Anesthesiology 1962;23:643–646.

17. Hunt JR, Rigor BM, Collins JR: The potential for contamination of continuous epidural catheters. Anesth Analg 1977;56:222–225.

18. Ross RM, Burday M, Baker T: Contamination of single dose of bupivacaine vials used repeatedly in the same patient [Abstract]. Anesth Analg 1992;74:S257.

19. Raedler C, Lass-Florl C, Puhringer F, et al: Bacterial contamination of needles used for spinal and epidural anaesthesia. Br J Anaesth 1999;83:657–658.

20. Edwards WB, Hingson RA: The present status of continuous caudal analgesia in obstetrics. N Y Acad Med Bull 1943;19:507–518.

21. Ferguson JF, Kirsch WM: Epidural empyema following thoracic extradural block. Case report. J Neurosurg 1974;41:762–764.

22. Saady A: Epidural abscess complicating thoracic epidural analgesia. Anesthesiology 1976;44:244–246.

23. Wenningsted-Torgard K, Heyn J, Willumsen L. Spondylitis following epidural morphine. Acta Anaesth Scand 1982;26:649–651.

24. McDonogh AJ, Cranney BS: Delayed presentation of an epidural abscess. Anaesth Intensive Care 1984;12:364–365.

25. Konig HJ, Schleep J, Krahling KH: Ein Fall von Querschnittsyndrom nach Kontamination eines Periduralkatheters. Reg Anaesth 1985;8:60–62.

26. Sollman W-P, Gaab MR, Panning B: Lumbales epidurales Hämatom und spinaler Abszess nach Periduralanästhesie. Reg Anaesth 1987;10:121–124.

27. Fine PG, Hare BD, Zahniser JC: Epidural abscess following epidural catheterization in a chronic pain patient: A diagnostic dilemma. Anesthesiology 1988;69:422–424.

28. Ready LB, Helfer D: Bacterial meningitis in parturients after epidural anesthesia. Anesthesiology 1989;71:988–990.

29. Berga S, Trierweiler MW: Bacterial meningitis following epidural anesthesia for vaginal delivery: A case report. Obstet Gynecol 1989;74:437–439.

30. Goucke CR, Graziotti P: Extradural abscess following local anaesthetic and steroid injection for chronic low back pain. Br J Anaesth 1990;65:427–429.

31. Lynch J, Zech D: Spondylitis without epidural abscess formation following short-term use of an epidural catheter. Acta Anaesthesiol Scand 1990;34:167–170.

32. Strong WE: Epidural abscess associated with epidural catheterization: A rare event? Report of two cases with markedly delayed presentation. Anesthesiology 1991;74:943–946.

33. Klygis LM, Reisberg BE. Spinal epidural abscess caused by group G streptococci. Am J Med 1991;91:89–90.

34. Dawson P, Rosenfeld JV, Murphy MA, et al: Epidural abscess associated with postoperative epidural analgesia. Anesth Intens Care 1991;19:569–591.

35. Ferguson CC: Infection and the epidural space: A case report. AANA J 1992;60:393–396.

36. NganKee WD, Jones MR, Thomas P, et al: Epidural abscess complicating extradural anaesthesia for caesarean section. Br J Anaesth 1992;69:647–652.

37. Sowter MC, Burgess NA, Woodsford PV, et al: Delayed presentation of an extradural abscess complicating thoracic extradural analgesia. Br J Anaesth 1992;68:103–105.

38. Shintani S, Tanaka H, Irifune A, et al: Iatrogenic acute spinal epidural abscess with septic meningitis: MR findings. Clin Neurol Neurosurg 1992;94:253–255.

39. Nordstrom O, Sandin R: Delayed presentation of an extradural abscess in a patient with alcohol abuse. Br J Anaesth 1993;70:368–369.

40. Davis L, Hargreaves C, Robinson PN: Postpartum meningitis. Anaesthesia 1993;48:788–789.

41. Ania BJ: Staphylococus aureus meningitis after short-term epidural analgesia. Clin Infect Dis 1994;18:844–845.

42. Borum SE, McLeskey CH, Williamson JB, et al: Epidural abscess after obstetric epidural analgesia. Anesthesiology 1995;82:1523–1526.

43. Liu SS, Pope A: Spinal meningitis masquerading as postdural puncture headache [Letter]. Anesthesiology 1996;85:1493–1494.

44. Dunn LT, Javed A, Findlay G, et al: Iatrogenic spinal infection following epidural anaesthesia: case report. Eur Spine J 1996;5:418–420.

45. Cooper AB, Sharpe MD: Bacterial meningitis and cauda equina syndrome after epidural steroid injections. Can J Anaesth 1996;43:471–475.

46. Barontini F, Conti P, Marello G, et al: Major neurological sequelae of lumbar epidural anesthesia. Report of three cases. Ital J Neurol Sci 1996;17:333–339.

47. Sarrubi FA, Vasquez JE: Spinal epidural abscess associated with the use of temporary epidural catheters: Report of two cases and review. Clin Infect Dis 1997;25:1155–1158.

48. Iseki M, Okuno S, Tanabe Y, et al: Methicillin-resistant *Staphylococcus aureus* sepsis resulting from infection in paravertebral muscle after continuous epidural infusion for pain control in a patient with herpes zoster. Anesth Analg 1998;87:116–118.

49. O'Brien DPK, Rawluk DJR: Iatrogenic *Mycobacterium* infection after an epidural injection. Spine 1999;24:1257–1259.

50. Halkic N, Blanc C, Corthesy ME, et al: Lumbar spondylodiscitis after epidural anaesthesia at a distant site [Letter]. Anaesthesia 2001;56:602–603.

51. Phillips JMG, Stedeford JC, Hartsilver E, et al: Epidural abscess complicating insertion of epidural catheters. Br J Anaesth 2002;89:778–782.

52. Royakkers AA, Willigers H, van der Ven AJ, et al: Catheter-related epidural abscesses—Don't wait for neurological deficits. Acta Anaesthesiol Scand 2002;46:611–61553.

53. Hagiwara N, Hata J, Takaba H, et al: Late onset of spinal epidural abscess after spinal epidural cathterization. No To Shinkei 2003;55:633–636.

54. Evans PR, Misra U: Poor outcome following epidural abscess complicating epidural analgesia for labour. Eur J Obstet Gynecol Reprod Biol 2003;109:102–105.

55. Yue WM, Tan SB: Distant skip level discitis and vertebral osteomyelitis after caudal epidural injection: A case report of a rare complication of epidural injections. Spine 2003;11:E209–E211.

56. Dawkins CJM: An analysis of the complications of extradural and caudal block. Anaesthesia 1969;24:554–563.

57. Dawson SJ: Epidural catheter infections. J Hosp Infect 2001;47:3–8.

58. Scott DB, Hibbard BM: Serious non-fatal complications associated with extradural block in obstetric practice. Br J Anaesth 1990;64:537–541.

59. Palot M, Visseaux H, Botmans C, et al: Epidemiologie des complications de l'analgesie peridurale obstetricale. Cah Anesthesiol 1994;42:229–233.

60. Eisen SM, Rosen N, Winesanker H, et al: The routine use of lumbar epidural anaesthesia in obstetrics: A clinical review of 9,532 cases. Can Anaesth Soc J 1960;7:280–289.

61. Holdcroft A, Morgan M: Maternal complications of obstetric epidural analgesia. Anaesth Intens Care 1976;4:108–112.

62. Abouleish E, Amortegui AJ, Taylor FH: Are bacterial filters needed in continuous epidural analgesia for obstetrics? Anesthesiology 1977;46:351–354.

63. Auroy Y, Benhamou D, Bargues L, et al: Major complications of regional anesthesia in France: The SOS Regional Anesthesia Hotline Service. Anesthesiology 2002; 97: 1274–1280.

64. Sethna NF, Berde CB, Wilder RT, et al: The risk of infection from pediatric epidural analgesia is low [Abstract]. Anesthesiology 1992;77(3A):A1158.

65. Darchy B, Forceville X, Bavoux E, et al: Clinical and bacteriologic survey of epidural analgesia in patients in the intensive care unit. Anesthesiology 1996;85:988–998.

66. McNeely JK, Trentadue NC, Rusy LM, et al: Culture of bacteria from lumbar and caudal epidural catheters used for postoperative analgesia in children. Reg Anesth 1997;22:428–431.

67. Abel MD, Horlocker TT, Messick JM, et al: Neurologic complications following placement of 4392 consecutive epidural catheters in anesthetized patients [Abstract]. Reg Anesth Pain Med 1998;23(Suppl 3):3.

68. Grass JA, Haider N, Group M, et al: Incidence of complications related to epidural catheterization and maintenance for postoperative analgesia [Abstract]. Reg Anesth Pain Med 1998;23:108.

69. Kost-Byerly S, Tobin JR, Greenberg RS, et al: Bacterial colonization and infection rate of continuous epidural catheters in children. Anesth Analg 1998;86:712–716.

70. Brooks K, Pasero C, Hubbard L, et al: The risk of infection associated with epidural analgesia. Infect Control Hosp Epidemiol 1995;16:725–726.

71. Holt HM, Andersen SS, Andersen O, et al: Infections following epidural catheterization. J Hosp Infect 1995;30:253–260.

72. Holt HM, Gahrn-Hansen B, Andersen SS, et al: Infections following epidural catheters [Letter]. J Hosp Infect 1997;35:245.

73. Stafford MA, Wilder RT, Berde CB: The risk of infection from epidural analgesia in children: A review of 1620 cases. Anesth Analg 1995;80:234–238.

74. Du Pen SL, Peterson DG, Williams A, et al: Infection during chronic epidural catheterization: Diagnosis and treatment. Anesthesiology 1990;73:905–909.

75. Zenz M, Piepenbrock S, Tryba M: Epidural opiates: Long-term experiences in cancer pain. Klin Wochenschr 1985;63:225–229.

76. Coombs DW: Management of chronic pain by epidural and intrathecal opioids: Newer drugs and delivery systems. Int Anesth Clin 1986;24:59–74.

77. Yaniv LG, Potasman I: Iatrogenic meningitis: An increasing role for resistant viridans streptococci? Case report and review of the last 20 years. Scand J Infect Dis 2000;32:693–696.

78. Corbett JJ, Rosenstein BJ: *Pseudomonas* meningitis related to spinal anesthesia. Report of three cases with a common source. Neurology 1971;21:946–950.

79. Siegel RS. Alicandri FP. Jacoby AW: Subgluteal infection following regional anesthesia [Letter]. JAMA 1974;229:268.

80. Beaudoin MG, Klein L: Epidural abscess following multiple spinal anaesthetics. Anaesth Intens Care 1984;12:163–164.

81. Abdel-Magid RA, Kotb HI: Epidural abscess after spinal anesthesia: A favorable outcome. Neurosurgery 1990;27:310–311.

82. Roberts SP, Petts HV: Meningitis after obstetric spinal anaesthesia. Anaesthesia 1990;45:376–377.

83. Lee JJ, Parry H: Bacterial meningitis following spinal anaesthesia for caesarean section. Br J Anaesth 1991;66:383–386.

84. Blackmore TK, Morley HR, Gordon DL: *Streptococcus mitis*–induced bacteremia and meningitis after spinal anesthesia. Anesthesiology 1993;78:592–594.

85. Ezri T, Szmuk P, Guy M: Delayed-onset meningitis after spinal anesthesia [Letter]. Anesth Analg 1994;79:606–607.

86. Mahendru V, Bacon DR, Lema MJ: Multiple epidural abscesses and spinal anesthesia in a diabetic patient. Case report. Reg Anesth 1994;19:66–68.

87. Gebhard JS, Brugman JL: Percutaneous disectomy for the treatment of bacterial discitis. Spine 1994;19:855–857.

88. Newton JA Jr, Lesnik IK, Kennedy CA: *Streptococcus salivarius* meningitis following spinal anesthesia [Letter]. Clin Infect Dis 1994;18:840–841.

89. Kaiser E, Suppini A, de Jaureguiberry JP, et al: Meningite aigue a *Streptococcus salivarius* après rachianesthesie. Ann Fr Anesth Reanim 1997;16:47–49.

90. Fernandez R, Paz I, Pazos C, et al: Meningitis producida por *Streptococcus* mitis tras anestesia intradural [Letter]. Enferm Infecc Microbiol Clin 1999;17:150.

91. Horlocker TT, McGregor DG, Matsushige DK, et al: A retrospective review of 4767 consecutive spinal anesthetics: Central nervous system complications. Perioperative Outcomes Group. Anesth Analg. 1997;84:578–584.

92. Evans FT: Sepsis and asepsis in spinal analgesia. Proc R Soc Med 1945;39:181–185.

93. Scarborough RA: Spinal anesthesia from the surgeon's standpoint. JAMA 1958;168:1324–1326.

94. Dripps RD, Vandam LD: Long-term follow-up of patients who received 10,098 spinal anesthetics. JAMA 1954;156:1486–1491.

95. Moore DC, Bridenbaugh LD: Spinal (subarachnoid) block. JAMA 1966;195:907–912.

96. Lund PC, Cwik JC: Modern trends in spinal anaesthesia. Can Anaesth Soc J 1968;15:118–134.

97. Sadove MS, Levin MJ, Rant-Sejdinaj I: Neurological complications of spinal anaesthesia. Can Anaesth Soc J 1961;8:405–416.

98. Arner O: Complications following spinal anesthesia. Their significance and a technique to reduce their incidence. Acta Chir Scand 1952;104:336–338.

99. Cascio M, Heath G: Meningitis following a combined spinal-epidural technique in a labouring term parturient. Can J Anaesth 1996;43:399–402.

100. Harding SA, Collis RE, Morgan BM: Meningitis after combined spinal-extradural anaesthesia in obstetrics. Br J Anaesth. 1994;73:545–547.

101. Stallard N, Barry P: Another complication of the combined extradural-subarachnoid technique [Letter]. Br J Anaesth 1995;75:370–371.

102. Aldebert S, Sleth JC: Meningite bacterienne après anesthesia rachidienne et peridurale combinee en obstetrique. Ann Fr Anesth Reanim 1996;15:687–688.

103. Dysart RH, Balakrishnan V: Conservative management of extradural abscess complicating spinal-extradural anaesthesia for caesarean section. Br J Anaesth 1997;78:591–593.

104. Schroter J, Wa Djamba D, Hoffmann V, et al: Epidural abscess after combined spinal-epidural block. Can J Anaesth 1997;44:300–304.

105. Bouhemad B, Dounas M, Mercier FJ, et al: Bacterial meningitis following combined spinal-epidural analgesia for labour. Anaesthesia 1998;53:290–295.

106. Peng PW, Chan VW: Local and regional block in postoperative pain control. Surg Clin North Am 1999;79:345–370.

107. Graf BM, Martin E: [Peripheral nerve block. An overview of new developments in an old technique]. Anaesthesist 2001;50:312–322.

108. Bergman BD, Hebl JR, Kent J, et al: Neurologic complications of 405 consecutive continuous axillary catheters. Anesth Analg 2003;96:247–252.

109. Meier G, Bauereis C, Heinrich C: [Interscalene brachial plexus catheter for anesthesia and postoperative pain therapy. Experience with a modified technique]. Anaesthesist 1997;46:715–719.

110. Nseir S, Pronnier P, Soubrier S, et al: Fatal streptococcal necrotizing fasciitis as a complication of axillary brachial plexus block. Br J Anaesth 2004;92:427–429.

111. Adam F, Jaziri S, Chauvin M: Psoas abscess complicating femoral nerve block catheter. Anesthesiology 2003;99:230–231.

112. Cuvillon P, Ripart J, Lalourcey L, et al: The continuous femoral nerve block catheter for postoperative analgesia: Bacterial colonization, infectious rate and adverse effects. Anesth Analg 2001;93:1045–1049.

113. Davlin LB, Aulicino PL: Osteomyelitis of the metacarpal head following digital block anesthesia. Orthopedics 1999;22:1187–1188.

114. Basu A, Bhalaik V, Stanislas M, et al: Osteomyelitis following a haematoma block. Injury 2003;34:79–82.

115. Dahlmann AH, Appaswamy S, Headon MP: Orbital cellulitis following sub-Tenon's anaesthesia. Eye 2002;16:200–201.

116. Redmill B, Sandy C, Rose GE: Orbital cellulitis following corneal gluing under sub-Tenon's local anaesthesia. Eye 2001;15:554–556.

117. Wildsmith JA: Regional anaesthesia requires attention to detail [Letter]. Br J Anaesth 1991;67:224–225.

118. Yentis SM: Wearing of face masks for spinal anaesthesia [Letter]. Br J Anaesth 1992;68:224.

119. Wildsmith JA: Wearing of face masks for spinal anaesthesia [Letter]. Br J Anaesth 1992;68:224.

120. O'Kelly SW, Marsh D: Face masks and spinal anaesthesia [Letter]. Br J Anaesth 1993;70:239.

121. Wildsmith JA: Face masks and spinal anaesthesia [Letter]. Br J Anaesth 1993;70:239.

122. Bromage PR: Postpartum meningitis [Letter]. Anaesthesia 1994;49:260.

123. Smedstad KG: Infection after central neuraxial block [Editorial]. Can J Anaesth 1997;44:235–238.

124. Panikkar KK, Yentis SM: Wearing of masks for obstetric regional anaesthesia. A postal survey. Anaesthesia 1996;51:398–400.

125. O'Higgins F, Tuckey JP: Thoracic epidural anaesthesia and analgesia: United Kingdom practice. Acta Anaesthesiol Scand 2000;44:1087–1092.

126. Sleth JC: Evaluation des mesures d'asepsie lors de la realisation d'un catheterisme epidural et perception de son risqué infectieux. Resultats d'une enquete en Languedoc-Roussillon. Ann Fr Anesth Reanim 1998;17:408–414.

127. Dawson SJ, Small H, Logan MN, et al: Case control study of epidural catheter infections in a district general hospital. Commun Dis Public Health 2000;3:300–302.

128. Philips BJ, Fergusson S, Armstrong P, et al: Surgical face masks are effective in reducing bacterial contamination caused by dispersal from the upper airway. Br J Anaesth 1992;69:407–408.

129. Chaiyakunapruk N, Veenstra DL, Lipsky BA, et al: Vascular catheter site care: The clinical and economic benefits of chlorhexidine gluconate compared with povidone iodine. Clin Infect Dis 2003;37(6):764–771.

130. Adam MN, Dinulescu T, Mathieu P, et al: Comparaison de l'efficacite de deux antiseptiques dans la prevention de l'infection liee aux catheters periduraux. Can Anesthesiol 1996;44:465–467.

131. Kasuda H, Fukuda H, Togashi H, et al: Skin disinfection before epidural catheterization: Comparative study of povidone-iodine versus chlorhexidine ethanol. Dermatology 2002;204(Suppl 1):42–46.

132. Kinirons B, Mimoz O, Lafendi L, et al: Chlorhexidine versus povidone iodine in preventing colonization of continuous epidural catheters in children. Anesthesiology 2001;94:239–244.

133. Sato S, Sakuragi T, Dan K: Human skin flora as a potential source of epidural abscess. Anesthesiology 1996;85:1276–1282.

134. Raad II, Hohn DC, Gilbreath BJ, et al: Prevention of central venous catheter-related infections by using maximal sterile barrier precautions during insertion. Infect Control Hosp Epidemiol 1994;15:231–238.

135. Centers for Disease Control and Prevention: Guidelines for the prevention of intravascular catheter-related infections. MMWR 2002;51(No. RR-10):1–36.

136. Pegues DA, Carr DB, Hopkins CC: Infectious complications associated with temporary epidural catheters. Clin Infect Dis 1994;19:970–972.

137. Green BGJ, Pathy GV: Ensuring sterility of opioids for spinal administration [Letter]. Anaesthesia 1999;54:511.

138. Boezaart AP, de Beer JF, du Toit C, et al: A new technique of continuous interscalene nerve block. Can J Anaesth 1999;46:275–281.

139. Cruse PJE, Foord R: The epidemiology of wound infection: A 10-year prospective study of 62 939 wounds. Surg Clin North Am 1980;60:27–40.

140. Schulz-Stübner S: First Experiences with a Regional Anesthesia Surveillance System (RASS). 13th WCA, Paris 2004 (Abstract).

141. Waldman SD: Cervical epidural abscess after cervical epidural nerve block with steroids. Anesth Analg 1991;72:717–718.

142. Mamourian AC, Dickman CA, Drayer BP, et al: Spinal epidural abscess: Three cases following spinal epidural injection demonstrated with magnetic resonance imaging. Anesthesiology 1993;78:204–207.

143. Tabo E, Ohkuma Y, Kimura S, et al: Successful percutaneous drainage of epidural abscess with epidural needle and catheter. Anesthesiology 1994;80:1393–1395.

144. Wang JS, Fellows DG, Vakharia S, et al: Epidural abscess—Early magnetic resonance imaging detection and conservative therapy. Anesth Analg 1996;82:1069–1071.

145. Laurila JJ, Kostamovaara PA, Alahuhta S: *Streptococcus salivarius* meningitis after spinal anesthesia. Anesthesiology 1998;89:1579–1580.

146. Rathmell JP, Garahan MB, Alsofrom GF: Epidural abscess following epidural analgesia. Reg Anesth Pain Med 2000;25:79–82.

73

Postdural Puncture Headache

Brian E. Harrington, MD

INTRODUCTION

Postdural puncture headache (PDPH) was perhaps the first recognized complication of regional anesthesia. Dr. August Bier noted this adverse effect in 1898 in the first patient to undergo successful spinal anesthesia, a 34-year-old laborer undergoing resection of an ulceration of the foot. Bier observed: "Two hours after the operation his back and left leg became painful and the patient vomited and complained of severe headache. The pain and vomiting soon ceased, but headache was still present the next day."[1]

The following week, Bier and his assistant, Dr. August Hildebrandt performed experiments on each other. Following the "cocainization of the spinal cord", Bier described first-hand his experience in the days to follow: "I had a feeling of very strong pressure on my skull and became rather dizzy

Portions of this text originally appeared in the following publication: Neal, Rathmell (eds): Complications in Regional Anesthesia and Pain Management, copyright 2006, published by Elsevier, Philadelphia, PA, USA, with permission.

when I stood up rapidly from my chair. All these symptoms vanished at once when I lay down flat, but returned when I stood up ... I was forced to take to bed and remained there for nine days, because all the manifestations recurred as soon as I got up ... The symptoms finally resolved nine days after the lumbar puncture."[1] Interestingly, since Bier's time, the clinical picture of PDPH has remained unchanged and it remains the most common complication of spinal anesthesia.

DIAGNOSIS

PDPH occurs following procedures that disrupt the integrity of the meninges. Most cases of PDPH are characterized by their typical onset, quality, and associated symptoms.

Onset

Onset of symptoms is generally delayed, with headache usually beginning 12–48 h (rarely > 5 days) following dural puncture. Following dural puncture, 65% experience symptoms within 24 h and 92% within 48 h.[2] An onset of symptoms within 1 h is suggestive of pneumocephalus, especially in the context of an epidural loss-of-resistance technique using air.[3]

Quality

The hallmark of PDPH is its postural nature, with symptoms worsening in the upright position and improving with recumbency. The International Classification of Headache Disorders further describes this positional quality as worsening within 15 min of sitting or standing and improving within 15 min after lying down.[4] Headache is nearly always bilateral, with a distribution that is frontal (25%), occipital (27%), or both (45%).[2] Headaches are typically described as "dull/aching," "throbbing," or "pressure-type" in nature.

Clinical Pearls

- PDPH occurs following procedures that disrupt the integrity of the meninges (ie dura and arachnoid mater)
- Onset of symptoms is generally delayed; 65% of patients experience symptoms within 24 h and 92% within 48 h.
- Onset of symptoms within 1 h is suggestive of pneumocephalus and not PDPH.
- The hallmark of PDPH is its postural nature, with symptoms worsening in the upright position and improving with recumbency.
- Pain and stiffness in the neck and shoulders are common and seen in nearly half of all patients experiencing PDPH.
- Nausea may be reported by a majority of patients.

The severity of PDPH symptoms is directly related to needle size. Larger needles are associated with more severe headaches[5] and a greater need for definitive treatment measures.[6] The severity of PDPH after spinal anesthesia varies from mild (11%) to moderate (23%), to severe (67%).[2]

Associated Symptoms

If headaches are severe, they are more likely to be accompanied by a variety of other symptoms. Pain and stiffness in the neck and shoulders is common and seen in nearly half of all patients experiencing PDPH.[7] With careful questioning, nausea may be reported by a majority of patients and can lead to vomiting.[2]

Uncommonly, patients may experience auditory or visual symptoms,[8] and the risk for either appears to be directly related to needle size.[9,10] In a large study of PDPH, these symptoms were present to a clinically significant degree in 0.4% of patients.[11] Auditory symptoms are frequently unilateral, and include hearing loss, tinnitus, and even hyperacousis. Subclinical hearing loss, especially in the lower frequencies, appears to be common following spinal anesthesia, even in the absence of PDPH.[10] Closely associated with auditory function, vestibular disturbances (dizziness or vertigo) may also occur. Visual problems include blurred vision, difficulties with accommodation, diplopia, and mild photophobia.[9] In contrast to headache complaints, nearly 80% of episodes of diplopia involve unilateral cranial nerve palsies.

Clinical Pearls

DIAGNOSIS OF POSTDURAL PUNCTURE HEADACHE

- History of known or possible dural puncture.
- Delayed onset of symptoms, but within 48 h.
- Bilateral headache (frontal, occipital, or both).
- Postural nature of symptoms.
- ± Associated symptoms.

Incidence

The reported incidence of PDPH varies considerably depending on the technique employed, patient population, definition of PDPH, and duration of follow-up. PDPH is primarily discussed in association with spinal anesthesia; however, it is also frequently observed following diagnostic lumbar puncture, myelography, and accidental dural puncture (ADP) during epidural techniques.

Rates of PDPH are particularly high (up to 10%) after myelography and diagnostic lumbar puncture, in which large-gauge needles are considered necessary due to the viscosity of contrast material and to facilitate the timely collection of cerebrospinal fluid (CSF).

Rates of PDPH following spinal anesthesia have steadily declined; from an incidence exceeding 50% in Bier's time, to around 10% in the 1950s,[11] until currently a rate of 1% or less can be reasonably expected. This reduction is clearly due to modifications in practice that have followed the identification of risk factors (discussed in the section on Risk Factors). In obstetric patients, a population known to be at high risk for PDPH, meta-analysis demonstrated an incidence of 1.7% using 27-gauge Whitacre needles.[12] Combined spinal-epidural techniques have also been associated with a low incidence of PDPH (1.6% in one study of over 2000 obstetric patients).[13] This observation may be due to several factors, including the ability to successfully use needles of very small diameters (ie, 27 gauge) with a noncutting tip design as well as possible tamponade provided by epidural infusions. Continuous spinal anesthesia using standard 20-gauge catheters (macrocatheters) has been reported by some to be associated with surprisingly low incidences of PDPH (3.4%) compared with single-dose spinal techniques using similar gauge needles.[14] This observation has been attributed to reaction to the catheter, which may promote better sealing of a breach in the meninges. However, deliberate continuous spinal anesthesia has usually been investigated in low-risk populations.

Epidural techniques are an attractive alternative to spinal anesthesia due to the perceived ability to avoid puncture of the dura. The problem is, however, that ADP cannot be reliably prevented and may be unrecognized at the time in over 25% of patients who eventually develop PDPH.[15] ADP is of greatest concern in the obstetric anesthesia setting, where the incidence may be up to 1.5%.[12] Of these patients, 52–80% will develop PDPH.

Medicolegal Considerations

PDPH is a significant source of concern and dissatisfaction for patients. In parturients who had experienced an ADP, 70% would not choose to have epidural analgesia again, and only 28% would recommend it to a friend or relative.[16] Iatrogenic headaches continue to represent a significant medicolegal liability, as noted by the high frequency of malpractice claims for headache in the American Society of Anesthesiologists Closed Claims Project database. For instance, for obstetric anesthesia claims, headache was the second most common maternal injury (after death) and resulted in payment in 56% of cases.[17,18] Similarly, headache following epidural steroid injections was the most common malpractice claim in pain management practices.[19] For these reasons, the potential for this complication necessitates a proper discussion and informed consent for any procedure that may result in PDPH.

Pathophysiologic Mechanisms Behind PDPH

Despite a great deal of research and observational data, the pathophysiology of PDPH remains incompletely understood.[20] It is generally accepted that PDPH results from a disruption of normal CSF homeostasis. CSF is produced primarily in the choroid plexus at a rate of approximately 0.35 mL/min and reabsorbed through the arachnoid villa. The total CSF volume in adults is maintained around 150 mL, of which approximately half is extracranial, and gives rise to normal lumbar opening pressures of 5 to 15 cm H_2O in the horizontal position (40–50 cm H_2O in the upright position). A sudden loss of CSF results in the development of typical PDPH symptoms, which resolve promptly with reconstitution of lost CSF volume.[21] It is thought that PDPH is due to the loss of CSF through a persistent leak in the meninges. In this regard, it has been postulated that the arachnoid mater may be at least as and perhaps more important than the dura mater in the genesis of PDPH.[22] However, the actual mechanism by which CSF hypotension generates headache is controversial and currently ascribed to a bimodal mechanism involving both loss of intracranial support and cerebral vasodilation (predominantly venous). Diminished hydrostatic support is thought to cause the brain to sag in the upright position, resulting in traction and pressure on pain-sensitive structures within the cranium (dura, cranial nerves, bridging veins, and venous sinuses). In addition. vasodilation may occur secondary to diminished intracranial CSF volume and reflexively secondary to traction on intracranial vessels.

Clinical Pearls

- The pathophysiology of PDPH is not well understood.
- It is generally accepted that PDPH results from a sudden loss of CSF.
- It is thought that the loss of CSF occurs through a persistent leak in the meninges.
- Diminished hydrostatic support causes the brain to sag in the upright position, resulting in traction and pressure on pain-sensitive structures within the cranium (dura, cranial nerves, bridging veins, and venous sinuses).
- Vasodilation may occur secondary to diminished intracranial CSF volume and reflexively secondary to traction on intracranial vessels.

The neural pathways primarily involved in PDPH include the ophthalmic branch of the facial nerve (CN V1) in frontal pain, cranial nerves IX and X in occipital pain, and cervical nerves C1 through C3 in neck and shoulder pain.[23] Nausea is attributed to vagal stimulation (CN X). Auditory and vestibular symptoms are secondary to the direct communication between the CSF and the perilymph via the cochlear aqueduct, which results in decreased perilymphatic pressures in the inner ear and an imbalance between the endolymph and perilymph.[8] Visual disturbances usually represent a transient palsy of the nerves that supply the extraocular muscles of the eye (CN III, IV, and, VI). The lateral rectus muscle is most often involved, attributed to the long, vulnerable intracranial course of the abducens nerve (CN VI).[9]

RISK FACTORS FOR DEVELOPING PDPH

Risk factors for PDPH can be broadly categorized into patient characteristics and procedural details.

Patient Characteristics

Although uncommon in children younger than 10 years of age, PDPH has a peak incidence in the teens and early 20s.[74] The incidence then declines over time, becoming infrequent in patients older than 50 years of age. Female gender has long been thought to impart an increased risk for PDPH.[11] However, gender has not always constituted an independent risk factor when age-matched nonpregnant populations are studied.[24] Pregnancy is generally regarded as a risk factor for PDPH,[11] but this consideration partially reflects the young age as well as the high incidence of ADP in the gravid population. Pushing during the second stage of labor, thought to promote the loss of CSF through a hole in the meninges, has been shown to be a significant risk factor for PDPH following ADP. Angle and colleagues noted that the cumulative

duration of bearing down correlated with the risk of developing PDPH in patients who had experienced an ADP and that patients who avoided pushing altogether (ie, proceeded to cesarean delivery prior to reaching second stage labor) had a much lower incidence of PDPH (10%) than those who pushed (74%).[25] Observed variations in the thickness of the dura (from 0.5 to nearly 2.0 mm) have also been proposed to influence the risk of PDPH, as punctures made where the dura is thicker appear to be less prone to allowing the loss of CSF.[26]

Clinical Pearl

- Patient age is the single most significant risk factor for developing PDPH.

PDPH appears to have an interesting association with other headaches. Patients who report having had a headache within the week prior to lumbar puncture have been observed to have a higher incidence of PDPH.[27] On further analysis, only those with chronic bilateral tension-type headaches were found to be at increased risk.[28] A history of unilateral headache[28] or migraine[29] has not been linked with an increased risk of PDPH. Menstrual cycle, a factor in migraine headaches, did not influence the rate of PDPH in one underpowered pilot study.[30] A small but statistically significant increased incidence of PDPH following spinal anesthesia has been reported if patients have a history of previous PDPH.[24] Patients with a history of ADP have been shown to have a slightly increased risk of another ADP (and subsequent PDPH).[31]

A number of other patient characteristics have been demonstrated to be minor risk factors for PDPH, including lower opening pressures,[32] lower patient body mass index,[27,33] low CSF substance P concentration,[34] and low baseline pain sensitivity.[35] Although such findings would appear to be of academic interest only, they may hold important keys to the future prevention and treatment of PDPH.

Risk Factors Related to the Procedure and Equipment

Needle size and tip design are the most important procedural factors.[5] Needle size is directly related to the risk of PDPH, with larger needles resulting in a higher incidence of symptoms.[11] "Noncutting" needles are associated with a reduced incidence of PDPH than occurs with "cutting" (eg, Quincke) needles of the same size. Noncutting needles, also referred to as pencil-point, blunt tip, atraumatic, or conical tip, include the Whitacre, Sprotte, European, Pencan, and Gertie Marx needles. Although originally thought to be less traumatic than cutting needles, electron microscopy has shown noncutting needles to produce a more traumatic hole in the dura, perhaps resulting in a better inflammatory healing response.[36] The influence of needle size on risk of PDPH appears to be less for noncutting needles than cutting needles (eg, the reduction in the incidence of PDPH between 22- and 26-gauge sizes is greater for cutting than noncutting needles). Some needles, such as the Greene and Atraucan, appear to be acceptable combinations of cutting and noncutting features.[37]

Inserting cutting needles with the bevel parallel to the long axis of the spine reduces the risk of PDPH.[24,38,39] This observation was for many years attributed to a "spreading" rather than cutting of longitudinally oriented dural fibers. However, scanning electron microscopy reveals the dura to be made of many layers of concentrically directed fibers,[40] and the importance of needle bevel insertion is most likely due to the longitudinal tension on the dura and its influence on CSF leakage through holes with differing orientations.

A greater number of dural punctures increases the rate of PDPH.[41] The angle of approach to the dura may be another important consideration, due to the dura–arachnoid relationship. Experimental and clinical evidence suggest that paramedian[42] (vs midline) and oblique[43] (vs 90-degree) approaches may allow for better sealing of a dural puncture, reducing CSF loss and resulting in a lower incidence of PDPH. The operator's experience, comfort, and skill are clearly associated with the incidence of ADP during epidural procedures, but have not consistently been a significant risk factor for other central neuraxial techniques. The possible contribution of operator fatigue, especially for ADP, remains to be determined.

A number of procedural details do not appear to influence the rate of development of PDPH, including patient position at the time of dural puncture,[27] bloody tap during spinal anesthesia,[44] addition of narcotics to spinal block,[45] and volume of spinal fluid removed (for diagnostic purposes).[27] The specific local anesthetic used may affect the rate of nonspecific headache but does not appear to influence the need for epidural blood patch (EBP).[46]

Practical Approach to Evaluating Patients Presenting with Headache After a Neuraxial Anesthetic

A careful history with a brief consideration of other possible diagnoses is usually sufficient to differentiate PDPH from other causes of headache (Table 73–1). Most nonpostward puncture headaches will not have a strong positional nature, as seen in PDPH. Vital signs (normal blood pressure and absence of fever) and a basic neurologic exam should be documented. Bilateral jugular venous pressure, briefly applied, tends to worsen headaches secondary to intracranial hypotension. Laboratory studies are usually not necessary for the diagnosis of PDPH and, if obtained, are generally unremarkable (most commonly, magnetic resonance imaging may show meningeal enhancement, and lumbar puncture reveal increased CSF protein and low opening pressures).

It should be noted that benign headaches are common in the perioperative setting, even in the absence of dural puncture, and have generally been noted to be less severe than PDPH[7] (causes may include anxiety, dehydration, hypoglycemia, anxiety, and caffeine withdrawal). It has even been proposed that some nonpostdural puncture headaches may be due to contamination of the central neuraxis with skin preparation solutions.[47] The majority of headaches following dural puncture will be benign nonspecific headaches. In a careful analysis of headache following spinal anesthesia using strict criteria for PDPH, Santanen and colleagues found an incidence of nonspecific headache of 18.5%, with an incidence of true PDPH of only 1.5%.[48] In an obstetric population, Grove noted postpartum headache in 23% of patients who had not had any regional anesthesia.[49]

Table 73–1.

Causes of Nonpostdural Puncture Headache Following Dural Puncture

Benign	Serious
Nonspecific headache	Meningitis
Exacerbation of chronic headache	Subdural hematoma
Hypertensive headache	Subarachnoid hemorrhage
Pneumocephalus	Preeclampsia/eclampsia
Sinusitis	Dural venous sinus thrombosis
Other	Other

Clinical Pearls

- Exclude nonpostdural puncture headaches.

- Non-PDPH headache will usually not have a strong positional nature.

- Benign headaches are common in the perioperative setting.

- Exacerbation of chronic headache (eg, tension, cluster, or migraine) is usually notable for a history of similar headaches.

- Lateralizing neurologic signs, fever/chills, seizures, or changes in mental status are not consistent with a diagnosis of PDPH.

- Maintain a high index of suspicion for subdural hematoma (SDH), which is often preceded by classic PDPH symptoms but progresses to lose its postural component and may include disturbances in mentation and focal neurologic signs.

- Dural venous sinus thrombosis (DVST) is usually seen in the postpartum obstetric population, in whom headache symptoms may progress to seizures, focal neurologic signs, and coma.

- Diagnosis of PDPH can be particularly challenging in patients who have undergone lumbar puncture as part of a diagnostic work-up for headache. In these situations, headache should have changed in quality, the most common difference being a new postural nature.

Exacerbation of chronic headache (eg, tension, cluster, or migraine) is usually notable for a history of similar headaches. Hypertensive headache has a clear association with significant hypertension. Pneumocephalus can produce a positional headache that does not respond to EBP and can be difficult to distinguish from PDPH, but is readily diagnosed with computed tomography.[50] Sinusitis may be associated with purulent nasal discharge and tenderness over the affected sinus and is often improved with assuming an upright position. A number of other benign causes are possible.

Serious causes of headache are rare but must be excluded. It is important to remember that lateralizing neurologic signs, fever/chills, seizures, or changes in mental status are not consistent with a diagnosis of PDPH. Meningitis tends to be associated with fever, leukocytosis, changes in mental status, and meningeal signs (eg, nuchal rigidity).[51] Subdural hematoma (SDH), long recognized as a potential complication of dural puncture, is believed due to intracranial hypotension resulting in excessive traction on cerebral vessels, leading to their disruption. Practioners should maintain a high index of suspicion for SDH, which is often preceded by classic PDPH symptoms but progresses to lose its postural component and may include disturbances in mentation and focal neurologic signs.[52] It has been proposed that early definitive treatment of severe PDPH may serve to pre-

vent SDH.[53] Subarachnoid hemorrhage, most commonly due to rupture of a cerebral aneurysm or arteriovenous malformation, is usually associated with the sudden onset of excruciating headache followed by a decreased level of consciousness or coma.[54] Preeclampsia/eclampsia often presents with headache and may only become evident in the postpartum period.[55,56] Dural venous sinus thrombosis (DVST) is usually seen in the postpartum obstetric population, in whom headache symptoms may progress to seizures, focal neurologic signs, and coma.[57] Predisposing factors for DSVT include hypercoagulability, toxemia, and dehydration. Reports of other intracranial pathology (intracranial tumor, intracerebral hemorrhage, etc) misdiagnosed as PDPH are extremely uncommon and will be detected with a thorough neurologic evaluation.[54]

Diagnosis of PDPH can be particularly challenging in patients who have undergone lumbar puncture as part of a diagnostic work-up for headache. In these situations, headache should have changed in quality, the most common difference being a new postural nature. Occasionally, if the benign diagnostic possibilities cannot be narrowed down with certainty, a favorable response to EBP can provide definitive evidence for a diagnosis of PDPH.

PREVENTION STRATEGIES

A number of recommendations can be made to decrease the risk of PDPH, but several long-standing practices, namely prolonged recumbency and aggressive hydration, do not appear to be useful.[58,59]

Subarachnoidal Needle Placement

Prevention of PDPH in the setting of spinal anesthesia involves appropriate patient selection and careful attention to technique. Patients younger than 40 years of age are at particularly high risk for PDPH, and alternatives to spinal anesthesia should perhaps be sought in these individuals unless the benefits are sufficiently compelling (as they appear to be in the obstetric population). Using needles with a lower risk of PDPH is the most important technical means of reducing the risk of PDPH with spinal anesthesia. As a rule, the smallest noncutting needles feasible should be employed. However, extremely small needles are more difficult to place, have a slow return of CSF, may be associated with multiple punctures of the dura, and may result in a higher rate of unsuccessful block. Therefore, it appears that the best compromise between the risk of PDPH and ease of placement is a 24- to 27-gauge noncutting needle. If cutting tip needles are used, the bevel should be directed parallel to the long axis of the spine.

It has been suggested that intravenous caffeine (500 mg caffeine sodium benzoate within 90 min after spinal anesthesia) reduces the incidence of moderate to severe headache.[60] However, the applicability of these data is questionable as this study involved the use of 22-gauge Quincke needles in a relatively young patient population.

Epidural Needle Placement

Unlike spinal anesthesia, patient selection appears to play a minimal role in the prevention of ADP during attempted epidural techniques. The use of a noncompressible medium (saline or local anesthetic) for loss-of-resistance generally results in a lower incidence of ADP than using air.[61] The risk of PDPH following ADP can probably also be reduced by always using the smallest gauge epidural needle possible (yet equipment options in this regard are limited with catheter techniques.

Optimal bevel orientation for epidural needle insertion remains a matter of debate. Although incidence of PDPH following ADP may be reduced by directing the needle bevel parallel to the long axis of the spine,[38] this technique necessitates a 90-degree rotation of the needle for catheter placement. Consequently, the possibility of dural trauma with needle rotation has prompted some to suggest always inserting epidural needles with the bevel facing the direction of desired catheter placement.[63]

Strategies to Reduce the Risk of PDPH After ADP

Since not all patients who experience an ADP will develop PDPH, and only a portion of those who do will require definitive treatment, a cautious approach in this regard is suggested. Several immediate measures following ADP have been proposed to prevent the development of PDPH. Replacing the stylet prior to needle withdrawal is a simple and possibly effective means of lowering the incidence of PDPH. This recommendation is based on observations of lumbar punctures performed using 21-gauge Sprotte needles and is theorized to decrease the possibility of an arachnoid mater "wick" through the dura.[64] Charsley and Abrams performed a subarachnoid injection of 10 mL of saline following ADP and noted a significantly reduced need for EBP in the treated group.[65] Their analysis is limited by the small number of patients studied, and further investigation is clearly indicated. Ayad and colleagues recommend placement of a subarachnoid catheter for 24 h following ADP.[66] In their obstetric population, catheter placement resulted in a rate of PDPH of only 6.2%, with an expected incidence under these conditions of over 50%. This impressive reduction in the incidence of PDPH, however, has not been noted in studies in which catheters have been left in place for less than 24 h.

Provided an epidural catheter can be successfully placed following ADP, prophylactic epidural saline has been used in hopes of reducing the incidence and severity of PDPH. Efforts have included both bolus (eg, 50 mL as a single injection or every 6 h for four doses) and continuous infusion techniques (commonly 600–1,000 mL over 24 h). In the largest analysis of this approach ($n = 241$), Stride and Cooper reported a reduction in the incidence of PDPH from 86% in a conservatively treated control group to 70% with epidural saline infusion.[67] Trivedi and colleagues noted a similar reduction in PDPH (from 87% to 67%) in 30 patients who received a single prophylactic "saline patch" (40–60 mL) following completion of the obstetric procedure.[68] Other studies of epidural saline have noted this modest decrease in the incidence of PDPH. Stride and Cooper also reported a lower incidence of severe headache (from 64% to 47%), but this effect has been inconsistently seen by other investigators, and there is no definitive evidence that epidural saline reduces the eventual need for EBP. Despite the paucity of data, a survey in North America published in 1998 reported 25% of tertiary care obstetrical centers using prophylactic epidural saline infusions.[69] Such observations appear to be due more to a desire to "do something" and the perceived safety of the practice rather than any proven efficacy. The 1999 National Obstetric Anesthetic Database in the United Kingdom reported epidural saline infusion/bolus used as immediate management in only 7% of cases of ADP.[7] Importantly, epidural saline does not appear to reduce the success rate of EBP. Although the epidural administration of saline is generally benign, transmitted pressure not uncommonly results in back and eye pain and has caused retinal hemorrhage.

Prophylactic Epidural Blood Patch: When, How, in Whom

The risk–benefit of prophylactic measures should be most favorable in those having the greatest likelihood of developing PDPH, such as obstetric patients experiencing an ADP with an epidural needle. However, investigations into the efficacy of the prophylactic EBP in this setting have yielded mixed results.[70] Scavone and colleagues, for example, in a prospective, randomized, double-blind study in an obstetric population found that the prophylactic EBP shortened the total duration of symptoms but failed to reduce the incidence of PDPH or subsequent need for EBP.[71] Currently, due to concerns of exposing patients to a potentially unnecessary and marginally beneficial procedure, most centers do not utilize the prophylactic EBP as a routine measure.[69]

If employed prophylactically, the EBP should be performed only after any spinal or epidural local anesthetic has worn off, as premature administration has been associated with excessive cephalad displacement of local anesthetic.[72] Residual epidural local anesthetic may also inhibit coagulation of blood, further decreasing the efficacy of EBP.[73]

TREATMENT STRATEGIES FOR PDPH

Once the diagnosis has been made, patients should be provided a straightforward explanation of the cause, natural history, and treatment options for PDPH. A treatment algorithm, based primarily on the severity of symptoms, can serve as a useful guide for management (Figure 73–1).

Time

PDPH is a complication that tends to resolve spontaneously. Prior to the introduction of definitive therapy for PDPH (ie, the EBP), the natural history of the disorder was documented

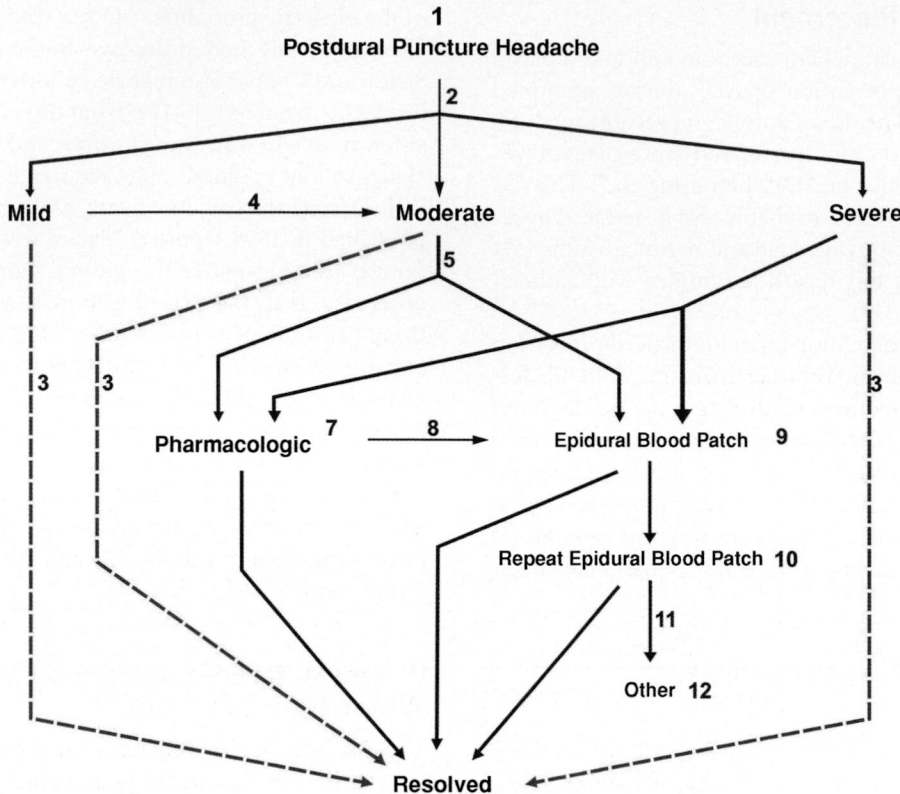

Figure 73–1. Treatment decision-making algorithm for postdural puncture headache.

1. When diagnosis is made, all patients should receive supportive measures (reassurance, bed rest, analgesics, hydration, quiet environment).
2. Severity of symptoms should be classified using VAS scale (mild 1–3, moderate 4–6, severe 7–10).
3. Virtually all patients will improve in time even without additional therapy. (dashed lines)
4. Symptoms worsen or fail to resolve within 5 days.
5. Patient preference dictates the choice between pharmacologic (less effective) and epidural blood patch (EBP).
6. In patients with severe symptoms, EBP is strongly suggested.
7. The most common pharmacologic measure is caffeine prescription.
8. The failure, worsening, or recurrence of symptoms after pharmacologic measures favors the use of EBP.
9. In addition to EBP, other epidural treatment options can be considered in select patients (eg, dextran, saline).
10. A period of 24 h should lapse before repeating EBP.
11. Failure of the second EBP should prompt reconsideration of the diagnosis and neurology consultation.
12. Insufficient data are available regarding the optimal treatment of the failed EBP. Further work-up in consultation with a neurologist or neurosurgeon is suggested.

From Neal, Rathmell (eds): Complications in Regional Anesthesia and Pain Management, copyright 2006, published by Elsevier, Philadelphia, PA, USA, with permission.

by Vandam and Dripps as they followed 1011 episodes of PDPH after spinal anesthesia using cutting needles of various sizes.[11] Although their analysis is flawed by a lack information on duration in 9% of patients, if one considers their observed data, spontaneous resolution of PDPH was seen in 59% of cases within 4 days and 80% within 1 week. More recently, Lybecker and coworkers followed 75 episodes of PDPH and, although providing an EBP to 40% of their patients, noted in the untreated patients a median duration of symptoms of 5 days with a range of 1 to 12 days.[2] These data, although generally reassuring, also illustrate the sometimes prolonged duration of untreated PDPH. Indeed, Vandam and Dripps noted 4% of patients still experiencing symptoms 7–12 months after spinal anesthesia.[11] Similar observations of prolonged symptoms have been reported following diagnostic lumbar puncture[74] and ADP.[75] A number of case reports

exist of successful treatment of PDPH months or years after known[76] or even occult dural puncture.[77]

Primarily due to the self-limited nature of PDPH, the optimal time course of treatment has not been well-defined. Although many practitioners have advocated 24–48 h of conservative therapy, the practicality of this approach is questionable, given the often severely disabling nature and prolonged duration of symptoms. Notably, the duration of PDPH appears to be directly related to needle size,[78] which would support early definitive therapy for severe headaches following dural punctures made with large (eg, epidural) needles.

Supportive Measures

Reassurance and supportive measures, although not expected to alter the duration of symptoms, are advised for all patients.

Most patients with severe PDPH will naturally seek a recumbent position for symptomatic relief. Although excessive hydration does not appear to influence the duration of symptoms,[59] patients should be encouraged to avoid dehydration. Oral analgesics (acetaminophen, NSAIDs, or narcotics) may be utilized, yet the relief obtained is often unimpressive, especially with severe headaches. Antiemetics and stool softeners should be prescribed when indicated. Abdominal binders can provide some degree of relief, but are uncomfortable and seldom used in modern practice.

Pharmacologic Treatments

A number of pharmacologic agents have been advocated as treatments for PDPH.[79] However, these options have generally been poorly studied and are of questionable efficacy due to the small numbers of patients treated, methodologic flaws in published reports, and the self-limited nature of PDPH.

Methylxanthines are used for their cerebral vasoconstrictive effects and include aminophylline,[80] theophylline, and the best studied, caffeine.[79] Caffeine has been used intravenously (500 mg caffeine sodium benzoate, which contains 250 mg caffeine) and orally (300 mg). Published studies of caffeine used for PDPH consistently demonstrate improvement at 1 to 4 h in over 70% of patients treated. However, a single oral dose of caffeine for treatment of PDPH was statistically no better than placebo at 24 h.[81] With a terminal half life of 6 h, repeated doses of caffeine would seem necessary for treatment of PDPH; however, no studies have evaluated more than two doses for efficacy or safety (of particular concern in the breastfeeding patient). Furthermore, there is no convincing evidence that caffeine reduces the eventual need for EBP. The temporary benefit observed with caffeine would indicate that it is perhaps most useful for relief of moderate symptoms while awaiting the spontaneous resolution of PDPH. The familiarity of caffeine for nonmedical purposes would argue for its general safety, but its use is contraindicated in patients with seizure disorders, pregnancy-induced hypertension, or a history of supraventricular tachyarrhythmias.

Sumatriptan, a serotonin type-1d receptor agonist that causes cerebral vasoconstriction, is commonly used for migraine headache and has also been used to treat PDPH. However, sumatriptan was not effective in a small randomized, prospective study for treatment of severe PDPH.[82] Corticosteroidogenics (ACTH and its synthetic form, cosyntropin/tetracosactin[83]) have also been proposed as treatments for PDPH. Reports of the successful use of these agents are intriguing, but their role in the management of PDPH awaits further study.

Epidural Interventions

Epidural Saline

Bolus injections of epidural saline (usually 20–30 mL, repeated as necessary if a catheter is present) have been reported to produce prompt and virtually universal relief of PDPH, yet the practice is plagued by an extremely high rate of headache recurrence. This transient effect is not surprising as increases in epidural pressure following bolus administration of saline have been shown to return to baseline within 10 min.[84] Favorable results achieved with this approach have been speculated to represent the mechanical reapproximation of a dural flap. A combination of saline bolus followed by infusion has occasionally been successful in the treatment of PDPH under exceptional circumstances.[85]

However, bolus administration of saline for treatment of PDPH is of questionable merit when compared with the EBP, especially when headaches are secondary to large-bore punctures of the dura.[86] Overall, epidural saline appears to be of limited value for established PDPH.

Epidural Blood Patch: When, Why, and How

During the past several decades, the EBP has emerged as the "gold standard" of treatment for PDPH.[44] This procedure has been well-described and consists of a sterile injection of autologous blood at or below the level of previous dural puncture (due to the preferential cephalad spread of blood in the lumbar epidural space[87]). The mechanism of the EBP, although not entirely understood, appears to be related to the ability to stop further CSF loss by the formation of clot over the defect in the dura as well as a tamponade effect with cephalad displacement of CSF (the "epidural pressure patch").[88]

A Cochrane Review (a systematic assessment of the evidence) of the EBP recently concluded that the role of this procedure in the prevention and treatment of PDPH was uncertain, primarily due to a lack of reliable data.[89] Reflecting this absence of adequately powered, randomized trials, a number of controversies surround the EBP.[90]

The optimal timing of the EBP is undetermined. A number of studies suggest that the procedure becomes more effective with the passage of time,[91–93] but this observation may simply be due to larger, harder to treat CSF leaks, which demand earlier attention. Although prophylactic use of the EBP does not appear to be warranted, there is little rationale for delaying EBP if symptoms are severe.

Clinical Pearls

EPIDURAL BLOOD PATCH PROCEDURE

- Obtain a written informed consent.
- Place the patient in a lateral decubitus position for greater comfort.
- Establish adequate venous access.
- Using standard sterile technique, place an epidural needle into the epidural space at or below the level of previous dural puncture.
- Using an 18-gauge needle (or through the saline lock previously placed), draw 20 mL of venous autologous blood using strict aseptic technique.

- Inject the blood steadily without delay while maintaining strict asepsis. The blood is injected until the patient complains of pressure or pain (usually in the back, buttocks, or head) or the entire 20 mL is used.

- Keep the patient recumbent for 1 to 2 h following injection. IV fluid may be administered during this time if adequate hydration is a concern.

ON DISCHARGE:

- Instruct the patient to avoid any heavy lifting, air travel, or Valsalva maneuvers for 24 to 48 hours.

- Advise the patient to utilize over-the-counter analgesics (eg, acetaminophen, ibuprofen) for any mild residual discomfort.

- Prescribe the patient stool softeners or cough suppressants if indicated.

- Give clear instructions on how to contact anesthesia personnel on call should they experience a recurrence or worsening of symptoms.

The ideal volume of blood for EBP is also unclear, as extensive epidural spread is visualized with volumes greater than 10 mL.[87] Currently, volumes of up to 20 mL are commonly employed, with the injection stopped when the patient complains of discomfort or fullness in the back, buttocks or head. There is no clear association between success rates for EBP and volume of blood used (between 10 and 20 mL), and there are few data to encourage the use of volumes greater than 20 mL.

Early observations of the EBP reported success rates well over 90%, but the true efficacy of the procedure appears to be significantly lower. Although the EBP is associated with nearly immediate symptomatic relief in approximately 90% of cases, follow-up reveals a significant number of patients experiencing incomplete relief, failure, and recurrence. In an analysis of 504 patients receiving EBP following dural puncture with needles of various sizes, Safa-Tisseront and colleagues noted complete relief in 75%, incomplete relief in 18%, and failure in 7%.[92] PDPH secondary to needles larger than 20 gauge were an independent risk factor for failure of EBP, an observation supported by studies in obstetric patients following ADP with epidural needles. Under these circumstances, Williams and colleagues noted complete relief of symptoms with EBP in only 33% of patients, partial relief in 50%, and no relief in 12%.[94] If performed, a second EBP resulted in complete relief in 50%, partial relief in 36%, and no relief in 14%. In a similar patient population, Banks and colleagues, despite initially observing complete or partial relief with EBP in 95% of patients, reported the return of moderate-to-severe symptoms in 31%, with a mean time to development of recurrent headache of 31.8 h (range 12–96 h).[93] The rates of repeat EBP for the Williams and Banks studies were 27% and 19%, respectively. These studies clearly demonstrate the reduced efficacy of the EBP following dural punctures made with large needles, which will not uncommonly make it necessary for clinicians to consider repeating the procedure. Success rates of a second EBP appear to be equal to that of a first.

Following the successful performance of an EBP, maintenance of the decubitus position for at least 1 and preferably 2 h may result in a more complete resolution of symptoms.[95] Avoidance of lifting, Valsalva maneuvers, and air travel for 24 to 48 h are commonly advised to minimize the risk of patch disruption. Finally, patients should be provided clear instructions for the provision of timely medical attention should they experience a recurrence of symptoms.

Contraindications and Risks

Contraindications to the EBP are similar to those of any epidural needle placement: patient refusal, coagulopathy, systemic sepsis, fever, and infection at the site. Theoretical concerns have been expressed regarding the possibility of neoplastic seeding of the central nervous system in patients with cancer.[96] Although not free of controversy,[97] the EBP has been safely provided to patients with HIV infection[98] and acute varicella.[99] The EBP may also be indicated and performed, with decreased volumes of blood, in the pediatric population[100] and at extralumbar (eg, cervical[101]) sites. Modifications of usual EBP technique have been suggested to accommodate the special needs of Jehovah's Witness patients.[102]

Minor side effects are common following the EBP. Patients should be warned to expect aching in the back, buttocks, or legs (seen in approximately 25% of patients).[93] Although usually short-lived, backache was noted to be persistent in 16% of patients following EBP, lasting 3–100 days (with a mean duration of 27.7 days).[103] Despite these lingering symptoms, patient satisfaction with the EBP is high. Other frequent but benign after effects of the EBP include transient neckache,[103] bradycardia,[104] and modest temperature elevation.[103] Significant risks of EBP are essentially the same as with other epidural procedures (infection, bleeding, nerve damage, and ADP). Occasionally, the temporary back and lower extremity radicular pain mentioned earlier has been reported to be severe. With proper technique, infectious complications are vanishingly rare. Although controversial, it appears that a previous EBP does not significantly influence the success of future epidural interventions.[105] Serious complications secondary to the EBP do occur but have usually consisted of isolated case reports and have often been associated with significant deviations from standard practice.[44]

Finally, a history of significant technical difficulties with attempted central neuraxial techniques, although not a contraindication to epidural treatments, should naturally encourage a trial of less invasive measures.

Other Epidural Treatments

A variety of alternatives to blood have been promoted as patch materials, including dextran-40,[106] hydroxyethyl starch,[107] gelatin,[107,108] and fibrin glue.[109] Although not without merit, these options remain poorly defined, and reports of their use should be considered preliminary.

NEUROLOGIC CONSULTATION: WHEN AND WHY

Neurologic consultation is indicated when serious non-PDPH is suspected or cannot reasonably be ruled out. Consultation is also appropriate for any headache with atypical features. As noted earlier, lateralizing neurologic signs, fever/chills, seizures, or change in mental status are not consistent with a diagnosis of PDPH. Proceeding with treatment measures directed toward PDPH under uncertain circumstances may hinder correct diagnosis, cause critical delays in proper treatment, and can prove harmful (the EBP, for example, by producing increases in intracranial pressure).

Persistent or recurrent headaches, although not necessarily requiring consultation, warrant follow-up and thoughtful reevaluation. As PDPH tends to resolve over time, headaches that worsen over time into headaches which no longer have a positional nature should be suspected to possibly be secondary to SDH (especially if there are focal neurologic signs or decreases in mental status).[53] Under these circumstances, a neurologic consultation should be obtained and diagnostic radiologic studies performed.

Although headache and most associated symptoms, including auditory symptoms,[10] resolve quickly following EBP, it should be noted that cranial nerve palsies generally resolve slowly (within 6 months).[9] Therefore, residual cranial nerve palsy, although usually not requiring any specific therapy, may appropriately prompt a neurology consult for reassurance and management.

Since the EBP has a reasonable success rate and PDPH tends to improve even without treatment, many practitioners seek neurologic consultation when symptoms have failed to resolve after a logical but arbitrary number of EBPs (commonly three).

SUMMARY

In summary, PDPH after neuraxial therapeutic, anesthetic, or diagnostic procedures continues to be a significant clinical concern. Prevention is obviously much preferable to the available treatment. PDPH of mild-to-moderate severity will resolve in a timely manner without specific treatment. Pharmacologic agents may be useful in the management of PDPH of mild-to-moderate severity. Despite proposed alternatives, the EBP remains the sole definitive treatment for PDPH, and its proper role in clinical practice continues to become more clearly defined. The prophylactic use of the EBP, for example, is of questionable value. PDPHs secondary to the use of large-gauge (ie, epidural) needles present a particular challenge, as they tend to be more severe, of longer duration, and more difficult to treat.

References

1. Bier A: Versuche über cocainisirung des rückenmarkes. Deutsche Z Chir 1899;51:361–368.
2. Lybecker H, Djernes M, Schmidt JF: Postdural puncture headache (PDPH): Onset, duration, severity, and associated symptoms. An analysis of 75 consecutive patients with PDPH. Acta Anaesthesiol Scand 1995;39:605–612.
3. Aida S, Taga K, Yamakura T, et al: Headache after attempted epidural block. The role of intrathecal air. Anesthesiology 1998;88:76–81.
4. International Headache Society: *International Classification of Headache Disorders,* 2nd ed. Cephalalgia 24 (Suppl 1), 2004.
5. Halpern S, Preston R: Postdural puncture headache and spinal needle design. Metaanalyses. Anesthesiology 1994;81:1376–1383.
6. Lambert DH, Hurley RJ, Hertwig L, et al: Role of needle gauge and tip configuration in the production of lumbar puncture headache. Reg Anesth 1997;22:66–72.
7. Chan TML, Ahmed E, Yentis SM, et al: Postpartum headaches: Summary report of the National Obstetric Anaesthetic Database (NOAD) 1999. Int J Obstet Anesth 2003;12:107–112.
8. Day CJE, Shutt LE: Auditory, ocular, and facial complications of central neural block. A review of possible mechanisms. Reg Anesth 1996;21:197–201.
9. Nishio I, Williams BA, Williams JP: Diplopia. A complication of dural puncture. Anesthesiology 2004;100:158–164.
10. Sprung J, Bourke DL, Contreras MG, et al: Perioperative hearing impairment. Anesthesiology 2003;98:241–257.
11. Vandam LD, Dripps RD: Long-term follow-up of patients who received 10,098 spinal anesthetics. Syndrome of decreased intracranial pressure (headache and ocular and auditory difficulties). JAMA 1956;161:586–591.
12. Choi PT, Galinski SE, Takeuchi L, et al: PDPH is a common complication of neuraxial blockade in parturients: A meta-analysis of obstetrical studies. Can J Anesth 2003;50:460–469.
13. Norris MC, Fogel ST, Conway-Long C: Combined spinal-epidural versus epidural labor analgesia. Anesthesiology 2001;95:913–920.
14. Horlocker TT, McGregor DG, Matsushige DK, et al: Neurologic complications of 603 consecutive continuous spinal anesthetics using macrocatheter and microcatheter techniques. Anesth Analg 1997;84:1063–1070.
15. Paech M, Banks S, Gurrin L: An audit of accidental dural puncture during epidural insertion of a Tuohy needle in obstetric patients. Int J Obstet Anesth 2001;10:162–167.
16. Costigan SN, Sprigge JS: Dural puncture: The patient's perspective. A patient survey of cases at a DGH maternity unit 1983–1993. Acta Anaesthesiol Scand 1996;40:710–714.
17. Chadwick HS, Posner K, Caplan RA, et al: A comparison of obstetric and nonobstetric anesthesia malpractice claims. Anesthesiology 1991;74:242–249.
18. Lee LA, Posner KL, Domino KB, et al: Injuries associated with regional anesthesia in the 1980s and 1990s. A closed claims analysis. Anesthesiology 2004;101:143–152.
19. Fitzgibbon DR, Posner KL, Domino KB, et al: Chronic pain management. American Society of Anesthesiologists Closed Claims Project. Anesthesiology 2004;100:98–105.
20. Levine DN, Rapalino O: The pathophysiology of lumbar puncture headache. J Neurol Sci 2001;192:1–8.
21. Kunkle EC, Ray BS, Wolff HG: Experimental studies on headache. Analysis of the headache associated with changes in intracranial pressure. Arch Neurol Psych 1943;49:323–358.
22. Bernards CM: Does the hole in the dura mater really matter: What's the evidence? Anesthesiology 101:556–558, 2004
23. Larrier D, Lee A: Anatomy of headache and facial pain. Otolaryngol Clin North Am 2003;36:1041–1053.
24. Lybecker H, Moller JT, May O, et al: Incidence and prediction of postdural puncture headache. A prospective study of 1021 spinal anesthesias. Anesth Analg 1990;70:389–394.

25. Angle P, Thompson D, Halpern S, et al: Second stage pushing correlates with headache after unintentional dural puncture in parturients. Can J Anesth 1999;46:861–866.

26. Dittmann M, Schafer HG, Ulrich J, et al: Anatomical re-evaluation of lumbar dura mater with regard to postspinal headache. Anaesthesia 1988;43:635–637.

27. Kuntz KM, Kokmen E, Stevens JC, et al: Post-lumbar puncture headaches: Experience in 501 consecutive procedures. Neurology 1992;42:1884–1887.

28. Hannerz J: Postlumbar puncture headache and its relation to chronic tension-type headache. Headache 1997;37:659–662.

29. Bader AM: The high risk obstetric patient. Neurologic and neuromuscular disease in the obstetric patient. Anesth Clin North Am 1998;16:459–476.

30. Echevarria M, Caba F, Rodriguez R: The influence of the menstrual cycle in postdural puncture headache. Reg Anesth Pain Med 1998;23:485–490.

31. Blanche R, Eisenach JC, Tuttle R, et al: Previous wet tap does not reduce success rate of labor epidural analgesia. Anesth Analg 1994;79:291–294.

32. Vilming ST, Schrader H, Monstad I: The significance of age, sex, and cerebrospinal fluid pressure in post-lumbar-puncture headache. Cephalalgia 1989;9:99–106.

33. Faure E, Moreno R, Thisted R: Incidence of postdural puncture headache in morbidly obese parturients. Reg Anesth 1994;19:361–363.

34. Clark JW, Solomon GD, Senanayake PD, et al: Substance P concentration and history of headache in relation to postlumbar puncture headache: Towards prevention. J Neurol Neurosurg Psychiatry 1996;60:681–683.

35. Gobel H, Schenkl S: Post-lumbar puncture headache: the relation between experimental suprathreshold pain sensitivity and a quasi-experimental clinical pain syndrome. Pain 1990;40:267–278.

36. Reina MA, de Leon-Casasola OA, Lopez A, et al.: An in vitro study of dural lesions produced by 25-gauge Quincke and Whitacre needles evaluated by scanning electron microscopy. Reg Anesth Pain Med 2000;25:393–402.

37. De Andres J, Valia JC, Errando C, et al: Subarachnoid anesthesia in young patients: a comparative analysis of two needle bevels. Reg Anesth Pain Med 1999;24:547–552.

38. Norris MC, Leighton BL, DeSimone CA: Needle bevel direction and headache after inadvertent dural puncture. Anesthesiology 1989;70:729–731.

39. Richman JM, Joe EM, Cohen SR, et al: Bevel direction and postdural puncture headache. A meta-analysis. Neurologist 2006;12:224–228.

40. Reina MA, Dittmann M, Garcia AL, et al: New perspectives in the microscopic structure of human dura mater in the dorsolumbar region. Reg Anesth 1997;22:161–166.

41. Seeberger MD, Kaufmann M, Staender S, et al: Repeated dural punctures increase the incidence of postdural puncture headache. Anesth Analg 1996;82:302–305.

42. Hatfalvi BI: Postulated mechanisms for postdural puncture headache and review of laboratory models. Clinical experience. Reg Anesth 1995;20:329–336.

43. Ready LB, Cuplin S, Haschke RH, et al: Spinal needle determinants of rate of transdural fluid leak. Anesth Analg 1989;69:457–460.

44. Harrington BE: Postdural puncture headache and the development of the epidural blood patch. Reg Anesth Pain Med 2004;29:136–163.

45. Devcic A, Sprung J, Patel S, et al: PDPH in obstetric anesthesia: Comparison of 24-gauge Sprotte and 25-gauge Quincke needles and effect of subarachnoid administration of fentanyl. Reg Anesth 1993;18:222–225.

46. Naulty JS, Hertwig L, Hunt CO, et al: Influence of local anesthetic solution on postdural puncture headache. Anesthesiology 1990;72:450–454.

47. Gurmarnik S, Kandror KV: Postdural puncture headache: The Betadine factor. Reg Anesth 1996;21:375–376.

48. Santanen U, Rautoma P, Luurila H, et al: Comparison of 27-gauge (0.41-mm) Whitacre and Quincke spinal needles with respect to post-dural puncture headache and non-dural puncture headache. Acta Anaesthesiol Scand 2004;48:474–479.

49. Grove LH: Backache, headache and bladder dysfunction after delivery. Br J Anaesth 1973;45:1147–1149.

50. Somri M, Teszler CB, Vaida SJ, et al.: Postdural puncture headache: An imaging-guided management protocol. Anesth Analg 2003;96:1809–1812.

51. Liu SS, Pope A: Spinal meningitis masquerading as postdural puncture headache. Anesthesiology 1996;85:1493–1494.

52. Davies JM, Murphy A, Smith M, et al.: Subdural haematoma after dural puncture headache treated by epidural blood patch. Br J Anaesth 2001;86:720–723.

53. Zeidan A, Farhat O, Maaliki H, et al: Does postdural puncture headache left untreated lead to subdural hematoma? Case report and review of the literature. Int J Obset Anesth 2006;15:50–58.

54. Bleeker CP, Hendriks IM, Booij LH: Postpartum post-dural puncture headache: Is your differential diagnosis complete? Br J Anaesth 2004;93:461–464.

55. Chames MC, Livingston JC, Ivester TS, et al: Late postpartum eclampsia: A preventable disease? Am J Obstet Gynecol 2002;186:1174–1177.

56. Van de Velde M, Corneillie M, Vanacker B, et al: Treatment for postdural puncture headache associated with late postpartum eclampsia. Acta Anaesth Belg 1999;50:99–102.

57. Borum SE, Naul LG, McLeskey CH: Postpartum dural venous sinus thrombosis after postdural puncture headache and epidural blood patch. Anesthesiology 1997;86:487–490.

58. Sudlow C, Warlow C: Posture and fluids for preventing post-dural puncture headache (Cochrane Review). In The Cochrane Library, Issue 4. Chichester, UK, John Wiley & Sons, 2004.

59. Dieterich M, Brandt T: Incidence of post-lumbar puncture headache is independent of daily fluid intake. Eur Arch Psychiatr Neurol Sci 1988;237:194–196.

60. Yucel A, Ozyalcin S, Talu GK, et al: Intravenous administration of caffeine sodium benzoate for postdural puncture headache. Reg Anesth Pain Med 1999;24:51–54.

61. Evron S, Sessler D, Sadan O, et al: Identification of the epidural space: loss of resistance with air, lidocaine, or the combination of air and lidocaine. Anesth Analg 2004;99:245–250.

62. Angle PJ, Kronberg JE, Thompson DE, et al: Dural tissue trauma and cerebrospinal fluid leak after epidural needle puncture. Anesthesiology 2003;99:1376–1382.

63. Duffy BL: "Don't turn the needle!" Anaesth Intens Care 1993;21:328–330.

64. Strupp M, Brandt T, Muller A: Incidence of post-lumbar puncture syndrome reduced by reinserting the stylet: A randomized prospective study of 600 patients. J Neurol 1998;245:589–592.

65. Charsley MM, Abram SE: The injection of intrathecal normal saline reduces the severity of postdural puncture headache. Reg Anesth Pain Med 2001;26:301–305.

66. Ayad S, Demian Y, Narouze SN, et al: Subarachnoid catheter placement after wet tap for analgesia in labor: Influence on the risk of headache in obstetric patients. Reg Anesth Pain Med 2003;28:512–515.

67. Stride PC, Cooper GM: Dural taps revisited. A 20-year survey from Birmingham Maternity Hospital. Anaesthesia 1993;48:247–255.

68. Trivedi NS, Eddi D, Shevde K: Headache prevention following accidental dural puncture in obstetric patients. J Clin Anesth 1993;5:42–45.

69. Berger CW, Crosby ET, Grodecki W: North American survey of the management of dural puncture occurring during labour epidural analgesia. Can J Anaesth 1998;45:110–114.

70. Vasdev GMS, Southern PA: Postdural puncture headache: The role of prophylactic epidural blood patch. Curr Pain Headache Rep 2001;5:281–283.

71. Scavone BM, Wong CA, Sullivan JT, et al: Efficacy of a prophylactic epidural blood patch in preventing post dural puncture headache in parturients after inadvertent dural puncture. Anesthesiology 2004;101:1422–1427.

72. Leivers D: Total spinal anesthesia following early prophylactic epidural blood patch. Anesthesiology 1990;73:1287–1289.

73. Tobias MD, Pilla MA, Rogers C, et al: Lidocaine inhibits blood coagulation: implications for epidural blood patch. Anesth Analg 1996;82:766–769.

74. Tohmo H, Vuorinen E, Muuronen A: Prolonged impairment in activities of daily living due to postdural puncture headache after diagnostic lumbar puncture. Anaesthesia 1998;53:296–307.

75. MacArthur C, Lewis M, Knox EG: Accidental dural puncture in obstetric patients and long term symptoms. Br Med J 1993;306:883–885.

76. Klepstad P: Relief of postural post dural puncture headache by an epidural blood patch 12 months after dural puncture. Acta Anaesthesiol Scand 1999;43:964–966.

77. Fine PG, Wong KC: Postdural puncture headache: An unusual case and review. Acta Anaesthesiol Sin 1996;34:33–35.

78. Kovanen J, Sulkava R: Duration of postural headache after lumbar puncture: Effect of needle size. Headache 1986;26:224–226.

79. Choi A, Laurito CE, Cunningham FE: Pharmacologic management of postdural puncture headache. Ann Pharmacother 1996;30:831–839.

80. Leibold RA, Yealy DM, Coppola M, et al: Post-dural-puncture headache: characteristics, management, and prevention. Ann Emerg Med 1993;22:1863–1870.

81. Camann WR, Murray RS, Mushlin PS, et al: Effects of oral caffeine on postdural puncture headache. A double-blind, placebo-controlled trial. Anesth Analg 1990;70:181–184.

82. Connelly NR, Parker RK, Rahimi A, et al: Sumatriptan in patients with postdural puncture headache. Headache 2000;40:316–319.

83. Canovas L, Barros C, Gomez A, et al: Use of intravenous tetracosactin in the treatment of postdural puncture headache: Our experience in forty cases. Anesth Analg 2002;94:1369.

84. Kroin JS, Nagalla SKS, Buvanendran A, et al: The mechanisms of intracranial pressure modulation by epidural blood and other injectates in a postdural puncture rat model. Anesth Analg 2002;95:423–429.

85. Stevens RA, Jorgensen N: Successful treatment of dural puncture headache with epidural saline infusion after failure of epidural blood patch. Acta Anaesthesiol Scand 1988;32:429–431.

86. Bart AJ, Wheeler AS: Comparison of epidural saline placement and epidural blood placement in the treatment of post-lumbar-puncture headache. Anesthesiology 1978;48:221–223.

87. Szeinfeld M, Ihmeidan IH, Moser MM, et al: Epidural blood patch: Evaluation of the volume and spread of blood injected into the epidural space. Anesthesiology 1986;64:820–822.

88. Vakharia SB, Thomas PS, Rosenbaum AE, et al: Magnetic resonance imaging of cerebrospinal fluid leak and tamponade effect of blood patch in postdural puncture headache. Anesth Analg 1997;84:585–590.

89. Sudlow C, Warlow C: Epidural blood patching for preventing and treating post-dural puncture headache (Cochrane Review). In The Cochrane Library, Issue 4. Chichester, UK, John Wiley & Sons, 2004.

90. Duffy PJ, Crosby ET: The epidural blood patch. Resolving the controversies. Can J Anesth 1999;46:878–886.

91. Loeser EA, Hill GE, Bennett GM, et al: Time vs. success rate for epidural blood patch. Anesthesiology 1978;49:147–148.

92. Safa-Tisseront V, Thormann F, Malassine P, et al: Effectiveness of epidural blood patch in the management of post-dural puncture headache. Anesthesiology 2001;95:334–339.

93. Banks S, Paech M, Gurrin L: An audit of epidural blood patch after accidental dural puncture with a Tuohy needle in obstetric patients. Int J Obstet Anesth 2001;10:172–176.

94. Williams EJ, Beaulieu P, Fawcett WJ, et al: Efficacy of epidural blood patch in the obstetric population. Int J Obstet Anesth 1999;8:105–109.

95. Martin R, Jourdain S, Clairoux M, et al: Duration of decubitus position after epidural blood patch. Can J Anesth 1994;41:23–25.

96. Bucklin BA, Tinker JH, Smith CV: Clinical dilemma: A patient with postdural puncture headache and acute leukemia. Anesth Analg 1999;88:166–167.

97. Newman P, Carrington D, Clarke J, et al: Epidural blood patch is contraindicated in HIV-positive patients. Int J Obstet Anesth 1994;3:167–169.

98. Tom DJ, Gulevich SJ, Shapiro HM, et al: Epidural blood patch in the HIV-positive patient. Anesthesiology 1992;76:943–947.

99. Martin DP, Bergman BD, Berger IH: Epidural blood patch and acute varicella. Anesth Analg 2004;99:1760–1762.

100. Janssens E, Aerssens P, Alliet P, et al: Post-dural puncture headaches in children. A literature review. Eur J Pediatr 2003;162:117–121.

101. Waldman SD, Feldstein GS, Allen ML: Cervical epidural blood patch. A safe effective treatment for cervical post-dural puncture headache. Anesth Review 1987;14:23–24.

102. Jagannathan N, Tetzlaff JE: Epidural blood patch in a Jehovah's Witness patient with post-dural puncture cephalgia. Can J Anaesth 2005;52:113.

103. Abouleish E, de la Vega S, Blendinger I, et al: Long-term follow-up of epidural blood patch. Anesth Analg 1975;54:459–463.

104. Andrews PJD, Ackerman WE, Juneja M, et al: Transient bradycardia associated with extradural blood patch after inadvertent dural puncture in parturients. Br J Anaesth 1992;69:401–403.

105. Hebl JR, Horlocker TT, Chantigian RC, et al: Epidural anesthesia and analgesia are not impaired after dural puncture with or without epidural blood patch. Anesth Analg 1999;89:390–394.

106. Aldrete JA: Persistent post-dural-puncture headache treated with epidural infusion of dextran. Headache 1994;34:265–267.

107. Souron V, Hamza J: Treatment of postdural puncture headaches with colloid solutions: An alternative to epidural blood patch. Anesth Analg 1999;89:1333–1334.

108. Ambesh SP, Kumar A, Bajaj A: Epidural gelatin (Gelfoam) patch treatment for post dural puncture headache. Anaesth Intens Care 1991;19:444–453.

109. Crul BJP, Gerritse BM, van Dongen RTM, et al: Epidural fibrin glue injection stops persistent postdural puncture headache. Anesthesiology 1999;91:576–577.

Does Regional Anesthesia
Make a Difference?

74

Pharmacoeconomics of Regional Anesthesia: Implications in Ambulatory Orthopedic Surgery, Hospital Admission, & Early Rehabilitation

Brian A. Williams, MD, MBA

INTRODUCTION

The analysis of the relationship of pharmaceutical and device costs to health care systems has been termed pharmacoeconomics, and four types of analytical techniques are commonly used for this purpose, namely cost-minimization, cost-benefit, cost-effectiveness, and cost-utility analyses.[1]

With diminishing payments from private and government-based health insurance programs worldwide, physicians and administrators are forced to focus attention toward cost-containment in order to maintain a profitable (or at least "break-even") enterprise. Cost analysis is an emerging tool in health care economics, which can help physicians and administrators meet these new challenges.

TYPES OF COST ANALYSES

Cost analysis examines health care expenditures, and the subtypes of cost analysis also examine factors that are inserted into a denominator of a cost equation. Such factors include monetary benefits (eg, cost-benefit analysis, or CBA), incremental changes of health-status variables (eg, cost-effectiveness analysis, or CEA), and patient-reported quality of life (eg, cost-utility analysis, or CUA).[2] If outcomes are determined to be equivalent regardless of the treatment program implemented, then a basic cost-minimization analysis is all that is required, since the denominators are equal and the only relevant comparison is between the cost numerators of the compared programs.[3]

Clinical Pearls

THE FOUR TYPES OF ANALYTICAL TECHNIQUES USED IN PHARMACOECONOMICS ARE

- Cost-minimization
- Cost-benefit analysis
- Cost-effectiveness analysis
- Cost-utility analysis

CEA is applicable when the effects of comparable health treatments or services share the same therapeutic goals, but have different degrees of effectiveness.[4] With CEA, the analyst can compare alternative treatment strategies so that results can be expressed in identical effectiveness units. CEA accounts for the effect of a treatment plan on all clinical outcomes and its economic implications, rather than considering only the cost of devices, supplies, and pharmaceuticals.[4] Effectiveness indicators, such as the number of adverse effects avoided or hospital stay reductions, are useful for comparing the different therapeutic alternatives considered. For this reason, CEA is one way of comparing treatment plans with the same desired effect but different outcome profiles, thus producing results expressed in terms of the number of adverse effects avoided. This approach implies weighting all adverse effects alike, or weighting the different adverse effects in the way deemed most suitable by the analyst.[4]

With respect to anesthesia selection, it is highly unlikely that comparing regional (RA) with general anesthesia/volatile agent (GAVA) techniques would show equal benefits or equal effectiveness (ie, life-years gained, days of disability avoided). RA significantly differs from GAVA, and the relevant side effect profiles and risks are quite different as well. In fact, in the past few years, it has become very clear in ambulatory procedures, for example, that the choices of the anesthetic and postoperative analgesic techniques have significant consequences on both the length of hospital stay and the frequency of unplanned hospitalization,[5,6] and consequently, the overall cost of the surgery. As a result, comparisons between RA and GAVA would require a cost-benefit, cost-utility, or cost-effectiveness analysis.

As physicians caring for individual patients, it is important to note that basing a clinical practice strictly on cost analysis is not well advised, since individual patients have individual needs. However, in the setting of identifiable patient and hospital benefits when RA is used instead of GAVA, proper patient education regarding the benefits of RA is a most necessary step before any patient or health system benefits can be enjoyed.

It is also important to note that the literature is not replete with conclusive evidence addressing cost-effectiveness of RA versus GAVA for surgical procedures in which both options are viable alternatives for patient care. Limited studies available can be used to apply cost analysis estimations for other studies that did not specifically address costs, but such approaches must be interpreted with caution.

ANESTHESIOLOGY INTERVENTIONS APPLIED TO COST ANALYSES

Selection of Techniques, Drugs, & Agents

Rationale for Avoiding General Anesthesia with Volatile Agents in Outpatients

When considering invasive outpatient orthopedic surgery, the routine use of GAVA without peripheral nerve blocks as the centerpiece of a multimodal analgesic plan is commonly associated with the following costly outcomes: (1) postanesthesia care unit (PACU) admission; (2) multiple nursing interventions for pain and postoperative nausea or vomiting (PONV); (3) PACU and same-day surgery discharge delays; and (4) unplanned hospital admission.[7–11] However, most hospital pharmacy and therapeutics committees are primarily focused on the pharmacy budget. Six percent or less of all hospital costs related to surgical care are attributed to pharmacy drug costs,[12] and examining drug costs in isolation without regard to patient outcomes is ill-advised. The "least expensive" outpatient GAVA technique, from the standpoint of drug acquisition for line items used for anesthesia induction and maintenance, would probably include thiopental, succinylcholine, opioids and volatile agents.

Postoperative Nausea & Vomiting & Comprehensive Multimodal Analgesia in Outpatient Regional Anesthesia Practice

Clinical Pearls

- General anesthesia with volatile agents causes postoperative nausea and vomiting (PONV).
- Opioids (including patient-controlled intravenous analgesia) cause PONV.
- Propofol and multimodal antiemesis prevent PONV.
- Multimodal analgesia minimizes opioid requirements.

A traditional GAVA plan (thiopental, succinylcholine, volatile agents, and opioids) is traditionally favored for these specific line-item budgets of the anesthesia department and the hospital pharmacy, but the technique is fraught with "downstream" expenses for the hospital and presents a common basis for patient dissatisfaction. It has been well documented that GA techniques that exclusively use propofol for induction and maintenance (or as an intravenous sedative technique combined with RA) has a significantly lower PONV rate than do GAVA techniques,[10,13,14] and volatile agents and opioids are considered to be the leading causes of PONV.[15] Exclusive use of propofol instead of volatile agents is considered to provide an important but incomplete method of prevention of PONV.[15] Three antiemetics of differing mechanisms are required to prevent equivalent PONV outcomes in GAVA patients versus propofol total intravenous technique patients.[16] RA techniques (without GA) are historically considered to be protective against PONV,[17] but recent research has indicated that there can be significant differences in PONV incidence when differing RA techniques are compared for the same type of surgical procedure.[18] In fact, patients undergoing single-injection peripheral nerve block (PNB) techniques that are later prescribed intravenous patient-controlled analgesia (IVPCA) do not appear to have significant benefit of PONV prevention versus similar patients undergoing GAVA with IVPCA,[17] whereas patients receiving sustained analgesia primarily with continuous PNBs obtain additional PONV prevention benefits.[17]

For simple knee arthroscopy (mean procedure time <30 min), GA with desflurane was compared with ipsilateral hyperbaric bupivacaine spinal anesthesia (4 mg) to assess PONV and a myriad of other outcomes.[19] Desflurane patients received PONV prophylaxis with dexamethasone and ondansetron if at least two risk factors were present (female, nonsmoker, PONV history, or motion sickness). Despite PONV prophylaxis in at-risk desflurane patients, all desflurane patients encountered significantly more PONV (6/32, 19%) than did selective spinal anesthesia patients (zero PONV, $p = 0.024$).[19] In addition, desflurane patients encountered significantly more pain in both phases of postoperative recovery and more "extreme tiredness" in phase II recovery than did patients receiving selective spinal anesthesia.[19]

Generally speaking, for outpatient orthopedic anesthesia routinely incorporating RA techniques: (1) GAVA should be avoided; (2) opioids should be minimized; and (3) at least two if not three antiemetics of differing mechanisms of antiemetic prophylaxis should be used. My suggested criteria for multimodal antiemetics in outpatient orthopedics are: (1) if the surgery duration is greater than 30 min; (2) if it is likely that opioids will be included in the postoperative anesthesia plan; (3) if intraarticular analgesic adjuncts are used that may increase PONV risk (eg, opioids, neostigmine); or (4) if GAVA is to be used. In outpatient orthopedics, use of a volatile agent alone is a sufficient sole risk factor for routine multimodal antiemetic prophylaxis, regardless of other risk factors. I suggest (1) oral perphenazine[18,20,21] (8 mg preoperatively, with consideration of a repeat 4-mg

oral dose postoperatively should breakthrough PONV symptoms occur, but avoided in patients with Parkinson disease or history of adverse extrapyramidal reactions to phenothiazines); (2) dexamethasone[18,22–26] (4 mg intravenously, perhaps avoided in diabetic patients); and (3) a 5-HT$_3$ serotoninergic antagonist. The combination of dexamethasone and a 5-HT$_3$ antagonist is more effective in preventing nausea and vomiting after discharge than is a 5-HT$_3$ antagonist used alone.[27]

It should be understood that opioids are commonly going to be used for RA procedure premedication, intraoperative management of nerve block onset latency, and postoperative analgesic rescue of symptomatic pain not covered by the peripheral block's nerve distribution. In addition, multimodal analgesic techniques, such as low-dose intravenous ketamine,[28–31] pre- and postoperative inhibitors of the cyclooxygenase type-2 enzyme,[32–35] and intraarticular injections by the surgeon to cover myriad mechanisms of the acute pain inflammatory cascade, also have the potential to be useful.[36–42] As of this writing, the United States Food and Drug Administration has issued advisories regarding celecoxib and valdecoxib, while rofecoxib and valdecoxib have already been withdrawn from the market by manufacturers, due to an increase of cardiovascular adverse events associated with long-term use, so caution is advised pending final regulatory declarations.

Minimizing Anesthesia-Controlled Time in the Operating Room

Clinical Pearl

■ Performing RA procedures in induction rooms may decrease both induction time and emergence time in the operating room (OR).

The potential value of the RA induction room should not be underestimated from the pharmacoeconomic perspective. Performing PNB techniques before OR entry has been shown to be associated with a time savings of approximately 9 min of OR time per case compared with using GAVA without blocks.[9] In general, when the patient enters the OR ready for surgical preparation, and has a faster emergence (and exit) due to the use of sedation versus GAVA, an OR with five cases can save 45 min/day. If the cost of a minute of OR time is estimated to be $30, then 1 day of this amount of time savings for five cases carries a potential cost reduction of $1350. A portion of this theoretical savings is likely "real" in centers operating at or above 80% capacity, in which forced overtime (of preoperative, intraoperative, and postoperative nursing/ancillary staff) is a major budgetary expenditure. The cost savings becomes even more significant when cases later in the day (eg, after 3 PM or 5 PM) are commonly "stacked" into fewer available staffed ORs, further lengthening already-long clinical days. Dexter and colleagues estimated that emergence which is 6 min faster than baseline likely translates to a per-case overtime reduction ranging from 1.3 to 2.6 min.[43] In a 50-case surgical pavilion, this translates to 65 to 130 min of overtime saved. How the reduction of anesthesia-controlled time influences OR staff retention is unknown. Repeated episodes of forced overtime for OR staff may lead to a loss of staff morale, which may translate to staff turnover. Staff turnover implies the replacement of departed, experienced staff with less experienced staff, associated training, and possible surgical process inefficiencies until training is complete and post-training experience is sufficient to resume an optimally efficient surgical process. Prolonged anesthesia-controlled time may also adversely affect staff morale in both phase 1 and phase 2 PACUs. No studies to date have correlated reduced anesthesia-controlled time and perioperative nursing or OR staff retention.

OR time savings for outpatient shoulder surgery, via shorter induction time and emergence time values has also been substantiated when interscalene nerve block was used alone without GAVA.[44] In this study, recovery room times and unplanned hospital admissions were also reduced in the patients treated with the interscalene block versus GAVA.[44]

Bypass of the Postanesthesia Care Unit in Ambulatory Surgery

Clinical Pearls

- Criteria exist to determine safe PACU bypass after regional and general anesthesia procedures.
- PACU bypass is achievable in up to 90% of RA patients.
- The implications for staffing in a high-volume PACU bypass program are significant.

In outpatient surgery, PACU bypass has been shown to be achievable in nearly 90% of patients receiving exclusively RA techniques (including neuraxial techniques if hemodynamic criteria are met).[10] To achieve PACU bypass in an institution where RA techniques are used in high volume, it is important to use tested criteria that incorporate both physiologic parameters and immediate symptomatic outcomes to determine PACU bypass eligibility and to use criteria that incorporate specific outcomes for both RA patients and GA patients.[45] Criteria that incorporate the original Regional Anesthesia PACU Bypass Criteria,[10] the traditional Modified Aldrete Score,[46] the White-Song Fast-Tracking Criteria,[47] and the Mayo Modified Discharge Scoring System have been recently proposed (Table 74–1).[45,48]

In surgical pavilions with large caseloads (eg, 50 cases/day), an 80% PACU bypass rate (compared with no PACU bypass) can lead to a PACU nurse full-time equivalent (FTE) staffing reduction of up to four FTE if the PACU nurses are full-time employees, or by 20 nursing hours if the PACU nurses are part-time employees.[43] When combined with forced overtime of OR staff and step-down recovery

staff, OR time savings and PACU bypass (documented to be achievable with exclusive use of RA) can present important cost-saving opportunities for the hospital.

In a patient population undergoing anterior cruciate ligament (ACL) reconstruction, PACU bypass is associated with hospital cost reduction of $420.[49] The cost savings component from the initial of $420 per PACU bypass patient (which excluded savings associated with nurse staffing reductions highlighted by Dexter and colleagues detailed earlier) were likely attributable to RA patients experiencing fewer symptoms than those receiving GAVA. Williams and coworkers also reported that throughout the multipavilion university hospital during peak use of PACU bypass (3000 outpatient orthopedics procedures per year), PACU nurse staffing requirements for 25,000 surgical patients per year (throughout all pavilions) consisted of 28 FTE PACU nurses.[49] When the main campus multipavilion hospital relocated outpatient orthopedics to another off-site hospital in the health system, PACU bypass was used on the main campus for monitored anesthesia care cases only. Soon after, PACU nurse staffing requirements increased to 36 FTE for the same annual caseload.[49] PACU bypass should not be underestimated as a potentially powerful cost management tool in ambulatory orthopedic anesthesia when nerve blocks are routinely used, not only from a staffing standpoint, but also with respect to overall symptom reduction and return to wakefulness during same-day recovery.

Successful Same-Day Discharge in Ambulatory Surgery

Clinical Pearls

- Hospital admission is costly.
- Additional materials costs for an RA program for outpatients are likely offset by significant overall hospital cost savings when reliably achieving PACU bypass and same-day discharge.

Woolhandler and Himmelstein have estimated that the cost of hospital admission (for all types of diagnoses and procedures) is $1050.[50] Williams and coworkers found that the hospital cost increment associated with an overnight admission after ACL reconstruction was $385.[49] The likely cost differences in the findings of Williams and coworkers versus those of Woolhandler and Himmelstein are likely related to the generally healthy status of outpatients presenting for ACL reconstruction. The key point is that it will always be less expensive for a patient to go home immediately after outpatient surgery than to be admitted overnight for observation.[51] That said, precautions are required to ensure that costs are not incurred later in the form of requiring hospital readmission for complications improperly managed during the initial admission, especially since these readmissions are often ineligible for third-party reimbursement. Indeed, refractory pain is the

Table 74–1.

Proposal for Standardized Postanesthesia Care Unit (PACU) Bypass/Discharge Criteria and Scoring System for Outpatients

Parameters below should be assessed only for patients who do not require any parenteral interventions for pain, nausea, vomiting, pruritus, shivering, or hypotension/orthostasis.[a]

Patient pain scores should not exceed 2–3 (out of 10) at the time of PACU bypass or PACU discharge.[b]

A score of 8 or above is recommended for PACU bypass or PACU discharge.[a]

Movement	Scores:
Purposeful movement of (at least) one lower and one upper extremity[a]	2
Purposeful movement of at least one upper extremity (but neither lower extremity)[a]	1
No purposeful movement[a,c−e]	0
	Movement Score:

Blood Pressure (sitting position assessment required after a supine assessment)[a]	Scores:
Within 20% of preoperative baseline[e] without orthostatic changes[a]	2
Between 20–40% of preoperative baseline[e] without orthostatic changes[a]	1
Less than 40% of preoperative baseline[e] or orthostatic changes[a]	0
	BP Score:

Level of Consciousness	Scores:
Awake,[a,c−e] follows commands;[a] easily aroused when called[e]	2
Arousable to stimuli, exhibits protective reflexes,[e] with or without following commands	1
Obtunded or persistently somnolent;[a,c−e] with or without protective reflexes	0
	LOC Score:

Respiratory Effort	Scores:
Coughs and deep-breathes freely,[c,d] or on command[a,e]	2
Only able to cough involuntarily, but not on command;[a] maintains airway without support[e]	1
Tachypnea, dyspnea or apnea,[a] and/or requiring airway maintenance[e]	0
	Respiratory Score:

Oxygen Saturation	Scores:
$Sao_2 \geq 95\%$[a] or $\geq$ (Preoperative reading minus 1) without supplemental oxygen[e]	2
$Sao_2 \geq 95\%$[a] or $\geq$ (Preoperative reading minus 1) with supplemental oxygen[e]	1
$Sao_2 \leq 94\%$[a] or < (Preoperative reading minus 1) with or without supplemental oxygen[e]	0
	Saturation Score:
	Total Score:

Adapted, with permission, from Williams BA: For outpatients, does regional anesthesia truly shorten the hospital stay, and how should we define postanesthesia care unit bypass eligibility? Anesthesiology 2004;101:3.

[a] Reference 10; [b] Reference 66; [c] Reference 46; [d] Reference 47; [e] Reference 48.

most common cause of hospital readmission after discharge, accounting for over one third of such readmissions.[52]

It is important to understand that the associated hospital cost reductions of $420 for PACU bypass and $385 for successful same-day discharge were calculated by using standard econometric techniques of multivariate regression analysis.[49] Thus, the associated cost savings captured in these values incorporate any and all expenditures related to OR time, additional RA equipment and medications used, prophylactic antiemetics, and postoperative parenteral nursing interventions required for symptoms. When specific time-resource and symptomatic outcomes were incorporated into the stated multivariate regression analysis, these covariates were not independent predictors of hospital costs, only PACU bypass and successful same-day discharge were independent predictors of hospital cost reductions. Thus, when deriving any cost analysis equation using these cost-saving values, it is important to use these values only for such analyses, pending the results of future, more detailed, economic studies. It would not be methodologically correct to simultaneously incorporate cost values from myriad other studies that calculate various itemized costs of events such as "minutes of PACU time," "minutes of phase 2 recovery time," or individual drug costs or labor costs. The use of cost estimate values from multiple studies is methodologically incorrect since "double-counting" would occur, which may artificially elevate incremental differences in cost, cost-benefit, cost-effectiveness, and cost-utility.

Successful Resource Management of Well-Trained RA Practitioners in the Ambulatory Surgery Setting

Clinical Pearls

- Routine use of PNBs in outpatient surgery is most efficient when patients are likely to encounter sufficient postoperative pain to justify their use.
- Important to categorize surgery as "sufficiently noninvasive" vs "sufficiently invasive" to justify nerve block use on a per-patient basis.

In ambulatory surgery, well-trained RA practitioners may be tempted to implement a comprehensive nerve block care algorithm for all surgical patients. This enthusiasm should be tempered by the consideration of the "opportunity cost" of providing labor-intensive nerve block anesthesia for patients who may not necessarily benefit from these procedures. For instance, in the study by Williams and colleagues,[11] 543 patients underwent "relatively noninvasive" outpatient knee surgery, while the remainder underwent "more invasive" knee surgery. Forty-three percent (253/543) of the patients undergoing the noninvasive procedure received femoral (with or without sciatic) nerve blocks, but the use of nerve blocks in these patients was not associated with a reduction in symptoms, nursing interventions, or unplanned hospital

admissions.[11] As a result, these authors concluded that based on this retrospective review of a significant clinical caseload of noninvasive knee surgery outpatients, nerve blocks should be reserved for patients who have significant refractory postoperative pain, or in other special situations such as a complicated pain history or intolerance to traditional oral analgesic techniques.

In the same review of 1200 consecutive knee surgery outpatients, 657 underwent more invasive knee surgery, and 527 of these 657 (80%) received femoral with or without sciatic nerve blocks.[11] In these patients, nerve block anesthesia and analgesia were significantly associated with reduced pain symptoms during recovery (therefore, fewer nursing interventions for pain management), and fewer unplanned hospital admissions. It is important to note that the selection of nerve block anesthesia–analgesia appears to be necessary but not sufficient to comprehensively reduce postoperative nursing interventions and unplanned hospital admissions: whenever GAVA was used (in the presence or the absence of nerve block anesthesia), the odds ratio of more associated symptoms after GAVA was 2.1 ($p < 0.001$), whereas the odds ratio of more associated unplanned hospital admissions after GAVA was 3.3 ($p = 0.001$).[11] Thus, nerve block anesthesia and analgesia for indicated (more invasive) procedures (ideally in the setting of a comprehensive multimodal analgesic care plan) and the avoidance of GAVA (for all procedures) will likely provide the anesthesia care team (and the hospital) with the fewest possible side effects and the greatest facilitation of successful same-day discharge. However, routine nerve blocks for noninvasive knee surgery may be an investment of RA practitioners' time (and risk) that may provide relatively little benefit, and that takes away opportunity for RA practitioners to engage in other value-adding activities. Such value-adding activity may include the placement of continuous nerve block catheters for select patients, when time may have been only available previously to administer a single-injection nerve block.

Pain Risk Stratification

Upper Extremity Surgery

Clinical Pearls

- Arthroscopic debridement and subacromial decompression of the shoulder are likely among the "least invasive" procedures with respect to postoperative pain.
- Rotator cuff repair and arthroplasty of the shoulder are likely among the "most invasive" procedures with respect to postoperative pain.
- Wrist and hand surgery can generate significant postoperative pain; however, the value of single-injection versus catheter techniques for these procedures requires further evaluation.

For outpatient shoulder or upper extremity surgery, there have been few substantiated, comprehensive recommendations for allocating nerve blocks (single-injection vs continuous infusion) based on anticipated postoperative pain, postoperative nursing interventions (with versus without), or unplanned hospital admissions.

In shoulder surgery, the comparison of single-injection blocks with GAVA has shown predictable findings. For arthroscopic acromioplasty of the shoulder performed under GAVA, Singelyn and colleagues showed that interscalene nerve block provided definitive recovery advantages over suprascapular nerve block, single-injection intraarticular local anesthetic, and controls.[53] For outpatient open surgery of the rotator cuff, Hadzic and coworkers reported that GAVA use (vs single-injection brachial plexus block with ropivacaine) led to increased postanesthesia care unit admissions (vs phase 1 recovery bypass), higher reports of postoperative pain, longer time to ambulation, longer time to same-day discharge, and higher risk of unplanned hospital admission.[54] In this study, no outcome differences occurred in follow-up from 24 h to 2 weeks after surgery, but this study was underpowered.

In a recent review, Boezaart suggested that an anterior approach to the brachial plexus is ideal for open-shoulder surgery, whereas a posterior (paravertebral) approach is well suited for arthroscopic surgery.[55] In this review, Boezaart explains that the anterior approach to the brachial plexus concomitantly provides reliable anesthesia to the overlying skin, but the posterior approach does not. Potential advantages to the posterior approach may include less frequent blockade of the phrenic nerve, but the posterior approach is also associated with less motor block. Arthroscopic shoulder surgery using the posterior approach, most commonly, must be accompanied by general anesthesia,[55] in order to provide sufficient analgesia to the overlying skin.

In two recent, separate studies of the efficacy of intraarticular analgesic infusions, some conclusions can be drawn regarding pain risk stratification in common outpatient shoulder procedures. One study by Harvey and associates showed that patients undergoing arthroscopic subacromial decompression of the shoulder receiving ropivacaine 0.2% in a continuous subacromial infusion experienced 34% lower pain scores than did saline controls.[56] Another study by Boss and coworkers[57] showed that patients receiving a continuous subacromial infusion of bupivacaine 0.25% after open acromioplasty and rotator cuff repair did not experience any difference in pain relief from those receiving saline placebo infusion. In one study by Klein and colleagues, patients undergoing open rotator cuff repair with an active treatment of local anesthetic infusion via an indwelling interscalene catheter had significantly improved pain management than did control patients receiving a saline placebo infusion.[58] Thus, the logical conclusion can be reached that open acromioplasty and rotator cuff repair likely creates more postoperative pain than does arthroscopic subacromial decompression, based on the lack of responsiveness of the former (more invasive) procedure to subacromial infusion analgesia, whereas the less invasive

procedure is responsive to subacromial infusion analgesia. However, open rotator cuff repair patients have favorable analgesic responses when a continuous interscalene catheter with local anesthetics is used.

A review by Chelly and associates[59] provides an overview that may guide practitioners for categories of postoperative shoulder pain, until more definitive evidence is available. In this review, shoulder procedures are clustered into a catheter-eligible category if the following procedures are involved: shoulder arthroplasty, rotator cuff repair, Bankart repair, and open reduction/internal fixation of the humerus. The benefit of continuous interscalene catheters for shoulder arthroplasty and rotator cuff repair is well documented.[58,60–65] Although logic would indicate similar effectiveness for less invasive procedures, there is little evidence at this time to indicate that interscalene brachial plexus catheters would be similarly useful for patients undergoing less invasive shoulder operations such as shoulder stabilization procedures, distal clavicle resection or acromioplasty, subacromial decompression, biceps tenodesis or tenotomy, or even routine debridement inside the glenohumeral joint, when compared with single-injection nerve blocks and perioperative multimodal oral analgesia. Thus, studies are needed to show the benefit of continuous nerve blocks (vs single-injection), and single-injection blocks (vs no blocks) for a wide variety of shoulder procedures that produce an uncertain magnitude of postoperative pain.

For outpatient wrist and hand surgery, Hadzic and coworkers addressed this patient population comparing chloroprocaine infraclavicular nerve block with GAVA, showing that GAVA use led to increased postanesthesia care unit admissions (vs phase 1 recovery bypass), higher reports of postoperative pain, longer time to ambulation, and longer time to same-day discharge.[66] However, there were no outcome differences in follow-up from 24 h to 2 weeks after surgery. This latter finding was underpowered and did not show statistical equivalence.[66] Chan and associates prospectively studied nonrandomized hand surgery patients ($n = 126$) undergoing either GAVA ($n = 39$), axillary block ($n = 42$), or Bier block ($n = 45$).[67] GAVA was associated with the most postoperative symptoms and nursing labor intensity, as well as the longest discharge times. Bier block patients had the fastest recovery times and lowest associated total perioperative costs, but also were at small risk for conversion of the anesthesia plan (2/45) to GAVA due to tourniquet pain. Gebhard and colleagues retrospectively studied hand surgery patients ($n = 62$) receiving GAVA ($n = 20$), Bier block ($n = 21$) or wrist block ($n = 21$).[68] They found that wrist block patients were discharged home soonest, and encountered (1) less hypertension than did Bier block patients; and (2) less hypotension than did GAVA patients.[68] McCartney and coworkers prospectively studied 100 hand surgery outpatients randomized to receive GAVA ($n = 50$) or brachial plexus block with lidocaine ($n = 50$). These authors found essentially similar if not identical findings to those reported by Hadzic (prospectively) and Chan (retrospectively) as mentioned earlier. McCartney and coworkers also concluded that there were no long-term (2-week) pain outcome differences, although the brachial plexus block group only received the short-acting local anesthetic lidocaine.[69]

For other (distal) upper extremity surgery, Chelly and associates state that PNB catheters are likely indicated for implantation procedures after trauma, as well as for open reduction/internal fixation of the hand or digits,[59] although a prospective randomized trial to definitively verify this intuitive concept may be difficult to achieve. Ilfeld and colleagues have shown that a continuous infraclavicular brachial plexus catheter (vs placebo catheter infusion) resulted in less postoperative dynamic pain and opioid consumption and fewer sleep disturbances.[70] The surgical procedures performed included open reduction/internal fixation (elbow, radius, or ulna), bony/capsular wrist procedures (carpectomy, capsulodesis, fusion, or shrinkage) metacarpal arthroplasty, suspensionplasty, and ulnar nerve transposition. Although all of these procedures are intuitively painful, the small study sample size (30 patients divided equally between two groups) prevents the practitioner from distinguishing relative postoperative pain scores per procedure.[70]

Less invasive upper extremity procedures (typically applicable to outpatients) have not been comprehensively studied with respect to potential the value of continuous catheters versus single-injection blocks. However, Rawal and coworkers[71] showed that an axillary continuous nerve block catheter with intermittent bolus dosing provided excellent wrist and hand analgesia for patients undergoing surgical procedures that may have been somewhat less invasive than those described earlier by Ilfeld and colleagues.[70] Rawal and coworkers' study included 60 patients who received a mepivacaine axillary block bolus and concomitant nerve block catheter placement and were undergoing carpal tunnel release ($n = 11$), finger fracture repair ($n = 11$), tendon repair ($n = 10$), finger joint arthrodesis ($n = 10$), wrist arthroscopy ($n = 8$), and tumor resection or other procedures ($n = 10$). This study neither studied a control group of patients undergoing no nerve block, nor a treatment group undergoing single-injection nerve block only. In fact, 3 of the 60 patients studied did not use the bolus dose function postoperatively. However, most every bolus treatment was prompted by patients achieving a verbal pain score of at least 5 (out of 10), and bolus treatments returned pain scores to around 3 (out of 10), thus providing clinically significant analgesia.[71] Patients in this study used all of their allotted boluses by the twelfth hour after surgery; as such, the reader may speculate that patients may simply benefit from a long-acting single-injection nerve block designed to provide 18 h of postoperative analgesia, instead of the technical complexity of a nerve block catheter. Rawal and coworkers found that the most common cause of patient dissatisfaction with the continuous catheter, intermittent–bolus technique was hand numbness.[71] Therefore, patient uncertainty and potential dissatisfaction associated with prominent numbness or motor block should likely be factored into the decision of which nerve block technique is selected when a single-injection versus a continuous catheter technique is considered.

To summarize, outpatient hand surgery often results in significant postoperative pain, with patient pain scores often reaching or exceeding VAS 5 (out of 10).[72] Retrospective reviews and prospective studies have demonstrated uniformly that patients receiving PNBs have significantly improved outcomes on the day of surgery compared with patients receiving GAVA. For shoulder surgery, the use of continuous brachial plexus catheters is sufficiently substantiated to recommend their routine placement (by trained practitioners) for invasive shoulder surgery. These findings also encourage the routine use (by trained practitioners) of all peripheral/regional techniques for upper extremity surgery, although further research is needed to determine outcome benefits of continuous versus single-injection nerve blocks in the days and weeks following mildly to moderately invasive shoulder and distal upper extremity surgery. The usefulness of intraarticular and incisional infusions after simple arthroscopic procedures of the shoulder has been documented, but these articular and incisional infusions do not appear to confer sufficient analgesia after more invasive, open, shoulder surgery.

Knee Surgery

> ## Clinical Pearls
>
> - Knee surgery has two tiers of postoperative pain considerations: the first is **extent of surgical trespass** on femoral versus sciatic nerve:
>   1. For least invasive procedures, blocks are probably not required.
>   2. For moderately invasive procedures, femoral nerve block are likely required.
>   3. For most invasive procedures, femoral and sciatic blocks are likely required.
> - The other tier is **likely pain duration:** short duration (likely manageable with single-injection nerve blocks), vs longer duration (manageable with continuous infusion blocks).

Recommendations for rational nerve block selection (single-injection, vs continuous catheter, vs none) in outpatient knee surgery have been recently suggested.[73] This guideline incorporates the resource management principles described earlier, and creates three major categories: (1) noninvasive, (2) more invasive, and (3) most invasive (Table 74–2). Noninvasive implies that routine use of nerve block analgesia is probably not necessary, as described previously.[11] "More invasive" implies that a routine femoral nerve block would be recommended, but that a sciatic nerve block is probably not necessary, since the vast majority of the postoperative pain is likely attributable to the femoral nerve distribution. "Most invasive" implies that the postoperative pain will be likely attributable to both femoral and sciatic nerve distributions, and both nerves would likely benefit from routine blockade. The more invasive and most invasive knee surgery categories are based on clustering moderate and severe into one category of surgical invasiveness.[11] This algorithm[73] also describes when

Table 74–2.

Algorithm for Recommended Nerve Block Analgesia for Knee Surgery

Category I (Noninvasive)

Types of Procedures: Knee arthroscopy with debridement, lateral release, meniscal surgery, simple meniscal repair, removal of superficial hardware, drop-out cast application

Care plan: No blocks unless unanticipated postoperative pain occurs

Category II (More invasive)—Femoral Nerve-Distributed Pain

IIA. Less painful Category II

Types of Procedures: Arthrotomy, deep hardware removal, microfracture, mosaicplasty/chondroplasty or cartilage transplant, complex meniscal surgery, ACL with allograft

Care plan: Single-injection femoral nerve block recommended: No sciatic block unless unanticipated pain refractory to femoral block.

IIB. More painful Category II

Types of Procedures: ACL patellar tendon autograft, femur osteotomy

Care plan: Continuous catheter recommended.

No sciatic block unless unanticipated pain refractory to femoral block

Category III (Most invasive)—Femoral and Sciatic Nerve-Distributed Pain

IIIA. Least painful Category III

Types of Procedures: Distal patella realignment, some complex meniscal repairs involving the posterior knee

Care plan: Single-injection femoral and sciatic nerve blocks

IIIB. More painful Category III

Types of Procedures: ACL hamstring autograft, meniscal reconstruction, unicompartmental knee arthroplasty

Care plan: Continuous femoral catheter and single-injection sciatic nerve block

IIIC. Most painful Category III

Types of Procedures: Total knee replacement, ACL hamstring autograft, meniscal reconstruction, high tibial osteotomy, multiligament reconstruction (including PCL, LCL, MCL, POL), posterolateral corner reconstruction, management of knee trauma involving multiple incisions affecting anterior and posterior knee

Care plan: Continuous femoral and sciatic nerve block catheters.

Do not block sciatic nerve via bolus or catheter infusion dose until dorsiflexion of the foot is documented postoperatively.

ACL = anterior cruciate ligament, PCL = posterior cruciate ligament, LCL = lateral collateral ligament, MCL = medial collateral ligament, POL = posterior oblique ligament

Adapted from Williams BA, Spratt D, Kentor ML: Continuous nerve blocks for outpatient knee surgery. Tech Reg Anesth Pain Manage 2004;8: 76.

a single-injection block would likely be sufficient, vs when a continuous nerve block catheter would likely be of greater benefit than a single injection.

Foot and Ankle Surgery

Clinical Pearls

- More studies are needed to delineate postoperative pain severity.
- Postoperative weight bearing and ambulation goals should be considered when deciding on the use of PNBs for postoperative pain management.

For outpatient foot and ankle surgery, few if any substantiated, comprehensive recommendations are available for allocating nerve blocks (single-injection vs continuous infusion) based on anticipated postoperative pain, postoperative nursing interventions (with vs without), or unplanned hospital admissions. Interestingly, few studies compared PNBs with GAVA for surgery below the knee. In addition, few studies have categorized postoperative foot and ankle pain as sufficiently manageable with a single-injection nerve block vs requiring an indwelling sciatic nerve catheter. Most studies evaluating the use of various approaches to the sciatic nerve block for foot and ankle surgery have either simply evaluated block success rate (with no comparative treatment group), compared varying popliteal/sciatic nerve block approaches (sometimes with neuraxial techniques), or compared continuous infusion strategies.

Singelyn and colleagues provided one of the first studies describing efficacy of the popliteal fossa block placed with nerve stimulator guidance, and reported a low 3% (15/507) rate of conversion to GAVA,[74] whereas Provenzano and coworkers reported a conversion rate to GAVA of 18% (84/467).[75] In the same study, Provenzano and coworkers reported a significant reduction in postoperative opioid requirements in patients with a successful popliteal fossa block compared with 367 patients who did not receive the block.[75]

When neuraxial techniques are being considered, Curatolo and associates provide important insight that epidural anesthesia for foot and ankle procedures is associated with a high (4.4%, 7/160) conversion rate to GAVA, although epidural success was correlated with larger per-segment doses.[76] Two studies have compared the efficacy of spinal anesthesia with popliteal fossa block, and both showed intraoperative efficacy of both techniques, although the in-hospital recovery after spinal anesthesia was more lengthy,[77,78] with an additional risk of urinary retention after spinal.[78] Generally speaking, meaningful postoperative analgesia should not be expected after neuraxial techniques, and analgesia after popliteal fossa block will depend on the local anesthetic agent (and additives) used. In addition, when the analgesic duration of the popliteal sciatic block (with long-acting local anesthetics) is compared with the durations of ankle block, foot block, or subcutaneous infiltration, one should expect doubling or tripling the analgesic duration with a sciatic-specific depot injection.[79]

Continuous sciatic nerve catheters have gained popularity in recent years. After being introduced by Singelyn and colleagues who described a complex Seldinger (catheter-over-guidewire) technique for catheter placement (achieving a 92% success rate),[80] authors have repeatedly found that continuous infusion nerve blocks lead to excellent analgesic outcomes when compared with single-injection blocks (or placebo catheters).[81-83] At this time, there are no definitive guidelines for the selection of single-injection vs continuous popliteal/sciatic techniques based on anticipated surgery, with the exception of recommendations implied by the myriad findings reported earlier. Others have suggested that for hardware removal from the foot and ankle, a single-injection block is sufficient, whereas for most other foot ankle procedures, the use of a continuous sciatic catheter may have additional benefits.[59] The ultimate decision about the use of single-injection vs continuous sciatic techniques may depend on realistic expectations by the surgeon regarding return to weight-bearing status. In this situation, the surgeon may not have an accurate impression of weight-bearing success rates in the setting of uncontrolled pain, but full weight-bearing in a the setting of a partially anesthetized sciatic nerve (via a continuous sciatic catheter) may be ill-advised.

Summary Statement Regarding Nerve Block Technique Allocation

The rational use of single vs continuous nerve block techniques in ambulatory surgery, that is, allocating the "scarce resource" of the well-trained RA practitioner and avoiding routine nerve blocks for patients who probably do not need them (or providing single-injection nerve blocks when a continuous catheter is not likely needed) will free up time to perform catheter techniques for patients undergoing indicated procedures. In OR settings that care for both outpatients and inpatients, this strategy allows the skilled RA practitioner to also dedicate time to nerve block catheter placement where it is most beneficial.

EFFECTS OF PNB TECHNIQUES ON POSTOPERATIVE LENGTH-OF-STAY & REHABILITATION OUTCOMES

The Need for Training & the Importance of Multimodal Analgesia

Clinical Pearls

- Pain is often undermanaged in the opinion of the general public.
- Many health care professionals feel they need more training in understanding analgesic methods and means to implement them.

Despite the evolution of multimodal analgesia and nerve block analgesia, little progress has been made with respect to patient perceptions of quality improvements in analgesia care. This has been documented in two studies almost a decade apart using similar methodologies by Warfield and Kahn[84] and Apfelbaum and coworkers.[85] Warfield and Kahn surveyed hospital patients from 300 hospitals (42% of which had acute pain management programs), and found that 77% of patients experienced pain after surgery, with 80% of these respondents categorizing their pain as moderate to severe. In the study by Apfelbaum and coworkers 8 years later, 80% of surveyed adults ($n = 250$) experienced pain after surgery, with 86% of these respondents characterizing the pain as moderate, severe, or extreme.[85] This latter study did not characterize the hospital-based acute pain management infrastructure where respondents underwent surgery.[85] Thus, the time between the first development of federal recommendations for acute pain management in 1992[86] and pain management mandates by the Joint Commission for Accreditation of Health Care Organizations in 2001[87] did not show perceptions of improvement in pain management after surgery in the general population.

One approach to making significant progress toward improving postoperative pain management is to properly educate clinical staff. One study by Loder and colleagues describe the surveying of the clinical staff of a rehabilitation hospital about their knowledge and attitudes regarding effective pain management.[88] This study showed that rehabilitation hospital staff hold generally progressive attitudes toward the treatment of pain, but with a substantial degree of ambivalence about the use of opioids in that treatment.[88] The same staff rated their own lack of education about pain management as one of the chief barriers to effective pain management, and a large percentage reported feeling uncomfortable with various technical aspects of pain care.[88] As pain management techniques continue to increase in both effectiveness and complexity, detailed planning and education is required for all health care providers, patients, and families (surgical hospital, rehabilitation hospital, outpatient rehabilitation facilities, and outpatients at home) to help make meaningful analgesia a successful endeavor.

Opioid protocols have been successfully implemented in rehabilitation hospital settings. Cheville and associates reported on the successful implementation of the use of controlled-release oxycodone for rehabilitation inpatients after unilateral total knee replacement surgery in a randomized controlled trial.[89] In this study ($n = 59$), patients were randomized to receive controlled-release oxycodone vs placebo every 12 h, with the opportunity to receive immediate-release oxycodone every 4 h as needed for breakthrough pain. Patients in the treatment group had lower pain scores, significantly better range of motion of the knee, and improved quadriceps strength than did the placebo group.[89] In addition, treatment group patients were discharged home from the inpatient rehabilitation facility 2.3 days sooner than placebo patients.[89] To summarize, a straightforward treatment intervention of a regularly scheduled controlled-release oral opioid led to significant outcome improvements and lower use of health care resources compared with the likely typical care plan of analgesics only as needed. However, such an approach may not gain widespread acceptance due to (likely unfounded) fears of opioid dependence and diversion. In addition, escalating doses of oral opioids are well associated with increasing side effects. Dose-dependent opioid-related side effects were well described recently in a study showing that the increase of daily opioid dosing by the equivalent of 4 mg of morphine is associated with one additional clinically meaningful opioid-related symptom, or one additional patient-day with an opioid-related clinically meaningful event.[90] These symptoms and events specifically included nausea, vomiting, constipation, urinary difficulty, difficulty with concentration, drowsiness, light-headedness, confusion, fatigue or weakness, pruritus, dry mouth, and headache.[90]

Logic would dictate that using multimodal analgesia, with a PNB technique as an integral component, will very likely help improve patient perceptions of pain relief after surgery, especially when the patients are no longer in a surgical hospital (eg, inpatient rehabilitation or discharged to home). Kehlet has reviewed important principles of multimodal analgesia on postsurgical physiology.[91] However, neuraxial regional anesthetic techniques are unlikely to be a meaningful contributor to postoperative analgesia out of the surgical hospital setting, for obvious reasons. PNB anesthesia, including continuous perineural infusions, will logically serve as a future centerpiece of multimodal analgesia outside the surgical hospital setting in the years to come, but significant progress will need to be made with respect to infusion technology; dose-response curve derivation; and education of clinical staff, patients, and family members when an anesthesiologist is not in immediate attendance.

Decreasing Role for Neuraxial Techniques

Clinical Pearls

- RA techniques have been traditionally associated with fewer thromboembolic complications.
- Newer anticoagulants have offset previous thromboembolic differences seen between regional and general anesthesia.
- Indwelling perineural catheters will emerge as the primary regional anesthetic technique for postoperative analgesia, given concerns about bleeding complications after neuraxial anesthesia in the anticoagulated patient.

For many years, neuraxial anesthesia was highly recommended as a technique of first choice for patients undergoing lower extremity total joint replacement or hip fracture repair. Much of this enthusiasm was based on the classic meta-analysis by Sorenson and Pace, which reported that the use of neuraxial vs general anesthesia was associated with a significant reduction in mortality (odds ratio = 0.67), and a 31%

reduction in deep venous thrombosis, for the repair of fractures of the femoral head.[92] Years later, the meta-analysis of several types of surgery (including orthopedics) by Rodgers and coworkers reported significant reductions in mortality (odds ratio = 0.70), pulmonary embolism (odds ratio = 0.45), deep vein thrombosis (odds ratio = 0.56), myocardial infarction (odds ratio = 0.67), renal failure (odds ratio = 0.57), pneumonia (odds ratio = 0.61), respiratory depression (odds ratio = 0.41), and transfusion requirements (odds ratio = 0.45 to 0.50) when neuraxial anesthesia was used instead of GAVA with postoperative intravenous patient-controlled opioid analgesia.[93]

Regional Anesthesia Techniques in the Setting of Modern Anticoagulants

Although the aforementioned studies would logically serve as landmarks for change in clinical practice, enthusiasm for neuraxial techniques has significantly decreased with the introduction of more potent and effective anticoagulants in routine clinical practice. Guidelines for neuraxial anesthetic use in the setting of systemic anticoagulation have been well publicized,[94,95] and the risks have been more accurately defined.[96] However, it seems less likely that patients will have neuraxial anesthesia available to them in these clinical settings in the near future, pending a long-term outcome study that describes the frequency of adverse events created (eg, hemorrhagic cerebral infarction[97]) versus adverse events prevented (eg, pulmonary embolism and death) by the use of newer antithrombotics and anticoagulant agents.

In a meta-analysis of outcomes after the use of fondaparinux (the first agent in the new class of factor Xa inhibitors) versus enoxaparin,[98] fondaparinux was shown to reduce the odds of venous thromboembolism by 55% compared with enoxaparin. Although fondaparinux was associated with higher "major bleeding," this did not translate to a clinically adverse outcome such as risk of reoperation or death. In addition, the use of fondaparinux appeared to offset any outcome benefits achieved by neuraxial anesthesia vs GAVA, specifically for the avoidance of venous thromboembolism. The likely loss of the availability of neuraxial techniques as surgeons focus on the prevention of venous thromboembolism, without regard for the other documented benefits of neuraxial anesthesia/analgesia (eg, on the cardiac, pulmonary, and renal organ systems), forces the well-trained RA practitioner to incorporate continuous PNBs to give patients any chance for meaningful postoperative analgesia after lower extremity joint replacement or fracture repair.

Evolving Role for CPNB in Lower Extremity Surgery

The use of continuous PNBs for joint replacement has been studied in recent years with uniformly positive results. In the early 1990s, outcomes were more equivocal, but many studies during that period addressed primarily single-injection techniques. In one study by Hirst and colleagues, patients receiving general anesthesia did not gain additional analgesic benefit from a femoral perineural infusion compared with patients who received a single-injection nerve block, although both groups required less postoperative opioid analgesia than did controls who received no block.[99] A study by J. G. Allen and associates showed that patients receiving femoral-sciatic single-injection blocks had better short-term (24 h) pain outcomes than did patients only receiving spinal.[100] Another single-injection block study for total knee replacement patients by H. W. Allen and colleagues showed that the addition of single-injection sciatic nerve block did not confer any additional benefit vs the use of femoral nerve block alone.[101] This latter finding has not been reproduced in any study with similar methodology.

In the late 1990s, two important studies from Europe examined rehabilitation outcomes after total knee replacement when a continuous femoral catheter was used (vs epidural catheter or control IVPCA device). These studies were predicated on the notion that continuous femoral nerve block analgesia (vs IVPCA) leads to not only better pain relief but also significantly better knee flexion, faster achievement of ambulation goals, and overall faster convalescence. Studies by Capdevila and coworkers[102] and Singelyn and associates[103] showed that total knee replacement patients undergoing general anesthesia with either continuous epidural analgesia or continuous femoral nerve block analgesia made faster progress meeting rehabilitation objectives and were discharged from the inpatient rehabilitation unit sooner than were patients receiving IVPCA. Patients receiving femoral nerve catheter infusions experienced fewer side effects than did epidural patients in both studies, and continuous femoral catheter patients were discharged home from inpatient rehabilitation units sooner by 20% (40 vs 50 days;[102] and 17 vs 21 days[103] in the femoral catheter vs IVPCA groups).

In the United States, a similar anesthetic treatment method was applied by Chelly and colleagues to total knee replacement patients.[104] All patients received GAVA and were randomized to receive IVPCA, epidural infusion, or single-injection femoral-sciatic blocks followed by a continuous femoral infusion. Patients with continuous femoral blocks (vs IVPCA patients) had an associated reduction of postoperative bleeding by 72% ($p < 0.05$), achieved better performance on continuous passive motion, had a 90% decrease in serious complications (including less blood loss), ambulated sooner (2.5 vs 3.5 days), and had a 20% decrease in the length of hospitalization (4 vs 5.5 days).[104] Duration of hospitalization did not include postoperative long-term rehabilitation (which is usually done on an outpatient basis in the United States)[104] as did the two previously listed European studies,[102,103] although early postoperative rehabilitation was aggressive.

The question of the need for a continuous sciatic catheter after total knee replacement was recently addressed in a prospective pilot study by Ben-David and coworkers.[105] In this study, 12 consecutive patients had continuous femoral and sciatic catheters placed preoperatively, but only the femoral catheters were dosed to allow for postoperative

evaluation of sciatic nerve function (specifically aiming to produce dorsiflexion). Sciatic catheters were dosed only if dorsiflexion was intact and postoperative knee pain was refractory to additional boluses through the femoral nerve catheter. Ten of these 12 patients required dosing of the sciatic catheters, with median pain scores of 7.5 (out of 10) before dosing, and 2.0 after dosing. This pilot study refutes the earlier finding by H. W. Allen and colleagues[101] with respect to the value of sciatic nerve block for total knee replacement.

For hip surgery, there has been less convincing evidence with respect to PNBs, pain management, and rehabilitation outcomes. From the Cochrane Database of Systematic Reviews (2002, with no updates since then), Parker and associates report that "Because of the small number of patients included in this review and the differing type of nerve blocks and timing of insertion, it is not possible to determine if nerve blocks confer any significant benefit when compared with other analgesic methods as part of the treatment of a hip fracture. Further trials with larger numbers of patients and full reporting of clinical outcomes would be justified."[106] However, this systematic review did not appear to include studies reported later in this section.

Fournier and coworkers reported that patients receiving single-injection femoral nerve block vs sham block had a 4-h delay in requests for first parenteral analgesic after prosthetic hip surgery, although pain outcomes were no different at 24 and 48 h.[107] Stevens and colleagues reported that patients undergoing total hip arthroplasty receiving lumbar plexus single-injection blocks had less pain for up to 6 h after surgery and less blood loss during and for up to 48 h after surgery.[108] Naja and associates reported (retrospectively) that elderly hip fracture patients receiving lumbar plexus and parasacral blocks (vs GAVA) encountered significantly less hypotension during surgery, were less likely to be admitted to the intensive care unit after surgery (0/30 vs 11/30), and had a shorter length of hospital stay (7 vs 14 days).[109] De Visme and colleagues ($n = 15$)[110] and Buckenmaier and coworkers ($n = 10$)[111] provided the first two reports of lumbar plexus and parasacral plexus blocks as the sole anesthetic for hip surgery (ie, coadministered GAVA or spinal anesthesia were not deemed necessary). Souron and associates found that patients receiving intrathecal morphine (0.1 mg) vs single-injection lumbar plexus block with ropivacaine had better overall analgesic outcomes with intrathecal morphine after primary hip arthroplasty, although intrathecal morphine patients had a 37% incidence of urinary retention (vs 11% for lumbar plexus block ($p < 0.05$).[112] Biboulet and colleagues compared single-injection femoral and lumbar plexus blocks with intravenous opioid PCA for patients undergoing total hip arthroplasty, and found that PCA was as efficient as the single-injection blocks used in overall outcome, even though the pain scores and opioid requirements were lowest in the lumbar plexus single-injection group during the first 4 h after surgery.[113] Kullenberg and coworkers prospectively studied 80 patients who underwent hip fracture repair and were randomized to receive single-injection femoral nerve block

($n = 40$, block placed postoperatively) or no block ($n = 40$).[114] This study found that nerve block patients had 15 h of meaningful pain relief and ambulated 13 h sooner (23 vs 36 h) than did patients who received no block.[114]

All of the above-mentioned studies particularly addressed single-injection nerve blocks for hip surgery and did not address continuous nerve block catheters. The following two studies did specifically address perineural infusions for such patients. Singelyn and Gouverneur prospectively evaluated 1338 patients undergoing total hip arthroplasty who chose either IVPCA, continuous femoral block, or patient-controlled epidural analgesia.[115] These authors reported that patients who received continuous femoral infusion had the highest satisfaction, fewest side effects, the lowest request rate for supplemental opioids, and the fewest technical problems, but pain scores themselves did not significantly differ.[115] In a randomized clinical trial Turker and coworkers compared patients receiving continuous lumbar plexus catheter ($n = 15$) with others receiving epidural catheter ($n = 15$) for hip hemiarthroplasty under GAVA and found that lumbar plexus catheter patients (1) had less motor block, (2) ambulated sooner, and (3) had significantly fewer overall complications.[116]

Based on the available evidence, femoral or lumbar plexus single-injection blocks have the potential to improve immediate postoperative analgesic outcome and possibly reduce hospital resource utilization in patients having invasive hip surgery. Unlike single-injection femoral nerve blocks, single-injection lumbar plexus blocks are commonly associated with a risk of epidural spread, which carries a risk of perioperative implications in a frail elderly patient with limited cardiovascular reserve. One theoretical strategy to avoid precipitous hypotension (from epidural spread with a single-injection lumbar plexus block) is to provide slow incremental doses via a continuous lumbar plexus catheter, helping to potentially prevent epidural spread. In this setting, the incremental doses can be stopped as soon as it appears that surgical anesthesia/analgesia seems to be in place, but still keeping the catheter injection port available to the anesthesia team during surgery in the event additional boluses are needed intraoperatively.

Other than epidural spread, the other potential concern for lumbar plexus blocks (specifically continuous catheters) is the risk of hematoma in an anticoagulated patient. Technically more challenging continuous lumbar plexus blocks have been associated with hematoma-related complications in three patients documented in two case reports.[117,118] In one patient who was fully anticoagulated and receiving aspirin (325 mg daily), three serial single-injection lumbar plexus blocks were given, the last of which was considered "difficult," and a retroperitoneal hematoma was diagnosed a few days later.[118] A second patient developed retroperitoneal hematoma in which significant vascular trauma was noted at the time the block was performed and the catheter placed.[117] A third patient developed retroperitoneal hematoma 2 days after the single-injection psoas compartment block was placed, and this patient was rendered supratherapeutic on intravenous

heparin throughout the 2 days after surgery.[117] In each of these three cases, the clinical situations could not be reasonably considered as routine, and all of these cases resolved without sequelae and without requiring surgical evacuation. Other than these three cases, there have been no reports of hemorrhagic complications in patients receiving lumbar plexus catheters in the setting of modern anticoagulation practice.[119] There have been no published data regarding the estimated risk of retroperitoneal hematoma associated with lumbar plexus catheter removal in patients receiving effective postoperative anticoagulant therapy for the prevention of deep venous thrombosis. More cases are required to establish the safety of such a protocol. When considering the risk of bleeding associated with the removal of a lumbar plexus catheter in patients who are anticoagulated for the prevention of DVT, it is also important to acknowledge that the consequences of such bleeding are less serious than the bleeding that may result from the placement or removal of an epidural catheter. Epidural hematoma has been associated with serious neurologic complications in over 50% of cases, whereas no serious neurologic complications have been associated with the development of a retroperitoneal hematoma. Nevertheless, the consensus of most clinicians who often utilize lumbar plexus and other continuous nerve block technique seems to be that removal of continuous nerve block catheters at this time need not receive the detailed scrutiny that has been deemed appropriate for epidural catheters.

Role of CNB Catheters & Effects on Rehabilitation in Upper Extremity Surgery

Data on the evaluation of physical therapy outcomes after major shoulder surgery performed with nerve block anesthesia are very limited. Two recent studies addressed in more detail the recovery of motor function, comparing different CNB infusion drugs and concentrations. Borgeat and colleagues studied hand motor function and the presence of paresthesias in the fingers after open-shoulder surgery, when pain was managed via a brachial plexus CNB. Two infusion drugs were compared: bupivacaine 0.15% and ropivacaine 0.2%.[62] Infusions were run via an electronic device at 5 mL/h, with a 4-mL bolus available with a 20-min lockout. Although both treatment groups' patients had equal analgesia and were equally satisfied, bupivacaine CNB patients had more hand weakness at 24, 48, and 54 h while reporting more finger paresthesias up to 48 h after the initial nerve block than did the ropivacaine patients.[62]

Another recent study addressing motor function was conducted by Casati and coworkers.[120] Patients who underwent open-shoulder surgery were assigned to one of two CNB infusion drugs: ropivacaine 0.2%, or levobupivacaine 0.125%. The infusion was run via an electronic device at 6 mL/h and allowed for a 2-mL bolus with a lockout of 15 min. There were no clinical differences in pain relief quality or motor function during the 24-h infusion period. Thus, it appears that ropivacaine 0.2% and bupivacaine/levobupivacaine 0.125% are equipotent in providing

CNB analgesia in the brachial plexus. The infusion rate of 5 to 6 mL/h while allowing for intermittent boluses of 2 to 4 mL with a 15- to 20-min lockout provides an optimal balance of analgesia and preserved motor function.

One important safety feature to consider in the postoperative recovery of patients receiving continuous interscalene analgesia is adequate ventilatory function. It is generally accepted that most patients undergoing brachial plexus nerve blocks for shoulder surgery will encounter simultaneous block of the phrenic nerve, which is responsible for proper function of the diaphragm.[121–124] Borgeat and associates measured respiratory function during use of a CNB dosing technique that used both a continuous infusion (ropivacaine 0.2%, 5 mL/h) and a CNB bolus function (3–4 mL with a 20-min lockout).[125] In this study, all patients received a preoperative bolus injection of ropivacaine 0.75%, 30 mL, and all patients underwent major shoulder surgery (rotator cuff repair, *n* = 26; arthroplasty, *n* = 7). The control group consisted of patients receiving IVPCA with opioids. Patients in the CNB group had better pain relief for up to 24 h after surgery than the patients who were randomized to the opioid PCA. An important new finding was that overall respiratory function was better in the CNB group than in the PCA group. Forced respiration (ie, movement in the diaphragm on the nonoperated side) was better in the CNB group at 24 and 48 h than in the PCA group. The rationale for this finding was that the pain control was better in the CNB group, and that there were fewer opioid-related side effects (eg, respiratory depression) in the CNB group, facilitating patients' forced respiratory efforts. Interestingly, forced diaphragmatic excursion on the side of surgery was not significantly different between the CNB and PCA groups at 24 and 48 h after surgery. This study showed that forced respiratory effort was improved up to 48 h after surgery in the CNB group, which when combined with better analgesia in the CNB group, provided an important safety validation in the evolution of same-day discharge of patients with CNB catheters and appropriate infusion devices after shoulder surgery.

To date, there do not appear to be any reviews regarding the role of no block, versus single-injection or continuous nerve blocks of the brachial plexus, as it relates to the timing of meeting physical therapy objectives. Generally speaking, rotator cuff repairs are associated with a very deliberate and conservative physical therapy course, in which full range of motion is not attempted until 6 weeks after surgery, allowing for the surgically augmented insertions to heal. Meanwhile, therapy objectives after total shoulder arthroplasty or hemiarthroplasty are somewhat less conservative, in which full range of motion is attempted at 4 weeks after surgery. For both rotator cuff repair and shoulder arthroplasty, heavy lifting is usually not permitted until 3 months after surgery. As a result, hand movement is the only available proxy indicator of physical therapy progress, and this entails typically only the first few days after surgery while an indwelling interscalene catheter is infusing. A similar absence of data also appears to be the case as it relates to physical therapy function of the elbow, wrist, and hand.

Cost Analysis Illustrations Based on Available Data

Cost-Minimization Analysis

For this analysis, we compare three anesthesia treatments for a traumatic, closed patellar fracture in one patient. The mathematical formulas described here can be applied to actual incidences of compared outcomes using weighted-average techniques derived from larger surgical population data.[126] For the individual patient in this example, GAVA is compared with two spinal anesthesia techniques, one of which uses a single-injection femoral nerve block (two-needle technique), the other which uses a femoral perineural catheter with single-injection sciatic nerve block (three-needle technique). Assumptions are as follows: (1) the GAVA patient will encounter a routine recovery room stay, then hospital admission for 2 days (pain management, antiemesis, and resolution of somnolence); (2) the two-needle patient will encounter an unplanned hospital admission to "23-h observation" after experiencing posterior knee pain treated with opioids and leading to PONV; and (3) the three-needle patient will be discharged home the same day with a disposable continuous infusion device after successfully bypassing the PACU. Based on cost assumptions (Table 74–3) described in previous reports,[8,49] the sole task of cost-minimization shows the incremental cost savings is roughly $800 for using the two-needle technique, and an additional $200 when the added cost of equipment and medication for the three-needle technique is offset by the cost savings of PACU bypass and the avoided hospital admission.

Cost-Effectiveness Analysis

For a hypothetical CEA analysis from the patient's (and the societal) perspective, we shall assume that patients are most interested in returning to nonstrenuous work as soon as possible, with sufficient cognitive function and pain control. In what should be interpreted as a strictly speculative illustration, the GAVA patient is assumed to require 10 days to return to work due to lingering effects of volatile agents, cumulative dose of opioids, and sedative effects of antiemetics. The two-needle patient would probably have less cognitive dysfunction from (1) avoiding volatile agents and (2) encountering less cumulative effects of opioids and antiemetics, whereas the three-needle patient is pain-free with the clearest cognition and is able to return to work on postoperative day 3 (with an infusing perineural catheter). The increments of improvement in the return-to-work parameter are calculated by determining the difference in days to return-to-work from the reference value of 10 days (for the GAVA patient). Then the incremental differences are inserted in the denominator, and the incremental hospital costs comprise the numerator. The ratio of incremental hospital cost savings to day of work saved for the patient (see Table 74–3) was most cost-effective (ie, the lowest cost effectiveness ratio) when the decision was made to use a femoral catheter and sciatic single-injection block (three-needle technique), instead of just a femoral block (two-needle technique). It

Table 74–3.

Cost Analysis Illustration–ORIF Patellar Fracture

Cost item	Anesthesia Care Plan for 3 Individual Patients					
	(1) GAVA	(2) Spi-Fem (2-needle)	(3) Spi-Fem Cath-Sci single-inj. (3-needle)	Incremental cost savings		
				2 v. 1	3 v. 2	3 v. 1
Base	$50	$60	$90			
Infusion device and drug	0	0	$200			
PACU Admission	$400	0	0			
Hospital Admission	$800 (2 d)	$400 (23 hr)	0	$790	$170	$960
Total Cost	$1250	$460	$290			
Effectiveness parameter				Incremental work days preserved		
Lost work days (nonstrenuous work)	10	8	2	2 v. 1	3 v. 2	3 v. 1
				2	6	8
Cost-Effectiveness Analysis: Ratio of incremental hospital costs to work days preserved				790/2	170/6	960/8
Incremental Cost-Effectiveness Ratios (hospital costs per day of work preserved for the patient)				$395: 1 day	$28: 1 day	$120: 1 day
Benefit parameter				Incremental wages preserved		
Lost wages at $200/day (strenuous work)	$2000	$1600	$400	2 v. 1	3 v. 2	3 v. 1
				$400	$1200	$1600
Cost–Benefit Analysis: Ratio of incremental hospital costs to wages preserved				790/400	170/1200	960/600
Incremental Cost-Benefit Ratios (hospital costs per dollar of wage preserved for the patient)				1.98	0.14	0.6
Utility parameter				Incremental utility units preserved		
Outcome units on QoR-40 anesthesia outcome survey on postoperative day 2 (max score = 200)	170	175	180	2 v. 1	3 v. 2	3 v. 1
				5	5	10
Cost–Utility Analysis: Ratio of incremental hospital costs to patient utility units preserved				790/5	170/5	960/10
Incremental Cost–Utility Ratios (hospital costs per preserved utility unit)				158	34	96

All values in U.S. dollars.
Base costs for GAVA and Spi-Fem based on Williams et al.[8]
PACU and hospital admission costs based on Williams et al.[49]
ORIF=open reduction and internal fixation, GAVA=general anesthesia with volatile agents, Spi-Fem=spinal anesthesia with single-injection femoral nerve block, Cath=perineural catheter, Sci single-inj.=single-injection sciatic nerve block, QoR-40=Quality of Recovery 40-item scale, as reported by Myles et al.[127]

should be understood that an isolated cost-effectiveness ratio is only meaningful in the context of comparative methods being evaluated. In addition, hospital costs for each anesthetic technique do not clearly reflect the costs associated with anesthesiologist labor because the incremental workload is increased from GAVA, to the two-needle technique, to the three-needle technique, respectively. One would hope that well-trained RA practitioners recognize the value of their services and compassionately care for patients in such a way that gives the patient the best chance for immediate return to work in a health care system that is otherwise optimized.

With respect to using more population-based return-to-work data for a given procedure in an institution, certainly, gaussian curves illustrating the 95% confidence intervals of actual return-to-work outcomes could be incorporated into the calculation, and similarly 95% confidence intervals of the cost-effectiveness ratio can be determined to evaluate the extent of overlap between techniques for the desired parameter of effectiveness. However, population-based return-to-work data after the wide variety of orthopedic procedures performed are scarce, and available population data are likely based currently only on a vast preponderance of cases being performed under GAVA without any PNB techniques.

Cost-Benefit Analysis

Using the design for the CEA example discussed earlier, the effectiveness variable for CBA analysis now takes on a monetary value in the denominator. In this analysis we will assume the patient requires reasonable ambulation capabilities at work as a factory foreman paid an hourly wage, who is not paid for time off for medical leave. The return to work benefit outcome takes the form of achieved wages. The return to work timeline remains the same as that described in the earlier CEA example (see Table 74–3). In this example, the reference value for 10 days of lost wages is $2000 (after receiving GAVA with no blocks). Patients receiving spinal anesthesia with femoral nerve block are assumed to return to work on postoperative day 8, incrementally reclaiming $400 of the lost $2000 in wages. Patients receiving spinal, femoral nerve block catheter, and single-injection sciatic block are assumed to return to work on postoperative day 3, thus reclaiming $1600 of the lost $2000 in wages. These reclaimed wages are inserted into the denominator of the incremental cost-benefit equations, with the respective hospital cost increments inserted into the numerator. The cost-benefit ratios (CBR, see Table 74–3) indicate that the selection of the three-needle technique provides a better (lower) CBR than does the two-needle technique, when the reference GAVA technique is considered as the standard for comparison.

CUA involves the insertion of a patient-reported effectiveness variable into the denominator of the cost analysis. We will use the QoR-40 of Myles and colleagues[127] as a measure of utility from the patient's perspective, again comparing the hospital costs of the GAVA patient ($1250 cost), vs $460 and $290 for spinal anesthesia patients receiving single-injection femoral nerve block vs continuous femoral and single-injection sciatic nerve blocks, respectively. The achieved utility scores based on the QoR-40 by Myles and colleagues (with possible highest score of 200) are assumed to be 170 (GAVA), 175 (two-needle), and 180 (three-needle), respectively. These QoR-40 scores are based on our unpublished data for 270 patients undergoing anterior cruciate ligament reconstruction with no nerve block, vs single-injection femoral block, vs continuous femoral infusion. The

incremental cost-utility ratios would be described as "hospital costs per preserved QoR-40 score unit (see Table 74–3). The two-needle technique shows an incremental cost-utility ratio of 158:1 versus GAVA, and the three-needle technique cost-utility ratio is 96:1 vs GAVA.

In both the cost-benefit and cost-utility illustrations, as with the cost-effectiveness illustration, the decision to use the three-needle technique instead of the two-needle technique provided the most impressive incremental pharmacoeconomic benefit. For the cost-effectiveness and cost-benefit analyses, the analyses showed that the selection of the three-needle technique vs the two-needle technique provided a magnitude of "patient/societal benefit" by a factor of 14 (in comparison with the selection of the two-needle technique vs GAVA), whereas the cost-utility benefit, the magnitude of benefit was a factor of almost 5 when comparing the same increments per technique. Indeed, it is conceivable that a win-win anesthetic technique (eg, total RA incorporating nerve block catheters) may provide much greater societal benefit than the patient may be able to recognize if using only symptom-specific patient satisfaction surveys.

Obviously, the preceding examples are quite simplistic and do not account for the significant variability in the care of many patients. However, the core structure of the analyses, including multiple variables that are important contributors to costs and outcomes, can be analyzed using decision analysis trees and weighted-average techniques, to provide meaningful comparisons of anesthesia care techniques.

SUMMARY & CONCLUSION

In the pharmacoeconomic analysis of the value of RA, several considerations are important. The first is to distinguish the objectives of outpatient surgery from the objectives for inpatient care. The second is to recognize that almost every decision made by the anesthesiologist may have a crucial influence on patient outcome not only in the short term, but also potentially in the long term. The third is for the skilled RA practitioner to rationally allocate his or her own labor-related resources to ensure that patient-specific and procedure-specific criteria are met for each and every patient being considered for regional anesthetic techniques, in order to minimize wasted effort on patients unlikely to benefit from these labor-intensive interventions. The fourth is that the anesthesiologist is likely the primary patient advocate with respect to analgesic outcome, due to less likelihood of expertise or even interest among surgical colleagues and other health care personnel. The fifth is that a coordinated effort is required to gain the surgeon's and patient's confidence in the anesthesia team while simultaneously guiding all other related health care personnel with education efforts to redefine policies and procedures. Finally, awareness of overall cost implications, to both the hospital and to society at large, is required to justify the expansion of (and reimbursement for) RA services to hospital administrators (and third-party payers or legislative entities).

References

1. White PF, Watcha MF: Pharmacoeconomics in anaesthesia: What are the issues? Eur J Anaesthesiol (Suppl) 2001;23:10–15.

2. Drummond MF, O'Brien B, Stoddart GL, et al: *Methods for the Economic Evaluation of Health Care Programmes*, 2d ed. Oxford University Press, 1997.

3. Williams BA, Kentor ML, Chelly JE: Cost-benefit and cost-utility analyses: Outpatient implications. In Steele SM, Nielsen KC, Klein SM (eds): *Ambulatory Anesthesia and Perioperative Analgesia*. McGraw-Hill, 2004.

4. Rodriguez-Monguio R, Otero MJ, Rovira J: Assessing the economic impact of adverse drug effects. Pharmacoeconomics 2003;21:623–650.

5. Pavlin DJ, Rapp SE, Polissar NL, et al: Factors affecting discharge time in adult outpatients. Anesth Analg 1998;87:816–826.

6. Pavlin DJ, Chen C, Penaloza DA, et al: Pain as a factor complicating recovery and discharge after ambulatory surgery. Anesth Analg 2002;95:627–634.

7. Williams BA, DeRiso BM, Engel LB, et al: Benchmarking the perioperative process: II. Introducing anesthesia clinical pathways to improve processes and outcomes, and reduce nursing labor intensity in ambulatory orthopedic surgery. J Clin Anesth 1998;10:561–569.

8. Williams BA, DeRiso BM, Figallo CM, et al: Benchmarking the perioperative process: III. Effects of regional anesthesia clinical pathway techniques on process efficiency and recovery profiles in ambulatory orthopedic surgery. J Clin Anesth 1998;10:570–578.

9. Williams BA, Kentor ML, Williams JP, et al: Process analysis in outpatient knee surgery: Effects of regional and general anesthesia on anesthesia-controlled time. Anesthesiology 2000;93:529–538.

10. Williams BA, Kentor ML, Williams JP, et al: PACU bypass after outpatient knee surgery is associated with fewer unplanned hospital admissions but more phase II nursing interventions. Anesthesiology 2002;97:981–988.

11. Williams BA, Kentor ML, Vogt MT, et al: Femoral-sciatic nerve blocks for complex outpatient knee surgery are associated with less postoperative pain before same-day discharge: A review of 1200 consecutive cases from the period 1996–1999. Anesthesiology 2003;98:1206–1213.

12. Macario A, Vitez TS, Dunn B, et al: Where are the costs in perioperative care? Analysis of hospital costs and charges for inpatient surgical care. Anesthesiology 1995;83:1138–1144.

13. Sneyd JR, Carr A, Byrom WD, et al: A meta-analysis of nausea and vomiting following maintenance of anaesthesia with propofol or inhalational agents. Eur J Anaesthesiol 1998;15:433–445.

14. Sinclair DR, Chung F, Mezei G: Can postoperative nausea and vomiting be predicted? Anesthesiology 1999;91:109–118.

15. Apfel CC, Roewer N: Postoperative nausea and vomiting. Anaesthetist 2004;53:377–389.

16. Apfel CC, Korttila K, Abdalla M, et al: A factorial trial of six interventions for the prevention of postoperative nausea and vomiting. N Engl J Med 2004;350:2441–2451.

17. Borgeat A, Ekatodramis G, Schenker CA: Postoperative nausea and vomiting in regional anesthesia: A review. Anesthesiology 2003;98:530–547.

18. Williams BA, Vogt MT, Kentor ML, et al: Nausea and vomiting after outpatient ACL reconstruction with regional anesthesia: Are lumbar plexus blocks a risk factor? J Clin Anesth 2004;16:276–281.

19. Korhonen AM, Valanne JV, Jokela RM, et al: A comparison of selective spinal anesthesia with hyperbaric bupivacaine and general anesthesia with desflurane for outpatient knee arthroscopy. Anesth Analg 2004;99:1668–1673.

20. Desilva PH, Darvish AH, McDonald SM, et al: The efficacy of prophylactic ondansetron, droperidol, perphenazine, and metoclopramide in the prevention of nausea and vomiting after major gynecologic surgery. Anesth Analg 1995;81:139–143.

21. Chestnutt WN, Clarke RS, Dundee JW: The influence of cyclizine and perphenazine on the emetic effect of meptazinol. Eur J Anaesthesiol 1986;3:27–32.

22. Splinter W, Roberts DJ: Prophylaxis for vomiting by children after tonsillectomy: Dexamethasone versus perphenazine. Anesth Analg 1997;85:534–537.

23. Coloma M, Duffy LL, White PF, et al: Dexamethasone facilitates discharge after outpatient anorectal surgery. Anesth Analg 2001;92:85–88.

24. Wang JJ, Ho ST, Lee SC, et al: The use of dexamethasone for preventing postoperative nausea and vomiting in females undergoing thyroidectomy: A dose-ranging study. Anesth Analg 2000;91:1404–1407.

25. Wang JJ, Ho ST, Lee SC, et al: The prophylactic effect of dexamethasone on postoperative nausea and vomiting in women undergoing thyroidectomy: A comparison of droperidol with saline. Anesth Analg 1999;89:200–203.

26. Coloma M, White PF, Markowitz SD, et al: Dexamethasone in combination with dolasetron for prophylaxis in the ambulatory setting: Effect on outcome after laparoscopic cholecystectomy. Anesthesiology 2002;96:1346–1350.

27. Gupta A, Wu CL, Elkassabany N, et al: Does the routine prophylactic use of antiemetics affect the incidence of postdischarge nausea and vomiting following ambulatory surgery? A systematic review of randomized controlled trials. Anesthesiology 2003;99:488–495.

28. Frizelle HP, Duranteau J, Samii K: A comparison of propofol with a propofol-ketamine combination for sedation during spinal anesthesia. Anesth Analg 1997;84:1318–1322.

29. Menigaux C, Fletcher D, Dupont X, et al: The benefits of intraoperative small-dose ketamine on postoperative pain after anterior cruciate ligament repair. Anesth Analg 2000;90:129–135.

30. Menigaux C, Guignard B, Fletcher D, et al: Intraoperative small-dose ketamine enhances analgesia after outpatient knee arthroscopy. Anesth Analg 2001;93:606–612.

31. Mortero RF, Clark LD, Tolan MM, et al: The effects of small-dose ketamine on propofol sedation: respiration, postoperative mood, perception, cognition, and pain. Anesth Analg 2001;92:1465–1469.

32. Malan TP Jr, Marsh G, Hakki SI, et al: Parecoxib sodium, a parenteral cyclooxygenase 2 selective inhibitor, improves morphine analgesia and is opioid-sparing following total hip arthroplasty. Anesthesiology 2003;98:950–956.

33. Tang J, Li S, White PF, et al: Effect of parecoxib, a novel intravenous cyclooxygenase type-2 inhibitor, on the postoperative opioid requirement and quality of pain control. Anesthesiology 2002;96:1305–1309.

34. Desjardins PJ, Shu VS, Recker DP, et al: A single preoperative oral dose of valdecoxib, a new cyclooxygenase-2 specific inhibitor, relieves post-oral surgery or bunionectomy pain. Anesthesiology 2002;97:565–573.

35. Joshi GP, Viscusi ER, Gan TJ, et al: Effective treatment of laparoscopic cholecystectomy pain with intravenous followed by oral COX-2 specific inhibitor. Anesth Analg 2004;98:336–342.

36. Cepeda MS, Uribe C, Betancourt J, et al: Pain relief after knee arthroscopy: Intra-articular morphine, intra-articular bupivacaine, or subcutaneous morphine? Reg Anesth 1997;22:233–238.

37. Soderlund A, Westman L, Ersmark H, et al: Analgesia following arthroscopy: A comparison of intra-articular morphine, pethidine and fentanyl. Acta Anaesthesiol Scad 1997;41:6–11.

38. Yang LC, Chen LM, Wang CJ, et al: Postoperative analgesia by intra-articular neostigmine in patients undergoing knee arthroscopy. Anesthesiology 1998;88:334–339.

39. Buerkle H, Boschin M, Marcus MA, et al: Central and peripheral analgesia mediated by the acetylcholinesterase-inhibitor neostigmine in the rat inflamed knee joint model. Anesth Analg 1998;86:1027–1032.

40. Gupta A, Axelsson K, Allvin R, et al: Postoperative pain following knee arthroscopy: The effects of intra-articular ketorolac and/or morphine. Reg Anesth Pain Med 1999;24:225–230.

41. Reuben SS, Connelly NR: Postoperative analgesia for outpatient arthroscopic knee surgery with intraarticular bupivacaine and ketorolac. Anesth Analg 1995;80:1154–1157.

42. Soderlund A, Boreus LO, Westman L, et al: A comparison of 50, 100 and 200 mg of intra-articular pethidine during knee joint surgery, a controlled study with evidence for local demethylation to norpethidine. Pain 1999;80:229–238.

43. Dexter F, Macario A, Manberg PJ, et al: Computer simulation to determine how rapid anesthetic recovery protocols to decrease the time for emergence or increase the phase I postanesthesia care unit bypass rate affect staffing of an ambulatory surgery center. Anesth Analg 1999;88:1053–1063.

44. Chelly JE, Greger J, Al Samsam T, et al: Reduction of operating and recovery room times and overnight hospital stays with interscalene blocks as sole anesthetic technique for rotator cuff surgery. Minerva Anestesiol 2001;67:613–619.

45. Williams BA: For outpatients, does regional anesthesia truly shorten the hospital stay, and how should we define postanesthesia care unit bypass eligibility? Anesthesiology 2004;101:3–6.

46. Aldrete JA: The post-anesthesia recovery score revisited. J Clin Anesth 1995;7:89–91.

47. White PF, Song D: New criteria for fast-tracking after outpatient anesthesia: A comparison with the modified Aldrete's scoring system. Anesth Analg 1999;88:1069–1072.

48. Jankowski CJ, Hebl JR, Stuart MJ, et al: A comparison of psoas compartment block and spinal and general anesthesia for outpatient knee arthroscopy. Anesth Analg 2003;97:1003–1009.

49. Williams BA, Kentor ML, Vogt MT, et al: The economics of nerve block pain management after anterior cruciate ligament reconstruction: Significant hospital cost savings via associated PACU bypass and same-day discharge. Anesthesiology 2004;100:697–706.

50. Woolhandler S, Himmelstein DU: Costs of care and administration at for-profit and other hospitals in the United States. N Engl J Med 1997;336:769–774.

51. Kitz DS, Slusary-Ladden C, Lecky JH: Hospital resources used for inpatients and ambulatory surgery. Anesthesiology 1988;69:383–386.

52. Coley KC, Williams BA, DaPos SV, et al: Retrospective evaluation of unanticipated admissions and readmissions after same day surgery and associated costs. J Clin Anesth 2002;14:349–353.

53. Singelyn FJ, Lhotel L, Fabre B: Pain relief after arthroscopic shoulder surgery: A comparison of intraarticular analgesia, suprascapular nerve block, and interscalene brachial plexus block. Anesth Analg 2004;99:589–592.

54. Hadzic A, Williams BA, Karaca PE, et al: For outpatient rotator cuff surgery, nerve block anesthesia provides superior same-day recovery over general anesthesia. Anesthesiology 2005;102:1001–1007.

55. Boezaart AP. Continuous interscalene block for ambulatory shoulder surgery. Best Pract Res Clin Anaesthesiol 2002;16:295–310.

56. Harvey GP, Chelly JE, Al Samsam T, et al: Patient-controlled ropivacaine analgesia after arthroscopic subacromial decompression. Arthroscopy 2004;20:451–455.

57. Boss AP, Maurer T, Seiler S, et al: Continuous subacromial bupivacaine infusion for postoperative analgesia after open acromioplasty and rotator cuff repair: Preliminary results. J Shoulder Elbow Surg 2004;13:630–634.

58. Klein SM, Grant SA, Greengrass RA, et al: Interscalene brachial plexus block with a continuous catheter insertion system and a disposable infusion pump. Anesth Analg 2000;91:1473–1478.

59. Chelly JE, Ben-David B, Williams BA, et al: Anesthesia and postoperative analgesia: Outcomes following orthopedic surgery. Orthopedics 2003;26:s865–s871.

60. Borgeat A, Schappi B, Biasca N, et al: Patient-controlled analgesia after major shoulder surgery: Patient-controlled interscalene analgesia versus patient-controlled analgesia. Anesthesiology 1997;87:1343–1347.

61. Borgeat A, Tewes E, Biasca N, et al: Patient-controlled interscalene analgesia with ropivacaine after major shoulder surgery: PCIA vs PCA. Br J Anaesth 1998;81:603–605.

62. Borgeat A, Kalberer F, Jacob H, et al: Patient-controlled interscalene analgesia with ropivacaine 0.2% versus bupivacaine 0.15% after major open shoulder surgery: The effects on hand motor function. Anesth Analg 2001;92:218–223.

63. Ilfeld BM, Morey TE, Wright TW, et al: Continuous interscalene brachial plexus block for postoperative pain control at home: A randomized, double-blinded, placebo-controlled study. Anesth Analg 2003;96:1089–1095.

64. Ilfeld BM, Morey TE, Wright TW, et al: Interscalene perineural ropivacaine infusion: A comparison of two dosing regimens for postoperative analgesia. Reg Anesth Pain Med 2004;29:9–16.

65. Singelyn FJ, Seguy S, Gouverneur JM: Interscalene brachial plexus analgesia after open shoulder surgery: Continuous versus patient-controlled infusion. Anesth Analg 1999;89:1216–1220.

66. Hadzic A, Arliss J, Kerimoglu B, et al: A comparison of infraclavicular nerve block versus general anesthesia for hand and wrist surgery in day-case surgery. Anesthesiology 2004;101:127–132.

67. Chan VW, Peng PW, Kaszas Z, et al: A comparative study of general anesthesia, intravenous regional anesthesia, and axillary block for outpatient hand surgery: Clinical outcome and cost analysis. Anesth Analg 2001;93:1181–1184.

68. Gebhard RE, Al-Samsam T, Greger J, et al: Distal nerve blocks at the wrist for outpatient carpal tunnel surgery offer intraoperative cardiovascular stability and reduce discharge time. Anesth Analg 2002;95:351–355.

69. McCartney CJ, Brull R, Chan VW, et al: Early but no long-term benefit of regional compared with general anesthesia for ambulatory hand surgery [erratum appears in Anesthesiology 101(4):1057, 2004]. Anesthesiology 2004;101:461–467.

70. Ilfeld BM, Morey TE, Enneking FK: Continuous infraclavicular brachial plexus block for postoperative pain control at home: A randomized, double-blinded, placebo-controlled study. Anesthesiology 2002;96:1297–1304.

71. Rawal N, Allvin R, Axelsson K, et al: Patient-controlled regional analgesia (PCRA) at home: Controlled comparison between bupivacaine and ropivacaine brachial plexus analgesia. Anesthesiology 2002;96:1290–1296.

72. Rawal N, Axelsson K, Hylander J, et al: Postoperative patient-controlled local anesthetic administration at home. Anesth Analg 1998;86:86–89.

73. Williams BA, Spratt D, Kentor ML: Continuous nerve blocks for outpatient knee surgery. Tech Reg Anesth Pain Manage 2004;8:76.

74. Singelyn FJ, Gouverneur JM, Gribomont BF: Popliteal sciatic nerve block aided by a nerve stimulator: A reliable technique for foot and ankle surgery. Reg Anesth 1991;16:278–281.

75. Provenzano DA, Viscusi ER, Adams SB Jr, et al: Safety and efficacy of the popliteal fossa nerve block when utilized for foot and ankle surgery. Foot Ankle Int 2002;23:394–399.

76. Curatolo M, Orlando A, Zbinden A, et al: Failure rate of epidural anaesthesia for foot and ankle surgery. A comparison with other surgical procedures. Eur J Anaesthesiol 1995;12:363–367.

77. Vloka JD, Hadzic A, Mulcare R, et al: Combined popliteal and posterior cutaneous nerve of the thigh blocks for short saphenous vein stripping in outpatients: An alternative to spinal anesthesia. J Clin Anesth 1997;9:618–622.

78. Casati A, Grispigni C, Aldegheri G, et al: Peripheral or central nerve blocks for foot surgery: A prospective, randomized clinical comparison. Foot Ankle Surg 2002;8:95.

79. McLeod DH, Wong DH, Claridge RJ, et al: Lateral popliteal sciatic nerve block compared with subcutaneous infiltration for analgesia following foot surgery. Can J Anaesth 1994;41:673–676.

80. Singelyn FJ, Aye F, Gouverneur JM: Continuous popliteal sciatic nerve block: An original technique to provide postoperative analgesia after foot surgery. Anesth Analg 1997;84:383–386.

81. White PF, Issioui T, Skrivanek GD, et al: The use of a continuous popliteal sciatic nerve block after surgery involving the foot and ankle: Does it improve the quality of recovery? Anesth Analg 2003;97:1303–1309.

82. Ilfeld BM, Morey TE, Wang RD, et al: Continuous popliteal sciatic nerve block for postoperative pain control at home: A randomized, double-blinded, placebo-controlled study. Anesthesiology 2002;97:959–965.

83. Chelly JE, Greger J, Casati A, et al: Continuous lateral sciatic blocks for acute postoperative pain management after major ankle and foot surgery. Foot Ankle Int 2002;23:749–752.

84. Warfield CA, Kahn CH: Acute pain management: Programs in U.S. hospitals and experiences and attitudes among U.S. adults. Anesthesiology 1995;83:1090–1094.

85. Apfelbaum JL, Chen C, Mehta SS, et al: Postoperative pain experience: Results from a national survey suggest postoperative pain continues to be undermanaged. Anesth Analg 2003;97:534–540.

86. Acute Pain Management Guideline Panel. *Acute Pain Management: Operative or Medical Procedures and Trauma. Clinical Practice Guideline.* AHCPR Pub No. 92-0032. Rockville, MD: Agency for Health Care Policy and Research, Public Health Service, U.S. Department of Health and Human Services, Feb. 1992.

87. Joint Commission on Accreditation of Healthcare Organizations. http://www.jcaho.org/accredited+organizations/hospitals/standards/revisions/index.htm Pain Management Standards, 2001.

88. Loder E, Witkower A, McAlary P, et al: Rehabilitation hospital staff knowledge and attitudes regarding pain. Am J Phys Med Rehabil 2003;82:65–68.

89. Cheville A, Chen A, Oster G, et al: A randomized trial of controlled-release oxycodone during inpatient rehabilitation following unilateral total knee arthroplasty [erratum appears in J Bone Joint Surg Am 83-A:915, 2001]. J Bone Joint Surg [Am] 2001;83:572–576.

90. Zhao SZ, Chung F, Hanna DB, et al: Dose-response relationship between opioid use and adverse effects after ambulatory surgery. J Pain Symptom Manage 2004;28:35–46.

91. Kehlet H: Multimodal approach to control postoperative pathophysiology and rehabilitation. Br J Anaesth 1997;78:606–617.

92. Sorenson RM, Pace NL: Anesthetic techniques during surgical repair of femoral neck fractures: A meta-analysis. Anesthesiology 1992;77:1095.

93. Rodgers A, Walker N, Schug S, et al: Reduction of postoperative mortality and morbidity with epidural or spinal anaesthesia: Results from overview of randomised trials. BMJ 2000;321:1493.

94. Horlocker TT, Wedel DJ, Benzon H, et al: Regional anesthesia in the anticoagulated patient: Defining the risks. Reg Anesth Pain Med 2004;29(2 Suppl):1.

95. Horlocker TT, Wedel DJ, Benzon H, et al: Regional anesthesia in the anticoagulated patient: Defining the risks (the second ASRA Consensus Conference on Neuraxial Anesthesia and Anticoagulation). Reg Anesth Pain Med 2003;28:172–197.

96. Mantilla CB, Horlocker TT, Schroeder DR, et al: Risk factors for clinically relevant pulmonary embolism and deep venous thrombosis in patients undergoing primary hip or knee arthroplasty. Anesthesiology 2003;99(3):552–560.

97. Dickinson LD, Miller LD, Patel CP, et al: Enoxaparin increases the incidence of postoperative intracranial hemorrhage when initiated preoperatively for deep venous thrombosis prophylaxis in patients with brain tumors. Neurosurgery 1998;43:1074–1081.

98. Turpie AG, Bauer KA, Eriksson BI, et al: Fondaparinux vs. enoxaparin for the prevention of venous thromboembolism in major orthopedic surgery: A meta-analysis of 4 randomized double-blind studies. Arch Intern Med 2002;162:1833–1840.

99. Hirst GC, Lang SA, Dust WN, et al: Femoral nerve block: Single injection versus continuous infusion for total knee arthroplasty. Reg Anesth 1996;21:292–297.

100. Allen JG, Denny NM, Oakman N: Postoperative analgesia following total knee arthroplasty: A study comparing spinal anesthesia and combined sciatic femoral 3-in-1 block. Reg Anesth Pain Med 1998;23:142–146.

101. Allen HW, Liu SS, Ware PD, et al: Peripheral nerve blocks improve analgesia after total knee replacement surgery. Anesth Analg 1998;87:93–97.

102. Capdevila X, Barthelet Y, Biboulet P, et al: Effects of perioperative analgesic technique on the surgical outcome and duration of rehabilitation after major knee surgery. Anesthesiology 1999;91:8–15.

103. Singelyn FJ, Deyaert M, Pendeville E, et al: Effects of intravenous patient-controlled analgesia with morphine, continuous epidural analgesia, and continuous three-in-one block on postoperative pain and knee rehabilitation after unilateral total knee arthroplasty. Anesth Analg 1998;87:88–92.

104. Chelly JE, Greger J, Gebhard R, et al: Continuous femoral blocks improve recovery and outcome of patients undergoing total knee arthroplasty. J Arthroplasty 2001;16:436–445.

105. Ben-David B, Schmalenberger K, Chelly JE: Analgesia after total knee arthroplasty: Is continuous sciatic blockade needed in addition to continuous femoral blockade? Anesth Analg 2004;98:747–749.

106. Parker MJ, Griffiths R, Appadu BN: Nerve blocks (subcostal, lateral cutaneous, femoral, triple, psoas) for hip fractures [update of Cochrane Database Syst Rev. 2001;(2):CD001159; PMID: 11405976]. Cochrane Database Syst Rev 1, 2002.

107. Fournier R, Van Gessel E, Gaggero G, et al: Postoperative analgesia with "3-in-1" femoral nerve block after prosthetic hip surgery. Can J Anaesth 1998;45:34–38.

108. Stevens RD, Van Gessel E, Flory N, et al: Lumbar plexus block reduces pain and blood loss associated with total hip arthroplasty. Anesthesiology 2000;93:115–121.

109. Naja Z, el Hassan MJ, Khatib H, et al: Combined sciatic-paravertebral nerve block vs. general anaesthesia for fractured hip of the elderly. Middle East J Anesthesiol 2000;15:559–568.

110. de Visme V, Picart F, Le Jouan R, et al: Combined lumbar and sacral plexus block compared with plain bupivacaine spinal anesthesia for hip fractures in the elderly. Reg Anesth Pain Med 2000;25:158–162.

111. Buckenmaier CC 3rd, Xenos JS, Nilsen SM: Lumbar plexus block with perineural catheter and sciatic nerve block for total hip arthroplasty. J Arthroplasty 2002;17:499–502.

112. Souron V, Delaunay L, Schifrine P: Intrathecal morphine provides better postoperative analgesia than psoas compartment block after primary hip arthroplasty. Can J Anaesth 2003;50:574–579.

113. Biboulet P, Morau D, Aubas P, et al: Postoperative analgesia after total-hip arthroplasty: Comparison of intravenous patient-controlled analgesia with morphine and single injection of femoral nerve or psoas compartment block. A prospective, randomized, double-blind study. Reg Anesth Pain Med 2004;29:102–109.

114. Kullenberg B, Ysberg B, Heilman M, et al: [Femoral nerve block as pain relief in hip fracture. A good alternative in perioperative treatment proved by a prospective study]. Lakartidningen 2004;101:2104–2107.

115. Singelyn FJ, Gouverneur JM: Postoperative analgesia after total hip arthroplasty: IV PCA with morphine, patient-controlled epidural analgesia, or continuous "3-in-1" block? A prospective evaluation by our acute pain service in more than 1,300 patients. J Clin Anesth 1999;11:550–554.

116. Turker G, Uckunkaya N, Yavascaoglu B, et al: Comparison of the catheter-technique psoas compartment block and the epidural block for analgesia in partial hip replacement surgery. Acta Anaesthesiol Scand 2003;47:30–36.

117. Weller RS, Gerancher JC, Crews JC, et al: Extensive retroperitoneal hematoma without neurologic deficit in two patients who underwent lumbar plexus block and were later anticoagulated. Anesthesiology 2003;98:581–585.

118. Klein SM, D'Ercole F, Greengrass RA, et al: Enoxaparin associated with psoas hematoma and lumbar plexopathy after lumbar plexus block. Anesthesiology 1997;87:1576–1579.

119. Hantler C, Despotis GJ, Sinha R, et al: Guidelines and alternatives for neuraxial anesthesia and venous thromboembolism prophylaxis in major orthopedic surgery. J Arthroplasty 2004;19:1004–1016.

120. Casati A, Borghi B, Fanelli G, et al: Interscalene brachial plexus anesthesia and analgesia for open shoulder surgery: A randomized, double-blinded comparison between levobupivacaine and ropivacaine. Anesth Analg 2003;96:253–259.

121. Urmey WF, McDonald M: Hemidiaphragmatic paresis during interscalene brachial plexus block: Effects on pulmonary function and chest wall mechanics. Anesth Analg 1992;74:352–357.

122. Urmey WF, Talts KH, Sharrock NE: One hundred percent incidence of hemidiaphragmatic paresis associated with interscalene brachial plexus anesthesia as diagnosed by ultrasonography. Anesth Analg 1991;72:498–503.

123. Urmey WF, Gloeggler PJ: Pulmonary function changes during interscalene brachial plexus block: Effects of decreasing local anesthetic injection volume. Reg Anesth 1993;18:244–249.

124. Urmey WF, Grossi P, Sharrock NE, et al: Digital pressure during interscalene block is clinically ineffective in preventing anesthetic spread to the cervical plexus. Anesth Analg 1996;83:366–370.

125. Borgeat A, Perschak H, Bird P, et al: Patient-controlled interscalene analgesia with ropivacaine 0.2% versus patient-controlled intravenous analgesia after major shoulder surgery: Effects on diaphragmatic and respiratory function. Anesthesiology 2000;92: 102–108.

126. Williams BA, Kentor ML: Making an ambulatory surgery center suitable for regional anaesthesia. Bailliere's Best Pract Res Clin Anaesthesiol 2002;16:175–194.

127. Myles PS, Weitkamp B, Jones K, et al: Validity and reliability of a postoperative quality of recovery score: The QoR-40. Br J Anaesth 2000;84:11–15.

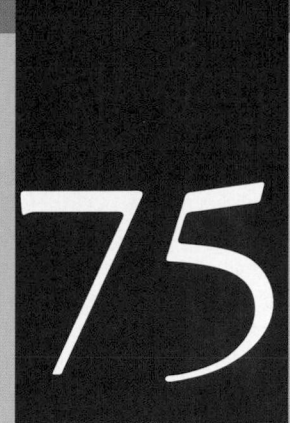

Effects of Regional Anesthesia & Analgesia on Perioperative Outcome

Christopher L. Wu, MD • Brian A. Williams, MD

INTRODUCTION

Patients with severe medical conditions who undergo surgery are at a higher risk for perioperative morbidity and mortality. These patients have limited physiologic reserves, which may be overwhelmed by the perioperative stress from the trauma of surgery. The use of perioperative regional anesthesia and analgesia may attenuate detrimental perioperative pathophysiology and potentially diminish the incidence of adverse patient outcomes including mortality and major morbidity.[1–4] Because only limited data are available on the effect of perioperative peripheral anesthesia and analgesia, this discussion, like much of the available data, focuses on the perioperative use of neuraxial, particularly epidural, anesthe-

sia and analgesia. Nevertheless, the general concepts behind the benefits of perioperative neuraxial anesthesia and analgesia may ultimately be applicable to peripheral anesthesia and analgesia.

In general, perioperative regional anesthesia and analgesia (as opposed to general anesthesia followed by systemic opioids for postoperative pain control), especially that using a local anesthetic-based solution, can provide superior analgesia and attenuate adverse perioperative pathophysiology, particularly the neuroendocrine stress response. These benefits potentially can translate into decreased incidence of morbidity and mortality and to improved convalescence. Curiously, however, trials did not consistently document an improvement in these outcomes with the perioperative use of regional anesthesia and analgesia. Although some data support the use of perioperative epidural anesthesia and analgesia to decrease postoperative pulmonary, gastrointestinal, and cardiovascular complications,[2–6] whether regional anesthesia is superior to general anesthesia in decreasing mortality is still controversial. Recent trials provide both supporting[1] and refuting[2,7] evidence. The various methodologic differences and problems present in available trial results influence both the interpretation and applicability of the trial results.[8]

INTRAOPERATIVE BENEFITS OF REGIONAL ANESTHESIA

A wide range of detrimental physiologic effects, such as the neuroendocrine stress response, hypercoagulation, immunosuppression, and impaired gastrointestinal and pulmonary function, occur as a result of surgical trauma. These effects contribute to the development of postoperative mortality and morbidity. Many of these adverse pathophysiologic responses begin in the intraoperative period and continue into the postoperative period, although the precise overall contribution of each period (intraoperative vs postoperative) to postoperative morbidity and mortality has not been fully evaluated. In a sense, these divisions (intraoperative vs postoperative) are artificial because most of these pathophysiologies follow a continuum from the intraoperative to postoperative period. However, elucidating the exact pathophysiology and differential contribution to postoperative morbidity and mortality would allow optimization of perioperative regional anesthesia and analgesia since different pathophysiologies will exhibit different peaks for the development of complications. For instance, the perioperative hypercoagulable state begins in the intraoperative period,[9] but the majority of thromboembolic events occur well into the postoperative period. Likewise, the incidence of other complications, such as myocardial infarction and delirium, often peak in the postoperative period (eg, second or third postoperative day).[10–12]

Clinical Pearls

- A recent meta-analysis of randomized studies examining the effect of intraoperative neuraxial vs general anesthesia on mortality demonstrated that use of perioperative neuraxial anesthesia reduced the overall mortality rate (primarily in orthopedic patients) by approximately 30%.
- The analysis also showed that perioperative neuraxial anesthesia and analgesia decreased the odds of the development of deep venous thrombosis by 44%, pulmonary embolism by 55%, pneumonia by 39%, and respiratory depression by 59% and decreased the need for transfusion by 55%.

Although many of the smaller randomized controlled trials failed to show a decrease in mortality rates with use of intraoperative regional anesthesia,[2,7,13,14] all of these trials were underpowered to assess a rare outcome, such as death. A meta-analysis of randomized data (up to 1997) examining the effect of intraoperative neuraxial vs general anesthesia on mortality included a total of 141 trials with 9559 subjects. Results demonstrated that the use of perioperative neuraxial anesthesia reduced the overall mortality rate (primarily in orthopedic patients) by approximately 30%.[1] Subgroup analysis showed that perioperative neuraxial anesthesia and analgesia decreased the odds of the development of deep venous thrombosis by 44%, pulmonary embolism by 55%, pneumonia by 39%, and respiratory depression by 59%, and reduced the need for transfusion by 55%. The majority of trials used in the meta-analysis compared intraoperative neuraxial anesthesia with general anesthesia, with only a few studies examining intraoperative epidural anesthesia followed by postoperative epidural analgesia.[1]

POSTOPERATIVE BENEFITS OF REGIONAL ANALGESIA

Although the majority of benefit trials focused on intraoperative neuraxial anesthesia vs general anesthesia, the role of postoperative regional analgesia on outcomes has not been evaluated extensively. As discussed previously, little data exist on the effect of postoperative peripheral analgesia on postoperative outcomes; the discussion here focuses primarily on postoperative epidural analgesia. Available data suggest that postoperative epidural analgesia may improve patient outcomes, including a decreased mortality rate.[2–6,15] An analysis of the Medicare claims database from 1997 through 2001 noted that the use of postoperative epidural analgesia was associated with a significant decrease in 7-day [odds ratio = 0.52 (95% confidence interval: 0.38–0.73), $p = 0.0001$] and 30-day [odds ratio = 0.74 (95% confidence interval: 0.63–0.89), $p = 0.0005$] mortality rates after a variety of surgical procedures.[15] Other benefits of perioperative epidural analgesia for decreasing morbidity are discussed later in this chapter; however, it must be kept in mind that some study design-related issues potentially limit the generalizability of these results to a broader surgical population.[16–18]

Cardiovascular Morbidity

Patients at risk for perioperative myocardial events have a higher incidence of myocardial ischemia and infarction. The stress of surgery or uncontrolled pain can activate the sympathetic nervous system, resulting in an imbalance between myocardial oxygen supply and demand and leading to myocardial ischemia and infarction.[19] In addition, postoperative hypercoagulability can contribute to the myocardial oxygen imbalance and be an important factor in the development of perioperative myocardial ischemia and infarction.[20]

Perioperative myocardial infarction and other cardiovascular events, such as congestive heart failure, ventricular arrhythmias, and sudden death, occur with greater frequency within the first 2–3 days after surgery.[12,21]

Clinical Pearl

■ Perioperative myocardial infarction and other cardiovascular events, such as congestive heart failure, ventricular arrhythmias, and sudden death, occur with greater frequency within the first 2–3 days after surgery.

Epidural analgesia may attenuate these adverse cardiovascular pathophysiologic events. Experimental studies demonstrate that thoracic epidural analgesia (TEA) will decrease cardiac sympathetic outflow; ease increases in heart rate, blood pressure, inotropy, and myocardial oxygen consumption; and result in a favorable myocardial supply and demand balance by improving coronary blood flow to subendocardial areas at risk for ischemia. These physiologic benefits were shown to reduce the anatomic extent of experimentally induced myocardial infarction and ischemia-induced malignant arrhythmias.[22–24] Clinically, the effect of postoperative epidural analgesia on the incidence of myocardial ischemia or infarction in randomized trials is not known with certainty,[13,25–29] although a meta-analysis revealed that the use of thoracic, but not lumbar, epidural analgesia significantly decreases the incidence of postoperative myocardial infarction.[3] The benefits of thoracic but not lumbar epidural analgesia in decreasing adverse cardiovascular events, such as myocardial infarction, corroborates the findings of the physiologic benefits of TEA in experimental studies.

Coagulation-Related Morbidity

Coagulation-related complications, such as deep venous thrombosis and pulmonary embolism, are a major cause of morbidity and mortality following surgery.[30,31] Patients are hypercoagulable postoperatively, in part, as a result of the neuroendocine stress response. Perioperative use of a local anesthetic-based neuraxial anesthetic and analgesic technique attenuate this hypercoagulable response by increasing peripheral blood flow, preserving fibrinolytic activity, easing increases in coagulation factors, and decreasing blood viscosity.[32] A number of randomized trials and meta-analyses indicate that the use of perioperative regional anesthesia and analgesia (vs general anesthesia) will decrease the incidence of postoperative hypercoagulability-related events, such as deep venous thrombosis, pulmonary embolism, and vascular graft thrombosis.[1,28,33,34] However, it is notable that many of these trial protocols did not use concurrent systemic thromboprophylaxis.

Clinical Pearl

■ Randomized trials and meta-analyses indicate that the use of perioperative regional anesthesia and analgesia decreases the incidence of postoperative hypercoagulability-related events, such as deep venous thrombosis, pulmonary embolism, and vascular graft thrombosis.

The effect of postoperative epidural analgesia per se on the development of hypercoagulability-related events is unclear. Some data demonstrate a lower incidence of deep venous thrombosis with use of postoperative epidural analgesia.[35,36] Experimental data indicate a lack of physiologic benefits (eg, increased blood flow) when continuing epidural analgesia into the postoperative period.[9] Similarly, Medicare claims analyses do not indicate that the presence of postoperative epidural analgesia will decrease the incidence of coagulation-related events.[15,37] Further study is needed to determine if the addition of perioperative neuraxial anesthesia and analgesia to systemic thromboprophylaxis will lower the incidence of coagulation-related events.

Gastrointestinal Morbidity

One of the most feared postoperative gastrointestinal complications is ileus, which results in increased postoperative pain, prolonged hospital stays, pulmonary complications, septic complications, and decreased wound healing.[6,38–42] The cause of postoperative ileus is multifactorial and includes the postoperative use of opioids, increases in sympathetic output (from the neuroendocrine stress response and uncontrolled pain), inputs from the systemic inflammatory response, and spinally mediated reflex arcs involving afferent stimuli (from somatic and visceral inputs) into the spinal cord and efferent stimuli from the sympathetic nervous system.[5,38,42] TEA using a local anesthetic-based analgesic regimen may assuage some of these detrimental pathophysiologic effects and increase gastrointestinal motility and intestinal blood flow.[5] TEA has many physiologic benefits, including increased gut mucosal blood flow,[28] with the possible reduction of ileus after bowel ischemia,[43] attenuation of somatic and visceral nociceptive afferent fibers of the spinal reflex arcs,[5] and exertion of a beneficial physiologic and analgesic effect after systemic absorption of local anesthetic.[44,45] In addition, epidural analgesia using a local anesthetic-based analgesic regimen decreases the amount of opioids used, which may facilitate return of gastrointestinal function.

Clinical Pearls

■ The cause of postoperative ileus is multifactorial and includes postoperative use of opioids, increases in sympathetic output (from the neuroendocrine stress response and uncontrolled pain), inputs from the systemic inflammatory response, and spinally mediated reflex arcs involving afferent stimuli (from somatic and visceral inputs) into the spinal cord and efferent stimuli from the sympathetic nervous system.

- Randomized controlled trial results suggest that when compared with systemic or neuraxial opioid analgesia, use of postoperative thoracic epidural analgesia with a local anesthetic-based regimen results in earlier return of gastrointestinal function.

Randomized controlled trial results suggest that when compared with systemic or neuraxial opioid analgesia, use of postoperative thoracic epidural analgesia with a local anesthetic-based regimen results in earlier return of gastrointestinal function. A systematic review of all randomized trial results demonstrated that epidural administration of local anesthetics (compared with systemic or epidural opioids) in patients undergoing abdominal surgery facilitates return of gastrointestinal function.[46] In addition, thoracic epidural analgesia with local anesthetics may provide earlier fulfillment of discharge criteria.[47,48] By contrast, use of epidural opioids, whether alone or in combination with local anesthetics, delays return of gastrointestinal motility compared with that seen in patients who receive epidural local anesthetics alone.[47,49–52]

Pulmonary Morbidity

Pulmonary complications, such as pneumonia and respiratory failure, are important causes of postoperative morbidity and mortality and are an important contributor to prolonged hospital and intensive care unit stays.[30,53] Altered pulmonary mechanics, inadequate analgesia, and systemic opioid analgesics contribute to perioperative respiratory complications, especially in patients receiving general anesthetic agents. These agents suppress the activation of respiratory muscles, resulting in uncoordination of respiratory muscle activity[54] and possibly decreased functional residual capacity (FRC) and atelectasis. In addition, spinal reflex inhibition of the phrenic nerve (with a resultant decrease in diaphragmatic function) also decreases FRC and can result in atelectasis. Finally, poor pain control can result in shallow breathing and interfere with the patient's ability to participate with respiratory therapy such as incentive spirometry.

Clinical Pearl

- Use of a local anesthetic-based epidural analgesia reduces reflexive spinal inhibition of diaphragmatic activity, preserves hypoxic pulmonary vasoconstriction in poorly ventilated segments of lung, and decreases the need for systemic opioids, all of which results in superior analgesia, allowing patients to more fully participate in rehabilitative physiotherapy.

Use of a local anesthetic-based epidural regimen may reduce some of these adverse pathophysiologic changes by attenuating reflexive spinal inhibition of diaphragmatic activity, preserving hypoxic pulmonary vasoconstriction in poorly ventilated segments of lung, and decreasing the use of systemic opioids. The regimen provides superior analgesia and allows patients to fully participate in rehabilitative physiotherapy.[55,56] Despite some controversy regarding the precise definition of pulmonary complications, randomized controlled trial results and meta-analyses demonstrated improved patient outcomes with the perioperative use of epidural techniques. Two meta-analyses demonstrated a decrease in the incidence of atelectasis, respiratory complications, and respiratory depression with perioperative use of regional anesthetic and analgesic techniques.[1,4] Use of epidural anesthesia–analgesia was superior to intercostal blocks, wound infiltration, or intrapleural analgesia in decreasing the incidence of pulmonary complications.[4] Recent findings of a large, randomized controlled trial corroborated the findings of these meta-analyses. In these trial results, high-risk patients undergoing abdominal surgery who had perioperative epidural anesthesia and analgesia (vs those without perioperative epidural analgesia) had a significantly lower incidence of respiratory failure.[3] Perioperative use of epidural analgesia also was shown to decrease pulmonary complications, decrease the incidence of dysrythmias, and facilitate postoperative extubation, resulting in a shorter length of intensive care unit stay for thoracic and cardiac bypass surgical patients.[57–59]

Patient-Oriented Outcomes

Assessment of patient-oriented outcomes, unlike that seen with "traditional" outcome studies, which focus on major morbidity and mortality, incorporates many different domains, including physiologic endpoints, adverse events, and psychosocial status. These "nontraditional" outcomes are recognized as valid and important outcome measurements in clinical care and research and reflect the global increased interest in patient-focused assessments. The perioperative use of regional anesthesia–analgesia (vs general anesthesia followed by systemic opioids) offers many advantages that may translate into improvements in many patient-oriented outcomes, including satisfaction, quality of recovery, and quality of life.[60] Compared with systemic opioids, epidural analgesia provides superior postoperative pain control. A systematic review, including nonrandomized trial results, revealed that intramuscular (IM) analgesia and intravenous patient-controlled analgesia (IVPCA) resulted in a higher incidence of moderate-to-severe and severe pain vs epidural analgesia (moderate-to-severe pain: 67.2% for IM, 35.8% for IVPCA, and 20.9% for epidural analgesia; severe pain: 29.1% for IM, 10.4% for IVPCA, and 7.8% for epidural analgesia).[61]

Clinical Pearls

- Perioperative use of regional anesthesia–analgesia (vs general anesthesia followed by systemic opioids) offers many advantages that may translate into improvements in patient-oriented outcomes such as satisfaction, quality of recovery, and quality of life.[60]

■ Compared with systemic opioids, epidural analgesia provides superior postoperative pain control.

These results were similar to meta-analysis findings in a review of randomized trials comparing epidural analgesia with systemic opioids. These trails found that epidural analgesia provided better overall postoperative analgesia than systemic opioids on each postoperative day up to 4 days after surgery.[56] When analyzed by types of surgery and pain assessments, all forms of epidural analgesia provided significantly better postoperative analgesia than systemic opioids, with the exception of thoracic epidural analgesia vs opioids for rest pain after thoracic surgery. Thus, it appears that epidural analgesia, regardless of analgesic agent, location of catheter placement, and type and time of pain assessment, provides superior postoperative analgesia to systemic opioids.[56]

The superior analgesia conferred by epidural (and presumably peripheral) analgesia may result in an improvement in patient-oriented outcomes. A systemic review examining the issue of patient satisfaction indicated that the use of both neuraxial and peripheral regional analgesic techniques resulted in higher patient satisfaction compared with those for systemic opioids.[62] In addition, when compared with systemic opioids, use of epidural analgesia is associated with an improved health-related quality of life (HRQL) in the postoperative period.[63,64] Despite the fact that patient satisfaction and quality of life are complex and difficult to measure properly, it appears that perioperative regional analgesia, in part because of the superior analgesia provided, improves patient-oriented outcomes such as patient satisfaction[62] and HCQL.[63,64]

"Epidural Analgesia" as a Generic Entity: Implications for Interpreting Its Effect on Patient Outcomes

Despite the affirmative data on improved patient outcomes with use of postoperative regional analgesia,[2–6] one of the major issues in the overall interpretation of results from these and other trials is the fact that "epidural analgesia" is commonly viewed as a generic entity. This is unfortunate because different parameters in the regional analgesic technique (ie, location of catheter placement, analgesic agents used, and duration of epidural analgesia) influence the efficacy of these techniques on patient outcomes. For example, the effect of postoperative epidural analgesia on outcomes is optimized with the use of a "catheter incision-congruent" technique, which implies placement of the epidural catheter in a location corresponding to the dermatomes of the surgical incision. Catheter incision-congruent (vs catheter incision-incongruent) catheter placement confers superior physiologic and analgesic benefits.[65,66]

Clinical Pearls

■ The effect of postoperative epidural analgesia on outcomes is optimized with the use of a catheter incision-congruent technique, which implies placement of the epidural catheter in a location corresponding to the dermatomes of the surgical incision.

■ Incorporating perioperative regional analgesia into a multimodal approach to patient convalescence appears to maximize the analgesic and physiologic benefits of the regional technique.

For example, high-risk cardiovascular patients undergoing upper abdominal or thoracic procedures may benefit from the use of TEA (catheter incision-congruent), which results in increases in coronary flow to subendocardial and ischemic areas and attenuation of sympathetically mediated coronary vasoconstriction,[23,67–69] both of which can contribute to decreased incidence of myocardial infarction.[3] In addition, for patients undergoing abdominal surgery, catheter incision-congruent (thoracic) catheter placement can result in the physiologic benefits of splanchnic sympathetic nervous system blockade, reduced inhibitory gastrointestinal tone, and increased intestinal blood flow,[5] all of which facilitate return of gastrointestinal function. Trial results consistently demonstrate a benefit from catheter incision-congruent epidural analgesia (vs systemic opioids) in the return of gastrointestinal function; however, these benefits do not appear in those studies that used catheter incision-incongruent epidural analgesia.[5] Thus, the differential physiologic and analgesic benefits of catheter incision-congruent analgesia improve patient outcomes.

In addition to the location of catheter placement, the specific analgesic agents (eg, opioids vs local anesthetics) influence patient outcomes. Despite the fact that neuraxial opioids are effective in controlling postoperative pain,[70] only epidural local anesthetics, through blockade of afferent and efferent signals to and from the spinal cord, suppression of the surgical stress response,[71] and prevention of spinal reflex inhibition of diaphragmatic and gastrointestinal function, have the ability to attenuate the adverse pathophysiologic responses that contribute to morbidity following surgery. Compared with neuraxial opioids, epidural local anesthetics may improve patient outcomes by allowing an earlier recovery of gastrointestinal motility after abdominal surgery[47,49–51] and reduced incidence of pulmonary complications.[4]

The duration of epidural analgesia may be another important factor in improving patient outcomes. Because many of the perioperative pathophysiologic responses that begin intraoperatively continue into the postoperative period, patients may not receive the full physiologic and analgesic benefits from epidural catheters that are prematurely removed or dislodged. For instance, facilitated return of gastrointestinal function was documented only in subjects that retained epidural analgesia for longer than 24 h compared with those who received epidural analgesia for less time.[5,72–75]

In addition, postoperative but not intraoperative epidural analgesia appears to decrease the incidence of myocardial infarction, which correlated to the peak incidence of myocardial infarction between 24 and 48 h after surgery.[3,21]

Finally, the incorporation of perioperative regional analgesia into a multimodal approach to patient convalescence appears to maximize the analgesic and physiologic benefits of the regional technique. By controlling perioperative pathophysiologic responses through attenuation of the neuroendocrine stress response, effective pain control, earlier mobilizing of patients, and facilitated return of gastrointestinal function to allow early enteral feeding, perioperative regional anesthetic and analgesic techniques are an important and integral part of a multimodal approach to patient convalescence.[76] A decrease in hormonal and metabolic stress and improvement in convalescence was demonstrated in patients undergoing other major procedures and participating in a perioperative multimodal pathway.[77] Study results indicate that postoperative regional analgesia as part of a multimodal approach to patient convalescence can result in a shorter time to extubation, superior analgesia, earlier return of bowel function, and earlier fulfillment of intensive care unit discharge criteria in patients undergoing abdominothoracic esophagectomy.[78] In addition, patients undergoing colon resection and receiving a multimodal approach to patient convalescence incorporating epidural analgesia had a reduced the length of hospitalization (from 6 to 10 days to a median of 2 days).[79] Thus, it appears that utilizing a multimodal approach to patient convalescence that incorporates perioperative regional anesthetic and analgesic techniques may control perioperative pathophysiologic responses and result in accelerated patient recovery and decreased length of hospitalization.[80]

COGNITIVE OUTCOME AFTER REGIONAL ANESTHESIA

Postoperative cognitive disorders (PCD) include a broad spectrum of impairments in cognitive function and memory or of consciousness with a common denominator of deficits in cognition and memory.[81] PCD can occur after surgery, with mental function typically reaching a nadir in the early postoperative period and returning to preoperative levels in the majority of patients at 1 week following surgery.[82,83] Certain patients are at higher risk for the development of PCD or long-term PCD. These populations include those undergoing certain types of surgery or those with coexisting medical diseases, preoperative cognitive dysfunction, and advanced age.[10,84] Recent data indicate that PCD in high-risk patients may occur more commonly than previously thought. A trial enrolling approximately 1200 patients older than age 60 years showed that PCD was present in 25.8% of patients 1 week postoperatively and 9.9% of patients 3 months after surgery, compared with 3.4% at 1 week and 2.8% at 3 months, respectively, for nonsurgical control patients.[84] Furthermore, postoperative delirium, a particularly problematic form of

PCD, may occur in 9% to 11% of elderly patients undergoing elective noncardiac surgery.[85,86] For instance, up to 37% of elderly patients undergoing hip fracture repair may experience PCD.[10]

The reason that PCD is especially significant is that its presence is an independent predictor of short- and long-term outcomes (eg, increased mortality, higher rates of major complications, longer lengths of stay, and higher rates of discharge to rehabilitative facilities), even after adjusting for age, comorbidities, and functional status.[87-90] Delirium in hospitalized patients contributes to an additional 17.5 million inpatient days and $4 billion in health care expenditures annually.[89] Decreased neurocognitive function results in a significant decrease in health-related quality of life, with an equally adverse social and financial effect for patients and their caregivers.[91] In addition, the presence of PCD may be a surrogate for the quality of the hospital care.[89] Finally, the incidence of PCD will continue to increase because the percentage of elderly people in the United States is estimated to increase to approximately 17% by 2020, with approximately 40% of all health care dollars spent on this population ($\approx$5% of the US gross domestic product).[92]

Although the precise cause of PCD is unknown, a multifactorial cause without a final common pathway appears to be the most reasonable explanation based on available studies.[93,94] In general, the most common hypotheses focus on a perioperative imbalance of neurotransmitters, especially of acetylcholine and serotonin, in the presence of a decreased neurophysiologic reserve, which is seen in elderly patients.[95-98] Others hypotheses revolve around the presence of inflammatory mediators, such as cytokines, in the development of PCD.[99] Thus, the trauma of surgery may disrupt normal neurotransmitter activity, release inflammatory mediators, and result in hormonal imbalances that contribute to the development of PCD, especially in vulnerable populations with decreased neurophysiologic reserves.[97]

Because PCD has a multifactorial cause, many risks factors may contribute to its development. Preoperatively, patients who are elderly[10,85,94] or those who have poor preoperative cognitive[10,85,94,100] or functional status[94,101] are at higher risk for developing PCD. The presence of a history of alcohol abuse or marked abnormalities in preoperative sodium, potassium, or glucose levels may also be predictors for the development of PCD.[94,102-104] Intraoperatively, certain types of surgical procedures (eg, cardiac surgery with cardiopulmonary bypass,[105] aortic aneurysm repair,[94] and orthopedic procedures in elderly patients[101,106,107]) are associated with higher rates of PCD. Cerebral hypoperfusion or abnormalities in intraoperative glucose and hematocrit levels do not appear to correlate with PCD.[108,109] The correlation of sustained and profound hypotension, hypoglycemia, anemia, or hypoxia to the development of PCD is unclear. A longer duration of surgery and anesthesia is associated with an increase in the incidence of PCD.[84,110] Postoperatively, the use of anticholinergic drugs, meperidine, and benzodiazepines, is associated with the development of PCD.[10,86,111] Complications, such as postoperative infections and respiratory complications, are also associated with the development of PCD.[84] Finally, increased levels of postoperative pain are associated with a higher incidence of PCD.[11,112,113]

POSTOPERATIVE COGNITIVE DYSFUNCTION & REGIONAL ANESTHESIA

Although the use of perioperative regional anesthesia and postoperative analgesia may be associated with a decrease in perioperative mortality and morbidity[1-4] in high-risk patients, the effect of perioperative regional anesthesia on PCD is unclear. Data from examination of the effect of peripheral nerve anesthesia and analgesia on PCD are limited, and the remainder of this discussion focuses on neuraxial techniques. Although a large number of randomized trials comparing intraoperative neuraxial with general anesthesia showed that the use of perioperative neuraxial anesthesia does not decrease the incidence of PCD, methodologic issues present in the study designs preclude a definitive answer about whether perioperative regional anesthesia influences the development of PCD.

A systematic review of the available published study results examining the effect of perioperative neuraxial anesthesia on cognitive function noted that of the 24 studies examined, 19 were randomized and 4 were nonrandomized trials.[114] Of the 19 randomized trials, 18 did not demonstrate a difference in cognitive function between intraoperative general anesthesia and neuraxial anesthesia. None of the five nonrandomized trials demonstrated a difference between in cognitive function as a result of intraoperative general anesthesia and those after neuraxial anesthesia. Based on this review, it appears that intraoperative neuraxial anesthesia alone does not have an effect on PCD; however, the presence of methodologic issues and the lack of examination of the effect of postoperative regional analgesia on the development of PCD are issues for future study.

All available studies have some degree of methodologic and study design issues, revolving around the definition of cognitive dysfunction, properties of the specific neuropsychological tests used, statistical considerations, and lack of control for postoperative pain, which may be confounding factors in interpreting these trial results.[115-117] The precise definition of cognitive dysfunction and the determination of how it is measured are important because cognitive function is an abstract concept consisting of domains of memory, attention, language, visual–spatial ability, abstraction, and psychomotor performance.[116] The definition of a postoperative cognitive deficit is not standardized and may be arbitrarily chosen based on a change in test performance (eg, 1 standard deviation).[115] The presence of a cognitive deficit may be based on just the presence of a change in one or two domains, which can easily occur when a large number of tests are used to assess PCD.[115,118] Using a large number of tests increases the chance of patient withdrawal and fatigue, which in itself may affect test results. Thus, the wide range in incidence of PCD may be due, in part, to the definition and

criteria of cognitive deficit chosen by the investigator. In addition, the neuropsychological tests used to assess PCD in the study may not be ideal in this setting because the majority of tests were designed for long-term cognitive performance in broader population-based studies or in subjects with dementing illnesses (eg, Alzheimer's disease).[117,119] Finally, the significance of the statistical analysis is limited because the accurate interpretation of large numbers of neuropsychological tests must be done with caution.[115,118]

Probably the area of most concern is the lack of control for postoperative analgesia in currently available trial results. In general, studies indicate that higher levels of postoperative pain are associated with a higher incidence of PCD (especially delirium).[11,113] Based on these results, it would seem that control of postoperative pain might theoretically decrease the incidence of PCD, which typically peaks within the first 3 postoperative days.[10] The implication here is that different analgesic regimens, which provide different levels of postoperative analgesia with varying side effects, may potentially result in a different incidence of PCD or level of postoperative cognitive function. This implication is especially important for postoperative regional (both neuraxial and peripheral) techniques because these analgesic regimens (especially the use of a local anesthetic-based solution) were shown to not only provide superior pain control versus systemic opioids[56,61] but also minimize the systemic effects of opioids, which may be associated with development of postoperative cognitive dysfunction.[94] In addition, epidural analgesia may decrease the incidence of postoperative respiratory complications,[1,4] which were shown to be associated with a higher incidence of PCD.[84] Thus, future evaluation of postoperative regional analgesia on PCD may be at least as important as the effects of intraoperative neuraxial anesthesia, particularly because the postoperative delirium peaks in the second or third postoperative day.

SUMMARY

In summary, PCD includes a broad assortment of disorders with many diverse clinical presentations and a multifactorial cause. PCD is an important marker for short- and long-term outcomes. The development of PCD has many risk factors, and certain surgical populations are at higher risk. Although the available data suggest that intraoperative neuraxial anesthesia does not decrease the incidence of PCD compared with general anesthesia, many methodologic and design issues affect the interpretation of some of these studies. Future work in this area should focus on the effect of various postoperative analgesia regimens and techniques on the development of PCD.

References

1. Rodgers A, Walker N, Schug S, et al: Reduction of postoperative mortality and morbidity with epidural or spinal anaesthesia: Results from overview of randomised trials. BMJ 2000;321:1493–1496.

2. Rigg JR, Jamrozik K, Myles PS, et al: Epidural anaesthesia and analgesia and outcome of major surgery: A randomised trial. Lancet 2002;359:1276–1282.

3. Beattie WS, Badner NH, Choi P: Epidural analgesia reduces postoperative myocardial infarction: A meta-analysis. Anesth Analg 2001;93:853–858.

4. Ballantyne JC, Carr DB, deFerranti S, et al: The comparative effects of postoperative analgesic therapies on pulmonary outcome: Cumulative meta-analyses of randomized, controlled trials. Anesth Analg 1998;86:598–612.

5. Hodgson PS, Liu SS: Thoracic epidural anaesthesia and analgesia for abdominal surgery: Effects on gastrointestinal function and perfusion. Balliere's Clin Anaesthesiol 1999;13:9–22.

6. Steinbrook RA: Epidural anesthesia and gastrointestinal motility. Anesth Analg 1998;86:837–844.

7. Norris EJ, Beattie C, Perler BA, et al: Double-masked randomized trial comparing alternate combinations of intraoperative anesthesia and postoperative analgesia in abdominal aortic surgery. Anesthesiology 2001;95:1054–1067.

8. Wu CL, Fleisher LA: Outcomes research in regional anesthesia and analgesia. Anesth Analg 2000;91:1232–1242.

9. Markel DC, Urquhart B, Derkowska I, et al: Effect of epidural analgesia on venous blood flow after hip arthroplasty. Clin Orthop Rel Res 1997;334:168–174.

10. Dyer CB, Ashton CM, Teasdale TA: Postoperative delirium: A review of 80 primary data-collection studies. Arch Intern Med 1995;155:461–465.

11. Lynch EP, Lazor MA, Gellis JE, et al: The impact of postoperative pain on the development of postoperative delirium. Anesth Analg 1998;86:781–785.

12. Badner NH, Knill RL, Brown JE, et al: Myocardial infarction after noncardiac surgery. Anesthesiology 1998;88:572–578.

13. Bode RH Jr, Lewis KP, Zarich SW, et al: Cardiac outcome after peripheral vascular surgery. Comparison of general and regional anesthesia. Anesthesiology 1996;84:3–13.

14. Christopherson R, Beattie C, Frank SM, et al: Perioperative morbidity in patients randomized to epidural or general anesthesia for lower extremity vascular surgery. Anesthesiology 1993;79:422–434.

15. Wu CL, Hurley RW, Herbert R, et al: Effect of perioperative epidural analgesia on patient mortality and morbidity following surgery in Medicare patients. Reg Anesth Pain Med 2004;29:525–533.

16. Andreae M: Underdosing the epidural invalidates a good clinical trial. Anesthesiology 2002;97:1026–1027.

17. Liu SS: An intensive, structured clinical trial can markedly reduce length of stay after abdominal surgery. Anesthesiology 2002;97:1025.

18. Amar D: Regional techniques and length of hospital stay after abdominal aortic surgery. Anesthesiology 2002;97:1029.

19. Johannsen UJ, Mark AL, Marcus ML: Responsiveness to cardiac sympathetic nerve stimulation during maximal coronary dilation produced by adenosine. Circ Res 1982;50:510–517.

20. Trip MD, Volkert MC, van Capelle FJ, et al: Platelet hyperreactivity and prognosis in survivors of myocardial infarction. N Engl J Med 1990;322:1549–1554.

21. Mangano DT, Hollenberg M, Fergert G, et al: Perioperative myocardial ischemia in patients undergoing noncardiac surgery—I: Incidence and severity during the 4 day perioperative period. J Am Coll Cardiol 1991;17:843–850.

22. Veering BT, Cousins MJ: Cardiovascular and pulmonary effects of epidural anaesthesia. Anaesth Intensive Care 2000;28:620–635.

23. Davis RF, DeBoer LW, Maroko PR: Thoracic epidural anesthesia reduces myocardial infarct size after size after coronary artery occlusion in dogs. Anesth Analg 1986;65:711–717.

24. Blomberg S, Ricksten SE: Thoracic epidural anaesthesia decreases the incidence of ventricular arrhythmias during acute myocardial ischaemia in the anesthetized rat. Acta Anaesthesiol Scand 1988;32:173–178.

25. Boylan JF, Katz J, Kavanagh BP, et al: Epidural bupivacaine–morphine analgesia versus patient-controlled analgesia following abdominal aortic surgery. Anesthesiology 1998;89:585–593.

26. Yeager MP, Glass DD, Neff RK, et al: Epidural anesthesia and analgesia in high-risk surgical patients. Anesthesiology 1987;66:729–736.

27. Boylan JF, Katz J, Kavanagh BP, et al: Epidural bupivacaine–morphine analgesia versus patient-controlled analgesia following abdominal aortic surgery: Analgesic, respiratory, and myocardial effects. Anesthesiology 1998;89:585–593.

28. Tuman KJ, McCarthy RJ, March RJ, et al: Effects of epidural anesthesia and analgesia on coagulation and outcome after major vascular surgery. Anesth Analg 1991;73:696–704.

29. Bois S, Couture P, Boudreault D, et al: Epidural analgesia and intravenous patient-controlled analgesia result in similar rates of postoperative myocardial ischemia after aortic surgery. Anesth Analg 1997;85:1233–1239.

30. Liu S, Carpenter RL, Neal JM: Epidural anesthesia and analgesia: their role in postoperative outcome. Anesthesiology 1995;82:1474–1506.

31. Clagett GP, Anderson FA, Heit J, et al: Prevention of venous thromboembolism. Chest 1995;108:312–334S.

32. Rosenfeld BA: Benefits of regional anesthesia on thromboembolic complications following surgery. Reg Anesth 1996;21:S9–12.

33. Sorenson RM, Pace NL: Anesthetic techniques during surgical repair of femoral neck fractures: A meta-analysis. Anesthesiology 1992;77:1095–1104.

34. Rosenfeld BA, Beattie C, Christopherson R, et al: The effects of different anesthetic regimens on fibrinolysis and the development of postoperative arterial thrombosis. Anesthesiology 1993;79:435–443.

35. Jorgensen LN, Rasmussen LS, Nielsen PT, et al: Antithrombotic efficacy of continuous extradural analgesia after knee replacement. Br J Anaesth 1991;66:8–12.

36. Dalldorf PG, Perkins FM, Totterman S, et al: Deep venous thrombosis following total hip arthroplasty: Effect of prolonged postoperative epidural anesthesia. J Arthroplasty 1994;9:611–616.

37. Wu CL, Anderson GF, Herbert R, et al: The effect of perioperative epidural analgesia on patient mortality and morbidity in the Medicare population undergoing total hip replacement. Reg Anesth Pain Med 2003;28:271–278.

38. Livingston EH, Passaro EP Jr: Postoperative ileus. Dig Dis Sci 1990;35:121–132.

39. Saito H, Trocki O, Alexander JW, et al: The effect of route of nutrient administration on the nutritional state, catabolic hormone secretion, and gut mucosal integrity after burn injury. JPEN: J Parenter Enteral Nutr 1987;11:1–7.

40. Moore FA, Feliciano DV, Andrassay RJ, et al: Early enteral feeding, compared with parenteral, reduces postoperative septic complications. Ann Surg 1992;216:172–183.

41. Shou J, Lappin J, Minnard EA, et al: Total parenteral nutrition, bacterial translocation, and host immune function. Am J Surg 1994;167:145–150.

42. Kehlet H, Holte K: Review of postoperative ileus. Am J Surg 2001;182 (Suppl):3–10S.

43. Udassin R, Eimerl D, Schiffman J, et al: Epidural anesthesia accelerates the recovery of postischemic bowel motility in the rat. Anesthesiology 1994;80:832–836.

44. Rimback G, Cassuto J, Wallin G, et al: Inhibition of peritonitis by amide local anesthetics. Anesthesiology 1988;69:881–886.

45. Groudine SB, Fisher HA, Kaufman RP, et al: Intravenous lidocaine speeds the return of bowel function, decreases postoperative pain, and shortens hospital stay in patients undergoing radical prostatectomy. Anesth Analg 1998;86:235–239.

46. Jorgensen H, Wetterslev J, Moiniche S, et al: Epidural local anaesthetics versus opioid-based analgesic regimens on postoperative gastrointestinal paralysis, PONV and pain after abdominal surgery. Cochrane Database Syst Rev 2000;4:CD001893.

47. Liu SS, Carpenter RL, Mackey DC, et al: Effects of perioperative analgesic technique on rate of recovery after colon surgery. Anesthesiology 1995;83:757–765.

48. de Leon-Casasola OA, Karabella D, Lema MJ: Bowel function recovery after radical hysterectomies: Thoracic epidural bupivacaine–morphine versus intravenous patient-controlled analgesia with morphine: A pilot study. J Clin Anesth 1996;8:87–92.

49. Scheinin B, Asantila R, Orko R: The effect of bupivacaine and morphine on pain and bowel function after colonic surgery. Acta Anaesthesiol Scand 1987;31:161–164.

50. Thoren T, Wattwil M: Effects on gastric emptying of thoracic epidural analgesia with morphine or bupivacaine. Anesth Analg 1988;67:687–694.

51. Thorn SE, Wickborn G, Philipson L, et al: Myoelectric activity in the stomach and duodenum after epidural administration of morphine or bupivacaine. Acta Anaesthesiol Scand 1996;40:773–778.

52. Jorgensen H, Fomsgaard JS, Dirks J, et al: Effect of epidural bupivacaine vs combined epidural bupivacaine and morphine on gastrointestinal function and pain after major gynaecological surgery. Br J Anaesth 2001;87:727–732.

53. Dales RE, Dionne G, Leech JA, et al: Preoperative prediction of pulmonary complications following thoracic surgery. Chest 1993;104:155–159.

54. Warner DO, Warner MA, Ritman EL: Human chest wall function during epidural anesthesia. Anesthesiology 1996;85:761–773.

55. Brimioulle S, Vachiery JL, Brichant JF, et al: Sympathetic modulation of hypoxic pulmonary vasoconstriction in intact dogs. Cardiovasc Res 1997;34:384–392.

56. Block BM, Liu SS, Rowlingson AJ, et al: Efficacy of postoperative epidural analgesia versus systemic opioids: A meta-analysis. JAMA 2003;290:2455–2463.

57. Turfrey DJ, Bay DA, Sutcliffe NP, et al: Thoracic epidural anaesthesia for coronary artery bypass graft surgery. Effects on postoperative complications. Anaesthesia 1994;52:1090–1095.

58. Stenseth R, Bjella L, Berg EM, et al: Effects of thoracic epidural analgesia on pulmonary function after coronary artery bypass surgery. Eur J Cardiothor Surg 1996;10:859–865.

59. Liu SS, Block BM, Wu CL: Effects of perioperative central neuraxial analgesia on outcome after coronary artery bypass surgery: A meta-analysis. Anesthesiology 2004;101:153–161.

60. Wu CL, Richman JM: Postoperative pain and quality of recovery. Curr Opin Anesthesiol 2004;17:455–460.

61. Dolin SJ, Cashman JN, Bland JM: Effectiveness of acute postoperative pain management: I. Evidence from published data. Br J Anaesth 2002;89:409–423.

62. Wu CL, Naqibuddin M, Fleisher LA: Measurement of patient satisfaction as an outcome of regional anesthesia and analgesia. Reg Anesth Pain Med 2001;26:196–208.

63. Carli F, Mayo N, Klubien K, et al: Epidural analgesia enhances functional exercise capacity and health-related quality of life after colonic surgery. Anesthesiology 2002;97:540–549.

64. Gottschalk A, Smith DS, Jobes DR, et al: Preemptive epidural analgesia and recovery from radical prostatectomy. JAMA 1998;279:1076–1082.

65. Broekema AA, Gielen MJ, Hennis PJ: Postoperative analgesia with continuous epidural sufentanil and bupivacaine: A prospective study in 614 patients. Anesth Analg 1996;82:754–759.

66. Kahn L, Baxter FJ, Dauphin A, et al: A comparison of thoracic and lumbar epidural techniques for post-thoracoabdominal esophagectomy analgesia. Can J Anaesth 1999;46(5 Pt 1):415–422.

67. Rolf N, Van de Velde M, Wouters PF, et al: Thoracic epidural anesthesia improves functional recovery from myocardial stunning in conscious dogs. Anesth Analg 1996;83:935–940.

68. Klassen GA, Bramwell RS, Bromage PR, et al: Effect of acute sympathectomy by epidural anesthesia on the canine coronary circulation. Anesthesiology 1980;52:8–15.

69. Kock M, Blomberg S, Emanuelsson H, et al: Thoracic epidural anesthesia improves global and regional left ventricular function during stress-induced myocardial ischemia in patients with coronary artery disease. Anesth Analg 1990;71:625–630.

70. Kehlet H: Modification of responses to surgery by neural blockade: Clinical implications. In Cousins MJ, Bridenbaugh PO (eds): *Neural Blockade in Clinical Anesthesia and Management of Pain*, 3rd ed. Lippincott-Raven, 1998, pp 129–175.

71. Rutberg H, Hakanson E, Anderberg B, et al: Effects of the extradural administration of morphine, or bupivacaine, on the endocrine response to upper abdominal surgery. Br J Anaesth 1984;56:233–238.

72. Wallin G, Cassuto J, Hogstrom S, et al: Failure of epidural anesthesia to prevent postoperative paralytic ileus. Anesthesiology 1986;65:292–297.

73. Kanazi GE, Thompson JS, Boskovski NA: Effect of epidural analgesia on postoperative ileus after ileal pouch–anal anastomosis. Am Surg 1996;62:499–502.

74. Hjortso NC, Neumann P, Frosig F, et al: A controlled study on the effect of epidural analgesia with local anaesthetics and morphine on morbidity after abdominal surgery. Acta Anaesthesiol Scand 1985;29:790–796.

75. Neudecker J, Schwenk W, Junghans T, et al: Randomized controlled trial to examine the influence of thoracic epidural analgesia on postoperative ileus after laparoscopic sigmoid resection. Br J Surg 1999;86:1292–1295.

76. Kehlet H: Multimodal approach to control postoperative pathophysiology and rehabilitation. Br J Anaesth 1997;78:606–617.

77. Brodner G, Van Aken H, Hertle L, et al: Multimodal perioperative management—combining thoracic epidural analgesia, forced mobilization, and oral nutrition—reduces hormonal and metabolic stress and improves convalescence after major urologic surgery. Anesth Analg 2001;92:1594–1600.

78. Brodner G, Pogatzki E, Van Aken H, et al: A multimodal approach to control postoperative pathophysiology and rehabilitation in patients undergoing abdominothoracic esophagectomy. Anesth Analg 1998;86:228–234.

79. Basse L, Jakobsen D, Billesbolle P, et al: A clinical pathway to accelerate recovery after colonic resection. Ann Surg 2000;232:51–57.

80. Kehlet H, Wilmore DW: Multimodal strategies to improve surgical outcome. Am J Surg 2002;183:630–641.

81. Rasmussen LS: Perioperative cognitive decline: The extent of the problem. Acta Anaesthesiol Belg 1999;50:199–204.

82. Riis J, Lomholt B, Haxholdt O, et al: Immediate and long-term mental recovery from general versus epidural anesthesia in elderly patients. Acta Anaesthesiol Scand 1983;27:44–49.

83. Edwards H, Rose EA, Schorow M, et al: Postoperative deterioration in pyschomotor function. JAMA 1981;245:1342–1343.

84. Moller JT, Cluitmans P, Rasmussen LS, et al: Long-term postoperative cognitive dysfunction in the elderly: ISPOCD1 study. Lancet 1998;351:857–861.

85. Marcantonio ER, Lee G, Orav JE, et al: The association of intraoperative factors with the development of postoperative delirium. Am J Med 1998;105:380–384.

86. Litaker D, Locala J, Franco K, et al: Preoperative risk factors for postoperative delirium. Gen Hosp Psychiatry 2001;23:84–89.

87. Francis J, Martin D, Kapoor WN: A prospective study of delirium in hospitalized elderly. JAMA 1990;263:1097–1101.

88. Marcantonio ER, Goldman L, Mangione CM, et al: A clinical prediction rule for delirium after elective noncardiac surgery. JAMA 1994;271:134–139.

89. Inuoye SK, Schlesinger MJ, Lydon TJ: Delirium: A symptom of how hospital care is failing older persons and a window to improve quality of hospital care. Am J Med 1999;106:565–573.

90. Marcantonio ER, Flacker JM, Michaels M, et al: Delirium is independently associated with poor functional recovery after hip fracture. J Am Geriatr Soc 2000;48:618–624.

91. Newman MF, Grocott HP, Matthew JP, et al: Report of the substudy assessing the impact of neurocognitive function on quality of life 5 years after cardiac surgery. Stroke 2001;32:2874–2881.

92. Anderson GF, Hussey PS: Population aging: A comparison among industrialized countries. Health Aff 2000;19:191–203.

93. Inouye SK, Charpentier PA: Precipitating factors for delirium in hospitalized elderly persons. Predictive model and interrelationship with baseline vulnerability. JAMA 1996;275:852–857.

94. Marcantonio ER, Juarez G, Goldman L, et al: The relationship of postoperative delirium with psychoactive medications. JAMA 1994;272:1518–1522.

95. Tune LE, Damlouji NF, Holland A, et al: Association of postoperative delirium with raised serum levels of anticholinergic drugs. Lancet 1981;2:651–653.

96. Bayindir O, Akpinar B, Can E, et al: The use of 5-HT3-receptor antagonist ondansetron for the treatment of postcardiotomy delirium. J Cardiothorac Vasc Anesth 2000;14:288–292.

97. Flacker JM, Lipsitz LA: Neural mechanisms of delirium: Current hypothesis and evolving concepts. J Gerontol 1999;54:B239–B246.

98. van der Mast RC: Pathophysiology of delirium. J Geriat Psych Neurol 1998;11:138–145.

99. van der Mast RC: Postoperative delirium. Dement Geriatr Cogn Disord 1999;10:401–405.

100. Ancelin ML, de Roquefeuil G, Ledesert B, et al: Exposure to anaesthetic agents, cognitive functioning and depressive symptomatology in the elderly. Br J Psychiatry 2001;178:360–366.

101. Zakriya KJ, Christmas C, Wenz JF Sr, et al: Preoperative factors associated with postoperative change in confusion assessment method score in hip fracture patients. Anesth Analg 2002;94:1628–1632.

102. Williams-Russo P, Urquhart BL, Sharrock NE, et al: Post-operative delirium: Predictors and prognosis in elderly orthopedic patients. J Am Geriat Soc 1992;40:759–767.

103. Galanakis P, Bickel H, Gradinger R, et al: Acute confusional state in the elderly following hip surgery: Incidence, risk factors and complications. Int J Geriatr Psychiatry 2001;16:349–355.

104. Parikh SS, Chung F: Postoperative delirium in the elderly. Anesth Analg 1995;80:1223–1232.

105. Arrowsmith JE, Grocott HP, Reves JG, et al: Central nervous system complications of cardiac surgery. Br J Anaesth 2000;84:378–393.

106. Fisher BW, Flowerdew G: A simple model for predicting postoperative delirium in older patients undergoing elective orthopedic surgery. J Am Geriatr Soc 1995;43:175–178.

107. Marcantonio ER, Flacker JM, Wright RJ, et al: Reducing delirium after hip fracture: A randomized trial. J Am Geriatr Soc 2001;49:516–522.

108. van Wermeskerken GK, Lardenoye JW, Hill SE, et al: Intraoperative physiologic variables and outcome in cardiac surgery. Part II: Neurologic outcome. Ann Thorac Surg 2000;69:1077–1083.

109. Abildstrom H, Hogh P, Sperling B, et al: Cerebral blood flow and cognitive dysfunction after coronary surgery. Ann Thorac Surg 2002;73:1174–1178.

110. Goldstein MZ, Young BL, Fogel BS, Benedict RH: Occurrence and predictors of short-term mental and functional changes in older adults undergoing elective surgery under general anaesthesia. Am J Geriat Psych 1998;6:42–52.

111. Berggren D, Gustafson Y, Eriksson B, et al: Postoperative confusion after anesthesia in elderly patients with femoral neck fractures. Anesth Analg 1987;66:497–504.

112. Schor JD, Levkoff SE, Lipsitz LA, et al: Risk factors for delirium in hospitalized elderly. JAMA 1992;267:827–831.

113. Duggleby W, Lander J: Cognitive status and postoperative pain: older adults. J Pain Sympt Manage 1994;9:19–27.

114. Wu CL, Hsu W, Richman JM, et al: Postoperative cognitive function as an outcome of regional anesthesia and analgesia. Reg Anesth Pain Med 2004;29:257–268.

115. Rasmussen LS, Larsen K, Houx P, et al: The assessment of postoperative cognitive function. Acta Anaesthesiol Scand 2001;45:275–289.

116. Morris MC, Evans DA, Hebert LE, et al: Methodological issues in the study of cognitive decline. Am J Epidemiol 1999;149:789–793.

117. Colsher PL, Wallace RB: Epidemiologic considerations in studies of cognitive function in the elderly: Methodology and nondementing acquired dysfunction. Epidemiol Rev 1991;13:1–27.

118. Miller LS, Rohling ML: A statistical interpretative method for neuropsychological test data. Neuropsychol Rev 2001;11:143–169.

119. Dijkstra JB, Jolles J: Postoperative cognitive dysfunction versus complaints: A discrepancy in long-term findings. Neuropsychol Rev 2002;12:1–14.

Regional Anesthesia & Acute Pain Management

Preemptive Analgesia, Regional Anesthesia, & the Prevention of Chronic Postoperative Pain

Scott S. Reuben, MD • Jeffrey Gadsden, MD

PREEMPTIVE ANALGESIA

Foundations

Preemptive analgesia as a concept began over 90 years ago, when Crile and Lower proposed that blocking noxious signals prior to a surgical incision may lead to some degree of central nervous system (CNS) protection against postoperative pain, though at that time the mechanism remained unclear.[1] Crile believed that a combination of locoregional blocks and general anesthesia (GA), especially when the blocks were performed in advance of the painful stimulus, favorably influenced postoperative recovery compared with GA alone. Crile concluded that "patients given inhalational anesthesia still need to be protected by regional anesthesia otherwise they might incur persistent central nervous system changes and enhanced postoperative pain."[2] The notion that the CNS "modulates" afferent pain signals before being perceived by the individual was furthered in 1965 when Melzack and Wall proposed their gate theory.[3] This landmark paper suggested that incoming pain signals are subject to inhibition by either competing nonpainful afferent input at the same spinal level or from supraspinal descending pathways. For example, rubbing one's foot after stubbing your toe lessens the perception of pain due to the "closure" of a theoretical gate in the substantia gelatinosa that allows for only one type of afferent impulse to be transmitted to the CNS. However, this theory did not incorporate long-term changes in the CNS following nociceptive input and to other external factors that impinge on the individual. It is now recognized that nociceptor function is dynamic and may be altered following tissue injury. Repetitive stimulation of small-diameter primary afferent fibers generates a progressive increase in action potential discharge and increased excitability of both peripheral and CNS neurons, an event termed *sensitization* or "wind-up." This is the mechanism by which pain may be prolonged beyond the duration normally expected with an acute insult. Furthermore, this increased excitability in the CNS has the capacity to permanently alter spinal cord function leading to the development of chronic pain following an acute injury. Preemptive analgesia has been proposed as a method of decreasing postoperative pain by the prevention or attenuation of this wind-up phenomenon.

Physiology of Central & Peripheral Sensitization

The perception of pain is not a hard-wired mechanism, wherein stimuli are always transmitted and processed in an identical manner each time. In fact the CNS exhibits a great deal of plasticity. The processing of pain signals is now recognized to be a complex physiologic cascade that involves dozens of different neurotransmitters and chemical substrates at several different anatomic locations. Operative procedures produce an initial afferent barrage of pain signals and generate a secondary inflammatory response, both of which contribute substantially to postoperative pain. The signals have the capacity to initiate prolonged changes in both the peripheral and central nervous system that will lead to the amplification and prolongation of postoperative pain. Peripheral sensitization, a reduction in the threshold of nociceptor afferent peripheral terminals, is a result of inflammation at the

site of surgical trauma.[4] Central sensitization, an activity-dependent increase in the excitability of spinal neurons, is a result of persistent exposure to nociceptive afferent input from the peripheral neurons.[5] Taken together, these two processes contribute to the postoperative hypersensitivity state ("spinal wind-up") that is responsible for a decrease in the pain threshold, both at the site of injury (primary hyperalgesia) and in the surrounding uninjured tissue (secondary hyperalgesia).

The perception of acute pain begins with the transduction of a mechanical, thermal, or chemical stimulus by peripheral nociceptors. These free nerve endings are not simply passive conductors of information, but are subject to modulation at the site of activation. Tissue injury (eg, surgical incision) results in several local responses that affect pain signal transduction and transmission. First, an inflammatory response is provoked by the release of contents from damaged cells. At the same time, nociceptor activation directly leads to the discharge of neuropeptides such as neurokinin A, calcitonin gene-related peptide (CGRP), and substance P from peripheral terminals of the primary nerve fibers.[6] These two processes contribute to the presence of a "sensitizing soup" of inflammatory mediators that includes bradykinin, serotonin, histamine, nitric oxide, and several others.[7] It is now known that these mediators act directly on the nociceptors themselves, causing an increase in spontaneous activity, a lowered threshold for activation, and increased and prolonged firing to a suprathreshold stimulus by the primary afferent neurons.[8] As a result of this peripheral sensitization, low-intensity stimuli that would normally not cause a painful response prior to sensitization now become perceived as pain, an effect termed *allodynia* (Figure 76–1).

Following transduction, nociceptive signals are carried by myelinated A-δ fibers and unmyelinated C fibers to the dorsal horn of the spinal cord, where they synapse with

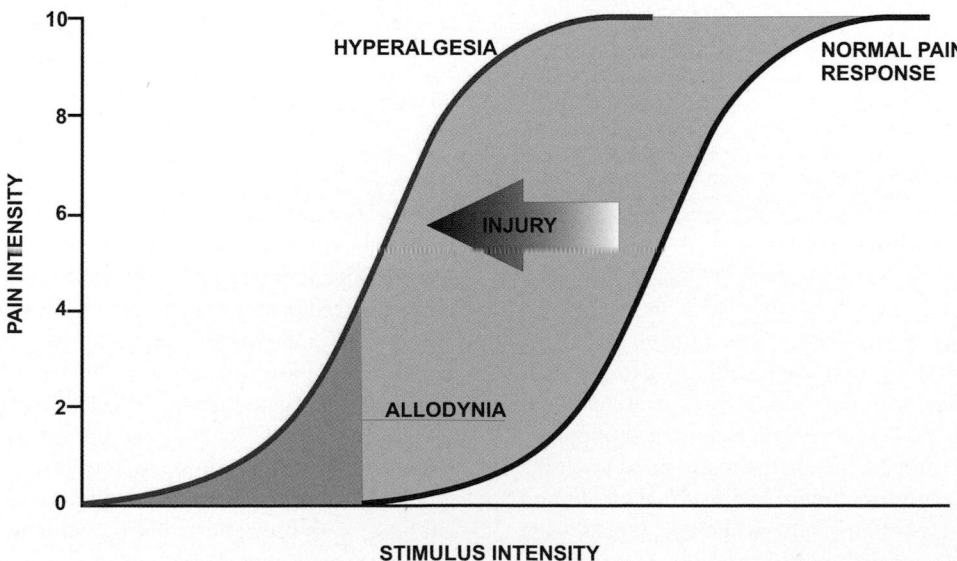

Figure 76–1. Allodynia—Low-intensity sensory stimuli that would normally not cause pain may become painful as a result of peripheral stimulation and its effect on lowering the threshold for activation of the peripheral nociceptors.

second-order neurons. The two different types of fibers typically exhibit specialization, with A-δ fibers responsible for the discrete, sharp response called "first pain," which is perceived almost immediately and is brief in duration. C fibers are slower to conduct and trigger a poorly localized, burning or aching type of pain ("second pain"), which tends to last beyond the termination of the acute stimulus and is associated with a growing region of hypersensitivity around the point where the noxious stimulus was applied.

These primary fibers terminate primarily in lamina I, II, and V[9] of the dorsal horn, where they synapse with second-order spinal neurons. Two forms of second-order neurons are important to the understanding of central sensitization. The first are called nociceptive-specific neurons and, as the name suggests, respond only to painful signals from A-δ and C fibers caused by a high-intensity stimulus. In contrast, wide dynamic range (WDR) neurons accept convergent input from a variety of nociceptive *and* nonnociceptive sources (eg, nonpainful touch). Normally, low-intensity nonpainful stimuli carried by A-β fibers to WDR neurons are interpreted (correctly) as inoffensive. However, under the constant barrage of nociceptive input that is associated with actual tissue damage, WDR neurons become sensitized and hyperresponsive. When this occurs, they may begin to discharge at a high rate following a normally innocuous stimulus, leading to allodynia and hyperalgesia.

In this manner, prolonged central sensitization has the capacity to lead to permanent alterations in the CNS that contribute to chronic pain long after the acute stimulus has been withdrawn. Sustained input from peripheral neurons can result in the death of inhibitory neurons, replacement with new afferent excitatory neurons, and the establishment of aberrant excitatory synaptic connections.[10] These alterations result in a prolonged state of sensitization resulting in intractable postsurgical pain that is unresponsive to many analgesics.[11] The incidence of postsurgical pain that persists well beyond what might be expected (ie, greater than 6–12 months) can be alarmingly high. A review of the current literature reveals estimates such as 6–12% after craniotomy,[12,13] 50–80% after leg amputation,[14–16] 50% after thoracotomy,[17,18] 11–57% after breast surgery,[19,20] 3–56% after laparoscopic cholecystectomy,[21–23] and 12% following inguinal herniorrhaphy.[24] Clearly there is significant variability in the incidence of chronic pain for each of these procedures, and specific risk factors for its development have been identified. These include, among others, preoperative pain of greater than 1 month's duration, intensity of acute postoperative pain, psychological vulnerability and anxiety, and a surgical approach with risk of nerve damage, such as posterolateral thoracotomy.[25] Interestingly, there is evidence that individual differences in the degree of endogenous modulation may predict one's likelihood of sustaining a prolonged painful state.[26] In other words, certain individuals may have heightened baseline pain sensitivity and reduced cortical-inhibitory modulation, rendering them more likely to develop chronic pain after surgery than individuals with "normal" pain processing.

Despite the identification of chronic postsurgical pain syndromes, little is known about the underlying mechanisms, natural history, and response to therapy of each syndrome.[27] However, as evidence continues to accumulate concerning the role of sensitization in the prolongation of postoperative pain, many researchers have focused on methods by which to not simply treat the symptoms as they occur, but prevent wind-up from occurring. This has led to the concept of preemptive analgesia.

Preemptive Analgesia

In 1988, Wall suggested that "we should consider the possibility that pre-emptive pre-operative analgesia has prolonged effects which long outlast the presence of drugs."[28] Some of the earliest experimental evidence supporting this theory noted that a painful stimulus in rats resulted in a distinct biphasic excitatory response in dorsal horn neurons—an immediate acute peak (at 0 to 10 min) and a subsequent, prolonged tonic phase lasting 20–65 min.[29] The study concluded that intrathecal opiates administered prior to the first-phase response but reversed with naloxone before the expected onset of the second-phase response were capable of preventing this latter stage. On the other hand, if the opiates were administered *after* the painful stimulus, the inhibitory effect on the second-phase pain response in the dorsal horn was greatly diminished. This experimental model was also used to investigate the role of local anesthetics in the dorsal horn response to pain. Coderre and colleagues showed that local anesthetics applied either at the site of injury or intrathecally prior (but not subsequent) to a subcutaneous formalin injection abolished the expression of the second tonic phase of the pain response in dorsal horn neurons.[30]

These early works lent support to the idea that sensitization may be preventable by pharmacologically inhibiting the action of these substances prior to the onset of the nociceptive onslaught. Since then, clinical studies have sought to test the hypothesis that preemptive analgesia provides for greater postoperative pain control than "traditional" intra- and postoperative analgesic regimens. A wide variety of drugs have been employed, such as nonsteroidal antiinflammatory agents (NSAIDs), opioids, α₂-agonists, and NMDA antagonists such as ketamine and dextromethorphan.[31] In addition, clinical investigators have attempted to target the sensitization process at one or more anatomic sites along the pathway, including the site of injury, peripheral nerve axon, dorsal horn of the spinal cord, and cerebral cortex (Figure 76–3).

Despite elegant demonstrations of its effect in some animal models, there exists some degree of controversy regarding the validity of preemptive analgesia in the clinical setting. Many studies have obtained equivocal results or have failed to clearly demonstrate that preemptive analgesia is efficacious. The reason for this may be related to the difference between the intensity and duration of the painful stimulus in early animal protocols compared with that experienced following a large surgical incision. In addition, some negative studies have been criticized for their methodology, especially

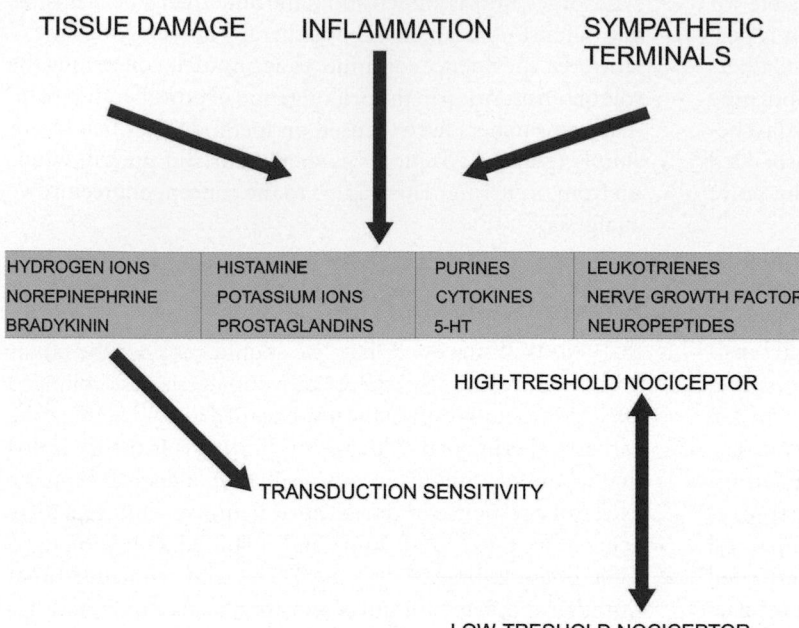

Figure 76–2. Pathophysiologic mechanisms leading to peripheral sensitisation.

in cases where the duration of the surgical pain far exceeds the experimental analgesic intervention. Studies that include pain as an outcome measure are often difficult to interpret given the subjective nature of the symptom and the tendency for confounding factors (eg, psychological elements) to play a role.

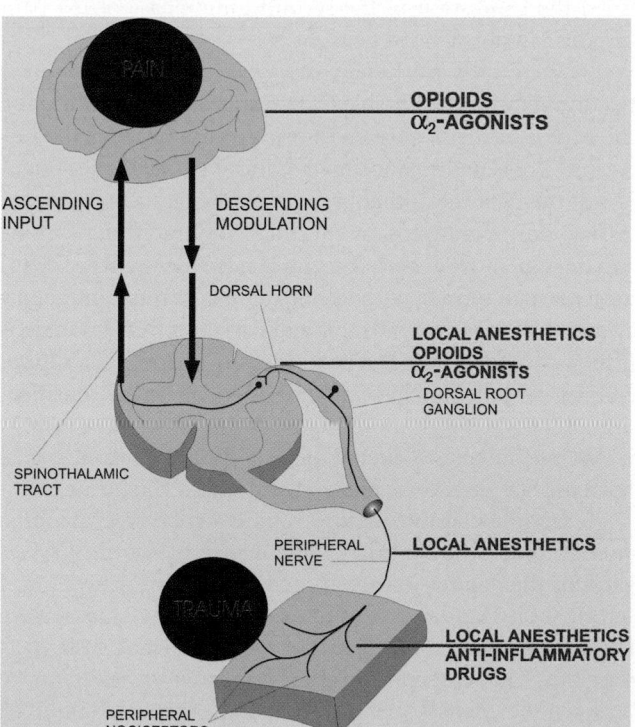

Figure 76–3. Pain pathways and levels at which pain transmission and perception can be modulated.

Since timing is thought to be the key issue, investigations into preemptive analgesia are best performed when a comparison is made between an intervention performed prior to incision with the same intervention performed after surgery has begun (eg, brachial plexus block before surgery *or* postoperatively). If preemptive analgesia is efficacious, then those patients who had their block placed preoperatively should have less pain than those who had their block placed after the incision but before the end of the procedure. Unfortunately, many studies of preemptive analgesia choose a methodology whereby a preincisional strategy is employed and compared with placebo (eg, local infiltration into the wound site before incision versus no infiltration). This study design does little to address the question of whether "pre- versus post-" makes a difference. Furthermore, the focus on demonstrating that pretreatment is more effective than the same treatment administered after incision or surgery has sidetracked progress since inclusion of a control group (eg, placebo administered before and after incision) has been ignored.[32] Two group studies that fail to demonstrate a superiority of the preincisional over the postincisional analgesic treatment intervention are inherently flawed because it is not known whether the absence of an effect reflects the relative efficacy of the postoperative blockade or the inefficacy of preoperative blockade in reducing central sensitization.[33]

Evidence in the Literature

In the last two decades, hundreds of studies of varied quality have been published relating to the efficacy and utility of preemptive analgesia strategies. The consensus is far from clear, with different reviewers reaching fundamentally dissimilar conclusions depending on the particular intervention used, the choice of control, the outcome measures, and so on. Two relatively recent meta-analyses attempted to clarify the picture by summarizing and analyzing data from high-quality, double-blinded, randomized controlled trials. Moiniche and coworkers included 80 randomized controlled trials (RCTs) representing 3761 patients published from 1983 to 2000.[34] Ong and associates analyzed 66 RCTs and 3261 patients that were published between 1987 and 2003.[35] Both sought to include only those papers in which an intervention was compared before *and* after surgical incision by the same route, and no placebo or dummy treatment was used. Also, the outcome measures that were extracted from the studies were standardized where possible. These were (1) pain intensity scores (eg, VAS), (2) time to first analgesic request or rescue dose, and (3) total supplemental analgesic dose.

These two meta-analyses represent the vast bulk of well-conducted clinical trials investigating preemptive analgesia in the current literature. The outcome measures chosen by the authors are traditional markers of analgesic efficacy in pain studies. In particular, pain intensity scores and total analgesic dose have been held up as the most reliable measures of a preemptive effect.[36,37] Given the broad range of analgesic strategies available (eg, local infiltration, neuraxial blocks, NSAIDs, etc), it is useful to review the existing evidence for each approach independently, using the combined results of these two meta-analyses and, where possible, any additional published evidence.

Local Wound Infiltration

Infiltrating local anesthetics into the skin and subcutaneous tissue prior to making an incision may be the simplest approach to preemptive analgesia. It is easy to perform by either surgeon or anesthesiologist, and with the appearance of a skin wheal, it provides a clear endpoint to the intervention. It is also a very safe procedure with few side effects, and low risk for toxicity. In the Moiniche and coworkers' study, 14 trials (736 patients) compared pre- vs postincisional wound infiltration for a variety of abdominal, thoracic, orthopedic, and head and neck procedures. Overall, no difference was found among study groups for all three outcome measures (see Table 76–1). On the other hand, Ong and associates looked at 15 RCTs (671 patients) addressing local infiltration and concluded that local anesthetic infiltration was clinically effective in reducing total analgesic use as well as prolonging the time to rescue analgesia, but did not achieve statistical significance with respect to reducing pain intensity compared with traditional methods.

Other recent randomized trials comparing pre- and postincisional local anesthetic infiltration also suggest no significant difference in pain outcomes. These include studies of infiltration of laparoscopic ports,[38,39] intraarticular sites,[40] laparotomy wounds,[41] and tonsillectomy wounds.[42]

Preincisional local wound infiltration appears to have little effect on postoperative pain scores compared with infiltration carried out at the conclusion of surgery. The data seem to suggest a potential benefit with respect to the amount of

Table 76–1.

Local Anesthetic Wound Infiltration

	Number of Trials (# of patients)	Pain Intensity	Time to First Analgesic	Supplemental Analgesic Demand/Use
Moiniche et al[34]	14 (n=736)	0	0	0
Ong et al[35]	15 (n=671)	?	+	+

+ = positive effect, 0 = no effect, ? = equivocal evidence.

postoperative analgesic use and time to rescue dose, but this is controversial. It remains unclear from these data whether local anesthetic infiltration into the wound provides long-term prevention of chronic incisional pain. Most of the studies terminated their assessment of effect at 24 to 48 h, well before the abatement of the acute postoperative pain. Since it is usually not a particularly challenging task to provide rescue analgesia in the immediate postoperative period, the utility of local infiltration prior to incision may be diminished.[43] However, the downside to the intervention is negligible, and there was no suggestion of a negative treatment effect. Also, there is evidence that local anesthetics possess antimicrobial properties when injected into a surgical wound[44] and are unlikely to negatively influence wound healing.[45]

REGIONAL ANESTHESIA

Peripheral Nerve Blocks

Peripheral nerve blocks (PNBs) are an attractive method of providing postoperative analgesia that, compared with general anesthesia alone, cut down on time to hospital discharge, reduce postoperative pain, and improve overall patient satisfaction.[46,47] Few clinicians would argue that a well-performed block provides for excellent pain control, but whether such blocks are best performed prior to incision or at the conclusion of surgery is still debated. A common belief is that it requires less analgesic to control pain before it starts than after the noxious input has begun, but few of studies directly address this issue.

Suresh and colleagues compared the effect of a preincisional great auricular block with 0.25% bupivacaine with postincisional block alone on postoperative pain in children undergoing tympanomastoid surgery.[48] There was no difference in postoperative analgesic requirements, time to first rescue dose, or vomiting. Another study of preemptive PNBs in the pediatric population was performed by Altintas and coworkers in which children undergoing hand surgery were randomized to receive an axillary block with 0.25% bupivacaine.[49] One group received the block after induction but before incision; the other received the block at the end of the procedure but while still under general anesthesia. The authors found essentially no difference between groups, except for significantly less isoflurane being used in the preincisional group. This methodology brings to the forefront the observation that it is generally deemed acceptable to carry out regional anesthetic techniques in anesthetized children, but not adults, although this attitude may be changing with the adoption of more objective measures of injection pressures when performing nerve blocks.[50]

Doyle and Bowler looked at the effect of preemptive intercostal blocks on postthoracotomy pain compared with blocks performed at the conclusion of surgery.[51] Patients were followed for a minimum of 12 months. Pain scores when taking a vital capacity breath during the first 48 h were somewhat decreased in the preincisional group, but no other measure showed a significant difference, including on VAS scores, extent and duration of intercostal nerve block, analgesic consumption, and the incidence of complications.

Huffnagle and associates investigated the efficacy of bilateral ilioinguinal and iliohypogastric nerve blocks when performed in conjunction with spinal anesthesia for cesarean delivery.[52] Patients were randomized to have the block performed before incision, after incision, or not at all. Although the results showed that postoperative patient satisfaction and morphine use did not differ amongst groups, the data may be hard to interpret, given a 50% block failure rate in the preincisional group.

Several studies examining the effect of intraneural[53] or perineural[54,55] catheters placed at the time of amputation showed little effect on long-term phantom pain, although the methodology was not appropriate for investigating preemptive analgesia.

In general, it appears to matter little whether a PNB used for postoperative pain is placed before or after incision. This again probably has to do with the duration of blockade following a painful surgical wound. For example, a patient having undergone rotator cuff repair with a single-shot brachial plexus block is likely to have significant pain on postoperative day 1. The widespread use of indwelling perineural catheters may change the balance of evidence in favor of preemptive placement, but this remains to be elucidated with clinical studies. Practical matters may play a more important role in the decision of when to administer the block, such as the availability of skilled staff to conduct the block in the recovery room or the wish to avoid a painful window period between the termination of general or neuraxial anesthesia and the onset of a block placed postoperatively.

Epidural & Caudal Analgesia

Epidural (and to a lesser extent caudal) analgesia is often carried through into the postoperative period by means of a catheter, which provides the potential advantage of an unbroken period of pain control from the operating room until the catheter is removed, usually 24–72 h later.[56] Combinations of local anesthetic, opioids, and other medications can be titrated to patient comfort and allow for an acceptable degree of motor function while still imparting a sensory block. Because a catheter can be placed in the epidural space preoperatively and utilized ad lib, epidural analgesia is a technique well suited to the study of any potential preemptive effect.

Moiniche and coworkers analyzed 10 studies of single-dose epidural analgesic regimens for procedures such as thoracotomy, laparotomy, hysterectomy, and lumbar laminectomy.[34] The results were inconsistent with a clear treatment effect. Likewise, of eight trials investigated for continuous epidural regimens, only three displayed significantly reduced VAS scores, whereas no differences were found in the other trials. Five studies comparing pre- and postincisional caudal blocks in children also revealed no clear difference between study groups with respect to any of the outcome measures.

Ong and associates' meta-analysis identified 13 studies (653 patients) comparing preincisional versus postincisional epidural analgesia.[35] Of these, seven favored pretreatment based on VAS scores, whereas the remaining six were found to be not significant. However, differences were found for total amount of supplemental analgesia—10 vs 3 studies came out in favor of preincisional epidural analgesia.

Both Beilin and colleagues[57] and Neustein and coworkers[58] studied the effect of preemptive epidural bupivacaine/fentanyl analgesia on pain outcomes following hysterectomy and thoracic surgery, respectively. The former trial reported significantly less severe postoperative pain in the preemptive group, as well as less elevated levels of both proinflammatory and antiinflammatory cytokines. In contrast, the study of analgesia following thoracic surgery revealed no treatment effect for the preincisional epidural blockade except for reduced isoflurane requirements.

Epidural anesthesia begun 18–72 h prior to amputation appears to provide no significant advantage in preventing phantom pain than standard opioid therapy, placebo, or local anesthetic via surgically placed perineural catheter.[59–62]

Although a centrally acting neural blockade such as epidural anesthesia should effectively block afferent pain impulses from being transmitted to the CNS, there is no substantial evidence that initiating the block prior to incision confers any considerable analgesic benefit once the epidural has been stopped. It appears that a case can be made for epidural analgesia in reducing the amount of analgesics required, at least while the epidural is operating. In addition, there is evidence that neuraxial anesthesia provides other salutary effects, such as improved gastric motility,[63] a blunted stress response to surgery,[64] and reduced thromboembolic complications.[65] Epidural and caudal analgesia may be clinically useful in prolonging the time to first analgesic request, but does not predictably reduce pain scores after surgery.

Nonsteroidal Antiinflammatory Drugs

Surgical trauma results in the induction of cyclooxygenase (COX), leading to the release of prostaglandins, which sensitize peripheral nociceptors and produce localized hyperalgesia (primary hyperalgesia), which can contribute to central sensitization in the postoperative period. Traditionally, nonsteroidal antiinflammatory drugs (NSAIDs) are thought to exert their analgesic effects by inhibiting the production of prostanoids from arachidonic acid, thus decreasing peripheral sensitization and the activation of peripheral nociceptor.[66] Considerable information has emerged in recent years regarding the involvement of prostaglandins and cyclooxygenases in the spinal cord.[67]

Recent evidence has suggested that COX-2 in the CNS may play a novel role in targeting nociceptive pathways.[68,69] This has been evidenced by a rapid upregulation of COX-2 expression in the CNS following peripheral trauma leading to central sensitization and pain hypersensitivity. The role of spinal COX in nociception has been implicated in several studies. First, intrathecal prostaglandin E_2 (PGE_2) causes hyperalgesia in rats.[70,71] It has been suggested that this inflammation-induced central sensitization is the result of an interaction of spinal prostaglandins and NMDA receptors.[70] Secondly, the intraspinal administration of COX-2 inhibitors significantly decreases centrally generated inflammatory pain hypersensitivity.[69] These results suggest that if COX-2 both inside and outside the brain is inhibited, then better pain relief is achieved.[72]

NSAIDs have been demonstrated as effective analgesics when administered at the conclusion of surgery.[73] In an attempt to further reduce pain hypersensitivity, clinical trials have examined the effect of administering NSAIDs prior to surgical incision. The preemptive analgesic effects of NSAIDs has been previously studied after a wide variety of surgical procedures demonstrating equivocal results.[7,34,35,74] Unfortunately, many methodologic problems have been encountered in these studies.[33] Reuben et al. were the first investigators to examine the analgesic effects of administering the same dose of an NSAID either before or after arthroscopic knee surgery.[75] The results of this study demonstrated that preoperative NSAID administration produced a significantly longer duration of postoperative analgesia, less 24 h opioid use, and lower incidental pain scores than did administering the same drug in the postoperative period.

A review of 18 randomized, single- or double-blinded studies that used an NSAID as the target intervention revealed that only 6 studies (33%) demonstrated a preemptive analgesic effect.[74] Furthermore, the beneficial effects of preemptive NSAIDs observed in most studies were minimal. The review by Moniche and coworkers included 20 clinical trials comparing preincisional with postincisional NSAID using a parallel or crossover design.[34] The authors concluded that some aspects of postoperative pain were improved by preemptive treatment in 4 of the 20 trials. Overall, the data demonstrated preemptive NSAIDs to be of no analgesic benefit when compared with postincisional administration of these drugs. In contrast, Ong and associates reviewed data from 16 randomized controlled trials with preemptive NSAIDs, concluding that these drugs improved analgesic

consumption and time to first analgesic request, but not postoperative pain scores.[35]

Although preemptive NSAIDs by themselves may be ineffective in eliminating pain following surgery, when utilized in combination with other analgesic drugs they may be effective in reducing the incidence of both acute and chronic pain.[76,77]

Opioids & Other Pharmacologic Agents

Although much of the focus of preemptive analgesia research has been on neural blockade—either through local infiltration, peripheral nerve blocks, or neuraxial anesthesia—there is great interest in expanding the understanding of other medications in preventing sensitization or wind-up following surgery. In addition to traditional agents such as opioids and NSAIDs, interest has been generated in the use of newer therapies such as *N*-methyl-D-aspartate (NMDA) receptor antagonists[78,79] and gabapentin.[80,81] Overall, the effect of preemptive opioids and NMDA receptor antagonists is unclear, with most studies in the two large meta-analyses showing no significant difference between groups. On the other hand, preemptive NSAIDs have been largely shown to reduce both analgesic consumption and the time to rescue analgesic following surgery.[35,75]

CHRONIC PAIN SYNDROMES FOLLOWING SURGERY

Despite its prevalence, our understanding of chronic postoperative pain and the potential means of risk reduction are somewhat deficient. We need to classify these chronic pain syndromes according to symptoms and mechanisms and greater emphasis needs to be placed on preventing its development. Preemptive analgesic techniques may play a role in reducing the incidence of certain chronic postsurgical pain syndromes,[82] and future large-scale randomized controlled trials are necessary to support these initial findings. Four chronic pain syndromes that are important clinically to the anesthesiologist are complex regional pain syndrome, phantom limb pain, chronic donor site pain, and postthoracotomy pain syndrome.

Complex Regional Pain Syndrome

Complex regional pain syndrome (CRPS) is a disorder characterized by the presence, following a noxious event, of regional pain and sensory changes such as temperature alterations, abnormal skin color, abnormal sudomotor activity, or edema.[83] Its onset is associated with a history of trauma (that is often innocuous) or immobilization, and there is typically no correlation between the severity of the initial injury and the ensuing painful syndrome.[84] The Consensus Conference of the International Association for the Study of Pain (IASP) has identified two forms of CRPS: CRPS type I (formerly known as reflex sympathetic dystrophy) and CRPS type II

Table 76–2.

CRPS Type I and II Characteristics

CRPS Type I

1. Type I is a syndrome that develops after an initiating noxious event.
2. Spontaneous pain or allodynia/hyperalgesia occurs, is not limited to the territory of a single peripheral nerve, and is disproportionate to the inciting event.
3. There is or has been evidence of edema, skin blood flow abnormality, or abnormal sudomotor activity in the region of the pain since the inciting event.
4. This diagnosis is excluded by the existence of conditions that would otherswise account for the degree of pain and dysfunction.

CRPS Type II

1. Type II is a syndrome that develops after a nerve injury. Spontaneous pain or allodynia/hyperalgesia occurs and is not necessarily limited to the territory of the injured nerve.
2. There is or has been evidence of edema, skin blood flow abnormality, or abnormal sudomotor activity in the region of the pain since the inciting event.
3. This diagnosis is excluded by the existence of conditions that would otherwise account for the degree of pain and dysfunction.

CRPS = complex regional pain syndrome.

(formerly known as causalgia).[85] The characteristics of each are summarized in Table 76–2.

Because there has been some debate regarding nomenclature and diagnostic standards, the IASP has also recently suggested a formal set of criteria for the diagnosis of CRPS.[86,87] Accordingly, patients should have:

1. At least one symptom in each of the following categories:
   a. Sensory (hyperesthesia)
   b. Vasomotor (temperature abnormalities or skin color abnormalities)
   c. Sudomotor/fluid balance (edema or sweating abnormalities)
   d. Motor (decreased range of movement, weakness, tremor or neglect)
2. And at least one sign within two or more of the following categories:
   a. Sensory (allodynia or hyperalgesia)
   b. Vasomotor (objective temperature abnormalities or skin color abnormalities)
   c. Sudomotor/fluid balance (objective edema or sweating abnormalities)
   d. Motor (objective decreased range of motion, weakness, tremor or neglect)

CRPS is often, but not always, associated with a state of sympathetically maintained pain (SMP).[88] This type of pain is sustained by sympathetic efferent innervation or by circulating catecholamines and is relieved by specific sympatholytic procedures such as nerve blocks. Sympathetically independent pain (SIP), in contrast, does not respond to sympatholytic blocks. Patients with CRPS may have varying elements of SMP or SIP throughout the course of the disease.[89]

CRPS is a potentially debilitating syndrome that leaves many patients without use of the affected limb. Once diagnosed, treatment should begin immediately. A multifocal approach is often recommended, including a combination of physiotherapy, antidepressant and anticonvulsant medications, steroids, sympathetic blocks, and, in some cases, spinal cord stimulation.[89]

The incidence of CRPS occurring after surgery varies and may be underreported.[90] Approximately 20% of CRPS patients who present to chronic pain clinics have a history of prior surgical procedures in the affected area.[91,92] There are accounts of CRPS after such procedures as breast surgery,[93,94] radial artery harvesting for cardiac surgery,[95] skin nevus excision,[96] and lumbar spine surgery.[97] However, perhaps not surprisingly, most reports of postoperative CRPS occur in the orthopedic population, especially after operations on the extremities. Estimates for various procedures include 2.3% following knee arthroscopy,[98] 2.1–5% following carpal tunnel release,[99–101] and 0.8–13% following total knee arthroplasty.[102–105] There is a wide range of reported incidences of this disorder after surgery, and this may be due to differences in methodology, particularly with respect to the interval at which the patients are assessed.[106] For example, patients assessed 3 months postoperatively are likely to have a different clinical presentation than those assessed 1 year out. Also, many of the reports originated before the definition of the syndrome was modified in the mid-1990s, so the external validity may be compromised for earlier investigations. Patients with CRPS who undergo surgery on the affected limb are thought to be at increased risk for recurrence or worsening of symptoms.[107,108]

Phantom Limb Pain

People who suffer the loss of a limb, either traumatically or surgically, almost always report some degree of perceived sensation in the lost limb. This phenomenon, first described over 400 years ago, was dubbed "phantom limb" in 1871 by S.W. Mitchell.[109] A distinction should be made between phantom limb pain (painful sensations referred to the absent limb), phantom limb sensation (any sensation in the absent limb, except pain), and stump pain (pain localized in the stump), although each of these may coexist in an individual patient at different times.[110]

Early studies reported that the incidence of phantom pain in amputees was below 5%.[111] Recent literature, however, suggests that the incidence is much higher and is probably between 50% and 80%.[112–114] The discrepancy may be explained by differences in methodologies. Early studies tended to base prevalence on the patient's request for pain relief, which may have underestimated the problem in patients who were reluctant to report pain to medical staff. Several risk factors have been identified for the development of phantom limb pain including the degree of preoperative pain, the magnitude of intraoperative noxious input, the intensity of postoperative pain, and psychological factors.[115,116]

Typically, phantom pain occurs early in the postamputation course with up to 70% of patients experiencing pain in the first several days after the injury.[117,118] Although phantom pain can be constant in some cases, it is predominantly intermittent in nature.[112] Some patients report a background low-intensity pain coupled with intermittent episodes of excruciating, debilitating pain.[119] It is often characterized as knife-like or stabbing, but sufferers frequently describe other varied sensations, such as shooting, squeezing, burning, aching, and throbbing.[119,120] Pain can be perceived anywhere along the absent limb, but is typically reported in distal areas (ie, hands and feet) as opposed to more proximal locations.[121] In prospective studies of the duration of phantom pain, patients tend to report an overall decrease in pain intensity and frequency of attacks over time, with some patients experiencing a complete remission. Unfortunately, this is the exception, and up to 60% of amputees are left with some degree of phantom pain 12–24 months after loss of the affected limb.[112,116,118]

The mechanisms of phantom pain are not completely clear. As is the case with other types of neuropathic pain, there are likely both peripheral and central nervous system factors at play. Increased spontaneous activity of both afferent peripheral nerves and dorsal root ganglion cells has been observed experimentally following the transection of a nerve. In addition, the sympathetic nervous system may have a role in sensitizing and maintaining the abnormal afferent output from damaged nerve fibers after amputation. It is now known that the CNS, including spinal cord, brainstem, thalamus, and cerebral cortex, undergoes significant functional reorganization following amputation. Studies using functional brain imaging have shown that areas of the somatosensory cortex corresponding to the amputated structure become responsive to neighboring cell assemblies as early as 10 days after the injury.[122] For example, a common finding in upper extremity amputees is a shift of the cortical representation of the mouth into the (deafferented) hand area.[123] The degree to which this reorganization occurs has been correlated with the magnitude of phantom limb pain, underscoring the role that CNS plasticity has in the generation and maintenance of neuropathic pain.[124]

The treatment of phantom limb pain remains challenging, despite the multitude of proposed treatments. A review of therapies for phantom pain published in 1980 reported over 40 different methods, but concluded that few provided consistent relief.[125] The majority of interventions are medical and consist of the same drugs used for the management of other neuropathic pain conditions, such as tricyclic antidepressants and anticonvulsants.[110] Other modalities include nonmedical options such as transcutaneous electrical nerve stimulation (TENS), massage, and acupuncture. Surgical therapies such as neurectomy, rhizotomy, and cordotomy are probably the least effective and may be best reserved for the most intractable cases.

Several investigations have focused on utilizing preventative regional analgesic techniques to reduce perioperative pain and long-term phantom pain following lower extremity amputation surgery.[126] Bach and colleagues[59] initially examined the effect of epidural morphine, epidural bupivacaine, or both in combination for 3 days before amputation ($n = 11$) or conventional analgesia ($n = 14$). All patients received epidural or spinal anesthesia for amputation and received conventional analgesics postoperatively. The incidence of phantom pain was reduced 6 months after amputation but not after 1 week or after 12 months in the epidural treatment group compared with the control group. Jahangiri and coworkers[60] confirmed the beneficial effects of perioperative epidural administration on preventing phantom pain following amputation surgery. These investigators examined the effect of an epidural infusion of bupivacaine, diamorphine, and clonidine ($n = 13$) preoperatively and maintained for at least 3 days postoperatively. For comparison, the control group ($n = 11$) received on-demand opioid analgesia. These authors observed a significant reduction in the incidence of phantom pain at 1 year following surgery. However, the largest prospective study ($n = 60$) to examine the effect of epidural analgesia on phantom pain failed to document any benefit at 7 days, 3 months, 6 months, and 12 months postoperatively. Similarly, clinical investigations evaluating the efficacy of continuous postoperative regional analgesia by nerve sheath block for amputation surgery have been equivocal, with some studies revealing beneficial effects,[54,127] and others demonstrating no long-term benefit.[53,55] It is interesting that perineural analgesia provided for a reduction in phantom pain in these two studies[54,127] since this technique is ineffective in blocking nociceptive inputs from the pre- or intraoperative periods. A later study investigated whether postamputation stump and phantom pain could be reduced by preoperative epidural block with bupivacaine and diamorphine compared with intraoperative placement of a perineural catheter infusing bupivacaine.[62] These investigators observed that both regional techniques were equally effective in preventing phantom pain, but the epidural analgesic technique was more effective in relieving stump pain in the immediate postoperative period.

Unfortunately, many of the regional analgesic studies evaluating the effect on reducing long-term phantom pain have significant design flaws, including that they were not prospective, randomized, or blinded; they utilized either no control group or historical controls; they investigated a heterogeneous study group; or they lacked sufficient power. The authors of a recent systematic review of the literature concluded that because of the poor quality and contradictory results, the randomized and controlled trials do not provide evidence to support any particular treatment of phantom limb pain in the acute perioperative period or later.[126]

In fact, a number of reports of peripheral nerve block and neuraxial techniques appear to have *caused* an exacerbation of phantom pain. These are seen primarily with lower limb amputations, although the phenomenon has been described following brachial plexus block for revision of an arm amputation.[128] This "reactivated" phantom pain associated with neural blockade is often severe and unresponsive to parenteral opioids. However, agents that are usually effective against neuropathic pain, such as lidocaine and carbemazepine, have been used effectively.[129] The mechanism by which regional anesthesia provokes this painful response is not completely understood. One possibility is that an absence of afferent sensory input after spinal anesthesia may decrease the level of inhibition and increase self-sustained neural activity that is common in the spinal cord following deafferentation.[130] Since a subanesthetic dose of thiopental (1 mg/kg) is effective at terminating the reactivation phantom pain, a central mechanism is implied.[131] Although some authors suggest avoiding spinal anesthesia in patients with a history of lower limb amputation,[132] the benefits of regional anesthesia must be weighed against the potential for this unusual and bizarre event to occur.

Chronic Donor Site Pain

The occurrence of chronic pain following spinal fusion surgery is not an uncommon complication. Autogenous bone grafts from the ilium are frequently harvested for the purposes of bone fusion in patients undergoing spinal stabilization surgery. Often, the pain from the donor site is more severe than that from the laminectomy incision.[133–136] Although this pain usually resolves over a period of several weeks, it may persist and represent a significant source of postoperative morbidity.[133–136] In fact, donor site pain has been reported in up to 39% of patients at 3 months, 38% at 6 months, 37% at 1 year, and 19% at 2 years after bone graft harvesting from the iliac crest.[135–137]

The precise mechanism of donor site pain remains obscure. It has been postulated to be muscular or periosteal in nature secondary to stripping of the abductors from the ilium.[133] In addition, the pain may be neuropathic in origin secondary to injury to small sensory nerves at the donor site. One nerve frequently injured while harvesting bone graft from the anterior ilium is the lateral femoral cutaneous nerve, which has been reported in up to 10% of cases.[134] Injury to the ilioinguinal nerve has also been reported, especially when the bone graft is harvested from the anterior ilium.[134] The superior cluneal nerves pierce the lumbodorsal fascia and cross the posterior iliac crest 8 cm lateral to the posterior superior iliac spine.[138] Injury to these nerves may occur while harvesting bone graft from the posterior ilium and may result in transient or permanent numbness and pain over the buttock area.

Two recent studies have demonstrated a significant reduction in the incidence of chronic donor site pain with the preemptive administration of analgesics.[77,137] Houghton and associates[139] have shown that the local application of a low dose of morphine can effectively block the development of hyperalgesia and allodynia in a rat model of bone damage. This

analgesic effect was considered to be mediated through μ-opioid receptor action in the bone. Reuben and colleagues[137] subsequently evaluated the analgesic effect of low-dose morphine administered to the site of bone graft harvesting in patients undergoing spinal fusion surgery. Sixty patients were randomized to receive either saline infiltration into the harvest site ($n = 20$), intramuscular morphine 5 mg ($n = 20$), or morphine 5 mg infiltrated into the harvest site ($n = 20$). This study revealed that morphine infiltrated into the bone graft harvest site resulted in a significant reduction in pain scores and opioid use for the first 24 h following surgery. Furthermore, the association of chronic donor site pain was significantly lower in the local morphine group (5%) than in the intramuscular morphine (37%) or saline infiltration (33%) groups. Another study from the same institution examined the analgesic effect of preemptive COX-2 administration for spinal fusion surgery.[77] It has been shown that COX-2 plays an integral role in the processes of peripheral and central sensitization,[140] and it is possible that early and sustained treatment with COX-2 inhibitors may thwart the progression of acute to chronic pain.[141] Eighty patients scheduled to undergo instrumented posterior spinal fusion were randomized to receive either celecoxib 400 mg 1 h prior to surgery and then 200 mg every 12 h postoperatively for the first 5 days or matching placebo at similar time intervals. Patients administered celecoxib reported lower pain scores and had less opioid use during the first 5 postoperative days. Chronic donor site pain was significantly higher in the placebo group (12/40, 30%) than in the celecoxib group (4/40, 10%) at 1 year following surgery.[77] The development of neuropathic pain following spinal fusion surgery may in part be mediated by central COX-2 expression resulting in central neuronal plasticity. Spinal COX-2 has been implicated in the development of allodynia after nerve injury in rats,[142] and peripheral prostaglandins have been implicated in the pathogenesis of neuropathic pain.[143] However, after the development of neurogenic inflammation, the responses to mechanical stimuli are not affected by spinal COX-2 inhibition.[142] Thus, spinal prostaglandin synthesis may be important for the induction and initial expression, but not for the maintenance of spinal cord hyperexcitability.[70] This may explain the lack of analgesic efficacy of NSAIDs for treatment of chronic donor site pain observed in the study by Reuben and colleagues.

These studies[77,137] highlight the importance of utilizing preemptive analgesics for pain management following spinal fusion surgery. It has been suggested that effective treatment of acute pain, particularly when accompanied by a neuropathic element, prevents the development of chronic postsurgical pain syndromes.[25,144–146] The reduction in chronic donor site pain may be attributed to a preemptive or preventative analgesic effect in which a reduction in spinal cord neuroplasticity derives from prompt reduction in the perioperative noxious afferent input associated with surgery. An early reduction in acute pain may facilitate early postoperative ambulation[147] and decrease fear-avoidance behaviors[148,149] also contributing to a reduction in chronic postsurgical pain.

Further studies are needed to assess the efficacy of preemptive analgesic techniques on reducing chronic donor site pain.

Postthoracotomy Pain Syndrome

Pain following thoracic surgery has been reported to be among the most intense clinical experiences known.[150] The nociceptive pathways responsible for postthoracotomy pain are still poorly understood.[151] Possible sources of nociceptive input that may contribute to postoperative pain following thoracic surgery are multiple and include the site of the surgical incision; disruption of the intercostal nerves; inflammation of the chest wall structures adjacent to the incision, pulmonary parenchyma, or pleura; and thoracostomy drainage tubes.[152] Unrelieved acute pain following thoracic surgery may contribute not only to postoperative pulmonary dysfunction,[153] but also to the development of postthoracotomy pain syndrome.[25,144–146]

Postthoracotomy pain syndrome is defined as pain that recurs or persists along a thoracotomy incision for at least 2 months following the surgical procedure.[154] The true incidence of postthoracotomy pain syndrome is difficult to determine, with a reported range from 5% to 80%.[155] Different definitions used to describe and assess pain, lack of large, prospective studies, small sample size, varying surgical techniques, varying perioperative management, and different periods of follow-up care have all contributed to the difficulty in determining the true incidence of this postsurgical pain syndrome.[155] Nonetheless, it has been estimated that half of all patients still alive 1–2 years after thoracotomy will suffer with persistent chest wall pain.[156] Furthermore, as much as 30% of patients might still experience pain 4–5 years after surgery.[156]

The exact mechanism for the pathogenesis of postthoracotomy pain syndrome is still unclear. Similar to chronic donor site pain, it has been suggested that both neuropathic and myofascial nociceptive pathways contribute to the development of postthoracotomy pain syndrome. Although damage to cutaneous or deep (muscle, joint, and viscera) tissue is typically associated with peripheral inflammation, damage to neural structures often leads to pathologic pain.[10] Damage to intercostal nerves during thoracic surgery leads to neural degeneration, neuroma formation, and the generation of spontaneous neural inputs.[10] Evidence suggests that although nociceptive and neuropathic pain depend on separate peripheral mechanisms, they are both significantly influenced by changes in CNS function.[10] The resultant neuroplastic changes in the CNS have the capacity to contribute to persistent pathologic pain following surgery.[10]

A variety of preemptive or preventative analgesic techniques have been utilized in an attempt to reduce sustained nociceptive input into the CNS and concomitant acute and chronic pain following thoracic surgery. In a retrospective review of 1000 thoracic surgery patients, Richardson and colleagues[157] assessed the efficacy of acute postoperative pain on the incidence of postthoracotomy pain syndrome at 2 months following surgery. The use of systemic opioids alone

was associated with a 23.4% incidence of postthoracotomy pain syndrome.[157] Interestingly, the use of intraoperative intercostal neurolysis with a cryoprobe increased the incidence of chronic pain to 31.6%.[157] In contrast, the use of continuous paravertebral infusion of bupivacaine in conjunction with systemic opioids decreased the incidence to 14.8%.[157] Furthermore, the addition of an NSAID to this analgesic regimen reduced the incidence of postthoracotomy pain syndrome to 9.9%.[157] These findings highlight the importance of utilizing a multimodal analgesic regimen for the prevention of acute and chronic postsurgical pain. In addition, even when a perioperative local anesthetic block is utilized, nociceptive afferent pathways to the CNS can still be activated leading to central sensitization.[157] There appears to be two forms of nociceptive input from peripheral inflamed tissue to the CNS.[140] The first is mediated by neural activity innervating the area of injury which may be reduced with local anesthetic neural blockade or peripherally acting COX-2 inhibitors. The second pathway is humorally mediated, in which interleukins reach the CNS via systemic pathways, resulting in upregulation of COX-2 in the CNS. This latter pathway is not affected by regional anesthesia and only blocked by centrally acting COX-2 inhibitors.[140] Thus it has been demonstrated that the addition of a centrally acting COX-2 inhibitor to a local anesthetic block can result in a significant decrease in CNS prostaglandin E2 (PGE2) levels and improved postoperative analgesia.[158] McCrory and coworkers[159] confirmed the analgesic benefit of adding a centrally acting COX-2 inhibitor with neuraxial analgesia for postthoracotomy pain. This randomized, prospective, double-blind study evaluated the analgesic efficacy of ibuprofen (peripherally acting NSAID), nimesulide (centrally acting NSAID), or placebo in conjunction with neuraxial analgesics. This study revealed a significant reduction in postoperative pain and opioid use with the centrally acting NSAID, nimesulide, compared with either ibuprofen or placebo. This pain reduction correlated with a significant reduction in PGE2 levels in the cerebrospinal fluid observed in the nimesulide group, which was not seen with either placebo or ibuprofen.

In a retrospective study of 159 patients undergoing posterolateral thoracotomy, Hu and associates[160] examined the effects of thoracic epidural analgesia on the incidence of postthoracotomy pain syndrome. Thoracic epidural anesthesia was given to 119 patients in conjunction with general anesthesia, and 40 patients received only general anesthesia. Thoracic epidural analgesia was initiated prior to surgical incision and maintained intraoperatively with an infusion of bupivacaine 0.5%. Following surgery, these patients were administered epidural morphine every 12 h for the first 3 days. These authors reported a similar incidence in postthoracotomy pain syndrome in the epidural analgesia group (42%) compared with the general anesthesia group (39%). In contrast to these findings, Obata and colleagues,[161] in a prospective, randomized, double-blind study, revealed a significant analgesic benefit when epidural analgesia was initiated prior to thoracic surgery. These investigators compared the analgesic effects of a continuous thoracic epidural infusion of mepivacaine initiated 20 min prior to surgery with one begun at the completion of surgery and continued for the first 3 postoperative days. This study revealed a significant reduction in both acute and chronic postthoracotomy pain at 6 months following surgery in the preincisional compared with the postincisional epidural analgesia group. The beneficial effects of epidural analgesia following thoracic surgery were confirmed in a more recent prospective, randomized, double-blind study performed by Senturk and coworkers.[162] These investigators compared the analgesic effects of three different analgesic techniques: (1) thoracic epidural analgesia initiated before, or (2) after surgical incision, and (3) intravenous patient controlled analgesia (PCA) on acute postoperative pain and the incidence of postthoracotomy pain syndrome 6 months following surgery. Patients in the prethoracic epidural group reported significantly less pain than those receiving the postthoracic epidural or the PCA groups for the first 48 h following surgery. The incidence of postthoracotomy pain syndrome was also significantly lower in the prethoracic epidural group (45%) than for those who received either the postthoracic epidural (63%) or the PCA (78%). Although both Obata and colleagues[161] and Senturk and coworkers[162] demonstrated a beneficial effect with the preemptive administration of epidural analgesia for thoracic surgery, Ochroch and associates[163] were unable to report similar findings. In a prospective, randomized, double-blind study of 157 patients, these investigators examined the analgesic efficacy of thoracic epidural analgesia initiated prior to surgical incision or at the time of rib approximation. Overall, there were no differences in pain scores or activity level during hospitalization or after discharge between the two groups. Furthermore, the number of patients reporting pain 1 year following surgery was similar for the two groups.

From these studies, it can be concluded that the method of perioperative pain management has a variable effect on the incidence of postthoracotomy pain syndrome. The reason for this variability may be explained by the multiple sources of nociceptive afferent pathways involved in the perception of pain following thoracic surgery.[152] These pain sources may be conveyed to the CNS via somatic nerves (intercostal nerves), phrenic nerve, cranial nerve (vagus nerve), the sympathetic nervous system, the parasympathetic system, and the brachial plexus.[155] It has been demonstrated that thoracic epidural analgesia is unable to abolish somatosensory evoked potential resulting from thoracic dermatomal stimulation, suggesting that this regional technique may be insufficient for blocking all nociceptive pain pathways.[164,165] Therefore, the use of regional blockade by itself is insufficient in providing complete pain relief and preventing central sensitization of the nervous system following thoracic surgery. A multimodal analgesic regimen, in which regional blocks are combined with NSAIDs and other analgesics, as described by Richardson and colleagues,[157] may provide for a reduction in both acute and chronic pain following thoracic surgery. Future prospective, randomized studies are needed to evaluate the efficacy of utilizing preventative multimodal analgesic techniques on the incidence of postthoracotomy pain syndrome.

MULTIMODAL PREEMPTIVE ANALGESIA

Despite major improvements in our understanding of acute pain physiology, sufficient pain relief that allows normal function has not been achieved during major surgical procedures without the risk of side effects. Optimal pain relief following surgery is difficult to achieve with the use of just one drug or regimen.[166] Many pain experts advocate the use of two or more classes of medications or techniques so as to reduce the side effect profile of any one drug and to make use of synergistic analgesic pathways or receptors. It is possible that, in the search for an ideal technique to provide true preemptive analgesia, a multimodal approach may be employed. There is already some clinical evidence that this can be an effective technique. Recently, Reuben and colleagues demonstrated that a preemptive multimodal regimen consisting of rofecoxib; acetaminophen; femoral nerve block; and an intraarticular injection of morphine, clonidine, and bupivacaine led to a reduction in the incidence of pain, opioid use, postoperative nausea and vomiting, length of stay, and unplanned admission to the hospital following anterior cruciate ligament surgery.[167] Furthermore, patients receiving this preemptive analgesic regimen demonstrated a significant reduction in long-term patellofemoral complications, including patellofemoral pain, flexion contracture, quadriceps weakness, and CRPS of the knee.[168] In addition, these patients were more likely to return to their preinjury level of activity including full sports participation.

Unfortunately the majority of studies evaluating the long-term benefits of utilizing preventative analgesic techniques failed to document any effect on wound hyperalgesia. Without such data, one cannot comment on the potential mechanisms responsible for a potential reduction in chronic postsurgical pain.[169] Recently, Lavand'homme and coworkers assessed the role of preventative multimodal analgesic techniques in reducing wound hyperalgesia and persistent postsurgical pain following major abdominal surgery.[170] In a randomized, double-blind trial these investigators examined the analgesic effects of thoracic epidural analgesia combined with ketamine following neoplastic colon resection. All patients received a thoracic epidural catheter, systemic ketamine (0.5 mg/kg and 0.25 mg/kg/h intraoperatively) and general anesthesia. Patients were allocated to four groups to receive intraoperative intravenous lidocaine-sufentanil-clonidine or epidural bupivacaine-sufentanil-clonidine followed postoperatively by either intravenous (lidocaine-morphine-clonidine) or epidural (bupivacaine-sufentanil-clonidine) PCA. These analgesics were administered by either intravenous or epidural route as a continuous infusion starting before incision until 72 h after surgery. This study revealed significantly higher analgesic requirements, pain scores, and area of wound hyperalgesia in the intravenous treatment group (intravenous–intravenous), and more patients reported residual pain from 2 weeks until 1 year (28%). Postoperative epidural treatment (intravenous–epidural) was less effective in preventing residual pain at 1 year (11%) than the intraoperative epidural (epidural–epidural and epidural–intravenous) groups (0%). This landmark study demonstrates a clear benefit of continuous epidural analgesia as a preventative treatment on the development of persistent postsurgical pain. Furthermore, intraoperative use of epidural analgesia seems to provide for more significant long-term prevention of residual pain. By demonstrating a reduction in mechanical hyperalgesia with these preventative analgesic techniques, this study highlights the major contribution of central sensitization in both short- and long-term incisional pain.

The pathophysiology of wind-up has yet to be completely defined, and as our understanding of the pathways involved is enhanced, the use of multiple agents to achieve a more complete and reliable preemptive blockade of sensitization is likely to occur.

CONCLUSION

Preemptive analgesia is a tempting concept for practitioners of anesthesia and perioperative pain medicine. However, despite the compelling experimental evidence, there has been a great deal of difficulty proving its existence in the clinical setting. This is probably related to multiple methodologic factors. Most importantly, the duration of the noxious afferent input from the surgical wound far exceeds those used for the original animal experiments. It is futile to attempt to manipulate a complex physiologic event such as postoperative pain with a single preoperative intervention that lasts only a few minutes or hours. Techniques that involve continuous infusions of local anesthetic such as epidurals hold the most promise in this area. In particular, continuous perineural catheters that are being used to prolong the effect of a peripheral nerve block are very exciting from the point of view of allowing a patient to be discharged home in comfort while at the same time potentially reducing the inflammatory sensitization that would otherwise occur in the spinal cord. As the popularity of these catheters grows, we are sure to see more clinical trials aimed at defining their role in preemptive analgesia.

Secondly, for a study to prove the efficacy, or even the existence, of preemptive analgesia, the intervention must be compared in three groups: preincision, postincision, and placebo. The use of a placebo vs a preincision intervention just serves to support the intuitive notion that "some pain medicine is better than none." Unfortunately, many studies are allowed to be conducted this way.

Whether or not the timing of an analgesic intervention in the perioperative period ends up being a critical part of the puzzle, the value of aggressive and comprehensive pain control for surgical patients should not be underestimated. Some clinicians are choosing to focus on providing "preventative," rather than simply "preemptive" analgesia. The term *preventative analgesia* was introduced to emphasize the fact that central neuroplasticity is induced by pre-, intra-, and postoperative nociceptive inputs.[171] Thus the goal of preventative analgesia is to reduce central sensitization that arises from noxious inputs arising throughout the entire perioperative period and not just from those occurring during the surgical incision. In other words, the provision of "intensive and prolonged, multimodal analgesic interventions"[34] may serve to insulate the susceptible neural pathways from a continuous barrage of nociceptive input over the long term, rather than as just a one-time treatment. Effective preventative analgesic techniques may not only be useful in reducing acute pain but also chronic postsurgical pain and disability.

As Gottshalk and Raja point out in their recent editorial, it is incumbent on anesthesiologists to "play a role in preventive medicine."[172] Preemptive analgesia is a good start, and though it remains a controversial subject at present, as our understanding of pain processing and the role of regional anesthesia in pain prevention improves, we can employ it to greater use in helping to keep our patients as comfortable as possible.

References

1. Crile GW, Lower WE: *Anoci-association.* WB Saunders, 1914.
2. Crile G: Phylogenetic association in relation to certain medical problems. Boston Med J 1910;163:893–904.
3. Melzack R, Wall PD: Pain mechanisms: A new theory. Science 1965;150:971–979.
4. Raja SN, Meyer RA, Campbell JN: Peripheral mechanisms of somatic pain. Anesthesiology 1988;68:571–590.
5. Woolf CJ: Evidence for a central component of post-injury pain hypersensitivity. Nature 1983;303:686–688.
6. Levine JD, Fields HL, Basbaum AI: Peptides and the primary afferent nociceptor. J Neurosci 1993;13:2273–2286.
7. Woolf CJ, Chong MS: Preemptive analgesia—Treating postoperative pain by preventing the establishment of central sensitization. Anesth Analg 1993;77:362–379.
8. LaMotte RH, Thalhammer JG, Torebjork HE, et al: J Neurosci. Peripheral neural mechanisms of cutaneous hyperalgesia following mild injury to heat 1982;2:765–781.
9. Light AR, Perl ER: Spinal termination of functionally identified primary afferent neurons with slowly conducting myelinated fibers. J Comp Neurol 1979;186:133–150.
10. Coderre TJ, Katz J, Vaccarino AL, et al: Contribution of central neuroplasticity to pathological pain: Review of clinical and experimental evidence. Pain 1993;52:259–285.
11. Woolf CJ, Salter MW: Neuronal plasticity: Increasing the gain in pain. Science 2000;288:1765–1768.
12. Kaur A, Selwa L, Fromes G, et al: Persistent headache after supratentorial craniotomy. Neurosurgery 2000;47:633–636.
13. Harner SG, Beatty CW, Ebersold MJ: Headache after acoustic neuroma excision. Am J Otol 1993;14:552–555.
14. Finch DR, Macdougal M, Tibbs DJ, et al: Amputation for vascular disease: The experience of a peripheral vascular unit. Br J Surg 1980;67:233–237.
15. Fisher K, Hanspal PS: Phantom pain, anxiety, depression, and their relation in consecutive patients with amputated limbs: Case reports. BMJ 1998;316:903–904.
16. Sherman RA, Sherman CJ, Parker L: Chronic phantom and stump pain among American veterans: Results of a survey. Pain 1984;18:83–95.
17. Bertrand PC, Regnard JF, Spaggiari L, et al: Immediate and long-term results after surgical treatment of primary spontaneous pneumothorax by VATS. Ann Thorac Surg 1996;61:1641–1645.
18. Katz J, Jackson M, Kavanagh BP, et al: Acute pain after thoracic surgery predicts long-term post-thoracotomy pain. Clin J Pain 1996;12:50–55.

19. Jung BF, Ahrendt GM, Oaklander AL, et al: Neuropathic pain following breast cancer surgery: Proposed classification and research update. Pain 2003;104:1–13.

20. Tasmuth T, von Smitten K, Kalso E: Pain and other symptoms during the first year after radical and conservative surgery for breast cancer. Br J Cancer 1996;74:2024–2031.

21. Stiff G, Rhodes M, Kelly A, et al: Long-term pain: Less common after laparoscopic than open cholecystectomy. Br J Surg 1994;81:1368–1370.

22. Ure BM, Troidl H, Spangenberger W, et al: Long-term results after laparoscopic cholecystectomy. Br J Surg 1995;82:267–270.

23. de Pouvourville G, Ribet-Reinhart N, Fendrick M, et al: A prospective comparison of costs and morbidity of laparoscopic versus open cholecystectomy. Hepatogastroenterology 1997;44:35–39.

24. Aasvang E, Kehlet H: Chronic postoperative pain: The case of inguinal herniorrhaphy. Br J Anaesth 2005;95:69–76.

25. Perkins FM, Kehlet H: Chronic pain as an outcome of surgery. Anesthesiology 2000;93:1123–1133.

26. Edwards RR: Individual differences in endogenous pain modulation as a risk factor for chronic pain. Neurology 2005;65:437–443.

27. Eisenberg E: Post-surgical neuralgia. Pain 2004;111:3–7.

28. Wall PD: The prevention of postoperative pain. Pain 1988;33:289–290.

29. Dickenson AH, Sullivan AF: Subcutaneous formalin-induced activity of dorsal horn neurons in the rat: differential response to an intrathecal opiate administered pre or post formalin. Pain 1987;30:349–360.

30. Coderre TJ, Vaccarino AL, Melzack R: Central nervous system plasticity in the tonic pain response to subcutaneous formalin injection. Brain Res 1990;535:155–158.

31. Dahl JB, Moiniche S: Pre-emptive analgesia. Br Med Bull 2004;71:13–27.

32. Katz J: Pre-emptive analgesia: Evidence, current status and future directions. Eur J Anesthesiol 1995;12:8–13.

33. Kissin I: Preemptive analgesia. Why its effect is not always obvious. Anesthesiology 1996;84:1015–1019.

34. Moiniche S, Kehlet H, Dahl J: A qualitative and quantitative systematic review of preemptive analgesia for postoperative pain relief-the role of timing of analgesia. Anesthesiology 2002;96:725–741.

35. Ong CK, Lirk P, Seymour RA, et al: The efficacy of preemptive analgesia for acute postoperative pain management: A meta-analysis. Anesth Analg 2005;100:757–773.

36. Moher D, Jadad AR, Nichol G, et al: Assessing the quality of randomized trials: An annotated bibliography of scales and checklists. Control Clin Trials 1995;16:62–73.

37. McQuay HJ: Pre-emptive analgesia. Br J Anaesth 1992;69:1–3.

38. Lam KW, Pun TC, Ng EH, et al: Efficacy of preemptive analgesia for wound pain after laparoscopic operations in infertile women: A randomised, double-blind and placebo control study. Br J Obstet Gynaecol 2004;111:340–344.

39. Lee IO, Kim SH, Kong MH: Pain after laparoscopic cholecystectomy: The effect and timing of incisional and intraperitoneal bupivacaine. Can J Anaesth 2001;48:545–550.

40. Fagan DJ, Martin W, Smith A: A randomized, double-blind trial of pre-emptive local anesthesia in day-case knee arthroscopy. Arthroscopy 2003;19:50–53.

41. Visalyaputra S, Sanansilp V, Pechpaisit N: Postoperative analgesic effects of intravenous lornoxicam and morphine with pre-emptive ropivacaine skin infiltration and preperitoneal instillation after transabdominal hysterectomy. J Med Assoc Thai 2002;85(Suppl 3):S1010–1016.

42. Podder S, Wig J, Malhotra SK, et al: Effect of pre-emptive analgesia on self-reported and biological measures of pain after tonsillectomy. Eur J Anaesthesiol 2000;17:319–324.

43. Hogan QH: No preemptive analgesia: is that so bad? Anesthesiology 2002; 96: 526–527.

44. Parr AM, Zoutman DE, Davidson JS: Antimicrobial activity of lidocaine against bacteria associated with nosocomial wound infection. Ann Plast Surg 1999;43:239–245.

45. Drucker M, Cardenas E, Arizti P, et al: Experimental studies on the effect of lidocaine on wound healing. World J Surg 1998;22:394–397.

46. Hadzic A, Williams BA, Karaca PE, et al: For outpatient rotator cuff surgery, nerve block anesthesia provides superior same-day recovery over general anesthesia. Anesthesiology 2005;102:1001–1007.

47. Hadzic A, Karaca PE, Hobeika P, et al: Peripheral nerve blocks result in superior recovery profile compared with general anesthesia in outpatient knee arthroscopy. Anesth Analg 2005;100:976–981.

48. Suresh S, Barcelona SL, Young NM, et al: Does a preemptive block of the great auricular nerve improve postoperative analgesia in children undergoing tympanomastoid surgery? Anesth Analg 2004;98:330–333.

49. Altintas F, Bozkurt P, Ipek N, et al: The efficacy of pre- versus postsurgical axillary block on postoperative pain in paediatric patients. Paediatr Anaesth 2000;10:23–28.

50. Gadsden J, Singh A, Iwata T, et al: Peripheral nerve blocks in heavily sedated patients. Abstract presented at the American Society of Regional Anesthesia and Pain Medicine Annual Spring Meeting and Workshops, Toronto, Canada, 2005.

51. Doyle E, Bowler GM: Pre-emptive effect of multimodal analgesia in thoracic surgery. Br J Anaesth 1998;80:147–151.

52. Huffnagle HJ, Norris MC, Leighton BL, et al: Ilioinguinal iliohypogastric nerve blocks—Before or after cesarean delivery under spinal anesthesia? Anesth Analg 1996;82:8–12.

53. Elizaga AM, Smith DG, Sharar SR, et al: Continuous regional analgesia by intraneural block: Effect on postoperative opioid requirements and phantom limb pain following amputation. J Rehabil Res Devel 1994;31:179–187.

54. Fisher V, Persen L, Lovlien M, et al: Continuous postoperative regional analgesia by nerve sheath block for amputation surgery: a pilot study. Anesth Analg 1991;72:300–303.

55. Pinzur M, Garla PG, Pluth T, et al: Continuous postoperative infusion of a regional anaesthetic after an amputation of the lower extremity. J Bone Joint Surg [Am] 1996;79:1752–1753.

56. Richman JM, Wu CL: Epidural analgesia for postoperative pain. Anesthesiol Clin North America 2005;23:125–140.

57. Beilin B, Bessler H, Mayhurd E: Effects of preemptive analgesia on pain and cytokine production in the postoperative period. Anesthesiology 2003;98:151–155.

58. Neustein SM, Kreitzer JM, Krellenstein D, et al: Preemptive epidural analgesia for thoracic surgery. Mt Sinai J Med 2002;69:101–104.

59. Bach S, Noreng MF, Tjellden NU: Phantom limb pain in amputees during the first 12 months following limb amputation, after preoperative lumbar epidural blockade. Pain 1988;33:297–301.

60. Jahangiri M, Bradley JWP, Jayatunga AP, et al: Prevention of phantom pain after major lower limb amputation by epidural infusion of diamorphine, clonidine and bupivacaine. Ann R Coll Surg Engl 1994;76:324–326.

61. Nikolajsen L, Ilkjaer S, Christensen JH, et al: Randomised trial of epidural bupivacaine and morphine in prevention of stump and phantom pain in lower-limb amputation. Lancet 1997;350:1353–1357.

62. Lambert AW, Dashfield AK, Cosgrove C, et al: Randomized prospective study comparing preoperative epidural and intraoperative perineural analgesia for the prevention of postoperative stump and phantom limb pain following major amputation. Reg Anesth Pain Med 2001;26:316–321.

63. Wattwil M, Thoren T, Hennerdal S, et al: Epidural analgesia with bupivacaine reduces postoperative paralytic ileus after hysterectomy. Anesth Analg 1989;68:353–358.

64. Brandt MR, Kehlet H, Binder C, et al: Effect of epidural analgesia on the glucoregulator endocrine response to surgery. Clin Endocrinol 1976;5:107–114.

65. Rodgers A, Walker N, Schug S, et al: Reduction of postoperative mortality and morbidity with epidural or spinal anesthesia: Results from overview of randomized trials. BMJ 2000;321:1–12.

66. McCormack K, Brune K: Dissociation between the antinociceptive and anti-inflammatory effects of nonsteroidal anti-inflammatory drugs. A survey of their analgesic efficacy. Drugs 1991;41:533–547.

67. Vanegas H, Schaible HG: Prostaglandins and cyclooxygenases in the spinal cord. Prog Neurobiol 2001;64:327–363.

68. Ferreira SH, Lorenzetti BB, Correa FMA: Central and peripheral antialgesic actions of aspirin-like drugs. Eur J Pharmacol 1978;53:39–48.

69. Samad TA, Moore KA, Sapirstein A, et al: Interleukin-1 -mediated induction of Cox-2 in the CNS contributes to inflammatory pain hypersensitivity. Nature 2001;410:471–475.

70. Vasquez E, Bär KJ, Ebersberger A, et al: Spinal prostaglandins are involved in the development but not the maintenance of inflammation-induced spinal hyperexcitability. J Neurosci 2001;21:9001–9008.

71. Yaksh TL, Malmberg AB: Spinal action of NSAIDs in blocking spinally mediated hyperalgesia: The role of cyclooxygenase products. Agents Actions Suppl 1993;41:89–100.

72. Bartfai T: Telling the brain about pain. Nature 2001;410:425–426.

73. Dahl JB, Kehlet H: Non-steroidal anti-inflammatory drugs: Rationale for use in severe postoperative pain. Br J Anaesth 1991;66:703–712.

74. Katz J: Pre-emptive analgesia: Importance of timing. Can J Anaesth 2001;48:105–114.

75. Reuben SS, Bhopatkar S, Maciolek H, et al: The preemptive analgesic effect of rofecoxib after ambulatory arthroscopic knee surgery. Anesth Analg 2002;94:55–59.

76. Reuben SS, Ekman E: The effect of cyclooxygenase-2 inhibition on analgesia and spinal fusion. J Bone Joint Surg [Am] 2005;87:536–542.

77. Reuben SS, Kuppinger J, Ekman EF: The effect of perioperative celecoxib administration on acute and chronic donor site pain following spinal fusion surgery. Anesth Analg 2005;100S:298.

78. Yeh CC, Jao SW, Huh BK, et al: Preincisional dextromethorphan combined with thoracic epidural anesthesia and analgesia improves postoperative pain and bowel function in patients undergoing colonic surgery. Anesth Analg 2005;100:1384–1389.

79. McCartney CJ, Sinha A, Katz J: A qualitative systematic review of the role of N-methyl-D-aspartate receptor antagonists in preventive analgesia. Anesth Analg 2004;98:1385–1400.

80. Pandey CK, Sahay S, Gupta D, et al: Preemptive gabapentin decreases postoperative pain after lumbar discoidectomy. Can J Anesth 2004;51:986–989.

81. Dahl JB, Mathiesen O, Moniche S: "Protective premedication": An option with gabapentin and related drugs? A review of gabapentin and pregabalin in the treatment of post-operative pain. Acta Anaesthesiol Scand 2004;48:1130–1136.

82. Reuben SS: The prevention of post-surgical neuralgia. Pain 2005;113:242–243.

83. Stanton-Hicks M, Janig W, Hassenbusch S, et al: Reflex sympathetic dystrophy: Changing concepts and taxonomy. Pain 1995;63:127–133.

84. Raja SN, Grabow TS: Complex regional pain syndrome I (reflex sympathetic dystrophy). Anesthesiology 2002;96:1254–1260.

85. Merskey KR, Bogduck N: *Classification of Chronic Pain: Description of Chronic Pin Syndromes and Definitions of Pain Terms,* 2nd ed. IASP press, 1994.

86. Bruehl S, Harden RN, Galer BS, et al: External validation of IASP diagnostic criteria for complex regional pain syndrome and proposed research diagnostic criteria. Pain 1999;81:147–154.

87. Harden RN, Bruehl S, Galer BS, et al: Complex regional pain syndrome: Are the IASP diagnostic criteria valid and sufficiently comprehensive? Pain 1999;83:211–219.

88. Roberts WJ: A hypothesis on the physiologic basis for causalgia and related pains. Pain 1986;24:297–311.

89. Birklein F: Complex regional pain syndrome. J Neurol 2005;252:131–138.

90. Reuben SS: Preventing the development of complex regional pain syndrome after surgery. Anesthesiology 2004;101:1215–1224.

91. Pak TJ, Martin GM, Magness JL, et al: Reflex sympathetic dystrophy: Review of 140 cases. Minn Med 1970;53:507–512.

92. Allen G, Galer BS, Schwartz L: Epidemiology of complex regional pain syndrome: A retrospective chart review of 134 patients. Pain 1999;80:539–544.

93. Papay FA, Verghese A, Stanton-Hicks M, et al: Complex regional pain syndrome of the breast in a patient after breast reduction. Ann Plast Surg 1997;39:347–352.

94. Graham LE, McGuigan C, Kerr S, et al: Complex regional pain syndrome post mastectomy. Rheumatol Int 2002;21:165–166.

95. Tang A, Ohri S: Reflex sympathetic dystrophy: An unusual complication of radial artery graft harvesting. J Cardiovasc Surg (Torino) 2002;43:49–50.

96. Prager JP, Csete M: An unusual cause of pain after nevus excision: Complex regional pain syndrome. J Am Acad Dermatol 1997;37:652–653.

97. Sachs BL, Zindrick MR, Beasley RD: Reflex sympathetic dystrophy after operative procedures on the lumbar spine. J Bone Joint Surg [Am] 1993;75:721–725.

98. Small NC: Complications in arthroscopic surgery performed by experienced arthroscopists. Arthroscopy 1998;4:215–221.

99. MacDonald RI, Lichtman DM, Hablon JJ, et al: Complications of surgical release for carpal tunnel syndrome. J Hand Surg 1978;3:70–76.

100. Lichtman DM, Florio RL, Mack GR: Carpal tunnel release under local anesthesia: Evaluation of the outpatient procedure. J Hand Surg 1979;4:544–546.

101. Shinya K, Lanzetta M, Conolly WB: Risk and complications in endoscopic carpal tunnel release. J Hand Surg 1995;20:222–227.

102. Harden RN, Bruehl S, Stanos S, et al: Prospective examination of pain-related and psychological predictors of CRPS-like phenomena following total knee arthroplasty: A preliminary study. Pain 2003;106:393–400.

103. Cameron HU, Park YS, Krestow M: Reflex sympathetic dystrophy following total knee replacement. Contemp Orthop 1994;29:279–281.

104. Katz MM, Hungerford DS, Krackow KA, et al: Reflex sympathetic dystrophy as a cause of poor results after total knee arthroplasty. J Arthroplasty 1986;1:117–124.

105. Ritter MA: Postoperative pain after total knee arthroplasty. J Arthroplasty 1997;12:337–339.

106. Bennett GJ, Harden RN: Questions concerning the incidence and prevalence of complex regional pain syndrome type I (RSD) (letter). Pain 2003;106:209–211.

107. Reuben SS, Rosenthal EA, Steinberg RB: Surgery on the affected upper extremity of patients with a history of complex regional pain syndrome: A retrospective study of 100 patients. J Hand Surg [Am] 2000;25:1147–1151.

108. Katz MM, Hungerford DS: Reflex sympathetic dystrophy affecting the knee. J Bone Joint Surg [Am] 1987;69:797–803.

109. Nathanson M: Phantom limbs as reported by S. Weir Mitchell. Neurology 1988;38:504–505.

110. Nikolajsen L, Jensen TS: Phantom limb pain. Br J Anaesth 2001;87:107–116.

111. Henderson WR, Smyth GE: Phantom limbs. J Neurol Neurosurg Psych 1948;11:88–112.

112. Wartan SW, Hamann W, Wedley JR, et al: Phantom pain and sensation among British veteran amputees. Br J Anaesth 1997;78:652–659.

113. Houghton AD, Nicholls G, Houghton AL, et al: Phantom pain: Natural history and association with rehabilitation. Ann R Coll Surg Engl 1994;76:22–25.

114. Kooijman CM, Dijkstra PU, Geertzen JHB, et al: Phantom pain and phantom sensations in upper limb amputees: An epidemiological study. Pain 2000;87:33–41.

115. Katz J: Prevention of phantom limb pain by regional anaesthesia. Lancet 1997;349:519–520.

116. Parkes CM: Factors determining the persistence of phantom pain in the amputee. J Psychosom Res 1973;17:97–108.

117. Nikolajsen L, Ilkjaer S, Jensen TS: Relationship between mechanical stimulation and postamputation pain: A prospective study. Eur J Pain 2000;4:327–334.

118. Jensen TS, Krebs B, Nielsen J, et al: Immediate and long-term phantom limb pain in amputees: Incidence, clinical characteristics and relationship to pre-amputation limb pain. Pain 1985;21:267–278.

119. Sherman RA, Sherman CJ: Prevalence and characteristics of chronic phantom limb pain among American veterans. Results of a trial survey. Am J Phys Med 1983;62:227–238.

120. Katz J, Melzack R: Pain 'memories' in phantom limbs: Review and clinical observations. Pain 1990;43:319–336.

121. Nikolajsen L, Ilkjaer S, Kroner K, et al: The influence of preamputation pain on postamputation stump and phantom pain. Pain 1997;72:393–405.

122. Weiss T, Miltner WH, Huonker R, et al: Rapid function plasticity of the somatosensory cortex following finger amputation. Exp Brain Res 2000;134:199–203.

123. Montoya P, Ritter K, Huse E: The cortical somatotopic map and phantom phenomena in subjects with congenital limb atrophy and traumatic amputees with phantom limb pain. Eur J Neurosci 1998;10:1095–1102.

124. Karl A, Birbaumer N, Lutzenberger W, et al: Reorganization of motor and somatosensory cortex in upper extremity amputees with phantom limb pain. J Neurosci 2001;21:3609–3618.

125. Sherman R: Published treatments of phantom limb pain. Am J Phys Med 1980;59:232–244.

126. Halbert J, Crotty M, Cameron ID: Evidence for the optimal management of acute and chronic phantom pain: A systematic review. Clin J Pain 2002;18:84–92.

127. Malawer MM, Buch R, Khurana JS, et al: Postoperative infusional continuous regional analgesia. A technique for relief of postoperative pain following major extremity surgery. Clin Orthop Relat Res 1991;266:227–237.

128. Lee E, Donovan K: Reactivation of phantom limb pain after combined interscalene brachial plexus block and general anesthesia: Successful treatment with intravenous lidocaine. Anesthesiology 1995;82:295–298.

129. Gentili ME: Recurrence of preoperative painful sensation during brachial plexus block. Anesthesiology 1998;88:281.

130. Mackenzie N: Phantom limb pain during spinal anaesthesia. Recurrence in amputees. Anaesthesia 1983;38:886–887.

131. Wajima Z, Shitara T, Inoue T, et al: Severe lightning pain after subarachnoid block in a patient with neuropathic pain of central origin: Which drug is best to treat the pain? Clin J Pain 2000;16:265–269.

132. Sellick BC: Phantom limb pain and spinal anesthesia. Anesthesiology 1985;62:801–802.

133. Summers BN, Eisenstein SM: Donor site pain from the ilium. A complication of lumbar spine fusion. J Bone Joint Surg [Br] 1989;71:677–680.

134. Kurz LT, Garfin SR, Booth RE: Harvesting autogenous iliac bone grafts. A review of complications and techniques. Spine 1989;14:324–331.

135. Fernyhough JC, Schimandle JJ, Weigel MC, et al: Chronic donor site pain complicating bone graft harvesting from the posterior iliac crest for spinal fusion. Spine 1992;12:1474–1480.

136. Goulet JA, Senunas LE, DeSilva GL, et al: Autogenous iliac crest bone graft: Complications and functional assessment. Clin Orthop 1997;339:76–81.

137. Reuben SS, Vieira P, Faruqi S, et al: Local administration of morphine for analgesia after iliac bone graft harvest. Anesthesiology 2001;95:390–394.

138. Goldstein LA: Lumbar spine. In Dickerson R: *Atlas of Orthopaedic Surgery*. Mosby, 1974, pp 450–453.

139. Houghton AK, Valdez JG, Westlund KN: Peripheral morphine administration blocks the development of hyperalgesia and allodynia after bone damage. Anesthesiology 1998;89:190–201.

140. Samad TA, Sapirstein A, Woolf CJ: Prostanoids and pain: Unraveling mechanisms and revealing therapeutic targets. Trends Molec Med 2002;8:390–396.

141. Gottschalk A, Smith DS: New concepts in acute pain therapy: Preemptive analgesia. Am Fam Physician 2001;63:1979–1984.

142. Zhao Z, Chen SR, Eisenach JC, et al: Spinal cyclooxygenase-2 is involved in the development of allodynia after nerve injury in rats. Neuroscience 2000;97:743–748.

143. Ma W, Eisenach JC: Morphological and pharmacological evidence for the role of peripheral prostaglandins in the pathogenesis of neuropathic pain. Eur J Neurosci 2002;15:1037–1047.

144. Cousins MJ, Power I, Smith G: 1996 Labat lecture: Pain—A persistent problem. Reg Anesth Pain Med 2000;25:6–21.

145. Macrae WA: Chronic pain after surgery. Br J Anaesth 2001;87:88–98.

146. Atkinson JH, Slater MA, Epping-Jordan JE: Identifying individuals at risk for chronicity. An opportunity to reexamine our treatment, timing, and targets. Pain Forum 1997;6:137–139.

147. Pellino T, Tluczek A, Collins M, et al: Increasing self-efficacy through empowerment. Preoperative education for orthopaedic patients. Orthop Nurs 1998;17:48–51.

148. Phillips HC: Avoidance behavior and its role in sustaining chronic pain. Behav Res Ther 1987;25:273–279.

149. Vlaeyen JWS, Linton SJ: Fear-avoidance and its consequences in chronic musculoskeletal pain: State of the art. Pain 2000;85:317–332.

150. Loan WB, Morrison JD: The incidence and severity of postoperative pain. Br J Anaesth 1967;39:695–698.

151. Conacher ID: Pain relief after thoracotomy. Br J Anaesth 1990;65:806–812.

152. Kavanagh BP, Katz J, Sandler AN: Pain control after thoracic surgery. A review of current techniques. Anesthesiology 1994;81:737–759.

153. Johnson WC: Postoperative ventilatory performance: Dependence upon surgical incision. Am Surg 1975;41:615–619.

154. Merskey H: Classification of chronic pain: Description of chronic pain syndromes and definitions of pain terms. Pain 1986;3S:138–139.

155. Karmakar MK, Ho AMH: Postthoracotomy pain syndrome. Thorac Surg Clin 2004;14:345–352.

156. Dajczman E, Gordon A, Kreisman H, Wolkove N: Long-term postthoracotomy pain. Chest 1991;99:270–274.

157. Richardson J, Sabanathan S, Mearns AJ, et al: Post-thoracotomy neuralgia. Pain Clin 1994;7:87–97.

158. Reuben SS, Buvenandran A, Kroin JS, et al: Effect of cyclooxygenase inhibitors on cerebrospinal fluid (CSF) prostaglandin E2 (PGE2) after surgery. Anesthesiology 2005;103:A1476.

159. McCrory C, Diviney D, Moriarty J, et al: Comparison between repeat bolus intrathecal morphine and epidurally delivered bupivacaine and fentanyl combination in the management of postthoracotomy pain with or without cyclooxygenase inhibition. J Cardioth Vasc Anesth 2002;16:607–611.

160. Hu JS, Lui PW, Wang H, et al: Thoracic epidural analgesia with morphine does not prevent postthoracotomy pain syndrome: A survey of 159 patients. Acta Anaesthesiol Sin 2000;38:195–200.

161. Obata H, Saito S, Fujita N, et al: Epidural block with mepivacaine before surgery reduces long-term post-thoracotomy pain. Can J Anaesth 1999;46:1127–1132.

162. Senturk M, Ozcan PE, Talu GK, et al: The effects of three different analgesia techniques on long-term postthoracotomy pain. Anesth Analg 2002;94:11–15.

163. Ochroch EA, Gottschalk A, Augostides J, et al: Long-term pain and activity during recovery from major thoracotomy using thoracic epidural analgesia. Anesthesiology 2002;97:1234–1244.

164. Lund C, Hansen OB, Mogensen T, et al: Effect of thoracic epidural bupivacaine 0.75% on somatosensory evoked potentials after dermatomal stimulation. Anesth Analg 1987;66:731–734.

165. Dahl JB, Rosenberg J, Lund C, et al: Effect of thoracic epidural bupivacaine 0.75% on somatosensory evoked potentials after dermatomal stimulation. Reg Anesth Pain Med 1990;15:73–75.

166. Kehlet H, Dahl JB: The value of "multimodal" or "balanced analgesia" in postoperative pain treatment. Anesth Analg 1993;77:1048–1056.

167. Reuben SS, Gutta SB, Maciolek H, et al: Effect of initiating a multimodal analgesic regimen upon patient outcomes after anterior cruciate ligament reconstruction for same-day surgery: A 1200-patient case series. Acute Pain 2004;6:87–93.

168. Reuben SS, Gutta SB, Maciolek H, et al: Effect of initiating a preventative multimodal analgesic regimen upon long-term patient outcomes after anterior cruciate ligament reconstruction for same-day surgery: A 1200-patient case series. Acute Pain 2005;7:65–73.

169. Brennan TJ, Kehlet H: Preventative analgesia to reduce wound hyperalgesia and persistent postsurgical pain. Anesthesiology 2005;103:681–693.

170. Lavand'homme P, De Kock M, Waterloos H: Intraoperative epidural analgesia combined with ketamine provides effective preventative analgesia in patients undergoing major digestive surgery. Anesthesiology 2005;103:813–820.

171. Kissin I: Preemptive analgesia: Terminology and clinical relevance. Anesth Analg 1994;79:809–810.

172. Gottschalk A, Raja SN: Severing the link between acute and chronic pain: The anesthesiologist's role in preventive medicine. Anesthesiology 2004;101:1063–1065.

The Role of Nonopioid Analgesic Techniques in the Management of Postoperative Pain

Paul F. White, MD

INTRODUCTION

An increasing number of complex operations are being performed on an outpatient basis for which the use of conventional opioid-based IV patient-controlled analgesia (IVPCA) and central neuraxial (spinal and epidural) analgesia are not practical techniques for pain management. For that and other reasons, effective treatment of acute postsurgical pain presents unique challenges for practitioners.[1] This expansion of outpatient surgery requires a perioperative analgesic regimen that is highly effective, has minimal side effects, is intrinsically safe, and can be easily managed away from the hospital or surgical center.[2]

Clinical Pearl

- Adequacy of postoperative pain control is one of the most important factors in determining when a patient can be safely discharged from a surgical facility and has a major influence on the patient's ability to resume the normal activities of daily living.

Adequacy of postoperative pain control is one of the most important factors in determining when a patient can be safely discharged from a surgical facility and has a major influence on the patient's ability to resume the normal activities of daily living.[3] Perioperative analgesia has traditionally been provided by opioid analgesics. However, extensive use of opioids is associated with a variety of perioperative side effects [eg, ventilatory depression, drowsiness and sedation, postoperative nausea and vomiting (PONV), pruritus, urinary retention, ileus, constipation] that can delay hospital discharge.[4] Intraoperative use of large bolus doses or continuous infusions of potent opioid analgesics may actually increase postoperative pain as a result of their rapid elimination or the development of acute tolerance.[5] In addition, it has been suggested by the Joint Commission on Accreditation of Healthcare Organizations (JCAHO) that excessive use of postoperative opioid analgesics leads to decreased patient satisfaction. Partial opioid agonists (eg, tramadol) are also associated with increased side effects (eg, nausea, vomiting, ileus) and patient dissatisfaction compared with those reported for both opioid[6] and nonopioid[7,8] analgesics.

Clinical Pearl

- Multimodal, or "balanced," analgesic techniques involving the use of smaller doses of opioids in combination with nonopioid analgesic drugs [eg, local anesthetics, ketamine, acetaminophen and nonsteroidal antiinflammatory drugs (NSAIDs)] are becoming increasingly popular approaches to preventing pain after surgery.

Therefore, in order to minimize the adverse effects of analgesic medications, anesthesiologists and surgeons are increasingly turning to nonopioid analgesic techniques as adjuvants for managing pain during the perioperative period. Multimodal, or "balanced," analgesic techniques involving the use of smaller doses of opioids in combination with nonopioid analgesic drugs [eg, local anesthetics, ketamine, acetaminophen and nonsteroidal antiinflammatory drugs (NSAIDs)] are becoming increasingly popular approaches to preventing pain after surgery (Table 77–1).[9–11] This review will discuss recent evidence supporting the use of nonopioid analgesic drugs and techniques for facilitating the recovery process during the perioperative period.

LOCAL ANESTHETIC TECHNIQUES

The routine use of peripheral nerve blocks and wound infiltration with long-acting local anesthetics as an adjuvant to local, regional, and general anesthetic techniques can improve postoperative pain management after a wide variety of surgical procedures (Table 77–2).[4] When administered before surgery, these simple techniques can also decrease anesthetic and analgesic requirements during surgery, as well as reduce the need for opioid-containing analgesics postoperatively. More effective pain relief in the early postoperative period, as a result of the residual sensory block produced by local anesthetics, facilitates recovery by enabling earlier ambulation and discharge home (ie, "fast-track" recovery).[12–14]

Table 77–1.

Commonly Used Nonopioid Drugs and Nonpharmacologic Techniques for Minimizing Pain after Ambulatory Surgery[a]

Local Anesthetics

Lidocaine, 0.5–2% SQ/IV
Bupivacaine, 0.125–0.5% SQ
Ropivacaine, 0.125–0.5% SQ
Levobuivacaine, 0.125–0.5% SQ

Nonsteroidal Antiinflammatory Drugs

Ketorolac, 15–30 mg PO/IM/IV
Diclofenac, 50–100 mg PO/IM/IV
Ibuprofen, 300–800 mg PO
Indomethacin, 25–50 mg PO/PR/IM
Naproxen, 250–500 mg PO
Celecoxib, 100–200 mg PO
Refecoxib, 25–50 mg PO

Miscellaneous Analgesic Compounds

Acetaminophen, 0.5–2g, PO/PR
Propacetamol, 0.5–2g, IV
Ketamine, 10–20 mg PO, IM/IV
Clonidine, 0.15–0.3 mg PO, IM/IV

Nonpharmacologic Therapies

Transcutaneous electrical nervce stimulation (TENS)
Transcutaneous acupoint electrical stimulation (TAES)
Acupuncture–like transcutaneous electrical nerve stimulation (ALTENS)

[a] *Routes of administration: PO = oral, PR = per rectum, SQ = subcutaneous/tissue, IM = intramuscular, IV = intravenous.*

In addition, use of local anesthetic-based techniques for preventing pain can decrease the incidence of PONV because of their opioid-sparing effects. However, these techniques are most effective for superficial procedures, and the duration of analgesia is only 6–8 h.

Clinical Pearl

- The routine use of peripheral nerve blocks and wound infiltration with long-acting local anesthetics as an adjuvant to local, regional, and general anesthetic techniques can improve postoperative pain management after a wide variety of surgical procedures.

Blockade of the ilioinguinal and iliohypogastric nerves significantly decreases opioid analgesic requirements in both children and adults undergoing inguinal herniorrhaphy by providing 6–8 h of postoperative pain relief.[15,16] Similarly,

Commonly Used Techniques for Administering Local Anesthesia During Ambulatory Surgery

Peripheral Nerve Blocks

Ilioinguinal/hypogastric (eg, herniorrhaphy)
Paracervical (eg, dilation/curettage, cone biopsy)
Penile (eg, circumcision)
Peroneal/femoral/saphenous/tibial/sural
(eg, podiatric)
Femoral/obturator/lateral femoral cutaneous/sciatic
(eg, leg)
Brachial plexus/axillary/ulnar/median/radial
(eg, arm/hand)
Peribulbar/retrobulbar (eg, ophthalmologic
procedures)
Mandibular/maxillary (eg, oral surgery)
IV regional (Bier block) (eg, arms, legs)

Tissue Infiltration and Wound Instillation

Cosmetic and wound procedures (eg, blepharoplasty,
nasal, septum, endosinus)
Excision of masses and biopsies (eg, breast, axilla,
lipomas)
Field blocks or "splash" technique (eg, hernia repair,
vasovasotomy)
Laparoscopic procedures (eg, cholecystectomy, tubal
ligation)
Arthroscopic procedures (eg, knees, shoulders)

Topical Analgesia

Eutectic mixture of local anesthetics (EMLA) (eg, skin
lesions)
Lidocaine spray (eg, bronchoscopy, endoscopy, hernia
repair)
Lidocaine gel or cream (eg, circumcision, urologic,
oral surgery)
Cocaine paste (eg, nasal, endosinus surgery)

a subcutaneous ring block of the penis provides effective perioperative analgesia for circumcision.[17] Local anesthetic infiltration of the mesosalpinx significantly decreases pain and cramping after laparoscopic tubal ligation.[18] Simple instillation of local anesthetic after removal of the gallbladder also reduced right upper quadrant and shoulder pain.[10,19] Pain after arthroscopic shoulder surgery was decreased significantly by a suprascapular nerve block,[20] and pain after knee surgery was minimized with a femoral nerve block.[21] However, more complete perioperative analgesia for painful shoulder and knee procedures requires use of interscalene brachial plexus,[22] and combined femoral, obturator, lateral femoral cutaneous, and sciatic nerve[23] blocks, respectively. Although additional preparation time may be required when major peripheral nerve blocks are performed before surgery,

these techniques can offer significant advantages over general and spinal anesthesia with respect to pain control in the postoperative period.[12,13,22,23]

It has been suggested that performing neural blockade with local anesthetics before surgical incision prevents the nociceptive input from altering excitability of the central nervous system by preemptively blocking the *N*-methyl-D-asparate- (NMDA) induced "wind up" phenomena and subsequent release of inflammatory mediators.[24] The concept of preemptive analgesia, or treating postoperative pain by preventing establishment of central sensitization, seems intuitively logical. However, the clinical relevance of preemptive analgesia has been questioned. Only a small number of well-controlled clinical studies have demonstrated any benefit of pre- vs postincisional analgesic administration.[25,26] A quantitative systematic review by Møiniche and colleagues[27] stated that evidence is still lacking to support the claim that the timing of single-dose or continuous postoperative pain treatment is critically important in the management of postsurgical pain. These investigators concluded that there was no convincing evidence that preemptive treatment with centrally or peripherally administered local anesthetics, NSAIDs, opioid analgesics, or ketamine offers any advantage with respect to postoperative pain relief when compared with a similar analgesic regimen administered after the surgical incision.[27] Nevertheless, preincisional local anesthetic administration offers an obvious advantage over infiltration at the end of surgery because it can provide supplemental intraoperative analgesia as well as effective analgesia in the early postoperative period after emergence from anesthesia.

Clinical Pearls

- The concept of preemptive analgesia, or treating postoperative pain by preventing establishment of central sensitization, seems intuitively logical.
- However, the clinical relevance of preemptive analgesia has been questioned.
- Only a small number of well-controlled clinical studies have demonstrated any benefit of pre- vs postincisional analgesic administration.

Preincisional infiltration of the surgical wound site with local anesthetics, combined with general anesthesia, is clearly superior to general or spinal anesthesia alone in reducing postoperative pain.[28,29] For example, preincisional infiltration of the tonsillar bed with bupivacaine decreased the intensity of both constant pain and pain on swallowing fluids for up to 5 days after tonsillectomy procedures.[29] Paracervical block with 0.5% bupivacaine also reduced pain and the need for opioid analgesics after vaginal hysterectomy under general anesthesia.[30] Preincisional ilioinguinal–iliohypogastric nerve block not only improves perioperative pain control for inguinal hernia repair, but reduces the need for oral opioid-containing analgesics in the postdischarge period.[16] Although local infiltration can reduce incisional pain after laparoscopic cholecystectomy,[31-34] some investigators have actually reported that infiltration of the trocar sites at the end of surgery provided better pain relief than when the local anesthetic was given before incision.[32] The overall analgesic efficacy of trocar wound infiltration after laparoscopic surgery remains controversial.[35]

Although preincisional infiltration of the operative site with local anesthetics remains popular for reducing the perioperative opioid analgesic requirement, other simpler local anesthetic delivery systems (eg, topical applications) have been described.[36-40] Topical analgesia with a lidocaine aerosol was effective in decreasing both pain and the opioid analgesic requirement after inguinal herniorrhaphy in adults,[36] and instillation of 0.25% bupivacaine before surgical closure compared favorably with an ilioinguinal–iliohypogastric nerve block in children undergoing hernia repair.[37] Furthermore, the simple application of topical lidocaine jelly or ointment, as well as eutectic mixture of local anesthesia (EMLA) cream, have been shown to be as effective as peripheral nerve blocks or parenteral opioids in providing pain relief after outpatient circumcision.[38-40] Use of a 5% lidocaine patch has also been reported to be effective in providing peripheral analgesia.[41] However, further studies are needed to define the role (if any) of this analgesic device in the postoperative period.

Intracavitary instillation of local anesthetics is another simple, yet effective, technique for providing pain relief during the early postoperative period after laparoscopic and arthroscopic procedures. For example, when 80 mL of lidocaine 0.5% or bupivacaine 0.125% was administered intraperitoneally at the start of the laparoscopic procedure, it significantly reduced postoperative scapular pain and the need for opioid analgesic during the first 48 h after surgery.[42] Compared with a control group receiving saline, use of intraperitoneal bupivacaine 0.5% (15–30 mL) also led to a larger percentage of patients going home on the day of surgery (79% vs 43%).[43] However, other studies involving intraperitoneal administration of local anesthetics during laparoscopy report inconsistent effects on postoperative pain and the need for opioid analgesics.[44-54] Some investigators have suggested that the beneficial effects of intraperitoneal bupivacaine are transient and have little effect on patient recovery.[49] Furthermore, when bupivacaine was injected at the preperitoneal fascial plane during extraperitoneal laparoscopic hernia repair, it also failed to reduce postoperative pain.[55] Subfascial infiltration with bupivacaine 0.5% at the trochar and incision sites reduced pain and the length of stay after laparoscopic nephrectomy procedures.[56] Yndgaard and coworkers[57] demonstrated that subfascially administered lidocaine was significantly more effective than subcutaneous injection in reducing pain after inguinal herniotomy. It is obvious that the location, volume, and timing of the local anesthetic administration are key factors in determining efficacy of intraperitoneal instillation in preventing pain after both superficial and laparoscopic surgery.[19,43,53]

Analogous to intraperitoneal administration, intrapleural instillation of local anesthetic solutions has been reported to improve pain control after laparoscopic surgery.[58-66] Some investigators report that interpleural bupivacaine produced more effective analgesia than intraperitoneal bupivacaine[66] and compared favorably with epidural bupivacaine[58] after laparoscopic cholecystectomy. Compared with standard opioid analgesics, intrapleural bupivacaine achieved better pain relief and greater improvement in postoperative pulmonary function.[59,64] In contrast, Oxorn and Whatley[65] reported that postoperative pulmonary mechanics were worsened after intrapleural bupivacaine. Adverse effects on pulmonary function (due to muscle weakness) and the risk of systemic local anesthetic toxicity (due to rapid systemic absorption) are the major concerns with this technique.[66,67] Although intercostal nerve blocks can also improve pain relief after cholecystectomy procedures, this does not necessarily lead to improved pulmonary function.[68]

Local anesthetics are also commonly injected into joint spaces to provide analgesia during and after arthroscopic procedures.[69,70] In a placebo-controlled study, intraarticular instillation of 30 mL of 0.5% bupivacaine reduced opioid requirements and facilitated early mobilization and discharge after knee arthroscopy.[70] In a follow-up study, a combination of intraarticular bupivacaine and systemic ketorolac (60 mg) further decreased pain in the early postoperative recovery period.[71] In addition to the local anesthetics, a wide variety of other adjuvants (eg, morphine, ketorolac, triamcinolone, and clonidine) have also been injected into the intraarticular space to decrease postarthroscopic pain.[72-77] Small-dose intraarticular morphine (0.5–1 mg), combined with bupivacaine, appears to provide the longest lasting and most cost-effective analgesia after knee arthroscopy.[76,77] Although administering intraarticular morphine before knee surgery was reported to provide a longer duration of analgesia and greater opioid-sparing effects than when it was given at the end of surgery,[77] the clinical advantage of preemptive intraarticular local anesthetic administration remains controversial.[27]

Clinical Pearls

- Local anesthetics decrease the severity of incisional pain in the early postoperative period.
- However, many patients still experience significant pain when the local anesthetic effect wears off.
- Continuous or intermittent perfusion of the surgical wound (or peripheral nerve) with local anesthetic solutions has been reintroduced as a way of extending local anesthetic-induced incisional pain relief into the postoperative period.

Although local anesthetic supplementation decreases the severity of incisional pain in the early postoperative period, many patients still experience significant pain when the local anesthetic effect wears off. Therefore, continuous[78,79] or intermittent perfusion[80,81] of the surgical wound (or peripheral nerve) with local anesthetic solutions has been reintroduced as a way of extending local anesthetic-induced incisional pain relief into the postoperative period. In a recent study by White and associates[82] infusion of 0.5% bupivacaine (4 mL/h) at the median sternotomy site reduced postoperative pain and opioid analgesic requirement after cardiac surgery. As a result of the opioid-sparing effect, these patients recovered bowel and bladder function more rapidly. Similarly, wound instillation with 0.2% ropivacaine (5 mL/h) improved pain control after spine fusion surgery.[83] These continuous local anesthetic infusion techniques can be modified to allow for patient-controlled local anesthetic administration after surgery.[84,85]

Investigators have failed to find consistent improvement in pain scores or opioid-sparing effects when the local anesthetic was infused at the incision site after abdominal surgery.[57,86–88] Efficacy of local anesthetic infusion systems is enhanced when the catheter is placed at the subfacial level or near a peripheral nerve. For example, a continuous popliteal-sciatic nerve block provides improved postoperative analgesia, decreased opioid use, and enhanced patient satisfaction after painful foot and ankle surgery.[89,90] Similarly, a continuous infraclavicular brachial plexus block provides highly effective pain control after discharge in patients undergoing shoulder surgery.[91] Although continuous local anesthetic infusions with concomitant IVPCA capability appears to be superior to a continuous infusion alone for prolonging nerve blocks,[92,93] many patients elect not to use the IVPCA function on their electronic pumps.[91]

When using a continuous local anesthetic infusion, analgesic efficacy is influenced by a wide variety of factors in addition to location to the catheter system, including the concentration and volume of the local anesthetic solution,[82] as well as the accuracy and consistency of the pumps.[94] The use of a disposable, nonelectronic infusion system may offer advantages over the electronic pump because its simplicity minimizes the need for trouble shooting.[95] However, accuracy of the infusion rate of the nonelectronic pumps can change over time.[94] Temperature changes also influence the infusion rate of elastomeric pumps, and battery life is a limiting factor for the electronic pumps.[94] With these catheter delivery systems, the risk of infection appears to be small. However, bacterial colonization of the catheter is a common occurrence.[96] Patient satisfaction and comfort when using these delivery systems outside the hospital is high, and over 90% of the patients are comfortable removing the catheter at home.[97] Finally, combining local anesthetic infusion techniques with other analgesic modalities as part of multimodal analgesic therapy further improves pain control throughout the perioperative period.[98]

Peripheral nerve block techniques are simple, safe, and highly effective approaches to providing perioperative analgesia. Use of long-acting local anesthetics for neural blockade techniques involving the upper (eg, interscalene brachial plexus block) and lower (eg, femoral-sciatic nerve block) extremities can facilitate an earlier discharge after major shoulder and knee reconstructive procedures, respectively.[99,100] Availability of long-acting local anesthetics that claim less

toxicity and greater selectivity with respect to sensory and motor blockade (eg, ropivacaine) may further enhance the benefits of local anesthetic supplementation after both major and minor surgery.

Although ropivacaine 0.2% provides better pain relief with less motor impairment than lidocaine 1% for continuous interscalene brachial plexus block,[101] its clinical advantages relative to equipotent concentrations of bupivacaine are less well established. Addition of adjuvants (eg, epinephrine, clonidine) that can prolong postoperative analgesia and facilitate recovery when using central and peripheral nerve blocks may be of greater clinical importance.[102,103] Interestingly, a more recent study[104] found that clonidine's use as an adjunct to ropivacaine as part of a continuous perineural infusion technique failed to reduce postoperative pain and oral analgesic usage or improve the patient's quality of sleep after upper extremity surgery when compared with the local anesthetic alone. Although pain control can be improved after orthopedic procedures by continuously infusing local anesthetic solutions,[89,90,105–107] availability of longer acting local anesthetic suspensions and "delayed release" formulations containing liposomes or polymer microspheres may minimize the need for continuous infusion catheter delivery system in the future.

NSAIDS

Oral NSAIDs have long been used for treating nonsurgical pain syndromes because of their well known antiinflammatory, antipyretic, and analgesic properties. When parenteral preparations of NSAIDs (eg, ketorolac, ketoprofen, diclofenac) became available, these drugs were more widely used in the management of acute perioperative pain. NSAIDs block the synthesis of prostaglandins by inhibiting cyclooxygenase (COX) types I and II, thereby reducing production of mediators of the acute inflammatory response. By decreasing the inflammatory response to surgical trauma, NSAIDs have been alleged to reduce peripheral nociception. Studies also suggest that the central response to painful stimuli is modulated by NSAID-induced inhibition of prostaglandin synthesis in the spinal cord.[27]

Clinical Pearl

- Oral NSAIDs have long been used for treating nonsurgical pain syndromes because of their well known antiinflammatory, antipyretic, and analgesic properties.

Early reports suggested that parenteral NSAIDs possessed analgesic properties comparable to those for traditional opioid analgesics[108–110] without opioid-related side effects.[111,112] Compared with the partial opioid agonist tramadol, diclofenac produced better postoperative pain relief with fewer side effects after cardiac surgery.[8] When administered as an adjuvant during outpatient anesthesia, ketorolac was associated with improved postoperative analgesia and patient comfort compared with fentanyl and the partial opioid agonist, dezocine.[112,113] Other investigators reported that ketorolac provided postoperative pain relief similar to that of fentanyl, but was associated with less nausea and somnolence, as well as an earlier return of bowel function.[114] In most studies, use of ketorolac has been associated with a less frequent incidence of PONV than the opioid analgesics. As a result, patients tolerate oral fluids and are fit for discharge earlier than those receiving only opioid analgesics during the perioperative period. Of interest, ketorolac (30 mg q6h) was superior to a dilute local anesthetic infusion (bupivacaine 0.125%) in supplementing epidural IVPCA hydromorphone in patients undergoing thoracotomy procedures.[115] Furthermore, it has been found that the injection of ketorolac (30 mg) at the incision site in combination with local anesthesia resulted in significantly less postoperative pain, a better quality of recovery, and earlier discharge compared with local anesthesia alone.[116] In fact, evidence exists for both a peripheral and central analgesic action of NSAIDs.[117] However, when ketorolac was substituted for, or combined with, fentanyl during minor gynecologic and laparoscopic procedures, beneficial effects of the NSAID were reduced.[118,119]

Using shock wave lithotripsy to evaluate the effect of NSAIDs on visceral pain, diclofenac produced only a marginal opioid-sparing effect.[120] However, when diclofenac (1 mg/kg IV) was administered before arthroscopic surgery, it was associated with similar pain scores to fentanyl (1 mcg/kg IV).[121] Preoperative diclofenac (50 mg) also decreased pain and the opioid analgesic requirements for 24 h after laparoscopic surgery.[122] Similarly, preoperative administration of ketorolac to patients undergoing laparoscopic cholecystectomy[119] decreased postoperative opioid requirements and improved some ventilatory variables during the early postoperative period. A perioperative ketorolac infusion (2 mg/h) also improved the quality of postoperative pain relief after abdominal surgery.[123] Ketorolac (30 mg IV) produced comparable analgesia to tramadol (100 mg IV), but with a 68% decreased incidence of PONV after maxillofacial surgery.[124] Of interest, diclofenac (1 mg/kg) is alleged to be a more cost-effective alternative to ketorolac (0.5 mg/kg).[125,126]

When diclofenac was administered preoperatively to pediatric patients, the incidence of both restlessness and crying, as well as the postoperative opioid requirements, were less than in patients treated with acetaminophen.[127] Similarly, oral ketorolac (1 mg/kg) was superior to small-dose acetaminophen (10 mg/kg) for pain in children undergoing bilateral myringotomy procedures.[128] In children undergoing inguinal hernia repair,[129] ketorolac (1 mg/kg IV) compared favorably with caudal bupivacaine 0.2% with respect to pain control and postoperative side effects. In addition, ketorolac-treated children had an improved recovery profile, including less vomiting, shorter times to voiding and ambulation, and earlier discharge home. Intraoperative administration of ketorolac as an adjuvant to general anesthesia in pediatric patients provided postoperative analgesia comparable

to morphine with less PONV.[130] When ketorolac or morphine is administered for pain control in pediatric patients, ketorolac-induced analgesia develops more slowly but lasts longer.[131]

Oral or rectal administration of NSAIDs is also effective and less costly in the prophylactic management of surgical pain.[132] For example, when oral naproxen was administered before laparoscopic surgery, postoperative pain scores, opioid requirements, and time to discharge were significantly reduced.[133] Furthermore, premedication with oral ibuprofen (800 mg) was associated with superior postoperative analgesia and less nausea than with fentanyl (75 mcg IV) after laparoscopic surgery.[134] However, the more important role for oral NSAIDs may be in the postdischarge period. Ibuprofen liquigel (400 mg PO) was significantly more effective than celecoxib (200 mg PO) in treating pain after oral surgery.[135] Ibuprofen (5 mg/kg PO) compared favorably with rofecoxib (0.625 mg/kg PO) for minimizing postoperative pain when used in combination with acetaminophen (20 mg/kg) prior to tonsillectomy procedures.[136] When used as part of a multimodal analgesic technique consisting of alfentanil, lidocaine, and ketorolac,[137] oral ibuprofen (800 mg q8h) was equianalgesic to paracetamol 800 mg in combination with codeine 60 mg (q8h) during the first 72 h after discharge and resulted in better global patient satisfaction and less constipation than opioid-containing oral analgesics. Ibuprofen (400 or 600 mg PO) appears to produce comparable analgesia to the combination tramadol (75–112.5 mg) and acetaminophen (650 or 975 mg) for acute postoperative pain relief.[138] To achieve the optimal benefit of using NSAIDs in the perioperative period, these compounds should be continued during the postdischarge period as part of a preventative pain management strategy.[98]

Despite the obvious benefits of using NSAIDs in the perioperative period, controversy still exists regarding their use because of the potential for gastrointestinal mucosal damage and renal tubular and platelet dysfunction.[139] Although some studies have found increased blood loss and risk of reoperation when ketorolac was administered to children undergoing tonsillectomy procedures,[140,141] a recent systematic review of the literature suggested that the evidence supporting an increase of bleeding was equivocal at best.[142]

COX 2 INHIBITORS

In an effort to minimize the potential for operative site bleeding complications, as well as gastrointestinal damage, associated with the classic nonselective NSAIDs such as ketorolac and diclofenac, the more highly selective COX-2 inhibitors are increasingly being used as nonopioid adjuvants for minimizing pain during the perioperative period (Table 77–3).[143] Early clinical studies in surgical patients evaluated the use of celecoxib, rofecoxib, and valdecoxib as preventative analgesics when administered for oral premedication.[144–148] Rofecoxib (50 mg PO) produced more effective and sustained analgesia than celecoxib (200 mg PO) after spinal surgery.[144] Celecoxib

Table 77–3.					
Dosage Recommendations and Duration of Action of COX-2 Inhibitors					
Drug (mg)	**Route of Administration**	**Onset (min)**	**Duration (h)**	**COX-2/COX-1 Activity**[a]	**Short-Term Administration Side Effects**
Celecoxib (100–200)	PO	30–50	4–8	8	Sulfonamide allergy (?)
Rofecoxib (12.5–50)	PO	30–50	12–24	35	Leg edema hypertension
Paracoxib (20–40)[b]	IM/IV	10–15	6–12	—	Not known
Valdecoxib (40–80)	PO	30–40	6–12	30	Not known
Etoricoxib (30–60)	PO	20–30	≥ 24	106	Not known

[a] *Data on file with Pharmacia (Skokie, IL) and Merck (West Point, PA).*
[b] *IV prodrug of valdecoxib (the active "analgesic" compound).*
COX-2 = cyclooxygenase-2.

(200 mg PO) was equivalent to acetaminophen (2 g PO) when administered before otolaryngologic operations.[145] However, the analgesic efficacy of celecoxib is dose-related, and 400 mg is the currently recommended dose for prevention of acute pain.[146] Rofecoxib (50 mg PO) produced significantly more effective analgesia than acetaminophen (2 g PO), and the pain relief was more sustained in the postdischarge period.[147] Premedication with rofecoxib also facilitated recovery by reducing postoperative pain and improving the quality of recovery from the patient's perspective.[148] It has also been suggested that the long-acting rofecoxib is more cost-effective than celecoxib in the perioperative period.[149] In a recent study,[143] a single preoperative dose of rofecoxib (25–50 mg PO) produced a 44–59% reduction in the PCA morphine requirement after major abdominal surgery.[150] However, clinical studies suggest a more sustained benefit can be achieved when the drug is administered both before and after surgery.[148,151] The recent withdrawal of rofecoxib from the market by its manufacturer because of an increased risk of cardiovascular side effects following prolonged use (>16 months) has led investigators to begin reevaluating other COX-2 inhibitors in the perioperative period.

Valdecoxib has been introduced recently for the prevention of postoperative pain, with doses of 20 to 40 mg reducing the opioid requirement by 25 to 50% after elective surgery.[152,153] In patients undergoing oral surgery and bunionectomy, premedication with valdecoxib 40 mg appears to produce the optimal analgesic effect in the postoperative period.[152] Valdecoxib is as rapidly acting and effective as oxycodone in combination with acetaminophen, but has a longer duration of action and fewer side effects when used for the management of pain after oral surgery. Valdecoxib (40 mg PO) was alleged to be even more effective than rofecoxib (50 mg PO) in treating pain after oral surgery.[154]

A parenterally active COX-2 inhibitor, parecoxib (a prodrug which is rapidly converted to valdecoxib), has been investigated as an alternative to the parenteral NSAIDs.[155–157]

However, to achieve equianalgesia with the IV prodrug, a higher dose may be required than of the orally active drug valdecoxib. Parecoxib is similar pharmacokinetically to both celecoxib and valdecoxib. Preliminary studies suggested that parecoxib (40–80 mg IV) is as effective and longer acting than ketorolac (30 mg IV) in reducing pain after oral[158] and laparotomy surgery.[159] Both preoperative and postoperative administration of this COX-2 inhibitor resulted in significant opioid-sparing effects, reduced adverse effects, and improved the quality of recovery and patient satisfaction with their postoperative pain management.[152,160] Unfortunately, a recent study in patients undergoing cardiac surgery suggested that perioperative use of parecoxib and valdecoxib as part of a 14-day analgesic treatment regimen increased adverse events, including sternal wound infections.[161] Another recent study found that when parecoxib (40 mg IV) was given at induction of anesthesia, it was less effective than ketorolac (30 mg IV) after tonsillectomy procedures.[141] A new more highly selective COX-2 inhibitor, etoricoxib (120 mg PO), provided rapid and long-lasting pain relief after dental surgery.[162] A recent study also suggested that etoricoxib was associated with fewer side effects than a standard opioid-containing oral analgesic. Current evidence suggest that the newer COX-2 inhibitors appear to offer minimal advantages over the first-generation COX-2 inhibitors and the nonselective NSAIDs.[163,164]

In addition to the growing controversy regarding the potential adverse cardiovascular risks of the COX-2 inhibitors, many orthopedic surgeons are also concerned about the negative influence of these compounds (as well as the traditional NSAIDs) on bone growth.[165,166] Since COX-2 activity appears to play an important role in bone healing,[167–169] some orthopedic surgeons have recommended that these drugs be avoided in the early postoperative period.[164,165] Since the effect on bone growth is dose-dependent and reversible,[166] COX-2 inhibitors should only be used for 3 to 5 days in the early postoperative period. Although several review articles on the COX-2 inhibitors have recently been published,[163,170–172] the question remains as to whether these compounds truly overcome the perceived *limitations* of the nonselective NSAIDs.[173]

ACETAMINOPHEN (PARACETAMOL)

Acetaminophen (also known as paracetamol) is perhaps the safest and most cost-effective nonopioid analgesic when it is administered in analgesic dosages. Although both parenteral and rectal acetaminophen produce analgesic effects in the postoperative period, concurrent use with an NSAID is superior to acetaminophen alone.[145,147] The addition of acetaminophen (1 g, q4h) to PCA morphine improved the quality of pain relief and patient satisfaction after major orthopedic procedures.[174] Although Watcha and colleagues[128] reported minimal analgesic-sparing effects after a 10 mg/kg oral dose of acetaminophen, Rusy and coworkers[140] found that a larger dose (35 mg/kg PR) was as effective as a ketorolac (1 mg/kg IV) in reducing pain after tonsillectomy procedures and was associated with less postoperative bleeding. Subsequently, Korpela and associates[175] demonstrated that the opioid-sparing effect of rectal acetaminophen was dose-related up to 60 mg/kg. The optimal dosing regimen for acetaminophen in children appears to consist of a preoperative initial dose of 30 to 40 mg/kg followed by a maintenance dose of 15 to 20 mg/kg every 6–8 h during the early postoperative period.[176] In adults, acetaminophen 2 g orally was equivalent to celecoxib 200 mg, but less effective than celecoxib 400 mg, rofecoxib 50 mg, or ketoprofen 150 mg in preventing pain after ambulatory surgery.[145–147]

Clinical Pearl

- Acetaminophen (also known as paracetamol) is perhaps the safest and most cost-effective nonopioid analgesic when it is administered in analgesic dosages.

An IV formulation of a prodrug of acetaminophen, propacetamol, has been administered to adults as an alternative to ketorolac in the perioperative period.[177,178] Propacetamol reduced IVPCA morphine consumption by 22% to 46% in patients undergoing major orthopedic surgery.[179,180] However, in patients undergoing cardiac surgery, propacetamol (2 g IV q6h for 3 days) failed to enhance analgesia, decrease opioid usage, or reduce adverse side effects in the postoperative period.[181] Propacetamol has become a popular adjuvant to opioid analgesics for postoperative pain control in Europe; however, this drug may soon be replaced when an investigational IV formulation of acetaminophen becomes available for clinical use.[182] Rectal acetaminophen (1.3 g) has also been successfully used as an adjuvant to NSAIDs and local anesthetics as part of a multimodal fast-tracking surgery recovery protocol.[183] Given the adverse effects associated with both NSAIDs and COX-2 inhibitors in patients with preexisting cardiovascular disease, acetaminophen may assume a greater role in postoperative pain management in the future.[184]

NMDA ANTAGONISTS

Ketamine is a unique IV anesthetic with analgesic-like properties that has been used for both induction and maintenance of anesthesia,[185] as well as an analgesic adjuvant during local anesthesia.[186,187] As a result of its well-known side effect profile (Table 77–4), ketamine fell into disfavor in the late

Table 77–4.

Potential Side Effects of Opioid and Nonopioid Analgesic Drugs

Opioids Analgesics

 Respiratory and cardiovascular depression
 Nausea, vomiting, retching and ileus
 Urinary hesitancy and retention
 Pruritus and skin rash
 Sedation and dizziness
 Tolerance and dependence

Local Anesthetics

 Residual motor weakness
 Peripheral nerve irritation
 Cardiac arrhythmias
 Allergic reactions
 Sympathomimetic effects (due to vasoconstrictors)

Nonsteroidal Antiinflammatory Drugs

 Operative-site bleeding
 Gastrointestinal bleeding
 Renal tubular dysfunction
 Allergic reactions and bronchospasm
 Hypertension
 Pedal edema

Acetaminophen

 Gastrointestinal upset
 Sweating
 Hepatotoxicity
 Agranulocytosis

Ketamine

 Hypertension
 Diplopia and nystagmus
 Dizziness and confusion
 Cardiac arrhythmias
 Nausea and vomiting
 Psychomimetic reactions

Nonpharmacologic Techniques

 Skin irritation/erythema
 Cutaneous discomfort

1980s. However, adjunctive use of small doses of ketamine (0.1–0.2 mg/kg IV) appears to be associated with opioid-sparing effects, a less frequent incidence of adverse events and greater patient and physician acceptance.[188] Several studies have described the use of small-dose ketamine in combination with local anesthetics or opioid analgesics.[189–199] However, when ketamine (1 mg/mL) was combined with morphine (1 mg/mL) for IVPCA after major abdominal surgery, it did not significantly improve pain relief and was associated with increased side effects (eg, vivid dreaming) compared with the opioid alone.[191] A recent study[192] supports use of an IVPCA morphine–ketamine combination in a 1:1 ratio with a lock-out interval of 8 min for pain control after major orthopedic procedures. Further studies are obviously needed to clarify ketamine's role as a supplemental analgesic.

Administration of ketamine (4–18 mcg/kg/min) in combination with propofol (30-90 mcg/kg/min) obviated the respiratory depression produced by commonly used sedative–opioid combinations, while producing positive mood effects after surgery, and may even provide for an earlier recovery of cognitive function.[186,187] In addition, a single bolus dose of ketamine (0.1–0.15 mg/kg IV), during surgery has been reported to produce significant opioid-sparing effects after painful orthopedic and intraabdominal procedures without increasing the incidence of side effects.[194–200] Ketamine (0.1 mg/kg IM) reduced swallowing-evoked pain after tonsillectomy procedures in children receiving a multimodal analgesic regimen.[198] Small doses of epidural ketamine (20–30 mg) enhanced epidural morphine-induced analgesia after major upper abdominal surgery.[199] Although it was alleged that ketamine possesses preemptive analgesic effects as a result of its ability to inhibit central NMDA receptors,[200] well-controlled clinical studies have failed to demonstrate significant preemptive analgesic effects.[201,202] Interestingly, a modest dose of ketamine (250 mcg/kg) after surgery was alleged to improve analgesia in the presence of opioid-resistant pain.[203] Acute tolerance to opioid-induced analgesia leading to long-lasting hyperalgesia may be prevented by repeat doses of this NMDA antagonist.[204]

Small doses of the *S*(+) and *R*(−) isomers of ketamine have been administered both IV and epidurally in an effort to decrease injury-induced hyperalgesia. Although *S*(+) ketamine (0.5 mg/kg IV followed by 0.125 to 1 mcg/kg/min) failed to improve pain control after arthroscopic knee surgery,[205] epidural *S*(+) ketamine (0.25 mg/kg) enhanced ropivacaine-induced analgesia after total knee arthroplasty.[206] Interestingly, transdermal nitroglycerin (5 mg) has been alleged to enhance the spinal analgesia produced by epidural *S*(+) ketamine (0.1–0.2 mg/kg).[207] Consistent with an early comparative clinical study involving the ketamine isomers.[208] *R*(-) ketamine (1 mg/kg IV) produced only a short-lasting analgesic effect in the postoperative period.[209]

Dextromethorphan, another NMDA receptor antagonist that inhibits wind-up and NMDA-mediated nociceptive responses in dorsal horn neurons, has been alleged to enhance opioid, local anesthetic, and NSAID-induced analgesia.

Premedication with dextromethorphan (150 mg PO) reduced the IVPCA morphine requirement in the early postoperative period after abdominal hysterectomy procedures, but failed to produce prolonged beneficial effects on wound hyperalgesia.[210] In patients undergoing laparoscopic cholecystectomy or inguinal herniorrhaphy procedures, dextromethorphan (90 mg PO) improved well-being and reduced analgesic consumption, pain intensity and sedation, as well as thermal-induced hyperalgesia.[211] Preincisional administration of dextromethorphan (40–120 mg IM) provided some evidence of preemptive analgesia in patients undergoing laparoscopic cholecystectomy and upper abdominal surgery.[212,213] Perioperative dextromethorphan (40–90 mg IM) reduced the opioid requirement or improved pain control (or both) after modified radical mastectomy.[214] Interestingly, in patients undergoing knee surgery, dextromethorphan (200 mg q8h) failed to significantly improve pain management.[215] Compared with ibuprofen (400 mg PO), dextromethorphan (120 mg PO) was significantly less effective in providing postoperative analgesia and was associated with increased nausea in the preoperative period.[216] In patients undergoing knee replacement surgery with epidural anesthesia, dextromethorphan (40 mg IM) also failed to produce any preemptive analgesic effect, but did enhance pain control in the postoperative period.[217]

Other NMDA antagonists are being actively investigated in the perioperative setting. Preoperative amantadine (200 mg IV) failed to enhance postoperative analgesia in patients undergoing abdominal hysterectomy procedures.[218] However, a more recent study reports that *perioperative* amantadine reduced the IVPCA morphine requirement after radical prostatectomy surgery.[219] Further clinical studies are clearly needed to better define the role of noncompetitive NMDA receptor antagonists in the perioperative setting.

ALPHA₂-ADRENERGIC AGONISTS

The α_2-adrenergic agonists, clonidine and dexmedetomidine, produce significant anesthetic and analgesic-sparing effects. Premedication with oral and transdermal clonidine decreased the IVPCA morphine requirement 50% after radical prostatectomy surgery.[220] Clonidine also improved and prolonged central neuroaxis[221,222] and peripheral nerve blocks[223] when administered as part of multimodal analgesic regimens. For example, epidural infusion of clonidine in combination with ropivacaine improved analgesia after major abdominal surgery in children.[224] Adding intrathecal clonidine (0.075 mg) to local anesthesia provided excellent analgesia for up to 8 h after urologic surgery.[225] Although clonidine (4 mcg/kg IV over 20 min) failed to reduce the IVPCA morphine requirement after lower abdominal surgery in adults, it did reduce pain, nausea, and vomiting while improving patient satisfaction with their pain relief.[226] However, when used to *treat* postoperative pain, clonidine (0.3 mg IV) was apparently ineffective.[227]

Dexmedetomidine is a pure α_2-agonist that also reduces postoperative pain and the opioid analgesic requirement.[228] However, its use was associated with increased postoperative sedation and bradycardia. When used for premedication before IV regional anesthesia,[229] dexmedetomidine (1 mcg/kg IV) reduced patient anxiety, sympathoadrenal responses, and intraoperative opioid analgesic requirement. Compared with propofol (75 mcg/kg/min), dexmedetomidine (1 mcg/kg followed by 0.4–0.7 mcg/kg/h) had a slower onset and offset of sedation, but was associated with improved analgesia and reduced morphine use in the postoperative period.[230] Administration of dexmedetomidine (1 mcg/kg followed by 0.4 mcg/kg/h) was also associated with a 66% reduction in IVPCA morphine use in the early postoperative period after major inpatient surgery.[231]

MISCELLANEOUS NONOPIOID COMPOUNDS

A diverse array of nonopioid pharmacologic compounds (eg, adenosine,[232,233] droperidol,[234] magnesium,[235] neostigmine,[236] gabapentin[237,238]) used during the perioperative period have been alleged to possess analgesic-sparing properties. Although such effects of these compounds have not been extensively evaluated and their use for acute postoperative pain management is considered investigational, the preliminary findings are nonetheless intriguing. For example, use of an adenosine infusion as an alternative to an opioid analgesic (remifentanil) for controlling acute autonomic responses during lower abdominal surgery resulted in a significant reduction in both postoperative pain scores and the requirement for opioid analgesics.[232]

Gabapentin (a structural analog of γ-aminobutyric acid; GABA) is an anticonvulsant that has proven useful in the treatment of chronic neuropathic pain and may also be a useful adjuvant in the management of acute postoperative pain.[237–242] For example, premedication with gabapentin (1.2 g PO) reduced postoperative analgesic requirement significantly without increasing side effects.[237] When gabapentin (1.2 g) was continued for 10 d after breast surgery[238] it reduced the postoperative opioid analgesic requirement and movement-related pain; however, the overall incidence of chronic pain was unaffected. Recent studies by Dierking and colleagues,[239] Turan and coworkers,[240] and Rorarius and associates[241] suggested that the improvement in postoperative pain control with gabapentin was not necessarily associated with a decrease in opioid-related side effects. Pregabalin, a related compound, has also been reported to possess analgesic potential comparable to ibuprofen in treating acute dental pain.[242] This review article discussed the potential role of gabapentin and pregabalin in "protective premedication."

Magnesium, a divalent cation, is also assumed to possess antinociceptive effects. For example, Kara and colleagues[235] reported that perioperative magnesium (30 mg/kg IV followed by an infusion of 0.5 g/h) yielded a significant reduction in the postoperative analgesic requirement after abdominal hysterectomy. A bolus dose of magnesium (50 mg/kg IV) at induction of anesthesia also led to improved pain control and better patient satisfaction with less opioid medication after major orthopedic surgery.[243] However, magnesium (50 mg/kg IV) failed to produce opioid-sparing effects after open cholecystectomy procedures.[244] In addition, a nonopioid multimodal analgesic regimen that included magnesium produced comparable postoperative pain relief with fewer side effects than fentanyl in obese patients undergoing gastric bypass surgery.[245] However, other investigators have failed to demonstrate a beneficial effect of magnesium (30–50 mg/kg followed by 10–15 mg/kg/h) with respect to reducing postoperative pain or the need for opioid analgesics.[246] Of interest, intrathecal magnesium was reported to prolong fentanyl analgesia.[247]

Neostigmine, a cholinesterase inhibitor, has been reported to possess analgesic properties when doses of 10 to 200 mcg were administered in the subarachnoid or epidural spaces.[236,248] Although peripherally administered neostigmine failed to produce postoperative analgesia, epidurally administered neostigmine (1 mcg/kg) produced more than 5 h of pain relief after knee surgery.[249] Neostigmine (10 mcg/kg) also enhanced epidural local analgesia.[250] Both epidural (60 mcg) and spinal (1–5 mcg) neostigmine enhanced morphine-induced neuraxial analgesia.[251–254] In patients undergoing knee replacement surgery with intrathecal bupivacaine, adjunctive use of neostigmine (50 mcg) was alleged to produce better postoperative analgesia than morphine (300 mcg).[255] In addition, transdermal nitroglycerin enhanced spinal neostigmine-induced postoperative analgesia without increasing perioperative side effects.[256] However, epidural neostigmine (75–300 mcg) alone produced only modest analgesia after cesarean delivery.[257] The primary adverse effects associated with neuraxial neostigmine appear to be mild sedation[257] and PONV (15–30%).[237,253]

Cannabinoids have been reported to reduce hyperalgesia and drug-induced allodynia. However, clinical studies have failed to demonstrate any evidence of postoperative analgesia.[258,259] A new antiinflammatory drug, inositol triphosphate, reduced postoperative pain and the need for opioid analgesics after cholecystectomy surgery.[260] However, additional well controlled clinical trials are needed with all of these novel adjunctive drugs.

NONPHARMACOLOGIC TECHNIQUES

Nonpharmacologic "electroanalgesic" techniques [eg, transcutaneous electrical nerve stimulation (TENS), acupuncture-like transcutaneous electrical nerve stimulation, percutaneous neuromodulation therapy] can also be useful adjuvants to pharmacologic compounds in the management of acute postoperative pain.[261] Given the inherent side effects produced by both opioid and nonopioid analgesics (see Table 77–4), it is possible that the use of nonpharmacologic approaches will assume a more prominent role in the future management of acute postoperative pain.[262]

Clinical studies suggest that electroanalgesia can reduce opioid analgesic requirements up to 60% after surgery.[263,264] In addition to reducing pain and the need for oral analgesics, Jensen and coworkers[265] reported a more rapid recovery of joint mobility after arthroscopic knee surgery. When used as an adjuvant to pharmacologic analgesia, TENS reduced the intensity of exercise-induced pain and facilitated ambulation after abdominal surgery.[266] In reviewing the medical literature, Carroll and associates[267] found conflicting results regarding the effect of TENS on the requirement for opioid analgesic medication and the quality of postoperative pain relief. Studies suggest that the location, intensity, timing, and frequency of electrical stimulation are all important variables influencing the efficacy of electroanalgesic therapies.[263,264,268] More recent studies have confirmed the importance of these variables in achieving improved pain relief with TENS therapy.[269]

Of interest, simple (mechanical) intradermal needles placed in the paravertebral region before abdominal surgery reduced postoperative pain and the opioid analgesic requirement, as well as PONV.[270] However, a "minute sphere"-induced acupressure technique (in which 1-mm stainless steel spheres are applied at known analgesic acupoints) failed to relieve pain after major abdominal surgery.[271] Other nonpharmacologic approaches that have been used as analgesic adjuvants in the perioperative period include cryoanalgesia,[272] ultrasound,[273] laser stimulation,[274] and hypnotherapy. However, well-controlled clinical studies are needed to establish benefits of these nonpharmacologic modalities on postoperative pain and patient outcomes after surgery.

SUMMARY

In summary, as more extensive and painful operations (eg, laparoscopic cholecystectomy, adrenalectomy, and nephrectomy procedures, as well as prostatectomy, laminectomy, shoulder and knee reconstructions, hysterectomy) are performed on an outpatient or short-stay basis, the use of multimodal perioperative analgesic regimens involving nonopioid analgesic therapies will likely assume an increasingly important role in facilitating the recovery process and improving patient satisfaction.[4] Pavlin and colleagues[275] recently confirmed the importance of postoperative pain on recovery after ambulatory surgery. Moderate-to-severe pain prolonged recovery room stay by 40 to 80 min. Use of local anesthetics and NSAIDs decreased pain scores and facilitated an earlier discharge home. Additional outcome studies are needed to validate the beneficial effect of these nonopioid therapeutic approaches with respect to important recovery variables (eg, resumption of normal activities [dietary intake, bowel function], return to work). Although many factors other than pain per se must be controlled in order to minimize postoperative morbidity and facilitate the recovery process,[1] pain remains a major concern of all patients undergoing elective surgical procedures.[276]

Opioid analgesics continue to play an important role in the management of moderate-to-severe pain after surgical procedures. However, adjunctive use of nonopioid analgesics will likely assume a greater role as minimally invasive ("key hole") surgery continues to expand.[2,4] In addition to the local anesthetics, NSAIDs, COX-2 inhibitors, acetaminophen, ketamine, dextromethorphan, α_2-agonists, gabapentin, magnesium, and neostigmine may all prove to be useful adjuncts in the management of postoperative pain in the future. Adjunctive use of droperidol[234] and glucocorticoid steroids[277,278] also appears to provide beneficial effects in the postoperative period. Use of analgesic drug combinations with differing mechanisms of action as part of a multimodal regimen will provide additive (or even synergistic) effects with respect to improving pain control, reducing the need for opioid analgesics and facilitating the recovery process.[279] Safer, simpler, and less costly analgesic drug delivery systems are needed to provide cost-effective pain relief in the post-discharge period as more major surgery is performed on an ambulatory (or short-stay) basis in the future.

The optimal nonopioid analgesic technique for postoperative pain management would therefore not only reduce pain scores and enhance patient satisfaction, but also facilitate earlier mobilization and rehabilitation by reducing pain-related complications after surgery. Recent evidence suggests that this goal can be best achieved by using a combination of preemptive techniques involving both centrally and peripherally acting analgesic drugs and devices.

References

1. Kehlet H, Dahl JB: Anaesthesia, surgery and challenges in postoperative recovery. Lancet 2003;362:1921–1928.
2. White PF: Ambulatory anesthesia advances into the new millennium. Anesth Analg 2000;90:1234–1235.
3. Chung F, Ritchie E, Su J: Postoperative pain in ambulatory surgery. Anesth Analg 1997;85:808–816.
4. White PF: The role of non-opioid analgesic techniques in the management of pain after ambulatory surgery. Anesth Analg 2002;94:577–585.
5. Guignard B, Bossard AE, Coste C, et al: Acute opioid tolerance: Intraoperative remifentanil increases postoperative pain and morphine requirement. Anesthesiology 2000;93:409–417.
6. Silvasti M, Svartling N, Pitkanen M, et al: Comparison of intravenous patient-controlled analgesia with tramadol versus morphine after microvascular breast reconstruction. Eur J Anaesthesiol 2000;17:448–455.
7. Rawal N, Allvin R, Amilon A, et al: Postoperative analgesia at home after ambulatory hand surgery: A controlled comparison of tramadol, metamizol, and paracetamol. Anesth Analg 2001;92:347–351.
8. Immer FF, Immer-Bansi AS, Tachesel N, et al: Pain treatment with a COX-2 inhibitor after coronary artery bypass operation: A randomized trial. Ann Thorac Surg 2003;75:490–495.
9. Eriksson H, Tenhunen A, Korttila K: Balanced analgesia improves recovery and outcome after outpatient tubal ligation. Acta Anaesthesiol Scand 1996;40:151–155.
10. Michaloliakou C, Chung F, Sharma S: Preoperative multimodal analgesia facilitates recovery after ambulatory laparoscopic cholecystectomy. Anesth Analg 1996;82:44–51.

11. Pavlin DJ, Horvath KD, Pavlin EG, et al: Preincisional treatment to prevent pain after ambulatory hernia surgery. Anesth Analg 2003;97:1627–1632.

12. Vloka JD, Hadzic A, Mulcare R, et al: Femoral and genitofemoral nerve blocks versus spinal anesthesia for outpatients undergoing long saphenous vein stripping surgery. Anesth Analg 1997;84:749–752.

13. Song D, Greilich NB, White PF, et al: Recovery profiles and costs of anesthesia for outpatient unilateral inguinal herniorrhaphy. Anesth Analg 2000;91:876–881.

14. Li S, Coloma M, White PF, et al: Comparison of the costs and recovery profiles of three anesthetic techniques for ambulatory anorectal surgery. Anesthesiology 2000;93:1225–1230.

15. Harrison CA, Morris S, Harvey JS: Effect of ilioinguinal and iliohypogastric nerve block and wound infiltration with 0.5% bupivacaine on postoperative pain after hernia repair. Br J Anesth 1994;72:691–693.

16. Ding Y, White PF: Post-herniorrhaphy pain in outpatients after preincision ilioinguinal-hypogastric nerve block during monitored anesthesia care. Can J Anaesth 1995;42:12–15.

17. Broadman LM, Hannallah RS, Belman AB, et al: Post-circumcision analgesia: A prospective evaluation of subcutaneous ring block of the penis. Anesthesiology 1987;67:399–402.

18. Baram D, Smith C, Stinson S: Intraoperative topical etidocaine for reducing postoperative pain after laparoscopic tubal ligation. J Reprod Med 1990;35:407–410.

19. Gharaibeh KI, Al-Jaberi TM: Bupivacaine instillation into gallbladder bed after laparoscopic cholecystectomy: Does it decrease shoulder pain? J Laparoendosc Adv Surg Tech A 2000;10:137–141.

20. Ritchie ED, Tong D, Chung F, et al: Suprascapular nerve block for postoperative pain relief in arthroscopic shoulder surgery: a new modality? Anesth Analg 1997;84:1306–12.

21. Tierney E, Lewis G, Hurtig JB, et al: Femoral nerve block with bupivacaine 0.25 per cent for postoperative analgesia after open knee surgery. Can J Anaesth 1987;34:455–458.

22. Brown AR, Weiss R, Greenberg C, et al: Interscalene block for shoulder arthroscopy: Comparison with general anesthesia. Arthroscopy 1993;9:295–300.

23. Casati A, Cappelleri G, Fanelli G, et al: Regional anaesthesia for outpatient knee arthroscopy: A randomized clinical comparison of two different anaesthetic techniques. Acta Anaesthesiol Scand 2000;44:543–547.

24. Woolf CJ, Chong MS: Preemptive analgesia—Treating postoperative pain by preventing the establishment of central sensitization. Anesth Analg 1993;77:362–379.

25. Ejlersen E, Andersen HB, Eliasen K, et al: A comparison between preincisional and postincisional lidocaine infiltration and postoperative pain. Anesth Analg 1992;74:495–498.

26. Reuben SS, Bhopatkar S, Maciolek H, et al: The preemptive analgesic effect of rofecoxib after ambulatory arthroscopic knee surgery. Anesth Analg 2002;94:55–59.

27. Møniniche S, Kehlet H, Dahl JB: A qualitative and quantitative systematic review of preemptive analgesia for postoperative pain relief—The role of timing of analgesia. Anesthesiology 2002;96:725–741.

28. Tverskoy M, Cozacov C, Ayache M, et al: Postoperative pain after inguinal herniorrhaphy with different types of anesthesia. Anesth Analg 1990;70:29–35.

29. Jebeles J, Reilly J, Gutierrez J, et al: The effect of preincisional infiltration of tonsils with bupivacaine on the pain following tonsillectomy under general anesthesia. Pain 1991;47:305–308.

30. O'Neal MG, Beste T, Shackelford DP: Utility of preemptive local analgesia in vaginal hysterectomy. Am J Obstet Gynecol 2003;189:1539–1541.

31. Bisgaard T, Klarskov B, Kristiansen VB, et al: Multi-regional local anesthetic infiltration during laparoscopic cholecystectomy in patients receiving prophylactic multimodal analgesia: A randomized, double-blinded, placebo-controlled study. Anesth Analg 1999;89:1017–1024.

32. Sarac AM, Aktan AO, Baykan N, et al: The effect of timing of local anesthesia in laparoscopic cholecystectomy. Surg Laparosc Endosc 1996;6:362–366.

33. Hasaniya NW, Zayed FF, Faiz H, et al: Preinsertion local anesthesia at the trocar site improves perioperative pain and decreases costs of laparoscopic cholecystectomy. Surg Endosc 2001;15:962–964.

34. Fong SY, Pavy TJ, Yeo ST, et al: Assessment of wound infiltration with bupivacaine in women undergoing day-case gynecological laparoscopy. Reg Anesth Pain Med 2001;26:131–136.

35. Moiniche S, Jorgensen H, Wetterslev J, et al: Local anesthetic infiltration for postoperative pain relief after laparoscopy: A qualitative and quantitative systematic review of intraperitoneal, port-site infiltration and mesosalpinx block. Anesth Analg 2000;90:899–912.

36. Sinclair R, Cassuto J, Hogstrom S, et al: Topical anesthesia with lidocaine aerosol in the control of postoperative pain. Anesthesiology 1988;68:895–901.

37. Casey WF, Rice LJ, Hannallah RS, et al: A comparison between bupivacaine instillation versus ilioinguinal/iliohypogastric nerve block for postoperative analgesia following inguinal herniorrhaphy in children. Anesthesiology 1990;72:637–639.

38. Tree-Trakarn T, Pirayavaraporn S: Postoperative pain relief for circumcision in children: Comparison among morphine, nerve block, and topical analgesia. Anesthesiology 1985;62:519–522.

39. Tree-Trakarn T, Pirayavaraporn S, Lertakyamee J: Topical analgesia for relief of post-circumcision pain. Anesthesiology 1987;67:395–399.

40. Choi WY, Irwin MG, Hui TWC, et al: EMLA® cream versus dorsal penile nerve block for postcircumcision analgesia in children. Anesth Analg 2003;96:396–399.

41. Gammaitoni AR, Alvarez NA, Galer BS: Safety and tolerability of the lidocaine patch 5%, a targeted peripheral analgesic: A review of the literature. J Clin Pharmacol 2003;43:111–117.

42. Narchi P, Benhamou D, Fernandez H: Intraperitoneal local anaesthetic for shoulder pain after day-case laparoscopy. Lancet 1991;338:1569–1570.

43. Paulson J, Mellinger J, Baguley W: The use of intraperitoneal bupivacaine to decrease the length of stay in elective laparoscopic cholecystectomy patients. Am J Surg 2003;69:275–278.

44. Rademaker BM, Kalkman CJ, Odoom JA, et al: Intraperitoneal local anaesthetics after laparoscopic cholecystectomy: Effects on postoperative pain, metabolic responses and lung function. Br J Anaesth 1994;72:263–266.

45. Joris J, Thiry E, Paris P, et al: Pain after laparoscopic cholecystectomy: Characteristics and effect of intraperitoneal bupivacaine. Anesth Analg 1995;81:379–384.

46. Scheinin B, Kellokumpu I, Lindgren I, et al: Effect of intraperitoneal bupivacaine on pain after laparoscopic cholecystectomy. Acta Anaesthesiol Scand 1995;39:195–198.

47. Raetzell M, Maier C, Schroder D, et al: Intraperitoneal application of bupivacaine during laparoscopic cholecystectomy—Risk or benefit? Anesth Analg 1995;81:967–972.

48. Pasqualucci A, de Angelis V, Contardo R, et al: Preemptive analgesia: Intraperitoneal local anesthetic in laparoscopic cholecystectomy. A randomized, double-blind, placebo-controlled study. Anesthesiology 1996;85:11–20.

49. Szem JW, Hydo L, Barie PS: A double-blinded evaluation of intraperitoneal bupivacaine vs saline for the reduction of postoperative pain and nausea after laparoscopic cholecystectomy. Surg Endosc 1996;10:44–48.

50. Mraovic B, Jurisic T, Kogler-Majeric V, et al: Intraperitoneal bupivacaine for analgesia after laparoscopic cholecystectomy. Acta Anaesthesiol Scand 1997;41:193–196.

51. Cunniffe MG, McAnena OJ, Dar JA, et al: A prospective randomized trial of intraoperative bupivacaine irrigation for management of shoulder-tip pain following laparoscopy. Am J Surg 1998;176:258–261.

52. Wallin G, Cassuto J, Hogstrom S, et al: Influence of intraperitoneal anesthesia on pain and the sympathoadrenal response to abdominal surgery. Acta Anaesthesiol Scand 1988;32:553–558.

53. Zmora O, Stolik-Dollberg O, Bar-Zakai B, et al: Intraperitoneal bupivacaine does not attenuate pain following laparoscopic cholecystectomy. JSLS 2000;4:301–304.

54. Maestroni U, Sortini D, Devito C, et al: A new method of preemptive analgesia in laparoscopic cholecystectomy. Surg Endosc 2002;16:1336–1340.

55. Saff GN, Marks RA, Kuroda M, et al: Analgesic effect of bupivacaine on extraperitoneal laparoscopic hernia repair. Anesth Analg 1998;87:377–381.

56. Ashcraft EE, Baillie GM, Shafizadeh SF, et al: Further improvements in laparoscopic donor nephrectomy: Decreased pain and accelerated recovery. Clin Transplant 2001;15:59–61.

57. Yndgaard S, Holst P, Bjerre-Jepsen K, et al: Subcutaneously versus subfascially administered lidocaine in pain treatment after inguinal herniotomy. Anesth Analg 1994;79:324–327.

58. Scott NB, Mogensen T, Bigler D, et al: Comparison of the effects of continuous intrapleural vs epidural administration of 0.5% bupivacaine on pain, metabolic response and pulmonary function following cholecystectomy. Acta Anaesthesiol Scand 1989;33:535–539.

59. Schroeder D, Baker P: Interpleural catheter for analgesia after cholecystectomy: The surgical perspective. Aust N Z J Surg 1990;60:689–694.

60. Frank ED, McKay W, Rocco A, et al: Interpleural bupivacaine for postoperative analgesia following cholecystectomy: A randomized prospective study. Reg Anesth 1990;15:26–30.

61. Stromskag KE, Minor BG, Lindeberg A: Comparison of 40 milliliters of 0.25% intrapleural bupivacaine with epinephrine with 20 milliliters of 0.5% intrapleural bupivacaine with epinephrine after cholecystectomy. Anesth Analg 1991;73:397–400.

62. Rademaker BM, Sih IL, Kalkman CJ, et al: Effects of interpleurally administered bupivacaine 0.5% on opioid analgesic requirements and endocrine response during and after cholecystectomy: A randomized double-blind controlled study. Acta Anaesthesiol Scand 1991;35:108–112.

63. Laurito CE, Kirz LI, VadeBoncouere TR, et al: Continuous infusion of interpleural bupivacaine maintains effective analgesia after cholecystectomy. Anesth Analg 1991;72:516–521.

64. Frenette L, Boudreault D, Guay J: Interpleural analgesia improves pulmonary function after cholecystectomy. Can J Anaesth 1991;38:71–74.

65. Oxorn DC, Whatley GS: Post-cholecystectomy pulmonary function following interpleural bupivacaine and intramuscular pethidine. Anaesth Intensive Care 1989;17:440–443.

66. Lee A, Boon D, Bagshaw P, et al: A randomized double-blind study of interpleural analgesia after cholecystectomy. Anaesthesia 1990;45:1028–1031.

67. Schulte-Steinberg H, Weninger E, Jokisch D, et al: Intraperitoneal *versus* interpleural morphine or bupivacaine for pain after laparoscopic cholecystectomy. Anesthesiology 1995;82:634–640.

68. Ross WB, Tweedie JH, Leong YP, et al: Intercostal blockade and pulmonary function after cholecystectomy. Surgery 1989;105:166–169.

69. Dahl MR, Dasta JF, Zuelzer W, et al: Lidocaine local anesthesia for arthroscopic knee surgery. Anesth Analg 1990;71:670–674.

70. Smith I, Van Hemelrijck J, White PF, et al: Effects of local anesthesia on recovery after outpatient arthroscopy. Anesth Analg 1991;73:536–539.

71. Smith I, Shively RA, White PF: Effects of ketorolac and bupivacaine on recovery after outpatient arthroscopy. Anesth Analg 1992;75:208–212.

72. Stein C, Comisel K, Haimerl E, et al: Analgesic effect of intraarticular morphine after arthroscopic knee surgery. N Engl J Med 1991;325:1123–1126.

73. Reuben S, Connelly NR: Postoperative analgesia for outpatient arthroscopic knee surgery with intraarticular bupivacaine and ketorolac. Anesth Analg 1995;80:1154–1157.

74. Wang JJ, Ho ST, Lee SC, et al: Intraarticular triamcinolone acetonide for pain control after arthroscopic knee surgery. Anesth Analg 1998;87:1113–1116.

75. Joshi W, Reuben SS, Kilaru PR, et al: Postoperative analgesia for outpatient arthroscopic knee surgery with intraarticular clonidine and/or morphine. Anesth Analg 2000;90:1102–1106.

76. Khoury GF, Chen ACN, Garland DE, et al: Intraarticular morphine, bupivacaine, and morphine/bupivacaine for pain control after knee videoarthroscopy. Anesthesiology 1992;77:263–266.

77. Reuben SS, Sklar J, El-Mansouri M: The preemptive analgesic effect of intraarticular bupivacaine and morphine after ambulatory arthroscopic knee surgery. Anesth Analg 2001;92:923–926.

78. Thomas DFM, Lambert WG, Williams KL: The direct perfusion of surgical wounds with local anaesthetic solution: An approach to postoperative pain? Ann R Coll Surg Engl 1983;65:226–229.

79. Gibbs P, Purushotam A, Auld C, et al: Continuous wound perfusion with bupivacaine for postoperative wound pain. Br J Surg 1988;75:923–924.

80. Levack ID, Holmes JD, Robertson GS: Abdominal wound perfusion for the relief of postoperative pain. Br J Anaesth 1986;58:615–619.

81. Gupta A, Thorn SE, Axelsson K, et al: Postoperative pain relief using intermittent injections of 0.5% ropivacaine through a catheter after laparoscopic cholecystectomy. Anesth Analg 2002;95:450–456.

82. White PF, Rawal S, Latham P, et al: Use of a continuous local anesthetic infusion for pain management after median sternotomy. Anesthesiology 2003;99:918–923.

83. Bianconi M, Ferraro L, Ricci R, et al: The pharmacokinetics and efficacy of ropivacaine continuous wound instillation after spine fusion surgery. Anesth Analg 2004;98:166–172.

84. Rawal N, Axelsson K, Hylander J, et al: Postoperative patient-controlled local anesthetic administration at home. Anesth Analg 1998:86:86–89.

85. Rawal N, Allvin R, Axelsson K, et al: Patient-controlled regional analgesia (PCRA) at home: Controlled comparison between bupivacaine and ropivacaine brachial plexus analgesia. Anesthesiology 2002;96:1290–1296.

86. Fredman B, Shapiro A, Zohar E, et al: The analgesic efficacy of patient-controlled ropivacaine instillation after Cesarean delivery. Anesth Analg 2000;91:1436–1440.

87. Fredman B, Zohar E, Tarabykin A, et al: Bupivacaine wound instillation via an electronic patient-controlled analgesia device and a double-catheter system does not decrease postoperative pain or opioid requirements after major abdominal surgery. Anesth Analg 2001;92:189–193.

88. Cameron AEP, Cross FW: Pain and morbidity after inguinal herniorrhaphy: ineffectiveness of subcutaneous bupivacaine. Br J Surg 1985;72:68–69.

89. Ilfeld BM, Morey TE, Wang RD, et al: Continuous popliteal sciatic nerve block for postoperative pain control at home: A randomized, double-blinded, placebo-controlled study. Anesthesiology 2002;97:959–965.

90. White PF, Issioui T, Skrivanek GD, et al: Use of a continuous popliteal sciatic nerve block for the management of pain after major podiatric surgery: does it improve quality of recovery? Anesth Analg 2003;97:1303–1309.

91. Ilfeld BM, Morey TE, Enneking FK: Continuous infraclavicular brachial plexus block for postoperative pain control at home: A randomized, double-blinded, placebo-controlled study. Anesthesiology 2002;96:1297–1304.

92. Singelyn FJ, Seguy S, Gouverneur JM: Interscale brachial plexus analgesia after open shoulder surgery: Continuous versus patient-controlled infusion. Anesth Analg 1999;89:1216–1220.

93. Singelyn FJ, Vanderelst PE, Gouverneus JM: Extended femoral nerve sheath block after total hip arthroplasty: Continuous versus patient-controlled techniques. Anesth Analg 2001;92:455–459.

94. Ilfeld BM, Morey TE, Enneking FK: Portable infusion pumps used for continuous regional analgesia: Delivery rate accuracy and consistency. Reg Anesth Pain Med 2003;28:424–432.

95. Capdevila X, Macaire P, Aknin P, et al: Patient-controlled perineural analgesia after ambulatory orthopedic surgery: A comparison of electronic *versus* elastomeric pumps. Anesth Analg 2003;96:414–417.

96. Cuvillon P, Ripart J, Lalourcey L, et al: The continuous femoral nerve block catheter for postoperative analgesia: bacterial colonization, infectious rate and adverse effects. Anesth Analg 2001;93:1045–1049.

97. Ilfeld BM, Esener DE, Morey TE, et al: Ambulatory perineural infusion: The patient's perspective. Reg Anesth Pain Med 2003;28:418–423.

98. Kehlet H, Dahl JB: The value of "multimodal" or "balanced analgesia" in postoperative pain treatment. Anesth Analg 1993;77:1048–1056.

99. Klein SM, Greengrass RA, Steele SM, et al: A comparison of 0.5% bupivacaine, 0.5% ropivacaine, and 0.75% ropivacaine for interscalene brachial plexus block. Anesth Analg 1998;87:1316–1319.

100. Mulroy MF, Larkin KL, Batra MS, et al: Femoral nerve block with 0.25% or 0.5% bupivacaine improves postoperative analgesia following outpatient arthroscopic anterior cruciate ligament repair. Reg Anesth Pain Med 2001;26:24–29.

101. Casati A, Vinciguerra F, Scarioni M, et al: Lidocaine versus ropivacaine for continuous interscalene brachial plexus block after open shoulder surgery. Acta Anaesthesiol Scand 2003;47:355–360.

102. Casati A, Magistris L, Fanelli G, et al: Small-dose clonidine prolongs postoperative analgesia after sciatic-femoral nerve block with 0.75% ropivacaine for foot surgery. Anesth Analg 2000 91:388–392.

103. Niemi G, Breivik H: Epinephrine markedly improves thoracic epidural analgesia produced by a small-dose infusion of ropivacaine, fentanyl, and epinephrine after major thoracic or abdominal surgery: A randomized, double-blinded crossover study with and without epinephrine. Anesth Analg 2002;94:1598–1605.

104. Ilfeld BM, Morey TE, Enneking FK: Continuous infraclavicular perineural infusion with clonidine and ropivacaine compared with ropivacaine alone: a randomized, double-blinded, controlled study. Anesth Analg 2003;97:706–712.

105. Klein SM, Greengrass RA, Grant SA, et al: Ambulatory surgery for multi-ligament knee reconstruction with continuous dual catheter peripheral nerve blockade. Can J Anaesth 2001;48:375–378.

106. Klein SM, Grant SA, Greengrass RA, et al: Interscalene brachial plexus block with a continuous catheter system and a disposable infusion pump. Anesth Analg 2000;91:1473–1478.

107. Ilfeld BM, Morey TE, Wright TW, et al: Continuous interscalene brachial plexus block for postoperative pain control at home: a randomized, double-blinded, placebo-controlled study. Anesth Analg 2003;96:1089–1095.

108. Yee JP, Koshiver JE, Allbon C, et al: Comparison of intramuscular ketorolac tromethamine and morphine sulphate for analgesia of pain after major surgery. Pharmacotherapy 1986;6:253–261.

109. O'Hara DA, Fragen RJ, Kinzer M, et al: Ketorolac tromethamine as compared with morphine sulfate for the treatment of postoperative pain. Clin Pharmacol Ther 1987;41:556–561.

110. Powell H, Smallman JMB, Morgan M: Comparison of intramuscular ketorolac and morphine in pain control after laparotomy. Anaesthesia 1990;45:538–542.

111. Murray AW, Brockway MS, Kenny GNC: Comparison of the cardiorespiratory effects of ketorolac and alfentanil during propofol anaesthesia. Br J Anaesth 1989;63:601–603.

112. Ding Y, White PF: Comparative effects of ketorolac, dezocine, and fentanyl as adjuvants during outpatient anesthesia. Anesth Analg 1992;75:566–571.

113. Ramirez-Ruiz M, Smith I, White PF: Use of analgesics during propofol sedation: a comparison of ketorolac, dezocine, and fentanyl. J Clin Anesth 1995;7:481–485.

114. Wong HY, Carpenter RL, Kopacz DJ, et al: A randomized double-blind evaluation of ketorolac tromethamine for postoperative analgesia in ambulatory surgery patients. Anesthesiology 1993;78:6–14.

115. Singh H, Bossard RF, White PF, et al: Effects of ketorolac versus bupivacaine coadministration during patient-controlled hydromorphone epidural analgesia after thoracotomy procedures. Anesth Analg 1997;84:564–569.

116. Coloma M, White PF, Huber PJ, et al: The effect of ketorolac on recovery after anorectal surgery: IV versus local administration. Anesth Analg 2000;90:1107–1110.

117. Romsing J, Moiniche S, Ostergaard D, et al: Local infiltration with NSAIDs for postoperative analgesia: Evidence for a peripheral analgesic action. Acta Anaesthesiol Scand 2000;44:672–683.

118. Ding Y, Fredman B, White PF: Use of ketorolac and fentanyl during outpatient gynecological surgery. Anesth Analg 1993;77:205–210.

119. Liu J, Ding Y, White PF, et al: Effects of ketorolac on postoperative analgesia and ventilatory function after laparoscopic cholecystectomy. Anesth Analg 1993;76:1061–1066.

120. Fredman B, Jedeikin R, Olsfanger D, et al: The opioid-sparing effect of diclofenac sodium in outpatient extracorporeal shock wave lithotripsy (ESWL). J Clin Anesth 1993;5:141–144.

121. McLoughlin C, McKinney MS, Fee JPH, et al: Diclofenac for day-care arthroscopy surgery: comparison with standard opioid therapy. Br J Anaesth 1990;65:620–623.

122. Gillberg LE, Harsten AS, Stahl LB: Preoperative diclofenac sodium reduces post-laparoscopy pain. Can J Anaesth 1993;40:406–408.

123. Varrassi G, Panella L, Piroli A, et al: The effects of perioperative ketorolac infusion on postoperative pain and endocrine-metabolic response. Anesth Analg 1994;78:514–519.

124. Zackova M, Taddei S, Calo P, et al: Ketorolac vs tramadol in the treatment of postoperative pain during maxillofacial surgery. Minerva Anesthesiol 2001;67:641–646.

125. Wilson YG, Rhodes M, Ahmed R, et al: Intramuscular diclofenac sodium postoperative analgesia after laparoscopic cholecystectomy: A randomized, controlled trial. Surg Laparosc Endosc 1994;4:340–344.

126. Fredman B, Olsfanger D, Jedeikin R: A comparative study of ketorolac and diclofenac on post-laparoscopic cholecystectomy pain. Eur J Anaesthesiol 1995;12:501–504.

127. Baer GA, Rorarius MGF, Kolehmainen S, et al: The effect of paracetamol or diclofenac administered before operation on postoperative pain and behavior after adenoidectomy in small children. Anaesthesia 1992;47:1078–1080.

128. Watcha MF, Ramirez-Ruiz M, White PF, et al: Perioperative effects of oral ketorolac and acetaminophen in children undergoing bilateral myringotomy. Can J Anaesth 1992;39:649–654.

129. Splinter WM, Reid CW, Roberts DJ, et al: Reducing pain after inguinal hernia repair in children: caudal anesthesia versus ketorolac tromethamine. Anesthesiology 1997;87:542–546.

130. Watcha MF, Jones MB, Lagueruela RG, et al: Comparison of ketorolac and morphine as adjuvants during pediatric surgery. Anesthesiology 1992;76:368–372.

131. Maunuksela EL, Kokki H, Bullingham RES: Comparison of IV ketorolac with morphine for postoperative pain in children. Clin Pharmacol Ther 1992;52:436–443.

132. Forse A, El-Beheiry H, Butler PO, et al: Indomethacin and ketorolac given preoperatively are equally effective in reducing early postoperative pain after laparoscopic cholecystectomy. Can J Surg 1996;39:26–30.

133. Comfort VK, Code WE, Rooney ME, et al: Naproxen premedication reduces postoperative tubal ligation pain. Can J Anaesth 1992;4:349–352.

134. Rosenblum M, Weller RS, Conard PL, et al: Ibuprofen provides longer lasting analgesia than fentanyl after laparoscopic surgery. Anesth Analg 1991;73:255–259.

135. Doyle G, Jayawardena S, Ashraf E, et al: Efficacy and tolerability of nonprescription ibuprofen versus celecoxib for dental pain. J Clin Pharmacol 2002;42:912–919.

136. Pickering AE, Bridge HS, Nolan J, et al: Double-blind, placebo-controlled analgesic study of ibuprofen on rofecoxib in combination with paracetamol for tonsillectomy in children. Br J Anaesth 2002;88:72–77.

137. Raeder JC, Steine S, Vatsgar TT: Oral ibuprofen versus paracetamol plus codeine for analgesia after ambulatory surgery. Anesth Analg 2001;92:1470–1472.

138. Edwards JE, McQuay HJ, Moore RA: Combination analgesic efficacy: Individual patient data meta-analysis of single-dose oral tramadol plus acetaminophen in acute postoperative pain. J Pain Symptom Manage 2002;23:121–130.

139. Souter A, Fredman B, White PF: Controversies in the perioperative use of nonsteroidal antiinflammatory drugs. Anesth Analg 1994;79:1178–1190.

140. Rusy LM, Houck CS, Sullivan LJ, et al: A double-blind evaluation of ketorolac tromethamine versus acetaminophen in pediatric tonsillectomy: analgesia and bleeding. Anesth Analg 1995;80:226–229.

141. Gunter JB, Varughese AM, Harrington JF, et al: Recovery and complications after tonsillectomy in children: a comparison of ketorolac and morphine. Anesth Analg 1995;81:1136–1141.

142. Moiniche S, Romsing J, Dahl JB, et al: Nonsteroidal antiinflammatory drugs and the risk of operative bleeding after tonsillectomy: a quantitative systematic review. Anesth Analg 2003;96:68–77.

143. FitzGerald GA, Patrono C: The coxibs, selective inhibitors of cyclooxygenase-2. N Engl J Med 2001;345:433–442.

144. Reuben SS, Connelly NR. Postoperative analgesic effects of celecoxib or rofecoxib after spinal fusion surgery. Anesth Analg 2000;91:1221–1225.

145. Issioui T, Klein KW, White PF, et al: The efficacy of premedication with celecoxib and acetaminophen in preventing pain after otolaryngologic surgery. Anesth Analg 2002;94:1188–1193.

146. Recart A, Issioui T, White PF, et al: The efficacy of celecoxib premedication on postoperative pain and recovery times after ambulatory surgery: a dose-ranging study. Anesth Analg 2003;96:1631–1635.

147. Issioui T, Klein KW, White PF, et al: Cost-efficacy of rofecoxib versus acetaminophen for preventing pain after ambulatory surgery. Anesthesiology 2002;97:931–937.

148. Ma H, Tang J, White PF, et al: Perioperative rofecoxib improves early recovery after outpatient herniorrhaphy. Anesth Analg 2004;98:970–975.

149. Watcha MF, Issioui T, Klein KW, et al: Costs and effectiveness of rofecoxib, celecoxib and acetaminophen for preventing pain after ambulatory otolaryngologic surgery. Anesth Analg 2003:96:987–994.

150. Sinatra RS, Shen QJ, Halaszynski T, et al: Preoperative rofecoxib oral suspension as an analgesic adjunct after lower abdominal surgery: the effects on effort-dependent pain and pulmonary function. Anesth Analg 2004;98:135–140.

151. Buvanendran A, Kroin JS, Tuman KJ, et al: Effects of perioperative administration of a selective cyclooxygenase 2 inhibitor on pain management and recovery of function after knee replacement: a randomized controlled trial. JAMA 2003;290:2411–2418.

152. Desjardins PJ, Shu VS, Recker DP, et al: A single preoperative oral dose of valdecoxib, a new cyclooxygenase-2 specific inhibitor, relieves post-oral surgery or bunionectomy pain. Anesthesiology 2002;97:565–573.

153. Joshi GP, Viscusi ER, Gan TJ, et al: Effective treatment of laparoscopic cholecystectomy pain with intravenous followed by oral COX-2 specific inhibitor. Anesth Analg 2004;98:336–342.

154. Fricke J, Varkalis J, Zwillich S, et al: Valdecoxib is more efficacious than rofecoxib in relieving pain associated with oral surgery. Am J Ther 2002;9:89–97.

155. Desjardins PJ, Grossman EH, Kuss ME, et al: The injectable cyclooxygenase-2-specific inhibitor parecoxib sodium has analgesic efficacy when administered preoperatively. Anesth Analg 2001;93:721–727.

156. Tang J, Li S, White PF, et al: Effect of parecoxib, a novel intravenous cyclooxygenase-2 inhibitor, on the postoperative opioid requirement and quality of pain control. Anesthesiology 2002;96:1305–1309.

157. Ng A, Smith G, Davidson AC: Analgesic effects of parecoxib following total abdominal hysterectomy. Br J Anaesth 2003;90:746–749.

158. Mehlisch DR, Desjardins PJ, Daniels S, et al: Single doses of parecoxib sodium intravenously are as effective as ketorolac in reducing pain after oral surgery. J Oral Maxillofac Surg 2003;61:1030–1037.

159. Barton SF, Langeland FF, Snabes MC, et al: Efficacy and safety of intravenous parecoxib sodium in relieving acute postoperative pain following gynecologic laparotomy surgery. Anesthesiology 2002;97:306–314.

160. Malan TP Jr, Marsh G, Hakki SI, et al: Parecoxib sodium, a parenteral cyclooxygenase 2 selective inhibitor, improves morphine analgesia and is opioid-sparing following total hip arthroplasty. Anesthesiology 2003;98:950–956.

161. Ott E, Nussmeier NA, Duke PC, et al: Efficacy and safety of cyclooxygenase 2 inhibitors parecoxib and valdecoxib in patients undergoing coronary artery bypass surgery. J Thorac Cardiovasc Surg 2003;125:1481–1492.

162. Malmstrom K, Kotey P, Coughlin H, et al: A randomized, double-blind, parallel-group study comparing the analgesic effect of etoricoxib to placebo, naproxen sodium, and acetaminophen with codeine using the dental impaction pain model. Clin J Pain 2004;20:147–155.

163. Romsing J, Moiniche S: A systematic review of COX-2 inhibitors compared with traditional NSAIDs, or different COX-2 inhibitors for postoperative pain. Acta Anaesthesiol Scand 2004;48:525–546.

164. Stichtenoth DO, Frolich JC: The second generation of COX-2 inhibitors: what advantages do the newest offer? Drugs 2003;63:33–45.

165. Glassman SD, Rose S, Matthew BE, et al: The effect of postoperative nonsteroidal antiinflammatory drug administration on spinal fusion. Spine 1998;23:834–838.

166. Einhorn TA: COX-2: Where are we in 2003? The role of cyclooxygenase-2 in bone repair. Arthritis Res Ther 2003;5:5–7.

167. Seidenberg AB, An YH: Is there an inhibitory effect of COX-2 inhibitors on bone healing? Pharm Res 2004;50:151–156.

168. Simon AM, Manigrasso MB, O'Connor JP: Cyclo-oxygenase 2 function is essential for bone fracture healing. J Bone Miner Res 2002;17:963–976.

169. Harder AT, An YH: The mechanisms of the inhibitory effects of nonsteroidal antiinflammatory drugs on bone healing: A concise review. J Clin Pharm 2004;43:807–815.

170. Gajraj NM: Cyclooxygenase-2 inhibitors. Anesth Analg 2003;96:1720–1738.

171. Gilron I, Milne B, Hong M: Cyclooxygenase-2 inhibitors in postoperative pain management. Anesthesiology 2003;99:1198–1208.

172. Cicconetti A, Bartoli A, Ripari F, et al: COX-2 selective inhibitors: A literature review of analgesic efficacy and safety in oral-maxillofacial surgery. Oral Surg Oral Med Oral Pathol Oral Radiol Endod 2004;97:139–146.

173. Hyllested M, Jones S, Pedersen JL, et al: Comparative effect of paracetamol, NSAIDs or their combination in postoperative pain management: A qualitative review. Br J Anaesth 2002;88:199–214.

174. Schug SA, Sidebotham DA, McGuinnety M, et al: Acetaminophen as an adjunct to morphine by patient-controlled analgesia in the management of acute postoperative pain. Anesth Analg 1998;87:368–372.

175. Korpela R, Korvenoja P, Meretoja OA: Morphine-sparing effect of acetaminophen in pediatric day-case surgery. Anesthesiology 1999;91:442–447.

176. Birmingham PK, Tobin MJ, Fisher DM, et al: Initial and subsequent dosing of rectal acetaminophen in children: A 24-hour pharmacokinetic study of new dose recommendations. Anesthesiology 2001;94:385–389.

177. Varrassi G, Marinangeli F, Agro F, et al: A double-blinded evaluation of propacetamol versus ketorolac in combination with

patient-controlled analgesia morphine: analgesic efficacy and tolerability after gynecologic surgery. Anesth Analg 1999;88:611–616.

178. Zhou TJ, Tang J, White PF: Propacetamol versus ketorolac for treatment of acute postoperative pain after total hip or knee replacement. Anesth Analg 2001;92:1569–1575.

179. Delbos A, Boccard E: The morphine-sparing effect of propacetamol in orthopedic postoperative pain. J Pain Symptom Manage 1995;10:279–286.

180. Hernandez-Palazon J, Tortosa JA, et al: Intravenous administration of propacetamol reduces morphine consumption alter spinal fusion surgery. Anesth Analg 2001;92:1473–1476.

181. Lahtinen P, Kokki H, Hendolin H, et al: Propacetamol as adjunctive treatment for postoperative pain after cardiac surgery. Anesth Analg 2002;95:813–819.

182. Moller PL, Juhl GI, Payen-Champenois C, et al: Ready-to-use IV paracetamol: comparable analgesic efficacy, but better local safety than its prodrug, propacetamol for postoperative pain after third molar surgery. Anesth Analg 2005;101:90–96.

183. Coloma M, Chiu JW, White PF, et al: The use of esmolol as an alternative to remifentanil during desflurane anesthesia for fast-track outpatient gynecologic laparoscopic surgery. Anesth Analg 2001;92:352–357.

184. Hillis WS: Areas of emerging interest in analgesia: Cardiovascular complications. Am J Ther 2002;9:259–269.

185. White PF, Way WL, Trevor AJ: Ketamine—Its pharmacology and therapeutic uses. Anesthesiology 1982;56:119–136.

186. Badrinath S, Avramov MN, Shadrick M, et al: The use of ketamine–propofol combination during monitored anesthesia care. Anesth Analg 2000;90:858–862.

187. Mortero RF, Clark LD, Tolan MM, et al: The effects of small-dose ketamine on propofol sedation: Respiration, postoperative mood, perception, cognition, and pain. Anesth Analg 2001;92:1465–1469.

188. Kohrs R, Durieux ME: Ketamine: Teaching an old drug new tricks. Anesth Analg 1998;87:1186–1193.

189. Blakeley KR, Klein KW, White PF, et al: A total IV anesthetic technique for outpatient facial laser resurfacing. Anesth Analg 1998;87:827–829.

190. Guillou N, Tanguy M, Seguin P, et al: The effects of small-dose ketamine on morphine consumption in surgical intensive care unit patients after major abdominal surgery. Anesth Analg 2003;97:843–847.

191. Reeves M, Lindholm DE, Myles PS, et al: Adding ketamine to morphine for patient-controlled analgesia after major abdominal surgery: A double-blinded, randomized controlled trial. Anesth Analg 2001;93:116–120.

192. Sveticic G, Gentilini A, Eichenberger U, et al: Combinations of morphine with ketamine for patient-controlled analgesia: A new optimization method. Anesthesiology 2003;98:1195–1205.

193. Suzuki M, Tsueda K, Lansing PS, et al: Small-dose ketamine enhances morphine-induced analgesia after outpatient surgery. Anesth Analg 1999;89:98–103.

194. Menigaux C, Fletcher D, Dupont X, et al: The benefits of intraoperative small-dose ketamine on postoperative pain after anterior cruciate ligament repair. Anesth Analg 2000;90:129–135.

195. Menigaux C, Guignard B, Fletcher D, et al: Intraoperative small-dose ketamine enhances analgesia after outpatient knee arthroscopy. Anesth Analg 2001;93:606–612.

196. Guignard B, Coste C, Costes H, et al: Supplementing desflurane–remifentanil anesthesia with small-dose ketamine reduces perioperative opioid analgesic requirements. Anesth Analg 2002;95:103–108.

197. Guillou N, Tanguy M, Seguin P, et al: The effects of small-dose ketamine on morphine consumption in surgical intensive care unit patients after major abdominal surgery. Anesth Analg 2003;97:843–847.

198. Elhakim M, Khalafallah Z, El-Fattah HA, et al: Ketamine reduces swallowing-evoked pain after paediatric tonsillectomy. Acta Anaesthesiol Scand 2003;47:604–609.

199. Taura P, Fuster J, Blasi A, et al: Postoperative pain relief after hepatic resection in cirrhotic patients: The efficacy of a single small dose of ketamine plus morphine epidurally. Anesth Analg 2003;96:475–480.

200. Fu ES, Miguel R, Scharf JE: Preemptive ketamine decreases postoperative narcotic requirements in patients undergoing abdominal surgery. Anesth Analg 1997;84:1086–1090.

201. Adam F, Libier M, Oszustowicz T, et al: Preoperative small-dose ketamine has no preemptive analgesic effect in patients undergoing total mastectomy. Anesth Analg 1999;89:444–447.

202. Dahl V, Ernoe PE, Steen T, et al: Does ketamine have preemptive effects in women undergoing abdominal hysterectomy procedures? Anesth Analg 2000;90:1419–1422.

203. Weinbroum AA: A single small dose of postoperative ketamine provides rapid and sustained improvement in morphine analgesia in the presence of morphine-resistant pain. Anesth Analg 2003;96:789–795.

204. Laulin JP, Maurette P, Corcuff JB, et al: The role of ketamine in preventing fentanyl-induced hyperalgesia and subsequent acute morphine tolerance. Anesth Analg 2002;94:1263–1269.

205. Jaksch W, Lang S, Reichhalter R, et al: Perioperative small-dose $S(+)$-ketamine has no incremental beneficial effects on postoperative pain when standard-practice opioid infusions are used. Anesth Analg 2002;94:981–986.

206. Himmelseher S, Ziegler-Pithamitsis D, et al: Small-dose $S(+)$-ketamine reduces postoperative pain when applied with ropivacaine in epidural anesthesia for total knee arthroplasty. Anesth Analg 2001;92:1290–1295.

207. Lauretti GR, Oliveira AP, Rodrigues AM, et al: The effect of transdermal nitroglycerin on spinal $S(+)$-ketamine antinociception following orthopedic surgery. J Clin Anesth 2001;13:576–581.

208. White PF, Ham J, Way WL, et al: Pharmacology of ketamine isomers in surgical patients. Anesthesiology 1980;52:231–239.

209. Mathisen LC, Aasbo V, Raeder J: Lack of preemptive analgesic effect of (R)-ketamine in laparoscopic cholecystectomy. Acta Anaesthesiol Scand 1999;43:220–224.

210. Ilkjaer S, Bach LF, Nielsen PA, et al: Effect of preoperative oral dextromethorphan on immediate and late postoperative pain and hyperalgesia after total abdominal hysterectomy. Pain 2000;86:19–24.

211. Weinbroum AA, Gorodezky A, Niv D, et al: Dextromethorphan attenuation of postoperative pain and primary and secondary thermal hyperalgesia. Can J Anaesth 2001;48:167–174.

212. Wu CT, Yu JC, Yeh CC, et al: Preincisional dextromethorphan treatment decreases postoperative pain and opioid requirement after laparoscopic cholecystectomy. Anesth Analg 1999;88:1331–1334.

213. Helmy SA, Bali A: The effect of the preemptive use of the NMDA receptor antagonist dextromethorphan on postoperative analgesic requirements. Anesth Analg 2001;92:739–744.

214. Wu CT, Yu JC, Yeh CC, et al: Postoperative intramuscular dextromethorphan injection provides pain relief and decreases opioid requirement after modified radical mastectomy. Int J Surg Invest 2000;2:145–149.

215. Wadhwa A, Clarke D, Goodchild CS, et al: Large-dose oral dextromethorphan as an adjunct to patient-controlled analgesia with morphine after knee surgery. Anesth Analg 2001;92:448–454.

216. Ilkjaer S, Nielsen PA, Bach LF, et al: The effect of dextromethorphan, alone or in combination with ibuprofen, on postoperative pain after minor gynaecological surgery. Acta Anaesthesiol Scand 2000;44:873–877.

217. Yeh CC, Hot ST, Kong SS, et al: Absence of preemptive analgesic effect of dextromethorphan in total knee replacement under epidural anesthesia. Acta Anaesthesiol Sin 2000;38:187–193.

218. Gottschalk A, Schroeder F, Ufer M, et al: Amantadine, a N-methyl-D-asparate receptor antagonist, does not enhance postoperative analgesia in women undergoing abdominal hysterectomy. Anesth Analg 2001;93:192–196.

219. Snijdelaar DG, Koren G, Katz J: Effects of perioperative oral amantadine on postoperative pain and morphine consumption in patients after radical prostatectomy. Anesthesiology 2004;100:134–141.

220. Segal IS, Jarvis DJ, Duncan SR, et al: Clinical efficacy of oral–transdermal clonidine combinations during the perioperative period. Anesthesiology 1991;74:220–225.

221. Singh H, Liu J, Gaines GY, et al: Effect of oral clonidine and intrathecal fentanyl on tetracaine spinal block. Anesth Analg 1994;79:1113–1116.

222. Milligan KR, Convery PN, Weir P, et al: The efficacy and safety of epidural infusions of levobupivacaine with and without clonidine for postoperative pain relief in patients undergoing total hip replacement. Anesth Analg 2000;91:393–397.

223. Singelyn FJ, Gouverneur JM, Robert A: A minimum dose of clonidine added to mepivacaine prolongs the duration of anesthesia and analgesia after axillary brachial plexus block. Anesth Analg 1996;83:1046–1050.

224. Klamt JG, Garcia LV, Stocche RM, et al: Epidural infusion of clonidine or clonidine plus ropivacaine for postoperative analgesia in children undergoing major abdominal surgery. J Clin Anesth 2003;15:510–514.

225. Santiveri X, Arxer A, Plaja I, et al: Anaesthetic and postoperative analgesic effects of spinal clonidine as an additive to prilocaine in the transurethral resection of urinary bladder tumours. Eur J Anaesthesiol 2002;19:589–593.

226. Jeffs SA, Hall JE, Morris S: Comparison of morphine alone with morphine plus clonidine for postoperative patient-controlled analgesia. Br J Anaesth 2002;89:424–427.

227. Striebel WH, Koenigs DI, Kramer JA: Intravenous clonidine fails to reduce postoperative meperidine requirements. J Clin Anesth 1993;5:221–225.

228. Aho MS, Erkola OA, Scheinin H, et al: Effect of intravenously administered dexmedetomidine on pain after laparoscopic tubal ligation. Anesth Analg 1991;73:112–118.

229. Jaakola ML: Dexmedetomidine premedication before intravenous regional anesthesia in minor outpatient hand surgery. J Clin Anesth 1994;6:204–211.

230. Arain SR, Ebert TJ: The efficacy, side effects, and recovery characteristics of dexmedetomidine versus propofol when used for intraoperative sedation. Anesth Analg 2002;95:461–466.

231. Arain SR, Ruehlow RM, Uhrich TD, et al: The efficacy of dexmedetomidine versus morphine for postoperative analgesia after major inpatient surgery. Anesth Analg 2004;98:153–158.

232. Zárate E, Sá Rêgo MM, White PF, et al: Comparison of adenosine and remifentanil infusions as adjuvants to desflurane anesthesia. Anesthesiology 1999;90:956–963.

233. Fukunaga AF, Alexander GE, Stark CW: Characterization of the analgesic actions of adenosine: comparison of adenosine and remifentanil infusions in patients undergoing major surgical procedures. Pain 2003;101:129–138.

234. Yamamoto S, Yamaguchi H, Sakaguchi M, et al: Preoperative droperidol improved postoperative pain relief in patients undergoing rotator-cuff repair during general anesthesia using intravenous morphine. J Clin Anesth 2003;15:525–529.

235. Kara H, Sahin N, Ulusan V, et al: Magnesium infusion reduces perioperative pain. Eur J Anaesthesiol 2002;19:52–56.

236. Lauretti GR, de Olivera R, Reis MP, et al: Study of three different doses of epidural neostigmine co-administered with lidocaine for postoperative analgesia. Anesthesiology 1999;90:1534–1536.

237. Dirks J, Fredensborg BB, Christensen D, et al: A randomized study of the effects of single-dose gabapentin versus placebo on postoperative pain and morphine consumption after mastectomy. Anesthesiology 2002;97:560–564.

238. Fassoulaki A, Patris K, Sarantopoulos C, et al: The analgesic effect of gabapentin and mexiletine after breast surgery for cancer. Anesth Analg 2002;95:985–991.

239. Dierking G, Duedahl TH, Rasmussen ML, et al: Effects of gabapentin on postoperative morphine consumption and pain after abdominal hysterectomy: A randomized, double-blind trial. Acta Anaesthesiol Scand 2004;48:322–326.

240. Turan A, Karamanlioglu B, Memis D, et al: Analgesic effects of gabapentin after spinal surgery. Anesthesiology 2004;100:935–938.

241. Rorarius MG, Mennander S, Suominen P, et al: Gabapentin for the prevention of postoperative pain after vaginal hysterectomy. Pain 2004;110:175–181.

242. Dahl JB, Mathiesen O, Moiniche S: "Protective premedication": An option with gabapentin and related drugs? A review of gabapentin and pregabalin in the treatment of post-operative pain. Acta Anaesthesiol Scand 2004;48:1130–1136.

243. Levaux C, Bonhomme V, Dewandre PY, et al: Effect of intraoperative magnesium sulphate on pain relief and patient comfort after major lumbar orthopaedic surgery. Anaesthesia 2003;58:131–135.

244. Bhatia A, Kashyap L, Pawar DK, et al: Effect of intraoperative magnesium infusion on perioperative analgesia in open cholecystectomy. J Clin Anesth 2004;16:262–5.

245. Feld JM, Laurito CE, Beckerman M, et al: Non-opioid analgesia improves pain relief and decreases sedation after gastric bypass surgery. Can J Anaesth 2003;50:336–341.

246. Ko S-H, Lim H-R, Kim D-C, et al: Magnesium sulfate does not reduce postoperative analgesic requirements. Anesthesiology 2001;95:640–646.

247. Buvanendran A, McCarthy RJ, Kroin JS, et al: Intrathecal magnesium prolongs fentanyl analgesia: a prospective, randomized, controlled trial. Anesth Analg 2002;95:661–666.

248. Tan P-H, Kuo J-H, Liu K, et al: Efficacy of intrathecal neostigmine for the relief of postinguinal herniorrhaphy pain. Acta Anaesthesiol Scand 2000;44:1056–1060.

249. Lauretti GR, de Loivera R, Perez MV, et al: Postoperative analgesia by intraarticular and epidural neostigmine following knee surgery. J Clin Anesth 2000;12:444–448.

250. Nakayama M, Ichinose H, Nakabayashi K, et al: Analgesic effect of epidural neostigmine after abdominal hysterectomy. J Clin Anesth 2001;13:86–89.

251. Turan A, Memis D, Basaran UN, et al: Caudal ropivacaine and neostigmine in pediatric surgery. Anesthesiology 2003;98:719–722.

252. Abdulatif M, El-Sanabary M: Caudal neostigmine, bupivacaine, and their combination for postoperative pain management alter hypospadias surgery in children. Anesth Analg 2002;95:1215–1218.

253. Almeida RA, Lauretti GR, Mattos AL: Antinociceptive effect of low-dose intrathecal neostigmine combined with intrathecal morphine following gynecologic surgery. Anesthesiology 2003;98:495–498.

254. Omais M, Lauretti GR, Paccola CA: Epidural morphine and neostigmine for postoperative analgesia after orthopedic surgery. Anesth Analg 2002;95:1698–1701.

255. Tan PH, Chia YY, Lo Y, et al: Intrathecal bupivacaine with morphine or neostigmine for postoperative analgesia alter total knee replacement surgery. Can J Anaesth 2001;48:551–556.

256. Lauretti GR, Oliveira AP, Juliano MC, et al: Transdermal nitroglycerine enhances spinal neostigmine postoperative analgesia following gynecological surgery. Anesthesiology 2000;93:943–946.

257. Kaya FN, Sahin S, Owen MD, et al: Epidural neostigmine produces analgesia but also sedation in women after cesarean delivery. Anesthesiology 2004;100:381–385.

258. Campbell FA, Tramer MR, Carroll D, et al: Are cannabinoids an effective and safe treatment option in the management of pain? A qualitative systematic review. BJM 2001;323:13–16.

259. Buggy DJ, Toogood L, Maric S, et al: Lack of analgesic efficacy of oral delta-9-tetrahydrocannabinol in postoperative pain. Pain 2003;106:169–172.

260. Tarnow P, Cassuto J, Jonsson A, et al: Postoperative analgesia by D-myo-inositol-1,2,6-trisphosphate in patients undergoing cholecystectomy. Anesth Analg 1998;86:107–110.

261. White PF, Li S, Chiu JW: Electroanalgesia: its role in acute and chronic pain management. Anesth Analg 2001;92:505–513.

262. White PF: Electroanalgesia: Does it have a place in the routine management of acute an chronic pain? Anesth Analg 2004;98:1197–1198.

263. Wang B, Tang J, White PF, et al: Effect of the intensity of transcutaneous acupoint electrical stimulation on the postoperative analgesic requirement. Anesth Analg 1997;85:406–13.

264. Hamza MA, White PF, Ahmed HE, et al: Effect of the frequency of transcutaneous electrical nerve stimulation on the postoperative opioid analgesic requirement and recovery profile. Anesthesiology 1999;91:1232–1238.

265. Jensen JE, Conn RR, Hazelrigg G, et al: The use of transcutaneous neural stimulation and isokinetic testing in arthroscopic knee surgery. Am J Sports Med 1985;13:27–33.

266. Rakel B, Frantz R: Effectiveness of transcutaneous electrical nerve stimulation on postoperative pain with movement. J Pain 2003;4:455–464.

267. Carroll D, Tramer M, McQuay H, et al: Randomization is important in studies with pain outcomes: Systematic review of transcutaneous electrical nerve stimulation in acute postoperative pain. Br J Anaesth 1996;77:798–803.

268. Chen L, Tang J, White PF, et al: The effect of the location of transcutaneous electrical nerve stimulation on postoperative opioid analgesic requirement: acupoint versus non-acupoint stimulation. Anesth Analg 1998;87:1129–1134.

269. Lin JG, Lo MW, Wen YR, et al: The effect of high and low frequency electroacupuncture in pain after lower abdominal surgery. Pain 2002;99:509–514.

270. Kotani N, Hashimoto H, Sato Y, et al: Preoperative intradermal acupuncture reduces postoperative pain, nausea and vomiting, analgesic requirement, and sympathoadrenal responses. Anesthesiology 2001;95:359–356.

271. Sakurai M, Suleman MI, Morioka N, et al: Minute sphere acupressure does not reduce postoperative pain with morphine consumption. Anesth Analg 2003;96:493–497.

272. Tovar EA, Roethe RA, Weissig MD, et al: One-day admission for lung lobectomy: an incidental result of a clinical pathway. Ann Thorac Surg 1998;65:803–806.

273. Hashish I, Hai HK, Harvey W, et al: Reduction of postoperative pain and swelling by ultrasound treatment: A placebo effect. Pain 1988;33:303–311.

274. Gam AN, Thorsen H, Lonnberg F: The effect of low-level laser therapy on musculoskeletal pain: a meta-analysis. Pain 1993;52:63–66.

275. Pavlin DJ, Chen C, Penaloza DA, et al: Pain as a factor complicating recovery and discharge after ambulatory surgery. Anesth Analg 2003;97:1627–1632.

276. Macario A, Weinger M, Carney S, et al: Which clinical anesthesia outcomes are important to avoid? The perspective of patients. Anesth Analg 1999;89:652–658.

277. Coloma M, Duffy LL, White PF, et al: Dexamethasone facilitates discharge after outpatient anorectal surgery. Anesth Analg 2001;92:85–88.

278. Aasboe V, Raeder JC, Groegaard B: Betamethasone reduces postoperative pain and nausea after ambulatory surgery. Anesth Analg 1998;87:319–323.

279. Kehlet H, Wilmore DW: Multimodal strategies to improve surgical outcome. Am J Surg 2002;183:630–641.

78

Acute Pain Service: Organization, Function, & Implementation

Narinder Rawal, MD, PhD

INTRODUCTION

Adequate perioperative analgesia is essential for the reduction of postoperative morbidity[1–4] and mortality.[2] Inadequately treated postoperative pain delays patient discharge and recovery and results in an inability to participate in rehabilitation programs, leading to poor patient outcomes. Recent studies[5] show that pain is inadequately treated despite the availability of drugs and techniques for pain management. The problem of inadequate pain relief is usually due to the lack of an appropriate department or service that utilizes available expertise and pharmacologic options, rather than the development of new medications or pain management modalities.

Although several authors in the late 1970s advocated the introduction of pain management teams to assume the responsibility for teaching and training in postoperative pain management, almost a decade passed before specialized in-hospital postoperative pain services eventually emerged. Recently, various medical and health care organizations have recommended the widespread introduction of an acute pain service (APS).[6–12] Having an APS is a prerequisite for accreditation for training by the Royal College of Anaesthetists in the United Kingdom and by the Australian and New Zealand College of Anaesthetists.[13]

Table 78–1 shows the prevalence of such services in Europe, North America, Australia, and New Zealand.[13–27]

Table 78–1.			
National Surveys of the Prevalence of Acute Pain Services			
Study	**Region/Country**	**Survey Year**	**Prevalence (n (%))**
Zimmerman[14]	Canada	1991	24/47 (53)
Goucke[15]	Australia, New Zealand	1992/1993	37/111 (33)
Rawal[16]	Europe	1993	37/105 (34)
Davies[17]	United Kingdom	1994	77/221 (35)
Windsor[18]	United Kingdom	1994 1990	151/354 (43) 10/358 (3)
Merry[19]	New Zealand	1994 1996	12/62 (19) 17/22d
Harmer[20]	United Kingdom	1995e	97/221 (44)
Ready[21]	United States	1995	236/324 (73)
Warfield[22]	United States	1995	126/300 (42)
Neugebauer[23]	Germany	1997	390/1000 (39)
Stamer[24]	Germany	1999	161/446 (36)
O'Higgins[25]	United Kingdom	2000	>49%
Goldstein[26]	Canada	2004	50/62 (93)
Powell[27]	United Kingdom	2004	270/325 (83)

Although the number of hospitals with an APS has increased worldwide, standards with respect to the structure and function of an APS are still lacking.[24] The nature of service provided, the staffing and facilities, the training and competence of personnel, and the effectiveness of an APS vary greatly. Many hospitals consider their current pain service adequate for their patients' needs, although they have only some but not all of the essential components of an APS.[20]

In 2004, a Canadian survey showed that the percentage of academic hospitals with an APS increased from 53% in 1993 to 92% in 2004.[26] However, an APS with anesthesiologists as sole pain management providers decreased from 36% to 22% in the same time span because of growing clinical demands and a reduced number of anesthesiologists. Only 44% of centers had a designated group of APS physicians, whereas nursing representation was 55%. An ongoing prospective data collection system was present in 29% of the hospitals surveyed. No information was obtained about the management of acute pain in patients who were not followed by an APS, which represented the majority of postoperative patients.[26] Furthermore, recent evidence indicates that some APSs provide only a limited service due to financial or logistical problems. These findings suggest that there is a compelling need to

develop APS standards with well-defined criteria for evaluating performance and comparing with national benchmarks.[27]

STRUCTURE & FUNCTION OF AN ACUTE PAIN SERVICE

The original organizational model for managing postoperative pain was largely catalyzed by an APS developed in the United States[21] and gradually introduced in the United Kingdom during the 1990s after the landmark report "Pain After Surgery."[7] However, implementation of APSs in hospitals since 1990 has been piecemeal and haphazard, with reports providing evidence of significant variation within and among hospitals in the structure and function of the service.[27]

Most major hospitals in the United States have an anesthesiology-based APS. The acute pain management team usually consists of staff and resident anesthesiologists, specially trained nurses, pharmacists, and physical therapists. Secretarial and billing personnel are also a part of a United States-style APS. Members of the pain management team regularly visit patients under the care of an APS. The anesthesiologist-based APS organization model usually provides a "high-tech" pain management service to patients receiving epidural analgesia or intravenous patient controlled analgesia (IVPCA). However, the costs of the United States-style APS are high and are being increasingly questioned by health care payers. In many institutions, surgeons have assumed management of IVPCA.

The need for new APS models that provide effective pain relief for all surgical patients is clear. As discussed later, the nurse-based, anesthesiologist-supervised APS model is an alternative to the conventional physician-based APS model. The United Kingdom Joint Colleges of Surgery and Anesthesia Working Party report[7] recommended that a multidisciplinary team including specialist nursing staff should run the APS. They further recommended that the APS should assume day-to-day responsibility for the management of postoperative pain, in-service training for nursing and medical staff, and research and auditing. Similar recommendations have been made by national expert committees in Australia,[6] the United States,[8,10] Germany,[9] Sweden,[11] and in an updated form by the American Society of Anesthesiologists (ASA) Task Force.[12] In the United Kingdom, two national surveys[14,15] were conducted to determine the extent to which the recommendations of the Working Party report had been implemented. Unfortunately, there appeared to be a large degree of variation in what was thought to constitute an APS, and some hospitals had only some of the elements recommended by the Working Party report.[18,20]

An ideal APS organization should provide optimal pain management for every surgical patient, including children and those undergoing outpatient surgical procedures. The Joint Commission for Accreditation of Healthcare Organizations (JCAHO), an independent not-for-profit organization that sets health care standards in the United States, recognizes the need for optimal pain management. JCAHO requires that hospitals assess, treat, and document pain, assures the competence of staff in pain assessment and management, and educate patients and their families about effective pain management. Hospitals must also consider ambulatory surgery patients' needs for information and provide guidelines for pain management after discharge from the hospital.[28]

One of the most important activities of an APS is to provide an ongoing review of institutional policies and practices regarding pain control and the mechanisms to deal with problems as they arise. The members of the APS should meet regularly to provide feedback and discuss opportunities for improvement. Such meetings are important for assessing the efficiency of the APS, highlighting practical problems, and finding solutions for inadequately functioning aspects of the APS.[29]

Although each institution may have different requirements for their own APS, modifications of published models may be necessary to accommodate local conditions. The main components of an APS should include the following:

1. Designated personnel responsible for providing 24-h APS (in small hospitals one or two individuals may be adequate).

2. Regular pain assessment (with appropriate scales for children and patients with cognitive impairment) at rest and movement, the maintenance of pain scores below a predetermined threshold, and regular documentation of pain scores ("make pain visible").

3. Active cooperation with surgeons and ward nurses for the development of protocols and critical pathways to achieve preset goals for postoperative mobilization and rehabilitation.

4. Ongoing teaching programs for ward nurses for the provision of safe and cost-effective analgesic techniques.

5. Patient education about pain monitoring and treatment options, goals, benefits, and adverse effects.

6. Regular audits of the cost-effectiveness of analgesic techniques and in- and outpatient service satisfaction.[28]

DOES AN ACUTE PAIN SERVICE IMPROVE OUTCOME?

It is believed that the introduction of an APS has led to an increase in the appropriate use of specialized analgesic techniques, such as IVPCA opioid, epidural, and perineural analgesia. The implementation of these techniques may represent a true advance in improving analgesia and patient well-being and in reducing postoperative morbidity.[12,13] An APS can reduce analgesic gaps that occur during the transition from IVPCA or epidural analgesia to oral analgesic therapy. Although evaluating the safety of analgesic techniques is an important objective of an APS, its role in preventing and reducing adverse events has not been well established. Wheatley and colleagues[30] reported a decrease from 1.3% to 0.4% in the incidence of lower respiratory tract infection after the introduction of an APS. Tsui and coworkers[31] investigated the benefits of an APS program in patients undergoing esophagectomy. The patients were cared for either by an APS ($n = 299$) or received conventional analgesic therapy in a non-APS setting ($n = 279$). In the APS group, patients received postoperative epidural or systemic opioid infusion, and the non-APS group received intermittent intramuscular injections of morphine. The APS group reported a significantly lower incidence of pulmonary and cardiac complications and a shorter hospital stay.[31] Other studies,[13,32,33] have not substantiated these findings.

Werner and associates[13] evaluated the effects of an APS on postoperative outcome in 44 audits and four clinical trials, which included 84,097 patients. Implementation of an APS was associated with a significant decrease in pain intensity. Additionally, the introduction of an APS was possibly associated with less postoperative nausea and vomiting and a decreased incidence of urinary retention. However, clear conclusions about the side effects of analgesic modalities, patient satisfaction, or postoperative morbidity could not be drawn due to a large variability in the studies regarding APS function and services provided.[13] McDonnell and colleagues[34] found that the implementation of an APS was associated with initiatives that are hallmarks of good postoperative pain management, but did not explore the effect of an APS on postoperative outcomes. Hospital administrators are more likely to invest in an APS if implementation of such a service results in measurable improvements in patient outcomes at an affordable cost.

COST-EFFECTIVENESS OF AN ACUTE PAIN SERVICE

Cost-benefit analyses are necessary to justify the need for an APS, but no such studies are available. Cost analyses of acute pain management are impeded by the lack of a well-defined baseline and outcome assessment. There is no valid method of assigning financial costs to differing levels of analgesia, and the effect of various analgesic techniques on economic outcomes has not been adequately examined.[13]

Cost-effectiveness analyses of postoperative pain management must consider not only the direct costs associated with analgesic drugs; devices; nursing and physician time; and duration of stay in the postanesthesia care unit, intensive care unit, or surgical ward, as well as postoperative morbidity; but also the indirect costs of improved analgesia and patient satisfaction.[13]

Brodner and coworkers[35] showed that the introduction of a multimodal program with improved pain relief, stress reduction, and early tracheal extubation decreased the number of patients who required a stay in an intensive care unit in the immediate postoperative period after major surgery. The hospital realized cost savings because of faster discharge from the high-dependency areas.[35] In an effort to reduce APS-related costs, several authors have advocated a low-cost, nurse-based, anesthesiologist-supervised model[5,36–38] as an alternative to the more expensive physician-based

multidisciplinary APS.[38–41] Currently, there is no evidence that a physician-based multidisciplinary APS is superior to a specialist nurse-based, anesthesiologist-supervised APS. Although cost-benefit studies are difficult to perform, there is a compelling need for such studies.

STRATEGIES FOR IMPLEMENTING AN ACUTE PAIN SERVICE

It is becoming increasingly clear that physicians must develop simple and less-expensive APS models for improving the quality of postoperative analgesia for every surgical patient (including day surgery patients) in a cost-effective way. At Orebro University Hospital in Orebro, Sweden, a pain specialist nurse-based, anesthesiologist-supervised model has been successfully implemented.[5] The first step to initiating a pain management program is organizing an interdisciplinary team of motivated individuals who represent diverse professional skills and approaches to patient care.

The anesthesiologist is responsible for both anesthetic care and postoperative pain management and selects the appropriate analgesic modality based on the departmental policy of using the "acute pain analgesic ladder" (Figure 78–1). A recent ASA practice guidelines publication[12] recommends similar therapeutic strategy. The publication suggests that, unless contraindicated, all patients should receive an around-the-clock regimen of nonsteroidal antiinflammatory drugs, cyclooxygenase inhibitors, or acetaminophen. In addition, anesthesiologists should consider performing regional blockade with local anesthetics. The choice of medication, dose, route, and duration of therapy however should be individualized.[12] During regular working hours, an anesthesiologist should be available for consultation and emergencies,

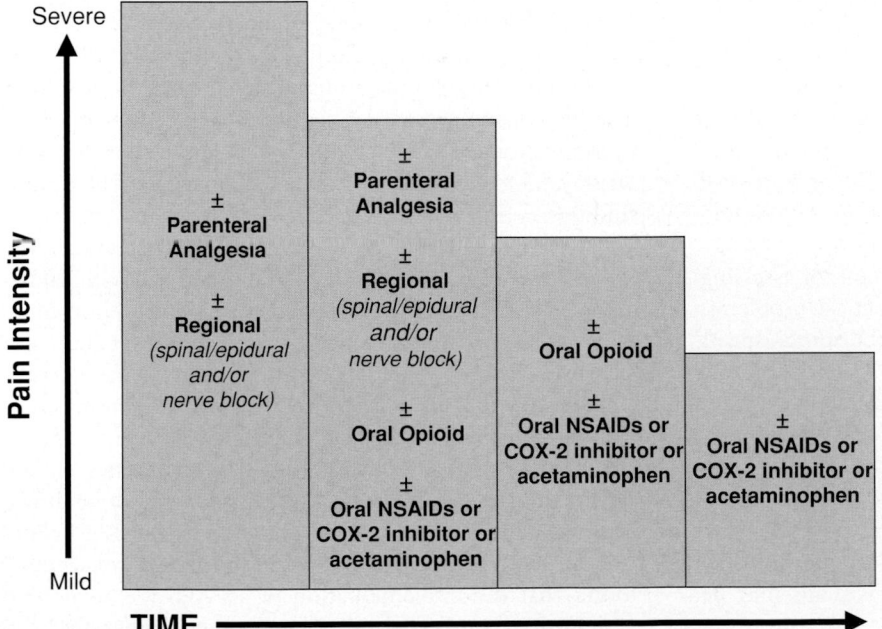

Figure 78–1. Management of postoperative (acute) pain: Choice of techniques and drugs based on the severity and timing of surgery. Acetaminophen is given to all patients irrespective of pain intensity or type of surgery.

Table 78–2.

Organization of Acute Pain Services at Orebro University Hospital, Orebro, Sweden

Healthcare Member Pain "Representatives"	Responsibilities
Director Acute Pain Service	Responsible for coordinating hospital-wide acute pain service and education
Anesthesiologists	Responsible for pre-, intra-, and postoperative care (including postoperative pain) for their surgical section
Pain "representative" ward surgeons	Responsible for pain management for their surgical ward; helps integration of analgesia techniques into clinical pathways for individual surgical procedures
Pain "representative" day/night nurses	Responsible for implementation of pain management guidelines and monitoring on the ward
Acute pain nurse (specialist pain nurse)	Daily rounds of all surgical wards
	Data collection for audits Trouble shoots technical problems Refers problem patients to section anesthesiologist (link between surgical ward and anesthesiologist) Bedside teaching of ward nurses

and after hours, the anesthesiologist on-call should assume the same function.

A specialist acute pain nurse (APN) plays an important role in the APS. Table 78–2 describes the duties of an APN, which include making daily visits to patients on all surgical wards. Postoperative pain therapy of individual patients is based on standard orders and protocols developed jointly by the anesthesiologist, surgeon, and ward nurse. The APN facilitates collaboration among anesthesiologists, surgeons, and nurses on surgical wards. The clinical nurse specialists or APN-educated ward nurses provide the necessary support and help initiate and supervise administration of analgesia, which empowers the ward nurses the flexibility to administer analgesics without delay and consult an anesthesiologist only when necessary.

Upgrading the Role of Ward Nurses

The APS model at Orebro University Hospital is based on the concept that postoperative pain relief can be greatly improved by providing in-service training for surgical nursing staff about the best use of IVPCA opioids and regional analgesia techniques.[5] Nurses on surgical wards are responsible for assessing the pain intensity, administering prescribed analgesic treatments, monitoring efficacy and adverse effects of treatment, and monitoring the extent of regional blockade. At Orebro University Hospital, ward nurses administer IV opioids, set up IVPCA devices, manage epidural analgesia, and change IVPCA and epidural analgesia drug administration parameters (within prescribed limits). Of note, the nurses did not have permission to do this at the time of implementation of an APS in 1991. Regular teaching and daily visits by the APN have resulted in effective and safe pain relief, confirmed by the annual audit data.

Patients are treated on the basis of standard orders and protocols developed jointly by the chiefs of anesthesiology, surgery, and nursing. Pain representatives meet every 3 months to discuss and implement necessary improvements.

The pain representatives from each surgical ward meet regularly with the anesthesiologist and APN to discuss improvements based on annual audit data.

Nurses must play a greater role in order to improve postoperative pain management on surgical wards. In many institutions, ward nurses cannot administer IV opioids, they are required to call an APS physician to obtain approval for administration of parenteral narcotics, and IVPCA and epidural analgesia dose adjustments. This is time-consuming, cost-ineffective, often unnecessary and leads to delay in alleviating pain. The restrictions for ward nurses are surprising in view of the increasing trends toward self-treatment by patients. Outside of hospitals, diabetic children self-administer insulin, and cancer patients self-administer epidural and intrathecal analgesics. There is increased acceptance of the use of home ventilators, home dialysis, home-PCA devices, perineural catheters, and opioids in noncancer pain. In many hospitals worldwide, midwives manage epidural analgesia for labor pain, but ward nurses cannot do the same for postoperative pain. There is convincing evidence from many countries and institutions that, with appropriate teaching and training, ward nurses can monitor and manage analgesic modalities such as IVPCA and epidural analgesia. Nurse education is widely recognized as an important priority in pain management.[5,20,28,29,39] Recent studies[5,20,39,40] have demonstrated the importance of the ward nurses in improving the efficacy of analgesic regimens. Surgeon and ward nurse participation is crucial in this model.

Defining Maximum Acceptable Pain Scores and "Making Pain Visible"

The ward nurse routinely documents the pain intensity of each patient using the Visual Analogue Scale (VAS) every 3 h and documents the adequacy of the treatment on a vital sign chart. The VAS assessment is the cornerstone of the APS model and includes pain at rest and during movement, both before and after an intervention. In the absence of a formal, documented pain assessment, much of the medical and nursing staff believes that patients who do not report pain do not feel pain. Alternatively, nurses inform patients that their pain will be maintained at or below a predefined threshold level (generally 3 on a 10-point VAS) and that pain scores in excess of the threshold will trigger interventions to reduce pain.[28] It is essential to define a maximally acceptable pain score and routinely document pain intensity before and after analgesic treatment. A VAS above 3 is promptly treated. Documentation also provides data for the audit and facilitates review and improvement of care. The APS should not ignore quality assurance measures.

Role of the Surgeon

Although all guidelines emphasize the importance of a multidisciplinary APS as a tool for improving postoperative pain relief, there is no distinction in the literature about the roles of individual members of the multidisciplinary team. The role of the surgeon is far more important than that of the pharmacist. An APS without the cooperation of the surgeon is doomed to failure. The surgeon must participate in the development of protocols for analgesic techniques, since most surgical patients do not need epidural analgesia or IVPCA techniques for effective analgesia. This is particularly true for patients having outpatient surgery, which includes 70% of all surgical operations. In this setting, the surgeon remains primarily responsible for clinical pathways to achieve preset goals for postoperative mobilization and rehabilitation to reduce hospital stay. In addition, the surgeons must assist in improving ward nurse compliance for the implementation of APS goals, including frequent pain assessment and documentation.[28]

Education

An APS must develop and implement educational programs for patients and health care providers. The educational process begins at the time of patient preoperative evaluation. Traditionally, patients assume that pain after surgery is inevitable, and are unlikely to be aware of the standard of care they can expect to receive and the potential benefits of effective pain relief. Education includes explaining the importance of adequate pain control, the commitment of hospital staff to providing effective pain control, the options available for managing postoperative pain, practical information about how to report pain intensity (eg, the VAS or a numerical scale), and how to participate in the pain management plan.[5,28,29]

Specialist Pain Nurse-Based APS: Does It Work?

In the APS model described, the only additional cost is that of two APNs. Orebro University Hospital performs approximately 16,000 surgical procedures each year. The design of this low-cost APS model benefits all patients (approximately €3 per patient, excluding drug and equipment costs). Regular audits have confirmed that the Orebro University Hospital APS achieves its goals of pain control in over 90% of patients. Anesthesiologist consultations have substantially decreased over time; currently it is in the range of one to two consultations per week.

The general principles for this organization model have been accepted and recommended for Swedish hospitals by the Swedish Medical Association.[11] Based on this model, Bardiau and associates[39] described the implementation of an APS in a 1005-bed Belgian general hospital, out of which 240 were surgical beds. The process was divided into eight stages over a 3-year period. This program anticipated an improvement in postoperative pain relief for all surgical inpatients and in the maintenance of this service over time. First, a pain management committee was formed, including anesthesiologists, surgeons, pharmacists, and nurses. Next, the committee conducted a survey of nurses' attitudes and knowledge of postoperative care using an anonymous 35-item questionnaire. Then, a 10-cm VAS scale was introduced for routine assessment of pain intensity. Over a 6-month period a baseline survey (survey I) was designed to analyze the current practices of pain treatment and a specialist nurse-based, anesthesiologist-supervised APS model was implemented. The pain management committee developed standardized treatment protocols, which included regular assessments of pain intensity using the VAS every 4 h and documentation of treatment efficacy by the APN, as well as the use of analgesic regimens. Three months later, a second survey (survey II) of 671 patients was conducted to assess the effect of an APS implementation. Finally, a third confirmation survey (survey III) of 2383 patients was conducted to investigate whether the initial improvements were maintained.

The initial survey of nurses identified the lack in knowledge and skills in assessing and managing pain effectively because of the absence of nursing guidelines and pain treatment protocols. However, pain relief improved significantly after the implementation of the APS. Interestingly, acetaminophen consumption increased significantly, whereas the use of nonsteroidal antiinflammatory drugs increased from 20% in survey I to 64% and 99% in surveys II and III, respectively. At the same time, opioid consumption decreased. The authors concluded that the standardization of analgesic therapies, nursing practice, and regular feedback on performance are essential factors to improving pain management. Organizing teams of anesthesiologists, surgeons, and nurses is necessary for this improvement. Cost-benefit analyses are now needed to further substantiate these results.[39]

AUDITS & CONTINUOUS QUALITY IMPROVEMENT OF THE ACUTE PAIN SERVICE

An audit is a monitoring and evaluation process that helps to recognize situations on which attention should be focused, and the analysis of specific aspects of clinical practice leads to the setting of standards against which future practice can be measured and evaluated. Regular audits will show whether the goals of an APS are achieved.[28] Audits of the APS are necessary for assessing the quality of pain management and for evaluating the adverse events of analgesic techniques such as IVPCA opioid, epidural analgesia, and peripheral nerve blocks. Such audits show problems with these techniques and the need for change in practice. An audit was performed in the northern and Yorkshire regions in the United Kingdom to assess postoperative pain management outcomes.[40] All patients undergoing surgical procedures over a 2-week period in 16 hospitals, ranging from large teaching hospitals with 5500 beds to smaller district general hospitals with fewer than 400 beds, were included in the study. Pain scores at rest and during movement were obtained in the recovery room, and at 24 h and 7 days postoperatively. Pain management modality data were also collected. The results showed that a large percentage of patients reported unacceptable levels of pain despite changes in practice and the development of an APS. Interestingly sites with pain management teams (ie, an APS) did not provide better pain management than those without an APS.[40] Stamer and colleagues[24] reviewed the literature on APS and concluded that despite the guidelines, most APS worldwide did not meet basic quality criteria, which were defined as regular assessment and documentation of pain scores at least once per day, written protocols for pain management, personnel assignment for an APS, and policies for postoperative pain management during nights and weekends. These studies emphasize the need for regular audits to address the problems of an APS and to justify the cost of the service. Unfortunately, the literature on APS audits and their effect is limited.

FUTURE PERSPECTIVES

The aims of the APS have expanded to promote postoperative comfort, rehabilitation, and quality of life. The widening of objectives, together with continuous elevation of standards and expectations, has placed a burden on an old order that is often ill equipped to serve the new ambitions.[41] Evidence that the standards of pain control are improving can be found in the way that pain is assessed. As pain control has improved, its evaluation has become more demanding. Although the goal of pain management remains a reduction in pain intensity, it is no longer sufficient to measure efficacy at rest but also on mobilization and on coughing for abdominal and thoracic surgery. Expanding the multidisciplinary approach could extend the role of an APS through the entire postoperative course, including patient rehabilitation. Such widening of the role might improve not only overall patient care, but also convince hospital managers that an APS is worthy of support.[41]

Central to concerns about after-hours care is the debate over whether the key role of an APS is to provide hands-on direct patient care or to provide a resource for education and training and the promotion of good clinical practice. Powell

and coworkers[27] argue that if an APS is well resourced and able to institute the widespread organizational and attitude required to overcome barriers to pain management, even a daytime APS would promote and maintain good clinical practice over the 24-h period.[27] Since many patients perceive nighttime pain as more severe,[42] the current "office hours" model of an APS that covers approximately 50 h of the 168 h in a week leaves many patients in pain.[27]

In the United Kingdom, there has been a debate about the future direction of the APS. Suggested developments include integrating the APS with other pain services (ie, chronic and palliative care), aligning the APS with critical care outreach teams, and developing comprehensive postoperative rehabilitation programs that would include an APS.[43] Integration of an APS with other pain services may not be ideal because the practical issues related to the management of postoperative pain differ from those related to chronic pain. The APS anesthesiologist is involved with the pre-, intra-, and postoperative phases, including performing, teaching, and training of regional anesthesia. However, not all chronic pain services include anesthesiologists. Even if the chronic pain physicians are anesthesiologists, they are rarely involved with the delivery of anesthesia and may not be familiar with the day-to-day practical issues of postoperative pain management on surgical wards. It is unclear whether the problems of postoperative pain can be solved by the development of a more comprehensive service.[27] At Orebro University Hospital, the APS is separate from the chronic pain service.

The APS plays a unique educational role, which can be expanded as other health care providers are incorporated into the team. The key role of the APS is to provide a resource for education and training, and promote effective pain control based on algorithms and protocols developed jointly by anesthesiologists, surgeons, and nurses. These protocols must be integrated into predefined clinical pathways for each surgical procedure. Furthermore, the integration of newly developed evidence-based, procedure-specific guidelines into an APS protocol should further optimize postoperative analgesia and outcome.[44–47] These guidelines allow practitioners to modify analgesic therapies based on local circumstances (eg, regulatory issues and the cost and availability of drugs).

SUMMARY

In summary, pain-free recovery is important for surgical patients, and the alleviation of pain contributes to improved clinical outcomes. Ineffective treatment of postoperative pain continues to be a major problem internationally. It is clear that the introduction of an APS has increased the awareness that adequate postoperative pain management contributes to the well-being of all patients. It is increasingly evident that an organized multidisciplinary team of dedicated physicians and nurses is a fundamental prerequisite for an effective APS program. Although controlled trials are not available, observational studies suggest that an APS is effective in reducing postoperative pain and analgesic adverse effects. In addition, the integration of the newer Internet-based, procedure-specific initiatives that provide evidence-based recommendations and allow the clinician to select appropriate analgesic techniques will inevitably further improve the efficacy of an APS.

The number of hospitals with an APS is increasing, but there is no consensus regarding the optimal structure and function of these services. The selection of an appropriate organizational structure may be as important to the success of the APS as the choice of analgesic modalities. In addition, there is an obvious need for developing well-defined criteria for evaluating the performance of an APS at an individual hospital and comparing it with national standards. It is important to recognize that the APS must tailor quality improvement to the local environment, because no single approach is guaranteed to be successful in all settings. An APS needs to document its value and demonstrate the justification of allotted resources and expertise. Finally, the integration of effective analgesia into surgical care is mandatory to improving outcome and will depend on close cooperation between surgeons and anesthesiologists.

References

1. Ballantyne J, Carr D, deFerranti S, et al: The comparative effects of postoperative analgesic therapies on pulmonary outcome: Cumulative meta-analyses of randomized, controlled trials. Anesth Analg 1998;86:598–612.

2. Rodgers A, Walker N, Schug S, et al: Reduction of postoperative mortality and morbidity with epidural or spinal anaesthesia: Results from overview of randomised trials. BMJ 2000;321:1493–1497.

3. Kehlet H, Holte K: Effect of postoperative analgesia reduces on surgical outcome. Br J Anaesth 2001;87:62–72.

4. Beattie W, Badner N, Choi P: Epidural analgesia reduces postoperative myocardial infarction: A meta-analysis. Anesth Analg 2001;93:853–858.

5. Rawal N, Berggren L: Organization of acute pain services—A low cost model. Pain 1994;57:117–123.

6. *Acute Pain Management Scientific Evidence.* National Health and Medical Research Council of Australia. Canberra, Australia, 1999.

7. *Pain After Surgery.* Surgeons of the Royal College (ed). Royal College of Surgeons and College of Anaesthetists Working Party on Pain after Surgery. London, 1990.

8. *Acute Pain Management: Operative and Medical Procedures and Trauma.* Agency for Health Care Policy and Research. US Department of Health and Human Services, Publication # 92-0032. Rockville (MD): AHCPR Publications, 1992.

9. Wulf H, Neugebauer E, Maier C: *Die behandlung akuter perioperativer und posttraumatischer schmerzen: Empfehlungen einer interdisziplinaeren expertenkommission.* G. Thieme, 1997 [in German].

10. *Hospital Accreditation Standards.* Joint Commission on Accreditation of Healthcare Organizations. 1992. Oakbrook, 2001.

11. *Behandling av postoperativ smirta rokTopp, guidelines, and quality indicators.* Svenska Lhkaresallskapet [Swedish Medical Association] Forlagshuset Gothia AB, Stockholm. Available at: www.gothia.nu. 2001.

12. Practice Guidelines for Acute Pain Management in the Perioperative Setting: An Updated Report by the American Society of Anesthesiologists Task Force on Acute Pain Management. Anesthesiology 2004;100:1573–1581.

13. Werner M, Seholm L, Rotbell-Nielsen P, et al. Does an acute pain service improve postoperative outcome? Anesth Analg 2002;95:1361–1372.

14. Zimmerman D, Stewart J: Postoperative pain management and acute pain service activity in Canada. Can J Anaesth 1993;40:568–575.

15. Goucke C, Owe H: Acute pain management in Australia and New Zealand. Anaesth Intensive Care 1995;23:715–717.

16. Rawal N, Allvin R for The EuroPain Acute Pain Working Party: Acute pain services in Europe: A 17-nation survey of 105 hospitals. Eur J Anaesthesiol 1998;15:354–363.

17. Davies K: Findings of a national survey of acute pain services. Nurs Times 1996;92:31–34.

18. Windsor A, Glynn C, Mason D. National provision of acute pain services. Anaesthesia 1996;51:228–231.

19. Merry A, Jugde M, Ready B: Acute pain services in New Zealand hospitals: A survey. N Z Med J 1997;110:233–235.

20. Harmer M, Davies K: The effect of education, assessment and a standardized prescription on postoperative pain management: The value of clinical audit in the establishment of acute pain services. Anaesthesia 1998;53:424.

21. Ready L: How many acute pain services are there in the United States, and who is managing patient-controlled analgesia (letter)? Anesthesiology 1995;82:322.

22. Warfield C, Kahn C: Acute pain management: Programs in US hospitals and experiences and attitudes among US adults. Anesthesiology 1995;83:1090–1094.

23. Neugebauer E, Hempel K, Sauerland S, et al: The status of perioperative pain therapy in Germany: Results of a representative, anonymous survey of 1,000 surgical clinics—Pain Study Group. Chirurg 1998;69:461–466.

24. Stamer U, Mpasios N, Stuber F, et al: A survey of acute pain services in Germany and a discussion of international survey data. Reg Anesth Pain Med 2002;27:125–131.

25. O'Higgins F, Tuckey J: Thoracic epidural anaesthesia and analgesia: United Kingdom practice. Acta Anaesthesiol Scand 2000;44:1087–1092.

26. Goldstein D, Van Den Kerkhof E, Blaine W: Acute pain management services have progressed albeit insufficiently in Canadian academic hospitals. Can J Anesth 2004;51:231–235.

27. Powell A, Davies H, Bannister J, et al: Rhetoric and reality on acute pain services in the UK: A national postal questionnaire survey. Br J Anaesth 2004;92:689–693.

28. Rawal N: Acute Pain Services revisited—Good from far, far from good? [Editorial]. Reg Anesth Pain Med 2002;27:117–121.

29. Blau W, Dalton A, Lindley C: Organization of hospital-based acute pain management programs. South Med J 1999;92:465–471.

30. Wheatley R, Madej T, Jackson U, et al: The first year's experience of an acute pain service. Br J Anaesth 1991;67:353–359.

31. Tsui S, Law S, Fok M, et al: Postoperative analgesia reduces mortality and morbidity after esophagectomy. Am J Sing 1997;173:472–478.

32. Lempa M, Gerards P, Koch G, et al: Efficacy of an acute pain service—A controlled comparative study of hospitals. Langenbecks Arch Chir Suppl Kongressbd 1998;115:673–676.

33. Rose D, Cohen M, Yee D: Changing the practice of pain management. Anesth Analg 1997;84:764–772.

34. McDonnell A, Nicholl J, Read S: Acute Pain Teams in England: current provision and their role in postoperative pain management. J Clin Nurs 2003;12:387–393.

35. Brodner G, Mertes N, Buerkle H, et al. Acute pain management. Analysis, implications, and consequences after prospective experience with 6349 surgical patients. Eur J Anaesthesiol 2000;17:566–575.

36. Coleman S, Booker-Milburn J: Audit of postoperative pain control: Influence of a dedicated acute pain nurse. Anaesthesia 1996;51:1093–1096.

37. Mackintosh C, Bowles S: Evaluation of a nurse-led acute pain service: Can clinical nurse specialists make a difference? J Adv Nurse 1997;25:30–31.

38. Bardiau F, Braeckman M, Seidel L, et al: Effectiveness of an acute pain service inception in a general hospital. J Clin Anesth 1999;11:583–589.

39. Bardiau F, Taviaux N, Albert A, et al: An intervention study to enhance postoperative pain management. Anest Analg 2003;96:179–185.

40. Taverner T. A regional pain management audit. Nurs Times 2003;99:34–37.

41. Bonnet F: Postoperative pain management: A continuing struggle. European Society of Anaesthesiologists Newsletter 2004;17:8–9.

42. Closs S, Briggs M, Everitt V: Implementation of research findings to reduce postoperative pain at night. Int J Nurs Stud 1999;36:21–31.

43. Counsell D: The acute pain service: A model for outreach critical care. Anaesthesia 2001;56:925–926.

44. Rosenquist R, Rosenberg J: Postoperative pain guidelines. Reg Anesth Pain Med 2003;28:279–288.

45. Rowlingson J, Rawal N: Postoperative pain guidelines—Targeted to the site of surgery. Reg Anesth Pain Med 2003;28:265–267.

46. Rawal N, McCloy R for the PROSPECT working group: Incisional and intraperitoneal local anaesthetics in laparoscopic cholecystectomy and abdominal hysterectomy: A systematic review. Reg Anesth Pain Med 2004;29:A307.

47. Fischer B, Camu F for the PROSPECT working group: Comparative benefits of epidural analgesia following hysterectomy and colonic resection. Reg Anesth Pain Med 2004;29:A309.

79

Organization of an Acute Pain Management Service Incorporating Regional Anesthesia Techniques

Eugene R. Viscusi, MD • Rehana Jan, MD • Leslie Schechter, PharmD • Suzanne Lenart, RNC • Paul H. Willoughby, MD

INTRODUCTION

The field of acute pain management has changed substantially in recent years. In the past, acute pain management consisted primarily of opioids given intermittently by intramuscular injection. In addition to pain on injection, this lead to undesirable "analgesic gaps" or periods of inadequate pain control between peak and trough opioid levels. Consequently, patients were often reluctant to request pain medications ordered "as needed."

To provide more continuous analgesia, intravenous patient controlled analgesia (IVPCA) was introduced in the 1980s, leading to the development of specialized pain management teams, most often under the direction of anesthesiologists. The application of intrathecal opioids and epidural analgesia for postoperative pain management heralded the first pain service in the United States.[1] In Europe, Narinder Rawal presented his experience introducing the role of nurses as valued members of the acute pain management team.[2] By the early 1990s, 40% of US hospitals had acute pain services.[3]

Table 79–1.

Key Points from the JCAHO Pain Management Standards

Patients have a right to pain management.

Pain must be asssessed at regular intervals. Pain should be reassessed soon following an intervention to treat pain to ensure a response.

Institutions are required to have policies and procedures for pain assessment and treatment.

Patient education for pain management is mandated.

Staff education concerning pain management is required.

Pain assessments are required as a discharge criterion.

JCAHO = Joint Commission on Accreditation of Healthcare Organizations.

The American Society of Anesthesiologists (ASA) Task Force first established practice guidelines for acute pain management in 1995.[4] These guidelines were revised in 2004, and the reader is encouraged to review this document.[5] The Joint Commission of Accreditation of Healthcare Organizations (JCAHO) established standards (Table 79–1) for pain management in January 2001.[6] These standards provided an impetus for hospitals to have an institution-wide commitment for policies and procedures to support effective pain management. This effort promoted the concept of pain as the "fifth vital sign" and established the patient's right to pain management. It also became evident that an effective pain management program can only be achieved with a strong institutional commitment. The revised ASA guidelines of 2004 highlighted the importance of multidisciplinary collaboration among anesthesiologists, surgeons, nurses, pharmacists, and other members of the healthcare team.

Early advances on this topic focused on safe application of aggressive techniques utilizing protocols and standing orders with the monitoring available on the ward. However, it is the PCA services that paved the way for the development of true acute pain management services providing on-demand systemic as well as epidural and intrathecal analgesia. The US model focused on physician management; the European model put a greater emphasis on the nursing role.

In recent years, regional anesthesia has gained popularity because if its contribution to postoperative pain management. Single and continuous peripheral neural blockade is increasingly practiced in both the inpatient and outpatient setting. However, effective application of these techniques requires adequate expertise, surveillance, and organization, not simply placing the particular block or catheter. Multidisciplinary acute pain teams can monitor and titrate these techniques to maximize pain relief and safety while minimizing side effects.

More aggressive techniques such as IVPCA, epidural analgesia, intrathecal opioids, and peripheral blocks find their best results when launched as part of a multimodal analgesic approach that incorporates nonsteroidal antiinflammatory agents (NSAIDs) and cyclooxygenase-2 (COX-2) inhibitors as well as other means of nonpharmacologic means to acute pain management (see Chapter 77, The Role of Nonopioid Analgesic Techniques in the Management of Postoperative Pain, for more information on nonpharmacologic means to pain management).[7,8] True multimodal analgesia targets multiple mechanisms of pain to effectively relieve both rest and dynamic pain.

A dedicated acute pain management team enhances implementation of these techniques for pain management. The primary goals of an acute pain management service are to offer a wide variety of services, provide a high level of patient surveillance, and integrate these services into the overall hospital setting. Optimal analgesia requires judicious dose adjustment to maximize the benefits and minimize the side effects of therapy. This can only occur if the patient is adequately monitored.

The purpose of this chapter is to provide strategies for effective postoperative pain management while enhancing safety and facilitating delivery of services. An organizational model for a nursing-based acute pain service is presented. Standard orders and protocols are also provided to facilitate implementation of the suggested principles and approaches. Finally, we provide many of the organizational tools and concepts we have found useful in the organizational design of our acute pain service.

INTRAVENOUS PATIENT-CONTROLLED ANALGESIA

IVPCA is commonly used as part of a multimodal approach to postoperative pain control. Sechzer[9] and Forrest[10] popularized the concept of PCA. Patients self-administer small doses of intravenous opioid at predetermined intervals (lockout), to maintain a minimum effective analgesic concentration (MEAC). This titration of the opioid provides a more constant plasma level of analgesic[11] and more consistent analgesia.[12] Maintaining opioid plasma levels within a tight range improves analgesia while reducing unwanted side effects that can occur with larger boluses. PCA pumps can be programmed to deliver opioids either by intermittent patient-controlled bolus doses alone or with a continuous background (or basal) infusion. PCA pumps are programmed to set the demand dose, lockout interval, hourly total dose, and basal infusion. Importantly, before starting PCA, analgesia must be established with an initial loading dose of opioid.[13] Without front loading, MEAC is not achieved for at least three elimination half-lives.[14] PCA is intended to *maintain* a level of pain control, not to initiate satisfactory analgesia. Therefore, if the PCA process is interrupted by pump failure, a faulty intravenous, or inadequate patient dosing, the patient will require bolus titration to achieve comfort before reinitiating PCA.

Clinical Pearls

- PCA advantages over intermittent injections include fewer analgesic gaps, maintaining analgesia with less total opioid consumption, fewer side effects, less use of nursing staff time, and improved patient satisfaction.
- Before starting PCA, analgesia must be established with an initial loading dose of opioid.

PCA advantages over intermittent injections include fewer analgesic gaps, maintaining analgesia with less total opioid consumption (thus with fewer side effects), less use of nursing staff time, and improved patient satisfaction. Patients can anticipate and proactively manage their pain, particularly before moving or coughing. There is also a psychological advantage because of the shortened interval between perception of pain and administration of medication.

In the opioid-naïve patient, the addition of a basal infusion to IVPCA has been shown not to improve analgesia, but increases the risks of this technique.[15] Without a basal infusion, the risk of clinically significant respiratory depression is generally low. Patients maintain normal levels of arterial CO_2 in the early postoperative period while receiving PCA therapy. Postoperative respiratory functions (forced expiratory volume, functional residual capacity, and peak flow rates) are not significantly different from those in patients receiving intramuscular injections of opioids.[16,17]

Clinical Pearls

- In the opioid-naïve patient, the addition of a basal infusion to IVPCA increases the risk of respiratory depression without the benefit of improving analgesia.
- Without a basal infusion, the risk of clinically significant respiratory depression with IVPCA is low.

The most common problem associated with IVPCA use is operator error, the most common cause of which is programming error and incorrect drug concentration.[18] When a medication error involves a PCA pump, the risk of patient harm increases 3.5 times.[19] The FDA's Manufacturer and User Facility Device Experience (MAUDE) Database for 2004 identified 21 deaths involving IVPCA pumps; 16 deaths were related to large-volume infusion pumps (LVP). Given that there are approximately 10 times as many LVPs as PCA pumps, it appears that the risk of a severe respiratory event from a PCA pump is at least 10 times greater than with an LVP.[20] To avoid these errors the nursing staff must understand the basis for therapy and be knowledgeable about the operational aspects of PCA pumps.

Clinical Pearls

COMMON PITFALLS WITH IVPCA USE
- Unfamiliarity with equipment.
- Equipment failure.
- Failure to understand usage by patients.
- Use of continuous opioid infusion in the opioid-naïve.

PRINCIPLES OF SAFE IVPCA USE
- Use standard equipotent PCA solutions.
- Avoid custom concentrations to reduce medication errors.
- Have defined protocols for respiratory and sedation monitoring.
- Utilize standard order forms or computer order entry to minimize prescribing errors.
- Include supplemental nursing boluses and side effect treatment as part of standard orders.
- Maintain a policy for naloxone antagonism of opioid-induced respiratory depression.
- Have PCA pump programming verified by two nurses.
- Reserve basal infusions of opioid for the opioid-tolerant patients only.

Patient-related PCA problems include failure to understand PCA therapy, intentional analgesic abuse, underutilization because of unwarranted fears of addiction, and PCA by proxy (operation by an individual other than the patient). Patients should be educated about PCA before surgery; the education should be frequently reinforced throughout treatment.

Morphine is the most commonly used PCA opioid. Hydromorphone and fentanyl are also favored because of their favorable metabolite profile. Meperidine has little place as an analgesic because of its neurotoxic metabolite, normeperidine. Table 79–2 summarizes the commonly used IVPCA equianalgesic opioid solutions.

An iontophoretic, transdermal drug-delivery system (ITS) has demonstrated the ability to provide needle-free patient-controlled delivery of fentanyl. This patient-controlled transdermal analgesia (PCTA) system is a preprogrammed and self-contained device about the size of a credit card. Clinical trials have demonstrated analgesic efficacy similar to that from standard morphine IVPCA.[21]

When converting between opioids, these conversion doses should be considered as an approximation because of incomplete cross tolerance. Patient responses may vary when converting from one opioid to another. Similar rules apply when converting the IV opioid therapy to the oral opioid analgesic therapy (Table 79–3).

Safe and effective use of PCA requires institution-wide protocols and standard orders (Figures 79–1 through 79–4).

Table 79–2.

Common IVPCA Equianalgesic Opioid Solutions

	Concentration mg/mL	Dose (mL)[a]	Lockout Interval (min)	Max Hourly Dose (mL)
Morphine sulfate	1	1–2	6	10–20
Hydromorphone (Dilaudid)	0.2	0.5–2	6–8	8–10
Fentanyl (Sublimaze)	0.01–0.02	1–2	6	10–20
Meperidine (Demorol)	10	1–2	6	10[b]

[a] *These doses are intended for opioid-naïve patients.*
IVPCA = intravenous patient-controlled analgesia.
[b] *Maximum 600 mg/day.*

Clinicians must have a thorough understanding of equianalgesic opioid doses (see Table 79–2).

PERIPHERAL NERVE BLOCKS

Peripheral nerve blocks are useful in providing surgical anesthesia and postoperative analgesia[22,23] with an acceptable side effect profile.[23,24] Single-injection techniques are limited in duration but can be extremely useful in the immediate

Table 79–3.

Equianalgesic Opioid Conversions from Intravenous to Oral Administration for Commonly Used Opioids

Drug	Intravenous Dose (mg)	Oral Dose (mg)
Morphine sulfate	10	30
Hydromorphone	1.5	7.5
Fentanyl	0.1–0.2	(Oral fentanyl is indicated for breakthrough pain. Hence no conversion is provided.)
Meperidine	100	300
Methadone	10	20[a]
Oxycodone	(not available)	15

[a] *In opioid naive patients.*

Table 79–4.

Indications for Peripheral Nerve Blocks

Upper Extremity Block	Indication
Interscalene block	Should surgery, rotator cuff repair
Axillary/infraclavicular block	Hand and wrist surgery
Lower Extremity Block	**Indication**
Lumbar plexus, femoral nerve	Hip and knee arthroscopy/arthroplasty ACL repair/knee surgery
Sciatic nerve, popliteal block/ankle block	Foot and ankle surgery

ACL = anterior cruciate ligament.

postoperative period. Continuous catheter techniques can extend the duration of analgesia to the desired length of time. The greatest hindrance to the catheter technique was the unavailability of appropriate equipment both for catheter insertion and drug delivery. Both of these obstacles have now been overcome. There are commercially available catheter insertion kits and drug delivery systems. The infusion pumps now available are small, portable, and lightweight. There is a large variety of commercially available PCA pumps with different characterists.[25] The introduction of these lightweight, portable infusion pumps has made home infusion possible, and it has been shown to be effective in randomized, double-blind, placebo-controlled studies.[26–28]

Numerous approaches have been described to the lumbar, sacral, and brachial plexuses and in the paravertebral space. The planned surgical procedure will determine the peripheral nerve block needed for postoperative analgesia. A brief example of common indications is listed in Table 79–4. The reader should refer to the respective chapters on individual nerve block techniques for in-depth discussion on indications and technical aspects of their use. In general, the peripheral nerve block techniques are indicated in patients expected to have moderate to severe postoperative pain that is not easily controlled with opioids or when opioid side effects are problematic.

Possible modes of local anesthetic infusion through these catheters include intermittent bolus, continuous infusion, or continuous infusion with PCA boluses. Infusion mode is often a matter of clinician preference. Continuous infusions and continuous infusion with PCA have been shown to be superior to the intermittent bolus technique.[29]

In an ambulatory setting, patient selection is critical. Only patients who are capable of accepting the additional responsibility of the catheter and infusion pump should be selected. Since some degree of cognitive dysfunction may occur in the early postoperative period, patients will benefit from a

Thomas Jefferson University Hospital
***J** Jefferson Health System*

MR#	
LW Acct#	
Name	

**Adult Patient Controlled Analgesia
(PCA) Order Form**

Complete or Imprint with Address-O-Plate

IMPORTANT: DO NOT WRITE IN MARGINS

1. Medication

☐ Morphine 1 mg/ml

☐ Hydromorphone (Dilaudid®) 0.2 mg/ml

☐ Fentanyl 10mcg/ml

☐ Other

2. Mode

☐ PCA only   ☐ PCA / Basal

3. Parameters

PCA Dose   _____ ml

Lockout Interval (delay)   _____ minutes

1 Hour Dose Limit   _____ ml

4. Continuous Basal Rate (if applicable)   _____ ml/hour

5. PRN nursing boluses (specify dose and interval)

6. Continuous IV solution:

(If none ordered, maintain 0.9% NaCl at 42 ml/hr).

7. Monitor respiratory rate, pain level, sedation level as follows:

• Upon arrival on the unit from PACU or upon initiation of PCA while on the unit:
q 1/2 hr x 2, q 1 hr x 2, then q 4 hrs for duration of therapy.

• In addition, if a bolus is given by the nurse (including boluses given at time PCA is initiated):
q 15 mins x 2.

8. Treatment of side effects:

1) Have naloxone available. Prior to administration, add naloxone 0.4mg to 0.9% NaCl to make a quantity of 10ml (0.04mg/ml) and notify APMS.

2) Nausea / vomiting _____

3) Pruritus _____

9. Call beeper_____ or primary service for:

1) Inadequate analgesia.

2) Nausea / vomiting, pruritus, uncontrolled by above measures.

3) RR < 10 or increasing somnolence.
In the event of **severe** respiratory depression (RR<5), house officer or nurse may administer naloxone diluted to 10ml with 0.9% NaCl for
final concentration of 0.04mg/ml. Administer 1ml (0.04mg) slowly over 1 minute, repeating 1ml doses as needed, up to 3ml over 3 minutes.

Physician Signature/Beeper #	Date	Time

Form 0197-00 (Rev. 01/02)   **White: Chart Copy • Yellow: Pharmacy Copy**   MUG 01.4252

Figure 79–1. Adult patient-controlled analgesia (PCA) order form.

Thomas Jefferson University Hospital
Jefferson Health System®

019600.1203

MR#

LW Acct#

Name

PCA/CADD Pump/Continuous
IV Infusion Analgesia Flow Sheet

Complete or Imprint with Address-O-Plate

Date	Time Started	Medication	Concentration (mg/ml)

| PCA Settings (note changes only) | | | q 4 Hrs | | Location | |

Date	Time	Dose	Delay	Basal	HR Limit	Pain Scale	Sed Scale	Resp (rate/min)	6am Total Volume	Adverse Effects	Alt Therapy	Syringe Change*	Initial*

PRN Nursing Bolus Dose Section

					15 Minutes			30 Minutes		
Date	Time	Initial	Pain Scale	Medication/Dose	Pain Scale	Sedation Scale	Resp Rate	Pain Scale	Sedation Scale	Resp Rate

Medication Wasted	Amount (mls)	RN	RN
Medication Wasted	Amount (mls)	RN	RN

Alternate Therapies

C	Cold	M	Massage
D	Distraction	MU	Music
GI	Guided Imagery	R	Relaxation
H	Heat	RP	Repositioning

Adverse Effects

A	Anxiety	IM	Immobility	P	Poor Appetite
C	Constipation	L	Decreased Loc	RD	Respiratory
CF	Confusion	N	Nausea		Depression
D	Depression	O	Orthostatic	U	Urinary Retention
I	Itching		Hypotension	V	Vomiting

Sedation Scale

1 Awake
2 Drowsy
3 Awakens Only When Aroused
4 Difficult to Arouse
5 Unresponsive

Init	Name

***ALL PCA SETTINGS AND SYRINGE CHANGES REQUIRE A CO-SIGNATURE.**

Pain Scale

(No Pain) 0 1 2 3 4 5 6 7 8 9 10 (Worst Pain Possible)

Yellow Copy/Pharmacy   Form 0196-00 (Rev. 12/03)   JG 03.3917

Figure 79–2. PCA/CADD pump/continuous IV infusion analgesia flow sheet.

IMPORTANT: DO NOT WRITE IN MARGINS

Thomas Jefferson University Hospital
Jefferson Health System

‖‖‖‖‖‖‖‖‖‖‖‖‖‖‖‖‖‖‖‖‖‖‖‖
* 2 4 0 9 0 0 . 1 2 9 9 *

MR#

LW Acct#

Name

Pain Assessment Sheet

Complete or Imprint with Address-O-Plate

Patient Goal

1. Where is your pain?

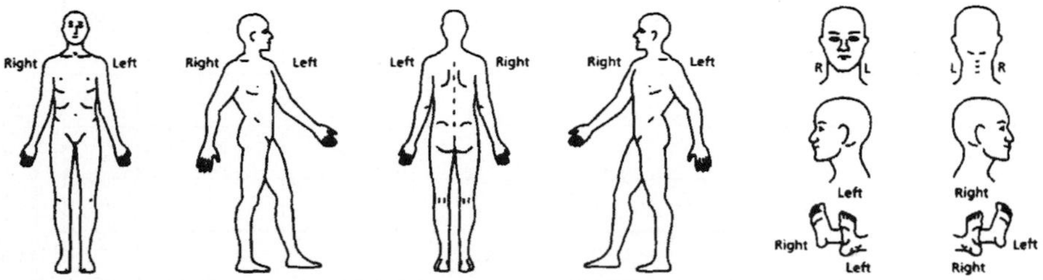

2. Which word/words describe your pain (you may check more than one)

☐ Aching   ☐ Gnawing   ☐ Penetrating   ☐ Shooting   ☐ Unbearable
☐ Burning   ☐ Nagging   ☐ Radiating   ☐ Stabbing   ☐ Other (describe):
☐ Exhausting   ☐ Numb   ☐ Sharp   ☐ Throbbing

Choose one:
☐ Occasional
☐ Continuous
☐ Intermittent

3. Rate your pain by circling the number that best describes your pain right now.

(No Pain)   0   1   2   3   4   5   6   7   8   9   10   (Worst Pain Possible)

4. How long have you had this pain?	5. What makes your pain better?	6. What makes your pain worse?

7. List the medications or therapies you are receiving for your pain? Circle the number to describe the amount of relief the treatment or medicine provides you. Zero=no relief; 10=complete relief

a)_____   0 1 2 3 4 5 6 7 8 9 10

b)_____   0 1 2 3 4 5 6 7 8 9 10

c)_____   0 1 2 3 4 5 6 7 8 9 10

8. What over the counter medications/herbs/vitamins have you taken on your own for your pain? Indicate amount of relief as indicated above.

a) _____ 0 1 2 3 4 5 6 7 8 9 10   d) _____ 0 1 2 3 4 5 6 7 8 9 10

b) _____ 0 1 2 3 4 5 6 7 8 9 10   e) _____ 0 1 2 3 4 5 6 7 8 9 10

c) _____ 0 1 2 3 4 5 6 7 8 9 10   f) _____ 0 1 2 3 4 5 6 7 8 9 10

9. Do you use alcohol for pain relief? ☐ Yes ☐ No If so, how much?	10. Do you smoke? ☐ Yes ☐ No If so, how much?

11. Circle the one number that describes how during the past week pain has interfered with your:

a. General Activity	Does Not Interfere	0	1	2	3	4	5	6	7	8	9	10		Completely Interferes
b. Mood	Does Not Interfere	0	1	2	3	4	5	6	7	8	9	10		Completely Interferes
c. Work	Does Not Interfere	0	1	2	3	4	5	6	7	8	9	10		Completely Interferes
d. Eating	Does Not Interfere	0	1	2	3	4	5	6	7	8	9	10		Completely Interferes
e. Sleep	Does Not Interfere	0	1	2	3	4	5	6	7	8	9	10		Completely Interferes
f. Enjoyment of Life	Does Not Interfere	0	1	2	3	4	5	6	7	8	9	10		Completely Interferes
g. Ability to Concentrate	Does Not Interfere	0	1	2	3	4	5	6	7	8	9	10		Completely Interferes
h. Relations with Other People	Does Not Interfere	0	1	2	3	4	5	6	7	8	9	10		Completely Interferes

Comments	Name

Form 240900 (Rev. 12/99)   M/UG 99.3772.3

Figure 79–3. Pain assessment sheet.

Pain Assessment Sheet

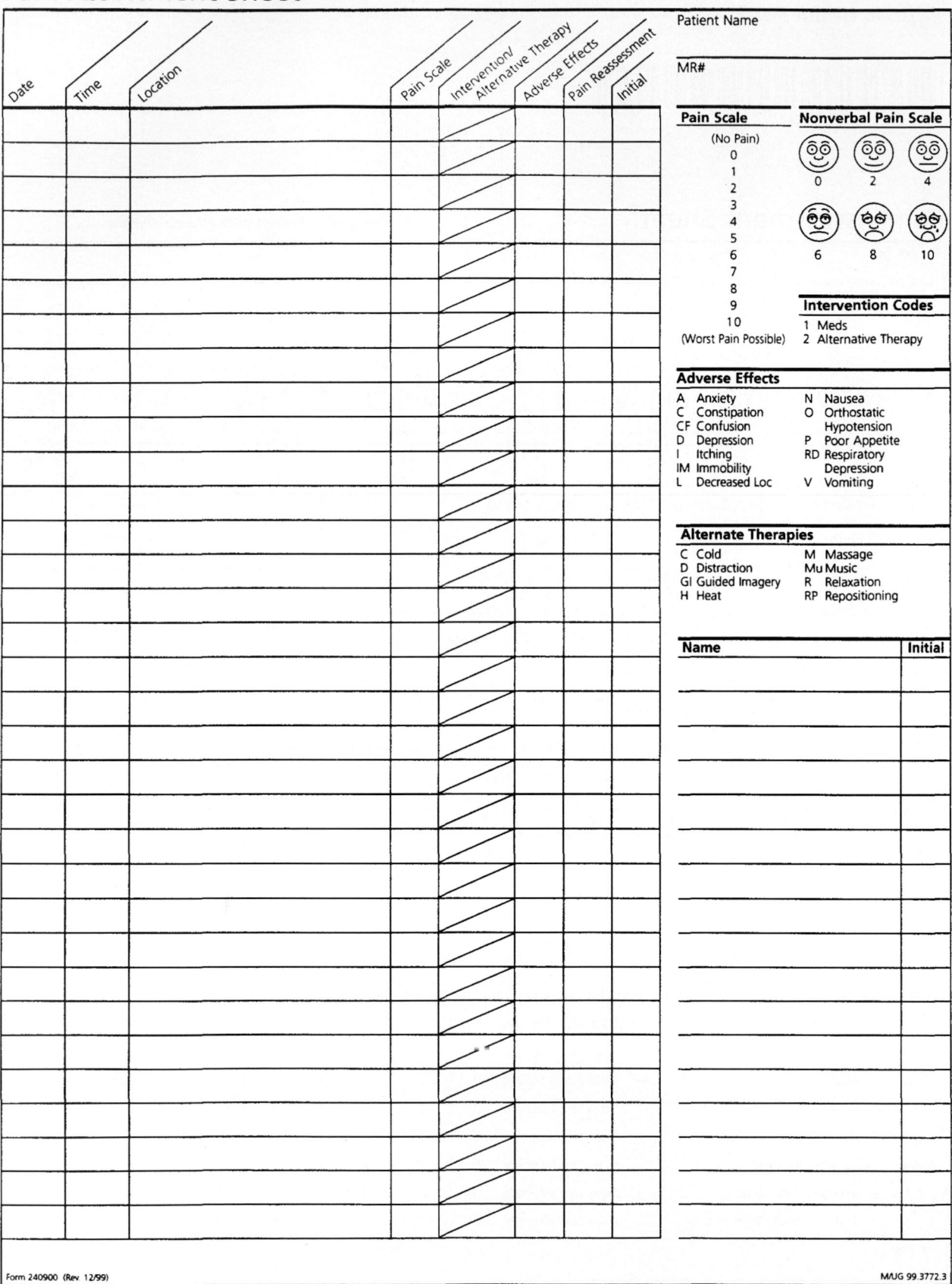

Figure 79–4. Pain assessment sheet.

caregiver at home for the first 24–48 h who can participate in patient care. To decrease the risk of local anesthetic toxicity, patients with hepatic or renal insufficiency should not be sent home with continuous catheters if they do not have a caregiver at home. Hence, patients without a caregiver, with baseline cognitive difficulties, with certain underlying medical problems, or patients living a distance from the medical facility may be poor candidates for ambulatory infusion techniques.

Recommendations for local anesthetic injection volume and catheter infusion rates are provided in the respective chapters. The reader should note that the suggested doses, volumes, concentrations, and infusion rates are only general guidelines and must be adjusted for individual patients. More in-depth discussion on these variables can be found in Chapters 10 (Local Anesthetic Solutions for Continuous Nerve Blocks) and 64 (Continuous Peripheral Nerve Blocks in Outpatients).

The successful use of peripheral catheters in the ambulatory setting requires patient education that should start in the preoperative area and extend into the postoperative period. Both patients and their caregiver must be involved. Instructions should be both verbal and written and include pager numbers and telephone numbers of responsible healthcare providers who will be available around the clock if problems occur. Although the surgeon is responsible for the overall care of the patient, the anesthesiologist providing the continuous regional technique must be responsible and available for catheter-related problems.

Key elements of patient instructions include:

- Protect the operative limb for the duration of the block.
- Keep the catheter site clean and dry.
- Do not operate machinery or drive a vehicle for the duration of the block.
- Approximate duration/resolution of the surgical block.
- Use of supplemental oral analgesics/opioids.
- Portable pump instructions.
- When and how to remove the catheter.
- Look for signs of catheter/local anesthetic infusion complications.
- Observe catheter site for swelling, tenderness, and drainage.

Careful follow-up is necessary with any continuous catheter technique. Visiting nurses may be helpful. Patients may benefit from daily telephone contact with specific questions about quality of analgesia, local anesthetic side effects, and possible catheter site infection. Documentation of these patient contacts should be made.

Clinical Pearls

- Successful use of peripheral catheters in the ambulatory setting requires patient education,
- Instructions should be both verbal and written and include pager numbers and telephone numbers of responsible healthcare providers who will be available around the clock if problems occur.

Patients may remove their peripheral infusion catheters at home, may return to the medical facility to have them removed, or a visiting nurse may remove the catheter. This may depend on the patients' abilities, the distance they must travel from the hospital, and their degree of mobility. Reusable infusion pumps may be mailed to the surgical facility in a padded envelope. With proper selection and education of patients, the incidence of injury to the blocked limb is very low.[30]

Complications of Continuous Catheter Techniques

1. Local anesthetic toxicity is a potential complication that can occur when large volumes or high concentrations of local anesthetics are used. Intravascular placement of catheters can be detected with epinephrine-containing local anesthetic test doses. Low concentrations of a long-acting local anesthetic with an acceptable safety profile are advisable. Ropivacaine, in 2 mg/mL concentration, infused in a continuous interscalene (brachial plexus) catheter at 6 to 9 mL/h has demonstrated safety.[31,32]

2. Patients should be instructed to look for signs of local infection at the catheter site, local tenderness, redness, and fever. These should be immediately reported to the healthcare providers. Even though infection at catheter sites is uncommon, one study reported 57% of femoral catheters showed bacterial colonization at 48 h.[33]

3. Although a rare occurrence, catheter migration must always be considered. Catheter failure is the most common sign of migration. Since the actual location of the local anesthetic infusion cannot be determined, failed catheters should always be removed promptly. Catheters may migrate into the intravascular compartment. Patients should be provided with a list of signs of intravascular infusion of local anesthetics: tinnitus, metallic taste in the mouth, and anxiety. Intramuscular migration of the catheter will result in either a decrease or complete cessation of analgesia. The infusion should be stopped since there is a theoretical risk of myositis.[34]

4. Careful dressing of the catheter site and use of surgical tape can reduce catheter dislodgment. Clear dressings are advantageous since they permit visualization of the insertion site. Commercially available skin preparations (similar to ostomy site skin preps) may increase adhesion while reducing skin breakdown. Adhesive surgical strips may be beneficial in regions that are difficult to secure. Catheters can also be secured by suturing or tunneling. This may be helpful for longer term placement.

5. Many varieties of infusion pumps are available for either continuous infusions or with patient-controlled boluses. The pump selection should be based on its accuracy of delivery, simplicity of use, and ability to allow for patient-initiated boluses. Cost should also be evaluated. Use of disposable pumps in the ambulatory setting is preferred, as patients are not required to return the equipment. Use of large-volume (250–400 mL) pumps will provide longer periods of analgesia. However, larger volumes of local anesthetic may increase the risk of systemic toxicity.

Table 79–5.

Applying Regional Anesthesia Techniques with Multimodal Therapy

Procedure	Regional	Multimodal
Thoracotomy	*Thoracic epidural* Site: T4 to T6 *Paravertebral blocks* Site: 1 level at incision + 2 levels up/down *Continuous paravertebral blocks* Site: 1–2 levels above and below incision	IVPCA opioids, NSAIDs, COX-2 inhibitor
Thoracoscopy	Thoracic epidural Site: T4 to T6 *Paravertebral blocks* Site: 1 level at incision + 2 levels up/down	PCA opioid, NSAIDs, COX-2 inhibitor
Upper abdominal cholecystectomy	Thoracic epidural Site: T9 to T10 *Paravertebral blocks* Site: 1 level at incision + 2 levels up/down	PCA opioid, NSAIDs, COX-2 inhibitor
Lower abdominal prostatectomy, cystectomy	Thoracic epidural Site: T11 to T12	PCA opioid, COX-2 inhibitor
Lower limb surgery TKR, peripheral vascular grafts, BKA, THR, ACL, distal patellar realignment	Lumbar epidural Site: L3 to L4 Lumbar plexus block Femoral nerve block Sciatic block	PCA opioid, COX-2 inhibitor, NSAIDs
Hernia repair (inguinal)	Field block, paravertebral block T12, L1 to L2	COX-2 inhibitors, NSAIDs
Foot surgery	Popliteal fossa nerve block and saphenous nerve block	COX-2 inhibitors, NSAIDs
Upper limb surgery Shoulder acromioplasty and/or arthroplasty, ORIF humerus Elbow procedures Distal forearm and hand procedures	Brachial plexus blocks Interscalane, infraclavicular Interscalene infraclavicular Axillary block Infraclavicular block Axillary block	Oral opioids COX-2 inhibitors, NSAIDs

IVPCA = intravenous patient-controlled analgesia, NSAIDs = nonsteroidal antiinflammatory drugs, COX-2 = cyclooxygenase 2, TKR = total knee replacement, BKA = below the knee amputation, ACL = anterior cruciate ligament, ORIF = open reduction, internal fixation.

Successful use of peripheral nerve catheter infusions requires an infrastructure consisting of anesthesiologists, surgeons, pharmacists, and nurses:

- A group of anesthesiologists with additional training in regional anesthesia.
- Around-the-clock coverage of the service by an anesthesiologist.
- Surgeons familiar and supportive of these techniques.
- Pharmacists familiar with the range of local anesthetic concentrations and infusion rates.
- Specially trained nurses to help maintain catheter infusions and provide patient education.
- Policies supporting attentive patient follow-up.

- Availability of infusion pumps.
- Proper patient selection and education.
- Institutional commitment to provide trained staff and equipment.
- Organizational tools, including standardized procedure note, order sets, and documentation records.

MULTIMODAL APPROACH TO ACUTE PAIN MANAGEMENT

Multimodal analgesia produces optimal pain relief by targeting pain at multiple pathways.[35] Combining analgesic techniques and drugs has a synergistic or additive effect and decreases the requirement for individual medication, thereby reducing the incidence of side effects.[36]

The surgical stress response produces endocrine and metabolic responses in the body. These pathways can be targeted pharmacologically at specific levels by adopting a multimodal approach to pain control.[37] The focus of the multimodal approach to acute postoperative pain management is to facilitate the patient's rehabilitation. Multimodal approaches combined with accelerated recovery protocols can reduce length of hospital stay.[38] This has been shown to work when the surgical team, anesthesiologists, nurses, and patients work together within established clinical pathways.[39]

Chronic pain has been identified as a consequence of surgery and poorly controlled acute pain.[40] Multimodal techniques may reduce central sensitization, improve pain control, and ultimately reduce long-term sequelae. The concepts of preemptive analgesia are discussed in Chapter 76 (Preemptive Analgesia, Regional Anesthesia, and the Prevention of Chronic Postoperative Pain). Local anesthetics and regional anesthesia techniques are critical components of multimodal analgesia. Potential uses are described in the following sections and in Table 79–5.

Opioids and nonsteroidal antiinflammatory drugs (NSAIDs) act both centrally and peripherally to decrease afferent impulses to the dorsal horn of the spinal cord. Ketamine, an N-methyl-D-aspartate (NMDA) receptor antagonist, when used in small doses (0.5–0.15 mg/kg IV) has been shown to improve pain relief if administered with opioids intravenously or epidurally.[41,42]

With appropriate patient selection, NSAIDs can be very effective. However, in some patients and situations NSAIDs can exert an antiplatelet effect that can cause surgical bleeding. They may also cause renal dysfunction. NSAIDs have an opioid-sparing effect[43] and can be administered orally or parentally. COX-2 inhibitors do not have an antiplatelet effect, making them desirable for postoperative pain management. Concern for cardiovascular problems has led to the withdrawal of certain COX-2 inhibitors from the market. However, this risk is associated with a duration of use longer than is indicated for most acute pain situations.

CONTINUOUS EPIDURAL ANALGESIA

Use of continuous epidural infusions of local anesthetic with or without opioids has become a cornerstone of multimodal analgesia.[44] The use of dilute local anesthetic solutions has been shown to decrease the incidence of deep venous thrombosis in the postoperative period.[45] It is an effective weapon in attenuating the endocrine metabolic response to surgical stress and to provide dynamic pain relief.[46] The epidural catheter must be functional and cover the dermatomal distribution of the surgical incision to be effective. Epidural catheters are best inserted at the middermatome of surgical trauma. Care must also be taken to advance between 3 and 5 cm of epidural catheter into the epidural space. A shallower insertion results in greater incidence of catheter dislodge-

ment, whereas an excessive length of catheter reduces efficacy and increases risk of catheter knotting. The routinely used nylon epidural catheters are difficult to direct in the epidural space, regardless of the direction of the epidural needle bevel. Hence, it is best to target a short length of catheter at the precise spinal cord level to cover surgical pain.

Clinical Pearl

- Use of continuous epidural infusions of local anesthetic with or without opioids has become a cornerstone of multimodal analgesia.

In a meta-analysis comparing epidural analgesia with parenteral opioids, epidural analgesia was found to provide more effective pain control.[47] Epidural opioids or local anesthetics either alone or in combination demonstrated superiority. Hence, when surgical pain is of high intensity and likely to last at least 48 h, epidural analgesia deserves consideration. Side effects of epidural analgesia include motor block, nausea and vomiting, pruritus, urinary retention, sedation, and respiratory depression. Epidural catheters in the presence of anticoagulation may increase the risk of epidural hematoma.

A number of other agents have demonstrated analgesic efficacy when administered by the epidural route either alone or in combination with other agents. These agents include anticholinergics, NMDA receptor antagonists (eg, ketamine) and α_2-adrenergic agonists. Epidural epinephrine, clonidine,[48] and dexmedetomidine[49] have demonstrated analgesic efficacy.

A standard epidural order form (Figures 79–5 and 79–6) and epidural procedure note (Figure 79–7) enhances documentation and reduces medication errors.

Clinical Pearls

EPIDURAL ANALGESIA

- Check patient's coagulation status before epidural insertion.
- Insert epidural needle at the middermatome of surgical trauma.
- Insert epidural catheter between 3 and 5 cm.
- Confirm epidural catheter is not intravascular or intrathecal.
- Obtain an anesthetic level and ensure epidural is functional *before* surgery.
- Activate the epidural during surgery (infusion or bolus).
- Be willing to accept a slightly lower blood pressure with epidural analgesia unless contraindicated.
- On emergence, administer epidural bolus to achieve patient comfort.

Thomas Jefferson University Hospital
Jefferson Health System

|‖|‖‖|‖|‖‖|‖|‖‖‖|‖|‖‖|‖|‖|‖‖|‖

* 0 1 9 4 0 0 . 0 1 0 2 *

MR# _____

LW Acct# _____

Name _____

Complete or Imprint with Address-O-Plate

Department of Anesthesia
Epidural / Intrathecal Analgesia Order Form

No administration (po, subq, IM or IV) of any narcotics, sedatives, hypnotics, tranquilizers, antiemetics or antihistamines unless part of this protocol or ordered by anesthesiology.

Allergies _____

1. This patient has ☐ Epidural catheter ☐ Intrathecal catheter ☐ Neither

2. This patient's primary mode of therapy is either *(choose a or b):*
   a. Continuous infusion of

   ☐ **Bupivacaine** _____ % (final concentration)   ☐ **Ropivacaine** _____ % (final concentration)

   ☐ **Fentanyl** _____ mcg/ml (final concentration)   ☐ **Morphine** _____ mg/ml (final concentration)

   ☐ **Hydromorphone** _____ mcg/ml (final concentration) ☐ **Epinephrine** _____

   ☐ **Other** _____

   Total volume _____ mls (qs using preservative free normal saline)
   to infuse at _____ **ml / hr** (Basal Rate).

   ☐ **Patient controlled epidural**   **PCA Dose** _____ **ml.**

   Lockout interval _____ **min.**

   Hourly Limit _____ **ml.**

   b. Single shot   ☐ **EPIDURAL**   ☐ **INTRATHECAL**   injection

   Medication _____ Dose _____ Time _____

3. Have naloxone 0.4mg available at bedside. Prior to administration, add naloxone 0.4mg to 0.9% NaCl
   to make a quantity of 10ml (0.04mg/ml) and notify APMS.

4. Heparin lock or IV at all times.

5. Please label patient's door and medication cardex **"Intraspinal Analgesia."**

6. For solutions containing narcotics, monitor resp. rate and sedation level as follows:

   Infusions   q _____ hr x _____, then q _____ hr for duration of therapy.

   Following Bolus   Resp. rate q 15 min. x 2.

7. For infusions containing local anesthetic, monitor motor score, B.P., and HR as follows:

   Infusions   q 4 hr. for duration of therapy.

   Following Bolus   q 5 min. x 4.

8. Monitor pain score q 4 hr.

9. **Treatment of side effects**

   Itching   Diphenhydramine Hydrochloride (Benadryl) 25–50 mg IVPB / IM q 4 hr. prn.

   Nausea/Vomiting _____

   Urinary Retention Straight cath. q 8hr. prn; may place foley cath if patient requires second straight cath.

10. For sleep *(if resp. rate > 12 / min. and patient is easily arousable):* Benadryl (diphenhydramine) 25–50 mg IVPB / IM / PO, qHS pm.

11. Call _____ pain service at beeper _____ for following:

    a. Resp. rate < 10. In the event of **severe** respiratory depression (RR<5), house officer or nurse may administer naloxone diluted to 10ml with 0.9%
    NaCl for final concentration of 0.04mg/ml. Administer 1ml (0.04mg) slowly over 1 minute, repeating 1ml doses as needed, up to 3ml over 3 minutes.

    b. Altered mental status or patient becomes difficult to arouse.

    c. Inadequate analgesia.

    d. Pruritus or Nausea and Vomiting not controlled by above measures.

    e. Problems with Intraspinal catheter.

    f. Increasing motor block.

12. Other _____

APMS RNs Only

☐ Follow thoracic epidural protocol

☐ Follow lumbar epidural protocol

☐ Alternate plans

  ☐ Epidural local and IV
     PCA opioid

  ☐ Other _____

  _____

  _____

  _____

  _____

  _____

IMPORTANT: DO NOT WRITE IN MARGINS

Signature	Date Ordered	Time Ordered

Form 0194-00 (Rev. 1/02)   **White: Chart Copy • Yellow: Pharmacy Copy**   MUG 01.4265

Figure 79–5. Epidural/intrathecal analgesia order form.

Thomas Jefferson University Hospital
Jefferson Health System

019500.0301

MR#

LW Acct#

Name

Epidural/PCEA/Intrathecal Analgesia Flow Sheet

Complete or Imprint with Address-O-Plate

Single Shot Injection (no catheter): ☐ Epidural   ☐ Intrathecal   Opioid ____   Dose ____   Time ____

Continuous Infusion
  Opioids: ☐ Fentanyl _____ mcg/ml   ☐ Morphine _____ mg/ml   ☐ Other (name/concentration) _____

  Local Anesthetics: ☐ Ropivicaine _____ %   Other Additives _____   Location _____

Nerve Blocks: ☐ Femoral Nerve Block   ☐ Brachial Plexus Catheter   Sed/Resp: q _____ hr 'til _____ then q _____ hr

Date	Time	Initial	Infusion Rate (ml/hr)	Opioid Conc.	LA Conc. (%)	Dose (ml)	Delay (min)	Basal (ml/hr)	Hour Limit	Pain Scale	Sedation Scale	Motor Scale	Resp Rate	BP	Heart Rate	Adverse Effects	Alt Therapy

Bolus Section: Instructions for vital signs after Bolus: **1)** Opioid Only: Record HR - BP - RR q 15 x 2   **2)** Local Anesthetic + Opioid: Record HR - BP - RR q 5 x 4

Date	Time	Pain Scale	Med/Conc/Dose	Time: HR - BP - RR	Pain Scale	Time: HR - BP - RR	Pain Scale	Time: HR - BP - RR	Pain Scale	Time: HR - BP - RR	Pain Scale

Medication Wasted	Amount (mls)		RN	RN
Medication Wasted	Amount (mls)		RN	RN

Alternate Therapies

C	Cold	M	Massage
D	Distraction	MU	Music
GI	Guided Imagery	R	Relaxation
H	Heat	RP	Repositioning

Pain Scale

(No Pain) 0 1 2 3 4 5 6 7 8 9 10 (Worst Pain Possible)

Adverse Effects

A	Anxiety	I	Itching
C	Constipation	IM	Immobility
CF	Confusion	L	Decreased Loc
D	Depression	N	Nausea
O	Orthostatic Hypotension		
P	Poor Appetite		
RD	Respiratory Depression		
V	Vomiting		

Sedation Scale

1	Awake
2	Drowsy
3	Awakens Only When Aroused
4	Difficult to Arouse
5	Unresponsive

Init ____ Name ____

Lower Extremity Motor Scale

5	Normal (Complete ROM vs Gravity w/ Full Resistance	2	Poor (Complete ROM w/Gravity Eliminated)
4	Good (Complete ROM vs Gravity w/ Some Resistance)	1	Trace (Evidence of Contraction. No Joint Movement)
3	Fair (Complete ROM vs Gravity)	0	Zero (No Evidence of Contraction)

Nonverbal Pain Scale

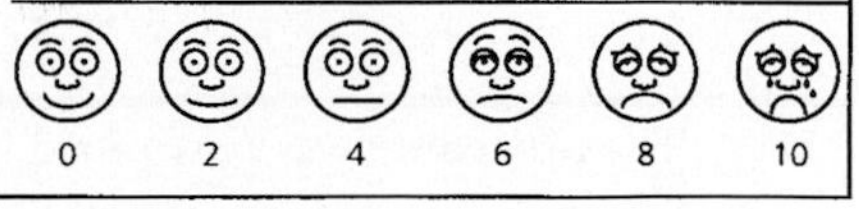

0 2 4 6 8 10

Form 0195-00 (Rev. 3/01)   M/UG 01.1472.2

Figure 79–6. Epidural/PCEA/intrathecal analgesia flow sheet. PCEA = patient-controlled epidural analgesia.

IMPORTANT: DO NOT WRITE IN MARGINS

Anesthesiology Procedure Note
NEURAXIAL BLOCKADE

Block(s) performed	Surgical site confirmed:
	☐ Left ☐ Right ☐ Midline

Patient Name

Medical Record #

Age   Sex

(Patient name plate stamp)

☐ **Anticoagulation/antithrombosis status was reviewed**

Indication: ☐ Analgesia ☐ Anesthesia   ☐ Specifically requested for management
Dx/pain location: of pain by Dr. _____

Date: _____/_____/20_____   **Start time** (:)   **End time** (:)

Pt Condition: Initial BP:_____/____ HR: ____O2 Sat: ____ **VAS Pain: 0 1 2 3 4 5 6 7 8 9 10**

    ☐ awake   ☐ sedate with meaningful contact maintained

    ☐ Performed under general anesthesia with the indication: _____

Preparation: ☐ drape   ☐ povidone-iodine ☐ chlorhexidine ☐ alcohol   ☐ iodophor/isopropyl

Position: ☐ LLD   ☐ RLD   ☐ sitting   ☐ prone

Technique: ☐ mid-line ☐ paramedian   ☐ loss of resistance to saline ☐ loss of resistance to air

    Approximate interspace: ☐ Thoracic: **T -T**   ☐ Lumbar: **L -L .**

    ☐ injection given through needle ☐ **Loss of resistance at depth:**   _____cm.

                      ☐ **Catheter insertion, mark at skin:**   _____cm.

Needle(s): ☐ Epidural needle gauge: _____   ☐ Needle length if not 3.5 inches:_____

    ☐ Spinal needle gauge: _____   ☐ Pencil-tip   ☐ Quincke ☐ introducer
    Manufacturer of neuraxial needle/catheter/ tray:

Injectate:

Spinal Local Anesthetic	Dose (mg)	Baricity	Adjuncts	Epinephrine

Epidural Local Anesthetic	Volume (ml)	Adjuncts	Epinephrine
			☐ 1/__00,000
			☐ not used

Narrative: **The test dose given was:**   **Action Taken**

Paresthesia encountered	☐ no	☐ yes	
CSF via catheter or epidural	☐ no	☐ yes	
Blood aspirated:	☐ no	☐ yes	
Intravenous/Spinal test:	☐ negative	☐ positive	
Pain on injection noted:	☐ no	☐ yes	

    Injection was made incrementally with constant monitoring and aspiration every _____ml's

Events: ☐ none: easy/ well tolerated ☐ difficult:

Success: **Block Level(s):**   ☐ failed   ☐ aborted   ☐ a full evaluation is pending

Pt Condition: Post BP:_____/____ HR: ____O2 Sat: ____ **VAS Pain: 0 1 2 3 4 5 6 7 8 9 10**

Sedation Given	Dose (mcg /mg)

☐ The procedure was performed by _____(sign). I was present and medically directed.

☐ I performed the procedure myself. **ATTENDING MD SIGNATURE:** _____

Figure 79–7. Anesthesiology procedure note, neuraxial blockade.

- If breakthrough pain occurs, assess the epidural level. This can easily be determined with cold (ice). Then, administer bolus with lidocaine 2% (3–5 mL).

- Reassess pain and anesthetic level; repeat if necessary if epidural is functioning. If no level is detected, replace epidural or establish another plan.

Commonly used solutions for epidural infusion and rates of administration are detailed in Tables 79–6 and 79–7.

The preprinted epidural analgesia forms are of vital importance to the efficacy, safety, time efficiency, and surveillance of the epidural analgesia program (Table 79–8).

Common problems and clinical dilemmas that occur during epidural infusion are presented in a decision-tree fashion in Figures 79–8 through 79–12. These decision-tree algorithms can be used to troubleshoot most of these issues on the ward.

Peripheral Nerve Blocks (& Multimodal Analgesia)

Peripheral neural blockade works best when it is part of a multimodal approach to pain control.[50] It may offer advantages over continuous catheter-based epidural analgesia in lower limb procedures, particularly when anticoagulation

Table 79–6.

Common Epidural Solutions

Lower Extremity (Lumbar Catheters)

Ropivacaine 0.2%/morphine 0.025 mg/mL
Ropivacaine 0.15%/morphine 0.025 mg/mL
Roivacaine 0.2% (plus PCA)

General Surgery (Thoracic Catheters)

Bupivacaine 0.125%/morphine 0.05 mg/mL
Bupivacaine 0.125%/morphine 0.025 mg/mL

Labor and Delivery (Lumbar Catheters)

Bupivacaine 0.1%/fentanyl 1.5 mcg/mL

PCA = patient-controlled analgesia.

Table 79–7.

Common Administration Rates of Epidural Infusions

Insertion Site	Common Rates (mL/h)
Thoracic catheter	3–6
Lumbar catheter	6–10

Table 79–8.

Important Elements of Epidural Analgesia Preprinted Orders

1. Drugs with concentrations
2. Instructions for administration
   a. If boluses
      i. Drug dose
      ii. Interval between injections
   b. If infusion
      i. Loading dose
      ii. Infusion rate
3. Instructions for treating breakthrough pain
4. Maintain IV route and access for emergency administration of drugs
5. A statement or warning that other CNS depressants should not be ordered on this patient unless approved by an anesthesiologist
6. Monitoring instructions
   a. Opioids
      i. Respiratory rate
      ii. Sedation level
      iii. Pain score
   b. Local anesthetics
      i. Bradycardia
      ii. Hypotension
      iii. Extensive sensory or motor block
7. Instructions for treatment of side effects
   a. Respiratory depression
   b. Nausea and/or vomiting
   c. Pruritus
   d. Urinary retention
8. Observations that should be communicated to the anesthesiologist
   a. Hypotension
   b. Uncontrolled nausea and vomiting
   c. Uncontrolled pruritus
9. Instructions for whom to contact if problems occur
10. Date, time, and signature of prescribing anesthesiologist

IV = intravenous, CNS = central nervous system.

is required for venous thromboembolism (VTE) prophalaxis. For single-injection techniques, adding epinephrine 1:200,000 or clonidine enhances the duration of the block. Since clonidine can cause sedation, bradycardia, and hypotension, it may not be a suitable agent for use in the ambulatory setting.

Infiltration with Local Anesthetics

Injecting the operative site with local anesthetic is a simple way to enhance pain control.[51] Local anesthetics can be injected or infused into joint spaces, surgical wounds, or in the vicinity of nerves near the surgical site. Local anesthetics are relatively inexpensive and remain the most useful and safe component of multimodal analgesia.

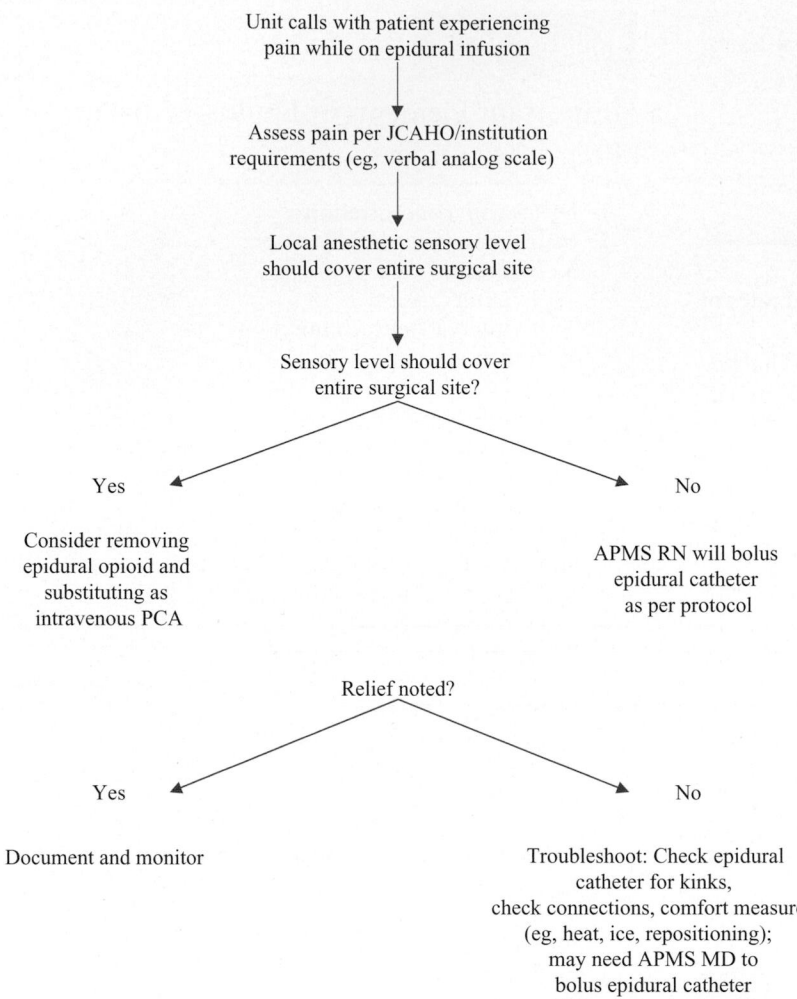

Figure 79–8. Troubleshooting diagram for patient experiencing pain while on epidural infusion. JCAHO = Joint Commission on Accreditation of Healthcare Organizations.

Acute Pain in the Patient with Chronic Pain

Patients with chronic pain present special challenges in the perioperative period. Their pain is typically poorly controlled by the routine administration of opioids alone. It is critical that such patients are identified in the preoperative period and an analgesia plan established before surgery[52] to avoid unnecessary prolonged periods of severe uncontrolled postoperative pain. Evidence from the literature supports that the opioid requirement in these patients can be much higher than in opioid-naïve patients.[53] These patients may present with a history of chronic opioid use, often at high doses and perhaps in conjunction with a variety of other pain medications. Following identification, these patients require careful assessment in the preoperative phase to fully describe the nature of their chronic pain, to quantify opioid requirements, and to document all current medications. Then, an analgesic plan must be formulated with the patient as an active participant.[54] Table 79–9 details practical approach to postoperative pain management in the patient with history of chronic pain.

Opioid-Tolerant Patients

Opioid-dependent patients may include patients with chronic pain,[55] active opioid abusers, or former addicts enrolled in long-term methadone maintenance programs. All of these patients have a high tolerance to the antinociceptive effects of opioids,[56] are pain-intolerant,[57] and can have opioid-induced hyperalgesia.[58]

It is important to identify these patients in the preoperative period and establish a sound pain management strategy before surgery. In the postoperative period these patients will often require more than twice their stable opioid dose. This rapid increase in opioid requirement has been termed *acute tolerance.* Patients should receive their daily maintenance opioid dose the morning of surgery. Even if regional anesthesia techniques are used, these patients must receive their minimum opioid requirement to prevent opioid withdrawal symptoms. In the immediate postoperative period, consider higher than routine doses of IVPCA with morphine or hydromorphone. (Hydromorphone and sufentanil are regarded as higher efficacy opioids and may be more helpful

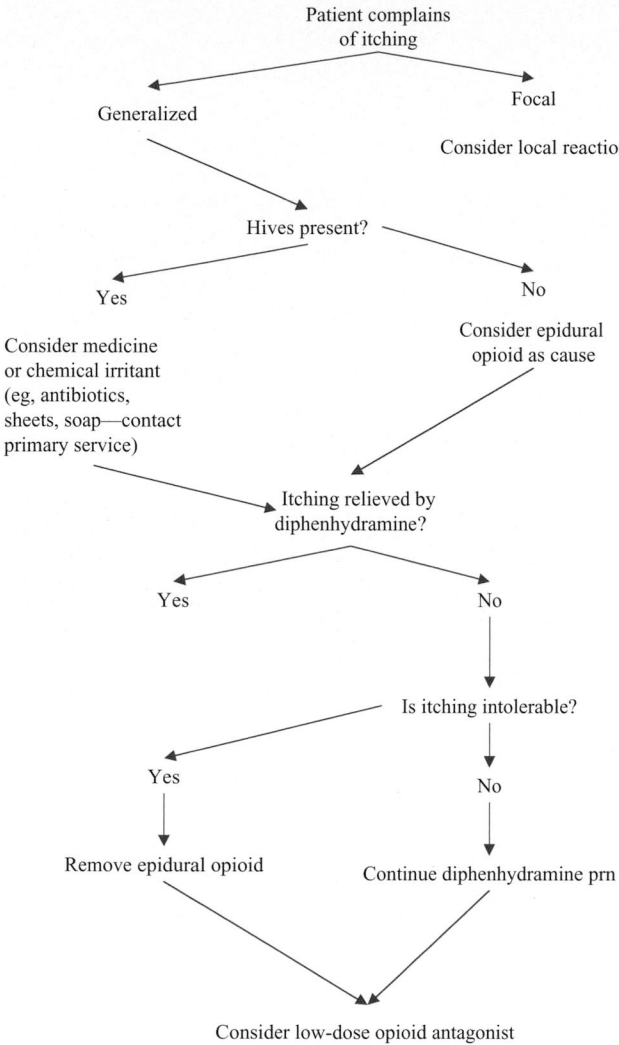

Figure 79–9. Troubleshooting diagram and management of the patient complaining of pruritus while on epidural infusion. prn = as needed.

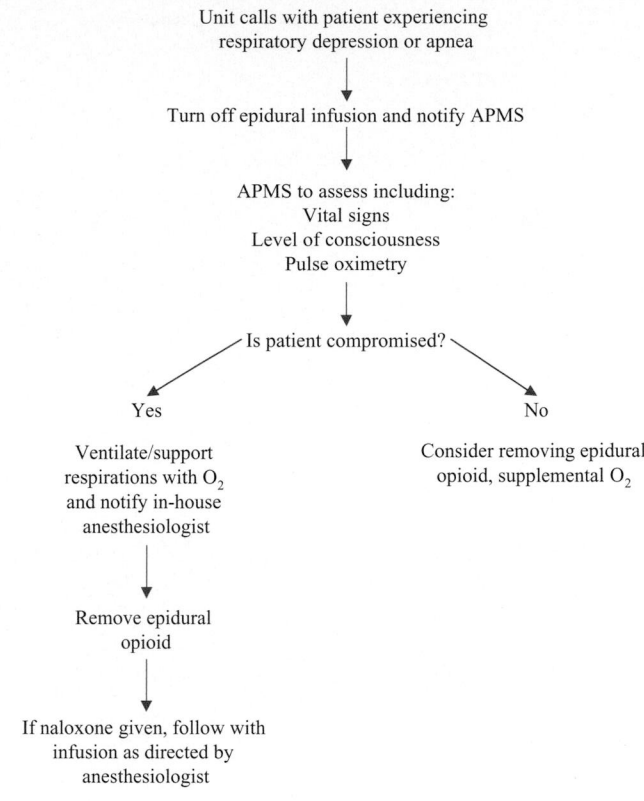

Figure 79–10. Management and troubleshooting in a patient with respiratory depression while on epidural infusion. APMS = acute pain management service.

Regional analgesia with local anesthetic and systemic opioid is a more efficient way of providing pain control than parenteral opioids alone. Use of an opioid with high intrinsic efficacy, such as sufentanil, is more effective[59] in the setting of opioid receptor down-regulation.[60] These patients

in opioid-tolerant patients.) With opioid tolerance, adding a basal IV opioid infusion to PCA may improve analgesia. The basal infusion may be dose-equivalent to a significant portion of the patient's maintenance requirement.

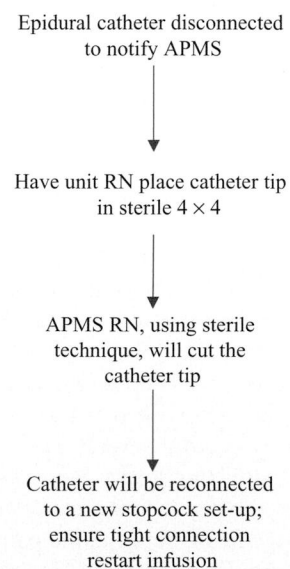

Figure 79–11. Decision tree in patient with disconnected epidural catheter. APMS = acute pain management service, RN = registered nurse.

Clinical Pearls

- Regional analgesia with local anesthetic and systemic opioid is a more efficient way of providing pain control than parenteral opioids alone.

- Use of an opioid with high intrinsic efficacy such as sufentanil is more effective in the opioid tolerant.

- Before and after hospital discharge, referral to a pain specialist can be very helpful in treating the opioid-dependent patient to help optimize pain management during rehabilitation and facilitate opioid dose tapering.

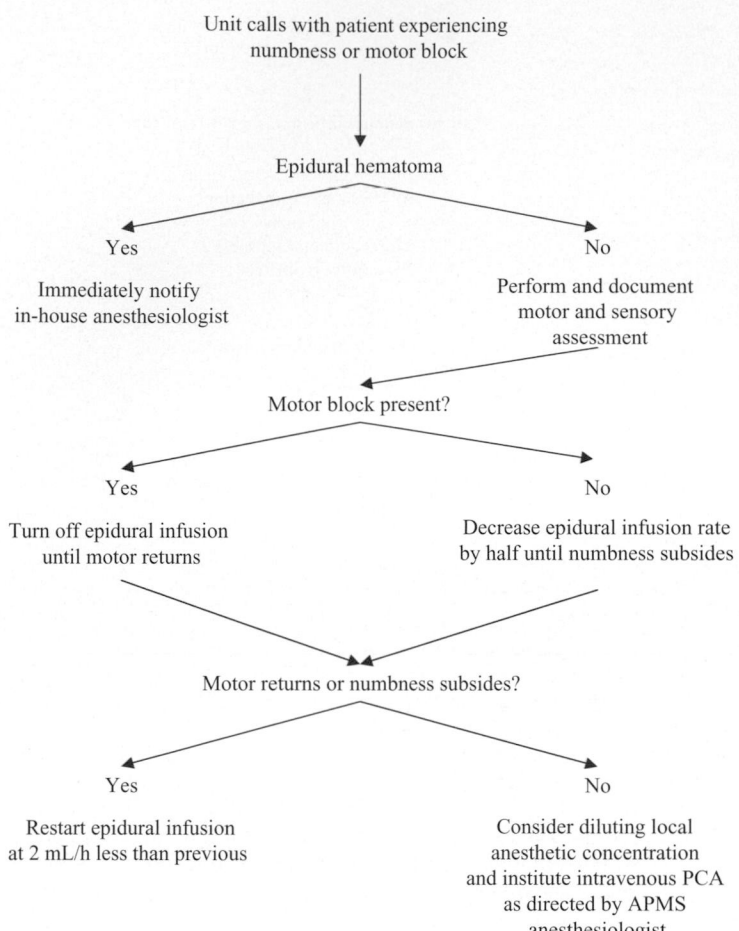

Figure 79–12. Decision tree in a patient with suspected epidural hematoma. APMS = acute pain management service, PCA = patient-controlled analgesia.

may benefit from the regional anesthesia, epidural, or parenteral opioids for a longer period of time than opioid-naïve patients.

In the postoperative period, converting opioid-tolerant patients to oral opioids can be quite challenging. One approach is to calculate the patient's 24-h opioid requirement from IVPCA and give two thirds that amount in the form of a long-acting oral opioid and one third in the form of a short-acting oral opioid to be used as needed. Table 79–8 provides an equianalgesic opioid conversion chart.

Baseline opioid doses should be tapered slowly to prevent withdrawal. Addition of other adjuncts such as α_2-adrenergic receptor agonists like clonidine, dexmedetomidine, NMDA receptor antagonists, and COX-2 inhibitors all help to decrease opioid need and improve analgesia. Tricyclic antidepressants may help with neuropathic pain, although these agents usually require several weeks to achieve efficacy. Membrane-stabilizing agents (eg, gabapentin) can be extremely helpful during the perioperative period in the presence of neurogenic or neuropathic pain. Routine doses of these agents should be continued. Surgery can cause new nerve injury and pain that may benefit from these agents.

Clinical Pearls

- In the postoperative period, converting opioid-tolerant patients to oral opioids can be quite challenging.
- One approach is to calculate the patient's 24-h opioid requirement from IVPCA and give two thirds that amount in the form of a long-acting oral opioid and one third in the form of a short-acting oral opioid to be used as needed.

Before and after hospital discharge, referral to a pain specialist can be very helpful in treating the opioid-dependent patient to help optimize pain management during rehabilitation and facilitate opioid dose tapering. Whenever possible, the pain specialist familiar with the patient's history should be involved in the postdischarge pain management. With patients chronically treated with opioids, patients may be better served by having a single opioid prescriber.

Considerations for managing the opioid-tolerant patient are presented in Table 79–10.

Table 79–9.

Management of Acute Pain in the Chronic Pain Patient

Preoperative Phase

1. Identify the chronic pain patient preoperatively
2. Assure the patient that pain control is a priority
3. Evaluate the location and character of chronic pain
4. Accurately determine the preoperative opioid requirement and identify all other pain medications
5. Formulate a multimodal analgesic plan (as part of the anesthetic plan) that incorporates the patient's preferences and cooperation
6. Communicate this plan to the primary anesthesia team and surgeon

Operative Phase

1. Ensure that patient has received morning doses of opioids and other pain medications and adequate preoperative sedation
2. Communicate with members of the surgical team the specific considerations for this patient
3. Incorporate a multimodal approach to the anesthetic (preoperative NSAID or COX-2 inhibitor, possible dose of membrane stabilizing agents, local anesthetics wherever practical, adequate intraoperative doses of opioids)
4. Ensure that patient is reasonably comfortable before leaving the operating room

Postoperative Phase

1. Inform recovery room nurse of plan and ensure that patient is comfortable prior to discharge from recovery room
2. Inform floor staff nurse of plan and provide individual or service to contact for pain issues
3. Maintain patient's routine pain medications throughout the perioperative period
4. Consider acute pain plan as an "overlay" on the patient's chronic pain management
5. Initiate oral therapy as soon as is practical
6. Utilize extended release oral opioids to reduce the analgesic "gaps" between doses of short acting opioids
7. Evaluate patient daily and adjust plan as needed
8. Pain medication requirements may change drastically during the weeks following discharge, so plan early for outpatient pain management

Table 79–10.

Considerations for Opioid Management in the Opioid-Tolerant Patient

1. Identify opioid requirements
2. Recognize that opioid requirements usually escalate with new acute pain on chronic pain (frequently two- to threefold increase)
3. Continue or start routine opioids as soon as possible after surgery, particularly extended release formulations
4. Add IVPCA to routine medications
5. A basal opioid background infusion may be indicated in the opioid tolerant
6. Larger than routine patient controlled doses are indicated
7. A rule of thumb is to provide approximately one-third to one-half the opioid requirement as basal or oral extended release and the remainder on demand. These doses may require frequent adjustment.
8. When converting to oral-only opioids, consider a "bridge" day:
   Calculate total opioid requirement (oral plus PCA).
   Provide a significant portion of opioid requirement as an oral extended-release agent (usually approximately half).
   Continue IVPCA patient demand dose only during this "bridge" day.
   On the following day, convert the total PCA opioid dose from the prior day to oral short-acting opioid.
   Continue that patient on this dose of oral short-acting plus extended-release opioid.
9. Patient will need careful follow-up after discharge to regulate opioid doses
10. High doses of opioids are usually well tolerated in patients who use opioids chronically. However, side effects still occur particularly at escalating doses so careful monitoring of the patient may be indicated.

Note: Opioids are only one aspect of the management! Remember to maximize the value of nonopioids during the perioperative period.
IVPCA = intravenous patient-controlled analgesia

EXTENDED-RELEASE EPIDURAL MORPHINE

Extended-release epidural morphine (EREM) (DepoDur, Endo Pharmaceuticals, Chadds Ford, PA) was approved by the US Food and Drug Administration in 2004 for postoperative pain management following major surgery. EREM is an extended-release formulation of morphine in a liposomal carrier, intended for epidural administration. EREM is approved for the treatment of postoperative pain by single-dose administration into the lumbar epidural space before major surgery or following umbilical cord clamping during cesarean section. EREM is not intended for intravenous, intrathecal, or intramuscular administration.

Recently published studies have demonstrated the safety and efficacy of EREM in a variety of surgical models. In a hip arthroplasty study, EREM provided analgesia for up to 48 h after surgery with a side effect profile similar to that for standard epidural opioid analgesia.[61] EREM demonstrated a marked reduction in the need for supplemental analgesia and delayed the time for first analgesic rescue. No additional analgesia was needed in 25% of EREM patients. Similarly, in the lower abdominal surgery study, EREM reduced the need for supplemental opioid analgesia and reduced pain scores.[62]

In a cesarean section study, EREM was compared with a standard epidural morphine dose of 5 mg.[63] Patients who received EREM at the 10- and 15-mg dose had both superior pain relief and extended analgesia for 48 h with less need for supplemental analgesia. To measure functionality of patients, an instrument was created to assess the effect of pain on common patient functions (resting in bed, sitting, waking, and using the rest room). Pain had significantly less impact on functional ability for 48 h after surgery in patients who received EREM at the 10- or 15-mg dose.

One must bear in mind that the doses in these initial studies employed opioids alone for analgesia. Consequently, opioid side effects were observed. In practice, most clinicians utilize multimodal analgesic techniques to reduce opioid requirements and their related side effects while optimizing pain relief. If clinicians use similar techniques with EREM, it is quite likely that lower doses may provide adequate analgesia while reducing typical opioid side effects, such as nausea, pruritus, sedation, and respiratory depression.

The potential of providing extended analgesia without an epidural catheter and epidural pump or IVPCA pump is very desirable. External pump technology is cumbersome for the patient, time-consuming for the nursing staff, and is associated with medication errors and pump programming errors. In many surgical settings, anticoagulation to prevent venous thromboembolis is now standard management. Consequently, indwelling epidural catheters may increase the risk of epidural hematoma formation. EREM may provide extended analgesia without the need for indwelling epidural catheters and without the difficulties associated with current epidural and IVPCA pumps.

ACUTE PAIN MANAGEMENT FROM A NURSING PERSPECTIVE

Nurses are a key component of an acute pain service. The pain nursing team may be composed of acute pain management nurses, pain resource nurses, and floor nurses. Acute pain management nurses are dedicated to promoting and providing care for patients in pain. In most settings, acute pain nurses work in collaboration with the department of anesthesiology. Acute pain management nurses operate best within an established framework of hospital-approved protocols and guidelines and through decision trees. Guidelines and protocols are intended to establish the basic standard of care and provide consistency in management.[64] Protocols prescribe methods of care in a less flexible way then guidelines,[65] but neither is a substitute for personal knowledge. Thoughtful application is essential if guidelines and protocols are to be safe and effective.

A nurse-driven acute pain service consists of a physician director and the nursing team. The physician determines the appropriate analgesic technique. The care team, consisting of an attending physician, resident, and an acute pain nurse, assesses patients on morning rounds and develops a comprehensive management plan. A standard daily clinical note will facilitate documentation (see Figures 79–3 and 79–4). The roles of the various team members are described in Table 79–11.

The pain management plan is communicated and coordinated by the acute pain nurse to the other members of the patient care team. The pain resource nurse is a floor nurse with special training in the assessment of pain and technical expertise in the various infusion devices. Optimally, every nursing unit has a pain resource nurse to provide peer support to other floor nurses and provide basic troubleshooting and assessment. Standard documentation sheets for pain assessment, epidural, and PCA are helpful (see Figures 79–3, 79–4, and 79–6).

A very specific process is followed so that protocols can be considered, approved, and eventually become part of a standard order set. The proposed protocols are then reviewed by the pharmacy and therapeutics (P&T) committee that makes recommendations resulting from evidence-based practice. The P&T committee is a multidisciplinary group composed of physicians, pharmacists, administrators, and nurses. Standard order sets then typically require the approval of a medical executive committee. Where computer physician order entry is employed (CPOE), standard order sets must be configured to maintain all necessary order details of the protocol. Thus, physicians are able to order a protocol of decision trees that allow the acute pain nurses to follow a defined path in the management of specific pain management scenarios.

With a nurse-driven acute pain service, the pain nurse is the first to respond to calls for the patient's pain issues. Pain nurses must possess astute assessment and critical thinking skills. This requires a background in critical care or postanesthesia care. Utilizing decision trees and critical

Table 79–11.

Description of Roles on an Acute Pain Service

APMS Director
- Determines direction of service
- Defines and coordinates clinical, educational, and research goals
- Develops policies and protocols for pain assessment and treatment
- Communicates with hospital administration, nursing service, and referring physicians
- Reviews quality assurance indicators

APMS Attending Staff
- Conducts daily patient rounds
- Performs and supervises regional anesthesia procedures
- Performs and supervises consultations
- Participants in educational and research goals

Residents and Fellows
- Daily patient rounds
- Responds to acute pain consults
- Performs various regional anesthetic techniques (epidurals, peripheral nerve blocks) both preoperative and postoperatively, as needed, for management of pain
- When "on-call": rounds with pain nurse late in the day to discuss management issues; available by pager for questions/consults throughout the night
- Participant in research and educational goals

Clinical Nurse Specialist (advance practice nurse)
- Coordinator of services provides continuity of care to APMS patients
- Designs and implements educational programs for the department of nursing and patient education
- Responsible for data collection and quality assurance activity
- Assists APMS director in development of goals, policies, protocols, and standards

Acute Pain Nurse
- Holds service pager and responds to calls for patients in pain or pain-related problems
- Conducts frequent proactive assessments of analgesia and its side effects
- Adjusts pain therapy or treatment of side effects according to a treatment algorithm and reassess efficacy of interventions
- Employs complementary techniques (ie, relaxation, imaging, distraction)
- Point-of-care peer support to staff nurses

Pain Resource Nurse
- Nurses specially trained in pain issues on each unit
- Pain management resource to peers in the unit
- Contact person with APMS
- Troubleshoots technical problems with infusion pumps
- Enhances hospital initiative to extend aggressive pain management for all patients

APMS = acute pain management service.

thinking, pain nurses are called on to manage pain and side effects of pain therapies, troubleshoot epidural and peripheral block catheters, titrating and bolusing as needed, and removing catheters when indicated. Pain nurses must be well trained at assessing hypotension, motor block, and excessive sedation. All actions and interventions of the pain nurse are entirely within the scope of institutional protocols. Figures 79–8 through 79–12 provide a number of practical decision trees for troubleshooting common clinical scenarios.

Pain nurses are the critical link in providing education and peer support to the various members of the nursing service. Nurse-driven acute pain services function proactively, closely monitoring and anticipating problems. The visible presence of pain nurses increases patient satisfaction, improves pain control and safety, and may improve patient outcome. Busy acute pain services utilizing aggressive regional anesthesia/analgesia techniques and opioid therapies may benefit from an organizational design that places nurse in key patient management positions. A nurse-driven acute pain service integrates the treatment of these patients into the overall hospital milieu and helps facility institutional consistency in the management of all pain issues within the facility.

PHARMACIST CONSIDERATIONS IN ACUTE PAIN MANAGEMENT

A pharmacist offers a unique perspective when establishing or expanding an acute pain service using regional anesthesia/analgesia techniques. Pharmacists have extensive training in pharmacology, pharmacokinetics, and pharmacoeconomics. In addition to the traditional role of the pharmacist in compounding and dispensing medications, a pharmacist can be a valued team member who provides clinical services in the areas of safe, rationale, and cost-effective drug therapy. Pharmacists may provide patient education and instruction, drug information, and alternative therapy options. Pharmacists may also be included in quality assurance data collection, proper pump selection, proper medication labeling, safety considerations, and the development of policies and procedures. Pharmacists can also be involved in hospital formulary medication decisions and have an important role in evaluating new products for formulary addition.

Pharmacy Considerations with Epidural Delivery

When the technique of epidural and intrathecal administration was developed, it was standard practice to administer medication as a single bolus or multiple as-needed bolus injections. Anesthesiologists generally prepared and administered the doses. This technique, however, may result in periods of inadequate pain control and has been associated with a higher frequency of adverse effects resulting from temporary peak levels of medications creating unwanted side effects.[66] Development of protocols for initial bolus doses followed by continuous infusions with or without patient-controlled epidural analgesia (PCEA) has revolutionized pain management.[65] Continuous infusions of epidural opioids or local anesthetics (or both) avoid the peaks and valleys of pain control and the need for multiple bolus injections.[66–68] Studies comparing continuous infusions and intermittent bolus administration have shown that continuous administration provides better analgesia with lower total doses administered.[67]

Pharmacists should be involved in the procurement and preparation of the epidural continuous infusion solutions. The preparation of epidural infusions must follow strict aseptic techniques outlined by the new standard of practice for compounding sterile preparations, published in Chapter 797 in the United States Pharmacopeia.[69] Epidural solutions are considered a "moderate risk level" for microbial contamination based on the fact that the solution contains no preservatives.[69] Appropriate labeling of epidural solutions and concentrations of commonly used epidural additive drugs are detailed in Tables 79–12 and 79–13.

Peripheral Nerve Blocks and Catheters

Peripheral anesthetic techniques have increased in popularity for the management of acute and chronic pain conditions.

Table 79–12.

Suggestions for Appropriate Epidural Labeling

1. All solution ingredients:
   a. Drug names
   b. Volumes
   c. Strength
2. Final concentration
3. Total volume
4. Rate of administration (mL/h)
5. Diluent used
6. Date of preparation and expiration
7. Time of expiration
8. Unique label stating "For Epidural Use Only"

Table 79–13.

Concentrations of Commonly Used Adjunctive Drugs in the Epidural Space

Drug	Concentration
Morphine	0.025–0.05 mg/mL
Fentanyl	2–5 mcg/mL
Sufentanil	1–2 mcg/mL
Hydromorphone	5–10 mcg/mL
Bupivacaine	0.1–0.15%
Ropivacaine	0.1–0.2%
Epinephrine	1:400,000

Studies have shown that patients who receive peripheral nerve blocks experience reduced postoperative pain and analgesia requirements and report more satisfaction with their pain management.[70] These techniques involve either bolus or intermittent doses, or continuous infusions of local anesthetics through a catheter near or around the nerve or nerve plexus that supplies the surgical area.[71,72]

A perineural placement of catheters for continuous local anesthetic is growing in popularity.[73–75] This technique of continuous peripheral nerve blocks or perineural local anesthetic infusions involves the percutaneous insertion of a catheter directly adjacent to the peripheral nerves or plexuses supplying an affected surgical site.[76] In the hospital setting, local anesthetic infusions can be prepared by the pharmacy, and the continuous infusion be accomplished with an infusion pump. In recent years, smaller electronic infusion pumps, syringe pumps, elastomeric pumps, and spring–powered pumps have been designed for use in the ambulatory setting. Because of the inherent risks of sending a patient home with an infusion device, most published studies limit ambulatory use of the pumps to patients expected to have moderate-to-severe postoperative pain of a duration more than 24 h and who will have difficulty managing the pain with oral opioids.[76] In addition, special consideration must be given to the caregiver's capability for managing the pump or the need for home care or visiting nurses to monitor, regulate, or discontinue the infusion.

An alternative to continuous regional blocks is continuous infusion of local anesthetic directly into the wound site.[77] A pump is attached to a catheter inserted near an incision site. The pump infuses a continuous flow of local anesthetic and may include the capability for patient control. For wound instillation devices, the local anesthetic may be added to the device in the sterile environment of the operating room or added into the device by pharmacy personnel using aseptic technique.

With the capability of infusing local anesthetics epidurally, intrathecally, peripherally, and topically, guidelines must be established for all healthcare providers to be aware of the type and route of local anesthetic administration. Unintentional administration of local anesthetic via two different routes may increase the risk for systemic toxicity. To prevent double administration, all local anesthetic administration should be documented in the patient chart. If CPOE is available, all orders should be entered into the computer. A warning screen should appear if duplicate local anesthetic orders are entered for a patient.

With the evolution of multimodal therapy, anesthesiologists and surgeons must communicate regarding all pain management therapy. In addition, pharmacists must review medication profiles and be aware of all local anesthetics dispensed and administered to patients. Pharmacists play a crucial role in monitoring the overall pharmacologic management of the patient.

Infusion Devices

Pharmacist involvement in the selection of infusion devices will offer a unique perspective on the advantages and disadvantages of various pumps. Many factors must be considered to determine the optimal device for a given clinical situation. Infusion devices should be safe, accurate, reliable, easy to use, and compatible with the drug delivery systems available.[68] For the management of acute pain, an external pump is standard. Several external devices are available on the market, including syringe pumps, peristaltic devices, and elastomeric reservoir pumps. When selecting a pump, several factors should be considered, including the acceptable infusion rate accuracy, PCA bolus capability, and total local anesthetic volume required.

Syringe pumps are used to deliver the contents of a syringe over a given period.[68] These devices can be programmed to deliver the contents of a syringe over several hours to several days. These pumps are commonly used for the delivery of opioids for IVPCA. Prefilled morphine and meperidine syringes are commercially available. Pharmacy personnel must compound other opioids or differing concentrations of commercially available products. Most of these devices must be locked to prevent patient manipulation and to prevent diversion of a controlled substance.

Peristaltic devices deliver a drug from a flexible reservoir via administration tubing that is mechanically squeezed.[68] These pumps are traditionally used to administer intravenous fluids. Some peristaltic devices have locked chambers to secure solutions. This would be of benefit for opioid infusions. Peristaltic pumps can accommodate larger volumes of solution. Flow rate capabilities range from 0.1 to 999 mL/h. Newer pumps have more sophisticated programming, allowing for minimum and maximum rates of any drug programmed into the device. Some programs also calculate infusion rates based on the patient's weight and the amount of drug to be administered per minute or hour. This new technology was developed to help prevent potential medication errors.

Elastomeric reservoir pumps force fluid through a flow regulator via elastomeric pressure of a balloon reservoir.[68] Depending on the brand, the reservoir volume varies, allowing for varying rates and length of therapy. This technology is used for continuous delivery of local anesthetics for continuous peripheral blocks or instillation directly into the wound.

Regardless of the type of infusion pump used, the maximum reservoir volume must be considered when establishing the use of epidural solutions or continuous nerve infiltrations. In addition, the range of administration rates is a critical factor in epidural delivery of medications.[68] Epidural infusion rates vary depending on the location of the epidural catheter and the drugs administered into the epidural space. Rates greater than 20 mL/h are generally not indicated. Table 79–7 provides a general guideline for epidural administration rates based on the placement of the epidural catheter.[77] Tables 79–12 and 79–13 provide useful information on epidural orders, labeling, and solutions. Figure 79–5 is a sample epidural order form.

When choosing an infusion device, consideration should be given to devices that allow for safe and secure administration of solutions while maximizing the time between refills or the interval between bag, syringe, or cassette changes. The potential for pump misidentification or confusion is ever-present, leading to medication errors or error in route of deliver. From a systems standpoint, rigorous policies are needed to prevent medication errors. This may include special labeling, route-specific tubing, and dedicated pumps for specific techniques, color-coding of labels and tubing, and two practitioner pump set-up checks. Representatives from the departments of biomedical engineering, nursing, anesthesiology, and pharmacy should all be involved in pump selection.

Solution Preparation, Stability, and Sterility

As described previously, pharmacists offer many valuable services to all areas of patient care. In regard to regional anesthesia, the most important contributions include accurate preparation and assurance of sterility and stability for all solutions prepared.

Any drug administered into the epidural or intrathecal space must be free of neurotoxic preservatives.[67,78] Agents containing preservatives such as methylparaben, benzyl alcohol, methylhydroxybenzoate, propylhydroxybenzoate, phenol, and formaldehyde must be avoided.[67,78] Standard epidural preparations guidelines call for the use of preservative-free solutions.

Although infection of the epidural or intrathecal space is rare, it can be fatal. Preparation of all epidural solutions must be performed with strict adherence to sterile aseptic technique. As of January 1, 2004, JCAHO officially surveyed accredited organizations for compliance with the United States Pharmacopeia (USP) general Chapter 797, Pharmaceutical Compounding-Sterile Preparations.[69] USP Chapter 797 details the procedures and requirements for compounding sterile preparations and sets standards that are applicable to all practice settings in which sterile preparations are compounded. Based on these guidelines, because epidural solutions contain no preservatives, they are considered to be a medium risk for microbial contamination. Certified pharmacy personnel using a laminar flow hood should prepare epidural, intrathecal solutions as well as solutions for continuous peripheral neural blockade.

The stability of morphine, fentanyl, hydromorphone, and fentanyl mixed with various local anesthetics in a variety of syringes and reservoirs has been studied.[79-82] Solutions studied maintained potency for at least 12 days. However, the risk of microbial contamination in preservative-free solutions is problematic. Current guidelines from the Centers for Disease Control and Prevention (CDC) recommend that preservative-free infusion solutions be completely used or discarded within 24 h of preparation when not refrigerated.[67,83,84] CDC guidelines also recommend that preservative-free solutions be stored under refrigeration for no more than 7 days.[83] Refrigeration must be continuous and occur immediately after mixing the solution. After the product is dispensed for patient use, a 24-h expiration date must be applied. USP Chapter 797 gives a medium risk level to preparations 30 h at room temperature and 7 days under refrigeration.[69] According to USP Chapter 797, if the product is not made in a laminar flow hood, it will be considered high risk and should be used within 24 h.[69] It would be prudent for institutions administering epidural, intrathecal, and continuous peripheral local anesthetic solutions to have the solutions prepared in accordance with USP Chapter 797.

Standardization of Regional Anesthesia Continuous Solutions

Standardizing epidural solution volumes, medications used, and drug concentrations are important considerations when establishing an epidural program. Consistency in prescribing and preparing epidural, intrathecal, and continuous peripheral local anesthetic solutions helps to reduce the potential for medication errors and simplifies the preparation process.[85-87] Having a limited number of concentrations for epidural solutions will prevent medication errors in prescribing, preparing, and administering epidurals. Pharmacists should work with anesthesiologists to determine dosing ranges for epidural drugs. Pharmacists should be familiar with the dosing ranges and should question orders that deviate from established guidelines. It would be beneficial to minimize the size of the solution bag for epidurals. If the rate of an epidural is mistakenly increased, a limited amount of epidural solution would be infused at the incorrect rate.

When initially establishing standard epidural solutions, physician preference and stability considerations should be assessed.[87] Decisions regarding standard epidural preparations must also take into consideration safety, cost, time, narcotic accountability, and reservoir volume of the infusion device.[85-87] When possible, using whole rather than partial ampules and vials and using available package sizes of the drugs will help to minimize waste.[87] This is beneficial in

helping to keep narcotic inventories as simple as possible. Although standard epidural solutions are usually adequate for most patients, it should be noted that these standard preparations might not be suitable for every patient. There may be instances when a patient requires a specialized preparation. The patient may have an allergy to one of the standard epidural components, or the patient may have a history of opioid tolerance and will require higher concentrations. If a nonstandard epidural is ordered, highlighting the concentrations may help to prevent confusion and errors.

- Standardization of epidural solutions may allow for batch preparation.
- Batch preparation helps to prevent a delay in starting an epidural and decreases the possibility of interrupting continuous pain therapy.
- Batching puts less stress on pharmacy personnel preparing solutions and on nurses in a need of a new solution bag.

Standardization of epidural solutions may allow for batch preparation. Batch preparation helps to prevent a delay in starting an epidural. In addition, depending on the infusion rate, more than one infusion bag may be needed per day. If an infusion is running dry, having batched solutions available prevents the possibility of interrupting continuous pain therapy. Batching puts less stress on pharmacy personnel preparing solutions and on nurses in a need of a new solution bag. However, maintenance of continuous pain relief therapy for the patient is the most important benefit. To provide the maximum expiration dating, certified individuals should do batch preparation of epidural solutions without preservative under strict aseptic conditions. Storage should be in accordance with the CDC and USP Chapter 797.[69]

Some pharmaceutical manufacturers provide compounding services for epidural and other solutions. Others manufacture standard concentrations. Expiration dating is extended beyond 7 days based on stability studies conducted by the pharmaceutical manufacturers. Institutions handling a large number of surgical and obstetric cases may find this service of use because compounding large amounts of epidurals requires additional staffing, supplies, and time. Therefore, the cost of the compounded products should be weighed against pharmacy considerations associated with preparing the solutions.[87]

Safety Considerations

Medication errors related to the use of opioid infusions and epidurals are among the most frequently reported.[85] To help prevent medication errors, it is imperative that all epidural solutions be labeled in a clear, concise, consistent manner.

Table 79–12 provides suggestions for the appropriate labeling of epidural solutions.[84] Labels should be legible and permanently affixed to the infusion bag or syringe in a manner that makes it easily readable.[84] The patient's name, date of preparation, and solution expiration should be clearly stated. The medication contents should be distinctly labeled with the name of the drugs and volumes used to prepare the solution. In addition, the final concentration and total volume should be clearly marked on the bag in bold lettering. Last, a bright auxiliary label reading *"For Epidural Use Only"* should be affixed to the bag or syringe.

Drugs intended for intravenous administration have been accidentally administered into the epidural or intrathecal space.[67,85–86] An error in the route of administration could have catastrophic consequences. The route of administration must be clearly noted on all order forms. Drug concentrations vary dramatically between intravenous, continuous peripheral block, epidural, and intrathecal routes. If an intravenous solution of morphine 1 mg/mL is administered epidurally, respiratory depression and death may result. In addition to anesthesiologists, nurses and pharmacists should be familiar with dosing ranges and standard concentrations for epidural and intrathecal preparations.

Proper labeling of the epidural tubing is also imperative. It is recommended that the distal ends of epidural and intravenous lines be labeled to clearly differentiate them.[85] A line dedicated to the administration of epidurals with port-free tubing should always be used to prevent accidental epidural administration of drugs intended for intravenous use.[85–86] It is also helpful to use single-chamber pumps dedicated to epidural infusions. Infusion pumps should also be labeled *"For Epidural Use Only."* If a multiple-chamber pump must be used for epidural administration, the other chambers should not be used for the infusion of any other medications. If an adjustment in rate or another medication is administered to the patient, nurses should always trace the tubing from the insertion site to a pump. If more than one pump is being used, placing the IV pump on the opposite side of the patient's bed from the epidural pump may help to prevent mistakes.[85]

Healthcare practitioners should be aware of the potential for error with hand-written orders. Only proper abbreviations should be accepted and clarification of any order completed prior to processing. The use of preprinted order forms has helped to reduce these types of errors. The ASA Task Force on Pain Management has established guidelines for the use of preprinted order forms in acute pain management.[88] The key elements for epidural analgesia preprinted order forms are listed in Table 79–8.

If a patient is receiving an epidural opioid, prescribing other sedative agents should be done with extreme caution. The service or anesthesiologist managing the epidural should be the only service prescribing other sedatives. If another service prescribes another sedative, the pharmacist should intervene and notify the service managing the opioid epidural. If CPOE is available, a warning screen should be displayed if a sedative is ordered.

Clinical Pearls

- In a patient receiving neuraxial opioids, prescribing other sedative agents should be done with extreme caution.
- The service or anesthesiologist managing the epidural should be the only service prescribing additional sedatives or narcotics.

The pharmacist's role in regional anesthesia may include reviewing patients' drug therapy, optimizing medication selection, and developing policies and procedures. Pharmacists also supervise and evaluate solution preparation, stability, storage, and safety issues. Additionally, the pharmacist can provide information on the cost of different mediation modalities, offering suggestions for the most cost-effective choices.

SUMMARY

Anesthesiologists, surgeons, pharmacists, and various members of the nursing team all have important roles when considering the organization of an acute pain service. Acute pain management requires a multimodal and multidisciplinary approach with a clear organizational framework. Regional anesthesia techniques for surgical anesthesia are a highly effective component of acute pain management. Maximizing the contributions of regional anesthesia to acute pain management requires integrating these techniques into the larger framework of patient care. Clinicians must regard their efforts as extending beyond the operating room and postanesthesia care unit. This requires an organizational framework that includes all members of the healthcare team, standard order sets, assessment and documentation forms, and institutionwide policies and procedures for the management of aggressive pain techniques. Strong institutional commitment is imperative.

References

1. Ready LB, Oden R, Chadwick HS, et al: Development of an anesthesiology-based postoperative pain management service. Anesthesiology 1988;68:100–106.
2. Rawal N, Berggren L: Organization of acute pain services: A low-cost model. Pain 1994;57(1):117–123.
3. Warfield CA, Kahn CH: Acute pain management. Anesthesiology 1995;83:1090–1094.
4. Anonymous: Practice guidelines for acute pain management in the Perioperative setting. A report by the American Society of Anesthesiologists Task Force on Pain Management, Acute Pain Section. Anesthesiology 1995;82:1071–1081.
5. An Updated Report by the American Society of Anesthesiologists Task Force on Acute Pain Management. Anesthesiology 2004;100:1573–1581.
6. Joint Commission on the Accreditation of Healthcare Organizations: Accreditation manual for hospitals. Oakbrook Terrace, IL: JCAHO, 2001.

7. Reuben SS, Connelly NR: Postoperative analgesic effects of celecoxib or rofecoxib after spinal fusion surgery. Anesth Analg 2000;91:1221–1225.

8. Kehlet H, Morgensen T: Hospital stay of 2 days after open sigmoidectomy with a multimodal rehabilitation programme. Br J Surg 1999;86:227–230.

9. Sechzer PH: Studies in pain with analgesic demand system. Anesth Analg 1971;50:1–10.

10. Forrest WH, Jr. Smithurst PW, Kienitz ME: Self-administration of intravenous analgesics. Anesthesiology 1970;33:363–365.

11. Dahlstrom B, Tamser A, Paalzow L, et al: Patient controlled analgesic therapy Part IV. Pharmacokinetics and analgesic plasma concentration of morphine. Clin Pharmacokinet 1982;7:266–279.

12. Ferrante FM, Orav EJ, Rocco AG, et al: A statistical model for pain in patients controlled analgesia and conventional intramuscular opioid regimens. Anesth Analg 1988;67:457–461.

13. White PF: Use of PCA for management of acute pain. JAMA 1988;259:243–247.

14. Gibaldi M, Perrier D: *Pharmacokinetics.* Marcel Dekker, 1975.

15. Parker RK, Holtmann B, White PF: Patient-controlled analgesia. Does a concurrent opioid infusion improve pain management after surgery? JAMA 1991;266(14):1947–1952.

16. Ellis R, Haines D, Shah R: Pain relief after abdominal surgery, comparison of IM morphine sublingual buprenorphine and self-administered IV pethadine. Br J Anaesth 1982;54:421–428.

17. Welcher EA: On demand analgesia a double-blind comparison of on demand IV fentanyl with IM morphine. Anesthesia 1983;38;19–25.

18. White PF: Mishaps with PCA. Anesthesiology 1987;66:81–83.

19. Sullivan M, Phillips MS: Patient-controlled analgesia pumps. USP Q R 2004;81:1–3.

20. Manufacturer and User Facility Device Experience Database (MAUDE). U.S. Food and Drug Administration, Center for Devices and Radiologic Health, Department of health and Human Services. Available on the web at: www.fda.gov/cdrh/maude.html.

21. Viscusi ER, Reynolds L, Chung F, et al: Patient-controlled transdermal fentanyl hydrochloride vs intravenous morphine pump for postoperative pain: a randomized controlled trial. JAMA 2004;291(11):1333–1141.

22. Ilfeld BM, Mory TE, Wright TW, et al: Continuous interscalene brachial plexus block for postoperative pain control at home. A randomized, double-blinded, placebo controlled study. Anesth Analg 2003;96:1089–1095.

23. Klein SM, Grant SA, Greengrass RA, et al: Interscalene brachial plexus block with continuous catheter insertion system and a disposable infusion pump. Anesth Analg 2000;91:1473–1478.

24. Ilfeld BM, Morey TE, Wang RD: Continuous popliteal sciatic nerve block for postop pain control at home. A double-blinded placebo controlled study. Anesthesiology 2000;97:959–965.

25. Ilfeld BM: Ambulatory perneural local anesthetic infusions: Portable pumps and dosing regimen selection. Tech Reg Anesth Pain Manage 2004;8(2):90–98.

26. Rawal N, Allvin R, Axelsson K: Patient-controlled regional anesthesia (PCRA) at home. Controlled comparison between bupivacaine and ropivacaine brachial plexus analgesia. Anesthesiology 2000;96:1290–1296.

27. Ilfeld BM, Morey TE, Enneking FK: Outpatient use of patient-controlled local anesthetic administration via a PSOAS compartment catheter to improve pain control and patient satisfaction after ACL reconstruction. Anesthesiology 2001;95:A38(abstract).

28. Klein SM: Beyond the hospital, continuous peripheral nerve blocks at home. Anesthesiology 2002;96:1283–1285.

29. Singelyn FJ, Seguy S, Gouverneur JM: Interscalene brachial plexus analgesia after open shoulder surgery: Continuous versus patient-controlled infusion. Anesth Analg 1999;89:1216–1220.

30. Klein SM, Nielsen KC, Greengrass RA, et al: Ambulatory discharge after long-acting peripheral nerve blockade: 2382 blocks with ropivacaine. Anesth Analg 2002;94:65–70.

31. Ekatodramis G, Borgeat A, Huledel G, et al: Continuous interscalene analgesia with Ropivacaine 2 mg/mL after major shoulder surgery. Anesthesiology 2003;98:143–150.

32. Klein SM, Nielsen KC: Brachial plexus blocks: Infusion and other mechanisms to provide prolonged analgesia. Curr Opin Anaesth 2003;16:393–399.

33. Cuvillon P, Ripart J, Lalourcey L, et al: The continuous femoral nerve block catheter for postop analgesia: Bacterial colonization infusion rate and adverse effects. Anesth Analg 2001:93:1045–1049.

34. Hogan Q, Dotson R, Erickson S, et al: Local anesthetics myotoxicity: A case and review. Anesthesiology 1994;80:942–947.

35. Kehlet H, Dahl JB: The value of multimodal or balanced analgesia in postoperative pain treatment. Anesth Analg 1993;77:1048–1056.

36. Gillies GWA, Kenny GNC, Bullingham RES: The morphine sparing effect of ketorolec tromethamine. Anesthesia 1987;42:727–731.

37. Kehlet H, Werner M, Perkins F: Balanced analgesia: What is it and what are its advantages in postoperative pain? Drugs 1999;58:793–797.

38. Kehlet H, Morgensen T: Hospital stay of 2 days after open sigmoidectomy with a multimodal rehabilitation programme. Br J Surg 1999;86:227–230.

39. Bradshaw BG, Liu S, Thirlby RC: Standardized perioperative care protocols and reduced length of stay after colon surgery. J Am Coll Surg 1998;186:501–506.

40. Perkins FM, Kehlet H: Chronic pain as an outcome of surgery. Anesthesiology 2000;93:1123–1133.

41. Lash V, Anderson K, Asenjo JF, et al: Low dose ketamine reduces morphine use after total knee arthroplasty. Can J Anaesth 2003;50:A5.

42. Taura P, Fuster J, Blasi A, et al: Postoperative pain relief after hepatic resection in cirrhotic patients: The efficacy of a single small dose of ketamine plus morphine epidurally. Anesth Analg 2003;96:475–580.

43. McCrory C, Lindahl S: Cyclooxygenase inhabitation for postoperative analgesia. Anesth Analg 2002;95:169–176.

44. Brodner G, Van Aken H, Hertle L, et al: Multimodal perioperative management—Combining thoracic epidural analgesia, forced mobilization, and oral nutrition-reduces hormonal and metabolic stress and improves convalescence after major urologic surgery. Anesth Analg 2001;2:1594–1600.

45. Hahnenkamp K, Theilmeier G, Van Aken H: The effects of local anesthetics in perioperative coagulation, inflammation and microcirculation. Anesth Analg 2002;94:1441–1447.

46. Kehlet H: Modification of responses to surgery by neural blockade. Clinical implications. In Cousins MJ, Brindenbaugh PO (eds): *Neural Blockade in Clinical Anesthesia and Management of Pain.* Lippincott Williams & Wilkins, pp 129–175.

47. Block BM, Liu SS, Rowlingson AJ, et al: Efficacy of postoperative epidural analgesia. JAMA 2003;290(18):2455–2463.

48. Sites B, Beech M, Biggs R: Intrathecal clonidine added to bupivacaine-morphine spinal anesthesia improves postoperative analgesia for total knee arthroplasty. Anesth Analg 2003;96:1083–1088.

49. Arain SR, Richlow RM, Uhrich TD: The efficacy of dexmedatomidine versus morphine for postoperative analgesia after major inpatient surgery. Anesth Analg 2004;98:153–158.

50. Singelyn FJ, Deyaert M, Joris D, et al: Effects of intravenous patient-controlled analgesia with morphine, continuous epidural analgesia, and continuous three-in-one rehabilitation after unilateral total knee arthroplasty. Anesth Analg 1998;87:88–92.

51. Pettersson N, Berggren P, Larsson N, et al: Pain relief by wound infiltration with bupivacaine or high-dose ropivacaine after inguinal hernia repair. Reg Anesth Pain Med 1999;24:569–575.

52. Carroll IR, Augst MS, Clark D: Management of perioperative pain in patients chronically consuming opioids. Reg Anesth Pain Med 2004;29(6):576–591.

53. de Leon-Casasola OA, Myers DP, Donaparthi S, et al: A comparison of postoperative epidural analgesia between patients with chronic cancer taking high doses of oral opioids versus opioid naïve patients. Anesth Analg 1993;76:302–307.

54. Mitra S, Sinatra RS: Perioperative management of acute pain in the opioid-dependent patient. Anesthesiology 2004;101:212–227.

55. Fishbain DA, Rosomoff HL, Rosomoff RS: Drug abuse, dependence, and addiction in chronic pain patients. Clin J Pain 1992;8:77–85.

56. Doverty M, Somogyi AA, White JM, et al: Methadone maintenance patients are cross-tolerant to the antinociceptive effects of morphine. Pain 2001;93:155–163.

57. Compton P, Charuvastra VC, Kintaudi K, et al: Pain responses in methadone-maintained opioid abusers. J Pain Symptom Manage 2000;20:237–245.

58. Angst MS, Koppert W. Pabh I, et al: Short term infusion of the mu-opioid agonist remifentanil in humans causes hyperalgesia during withdrawal. Pain 2003;106:49–57.

59. deLeon-Casasola OA, Lema MJ: Epidural sufentanil for acute pain control in a patient with extreme opioid dependency. Anesthesiology 1992;76:853–856.

60. Sosnowski M, Yaksh TL: Differential cross-tolerance between intrathecal morphine and sufentanil in the rat. Anesthesiology 1990;73:1141–1147.

61. Viscusi ER, Martin G, Hartrick CT, et al: Forty-eight hours of postoperative pain relief after total hip arthroplasty with a novel, extended-release epidural morphine formulation. Anesthesiology 2005;102:1014–1022.

62. Gamgling D, Hughes T, Martin G, et al: A comparison of DepoDur, a novel, single-dose extended-release epidural morphine, with standard epidural morphine for pain relief after lower abdominal surgery. Anesth Analg 2005;100:1065–1074.

63. Garvalho B, Riley E, Cohen SE, et al: Single-dose, sustained-release epidural morphine in the management of postoperative pain after elective cesarean delivery: Results of a multicenter randomized controlled study. Anesth Analg 2005;100:1150–1158.

64. www.worldwidewounds.com

65. Fletcher J: Framework guidelines for wound care. Prof Nurse 2000;17(2):917–921.

66. Mulroy MF: Epidural opioid delivery methods: Bolus, continuous infusion, and patient-controlled epidural analgesia. Reg Anesth 1996;21:100–104.

67. Littrell RA: Epidural analgesia. Am J Hosp Pharm 1991;48:2460–2474.

68. Kwan JW: Use of infusion devices for epidural or intrathecal administration of spinal opioids. Am J Hosp Pharm 1990;47:S18–S23.

69. Pharmaceutical considerations—sterile preparations (general information chapter 797). In *The United States Pharmacopeia*, 27th rev, and *The National Formulary*, 22nd ed. Rockville, MD: The United States Pharmacopeial Convention, 2004, pp 2350–2370.

70. Murauski JD, Gonzalez, KR: Peripheral nerve blocks for postoperative analgesia. AORN J 2002;75(1):136–147.

71. Holder KA, Dougherty TB, Porche VH, et al: Postoperative pain management. Int Anesthesiol Clin 1998;36:71–86.

72. Peng PWH, Chan VWS: Local and regional block in postoperative pain control. Surg Clin North Am 1999;79:345–370.

73. Liu SS, Salinas FV: Continuous plexus and peripheral nerve blocks for postoperative analgesia. Anesth Analg 2003;96:263–272.

74. Rawal N, Axelsson K, Hylander J, et al: Postoperative patient-controlled local anesthetic administration at home. Anesth Analg 1998;86:86–89.

75. Ilfeld, BM, Enneking FK: Continuous peripheral nerve blocks at home: A review. Anesth Analg 2005;100(6):1822–1833.

76. Zohar E, Fredman B, Phillipov A, et al: The analgesic efficacy of patient-controlled bupivacaine wound instillation after total abdominal hysterectomy with bilateral salpingo-oophorectomy. Anesth Analg 2002;93(2):482–487.

77. Carfagno ML, Schechter LN: Regional anesthesia and acute pain management: A pharmacist's perspective. Tech Reg Anesth Pain Manage 2002;6(2):77–86.

78. Shafer AL, Donnelly AJ: Management of postoperative pain by continuous epidural infusions of analgesics. Clin Pharm 1991;10:745–764.

79. Stiles ML, Tu YH, Allen LV: Stability of morphine sulfate in portable pump reservoirs during storage and simulated administration. Am J Hosp Pharm 1989;46:1404–1407.

80. Tu YH, Stiles ML, Allen LV: Stability of fentanyl citrate and bupivacaine hydrochloride in portable pump reservoirs. Am J Hosp Pharm 1990;40:2037–2040.

81. Altman L, Hopkins RJ, Bolton S: Stability of morphine sulfate in Cormed III (Kalex) intravenous bags. Am J Hosp Pharm 1990;47:2040–2042.

82. Duafala ME, Kleinberg MI, Nacov C, et al: Stability of morphine sulfate in infusion devices and containers for intravenous administration. Am J Hosp Pharm 1990;47:143–146.

83. Centers for Disease Control and Prevention: Guideline for the prevention of intravascular device-related infections. Am J Infect Control 1996;24:262–293.

84. American Society of Health-System Pharmacists: ASHP guideline on quality assurance for pharmacy-based sterile products. Am J Health Sys Pharm 2000;57:1150–1169.

85. ISMP Canada Safety Bulletin: Reports of epidural infusion errors. ISMP Medication Safety Alert 2003;3(1):1.

86. Wheeler SJ, Wheeler DW: Medication errors in anaesthesia and critical care. Anaesthesia 2005;60:257–273.

87. Dollard JV, Python JP: Standardization of epidural preparations for postoperative analgesia. Am J Health-Sys Pharm 1995;52:2565–2567.

88. American Society of Anesthesiologists Task Force on Pain Management: Practice guidelines for acute pain management in the perioperative setting. Anesthesiology 1995;82:1071–1081.

Documentation & Training of Regional Anesthesia

80

Documentation of Regional Anesthesia Procedures

J. C. Gerancher, MD

I. INTRODUCTION

II. DOCUMENTATION OF PERFORMANCE

III. DOCUMENTATION OF INFORMED CONSENT

IV. SUMMARY

INTRODUCTION

Regional anesthesia practices are expanding and multiple techniques and approaches, with increasingly sophisticated equipment and medications, are currently being utilized. Automated[1-3] and hand-held computerized[4,5] medical record documentation for anesthetics are being developed, promoted, and instituted. These changes are occurring in a climate where documentation must meet the burden of legal, billing, and regulatory compliance. At present, basic standards for the documentation of regional anesthesia procedures (even those for the established paper-based anesthesia record) are lacking. Most formats for documentation of our anesthesia practices have evolved largely out of our practices for delivery of general anesthesia.[6]

In short, the demands for documentation of regional anesthesia are growing while the utility of our traditional approaches become less adequate. The first goal of this chapter is to provide the reader with two newly designed templates to guide documentation of the performance of regional anesthesia procedures and to review the very limited literature on established paper- or computer-based records in this area. The second goal is to scrutinize documentation of the consent process for regional anesthesia and provide a similar example of a comprehensive consent form.

DOCUMENTATION OF PERFORMANCE

Recently, collective expertise of individuals from several North American academic institutions was pooled to create a peripheral nerve block (PNB) form.[7] The form represents a consensus reached by the authors and is based on available evidence in the literature, each of the author's knowledge of clinical practice, development of their own equipment and practices, medicolegal considerations, familiarity with billing and regulatory compliance, and experience with development of PNB procedure notes at their home institutions (Figure 80–1).[7]

Anesthesiology Procedure Note

PERIPHERAL NERVE BLOCKADE

Peripheral Nerve Block(s) performed

Patient Name

Medical Record #

Age   Sex

(Patient name plate stamp)

Approach: _____ ☐ **Left** ☐ **Right** side confirmed

Indication: ☐ Analgesia ☐ Surgical anesthesia   Dx/pain location:_____

☐ Specifically requested for management of pain by Dr. _____

Date: _____/_____/20_____ **Start time** (:) **End time** (:)

Pt Condition: **Initial BP:**_____/_____ **HR:** ____ **VAS Pain score: 0 1 2 3 4 5 6 7 8 9 10**

☐ awake   ☐ sedate with meaningful contact maintained

☐ PNB performed under spinal / epidural / general anesthesia. Indication: _____

Preparation: ☐ povidone-iodine ☐ chlorhexidine ☐ iodophor/isopropyl ☐ alcohol   ☐ drape

Position: ☐ supine   ☐ prone   ☐ LLD   ☐ RLD   ☐ sitting

Needle(s):   ☐ short-bevel   ☐ Tuohy   ☐ long-bevel   ☐ pencil-tipped

Manufacturer, length, gauges: _____

Technique: ☐ injection through needle   ☐ catheter placement   **(depth at skin_____cm).**

☐ nerve stimulation   ☐ infiltration   ☐ ultrasound

☐ paresthesia. describe quality of paresthesia :_____

Motor response or paresthesia obtained	mA	mS	depth (cm)	Sedation Given	mg/mcg
				Midazolam	
				Fentanyl	

Injectate: ☐ **bupivacaine**   ☐ **ropivacaine**   ☐ **mepivacaine**   ☐ **lidocaine**   ☐ **2-CP**

Concentration (%)	Volume (mL)	Adjunct	Epinephrine
			☐ 1/___00,000
			☐ not used

Narrative: Injection was made incrementally with constant monitoring and aspiration every _____ ml's.

		Action Taken	
Blood aspirated:	☐ no	☐ yes	
Intravenous test using epinephrine:	☐ negative	☐ positive	
Pain on injection noted:	☐ no	☐ yes	
Resistance on injection	☐ normal	☐ high	

Events: ☐ none: easy and well tolerated   ☐ difficult:

Success: ☐ complete ☐ partial   ☐ failed   ☐ aborted   ☐ full evaluation pending

Pt Condition: **Post BP:**_____/_____ **HR:** ____ **VAS Pain score: 0 1 2 3 4 5 6 7 8 9 10**

☐ The procedure was performed by _____(sign). I was present and medically directed.

☐ I performed the procedure myself. **ATTENDING MD SIGNATURE:** _____

Figure 80–1. Anesthesia procedure note for peripheral nerve block.

Prior to this description, an example of a regional anesthesia procedure note could not be found in the literature. Starting almost 40 years ago, publications have described the development and evaluation of individual anesthesia records.[6,8,9] Authors have developed forms for documenting anesthetics with pooled expertise at a single practice[6,8] and multiple institutions.[9] Most anesthesia forms in use today likely have elements derived from these forms or have formats and content developed in parallel many years ago. Common to most of these efforts is a lack of emphasis on the documentation of regional techniques. In surveys of anesthesia records, space or narrative details of regional anesthetics have been noted in only 2–30%.[10–12] This lack of emphasis on regional anesthesia leads to sparse documentation of these procedures. We do not really know how often regional anesthetics are well or are poorly documented, but we know in general that documentation of anesthesia is often lacking[13–19] and that many malpractice suits are difficult to defend because of inadequacies of the medical record.[16,20]

Since the publication of the PNB form above, another similar form documenting the performance of neuraxial blockade has been devised (Figure 80–2).[21] Both these forms were created using the expertise of many individuals at several institutions. Furthermore, both efforts shared the goal of providing documentation of sound clinical care in the format of a robust medicolegal, billing, and regulatory-compliant form. The authors of both forms used the literature to find support for including or excluding each proposed entry prior to compiling the form. If an entry was included it was believed to be a key element of clinical care, and legal, billing, or regulatory compliance. Neither of these documents will be ideal for every institution. When formulating a procedure note, keep the following five suggestions in mind:

Clinical Pearls

- Guide the anesthesia practitioner to meet the standard of care in every interaction. Do so through the format of the form. Using Figure 80–1 as an example, the practitioner can simply check a box if he has performed an IV test with epinephrine, but must record the rationale when he does not. The practitioner must document corrective actions for untoward events such as encountering blood in the needle or pain or high pressure with injection.

- Encourage efficiency while ensuring thoughtfulness. Anesthesiologists might be able to simply check boxes for routine aspects of procedures, but the form should also require written contributions for decisions that need individualization. For example in Figure 80–2, the anesthesiologist must fill in the drug choices and adjuvants for neuraxial blockade and record the parameters that elicit a motor response when using a nerve stimulator or paresthesia on completing the form in Figure 80–1.

- Require documentation to safeguard against common medicolegal challenges.

For example, both figures are formatted to require the practitioner to characterize the patient's state of consciousness, in part because current medicolegal disputes may center on the patient's level of consciousness. Furthermore, although there is no evidence in the literature that level of consciousness has any relevance to the risk of nerve injury, such documentation may offer clues for future analysis of risk factors for nerve block-related complications. Figure 80–2 requires documentation of conformation of antithrombisis–anticoagulation status, in part for similar reasons.

- Document compliance with initiatives adopted by regulatory agencies. Both Figure 80–1 and Figure 80–2 allow adequate space for patient identification, recognition of site and side of surgery, and acknowledge the importance of assessment of analgesia using pain scores. (Again, this is sound clinical judgment but also represents a good approach to regulatory compliance).

- Facilitate successful and accurate billing. For example, both Figures 80–1 and 80–2 include boxes that should be checked to indicate that the surgeon has requested certain PNBs for postoperative pain management, and these blocks are clearly listed and named. Without this documentation, the insurer may be less likely to reimburse. The procedure note should also ensure that an anesthesiologist medically directs each block, which is important in a residency or other training program.

Used at St. Lukes-Roosevelt Hospital for a number of years. Documentation at this institution incorporates numerical information on injection pressure (see Figure 80–3).[22] This is a good example of individualization of documentation for the needs of a particular institution. The authors of this form collect data on injection pressure during PNBs. These authors are in the process of using data on injection pressure to create a database in which a correlation between injection pressures and neurapraxia is being sought.[23] The association between regional anesthesia practices and peripheral nerve injuries is a particularly complex and rapidly changing subject, with patient care as well as economic, legal, and public relations ramifications. Documentation of regional anesthesia procedures may be especially helpful in improving our understanding of these associations. Furthermore, documentation is likely to provide the clinician with medicolegal protection. For example, the authors of Figure 80–3 note that although the practice of injection pressure monitoring has not yet become standard,[7] objective monitoring and documentation of injection pressure may serve as strong medicolegal evidence that the anesthesia provider avoided an injection force capable of injuring a fascicle (greater than 20 PSI) by using all available knowledge and technology to do so.[23] When neurologic complications do occur, these complications may be attributed to regional anesthesia procedures by patients, clinicians, hospital administrators, and lawyers in spite of the fact that surgery and positioning during surgery may be the

Anesthesiology Procedure Note
NEURAXIAL BLOCKADE

Block(s) performed	Surgical site confirmed:

☐ Left ☐ Right ☐ Midline

Patient Name
Medical Record #
Age   Sex

(Patient name plate stamp)

☐ **Anticoagulation/antithrombosis status was reviewed**

Indication: ☐ Analgesia ☐ Anesthesia   ☐ Specifically requested for management
Dx/pain location: of pain by Dr. _____

Date: _____/_____/20_____   **Start time** (:)   **End time** (:)

Pt Condition: Initial BP:_____/_____ HR:_____O2 Sat: _____ VAS Pain: 0 1 2 3 4 5 6 7 8 9 10

☐ awake   ☐ sedate with meaningful contact maintained

☐ Performed under general anesthesia with the indication: _____

Preparation: ☐ drape   ☐ povidone-iodine ☐ chlorhexidine ☐ alcohol   ☐ iodophor/isopropyl

Position: ☐ LLD   ☐ RLD   ☐ sitting   ☐ prone

Technique: ☐ mid-line ☐ paramedian   ☐ loss of resistance to saline ☐ loss of resistance to air

Approximate interspace: ☐ Thoracic: **T -T**   ☐ Lumbar: **L -L .**

☐ injection given through needle ☐ **Loss of resistance at depth:** _____cm.

☐ **Catheter insertion, mark at skin:** _____cm.

Needle(s): ☐ Epidural needle gauge: _____ ☐ Needle length if not 3.5 inches:_____

☐ Spinal needle gauge: _____ ☐ Pencil-tip   ☐ Quincke ☐ introducer
Manufacturer of neuraxial needle/catheter/ tray:

Injectate:

Spinal Local Anesthetic	Dose (mg)	Baricity	Adjuncts	Epinephrine

Epidural Local Anesthetic	Volume (ml)	Adjuncts	Epinephrine
			☐ 1/__00,000
			☐ not used

Narrative: **The test dose given was:**   **Action Taken**

Paresthesia encountered	☐ no	☐ yes	
CSF via catheter or epidural	☐ no	☐ yes	
Blood aspirated:	☐ no	☐ yes	
Intravenous/Spinal test:	☐ negative	☐ positive	
Pain on injection noted:	☐ no	☐ yes	

Injection was made incrementally with constant monitoring and aspiration every _____ml's.

Events: ☐ none: easy/ well tolerated ☐ difficult:

Success: **Block Level(s):** _____ ☐ failed   ☐ aborted   ☐ a full evaluation is pending

Pt Condition: Post BP:_____/_____ HR:_____O2 Sat: _____ VAS Pain: 0 1 2 3 4 5 6 7 8 9 10

Sedation Given	Dose (mcg /mg)

☐ The procedure was performed by _____(sign). I was present and medically directed.

☐ I performed the procedure myself. **ATTENDING MD SIGNATURE:** _____

Figure 80–2. Anesthesia procedure note for neuraxial blockade.

principal and much more commonly encountered reasons for nerve deficit. Therefore, a lack of objective documentation of regional anesthesia may place pracitioners in a uniquely vulnerable position in cases of adverse neurologic outcome. Although this may be less of an issue for institutions where regional anesthesia has become established, it can present a significant obstacle to establishing regional anesthesia in others.

Ideally, more widespread use of procedure forms to document regional anesthesia and the sound medical care that is part of the regional anesthetic, may even result in more widespread use of these procedures. Hopefully, this will occur when the forms we use result in easier documentation, more standardization of care, and better regulatory and medicolegal protection for the clinician, while at the same time giving the researcher a tool for collecting data to adapt our practices for the future.

Peripheral nerve injury with PNBs is a particularly complex and rapidly changing subject, with patient care, economic, legal and public relations ramifications. It is well accepted that neurologic complications are more commonly caused by an injury during surgery and involving positioning rather than resulting from the use of PNBs. However, because the nature of the nerve block procedure involves placing a needle in the vicinity of the nerves and plexuses, it is often assumed that a PNB procedure is a cause for any neurologic symptoms following surgery. The current lack of monitoring tools during PNBs and objective documentation of PNBs places regional anesthesia practitioners in a uniquely vulnerable position in cases of adverse neurologic outcome. Although this may be less of a problem in institutions with tradition of using regional anesthesia, it can present a significant obstacle in practices wishing to introduce PNB procedures. Adherence to the suggested PNB documentation coupled with more objective monitoring of various aspects of PNB procedure is likely to result in both a reduction of the risk of neurologic injury and a more widespread use of PNB procedures in clinical practice.

DOCUMENTATION OF INFORMED CONSENT

Informed consent is a process that consists of three steps: (1) disclosure of medical information, (2) patient understanding (or competency), and (3) mutual decision-making.[24] Documenting the adequacy of the informed consent process is difficult if not impossible for any medical treatment including regional anesthesia. However, using a written form to document the conduct of the informed consent process as it relates to regional anesthesia may have advantages for all three steps of the consent process. Furthermore written consent may have benefits beyond relying on verbal informed consent alone. First, a well-constructed informed consent form may guide the process by providing scripted information. For example, most state legislatures in the United States have upheld the idea that the disclosure of risk during the informed consent process should cover those risks that are common and those that are the most serious.[24] A document can be used to guide

disclosure as a matter of routine. Disclosing information in this way has not been found to alarm patients.[25] Second, written consent has been shown to improve patient recall of risks and benefits, which may improve patient understanding of medical therapy.[25] Third, because regional anesthesia is often viewed as an optional therapy in addition to or beyond general anesthesia, patients' and physicians' medical decision making must incorporate a discussion of both benefits and risks. A written consent form that documents both may help establish that this process truly occurred. Such a form could in itself be viewed as a patient education document: When a physician reviews the form (Figure 80–4) with the patient, the document becomes an integral part of the informed consent process in addition to the documentation of the process.

All but one study of informed consent have focused on therapies besides regional anesthesia. Most studies[26–32] examining informed consent in medicine have centered on the issue of patient recall. Recall of information is, of course, not the same as understanding of the information, but it is the one objective measure of competency we have. These studies have generally demonstrated poor rates of recall. With verbal consent, recall has been found to be adversely effected by the style of presentation.[33] With written consent, recall has been found to depend on format of the form. Written consent has been found to be recalled best when the consent form is a brief one,[34] the patient is given an opportunity to discuss it with the anesthesiologist, and the patient is given a copy of the signed consent document.[35]

Similarly to the two examples of regional anesthesia procedure notes, the example of an anesthesia risk disclosure form will not be ideal for each practice. For that reason, I recommend that the reader adapt the forms to his or her practice.

Clinical Pearls

When obtaining informed consent keep the following five suggestions in mind:

- Be brief. Figure 80–4 uses a table type format to help avoid the appearance of a document with multiple paragraphs of text. Brevity enhances recall.

- Include major and common risks but do so along with specific benefits or expected outcomes. If only risks are disclosed without discussion of benefits, the patient cannot make an informed decision. The patient will not understand why these risks should be undertaken.

- Educate and document at the same time. Written as well as verbal discussion has been shown to best enhance recall of consent. Obtaining written consent without discussion is neither medically or legally valid.

- Indicate both the common practices of the practitioner and the preferences of the patient. Figure 80–4 is geared to the practice of regional anesthesia, incorporating a check box system to indicate what has been discussed with each patient.

- Offer a copy of the form to the patient. This simple intervention has been shown to improve recall of information.

NERVE BLOCK PROCEDURE: Block Procedure Description

BLOCK PROCEDURE:
☐ Cervical Block (Superficial)
☐ Cervical Block (Deep)
☐ Interscalene Block
☐ Supraclavicular Block
☐ Interscalene Block
☐ Infraclavicular Block
☐ Axillary Block
☐ Paravertebral Block

☐ Lumbar Plexus Block
☐ Sciatic Block
☐ Popliteal Block
☐ Femoral Block
☐ Saphenous Block
☐ Ankle Block
☐ Other: Specify

BLOCK PRIMARILY USED FOR:

☐ Postoperative Pain Management

☐ Surgery

TECHNIQUE:
☐ Classical
☐ Single Injection
☐ Multiple Injection:
    Specify:_____
☐ Nerve Stimulator Current_____mA
☐ Motor Response:
    Specify: _____
☐ Number of Attempts:
    Specify: _____
☐ Paresthesia

☐ Trans-Arterial
☐ Sterile
☐ Continuous
☐ Air Aspirated
☐ No Blood Aspirated
☐ No Pain on Injection
☐ No resistance on Injection
☐ Injection pressure < 20psi
    Specify: _____psi

NEEDLE:
☐ Stimuplex 22 G 5 cm, short bevel
☐ Stimuplex 22 G 10cm, short bevel
☐ Stimuplex 22 G 3cm, short bevel
☐ Stimulating 18 G Tuohy 2"
☐ Stimulating 18 G Tuohy 4"
☐ Quincke 22 G 4"
☐ Other
    Specify:_____

LOCAL ANESTHETIC:
☐ Ropivacaine 0.75% (_)ml
☐ Ropivacaine 0.5% (_) ml
☐ Lidocaine 2% + 1:300,000 Epi
    +HCO3 (_) ml
☐ Mepivacaine 1.5% (_) ml
☐ Mepivacaine 1.5% + 1:300,000
    Epi +HCO3 (_) ml
☐ Chloroprocaine 3% (_) ml
☐ Chloroprocaine 3% +1:300,000
    Epi + HCO3 (_) ml
☐ Other:
    Specify _____

Figure 80–3. Automated menu-driven nerve block documentation form.

SUMMARY

In summary, the modern area of widespread application of regional anesthesia requires similar reevaluation and improvement of the medical record keeping. Whether they are paper or electronic, anesthesia records need to emphasize regional anesthesia in our documentation of the medical practice of anesthesia and in documentation of the process of informed consent. Future developments in this area will inevitably see introduction of objective monitors both for decreasing the risk of neurologic injury and better documentation of regional anesthesia procedures.

(Patient name label)

ANESTHESIA REQUEST RISK DISCLOSURE FORM

We select the type of anesthesia based on what we normally plan for your surgery, your medical condition, and what your surgeon prefers. Anesthesia is also planned based on what you want. Please use this form to understand what we do as part of your anesthesia and to show that you give consent.

An Explanation of Anesthesia and Pain Relief

☐ **General Anesthesia** (with or without a breathing tube)	Technique	Medicines put into your IV will make you unconscious. A breathing tube may be put into your windpipe or throat after you are unconscious. Medicine breathed through this tube will keep you unconscious while a machine may breathe for you. If numbing medicines are used to keep you comfortable, you will likely not need a breathing tube, medicines breathed in, or a breathing machine. Instead, constant IV medicines will keep you asleep.
	Expected Result	You will not be aware during surgery.
	Specific Risks	Nausea and vomiting, mouth or throat pain, hoarseness, injury to mouth, teeth or eye, breathing stomach contents into the lungs, Pneumonia, permanent weakness, numbness, or pain from a nerve injury. Becoming aware of what's going on during surgery.
☐ **Epidural, Spinal, or Caudal Anesthesia**	Technique	Medicine put through a needle or tube between the bones of your back will numb your body.
	Expected Result	You will temporarily lose feeling and movement to the lower part of your body, or to your chest and belly. You will have pain relief for a period of time after surgery.
	Specific Risks	Nausea and vomiting, headache, backache, or having a seizure, permanent weakness, numbness, or pain from a nerve injury.
☐ **Peripheral Nerve Block**	Technique	Medicine put through a needle or tube near nerves of your arm, leg, chest, or belly will numb your body.
	Expected Result	You will temporarily lose feeling and movement of all or part of a limb, your chest, or belly. You will have pain relief for a period of time after surgery.
	Specific Risks	Soreness or bruising, injury to a blood vessel, having a seizure, permanent weakness, numbness, or pain from a nerve injury. Lung collapse with specific types of peripheral nerve blocks.
☐ **Bier Block**	Technique	Medicine put through an IV into a vein of your arm.
	Expected Result	You will lose feeling and movement of an arm during surgery.
	Specific Risks	Having a seizure, injury to blood vessels, or permanent weakness, numbness, or pain from a nerve injury.
☐ **Sedation**	Technique	Medicine put into your bloodstream through an IV will make you less aware.
	Expected Result	You will be less aware and less anxious during surgery.
	Specific Risks	Nausea and vomiting, slowed breathing, injury to a blood vessel.

Figure 80–4. Anesthesia request risk disclosure form.

An Explanation of Special Procedures

	Technique	☐ a tube put in an artery of your arm or leg to monitor pressures
☐ **Arterial Line**		☐ a tube put in a vein of your neck or chest to monitor pressures
☐ **Central Line**		☐ a tube put in your neck or chest to monitor heart pressures
☐ **Pulmonary Artery Line**		☐ an ultrasound probe put into your throat to monitor your heart
		☐ a tube put between the bones of your back to remove spinal fluid
☐ **TEE**		☐ a breathing tube put in with you awake or sedated for your safety
		☐ a breathing tube left in after surgery for your safety
☐ **Lumbar Drain**	Expected Result	Better safety of anesthesia or surgery care, monitoring, blood sampling, or putting medicines into veins
☐ **Awake Intubation**	Specific Risks	☐ Injury to blood vessels and heart.
		☐ Lung collapse.
		☐ Irregular heart rhythm.
☐ **Postoperative Ventilation**		☐ Mouth or throat pain, hoarseness, injury to mouth or teeth.
		☐ Headache, backache, or permanent weakness, numbness, or pain from nerve injury.

Consent for the Transfusion Blood or Blood Components

☐ **I hereby authorize and consent to the transfusion of blood or blood components during my treatment.** ☐ **I will not accept a blood transfusion as a life saving measure.**	I hereby acknowledge that I understand the following list of items or that they have been explained to me: • I understand that I may need a transfusion of blood or one of its components in the interest of my health and proper medical care. I understand what a transfusion is and the procedures that will be involved. • Although the blood has been carefully tested, I understand there are possible risks such as unexpected reactions or transmission of viral hepatitis, AIDS, and other infectious agents. • Alternatives to blood transfusion, if any, have been explained to me. • I understand that no guarantee as to the outcome of these transfusions has been made. • I understand that I may revoke this consent for a transfusion at any time.

All types of anesthesia carry some risk of severe complications. Although rare, these include infection, drug reactions, blood clots, paralysis, stroke, heart attack, brain damage, and death. Anesthesia could injure a fetus if you are pregnant. Sometimes, the type of anesthesia may need to be changed during surgery to better care for you or aid the surgeon's task.

I have read this form or had it read to me. I understand what it says. I have been given a chance to ask questions and have them answered. Types of anesthesia, special procedures, and transfusions have all been explained. I have enough information to give my permission to use these as needed.

_____

Signature of the patient (or the patient's legal representative authorized to sign for the patient)

Witness (only necessary in the event of telephone consent or if the patient signs with an "X" mark)

I have discussed the contents of this form with the patient (or legal representative authorized to sign).

_____   _____   ____/____/____   (____:____)

Person obtaining the signature   Physician obtaining consent   Date   Time

Figure 80–4. *(Continued)*

References

1. Merry AF, Webster CS, Mathew DJ: A new, safety-oriented, integrated drug administration and automated anesthesia record system. Anesth Analg 2001;93:385–390.

2. Quinzio L, Junger A, Gottwald B, et al: User acceptance of an anaesthesia information management system. Eur J Anaesthesiol 2003;20:967–972.

3. Bicker AA, Gage JS, Poppers PJ: An evolutionary solution to anesthesia automated record keeping. J Clin Monit Comput 1998;14:421–424.

4. Hammond EJ, Sweeney BP: Electronic data collection by trainee anaesthetists using palm top computers. Eur J Anaesthesiol 2000;17:91–98.

5. Fu Q, Xue Z, Zhu J, et al: Anaesthesia record system on handheld computers—Pilot experience and uses for quality control and clinical guidelines. Comput Methods Programs Biomed 2005;77:155–163.

6. Fisher JA, Bromberg IL, Eisen LB: On the design of anaesthesia record forms. Can J Anaesth 1994;41:973–983.

7. Gerancher JC, Viscusi ER, Liguori GA, et al: Development of a standardized peripheral nerve block procedure note form. Reg Anesth Pain Med 2005;30:67–71.

8. Jackson CJ, Scott RJ: A new comprehensive anaesthetic record. Anaesth Intensive Care 1989;17:475–481.

9. Biddle C, Bauer L, Dosch M, et al: Analysis of noteworthy indicators on the anesthesia record: A prospective, multiregional study. AANA J 2001;69:407–410.

10. Seed RF, Welsh EA: Anaesthetic records in Great Britain and Ireland. Anaesthesia 1976;31:1199–1210.

11. Roach VJ, Lau TK, Kee WD, et al: Perioperative documentation: Are we doing enough? Aust N Z J Obstet Gynaecol 1998;38:166–169.

12. Bembridge M, Bembridge JL: A survey of anaesthetic charts. Anaesthesia 1988;43:690–693.

13. Rowe L, Galletly DC, Henderson RS: Accuracy of text entries within a manually compiled anaesthetic record. Br J Anaesth 1992;68:381–387.

14. Simmonds M, Petterson J: Anaesthetists' records of pre-operative assessment. Clin Perform Qual Health Care 2000;8:22–27.

15. Feldman JM: Do anesthesia information systems increase malpractice exposure? Results of a survey. Anesth Analg 2004;99:840–843.

16. Nicopoullos JD, Karrar S, Gour A, et al: Significant improvement in quality of caesarean section documentation with dedicated operative proforma-completion of the audit cycle. J Obstet Gynaecol 2003;23:381–386.

17. Galletly DC, Rowe WL, Henderson RS: The anaesthetic record: A confidential survey on data omission or modification. Anaesth Intensive Care 1991;19:74–78.

18. Moody ML, Kremer MJ: Preinduction activities: A closed malpractice claims perspective. AANA J 2001;69:461–465.

19. Devitt JH, Rapanos T, Kurrek M, et al: The anesthetic record: Accuracy and completeness. Can J Anaesth 1999;46:122–128.

20. Campion FX: Good medical records can be strongest malpractice defense. In *Grand Rounds on Medical Malpractice.* American Medical Association, 1990.

21. Viscusi ER, Gerancher JC, Weller, R, et al: "Not Documented? Not Done! A Proposed Procedure Note for Neuraxial Blockade." American Society of Regional Anesthesia and Pain Medicine 2005 Annual Spring Meeting April 21–24, 2005, Toronto, Canada.

22. Hadzic A, Vloka J: Neurologic complications of peripheral nerve blocks and methods to prevent them. In Hadzic A, Vloka J (eds): *Peripheral Nerve Blocks: Principles and Practice,* McGraw-Hill, 2003.

23. Hadzic A, Dilberovic F, Shah S, et al: Combination of intraneural injection and high injection pressure leads to fascicular injury and neurologic deficits in dogs. Reg Anesth Pain Med 2004;29:417–423.

24. Meisel A, Roth LH: What we do and do not know about informed consent. JAMA 1981;246:2473–2477.

25. Gerancher JC, Grice SC, Dewan DW, et al: An evaluation of informed consent prior to epidural analgesia for labor and delivery. Int J Obstet Anaesth 2000;9:168–173.

26. Robinson G, Merav A: Informed consent: Recall by patients tested postoperatively. Ann Thorac Surg 1976;22:209–212.

27. Cassileth BR, Zupkis RV, Sutton-Smith K, et al: Informed consent—Why are its goals imperfectly realized? N Engl J Med 1980;302:896–900.

28. Taub HA, Baker MT: The effect of repeated testing upon comprehension of informed consent materials by elderly volunteers. Exp Aging Res 1983;9:135–138.

29. Clark SK, Leighton BL, Seltzer JL: A risk-specific anesthesia consent form may hinder the informed consent process. J Clin Anesth 1991;3:11–13.

30. Leighton BL, Bauman J, Seltzer J: The effect of a detailed anesthesia consent form on patient recall and anxiety. Anesthesiology 1987;67:A567.

31. Done ML, Lee A: The use of a video to convey preanesthetic information to patients undergoing ambulatory surgery. Anesth Analg 1998;87:531–536.

32. Zvara DA, Nelson JM, Brooker RF, et al: The importance of the postoperative anesthetic visit: Do repeated visits improve patient satisfaction or physician recognition? Anesth Analg 1996;83:793–797.

33. Dawes PJ, O'Keefe L, Adcock S: Informed consent: Using a structured interview changes patients' attitudes towards informed consent. J Laryngol Otol 1993;107:775–779.

34. Williams RL, Rieckmann KH, Trenholme GM, et al: The use of a test to determine that consent is informed. Mil Med 1977;141:542–545.

35. Morrow G, Gootnick J, Schmale A: A simple technique for increasing cancer patients knowledge of informed consent to treatment. Cancer 1978;42:793–799.

81

Teaching Regional Anesthesia

Susan B. McDonald, MD • Joseph M. Neal, MD

INTRODUCTION

Over the past 20 years, the importance of training anesthesiologists in regional anesthesia has become recognized worldwide. More practitioners use regional anesthetic blocks for their patients and choose regional anesthesia for themselves when they undergo surgery. Documented improved outcomes (eg, obstetric anesthesia, acute pain management, ambulatory surgery, etc) have also contributed to the increase in popularity and use of regional anesthesia in the recent years. Despite this trend, the quality of training in regional anesthesia is less than needed for residents and fellows, as well as for practicing anesthesiologists. Quality training in regional anesthesia is necessary to promote not only clinical competence but also practitioner confidence in the ability to perform the skill proficiently and safely. Surveys of residency programs demonstrate narrowing variability in training, and recent consensus-based regional anesthesia fellowship guidelines may further improve training at all levels. Academic programs have employed conventional and unconventional methods to compliment the exposure to regional anesthesia opportunities that residents and fellows receive in the operating room, obstetric suite, and pain clinic. In this chapter, these teaching concepts will be discussed as well as future goals for improving regional anesthesia training for all anesthesiologists.

PAST & CURRENT TRAINING EXPERIENCE

Evolution of Regional Anesthesia Training

As early as the 1920s, there were dedicated teachers of regional anesthesia. In the United States, both Gaston Labat and John S. Lundy offered 3-month courses in the basics to interested practitioners. Of note, such teaching influenced many renowned anesthesiologists of the time, including Ralph

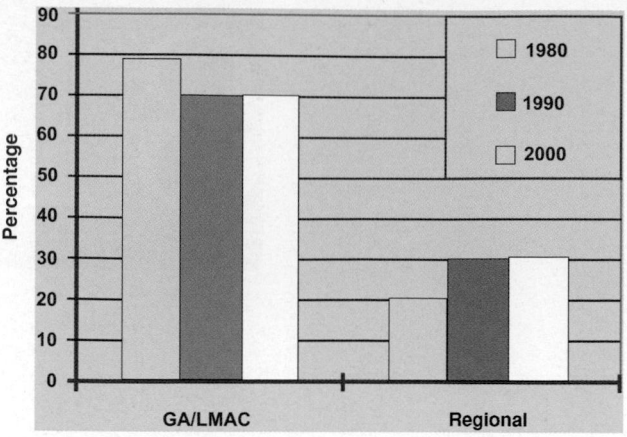

Figure 81–1. The use of regional anesthesia in residency training programs compared with general or local anesthesia for cases in 1980 (21.3%), 1990 (29.8%), and 2000 (30.2%). (Reprinted with permission from Kopacz DJ, Neal JM: Regional anesthesia and pain medicine: Residency training—the year 2000. Reg Anesth Pain Med 2002;27:9–14.)

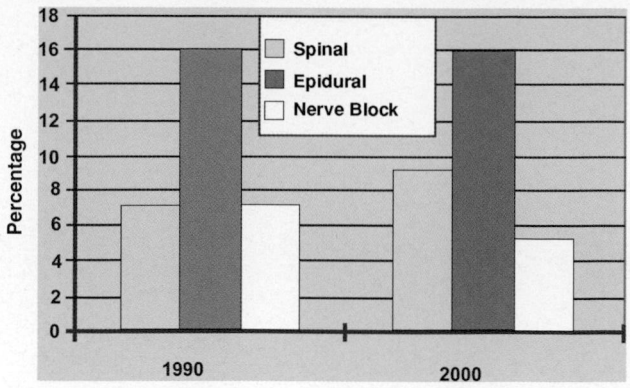

Figure 81–2. Distribution of types of regional anesthesia in residency training programs did not change significantly between 1990 and 2000 ($p = 0.75$). (Reprinted with permission from Kopacz DJ, Neal JM: Regional anesthesia and pain medicine: Residency training—the year 2000. Reg Anesth Pain Med 2002;27:9–14.)

Waters and Emery Rovenstine.[1] At that time, a few experts promoted regional anesthesia, including the members of the first American Society of Regional Anesthesia, which was founded by Labat. Nevertheless, prior to the last quarter century, only a few residency programs had officially incorporated regional anesthesia as part of their educational curriculum.

It was not until 1996 that the Anesthesiology Residency Review Committee (RRC) of the Accreditation Council for Graduate Medical Education (ACGME) formally listed a minimal number of regional anesthetic blocks as a requirement of training in anesthesiology.[2] Prior to that time, regional anesthesia training varied widely in residency programs. For instance, a survey conducted in 1980 showed that regional anesthesia use ranged from 2.8 to 55.7% among responding training programs, with approximately 21% of all cases using regional anesthesia.[3] Indeed, students of well-respected programs could graduate having performed fewer than a handful of spinal anesthetics. These numbers improved somewhat by 1990, but although regional anesthesia was utilized in more cases (29.8%), primarily reflecting increases in obstetric and pain management applications of regional techniques, the large discrepancy continued, with 2.8 to 58.5% total caseload experience.[4] By the year 2000, the number of surgical cases with regional anesthetics did not significantly increase (30.2%) nor did the distribution of the types of anesthetics (Figures 81–1 and 81–2), but there was much less disparity in usage by training programs nationwide.[5]

Accreditation Agency Requirements

As the current RRC program requirements state, residents must perform 50 epidural, 50 spinal, and 40 peripheral nerve blocks plus an additional 25 nerve blocks for pain management.[2] The most recent survey shows that nearly all residents meet the requirement for neuraxial blocks, which does not stratify between lumbar and thoracic epidurals or account for continuous spinal or combined spinal-epidural experience. Indeed, although most residents exceed that required number, nearly half of their regional anesthesia training still occurs in the obstetric suite.[5] These data are encouraging, since studies of clinical competence show it takes between 60 and 90 epidural blocks to reach at least 80% success[6–8] (Figure 81–3). Achieving a level of competency is reflected in resident confidence, as surveys of graduating residents showed more than 94% were very confident in their lumbar epidural skills.[8–10] Similar evidence exists for spinal blocks. Surveyed residents felt very confident in their ability to perform spinal anesthesia.[9] Kopacz and colleagues demonstrated that at least 45 spinal anesthetics had to be performed before at least a 90% success rate was attained,[7] a number much closer to the RRC requirement.

The data for peripheral nerve block performance, however, is disappointing. Approximately 40% of all residents in the year 2000 had inadequate experience in peripheral nerve blocks.[5] Not only is this unfortunate from an education standpoint, but it may present a patient safety issue. Residents not adequately trained in a particular block are unlikely to use that block in practice;[11] or worse, they may be asked to provide nerve block services without the necessary skills.[9,12] Multiple surveys have demonstrated that graduating residents do not feel confident in their peripheral nerve block skills[9] (Figure 81–4). This may be especially true for lower extremity nerve blocks[12,13] (Figure 81–5). Furthermore, the vagueness of "40 peripheral blocks" allows this discrepancy between block types to occur. Indeed, 40 performances of any *one* nerve block will satisfy the training requirements by the RRC, but it will be inadequate to attain competency in other block techniques. Konrad and coworkers demonstrated that 70 axillary blocks are needed before an 85% success rate can be achieved[6] (Figure 81–6). Rosenblatt and associates showed that more than 10 interscalene blocks are necessary before

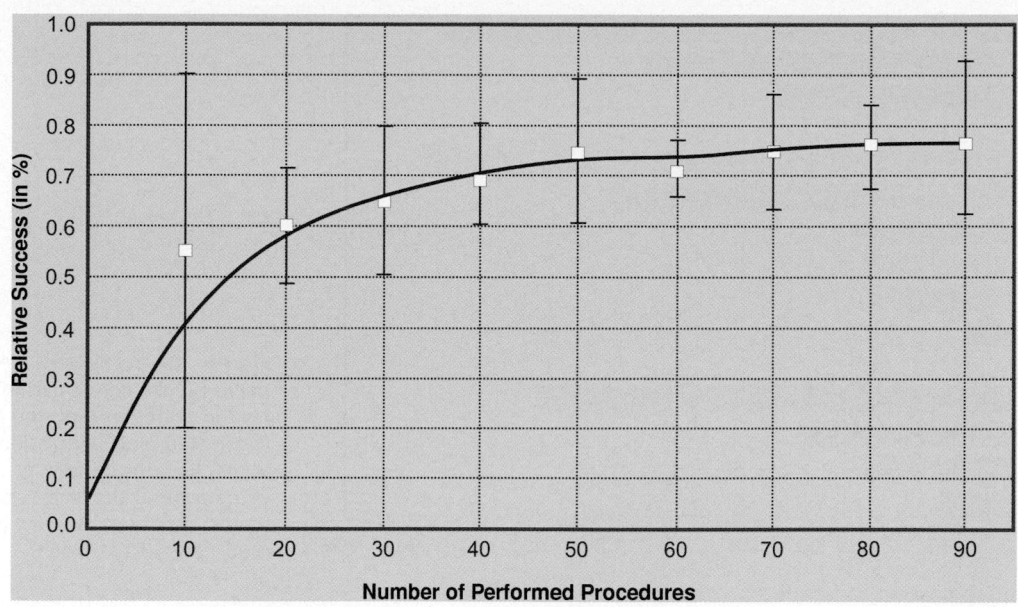

Figure 81–3. The learning curve for epidural anesthesia: demonstrating a minimum of 90 blocks to reach 80% success rate. (Reprinted with permission from Konrad C, Schuepfer G, Wietlisbach M, et al: Learning manual skills in anesthesiology. Is there a recommended number of cases for anesthetic procedures? Anesth Analg 1998;86:635–639.)

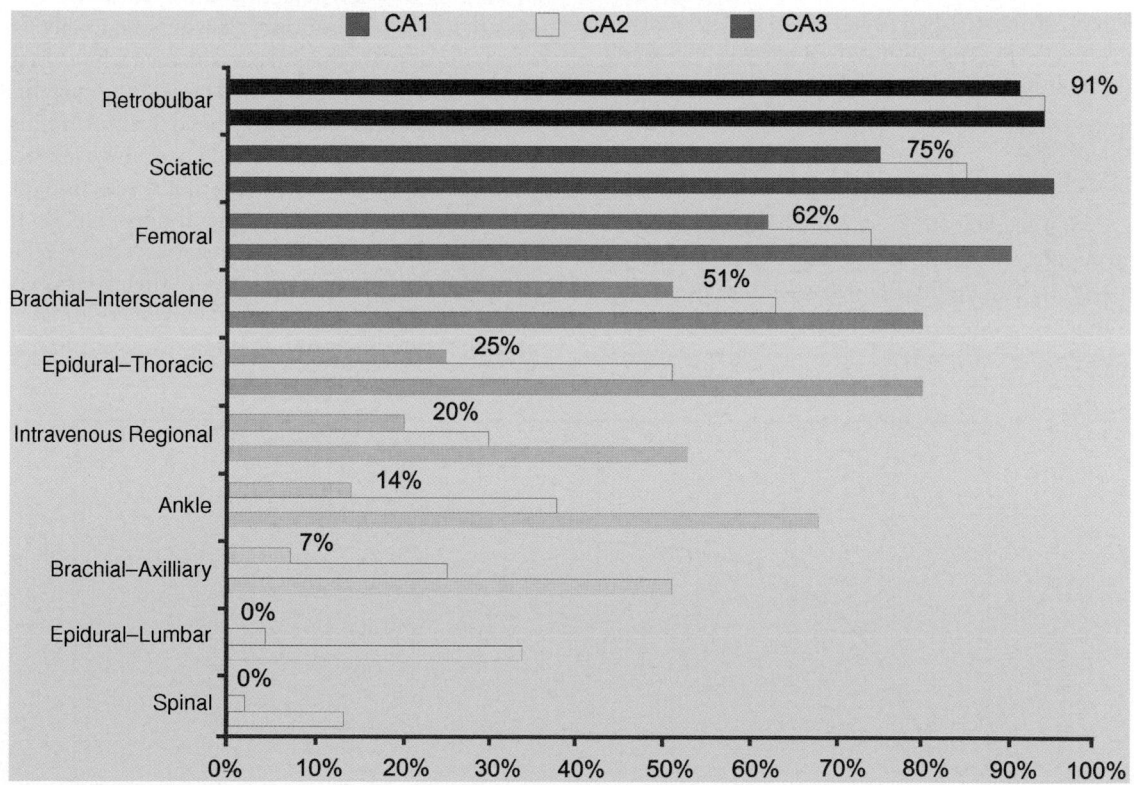

Figure 81–4. The percentage of residents, per training year, who categorized themselves as "not confident" in performing a particular block. Exact percentages are listed for the CA-3 resident class. Residents felt least confident with peripheral nerve blocks, and no CA-3 resident admitted to being "not confident" for spinal or lumbar epidural anesthesia. (Reprinted with permission from Smith MP, Sprung J, Zura A, et al: A survey of exposure to regional anesthesia techniques in American anesthesia residency training programs. Reg Anesth Pain Med 1999;24:11–16.)

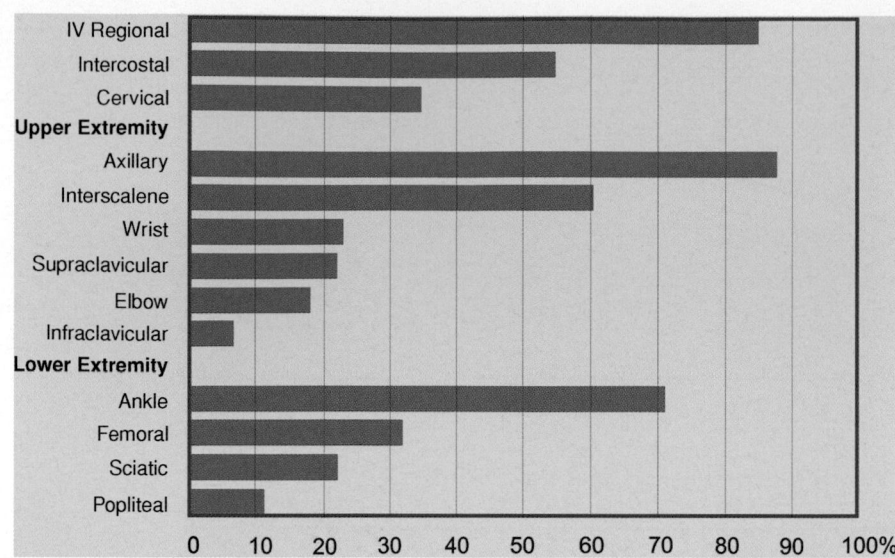

Figure 81–5. Percentage of peripheral nerve blocks performed in practice in the United States, as reported by practitioners. (Reprinted with permission from Hadzic A, Vloka JD, Kuroda MM et al: The practice of peripheral nerve blocks in the United States: A national survey. Reg Anesth Pain Med 1998;23:241–246.)

the resident attains at least 50% autonomy.[14] Therefore, it is unlikely that many residents are developing the necessary proficiency because they are not performing enough peripheral nerve blocks. Furthermore, many teaching departments have fewer regional anesthesia teachers than they would prefer. A 2004 survey of department chairs noted that on average they would ideally hire two additional regional anesthesia specialists on their faculty.[15]

Clinical Pearl

- Anesthesiology residents trained in the United States are much more likely to fulfill accrediting agency requirements for spinal and epidural anesthesia than those for peripheral nerve blocks.

ENRICHING THE EDUCATIONAL EXPERIENCE

Assessing Competency

In addition to a skilled faculty and a culture of using regional anesthesia for surgical cases, learning regional anesthesia requires much more than mastering the technical aspects of directing a needle to the intended target. The current RRC focus on the number of blocks performed during training does little to assess actual technical competence, much less nontechnical proficiency, such as consulting skills, selection, and perioperative management of peripheral nerve blocks. Resident or fellow confidence in the technical aspects of regional anesthesia may not be at all reflective of their overall competence. Indeed, inexperienced trainees may overestimate their technical skills, but be incompetent in the nontechnical aspects of

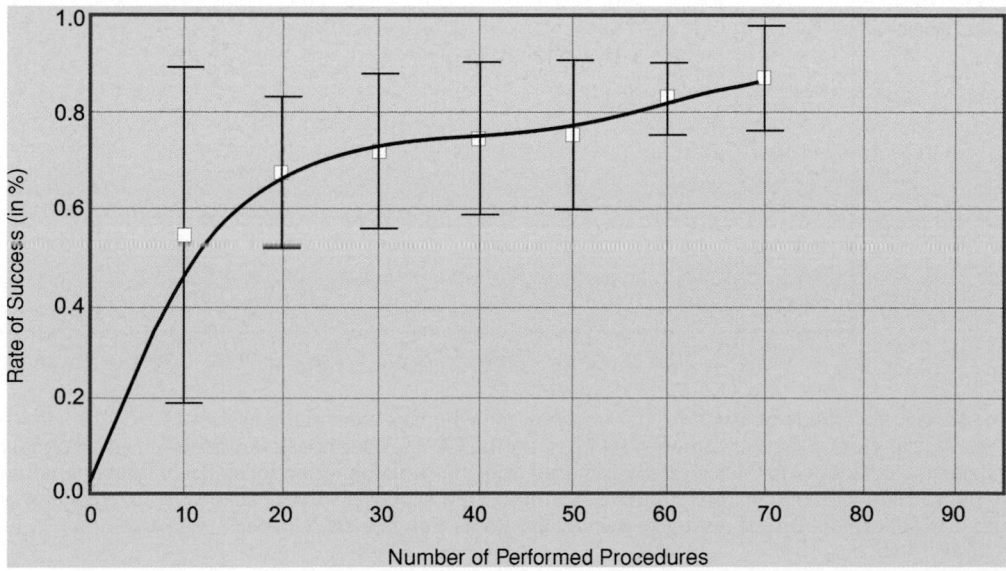

Figure 81–6. The learning curve for brachial plexus anesthesia: Demonstrating a minimum of 70 blocks to reach 85% success rate. (Reprinted with permission from Konrad C, Schuepfer G, Wietlisbach M, et al: Learning manual skills in anesthesiology. Is there a recommended number of cases for anesthetic procedures? Anesth Analg 1998;86:635–639.)

regional anesthesia. The actual number of blocks performed says little about the trainee's mastery of the physiology and pharmacology of regional anesthesia, intraoperative sedation skills, awareness and management of complications, or overall judgment in selecting which patients should be offered regional techniques. Although competence in these areas can be assessed to some degree by written and oral certifying examinations, the teaching and assessment of the nontechnical aspects of regional anesthesia remains a challenge. Indeed, even former regional anesthesia fellows have expressed their disappointment that nontechnical components were not better addressed during their training.

Alternatives to Bedside Teaching

Many residency programs feel the necessity to increase the individual resident's block experience but do not have the surgical case load or operating room logistics to accommodate this goal. In efforts to improve education in regional anesthesia, faculty members have devised other ways to teach blocks. More modern methods include interactive graphics on CD-ROM, a learning tool that is readily at hand (literally, as handheld devices can carry the software) and increasingly popular among residents. Outstanding DVD tutorials have recently become available that allow the student to learn the relevant anatomy and block placement in a three-dimensional mode.[16] Others use cadaveric models and simulators to practice blocks and learn anatomy. Invaluable experience in the placement of continuous perineural catheters can be gained in anesthetized pigs and other animals. Some teachers advocate videotaping residents while they perform regional anesthesia procedures, believing such immediate visual feedback coupled with expert goal-directed critique can help improve skills.[17] Recently, some have described using ultrasound as a visual aid to teach correct needle placement for obstetric lumbar epidural blocks, as such guidance has been shown to improve residents' learning curve.[18] Virtual reality teaching models are currently being developed, but are not yet commercially available.

Unconventional models can be created with everyday household objects. For example, one model was created with a banana, some slices of bread, and a balloon. As the resident passes the needle through the banana using loss of resistance technique, the fruit mimics the feel of the subcutaneous tissues and ligamentum flavum, and if they should advance too far through the bread (epidural space), the balloon (dura) will pop.[19] A foam-block model can be used to teach residents how minimally changing the angle of the needle at the skin greatly affects where the tip of the needle is ultimately placed.[7]

Residents can also learn from receiving regional anesthesia themselves. Residents participating in compensated volunteer studies learned aspects of regional anesthesia that cannot be taught. After the experience, residents acknowledge that they learned to be more sensitive to patient concerns and to be better communicators with their patients regarding regional anesthesia. Other common observations included the value of sedation, the concept of gentle vs rough touch, and the discomfort caused by local anesthesia infiltration, nerve stimulators, and paresthesias.[20]

Some programs have created "block rotations" as a means of increasing the number of blocks, especially peripheral nerve blocks, to which residents are exposed.[21] Theoretically, although the total number of cases suitable for blocks remains the same, the actual provision of regional anesthesia to patients increases because of heightened resident awareness and confidence in choosing such techniques as part of their anesthetic plan. During these rotations, residents are assigned to a preoperative block area where they perform or teach (or both) all available blocks. This arrangement has the advantage of the residents being able to repeat many blocks in a short period of time, thus reinforcing their skills, although these skills may then atrophy when the residents are no longer assigned to the block rotation. A disadvantage to this approach to teaching is that residents do not then follow their blocks into the operating room, do not intraoperatively manage blocks, and thus do not learn to manage the failed or partial block or the complications and side effects of their blocks. In other words, the downside of the block rotation is that residents may not appreciate that there is far more to regional anesthesia than proper needle placement. Nevertheless, "block rotations" are becoming increasingly popular as a way for residency programs to teach regional anesthesia outside of the obstetric suite and pain clinic.

Regional Anesthesia Fellowship Training

The ultimate means for a resident to become a highly skilled regional anesthesiologist is to enroll in a fellowship program. In 2005, approximately 12 active fellowship programs existed in the United States and Canada.[15] That is considerably increased from the two or three training programs that were available prior to the mid 1990s[22] and represents an encouraging statistic for regional anesthesia education. Unlike pain medicine, regional anesthesia fellowships are not ACGME-accredited. Thus, the training experience and clinical focus has varied considerably among programs.[15,22] Recent efforts from fellowship program directors has resulted in consensus-based guidelines for regional anesthesia fellowships in North America to ensure that fellows receive the quality and quantity of regional anesthesia experience they need to become true experts in the field.[22]

Continuing Education Opportunities

A final challenge is how best to train postgraduate anesthesiologists in emerging regional techniques. The time-honored method of learning new techniques on patients is less than ideal. To a great extent, continuing medical education programs such as those offered by the American Society of Regional Anesthesia and Pain Medicine and by a number of institutions with tradition in teaching regional anesthesia serve a valuable role in updating anesthesiologists on the nontechnical aspects of regional anesthesia and pain medicine advances. Unfortunately, technical training is incompletely accomplished in workshop settings. However, the increased availability of cadaver-based anatomy courses and workshops, animal labs, computer-generated imaging technologies, and websites that teach regional anesthesia are encouraging as future generations of anesthesiologists strive to maintain their skills in an ever-changing subspecialty.

Clinical Pearls

- The number of blocks performed or consistently placing a needle near the target nerve are not entirely satisfactory measures of regional anesthesia competency.

- Innovative teaching methods must be developed not only for resident and fellow training, but for the continuing education of postgraduate practitioners.

FUTURE DIRECTIONS

Training residents and postgraduates in regional anesthesia has improved remarkably over the past two decades, but many challenges remain. Current research in how regional techniques affect perioperative outcome, as well as the rapid development of continuous perineural catheters, extended-duration local anesthetic and opioid preparations, and ultrasound-assisted nerve localization all point to future anesthesiologists becoming more involved in regional anesthesia, not less. At the time of this writing, the Anesthesiology RRC/ACGME is considering increasing the numbers of blocks that residents must perform if their programs are to remain accredited. Some training programs may be challenged to provide this clinical experience and suitable numbers of expert faculty. Nonpatient training techniques such as virtual reality, interactive learning programs, and animal labs will likely play an increasing role in the education of future residents and postgraduates alike.

References

1. Bacon DR: Gaston Labat, John Lundy, Emery Rovenstine, and the Mayo Clinic: The spread of regional anesthesia in America between the World Wars. J Clin Anesth 2002;14:315–320.
2. Accreditation Council for Graduate Medical Education: Program requirements for graduate medical education in anesthesiology. www.acgme.org/acWebsite/RRC. Accessed December 22, 2004.
3. Bridenbaugh LD: Are anesthesia resident programs failing regional anesthesia? Reg Anesth 1982;7:26–28.
4. Kopacz DJ, Bridenbaugh LD: Are anesthesia residency programs failing regional anesthesia? The past, present, and future. Reg Anesth 1993;18:84–87.
5. Kopacz DJ, Neal JM: Regional anesthesia and pain medicine: Residency training—The year 2000. Reg Anesth Pain Med 2002;27: 9–14.
6. Konrad C, Schuepfer G, Wietlisbach M, et al: Learning manual skills in anesthesiology. Is there a recommended number of cases for anesthetic procedures? Anesth Analg 1998;86:635–639.
7. Kopacz DJ, Neal JM, Pollock JE: The regional anesthesia "Learning Curve": What is the minimum number of epidural and spinal blocks to reach consistency? Reg Anesth 1996;21:182–190.
8. Schuepfer G, Konrad C, Schmeck J, et al: Generating a learning curve for pediatric caudal epidural blocks: An empirical evaluation of technical skills in novice and experienced anesthetists. Reg Anesth Pain Med 2000;25:385–388.
9. Smith MP, Sprung J, Zura A, et al: A survey of exposure to regional anesthesia techniques in American anesthesia residency training programs. Reg Anesth Pain Med 1999;24:11–16.
10. Blumenthal D, Gokhale M, Campbell EG, et al: Preparedness for clinical practice: Reports of graduating residents at academic health centers. JAMA 2001;286:1027–1034.
11. Buffington CW, Ready LB, Horton WG: Training and practice factors influencing the use of regional anesthesia: Implications for resident education. Reg Anesth 1986;11:2–6.
12. Hadzic A, Vloka JD, Kuroda MM, et al: The practice of peripheral nerve blocks in the United States: A national survey. Reg Anesth Pain Med 1998;23:241–246.
13. Bouaziz H, Mercier FJ, Narchi P, et al: Survey of regional anesthetic practice among French residents at time of certification. Reg Anesth 1996;22:218–222.
14. Rosenblatt MA, Fishkind D: Proficiency in interscalene anesthesia-how many blocks are necessary? J Clin Anesth 2003;15:282–288.
15. Neal JM, Kopacz DJ, Liguori GA, et al: The training and careers of regional anesthesia fellows—1983–2002. Reg Anesth Pain Med 2005;30:226–230.
16. Delbac A, Eisenach JC, Albert N, et al: *Peripheral Nerve Blocks on DVD: Upper and Lower Limb Package* [computer program]. Version 2.0. Lippincott Williams & Wilkins, 2005.
17. Birnbach DJ, Santos AC, Bourlier RA, et al: The effectiveness of video technology as an adjunct to teach and evaluate epidural anesthesia performance skills. Anesthesiology 2002;96:5–9.
18. Grau T, Bartusseck E, Conradi R, et al: Ultrasound imaging improves learning curves in obstetric epidural anesthesia: A preliminary study. Can J Anaesth 2003;50:1047–1050.
19. Leighton BL: A greengrocer's model of the epidural space (correspondence). Anesthesiology 1989;70:368–369.
20. McDonald SB, Thompson GE: "See one, do one, teach one, have one": A novel variation on regional anesthesia training. Reg Anesth Pain Med 2002;27:456–459.
21. Martin G, Lineberger CK, MacLeod DB, et al: A new teaching model for resident training in regional anesthesia. Anesth Analg 2002;95:1423–1427.
22. Hargett MJ, Beckman JD, Liguori GA, et al: Guidelines for regional anesthesia fellowship training. Reg Anesth Pain Med 2005;30:218–225.

82

Regional Anesthesia Fellowships

James Beckman, MD • Gregory A. Liguori, MD

INTRODUCTION

Fellowship training is essential to the advancement of any subspecialty. Graduates of fellowship programs are likely to become the future custodians of clinical, educational, administrative, and research efforts in that specialty. The role of basic residency training in any medical specialty is to obtain a degree of comfort and proficiency in that particular field. Proficiency, defined as the "advancement in knowledge" or skill in a field of medicine,[1] should be the minimum goal of any postgraduate training program. Indeed, the Program Requirements for Residency Education in Anesthesiology states that residency programs must "promote the acquisition of the knowledge, skills, clinical judgment, and attitudes essential to the practice of anesthesiology".[2]

Subspecialization can be defined as the process by which each generation is able to provide better patient care and to conduct research and educational missions more effectively than the previous generation.[3] The Program Requirements for Residency Training in the Subspecialties of Anesthesiology define "advanced training" as an educational experience of at least 1 year, designed to develop advanced knowledge and skills in a specific clinical area.[4] This expertise, or special skill and knowledge representing mastery of a particular subject, is the goal of every fellowship program.

Table 82–1.
Recognized Subspecialties of Anesthesia
Pain management
Critical care
Pediatric anesthesia
Cardiac anesthesia
Obstetrical anesthesia
Ambulatory anesthesia
Neuroanesthesia
Regional anesthesia

In 1995[5] the American Society of Anesthesiologists (ASA) newsletter reported the findings of the ASA Committee on Anesthesia Subspecialties. This committee was formed in response to a growing trend of subspecialization within the field. Currently, several areas of subspecialty training are available in the field of anesthesiology (Table 82–1).

Of these, only pain management, critical care, and pediatric anesthesia are officially accredited by the American College of Graduate Medical Education (ACGME). In addition, critical care and pain management offer graduates certification via an examination process. Graduates of other subspecialty programs are presented with a certificate of completion; however, these programs receive no specific recognition from the American Board of Anesthesiology (ABA). Although proficiency in each of these subspecialty fields is often gained during the course of an anesthesia residency, by and large, true expertise can only be accomplished with fellowship training in that given specialty.

The extent to which the fundamentals of regional anesthesia are taught during residency varies widely among training programs. In many cases, the level of training may well be inadequate.[6,7] Fellowship training should ideally be concerned with the development of expertise in the practice and theory of regional anesthesiology. It is interesting to note, that although the medical and surgical applications of regional anesthesia began over a century ago, and the formalization of the subspecialty by the modern-day American Society of Regional Anesthesia (ASRA) began over three decades ago, fellowship training in regional anesthesia is a relatively new endeavor.

HISTORY

The birth of regional anesthesia as a science dates to the late nineteenth century. In 1884, Koller, often credited with one of the first applications of local anesthetics to produce

anesthesia, described the application of cocaine to the cornea in order to produce a surgical anesthetic state.[8] Corning (1888) and Bier (1899) were the first to apply local anesthetics to the spinal cord to produce anesthesia.[9] Of course, none of these three were anesthesiologists because the formalization of the specialty had not yet come into existence.

The first formal organization of regional anesthesiologists was the original American Society of Regional Anesthesia (ASRA). This organization, founded in 1923, consisted of general surgeons, neurosurgeons, and other physicians practicing anesthesia.[8] Formal certification in anesthesiology occurred in the mid-1930s when the first fellowship certificates were issued to American anesthesiologists by the New York Society of Anesthetists (NYSA). This organization would later become the American Society of Anesthesiologists (ASA). Certification was offered in order to "protect the public against irresponsible and unqualified practitioners who profess to be specialists in anesthesiology".[9] In the early 1940s, the original ASRA was incorporated into the ASA.

In 1974, the American Society of Regional Anesthesia was "reintroduced" by a group of physicians known today as "founding fathers" of the current subspecialty society. It is noteworthy that although each of these physicians (L. Donald Bridenbaugh, Harold Carron, Jordan Katz, P. Prithvi Raj, and Alon P. Winnie) was a trained anesthesiologist, none completed a formal regional anesthesia fellowship program because formal subspecialty training in regional anesthesia did not exist at the time. Although ASRA itself has not formally endorsed fellowship training in regional anesthesia, it has cultivated an environment in which individuals dedicated to fellowship training have been able to collaborate on a common goal.

Very little information is written about the first formalized regional anesthesia fellowships. It appears that Brigham and Women's Hospital under the leadership of Benjamin Covino. and Virginia Mason Medical Center led by Daniel Moore, offered the earliest formal training programs in the subspecialty of regional anesthesia circa 1980. During the following two decades, several additional fellowship programs developed throughout the United States and Canada, offering advanced training in regional anesthesia lasting 3–6 months. These rotations, although then termed *fellowships*, did not fulfill the current criteria for fellowship training. Currently, the ASRA Website advertises 11 formal fellowship programs in regional anesthesia in the United States and Canada (Table 82–2). In addition, several other regional anesthesia fellowship programs not posted on the ASRA Website are currently functioning or in development (Table 82–3).

Fellowship training in regional anesthesia has been clearly gaining in the popularity over the last decade. A survey of regional anesthesia fellowship graduates found that this increase correlated with both the number of residency graduates and the number of those graduates seeking fellowship training in all subspecialties.[10] Alternatively, the number of graduates seeking fellowship training in other anesthesia subspecialties has fluctuated. This observation has been influenced by a variety of factors over the years. For those who

Table 82–2.

Regional Anesthesia Fellowship Programs Featured on the ASRA Website

Program	Location
Dartmouth-Hitchcock Medical Center	Lebanon, NH, USA
Duke University Medical Center	Durham, NC, USA
Hospital for Special Surgery	New York, NY, USA
St. Luke's-Roosevelt Hospital Center	New York, NY, USA
University of Florida	Gainesville, FL, USA
University of Ottawa	Ottawa, ON, CANADA
University of Pittsburgh	Pittsburgh, PA, USA
University of Toronto	Toronto, ON, CANADA
Virginia Mason Medical Center	Seattle, WA, USA
Walter Reed Army Medical Center	Washington, DC, USA
Yale University School of Medicine	New Haven, CT, USA

Table 82–3.

Other Regional Anesthesia Fellowships in Existence or in Development

Program	Location
Brigham and Women's Hospital	Boston, MA, USA
Children's Hospital of Philadelphia	Philadelphia, PA, USA
Columbia University	New York, NY, USA
Johns Hopkins University	Baltimore, MD, USA
Mayo Clinic	Rochester, MN, USA
McGill University	Montreal, Quebec, CANADA
University of Iowa	Iowa City, IA, USA
University of Kentucky	Louisville, KT, USA
University of Manitoba	Winnipeg, Manitoba, CANADA
University of Texas	Houston, TX, USA

began their residency training in or after 1986, the program duration increased from 2 to 3 years. As a consequence, the number of graduates finishing residency training in 1986 declined (Figure 82–1). This is the most likely explanation for the decline in fellows trained at that time. Other fluctuations in numbers of trainees are likely driven by job market forces and developments in the field. Despite the short decline in numbers, it is interesting to note that the percentage of anesthesia residents seeking 12-month subspecialty training programs has actually expanded steadily since 1989 when anesthesia residency training increased from 3 to 4 years including

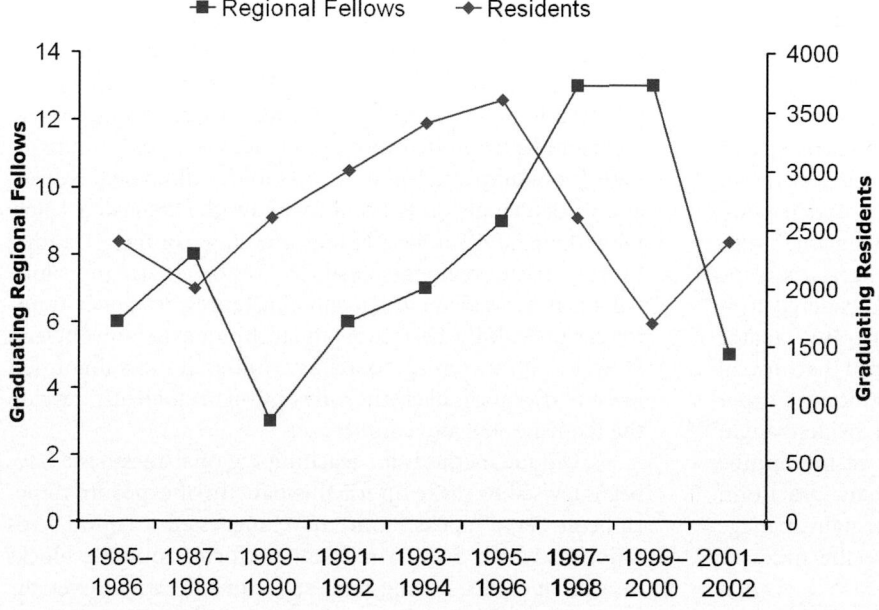

Figure 82–1. Relationship of regional anesthesia fellowship graduates to US anesthesiology residency graduates. The number of 1988 residency graduates and 1989–1990 fellowship graduates is reduced as a consequence of anesthesiology training increasing from 2 to 3 clinical anesthesia years, with the class that began residency training July 1986. Data are summed over 2 years to decrease variation. Regional anesthesia fellow data represent respondents to survey. (Reprinted, with permission, from: Neal JM, Kopacz DJ, Liguori GA, et al: The training and careers of regional anesthesia fellows—1983-2002. Reg Anesth Pain Med 2005;30:226-232).

internship.[10] Although this report did not specifically examine fellowships in regional anesthesia, the authors[11] noted a shift in the disciplines in which the graduating residents seek further training. Significant decreases were seen in numbers pursuing critical care and research tracks, whereas large increases are seen in those seeking pain management and cardiac anesthesia training fellowships.

Decreases in research fellowships are not surprising as anesthesiology receives only a small percentage of government-funded research dollars.[11] Presumably, as departments have felt the constraints of decreasing reimbursements, fewer positions are available for researchers who cannot support themselves with extramural funding. In the case of pain management, one can speculate two reasons for the increase in interest in this subspecialty: the ability to have one's own practice and an increased control over scheduling.

Cardiac anesthesia is widely recognized as excellent preparation in caring for the critically sick in the operating room, for both cardiac and noncardiac surgery. It will be interesting and informative to observe the trends in numbers of residency graduates seeking subspecialty training in cardiac anesthesia as the number of open-heart procedures continues to decline secondary to advances in interventional cardiology and more conservative medical management.

In summary, although the specialty of regional anesthesia has existed for over a century, formal fellowship training is only in its infancy. It is only during the last two decades that these fellowship programs have flourished in response to the growing influence of regional anesthesia on the practice as a whole.

RAISON D'ETRE

Various personal or professional factors can motivate undertaking any subspecialty training. They may include obtaining expertise in a narrow field in order to provide superior patient care or accomplishing a personal sense of mastery in a subspecialty field. Other motives may include job security in a particular institution, marketing advantages, and enhanced income.[3] In essence, however, a fellowship trainee is primarily working to develop an expertise in a focused clinical area. This expertise should be considered distinctly different from proficiency. In recently published updated ASA guidelines for acute postoperative pain management,[12] three modalities, including IVPCA, neuraxial analgesia, and peripheral nerve blocks and catheters, were considered to be particularly effective in the setting of postoperative analgesia. Importantly, these guidelines recommended that an analgesic modality be chosen based on the practitioner's expertise. If indeed, as suggested by Kopacz and Bridenbaugh,[6] many graduating residents are falling short of the number of blocks necessary to achieve proficiency, many practitioners will be limited in their choices for acute pain management because they will be unlikely to have the necessary expertise.

Residency training is charged with providing the skills necessary to practice safely across a broad range of experiences. Kopacz and Bridenbaugh,[6] in an article entitled "Are Anesthesia Residency Programs Failing Regional Anesthesia? The Past, Present and Future," examine basic training in regional anesthesia. In a study performed using a survey of residents, an estimate is made of trainees' exposure to regional anesthetic techniques. The authors cite an increase in regional techniques as a total percentage of anesthetics delivered by the residents from 21.3% in 1980 to 29.8% in 1990. However, this 50% increase was due mainly to increased numbers of lumbar epidurals. In many cases, peripheral nerve blocks (PNB) make up only a small percentage of a resident's training. The authors' calculations suggest that some residents completed their training having performed as few as seven peripheral nerve blocks. Hadzic and colleagues[13] surveyed practicing anesthesiologists regarding their use of regional techniques. Notably, 50% of the respondents reported performing fewer than five PNBs per month. In a survey of residents in training, Smith and coworkers[7] asked the residents to rate their level of confidence in regional techniques. Respondents commonly reported no confidence in techniques in which the median number performed during residency was fewer than 10. Large numbers of residents reported that they lacked confidence when performing femoral, interscalene, and sciatic blocks; however, more than 90% of CA-3 residents felt very confident in performance of spinals and epidurals. Certainly, the practitioner's level of confidence in a technique will affect his or her tendency to use that specific technique in practice. It is clear from these reports that many residency programs struggle, and in some cases even fail, to provide the necessary experience to achieve proficiency in regional anesthetics, let alone expertise. It is natural for those physicians who possess some motivation to become an expert in regional anesthesia to pursue fellowship training.

A number of investigators have attempted to ascertain the frequency that certain procedures must be performed in order to develop proficiency.[14,15] Estimates of the number of procedures needed to achieve 90% success rates varied from 60 to 90 lumbar epidurals, 45 to 70 spinals, and more than 50 intubations. The percent of successful completions of a technique is an aggregate number from a group of residents and may underestimate the actual needs of individuals to obtain proficiency. As previously discussed, Kopacz and Bridenbaugh[6] noted that many residents may complete fewer than these numbers in their training. For those wanting to truly master regional anesthesia, residency training alone will likely be inadequate. In some instances, residency training can provide the basic tools and techniques to be proficient. However, if one wishes to act as a full-scale consultant, fellowship training is likely the only option to efficiently develop the requisite skill and confidence.

Unique methods for teaching regional anesthesia have been devised to make up for this paucity of exposure to peripheral nerve blocks. Some have suggested a regional rotation in which a CA-3 resident performs multiple blocks in a preoperative setting and, subsequently, turns over the intraoperative management to another anesthesia provider.[16] In so doing, the residents increased the frequency of certain blocks performed by two to four times. Although this program may address some of the issues related to providing adequate frequency for achieving proficiency, this form of training may have its shortcomings. The main problem is that following block placement, trainees no longer manage the intraoperative portion of the regional anesthetic. A variety of intraoperative complications often occur during the course of an anesthetic that must also be anticipated and recognized in a timely fashion. Therefore, the development of a true expertise in the field relies on specific aspects of the intraoperative care and the ability to anticipate, recognize, and treat the accompanying perturbations such as the hemodynamic and respiratory effects of regional anesthetics.

The debate for and against subspecialization is deeply rooted in medicine. The need for specialization driven by the expansion of medical science is articulately reported to The American Medical Association (AMA) Committee on Specialties in 1869. In a report from The ASA Committee on Anesthesia Subspecialties, subspecialization offers a number of beneficial developments to the specialty at large.[5] Among these advances are subspecialty-oriented research, formation of subspecialty organizations, subspecialty-oriented scientific publications, and subspecialty education. The field of regional anesthesia has certainly thrived with regard to each of these developments. ASRA, along with its international counterparts, the European (ESRA), Asian and Oceanic (AOSRA), and Latin American (LASRA) Societies of Regional Anesthesia are vital organizations dedicated to the advancement of the specialty. The journal *Regional Anesthesia and Pain Medicine* is the official journal for aforementioned societies and highlights regional anesthesia-oriented research. Furthermore, two other major anesthesia journals, *Anesthesiology* and *Anesthesia and Analgesia*, both contain subspecialty sections dedicated to publishing information on research and clinical advances in regional anesthesia. Therefore, subspecialty education, in the form of regional anesthesia fellowships is a natural extension of the development of the subspecialty.

Other anesthesia subspecialties have had similar developmental histories. In 1997, the ACGME, in response to strong research and organizational developments, recognized pediatric anesthesia fellowship training. In developing a core curriculum for fellowship training in pediatric anesthesiology, the developers did not intend to influence the guidelines laid out by the Residency Review Committee (RRC) for training during residency,[17] but rather to have a consistent core curriculum to provide a basis for uniformity in training from program to program. The subspecialty training in pediatric anesthesiology confers a relatively well defined clinical benefit.[18] Patients of anesthesiologists who had undergone fellowship training in pediatrics (or an equivalent experience) had fewer anesthesia-related cardiac arrests, an apparent improvement in outcome that has been noted by others.[19] A controversial debate may arise when considering the ramifications of the Keenan study.[18] It is certainly not practical to suggest that all pediatric anesthesia be delivered

by pediatric fellowship-trained anesthesiologists. Similarly, a few would suggest that only those anesthesiologists who have completed regional anesthesia fellowships be allowed to perform neuraxial blocks. What this may suggest, however, is that in institutions where anesthesiologists with subspecialty training or equivalent experiences are present, a clinical advantage may by conferred by directing practitioners toward their area of expertise, particularly in more difficult cases. In addition, the scope and complexity of practice of regional anesthesia has vastly expanded over the last decade, making it very difficult to keep up with advances in the field and adopt new procedures for practitioners without concentrated training in regional anesthesia. Such training is not only necessary to ensure the success rate, but also to avoid the risk of complications with advanced regional anesthesia procedures.

In the case of regional anesthesia, residency training is expected to provide the solid foundation required by general practitioners. Indeed, as noted by Smith and colleagues,[7] the vast majority of residency graduates feel confident with their instruction in spinals, epidurals, and axillary blocks. One must then consider the true meaning of expertise in regional anesthesia afforded by fellowship training. The first consideration relates to refining one's skills in performing basic techniques such as spinals and epidurals. Developing high or near-perfect success rates may be considered a goal of fellowship training. Furthermore, performing these blocks on morbidly obese individuals, patients with ankylosing spondylitis or scoliosis, and patients with other medical or surgical comorbidities may be considered beyond the scope of proficiency during residency training.

The second consideration relates to developing skills in advanced regional anesthetic blocks and techniques. Hadzic and coworkers[20] separate regional blocks into basic, intermediate, and advanced categories (http://www.nysora.com/techniques/). Although residents are expected to become proficient in the basic and intermediate techniques, it is often during a fellowship that the advanced techniques can be mastered. Furthermore, new nerve localization techniques such as ultrasound-guided peripheral nerve blocks cannot be introduced during most residency programs. The future experts in ultrasound-guided needle localization will most likely come from fellowship training programs.

The final considerations relate to performing regional anesthesia in complicated cases, complex procedures, or in specialized areas of anesthesia practice, such as outpatient surgery. Consider the case of a patient with significant aortic stenosis for hip surgery.[21] Conventional teaching would suggest that neuraxial blockade would be contraindicated. However, a properly executed neuraxial block may be an excellent alternative to general anesthesia. Careful perioperative fluid management with radial and pulmonary artery catheters followed by a neuraxial block that was brought on gradually may be a superior method for avoiding the hemodynamic perturbations often experienced during general anesthesia. In this case, an anesthesiologist with significant experience managing an otherwise routine block may prove advantageous. Alternatively, we may consider the case of a healthy patient

Table 82–4.

Clinical Considerations for Regional Anesthesia Fellowship Training

Redefining skills in performing basic blocks
Developing skills in advanced regional techniques
Developing expertise in regional anesthesia for complex patients
Developing expertise in complex regional anesthetic techniques

having a total hip replacement under hypotensive epidural anesthesia (HEA). In this instance, the technique itself rather than the patient is what requires expertise and experience to ensure a safe outcome.[22] The knowledge of pharmacokinetics of local anesthetics and the wherewithal to recognize signs of hypovolemia as well as a familiarity with the procedure being performed are essential to timely intervention.[23] These clinical considerations are summarized in Table 82–4.

The goals of fellowship training in regional anesthesia extend beyond clinical considerations. Graduates of fellowship programs should also be the beneficiaries of a rigorous didactic program. Theoretic considerations such as complications of various techniques, local anesthetic pharmacology, and outcomes analysis are as important as clinical expertise. Finally, exposure to academic and research initiatives is essential. It is these objectives that led to the development of formal guidelines for fellowship training in regional anesthesia.

ORGANIZATION

In 2002, directors of several regional anesthesia fellowship programs assembled to develop a set of formal guidelines intended to build a foundation for current and future fellowship training in the subspecialty. At the time, several programs had individual guidelines, but no uniform standard existed. It was perceived that the potential existed for such guidelines to improve training in terms of academic, clinical, and administrative aspects of regional anesthesia fellowships. Anesthesiologists who had interest in regional anesthesia, but were not associated with fellowship programs were also invited to participate in the development of the guidelines.

Over the course of the next 2 years, clinical curricula, educational programs, and academic initiatives were debated and discussed at a series of meetings. In October 2003, the Guidelines for Regional Anesthesia Fellowship Training (reproduced at the end of this chapter) were finalized and formally approved by the group.[24] In developing this set of guidelines for regional anesthesia fellowship programs, a number of general and specific recommendations were made

concerning organization of a fellowship. The goal was to provide a strong foundation in the clinical practice of regional anesthesia, offer a solid didactic program, and provide the opportunity for academic initiatives. These goals should be realized while allowing enough flexibility for individual institutions to highlight their particular strengths in this extremely broad subspecialty field. Although the guidelines make certain recommendations regarding structure, it is common for different institutions to vary in their focus and style, therefore offering an individualized and unique training experience.

Because of these different practice environments, a minimum number of blocks required for fellows to establish an expertise is conspicuously absent from the guidelines. Although a significant body of literature does exist on numbers of procedures necessary for achieving proficiency, program directors did not believe that minimum numbers were seminal to training experts. It was agreed that no program could ensure its fellows perform large numbers of every block, but that an in-depth command of different techniques listed in categories would serve as the cornerstone of clinical training.[20]

The organization of the fellowships does require, however, that fellows have a formal rotation on an acute pain service. As noted earlier, PCIVA, peripheral nerve catheters, and patient-controlled epidural analgesia are the recognized modalities for an acute pain service. The fellows' extensive exposure to nerve blocks and neuraxial anesthesia, combined with a rotation in acute pain management, as part of the curriculum makes graduates of regional anesthesia-training programs uniquely suited for managing an acute pain service.

Among the organizational stipulations, it is essential that programs have an affiliation (either directly or through written agreement) with an institution that has an accredited residency. Furthermore, program directors must be board-certified and have completed a regional anesthesia fellowship or possess the appropriate advanced clinical experience.

To safeguard the academic advancement of the subspecialty, programs must have a formal didactic program. This should include a portion of their grand rounds dedicated to regional topics. Furthermore, fellows must participate in some form of scholarly activity, including clinical research, case reports submitted to peer-reviewed journals, or authoring a book chapter or review article. These efforts will give the fellows in training an opportunity to study a segment of the literature in depth and further hone their expertise.

The benefit of the latitude allowed within these guidelines is that it permits excellent and distinctly different institutions to train regional anesthesiologists. Moreover, those interested in pursuing fellowships in regional anesthesia may make choices based on location, institutional style, and other intangibles and still be assured an optimal educational experience. Department chiefs consider training in regional anesthesia a desirable attribute.[10] When recruiting graduates of programs that subscribe to these guidelines, they can reasonably expect certain basic abilities in common.

CONCLUSION

Regional anesthesia is an increasingly popular anesthetic and analgesic option for a wide variety of surgical procedures. At the conclusion of residency training, all anesthesiologists should be proficient in basic regional techniques. That goal may or may not be accomplished on a universal basis. However, except in rare circumstances, true expertise in the field will often be obtained only during fellowship training. The public and professional interest in regional anesthesia will continue to expand. An increasing number of experts in the field will likely be required to accommodate this expansion. The mission and well-being of fellowships in regional anesthesia will certainly reflect the well-being of the subspecialty for years to come.

GUIDELINES FOR REGIONAL ANESTHESIA FELLOWSHIPS

A Consensus Document from the Directors of Regional Anesthesia Fellowship Programs

Mission Statement

> The purpose of this endeavor is to develop a set of standards for subspecialty training in regional anesthesia.
>
> These fellowship programs will ensure the ongoing development of regional anesthesia as a defined subspecialty.
>
> Research activities, educational curricula, and most importantly, clinical care will be emphasized.

Program Requirements for Fellowship Training in Regional Anesthesia

Outline

  I. Scope and Duration of Training
 II. Institutional Organization
III. Program Director and Faculty
 IV. Facilities and Resources
  V. The Educational Program
 VI. Scholarly Activity
VII. Consultant Skills
VIII. Evaluation
 IX. Board Certification

I. Scope and Duration of Training

Scope of Training

Regional anesthesia training is a subspecialty focused on the perioperative management of patients receiving neuraxial or peripheral neural blockade for anesthesia or analgesia. Fellowship training should be concerned with the development of expertise in the practice and theory of regional anesthesiology.

Duration of Training

The time required for sub-specialty training in regional anesthesia shall be 12 months. There should be enough flexibility to allow the Program Director to tailor the program to meet the individual needs of their fellows. Specialized clinical rotations of less than 12 months may be made available but the minimum amount of training necessary to use fellowship in the diploma language is 1 year.

II. Institutional Organization

Relationship to a Core Program

Institutions with sub-specialty training in regional anesthesia must have a direct affiliation with an ACGME (or similar, eg, RCPC or RCA) accredited residency in anesthesiology. If the institution in which the fellowship is based is other than the primary institution of an accredited residency, a written agreement linking the two, and an evaluation protocol consistent with ACGME (or equivalent) approved standards for residency programs must be prerequisites.

Institutional Policy and Resources

The fellowship must be recognized and approved by the institution's division of Medical Education.

III. Program Director and Faculty

Program Director

The Director of the fellowship training program must be an ABA Board-Certified anesthesiologist (or equivalent, eg, FRCPC, FRCA) who has completed 1 year of fellowship training in regional anesthesia or is a dedicated and skilled practitioner of regional anesthesia. The Program Director must also have an academic and/or clinical affiliation with an ACGME (or recognized equivalent) accredited institution.

Faculty

The majority of the faculty in the training program must be Board-Certified (or equivalent) in Anesthesiology. A division of the faculty in the training program must also demonstrate an expertise in regional anesthesiology and/or related disciplines such as acute pain medicine. The number of faculty in a program may vary based on the number of fellows in training; however, a minimum of two regional anesthesia faculty must be maintained.

IV. Facilities and Resources

Equipment

Suitable equipment for the performance of a wide variety of regional anesthetic techniques must be available. Such equipment must include nerve simulators, neuraxial and peripheral block supplies, catheter systems, and the basic requirements for conducting general anesthesia, according to the ASA standards.

Dedicated and acceptable on-call facilities must also be maintained if fellows are expected to take in-house call.

Support Services

Appropriate support services, which may include, but are not limited to anesthesia technical and pharmacy support should be available as needed by the program.

Library

A departmental library, or portion of the institutional library, dedicated to anesthesiology with literature specific to the practice of regional anesthesia must be maintained.

V. The Educational Program

Clinical Education

The clinical program will serve as the cornerstone of the fellowship training in regional anesthesia. In order to achieve the necessary level of expertise, fellows should be familiar with the indications, contraindications, techniques, and complications of the techniques listed on the following pages:

Basic Techniques

- Superficial cervical plexus block
- Axillary brachial plexus block
- Intravenous regional anesthesia (Bier block)
- Wrist block
- Digital nerve block
- Intercostobrachial nerve block
- Saphenous nerve block
- Ankle block
- Spinal anesthesia
- Lumbar epidural anesthesia
- Combined spinal-epidural anesthesia
- Femoral nerve block

Intermediate Techniques

- Deep cervical plexus block
- Interscalene block
- Supraclavicular block
- Infraclavicular block
- Sciatic nerve block: posterior approach
- Genitofemoral nerve block
- Popliteal block: all approaches
- Suprascapular nerve block
- Intercostal nerve block
- Thoracic epidural anesthesia

Advanced Techniques

- Continuous interscalene block
- Continuous infraclavicular block
- Continuous axillary block
- Thoracolumbar paravertebral block: single injection or continuous

- Lumbar plexus block
- Combined lumbar plexus/sciatic block
- Continuous femoral nerve block
- Sciatic nerve block: anterior approach and parafemoral technique
- Obturator nerve block
- Continuous sciatic nerve block
- Continuous popliteal block: all approaches
- Cervical epidural anesthesia
- Cervical paravertebral block
- Maxillary nerve block
- Mandibular nerve block
- Retrobulbar and peribulbar nerve block

Fellows will be required to complete a formal rotation in acute pain management. This rotation will include multimodal analgesic techniques such as neuraxial and peripheral nerve catheters, local anesthetics and narcotic infusions, and nonnarcotic analgesic adjuvants. Indications, contraindications, side effects, potential complications, and daily management of patients on the acute pain service should be stressed.

Fellows should complete daily case logs to track their clinical experience. These logs should be reviewed regularly with the appropriate faculty advisor.

Fellows must be able to show competency in the following areas:

- Demonstrate rational selection of regional anesthesia for specific clinical situations
- Demonstrate effective anxiolysis of patients by both pharmacological and interpersonal techniques
- Demonstrate cost-effective management decision
- Demonstrate ability to rescue failed regional anesthesia techniques
- Demonstrate effective management of isolated peripheral nerve and central neuraxial blocks with respect to the physiologic consequences both intraoperatively and postoperatively
- Demonstrate successful use of a peripheral nerve stimulator for neuronal blocks
- Demonstrate effective management of regional anesthesia in critically ill patients
- Demonstrate knowledge of practice management principles as they relate to regional anesthesia

Exposure to regional anesthetic techniques involving pediatric and ambulatory surgery patients is strongly encouraged. Access to cadavers and/or electronic models would greatly enhance the educational program experience, as would exposure to advanced localization techniques for block placement (eg, ultrasound), where feasible. Physiologic and pharmacologic consequences of regional anesthesia must be stressed. Particular attention should be focused on the potential respiratory and hemodynamic perturbations which accompany performance of neuraxial and peripheral nerve blocks.

Didactic Educational Program

A didactic and educational program specifically dedicated to regional anesthesia practice must also be a part of fellowship training.

1. A lecture series or Grand Rounds which covers topics relevant to, but not limited to, regional anesthesia, shall be held no fewer than 12 times per year. A "Journal Club" (current literature review) should be held at least once monthly. Fellows should present articles at least twice in 12 months under the supervision of an attending anesthesiologist. A case conference specifically designed for fellows and supervised, or given, by a qualified faculty member shall occur at least once per month.
2. Fellows shall be expected to deliver a Grand Rounds lecture, including a relevant literature review at least once during the course of the fellowship.
3. Fellows should appreciate the practice of regional anesthesia from a multidisciplinary approach including joint conferences with surgical or medical colleagues.
4. Fellows should have the opportunity to learn teaching techniques by educating junior residents during the academic year.

By completion of the accredited program, the fellow is expected to have a working knowledge base consisting of the following:

- Understands general attributes of local anesthetic pharmacology
- Understands specific clinical attributes of various local anesthetics, including onset, duration, motor/sensory differentiation, toxicity, and treatment
- Understands principles and indications for various local anesthetic adjuvants, including epinephrine, phenylephrine, opioids, sodium bicarbonate, and clonidine
- Understands principles of and options for regional anesthetic procedures
- Understands complications of regional anesthetic techniques
- Understands principles of regional anesthesia as they apply to pain management
- Understands outcome studies related to the influence of regional anesthesia on perioperative outcome
- Develops familiarity with major scientific studies related to regional anesthesia

VI. Scholarly Activity

Expectations for Fellows

Fellows shall have the opportunity to participate in clinical and/or laboratory research and be given appropriate nonclinical time to fulfill these goals. There will be opportunities for the fellow to become involved in research already in progress or to develop an original project. In either case, an appropriate attending anesthesiologist will be appointed to mentor and assist the fellow to facilitate these goals. The types of activities that would suffice as academic projects include a research

paper and/or case report submitted to a peer-review journal and presented; a clinical chart review or a review article submitted to, and accepted by, a peer-reviewed journal; a book chapter; or other endeavor.

Expectations for Faculty

The quality of the educational environment of the parent and integrated institutions is of paramount importance to the program. Adequate documentation of scholarly activity on the part of the program director and the teaching faculty at the parent and integrated institutions must be submitted at the time of the program review. Scholarly activity at affiliated institutions cannot account for or substitute for the educational environment of the parent and integrated institutions.

Documentation of scholarly activities is based on:

1. Active participation of the faculty in clinical discussions, rounds, and conferences in a manner that promotes a spirit of inquiry and scholarship. Scholarship implies an in-depth understanding of basic mechanisms of normal and abnormal states and the application of current knowledge to practice.
2. Participation in journal clubs and research conferences.
3. Participation in research, particularly in projects funded following peer review that result in publications or presentations at regional and national scientific meetings.
4. Active participation in regional or national professional and scientific societies, particularly through presentations at organizations' meetings and publications in their journals.
5. Offering of guidance and technical support (eg, research design, institutional committee protocol approval, statistical analysis) for fellows involved in scholarly activities.

While not all members of a teaching faculty can be investigators, clinical and/or basic science research must be ongoing in the department of anesthesiology of the parent and integrated institution(s). The faculty, as a whole, must document active involvement in all phases of scholarly activity as defined above in order to be considered adequate to conduct a program of graduate education in anesthesiology.

VII. Consultant Skills

Communication Skills

Fellows should possess communication skills sufficient to solicit and impart information. The fellow must be able to clearly delineate options available to the patient regarding regional anesthesia as well as the risks and benefits in a manner that is understandable to the patient.

Collaboration Skills

Fellows must be able to work in a team environment, communicating and cooperating with surgeons, nurses, pharmacists, physical therapists, and all members of the perioperative team.

By the end of the fellowship, successful graduates will be able to:

- Appreciate the roles of other members of the team
- Communicate clearly in a collegial manner that facilitates the achievement of care goals
- Help other members of the team to enhance the sharing of important information
- Formulate care plans that utilize the multidisciplinary team skills, such as a plan for facilitated recovery

VIII. Evaluation

As per ACGME Residency Guidelines, the attending faculty will be evaluated by the fellows twice annually.

Written evaluations of fellows by all faculty with whom they have worked shall occur quarterly. The results of these evaluations shall be recorded and reviewed with the fellows by the program director no less often than every 6 months.

References

1. *Merriam-Webster's Collegiate Dictionary,* 10th ed. Merriam-Webster, Incorporated, 2002.
2. http://www.acgme.org/acWebsite/downloads/RRC_progReq/040pr703_u804.pdf
3. Bailey BJ: Fellowship proliferation. Impact and long-range implications. Arch Otolaryngol Head Neck Surg 1994;120:1065–1070.
4. Memon Z: Resident's Review: Anesthesia Fellowships on the Rise—New Wave or Dinosaur That Won't Die?, American Society of Anesthesiologists Newsletter, 1996.
5. Reves JG: Anesthesia Subspecialization—Current and Future Trends, American Society of Anesthesiologists Newsletter, 1995, pp 6–9.
6. Kopacz DJ, Bridenbaugh LD: Are anesthesia residency programs failing regional anesthesia? The past, present, and future. Reg Anesth 1993;18:84–87.
7. Smith MP, Sprung J, Zura A, et al: A survey of exposure to regional anesthesia techniques in American anesthesia residency training programs. Reg Anesth Pain Med 1999;24:11–16.
8. Raj PP: Historical aspects of regional anesthesia. In Raj PP (ed): *Textbook of Regional Anesthesia.* Churchill Livingstone, 2002, pp 12–13.
9. Rosenthal MH, Hughes FP: Certification in Anesthesiology: Where It's Been and Where it's Going, American Society of Anesthesiologists Newsletter, 2004.
10. Neal JM, Kopacz DJ, Liguori GA, et al: The training and careers of regional anesthesia fellows-1983–2002. Reg Anesth Pain Med 2005;30:226–232.
11. Havidich JE, Haynes GR, Reves JG: The effect of lengthening anesthesiology residency on subspecialty education. Anesth Analg 2004;99:844–856.
12. Practice guidelines for acute pain management in the perioperative setting: An updated report by the American Society of Anesthesiologists Task Force on Acute Pain Management. Anesthesiology 2004;100:1573–1581.
13. Hadzic A, Vloka JD, Kuroda MM, et al: The practice of peripheral nerve blocks in the United States: A national survey. Reg Anesth Pain Med 1998;23:241–246.
14. Konrad C, Schupfer G, Wietlisbach M, et al: Learning manual skills in anesthesiology: Is there a recommended number of cases for anesthetic procedures? Anesth Analg 1998;86:635–639.
15. Kopacz DJ, Neal JM, Pollock JE: The regional anesthesia "learning curve." What is the minimum number of epidural and spinal blocks to reach consistency? Reg Anesth 1996;21:182–190.
16. Martin G, Lineberger CK, MacLeod DB, et al: A new teaching model for resident training in regional anesthesia. Anesth Analg 2002;95:1423–1427.
17. Rockoff MA, Hall SC: Subspecialty training in pediatric anesthesiology: What does it mean? Anesth Analg 1997;85:1185–1190.
18. Keenan RL, Shapiro JH, Dawson K: Frequency of anesthetic cardiac arrests in infants: Effect of pediatric anesthesiologists. J Clin Anesth 1991;3:433–437.
19. Culling RD: Frequency of anesthetic cardiac arrest in infants: Effect of pediatric anesthesiologists. J Clin Anesth 1992;4:343–346.
20. Hadzic A, Vloka JD, Koenigsamen J: Training requirements for peripheral nerve blocks. Curr Opin Anaesthesiol 2002;15:669–673.
21. Collard CD, Eappen S, Lynch EP, et al: Continuous spinal anesthesia with invasive hemodynamic monitoring for surgical repair of the hip in two patients with severe aortic stenosis. Anesth Analg 1995;81:195–198.
22. Sharrock NE, Salvati EA: Hypotensive epidural anesthesia for total hip arthroplasty: A review. Acta Orthop Scand 1996;67:91–107.
23. Sharrock NE: Asystole under hypotensive epidural anesthesia. Anesth Analg 1998;87:982.
24. Hargett MJ, Beckman JD, Liguori GA, et al: Guidelines for regional anesthesia fellowship training. Reg Anesth Pain Med 2005;30:218–225.

83

Principles of Statistical Methods for Research in Regional Anesthesia

Maxine M. Kuroda, PhD, MPH

NECESSARY BASICS

Anesthesiologists treat thousands of patients in their busy clinical careers; they also save thousands of lives. However, anesthesiologists also have a place in research where their work is far-reaching and affects untold millions of people worldwide. This chapter is dedicated to those anesthesiologists who actively undertake research and who keep abreast of the research literature in order to better serve their patients.

The chapter begins with some very basic principles of statistics that form the foundation for those methods most frequently used in regional anesthesia research. The basic principles, albeit more theoretical, are included in the hopes of offering more than a cookbook approach to the statistical procedures. Indeed, most statistical packages willingly "crunch data," so I include only a limited number of calculations; preferring instead to emphasize appropriate application of methods and interpretation of results. It is hoped that this chapter will foster more effective dialogue between anesthesiologist and statistician. That is, by the end of the chapter, the reader should have a better understanding of what a statistician needs to know about studies and why this information is crucial to reaching valid research conclusions.

What Is Statistics?

Sir Ronald A. Fisher (1890–1962), the father of statistics, considered the science of statistics to be mathematics applied to observational data: "Statistics may be regarded as (i) the study of populations, (ii) as the study of variation, (iii) as the study of methods of the reduction of data."[1] His definition has three important implications for research:

1. Investigators would like to apply their research findings to vast populations, but it is seldom feasible to study an entire population, so they must study samples from it.
2. Each sample studied will be slightly different, ie, there is variation among samples. Thus there will be differences among samples even from studies that have used the same design and methods.
3. Investigators summarize and test the data from their study sample in order to reach reasonable conclusions about the parent population that they can communicate to colleagues, journal editors, and to the public.

Types of Data

The types of data collected in a study determine the type of statistical analyses. Table 83–1 describes the three types of data, what they represent, their typical level of measurement, and their properties.[2]

Quantitative data are on a scale that has equal intervals, eg, the difference between 50 and 60 years of age is the same as the difference between 60 and 70 years of age. When the scale has a true zero point, it is possible to look at the ratio of measurements, eg, a 60-year-old patient is twice as old as a 30-year-old patient.

Table 83–1.

Properties of Three Types of Data

Type	Numbers Are	Typical Level of Measurement and Properties
Quantitative	Amount or count	Cardinal True zero Equal intervals Order Classification Frequency distribution
Ranked	Relative standing	Ordinal Order Classification No frequency distribution
Qualitative	Class membership	Nominal Classification Frequency distribution

Ranked data indicate relative standing. For instance, ASA physical status is assigned to each patient prior to surgery as an indicator of anesthetic risk. Although there is order, we can *not* say that an ASA physical status IV patient has twice the risk of an ASA physical status II patient.

Qualitative data indicate class membership. For example, women delivering vaginally are in a different category from women delivering by cesarean section. It should be noted that with qualitative data, one category is no better than another. Thus, in this example, the vaginal and cesarean section categories merely reflect class membership; they do not reflect increased risk that may accompany women delivering by either method.

Although seemingly elementary, it is often surprisingly difficult to determine what type or types of data your variables represent. It is always a wise idea to keep a data dictionary. Table 83–2 illustrates the setup for such a data dictionary with examples of possible variables that might be included. A field for comments (an alphanumeric string variable) is quite useful for recording remarks on individual patients, eg, "Intraoperative time lengthened because electrocautery device malfunctioned."

Basic Study Designs

Study design plays an important role in ensuring the validity of a study. Table 83–3 describes the four basic study designs.[3] The hallmark of the experimental design is that the investigator manipulates the exposure (independent variable) to assess its effect on outcome (dependent variable). The cross-sectional, retrospective, case-control, and prospective cohort designs are primarily observational in that the investigator does not manipulate exposure(s) because of research intent

Table 83–2.

Data Dictionary

Variable	Label	Definition	Type	Values	Comments
gender	Gender		N	0 = Female 1 = Male	
race	Race		N	1 = White 2 = Black 3 = Hispanic 8 = Other 9 = Unknown	Include "mixed" race in "other" category
dos	Date of surgery		D		Not date of preop visit
induct	Induction time	Anesthesia start to anesthesia completed, eg, spinal anesthetic injected	N (min)		Missing for MAC patients
vas36hr	VAS 36 h	VAS 36 h after PACU discharge	N	1–100	Not available on patients who bypassed PACU
vas2wk	VAS 2 weeks	VAS 2 weeks after hospital discharge	N	1–10	Obtained by phone interview
comments	Comments		S		Miscellaneous notes on patients

N = numeric, D = date, S = string (alphanumeric).

or ethical prohibitions. For instance, a researcher may want to know whether family infrastructure affects time to return to work following surgery. Since patients cannot be assigned to supportive or nonsupportive families, data must be obtained through interviews or other observational techniques.

There are many other study designs, most of which are variants of these basic ones, and many studies will include a combination of designs. As each design has its advantages and limitations, choice of design depends on the research question or hypothesis as well as feasibility and cost. Even the experimental design, considered to be the "gold standard," is not always ethical, and results are only generalizable to patients like those who participated in the study. Moreover, no study is immune to bias, ie, any systematic error that threatens the validity of research findings.[4] For instance, a study's recruitment methods may enroll predominantly employed, upper middle class participants. These subjects tend to be more health conscious and perhaps get their health problems detected earlier when their disease is not so severe. Therefore, depending on the particular exposure and outcome being studied, the research findings may be biased by the inclusion of numerous subjects with these characteristics. There are endless ways in which a study can contain such systematic errors. Your past experience (or that of colleagues) may allow you to anticipate certain features of a study that would make it vulnerable to bias. Incorporate this information into your study design to avoid bias because, once a study is biased, its data cannot be "fixed" through statistical wizardry.

Studies in regional anesthesia will often follow the protocols of the experiment or clinical trial. The investigator will typically begin by randomly assigning patients to the "arms" of the experiment. For instance, in order to compare the effectiveness of a new anesthetic with an established standard, an investigator would randomly assign patients to receive one *or* the other of these medications. Similarly, patients might be randomly assigned to receive a novel combination of anesthetics to see whether the new cocktail is more effective or has fewer side effects than standard combinations of the medications.

Table 83–3.

Basic Study Designs

1. Experimental (clinical trial)
   Exposure manipulated by the researcher
2. Cross-sectional
   Exposure and disease/outcome obtained at the same time or within a short period of time
3. Retrospective case-control
   Cases and controls selected and past exposures ascertained through interviews, medical records
4. Prospective cohort
   Exposed and unexposed individuals selected and followed to disease/outcome

Clinical Pearls

- Random assignment ensures that likelihood of assignment is equivalent for the treatment arms.

- Because patients are not more likely to be assigned to one arm of the trial than another, the overall effect of random assignment is to reduce confounding by extraneous factors.

Random assignment ensures that likelihood of assignment is equivalent for the treatment arms. Because patients are not more likely to be assigned to one arm of the trial than another, the overall effect of random assignment is to reduce confounding by extraneous factors. However, random assignment can occasionally produce atypical groups. It is possible to assign high-BMI patients to one group and low-BMI patients to another. If such groups occur following random assignment, subjects should not be reassigned by the investigator. Fortunately, random assignment typically creates groups that are similar with respect to known (and even unrecognized) confounders.[5]

Random assignment is conducted in several ways. For simple randomization, one of the more popular methods is to use sealed envelopes. After consent to participate in the study has been given by the patient, the investigator or an assistant randomly picks an envelope that contains the group assignment for the patient. An equally valid method of random assignment involves the use of a printed table of random numbers (found in many statistics books) or computer-generated random numbers (an option in many statistical packages). A number in the table is pointed to with eyes closed. After this starting point is established by "blind stab," the numbers are consecutively followed in a prespecified direction (top to bottom, left to right, or even diagonally). Numbers are taken in groups of 2s, 3s, or 4s, depending on whether ≤99, 100–999, or 1000+ patients are to be included in the study. If even numbers have been prespecified as the placebo group and odd numbers as the treatment group, any patient who consents when the number is even is assigned to the placebo group. If the next number is odd, the next patient who consents is assigned to the treatment group; however, if the next number is even, that patient becomes the second individual assigned to the placebo group. The process continues until all consenting patients are assigned to a group and may produce unequal numbers in the groups. Modifications to this scheme are incorporated depending on whether three or more groups are being studied. For example, numbers 01–33 could be assigned to the first group, 34–66 to the second group, and 67–99 to the third group.[5]

Other methods, such as blocked, stratified, weighted, or cluster randomization, may be useful[5] and will be mentioned briefly. Blocked randomization is used when the investigator wishes to keep the number of subjects in each group very similar throughout the randomization process. Blocks are developed in which each treatment arm occurs the same number of times but in different orders. Because patients are then assigned in blocks, each treatment arm will have the same number of subjects. Stratified randomization is used when there is prior knowledge that it is important to balance a particular characteristic among groups. For example, to study the effects of two different epidurals on laboring women, the researcher may want to assign women by parity status to ensure similar numbers of primiparous and multiparous women. Within each of these strata, parturients are assigned to receive one of the two epidurals using the blocked method just described. Weighted randomization is used when there is a reason to have unequal numbers of subjects in the groups (perhaps more subjects are needed in a particular group in order to obtain a precise estimate of a key variable). This is easily accomplished by adapting the methods of simple randomization, eg, numbers 01–66 could be assigned to the first group and 67–99 to the second group. Finally, cluster randomization is used to allocate treatments to geographic areas rather than to individual subjects. Its relevance to regional anesthesia would include multicenter clinical trials.

Difference Between Descriptive & Inferential Statistics

There are two main subdivisions of statistics. Descriptive statistics portray features of the data that are of interest by organizing and summarizing the collection of observations.[6] How this is done depends on the type of data collected. For example, types of peripheral nerve block (PNB) with respect to age of patient in years (a quantitative amount) will likely be presented as a mean and standard deviation of age for each of the blocks; however, frequency of blocks by peripheral vs neuraxial, by upper vs lower extremity surgery, or by gender of patient will likely be presented as numbers and percentages, as these qualitative data indicate class membership.

Inferential statistics uses information from study samples to test hypotheses about effects that are thought to be true in the population as a whole.[6] Inferential statistics can be used to answer such questions as whether length of stay in the postanesthesia care unit (PACU) is significantly longer for patients who received femoral or sham block for anterior cruciate ligament repair.

Both areas of statistics are important. The distributional characteristics (ie, central tendency, spread, and shape) that constitute descriptive statistics are the very foundation of the more "glamorous" inferential statistics. Moreover, because descriptive statistics characterize key features of the data, it is an important tool for data cleaning. Are there missing values? If so, how much information is missing and why? Do the data make sense? Although an equal number of male and female patients may be expected to receive neuraxial anesthesia for lower extremity surgery, it would be an error to find a male receiving an epidural prior to delivery. Are there outliers; if so, are they true outliers or simply typographical errors? Did the patient weigh 702 lb or was weight written sloppily and the patient actually weighed 202 lb? By the end of this chapter, it should also be clear that the assumptions that must be met in order to apply inferential statistics properly are based on the distributional characteristics of descriptive statistics. Finally, statisticians will look at these characteristics to decide whether data need to be transformed before inferential statistics can be applied.

Measures of Central Tendency

The three most commonly used measures of central tendency are the mean, median, and mode.[6] The mean is the balance point of the distribution and is responsive to the exact position of each score in the distribution. It is an indicator of skewness (ie, nonbell shapes) when used in conjunction with the median. However, because it is sensitive to each score in the distribution, the mean is more easily influenced by extreme scores than the median and the mode.

The median is the point that divides the upper and lower halves of a scale of ordered scores. Since it is not responsive to the exact value of the scores, it is less affected by extreme scores than the mean, and is often a better choice than the mean when describing central tendency for strongly skewed distributions. In fact, it is the only relatively stable measure for open-ended distributions.

The mode is simply the most frequently occurring score or the class interval that contains the largest number of subjects. The mode is easily "calculated" and is the only measure suitable for qualitative (class membership) data. Nonetheless, the mode is of little use beyond the descriptive level.

Measures of Spread

The three most commonly used measures of spread are the range, variance, and standard deviation.[6] The range is simply the distance spanned by the highest and lowest scores in an ordered distribution. Thus it does not account for scores that fall between these two extremes. The range is easily "calculated" but is of little use beyond the descriptive level.

As noted by Fisher, variance is a key concept in statistics. Simply put, variance is the mean of squared deviations from the mean, $S^2 = [\sum (X - \bar{X})^2]/n$. Each score or observation in a sample is subtracted from the sample mean. These differences (deviations) are squared and summed, and the total is divided by the number of scores. Although vital to statistical inference, variance is of little use for descriptive purposes because people generally find it too difficult to think in terms of squares.

It is easier to think in terms of the standard deviation, which is merely the square root of the variance, $S = \sqrt{[\sum (X - \bar{X})^2]/n}$. The standard deviation is not only the most important measure to describe spread, but is of great use in inferential statistics. It is responsive to the exact position of each score in the distribution, but is quite resistant to sampling variation. As shown in the preceding formula, the standard deviation decreases as sample size increases.

Measures of Shape

Distributions come in many shapes, eg, rectangular, J-shaped, U-shaped. Shape can be described in terms of skewness and kurtosis.[6] A distribution is positively skewed if its values appear to be pulled toward the higher end of the scale; conversely, a distribution is negatively skewed if its values appear to be pulled toward the lower end of the scale (as shown in 5 and 6, respectively, in Figure 83–1). The visual analogue scores (VAS) that are used to record patient ratings of pain are often positively skewed, indicating that most patients are comfortable and rate their pain at the low end of the distribution. Because the shape of the VAS distribution is not symmetrical and bell-shaped, it would be appropriate to categorize pain levels into discrete, reasonable ranges, eg, 0–3 none to mild pain, 4–7 moderate pain, and 8–10 excruciating pain. Nonparametric statistical procedures can be applied to

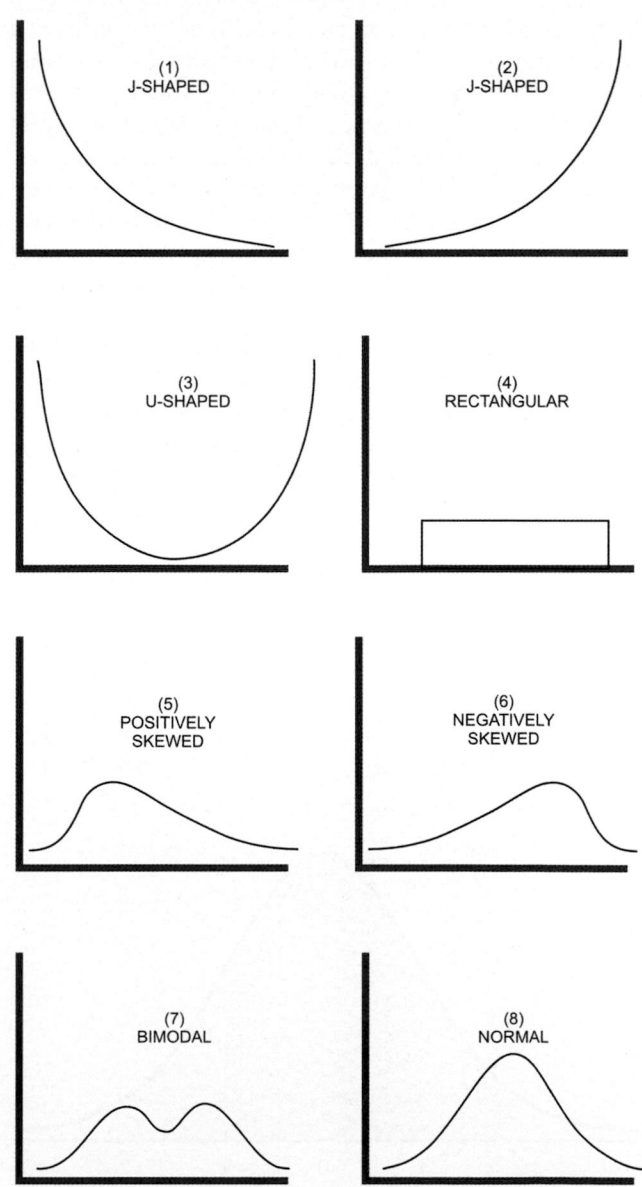

Figure 83–1. A few common distributional shapes.

test associations of interest that include these categories of pain.

Kurtosis describes peakedness. Leptokurtic distributions have many values in the center and fewer in the tails of the distribution, giving them a peaked shape with "skinny" tails. In contrast, platykurtic distributions are less peaked so more values reside in the tails of the distribution, giving them a flatter shape with "fatter" tails. Finally, the mesokurtic distribution has more of a bell shape that approaches that of the normal curve.

The Normal Curve

There is only one standard normal curve. This gaussian curve, named for Carl Friedrich Gauss, a German mathematician (1777–1855), has particular distributional characteristics that are important for inferential statistics. It is symmetrical, bell-shaped, and has a mean of 0 and a standard deviation of 1. As shown in Figure 83–2, its tails do not touch the horizontal axis because the distribution continues to infinity. Nonetheless, approximately 68% of the scores fall within $\pm$ 1 standard deviation of the mean, and roughly 95% of the scores fall within $\pm$ 2 standard deviations of the mean; hence, few drawings of the normal curve need to continue beyond $\pm$ 3 standard deviations. Table 83–4 gives areas under the standard normal curve for values of z. In particular, note that z scores of $\pm$ 1.96 correspond to 2.5% in each tail of the curve.

The convenient distributional characteristics of the gaussian curve allow us to calculate standard, or z scores, ie, $z = (X - \bar{X})/S$. In effect, this simple calculation of score minus mean divided by standard deviation gives individual scores their addresses on the normal curve. As scores have been standardized to the same curve, we can compare performance on different measures. For example, a score of 95 on an English exam and a score of 75 on a math exam does not necessarily mean that the student performed better on the English than on the math exam. If the mean for the English exam was 100 with a standard deviation of 7.5, the student's score of 95 is two-thirds of a standard deviation *below* the mean. If the mean for the math exam was 60 with a standard deviation of 10, the student's score of 75 is 1.5 standard devi-

ations *above* the mean. Thus this student actually performed better on the math exam than on the English exam.

Sampling Distribution of the Mean

Recall that it is rarely possible to study an entire population, so we must look at a sample taken from the population and draw conclusions based on our particular sample. But in order to do this, we must first look at the notion of the sampling distribution of the mean. Instead of individual scores, the sampling distribution of the mean consists of the *means* of all samples of a specified size taken from the entire population.[2] We then determine our particular sample's "address" in this distribution.

The hypothetical parent population at the top of Figure 83–3 consists of four scores. The means of every possible sample of size 2 are calculated and distributed into the sampling distribution of the mean at the bottom of the illustration. From this sampling distribution we are able to determine the address of any sample mean (here, of size 2) that we might obtain. Thus a sample mean of 4.5 has an address approximately three-quarters of a standard deviation above the mean on this sampling distribution.

Central Limit Theorem

In order for the concept of sampling distribution of the mean to be useful, we must also consider the third distributional characteristic, shape. Here, we are fortunate to have an ally known as the central limit theorem. It states that the shape of the sampling distribution of the mean approximates a normal curve if sample size is sufficiently large. So, the question becomes "what is sufficiently large?" This depends on the shape of the parent population. If the parent population is normal, any sample size is sufficiently large. Depending on the extent of abnormality in the parent population, sample sizes between 25 and 100 are typically large enough for the sampling distribution of the mean to obtain the symmetrical bell shape with central peak and tapered flanks on either side.

Null Hypothesis

The null hypothesis (denoted as H_0) is a statement that there is no effect (eg, there is no difference in length of PACU stay between patients given regional anesthesia and patients given general anesthesia). H_0 is presumed true until proven false. We must decide whether to reject or retain H_0 based on samples of patients given regional or general anesthesia. Our decision depends on the address of the test statistic on its sampling distribution (Figure 83–4). A test statistic whose address is in the extreme tails of the distribution is likely to have arisen from a distribution dissimilar to that described by the null hypothesis, and the conclusion would be to reject H_0. Conversely, a test statistic whose address is in the middle of the distribution is likely to have arisen from a parent population similar to that described by the null hypothesis, and the conclusion would be to retain H_0. *P*-values indicate how extreme a test statistic is and are used as a guide to rejecting or retaining the null hypothesis.

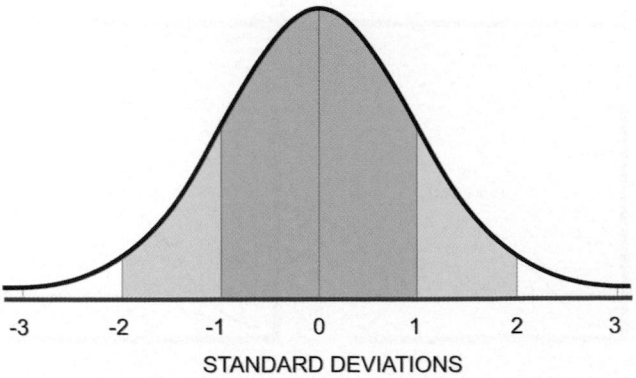

Figure 83–2. The gaussian (standard normal) curve.

STANDARD DEVIATIONS

-3   -2   -1   0   1   2   3

Table 83–4.

Proportions (of Area) Under Standard Normal Curve for Values of z

A	B	C	A	B	C	A	B	C
z			z			z		
0.00	.0000	.5000	0.56	.2123	.2877	1.12	.3686	.1314
0.01	.0040	.4960	0.57	.2157	.2843	1.13	.3708	.1292
0.02	.0080	.4920	0.58	.2190	.2810	1.14	.3729	.1271
0.03	.0120	.4880	0.59	.2224	.2776	1.15	.3749	.1251
0.04	.0160	.4840	0.60	.2257	.2743	1.16	.3770	.1230
0.05	.0199	.48Q1	0.61	.2291	.2709	1.17	.3790	.1210
0.06	.0239	.4761	0.62	.2324	.2676	1.18	.3810	.1190
0.07	.0279	.4721	0.63	.2357	.2643	1.19	.3830	.1170
0.08	.0319	.4681	0.64	.2389	.2611	1.20	.3849	.1151
0.09	.0359	.4641	0.65	.2422	.2578	1.21	.3869	.1131
0.10	.0398	.4602	0.66	.2454	.2546	1.22	.3888	.1112
0.11	.0438	.4562	0.67	.2486	.2514	1.23	.3907	.1093
0.12	.0478	.4522	0.68	.2517	.2483	1.24	.3925	.1075
0.13	.0517	.4483	0.69	.2549	.2451	1.25	.3944	.1056
0.14	.0557	.4443	0.70	.2580	.2420	1.26	.3962	.1038
0.15	.0596	.4404	0.71	.2611	.2389	1.27	.3980	.1020
0.16	.0636	.4364	0.72	.2642	.2358	1.28	.3997	.1003
0.17	.0675	.4325	0.73	.2673	.2327	1.29	.4015	.0985
0.18	.0714	.4286	0.74	.2704	.2296	1.30	.4032	.0968
0.19	.0753	.4247	0.75	.2734	.2266	1.31	.4049	.0951
0.20	.0793	.4207	0.76	.2764	.2236	1.32	.4066	.0934
0.21	.0832	.4168	0.77	.2794	.2206	1.33	.4082	.0918
0.22	.0871	.4129	0.78	.2823	.2177	1.34	.5099	.0901
0.23	.0910	.4090	0.79	.2852	.2148	1.35	.4115	.0885
0.24	.0948	.4052	0.80	.2881	.2119	1.36	.4131	.0869
0.25	.0987	.4013	0.81	.2910	.2090	1.37	.4147	.0853
0.26	.1026	.3974	0.82	.2939	.2061	1.38	.4162	.0838
0.27	.1064	.3936	0.83	.2967	.2033	1.39	.4177	.0823
0.28	.1103	.3897	0.84	.2995	.2005	1.40	.4192	.0808
0.29	.1141	.3859	0.85	.3023	.1977	1.41	.4207	.0793
0.30	.1179	.3821	0.86	.3051	.1949	1.42	.4222	.0778
0.31	.1217	.3783	0.87	.3078	.1922	1.43	.4236	.0764
0.32	.1255	.3745	0.88	.3106	.1894	1.44	.4251	.0749
0.33	.1293	.3707	0.89	.3133	.1867	1.45	.4265	.0735
0.34	.1331	.3669	0.90	.3159	.1841	1.46	.4279	.0721
0.35	.1368	.3632	0.91	.3186	.1814	1.47	.4292	.0708
0.36	.1406	.3594	0.92	.3212	.1788	1.48	.4306	.0694
0.37	.1443	.3557	0.93	.3238	.1762	1.49	.4319	.0681
0.38	.1480	.3520	0.94	.3264	.1736	1.50	.4332	.0668
0.39	.1517	.3483	0.95	.3289	.1711	1.51	.4345	.0655
0.40	.1554	.3446	0.96	.3315	.1685	1.52	.4357	.0643
0.41	.1591	.3409	0.97	.3340	.1660	1.53	.4370	.0630
0.42	.1628	.3372	0.98	.3365	.1635	1.54	.4382	.0618
0.43	.1664	.3336	0.99	.3389	.1611	1.55	.4394	.0606
0.44	.1700	.3300	1.00	.3413	.1587	1.56	.4406	.0594
0.45	.1736	.3264	1.01	.3438	.1562	1.57	.4418	.0582
0.46	.1772	.3228	1.02	.3461	.1539	1.58	.4429	.0571
0.47	.1808	.3192	1.03	.3486	.1515	1.59	.4441	.0559
0.48	.1844	.3156	1.04	.3508	.1492	1.60	.4452	.0548
0.49	.1879	.3121	1.05	.3531	.1469	1.61	.4463	.0537
0.50	.1915	.3085	1.06	.3554	.1446	1.62	.4474	.0526
0.51	.1950	.3050	1.07	.3577	.1423	1.63	.4484	.0516
0.52	.1985	.3015	1.08	.3599	.1401	1.64	.4495	.0505
0.53	.2019	.2981	1.09	.3621	.1379	1.65	.4505	.0495
0.54	.2054	.2946	1.10	.3643	.1357	1.66	.4515	.0485
0.55	.2088	.2912	1.11	.3665	.1335	1.67	.4525	.0475

A′	B′	C′	A′	B′	C′	A′	B′	C′
$-z$			$-z$			$-z$		

(cont.)

Table 83–4.

(Continued)

A	B	C	A	B	C	A	B	C
z			z			z		
1.68	.4535	.0465	2.24	.4875	.0125	2.80	.4974	.0026
1.69	.4545	.0455	2.25	.4878	.0122	2.81	.4975	.0025
1.70	.4554	.0446	2.26	.4881	.0119	2.82	.4976	.0024
1.71	.4564	.0436	2.27	.4884	.0116	2.83	.4977	.0023
1.72	.4573	.0427	2.28	.4887	.0113	2.84	.4977	.0023
1.73	.4582	.0418	2.29	.4890	.0110	2.85	.4978	.0022
1.74	.4591	.0409	2.30	.4893	.0107	2.86	.4979	.0021
1.75	.4599	.0401	2.31	.4896	.0104	2.87	.4979	.0021
1.76	.4608	.0392	2.32	.4898	.0102	2.88	.4980	.0020
1.77	.4616	.0384	2.33	.4901	.0099	2.89	.4981	.0019
1.78	.4625	.0375	2.34	.4904	.0096	2.90	.4981	.0019
1.79	.4633	.0367	2.35	.4906	.0094	2.91	.4982	.0018
1.80	.4641	.0359	2.36	.4909	.0091	2.92	.4982	.0018
1.81	.4649	.0351	2.37	.4911	.0089	2.93	.4983	.0017
1.82	.4656	.0344	2.38	.4913	.0087	2.94	.4984	.0016
1.83	.4664	.0336	2.39	.4916	.0084	2.95	.4984	.0016
1.84	.4671	.0329	2.40	.4918	.0082	2.96	.4985	.0015
1.85	.4678	.0322	2.41	.4920	.0080	2.97	.4985	.0015
1.86	.4686	.0314	2.42	.4922	.0078	2.98	.4986	.0014
1.87	.4693	.0307	2.43	.4925	.0075	2.99	.4986	.0014
1.88	.4699	.0301	2.44	.4727	.0073	3.00	.4987	.0013
1.89	.4706	.0294	2.45	.4929	.0071	3.01	.4987	.0013
1.90	.4713	.0287	2.46	.4931	.0069	3.02	.4987	.0013
1.91	.4719	.0281	2.47	.4932	.0068	3.03	.4988	.0012
1.92	.4726	.0274	2.48	.4934	.0066	3.04	.4988	.0012
1.93	.4732	.0268	2.49	.4936	.0064	3.05	.4989	.0011
1.94	.4738	.0262	2.50	.4938	.0062	3.06	.4989	.0011
1.95	.4744	.0256	2.51	.4940	.0060	3.07	.4989	.0011
1.96	.4750	.0250	2.52	.4941	.0059	3.08	.4990	.0010
1.97	.4756	.0244	2.53	.4943	.0057	3.09	.4990	.0010
1.98	.4761	.0239	2.54	.4945	.0055	3.10	.4990	.0010
1.99	.4767	.0233	2.55	.4946	.0054	3.11	.4991	.0009
2.00	.4772	.0228	2.56	.4948	.0052	3.12	.4991	.0009
2.01	.4778	.0222	2.57	.4949	.0051	3.13	.4991	.0009
2.02	.4783	.0217	2.58	.4951	.0049	3.14	.4992	.0008
2.03	.4788	.0212	2.59	.4952	.0048	3.15	.4992	.0008
2.04	.4793	.0207	2.60	.4953	.0047	3.16	.4992	.0008
2.05	.4798	.0202	2.61	.4955	.0045	3.17	.4992	.0008
2.06	.4803	.0197	2.62	.4956	.0044	3.18	.4993	.0007
2.07	.4808	.0192	2.63	.4957	.0043	3.19	.4993	.0007
2.08	.4812	.0188	2.64	.4959	.0041	3.20	.4993	.0007
2.09	.4817	.0183	2.65	.4960	.0040	3.21	.4993	.0007
2.10	.4821	.0179	2.66	.4961	.0039	3.22	.4994	.0006
2.11	.4826	.0174	2.67	.4962	.0038	3.23	.4994	.0006
2.12	.4830	.0170	2.68	.4963	.0037	3.24	.4994	.0006
2.13	.4834	.0166	2.69	.4964	.0036	3.25	.4994	.0006
2.14	.4838	.0162	2.70	.4965	.0035	3.30	.4995	.0005
2.15	.4842	.0158	2.71	.4966	.0034	3.35	.4996	.0004
2.16	.4846	.0154	2.72	.4967	.0033	3.40	.4997	.0003
2.17	.4850	.0150	2.73	.4968	.0032	3.45	.4997	.0003
2.18	.4854	.0146	2.74	.4969	.0031	3.50	.4998	.0002
2.19	.4857	.0143	2.75	.4970	.0030	3.60	.4998	.0002
2.20	.4861	.0139	2.76	.4971	.0029	3.70	.4999	.0001
2.21	.4864	.0136	2.77	.4972	.0028	3.80	.4999	.0001
2.22	.4868	.0132	2.78	.4973	.0027	3.90	.49995	.00005
2.23	.4871	.0129	2.79	.4974	.0026	4.00	.49997	.00003
A′	B′	C′	A′	B′	C′	A′	B′	C′
−z			−z			−z		

Data from Witte RS, Witte JS: Appendix D: Table A—Proportions under normal curve for values of z. In Witte RS, Witte JS: Statistics, 7th ed. John Wiley & Sons, 2003.

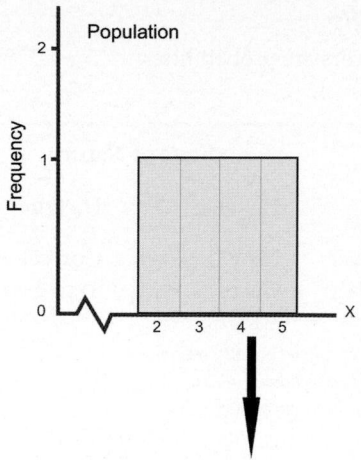

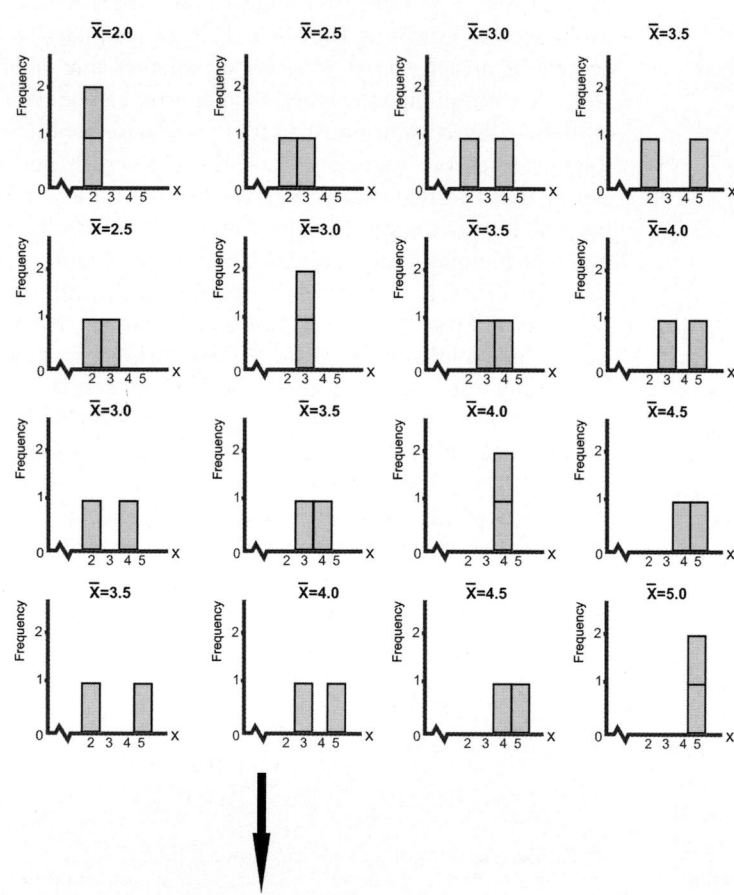

All Possible (16) Samples of Size Two

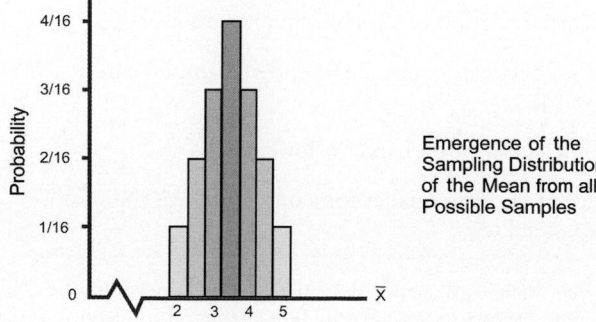

Sampling Distribution of the Mean

Emergence of the Sampling Distribution of the Mean from all Possible Samples

Figure 83–3. A sampling distribution of the mean.

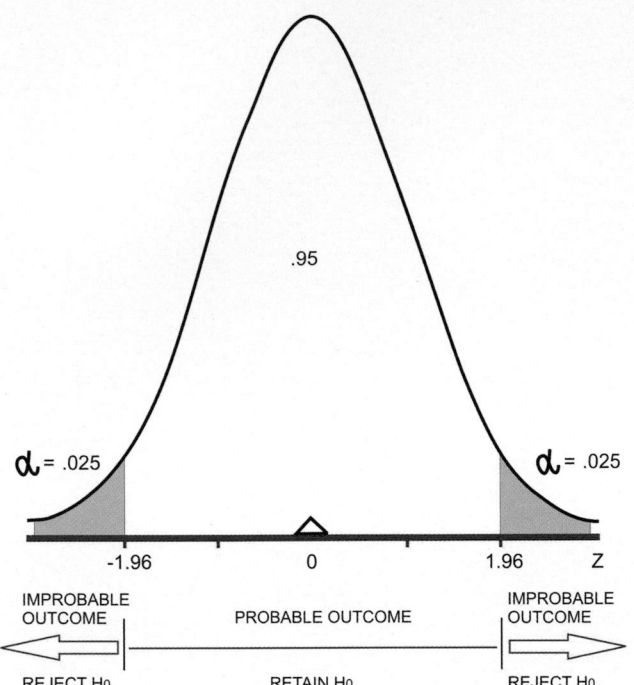

Figure 83–4. Hypothesized sampling distribution of z.

Alternative Hypothesis

The null hypothesis always makes a claim about one specific value. For example, if we test that there is no difference in time to onset of two anesthetics, we are testing that the difference in onset time between the two anesthetics is literally 0.0000. The alternative, or research, hypothesis (denoted as H_1 or sometimes as H_A) generally complements the null hypothesis and makes a claim about a range of values. Since it is impossible to test infinitesimally every value in a range, we always test the null hypothesis despite our very real research interest in the alternative hypothesis.

The alternative hypothesis comes in three forms: two-sided, one-sided with lower tail critical, one-sided with upper tail critical. If we state that the effect of a new anesthetic on intraoperative blood pressure is different from that of the more established anesthetic, we have not indicated directionality (the new anesthetic may either raise or lower intraoperative blood pressure), so the alternative hypothesis is two-sided. If we state that the effect of a new anesthetic is to lower or to raise intraoperative blood pressure, the alternative hypothesis is one-sided with lower tail critical or upper tail critical, respectively. Choice of the one-sided alternative hypothesis should be stated when your sole concern is about deviations in one direction. However, for most studies, the two-sided alternative hypothesis should be stated.

The null hypothesis and *one* of these alternative hypotheses is stated for each research aim of a study. These hypotheses are not questions and should not be written as such. They should not be influenced by preliminary peeks at the data, and ideally should be stated before data are even collected. Once statements about H_0 and H_1 are made, they cannot be changed to accommodate the empirical findings of the study.

Type I & Type II Errors

The type I and type II errors are probabilities:

		State of Nature	
		H_0 false	H_0 true
Decision	Retain H_0	Type II $(\beta)^a$	Correct
	Reject H_0	Correct[b]	Type I $(\alpha)^c$

[a] *"Missing the boat," or failing to convict a guilty person*
[b] *"Power" or rejecting H_0 when H_0 is false $(1 - \beta)$*
[c] *"False alarm" or convicting an innocent person*

The type I error is the probability of rejecting H_0 when H_0 is, in fact, true (there actually is no effect). The type II error is the probability of accepting H_0 when H_0 is, in fact, false (there actually is an effect). At issue is not whether one error is worse to commit than the other. Neither error can be avoided entirely, so investigators must decide how much error they can tolerate. Is it more important to avoid a type I error (perhaps stating that a particular anesthetic can be used at a lower dose because it provides excellent pain relief when it really does not, which might result in undue pain for the patient) or is it more important to avoid a type II error (perhaps stating that a particular anesthetic does not cause bradycardia when it really does, which might endanger the patient during surgery)?

After due consideration, the investigator sets the tolerable type I error by specifying α. Typically, this is .05, that is, the investigator is willing to take a 5% chance of committing the type I error. Things are a bit more complex with the type II error inasmuch as a number of factors can affect the size of the type II error. The factor over which the investigator has most control is sample size. Studying a larger sample lowers the probability of committing the type II error (Table 83–5).

Table 83–5.

Factors Affecting Type II Error (β)

Sample size: Larger sample size lowers β.

Discrepancy between what is hypothesized and what is true: Larger discrepancy lowers β.

Standard deviation of variable: Smaller σ lowers β.

Relation between samples: Dependent samples can lower β.

Level of significance: Larger α lowers β.

Choice of H_1: β is smaller for a one-sided test than for a two-sided test.

Data from Minium EW: Statistical Reasoning in Psychology and Education, 2nd ed. John Wiley & Sons, 1978.

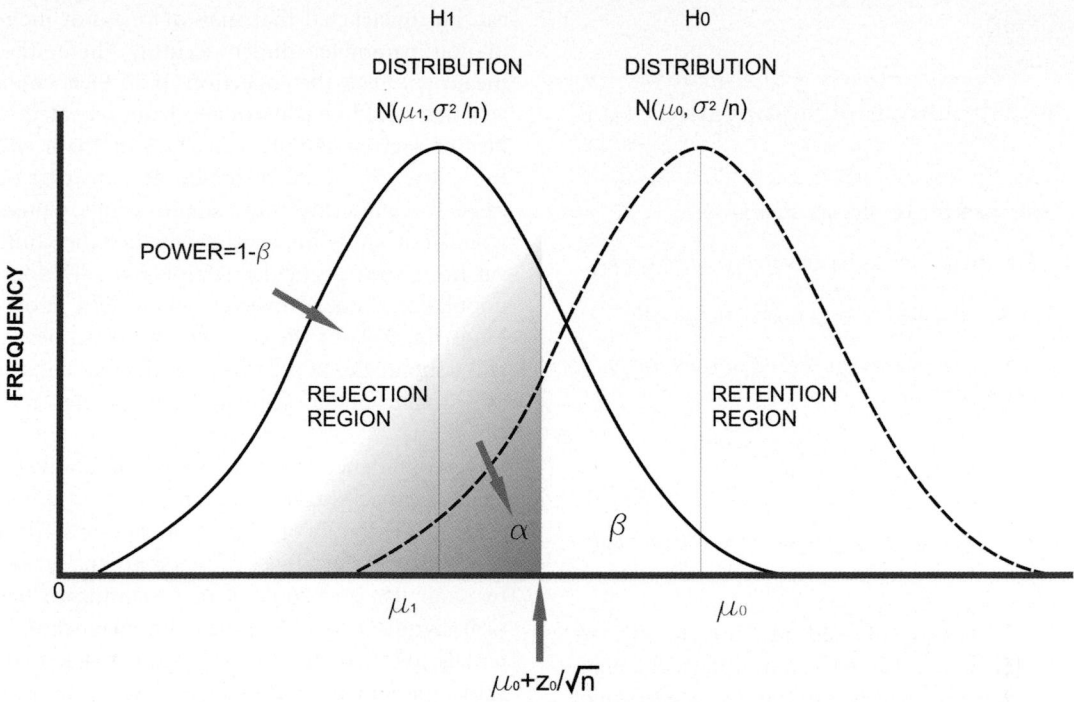

Figure 83–5. Sample size estimation.

Principle of Sample Size Estimation

Figure 83–5 shows the underlying sampling distribution of the population means under both the null and alternative hypotheses. For simplicity, only one curve (that for a one-sided lower tail critical test) is shown for the alternative hypothesis. If the researcher has decided to set the type I error at, say, .05, the critical value ("address"), denoted in the figure as $\mu_0 + z_\alpha \ \sigma\sqrt{n}$, is -1.64 for the z statistic (see Table 83–4). Therefore, test statistics with addresses to the right of this critical value would result in retention of the null hypothesis, and addresses to the left of the critical value would result in rejection of the null hypothesis.

Power $(1 - \beta)$ is determined by the sampling distribution of the alternative hypothesis. As previously mentioned, increasing sample size decreases variability. Thus, if the usual control over β is exercised (ie, increasing sample size), both curves pull apart, resulting in less overlap of their tails. The probability of committing a type II error (β) is lessened as the two curves pull apart. This is why it is important to obtain a reasonable estimate of the number of subjects needed in research studies. With too few subjects, the overlap of the curves may be so considerable that it may be impossible to detect a difference, even a sizeable one. With too many subjects, the overlap of the curves may be so slight that a small, clinically unimportant difference can meet or exceed the criterion for statistical significance. Factors that affect sample size are summarized in Table 83–6.

Degrees of Freedom

As the name implies, degrees of freedom (df) are the number of values, within a given set of values, that are free to vary. For example, in order to estimate the population variance (σ^2) from the standard deviation (S) of a sample of values, one of the scores cannot vary. Why? It is a mathematical truth that differences from a mean must sum to zero, that is, $\sum (X_i - \bar{X}) = 0$. So, given three scores (X_1, X_2, X_3 in the sample, the first deviation ($X_1 - \bar{X}$) might be $+4$, and the second deviation ($X_2 - \bar{X}$) might be -5. The third deviation ($X_3 - \bar{X}$) must therefore be $+1$. That is, the score X_3 is not free to vary because it must take a value that will produce a deviation of $+1$.

In general, a degree of freedom is used whenever a parameter is estimated, such as the population variance that was

Table 83–6.

Factors Affecting Sample Size (n)

n increases as variance (σ^2) increases.

n increases as the significance level is made smaller (ie, as α decreases).

n increases as the required power is made larger (ie, as $1 - \beta$ increases).

n decreases with larger absolute value of the distance between the null and alternative means (that is, as $|\mu_0 - \mu_1|$ increases).

n is larger for two-sided than for one-sided tests.

Data from Minium EW: Statistical Reasoning in Psychology and Education, 2nd ed. John Wiley & Sons, 1978.

Table 83–7.

Guidelines for Judging the Significance of a *p*-Value

If $.01 \leq p < .05$, then the results are *significant*.

If $.001 \leq p < .01$, then the results are *highly significant*.

If $p < .001$, then the results are *very highly significant*.

If $p > .05$, then the results are considered *not significant* (sometimes denoted by NS).

However, if $.05 \leq p < .10$, then a trend toward statistical significance is sometimes noted.

Data from Rosner B: Fundamental of Biostatistics, *5th ed. Duxbury 2000.*

illustrated. Similarly, a degree of freedom is used to estimate each treatment effect being studied in a multifactorial analysis of variance procedure and to estimate each coefficient in a multiple regression model. This is the primary reason that statisticians are concerned about having sufficiently large sample sizes in research studies.

p-Value

The *p*-value can be viewed from two very similar perspectives. Thus far, no formal statistical testing has been conducted; however, the concept of critical values has been described: A test statistic is computed and compared with an "address" determined by the tolerable type I error. Thus the *p*-value is the level of significance at which the test statistic is on the borderline between the retention and rejection regions of H_0. This is frequently .05 (or .025 in both tails for the two-sided test). Although statisticians are not certain how Fisher chose the critical *p*-value of .05, he may have felt that this is the extent of type I error that most researchers could comfortably accept (Table 83–7).

The *p*-value can also be viewed as the probability of obtaining a test statistic as extreme as or more extreme than the actual test statistic obtained given that H_0 is true. Most statistical software programs automatically provide *p*-values. The computer printout will contain notations attached to test statistics, such as $p = .036$, indicating that the probability of obtaining a test statistic at least as extreme as the one obtained is only 3.6%. And, as this is rather rare, H_0 would be rejected. Note that the *p*-value of .036 should not be interpreted as a 96.4% chance that H_0 is wrong. Put another way, *p*-values are calculated on the assumption that H_0 is true, *but they do not tell us whether that assumption is correct.*[7]

Confidence Intervals

Confidence intervals expand our view beyond *p*-values. Figure 83–6 illustrates that for samples of a given size, intervals

can be constructed that may or may not include the population parameter under scrutiny (here, the population mean, μ). Over the collection of all 95% confidence intervals that could be constructed from repeated random samples of a given sample size, 95% of them will contain μ. In reality, you would be unable to construct this figure because you will study only a single sample. Consequently, you would not know for certain whether the confidence interval from your particular sample actually does include the population value. However, you would know that, in the long run, 95% of the intervals from studies such as yours will contain the population parameter. Thus you will have an estimate of the population parameter with reasonable certainty.

Confidence intervals have several advantages. The *p*-value approach makes a statement about a derived statistic (usually the family of *F*, *r*, or chi-square statistics). This approach merely produces a yes or no answer about whether to retain H_0 and could lead to confusion between statistical significance and clinical importance. Confidence intervals, on the other hand, make a statement about the actual parameter of interest. That is, an estimate of the likely value of the population parameter is produced along with an idea of the precision with which this estimate was made. If the confidence interval is narrow, the estimate was based on a sizeable number of subjects and precision is good; conversely, if the confidence interval is wide, the estimate was based on fewer subjects and precision is not as good.

Parametric & Nonparametric Statistical Tests & When to Use Them

A parameter is a characteristic of a population. One of the parameters that we are often interested in is the population mean, μ. Parameters are usually denoted by Greek letters, whereas characteristics of samples are usually denoted by Roman letters (eg, a sample mean is denoted as $\bar{X}$). Parametric tests evaluate specific differences among population parameters, such as population means or variances, but nonparametric tests evaluate hypotheses for *entire* population distributions.

Parametric tests are used with quantitative data and require assumptions about the precise form of the population distribution, eg, normality and equal variance (also known as homogeneity of variance). Nonparametric tests are used with quantitative, ranked, or qualitative data and require no assumptions about the precise form of the population distribution. These "distribution-free" tests can be used with quantitative data that have nonnormal distributions and when variances of the groups are not equal, but they must be used with ranked or qualitative data.

When it is believed that the normality and homogeneity assumptions are met, parametric tests are more powerful than nonparametric tests. However, when sample size is small (say, less than 10), there is a very good possibility that the assumption of normality has been violated; furthermore, when

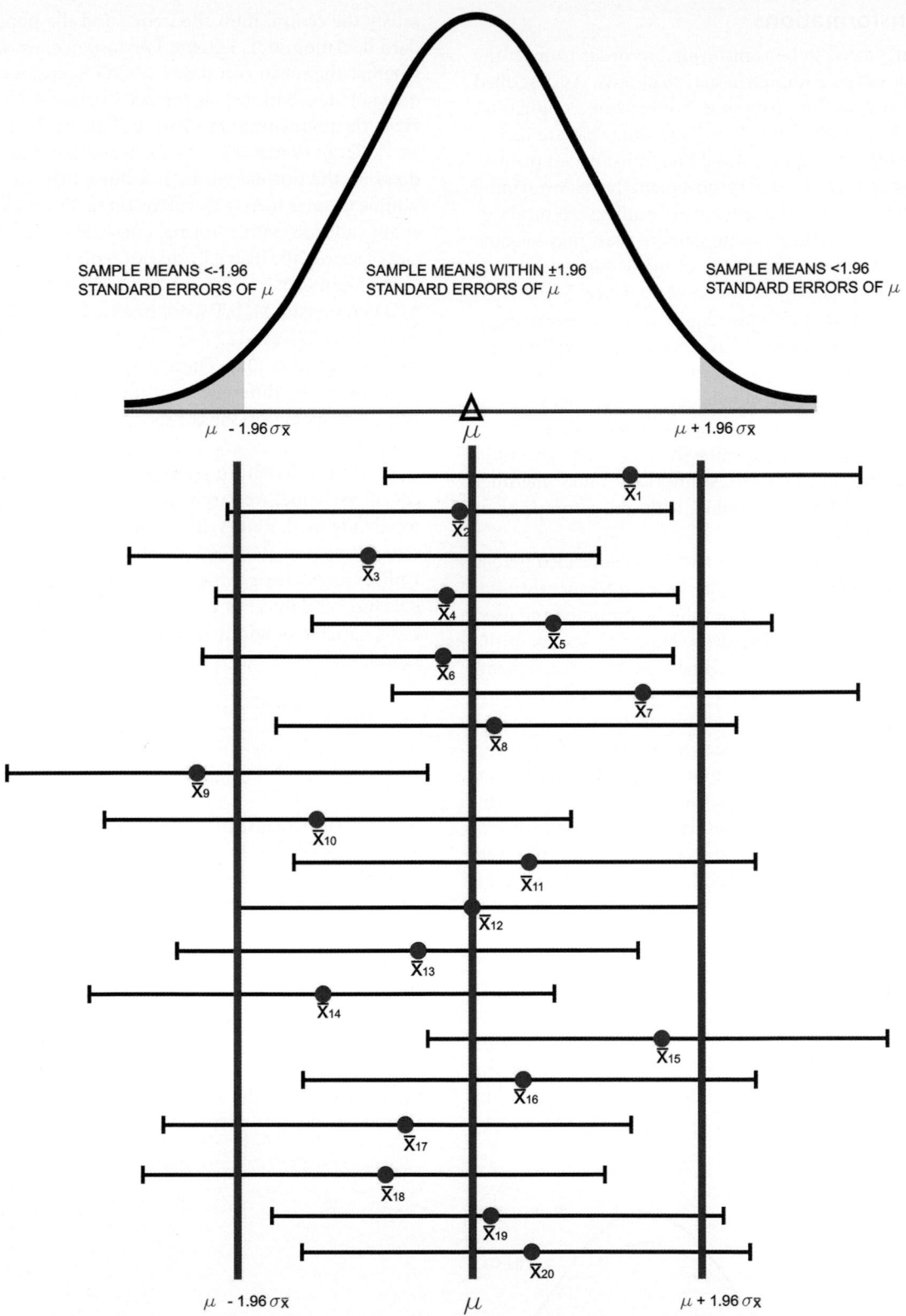

Figure 83–6. Several 95% confidence intervals arising from the sampling distribution of the mean.

sample sizes are small and unequal, there is a very good possibility that the assumption of equal variance has been violated. Under these circumstances, the nonparametric tests should probably be used. We have already discussed an example of

nonnormality with the VAS scores. It was suggested that perhaps the scores should be categorized into levels of pain and submitted to nonparametric tests (as will be discussed in the section on Nonparametric Tests).

Data Transformations

Raw data may need to be transformed in order to meet the assumptions of the parametric statistical tests. As described throughout this section, data must come from a population with normally distributed values. Thus data that are inconsistent with this assumption should be transformed prior to conducting a statistical test. It is convenient that transforming to normality can reduce the influence of outliers (atypical values) on the analysis, thus a nonparametric test may become unnecessary. Another assumption of many parametric tests is that different groups have the same variance; hence, violations to this assumption may require data transformation. A third assumption applies to regression (and will be covered in Parametric Tests). It states that the model must be a linear combination of variables; hence, transformation must be considered if regression coefficients or raw data suggest a violation. It is indeed fortunate that the same transformation often helps to meet the first two assumptions (and sometimes even the third), rather than dealing with one assumption at the expense of the other two.

The only transformation that will be described here is the log transformation as it is by far the most frequently used. Simply, the logarithm of each raw value is computed and used in the inferential statistical analysis. However, results of the analysis are presented in the original scale of measurement. Other transformations require that the square root, reciprocal, square, or even the arcsine of the raw data are obtained prior to analysis. Statistical advice is necessary when using transformations, as certain conditions apply. For instance, a statistician may note that variance increases as the mean of the groups increases (producing a rather funnel-shaped scatterplot) and is likely to suggest the log transformation. However, the statistician will also know that this transformation can be used only if the outcome variable takes no negative values.

PARAMETRIC TESTS

Our foray into inferential statistics begins with the z test for a single population mean, the most fundamental of the inferential tests. This test is accurate only when the population is normally distributed (or the sample size is large enough to satisfy the central limit theorem), and the population standard deviation, σ, is known. For instance, we wish to know whether the mean composite MCAT scores for college students in New York equals the 2005 national average of 24.5. Here, the population standard deviation is known ($\pm\,6.5$).

Recall that $z = (X - \bar{X})/S$ and provides a *score*'s address on the normal curve. It follows that the z score for a sample mean is merely an extension that provides the sample *mean*'s address on the normal curve. So, instead of frequencies of scores, the distribution now consists of frequencies of all sample means $z = (\bar{X} - \mu)/\sigma_{\bar{X}}$ where $\sigma_{\bar{X}} = \sigma/\sqrt{n}$. If the mean composite MCAT score from a sample of 30 New York students is 27, $z = (27 - 24.5)/(6.5/\sqrt{30}) = 2.1$, which is significant at $p = .018$. Therefore, we reject H$_0$ that New York students are no different from the national average (in fact, they score higher on the composite MCAT than the national average).

Unfortunately, in regional anesthesia and in other areas of medicine, we rarely know σ, so the z statistic is not frequently used. Rather, it was included here because it is instructive to note the difference between the z and t statistics. Unlike the z statistic, which has a known population standard deviation and thus has a constant denominator, the t statistic has a variable denominator that depends on the size of the sample.

$$z = \frac{(\text{normally distributed variable}) - (\text{constant})}{(\text{constant})}$$

$$= \frac{\bar{X} - \mu}{\sigma_{\bar{X}}} \quad \text{where} \quad \sigma_{\bar{X}} = \frac{\sigma}{\sqrt{n}}$$

$$t = \frac{(\text{normally distributed variable}) - (\text{constant})}{(\text{variable})}$$

$$= \frac{\bar{X} - \mu}{s_{\bar{X}}} \quad \text{where} \quad s_{\bar{X}} = \frac{s}{\sqrt{n}}$$

This is because there is a whole family of t curves, one curve for each sample size. As shown in Figure 83–7, although each curve is bell-shaped, the area of the curve in the tails increases as sample size decreases. Thus the z score address on a curve with few degrees of freedom must be higher (in the upper tail) and lower (in the lower tail) than the address on a curve with many degrees of freedom. This is to accommodate the

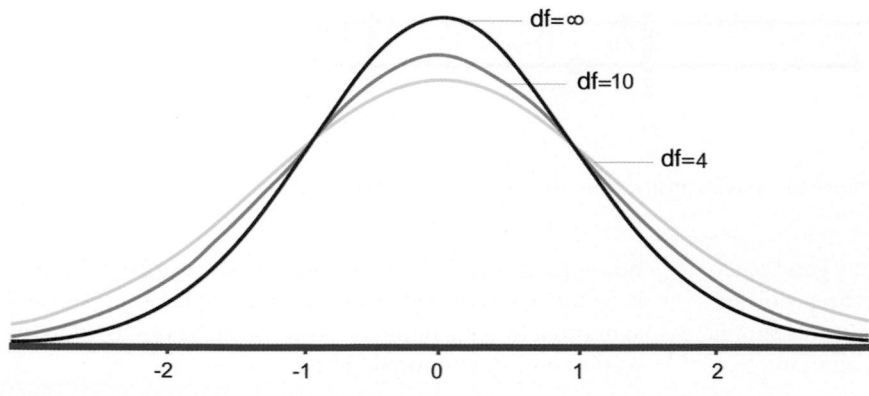

Figure 83–7. A couple of t distributions.

former's thicker tails. For the curves shown in the figure, the z scores are ± 2.776 and ± 2.228 with 4 and 10 df, respectively, for 2.5% in each tail.

The difference between the t and standard normal distributions is greatest for small sample size (usually <30). As sample size increases, the curves converge to that of the standard normal curve because the sample variance (s^2) becomes less variable, and s^2 is better able to approximate the population variance (σ^2). In fact, tables of critical values for the t statistic rarely include degrees of freedom beyond 120, as critical values beyond 120 are virtually the same as those in the table for the z statistic (in which degrees of freedom are infinite).

It should also be noted that the sample variance, s^2, is now being denoted with a lower case s, as opposed to the upper case S used in the descriptive statistics section of this chapter. Deviations of scores from their sample mean, $\bar{X}$, tend to be smaller than deviations from other values, such as the population mean, μ. Thus for inferential statistics, a better estimate of the population variance, σ^2, is necessary. In order to offset a sum of squared deviations that is too small, the number of scores in the denominator of s^2 is reduced by 1. The sample variance, s^2, calculated with $n-1$ in the denominator, is denoted by the lower case s in order to distinguish it from the sample variance, S^2, used in descriptive statistics (which has n in the denominator).

For our example of the t test for a single sample, we wish to know whether the heart rate of patients undergoing interscalene brachial plexus block differs from the adult norm of 72. Heart rate is recorded on 18 patients (mean 75 bpm ± 8.8). We calculate $t_{df=17} = (75 - 72)/(8.8/\sqrt{18}) = 1.45$, which is not significant at $p > .05$. Thus heart rate in our sample of patients undergoing interscalene brachial plexus block does not differ from the adult norm of 72 bpm. Note that the test is with 17 df because a degree of freedom was lost estimating $s_{\bar{x}}$.

Student's *t* Test

The Student's t test compares two independent groups with respect to some continuous variable. The test was named for William S. Gosset, a British chemist and statistician (1876–1937) who worked out the mathematics for the family of t distributions and wrote under the penname of Student. The groups must be independent, so a patient cannot contribute more than one value to a group nor can a patient contribute values to both groups. The formula to test is basically the same as that for the one sample case, in which the sample mean has been replaced by the mean difference, $(\bar{X}_1 - \bar{X}_2)$, the population mean by the population mean difference, $(\mu_1 - \mu_2)$, and the sample standard deviation by the standard error of the mean difference, $s_{\bar{X}_1 - \bar{X}_2}$. It should be noted that $(\mu_1 - \mu_2)$ is regarded as 0 whenever the null hypothesis posits no difference between the groups. It should also be noted that the standard error is essentially a standard deviation; the term *error* is often used to describe variability of computed measures, such as a sample mean.

For our example, we wish to know whether postoperative heart rate measured in the recovery room differs between patients who receive general and those who receive spinal anesthesia. Postoperative heart rate on 10 patients who received general anesthesia (87.7 ± 8.8) is compared with that of 10 patients who received spinal anesthesia (72.7 ± 7.1), $t_{df=18} = 4.2$, $p = .001$. Thus postoperative heart rate differs by anesthetic technique; it is higher in patients who receive general anesthesia. Note that 2 df were lost estimating s_1 and s_2.

$$t = \frac{(\bar{X}_1 - \bar{X}_2) - (\mu_1 - \mu_2)}{s_{\bar{X}_1 - \bar{X}_2}}$$

where $s^2_{pooled} = \dfrac{(n_1 - 1)s_1^2 + (n_2 - 1)s_2^2}{(n_1 - 1)(n_2 - 1)}$,

$$s_{\bar{X}_1 - \bar{X}_2} = \sqrt{\frac{s^2_{pooled}}{n_1} + \frac{s^2_{pooled}}{n_2}}, \text{ and}$$

$$df = (n_1 - 1) + (n_2 - 1).$$

Since

$$s_p^2 = \frac{(10 - 1)(8.8^2) + (10 - 1)(7.1^2)}{(10 - 1)(10 - 1)} = 63.925 \quad \text{and}$$

$$s_{\bar{X}_1 - \bar{X}_2} = \sqrt{\frac{63.925}{10} + \frac{63.925}{10}} = 3.576,$$

$$\therefore t = \frac{(87.7 - 72.7) - 0}{3.576} = 4.2 \; (p = .001)$$

Dependent (Paired) *t* Test

Groups are not independent if subjects are matched on some variable or the same subjects are tested before and then after some intervention. For our example, we wish to know whether heart rate differs between patients who received epidural anesthesia at the T1 level before and after a bolus of 15 mL of 2% lidocaine. Heart rate prior to bolus (78.7 ± 7.4) is compared with heart rate subsequent to bolus administration (69.6 ± 6.7) in the same patients, $t_{df=9} = -10.4$, $p < .001$. Heart rate before bolus differs from heart rate after bolus; it is lower following bolus administration. Note the similarity with the Student's t formula: The sample mean difference, $(\bar{X}_1 - \bar{X}_2)$, has been replaced by the mean difference between scores, $\bar{D}$, the population mean difference, $(\mu_1 - \mu_2)$, has been replaced by the population difference, μ_D, and the standard error of the mean difference, $s_{\bar{X}_1 - \bar{X}_2}$, by $s_{\bar{D}}$. It should also be noted that μ_D is again regarded as 0 because the null hypothesis posits no difference in heart rate before and after boluses of lidocaine.

$$t = \frac{\bar{D} - \mu_D}{s_{\bar{D}}}, \text{ where } s_D = \sqrt{\frac{n(\sum D^2) - (\sum D)^2}{n(n - 1)}},$$

$$s_{\bar{D}} = \frac{s_D}{\sqrt{n}}, \text{ and } df = (pairs - 1).$$

Given $\Sigma\, D = -91$, $\Sigma\, D^2 = 897$ (calculations not shown),

$$\bar{D} = \frac{-91}{10} = -9.1,\ s_D = \sqrt{\frac{10(897) - (-91)^2}{10(10-1)}} = 2.7669,$$

$$\text{and } s_{\bar{D}} = \frac{2.7669}{\sqrt{10}} = 0.87496$$

$$\therefore t = \frac{-9.1}{0.87496} = -10.4\ (p < .001)$$

One-Way Analysis of Variance

One-way analysis of variance (ANOVA) extends the Student's *t* test of two population means to three (or more) population means. Whereas the difference in postoperative heart rate between patients randomly assigned to receive one of two different anesthetic techniques might be tested with the Student's *t* test, one-way ANOVA could be used to test differences in postoperative heart rate between patients randomly assigned to receive one of three (or more) different anesthetic techniques. The assumptions in ANOVA are the same as those for Student's *t*, ie, all underlying populations are normally distributed with equal variance.

Deviations reflecting random error and the effect of treatment are calculated and compared as a ratio of two variances, known as the *F* ratio in honor of Fisher. When the null hypothesis is true and there is no treatment effect, both the numerator and denominator of the ratio will merely reflect deviations caused by random error. As these will tend to be similar, the *F* ratio will vary about a value of 1.0. Conversely, when the null hypothesis is false and there is a treatment effect, the groups will differ from each other. The deviations that are due to treatment enlarge the numerator sums of squares, and the *F* ratio will become greater than 1.0. In order to determine whether the *F* ratio has become large enough to conclude that the groups actually do differ beyond chance fluctuation, its address is located on the *F* distribution (a sampling distribution of variance ratios). If its address falls beyond the critical value into the improbable region, the null hypothesis of no effect is rejected. That is, the anesthetic techniques do differ in how they affect postoperative heart rate. Conversely, if the *F* ratio's address falls in the probable region, the null hypothesis is retained (ie, the anesthetic techniques do not differ in how they affect postoperative heart rate). Like the *t* distributions, there is a whole family of *F* distributions, and the critical values are looked up by the appropriate number of degrees of freedom in the numerator and denominator or are provided by the statistical program.

For our example, we wish to know whether postoperative heart rate differs among patients who received general, spinal, or PNB for knee arthroplasty surgery. Postoperative heart rate is studied in patients who are randomly assigned to receive one of the three anesthetic techniques (20 patients per group). We find from the ANOVA that postoperative heart rate differs significantly by anesthetic technique (the critical value for *F* with 2 and 57 df is approx-

imately 5.0 for $p = .01$ and is exceeded by the obtained *F* ratio of 6.5). Subsequent pairwise comparisons reveal that postoperative heart rate is lower in patients given spinal anesthesia (72 bpm) than in those given general anesthesia (88 bpm) but does not differ from that of patients given PNB (78 bpm).

ANOVA Table

Source of Variation	*df*	Sum of Squares	Mean Square	*F*	*p*-Value
Treatment (anesthetic technique)	2	115.6	57.8	6.5	<.01
Error	57	507.4	8.9		
Total	59	623			

Factorial ANOVA

Even though we studied three groups in the one-way ANOVA example and could have studied more, we still only looked at a single independent variable (eg, anesthetic technique). A researcher who wishes to look at more than one independent variable turns to factorial ANOVA. For instance, a researcher interested in the effects of three anesthetic techniques (general, spinal, or PNB) *and* intake of a beta-blocker (yes/no) on postoperative heart rate would use a 3×2 factorial ANOVA. More complex multidimensional designs, such as a four factor $5 \times 4 \times 3 \times 6$ design, are discouraged as they are far too complex for most people to comprehend. Nonetheless, factorial designs are a statistical "best buy." In our example, the researcher can look not only at the effects of the first factor (anesthetic technique) and the effect of the second factor (intake of beta-blocker), but can also look at the effects of any interactions between these two independent variables. Moreover, these analyses are all possible using the same subjects.

Factorial ANOVA has the same assumptions as one-way ANOVA. However, with one-way ANOVA, there is not much to fear about violating assumptions as long as the group sample sizes are equal and fairly large (>10 per group). Factorial ANOVA is not as robust for unequal sample sizes of the groups. Even small departures from equal sample sizes could cause extensive computational and interpretation problems.

Interaction

Interaction occurs when the measure of effect (between exposure and outcome) is modified by the presence of another variable. For our example, the interaction between anesthetic technique and intake of a beta-blocker is significant.

ANOVA Table

Source of Variation	df	Sum of Squares	Mean Square	F	p-Value
Treatment (anesthetic technique)	2	97	48.5	6.1	<.01
Beta blocker (yes/no)	1	39.6	39.6	5.0	<.05
Interaction (technique × blocker)	2	114	57	7.2	<.01
Error	54	426.6	7.9		
Total	59	677.2			

This is illustrated in Figure 83–8. Patients who receive beta-blockers and spinal anesthesia or PNB have a substantially decreased postoperative heart rate compared with those who do not receive beta-blockers, but postoperative heart

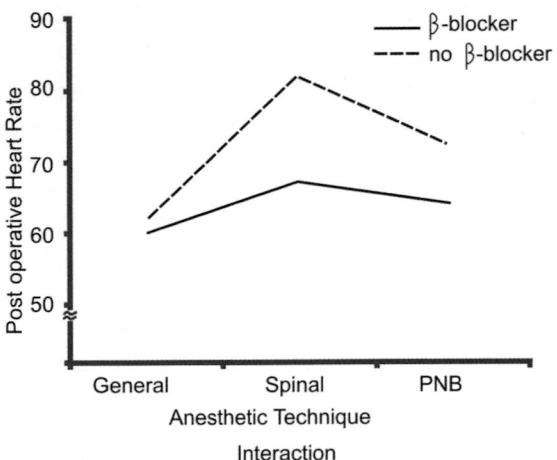

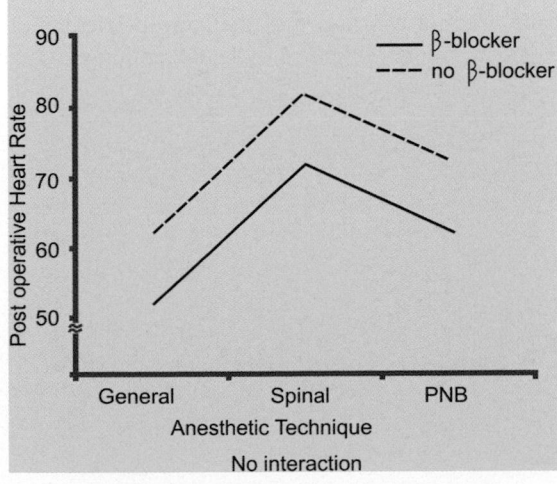

Figure 83–8. Interaction vs no interaction.

rate is only minimally decreased in patients who receive beta-blockers and general anesthesia. Note that when interaction is found, it is the interaction that is of interest and thus described in the report. In our example, the main effects of anesthetic technique and intake of beta-blocker are also statistically significant, but they no longer have "center stage." On the other hand, if there had been *no* interaction, the main effects would have been reported separately as both are statistically significant, eg, postoperative heart rate differs by anesthetic technique and is decreased in patients who receive beta-blockers prior to surgery. Moreover, the lines for intake/no intake of beta-blocker would have been fairly parallel (as is also illustrated in Figure 83–8).

Multiple Comparisons

We return to the one-way ANOVA example of the effects of three different anesthetic techniques on postoperative heart rate. If our *F* ratio is statistically significant, we know that the three sample means come from different populations, ie, the anesthetic techniques differ in how they affect postoperative heart rate. However, a significant *F* ratio does not tell us which group or groups are different. Is postoperative heart rate in patients who receive general anesthesia different from that of patients who receive spinal anesthesia, but not different from that of patients who receive PNB? If specific interest in a comparison (say, between general and spinal anesthetic techniques) had been stated *before looking at the data*, the difference in postoperative heart rate between these two techniques could be followed by the Student's *t* test. However, when such a priori comparisons have not been expressed, several comparisons among the groups must be conducted to determine where the significant difference(s) lie. These comparisons are considered post hoc because they involve data that have already been reviewed and analyzed (here, by one-way ANOVA). The problem is the greater the number of statistical tests run, the greater the risk of committing a type I error (saying there is a difference when there really is none). This is because a null hypothesis rejected at $\alpha = .05$ on a *single* test confers a 5% chance of committing a type I error, but as more and more multiple comparisons are made, the experiment-wise α rises, and it can rise very fast.

Fortunately, a number of tests are designed to help control the experiment-wise error. Three methods are commonly used when the investigator wishes to compare all pairs of means: the Bonferroni approach, the Tukey honestly significant difference test, and the Student–Newman–Keuls comparison test. In the Bonferroni approach, the α level is divided by the number of all possible *pairs* of groups to be compared. For three groups in the experiment (here, simply designated as A, B, and C), α would be divided by 3 (AB, AC, BC); for four groups (A, B, C, D), α would be divided by 6 (AB, AC, AD, BC, BD, CD). Group differences are tested by the Student's *t* test using the pooled estimate of the variance (error mean square from the one-way ANOVA). The *t* statistic for each comparison must then exceed the more stringent adjusted α in order to be declared statistically significant. The Bonferroni approach

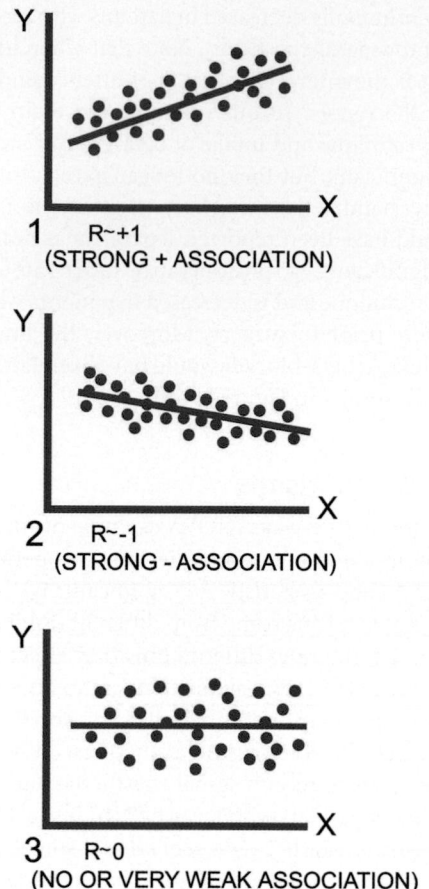

1 R~+1
(STRONG + ASSOCIATION)

2 R~-1
(STRONG - ASSOCIATION)

3 R~0
(NO OR VERY WEAK ASSOCIATION)

Figure 83–9. Pearson's product moment correlation coefficient (*r*).

control group to each of the other treatment groups. Scheffé's method is useful if the investigator is interested in elaborate comparisons (known as contrasts), eg, the mean of (A + B + C) vs D; however, it is more conservative than other post hoc tests. Clearly, statistical expertise should be sought when multiple comparison decisions need to be made.

Correlation

Numerous statistics can be calculated to assess the extent of association between variables, eg, φ coefficient, biserial, point biserial. However, the most well-known and frequently used is the Pearson product-moment correlation coefficient (simply denoted as *r*). Pearson's *r*, named for the British mathematician, Karl Pearson (1857–1936), is a measure of association between two continuous variables, both obtained on separate subjects (Figure 83–9). The coefficient ranges from +1 (perfect positive association) to –1 (perfect negative association). Values around 0 indicate that the two variables are not associated, eg, height of patient and duration of block. As *r* approaches +1, an individual with a high value for one variable is likely to have a high value for the other; similarly, an individual with a low value for one variable is likely to have a low value for the other. For instance, intensity of current at which the sciatic nerve is stimulated is positively correlated with time to anesthesia onset. Conversely, as *r* approaches –1, an individual with a high value for one variable is likely have a low value for the other and vice versa. For instance, when performing PNBs with stimulating currents below 0.25 mA, intensity of current is negatively correlated with percent of successful blockades.

It is important to note, however, that Pearson's *r* does not measure several things:[8]

- *r* makes no statement about causality. Even though two variables are strongly associated (either positively or negatively), one did not *cause* the other.
- *r* is not a measure of the magnitude of the slope of the regression line (Figure 83–10). Both lines indicate perfect association, however, the slope is only impressive for the panel on the left.
- Finally, *r* is not a measure of the appropriateness of the straight-line model (Figure 83–11). Regardless of a high or

tends to be conservative (less powerful) and should be used only when testing a few pairs of means (ie, not more than five groups). The Tukey and Student–Newman–Keuls tests use range tests to identify homogeneous subsets of means that are not different from one another. They make all possible comparisons between groups and are more powerful when testing a large number of pairs of means. Other popular post hoc comparison methods include the Dunnett's test, which is useful when the investigator is not interested in comparing groups among themselves, but instead wishes to compare one

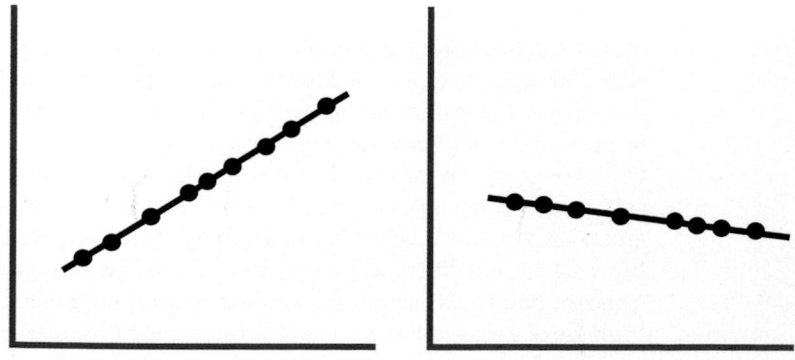

r=1; slope impressive   r=1; slope not impressive   **Figure 83–10.** *r* is not a measure of slope.

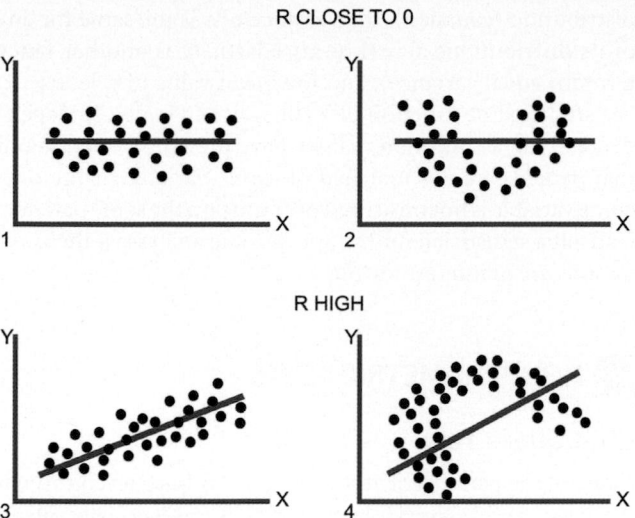

Figure 83–11. *r* is not a measure of appropriateness of straight-line model.

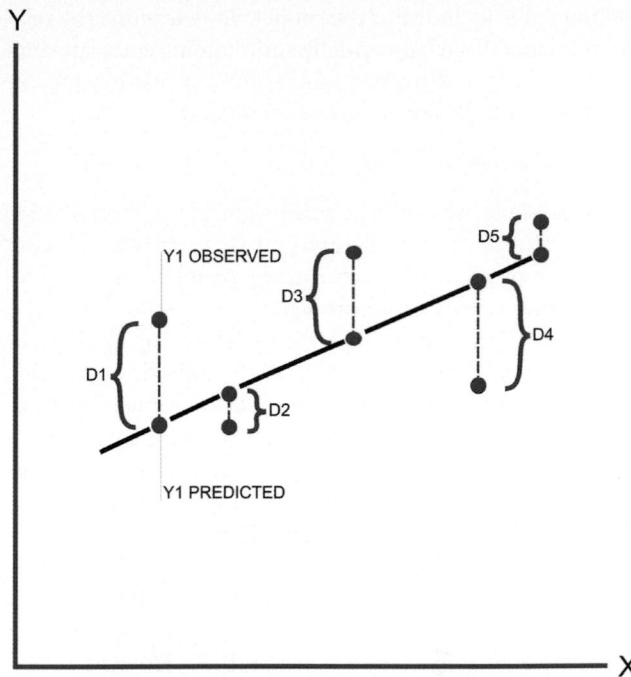

Figure 83–12. Least squares regression.

low *r*, there could be a nonlinear association in the data that would not be discerned simply by considering the value of *r*. A picture is worth a 1000 words!

We will not derive the level of significance associated with values of Pearson's *r*. Suffice it to say, that Pearson's *r* computed from a sample is used to test the null hypothesis that the population correlation (ρ) is zero (ie, H_0: $\rho = 0$) or to test the null hypothesis that the population correlation is some value suggested from past experience or theory (ie, H_0: $\rho = \rho_0$ where $\rho_0 \neq 0$). A statistician will be able to test these hypotheses and construct the appropriate confidence intervals. Moreover, statistical expertise is advised if your research interest lies in testing the equality of two correlations from independent random samples (ie, H_0: $\rho_1 = \rho_2$) or two correlations of different variables within the same sample (eg, H_0: $\rho_{12} = \rho_{13}$).

Least Squares Regression

When the correlation coefficient is 0, we know that *x* is useless in predicting *y*. When the correlation coefficient is +1 or −1, we know that *x* is exactly correct in predicting *y*. However, the value of the correlation coefficient, in and of itself, does not tell us how to go about making the prediction. So, on what structure can prediction be based? If the *x* and *y* variables have a linear relationship, the structure can be a line through the scatterplot of points, in which each dot represents the intersection of a subject's *x* and *y* values. The problem is that innumerable lines could be drawn through the scatterplot. Which is the "best fitting" one? Pearson solved this problem by determining the line in such a way that the sum of the squared differences (d_i's) between each scatterplot dot and the line is as small as possible (hence the term, *least squares regression*). That is, the sum of squared discrepancies shown in Figure 83–12 is at a minimum. No other line through that scatterplot has a lower sum of squares.

With bivariate (simple) linear regression, a continuous variable *y* is predicted from a continuous variable *x* based on the equation for a straight line, $y = \alpha + \beta x + \varepsilon$. Thus the components that predict *y* are a constant that indicates the value of *y* when *x* is 0 (known as the intercept of the line, α), a coefficient that indicates the change in *y* for each 1 unit change in *x* (known as the slope, β), and an error term that indicates variability of the observed values from the regression line (ε). For our example, we wish to predict duration of femoral nerve blockade from the concentration of 0.5% lidocaine administered. Duration of femoral nerve blockade (in minutes) is measured in 24 patients receiving 0.5%, 1.0%, 1.5%, or 2.0% lidocaine. The model produced (calculations not shown) is $y = -2.5 + 124x = -2.5 + 124(.5) = 59.5$, indicating an increase of approximately 60 min in duration of femoral nerve blockade for every unit increase of 0.5% lidocaine.

With multiple linear regression, a continuous variable *x* is used to predict a continuous variable *y, while controlling or adjusting for the influence of one or more potentially confounding variables.* When mixed with the exposure and outcome, confounders can strengthen, weaken, or otherwise distort the true association between exposure and outcome.[9] As an example, we found from bivariate linear regression that a concentration of 0.5% lidocaine is predictive of duration of femoral blockade. However, concentration of local anesthetic may predict a duration of femoral blockade that is substantially longer than 60 min when a variable reflecting presence or absence of preexisting neuropathy (eg, diabetic neuropathy) is also included in the model. On the other hand, concentration of local anesthetic may *not* predict duration of femoral blockade when stimulating current at which motor response is observed is included in the model. To determine the relative influence of such potentially confounding covariates and to take a more undisturbed look at the x–y relationship, we construct multiple linear regression models,

$$y = \alpha + \beta_1 x_1 + \beta_2 x_2 + \beta_3 x_3 + \cdots + \beta_i x_i + \varepsilon$$

In our example, we would be able to look at the effect of 0.5% lidocaine concentration on duration of femoral blockade after the effects of preexisting neuropathy or intensity of nerve-stimulating current are controlled.

Covariates can be discrete variables (eg, gender) or continuous variables (eg, age). With multiple regression, quadratic terms can be added to model nonlinear relationships (eg, x_1^2), and product terms can be added to model interactions (eg, $x_2 x_3$). If these nonlinear and interaction terms are included in the model, the component terms (x_1, x_2, x_3) should also be included in the model, eg,

$$y = \alpha + \beta_1 x_1 + \beta_2 x_2 + \beta_3 x_3 + \beta_4 x_1^2 + \beta_5 x_2 x_3 + \varepsilon$$

Assumptions for the Straight-Line Model

Whether we are constructing a bivariate or multivariable regression model, five assumptions must be met. Students of statistics remember them by the acronym, HEIL Gauss (homoscedasticity, existence, independence, linearity, and normal distribution), even though it seems more logical to describe these assumptions in a different order.[8] So, referring to Figure 83–13, let us begin with "existence." This assumption states that, at any given fixed value of the variable x, there exists a random variable y, and that this random variable y has a probability distribution with finite mean and variance. The distribution of y for any fixed value of x has a normal

distribution (gaussian), the variance of y is the same for any of its distributions at x (homoscedasticity is another fancy term for equal variance), and the mean value of y, ie, $\mu y \mid x$, is a straight-line function of x (linearity). Finally, "independence" is an assumption that we have previously met. Recall that patients are not matched on some variable or the outcome variable is not measured over time on the same patients. Consult a statistician for the appropriate analyses if these situations are of interest to you.

NONPARAMETRIC TESTS

Chi-Square Test

Many of the parametric tests are quite "robust" even though their assumptions are violated, and they are especially robust when the sample size is moderate or large. However, if the violations are sizeable and the sample size is small or, if the data are ranks or are qualitative, we turn to the nonparametric tests.

One of the most popular of the nonparametric tests is the chi-square (χ^2) test. It requires that observations are independent, ie, each subject is counted in one, and only one, cell of a contingency table. It also requires that expected frequencies are sufficiently large. So, how are expected frequencies obtained, and what is "sufficiently large?" An expected frequency for a given cell is obtained by multiplying the row and column marginals for that cell and dividing the product by n. Thus the expected frequency for the upper left-hand cell with its observed frequency a is $[(a + b)(a + c)]/n$. This process is repeated for each of the remaining three cells. An expected frequency of 5 typically suffices for the test. The Fisher's

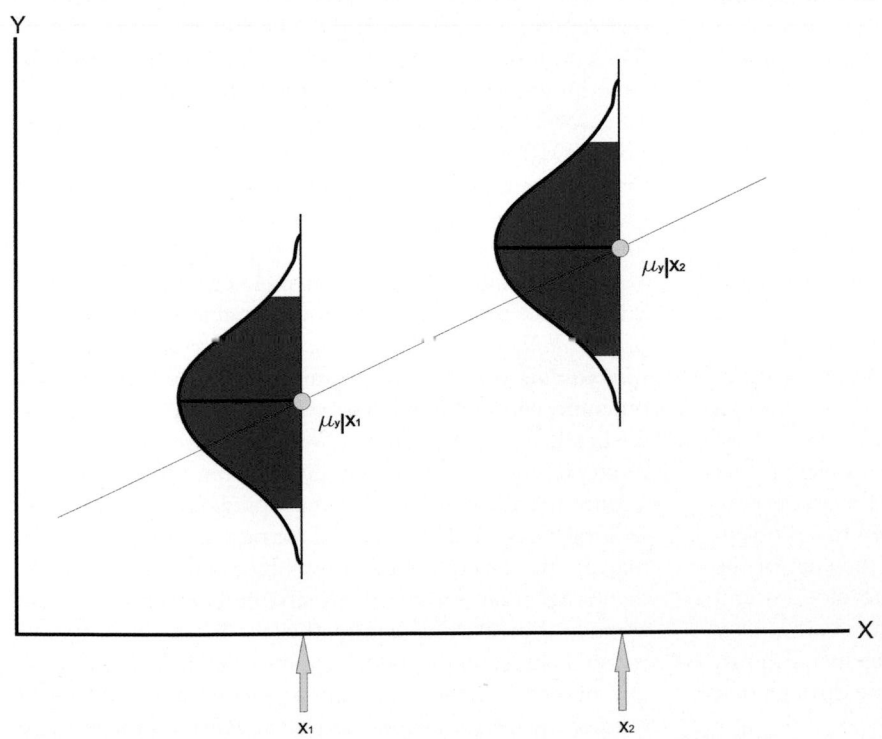

Figure 83–13. HEIL Gauss.

exact test (described in the following section) is typically used instead of χ^2 when any cell has an expected frequency less than 5.

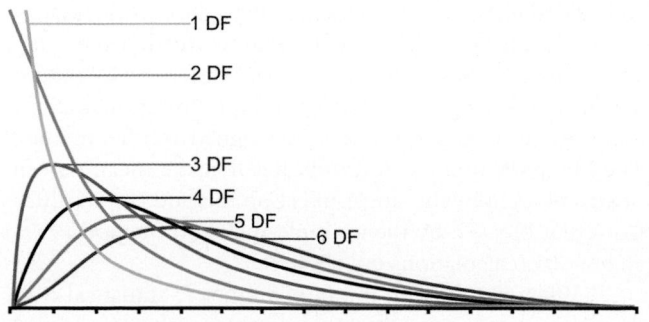

In the numerator for each cell, a constant 0.5, known as Yates' correction, is subtracted from the absolute difference between observed and expected frequencies because the continuous χ^2 distribution is being used to represent the discrete distribution of sample frequencies. Numerators are squared and divided by the expected frequencies of the respective cells, and the proportions summed over all cells. In short, the χ^2 statistic reflects the size of the discrepancies between observed and expected frequencies as a proportion of the expected frequency. So, large χ^2's indicate differences generated by associations that are not likely to be due to chance; conversely, small χ^2's indicate differences that could be accounted for by chance. As with the t distributions, there is a whole family of χ^2 distributions. Their shapes differ depending on the degrees of freedom (Figure 83–14). Hence the critical values for statistical significance that correspond to rejection regions for various values of α will also differ according to the χ^2 statistic's degrees of freedom, calculated as (rows – 1)(columns – 1).

Our example evaluates the association between parity and requests for epidurals during labor. In this example, 70% of primiparous women opt for epidurals compared with 55% of multiparous women. Following the calculations just described, the χ^2 statistic has a value of almost 9. Is this large enough to conclude that the sample did not produce a chance finding? The test statistic exceeds the .01 level of significance but not the .001 level of significance with 1 df, thus requests for epidurals is associated with parity. It should be noted that, although χ^2 is an excellent measure of the statistical *significance* of an association, it does not measure the *extent* of association.[10] Thus it would be wrong to conclude that

primiparous women are about 9 times more likely to opt for epidurals than multiparous women.

| | | Epidural | | |
		Yes	No	Total
Parity	Primiparous	140	60	200
	Multiparous	110	90	200
	Total	250	150	400

$$\chi^2 = \sum \frac{(|f_O - f_E| - 0.5)^2}{f_E} = \frac{(|140 - 125| - 0.5)^2}{125}$$
$$+ \frac{(|60 - 75| - 0.5)^2}{75} + \frac{(|110 - 125| - 0.5)^2}{125}$$
$$+ \frac{(|90 - 75| - 0.5)^2}{75} = 8.97$$

where $f_E = (200)(250)/400 = 125$ for cells a and c, and $(200)(150)/400 = 75$ for cells b and d, and df = (rows – 1)(columns – 1) = (2 – 1)(2 – 1) = 1.

Consult with a statistician when conducting χ^2 tests that involve more than the 2 × 2 table. For example, you may wish to calculate the χ^2 statistic for larger tables, such as a 4 × 5 table, following the principles described in the preceding figure. However, if the overall χ^2 statistic is significant, you must conduct several comparisons to determine which cells are different from each other, and you would again be faced with the issue of multiple comparisons. In other instances, you may wish to examine the association of a variable among categories of another variable that has an intrinsic order. For instance, you may wish to examine the association of position of patient (supine vs sitting) by level of spinal anesthesia, which has an intrinsic quantitative order (eg, <L1, L1 ≤ T8, >T8). Or, you may wish to examine the association of nerve localization method (eg, nerve stimulator vs "blind") by PNB success, which has an intrinsic qualitative order (eg, failed, incomplete, complete). A statistician will be able to conduct the χ^2 tests that are appropriate for these situations.

Fisher's Exact Test

The "exact" test (more properly, the Fisher–Irwin exact test) applies when the expected value of at least one cell in a 2 × 2 table is <5. Recall that expected frequencies are based on marginal frequencies; but marginals that are small are less precise and may lead to an inaccurate test of significance based on the χ^2 distribution. Thus the exact test uses a different kind of probability distribution (the hypergeometric) to derive an exact probability (P_{obs}) that is associated with the cell frequencies in the observed table. The calculations are repeated for all other tables that can possibly be constructed using the same marginal frequencies as those in the observed table. Finally, any exact probabilities that are less than or equal to P_{obs} are summed. This sum is the Fisher's exact p-value. As is typical, Fisher's exact p-values <.05 are considered statistically significant.

Figure 83–14. A family of χ^2 distributions.

McNemar's Chi-Square

In the χ^2 tests described thus far, subjects are independent, ie, each patient falls in one, and only one, cell. McNemar's χ^2 applies to situations in which patients are matched or in which their before–after scores are tested. In the example depicted, we wish to know whether block success differs by type of catheter. Interscalene blocks are induced by boluses of local anesthetic through stimulating or nonstimulating catheters. The procedures are performed 2 weeks apart in the same ($n = 20$) volunteers. Intuitively, it can be appreciated that the concordant cells (a and d) do not give us any information about differences in block success by type of catheter. So, we look to the discordant cells (b and c) for the test. The value of the McNemar's χ^2 test statistic is a mere 0.2. The statistic is referred to the χ^2 critical value of 3.84 with 1 df and is not significant. There is no association between type of catheter and interscalene block success.

		Non-stimulating catheter	
		Success	Failure
Stimulating catheter	Success	$a = 5$	$b = 7$
	Failure	$c = 5$	$d = 3$

$$\chi^2_{\text{McNemar}} = \frac{(|b - c| - 0.5)^2}{b + c} = \frac{(|7 - 5| - 0.5)^2}{7 + 5}$$
$$= 0.1875 \text{ (NS)}$$

Spearman's Rho

Spearman's rho (ρ) (sometimes denoted as r_s) was named for British psychologist, Charles E. Spearman (1863–1945) and is the nonparametric counterpart to the Pearson r. It is used to examine the association between two variables when one or both are ordinal or has a very nonnormal shape. Spearman's ρ reflects the degree of regularity among pairs of ranks instead of pairs of scores. In fact, if Pearson's r is calculated on ranked data, its value would be equivalent to that of Spearman's ρ. Although Spearman's ρ varies between $+1$ and -1 (as does Pearson's r), it is not as responsive to the available information in that it is computed on the relative standing of scores within a set of observations (ie, their ranks) rather than on the quantitative score values themselves.

For our example, we wish to know whether Apgar scores recorded at 1 and 5 min after birth are correlated. As Apgar scores tend to be negatively skewed (most newborns have high Apgar scores), we decide to calculate a Spearman's ρ. We find that its value is 0.639 based on the 1- and 5-min Apgar scores of 20 randomly selected babies ($p = .02$, calculations not shown). Thus high Apgar scores at 1 min are associated with high Apgar scores at 5 min, and low Apgar scores at 1 min are associated with low Apgar scores at 5 min. The statistical test for significance is based on the t distribution with $n - 2$ df when $n \geq 10$. If $n < 10$, the t distribution cannot be used, and a table of exact significance levels must be consulted with the help of your statistician.

Some Other Nonparametric Tests Commonly Used in Regional Anesthesia Research

Mann–Whitney U (Wilcoxon Ranked Sum Test)

Several nonparametric counterparts to the Student's t test can evaluate whether two independent samples come from the same population. The most popular of these is the Mann–Whitney U, a test which is fundamentally equivalent to the Wilcoxon ranked sum test. Like the Student's t test, these tests assume that the groups are independent; however, they are immune to violations to normality and equal variance assumptions. As noted earlier, the nonparametric tests consider entire population distributions rather than differences among population parameters, such as the difference between two population means. Nevertheless, if the two population distributions are even moderately similar in shape and variability, the nonparametric tests are excellent tests of central tendency. Since these tests are based on ranks, investigators often interpret their results in terms of a comparison of medians.

For the Mann–Whitney U test, observations from both groups are combined, and ranks are assigned in ascending order. (Average rank is assigned whenever scores are tied; however, the number of ties should be small compared with the total number of observations.) The collective ranks for each group would be similar if there is no difference between the underlying populations, ie, the samples come from the same or similar populations (H_0 is true). Conversely, the collective ranks for each group would be dissimilar if the underlying populations are different, ie, the samples come from different populations (H_0 is not true). The statistic U is the *smaller of* the number of times a value in the first group precedes a value in the second group and the number of times a value in the second group precedes a value in the first group. Thus, if sample sizes are n_1 and n_2, the quantity $U/n_1 n_2$ is the estimated proportion or probability that a new observation sampled from the first population will be less than a new observation sampled from the second population. This interpretation may be helpful in describing the results of a research study. When the sample size of either group exceeds 20, U can be used to approximate a z ratio that has the standard normal distribution. Statistical significance is then estimated from the standard normal distribution. Thus at the .05 level of significance, the null hypothesis is rejected if the observed z is more negative than or equal to -1.96 (two-sided test) or -1.65 (one-sided test); otherwise the null hypothesis is retained.

For our example, we wish to know whether the extent of reliable anesthesia for hand surgery differs by method of axillary block (single-injection vs multiple-injection method) administered to patients randomly assigned to either method. The Mann–Whitney U test indicates that the mean percent of arm blocked by the single-injection method (85%) differs from that blocked by the multiple-injection method (95%) at $p < .05$ (calculations not shown).

When conducting the nonparametric statistical tests, there are several important reasons to consult a statistician. For instance, consult a statistician if many ties occur in your data; complicated corrections should be applied when there are too many ties (say, as many as a third of all scores are tied). Moreover, although computer packages should automatically adjust for tied ranks, not all do. If your sample is small (<10) exact probabilities should be calculated. However, computer packages may use the large-sample normal approximation to calculate statistical significance even for small samples. Statistical programs also differ in how the statistic is reported in the printout. For example, when reporting the Wilcoxon ranked sum test, SPSS for Windows (11.0.1) will display the rank sum of the smaller sample (or the rank sum of the first designated group if the samples are equal), whereas Minitab (release 6.1) calculates the Wilcoxon ranked sum test for the first designated sample (which is not necessarily the smaller sample).

Sign Test

The sign test and Wilcoxon signed ranks test are nonparametric counterparts to the paired or dependent t test. They apply to studies in which subjects are matched on a potentially confounding variable (and then assigned to treatment groups) or the same subjects are assessed at two separate times (eg, before and after treatment). The sign test assumes that the paired differences are randomly drawn from the population of difference scores (and sampling is with replacement). An additional assumption is that no difference is exactly zero (even though the test is reasonably robust provided the number of zeros is small). Each difference between paired measurements is assigned either a plus ($+$) or a minus ($-$) sign, depending on the direction of the difference. The number of pluses and minuses would be similar if the matched pairs or the before–after groups come from the same population. The observed and expected (ie, half of the subjects are expected to have positive differences and half to have negative differences) frequencies are submitted to a χ^2 test with 1 df to determine whether the difference is beyond chance fluctuation. This will be reasonably accurate for 10 or more pairs of scores; smaller numbers of pairs require a small-sample approach (the binomial test). Unfortunately, the sign test responds only to the direction of the difference between pairs of scores and is likely to have little utility in regional anesthesia studies.

Wilcoxon Signed Ranks Test

The Wilcoxon signed ranks test is another nonparametric counterpart to the paired or dependent t test. Unlike the sign test, it uses information about the size of the difference as well as directionality. For our example, we wish to know whether the extent of reliable anesthesia for hand surgery differs by method of axillary block (single-injection vs multiple-injection) administered to 20 volunteers in randomized order 2 weeks apart. Thus the same volunteers receive each of the injection methods. The mean percent of arm blocked by the single-injection method (85%) differs from that blocked by the multiple-injection method (97%) at $p < .05$ (calculations not shown).

In addition to the assumptions of the sign test, the Wilcoxon signed ranks test also assumes that there are no ties in rank (even though the test is reasonably robust provided the number of ties is small) and that the *differences* between pairs of scores have a symmetrical distribution. This last assumption makes the Wilcoxon signed ranks test the only nonparametric method whose results can be affected by data transformations. In the case of the Wilcoxon, a transformation should be used only if it makes the distribution of the differences more symmetrical. Thus a statistician should be consulted to determine whether data transformations are appropriate for your data. If the number of nonzero differences is >15, the Wilcoxon can be used to approximate a z ratio that has the standard normal distribution. However, the value of the observed z will always be negative (or equal to zero). Thus, at the .05 level of significance, the null hypothesis is rejected if the observed z is more negative than or equal to -1.96 (two-sided test) or -1.65 (one-sided test); otherwise the null hypothesis is retained. Special small-sample methods are used if the number of nonzero differences is ≤15, and a statistician should be consulted.

Kruskal–Wallis H

This nonparametric counterpart to one-way ANOVA tests whether three or more independent samples are from the same population. It is an extension of the Mann–Whitney U and has the same assumptions (ie, independence and no ties in rank). Scores from all subgroups are combined and ranked in ascending order. Ties are assigned the mean rank of the scores that are tied. Once ranks have been assigned in the combined group, the subgroups are reconstructed, and the mean rank for each subgroup is compared with the mean rank for the combined group. If the subgroup samples come from identical populations, their mean ranks are similar to the overall mean rank. If the samples come from different populations, their mean ranks vary more widely about the overall mean rank. The Kruskal–Wallis H compares the total magnitude of these discrepancies with what might be expected by chance. Exact probabilities have been worked out for tiny samples. However, in most cases (eg, with three groups and four or more subjects in each), the χ^2 distribution may be used to evaluate the statistic H with good approximate results. Like χ^2, H is nondirectional because it reflects the magnitude of the discrepancies without regard to their direction. So, like χ^2, the region of rejection appropriately lies in the upper tail of the distribution. Finally, as with ANOVA, it is possible to make multiple comparisons among the groups compared by the Kruskal–Wallis H. As always, inflation of the experiment-wise type I error must be considered.

For our example, we wish to know whether the extent of reliable anesthesia for hand surgery differs by method of axillary block (one-, two-, three-, or four-injection) administered to patients randomly assigned to each of the four methods. The mean percent of arm blocked differs by injection method (85%, 90%, 95%, and 99%, respectively) at $p < .05$. Post-hoc comparisons indicate that the extent of reliable anesthesia for hand surgery by the single-injection method differs from that of the combined multiple-injection methods (calculations not shown).

Logistic Regression

As discussed in the section on Parametric Tests, multiple linear regression models contain explanatory covariates (independent variables) in order to predict a continuous outcome (dependent variable). It is, however, often the case that the outcome of interest is a dichotomous variable, eg, the presence or absence of a disease. Logistic regression applies in such instances. Why? If an outcome variable can only take numerical values of 0 or 1, then the mean of these values in a sample of patients is the proportion of patients with the disease (or equivalently, the probability that a patient has the disease of interest). Thus instead of predicting a continuous outcome, the task of the regression model is to predict the *proportion* of patients with the outcome for given combinations of the explanatory variables contained in the model. Unfortunately, this can produce impossible probabilities outside the range of 0 to 1, so it is useful to work with a *transformation* of the proportion to be predicted. Logistic regression uses the logit transformation, ie, the natural logarithm of the odds of the outcome, $\text{logit}(p) = \log_e(p/[1-p])$, where p is the proportion of patients with the outcome and always lies in the range 0 and 1.

Unlike least squares regression, the intercept and coefficients in a logistic regression model are obtained through an interative process that results in a unique set of maximum likelihood estimates. Among all possible values that could describe the parent population from which the sample emerged, the maximum likelihood estimates are those values that most likely gave rise to the observed data. For our example, logistic regression is used to estimate the risk for severe hypotension (decrease in blood pressure >30% of baseline) vs no severe hypotension following neuraxial blockade. A single binary predictor (dry mucosa vs no dry mucosa) is included in the model. The analysis yields a maximum likelihood coefficient, $b_{\text{dry mucosa}} = 0.6931$, with standard error$_{\text{dry mucosa}} = 0.1119$. For binary predictors coded 0 or 1, the odds ratio (a widely used measure of risk) can be directly estimated by exponentiating the logistic regression coefficient, ie, $\text{OR} = e^b$. Thus if patients without dry mucosae are coded as 0 and patients with dry mucosae as 1, exponentiation of the coefficient, $e^{0.6931} = 2$, indicates a twofold risk for severe hypotension for patients with dry mucosae. Moreover, a confidence interval can be constructed, ie, $e^{[b \pm (z_{\alpha/2})(\text{s.e.}_b)]}$, which yields $e^{[0.6931-(1.96)(0.1119)]} = 1.6$ and $e^{[0.6931+(1.96)(0.1119)]} = 2.5$ as the lower and upper 95% confidence limits, respectively. Compared with patients without dry mucosae, risk for severe hypotension for patients with dry mucosae is likely to be increased at least 60% but no greater than 2.5-fold.

Another expression for the estimated probability of disease, $p = 1/(1 + e^{-(\alpha + \beta_1 x_1 + \cdots + \beta_i x_i)})$, can be rearranged in terms of the log odds of disease, ie, $\text{logit}(p) = \alpha + \beta_1 x_1 + \cdots + \beta_i x_i$, which is reminiscent of the multiple linear regression model, but will always yield values of p that are between 0 and 1. The coefficients (b_i's) denote the amount of increase or decrease in the logs odds of the outcome associated with a unit change in the predictor. For instance, a model for the

Table 83–8.

Severe Hypotension Associated with Neuroxial Blockade: An Example of a Patient with Specific Clinical Characteristics

Predictor	Coefficient	Patient
Intercept	−4.5799	
Age (10-year increments)	0.0296	60 years old
Preop urine output (>100 mL/h = 0 vs ≤ 100 mL/h = 1)^a	−0.6931	>100 mL/h
Hypovolemia (No = 0, Yes = 1)	1.6094	Yes
Preop heart rate (10 bpm increments over 72 bpm)	0.6900	82 bpm
Dry mucosa (No = 0, Yes = 1)	0.5878	No

^{a} *The coefficient for preop urine output is negative as the riskier condition (>100 mL/h) is coded as 0.*

probability of severe hypotension associated with neuraxial blockade might contain the following predictors and their coefficients (Table 83–8).

The log odds for severe hypotension in a 60-year-old hypovolemic patient with preoperative urine output >100 mL/h, preoperative heart rate of 82 bpm, and no dry mucosa is

$$\text{logit}(p) = -4.5799 + (0.0296 \times 6) + (-0.6931 \times 0)$$
$$+ 1.6094 + (0.6900 \times 1) + (0.5878 \times 0)$$
$$= -2.1029$$

This patient's probability of severe hypotension is $1/(1 + e^{-(-2.1029)})$ or about 11%.

It is possible to compare the risk profiles of two patients using the coefficients in the model. For instance, $\text{logit}(p_1)$ for a patient with dry mucosa can be compared with the $\text{logit}(p_2)$ for a patient without dry mucosa (all other predictive characteristics being the same between these patients). That is,

$$\text{logit}(p_1) - \text{logit}(p_2) = \log\left(\frac{p_1}{1-p_1}\right) - \log\left(\frac{p_2}{1-p_2}\right)$$
$$= \log\left[\frac{p_1(1-p_2)}{p_2(1-p_1)}\right]$$

For our example, the coefficients for the intercept, age, preoperative urine output, hypovolemia, and preoperative heart rate cancel out between these two patients as they are the same for both patients. This results in $\text{logit}(p_1) = 0.5878$ for the patient with dry mucosa and $\text{logit}(p_2) = 0$ for the patient without dry mucosa. When the difference, $\text{logit}(p_1) - \text{logit}(p_2) = 0.5878$, is exponentiated, $e^{0.5878} = 1.8$, we obtain the odds ratio (risk) for severe hypotension due to dry mucosa that has been *adjusted for* age, preoperative urine output, hypovolemia, and preoperative heart rate. The adjusted odds ratio appears to be slightly lower than the unadjusted odds ratio (2.0) calculated earlier.

Clinical Pearls

1. Know your data. Know the types of variables that you are measuring.
   - Keep a data dictionary.

2. Consult with your statistician at the planning stage of your research study.
   - Strive to use the least complex study design and statistical analyses that will answer your research questions.

3. Remember that bias typically cannot be corrected through statistical methods. So, think carefully and thoroughly about features of your study design that may lead to systematic errors, in particular with respect to (a) ascertainment and selection of your subjects, and (b) measurement of your exposure variables (eg, vulnerability to recall or interviewer bias).

4. Have clear specific aims and hypotheses prepared. Null and alternative hypotheses are not questions, so *write* clear, declarative statements for your null and alternative hypotheses. Once stated, they should not be changed to fit the research findings. The two-sided alternative hypothesis is generally more appropriate than the one-sided alternatives, especially so for new areas of research.

5. Have a reasonable idea of the type I and type II error probabilities that you would be willing to tolerate based on your area of research interest.

6. Have some idea of the difference that is clinically meaningful to detect. A literature review may help you estimate this difference and may provide an estimate of variability in the outcome of interest. (If not available, you may need to conduct a preliminary study to estimate these parameters.) Your statistician will use this information to calculate the sample size required to detect the desired difference at your specified probability of committing a type I error (α) and with sufficient power ($1 - \beta$).

7. Potential confounding variables must be included during the design phase of the study. Their choice and accuracy of measurement directly affects the extent to which confounding can be controlled by statistical procedures. During your background literature review, consider factors that other investigators have included in their studies. Did they feel that these factors could have influenced their findings? Did they suspect other factors that were not included (or could not be included) in their studies but perhaps should have been?

8. With the help of your statistician, choose between parametric and nonparametric alternatives. You will usually perform one (not both) of these methods to test a given variable. For quantitative data, this will typically be a parametric method unless there are clear indications that the underlying assumptions are not met. If violations to these assumptions are noted, your statistician will offer advice with respect to data transformations that may be appropriate for your study prior to running a parametric test. For ranked or qualitative data, descriptive or nonparametric methods must be used.

9. Discuss multiple comparisons with your statistician. If numerous comparisons or contrasts are included in your study, what adjustments are necessary?

10. With the help of your statistician, plan the best ways to present your findings. Should your data simply be stated in the text or should selected findings be featured in tables and figures?

OBSERVATIONS FROM REVIEWING MANUSCRIPTS SUBMITTED TO ANESTHESIOLOGY JOURNALS

This section describes several common errors found while reviewing manuscripts that have been submitted for publication in anesthesiology journals. Comments pertain to the research (nonclinical) perspective.

Clinical Relevance & Conceptualization

Research questions arise primarily from clinical need, and clinical relevance dictates the choice of study parameters. Authors must not assume that clinical utility obviates the need to sell their studies to the anesthesiology community. For example, researchers embarking on a study of catheter shearing during removal would have to substantiate the importance of focusing on an occurrence that is exceedingly rare (and perhaps of little clinical interest). Moreover, these researchers must be careful to use forces that could actually be encountered in the clinical setting.

Authors often neglect to explain their choice of study parameters. For instance, if patients must be older than 50 years of age in order to be eligible for a study of cervical plexus block, the authors should provide the reason for this inclusion criterion. Is it because the surgery for which cervical plexus block is appropriate is rarely performed in individuals younger than 50 years of age? Similarly, choice of drugs is universally explained, but the rationale for choosing specific doses to be studied is sometimes neglected.

Clinical relevance dictates conceptualization of a study in other, often subtle, ways. For instance, when studying ultrasound-guided peripheral nerve block of the sciatic nerve using different landmarks, it is important to establish the level of experience of the anesthesiologists participating in the study. However, as their experience is likely to be more extensive in the brachial plexus and femoral nerve blocks than in the sciatic nerve block, it is not sufficient to tell the readers that each anesthesiologist has completed more than 50 ultrasound-guided peripheral nerve blocks. The readers should also be told how much of this experience was specifically with the *sciatic nerve* block as this is the focus of the study.

Methodology

The two most common problems in methodology are inadequate control for potential confounding variables and inaccuracies in measurement. For instance, a study comparing the length of postoperative analgesia between two local anesthetics administered by popliteal nerve block would have to control for physiologic attributes of the patient (eg, age, presence of diabetic neuropathy) that could be associated with effectiveness of the drugs and postoperative analgesia. In regional anesthesia studies, this is typically accomplished by randomly assigning patients to receive one or the other of the two local anesthetics. For follow-up, patients are often phoned at home and asked the time that they took their first analgesic and VAS scores at specific times following discharge. But even patients discharged with detailed, written directions could misunderstand or fail to record this information. Moreover, accuracy depends heavily on the interviewer's skill with neutral probing as the patient attempts to recall the requested information. Thus it is necessary to work closely with the patients (providing them with easy-to-follow directions and questionnaires) as well as with well-trained research assistants in order to collect data as accurately as possible.

Statistics

Although it is assumed that the appropriate statistical procedures were conducted with the help of a statistician, a number of problems pertain to the reporting of the statistical methods. For instance, a paper may report a gender difference among three PNBs studied or differences in duration of surgery among these blocks, but fail to mention the statistical tests used to assess these differences. If a nonparametric statistical procedure is performed instead of a parametric one, it is useful to explain why the nonparametric counterpart was chosen. For instance, VAS scores may have been categorized and submitted to a χ^2 analysis because of nonnormality of the distribution. Moreover, if a figure is included, the categories of VAS should be graphed in a histogram, ie, VAS should not be illustrated in a line graph indicative of a continuous variable.

Papers have included statements that adjustments were made for multiple comparisons without describing the results of these comparisons. For instance, a statement that "repeated measures ANOVA with Tukey post hoc pair-wise testing" is a bit of overkill if no such comparisons were actually made. Papers have also stated a one-sided alternative hypothesis where

the two-sided alternative hypothesis is clearly warranted. This is problematic because a statistic could exceed the critical value of a one-sided test, but fail to exceed the more extreme critical value of the two-sided test. A false claim of statistical significance is made because it is based on an inappropriate alternative hypothesis.

Presentation of Results

Errors of presentation often revolve around the confusion between statistical significance and clinical importance. Writers mistakenly refer to a nonsignificant or insignificant effect when describing an effect that is "clinically unimportant" or "has little clinical impact."

Tables

- Tables are often recited to the readership. As readers can read for themselves, short summaries of the table contents are more useful. For instance, if a table includes the information that in the United States, 37% of patients received general anesthesia and 63% received peripheral nerve blocks in 2004, the authors can summarize this by stating, "Nearly twice as many patients received peripheral nerve blocks than general anesthesia in 2004, an increase of 200,000 from 2000."

- Often the converse is true, that is, authors include too much verbiage that could be more clearly presented in a table. For instance, stating "Surgical procedures included open-shoulder stabilization ($n = 5$), hemiarthroplasty ($n = 10$), rotator cuff surgery/decompressions ($n = 5$), other shoulder procedures including W, X, Y, Z ($n = 5$)" could be appreciated better as part of the patient demographic characteristics table. The readers can easily do a quick check that the total number of patients (here, $n = 25$) is accounted for.

- Tables often contain unnecessary information, eg, both standard deviations and ranges when one of these measures of variability usually suffices, a column or row of zeroes to indicate that no block failures occurred when this is in the text and a series of zeroes just looks silly, and n (%) for each gender when n (%) male *or* female suffices. Moreover, if only ASA physical status 1 or 2 patients are eligible for a study, it is not necessary to give the n (%) of patients in each of these two categories, especially if no comparisons between these categories are relevant to the study. The ASA physical status breakdown in the table becomes superfluous.

- Occasionally, variables that are not continuous measures are presented as though they are. For instance, T11.25 and T9.75 for thoracic positions in the longitudinal plane could be misleading if whole vertebrae were measured and not parts of them.

- Sometimes it is unclear what comparisons a p-value refers to in a table. For instance, a table may include measurements on several dorsal locations and several nondorsal locations. Yet it is unclear that the p-value refers to a comparison of the *mean* measurements of all dorsal locations against the mean measurements of all nondorsal locations.

- Notations contained in the table may not be explained in the footnotes (and sometimes not even in the text). For instance, asterisks in the table indicate that a footnote applies, but no footnote or legend is included as part of the table.

Figures

- Papers often include an excessive number of figures, many of which are simply unnecessary. The idea is not to present the same results in different ways. Moreover, a finding can often be described in a single sentence, and each sentence does not need a figure.
- The wrong type of graph may be used to portray the data. For instance, a bar graph (small spaces between bars) is appropriate for nominal categories (eg, a series of different types of PNBs), whereas a histogram (flush bars) is appropriate for categories of a continuous variable (eg, age groups).
- Figures are not always consistent with the text. For instance, the text may state that lidocaine kinetics were completed on 15 patients, but the figure may include values for only 10 patients.

Discussion & Conclusions

Overoptimism appears to be the bane of discussion and concluding statements. Not only do authors have a tendency to *re*state their findings, but they are often tempted to *over*state their findings. For instance, a statement to the effect that 0.5% ropivacaine *is superior to* 1% mepivacaine for a particular block may not be warranted if the study only looked at length of postoperative analgesia. Many other factors go into making one drug "superior" to another (eg, speed of onset, success rate). The authors should simply state that 0.5% ropivacaine provided longer postoperative analgesia than 1% mepivacaine.

Authors are often tempted to overstep the boundaries of their study. For instance, the conclusion that "Dose of remifentanil for sedation during carotid endarterectomy under cervical plexus block should be reduced in patients older than 70 years of age" may not be warranted if effects of the drug at lower doses were not tested in the study. This is because satisfactory block may not be achieved in patients older than 70 years of age if the drug is given at lower doses. Similarly, it could not be concluded that "The 12.5-mcg dose of fentanyl is optimal in terms of surgical anesthesia, hemodynamic stability, and reliability of block" if the 12.5-mcg dose was the highest dose tested. This is because higher doses may be even more "optimal."

Misleading statements are not easy to detect. For instance, stating that the tensile strength of 19- and 20-gauge Brand X epidural catheters differed at *varying* temperatures implies that the catheters were tested on a gradient of temperatures. If only two temperatures were studied, the statement should be revised to reflect that fact (eg, the tensile strength of 19- and 20-gauge Brand X epidural catheters differed at the two temperatures studied). Similarly, stating that significantly more "technical failures" (eg, impossible nerve stimulation) occurred in a specific group may be misleading if the so-called technical failures were only a portion of the total number of block failures that occurred. This is because the total number of block failures may be the primary outcome and may be similar among the groups, but the readers would be left with the impression that one group had more failures (overall) than the others. Finally, it would be misleading to omit some of the parameters tested in a study. For instance, when comparing two approaches to the sciatic nerve block in emergency situations, time to establish landmarks may be significantly (statistically) shorter by approach A, yet time to perform the block may be slightly (nonsignificantly) shorter by approach B, and time to block onset may not differ at all between the approaches. It would be misleading to conclude that approach A is faster than approach B, especially if difference in time to establish landmarks is only a few "statistically significant" minutes shorter by approach A and could easily be offset by approach B's slightly shorter time to perform the block.

References

1. Fisher RA: *Statistical Methods for Research Workers.* Hafner Publishing Company, 1948.
2. Witte RS: *Statistics.* Holt, Rinehart and Winston, 1980.
3. Lilienfeld AM, Lilienfeld DE: *Foundations of Epidemiology.* Oxford University Press, 1980.
4. Mausner JS, Kramer S: *Epidemiology—An Introductory Text,* 2nd ed. WB Saunders, 1985.
5. Altman DG: *Practical Statistics for Medical Research.* Chapman & Hall, 1991.
6. Minium EW: *Statistical Reasoning in Psychology and Education,* 2nd ed. John Wiley & Sons, 1978.
7. Motulsky H: *Intuitive Biostatistics.* Oxford University Press, 1995.
8. Kleinbaum DG, Kupper LL, Muller KE: *Applied Regression Analysis and Other Multivariable Methods,* 2nd ed. Duxbury Press, 1988.
9. Kelsey JL, Thompson WD, Evans AS: *Methods in Observational Epidemiology. Monographs in Epidemiology and Biostatistics,* vol. 10. Oxford University Press, 1986.
10. Fleiss JL: *Statistical Methods for Rates and Proportions,* 2nd ed. John Wiley & Sons, 1981.

Index